SAUNDERS

COMPREHENSIVE
REVIEW *for the*
NCLEX-PN®
EXAMINATION

SAUNDERS

COMPREHENSIVE REVIEW *for the*
NCLEX-PN®
EXAMINATION

LINDA ANNE SILVESTRI, MSN, RN

Instructor of Nursing
Salve Regina University
Newport, Rhode Island;
President
Nursing Reviews, Inc.,
and
Professional Nursing Seminars, Inc.
Charlestown, Rhode Island

Third Edition

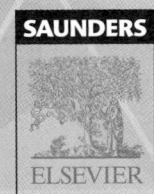

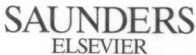

11830 Westline Industrial Drive
St. Louis, Missouri 63146

SAUNDERS COMPREHENSIVE REVIEW FOR THE NCLEX-PN®
EXAMINATION
Copyright © 2006, Elsevier Inc.

ISBN-13: 978-1-4160-0052-5
ISBN-10: 1-4160-0052-6

NCLEX-PN® is a registered trademark and service mark of the National Council of State Boards of Nursing, Inc.

Previous editions copyrighted 2003, 2000

ISBN-13: 978-1-4160-0052-5
ISBN-10: 1-4160-0052-6

Managing Editor: Nancy O'Brien
Associate Developmental Editor: Charlene R.M. Ketchum
Publication Services Manager: John Rogers
Project Manager: Doug Turner
Designer: Jyotika Shroff

Printed in the United States of America

Last digit is the print number: 9 8 7 6 5 4 3 2 1

To my parents
my mother, **Frances Mary,**
and in loving memory of my father, **Arnold Lawrence,**
who taught me to always love, care, and be the best that I could be!

To my grandmother
Beatrice Elizabeth Profiglio
my memories of her caring and love will remain in my heart forever.

About the Author

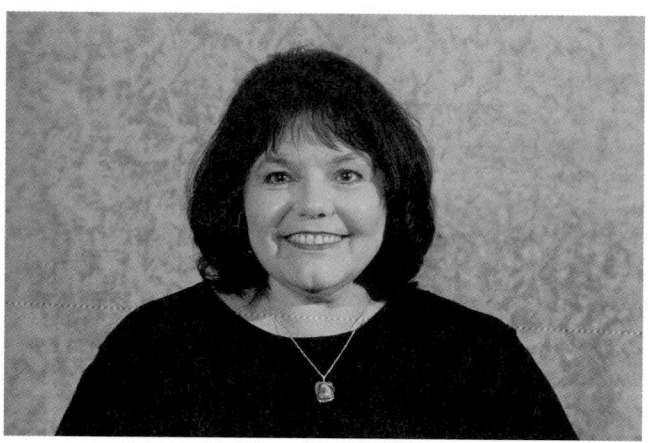

Linda Anne Silvestri received her diploma in nursing at Cooley Dickinson Hospital School of Nursing in Northampton, Massachusetts. Afterwards, she worked at Baystate Medical Center in Springfield, Massachusetts, in acute medical-surgical units, the intensive care unit, the emergency department, pediatric units, and other acute care units. She later received an associate degree from Holyoke Community College in Holyoke, Massachusetts, and then received her Bachelor of Science degree in nursing from American International College in Springfield, Massachusetts.

A native of Springfield, Massachusetts, Linda began her teaching career as an instructor of medical-surgical nursing and leadership-management nursing at Baystate Medical Center School of Nursing in 1981. In 1985, she earned her Master of Science degree in nursing from Anna Maria College in Paxton, Massachusetts, with a dual major in Nursing Management and Patient Education. Linda is a member of Sigma Theta Tau.

Linda relocated to Rhode Island in 1989 and began teaching advanced medical-surgical nursing and psychiatric nursing to RN and LPN students at the Community College of Rhode Island. While she was teaching at the Community College of Rhode Island, a group of students asked Linda to help them prepare for the NCLEX examination. Based on her experience as a nursing educator and as an NCLEX item writer, she developed a comprehensive review course to prepare nursing graduates for the NCLEX examination. In 1994, Linda began teaching medical-surgical nursing at Salve Regina University in Newport, Rhode Island. She also prepares nursing students at Salve Regina University for the NCLEX-RN examination.

In 1991, Linda established Professional Nursing Seminars, Inc., and in 2000, she established Nursing Reviews, Inc. Both companies are dedicated to conducting NCLEX-RN and NCLEX-PN review courses and assisting nursing graduates to achieve their goals of becoming registered nurses and/or licensed practical/vocational nurses.

Today, Linda Silvestri's companies conduct NCLEX review courses throughout New England. She is the successful author of numerous NCLEX-RN and NCLEX-PN review products, including *Saunders Comprehensive Review for the NCLEX-RN Examination, Saunders Q&A Review for the NCLEX-RN Examination, Saunders Computerized Review for the NCLEX-RN Examination, Saunders Strategies for Success for the NCLEX-RN Examination, Saunders Instructor's Resource Package for NCLEX-RN, Saunders Comprehensive Review for the NCLEX-PN Examination, Saunders Q&A Review for NCLEX-PN Examination, Saunders Review Cards for the NCLEX-PN Examination,* and *Saunders Instructor's Resource Package for NCLEX-PN.* Linda has also written several online products including the online specialty tests titled *Adult Health, Mental Health, Maternal-Newborn, Pediatrics, and Pharmacology,* and the *Saunders Online Review Course for the NCLEX-RN Examination.*

Contributors

Stephanie A. Dupler, LPN
Graduate
Lebanon County Career and Technology Center
Lebanon, Pennsylvania

Laurent W. Valliere, BS
Vice President
Professional Nursing Seminars, Inc.
Charlestown, Rhode Island

The author and publisher would also like to acknowledge the following individuals for their contributions to the previous editions of this book:

Alicia M. Adams, MN, RN, CEN
Director
Practical Nursing and Allied Health
Uintah Basin Applied Technology Center
Roosevelt, Utah

Carol Boswell, EdD, RN
Chairperson
Odessa College Nursing Program
Odessa, Texas

Sharen Brady, MSN, RN
Early Intervention Specialist
Associate Professor of Nursing in PN/ADN Program
Weber State University
Ogden, Utah

Brenda E. Caranicas, MS, RN
Director
Practical Nursing Program
Fort Berthold Community College
New Town, North Dakota

Jean DeCoffe, MSN, RN
Assistant Professor of Nursing
Curry College
Milton, Massachusetts

Mary Ann Hogan, MSN, RN, CS
Clinical Assistant Professor
University of Massachusetts
Amherst, Massachusetts

Lisa Ivers, BSN, RN
Instructor
Indiana University
Butler County Program of Practical Nurse Education
Hamilton, Ohio

Lula Johnson, MSN, RN
Director
JTPA School of Practical Nursing
Detroit, Michigan

Mary T. Kowalski, MSN, BA, RN
Director of Vocational Nursing and Health Career
    Programs
Cerro Coso Community College
Ridgecrest, California

Beverly McNeese, RN
Department Head
Practical Nursing Program
Louisiana Technical College, Baton Rouge Campus
Baton Rouge, Louisiana

Jan H. Mearkle, MSN, RN, CSNP
Instructor
Southwest Mississippi Community College
Summit, Mississippi

Jo Ann Barnes Mullaney, PhD, RN, CS
Professor of Nursing
Salve Regina University
Newport, Rhode Island

Joann E. Potts Peuterbaugh, MSN, RN
LPN Coordinator
F.W. Olin Vocational School of Practical Nursing
Alton, Illinois

Ann Leiphart Unholz, MS, RN
Director, Henrico County
St. Mary's Hospital School of Practical Nursing
Highland Springs, Virginia

Paula A. Viau, PhD, RN
Associate Dean of Nursing
College of Nursing, University of Rhode Island
Kingston, Rhode Island

Margaret Wafstet, MN, RN
Director
Practical Nursing Program
University of Montana/College of Technology,
   Missoula
Missoula, Montana

Mary Louise White, MSN, RN
Clinical Nurse Specialist
Delta College
University Center, Michigan

REVIEWERS

Brigitte L. Casteel, BSN, RN
Assistant Professor
Program Director, Practical Nursing Program
Mountain Empire Community College
Big Stone Gap, Virginia

Dolores Cotton, MS, BSN, RN
Practical Nursing Coordinator
Meridian Technology Center
Stillwater, Oklahoma

Sally Flesch, PhD, MA, BSN, RN
Professor
Black Hawk College
Moline, Illinois

Margaret M. Gingrich, MSN, RN
Associate Professor
Harrisburg Area Community College
Harrisburg, Pennsylvania

Allen Hamilton, MS, BSN, RN
Nursing Instructor, Retired
McLennan Community College
Waco, Texas

Rosemary Macy, PhDc, RN
Assistant Professor
Boise State University
Boise, Idaho

Nancy K. Maebius, PhD, RN
Consultant
Galen Health Institute School of Nursing
San Antonio, Texas

Collette Moreno, MSN, RN
Nursing Faculty
Galen Health Institute School of Nursing
San Antonio, Texas

Lorene Payne, MSN, RN
Professor of Nursing
Tomball College
Tomball, Texas

STUDENT REVIEWERS

Anita Buss
Lebanon County Career & Technology Center
Lebanon, Pennsylvania

April Oland Childs
Salve Regina University
Newport, Rhode Island

Doris Pence
Lebanon County Career & Technology Center
Lebanon, Pennsylvania

Mary Propst
Lebanon County Career & Technology Center
Lebanon, Pennsylvania

Rhonda Singer
Lebanon County Career & Technology Center
Lebanon, Pennsylvania

Katie Weik
Lebanon County Career & Technology Center
Lebanon, Pennsylvania

Preface

Welcome to *Saunders Pyramid to Success!*

The *Saunders Comprehensive Review for the NCLEX-PN® Examination* is one of a series of products designed to assist you in achieving your goal of becoming a licensed practical/vocational nurse. The *Saunders Comprehensive Review for the NCLEX-PN® Examination* will provide you with a comprehensive review of all of the nursing content areas specifically related to the new 2005 NCLEX-PN test plan implemented by the National Council of State Boards of Nursing.

ORGANIZATION

The *Saunders Comprehensive Review for the NCLEX-PN® Examination* contains 20 units and 66 chapters. The chapters are designed to identify specific components of nursing content. The chapters contain practice questions reflective of the chapter content and of the 2005 NCLEX-PN test plan.

The new test plan identifies a framework based on *Client Needs*. These Client Needs categories include Safe, Effective Care Environment; Health Promotion and Maintenance; Psychosocial Integrity; and Physiological Integrity. *Integrated Processes* are also identified as a component of the test plan. These include Caring; Clinical Problem-Solving Process (Nursing Process); Communication and Documentation; and Teaching/Learning. All of the chapters address the components of the test plan framework.

UNIT I: NCLEX-PN® PREPARATION

Chapter 1 addresses all of the information about the 2005 NCLEX-PN test plan and the testing procedures related to the examination. This chapter answers all of those questions that you may have regarding the testing procedures.

Chapter 2 provides information to the foreign-educated nurse about the process of obtaining a license to practice as a licensed practical/vocational nurse in the United States.

Chapter 3 discusses the issue of NCLEX-PN preparation from a nonacademic view and provides an emphasis on a holistic approach for your individual test preparation. This chapter identifies the components of a structured study plan and pattern, anxiety reduction techniques, and personal focus issues.

Nursing students want to hear what other students have to say about their experiences with the NCLEX-PN examination. Students seek a view of what it is really like to take an NCLEX-PN examination. Chapter 4 is written by a nursing student who recently took the NCLEX-PN examination. The chapter addresses the issue of what the examination is all about, and includes the student's story of success.

Test-taking strategies are an important component of success in taking such an important examination. Chapter 5, *Test-Taking Strategies*, includes all of those important strategies that will help teach you how to read a question, how not to read into a question, and how to use the process of elimination and various other strategies to select the correct response from the choices presented.

UNIT II: ISSUES IN NURSING

Unit II addresses relevant nursing issues reflective of the components of the NCLEX-PN test plan. Chapter 6, *Cultural Diversity*, identifies cultures and the related factors that promote maintenance of cultural identity when caring for culturally diverse clients. Alternative and complementary therapies are also reviewed in this chapter. Chapter 7, *Ethical and Legal Issues*, provides a review of the ethical and legal considerations important to the practice of nursing and relevant to the components of the test plan. Chapter 8, *Delegating, Managing, and Prioritizing Client Care*, identifies the leadership and management issues pertinent to the practice of nursing. This chapter emphasizes content related to time management, prioritizing, and assignment-making and the principles related to delegation. Disaster planning and triage are also reviewed.

UNIT III: NURSING SCIENCES

The chapters in this unit specifically address areas that students have identified as areas of concern requiring review. Chapter 9, *Fluids and Electrolytes*, and Chapter 10, *Acid-Base Balance*, highlight the key components of human physiology, then introduce the necessary data collection and nursing interventions required in caring for a client with an alteration or imbalance. Chapter 11, *Laboratory Values*, identifies common laboratory studies, normal values, and significant information related to specific laboratory tests. Chapter 12, *Nutritional Components of Care*, addresses the various food groups and important nutritional components of specific diet therapy. This chapter will assist in your review of the selection of the correct food or the foods to avoid with certain physiological conditions, because these types of questions are certainly addressed in the NCLEX-PN examination. Chapter 13, *Intravenous Therapy and Blood Administration*, focus on the nurse's role in monitoring these therapies and complications.

UNIT IV: FUNDAMENTAL SKILLS

Chapter 14, *Hygiene and Safety*, addresses nursing care specific to client safety and the measures that promote environmental safety. Standard precautions, transmission-based precautions, and radiation precautions are reviewed. Additionally, chemical and biological warfare agents and their potentially fatal effects are reviewed. Chapter 15, *Medication and Intravenous Administration*, includes the important components related to conversion tables, calculation of medication dosages, and intravenous (IV) solutions and flow rates. Chapter 16, *Basic Life Support*, has been included to assist you in reviewing the steps in cardiopulmonary resuscitation and the Heimlich maneuver and to refresh your memory on the priorities to be addressed in emergency situations. Chapter 17, *Perioperative Nursing Care*, addresses the key components related to caring for the client requiring surgery. Chapter 18, *Positioning Clients*, identifies safe client positions specific to various surgical and diagnostic procedures. Chapter 19, *Care of a Client with a Tube*, addresses the common types of tubes used in the clinical setting, such as chest, gastrointestinal, and renal tubes, which have always been very confusing to students, particularly in terms of their purpose and nursing care involved.

UNITS V, VI, AND VII: MATERNITY NURSING, GROWTH AND DEVELOPMENT ACROSS THE LIFE SPAN, AND PEDIATRIC NURSING

Unit V, *Maternity Nursing*, includes chapters that address maternity issues, the care of the newborn, and maternity and newborn medications. Unit VI, *Growth and Development Across the Life Span*, addresses the common theories of growth and development used in the profession of nursing, developmental stages and transitions, and content related to caring for the older client. Unit VII, *Pediatric Nursing*, focuses on pediatric care and the specifics related to administering medication to the child.

UNIT VIII THROUGH XVIII: ADULT HEALTH

Units VIII through XVIII address the components of adult health and are divided based on specific body systems including the integumentary, endocrine, gastrointestinal, respiratory, cardiovascular, renal, eye and ear, neurological, musculoskeletal, and immune systems. Oncology nursing is also addressed. These chapters incorporate the Integrated Processes and all of the Client Needs components of the NCLEX-PN test plan, with a particular emphasis on Physiological Integrity. Each unit includes a pharmacology chapter that provides a comprehensive review of the medications specific to that body system.

UNIT XIX: MENTAL HEALTH NURSING

This unit primarily addresses the Psychosocial Integrity category of the Client Needs component of the test plan. Specific mental health disorders are addressed. This unit includes a chapter that provides a comprehensive review of psychiatric medications.

UNIT XX: COMPREHENSIVE TEST

Unit XX contains a comprehensive examination with practice questions related to all of the content areas addressed in this book. It consists of 85 questions representative of the percentages identified in the NCLEX-PN test plan. Multiple choice questions and questions in the alternate test question format are included in this test, as well as in the practice tests found at the end of each chapter in this book.

SPECIAL FEATURES OF THE BOOK
PYRAMID TERMS

Each content area, either a chapter or unit, begins with *Pyramid Terms* and their definitions. These important terms are significant to the content contained in the chapter. In addition, the *Pyramid Terms* are in bold type throughout the content section.

PYRAMID TO SUCCESS

The *Saunders Pyramid to Success*, a unit or chapter introduction, provides you with an overview of the chapter, guidance and direction regarding the focus of review in the particular content area, and its relative importance to the 2005 NCLEX-PN test plan. Specific nursing content areas, as specified in the test plan, are identified. The *Saunders Pyramid to Success* reviews the Client Needs and the Integrated Processes as they pertain to the content in that unit or chapter. These points are the specific components to keep in mind as you review the chapter outline.

PYRAMID POINTS

Pyramid Points are the bullets that are placed at specific content areas throughout the chapters. The *Pyramid Points* provide you with immediate recognition of content that is important in preparation for the NCLEX-PN examination. These bullets identify areas of content that typically appear on the NCLEX-PN examination.

PRACTICE QUESTIONS

While preparing for the NCLEX-PN examination, it is crucial for students to answer the practice questions. This book contains 1500 practice questions in NCLEX format. The accompanying software includes all of the questions from the book, plus an additional 2000 questions, for a total of 3500 questions.

MULTIPLE CHOICE AND ALTERNATE FORMAT QUESTIONS

Each content chapter is followed by a practice test. Each practice test contains several multiple choice questions and one *Alternate Format Question*. The *Alternate Format Question* may be presented as a fill-in-the blank, multiple response, prioritizing (ordered response), or chart/exhibit question. These questions provide you with practice in prioritizing and decision-making.

IMAGE QUESTIONS

The accompanying software contains *Image Questions* representative of the 2005 NCLEX-PN test plan. These questions are in NCLEX format, and each question presents an image, figure, or illustration (hot spots) as a component of the question.

ANSWER SECTION

The answer section for each practice question include the correct answer, rationale, test-taking strategy, question categories, and reference source. The structure for the answer section is unique and provides the following information:

The Rationale: The rationale provides you with the significant information regarding both correct and incorrect options.

Test-Taking Strategy: The test-taking strategy provides you with the logical path in selecting the correct option and assists you in selecting an answer to a question on which you must guess. Specific suggestions for review are identified in the test-taking strategy.

Question Categories: Each question is identified based on the categories used by the NCLEX-PN test plan. Additional content categories are provided with each question to assist you in identifying areas in need of review. The categories identified with each practice question include Level of Cognitive Ability, Client Needs, Integrated Process, and the specific nursing Content Area. All categories are identified by their full names so that you do not need to memorize codes or abbreviations.

Reference: A reference, including a page number, is provided so you can easily find the information that you need to review in your nursing textbooks.

PHARMACOLOGY AND MEDICATION CALCULATIONS REVIEW

Students consistently say that pharmacology is an area in which they need assistance. The 2005 NCLEX-PN test plan incorporates pharmacology in the examination to a greater extent than in the past. Therefore, pharmacology chapters have been included for your review and practice. This book includes 13 pharmacology chapters, a medication and intravenous (IV) calculation chapter, and a pediatric medication calculation chapter. Each of these chapters is followed by a practice test using the same question format described earlier. This book and accompanying software contains over 400 pharmacology questions.

NCLEX-PN® REVIEW SOFTWARE

You will find a CD-ROM containing NCLEX-PN review software packaged in the back of this book. This software contains 3500 practice questions. It also includes the alternate format questions and the image practice questions. This Windows- and Macintosh-compatible CD-ROM offers the following testing modes for review:

Quiz: Ten randomly chosen questions in a specific selected content area. The answer, rationale, test-taking strategy, question categories, reference source, and results appear after you have answered all 10 questions.

Study: All questions in a specific selected content area. The answer, rationale, test-taking strategy, question categories, and reference source appear after you have answered each question.

Examination: One hundred randomly chosen questions from the entire pool of more than 3500 questions. The answer, rationale, test-taking strategy, question categories, reference source, and results appear after you have answered all 100 questions.

HOW TO USE THIS BOOK

Saunders Comprehensive Review for the NCLEX-PN® Examination is especially designed to help you with your successful journey to the peak of the *Saunders Pyramid to Success*, becoming a licensed practical/vocational nurse. As you begin your journey through this book, you will be introduced to all of the important points regarding the 2005 NCLEX-PN examination, the process of testing, and the unique and special tips regarding how to prepare yourself for this very important examination.

You should begin your process through the *Saunders Pyramid to Success* by reading all of Unit I and becoming familiar with the important points regarding the NCLEX-PN examination. Read the chapter from the nursing graduate who recently passed the examination and note what this graduate has to say about the examination. The test taking–strategy chapter will provide you with important strategies that will help you select the correct answer or narrow your choices when you must guess. Read this chapter and practice these strategies as you proceed through your journey with this book. Continue your journey by reading each of the chapters and content areas. Review the *Pyramid Terms* and the *Saunders Pyramid to Success* and identify the Client Needs and Integrated Processes specific to the test plan in that area. Read each of the content areas focusing on the *Pyramid Points* that identify those areas most likely to be tested on the NCLEX-PN examination.

As you read each chapter, identify your strengths and those areas in need of further review. Highlight these areas and test your strengths and abilities by taking all of the practice tests provided at the end of the chapters. Be sure to read all of the rationales and the test-taking strategies. The rationale provides you with the significant information regarding both the correct and incorrect options. The test-taking strategy offers you the logical path to selecting the correct option. The strategy also identifies content area that you need to review if you had difficulty with the question. Use the reference source listed so you can easily find the information that you need to review.

After reviewing all of the chapters in the book, turn to Unit XX, the Comprehensive Test. Take this examination and then review each question, answer, and rationale. Identify any areas requiring further review; then take the time to review those areas again.

After using this book to review specific content areas, continue on your journey through the *Saunders Pyramid*

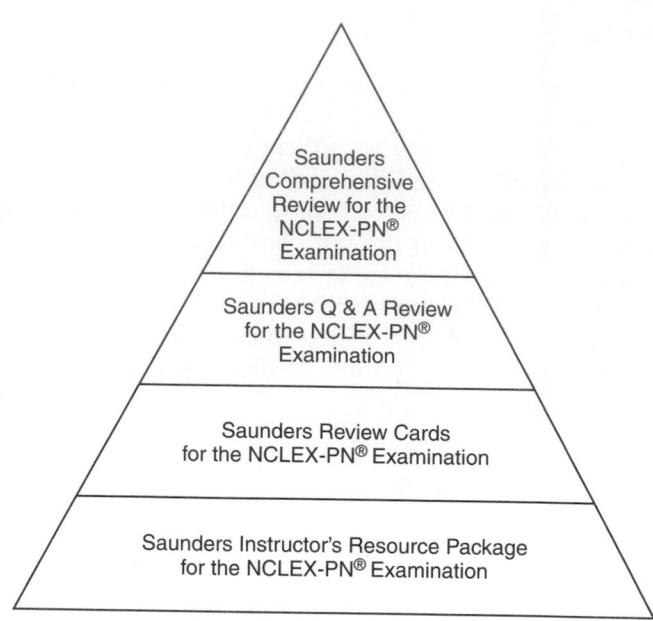

to *Success* with the companion book, *Saunders Q & A Review for the NCLEX-PN® Examination*, for additional practice questions. The companion book and its accompanying software offer you over 3000 practice questions on specific areas outlined by the 2005 NCLEX-PN test plan. With practice questions uniquely focused on the Client Needs and the Integrated Processes, you can assess your level of competence.

An additional component of the *Saunders Pyramid to Success* is the *Saunders Review Cards for the NCLEX-PN® Examination*. This product provides you with over 900 practice test questions, including multiple-choice questions and the new alternative test items, such as fill-in-the-blank, multiple response, prioritizing (ordered response), and image (hot spot) questions. The practice question is located on one side of the review card. The reverse side of the review card contains the correct answer, rationale, and question categories for the practice question on the front of the card.

A final component of the *Saunders Pyramid to Success* is the *Saunders Instructor's Resource Package for the NCLEX-PN® Examination*. This manual and CD-ROM accompany the Saunders program of NCLEX-PN review products. Be sure to ask your nursing program director and nursing faculty about this CD-ROM and its use for a review course or a self-paced review in your school's computer laboratory.

Good luck with your journey through the *Saunders Pyramid to Success*. I wish you continued success throughout your new career as a licensed practical/vocational nurse!

Linda Anne Silvestri, MSN, RN

Acknowledgments

Sincere appreciation and warmest thanks are extended to the many individuals who in their own way have contributed to the publication of this book.

First, I want to thank all of my nursing students at the Community College of Rhode Island in Warwick who approached me in 1991 and persuaded me to assist them in preparing to take the NCLEX examination. Their enthusiasm and inspiration led to the commencement of my professional endeavors in conducting NCLEX review courses for nursing students. I also thank the numerous nursing students who have attended my review courses for their willingness to share their needs and ideas. Their input has certainly added a special uniqueness to this publication.

I wish to acknowledge all of the nursing faculty who taught in my NCLEX review courses. Their commitment, dedication, and expertise has certainly assisted nursing students in achieving success with the NCLEX examination. Additionally, I want to acknowledge Laurent W. Valliere for his contribution to this publication, for teaching in my NCLEX review courses, and for his commitment and dedication in assisting my nursing students to prepare for the NCLEX examination from a nonacademic point of view.

I sincerely acknowledge and thank two very important individuals from Elsevier Health Sciences. I thank Nancy O'Brien, Managing Editor, for all of her assistance throughout the preparation of this edition and for her continuous enthusiasm, support, and expert professional guidance. And I thank Charlene Ketchum, Associate Developmental Editor, for her continuous assistance and support and for keeping me on schedule with manuscript submission. Charlene's expert organizational skills maintained order for all of the work that I submitted for manuscript production.

A special thank you and acknowledgment goes to two important individuals, Dianne E. Ventrice and Lawrence Fiorentino. They provided continuous support and dedication to my work in both the NCLEX review courses and in reference support for the third edition of this book.

I want to acknowledge all of the staff at Elsevier Health Sciences for their tremendous assistance throughout the preparation and production of this publication. A special thank you to all of them.

I thank all of the special people in the production department, John Rogers, Publication Services Manager; Doug Turner, Project Manager; Jyotika Shroff, Senior Designer; and Dave Rushing, Multimedia Producer, all of whom assisted in finalizing this publication.

I sincerely thank Bob Boehringher, Director of Nursing Marketing, and Andrew Eilers, Marketing Manager, whose support, hard work, and special creativity assisted with this publication.

I would also like to acknowledge Patricia Mieg, Educational Sales Representative, who encouraged me to submit my ideas and initial work for the first edition of this book to the W.B. Saunders Company.

I want to acknowledge my parents who opened my door of opportunity in education. I thank my mother, Frances Mary, for all of her love, support, and assistance as I continuously worked to achieve my professional goals. I thank my father, Arnold Lawrence, who always provided insightful words of encouragement. My memories of his love and support will always remain in my heart.

I also thank my sister, Dianne Elodia; my brother, Lawrence Peter; and my niece, Gina Marie, who were continuously supportive, giving, and helpful during my research and preparation of this publication.

I want to acknowledge all of the contributors who provided many of the practice questions contained in this publication and to the many faculty and student reviewers for their thoughts and ideas.

A special thank you goes to Stephanie Dupler, LPN, for providing a chapter to this publication regarding her experiences with the NCLEX-PN examination.

I also need to thank Salve Regina University for the opportunity to educate nursing students in the baccalaureate nursing program and for its support during my research and writing of this publication. I would like to especially acknowledge my colleagues, Dr. Sandra Solem, Dr. JoAnn Mullaney, Dr. Ellen McCarty, Dr. Jane McCool, Dr. Peggy Matteson, and Dr. Bethany Sykes for all of their support and encouragement.

I wish to acknowledge the Community College of Rhode Island, which provided me the opportunity to educate nursing students in the Associate Degree of Nursing Program, and a special thank you to Patricia Miller, MSN, RN, and Michelina McClellan, MS, RN, from Baystate Medical Center, School of Nursing, in Springfield, Massachusetts, who were my first mentors in nursing education.

Lastly, a very special thank you to all of my nursing students—past, present, and future. Your love and dedication to the profession of nursing and your commitment to provide health care will bring never-ending rewards!

Linda Anne Silvestri, MSN, RN

Contents

NCLEX-PN® Preparation

The NCLEX-PN® Examination

THE PYRAMID TO SUCCESS

Welcome to the Pyramid to Success!

Saunders Comprehensive Review for the NCLEX-PN® Examination is specially designed to help you begin your successful journey to the peak of the Pyramid, becoming a Licensed Practical/Vocational Nurse!

As you begin your journey, you will be introduced to all the important points regarding the NCLEX-PN examination, the process of testing, and the unique and special tips regarding how to prepare yourself for this very important examination. All these important test-taking strategies are detailed. These details will guide you in selecting the correct option or in making a logical guess when you are unsure of the answer. Also, you will read what a nursing graduate, who recently passed the NCLEX-PN, has to say about the examination.

Each content area in this book begins with the Pyramid to Success. The Pyramid to Success addresses specific points related to the NCLEX-PN, including the Pyramid Terms, the Client Needs, and the Integrated Processes, as identified in the test plan framework for the examination. Pyramid Terms are key words that are defined and boldfaced throughout each chapter to direct your attention to those significant NCLEX-PN points. The Client Needs and the Integrated Processes specific to the content of the chapter are identified.

Throughout each chapter, you will find the Pyramid Point bullets that identify areas most likely to be tested on the NCLEX-PN. Read each chapter and identify your strengths and areas in need of further review. Test your strengths and abilities by taking all the practice tests provided in this book. Be sure to read all the rationales and test-taking strategies. The rationale provides you with significant information regarding both the correct and incorrect options. The test-taking strategy provides you with the logical path for selecting the correct option. The test-taking strategy also identifies the content area to review, if required. The reference source and page number are provided so that you can easily locate the information you need to review. Each question is coded based on the Level of Cognitive Ability, the Client Needs, the Integrated Process, and the nursing content area.

After completing your comprehensive review in this book, continue on your journey through the Pyramid to Success with the companion book, *Saunders Q & A Review for the NCLEX-PN Examination*, which provides you with over 3000 practice questions based on the NCLEX-PN test plan, and *Saunders Review Cards for the NCLEX-PN Examination*, which provides you with over 900 additional practice questions. These additional products in the Saunders Pyramid to Success can be obtained online at www.elsevierhealth.com/reviewand testing.

Let's begin our journey through the Pyramid to Success!

THE EXAMINATION PROCESS

An important step in the Pyramid to Success is to become as familiar as possible with the examination process. A significant amount of anxiety can occur in candidates facing the challenge of this examination. Knowing what the examination is about and knowing what you will encounter during the process of testing will assist in alleviating fear and anxiety. The information in this chapter addresses the procedures related to the development of the NCLEX-PN test plan, the components of the test plan, and the answers to the questions most commonly asked by nursing students and graduates preparing to take the NCLEX-PN.

The information in this chapter related to the test plan was obtained from the National Council of State Boards of Nursing (NCSBN) Web site (www.ncsbn.org) and from the *NCLEX-PN Examination Detailed Test Plan for the National Council Licensure Examination for Licensed Practical/Vocational Nurses*, National Council of State

Boards of Nursing, Chicago (2005). Additional information regarding the test and its development can be obtained by accessing the NCSBN Web site or by writing to the National Council of State Boards of Nursing, 111 East Wacker Drive, Suite 2900, Chicago, IL 60601.

NCLEX-PN®

The term *NCLEX-PN* stands for National Council Licensure Examination for Practical/Vocational Nurses. The NCLEX-PN is a computer-administered examination that the nursing graduate must take and pass in order to practice in the role as a practical/vocational nurse. This examination measures the competency needed to practice safely and effectively as a newly licensed entry-level practical/vocational nurse.

DEVELOPMENT OF THE TEST PLAN

As an initial step in the test development process, the NCSBN considers the legal scope of nursing practice as governed by state laws and regulations, including the Nurse Practice Act. The NCSBN uses these laws to define the areas on the NCLEX-PN that will assess the competence of candidates for nurse licensure.

The NCSBN also conducts a Practice Analysis study to determine the framework for the test plan for the NCLEX-PN. The participants in this study include newly licensed practical and vocational nurses. The participants are provided with a list of nursing activities and are asked about the frequency of performing these specific activities, their impact on maintaining client safety, and the setting where the activities are performed. The analysis of the data obtained from this study guides the development of a framework for entry-level nurse performance that incorporates specific client needs and the processes fundamental to the practice of nursing. The NCLEX-PN test plan is derived from this framework. Because nursing practice continues to change, this study is conducted every 3 years. The results of this study, most recently conducted in 2003, provided the structure for the test plan implemented in April 2005.

THE TEST PLAN

The content of the NCLEX-PN reflects the activities that an entry-level practical and vocational nurse must be able to perform to provide clients with safe and effective nursing care. The questions are written to address the Levels of Cognitive Ability, Client Needs, and Integrated Processes as identified in the test plan.

Levels of Cognitive Ability

The NCLEX-PN examination consists primarily of multiple-choice questions written at the cognitive levels of knowledge, comprehension, application, and analysis.

However, the majority of questions address the application and analysis level. See Box 1-1 for an example of a question at the cognitive level of analysis.

Client Needs

In the new test plan, implemented in April 2005, the NCSBN identified a test plan framework based on Client Needs. This framework was selected on the basis of the findings in the Practice Analysis study. Additionally, using Client Needs provides a structure for defining nursing actions and competencies across all settings for all clients and meets requirements specified by state laws and statutes. The NCSBN has identified four major categories of Client Needs. Some are further divided into subcategories and the percentage of test questions in each subcategory is identified. Table 1-1 identifies these categories and subcategories and the associated percentage of test questions.

Safe, Effective Care Environment

The Safe, Effective Care Environment category includes two subcategories, Coordinated Care, and Safety and Infection Control. Coordinated Care (11% to 17%) addresses content related to facilitating effective client care through collaboration with other health care team members. Safety and Infection Control (8% to 14%) addresses content that tests the knowledge, skills, and ability required to protect clients and health care personnel from environmental hazards. Box 1-2 presents examples of questions that address these two subcategories.

BOX 1-1

Level of Cognitive Ability

The nurse is collecting data from a perinatal client with a history of left-sided heart failure and notes that the client is experiencing unusual episodes of a cough on minimal exertion. The nurse recognizes this finding as significant and associated with the first indicator of which cardiac problem?

1. Orthopnea
2. Decreased blood volume
3. Right-sided heart failure
4. Pulmonary edema

Answer: 4

This question requires the test-taker to analyze the data provided in order to recognize the client's problem. The test-taker needs to know the complications of left-sided heart failure and the signs and symptoms of pulmonary edema. The analysis of the data provided in the question directs the test-taker to the correct option.

LEVEL OF COGNITIVE ABILITY: ANALYSIS

TABLE 1-1

Client Needs and the Percentage of Test Questions

Client Needs	Percentage of Test Questions
SAFE, EFFECTIVE CARE ENVIRONMENT	
Coordinated Care	11%-17%
Safety and Infection Control	8%-14%
HEALTH PROMOTION AND MAINTENANCE	7%-13%
PSYCHOSOCIAL INTEGRITY	8%-14%
PHYSIOLOGICAL INTEGRITY	
Basic Care and Comfort	11%-17%
Pharmacological Therapies	9%-15%
Reduction of Risk Potential	10%-16%
Physiological Adaptation	12%-18%

From National Council of State Boards of Nursing (eds.). (2005). *Detailed test plan for the National Council licensure examination for practical/vocational Nurses.* Chicago: National Council of State Boards of Nursing.

BOX 1-2

Safe, Effective Care Environment

COORDINATED CARE
The nurse observes that a client becomes agitated and incoherent and suspects that the client is experiencing a reaction to medication. In planning a safe environment for this client, the nurse should:
1. Request that the physician order restraints and sedation
2. Ask the family to stay with the client
3. Ask a nursing assistant to stay with the client
4. Collaborate with the registered nurse
Answer: 4
This question addresses the subcategory Coordinated Care in the Client Needs category Safe, Effective Care Environment. The nurse has the responsibility to facilitate safe and effective client care through collaboration with other health care team members.

SAFETY AND INFECTION CONTROL
The nurse is assigned to care for a client receiving an intravenous (IV) infusion. While caring for the client, the nurse implements which action to decrease the risk for infection?
1. Takes the vital signs at 4-hour intervals
2. Changes the IV dressing every shift
3. Uses aseptic technique when handling the intravenous solution and tubing
4. Administers acetaminophen (Tylenol) every 4 hours
Answer: 3
This question addresses the subcategory, Safety and Infection Control, in the Client Needs category, Safe, Effective Care Environment. It addresses content related to surgical asepsis and protecting the client from infection.

BOX 1-3

Health Promotion and Maintenance

The nurse is assisting in planning a health maintenance program for a group of older adults. Which activity would best promote health and maintenance in this group?
1. Gardening every day for an hour
2. Walking three to five times a week for 30 minutes
3. Sculpting once a week for 40 minutes
4. Cycling three times a week for 20 minutes
Answer: 2
This question addresses the Client Needs category Health Promotion and Maintenance and addresses the aging process. Exercise and activity are essential for health promotion and maintenance in the older adult and for achieving an optimal level of functioning. One of the best exercises for an older adult is walking, progressing to 30-minute sessions three to five times each week.

Health Promotion and Maintenance

The Health Promotion and Maintenance category (7% to 13%) addresses the principles related to growth and development and the aging process. This Client Needs category also addresses content that tests the knowledge, skills, and ability required to assist the client, family members, and/or significant others to prevent health problems, recognize alterations in health, and develop health practices that promote and support wellness. Box 1-3 presents an example of a question in this Client Needs category.

Psychosocial Integrity

The Psychosocial Integrity category (8% to 14%) addresses content that tests the knowledge, skills, and ability required to promote and support the ability of the client, family, and/or significant others to cope, adapt, and/or problem-solve during stressful events. This Client Needs category also addresses the emotional, mental, and social well-being of the client, family, and significant other, and the knowledge, skills, and ability required to care for the client with an acute or chronic mental illness. See Box 1-4 for an example of a question in this Client Needs category.

Physiological Integrity

The Physiological Integrity category includes four subcategories, Basic Care and Comfort, Pharmacological Therapies, Reduction of Risk Potential, and Physiological Adaptation. Basic Care and Comfort (11% to 17%) addresses content that tests the knowledge, skills, and ability required to provide comfort and assistance in the performance of the activities of daily living. Pharmacological Therapies (9% to 15%) addresses content that tests the knowledge, skills, and ability required to provide care related to the administration of medications and monitoring clients receiving parenteral therapies. Reduction of Risk Potential (10% to 16%)

BOX 1-4

Psychosocial Integrity

The nurse is assigned to care for a client with ovarian cancer. While giving morning care, the client says, "If I can just live long enough to attend my daughter's graduation, I'll be ready to die." Which phase of coping is this client experiencing?

1. Isolation
2. Bargaining
3. Depression
4. Acceptance

Answer: 2

This question addresses the Client Needs category Psychosocial Integrity, and the content addresses coping mechanisms. Bargaining is the phase of coping in which the dying person tries to negotiate, as in this case, making a deal with God or fate.

addresses content that tests the knowledge, skills, and ability required to reduce the client's potential for developing complications or health problems related to existing conditions, treatments, or procedures. Physiological Adaptation (12% to 18%) addresses content that tests the knowledge, skills, and ability required to participate in providing care to clients with acute, chronic, or life-threatening physical health conditions. See Box 1-5 for examples of questions in this Client Needs category.

Integrated Processes of the Test Plan

The NCSBN has identified four processes fundamental to the practice of nursing. These processes are a component of the test plan and are integrated throughout the categories of Client Needs (Box 1-6).

TYPES OF QUESTIONS ON THE EXAMINATION

The types of questions that may be administered on the examination include multiple choice, fill in the blank, multiple response, prioritizing (ordered response), chart/exhibit, and those that contain a figure or illustration (hot spots). Some questions may require you to use the mouse component of the computer system. For example, you may be presented with a visual that displays the arterial vessels of an adult client. In this visual, you may be asked to "point and click" (using the mouse) on the area where the dorsalis pedis pulse can be felt. With these questions, the NCSBN provides specific directions to guide you in the testing process. Be sure to read these directions as they appear on the computer screen.

Multiple-Choice Questions

Most of the questions that you are asked to answer are in the multiple-choice format. These questions provide you with data about a particular client situation and give four answers or options.

Fill in the Blank

These types of questions may ask you to perform a medication calculation, determine an intravenous flow rate, or calculate an intake or output record on a client. You need to type in your answer. See Box 1-7 for an example.

Multiple Response

In this type of question, you are asked to select or check all the options, such as nursing interventions, that relate to the information in the question. There is no partial credit given for correct selections. See Box 1-8 for an example.

Prioritizing (Ordered Response)

These questions may ask you to number or place (drag and drop) your nursing actions in order of priority. Information will be presented in a question and, based on the data, you need to determine what you will do first, second, third, and so forth. See Box 1-9 for an example.

Figure or Illustration (Hot Spot)

This type of question provides you with a figure or illustration and asks you to answer the question based on it. The question could contain a chart, table, figure, or illustration. You may also be asked to use the computer mouse and point and click on a specific area (hot spot) in the visual. A visual or image may appear in any type of question, including a multiple-choice question. See Box 1-10 for an example.

Chart/Exhibit

In this type of question, you are presented with a problem and a chart/exhibit. You need to refer to the information in the chart/exhibit to answer the question. See Box 1-11 for an example.

COMPUTERIZED ADAPTIVE TESTING (CAT)

The acronym *CAT* stands for computerized adaptive testing. This means that the examination is created as the test-taker answers each question. All the test questions are categorized on the basis of the test plan structure and the level of difficulty of the question. As you answer a question, the computer determines your competency based on the answer that you selected. If you selected the correct answer to a question, the computer scans the question bank and selects a more difficult question. If you selected an incorrect answer, the computer scans the question bank and selects an easier question.

BOX 1-5

Physiological Integrity

BASIC CARE AND COMFORT

A nurse provides instructions to a client about the use of a cane and watches as the client uses the device. Which observation by the nurse indicates the need to provide additional instructions to the client?
1. The client holds the cane on the strong side.
2. The client holds the cane approximately 6 inches to the side of the foot.
3. The client flexes the elbow at a 15- to 30-degree angle when holding the cane in place.
4. The client moves the cane and the stronger leg forward first, and then moves the weaker leg forward.

Answer: 4

This question addresses the subcategory Basic Care and Comfort in the Client Needs category Physiological Integrity, and addresses client mobility and promoting assistance in an activity of daily living. Note the issue of the question—the need for the nurse to provide additional instructions. Visualize each options in terms of its safety in performing ambulation with regard to the use of a cane. This will direct you to option 4, the option that is unsafe.

PHARMACOLOGICAL THERAPIES

A client is taking capreomycin sulfate (Capastat Sulfate), a second-line tuberculosis medication, as a component of pharmacological treatment for tuberculosis. The client calls the nurse at the physician's office and tells the nurse that he is experiencing ringing in his ears. The nurse appropriately tells the client that:
1. He should speak with the physician about the problem
2. Ringing in the ears is an expected effect of the medication
3. He should discontinue the medication
4. Ringing in the ears is a harmless effect of the medication

Answer: 1

This question addresses the subcategory Pharmacological Therapies in the Client Needs category Physiological Integrity. Capreomycin is a second-line antituberculosis medication that is administered in conjunction with a first-line medication to treat tuberculosis. It can cause damage to cranial nerve VIII (ototoxicity), resulting in hearing loss, tinnitus, and disturbance of balance. Ototoxicity is not an expected or harmless effect of the medication and, if it occurs, the physician needs to be notified. The nurse does not adjust a medication dosage or discontinue a medication.

REDUCTION OF RISK POTENTIAL

The nurse is assigned to assist in caring for a client who has undergone cystoscopy. The nurse recognizes that which of the following is an abnormal sign, if noted during the first few hours after the procedure?
1. Pink-tinged urine
2. Grossly bloody urine with clots
3. Clear yellow urine
4. Yellow-colored urine

Answer: 2

This question addresses the subcategory Reduction of Risk Potential in the Client Needs category Physiological Integrity. It relates to a potential complication of a procedure. Grossly bloody urine with clots is always an abnormal finding and should be reported immediately.

PHYSIOLOGICAL ADAPTATION

The nurse is assigned to care for a client with a diagnosis of pheochromocytoma. The nurse notes in the laboratory report that the client's magnesium level is 7 mEq/L. Based on this laboratory result, the nurse recognizes which of the following signs as significant?
1. Drowsiness
2. Hypertension
3. Hyperpnea
4. Hyperactive reflexes

Answer: 1

This question addresses the subcategory Physiological Adaptation in the Client Needs category Physiological Integrity. It addresses an alteration in body systems. Neurological manifestations begin to occur at magnesium levels of 6 to 7 mEq/L and are noted as symptoms of neurological depression, such as drowsiness, sedation, lethargy, respiratory depression, muscle weakness, and areflexia.

This process continues until the test plan requirements are met and a reliable pass-or-fail decision is made.

When a test question is presented on the computer screen, it must be answered or the test will not move on. This means that you are not able to skip questions, go back and review questions, or go back and change answers. Remember, in a CAT examination, once an answer is recorded, all subsequent questions administered depend, to an extent, on the answer selected for that question. Skipping and returning to earlier questions are not compatible with the logical methodology of a computerized adaptive test. The inability to skip questions or go back to change previous answers is not a disadvantage to you. Actually, you will not fall into the "trap" of changing a correct answer to an incorrect one with the CAT system.

If you are faced with a question that contains unfamiliar content, you may need to guess at the answer. There is no penalty for guessing on this examination. Remember, with the majority of the questions, the answer is right there in front of you. If you need to guess, use your nursing knowledge to its fullest extent, as well as all the test-taking strategies that you have practiced in this review program.

BOX 1-6

Integrated Processes of the Test Plan

Caring
Clinical Problem-Solving Process (Nursing Process)
Communication and Documentation
Teaching/Learning

BOX 1-7

Fill in the Blank

A physician orders an intramuscular dose of 200,000 units of penicillin G benzathine (Bicillin). The label on the ampule sent from the pharmacy reads penicillin G benzathine (Bicillin), 300,000 units/mL. The nurse prepares how much medication to administer the correct dose? (Round to the nearest tenth.)

Answer: 0.7

In this question, you need to use the formula for calculating a medication dose. Once the dose is determined, you must type in your answer. In this question, you are asked to round to the nearest tenth. Always follow the specific directions noted on the computer screen when answering the question. Also, remember that there will be an on-screen calculator on the computer for your use, if needed.

BOX 1-8

Multiple Response

A hospitalized client who was diagnosed with a cerebral aneurysm is placed on aneurysm precautions. Select all nursing interventions that apply for these precautions.
Answer:

___ Allow the client to perform activities of daily living independently, including bathing and dressing.

___ Encourage the client to dress in street clothes and shoes every day.

_X_ Encourage restful activities such as listening to quiet music.

___ Keep the room well lit, especially during the daytime hours.

_X_ Administer stool softeners to the client.

_X_ Restrict visitors and keep visits short.

In a multiple-response question, you are asked to select or check all the options, such as nursing interventions, that relate to the information in the question. To answer this question, recalling the pathophysiology associated with a cerebral aneurysm and that a primary concern is rupture of the aneurysm assist in identifying the appropriate nursing interventions. Remember, follow the specific directions noted on the computer screen.

BOX 1-9

Prioritizing (Ordered Response)

A nurse prepares to care for an older client admitted to the hospital with a diagnosis of dehydration. On data collection, the nurse notes that the client is weak when ambulating, is intermittently confused, and her skin is dry. The client reports that she has been able to eat and drink small amounts but that the diarrhea will not stop. The client also tells the nurse that she lives alone and cannot socialize much because she does not drive and does not have family close by who can visit her. The nurse reviews the client's plan of care and notes that four nursing diagnoses are listed. Prioritize the nursing diagnoses (using the numbers 1, 2, 3, 4, 5) from highest priority (number 1) to lowest priority (number 5).

___ Deficient fluid volume
___ Risk for impaired skin integrity
___ Acute confusion
___ Risk for injury
___ Risk for social isolation

Answer: 14235

This question asks you to prioritize the nursing diagnoses identified for this client in order of importance and provides you with directions regarding numbering from highest priority to lowest priority. Remember, read the directions on the computer screen to guide you in answering this type of question. The nursing diagnosis most appropriate (highest priority) for the client who is dehydrated is deficient fluid volume. Because the nursing diagnosis acute confusion is an actual client problem, and because confusion could place the client at risk for injury, acute confusion would be the second priority. Risk for injury, risk for impaired skin integrity, and risk for social isolation are potential but not actual problems. Risk for injury would be the third priority because of the client's problem with acute confusion. Risk for impaired skin integrity is the fourth priority because it is a physiological need. This would be followed by risk for social isolation, a psychosocial need.

You do not need any computer experience to take this examination. A keyboard tutorial is provided and administered to all test-takers at the start of the examination. The tutorial will instruct you on the use of the on-screen optional calculator, the use of the mouse, and how to record an answer. In addition to the traditional four-option multiple-choice question, the tutorial also provides instructions on how to respond to different question formats. A proctor is present to help explain the use of the computer to ensure that you fully understand how to proceed.

REGISTERING TO TAKE THE EXAMINATION

The initial step in the registration process is to submit an application to the state board of nursing in the state in which you intend to obtain licensure. You need to obtain information from the board of nursing regarding

BOX 1-10

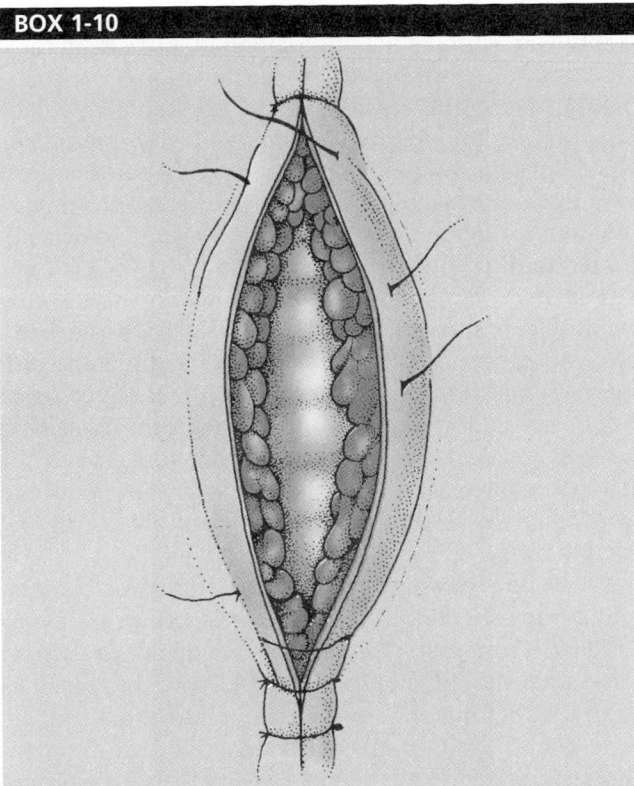

FIG. 1-1 (From Ignatavicius, D., & Workman, M. [2002]. *Medical surgical nursing: Critical thinking for collaborative care* (4th ed.) Philadelphia: W.B. Saunders.)

A nurse is changing an abdominal dressing on a client who has had abdominal surgery. After removing the old dressing, the nurse assesses the surgical site. The nurse takes which initial action if this wound appearance has been observed?

1. Redress the wound with a dry sterile dressing.
2. Document the findings.
3. Apply a sterile, nonadherent dressing.
4. Ask the client to cough to assess for protrusion of the internal structures.

Answer: 3

In this question, you are provided with an illustration and asked for the initial nursing action based on your observation. Wound dehiscence is a partial or complete separation of the outer layers of the wound. From the options provided, the nurse would apply a sterile, nonadherent dressing to the wound. A dry dressing could disrupt the integrity of the underlying tissues. The nurse would document the findings, but this would not be the initial action. Asking the client to cough could cause an extension of the outer layers of the wound.

BOX 1-11

Chart/Exhibit

CLIENT'S CHART
TAB: LABORATORY
Sodium 150 mEq/L
Potassium 4.0 mEq/L
Chloride 102 mEq/L
Bicarbonate 26 mEq/L

The nurse reviews the client's laboratory results for electrolyte levels. The nurse reports which abnormal result?

1. Sodium
2. Potassium
3. Chloride
4. Bicarbonate

Answer: 1

In this question, you are provided with the client's chart and laboratory results. You need to refer to the laboratory results to answer the question. On the NCLEX-PN examination, you will need to use the computer mouse and click on the appropriate Tab noted on the client's chart. In this question, you would click on the Tab: Laboratory. Normal levels are the following: sodium, 135 to 145 mEq/L; potassium, 3.5 to 5.1 mEq/L; chloride, 98 to 107 mEq/L; and bicarbonate, 22 to 29 mEq/L.

the specific registration process, because the process may vary from state to state. In most states, you may register for the examination through the Internet, by mail, or by telephone. The NCLEX candidate Web site is www.vue.com/nclex. It is very important that you follow the registration instructions and complete the registration forms precisely and accurately. Registration forms that are not properly completed or not accompanied by the proper fees in the required method of payment will be returned to you and delay testing. There is a fee for taking the examination, and you may also have to pay additional fees to the board of nursing in the state in which you are applying. You will be sent a confirmation indicating that your registration was received. If you do not receive a confirmation within 4 weeks of submitting your registration, you should contact the NCLEX candidate services. Information regarding this contact can be obtained at the NCLEX candidate Web site at www.vue.com/nclex.

AUTHORIZATION TO TEST FORM

Once your eligibility to test has been determined by the board of nursing in the state in which licensure is requested, your registration form is processed and an Authorization to Test (ATT) form will be sent to you. You cannot make an appointment until the state board of nursing declares eligibility and you receive an ATT form. The examination is given at a Pearson Professional Center, and an appointment can be made through the Internet (www.vue.com/nclex) or by telephone. The ATT form will list the telephone numbers of all Pearsons Professional Centers in the nation. You can schedule an appointment at any Pearson Professional Center. You do not have to take the examination in the same state in which you are seeking licensure. A confirmation of your appointment will be sent to you.

The ATT form contains important information, including your test authorization number, candidate identification number, and expiration date. Note the expiration date on the form because you must test by this date. You also need to take your ATT form to the test center on the day of your examination. You will not be admitted to the examination if you do not have it.

If for any reason you need to cancel or reschedule your test appointment, you can make the change on the candidate Web site (www.vue.com/nclex) or by calling candidate services. The change needs to be made one full business day (24 hours) before your scheduled appointment. If you fail to arrive for the examination or to reschedule or cancel your appointment to test without providing appropriate notice, you forfeit your examination fee and your ATT is invalidated. This information is reported to the board of nursing in the state in which you have applied for licensure, and you will be required to register and pay the testing fees again.

It is important that you arrive at the testing center at least 30 minutes before the test is scheduled. If you arrive late for the scheduled testing appointment, you may be required to forfeit your examination appointment. If it is necessary for the appointment to be forfeited, you need to reregister for the examination and pay an additional fee. The board of nursing is notified that you did not test. A few days before your scheduled date of testing, take the time to drive to the testing center to determine its exact location, the length of time required to arrive there, and any potential obstacles that might delay you, such as road construction, traffic, or parking.

SPECIAL TESTING CIRCUMSTANCES

A test-taker with needs who requires special testing accommodations should contact the board of nursing before submitting a registration form. The board of nursing, which must authorize special testing accommodations, will provide the procedures for the request. Following board of nursing approval, the NCSBN reviews the requested accommodations and must also approve the request. If the request is approved, the testing appointment must be made by the NCLEX Program Coordinator, who can be contacted by calling NCLEX candidate services. Canceling or rescheduling an appointment must be done through the NCLEX Program Coordinator.

THE TESTING CENTER

The test center is designed to ensure complete security of the testing process. Strict candidate identification requirements have been established. To be admitted to the testing center, it is imperative that you bring the ATT form, along with two forms of identification. Both forms of identification must be signed, current or nonexpired, and one must contain your recent photograph. The name on the photograph identification must be exactly the same as the name on the ATT form. A digital fingerprint, signature, and photograph will be obtained at the test center and will accompany the NCLEX results to confirm your identity. Additionally, if you leave the testing room for any reason, you are required to have your fingerprint taken again to be readmitted to the room.

Personal belongings are not allowed in the testing room. Secure storage is provided for the candidate; however, storage space is limited, so you must plan accordingly. In addition, the testing center does not assume responsibility for your personal belongings. The testing waiting areas are generally small; therefore, friends or family members who accompany you are not permitted to wait in the testing center while you are taking the examination.

Once you have completed the admission process and a brief orientation, the proctor escorts you to your assigned computer. You are seated at an individual table area with an appropriate work space that includes computer equipment, appropriate lighting, an erasable note board, and a marker. No items, including unauthorized scratch paper, are allowed into the testing room. Electronic devices such as watches, beepers, or cell phones are not allowed into the testing room. Eating, drinking, or the use of tobacco is not allowed in the testing room. You will be observed at all times by the test proctor while taking the examination. Additionally, there is video and audio recording of all test sessions. Pearson Professional Centers has no control over the sounds made by typing on the computer. If these sounds are distracting, raise your hand to summon the proctor. Earplugs are available on request.

You must follow the directions given by the test center staff and must remain seated during the test, except when authorized to leave. If you believe you have a problem with the computer, need more scratch paper, need to take a break, or need the test proctor for any reason, you must raise your hand.

TESTING TIME

The maximum testing time is 5 hours, and this time period includes the tutorial, the sample items, all breaks, and the examination. All breaks are optional. You must leave the testing room during breaks and, when you return, you will be required to provide a fingerprint to be readmitted to the testing room.

LENGTH OF THE EXAMINATION

The minimum number of questions that you need to answer is 85. Of these 85 questions, 60 are operational (scored) questions and 25 are pretest (unscored) questions. The maximum number of questions in the test is 205. Of the total number of questions that you need to answer, 25 are pretest (unscored) questions.

The pretest questions are questions that may be presented as scored questions on future examinations. These pretest questions are not identified as such. In other words, you do not know which questions are the pretest (unscored) questions.

PASS OR FAIL DECISIONS

All the examination questions are categorized by test plan area and level of difficulty. This is an important point to keep in mind when considering how a pass or fail decision is made by the computer, because a pass or fail decision is not based on a percentage of correctly answered questions. After the minimum number of questions have been answered (85 questions), the computer compares the test-taker's ability level to the standard required for passing. The standard required for passing is set based on the expert judgment of several individuals appointed by the National Council of State Boards of Nursing. If the test-taker is clearly above the passing standard, then the test-taker passes the examination. If the test-taker is clearly below the passing standard, then the test-taker fails the examination. If the computer is not able to clearly determine if the test-taker has passed or failed because the test-taker's ability is close to the passing standard, then the computer continues asking questions. After each question, the test-taker's ability is determined, and when it becomes clear on which side of the passing standard that the test-taker falls (above the standard or below the standard), the examination ends. If the test-taker is administered the maximum number of questions (205 questions), the computer will make a pass or fail decision by recomputing the test-taker's final ability level, based on every question answered, and comparing it with the passing standard. If the ability level is above the passing standard, the test-taker passes. If it is not above the passing standard, the test-taker fails.

If the examination ends because you have run out of time, the computer may not have enough information to make a clear pass or fail decision. If this is the situation, the computer will review the test-taker's performance during testing. If the test-taker's ability was consistently above the passing standard, the test-taker passes. If the test-taker's ability falls to or below the passing standard, even once, the test-taker fails.

COMPLETING THE EXAM

Once the test is completed, you will complete a brief computer-delivered questionnaire about your testing experience. After this questionnaire is completed, you need to raise your hand to summon the test proctor. The test proctor will collect and inventory all note boards and then permit you to leave.

PROCESSING RESULTS

Every computerized examination is scored twice: once by the computer at the testing center and then again after the examination is transmitted to Pearson Professional Centers. No results are released at the test center. The board of nursing will mail your results to you approximately one month after taking the examination. You should not telephone Pearson Professional Centers, the National Council of State Boards of Nursing, candidate services, or the state board of nursing for results.

CANDIDATE PERFORMANCE REPORT

A candidate performance report is provided to a test-taker who failed the examination. This report provides the test-taker with information about their strengths and weaknesses in relation to the test plan and provides a guide for studying and retaking the examination. The test-taker should refer to the state board of nursing in the state in which licensure is sought for procedures regarding the time period for retaking the examination.

INTERSTATE ENDORSEMENT

Because the NCLEX-PN examination is a national examination, you can apply to take the examination in any state. Once licensure is received, you can apply for Interstate Endorsement. The procedures and requirements for Interstate Endorsement may vary from state to state, and these procedures can be obtained from the state board of nursing in the state in which endorsement is sought.

STATE BOARDS OF NURSING

Contact information was obtained from the National Council of State Boards of Nursing, Inc., Web site (http://www.ncsbn.org/). Because contact information may change, access this Web site if necessary.

Alabama Board of Nursing
770 Washington Avenue
RSA Plaza, Suite 250
Montgomery, AL 36130-3900
Phone: (334) 242-4060
Web site: http://www.abn.state.al.us/

Alaska Board of Nursing
550 West Seventh Avenue, Suite 1500
Anchorage, AK 99501-3567
Phone: (907) 269-8161
Web site: http://www.dced.state.ak.us/occ/pnur.htm

American Samoa Health Services Regulatory Board
LBJ Tropical Medical Center
Pago Pago, AS 96799
Phone: (684) 633-1222

Arizona State Board of Nursing
1651 East Morten Avenue, Suite 210
Phoenix, AZ 85020
Phone: (602) 889-5150
Web site: http://www.azboardofnursing.org/

Arkansas State Board of Nursing
University Tower Building
1123 South University, Suite 800
Little Rock, AR 72204-1619
Phone: (501) 686-2700
Web site: http://www.state.ar.us/nurse

California Board of Vocational Nurse and Psychiatric Technicians
2535 Capitol Oaks Drive, Suite 205
Sacramento, CA 95833
Phone: (916) 263-7800
Web site: http://www.bvnpt.ca.gov/

Colorado Board of Nursing
1560 Broadway, Suite 880
Denver, CO 80202
Phone: (303) 894-2430
Web site: http://www.dora.state.co.us/nursing/

Connecticut Board of Examiners for Nursing
Department of Public Health
410 Capitol Avenue, MS# 13PHO
P.O. Box 340308
Hartford, CT 06134-0328
Phone: (860) 509-7624
Web site: http://www.state.ct.us/dph/

Delaware Board of Nursing
861 Silver Lake Blvd.
Cannon Building, Suite 203
Dover, DE 19904
Phone: (302) 739-4522
Web site: http://www.professionallicensing.state.de.us/boards/nursing/index.shtml

District of Columbia Board of Nursing
Department of Health
717 14th Street NW, Suite 600
Washington, DC 20005
Phone: (202) 724-4900
Web site: http://www.dchealth.dc.gov

Florida Board of Nursing
Mailing Address:
4052 Bald Cypress Way, BIN C02
Tallahassee, FL 32399-3252
Street Address:
4042 Bald Cypress Way, Room 120
Tallahassee, FL 32399
Phone: (850) 245-4125
Web site: http://www.doh.state.fl.us/mqa/

Georgia State Board of Licensed Practical Nurses
237 Coliseum Drive
Macon, GA 31217-3858
Phone: (478) 207-1640
Web site: http://www.sos.state.ga.us/plb/lpn

Guam Board of Nurse Examiners
Mailing Address:
P.O. Box 2816
Hagatna, Guam 96932
Street Address (for FedEx and UPS)
651 Legacy Square Commercial Complex, Suite 9
South Route 10
Mangilao, Guam 96913
Phone: (671) 735-7406; (671) 725-7411
Web site: http://www.dphss.govguam.net/hplo.htm

Hawaii Board of Nursing
King Kalakaua Building
335 Merchant Street, 3rd Floor
Honolulu, HI 96813
Phone: (808) 586-3000
Web site: http://www.state.hi.us/dcca/pvl/areas_nurse.html

Idaho Board of Nursing
280 North 8th Street, Suite 210
P.O. Box 83720
Boise, ID 83720
Phone: (208) 334-3110
Web site: http://www.state.id.us/ibn/ibnhome.htm

Illinois Department of Professional Regulation
Chicago office
James R. Thompson Center
100 West Randolph, Suite 9-300
Chicago, IL 60601
Phone: (312) 814-2715
Web site: http://www.dpr.state.il.us/

Springfield office
320 West Washington Street, 3rd Floor
Springfield, IL 62786
Phone: (217) 782-8556

Indiana State Board of Nursing
Health Professions Bureau
402 West Washington Street, Room W066
Indianapolis, IN 46204
Phone: (317) 234-2043
Web site: http://www.state.in.us/hpb/boards/isbn/

Iowa Board of Nursing
RiverPoint Business Park
400 SW 8th Street, Suite B
Des Moines, IA 50309-4685
Phone: (515) 281-3255
Web site: http://www.state.ia.us/government/nursing/

Kansas State Board of Nursing
Landon State Office Building
900 SW Jackson, Suite 1051
Topeka, KS 66612
Phone: (785) 296-4929
Web site: http://www.ksbn.org/

Kentucky Board of Nursing
312 Whittington Parkway, Suite 300
Louisville, KY 40222
Phone: (502) 429-3300
Web site: http://www.kbn.ky.gov/

Louisiana State Board of Practical Nurse Examiners
3510 North Causeway Boulevard, Suite 501
Metairie, LA 70002
Phone: (504) 838-5791
Web site: http://www.lsbpne.com/

Maine State Board of Nursing
158 State House Station
Augusta, ME 04333
Phone: (207) 287-1133
Web site: http://www.maine.gov/boardofnursing/

Maryland Board of Nursing
4140 Patterson Avenue
Baltimore, MD 21215
Phone: (410) 585-1900
Web site: http://www.mbon.org

Massachusetts Board of Registration in Nursing
Commonwealth of Massachusetts
239 Causeway Street Suite 500
Boston, MA 02114
Phone: (617) 727-9961
Web site: http://www.state.ma.us/reg/boards/rn/

Michigan/DCH/Bureau of Health Professions
Ottawa Towers North
611 West Ottawa, 1st Floor
Lansing, MI 48933
Phone: (517) 335-0918
Web site: http://www.michigan.gov/healthlicense

Minnesota Board of Nursing
2829 University Avenue SE, Suite 500
Minneapolis, MN 55414
Phone: (612) 617-2270
Web site: http://www.nursingboard.state.mn.us/

Mississippi Board of Nursing
1935 Lakeland Drive, Suite B
Jackson, MS 39216-5014
Phone: (601) 987-4188
Web site: http://www.msbn.state.ms.us/

Missouri State Board of Nursing
3605 Missouri Blvd.
P.O. Box 656
Jefferson City, MO 65102-0656
Phone: (573) 751-0681
Web site: http://pr.mo.gov/nursing.asp

Montana State Board of Nursing
301 South Park
P.O. Box 200513
Helena, MT 59620-0513
Phone: (406) 841-2340
Web site: http://www.discoveringmontana.com/dli/
bsd/license/bsd_boards/nur_board/board_page.htm

Nebraska Department of Health and Human Services Regulation and Licensure
301 Centennial Mall South
Lincoln, NE 68509-4986
Phone: (402) 471-4376
Web site: http://www.hhs.state.ne.us/crl/nursing/
nursingindex.htm

Nevada State Board of Nursing
5011 Meadowood Mall #201
Reno, NV 89502-6547
Phone: (775) 688-2620
Web site: http://www.nursingboard.state.nv.us/

New Hampshire Board of Nursing
21 South Fruit Street, Suite 16
Concord, NH 03301-2341
Phone: (603) 271-2323
Web site: http://www.state.nh.us/nursing/

New Jersey Board of Nursing
P.O. Box 45010
124 Halsey Street, 6th Floor
Newark, NJ 07101
Phone: (973) 504-6586
Web site: http://www.state.nj.us/lps/ca/medical.htm

New Mexico Board of Nursing
6301 Indian School Road NE, Suite 710
Albuquerque, NM 87110
Phone: (505) 841-8340
Web site: http://www.state.nm.us/clients/nursing

New York State Board of Nursing
Education Building
89 Washington Avenue, 2nd Floor, West Wing
Albany, NY 12234
Phone: (518) 474-3817 Ext. 280
Web site: http://www.nysed.gov/prof/nurse.htm

North Carolina Board of Nursing
3724 National Drive, Suite 201
Raleigh, NC 27602
Phone: (919) 782-3211
Web site: http://www.ncbon.com/

North Dakota Board of Nursing
919 South 7th Street, Suite 504
Bismarck, ND 58504
Phone: (701) 328-9777
Web site: http://www.ndbon.org/

Northern Mariana Islands
Commonwealth Board of Nurse Examiners
P.O. Box 501458
Saipan, MP 96950
Phone: (670) 664-4812

Ohio Board of Nursing
17 South High Street, Suite 400
Columbus, OH 43215-3413
Phone: (614) 466-3947
Web site: http://www.nursing.ohio.gov

Oklahoma Board of Nursing
2915 North Classen Blvd., Suite 524
Oklahoma City, OK 73106
Phone: (405) 962-1800
Web site: http://www.youroklahoma.com/nursing

Oregon State Board of Nursing
800 NE Oregon Street, Box 25, Suite 465
Portland, OR 97232
Phone: (503) 731-4745
Web site: http://www.osbn.state.or.us/

Pennsylvania State Board of Nursing
P.O. Box 2649
Harrisburg, PA 17105-2649
Phone: (717) 783-7142
Web site: http://www.dos.state.pa.us/bpoa/cwp/
view.asp?a=1104&q=432869

Puerto Rico Board of Nurse Examiners
Commonwealth of Puerto Rico
800 Roberto H. Todd Avenue, Room 202, Stop 18
Santurce, PR 00908
Phone: (787) 725-7506

**Rhode Island Board of Nurse Registration
and Nursing Education**
105 Cannon Building, Three Capitol Hill
Providence, RI 02908
Phone: (401) 222-5700
Web site: http://www.healthri.org/hsr/professions/
nurses.htm

South Carolina State Board of Nursing
110 Centerview Drive, Suite 202
Columbia, SC 29210
Phone: (803) 896-4550
Web site: http://www.llr.state.sc.us/pol/nursing

South Dakota Board of Nursing
4305 South Louise Avenue, Suite 201
Sioux Falls, SD 57106-3115
Phone: (605) 362-2760
Web site: http://www.state.sd.us/doh/nursing/

Tennessee State Board of Nursing
425 Fifth Avenue North, 1st Floor
Cordell Hull Building
Nashville, TN 37247
Phone: (615) 532-5166
Web site: http://www.tennessee.gov/health

Texas Board of Nurse Examiners
333 Guadalupe, Suite 3-460
Austin, TX 78701
Phone: (512) 305-7400
Web site: http://www.bne.state.tx.us/

Utah State Board of Nursing
Heber M. Wells Bldg., 4th Floor
160 East 300 South
Salt Lake City, UT 84111
Phone: (801) 530-6628
Web site: http://www.commerce.state.ut.us/

Vermont State Board of Nursing
81 River Street
Heritage Building
Montpelier, VT 05609-1106
Phone: (802) 828-2396
Web site: http://www.vtprofessionals.org/opr1/nurses/

Virgin Islands Board of Nurse Licensure
Veterans Drive Station
St. Thomas, VI 00803
Phone: (340) 776-7397
Web site: http://www.ribnl.org

Virginia Board of Nursing
6603 West Broad Street, 5th Floor
Richmond, VA 23230-1712
Phone: (804) 662-9909
Web site: http://www.dhp.virginia.gov/

Washington State Nursing Care Quality Assurance Commission
Department of Health, HPQA #6
310 Israel Road SE
Tumwater, WA 98501-7864
Phone: (360) 236-4700
Web site: https://wws2.wa.gov/doh/hpqa-licensing/HPS6/Nursing/default.htm

West Virginia State Board of Examiners for Licensed Practical Nurses
101 Dee Drive
Charleston, WV 25311
Phone: (304) 558-3572
Web site: http://www.lpnboard.state.wv.us/

Wisconsin Department of Regulation and Licensing
1400 East Washington Avenue, RM 173
Madison, WI 53708
Phone: (608) 266-0145
Web site: http://www.drl.state.wi.us/

Wyoming State Board of Nursing
2020 Carey Avenue, Suite 110
Cheyenne, WY 82002
Phone: (307) 777-7601
Web site: http://nursing.state.wy.us/

REFERENCES

Chernecky, C., & Berger, B. (2004). *Laboratory tests and diagnostic procedures* (4th ed.). Philadelphia: W.B. Saunders.

DeWit, S. (2005). *Fundamental concepts and skills for nursing* (2nd ed.). Philadelphia: W.B. Saunders.

Hill, S., & Howlett, H. (2005). *Success in practical/vocational nursing: From student to leader* (5th ed.). Philadelphia: W.B. Saunders.

Hodgson, B., & Kizior, R. (2005). *Saunders nursing drug handbook 2005*. Philadelphia: W.B. Saunders.

Ignatavicius, D., & Workman, M. (2002). *Medical-surgical nursing: Critical thinking for collaborative care* (4th ed.). Philadelphia: W.B. Saunders.

Linton, A.., & Maebius, N. (2003). *Introduction to medical-surgical nursing* (3rd ed.). Philadelphia: W.B. Saunders.

Malarkey, L., & McMorrow, M. (2005). *Nursing guide to laboratory and diagnostic tests*. Philadelphia: W.B. Saunders.

Morrison-Valfre, M. (2005). *Foundations of mental health care* (3rd ed.). St. Louis: Mosby.

National Council of State Boards of Nursing (eds.) (2005). *Detailed Test Plan for the National Council Licensure Examination for Practical/Vocational Nurses*. Chicago: National Council of State Boards of Nursing.

National Council of State Boards of Nursing, Inc. Web site: http://www.ncsbn.org/

Potter, P., & Perry, A. (2005) *Fundamentals of nursing* (6th ed.). St. Louis: Mosby.

Wold, G. (2004). *Basic geriatric nursing* (3rd ed.). St. Louis: Mosby.

Preparation for the NCLEX-PN® Examination: Transitional Issues for the Foreign-Educated Nurse

INTRODUCTION

This chapter is written to provide you with information regarding the certification processes that you will have to pursue to become a licensed practical/vocational nurse in the United States. An important factor to consider as you pursue this process is that some of the requirements may vary from state to state. Therefore, as a first step in the process, it is important to contact the board of nursing in the state in which you are planning to obtain licensure. To assist you in making a contact with the state board of nursing, refer to Chapter 1 in this book. At the end of the chapter, you will find the addresses, telephone numbers, and Web site address of each state, if a Web site is available. You can also access this information through the National Council of State Boards of Nursing (NCSBN) Web site at http://www.ncsbn.org. Once you have accessed the NCSBN Web site, select the link titled "Boards of Nursing." Additionally, you can write to the NCSBN regarding the NCLEX-PN examination; the address is 111 East Wacker Drive, Suite 2900, Chicago, IL 60601. The telephone number for the NCSBN is (312) 525-3600; the fax number is (312) 279-1032.

VISASCREEN

U.S. immigration law requires that foreign-educated nurses successfully complete a screening program before receiving an occupational visa (Section 343 of the Illegal Immigration Reform and Immigration Responsibility Act of 1996). Therefore, you are required to obtain a VisaScreen certificate.

The Commission on Graduates of Foreign Nursing Schools (CGFNS) is the organization that offers this federal screening program. The International Commission on Health Care Professions (ICHP), a division of the Commission on Graduates of Foreign Nursing Schools, administers the VisaScreen. The VisaScreen components include an educational analysis, license verification, assessment of proficiency in the English language, and an examination that tests nursing knowledge. Each component is described below. Once all the components have been successfully achieved, the applicant is presented with a VisaScreen certificate. Information related to the VisaScreen can be obtained from the CGFNS Web site at http://cgfns.org.

Educational Analysis

The educational analysis does the following:
1. Ensures that the applicant's education meets all statutory and regulatory requirements for the profession and is comparable to the education of a U.S. graduate seeking licensure
2. Requirements may include the following:
   a. Proof of completion of a senior secondary school or high school education
   b. Proof of completion from a government-approved professional health care nursing program
   c. Documentation of completion of a specified number of clock and/or credit hours in specific theoretical and clinical areas while in nursing school

Licensure Verification

The applicant must present all current and past licensure for review.

Proficiency in the English Language

The applicant must submit proof of a passing score on an approved U.S. Department of Education and Department of Health and Human Services English language proficiency examination. (See Box 2-1 for a list of the English proficiency examination and testing organizations.)

BOX 2-1

English Language Proficiency Examination and Testing Organizations

TESTS ADMINISTERED BY THE EDUCATIONAL TESTING SERVICE (ETS) WORLDWIDE
Test of English as a Foreign Language (TOEFL)
Test of English for International Communication (TOEIC)
Contact Information:
Educational Testing Service (ETS)
P.O. Box 6151
Princeton, NJ 08541-6151
Telephone: (609) 771-7100
E mail: toefl@ets.org

INTERNATIONAL ENGLISH LANGUAGE TESTING SYSTEM (IELTS), JOINTLY MANAGED BY BRITISH COUNCIL AND IELTS AUSTRALIA
Contact Information:
International English Language Testing System (IELTS)
IELTS Administrator
Cambridge Examinations and IELTS International
100 East Corson Street, Suite 200
Pasadena, CA 91103
Telephone: (626) 564-2954
E mail: ielts@ceii.org
Web site: www.ielts.org

Examination to Test Nursing Knowledge

1. The Qualifying Examination that is administered as part of the process for obtaining a CGFNS certificate tests nursing knowledge; therefore, a CGFNS certificate provides proof of adequate nursing knowledge. This Qualifying Examination is described below under "Components of the CGFNS Certification Program."
2. A foreign-educated nurse who is currently licensed and practicing nursing in the United States is also required to obtain a VisaScreen; if the nurse does not have a CGFNS certificate, the nurse may be granted eligibility to take the NCLEX-PN examination to provide proof of nursing knowledge. The Candidate Bulletin for NCLEX-PN for VisaScreen can be obtained at the National Council of State Boards of Nursing Web site at www.ncsbn.org.

STATE REQUIREMENTS

Most states in the United States require that you receive certification from CGFNS before you are eligible to take the NCLEX-PN examination. If the state in which you intend to obtain licensure does not require CGFNS certification, it may require submission of some of the same documents that CGFNS requires. Therefore, in addition to what CGFNS requires, a state may require the following:
1. Proof of citizenship or lawful alien status
2. Official transcripts of educational credentials sent directly to the board of nursing from the school of nursing

3. Validation of theoretical instruction and clinical practice in a variety of nursing areas, including medical nursing, surgical nursing, pediatric nursing, maternity and newborn nursing, and mental health nursing
4. Copy of nursing license and/or diploma
5. Proof of proficiency in the English language
6. Photographs of the applicant
7. Application fees

COMMISSION ON GRADUATES OF FOREIGN NURSING SCHOOLS

The Commission on Graduates of Foreign Nursing Schools (CGFNS) provides a certification program for nurses educated and licensed outside the United States. The Certification Program offered by CGFNS is a requirement of most state boards of nursing, and the certificate may be required before you can take the NCLEX-PN examination. This program ensures that you are eligible and qualified to meet licensure and other practice requirements in the United States, and it also predicts your success on the NCLEX-PN examination. This program also assists you in obtaining your VisaScreen certificate. Additional information relating to CGFNS and its Certification Program can be obtained through its Web site at http://www.cgfns.org.

Eligibility for the CGFNS Certification Program

The CGFNS Certification Program is designed for nurses educated in nursing outside the United States who hold both an initial and current registration or licensure as a nurse. According to CGFNS, the foreign-educated nurse must have obtained theoretical instruction and clinical practice in a variety of nursing areas. These nursing areas include medical nursing, surgical nursing, pediatric nursing, maternity and newborn nursing, and mental health nursing. If the nurse educated outside the United States does not meet these requirements, he or she is not eligible for the Certification Program.

Components of the CGFNS Certification Program

The CGFNS Certification Program contains three parts, and all parts must be successfully completed in order to be awarded a CGFNS certificate. The three parts include a credentials review, a qualifying examination that tests nursing knowledge, and an English language proficiency examination. The qualifying examination and the English language proficiency examination can be taken at various locations throughout the world. This provides the applicant the opportunity to obtain the CGFNS certificate before traveling to the Unites States or another country to take the NCLEX-PN examination. The three parts of the Certification Program are described on p.18.

Credentials Review

CGFNS requires validation of education and a licensing history of the applicant to ensure that the applicant has the appropriate credentials to seek certification. Transcripts and validation documents must be received by CGFNS from the nursing program and licensing agency. Transcripts and validation documents will not be accepted from the applicant. The specific credentialing requirements are similar to those needed for the VisaScreen certificate and include the following:

1. Completed a senior secondary school or high school education
2. Graduated from a government-approved nursing program
3. Obtained theoretical instruction and clinical practice in the areas of medical nursing, surgical nursing, pediatric nursing, maternity and newborn nursing, and mental health nursing
4. Holds a full, unrestricted, current license or registration to practice in the country where he or she completed their general nursing education

Qualifying Examination

The Qualifying Examination tests the applicant's knowledge in nursing in a variety of areas, such as adult health, pediatrics, maternity and newborn care, and mental health. The examination is designed to ensure that the applicant has the knowledge to provide nursing care to various client groups at the same level as recent U.S. nursing graduates.

English Language Proficiency Examination

The applicant must take and pass an English language proficiency examination, which can be taken before or after the Qualifying Examination. This examination needs to be taken from a testing organization that is approved by CGFNS, and the applicant must apply directly to the testing organization to take the examination. The examination scores must be sent directly to CGFNS from the testing organization. CGFNS will not accept test scores from the applicant. See Box 2-1 for the types of English language proficiency examinations, approved testing organizations, and their contact information.

CGFNS identifies certain applicants as exempt from the English language proficiency requirement. In order for an applicant to be exempt, he or she must meet all the following criteria: native language is English; country of nursing education was Australia, Canada (except Quebec), New Zealand (or the United Kingdom), Trinidad and Tobago; and language of instruction and language of textbooks was English.

Once you have successfully met each of the three required components of the CGFNS Certification Program, CGFNS will issue a certificate of completion. Unless the state in which you intend to obtain licensure indicates additional requirements, if you have received your VisaScreen certificate, you will be eligible to take the NCLEX-PN examination.

REGISTERING TO TAKE THE NCLEX-PN EXAMINATION

The initial step in the registration process is to submit an application to the state board of nursing in the state in which you intend to obtain licensure. You need to obtain information from the board of nursing regarding the specific registration process, because the process may vary from state to state. In most states, you can register for the examination through the Internet, by mail, or by telephone. The NCLEX-PN candidate Web site is www.vue.com/NCLEX-PN. It is very important that you follow the registration instructions and complete the registration forms precisely and accurately. Registration forms not properly completed, or not accompanied by the proper fees in the required method of payment, will be returned to you and will delay testing. There is a fee for taking the examination, and you may also have to pay additional fees to the board of nursing in the state in which you are applying. You will be sent a confirmation indicating that your registration has been received. If you do not receive a confirmation within 4 weeks of submitting your registration, you should contact the candidate services. Information regarding this contact can be obtained at the NCLEX-PN candidate Web site at www.vue.com/NCLEX-PN.

Once your eligibility to take the NCLEX-PN examination has been verified by the board of nursing in the state in which licensure is requested, your registration form is processed and an Authorization to Test form will be sent to you. You cannot make an appointment until the board of nursing declares your eligibility and you receive an Authorization to Test form. The examination will take place at one of the Pearson Professional Centers, and an appointment can be made through the Internet or by telephone. You can schedule an appointment at any of the Pearson Professional Centers. You do not have to take the examination in the same state in which you are seeking licensure. A confirmation of your appointment will be sent to you. For additional information regarding the NCLEX-PN examination and testing procedures, see Chapter 1.

PREPARING TO TAKE THE NCLEX-PN EXAMINATION

The challenge presented to you is one that requires patience and endurance. The positive result of your endeavor will certainly reward you professionally and give you the personal satisfaction of knowing that you have become part of a family of highly skilled professionals, the Licensed Practical/Vocational Nurse. You have successfully completed the requirements to become eligible to take the NCLEX-PN examination, and now you have one more important goal to achieve, passing the NCLEX-PN examination.

I highly recommend adequate preparation for the NCLEX-PN examination, because the examination is difficult. An important step that you have taken in preparing is that you are using this book, *Saunders Comprehensive Review for the NCLEX-PN® Examination.* Once you have reviewed the content and answered the practice questions, the next step in your journey to success is to use the companion book, *Saunders Q & A Review for the NCLEX-PN® Examination.* This book also provides you with over 3000 practice questions based on the NCLEX-PN test plan. Also available for your preparation for the NCLEX-PN examination is the *Saunders Review Cards for the NCLEX-PN® Examination,* which contains over 900 practice questions based on the NCLEX-PN test plan.

Lastly, never lose sight of your goal. Patience and dedication will contribute significantly to your achieving the status of Licensed Practical/Vocational Nurse. Remember, success is climbing a mountain, facing the challenge of obstacles, and reaching the top of the mountain. I wish you the best success in your career as a licensed practical/vocational nurse in the United States of America!

REFERENCES

Commission on Graduates of Foreign Nursing Schools. Web site: http://www.cgfns.org.

Commission on Graduates of Foreign Nursing Schools. *Fact Sheet.* Retrieved April 3, 2005, from http://www.cgfns.org/fact-cert.shtml.

Commission on Graduates of Foreign Nursing Schools. *VisaScreen.* Retrieved April 3, 2005, from http://www.cgfns.org/prog-visa.shtml.

Commission on Graduates of Foreign Nursing Schools. *Certification Program.* Retrieved April 3, 2005, from http://www.cgfns.org/prog-cert.shtml.

Educational Testing Service, Princeton, NJ. Web site: http://ets.org/. E mail: toefl@ets.org.

International English Language Testing System. Web site: www.ielts.org. E mail: ielts@ceii.org.

National Council of State Boards of Nursing. Web site: http://www.ncsbn.org.

National Council of State Boards of Nursing. (2005). *2005 NCLEX-PN® for VisaScreen Candidate Bulletin.* Chicago: Author.

National Council of State Boards of Nursing. (2005). *2005 NCLEX-PN® Examination Candidate Bulletin.* Chicago: Author.

Pathways to Success

LAURENT W. VALLIERE, B.S.

PYRAMID TO SUCCESS

Preparing to take the NCLEX-PN examination can produce a great deal of anxiety. You may be thinking that NCLEX-PN is the most important examination that you will ever have to take and that it reflects the culmination of everything that you have worked so hard for. NCLEX-PN is an important examination because receiving that nursing license means that you can begin your career as a licensed practical/vocational nurse. Your success on the NCLEX-PN involves expelling all thoughts that might allow this examination to appear overwhelming and intimidating. Such thoughts will take complete control over your destiny. A positive attitude, a structured plan for preparation, and maintaining control in your pathway to success will ensure achievement in reaching the peak of the Pyramid to Success (Box 3-1).

THE FOUNDATION

The foundation of the Pyramid to Success begins with a positive attitude and developing short- and long-term goals. Both a positive attitude and a list of goals will lead you toward achievement and success. Without these components, the Pyramid to Success leads to nowhere and has no end point. You will expend energy and valuable time and experience exhaustion without any accomplishment. Therefore, it is imperative that you take the time to develop that positive attitude and to establish your short- and long-term goals.

Where do you start? To begin this process, find a location that offers solitude. Sit or lie in a comfortable position, close your eyes, relax, inhale deeply, hold your breath to a count of 4, exhale slowly and, again, relax. Repeat this breathing exercise several times until you begin to feel relaxed and free from anxiety. Allow your mind to become void of all chatter. Now you are in control and your mind can see for miles. Your highway of life has a multitude of destinations to which you

may travel. It is now time for you to plan the order of your journey to the Pyramid to Success.

THE LIST

It is time to create "The List." The List is your set of goals. Right now, you may or may not have a scheduled date for taking the NCLEX-PN examination. Begin by developing the goals you wish to accomplish today, tomorrow, and into the future. Allow yourself the opportunity to list all that is flowing from your mind. Write your goals on a piece of paper. When the List is complete, it is time to store it away for 2 or 3 days. Then, retrieve and review the List and begin the process of planning to prepare for the NCLEX-PN examination.

THE PLAN

Now that you have the List in order, look at the goals that relate to your studying for the licensing exam. The first task is to decide what study pattern works best for you. Take the time to review what has worked most successfully for you in the past. There are questions that must be addressed in order to develop your plan for study (Box 3-2).

"The Plan" must include how you will manage your study needs and the demands of your family and friends. Take time to think about how you will balance your everyday commitments with your plan for study. Your family and friends are key players in your life and are going to become a part of your Pyramid to Success. After you have established your study needs, communicate your needs and the importance of your study plan in achieving your goal of becoming a licensed practical/vocational nurse to your family and friends.

The Plan must include a schedule. Establish a realistic schedule that includes your daily, weekly, and future goals, and adhere to it. This consistency will provide

BOX 3-1

Pathways to Success

THE FOUNDATION
Maintain a positive attitude
Think about short- and long-term realistic goals
Develop control

THE LIST
Document short- and long-term realistic goals
Maintain control

THE PLAN
Develop a study plan and schedule
Decide on the place to study
Balance personal and work obligations with the study schedule
Share your study schedule and personal needs with others
Implement the study plan

POSITIVE PAMPERING
Establish healthy eating habits
Plan time for exercise and fun activities
Include activities in the schedule that provide positive mental stimulation

FINAL PREPARATION
Review goals
Identify goals achieved
Remain focused to complete the plan of study
Write down the date and time of the examination and post it next to your name with the letters LPN or LVN following, and the word "*YES!*"
Plan a test drive to the testing center
Enjoy relaxing activities on the day before the examination

THE DAY OF THE EXAMINATION
Groom yourself for success
Eat a healthy and nutritious breakfast
Maintain a confident and positive attitude
Maintain control
Meet the challenges of the day
Reach the peak of the Pyramid to Success

BOX 3-2

Developing a Plan for Study

Do I work better alone or in a group study environment?
If I work best in a group, does the group consist of one, two, or more study partners?
Who are these study partners?
How long should my study sessions last?
Does the time of day that I study make a difference for me?
Do I retain more if I study in the morning?
How does my work schedule affect my study pattern?
How do I balance my family obligations with my need to study?
Do I have a comfortable study area at home, or do I need to find another environment that is more conducive to my study needs?

Your friend may say, "Come on. Take some time off. You have plenty of time to study. Study later when we get back!" Then you are faced with a decision. You must weigh all the factors carefully. You must keep your goals in mind and remember that your need for positive momentum is critical. Your decision may not be an easy one, but it must be one to help you ensure that your goal of becoming a licensed practical/vocational nurse is achieved. Remember, positive momentum and a goal achievement plan need to be shared by all who support you.

POSITIVE PAMPERING

Positive momentum can be maintained only if you are properly balanced. This means that you must continue to care for yourself. Proper exercise, diet, and positive mental stimulation are critical to achieving your goal of becoming a licensed practical/vocational nurse. Just as you have developed a schedule for study, you should have a schedule that includes some fun and some form of physical activity. It is your choice—aerobics, running, weight lifting, bowling, or whatever makes you feel good about yourself. Time spent away from the difficult study schedule and devoted to some form of fun and physical exercise pays back 100-fold in its rewards. You will feel alive and more energetic with a schedule that includes these activities.

Establish healthy eating habits. Stay away from fatty foods, because they will slow you down. Eat lighter meals and eat more frequently. Include complex carbohydrates in your diet for energy, and be careful not to include too much caffeine in your daily diet. Continue to feel good about yourself, because you are in control.

Also, take the time to pamper yourself with activities that make you feel even better about who you are. Make dinner reservations at your favorite restaurant with someone who is special and is supporting your goal to become a licensed practical/vocational nurse. Take walks

advantages to you and to those supporting you. A daily schedule allows you to plan your topic areas for study more carefully. Adherence to the Plan helps you develop a rhythm that can only enhance your retention skills and positive momentum. Those who are supporting you will share this rhythm and will be able to schedule their activities and lives better, because you are consistent with your study schedule. You are moving forward, and you are in control!

A difficult part of the Plan might be how you will deal with those family and friends who choose not to participate in your Pyramid to Success. What if an individual (or individuals) decides not to be part of the Pyramid? For example, what do you do if a friend asks you to go to a movie and it is your scheduled study time.

in a place that has a particular tranquility, where you can reflect on the positive momentum that you have achieved and maintained. Whatever it is, wherever it takes you, allow yourself the time to do some Positive Pampering.

FINAL PREPARATION

You have established the foundation of your Pyramid. You have developed your list of goals and your study plan, and have maintained your positive momentum. You are moving forward, and you are in control. When you receive your date and time for the NCLEX-PN examination, you may immediately think, "I am not ready!" Stop! Reflect on all that you have achieved. Think about your goal achievement and the organization of the positive life momentum with which you have surrounded yourself. Think about all those individuals who love and support your efforts to become a licensed practical/vocational nurse. Believe that the challenge awaiting you is one that you have successfully prepared for, and that will lead you to your goal, becoming a licensed practical/vocational nurse.

Take a deep breath, and organize your remaining days so that your educational and personal needs are fulfilled. Support your positive momentum with a visual technique. Write your name in large letters, and write the letters "LPN" or "LVN" after it. Post one or more of these visual reinforcements in areas that you frequent. This form of motivational technique works for many individuals preparing for this examination.

Through all that you have accomplished to this point, it is imperative that you not fall into the trap of expecting too much of yourself. The idea of perfection must not drive you to a point that causes your positive momentum to slow down or hesitate. You must believe in who you are, as you are, and stay focused on your goal. Allow yourself the opportunity to continue to carry out your plan in a manner that is most agreeable with who you are, not someone else. The date and time are in hand. Write down the date and time, and underneath write the word "YES!" Post this next to your name, plus LPN or LVN.

You must ensure that you know how to get to the testing center. A test run is a must. Time the drive, and allow for road construction or whatever might occur to slow down traffic. On the test run, when you arrive at the test facility, it might help for you to go inside. Walk in and become familiar with the lobby and the surroundings. This might help alleviate some of the peripheral nervousness associated with entering an unknown building. Remember, you must do whatever it takes to keep yourself in control. If familiarizing yourself with the facility helps you maintain positive momentum, by all means be sure to do so. Who is in control? You are!

It is time to check your study plan and make the necessary adjustments now that a firm date and time have been set. Adjust your review so that it flows to your needs and your study plan ends 2 days before the examination. Remember that the mind is like a muscle: if it is overworked, it has no strength or stamina. Your strategy is to rest your body and mind on the day before the examination. Your strategy is to stay in control and allow yourself the opportunity to be absolutely fresh and attentive on the day of the examination. This will help you control the nervousness that is natural, achieve the clear thought processes required, and feel confident that you have done all that is necessary to prepare and conquer this challenge. The day before the examination is to be one of pleasure. Treat yourself to what you enjoy the most.

Relax! You have prepared yourself well for the challenge of tomorrow. Allow yourself a good night's sleep, and wake up on the day of the examination knowing that you are absolutely ready to succeed. Look at your name with LPN or LVN after it and the word "YES!"

THE DAY OF THE EXAMINATION

Wake up believing in yourself, and that all you have accomplished is about to propel you to the professional level of licensed practical/vocational nurse. Allow yourself plenty of time, eat a nutritious breakfast, and groom yourself for success. You are ready to meet the challenges of the day and overcome any obstacle that may face you. Today will soon be history, and tomorrow will bring you the envelope on which you read your name and the words "Licensed Practical/Vocational Nurse" after it.

Be proud and confident of your achievements. You have worked hard to achieve your goal of becoming a licensed practical/vocational nurse. If you believe in yourself and your goals, no one person or obstacle can move you off the pathway that leads to success, to the peak of the Pyramid.

Congratulations, and I wish you the very best in your career as a licensed practical/vocational nurse!

The NCLEX-PN® Examination: From a Student's Perspective

STEPHANIE A. DUPLER, LPN

The progression toward becoming a licensed practical nurse starts slowly. During nursing school, my instructors taught me step by step how to think, problem-solve, and act differently—all of the most important building blocks to becoming a competent and professional nurse. At the beginning of nursing school, I never really understood the reasoning behind this. Now, as a licensed practical nurse, I am grateful for the skills that I inadvertently did not realize I had learned. Although all this learning is important, it's almost all in vain if you cannot complete the one last step successfully, and that is passing the dreaded NCLEX-PN licensing examination.

With all the hard work and the long, busy days of working, studying, and attending clinicals, you just don't think about the fact that you will need to take the NCLEX-PN examination. Every student knows that the examination needs to be taken and passed, but you just don't focus on it or think that it's ever going to happen. It all becomes a reality when you are faced with the challenge of preparing for it.

I started preparing for the NCLEX-PN examination slowly, about 5 months before graduation from nursing school. I purchased an NCLEX-PN preparation book, and during some of my rare free time, I read through the questions slowly to see if I could really "perform on the spot," if needed. I felt like I had all the time in the world to prepare for this examination, although in reality I didn't. The fact that I needed to take this examination didn't really hit me until graduation.

The day I received my nursing diploma was the day I was no longer a student and the day that taking the NCLEX-PN examination was really becoming a reality. After graduation, I took about 2 weeks to regroup, relax, and focus on my goals and what I thought I really needed to accomplish up until the day of the examination. I had been told many things over the past year about the ways to prepare for this examination, but I needed to figure out what was best for me and what would work for me.

I decided that I would spend approximately 2 hours a day, divided between reviewing nursing content from my NCLEX-PN review book that was still a little sketchy for me, and answering practice questions from the book. The book I purchased also had a CD, and I highly recommend a review book that has a CD and the capability of providing various testing formats. With this type of product, you can take practice tests, time yourself, and then review your overall performance at the end of the test. Taking these practice tests really helped my self-esteem on the days when I was thinking that there was no way I was ever going to pass this examination. As I prepared to take the examination, I reminded myself every day that all the information I had tried so hard to learn during nursing school was still there; I just had to relax and let my mind take over.

I was really nervous on examination day, the way I expected to be. It should have felt like the first day of the rest of my life and career; instead, it felt like the end of it. During the examination, I tried different relaxation techniques. The technique that worked best for me was to block all noise, environmental factors, and other test-takers out of my world. The testing environment is stressful, really stressful. I took my time during the examination to assure myself that I wasn't rushing just to get out of this testing situation. I didn't want my examination to end at the minimum number of questions, but at the same time I had hoped it would. It did end at the minimum number of questions. I wanted to yell at the computer, convinced that I had failed, and I wanted more questions to prove that I really could pass this examination, but that wasn't going to happen. I already had my chance, so I left the center.

Every day following my examination, at least once and sometimes several times a day, I went to the state department of nursing Web site to find out if my name was listed, with a license number issued. Although it took only a few days for my name and license number to be listed, it felt like years. I received my actual nursing license in the mail about a week or so after I took the examination.

There are several pieces of advice that I can give to students attending nursing school, but the most important piece is to always look and listen during your learning experiences. You can learn from anyone and everyone, and every day is a learning experience in one way or another. Relax, and trust in yourself. You have worked so hard to reach your goal. Trust in yourself that you have everything you need to be successful. Good luck to you in whatever you may do!

Test-Taking Strategies

I. PYRAMID TO SUCCESS (Box 5-1)

II. HOW TO AVOID READING INTO THE QUESTION (Box 5-2)

A. Pyramid points
   1. Read every word in the question and specifically determine what the question is asking
   2. Focus only on the information in the question and avoid asking yourself "Well, what if . . . ?"
   3. Look for the key words in the question, such as *early signs* or *late signs*
   4. In multiple-choice questions, multiple-response questions, chart/exhibit questions, or questions that require you to number in order of priority, read every choice or option presented
   5. Use the process of elimination when choices or options are presented; reread the question and what the question is specifically asking to assist you in determining your final choice(s)
   6. With questions that require you to fill in the blank, focus on the information in the question and determine what the question is asking; if the question requires you to calculate a medication dose, an intravenous flow rate, or intake and output amounts, recheck your work in calculating to verify the answer
   7. Remember, focus on the information in the question and specifically on what the question is asking

B. The parts of a question (Box 5-3)
   1. The question will consist of a case situation, question stem, and options; a fill-in-the blank question will not contain options, and some figure or illustration (hot spot) questions may or may not contain options
   2. The case situation provides you with the information about the client and the information you need to consider in answering the question

---

BOX 5-1

Pyramid to Success

Read the question and every option thoroughly and carefully.
Ask yourself, "What is the question specifically asking?"
Be alert to key words and true and false response questions.
Eliminate the incorrect options.
Use all your nursing knowledge, your clinical experiences, and your test-taking skills and strategies to answer the question.

BOX 5-2

Practice Question: Avoid Reading into the Question

A client with metastatic cancer is receiving morphine sulfate to alleviate pain. The nurse monitors the client for which *adverse* or *toxic effect* of the medication?
   1. Dizziness
   2. Sedation
   3. Skeletal muscle flaccidity
   4. Nausea

Answer: 3

TEST-TAKING STRATEGY

Read every word in the question and specifically determine what the question is asking. The question is asking about the adverse or toxic effect of morphine sulfate. Dizziness, sedation, and nausea are side effects of morphine sulfate that the client may experience, but these are not toxic effects. Remember, focus on the information in the question and what the question is asking.

Multiple-Choice Question: Case Situation, Question Stem, and Options

CASE SITUATION
The nurse is monitoring a child for bleeding following surgery for removal of a brain tumor. The nurse checks the head dressing for the presence of blood and notes a colorless drainage on the back of the dressing.

QUESTION STEM
Which of the following is the most appropriate nursing intervention?

OPTIONS
1. Circle the area of drainage and continue to monitor
2. Reinforce the dressing
3. Notify the registered nurse
4. Document the findings and continue to monitor
Answer: 3

3. The question stem asks something specific about the case situation
4. The options are all of the answers
5. In a multiple-choice question, there will be four options and you must select one; read every option carefully, and always use the process of elimination
6. In a multiple-response question, there will be several options, and you must select all options that apply to the situation in the question; read each option carefully; visualize the situation, and use your nursing knowledge to answer the question
7. In a prioritizing (ordered response) question, you will be required to list in order of priority certain nursing interventions; visualize the situation, and use your nursing knowledge to answer the question
8. A chart/exhibit question will most likely contain options; read the question carefully and all the information in the chart/exhibit to answer the question

III. LOOK FOR KEY WORDS (Boxes 5-4 and 5-5)
A. Key words focus your attention on a specific or critical point to consider when answering the question
B. Some key words may indicate that all the options are correct, and that it will be necessary to prioritize to select the correct option
C. As you read the question, look for the key words; key words will make a difference with regard to how you will answer the question

IV. THE ISSUE OF THE QUESTION (Box 5-6)
A. The issue of the question is the specific subject content that the question is asking about

Common Key Words

Early or late
Best
First
Initial
Immediately
Most likely or least likely
Most appropriate or least appropriate

Practice Question: Look for the Key Words

A nurse is assisting in caring for a client who just returned from the recovery room after undergoing abdominal surgery. The nurse monitors the client for which *early sign* of hypovolemic shock?
    1. Increased pulse rate
    2. Increased depth of respiration
    3. Lethargy
    4. Increased orientation to surroundings
Answer: 1

TEST-TAKING STRATEGY
Note the key words, *early sign*. Focusing on these key words and recalling that the earliest clinical signs of hypovolemic shock are cardiovascular changes will direct you to the correct option. Increased orientation to surroundings is expected as the effects of anesthesia resolve. Although increased depth of respirations and lethargy occur in hypovolemic shock, these are not early signs. Rather, they occur as the shock progresses. Remember to look for key words.

The Issue of the Question

A nurse administers a dose of scopolamine to a preoperative client. The nurse monitors the client for which side effect of this medication?
    1. Excessive urination
    2. Diaphoresis
    3. Dry mouth
    4. Pupillary constriction
Answer: 3

TEST-TAKING STRATEGY
Focus on the issue, the side effect of a medication. Use your nursing knowledge, clinical experiences, and test-taking skills and strategies to answer the question. Recalling that scopolamine is an anticholinergic medication that frequently causes the side effects of dry mouth, urinary retention, decreased sweating, and pupil dilation will direct you to the correct option.

BOX 5-7

Practice Question: True Response

A client with suspected meningitis is being scheduled for diagnostic tests. The nurse anticipates that which of the following diagnostic tests will *most likely* be prescribed to *confirm* the diagnosis?
  1. Serum electrolytes
  2. Electromyography
  3. White blood cell count
  4. Lumbar puncture

Answer: 4

TEST-TAKING STRATEGY

This question identifies an example of a true response question. Note the key words, *most likely* and *confirm*. Focus on the diagnosis presented in the question and the associated pathophysiology to assist in directing you to option 4. Remember, meningitis is an acute or chronic inflammation of the meninges and the cerebrospinal fluid. The key diagnostic test used in meningitis is the lumbar puncture. A white blood cell count and serum electrolyte test may also be performed. Electromyography is not a key diagnostic test. Remember that true response questions ask you to select an option that is accurate.

BOX 5-8

Practice Question: False Response

A nurse has reinforced discharge instructions to a client who underwent a right mastectomy with axillary lymph node dissection. Which statement by the client indicates a *need for further instruction* regarding home care measures?
  1. "I need to be sure to wear thick mitt covers or use thick pot holders when I am cooking."
  2. "I should inform all of my other health care providers that I have had this surgical procedure."
  3. "It is all right to use a straight razor to shave under my arms."
  4. "I need to be sure that I do not have blood pressures or blood drawn from my right arm."

Answer: 3

TEST-TAKING STRATEGY

This question identifies an example of a false response question. Note the key words, *need for further instruction*. These key words indicate that you need to select an option that identifies an incorrect client statement. Recalling that edema and infection are the concerns with this client, and that the client needs to be instructed in the measures that will avoid trauma to the affected arm, will direct you to the correct option.

B. Identifying the issue of the question will assist in eliminating the incorrect options and direct you to selecting the correct option
C. The issue of the question can include:
   1. A medication or effect of intravenous (IV) therapy
   2. A side effect of a medication
   3. An adverse or toxic effect of a medication
   4. A treatment or procedure
   5. A complication of a health care problem, treatment, or procedure
   6. A specific nursing action

V. TRUE AND FALSE RESPONSE QUESTIONS
(Boxes 5-7 and 5-8)
A. True response questions use key words that ask you to select an option that is accurate regarding the information in the question
B. False response questions use key words that ask you to select an option that is not accurate regarding the information in the question
C. Read every word in the question, and be especially alert in noting key words that ask you to select an option that is not accurate regarding the information in the question

VI. QUESTIONS THAT REQUIRE PRIORITIZING
A. Questions in the examination may require you to use the skill of prioritizing nursing actions
B. Look for the key words in the question that indicate the need to prioritize (Box 5-9)

BOX 5-9

Common Key Words that Indicate the Need to Prioritize

Best
Essential
First
Highest priority
Immediate
Initial
Most important
Next
Primary
Vital

C. Remember, when a question requires prioritization, all options may be correct, and you need to determine the correct order of action
D. Guidelines to use include the ABCs—airway, breathing, and circulation; Maslow's Hierarchy of Needs theory; and the steps of the nursing process (clinical problem-solving process)
E. The ABCs (Box 5-10)
   1. Use the ABCs—airway, breathing, and circulation—when selecting an answer or determining the order of priority
   2. Remember the order of priority: airway, breathing, and circulation
   3. Airway is always the first priority!

F. Maslow's Hierarchy of Needs theory (Box 5-11)
 1. Use Maslow's Hierarchy of Needs theory as a guide to prioritize
 2. Physiological needs are the priority; therefore, select an option or determine the order of priority by addressing physiological needs first
 3. When a physiological need is not addressed in the question or noted in one of the options, continue to use Maslow's Hierarchy of Needs theory as a guide and look for the option that addresses safety
G. Steps of the nursing process (clinical problem-solving process) to prioritize

---

Practice Question: Use of the ABCs

The client with a diagnosis of cancer is receiving morphine sulfate 10 mg subcutaneously every 3 to 4 hours for pain. When assisting in planning care for the client, the nurse includes which *priority* action?
 1. Monitor stools
 2. Monitor the urine output
 3. Encourage the client to cough and take deep breaths
 4. Encourage fluid intake

Answer: 3

TEST-TAKING STRATEGY

Use the ABCs—airway, breathing, and circulation—as a guide to direct you to the correct option. Recall that morphine sulfate suppresses the cough reflex and the respiratory reflex. Although options 1, 2, and 4 are components of the plan of care, the correct option addresses airway. Remember, use the ABCs—airway, breathing, and circulation—to prioritize.

BOX 5-11

Practice Question: Maslow's Hierarchy of Needs Theory

A client in a long-term care facility has had a series of gastrointestinal (GI) diagnostic tests, including an upper GI series and endoscopies. On the client's return to the long-term care facility, the *highest priority* is to collect data regarding the client's:
 1. Level of consciousness
 2. Ability to ambulate independently
 3. Hydration and nutrition status
 4. Orientation level

Answer: 3

TEST-TAKING STRATEGY

Note the key words, *highest priority*. Use Maslow's Hierarchy of Needs theory to prioritize, remembering that physiological needs come first. Using this guideline will direct you to option 3. Hydration and nutrition status are physiological needs. Remember, physiological needs are the priority!

---

 1. Use the steps of the nursing process (clinical problem-solving process) to prioritize
 2. The steps include data collection, planning, implementation, and evaluation and are followed in this order
 3. Data collection
   a. Data collection questions address the process of gathering subjective and objective data relative to the client, communicating and documenting information gained in data collection, and contributing to the formulation of nursing diagnoses
   b. Remember that data collection is the first step in the nursing process (clinical problem-solving process)
   c. When you are asked a question regarding your initial or first nursing action, look for key words in the options that reflect the collection of data relative to the client (Box 5-12)
   d. If an option contains the concept of collection of client data, it is best to select that option (Box 5-13)
   e. If a data collection action is not one of the options, follow the steps of the nursing process (clinical problem-solving process) as your guide in selecting your initial or first action
   f. Possible exception to the guideline: If the question presents an emergency situation, read carefully; in an emergency situation, an intervention may be the priority!
 4. Planning (Box 5-14)
   a. Planning questions require providing input into plan development, assisting in the formulation of the goals of care, and assisting in the development of a plan of care
   b. Remember that this is a nursing examination and the answer to the question most likely involves something that is included in the nursing care plan, rather than the medical plan
 5. Implementation (Box 5-15)
   a. This exam is about NURSING, so focus on the nursing action rather than on the medical

---

BOX 5-12

Data Collection: Key Words

Check
Collect
Determine
Find out
Gather
Identify
Monitor
Observe
Obtain information
Recognize

action, unless the question is asking you what prescribed medical action is anticipated

b. Implementation questions address the process of assisting with organizing and managing care, providing care to achieve established goals, and communicating and documenting nursing interventions thoroughly and accurately

c. On NCLEX-PN, the only client that you need to be concerned about is the client in the question that you are answering

d. When you are answering a question, remember that this client is your only assigned client

e. Answer the question as if the situation were textbook and ideal, and the nurse has all the time and resources needed and readily available at the client's bedside

6. Evaluation (Box 5-16)

a. Evaluation questions focus on comparing the actual outcomes of care with the expected outcomes, and communicating and documenting findings

---

BOX 5-13

Practice Question: The Nursing Process/Data Collection

A nurse is caring for a client with chronic obstructive pulmonary disease who suddenly complains of increased dyspnea. The client is on oxygen at 2 L/minute and the respiratory rate is 22 breaths per minute. The nurse should take which action *first*?

1. Increase the liter flow of oxygen
2. Check the client's respiratory status
3. Contact a respiratory therapist
4. Tell the client that there is no need to worry

Answer: 2

TEST-TAKING STRATEGY

Note the key word, *first,* and use the steps of the nursing process. Data collection is the first step. Of the four options presented, the only option that reflects the process of data collection is option 2. Options 1, 3, and 4 identify the implementation step of the nursing process. Remember data collection in the first step of the nursing process!

BOX 5-14

Practice Question: The Nursing Process/Planning

A nurse is preparing to assist with the care of a client following a gastroscopy procedure. The nurse suggests including which nursing intervention in the *plan of care*?

1. Place the client in a supine position to provide comfort
2. Monitor the client's vital signs every hour for 4 hours
3. Provide saline gargles immediately on return to the nursing unit to aid in comfort
4. Check the gag reflex by using a tongue depressor to stroke the back of client's throat

Answer: 4

TEST-TAKING STRATEGY

Planning questions require providing input into plan development, assisting in the formulation of the goals of care, and assisting in the development of a plan of care. Use of the ABCs—airway, breathing, and circulation—will also assist in answering this question. Option 4 is the only option that addresses airway. Remember, planning is the second step of the nursing process.

BOX 5-15

Practice Question: The Nursing Process/Implementation

A nurse is assisting in caring for a client with preeclampsia who is at risk for eclampsia. The nurse understands that, if the client progresses from preeclampsia to eclampsia, the *first action* is to:

1. Prepare for the administration of intravenous magnesium sulfate
2. Check the client's blood pressure and fetal heart tones
3. Clear and maintain an open airway
4. Administer oxygen by face mask

Answer: 3

TEST-TAKING STRATEGY

Implementation questions address the process of organizing and managing care. This question also requires that you prioritize the nursing actions. Use the ABCs—airway, breathing, and circulation—to answer the question. The first action is to clear and maintain an open airway. Remember, implementation is the third step of the nursing process.

BOX 5-16

Practice Question: The Nursing Process/Evaluation

A client with multiple sclerosis has been taking oxybutynin (Ditropan). The nurse *determines the degree of effectiveness* of the medication by asking the client about changes in:

1. Extent of muscle spasms
2. Level of fatigue
3. Bowel movements
4. Patterns of urination

Answer: 4

TEST-TAKING STRATEGY

This is an evaluation question. Note the key words, *determines the degree of effectiveness.* Oxybutynin is an antispasmodic used to relieve symptoms of urinary urgency, frequency, nocturia, and incontinence in clients with an uninhibited or reflex neurogenic bladder. Recalling that this medication is used to treat bladder dysfunction will direct you to option 4. Remember, evaluation is the fourth step of the nursing process.

b. These questions focus on assisting in determining the client's response to care, and identifying factors that may interfere with implementation of the plan of care

c. In an evaluation question, be alert to false response questions because they are frequently used in evaluation-type questions, and the question may ask for a client statement that indicates either accurate or inaccurate information related to the issue of the question

VII. CLIENT NEEDS

A. Safe, Effective Care Environment

1. These questions address the provision that the nurse provides nursing care, collaborates with other health care team members to facilitate effective client care, and protects clients, significant others, and health care personnel from environmental hazards

2. Be alert to safety needs addressed in a question, and remember the importance of hand washing, call bells, bed positioning, and the appropriate use of side rails

B. Physiological Integrity

1. These questions address the provision that the nurse provides comfort and assistance in the performance of activities of daily living, provides care related to the administration of medications, and monitors clients receiving parenteral therapies

2. These questions also address the nurse's ability to reduce the client's potential for developing complications or health problems related to treatments, procedures, or existing conditions, and the nurse's role in participating in providing care to clients with acute, chronic, or life-threatening physical health conditions

3. Use Maslow's Hierarchy of Needs theory, and remember that physiological needs are a priority and are addressed first

4. Use the ABCs—airway, breathing, and circulation—and the steps of the nursing process (clinical problem-solving process) when selecting an option addressing physiological integrity

C. Psychosocial Integrity

1. These questions address the provision that the nurse provides nursing care that promotes and supports the emotional, mental, and social well-being of the client and significant other(s)

2. Content addressed in these questions relates to promoting the client's or significant other(s)' ability to cope, adapt, or problem-solve in situations such as illnesses, disabilities, or stressful events

3. Content also includes the nurse's role in recognizing and providing care for clients with maladaptive behavior, and assisting with behavior

management of the client with an acute and/or chronic mental illness or a cognitive psychosocial disturbance

4. In this Client Needs category, you may be asked communication-type questions that relate to how you would respond to a client, a client's family member or significant other, or other health care team members

5. Use therapeutic communication techniques to answer communication questions because of their effectiveness in the communication process

6. Remember to select the answer that focuses on the client's, client's family member's, or significant other's feelings, concerns, anxieties, or fears (Box 5-17)

D. Health Promotion and Maintenance

1. These questions address the provision that the nurse provides and assists in directing nursing care to promote and maintain health

2. Content addressed in these questions relates to assisting the client and significant other(s) during the normal expected stages of growth and development, from conception through advanced old age, and providing client care related to the prevention and early detection of health problems

3. Use the Teaching/Learning Theory if the question addresses client education, remembering that client motivation and client readiness to learn is the first priority

4. Be alert to false response questions that address health promotion and maintenance and client education

---

BOX 5-17

Practice Question: Communication

A mother says to the nurse, "I am afraid that my child might have another seizure." The nurse states which therapeutic response to the mother?

1. "Why worry about something that you cannot control?"
2. "Most children will never experience a second seizure."
3. "Tell me what frightens you the most about seizures."
4. "Acetaminophen (Tylenol) can prevent another seizure from occurring."

Answer: 3

TEST-TAKING STRATEGY

Option 3 is the only option that addresses the mother's fears. Option 1 blocks communication because it states that the mother should not worry. Options 2 and 4 are incorrect because the nurse is giving false assurance that a seizure will not recur or can be prevented in this child. Remember, focus on feelings, concerns, anxieties, or fears.

VIII. ELIMINATING SIMILAR OPTIONS (Box 5-18)

A. When answering the question, use the process of elimination and look for similar options

B. If any of the options include the same idea, then they are incorrect and can be eliminated

C. Remember that there is only one correct option, and the answer to the question is the option that is different

IX. ELIMINATE OPTIONS THAT CONTAIN ABSOLUTE WORDS (Box 5-19)

A. As you read each option, look for absolute words

B. Absolute words tend to make an option incorrect and, if you note an absolute word in an option, eliminate that option

C. Some of these absolute words include *all,* *always,* *every,* *must,* *none,* *never,* and *only*

X. LOOK FOR THE UMBRELLA OPTION (Box 5-20)

A. When answering a question, if you note that more than one option appears to be correct, look for the umbrella option (also known as global option or comprehensive option)

B. The umbrella option is one that is a general statement and may contains the ideas of the other options within it

C. The umbrella option will be the correct answer

XI. USE THE GUIDELINES FOR DELEGATING AND ASSIGNMENT-MAKING (Box 5-21)

A. You may be asked a question that will require you to decide how you delegate a task or assign clients to other health care providers

B. Focus on the information in the question and on what task or assignment is to be delegated

C. Once you have determined what task or assignment is to be delegated, consider the client's needs, and match the client's needs with the scope of practice of the health care providers identified in the question

D. The nurse practice act and any practice limitations define which aspects of care can be delegated and which must be performed by a nursing assistant, a licensed practical/vocational nurse, and/or a registered nurse

---

BOX 5-18

Practice Question: Eliminate Similar Options

A licensed practical nurse is assigned to care for a group of clients. On review of the clients' medical records, the nurse determines that which client is at risk for excess fluid volume?
1. The client with an ileostomy
2. The client on diuretics
3. The client on gastrointestinal suctioning
4. The client with renal failure

Answer: 4

TEST-TAKING STRATEGY

Focus on what the question is asking, the client at risk for excess fluid volume. Think about the pathophysiology associated with each condition identified in the options. The only client that retains fluid is the client with renal failure. The client with an ileostomy, the client on diuretics, and the client on gastrointestinal suctioning all lose fluid. Remember, eliminate similar options.

BOX 5-19

Practice Question: Eliminate Options that Contain Absolute Words

A nurse is instructing a postpartum client about infection prevention. The nurse determines that the client understands the instructions when the client states which of the following?
1. "I must not allow my toddler near the baby."
2. "I will use a clean towel to dry my perineal area."
3. "I must wash my nipples with a mild antibacterial soap before and after breast-feeding."
4. "I must wash my clothing separately from the family's until my bleeding has stopped."

Answer: 2

TEST-TAKING STRATEGY

Eliminate options that contain absolute words. Options 1, 3, and 4 contain the absolute word *must*. Remember that absolute words tend to make an option incorrect.

BOX 5-20

Practice Question: Look for the Umbrella Option

A male client who is admitted to the hospital for an unrelated medical problem is diagnosed with urethritis caused by a chlamydial infection. The nurse assigned to the client understands that what measures are necessary to prevent contraction of the infection during care?
1. Enteric precautions
2. Contact isolation
3. Standard precautions
4. Gloves and a mask when in the client's room

Answer: 3

TEST-TAKING STRATEGY

Recall that this infection is sexually transmitted. Also, note that option 3 is the umbrella (global) option. Remember, the umbrella option includes the ideas of the other options within it.

Practice Question: Use the Guidelines for Delegating and Making Assignments

A nurse is planning the client assignments for the day and has a licensed practical nurse (LPN) and a nursing assistant on the nursing team. Which client would the nurse most appropriately assign to the LPN?
1. A client with stable congestive heart failure who has early-stage Alzheimer's disease
2. A client who is weak and needs assistance with bathing
3. A client with emphysema who is receiving oxygen, 2 L by nasal cannula, and becomes dyspneic on exertion
4. A client who is scheduled for a visit from the physical therapist

Answer: 3

TEST-TAKING STRATEGY
The nurse would most appropriately assign the client with emphysema to the LPN. This client has an airway problem and has the highest priority needs of the clients presented in the options. The clients described in options 1, 2, and 4 can appropriately be cared for by the nursing assistant. Remember, match the client's needs with the scope of practice of the health care provider.

E. Generally noninvasive interventions such as skin care, range-of-motion exercises, ambulation, grooming, and hygiene measures can be assigned to a nursing assistant
F. A licensed practical/vocational nurse can perform the tasks that a nursing assistant can perform and can also perform certain invasive tasks, such as dressings, suctioning, urinary catheterization, and administering oral, subcutaneous, and intramuscular injections
G. The registered nurse can perform the tasks that a licensed practical/vocational nurse can perform, and is responsible for assessment and planning care, supervising care, initiating teaching, and administering intravenous medications

XII. ANSWERING PHARMACOLOGY QUESTIONS (Box 5-22)

A. If you are familiar with the medication, use nursing knowledge to answer the question
B. Remember that the question will identify both the generic name and the trade name of the medication
C. If the question identifies a medical diagnosis, then try to establish a relationship between the medication and the diagnosis; for example, you can determine that cyclophosphamide (Cytoxan) is an antineoplastic medication if the question refers to a client with breast cancer who is taking this medication
D. Try to determine the classification of the medication being considered to assist in answering the question;

Practice Question: Answering Pharmacology Questions

Oral levothyroxine (Synthroid), 50 µg (micrograms) daily is prescribed for a client with hypothyroidism. The nurse provides medication instructions to the client and tells the client to take the medication:
1. Just after breakfast
2. With a snack at 3:00 PM
3. In the morning on an empty stomach
4. With food

Answer: 3

TEST-TAKING STRATEGY
Note that a medical diagnosis is presented in the question. This will assist you in determining that the medication is used to treat this condition. Additionally, most thyroid replacement medications contain "-thy-" in their names. Also, use the strategy of eliminating similar options. Note that options 1, 2, and 4 are similar and indicate that the medication should be taken with food. Remember, with pharmacology questions, focus on the information in the question and on the classification of the medication.

identifying the classification will assist in determining a medication action and/or side effects—for example, diltiazem (Cardizem) is a cardiac medication
E. Recognize the common side effects associated with each medication classification and then relate the appropriate nursing interventions to each side effect; for example, if a side effect is hypertension, then the associated nursing intervention would be to monitor the blood pressure
F. Learn medications that belong to a classification by commonalities in their medication names; for example, medications that are xanthine bronchodilators end with "-line" (e.g., theophylline)
G. Look at the medication name and use medical terminology to help determine the medication action; for example, *Lopressor* lowers (*Lo*) the blood pressure (*pressor*)
H. If the question requires a medication calculation, remember that a calculator is available on the computer; talk yourself through each step to be sure that the answer makes sense, and recheck the calculation before answering the question, particularly if the answer seems like an unusual dosage
I. Pyramid points to remember
1. Generally, the client should not take an antacid with medication, because the antacid will affect the absorption of the medication
2. Enteric-coated and sustained-release tablets should not be crushed; capsules should not be opened
3. The client should never adjust or change a medication dose or abruptly stop taking a medication
4. The nurse never adjusts or changes the client's medication dosage and never discontinues a medication

5. The client needs to avoid taking any over-the-counter medications or any other medications such as herbal preparations, unless they are approved for use by the health care provider

6. The client needs to avoid alcohol and smoking

7. Medications are never administered if the order is difficult to read or is unclear, or identifies a medication dose that is not a normal dose

REFERENCES

Christensen, B., & Kockrow, E. (2003). *Foundations of nursing* (4th ed.). St. Louis: Mosby.

DeWit, S. (2005). *Fundamental concepts and skills for nursing* (2nd ed.). Philadelphia: W.B. Saunders.

Harkreader, H., & Hogan, M.A. (2004). *Fundamentals of nursing: Caring and clinical judgment.* (2nd ed.). Philadelphia: W.B. Saunders.

Hill, S., & Howlett, H. (2005). *Success in practical/vocational nursing: From student to leader.* (5th ed.). Philadelphia: W.B. Saunders.

Morrison-Valfre, M. (2005). *Foundations of mental health care* (3rd ed.). St. Louis: Mosby.

National Council of State Boards of Nursing (Eds.). (2005). *NCLEX-PN® examination: Detailed test plan for the National Council licensure examination for licensed practical/vocational nurses.* (Effective Date: April 2005). Chicago: Author.

Potter, P., & Perry, A. (2003). *Basic nursing: Essentials for practice* (5th ed.). St. Louis: Mosby.

Price, D., & Gwin, J. (2005). *Thompson's pediatric nursing* (9th ed.). Philadelphia: W.B. Saunders.

Issues in Nursing

Cultural Diversity

PYRAMID TERMS

acculturation Process of learning norms, beliefs, and behavioral expectations of a group other than one's own group.

belief Something accepted as true by a culture.

cultural assimilation Process in which individuals from a minority group are absorbed by the dominant culture and take on the characteristics of the dominant culture.

cultural competence The acquisition of knowledge, understanding, and appreciation of a culture that facilitates the provision of culturally appropriate health care.

cultural diversity The differences among groups of people that result from ethnic, racial, and cultural variables.

cultural imposition The tendency to impose one's own beliefs, values, and patterns of behavior on individuals from another culture.

culture The dynamic network of knowledge, beliefs, patterns of behavior, ideas, attitudes, values, and norms that are unique to a particular group of people.

dominant culture The group whose values prevail within a society.

ethnic group A group of people within a culture who share an identity based on race, religion, color, national origin, or language.

ethnicity An individual's identification of self as part of an ethnic group.

ethnocentrism An assumption of cultural superiority and an inability to accept another culture's ways.

minority group An ethnic, cultural, racial, or religious group that constitutes less than a numerical majority of the population.

oppression The imposition of the cultural ways of one group on another group.

race A grouping of people that is based on biological similarities. Members of a racial group have similar physical characteristics, such as blood group, facial features, and color of skin, hair, and eyes.

racism Discrimination directed toward individuals or groups who are perceived to be inferior because of biological differences; often accompanied by oppression.

stereotyping An expectation that all people within the same racial, ethnic, or cultural group act alike and share the same beliefs and attitudes.

subculture A group of people with characteristic patterns of behavior that distinguish the group from the larger culture or society.

values Principles and standards that have meaning and worth to an individual, family, group, community, or culture.

PYRAMID TO SUCCESS

Often, nurses care for clients who come from ethnic, cultural, or religious backgrounds that are different from their own. Awareness of, and sensitivity to, the unique health and illness beliefs and practices of others are essential in the delivery of safe and effective care. Acknowledgment and acceptance of cultural differences with a nonjudgmental attitude are essential in providing culturally sensitive care. The belief underlying the NCLEX-PN test plan is that people are unique individuals and define their own systems of daily living, which reflect their values, motives, and lifestyles. The Integrated Processes addressed in this chapter are Caring, Clinical Problem-Solving Process (Nursing Process), Communication and Documentation, and Teaching/Learning.

CLIENT NEEDS
Safe, Effective Care Environment

Acting as a client advocate

Client's rights

Communicating the need for referrals to members of the health care team

Confidentiality

Continuity of care

Establishing priorities

Ethical practice

Legal responsibilities

Respecting the client's control of personal environment/ property

Health Promotion and Maintenance

Aging process
Disease prevention
Family planning and family systems
Growth and development
Health and wellness
Health screening
Lifestyle choices

Psychosocial Integrity

Coping mechanisms
Cultural diversity
End of life
Family dynamics
Religious and spiritual influences on health
Support systems
Therapeutic communications

Physiological Integrity

Alternative and complementary therapies
Blood and blood products
Illness management
Nonpharmacological comfort interventions
Nutrition and oral hydration (Boxes 6-1 and 6-2)
Palliative/comfort care
Therapeutic procedures

BOX 6-1

Dietary Preferences of Ethnic Groups

AFRICAN AMERICANS
Fried foods
Pork, greens, rice
Some pregnant African-American women engage in pica

ASIAN AMERICANS
Soy sauce
Raw fish
Rice

EUROPEAN (WHITE)-ORIGIN AMERICANS
Carbohydrates (potatoes)
Red meat

HISPANIC AMERICANS
Beans
Fried foods
Spicy foods
Tortillas
Carbonated beverages

AMERICAN INDIANS, ALEUTS, ESKIMOS
Blue cornmeal
Fish
Game
Fruits and berries
Navajos prefer meat and blue cornmeal and tend to avoid consumption of milk

---

I. AFRICAN AMERICANS

A. Communication
  1. Competent in standard English and in Black English, a variation based on pronunciation, grammar, and vocabulary
  2. Head nodding does not necessarily mean agreement
  3. Direct eye contact may be interpreted as rudeness or aggressive behavior
  4. Nonverbal communication is very important
  5. Personal questions asked on initial contact with a person may be viewed as intrusive
B. Time orientation and personal space preferences
  1. Time orientation varies according to age, socioeconomics, and subgroups and may include past, present, or future orientation
  2. May be late for an appointment because relationships and events may be deemed more important than being on time
  3. Comfortable with close personal space when interacting with family and friends
C. Social roles
  1. Large extended-family networks are important; the elderly are respected
  2. Many single-parent, female-headed households

  3. Religious **beliefs** and church affiliation are sources of strength
D. Health and illness
  1. Religious **beliefs** profoundly affect ideas about health and illness
  2. Illness can be prevented by nutritious meals, rest, and cleanliness
E. Health risks
  1. Sickle cell anemia
  2. Hypertension
  3. Heart disease
  4. Cancer
  5. Lactose intolerance
  6. Diabetes mellitus
F. Interventions
  1. Recognize the presence of many individual and subgroup variations
  2. Build a relationship based on trust
  3. Clarify meaning of client's verbal and nonverbal behavior
  4. Be flexible and avoid rigidity in scheduling care
  5. Encourage family involvement
  6. Alternative modes of healing may include herbs, prayer, and laying on of hands

BOX 6-2

Religions and Dietary Preferences

SEVENTH-DAY ADVENTIST (CHURCH OF GOD)
Alcohol, coffee, and tea prohibited
Some groups prohibit meat

BUDDHISM
Alcohol and drug use discouraged
Some sects are vegetarian

ROMAN CATHOLICISM
Avoid meat on Ash Wednesday and Good Friday
Optional fasting during Lent season
During Lent, discourage meat on Friday
Children and the ill are exempt from fasting

CHURCH OF JESUS CHRIST OF LATTER-DAY SAINTS (MORMON)
Alcohol, coffee, and tea prohibited
Limited consumption of meat
First Sunday of the month is time for fasting

HINDUISM
Beef and veal prohibited
Many individuals are vegetarians
Limited consumption of meat
Fasting occurs on specific days of the week according to
   which god the person worships
Children are not allowed to participate in fasting
Fasting rituals vary from complete abstinence to
   consumption of only one meal per day

ISLAM
Pork prohibited
Any meat product not ritually slaughtered is prohibited
Avoidance of alcohol or drugs

During Ramadan (ninth month of Mohammedan year),
   fasting occurs during daytime

JEHOVAH'S WITNESS
Prohibition of any foods to which blood has been added
Can consume animal flesh that has been drained

JUDAISM
Dietary kosher laws must be adhered to by Orthodox
   believers
Meats allowed include animals that are vegetable eaters,
   cloven-hoofed animals, and animals that are ritually
   slaughtered
Fish that have scales and fins are allowed
Any combination of meat and milk is prohibited
During Yom Kippur, 24-hour fasting
Pregnant women and those who are seriously ill are
   exempt from fasting
During Passover, only unleavened bread is eaten

PENTECOSTAL (ASSEMBLY OF GOD)
Alcohol is prohibited
Avoid consumption of anything to which blood has been
   added
Some individuals avoid pork

RUSSIAN ORTHODOX
Abstention from meat and dairy products on Wednesday,
   Friday, and during Lent
During Lent, all animal products, including dairy products,
   are forbidden
Fasting during Advent
Exceptions from fasting include illness and pregnancy

II. ASIAN AMERICANS

A. Communication
   1. Languages include Chinese, Japanese, Korean, Vietnamese, English
   2. Silence is valued
   3. Eye contact may be considered inappropriate or disrespectful
   4. Criticism or disagreement is not expressed verbally
   5. Head nodding does not necessarily mean agreement
   6. The word "no" may be interpreted as disrespect for others

B. Time orientation and personal space preferences
   1. Time orientation reflects respect for the past, but includes emphasis on the present and the future
   2. Prefer a formal personal space, except with family and close friends
   3. Usually do not touch others during conversation
   4. Touching is unacceptable with members of opposite sex
   5. The head is considered to be sacred; therefore touching someone on the head is disrespectful

C. Social roles
   1. Devoted to tradition
   2. Large extended-family networks
   3. Loyalty to immediate and extended family and honor are valued
   4. Family unit is very structured and hierarchical
   5. Men have the power and authority, and women are expected to be obedient
   6. Education is viewed as important
   7. Religions include Taoism, Buddhism, Islam, Christianity
   8. Social organizations are strong within the community

D. Health and illness
   1. Health is a state of physical and spiritual harmony with nature and a balance between positive and negative energy forces (yin and yang)

2. A healthy body is viewed as a gift from ancestors
3. Illness is viewed as an imbalance between yin and yang
4. Yin foods are cold and yang foods are hot; cold foods are eaten when one has a hot illness, and hot foods are eaten when one has a cold illness
5. Illness is attributed to prolonged sitting or lying, or to overexertion

E. Health risks
   1. Hypertension
   2. Heart disease
   3. Cancer
   4. Lactose intolerance
   5. Thalassemia

F. Interventions
   1. Avoid physical closeness and excessive touching; only touch a client's head when necessary, informing the client before doing so
   2. Limit eye contact
   3. Avoid gesturing with hands
   4. If possible, a female client prefers a female health care provider
   5. Clarify responses to questions and expectations of health care provider
   6. Be flexible and avoid rigidity in scheduling care
   7. Encourage family involvement
   8. Alternative modes of healing may include herbs, acupuncture, restoration of balance with foods, massage, and offering prayers and incense

III. EUROPEAN (WHITE)-ORIGIN AMERICANS

A. Communication
   1. Languages include national languages, English
   2. Silence can be used to show respect or disrespect for another, depending on situation
   3. Eye contact is viewed as indicating trust-worthiness

B. Time orientation and personal space preferences
   1. Future oriented
   2. Time is valued; tend to be on time and to be impatient with people who are not on time
   3. May be aloof and tend to avoid close physical contact
   4. Handshakes may be used for formal greetings

C. Social roles
   1. The nuclear family is the basic unit; the extended family is also important
   2. The man is the dominant figure, but variation of gender roles exists within families and relationships
   3. Religion includes Judeo-Christian **beliefs**
   4. Community social organizations are important

D. Health and illness
   1. Health is usually viewed as an absence of disease or illness
   2. Have a tendency to be stoical when expressing physical concerns

3. Primarily rely on modern Western health care delivery system

E. Health risks
   1. Cancer
   2. Heart disease
   3. Diabetes mellitus
   4. Injury

F. Interventions
   1. Monitor client's body language
   2. Respect client's personal space

IV. HISPANIC AMERICANS

A. Communication
   1. Languages include Spanish and Portuguese
   2. Tend to be verbally expressive, yet confidentiality is important
   3. Avoiding eye contact with a person in authority indicates respect and attentiveness
   4. Direct confrontation is disrespectful, and the expression of negative feelings is impolite
   5. Dramatic body language, such as gestures or facial expressions, is used to express emotion or pain

B. Time orientation and personal space preferences
   1. Oriented more to the present
   2. May be late for an appointment, because relationships and events are valued more than being on time
   3. Comfortable when in close proximity with family, friends, and acquaintances
   4. Very tactile and use embraces and handshakes
   5. Value the physical presence of others
   6. Politeness and modesty are essential

C. Social roles
   1. The nuclear family is the basic unit; also, there are large extended-family networks
   2. The extended family is highly regarded
   3. Needs of the family take precedence over individual family members' needs
   4. Depending on age and **acculturation** factors, men are the decision makers and breadwinners, and women are the caretakers and homemakers
   5. Religions include Catholicism, Evangelical Christianity, Jehovah's Witness, Mormonism
   6. Strong church affiliation
   7. Social organizations strong within the community

D. Health and illness
   1. Health may be a reward from God or a result of good luck
   2. Health results from a state of balance between "hot and cold" forces and "wet and dry" forces
   3. Illness may be viewed as a result of God's punishment for sins
   4. Folk medicine traditions

E. Health risks
   1. Lactose intolerance

2. Diabetes mellitus
3. Parasites
4. Hypertension
5. Heart disease
F. Interventions
1. Allow time for the client to discuss treatment options with family members
2. Protect privacy
3. Offer to call clergy because of the significance of religious practices related to illnesses
4. Ask if it would be all right to touch a child before examining him or her
5. Be flexible regarding time of arrival for appointments, and avoid rigidity in scheduling care
6. Alternative modes of healing include herbs, consultation with lay healers, restoration of balance with hot or cold foods, prayer, and religious medals

V. NATIVE AMERICANS
A. Communication
1. Languages include English, Navajo, other tribal languages
2. Silence indicates respect for the speaker
3. Speak in a low tone of voice and expect others to be attentive
4. Eye contact is viewed as a sign of disrespect
5. Body language is important
B. Time orientation and personal space preferences
1. Oriented more to present
2. Personal space is very important
3. Will lightly touch another person's hand during greetings
4. Massage is used for the newborn infant to promote bonding between infant and mother
5. Touching a dead body may be prohibited in some tribes
C. Social roles
1. Very family oriented
2. Basic family unit is the extended family, which often includes people from several households
3. In some tribes, grandparents are viewed as family leaders
4. Elders are honored
5. Children are taught to respect traditions
6. The father does all the work outside the home, and the mother assumes responsibility for domestic duties
7. Sacred myths and legends provide spiritual guidance
8. Religion and healing practices are integrated
9. Community social organizations are important
D. Health and illness
1. Health is a state of harmony between the person, the family, and the environment

2. Illness is caused by supernatural forces and by disequilibrium between person and environment
3. Traditional health and illness **beliefs** may continue to be observed; natural and religious folk medicine tradition
E. Health risks
1. Alcohol abuse
2. Injury
3. Heart disease
4. Diabetes mellitus
5. Tuberculosis
6. Arthritis
7. Lactose intolerance
8. Gallbladder disease
9. American Eskimos are susceptible to glaucoma
F. Interventions
1. Clarify communication
2. Understand that the client may be attentive, even when eye contact is absent
3. Be attentive to own use of body language
4. Obtain input from members of extended family
5. Encourage client to personalize space in which health care is delivered; for example, encourage client to bring personal items or objects to the hospital
6. In the home, check for the availability of running water, and modify infection control and hygiene practices as necessary
7. Alternative modes of healing include herbs, restoration of balance between the person and the universe, consultation with traditional healers

VI. THE AMISH SOCIETY (Box 6-3)

VII. END-OF-LIFE ISSUES (Box 6-4)
A. Christian Science religion is unlikely to use medical means to prolong life
B. Jewish faith generally opposes prolonging life after irreversible brain damage
C. Autopsy may be prohibited, opposed, or discouraged by Eastern Orthodox religions, Muslims, Jehovah's Witnesses, and Orthodox Jews
D. Organ donation is prohibited by Jehovah's Witnesses and Muslims
E. Buddhists in the United States encourage organ donation and consider it an act of mercy
F. Cremation is discouraged, opposed, or prohibited by the Mormon, Eastern Orthodox, Islamic, and Jewish faiths
G. Hindus prefer cremation and casting the ashes into a holy river
H. Hispanic and Latino groups
1. The family generally makes decisions and may withhold the diagnosis or prognosis from the client

BOX 6-3

The Amish Society: Beliefs and Practices

Maintain a culture distinct and separate from the non-Amish

Usually speak a German dialect called Pennsylvania Dutch

German language is used during worship; English is learned in school

Men follow the laws of the Hebrew Scriptures with regard to beards (mustaches are not grown because of the long association of mustaches with the military)

Men usually dress in a plain, dark suit; women usually wear a plain dress with long sleeves, bonnet, and apron

Women are not allowed to hold positions of power in the congregational organization

Marriage outside the faith is not allowed

Family life has a patriarchal structure

Although the roles of the women are considered equally important to those of men, they are very unequal in terms of authority

Unmarried women remain under the authority of their father

Wives are submissive to their husbands

Generally remain separate from the rest of the world, physically and socially

Reject materialism and worldliness

Amish do not allow themselves to be photographed

Value living simply; may choose to avoid technology, such as electricity and cars

Highly value responsibility, generosity, and helping others

Often work as farmers, builders, quilters, and homemakers

Use traditional health care and alternative health care, such as healers, herbs, and massage

Believe that health is a gift from God, but that clean living and a balanced diet help maintain it

Many choose not to have health insurance, and mutual aid funds for Amish members are maintained to help with medical costs

Funerals are conducted in the home without a eulogy, flower decorations, or any other display; caskets are plain and simple without adornment

At death, women are usually buried in their bridal dress

One is believed to live on after death, with either eternal reward in heaven or punishment in hell

BOX 6-4

Religion and End-of-Life Care

CHRISTIANITY
Catholic and Eastern Orthodox
Anointing of the sick by a priest
Other sacraments before death include reconciliation and holy communion
Protestant
No last rites (anointing of the sick is accepted by some groups)
Prayers are given to offer comfort and support
Church of Jesus Christ of Latter-Day Saints (Mormon)
May administer a sacrament if the client requests
Jehovah's Witness
Do not believe in sacraments
Will be excommunicated if they receive a blood transfusion

ISLAM
Second-degree male relatives such as cousins or uncles should be the contact person and determine whether the client and/or family should be given information about the client
Client may choose to face Mecca (west or southwest in the United States)
The head should be elevated above the body
Discussions about death are not usually welcomed
Stopping medical treatment is against the will of Allah (Arabic word for God)
Grief may be expressed through slapping or hitting the body
If possible, only a same-sex Muslim should handle the body after death; if not possible, non-Muslims should wear gloves so as not to touch the body

JUDAISM
Prolongation of life is important (life support must be maintained on a client until death)
A dying person should not be left alone (a rabbi's presence is desired)
Autopsy and cremation are forbidden

HINDUISM
Rituals include tying a thread around the neck or wrist of the dying person, sprinkling the person with special water, or placing a leaf of basil on their tongue
After death, the sacred threads are not removed and the body is not washed

BUDDHISM
A shrine to Buddha may be placed in the client's room
Time for meditation at the shrine is important and should be respected
Clients may refuse medications that could alter their awareness (such as opioids)
After death, a monk may recite prayers for 1 hour (need not be done in the presence of the body)

2. Extended family members are often involved in end-of-life care (pregnant women may be prohibited from caring for the dying or attending funerals)
3. Several family members may be at the dying client's bedside
4. Vocal expression of grief and mourning is acceptable and expected
5. Refuse procedures that alter the body, such as organ donation or autopsy
6. Prefer to die at home

I. African Americans
   1. Discuss issues with the spouse or older family member (elders are held in high respect)

2. Family is highly valued and is central to the care of the terminally ill
3. Open displays of emotion are common and accepted
4. Organ and blood donation are usually not allowed
5. Prefer to die at home

J. Chinese Americans
1. Family members may make decisions about care and often do not tell the client their diagnosis or prognosis
2. Dying at home may be considered bad luck

K. Native Americans
1. Family meetings may be held to make decisions about end-of-life issues and the type of treatments that should be pursued
2. Some tribes avoid contact with the dying (may prefer to die in the hospital)

VIII. COMPLEMENTARY AND ALTERNATIVE THERAPIES

A. Description
1. Therapies used in addition to conventional treatment that provide healing resources and focus on the mind-body connection
2. Includes high-risk therapies (some that are invasive) and low-risk therapies (those that are noninvasive)
3. The National Center for Complementary and Alternative Medicine (NCCAM) has proposed a classification system that includes five categories of complementary and alternative types of therapy (Box 6-5)

B. Alternative medical systems
1. Environmental medicine: Focuses on preventing the harmful effects of environmental toxins; interventions include teaching, therapeutic diets, detoxification, immunotherapy, counseling, and use of environmentally safe products
2. Traditional Chinese medicine: Focuses on restoring and maintaining a balanced flow of vital energy and interventions, including acupressure, acupuncture, herbal therapies, diet, meditation, and Tai Chi and Qigong (exercises that focus on breathing, visualization, and movement)
3. Ayurveda: Focus is on the balance of mind, body, and spirit; interventions include diet, medicinal herbs, detoxification, breathing exercises, meditation, and yoga
4. Homeopathy: Focuses on healing; interventions consist of small doses of specially prepared plant and mineral extracts that assist in the body's innate healing process
5. Naturopathy: Focuses on enhancing the body's natural healing responses; interventions include nutrition, herbology, hydrotherapy, homeopathy, acupuncture, physical therapies, and counseling and psychotherapy

C. Mind-body interventions
1. Focuses on controlling physical functions through positive mental processes
2. Interventions include biofeedback, hypnosis, relaxation therapy, meditation, music or art therapy, Qigong, prayer, and mental healing

D. Biologically based therapies (Box 6-6)
1. Include natural and biologically derived products, interventions, and practices
2. Interventions include aromatherapy, herbal therapies, macrobiotic diet, and orthomolecular therapy

E. Manipulative and body-based interventions
1. Involve manipulation and movement of the body by a therapist
2. Includes acupressure, movement reeducation techniques, chiropractic therapy, and therapeutic massage

F. Energy therapies
1. Focus on energy originating within the body or on energy from other sources
2. Interventions include therapeutic touch and magnetic therapy

---

BOX 6-5

Categories of Complementary and Alternative Therapies

Alternative Medical Systems
Mind-Body Interventions
Biological-Based Therapies
Manipulative and Body-Based Methods
Energy Therapies

BOX 6-6

Biological-based therapies

AROMATHERAPY
The use of topical or inhaled oils (plant extracts) that will promote and maintain health

HERBAL THERAPIES
The use of herbs derived from mostly plant sources that will maintain and restore balance and health

MACROBIOTIC DIET
Diet high in whole-grain cereals, vegetables, beans, sea vegetables, and vegetarian soups
Meat, animal fat, eggs, poultry, dairy products, sugars, and artificially produced foods are eliminated from the diet

ORTHOMOLECULAR THERAPY
Focuses on nutritional balance and includes the use of vitamins, essential amino acids, essential fats, and minerals

IX. HERBAL THERAPIES (Box 6-7)

A. Description: The use of herbs (plant or a plant part) for therapeutic value on health

B. Some herbs have been determined to be safe, yet some herbs, even in small amounts, can be toxic

C. If the client is taking prescription medications, the client should consult with the health care provider regarding the use of herbs, because serious herb-medication interactions can occur

D. Client teaching points

1. Discuss herbal therapies with health care provider before use

---

BOX 6-7

Commonly Used Herbs

Aloe: Anti-inflammatory and antimicrobial effect; accelerates wound healing

Angelica: Antispasmodic and vasodilator; balances the effects of estrogen

Bilberry: Improves microcirculation in the eyes

Black cohosh: Produces estrogen-like effects

Cat's claw: Antioxidant; stimulates the immune system, lowers the blood pressure

Chamomile: Antispasmodic and anti-inflammatory; produces a mild sedative effect

Dehydroepiandrosterone (DHEA): Converts to androgens and estrogen; slows the effects of aging, and is used for erectile dysfunction

Echinacea: Stimulates the immune system

Evening primrose: Assists with the metabolism of fatty acid

Feverfew: Anti-inflammatory; used for migraine headaches, arthritis, and fever

Garlic: Antioxidant; used to lower cholesterol levels

Ginger: Antiemetic; used for nausea and vomiting

Ginkgo biloba: Antioxidant; used to improve memory

Ginseng: Increases physical endurance and stamina; used for stress and fatigue

Glucosamine: Amino acid that assists in the synthesis of cartilage

Goldenseal: Anti-inflammatory and antimicrobial; used to stimulate the immune system; has an anticoagulant effect and may increase blood pressure

Kava: Antianxiety and skeletal muscle relaxant; produces a sedative effect

Melatonin: Hormone that regulates sleep; used for insomnia

Milk thistle: Antioxidant; stimulates the production of new liver cells, reduces liver inflammation, and is used for liver and gallbladder disease

Peppermint oil: Antispasmodic; used for irritable bowel syndrome

St. John's wort: Antibacterial, antiviral, and antidepressant

Saw palmetto: Antiestrogen activity; used for urinary tract infections and benign prostatic hypertrophy

Valerian: Used to treat nervous disorders such as anxiety, restlessness, and insomnia

Zinc: Antiviral; stimulates the immune system

---

2. Contact the physician if any side effects of the herbal substance occur

3. Contact the health care provider before stopping the use of a prescription medication

4. Avoid using herbs to treat a serious medical condition such as heart disease

5. Avoid taking herbs if pregnant or attempting to get pregnant or if nursing

6. Do not give herbs to infants or young children

7. Purchase herbal supplements only from a reputable manufacturer; the label should contain the scientific name of the herb, name and address of the manufacturer, batch or lot number, date of manufacture, and expiration date

8. Adhere to the recommended dose; if herbal preparations are taken in high doses, they can be toxic

9. Moisture, sunlight, and heat may alter the components of herbal therapy

10. If surgery is planned, the herbal therapy may need to be discontinued 2 to 3 weeks before surgery

X. LOW-RISK THERAPIES

A. Description: Therapies that have no adverse effects that the nurse can use when implementing care

B. Common low-risk therapies

1. Meditation
2. Relaxation techniques
3. Imagery
4. Music therapy
5. Massage
6. Touch
7. Laughter and humor
8. Spiritual measures such as prayer

XI. NURSING CONSIDERATIONS

A. Principle: If health care recommendations, interventions, or treatments do not fit within the client's **cultural value** system, they will not be followed

B. Data collection skills: Be alert to cues regarding eye contact, personal space, time concepts, and understanding of the recommended plan of care

C. Knowledge: Learn about the **cultures** of clients with whom you will be working; additionally, learn from your clients about their health care practices

D. Flexibility: Allow for variation in accomplishing goals of health care; negotiate with the client until a mutually agreeable plan is established

E. Communication principles

1. Treat each client and those accompanying the client with respect
2. Appreciate the differences and diversity of **beliefs** about health, illness, and treatment modalities
3. Ask the client who has been consulted about the illness or condition and what treatments were recommended by the consultant

4. Clarify perception of what the client has said or done and perception about the client's expectations of the health care provider
5. If language barriers pose a problem, seek an interpreter; avoid using family members as interpreters except as a last resort

PRACTICE QUESTIONS

1. A nurse is assisting in collecting data on an African-American client admitted to the ambulatory care unit who is scheduled for a hernia repair. Which of the following information about the client is of least priority during the data collection?
   1. Cardiovascular
   2. Neurological
   3. Respiratory
   4. Psychosocial

2. A nursing instructor is providing a session on cultural beliefs related to health and illness. Following the session, the instructor asks a nursing student to describe the beliefs of an African American in regard to illness. Which statement describes the beliefs of an African American in regard to illness?
   1. "Illness is due to an imbalance between yin and yang."
   2. "Illness is due to prolonged sitting."
   3. "Illness is a disharmonious state that may be caused by demons and spirits."
   4. "Illness is due to lack of exercise."

3. A nurse is planning to reinforce instructions to the African-American client about nutrition. When developing the plan, the nurse is aware that a common dietary practice of African Americans is to eat:
   1. Fried foods
   2. Rice as the basis for all meals
   3. Red meat
   4. Raw fish

4. A nurse is assigned to care for an Asian-American client. The nurse plans care knowing that which of the following describes the Asian-American's view of illness?
   1. Illness is caused by supernatural forces
   2. Illness is a punishment for sins
   3. Illness is a disharmonious state that may be caused by demons and spirits
   4. Illness is due to an imbalance between yin and yang

5. A nursing student is discussing cultural diversity issues in a clinical conference. The nursing instructor asks a student to describe ethnocentrism. Which statement indicates a lack of understanding of the issue of ethnocentrism?
   1. "It is a tendency to view one's own ways as best."
   2. "It is acting in a manner that is superior to other cultures."
   3. "It is believing that ones' own ways are the only acceptable way."
   4. "It is imposing one's beliefs on individuals from another culture."

6. A nurse consults with a nutritionist regarding the dietary preferences of an Asian-American client. Which of the following foods would the nurse plan to include in the diet plan?
   1. Red meat
   2. Rice
   3. Fried foods
   4. Fruits

7. An antihypertensive medication has been prescribed for a client with hypertension. The client tells the nurse that she would like to take an herbal substance to help lower her blood pressure. The nurse should:
   1. Tell the client that if she takes the herbal substance she will need to have her blood pressure checked frequently
   2. Advise the client to discuss the use of an herbal substance with the physician
   3. Teach the client how to take her blood pressure so that it can be monitored closely
   4. Tell the client that herbal substances are not safe and should never be used

8. A Hispanic-American mother brings her child to the clinic for an examination. Which of the following is important when gathering data about the child?
   1. Avoiding eye contact
   2. Touching the child during the examination
   3. Avoiding speaking to the child
   4. Using body language only

9. A client is diagnosed with cancer and is told that surgery followed by chemotherapy will be necessary. The client states to the nurse, "I have read a lot about complementary therapies. Do you think that I should try it?" The nurse responds by making which appropriate statement?
   1. "No, because it will interact with the chemotherapy."
   2. "You need to ask your physician about it."
   3. "I would try anything that I could if I had cancer."
   4. "There are many different forms of complementary therapies. Let's talk about these therapies."

10. A nurse is preparing to assist a Jewish client with eating lunch. A kosher meal is delivered to the client. Which nursing action is most appropriate in assisting the client with the meal?
   1. Carefully transferring the food from the paper plates to glass plates
   2. Unwrapping the eating utensils for the client
   3. Replacing the plastic utensils with metal eating utensils
   4. Asking the client to unwrap the eating utensils and allowing the client to prepare the meal for eating

ALTERNATE FORMAT QUESTION: MULTIPLE RESPONSE

A nursing student is asked to identify the practices and beliefs of the Amish society. Select all practices and beliefs of the Amish society.
____ The authority of women is equal to men
____ Remain secluded and avoid helping others
____ Use traditional health care and alternative health care, such as healers, herbs, and massage
____ Believe that health is a gift from God
____ Many choose not to have health insurance
____ Funerals are conducted in the home without a eulogy, flower decorations, or any other display; caskets are plain and simple without adornment

ANSWERS

1. Answer: **4**
Rationale: The psychosocial data is the least priority during the initial admission data collection. In the African-American culture, it is considered intrusive to ask personal questions on the initial contact or meeting. Additionally, cardiovascular, neurological, and respiratory data include physiological assessments that would be the priority.
Test-Taking Strategy: Note the key words, *least priority*. Use Maslow's Hierarchy of Needs theory to answer the question. Options 1, 2, and 3 address physiological needs. Review the characteristics of the African-American culture if you had difficulty with this question.
Level of Cognitive Ability: Comprehension
Client Needs: Physiological Integrity
Integrated Process: Nursing Process/Data Collection
Content Area: Fundamental Skills
Reference: Potter, P., & Perry, A. (2005), *Fundamentals of nursing* (6th ed.). St. Louis: Mosby, pp. 124, 393-394.

2. Answer: **3**
Rationale: In the African-American culture, illness is viewed as a disharmonious state that may be caused by demons and spirits. The goal of treatment, from the traditional African perspective, is to remove the harmful spirit from the body of the ill person. Asian-Americans believe that illness is due to an imbalance between yin and yang and caused by prolonged sitting or lying, or overexertion.
Test-Taking Strategy: Knowledge regarding the beliefs related to health and illness in the various cultures assists in answering the question. From this point, use the process of elimination to determine the correct option. Review the characteristics of the African-American culture if you had difficulty with this question.
Level of Cognitive Ability: Comprehension
Client Needs: Psychosocial Integrity
Integrated Process: Teaching/Learning
Content Area: Fundamental Skills
Reference: Potter, P., & Perry, A. (2005), *Fundamentals of nursing* (6th ed.). St. Louis: Mosby, p. 124.

3. Answer: **1**
Rationale: African-American food preferences include chicken, pork, greens, rice, and fried foods. Asian Americans eat raw fish, rice, and soy sauce. Hispanic Americans prefer beans, fried foods, spicy foods, chili, and carbonated beverages. European Americans prefer carbohydrates and red meat.
Test-Taking Strategy: Use the process of elimination. Recalling that African Americans are at risk for hypertension and coronary artery disease will assist in directing you to option 1. Review the food preferences of the African-American culture if you had difficulty with this question.
Level of Cognitive Ability: Comprehension
Client Needs: Physiological Integrity
Integrated Process: Nursing Process/Planning
Content Area: Fundamental Skills
References: Nix, S. (2005). *Williams' basic nutrition and diet therapy* (12th ed.). St. Louis: Mosby, pp. 252-254. Peckenpaugh, N. (2003). *Nutrition essentials and diet therapy* (9th ed.). Philadelphia: W.B. Saunders, p. 9.

4. Answer: **4**
Rationale: Asian Americans believe that illness is caused by an imbalance between yin and yang, by prolonged sitting or lying, or by overexertion. In the African-American culture, illness is viewed as a disharmonious state that may be caused by demons and spirits. Native Americans believe that illness is caused by supernatural forces.
Test-Taking Strategy: Knowledge regarding the beliefs related to health and illness of the various cultures assists in answering the question. From this point, use the process of elimination to determine the correct option. Review the characteristics of the Asian-American culture if you had difficulty with this question.
Level of Cognitive Ability: Comprehension
Client Needs: Psychosocial Integrity
Integrated Process: Nursing Process/Planning
Content Area: Fundamental Skills
References: Jarvis, C. (2004). *Physical examination and health assessment* (4th ed.). Philadelphia: W.B. Saunders, pp. 44-45. Potter, P., & Perry, A. (2005). *Fundamentals of nursing* (6th ed.). St. Louis: Mosby, p. 921.

5. Answer: **4**
Rationale: Ethnocentrism is a tendency to view one's own ways of life as the most desirable, acceptable, or best, and to act in a superior manner toward another culture. Cultural imposition is the tendency to impose one's own beliefs, values, and patterns of behavior on individuals from another culture.
Test-Taking Strategy: Use the process of elimination and note the key words, *indicates a lack of understanding*, in the stem of the question. Also, note the similarity in options 1, 2, and 3. If you had difficulty with this question, review culturally related concepts.
Level of Cognitive Ability: Comprehension
Client Needs: Psychosocial Integrity
Integrated Process: Teaching/Learning

Content Area: Fundamental Skills
Reference: Jarvis, C. (2004). *Physical examination and health assessment* (4th ed.). Philadelphia: W.B. Saunders, p. 40.

6. Answer: **2**
Rationale: Asian-American food preferences include raw fish, rice, and soy sauce. African-American food preferences include chicken, pork, greens, rice, and fried foods. Hispanic Americans prefer beans, fried foods, spicy foods, chili, and carbonated beverages. European Americans prefer carbohydrates and red meat.
Test-Taking Strategy: Knowledge regarding the food practices and preferences related to the various cultures is required to answer the question. Correlate rice with Asian Americans to answer questions similar to this one. Review the food preferences associated with the Asian-American culture if you had difficulty with this question.
Level of Cognitive Ability: Comprehension
Client Needs: Physiological Integrity
Integrated Process: Nursing Process/Planning
Content Area: Fundamental Skills
Reference: Nix, S. (2005). *Williams' basic nutrition & diet therapy* (12th ed.). St. Louis: Mosby, p. 255.

7. Answer: **2**
Rationale: Although herbal substances may have some beneficial effects, not all herbs are safe to use. Clients who are being treated with conventional medication therapy should be advised to avoid herbal substances with similar pharmacological effects, because the combination may lead to an excessive reaction or to unknown interaction effects. Therefore, the nurse would advise the client to discuss the use of the herbal substance with the physician.
Test-Taking Strategy: Use the process of elimination. Eliminate option 4 first because of the absolute word *never*. Next, eliminate options 1 and 3 because they are similar. Review the limitations associated with the use of herbal substances if you had difficulty with this question.
Level of Cognitive Ability: Application
Client Needs: Physiological Integrity
Integrated Process: Nursing Process/Implementation
Content Area: Fundamental Skills
References: Lewis, S., Heitkemper, M., & Dirksen, S. (2004). *Medical-surgical nursing: Assessment and management of clinical problems* (6th ed.). St. Louis: Mosby, p. 101.
Skidmore-Roth, L. (2001). *Mosby's handbook of herbs and natural supplements*. St. Louis: Mosby, p. 182.

8. Answer: **2**
Rationale: In the Hispanic-American culture, eye behavior is significant. The "bad (evil) eye" can be given to a child if a person looks at and admires the child without touching the child. Therefore, touching the child during the examination is very important. Although avoiding eye contact indicates respect and attentiveness, this is not the most important intervention. Avoiding speaking to the child, and using body language only, are not therapeutic interventions.
Test-Taking Strategy: Use the process of elimination. Eliminate options 3 and 4 first because they are similar. From the remaining options, select the intervention that is most

therapeutic, which is touch. Review the characteristics of the Hispanic-American culture if you had difficulty with this question.
Level of Cognitive Ability: Application
Client Needs: Psychosocial Integrity
Integrated Process: Nursing Process/Data Collection
Content Area: Fundamental Skills
References: Jarvis, C. (2004). *Physical examination and health assessment* (4th ed.), Philadelphia: W.B. Saunders, p. 70.
Potter, P., & Perry, A. (2005). *Fundamentals of nursing* (6th ed.). St. Louis: Mosby, p. 913.

9. Answer: **4**
Rationale: Complementary (alternative) therapies include a wide variety of treatment modalities that are used in addition to conventional treatment to treat a disease or illness. These therapies complement conventional treatment but should be approved by the person's health care provider to ensure that the treatment does not interact with prescribed therapy. Although the physician should approve the use of a complementary therapy, and although some of these therapies can interact with the prescribed treatment plan, the statements in options 1 and 2 are inappropriate. Similarly, option 3 is an inappropriate response to the client. Option 4 addresses the client's question and encourages discussion.
Test-Taking Strategy: Use therapeutic communication techniques. Eliminate options 1, 2, and 3 because they are nontherapeutic. Option 4 is the only option that addresses the client's question and encourages discussion. Review therapeutic communication techniques if you had difficulty with this question.
Level of Cognitive Ability: Application
Client Needs: Physiological Integrity
Integrated Process: Communication and Documentation
Content Area: Fundamental Skills
References: Lewis, S., Heitkemper, M., & Dirksen, S. (2004). *Medical-surgical nursing: Assessment and management of clinical problems* (6th ed.). St. Louis: Mosby, p. 94.
Potter, P., & Perry, A. (2005). *Fundamentals of nursing* (6th ed.). St. Louis: Mosby, p. 437.

10. Answer: **4**
Rationale: Kosher meals arrive on paper plates and with plastic utensils sealed. Health care providers should not unwrap the utensils or transfer the food to another serving dish. Although the nurse may want to be helpful in assisting the client with the meal, the only appropriate option for this client is option 4.
Test-Taking Strategy: Use the process of elimination and knowledge regarding the rituals associated with kosher meals. Options 1 and 3 are similar and can be eliminated first. To choose from the remaining options, it is necessary to be familiar with kosher rituals. If you had difficulty with this question, review the dietary practices of this Jewish client.
Level of Cognitive Ability: Application
Client Needs: Psychosocial Integrity
Integrated Process: Nursing Process/Implementation
Content Area: Fundamental Skills
Reference: Nix, S. (2005). *Williams' basic nutrition and diet therapy* (12th ed.). St. Louis: Mosby, p. 249.

ALTERNATE FORMAT QUESTION: MULTIPLE RESPONSE

Answers:

Use traditional health care and alternative health care, such as healers, herbs, and massage

Believe that health is a gift from God

Many choose not to have health insurance

Funerals are conducted in the home without a eulogy, flower decorations, or any other display; caskets are plain and simple without adornment

Rationale: The Amish society maintains a culture distinct and separate from the non-Amish and generally remain separate from the rest of the world, physically and socially. Men usually dress in a plain, dark suit; women usually wear a plain dress with long sleeves, bonnet, and apron. Women are not allowed to hold positions of power in the congregational organization. Family life has a patriarchal structure and, although the roles of the women are considered equally important to those of men, they are very unequal in terms of authority. Marriage outside the faith is not allowed, and unmarried women remain under the authority of their father. The Amish society rejects materialism and worldliness, values living simply, and may choose to avoid technology, such as electricity and cars. They highly value responsibility, generosity, and helping others, and often work as farmers, builders, quilters, and homemakers. The Amish use traditional health care and alternative health care, such as healers, herbs, and massage, and believe that health is a gift from God, but that clean living and a balanced diet help maintain it. They may choose not to have health insurance and maintain mutual aid funds for Amish members to help with medical costs.

Funerals are conducted in the home without a eulogy, flower decorations, or any other display; caskets are plain and simple, without adornment. At death, women are usually buried in their bridal dress. The Amish believe that one lives on after death, either receiving eternal reward in heaven or being punished in hell.

Test-Taking Strategy: Specific knowledge regarding the practices and beliefs of the Amish society is needed to answer this question. Review the characteristics of this group of people if you had difficulty with this question.

Level of Cognitive Ability: Comprehension

Client Needs: Psychosocial Integrity

Integrated Process: Teaching/Learning

Content Area: Fundamental Skills

References: Harkreader, H., & Hogan, M.A. (2004). *Fundamentals of nursing: Caring and clinical judgment.* (2nd ed.). Philadelphia: W.B. Saunders, p. 900.

REFERENCES

Harkreader, H., & Hogan, M.A. (2004). *Fundamentals of nursing: Caring and clinical judgment* (2nd ed.). Philadelphia: W.B. Saunders.

Jarvis, C. (2004). *Physical examination and health assessment* (4th ed.). Philadelphia: W.B. Saunders.

Lewis, S., Heitkemper, M., & Dirksen, S. (2004). *Medical-surgical nursing: Assessment and management of clinical problems* (6th ed.). St. Louis: Mosby.

National Council of State Boards of Nursing (2005). *Detailed test plan for the National Council licensure examination for practical/vocational nurses.* Chicago: Author.

Nix, S. (2005). *Williams' basic nutrition and diet therapy* (12th ed.). St. Louis: Mosby.

Peckenpaugh, N. (2003). *Nutrition essentials and diet therapy* (9th ed.). Philadelphia: W.B. Saunders.

Potter, P., & Perry, A. (2005). *Fundamentals of nursing* (6th ed.). St. Louis: Mosby.

Skidmore-Roth, L. (2001). *Mosby's handbook of herbs and natural supplements.* St. Louis: Mosby.

The Amish: Practices of various groups. Retrieved April 23, 2005, from www.religioustolerance.org/amish.htm.

Ethical and Legal Issues

PYRAMID TERMS

advance directive   Written document, recognized by state law, that provides directions concerning the provision of care when a person is unable to make his or her own treatment choices.

advocacy   Acting on behalf of the client, and protecting the client's right to make his or her own decisions.

consent   Voluntary act by which a person agrees to allow someone else to do something.

ethics   Concerns the distinction between right and wrong on the basis of a body of knowledge, not just on the basis of opinions.

informed consent   The client understands the reason for the purposed intervention, with its benefits and risks, and agrees to the treatment by signing a consent form.

law   A system composed of general rules governing conduct and the procedures for resolving disputes when rules are not followed.

malpractice   Failure to meet the standards of acceptable care, which results in harm to another person.

negligence   Failure to provide care that a reasonable person would ordinarily use in a similar circumstance.

client's Bill of Rights   Includes the rights and responsibilities of clients receiving care.

values   Beliefs and attitudes that may influence behavior and the process of decision making.

PYRAMID TO SUCCESS

Across all settings in the practice of nursing, nurses are frequently confronted with ethical and legal issues related to client care. It is the responsibility of the professional nurse to be aware of the ethical principles, laws, and guidelines related to providing safe and quality care to clients. In the Pyramid to Success, focus on ethical practices; the Nurse Practice Act, client's rights, particularly confidentiality and informed consent; advocacy, documentation, and advance directives; and cultural, religious, and spiritual issues. The Integrated Processes addressed in this chapter are Caring, Clinical Problem-Solving Process (Nursing Process), Communication and Documentation, and Teaching/Learning.

CLIENT NEEDS
Safe, Effective Care Environment

Acting as an advocate
Advance directives
Client's rights
Confidentiality
Continuous quality improvement
Establishing priorities
Ethical practice
Incident reports
Informed consent
Legal responsibilities
Resource management

Health Promotion and Maintenance

Developmental stages and transitions
Family systems
Lifestyle choices

Psychosocial Integrity

Abuse/neglect
Chemical dependency
Coping mechanisms
Cultural, spiritual, and religious issues
End of life
Grief and loss
Support systems

Physiological Integrity

Alterations in body systems
Palliative/comfort care
Unexpected responses to therapies

I. ETHICS

A. **Description:** The branch of philosophy that concerns the distinction between right and wrong on the basis of a body of knowledge, not just on the basis of opinions

B. **Morality:** Behavior in accordance with customs or tradition, usually reflecting personal or religious beliefs

C. **Ethical principles:** Codes that direct or govern nursing actions (Box 7-1)

D. **Values:** Beliefs and attitudes that may influence behavior and the process of decision-making

E. **Values clarification:** Process of analyzing one's own **values** to better understand what is truly important

F. Ethical codes
   1. Provide broad principles for determining and evaluating client care
   2. Are not legally binding, but in most states, the Board of Nursing has authority to reprimand nurses for unprofessional conduct that results from violation of the ethical codes
   3. Specific ethical codes
      a. National Federation of Licensed Practical Nurses (NFLPN) Code for Licensed Practical/Vocational Nurses
      b. NFLPN Nursing Practice Standards
      c. NFLPN Specialized Nursing Practice Standards
      d. National Association of Practical Nurse Education and Service (NAPNES) Code of Ethics
      e. NAPNES Standards of Practice for Practical/Vocational Nurses

G. Ethical dilemma
   1. Occurs when there is a conflict between two or more ethical principles
   2. There is no correct decision
   3. The nurse must make a choice between two alternatives that are equally unsatisfactory

---

BOX 7-1

Ethical Principles

Autonomy: Respect for an individual's right to self-determination

Nonmaleficence: The obligation to do or cause no harm to another

Beneficence: The duty to do good to others and to maintain a balance between benefits and harms; paternalism is an undesirable outcome of beneficence, in which the health care provider decides what is best for the client and attempts to encourage the client to act against his or her own choices

Justice: The equitable distribution of potential benefits and tasks; determining the order in which clients should be cared for

Veracity: The obligation to tell the truth

Fidelity: The duty to do what one has promised

---

   4. May occur as a result of differences in cultural or religious beliefs
   5. Ethical reasoning is the process of thinking through what one ought to do in an orderly and systematic manner to provide justification for actions on the basis of principles

H. Advocate
   1. A person who speaks up for or acts on the behalf of the client, protects the client's right to make his or her own decisions, and upholds the principle of fidelity
   2. Represents the client's viewpoint to others
   3. Avoids letting personal **values** influence **advocacy** for the client
   4. Supports the client's decision, even when it conflicts with his or her own preferences or choices

I. **Ethics** committees
   1. Multidisciplinary approach to facilitate dialogue regarding ethical dilemmas
   2. Develop and establish policies and procedures for the prevention and resolution of dilemmas

---

II. REGULATION OF NURSING PRACTICE

A. Nurse practice act
   1. A series of statutes enacted by each state legislature to regulate the practice of nursing in that state
   2. Nurse practice acts set educational requirements for the nurse, distinguish between nursing practice and medical practice, and define the scope of nursing practice
   3. Additional issues covered by nurse practice acts include licensure requirements for protection of the public, grounds for disciplinary action, rights of the nurse licensee if a disciplinary action is taken, and related topics
   4. All nurses are responsible for knowing the provisions of the act for the state or province in which they work

B. Standards of care
   1. Guidelines by which the nurse should practice
   2. Guidelines for determining whether nurses have performed duties in an appropriate manner
   3. If a nurse does not perform duties within accepted standards of care, the nurse places himself or herself in jeopardy of legal action
   4. If a nurse is named as a defendant in a **malpractice** lawsuit and it is shown that neither the accepted standards of care outlined by the state or province nursing practice act nor the policies of the employing institution were followed, the nurse's legal liability is clear

C. Employee guidelines
   1. Respondent superior: Employer will be held liable for any negligent acts of an employee if the alleged negligent act occurred during the employment

relationship and was within the scope of the employee's responsibilities
2. Contracts
   a. Nurses are responsible for carrying out the terms of contractual agreement with the employee agency and the client
   b. The nurse employee relationship is governed by established employee handbooks and by client care policies and procedures that create obligations, rights, and duties between those parties
3. Institutional policies
   a. Written policies and procedures of the employing institution that detail how nurses are to perform their duties
   b. Policies and procedures are usually quite specific and are located in manuals in most health care facilities
   c. Although policies are not laws, courts generally rule against nurses who violate policies
   d. If the nurse practices nursing in accordance with the client care policies and procedures established by the employer, functions within the job responsibility, and provides care consistently in a non-negligent manner, the potential for liability is minimized
D. Hospital staffing
   1. Nurses should not walk out when staffing is inadequate, because charges of abandonment can be made
   2. Nurses in short-staffing situations are obligated to make a report to nursing administration
E. Floating
   1. An acceptable legal practice used by hospitals to solve their understaffing problems
   2. Legally, a nurse cannot refuse to float unless a union contract guarantees that the nurse can work only in a specified area or the nurse can prove lack of knowledge for the performance of assigned tasks
   3. Nurses in a floating situation must not assume responsibility beyond their level of experience or qualification
   4. Nurses who float should inform the supervisor of any lack of experience in caring for the type of clients on the new nursing unit
   5. The nurse should request and be given orientation to the new unit
F. Disciplinary action
   1. Boards of nursing may deny, revoke, or suspend any license to practice as a practical/vocational nurse, in accordance with their statutory authority
   2. Causes for disciplinary action
      a. Unprofessional conduct
      b. Conduct that could adversely affect the health and welfare of the public
      c. Breach of client confidentiality

d. Failure to use sufficient knowledge, skills, or nursing judgment
e. Physically or verbally abusing a client
f. Assuming duties without sufficient preparation
g. Knowingly delegating nursing care to unlicensed personnel that places the client at risk for injury
h. Failure to accurately maintain a record for each client
i. Falsifying a client's record
j. Leaving a nursing assignment without properly notifying appropriate personnel

III. LEGAL LIABILITY
A. **Laws**
   1. Nurses are governed by civil and criminal **law** in roles as providers of services, employees of institutions, and private citizens
   2. A nurse has a personal and legal obligation to provide a standard of client care expected of a reasonably competent professional nurse
   3. Nurses are held responsible (liable) for harm resulting from their negligent acts or their failure to act
B. Types of **laws** (Box 7-2)
C. **Negligence** and **malpractice**
   1. Conduct that falls below the standard of care
   2. Can include acts of commission as well as acts of omission
   3. If a nurse gives care that does not meet appropriate standards, he or she may be held liable for **negligence**
   4. **Malpractice** is **negligence** on the part of a nurse
   5. **Malpractice** is determined if the nurse owed a duty to the client and did not carry out the duty and the client was injured because the nurse failed to perform the duty

---

BOX 7-2

Types of Laws

Contract law: Concerned with enforcement of agreements among private individuals
Civil law: Concerned with relationships among people and the protection of a person's rights; violation may cause harm to an individual or property, but no grave threat to society exists
Criminal law: Concerned with relationships between individuals and governments and with acts that threaten society and its order; a crime is an offense against society that violates a law and is defined as a misdemeanor (less serious nature) or felony (serious nature)
Tort law: Civil wrong, other than a breach in contract, in which the law allows an injured person to seek damages from a person who caused the injury

6. Proof of liability
   a. Duty: At the time of injury, a duty existed between the plaintiff and the defendant
   b. Breach of duty: The defendant breached duty of care to the plaintiff
   c. Proximate cause: The breach of the duty was the legal cause of injury to the client
   d. Damage or injury: The plaintiff experienced injury or damages or both and can be compensated by law
D. Professional liability insurance
   1. Nurses need their own liability insurance for protection against **malpractice** lawsuits
   2. Having his or her own insurance provides the nurse protection as an individual and allows the nurse to have an attorney present who has only the nurse's interests in mind
E. Good Samaritan laws
   1. Passed by a state legislature; laws may vary from state to state
   2. Encourage health care professionals to assist in emergency situations without fear of being sued for the care provided
   3. These laws limit liability and offer legal immunity for people helping in an emergency, providing they give reasonable care
   4. Immunity from suit applies only when all conditions of the state **law** are met; for example, the health care provider receives no compensation for the care provided and the care given is not intentionally negligent
F. Controlled substances
   1. Adhere to facility policies and procedures concerning administration of controlled substances, which are governed by federal and state laws
   2. Controlled substances must be kept securely locked, and only authorized personnel should have access to them

IV. COLLECTIVE BARGAINING

A. Formalized decision-making process between representatives of management and representatives of labor to negotiate wages and conditions of employment
B. When collective bargaining breaks down because an agreement cannot be reached, the employees usually call a strike
C. Striking presents a moral dilemma to many nurses, because nursing practice is a service to people

V. LEGAL RISK AREAS

A. Assault
   1. Occurs when a person puts another person in fear of a harmful or offensive contact
   2. The victim fears and believes that harm will result as a result of the threat

B. Battery: An intentional touching of another's body without the other's consent
C. Invasion of privacy: Includes violating confidentiality, intruding on private client or family matters, and sharing client information with unauthorized persons
D. False imprisonment
   1. Occurs when a client is not allowed to leave a health care facility when there is no legal justification to detain the client
   2. Occurs when restraining devices are used without an appropriate clinical need
   3. A client can sign an "Against Medical Advice" form when the client refuses care and is competent to make decisions
   4. Document circumstances in the medical record to avoid allegations by the client that cannot be defended
E. Defamation: A false communication or a careless disregard for the truth that causes damage to someone's reputation, either in writing (libel) or verbally (slander)
F. Fraud: Results from a deliberate deception intended to produce unlawful gains

VI. CLIENT'S RIGHTS

A. Description
   1. A document that reflects acknowledgment of a client's right to participate in his or her health care, with an emphasis on client autonomy
   2. Provides a list of the rights of the client and responsibilities that the hospital cannot violate (Box 7-3)
   3. The client's rights affect the relationship between the client and health care provider and between the client and health care delivery system, and protect the client's ability to determine the level and type of care received
   4. Laws and standards (Box 7-4)
B. Rights for the mentally ill (Box 7-5)
   1. Mental Health Systems Act (MHSA) of 1980 created rights for the mentally ill
   2. Joint Commission on Accreditation of Healthcare Organization (JCAHO) developed policy statements on the rights of the mentally ill
   3. Psychiatric facilities are required to have a **client's Bill of Rights** posted in a visible area
C. Organ donation and transplantation
   1. Client has the right to decide to become an organ donor and a right to refuse an organ transplant as a treatment option
   2. An individual who is at least 18 years of age may indicate their wish to become a donor on their driver's license (state specific) or in an advance directive
   3. The Uniform Anatomical Gift Act provides a list of individuals who can provide informed consent for the donation of a deceased individual's organs

BOX 7-3

Patient's Rights When Hospitalized

- Right to considerate and respectful care
- Right to be informed about illness, possible treatments, and likely outcome, and to discuss this information with the physician
- Right to know the names and roles of the people who are involved in care
- Right to consent or refuse a treatment
- Right to have an advance directive
- Right to privacy
- Right to expect that medical records are confidential
- Right to review the medical record and to have information explained
- Right to expect that the hospital will provide necessary health care services
- Right to know if the hospital has relationships with outside parties that may influence treatment or care
- Right to consent or refuse to take part in research
- Right to be told of realistic care alternatives when hospital care is no longer appropriate
- Right to know about hospital rules that affect treatment and about charges and payment methods

Modified from Christensen, B., & Kockrow, E. (2003). *Foundations of nursing* (4th ed.). St. Louis: Mosby.

BOX 7-4

Laws and Standards

American Hospital Association: Issued a patient's bill of rights

American Nurses Association: Developed the Code for Nurses, which defines the nurse's responsibility for upholding the client's rights

Mental Health Systems Act: Developed rights for the mentally ill client

Joint Commission on the Accreditation of Healthcare Organizations (JCAHO): Developed policy statements on the rights of the mentally ill

BOX 7-5

Rights for the Mentally Ill

- Right to be treated with dignity and respect
- Right to communicate with people outside the hospital
- Right to keep clothing and personal effects with them
- Right to religious freedom
- Right to be employed
- Right to manage property
- Right to execute wills
- Right to enter into contractual agreements
- Right to make purchases
- Right to education
- Right to habeas corpus (written request for release from the hospital)
- Right to an independent psychiatric examination
- Right to civil service status, including the right to vote
- Right to retain licenses, privileges, or permits
- Right to sue or be sued
- Right to marry or divorce
- Right to treatment in the least restrictive setting
- Right not to be subject to unnecessary restraints
- Right to privacy and confidentiality
- Right to informed consent
- Right to treatment and to refuse treatment
- Right to refuse participation in experimental treatments or research

Modified from Stuart, G., & Laraia, M. (2005). *Principles and practice of psychiatric nursing* (8th ed.). St. Louis: Mosby.

4. Criteria for organ donations are set by the United Network for Organ Sharing (UNOS)
5. Some organs such as the heart, lungs, and liver can only be obtained from a person who was on mechanical ventilation and has suffered brain death, whereas other organs or tissues can be removed several hours after death
6. Donor must be free of infectious disease and cancer
7. Requests to the family for organ donation from a deceased family member are usually done by the physician or nurse specially trained for making such requests
8. Donation of organs does not delay funeral arrangements, there is no obvious evidence that the organs were removed from the body when the body is dressed, and there is no cost to the family for removal of the organs donated

D. Religious beliefs: Organ donation and transplantation
   1. Catholic Church: Organ donation and transplants are acceptable
   2. Eastern Orthodox Church: Discourages organ donation
   3. Islam: Body parts may not be removed or donated for transplantation
   4. Jehovah's Witness: An organ transplant may be accepted, but the organ must be cleansed with a nonblood solution before transplantation
   5. Orthodox Judaism
      a. All body parts removed during autopsy must be buried with the body, because it is believed that the entire body must be returned to the earth
      b. Organ transplantation may be allowed with the rabbi's approval

VII. INFORMED CONSENT

A. Description
   1. Consent is a client's approval (or that of the client's legal representative) to have the client's body touched by a specific individual
   2. Consents, or releases, are legal documents that indicate the client's permission to perform

BOX 7-6

Types of Consents

Admission agreement: Obtained at the time of admission; identifies the health care agency's responsibility to the client

Blood transfusion consent: Indicates that the client was informed of the benefits and risks of the transfusion; some clients hold religious beliefs that would prohibit receiving a blood transfusion, even in a life-threatening situation

Surgical consent: Obtained for all surgical or invasive procedures or diagnostic tests that are invasive; the physician, surgeon, or anesthesiologist who performs the surgical or other procedure is responsible for explaining the procedure, its risks, benefits, and possible alternative options

Research consent: Obtains permission from the client regarding participation in a research study; informs the client about the possible risks, consequences, and benefits of the research

Special consents: Required for the use of restraints, photographing the client, disposal of body parts during surgery, donating organs after death, or performing an autopsy

BOX 7-7

Mentally or Emotionally Incompetent Clients

Declared incompetent
Unconscious
Under the influence of alcohol or drugs
Chronic dementia or other mental deficiency

surgery, perform a treatment, or give information to a third party

3. Types of consents (Box 7-6)

4. **Informed consent** indicates the client's participation in the decision regarding health care

5. The client must be informed, in understandable terms, of the risks and benefits of the surgery or treatment, what the consequences are for not having the surgery or procedure performed, treatment options, and the name of the health care provider performing the surgery or procedure

6. A client's questions about the surgery or procedure must be answered before signing the consent

7. A consent must be freely signed by the client without threat or pressure and must be witnessed by another adult

8. A client who has been medicated with sedating medications or any other medications that can affect his or her cognitive abilities should not be asked to sign a consent

9. Legally, the client must be mentally and emotionally competent to give consent

10. If a client is declared mentally or emotionally incompetent, the next of kin, appointed guardian (appointed by the court), or durable power of attorney has legal authority to give consent (Box 7-7)

11. A competent client over 18 years of age must sign the consent

12. In most states, when a nurse is involved in the **informed consent** process, the nurse is only

witnessing the signature of the client on the **informed consent** form

13. An **informed consent** can be waived for urgent medical or surgical intervention as long as institutional policy so indicates

14. A client has the right to refuse information, waive the **informed consent**, and undergo treatment, but this decision must be documented in the medical record

15. A client may withdraw his or her consent at any time

B. Minors

1. A minor is a client under legal age as defined by state statute (usually younger than 18 years old)

2. A minor may not give legal consent, and consent must be obtained by a parent or the legal guardian

3. Parental or guardian consent should be obtained before treatment is initiated for a minor except in an emergency; in situations in which the consent of the minor is sufficient, such as treatment related to substance abuse, treatment of a sexually transmitted disease, human immunodeficiency virus testing and acquired immunodeficiency syndrome (AIDS) treatment, birth control services, pregnancy, or psychiatric services; emancipated minor; or if a court order or other legal authorization has been obtained (state laws need to be followed)

C. Emancipated minor

1. A minor who has established independence from the parents through marriage, pregnancy, service in the armed forces, or by a court order

2. An emancipated minor is considered legally capable of signing an **informed consent**

VIII. HEALTH INSURANCE PORTABILITY AND ACCOUNTABILITY ACT (HIPAA)

A. Description

1. Describes how personal health information (PHI) may be used and how the client can obtain access to the information

2. PHI includes individually identifiable information that relates to the client's past, present, or future health, treatment, and payment for health care services

3. HIPAA requires health care agencies to keep PHI private, provides information to the client about

the legal responsibilities regarding privacy, and explains the client's rights with respect to PHI

4. The client has various rights as a consumer of health care under HIPAA, and any client requests may need to be placed in writing; a fee may be attached to certain client requests
5. The client may file a complaint if he or she believes that privacy rights have been violated

B. Client's rights
  1. To request a copy of PHI
  2. To ask the health care agency to amend the PHI that is contained in a record if the PHI is inaccurate
  3. To request a list of disclosures made regarding the PHI as specified by HIPAA
  4. To request to restrict the way the health care agency uses or discloses PHI regarding treatment, payment, or health care services unless information is needed to provide emergency treatment
  5. To request that the health care agency communicates with the client in a certain way or at a certain location; the request must specify how or where the client wishes to be contacted
  6. To request a paper copy of the HIPAA notice

C. Health care agency use and disclosure of PHI
  1. The health care agency obtains PHI in the course of providing and/or administering health insurance benefits for the client and may use or disclose PHI in administering benefits
  2. Use or disclosure of PHI may be done for:
    a. Health care payment purposes
    b. Health care operations purposes
    c. Treatment purposes
    d. Providing information about health care services
    e. Data aggregation purposes to make health care benefit decisions
    f. Administering health care benefits
  3. Additional uses or disclosures of PHI (Box 7-8)

IX. CLIENT PRIVACY
A. Client's right to protection against unreasonable and unwarranted interference into his or her private affairs
B. Violations (Box 7-9)

X. CONFIDENTIALITY
A. Description
  1. Client's right to privacy in the health care system
  2. A special relationship exists between the client and nurse, in which information discussed will not be shared with a third party who is not directly involved in the client's care
B. Nurse's responsibility
  1. Nurses are bound to protect client confidentiality by most nurse practice acts, by ethical principles and standards, and by institutional and agency policies and procedures

---

BOX 7-8

Uses or Disclosures of PHI

- Compliance with legal proceedings or for limited law enforcement purposes
- May be disclosed:
  - To a family member or significant other in a medical emergency
  - To a personal representative appointed by the client or designated by law
  - For research purposes in limited circumstances
  - To a coroner, medical examiner, or funeral director about a deceased person
  - To an organ procurement organization in limited circumstances
  - To avert a serious threat to the client's health or safety or the health or safety of others
  - To a governmental agency authorized to oversee the health care system or government programs
  - To the U.S. Department of Health and Human Services for the investigation of compliance with HIPAA or to fulfill another lawful request
  - To federal officials for lawful intelligence or national security purposes
  - To protect health authorities for public health purposes
  - To appropriate military authorities if a client is a member of the armed forces
  - In accordance with a valid authorization signed by the client

Modified from Combined Life Insurance of New York. (2003). *HIPAA notice of privacy practices for personal health information.* Web site: http://www.keio.edu/parents/hippa.html.

BOX 7-9

Invasion of Privacy

- Taking photographs of the client
- Release of medical information to an unauthorized person, such as a member of the press, family, friend, or neighbor of the client, without the client's permission
- Use of the client's name or picture for the health care agency's sole advantage
- Intrusion by the health care agency regarding the client's affairs
- Publication of information about the client
- Publication of embarrassing facts
- Public disclosure of private information
- Leaving the curtains or room door open while a treatment or procedure is being performed
- Allowing individuals to observe a treatment or procedure without the client's consent
- Leaving a confused or agitated client sitting in the nursing unit hallway
- Interviewing a client in a room with only a curtain between clients, or where conversation can be overheard
- Accessing medical records when unauthorized to do so

2. Disclosure of confidential information exposes the nurse to liability for invasion of the client's privacy

3. The nurse needs to protect the client from indiscriminate disclosure of health care information that may cause harm (Box 7-10)

C. Medical records

1. Medical record is confidential

2. Client has the right to read the medical record and have copies of the record

3. Only staff directly involved in care have legitimate access to a client's record and may include physicians and nurses caring for the client, technicians, therapists, social workers, unit secretaries, client advocates, administrators (for statistical analysis, staffing, quality care review); others must ask permission from the client to review a record

4. The medical record is sent to the hospital records or health information department after hospital discharge

D. Computerized medical records

1. Health care employees should have access only to the client's record in the nursing unit or work area

2. Confidentiality can be protected by the use of special computer access codes to limit what employees can find in computer systems

3. The use of a password or identification code is needed to enter and sign off a computer system

4. A password or identification code should never be shared with another person

5. Personal passwords should be periodically changed to prevent unauthorized computer access

E. Research: Any information provided by the client will not be reported in any manner that could identify the client and will not be made accessible to anyone outside the research team

XI. LEGAL SAFEGUARDS

A. Risk management

1. A planned method to identify, analyze, and evaluate risks, followed by a plan for reducing the frequency of accidents and injuries

2. Programs are based on a systematic reporting system for incidents or unusual occurrences

B. Incident reports (Box 7-11)

1. A tool used as a means of identifying risk situations and improving client care

2. Follow specific documentation guidelines

3. Fill out completely, accurately, and factually

4. The report form should not be copied or placed in the client's record

5. No reference should be made to the incident report form in the client's record

6. Not a substitute for a complete entry in the client's record regarding the incident

C. Safeguarding valuables

1. Client's valuables should be given to a family member or secured for safekeeping in a stored and locked designated location, such as the agency's safe, and the location of the client's valuables is documented per agency policy

2. Many health care agencies require a client to sign a release to free the agency of the responsibility for lost valuables

3. A client's wedding band can be taped in place unless there is a risk for swelling of the hand or fingers

4. Religious items, such as scapulas or religious medals, may be pinned to the client's gown if allowed by agency policy

D. Physician's orders

1. A nurse is obligated to carry out a physician's order except when the nurse believes an order to be inappropriate

2. A nurse carrying out an inaccurate order may be legally responsible for any harm suffered by the client

3. Clarify an unclear or inappropriate order, or an order in question, with the physician

4. If no resolution occurs regarding the order in question, contact the nurse manager or supervisor

5. Telephone orders: Follow agency policy (Box 7-12)

6. Medication orders (Box 7-13)

E. Documentation

1. Legally required by accrediting agencies, state licensing laws, and state nurse and medical practice acts

---

BOX 7-10

Maintaining Confidentiality

- Not discussing client issues with other clients or staff uninvolved in the client's care
- Health care information is not shared with others without the client's consent (includes family members or friends of the client)
- Keeping all information about a client private and not revealing it to someone not directly involved in care
- Client information is shared in private and secluded areas
- Protecting the medical record from all unauthorized readers

---

BOX 7-11

Incidents That Need to Be Reported

Accidental omission of ordered therapies
Circumstances that led to injury or a risk for client injury
Client falls
Medication administration errors
Needlestick injuries
Procedure-related or equipment-related accidents
A visitor having symptoms of an illness

BOX 7-12

Telephone Orders

Date and time the entry
Repeat the order to the physician and record the order
Sign the order; begin with t.o. (telephone order), write the physician's name, and then add your signature to the order
If another nurse witnessed the order, that signature follows
The physician needs to countersign the order within a time frame according to agency policy

---

BOX 7-13

Components of a Medication Order

Date and time when the order was written
Medication name
Medication dosage
Route of administration
Frequency of administration
Physician or health care provider's signature

---

2. Follow agency guidelines and procedures (Box 7-14)
F. Client/family teaching
   1. Provide complete instructions in a language that client or family can understand
   2. Document client and family teaching, what was taught, evaluation of understanding, and who was present during the teaching session
   3. Inform client of what would happen if information shared during teaching is not followed

XII. LEGAL DOCUMENTS

A. Advance directives
   1. Written document (sometimes called a living will) recognized by state **law** that provides directions concerning the provision of care when a client is unable to make his or her own treatment choices
   2. May also include naming a relative or friend (health care proxy), who will make health care decisions in the event of the client's incapacitation
B. Patient Self-Determination Act
   1. Became a law in the United States in 1990 and was implemented in all health care institutions
   2. A client must be provided with information about their rights to identify written directions about the care they wish to receive in the event that he or she becomes incapacitated and is unable to make health care decisions
   3. On admission to a health care facility, the client is asked about the existence of an **advance directive**; if one exists, it must be documented and included as part of the medical record

---

BOX 7-14

Documentation Guidelines

NARRATIVE DOCUMENTATION
Use a black-colored ink pen
Date and time entries
Provide objective, factual, and complete documentation
Document care, medications, treatments, and procedures as soon as possible after completion
Document client's responses to interventions
Document consent for or refusal of treatments
Document calls made to other health care providers
Do not document for others or change documentation for other individuals
Sign and title each entry
Use quotes as appropriate for subjective data
Use correct spelling, grammar, and punctuation
Avoid unacceptable abbreviations
Avoid judgmental or evaluative statements, such as "uncooperative client"
Do not leave blank spaces on documentation forms
Follow agency policies when an error is made (draw one line through the error, initial, and date)
Follow agency guidelines regarding late entries

COMPUTERIZED DOCUMENTATION
Use only the user identification (ID) code, name, or password
Never lend access ID to another
Maintain privacy and confidentiality of documented information printed from the computer

---

   4. If the client signs an **advance directive** at the time of admission, it must be documented in the client's medical record
C. Living will
   1. An **advance directive** document that lists the medical treatment a client chooses to omit or refuse if the client becomes unable to make decisions and is terminally ill
   2. States have their own requirements for executing living wills but, generally, two witnesses, neither of whom can be a relative or physician, are needed when the client signs the living will
D. Durable power of attorney: A legal document that appoints a person (health care proxy) chosen by the client to carry out his or her wishes as expressed in the **advance directive**, or to make decisions on their behalf if and when they can no longer do so
E. "Do Not Resuscitate" (DNR) orders
   1. Orders written by a physician when a client has indicated a desire to be allowed to die if he or she stops breathing or his or her heart stops beating
   2. The client or his or her legal representative must provide **informed consent** for the DNR status
   3. The DNR order must be clearly defined so that other treatment, not refused by the client, will be continued

4. The DNR order must be reviewed on a regular basis according to agency policy (usually every 3 days for hospitalized clients and every 60 days for clients in residential health care facilities)

5. All health care personnel must know if a client has a DNR order

6. A nurse who attempts to resuscitate a client who has a DNR order would be acting without the client's consent and committing battery

7. Specific agency guidelines must be followed regarding when and under what circumstances a verbal DNR order is acceptable

F. The nurse's role

1. Discussing advance directives with the client opens the communication channel to establish what is important to the client and what he or she may view as promoting life versus prolonging dying

2. The nurse needs to ensure that the client was provided with information about his or her right to identify written directions about the care they wish to receive

3. On admission to a health care facility, the nurse determines if an advance directive exists and ensures that it is part of the medical record

4. The nurse ensures that the physician was notified of the presence of an **advance directive**

5. All health care workers need to follow the directions of an **advance directive** to be immune from liability

6. Some agencies have specific policies that prohibit a nurse from signing as a witness to a legal document, such as a living will

7. If a nurse witnesses a legal document, he or she must document the event and the factual circumstances surrounding the signing in the medical record

8. Documentation as a witness should include who was present, any significant comments by the client, and the nurse's observations of the client's conduct during this process

XIII. REPORTING RESPONSIBILITIES

A. Requirements: Nurses are required to report certain communicable diseases or criminal activities, such as abuse, gunshot or stab wounds, assaults, homicides, and suicides, to the appropriate authorities

B. The impaired nurse

1. If a nurse suspects that a coworker is abusing chemicals, the nurse must report the individual to the nursing administration in a confidential manner, with the goal of treatment being the priority issue

2. Nursing administration then notifies the board of nursing regarding the nurse's behavior

C. Occupational Safety and Health Act (OSHA)

1. Requires that an employer provide a safe workplace for employees, according to regulations

2. Employees can confidentially report working conditions that violate regulations

3. An employee who does not report unsafe working conditions can be retaliated against by the employer

D. Sexual harassment

1. Prohibited by state and federal laws

2. Includes unwelcome conduct of a sexual nature

3. Follow agency policies and procedures to handle reporting a concern or complaint

PRACTICE QUESTIONS

1. A nurse enters a client's room and finds the client lying on the floor. The nurse checks the client and then calls the nursing supervisor and the physician to inform them of the occurrence. The nursing supervisor instructs the nurse to complete an incident report. The nurse completes the incident report, understanding that it allows the analysis of adverse client events through:

1. A method of promoting quality care and risk management

2. Determining the effectiveness of interventions in relation to outcomes

3. The appropriate method of reporting to local, state, and federal agencies

4. Providing clients with necessary stabilizing treatments

2. A nurse observes that a client received pain medication 1 hour ago from another nurse but that the client still has severe pain. The nurse has previously observed this same occurrence. Based on the nurse practice act, the observing nurse plans to do which of the following?

1. Talk with the nurse who gave the medication

2. Report the information to a nursing supervisor

3. Call the Impaired Nurse Organization

4. Report the information to the police

3. A client has died, and a nurse asks a family member about the funeral arrangements. The family member refuses to discuss the issue. The nurse's most appropriate action is to:

1. Provide information needed for decision making

2. Suggest a referral to a mental health professional

3. Show acceptance of feelings

4. Remain with the family member without discussing funeral arrangements

4. A client arrives in the emergency room and is staggering, confused, and verbally abusive. The client complains of a headache from drinking alcohol and is asking for medication. The nurse explains to the client that the physician will need to perform an assessment before the administration of medication. When the client becomes verbally abusive, the nurse threatens to place the client in restraints. With which of the following can the client legally charge the nurse as a result of the nursing action?

1. Assault

2. Battery

3. Negligence

4. Invasion of privacy

5. A nurse lawyer provides an education session to the nursing staff regarding client rights. A nurse asks the lawyer to describe an example that might relate to invasion of client privacy. A nursing action that indicates a violation of this right is:

   1. Taking photographs of the client without consent

   2. Telling the client that he or she cannot leave the hospital

   3. Threatening to place a client in restraints

   4. Performing a surgical procedure without consent

6. A nurse calls the physician of a client scheduled for a cardiac catheterization because the client has numerous questions regarding the procedure and has requested to speak to the physician. The physician is very upset and arrives at the unit to visit the client after prompting by the nurse. The nurse is outside the client's room and hears the physician tell the client in a derogatory manner that the nurse "doesn't know anything." The nurse plans to address the physician's remark, understanding that the physician has violated which legal tort?

   1. Libel

   2. Slander

   3. Assault

   4. Negligence

7. A nurse employed in a long-term care facility calls the physician regarding a new medication order because the dose prescribed is higher than the recommended dosage. The nurse is unable to locate the physician, and the medication is due to be administered. Which of the following actions does the nurse take?

   1. Holds the medication until the physician can be contacted

   2. Administer the dose prescribed

   3. Administers the recommended dose until the physician can be located

   4. Contacts the nursing supervisor

8. A nurse enters a client's room and finds the client sitting on the floor. The nurse checks the client thoroughly and then assists the client back to bed. The nurse completes an incident report and notifies the nursing supervisor and physician of the incident. Which of the following is the next nursing action regarding the incident?

   1. Make a copy of the incident report for the physician

   2. Place the incident report in the client's chart

   3. Document a complete entry in the client's record concerning the incident

   4. Document in the client's record that an incident report has been completed

9. A nursing graduate who recently passed NCLEX-PN is employed as a licensed practical nurse (LPN) in a local hospital. During orientation, the nurse educator asks the LPN about his or her understanding of the need to obtain professional liability insurance. The appropriate response by the LPN is:

   1. "The hospitals liability insurance will cover my actions."

   2. "It is very expensive and not necessary."

   3. "Nurses are encouraged to have their own malpractice insurance."

   4. "The majority of suits are filed against physicians and the hospital."

10. A nurse witnesses an automobile accident and provides care at the scene of the accident to an open wound on a young child. The family is extremely grateful and insists that the nurse accept monetary compensation for the care provided to the child. Because of the family's insistence, the nurse accepts the compensation to avoid offending the family. The child develops an infection and sepsis and is hospitalized. The family files suit against the nurse who provided care to the child at the scene of the accident. The nurse understands that which of the following is accurate regarding immunity from this suit?

    1. The Good Samaritan law will protect the nurse

    2. The Good Samaritan law will protect the nurse if the care given at the scene was not negligent

    3. The Good Samaritan law will not provide immunity from suit if the nurse accepted compensation for the care provided

    4. The Good Samaritan law protects laypersons and not professional health care providers

11. A client is brought to the emergency room after a serious accident, is unconscious, and is bleeding profusely. Surgery is required immediately to save the client's life. In regard to informed consent for the surgical procedure, which of the following is the best action?

    1. Try calling the client's spouse to obtain telephone consent before the surgical procedure

    2. Transport the client to the operating room immediately, as required by the physician, without obtaining an informed consent

    3. Ask the friend who accompanied the client to the emergency room to sign the consent form

    4. Call the nursing supervisor to initiate a court order for the surgical procedure

12. A nurse arrives at work and is told to report (float) to the pediatric unit for the day because the unit is understaffed and needs additional nurses to care for the children. The nurse has never worked in the pediatric unit. Which of the following is the appropriate nursing action?

    1. Refuse to float to the pediatric unit

    2. Call the hospital lawyer

3. Call the nursing supervisor
4. Report to the pediatric unit and identify tasks that can be safely performed

13. A nurse enters a client's room and notes that the client's lawyer is present and that the client is preparing a living will. The living will requires that the client's signature be witnessed, and the client asks the nurse to witness the signature. Which of the following is the appropriate nursing action?
    1. Sign the will as a witness to signature only
    2. Sign the will clearly identifying credentials and employment agency
    3. Decline from signing the will
    4. Call the hospital lawyer before signing the will

14. An older woman is brought to the emergency room. When caring for the client, the nurse notes old and new ecchymotic areas on both arms and buttocks. The nurse asks the client how the bruises were sustained. The client, although reluctant, tells the nurse in confidence that her daughter frequently hits her if she gets in the way. Which of the following is the appropriate nursing response?
    1. "I promise I will not tell anyone but let's see what we can do about this."
    2. "I have a legal obligation to report this type of abuse."
    3. "Let's talk about ways that will prevent your daughter from hitting you."
    4. "This should not be happening, and if it happens again you must call the emergency room."

15. A client tells the nurse of his decision to refuse external cardiac massage. Which of the following would be the appropriate initial nursing action?
    1. Notify the physician of the client's request
    2. Document the client's request in the client's record
    3. Conduct a client conference to share the client's request
    4. Discuss the client's request with the family

ALTERNATE FORMAT QUESTION: MULTIPLE RESPONSE

Select all correct guidelines related to narrative documentation.
_____ Use a blue-colored ink pen
_____ Date and time entries
_____ Document judgmental information completely
_____ Sign and title each entry
_____ Do not leave blank spaces on documentation forms
_____ Avoid judgmental and evaluative statements

ANSWERS

1. *Answer:* **1**
Rationale: Proper documentation of unusual occurrences, incidents, and accidents, and the nursing actions taken as a result of the occurrence, are internal to the institution or agency. Documentation on the incident report allows the nurse and administration to review the quality of care and determine any potential risks present. Options 2, 3, and 4 are incorrect.
Test-Taking Strategy: Use the process of elimination. Eliminate options 2 and 4 because incident reports are not routinely filled out for interventions or treatment measures. Eliminate option 3 because incident reports are not used to report occurrences to other agencies. Medical records are used for this purpose. Review the purpose of incident reports if you had difficulty with this question.
Level of Cognitive Ability: Application
Client Needs: Safe, Effective Care Environment
Integrated Process: Nursing Process/Implementation
Content Area: Fundamental Skills
Reference: Potter, P., & Perry, A. (2005). *Fundamentals of nursing* (6th ed.). St. Louis: Mosby, pp. 419, 497.

2. *Answer:* **2**
Rationale: Nurse practice acts require reporting the suspicion of impaired nurses. The Board of Nursing has jurisdiction over the practice of nursing and may develop plans for treatment and supervision. This suspicion needs to be reported to the nursing supervisor, who will then report to the Board of Nursing. Option 1 may cause a conflict. Options 3 and 4 are inappropriate.
Test-Taking Strategy: Use the principles related to following the channels of communication in a health care agency when answering this question. By reporting the information, the nurse alerts the institution to the potential problem and sets the stage for further investigation and appropriate action. Review the actions to take regarding reporting the suspicion of an impaired nurse if you had difficulty with this question.
Level of Cognitive Ability: Application
Client Needs: Safe, Effective Care Environment
Integrated Process: Nursing Process/Planning
Content Area: Fundamental Skills
Reference: Potter, P., & Perry, A. (2005). *Fundamentals of nursing* (6th ed.). St. Louis: Mosby, p. 407.

3. *Answer:* **4**
Rationale: The family member is exhibiting the first stage of grief–denial and the nurse should remain with the family member. Option 1 may be an appropriate intervention for the bargaining stage. Option 2 may be an appropriate intervention for depression. Option 3 is an appropriate intervention for the acceptance or reorganization and restitution stage.
Test-Taking Strategy: Use therapeutic communication techniques to direct you to option 4. Remember to address client and family feelings first. Review the grieving process and therapeutic communication techniques if you had difficulty with this question.

Level of Cognitive Ability: Application
Client Needs: Psychosocial Integrity
Integrated Process: Caring
Content Area: Fundamental Skills
Reference: Potter, P., & Perry, A. (2005). *Fundamentals of nursing* (6th ed.). St. Louis: Mosby, pp. 570-571.

4. *Answer:* **1**
Rationale: An assault occurs when a person puts another person in fear of a harmful or offensive contact. For this intentional tort to be actionable, the victim must be aware of the threat of harmful or offensive contact. Battery is the actual contact with one's body. Negligence involves actions below the standards of care. Invasion of privacy occurs when the individual's private affairs are unreasonably intruded into.
Test-Taking Strategy: Use the process of elimination. Note the key word, *threatens*, in the question. This will direct you to option 1. Review the descriptions associated with each term in the options if you had difficulty with this question.
Level of Cognitive Ability: Comprehension
Client Needs: Safe, Effective Care Environment
Integrated Process: Nursing Process/Implementation
Content Area: Fundamental Skills
Reference: Potter, P., & Perry, A. (2005), *Fundamentals of nursing* (6th ed.). St. Louis: Mosby, p. 413.

5. *Answer:* **1**
Rationale: Invasion of privacy takes place when an individual's private affairs are intruded on unreasonably. Not allowing a client to leave the hospital constitutes false imprisonment. Threatening to place a client in restraints constitutes assault. Performing a surgical procedure without consent is an example of battery.
Test-Taking Strategy: Use the process of elimination. Note the key words, *invasion of client privacy*. These words should direct you to option 1. Review those situations that include invasion of client privacy if you had difficulty with this question.
Level of Cognitive Ability: Comprehension
Client Needs: Safe, Effective Care Environment
Integrated Process: Nursing Process/Implementation
Content Area: Fundamental Skills
Reference: Potter, P., & Perry, A. (2005). *Fundamentals of nursing* (6th ed.). St. Louis: Mosby, p. 413.

6. *Answer:* **2**
Rationale: Defamation is a false communication or careless disregard for the truth that causes damage to someone's reputation, either in writing (libel) or verbally (slander). An assault occurs when a person puts another person in fear of a harmful or an offensive contact. Negligence involves the actions of professionals that fall below the standard of care for a specific professional group.
Test-Taking Strategy: Use the process of elimination and focus on the information in the question. You can easily eliminate options 3 and 4, first recalling the definitions of these terms. From the remaining options, recalling that slander constitutes verbal defamation will direct you to option 2. Review the torts identified in the options if you had difficulty with this question.
Level of Cognitive Ability: Application
Client Needs: Safe, Effective Care Environment

Integrated Process: Nursing Process/Planning
Content Area: Fundamental Skills
Reference: Potter, P., & Perry, A. (2005). *Fundamentals of nursing* (6th ed.). St. Louis: Mosby, p. 414.

7. *Answer:* **4**
Rationale: If the physician writes an order that requires clarification, it is the nurse's responsibility to contact the physician for clarification. If there is no resolution regarding the order, because the physician cannot be located, or because the order remains as it was written after talking with the physician, the nurse should then contact the nurse manager or supervisor for further clarification as to what the next step should be. Under no circumstances should the nurse proceed to carry out the order until clarification has been obtained.
Test-Taking Strategy: Use the process of elimination. Eliminate options 2 and 3 first because they are similar and are unsafe actions. Holding the medication can result in client injury. The nurse needs to take action. Option 4 clearly identifies the required action in this situation. Review nursing responsibilities related to the physician's orders if you had difficulty with this question.
Level of Cognitive Ability: Application
Client Needs: Safe, Effective Care Environment
Integrated Process: Nursing Process/Implementation
Content Area: Fundamental Skills
Reference: Potter, P., & Perry, A. (2005). *Fundamentals of nursing* (6th ed.). St. Louis: Mosby, p. 419.

8. *Answer:* **3**
Rationale: The incident report is confidential and privileged information and should not be copied, placed in the chart, or have any reference made to it in the client's record. The incident report is not a substitute for a complete entry in the client's record concerning the incident.
Test-Taking Strategy: Use the process of elimination. Eliminate options 2 and 4 first because they are similar. Recalling that incident reports should not be copied will direct you to option 3. Review nursing responsibilities related to incident reports if you had difficulty with this question.
Level of Cognitive Ability: Application
Client Needs: Safe, Effective Care Environment
Integrated Process: Nursing Process/Implementation
Content Area: Fundamental Skills
Reference: Potter, P., & Perry, A. (2005). *Fundamentals of nursing* (6th ed.). St. Louis: Mosby, p. 497.

9. *Answer:* **3**
Rationale: Nurses need their own liability insurance for protection against malpractice lawsuits. Nurses erroneously assume that they are protected by an agency's professional liability policies. Usually, when a nurse is sued, the employer is also sued for the nurse's actions or inactions. Even though this is the norm, nurses are encouraged to have their own malpractice insurance.
Test-Taking Strategy: Note that the issue of the question relates to "professional liability insurance." Focusing on this issue should direct you to option 3. Review liability related to malpractice insurance if you had difficulty with this question.
Level of Cognitive Ability: Comprehension

Client Needs: Safe, Effective Care Environment
Integrated Process: Nursing Process/Implementation
Content Area: Fundamental Skills
Reference: Potter, P., & Perry, A. (2005). *Fundamentals of nursing* (6th ed.). St. Louis: Mosby, pp. 411-412.

10. *Answer:* **3**
Rationale: A Good Samaritan law is passed by a state legislature to encourage nurses and other health care providers to provide care to a person when an accident, emergency, or injury occurs, without fear of being sued for the care provided. Called immunity from suit, this protection usually applies only if all the conditions of the law are met; for example, the health care provider receives no compensation for the care provided, and the care given is not willfully or wantonly negligent.
Test-Taking Strategy: Read the question carefully and note the key words, *accepts monetary compensation.* This will direct you to option 3. Additionally, options 1, 2, and 4 are similar. Review the Good Samaritan law if you had difficulty with this question.
Level of Cognitive Ability: Comprehension
Client Needs: Safe, Effective Care Environment
Integrated Process: Nursing Process/Implementation
Content Area: Fundamental Skills
Reference: Potter, P., & Perry, A. (2005). *Fundamentals of nursing* (6th ed.). St. Louis: Mosby, pp. 411-412.

11. *Answer:* **2**
Rationale: Generally, there are only two instances in which the informed consent of an adult client is not needed. One instance is when an emergency is present and delaying treatment for the purpose of obtaining informed consent would result in injury or death to the client. The second instance is when the client waives the right to give informed consent. Options 1, 3, and 4 are inappropriate.
Test-Taking Strategy: Use the process of elimination. Option 3 can be easily eliminated first. Note the key words, *surgery is required immediately.* Options 1 and 4 would delay treatment and should be eliminated. Review the issues surrounding informed consent if you had difficulty with this question.
Level of Cognitive Ability: Application
Client Needs: Safe, Effective Care Environment
Integrated Process: Nursing Process/Implementation
Content Area: Fundamental Skills
References: Brent, N. (2001). *Nurses and the law* (2nd ed.). Philadelphia: W.B. Saunders, p. 210.
Potter, P., & Perry, A. (2005). *Fundamentals of nursing* (6th ed.). St. Louis: Mosby, p. 416.

12. *Answer:* **4**
Rationale: Floating is an acceptable legal practice used by hospitals to solve their understaffing problems. Legally, a nurse cannot refuse to float unless a union contract guarantees that the nurse can only work in a specified area or the nurse can prove the lack of knowledge for the performance of assigned tasks. When encountered with this situation, the nurse should identify potential areas of harm to the client.
Test-Taking Strategy: Use the process of elimination. Options 1 and 2 can be eliminated first because they are inappropriate. From the remaining options, eliminate option 3 because it is premature to call the nursing supervisor. Review nursing responsibilities related to floating if you had difficulty with this question.
Level of Cognitive Ability: Application
Client Needs: Safe, Effective Care Environment
Integrated Process: Nursing Process/Implementation
Content Area: Fundamental Skills
Reference: Potter, P., & Perry, A. (2005). *Fundamentals of nursing* (6th ed.). St. Louis: Mosby, pp. 418-419.

13. *Answer:* **3**
Rationale: Living wills are required to be in writing and signed by the client. The client's signature either must be witnessed by specified individuals or notarized. Many states prohibit any employee, including a nurse in a facility where the client is receiving care, from being a witness.
Test-Taking Strategy: Use the process of elimination. Options 1 and 2 are similar and should be eliminated first. From the remaining options, option 3 is the appropriate action. Review legal implications associated with wills if you had difficulty with this question.
Level of Cognitive Ability: Application
Client Needs: Safe, Effective Care Environment
Integrated Process: Nursing Process/Implementation
Content Area: Fundamental Skills
Reference: Brent, N. (2001). *Nurses and the law* (2nd ed.). Philadelphia: W.B. Saunders, p. 217.

14. *Answer:* **2**
Rationale: Confidential issues are not to be discussed with nonmedical personnel or with the person's family or friends without the client's permission. Clients should be assured that information is kept confidential, unless it places the nurse under a legal obligation. The nurse must report situations related to child or elderly abuse, gunshot wounds, stabbings, and certain infectious diseases.
Test-Taking Strategy: Use the process of elimination. Option 4 can be eliminated first because this action does not protect the client from injury. Options 1 and 3 are similar and should be eliminated next. Review the nursing responsibilities related to reporting obligations if you had difficulty with this question.
Level of Cognitive Ability: Application
Client Needs: Psychosocial Integrity
Integrated Process: Communication and Documentation
Content Area: Fundamental Skills
References: Brent, N. (2001). *Nurses and the law* (2nd ed.). Philadelphia: W.B. Saunders, p. 288.
Potter, P., & Perry, A. (2005). *Fundamentals of nursing* (6th ed.). St. Louis: Mosby, p. 433.

15. *Answer:* **1**
Rationale: External cardiac massage is one type of treatment that a client can refuse. The appropriate initial action is to notify the physician because a written "Do Not Resuscitate" (DNR) order from the physician must be present. The DNR order must be reviewed or renewed on a regular basis per agency policy.
Test-Taking Strategy: Use the process of elimination. Note the key words, *appropriate initial action.* Although options 2, 3, and 4 may be appropriate, remember that first a written

physician's order is necessary. Review DNR procedures if you had difficulty with this question.

Level of Cognitive Ability: Application
Client Needs: Safe, Effective Care Environment
Integrated Process: Nursing Process/Implementation
Content Area: Fundamental Skills
References: Brent, N. (2001). *Nurses and the law* (2nd ed.). Philadelphia: W.B. Saunders, p. 257.
Potter, P., & Perry, A. (2005). *Fundamentals of nursing* (6th ed.). St. Louis: Mosby, p. 410.

ALTERNATE FORMAT QUESTION: MULTIPLE RESPONSE

Answers:
Date and time entries
Sign and title each entry
Do not leave blank spaces on documentation forms
Avoid judgmental and evaluative statements
Rationale: The nurse uses a black-colored ink pen to document because black ink allows the chart to be duplicated with adequate readability for long-term storage. The nurse always dates and times entries and signs and titles each entry. The nurse provides objective, factual, and complete documentation and avoids subjective, judgmental, and evaluative statements. Quotes are used to relate what the client actually said. The nurse avoids leaving blank spaces on documentation forms, because this allows for an area in which notes can be entered by others at a later time. Recording of information on the client's record must be sequential.

Test-Taking Strategy: Read each item carefully. Think about the legal responsibilities related to documentation to select the correct guidelines. Review these guidelines if you had difficulty with this question.

Level of Cognitive Ability: Application
Client Needs: Safe, Effective Care Environment
Integrated Process: Communication and Documentation
Content Area: Fundamental Skills
Reference: Harkreader, H., & Hogan, M.A. (2004). *Fundamentals of nursing: Caring and clinical judgment* (2nd ed.). Philadelphia: W.B. Saunders. pp. 219-221.

REFERENCES

Brent, N. (2001). *Nurses and the law* (2nd ed.). Philadelphia: W.B. Saunders.

Christensen, B., & Kockrow, E. (2003). *Foundations of nursing* (4th ed.). St. Louis: Mosby.

Combined Life Insurance of New York. (2003). *HIPAA notice of privacy practices for personal health information.* Retrieved January 2004 from http://www. keio.edu/parents/hippa.html.

Harkreader, H., & Hogan, M.A. (2004). *Fundamentals of nursing: Caring and clinical judgment* (2nd ed.). Philadelphia: W.B. Saunders.

National Council of State Boards of Nursing. (2005). *Detailed test plan for the National Council licensure examination for practical/vocational nurses.* Chicago: Author.

Potter, P., & Perry, A. (2005). *Fundamentals of nursing* (6th ed.). St. Louis: Mosby.

Stuart, G., & Laraia, M. (2005). *Principles and practice of psychiatric nursing* (8th ed.). St. Louis: Mosby.

Delegating, Managing, and Prioritizing Client Care

PYRAMID TERMS

accountability A moral concept that involves acceptance by the professional nurse of the consequences of a decision or action.

case management Represents an interdisciplinary health care delivery system designed to promote appropriate use of hospital personnel and material resources to maximize hospital revenues while providing for optimal outcome of care.

critical paths Provide effective clinical management systems for monitoring care and for reducing or controlling the length of hospital stay.

delegation Process of transferring a selected nursing task in a situation to an individual who is competent to perform that specific task.

empowerment An interpersonal process of enabling others to do for themselves.

leadership An interpersonal process that involves motivating and guiding others to achieve goals.

management The accomplishment of tasks either by one's self or by directing others.

prioritizing Deciding which needs or problems require immediate action and which could be delayed until a later time because they are not urgent.

responsibility The duty to act.

variances Actual deviations or detours from the critical paths.

▲ PYRAMID TO SUCCESS

The nurse is both a leader and a manager. As described in the NCLEX-PN test plan, the nurse needs to collaborate with other members of the multidisciplinary health care team to facilitate effective care. Pyramid points focus on the concepts of management and supervision, leadership responsibilities, case management, resource management, making client care assignments, the process of delegation, establishing priorities among a group of clients, and the principles of time management. The Integrated Processes addressed in this chapter include Caring, Clinical Problem-Solving Process (Nursing Process), Communication and Documentation, and Teaching/Learning.

CLIENT NEEDS
Safe, Effective Care Environment

Client care assignments
Concepts of management and supervision
Cost-effective measures when providing nursing care
Consultation with members of the health care team
Delegation of client care
Establishing priorities of care
Identifying practice limitations
Performance improvement (quality assurance)
Resource management
Supervising the delivery of client care
Variance reports

Health Promotion and Maintenance

Client's ability to perform self-care
Disease prevention
Family systems
Health and wellness
Health screening
Health promotion programs

Psychosocial Integrity

Cultural, spiritual, and religious issues
Support systems
Therapeutic interactions

Physiological Integrity

Ensuring that palliative/comfort care is provided to the client

Potential for alterations in body systems
Unexpected responses to therapy

I. HEALTH CARE DELIVERY

A. Managed care
1. Designed to control the cost of health services and promote a continuum of care through the development and use of integrated services
2. Uses a select group of providers who agree to a predetermined payment before delivering care
3. Client care is outcome driven and is managed by a **case management** process
4. Emphasizes the promotion of health, client education and responsible self-care, early identification of disease, and the use of health care resources

B. **Case management**
1. An organized system for delivering health care to an individual client or a group of clients through their illness
2. Includes assessment and development of a plan of care, coordination of all services, referral, and follow-up

C. Case manager
1. A registered nurse who assumes responsibility for coordinating the client's care from the time of admission and following discharge
2. Establishes a plan of care with the client, coordinates any consultations and referrals, and facilitates discharge

D. **Critical paths**
1. A multidisciplinary treatment plan that identifies the clinical interventions over a projected length of stay or a projected time frame for specific case types
2. All members of the health care team work with one plan to achieve the same client outcomes
3. The goal of a **critical paths** to anticipate and recognize negative **variance** early so that appropriate action can be taken and better client outcomes can result
4. **Variances**
   a. Actual deviations or detours from the **critical path**
   b. Positive **variance** occurs when a client achieves maximum benefit and is discharged earlier than anticipated on his or her **critical path**
   c. Negative **variance** occurs when untoward events prevent a timely discharge and the length of hospital stay is longer than planned for a client on a specific **critical path**
   d. **Variance** analysis occurs continually as the case manager and other caregivers monitor client outcomes against the **critical path**
   e. Accurate monitoring of **critical path** with variance analysis can estimate the financial impact of client care
   f. If the variance is predictable, negotiation with insurers for an additional length of hospital stay can maximize client care revenues

E. Care maps
1. Initially developed at the New England Medical Center in Boston
2. A model for a **critical path**
3. Incorporates day-to-day expected client outcomes and those outcomes anticipated at discharge or at the end of a treatment phase
4. Outlines clinical assessments, treatments and procedures, dietary interventions, activity and exercise therapies, client education, discharge planning

F. Nursing care plan
1. A written guideline and communication tool that identifies the client's pertinent assessment data, problems and nursing diagnoses, goals, interventions, and expected outcomes
2. Enhances continuity of care by identifying specific nursing actions necessary to achieve the goals of care
3. The client and family are involved in developing the plan of care, and both short-term and long-term goals are identified
4. Client problems, goals, interventions, and expected outcomes are documented in the care plan, and the plan provides a framework for evaluation of the client's response to nursing actions

II. FORMAL ORGANIZATIONS

A. Mission statement: Communicates in broad terms an organization's reason for existence, the geographic area the organization serves, and attitudes, beliefs, and values within which the organization functions
B. Goals and objectives: Measurable activities specific to the development of designated services and programs of an organization
C. Organizational chart: Depicts and communicates how activities are arranged, how authority relationships are defined, and how communication channels are established
D. Procedures and protocols
1. Guides that define appropriate courses of action
2. Procedure defines a task
3. Protocol signifies the definition of a clinical process
E. Centralization: When decisions are made by a limited number of individuals at the top of the organization, or by managers of a department or unit, and thereafter communicated to the employees
F. Decentralization: Authority is distributed throughout the organization to allow for increased **responsibility** and **delegation** in decision making

III. CONTINUOUS (TOTAL) QUALITY IMPROVEMENT

A. A program that focuses on processes or systems that significantly contribute to effective client care outcomes

B. When total quality improvement is part of a health care agency's philosophy, every staff member becomes involved in ways to improve care and outcomes

C. Quality of a health care organization is defined in its mission statement and in the philosophy of the nursing department; these statements identify how nurses are to perform, identify the services that are made available to the client, and provide directions for professional standards and care guidelines that should guarantee excellent client outcomes

D. The Joint Commission on Accreditation of Healthcare Organizations (JCAHO) describes quality improvement as an approach to the continuous assessment and improvement of the methods of providing health care to meet the needs of others

E. The quality improvement process is similar to the nursing process and involves a multidisciplinary process

F. An outcome indicates whether the interventions are effective, if the client progressed, how well standards are met, and if changes are necessary

G. The evaluation of health care is a process used to determine the quality of care and service provided to clients

H. The nurse has the responsibility to recognize trends in nursing practice, identify when recurrent problems occur, and initiate opportunities to improve the quality of care

IV. NURSING DELIVERY SYSTEMS

A. Functional nursing
1. Involves a task approach to client care, with major tasks being delegated by the charge nurse to individual members of the team
2. Goals are concerned with work productivity at the lowest possible cost
3. Tasks are generally assigned to the lowest skilled paid workers available to do the work

B. Team nursing
1. The team is generally led by a registered nurse who is responsible for assessing, developing nursing diagnoses, planning, and evaluating each client's plan of care
2. Each staff member works fully within the realm of his or her educational and clinical expertise
3. Each staff member is **accountable** for client care and outcomes of care delivered in accordance with the licensing and practice scope as determined by hospital policy and state law

4. Characterized by a high degree of respect for and maturity of team members, and by a high degree of communication and collaboration among members

C. Primary nursing
1. Focuses on client outcomes as opposed to nursing tasks
2. Concerned with keeping the nurse at the bedside, actively involved in client care, while planning goal-directed, individualized care

V. PROFESSIONAL RESPONSIBILITIES

A. **Accountability**
1. The process that mandates that individuals are answerable for their actions and have an obligation (or duty) to act
2. Involves assuming only the responsibilities that are within one's scope of practice and not assuming **responsibility** for activities in which competence has not been achieved
3. Involves admitting mistakes rather than blaming others, and evaluating the outcomes of one's own actions
4. Includes a **responsibility** to the client to be competent, to render nursing services in accordance with standards of nursing practice, and to adhere to the professional ethics code

B. **Leadership**
1. The interpersonal process that involves motivating and guiding others to achieve goals
2. A method of modeling accountable behavior to others

C. **Leadership** styles
1. Autocratic
   a. Leader focused
   b. Leader maintains strong control, makes the decisions, and solves all problems
   c. Leader dominates the group and commands rather than makes suggestions or seeks input
2. Democratic
   a. Also called participative **leadership**
   b. Based on the belief that every group member should have input into the development of goals and problem solving
   c. Leader acts primarily as a facilitator and a resource person
   d. Leader is concerned for each member of the group
   e. A more participative style and much less authoritarian than the autocratic **leadership** style
3. Laissez-faire
   a. Leader assumes a passive, nondirective, and inactive approach
   b. **Leadership** responsibilities are either assumed by the members of the group or completely relinquished

c. All decision making is left to the group, with the leader giving little if any guidance, support, or feedback

d. Behavior by the group may be permissible as a result of the leader's lack of limit setting and stated expectations

4. Situational

a. Using a combination of styles based on current circumstances and events

b. Leadership styles are assumed according to the needs of the group and the tasks to be achieved

D. **Leadership** qualities (Box 8-1)

E. **Management:** The accomplishment of tasks either by oneself or by directing others

F. Problem-solving process

1. Involves obtaining information and using it to reach an acceptable solution to a problem

2. Steps of the problem solving process are similar to the steps of the clinical problem-solving process (nursing process) (Table 8-1)

VI. EMPOWERMENT

A. An interpersonal process of enabling others to do for themselves

B. Occurs when individuals are better able to influence what happens to them

C. Involves open communication, mutual goal setting, and decision making

D. Nurses can **empower** clients through advocacy

VII. CONFLICT

A. Description: Arises from a perception of incompatibility or difference in beliefs, attitudes, values, goals, priorities, or decisions

B. Types of conflict

1. Intrapersonal: Occurs within a person

2. Interpersonal: Occurs between and among clients, nurses, and other staff members

3. Organizational: Occurs when an employee confronts policies and procedures of the organization

C. Modes of conflict resolution

1. Avoiding

a. Is unassertive and uncooperative

b. The individual neither pursues his or her needs, goals, or concerns nor assists others to pursue theirs

c. Postpones the issue

2. Accommodating

a. The individual neglects his or her own needs, goals, or concerns (unassertive) while trying to satisfy those of others

b. The individual obeys and serves others and often feels resentment and disappointment, because he or she "gets nothing in return"

3. Competing

a. The individual pursues his or her own needs and goals at the expense of others

b. May also take the form of standing up for rights and defending important principles

4. Compromising

a. Is assertive and cooperative

b. Individuals work creatively and openly to find the solution that most fully satisfies all important goals and concerns to be achieved

VIII. ROLES OF HEALTH TEAM MEMBERS

A. Nurse

1. Promotes health and disease prevention

2. Provides comfort and care to clients

3. Makes decisions

4. Acts as a client advocate

5. Manages client care

6. Communicator

7. Teaches clients and others

8. Acts as a resource person

9. Allocates resources in a cost-effective manner

B. Physician: Diagnoses and treats disease

C. Physician assistant

1. Provides assistance to the physician

2. Conducts physical examinations, performs diagnostic procedures, assists in the operating room and emergency room, performs treatments

D. Physical therapist: Assists in examining, testing, and treating the physically disabled

---

BOX 8-1

Leadership Qualities

Communication
Credibility
Critical thinking
Initiating action
Risk taking

TABLE 8-1

Problem-Solving Processes

Problem-Solving Process	Clinical Problem-Solving Process (Nursing Process)
Identifying a problem and collecting data about the problem	Data collection
Determining a plan of action	Planning
Carrying out the plan	Implementation
Evaluating the plan	Evaluation

E. Occupational therapist: Develops adaptive devices that help chronically ill or handicapped clients perform activities of daily living

F. Respiratory therapist: Delivers treatments designed to improve the client's ventilation and oxygenation status

G. Nutritionist: Assists in planning dietary measures to improve or maintain a client's nutritional status

H. Continuing care nurse: Coordinates discharge plans for the client

I. Assistive personnel/nursing assistant: Provides assistance to the nurse with specified tasks and functions

J. Pharmacist: Formulates and dispenses medications

K. Social worker: Counsels clients and families

L. Pastoral care provider: Offers spiritual support and guidance to clients and families

M. Secretarial staff: Provides support to the health care team, organizes and schedules diagnostic tests and procedures, and arranges for services needed by the client and family

IX. HEALTH CARE TEAM COMMUNICATION

A. Client care planning can be accomplished through referral to or consultation with other health care specialists and through client care conferences, which involve members from all health care disciplines

B. Reports
   1. Should be factual, accurate, current, complete, and organized
   2. Should include essential background information, subjective data, objective data, any changes in the client's status, nursing diagnoses, treatments and procedures, medication administration, client teaching, discharge planning, family information, the client's response to treatments and procedures, and the client's priority needs
   3. Change of shift report
      a. Provides continuity of care among nurses who are caring for a client
      b. May be given orally, by audiotape, or by walking rounds at the client's bedside
      c. Describes the client's health status and informs the nurse on the next shift about the client's needs and priorities for care
   4. Telephone reports
      a. Purposes
         (1) To inform a physician of a client's change in status
         (2) To communicate information about a client's transfer to or from another unit or facility
         (3) To obtain results of laboratory or diagnostic tests
      b. The telephone report should be documented and should include when the call was made,

who made the call, who was called, to whom information was given, what information was given, and what information was received
   5. Transfer reports
      a. To provide continuity of care; may be given by phone or in person (Box 8-2)
      b. The receiving nurse needs to be provided an opportunity to ask questions about the client's status

BOX 8-2

Transfer Reports

Client's name, age, physician, and diagnosis
Current health status and current plan of care
Client's needs and priorities for care
Any data collection or interventions that need to be done after transfer, such as laboratory tests, medication administration, or dressing changes
Need for any special equipment
Any additional considerations, such as resuscitation status, precautionary considerations, or family issues

X. CONSULTING WITH THE HEALTH CARE TEAM

A. Process in which a specialist is sought to identify methods of care or treatment plans to meet the needs of a client

B. Consultation is needed when the nurse encounters a problem that cannot be solved using nursing knowledge, skills, and available resources

C. Consultation is also needed when the exact problem remains unclear; a consultant can objectively and more clearly assess and identify the exact nature of the problem

XI. DISCHARGE PLANNING

A. Begins when the client is admitted to the hospital or health care facility

B. Is a multidisciplinary process that ensures that the client has a plan for continuing care after leaving the health care facility and assists in the client's transition from one environment to another

C. All caregivers need to be involved in discharge planning, and referrals to other health care professionals or agencies may be needed; a physician's order may be needed for the referral and the referral needs to be approved by the client's insurer

D. The nurse should anticipate the client's discharge needs and suggest making the referral as soon as possible (involve the client and family in the referral process)

E. The nurse needs to reinforce client and family teaching regarding care at home (Box 8-3)

BOX 8-3

Discharge Teaching

How to administer prescribed medications
Side effects of medications that need to be reported to the physician
Prescribed dietary and activity measures
Complications of the medical condition that need to be reported to the physician
How to perform prescribed treatments
How to use any special equipment prescribed for the client
Schedule for any home care services that are planned
How to access available community resources
When to obtain follow-up care

BOX 8-4

Principles and Guidelines of Delegating

Delegate the right task to the right delegatee: be familiar with the experience of the delegatee, their scope of practice, their job description, agency policy and procedures, and the state nurse practice act
Provide clear directions about the task, and ensure that the delegatee understands the expectations
Determine the degree of supervision that may be required
Provide the delegatee with the authority to complete the task; provide a deadline for completion of the task
Evaluate the outcome of care that has been delegated
Provide feedback to the delegatee regarding their performance
Generally noninvasive interventions such as skin care, range-of-motion exercises, ambulation, grooming, and hygiene measures can be assigned to a nursing assistant
An LPN can perform the tasks that a nursing assistant can perform and can also carry out certain invasive tasks, such as applying dressings, suctioning, urinary catheterization, and administering oral, subcutaneous, and intramuscular injections
The RN can perform the tasks that an LPN can perform and is responsible for assessment and planning care, initiating teaching, and administering intravenous medications

---

XII. PERFORMANCE IMPROVEMENT (QUALITY ASSURANCE)

A. Description
  1. Process of evaluating the outcome of care measured against predetermined standards
  2. Aspects of care that represent the predetermined standards are selected, criteria for achievement of the standards are identified, and methods of monitoring are defined
  3. Compliance in achieving the predetermined standards is measured and ways to improve compliance are sought, if needed
B. Retrospective audit: An evaluation method to inspect the medical record for documentation of compliance with the standards
C. Concurrent audit: An evaluation method to inspect the nursing staff's compliance with predetermined standards and criteria while the nurses are providing care
D. Quality assurance staff, charge nurse, or nurse educator may perform the review; a peer review approach may be implemented in which all members of the nursing staff are involved

XIII. DELEGATION AND ASSIGNMENTS

A. **Delegation**
  1. Process of transferring a selected nursing task in a situation to an individual who is competent to perform that specific task
  2. Involves achieving outcomes and sharing activities with other individuals who have the authority to accomplish the task
  3. The Nurse Practice Act and any practice limitations define which aspects of care can be delegated and which must be performed by the registered nurse, the licensed practical/vocational nurse, and unlicensed personnel
  4. Even though a task may be delegated to someone, the nurse who delegates maintains **accountability** for the overall nursing care of the client

  5. Only the task, not the ultimate **accountability**, may be delegated to another
B. Principles and guidelines of delegating (Box 8-4)
C. Assignments
  1. Description: Transferring **responsibility** and **accountability**
  2. Guidelines for client care assignments
    a. Always ensure client safety
    b. Be aware of individual variations in work abilities
    c. Determine which tasks can be delegated and to whom
    d. Match the task to the delegatee on the basis of the Nurse Practice Act and appropriate position descriptions
    e. Provide directions that are clear, concise, accurate, and complete
    f. Validate the person's understanding of the directions
    g. Communicate a feeling of confidence to the delegatee, and provide feedback promptly after the task is performed
    h. Maintain continuity of care as much as possible when assigning client care

XIV. TIME MANAGEMENT

A. Description
  1. A technique designed to assist in completing tasks within a definite time period

2. Learning how, when, and where to use one's time and establishing personal goals and time frames
3. Requires an ability to anticipate the day's activities, to combine activities when possible, and to be uninterrupted by nonessential activities
4. Involves efficiency in completing tasks as quickly as possible, effectiveness in deciding on the most important task to do, and doing it correctly

B. Principles and guidelines
1. Identify tasks, obligations, and activities, and write them down
2. Organize the workday; identify which tasks must be completed in specified time frames
3. Prioritize client needs according to importance
4. Anticipate the needs of the day, and provide time for unexpected and unplanned tasks that may arise
5. Focus on beginning the daily tasks, working on the most important first, while keeping goals in mind; look at the final goal for the day, which will help break down tasks into manageable parts
6. Begin client rounds at the beginning of the shift, collecting data on each assigned client
7. Delegate tasks when appropriate
8. Keep a daily hour-by-hour log to assist in providing structure to the tasks that must be accomplished, and cross tasks off the list as they are accomplished
9. Use hospital resources wisely, anticipating resource needs, and gather the necessary supplies before beginning the task
10. Organize paperwork, and continuously document task completion and necessary client data throughout the day
11. At the end of the day, evaluate the effectiveness of time **management**

XV. PRIORITIZING CARE

A. **Prioritizing:** Deciding which needs or problems require immediate action and which ones may be delayed until a later time, because they are not urgent
B. Guidelines for **prioritizing** (Box 8-5)
C. Setting priorities for reinforcing client teaching
1. Determine client's immediate needs
2. Review the learning objectives established for the client
3. Determine what the client perceives as important
4. Determine the client's anxiety level and the time available to teach
D. **Prioritizing** when caring for a group of clients
1. Identify the problems of each client
2. Review nursing diagnoses
3. Determine which client problems are most urgent on the basis of basic needs, the client's

---

BOX 8-5

Guidelines for Prioritizing

The nurse and the client mutually rank the client's needs in order of importance on the basis of the client's physical and psychological needs, safety, and the client's own needs and expectations; what the client sees as his or her priority needs may be different from what the nurse sees as the priority

Priorities are classified as high, intermediate, or low

Client needs that are life threatening or that could result in harm to the client if they are left untreated are high priorities

Nonemergency and non–life-threatening client needs are intermediate priorities

Client needs that are not directly related to the client's illness or prognosis are low priorities

When providing care, the nurse needs to decide which needs or problems require immediate action and which ones could be delayed until a later time because they are not urgent

Client problems that involve actual or life-threatening concerns are considered prior to potential health-threatening concerns

When prioritizing care, the nurse must consider time constraints and available resources

Problems identified as important by the client must be given high priority

The ABCs—airway, breathing, and circulation—can be used as a guide when determining priorities; client needs related to maintaining a patent airway are always the priority

Maslow's Hierarchy of Needs theory can be used as a guide in determining priorities; identifies the levels of physiological needs, safety, love and belonging, self-esteem, and self-actualization (basic needs are met before moving to other needs in the hierarchy)

The steps of the clinical problem-solving process (nursing process) can be used as a guide in determining priorities; remember that data collection is the first step of the nursing process

---

changing or unstable status, and complexity of the client's problem
4. Anticipate the time that it might take to care for the priority needs of the client
5. Combine activities, if possible, to resolve more than one problem at a time
6. Involve the client in the care as much as possible

XVI. DISASTERS AND DISASTER PLANNING

A. Description
1. A disaster is any human-made or natural event that causes destruction and devastation that requires assistance from others (Box 8-6)

BOX 8-6

Types of Disasters

HUMAN-MADE DISASTERS

Dam failures resulting in flooding

Hazardous substance accidents, such as pollution, chemical spills, or toxic gas leaks

Accidents that result in the release of radiological materials

Resource shortages, such as food, water, and electricity

Structural collapse, fire, or explosions

Terrorist attacks, such as bombing, riots, and bioterrorism

Transportation accidents

NATURAL DISASTERS

Blizzards

Communicable disease epidemics

Cyclones

Droughts

Earthquakes

Floods

Forest fires

Hailstorms

Hurricanes

Landslides

Mudslides

Tornadoes

Tsunamis (tidal waves)

Volcanic eruptions

2. In regard to a health care agency, a disaster can be external or internal; external disasters include those that occur outside of the health care agency, and internal disasters include those that occur inside the health care agency
3. A disaster preparedness plan is a formal plan of action for coordinating the response of a health care agency's staff in the event of a disaster in the health care agency or surrounding community

B. American Red Cross (ARC)

1. Has been given authority by the federal government to provide disaster relief
2. All ARC disaster relief assistance is free; local offices are located across the United States
3. Participates with the government in developing and testing community disaster plans
4. Identifies and trains personnel for disaster response
5. Works with businesses and labor organizations to identify resources and people for disaster work
6. Educates the public about ways to prepare for a disaster
7. Operates shelters, provides assistance to meet immediate emergency needs, and provides disaster health services, including emotional and mental health support
8. Handles inquires from family members

9. Coordinates relief activities with other agencies
10. Nurses are directly involved with the ARC and assume such functions as managers, supervisors, and educators of first aid; they also participate in disaster preparedness and disaster relief programs, and provide services such as disaster relief, blood collection drives, and immunization programs

C. Phases of disaster management

1. The Federal Emergency Management Agency (FEMA) identifies four disaster management phases: mitigation, preparedness, response, and recovery

   a. Mitigation
      (1) Refers to actions or measures that can either prevent the occurrence of a disaster or reduce the damaging effects of a disaster
      (2) Involves determining the community hazards and community risks (actual and potential threats) if a disaster occurs
      (3) Involves awareness of available community resources and community health personnel, which will facilitate mobilization of activities and minimize chaos and confusion if a disaster occurs
      (4) Includes determining the resources available for care to infants, the older client, the disabled, and those with chronic health problems

   b. Preparedness
      (1) Involves plans for rescue, evacuation, and caring for disaster victims
      (2) Involves plans for training disaster personnel and gathering resources, equipment, and other materials needed for dealing with the disaster
      (3) Includes identifying specific responsibilities for various disaster response personnel
      (4) Includes establishing a community disaster plan and an effective public communication system
      (5) Involves setting up an emergency medical system and a plan for activation
      (6) Includes checking proper functioning of emergency equipment
      (7) Involves making anticipatory provisions and setting up a location for distributing food, water, clothing, shelter, other supplies, and needed medicine
      (8) Includes checking supplies on a regular basis and replenishing outdated supplies
      (9) Includes practicing community disaster plans (mock disaster drills)

   c. Response
      (1) Includes putting disaster planning services into action and includes the actions taken to save lives and prevent further damage

(2) Primary concerns include safety, physical health, and mental health of both the victims and members of the disaster response team

d. Recovery

(1) Includes actions taken to return to a normal situation following the disaster

(2) Includes preventing debilitating effects and restoring personal, economic, and environmental health and stability to the community

D. Levels of disaster: FEMA identifies three levels of disaster, and the level determines the FEMA response (Box 8-7)

1. Once a federal emergency has been declared, the Federal Response Plan (FRP) may take effect and activate emergency support functions (ESFs)

2. ESFs of the ARC includes sheltering, feeding, performing emergency first aid, providing a disaster welfare information system, and coordinating bulk distribution of emergency relief supplies

3. Disaster medical assistant teams (DMATs), teams of specially trained personnel, can be activated and sent to a disaster site to provide triage and medical care to victims until they can be evacuated to a hospital

▲ E. Nurse's role in disaster planning

1. Personal and professional preparedness

a. Make personal and family preparations (Box 8-8)

b. Be aware of the disaster plan at the place of employment and in the community

c. Maintain certification in disaster training and in cardiopulmonary resuscitation

d. Participate in mock disaster drills

e. Prepare professional emergency response items, such as a copy of the nursing license, personal health care equipment such as a stethoscope, cash, warm clothing, record-keeping materials, and other nursing care supplies

2. Disaster response

a. In the heath care agency setting, if a disaster occurs, the agency disaster preparedness plan (emergency response plan) is immediately activated and the nurse responds by following the directions identified in the plan

b. In the community setting, if the nurse is the first responder to a disaster, the nurse cares for the victims by attending to those with life-threatening problems first; once rescue workers arrive at the scene, immediate plans for triage should begin

F. Triage   ▲

1. In a disaster or war: Classifying victims according to the severity of the injury, urgency of treatment, and place for treatment

2. In an emergency department: Classifying clients according to their need for care and establishing priorities of care—the type of illness, the severity of the problem, and the resources available govern the process

a. Triage rating systems: Various rating systems categories are used in clinical settings; the nurse must be familiar with the rating system in the health care agency in which he or she is employed (Box 8-9)

b. Emergency department triage system   ▲

(1) A commonly used rating system in an emergency department is a three-tiered system

---

BOX 8-7

Levels of Disaster

LEVEL III DISASTER
Considered a minor disaster and involves a minimal level of damage, but could result in a presidential declaration of an emergency

LEVEL II DISASTER
Considered a moderate disaster; will likely result in a presidential declaration of an emergency, with moderate federal assistance

LEVEL I DISASTER
Considered a massive disaster, involves significant damage, and results in a presidential disaster declaration, with major federal involvement and full engagement of federal, regional, and national resources

---

BOX 8-8

Emergency Plans and Supplies

Plan a meeting place for family members
Identify where to go if an evacuation is necessary
Determine when and how to turn off water, gas, and electricity at main switches
Locate the safe areas in the home for each type of disaster
Have a 3-day supply of water available (1 gallon per person per day)
Have a 3-day supply of nonperishable food available
Replace water supply every 3 months and food supply every 6 months
Emergency supplies: clothing and blankets; first-aid kit; adequate supply of prescription medication; battery-operated radio; flashlight and batteries; credit card, cash, or traveler's checks; extra set of car keys and full tank of gas in the car; sanitation supplies for washing, toileting, and disposing of trash; extra pair of eyeglasses, special items for infants, the older client, or the disabled; pet supplies, such as food, water, leash, kitty litter and pan; important documents in a waterproof case

BOX 8-9
Triage Rating Systems

FIVE-TIER SYSTEM (MOST OFTEN USED IN MILITARY TRIAGE)
Victim is dead or will die
Life threatening (emergent): Victim has life-threatening injuries, but they are readily correctible
Urgent: Victim must be treated within 1 to 2 hours
Delayed (nonurgent): Victim is noncritical or ambulatory; victim has no injury and no treatment is necessary
No injury: No treatment is necessary

FOUR-TIER SYSTEM
Immediate (emergent): Victim is seriously injured but has a reasonable chance for survival
Delayed (nonurgent): Victim can wait for care after simple first aid is given
Expectant: Victim is extremely critical and dying
Minimal (nonurgent): Victim has no impairment of function and can either treat self or be treated by a nonprofessional

THREE-TIER SYSTEM (COMMONLY USED IN HEALTH CARE AGENCIES)
Life threatening (emergent): Victim has life-threatening injuries, but they are readily correctible
Urgent: Victim must be treated within 1 to 2 hours
Delayed (nonurgent): Victim has no injury, is noncritical or ambulatory

TWO-TIER SYSTEM
Immediate: Includes victims that have life-threatening injuries that are readily correctable on the scene (emergent) and victims who must be treated within 1 to 2 hours (urgent)
Delayed (nonurgent): Victims who have no injuries, have noncritical injuries, are ambulatory, dying, or dead

Modified from *Mosby's medical, nursing, and allied health dictionary* (6th ed.). (2002). St. Louis: Mosby, p. 1747.

BOX 8-10
Emergency Department Triage System

EMERGENT (RED): PRIORITY 1 (HIGHEST)
Given to clients who have life-threatening injuries and need immediate attention and continuous evaluation, but who have a high probability for survival once stabilized
Such clients include those with trauma, chest pain, severe respiratory distress or cardiac arrest, limb amputation, and/or acute neurological deficits, and those who have sustained chemical splashes to the eyes

URGENT (YELLOW): PRIORITY 2
Given to clients who require treatment and whose injuries have complications that are not life threatening, provided that they are treated within 1 to 2 hours; these clients require continuous evaluation every 30 to 60 minutes thereafter
Such clients include those with a simple fracture, asthma without respiratory distress, fever, hypertension, abdominal pain, or a renal stone

NONURGENT (GREEN): PRIORITY 3
Given to clients with local injuries who do not have immediate complications and who can wait several hours for medical treatment; these clients require evaluation every 1 to 2 hours thereafter
Such clients include those with conditions such as a minor laceration, sprain, or cold symptoms

that uses the categories of emergent, urgent, and nonurgent; may also identify these categories by color coding or numbers (Box 8-10)
  (2) The nurse needs to be familiar with the health care agency's triage system
  (3) When caring for the client who has died, the nurse needs to recognize the importance of family rituals and provide support to loved ones
  (4) Organ donation procedures of the health care agency need to be addressed if appropriate
G. Client data collection in the emergency department
  1. Primary data collection
    a. The purpose is to identify any client problem that poses an immediate or potential threat to life
    b. Information is gathered primarily through objective data and, if any abnormalities are found, immediate interventions are initiated
    c. The nurse uses the ABCs—airway, breathing, and circulation—as a guide in assessing the client's needs and also assesses the client who sustained a traumatic injury for signs of a head injury or cervical spine injury
  2. Secondary data collection
    a. Performed following the primary data collection and after treatment for any problems identified
    b. Performed to identify any other life-threatening problems that the client might be experiencing
    c. Both subjective and objective data are obtained; include a history, general overview, vital sign measurement, neurological assessment, pain assessment, and complete or focused physical assessment

PRACTICE QUESTIONS

1. A nurse is assigned to care for four clients. In planning client rounds, which client would the nurse collect data on first?
  1. A client receiving oxygen via nasal cannula who had difficulty breathing during the previous shift

  2. A postoperative client preparing for discharge
  3. A client scheduled for a chest x-ray
  4. A client requiring daily dressing changes

2. A nurse is assisting in reviewing the critical paths of the clients on the nursing unit. In performing a variance analysis, which of the following would indicate the need for further action and analysis?
  1. Clear breath sounds in a client with congestive heart failure
  2. A postoperative client develops a cough and a fever
  3. The absence of a wound infection in a client who had a coronary artery bypass graft
  4. A client with diabetes mellitus demonstrating accurate use of a glucometer following teaching

3. A licensed practical nurse (LPN) is attending anagency orientation regarding the nursing model of practice implemented in the facility. The nurse is told that the nursing model is a team nursing approach. The nurse understands that which of the following is a characteristic of this type of nursing model of practice?
  1. A task approach method is used to provide care to clients
  2. A single registered nurse (RN) is responsible for providing nursing care to a group of clients
  3. Managed care concepts and tools are used in providing client care
  4. Nursing personnel are led by an RN leader in providing care to a group of clients

4. A client experiences a cardiac arrest. The nurse leader quickly responds to the emergency and assigns clearly defined tasks to the work group. In this situation, the nurse is implementing which leadership style?
  1. Autocratic
  2. Situational
  3. Laissez-faire
  4. Democratic

5. A nurse has delegated several nursing tasks to staff members. The nurse's primary responsibility following delegation of the tasks is to:
  1. Allow each staff member to make judgments when performing the tasks
  2. Perform follow-up with each staff member regarding the performance of the task and the outcomes related to implementing the task
  3. Document that the task was completed
  4. Assign the tasks that were not completed to the next nursing shift

6. A nurse is planning the client assignments. Which of the following is the least appropriate assignment for the nursing assistant?
  1. Assist a child who is profoundly developmentally disabled to eat lunch
  2. Obtain frequent oral temperatures on a client
  3. Accompany a 51-year-old man, being discharged to home following a bowel resection 8 days ago, to his transportation

  4. Collect a urine specimen from a 70-year-old woman admitted 3 days ago

7. A licensed practical nurse is planning the client assignments for the day. Which of the following is the most appropriate assignment for the nursing assistant?
  1. A client requiring frequent vital signs following a cardiac catheterization
  2. A client who requires frequent ambulation
  3. A client requiring a wound irrigation
  4. A client receiving continuous tube feedings

8. A nurse employed in a long-term care facility is planning the client assignments for the shift. Which of the following clients would the nurse appropriately assign to the nursing assistant?
  1. A client requiring twice-daily dressing changes
  2. A client requiring a 24-hour urine collection
  3. A client on a bowel management program requiring rectal suppositories and a daily enema
  4. A diabetic client requiring daily insulin and reinforcement of dietary measures

9. A nurse is assigned to care for four clients. In planning client rounds, which client would the nurse check first?
  1. A client admitted on the previous shift who has a diagnosis of gastroenteritis
  2. A client in skeletal traction
  3. A client on a ventilator
  4. A postoperative client preparing for discharge

10. A nurse employed in an emergency department is assigned to assist in triage for clients arriving to the emergency room for treatment on the evening shift. The nurse would assign highest priority to which of the following clients?
  1. A client with chest pain who states that he just ate pizza that was made with a very spicy sauce
  2. A client with a minor laceration on the index finger sustained while cutting an eggplant
  3. A client complaining of muscle aches, a headache, and malaise
  4. A client who twisted her ankle when she fell while rollerblading

ALTERNATE FORMAT QUESTION: PRIORITIZING (ORDERED RESPONSE)

The nurse on the day shift is assigned to care for the following three clients. List in order of priority how the nurse would plan to check the assigned clients. (Number 1 is the client who the nurse would check first.)

____ Client is scheduled for a cardiac catheterization at 10:00 AM

____ Client was newly diagnosed with diabetes mellitus and is scheduled for discharge to home

____ Client with a tracheostomy and is on a mechanical ventilator

ANSWERS

1. *Answer:* 1

Rationale: The airway is always a high priority, and the nurse would attend to the client who has been experiencing an airway problem first. The clients described in options 2, 3, and 4 would be an intermediate priority.

Test-Taking Strategy: Use Maslow's Hierarchy of Needs theory and the ABCs—airway, breathing, and circulation—to answer the question. Remember that the airway is always the first priority. Review these prioritizing principles if you had difficulty with this question.

Level of Cognitive Ability: Application
Client Needs: Safe, Effective Care Environment
Integrated Process: Nursing Process/Planning
Content Area: Delegating/Prioritizing
References: Christensen, B., & Kockrow, E. (2003). *Foundations of nursing* (4th ed) St. Louis: Mosby, p. 1042.
Linton, A., & Maebius, N. (2003). *Introduction to medical-surgical nursing* (3rd ed.). Philadelphia: W.B. Saunders, p. 500.

2. *Answer:* 2

Rationale: Variances are actual deviations or detours from the critical paths. Variances can be positive or negative, avoidable or unavoidable, and can be caused by a variety of factors. Positive variance occurs when the client achieves maximum benefit and is discharged earlier than anticipated. Negative variance occurs when untoward events prevent a timely discharge. Variance analysis occurs continuously to anticipate and recognize negative variance early, so that appropriate action can be taken. A postoperative client who develops a cough and a fever identifies a negative outcome.

Test-Taking Strategy: Use the process of elimination noting the key words, *indicate the need for further action and analysis.* Options 1, 3, and 4 identify positive outcomes. Option 2 identifies a negative outcome. Review the purpose of variance analysis if you had difficulty with this question.

Level of Cognitive Ability: Analysis
Client Needs: Safe, Effective Care Environment
Integrated Process: Nursing Process/Evaluation
Content Area: Leadership/Management
Reference: Potter, P., & Perry, A. (2005). *Fundamentals of nursing* (6th ed.). St. Louis: Mosby, pp. 485-487.

3. *Answer:* 4

Rationale: In team nursing, nursing personnel are led by an RN leader when providing care to a group of clients. Option 1 identifies functional nursing. Option 2 identifies primary nursing. Option 3 identifies a component of case management.

Test-Taking Strategy: Note that the issue of the question relates to team nursing. Keep this issue in mind and use the process of elimination. Option 4 is the only option that identifies the concept of a team approach. Review the various types of nursing delivery systems if you had difficulty with this question.

Level of Cognitive Ability: Comprehension
Client Needs: Safe, Effective Care Environment
Integrated Process: Nursing Process/Implementation
Content Area: Leadership/Management
Reference: Christensen, B., & Kockrow, E. (2003). *Foundations of nursing* (4th ed.). St. Louis: Mosby, p. 1041.

4. *Answer:* 1

Rationale: Autocratic leadership is an approach wherein the leader retains all authority and is primarily concerned with task accomplishment. It is an effective leadership style to implement in an emergency or crisis situation. The leader assigns clearly defined tasks and establishes one-way communication with the work group, making all of the decisions alone. Situational leadership is a comprehensive approach that incorporates the leader's style, the maturity of the work group, and the situation at hand. Laissez-faire is a permissive style of leadership in which the leader gives up control and delegates all decision making to the work group. Democratic leadership is a people-centered approach that is primarily concerned with human relations and teamwork. This leadership style facilitates goal accomplishment and contributes to the growth and development of the staff.

Test-Taking Strategy: Use the process of elimination. Focusing on the data in the question and the nurse leader's actions will direct you to option 1. Review the various leadership styles if you had difficulty with this question.

Level of Cognitive Ability: Application
Client Needs: Safe, Effective Care Environment
Integrated Process: Nursing Process/Implementation
Content Area: Leadership/Management
Reference: Zerwekh, J., & Claborn, J. (2003). *Nursing today: Transitions and trends* (4th ed.). Philadelphia: W.B. Saunders, p. 103.

5. *Answer:* 2

Rationale: The ultimate responsibility for a task lies with the person who delegated it. Therefore, it is the nurse's primary responsibility to follow up with each staff member regarding the performance of the task and the outcomes related to implementing the task. Not all staff members have the education, knowledge, and ability to make judgments about tasks being performed. The nurse documents that the task has been completed, but this would not be done until follow-up was implemented and outcomes were identified. It is not appropriate to assign the tasks that were not completed to the next nursing shift.

Test-Taking Strategy: Use the process of elimination noting the key words, *primary responsibility.* Recalling that the ultimate responsibility for a task lies with the person who delegated it will direct you to option 2. Review the guidelines related to delegating if you had difficulty with this question.

Level of Cognitive Ability: Application
Client Needs: Safe, Effective Care Environment
Integrated Process: Nursing Process/Implementation
Content Area: Leadership/Management
Reference: Potter, P., & Perry, A. (2005). *Fundamentals of nursing* (6th ed.). St. Louis: Mosby, p. 379.

6. *Answer:* 1

Rationale: The nurse must determine the most appropriate assignment based on the skills of the staff member and the needs of the client. In this case, the least appropriate assignment for the nursing assistant would be assisting with feeding a profoundly developmentally disabled child. The child is likely to have difficulty eating, and therefore has a higher potential for complications, such as choking and aspiration.

The remaining options do not include data indicating that these tasks carry any unforeseen risk.

Test-Taking Strategy: Note the key words, *least appropriate.* Use the ABCs—airway, breathing, and circulation—and recall the principles of delegation and supervision of the work of others in answering the question. Remember that work delegated to others must be done consistent with the individual's level of expertise and licensure or lack of licensure. Review the principles related to assignments and delegation if you had difficulty with this question.

Level of Cognitive Ability: Application
Client Needs: Safe, Effective Care Environment
Integrated Process: Nursing Process/Implementation
Content Area: Leadership/Management
Reference: Christensen, B., & Kockrow, E. (2003). *Foundations of nursing* (4th ed.). St. Louis: Mosby, p. 1041.

7. Answer: 2
Rationale: The nurse must determine the *most appropriate* assignment based on the skills of the staff member and the needs of the client. In this case, the most appropriate assignment for a nursing assistant would be to care for the client who requires frequent ambulation. The nursing assistant is skilled in this task. The client who had a cardiac catheterization will require specific monitoring in addition to vital signs. Wound irrigations and tube feedings are not performed by unlicensed personnel.

Test-Taking Strategy: Note the key words *most appropriate.* Use the process of elimination recalling the principles of delegation and supervision of the work of others. Remember that work delegated to others must be done consistent with the individual's level of expertise and licensure or lack of licensure. Review the principles of delegation if you had difficulty with this question.

Level of Cognitive Ability: Application
Client Needs: Safe, Effective Care Environment
Integrated Process: Nursing Process/Planning
Content Area: Leadership/Management
Reference: Potter, P., & Perry, A. (2005). *Fundamentals of nursing* (6th ed.). St. Louis: Mosby, pp. 42, 378-379, 418.

8. Answer: 2
Rationale: Assignment of tasks needs to be implemented based on the job description of the individual, the level of clinical competence, and state law. Options 1, 3, and 4 involve care that requires the skill of a licensed nurse.

Test-Taking Strategy: Use the process of elimination and knowledge regarding tasks that can be safely delegated to the nursing assistant. Eliminate options 1, 3, and 4 because these clients require care that needs to be provided by a licensed nurse. Review the principles related to assignments and delegation if you had difficulty with this question.

Level of Cognitive Ability: Application
Client Needs: Safe, Effective Care Environment
Integrated Process: Nursing Process/Planning
Content Area: Leadership/Management
Reference: Christensen, B., & Kockrow, E. (2003). *Foundations of nursing* (4th ed.). St. Louis: Mosby, p. 1041.

9. Answer: 3
Rationale: The airway is always a high priority, and the nurse first checks the client on a ventilator. The clients described in options 1, 2, and 4 have needs that would be identified as intermediate priorities.

Test-Taking Strategy: Use Maslow's Hierarchy of Needs theory and the ABCs—airway, breathing, and circulation—to answer the question. Remember that the airway is always the first priority. Review principles related to prioritizing if you had difficulty with this question.

Level of Cognitive Ability: Application
Client Needs: Safe, Effective Care Environment
Integrated Process: Nursing Process/Planning
Content Area: Delegating/Prioritizing
Reference: Potter, P., & Perry, A. (2005). *Fundamentals of nursing* (6th ed.). St. Louis: Mosby, p. 319.

10. Answer: 1
Rationale: In an emergency department, triage involves classifying clients according to their need for care and includes establishing priorities of care. The type of illness, the severity of the problem, and the resources available govern the process. Clients with trauma, chest pain, severe respiratory distress or cardiac arrest, limb amputation, or acute neurological deficits, and those who sustained a chemical splash to the eyes, are classified as emergent and are the number 1 priority. Clients with conditions such as a simple fracture, asthma without respiratory distress, fever, hypertension, abdominal pain, or the client with a renal stone, have urgent needs and are classified as the number 2 priority. Clients with conditions such as a minor laceration, sprain, or cold symptoms are classified as nonurgent and are the number 3 priority.

Test-Taking Strategy: Note the key words, *highest priority.* Use the ABCs—airway, breathing, and circulation—to direct you to option 1. A client experiencing chest pain is always classified as priority number 1 until a myocardial infarction has been ruled out. Review the triage classification system commonly used in a hospital emergency department if you had difficulty with this question.

Level of Cognitive Ability: Application
Client Needs: Safe, Effective Care Environment
Integrated Process: Nursing Process/Implementation
Content Area: Delegating/Prioritizing
Reference: Lewis, S., Heitkemper, M., & Dirksen, S. (2004). *Medical-surgical nursing: Assessment and management of clinical problems* (6th ed.). St. Louis: Mosby, p. 1846.

ALTERNATE FORMAT QUESTION: PRIORITIZING (ORDERED RESPONSE)
Answer: 231
Rationale: The airway is always a high priority and the nurse first assesses the client who has a tracheostomy and is on a mechanical ventilator. The nurse next assesses the client scheduled for the cardiac catheterization at 10:00 AM, because the client may have needs that must be met or preprocedure orders that need to be carried out. Finally, the nurse checks the client scheduled for discharge.

Test-Taking Strategy: Use Maslow's Hierarchy of Needs theory and the ABCs—airway, breathing, and circulation. Focus only on the data identified in the question. Remember that airway is always the first priority. Review principles related to prioritizing if you had difficulty with this question.
Level of Cognitive Ability: Application

Client Needs: Safe, Effective Care Environment
Integrated Process: Nursing Process/Planning
Content Area: Delegting/Prioritizing
Reference: Potter, P., & Perry, A. (2005). *Fundamentals of nursing* (6th ed.). St. Louis: Mosby, p. 319.

REFERENCES

Christensen, B., & Kockrow, E. (2003). *Foundations of nursing* (4th ed.). St. Louis: Mosby.

Lewis, S., Heitkemper, M., & Dirksen, S. (2004). *Medical-surgical nursing: Assessment and management of clinical problems* (6th ed.). St. Louis: Mosby.

Linton, A. & Maebius, N. (2003). *Introduction to medical-surgical nursing* (3rd ed.). Philadelphia: W.B. Saunders.

Mosby's medical, nursing, and allied health dictionary (6th ed.). St. Louis: Mosby.

National Council of State Boards of Nursing (2005). *Detailed test plan for the National Council licensure examination for practical/vocational nurses.* Chicago: Author.

Potter, P., & Perry, A. (2005). *Fundamentals of nursing* (6th ed.). St. Louis: Mosby.

Zerwekh, J., & Claborn, J. (2003). *Nursing today: Transitions and trends* (4th ed.). Philadelphia: W.B. Saunders.

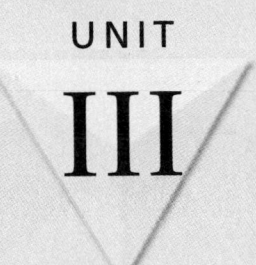

Nursing Sciences

Fluids and Electrolytes

PYRAMID TERMS

calcium A mineral element needed for the process of bone formation, coagulation of blood, excitation of cardiac and skeletal muscle, maintenance of muscle tone, conduction of neuromuscular impulses, and synthesis and regulation of the endocrine and exocrine glands.

fluid volume deficit Dehydration in which the body's fluid intake is not sufficient to meet the body's fluid needs.

fluid volume excess Fluid intake or fluid retention exceeds the body's fluid needs; also called overhydration or fluid overload.

homeostasis The tendency of biological systems to maintain relatively constant conditions in the internal environment while continuously interacting with and adjusting to changes originating within or outside the system.

hypercalcemia A serum calcium level that exceeds 10 mg/dL.

hyperkalemia A serum potassium level that exceeds 5.1 mEq/L.

hypermagnesemia A serum magnesium level that exceeds 2.6 mg/dL.

hypernatremia A serum sodium level that exceeds 145 mEq/L.

hyperphosphatemia A serum phosphorus level that exceeds 4.5 mg/dL.

hypocalcemia A serum calcium level below 8.6 mg/dL.

hypokalemia A serum potassium level below 3.5 mEq/L.

hypomagnesemia A serum magnesium level below 1.6 mg/dL.

hyponatremia A serum sodium level below 135 mEq/L.

hypophosphatemia A serum phosphorus level below 2.7 mg/dL.

magnesium Concentrated in the bone, cartilage, and within the cell itself and is required for the use of adenosine triphosphate (ADP) as a source of energy. It is necessary for the action of numerous enzyme systems, such as carbohydrate metabolism, protein synthesis, nucleic acid synthesis, and contraction of muscular tissue. It also regulates neuromuscular activity and the clotting mechanism.

potassium A principal electrolyte of intracellular fluid and the primary buffer within the cell itself; needed for nerve conduction, muscle function, acid-base balance, and osmotic pressure. Along with calcium and magnesium, it controls the rate and force of contraction of the heart and, thus, cardiac output.

phosphorus Needed for generation of bony tissue; functions in the metabolism of glucose and lipids, in the maintenance of acid-base balance, and in the storage and transfer of energy from one site in the body to another. Phosphorus levels are evaluated in relation to calcium levels because of their inverse relationship: when calcium levels are decreased, phosphorus levels are increased, and when phosphorus levels are decreased, calcium levels are increased.

sodium An abundant electrolyte that maintains osmotic pressure and acid-base balance and transmits nerve impulses.

PYRAMID TO SUCCESS

Pyramid points focus primarily on data collection related to a fluid and electrolyte imbalance, interventions, and evaluating the expected outcomes. Fluid and electrolytes constitute a content area that is complex and sometimes difficult to understand. It is important to understand cell functions and properties and the concepts related to body fluids as outlined in this chapter. Review this content. Pyramid points also focus on the common fluid and electrolyte disturbances. Focus on the pyramid points related to the causes, data collection, and related treatments. Integrated Processes addressed in this chapter are Nursing Process (Clinical Problem Solving Process), Caring, Communication and Documentation, and Teaching/Learning.

CLIENT NEEDS
Safe, Effective Care Environment

Accident prevention and protection and safety of the client when an imbalance exists, particularly when changes in cardiovascular, respiratory, gastrointestinal (GI), neuromuscular, renal, or central nervous system (CNS) occur, or when the client is at risk for complications such as seizures, respiratory depression, or dysrhythmias

Consultation with members of the health care team

Establishing priorities

Handling hazardous and infectious materials to prevent injury to self, health care personnel, and others

Medical and surgical asepsis and preventing infection in the client when samples for laboratory studies are obtained or when intravenous fluids are administered

Standard, transmission-based, and other precautions to prevent transmission of infection to self and others

Health Promotion and Maintenance

Health screening and the potential risk for a fluid and electrolyte imbalance

Reinforcing instructions related to medication and diet management

Reinforcing instructions related to the potential risk for a fluid and electrolyte balance, measures to prevent an imbalance, signs and symptoms of an imbalance, and actions to take if signs and symptoms develop

Psychosocial Integrity

Providing support and continuously informing the client of the purposes for prescribed interventions

Providing reassurance to the client who is experiencing a fluid or electrolyte imbalance

Physiological Integrity

Identifying clients at risk for a fluid or electrolyte imbalance

Monitoring laboratory values

Monitoring for complications related to the imbalance

Assisting in managing emergencies

Identifying the expected and unexpected responses to treatment and documenting accordingly

I. CELL PROPERTIES (Box 9-1)

II. CONCEPTS OF FLUID AND ELECTROLYTE BALANCE

A. Electrolytes
1. Description: When a substance is dissolved in solution and some of its molecules split or dissociate into electrically charged atoms or ions (see Box 9-1)
2. Measurement
   a. To measure volumes of fluids, the metric system is used: liters (L) or milliliters (mL)
   b. The unit of measure that expresses the combining activity of an electrolyte is the milliequivalent (mEq)

Cell Properties

Atom: The smallest part of an element that still has the properties of the element, composed of particles known as the proton (positive charge), neutron (neutral), and electron (negative charge). Protons and neutrons are in the nucleus of the atom; therefore, the nucleus is positively charged. Electrons carry a negative charge and revolve around the nucleus. As long as the number of electrons is the same as the number of protons, there is no net charge on the atom—that is, it is neither positive nor negative. Atoms may gain, lose, or share electrons, and then are no longer neutral.

Molecule: When two or more atoms combine to form a substance.

Ion: An atom that carries an electrical charge because it has either gained or lost electrons. Some ions carry a negative electrical charge, and some carry a positive charge.

Cation: An ion that carries a positive charge because it has given away or lost electrons. The result is fewer electrons than protons and a positive charge.

Anion: An ion that has gained electrons and therefore carries a negative charge. When an ion has gained or taken on electrons, it assumes a negative charge, and the result is a negatively charged ion.

B. Body fluid compartments (Box 9-2)
1. Description
   a. Fluid in each of the body compartments contains electrolytes
   b. Each compartment has a particular composition of electrolytes, which differs from that of other compartments
   c. To function normally, body cells must have fluids and electrolytes in the right compartments and in the right amounts
   d. Whenever an electrolyte moves out of a cell, another electrolyte moves in to take its place
   e. Compartments are separated by semipermeable membranes

C. Third-spacing
1. The accumulation and sequestration of trapped extracellular fluid in an actual or potential body space as a result of disease or injury
2. The trapped fluid represents a volume loss and is unavailable for normal physiological processes
3. Fluid may be trapped in body spaces such as the pericardial, pleural, peritoneal, or joint cavities; the bowel; or the abdomen; or within soft tissues after trauma or burns
4. Assessing the intravascular fluid loss is difficult; it may not be reflected in weight changes or intake and output (I&O) records, and may not become apparent until after organ malfunction occurs

D. Edema
  1. An excess accumulation of fluid in the interstitial spaces
  2. Localized edema occurs as a result of traumatic injury from accidents or surgery, local inflammatory processes, or burns
  3. Generalized edema, also called anasarca, is an excessive accumulation of fluid in the interstitial space throughout the body as a result of a condition such as cardiac, renal, or liver failure
E. Body fluid
  1. Description
    a. Provides transportation of nutrients to the cells and carries waste products from the cells
    b. Total body fluid amounts to about 60% of body weight
    c. A loss of 10% of body fluid in the adult is serious
    d. A loss of 20% of the body fluid in the adult is fatal
  2. Constituents of body fluids
    a. Body fluids consist of water and dissolved substances
    b. The largest single fluid constituent of the body is water
F. Body fluid transport
  1. Diffusion
    a. The movement of particles in all directions through a solution
    b. Diffusion occurs within fluid compartments and from one compartment to another, if the barrier between the compartments is permeable to the diffusing substances
    c. Diffusion of a solute (substance that is dissolved) spreads the molecules from an area of high concentration to an area of lower concentration
    d. A permeable membrane allows substances to pass through it without restriction
    e. A selectively permeable membrane allows some solutes to pass through without restriction but prevents other solutes from passing freely
  2. Osmosis
    a. Osmotic pressure is the force that draws the water from a less concentrated solution through a selectively permeable membrane into a more concentrated solution
    b. If a membrane is permeable to water but not to all the solutes present, it is a selective or semipermeable membrane
    c. When the solvent (solution in which the solvent is dissolved) or water moves across the membrane, the process is called osmosis
  3. Filtration
    a. Filtration is the movement of solutes and solvents by hydrostatic pressure
    b. Hydrostatic pressure is the force exerted by the weight of a solution
    c. The movement is from an area of greater pressure to an area of lesser pressure
  4. Osmolality
    a. Refers to the number of osmotically active particles per kilogram of water
    b. In the body, osmotic pressure is measured in milliosmols (mOsm)
    c. The normal osmolality of plasma is 280 to 294 mOsm/kg
  5. Hydrostatic pressure
    a. The force exerted by the weight of a solution
    b. When there is a difference in the hydrostatic pressure on two sides of a membrane, water and diffusible solutes move out of the solution that has the higher hydrostatic pressure by the process of filtration
    c. At the arterial end of the capillary, the hydrostatic pressure is greater than the osmotic pressure; therefore, fluids and diffusible solutes move out of the capillary
    d. At the venous end, the osmotic pressure or pull is greater than the hydrostatic pressure, and fluids and some solutes move into the capillary
    e. The excess fluid and solutes remaining in the interstitial spaces are returned to the intravascular compartment by the lymph channels
G. Movement of body fluid
  1. Description
    a. Cell membranes separate the interstitial fluid from the intravascular fluid
    b. Cell membranes are selectively permeable; that is, the cell membrane and the capillary wall allow water and some solutes free passage through them
    c. Several forces affect the movement of water and solutes through the walls of cells and capillaries
    d. The greater the number of particles in the concentrated solution, the more pull there will be to move the water through the membrane
    e. If the body loses more electrolytes than fluids, as can happen in diarrhea, then the extracellular fluid will contain fewer electrolytes or less solute than the intracellular fluid (ICF)

f. Fluids and electrolytes must be kept in balance for health; when they remain out of balance, death can occur

2. Isotonic solutions (Table 9-1)

a. When the solutions on both sides of a selectively permeable membrane have established equilibrium or are equal in concentration, they are then isotonic

b. Isotonic solutions are isotonic to human cells, and thus there will be very little osmosis

3. Hypotonic solutions (see Table 9-1)

a. When a solution contains a lower concentration of salt or solute than other solutions, it is hypotonic

b. A hypotonic solution has less salt or more water than an isotonic solution

c. Hypotonic solutions are hypotonic to the cells; therefore, osmosis would continue in an attempt to bring about balance or equality

4. Hypertonic solutions: A solution that has a higher concentration of solutes than another solution is a hypertonic solution (see Table 9-1)

5. Osmotic pressure

a. The force that draws the solvent from a solution with more solvent activity through a selectively permeable membrane to a solution with less solvent activity

b. When the solutions on each side of a selectively permeable membrane are equal in concentration, they are isotonic

c. A hypotonic solution has less solute than an isotonic solution, whereas a hypertonic solution contains more solute

6. Active transport

a. If an ion is to move through a membrane from an area of low concentration to an area of higher concentration, an active transport system is necessary

b. An active transport system moves molecules or ions uphill against concentration and osmotic pressure

c. Metabolic processes in the cell supply the energy for active transport

d. Substances that are actively transported through the cell membrane include ions of sodium, potassium, calcium, iron, and hydrogen, some sugars, and amino acids

H. Body fluid excretion (Box 9-3)

1. Description

a. Fluids leave the body by several routes, including the skin, lungs, gastrointestinal (GI) tract, and kidneys

b. The kidneys excrete the largest quantity of fluid

c. As long as all organs are functioning normally, the body can maintain balance in its fluid content

2. Skin

a. Water is lost through the skin by diffusion in the amount of approximately 400 mL/day and by perspiration

b. The amount of water lost by perspiration will vary according to the temperature of the environment and of the body, but the average amount of loss is 100 mL/day

c. Water lost through the skin by diffusion is called insensible loss (individual is unaware of losing that water)

3. Lungs

a. Water is lost from the lungs through expired air that is saturated with water vapor

b. The amount of water lost from the lungs will vary with the rate and the depth of respiration

c. The average amount of water lost from the lungs is approximately 350 mL/day

d. Water lost from the lungs is called insensible loss

4. GI tract

a. Large quantities of water are secreted into the GI tract, but almost all this fluid is reabsorbed

b. A very large volume of electrolyte-containing liquids moves into the GI tract and then returns again into the extracellular fluid (ECF)

c. The average amount of water lost in the feces is 150 mL/day, equal to the amount of water gained through the oxidation of foods

d. Severe diarrhea will result in the loss of large quantities of fluids and electrolytes

5. Kidneys

a. Play a major role in regulating fluid and electrolyte balance

TABLE 9-1

Tonicity of Intravenous Fluids

Solution	Tonicity
0.45% saline (½ normal saline [NS])	Hypotonic
0.9% saline (NS)	Isotonic
5% dextrose in water (5% D/W)	Isotonic
5% dextrose in 0.225% saline (5% D/¼ NS)	Isotonic
Lactated Ringer's solution	Isotonic
5% dextrose in lactated Ringer's solution	Hypertonic
5% dextrose in 0.45% saline (5% D/½ NS)	Hypertonic
5% dextrose in 0.9% saline (5% D/NS)	Hypertonic
10% dextrose in water (10% D/W)	Hypertonic

BOX 9-3

Daily Body Fluid Excretion or Loss

WHERE FLUID IS LOST OR EXCRETED	AMOUNT LOST OR EXCRETED (mL)
Skin (by diffusion)	400
Skin (by perspiration)	100
Lungs	350
Feces	150
Kidneys	1500

b. Normal kidneys can adjust the amount of water and electrolytes leaving the body

c. The quantity of fluid excreted by the kidneys is determined by the amount of water ingested and the amount of waste and solutes excreted

d. The usual urine output is approximately 1500 mL/day; however, this will vary greatly, depending on fluid intake, amount of perspiration, and other factors

I. Body fluid replacement

   1. Description: Water enters the body through three sources: oral liquids, water in foods, and water formed by oxidation of foods

   2. Amounts

     a. The average total amount of water taken into the body by all three sources is 2500 mL/day

     b. About 10 mL of water is released by the metabolism of each 100 calories of fat, carbohydrates, or proteins

   3. Electrolytes

     a. Electrolytes are present in both foods and liquids

     b. With a normal diet, an excess of essential electrolytes is taken in and the unused electrolytes are excreted

J. Maintaining fluid and electrolyte balance

   1. Description

     a. Homeostasis is a term that indicates the relative stability of the internal environment

     b. Concentration and composition of body fluids must be nearly constant

     c. In a client, when one of the substances, either fluid or electrolyte, is deficient, it must be replaced normally by the intake of food and water or by therapy such as intravenous (IV) administration and/or medications

     d. When the client has an excess of fluid or electrolytes, therapy is directed toward assisting the body to eliminate the excess

   2. Kidneys: Play a major role in controlling all types of balance in fluid and electrolytes

   3. Adrenal glands: Through the secretion of aldosterone, the adrenal glands also aid in controlling extracellular fluid volume by regulating the amount of **sodium** reabsorbed by the kidneys

   4. Antidiuretic hormone (ADH): ADH from the pituitary gland regulates the osmotic pressure of extracellular fluid by regulating the amount of water reabsorbed by the kidney

III. FLUID VOLUME DEFICIT

A. Description

   1. Dehydration in which the body's fluid intake is not sufficient to meet the body's fluid needs

   2. The goal of treatment is to restore fluid volume, replace electrolytes as needed, and eliminate the cause of the **fluid volume deficit**

B. Causes

   1. Vomiting and/or diarrhea

   2. Continuous GI irrigation

   3. GI suctioning

   4. Ileostomy or colostomy drainage

   5. Draining wounds, burns, or fistulas

   6. Increased urine output from the use of diuretics

C. Data collection

   1. Thirst

   2. Poor skin turgor and dry mucous membranes

   3. Increased heart rate, thready pulse, postural hypotension

   4. Rapid weight loss

   5. Flat neck or hand veins

   6. Dizziness or weakness

   7. Decrease in urine volume and dark, concentrated urine

   8. Increased specific gravity of the urine

   9. Confusion

   10. Increased hematocrit

D. Interventions

   1. The cause of the fluid volume deficit is treated and fluids are replaced (lactated Ringer's solution, 0.9% normal saline) as prescribed

   2. Monitor vital signs

   3. Check mucous membranes and skin turgor

   4. Monitor weight daily

   5. Monitor I&O (intake and output)

   6. Test urine for specific gravity

   7. Monitor hematocrit and electrolyte levels

IV. FLUID VOLUME EXCESS

A. Description

   1. Fluid intake or fluid retention exceeds the body's fluid needs

   2. Also called overhydration or fluid overload

   3. The goal of treatment is to restore fluid balance, correct electrolyte imbalances, if present, and eliminate or control the underlying cause of the overload

B. Data collection

   1. Cough and dyspnea

   2. Lung crackles

   3. Increased respirations and heart rate

   4. Increased blood pressure and bounding pulse

   5. Pitting edema

   6. Weight gain

   7. Neck and hand vein distention

   8. Decreased hematocrit

   9. Confusion

C. Interventions

   1. Monitor vital signs

   2. Position client in semi-Fowler's position

   3. Check for edema

4. Monitor I&O
5. Monitor weight
6. Administer diuretics as prescribed
7. Monitor hematocrit and electrolyte levels
8. Restrict fluids as prescribed
9. Provide a low-**sodium** diet as prescribed

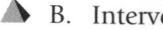

V. HYPOKALEMIA (Table 9-2)

A. Description (Box 9-4)
   1. A serum **potassium** level below 3.5 mEq/L
   2. **Potassium** deficit is the most common electrolyte imbalance and is potentially life threatening
B. Interventions
   1. Monitor vital signs
   2. Monitor neuromuscular activity
   3. Monitor I&O
   4. Check renal function before administering **potassium**
   5. Administer **potassium** supplements as prescribed (orally or monitor by IV)
   6. Oral potassium chloride has an unpleasant taste and should be taken with juice or other desired liquid

7. Oral **potassium** preparations can cause GI irritation and should not be taken on an empty stomach
8. If the client complains of abdominal pain, distention, nausea, vomiting, diarrhea, or GI bleeding, the oral **potassium** may need to be discontinued
9. When **potassium** is added to an IV solution, shake the bag and invert it to ensure that the **potassium** is evenly distributed
10. An IV bolus injection of **potassium** is never administered; it is always diluted
11. A client receiving more than 10 mEq/hour should be placed on a cardiac monitor; the infusion is controlled by an infusion device
12. Monitor for cardiac changes during the administration of **potassium**
13. Monitor electrolyte values
14. Monitor the IV site; if phlebitis or infiltration occurs, the IV should be stopped immediately and restarted at another site
15. Instruct client not to use salt substitutes containing **potassium** unless prescribed by the physician

VI. HYPERKALEMIA (see Table 9-2)

A. Description: A serum **potassium** level that exceeds 5.1 mEq/L (see Box 9-4)
B. Interventions
   1. Monitor vital signs
   2. Monitor for cardiac changes
   3. Decrease **potassium** intake
   4. Administer **potassium**-excreting diuretics as prescribed

TABLE 9-2

Potassium Imbalances

Hypokalemia	Hyperkalemia
CAUSES	**CAUSES**
Use of non–potassium-sparing diuretics	Renal failure
Diarrhea	Intestinal obstruction
Vomiting	Cell damage
Inadequate intake of potassium	Excessive oral or parenteral administration of potassium
Excessive gastric suction	Metabolic acidosis
Excessive fistula drainage	Addison's disease
Cushing's syndrome	Excessive use of potassium-based salt substitutes
Chronic use of corticosteroids	Transfusion of stored blood (breakdown of older red blood cells release potassium)
Renal disease	
Total parenteral nutrition	
Uncontrolled diabetes	
Alkalosis	
SIGNS AND SYMPTOMS	**SIGNS AND SYMPTOMS**
Leg and abdominal cramps	Muscle weakness
Lethargy and weakness	Paresthesias
Shallow respirations and thready pulse	Hypotension
Confusion	Diarrhea
Decreased or absent reflexes	Hyperactive bowel sounds
Hypoactive bowel sounds and ileus	Wide, flat P waves, widened QRS complex, prolonged PR interval, depressed ST segment, and narrow, peaked T waves
Postural hypotension	
Peaked P waves, flat T waves, depressed ST segment and U waves	

BOX 9-4

Potassium

NORMAL VALUE
3.5 to 5.1 mEq/L

COMMON FOOD SOURCES
Avocado
Bananas
Cantaloupe
Carrots
Fish
Mushrooms
Oranges
Potatoes
Pork, beef, veal
Raisins
Spinach
Strawberries
Tomatoes

5. Monitor I&O
6. Monitor laboratory values
7. Emergency treatment includes rapid IV administration of dextrose with regular insulin to move excess **potassium** into the cells
8. Administer **sodium** polystyrene sulfonate (Kayexalate) orally or by enema as prescribed, which releases **sodium** ions in exchange for primarily **potassium** ions and absorbs the **potassium** into the GI tract for excretion
9. Monitor for **calcium** and **magnesium** loss when using Kayexalate
10. Monitor renal function
11. Prepare for peritoneal or hemodialysis as prescribed
12. When blood transfusions are prescribed for a client with a **potassium** imbalance, the client should receive fresh blood, if possible, because transfusions of stored blood may elevate the **potassium** level as the breakdown of older blood cells releases **potassium**
13. Instruct client to avoid foods high in **potassium**
14. Instruct client to avoid the use of salt substitutes or other **potassium**-containing substances

VII. HYPONATREMIA (Table 9-3)
A. Description: A serum **sodium** level below 135 mEq/L (Box 9-5)
B. Interventions
   1. Monitor vital signs
   2. Monitor I&O
   3. Monitor weight
   4. Assess skin turgor and mucous membranes
   5. Restrict water intake and avoid tap water enemas
   6. Use normal saline solution rather than sterile water for irrigation
   7. Administer **sodium** replacement as prescribed and monitor electrolyte values
   8. Encourage foods high in **sodium**
   9. If the client is taking lithium, monitor lithium level, because **hyponatremia** can cause diminished lithium excretion, resulting in toxicity

VIII. HYPERNATREMIA (see Table 9-3)
A. Description: A serum **sodium** level that exceeds 145 mEq/L (see Box 9-5)
B. Interventions
   1. Monitor vital signs
   2. Monitor I&O
   3. Monitor electrolyte levels
   4. Increase water intake orally; provide water between meals or tube feedings and encourage the client to drink 8 to 10 glasses of water daily

TABLE 9-3

Sodium Imbalances

Hyponatremia	Hypernatremia
CAUSES	**CAUSES**
Inadequate sodium intake (Nothing by mouth [NPO], low-sodium diet)	Decreased water intake or excessive loss of water
Gastrointestinal suction	Fever
Excessive intake of water	Excessive perspiration
Irrigation of GI tubes with plain water	Dehydration
	Hyperventilation
Potent diuretics	Watery diarrhea
Increased perspiration	Enteral nutrition and total parental nutrition (TPN) deplete the cells of water
Draining skin lesions	
Burns	Diabetes insipidus
Nausea and vomiting	Cushing's syndrome
Diabetic ketoacidosis (DKA)	Impaired renal function
Syndrome of inappropriate antidiuretics hormone secretion (SIADH)	Use of corticosteroids
	Excessive administration of sodium bicarbonate
Retention of fluid, such as with kidney or heart failure	
SIGNS AND SYMPTOMS	**SIGNS AND SYMPTOMS**
Rapid, thready pulse	Dry mucous membranes
Postural blood pressure changes	Loss of skin turgor
Weakness	Thirst
Abdominal cramping	Flushed skin
Poor skin turgor	Elevated temperature
Muscle twitching and seizures	Oliguria
Apprehension	Muscle twitching
	Fatigue
	Confusion
	Seizures

BOX 9-5

Sodium

NORMAL VALUE
135 to 145 mEq/L

COMMON FOOD SOURCES
Bacon
Butter
Canned food
Cheese, such as American or cottage cheese
Hot dogs
Ketchup
Lunch meat
Milk
Mustard
Processed food
Snack food
Soy sauce
Table salt
White and whole-wheat bread

IX. HYPOCALCEMIA (Table 9-4)

A. Description: A serum **calcium** level below 8.6 mg/dL (Box 9-6)
B. Interventions
   1. Monitor vital signs
   2. Monitor for the presence of Chvostek's and Trousseau's signs
   3. Provide a quiet environment and avoid over-stimulation
   4. Initiate seizure precautions
   5. Administer **calcium** orally or monitor IV **calcium** administration as prescribed
   6. Administer vitamin D as prescribed to aid in the absorption of **calcium** from the intestinal tract
   7. Administer **calcium** supplements 1 to 2 hours after meals to maximize intestinal absorption
   8. Keep 10% **calcium** gluconate available for acute **calcium** deficit
   9. Monitor **calcium** levels closely after thyroid surgery
   10. Instruct client taking **calcium**-excreting medications to have serum **calcium** levels checked periodically
   11. Teach the client about the proper use of antacids or laxatives
   12. Instruct the client to consume foods high in **calcium**

X. HYPERCALCEMIA (see Table 9-4)

A. Description: A serum **calcium** level that exceeds 10 mg/dL (see Box 9-6)
B. Interventions
   1. Monitor vital signs
   2. Monitor for dysrhythmias
   3. Restrict **calcium** intake
   4. Increase mobility
   5. Assist with passive range-of-motion exercises when ambulation is not possible
   6. Move clients carefully
   7. Monitor for the development of pathological fractures
   8. Monitor for severe flank or abdominal pain and strain urine to check for urinary stones
   9. Monitor level of consciousness
   10. Monitor for confusion and neurological changes
   11. Avoid large doses of vitamin D supplements
   12. Avoid the use of thiazide diuretics
   13. Prepare for administration of phosphate as prescribed

TABLE 9-4

Calcium Imbalances

Hypocalcemia	Hpercalcemia
CAUSES	**CAUSES**
Inadequate dietary intake of calcium	Excessive intake of calcium supplements, milk, and antacid products containing calcium
Increased absorption of calcium from intestinal tract	
Inadequate vitamin D consumption	Excessive intake of vitamin D
Diarrhea	Increased bone reabsorption or destruction from conditions such as bone tumors, fractures, osteoporosis, immobility
Long-term immobilization and bone demineralization	
Excessive GI losses from diarrhea or wound draining	
End-stage renal disease	Decreased excretion of calcium
Calcium-excreting medications such as diuretics, caffeine, anticonvulsants, heparin, laxatives, nicotine	Renal failure
	Use of thiazide diuretics
	Hyperparathyroidism
Decreased secretion of parathyroid hormone	Use of lithium
	Use of glucocorticoids
Acute pancreatitis	Adrenal insufficiency
Crohn's disease	
Excessive administration of blood	
SIGNS AND SYMPTOMS	**SIGNS AND SYMPTOMS**
Tachycardia	Increased heart rate and blood pressure
Hypotension	
Paresthesias	Bounding pulse
Twitching	Bradycardia (late stage)
Cramps	Shortened QT interval and widened T wave
Tetany	
Positive Chvostek's or Trousseau's sign	Muscle weakness (hypotonicity)
Diarrhea	Diminished deep tendon reflexes
Hyperactive bowel sounds	
Prolongation of QT interval	Nausea and vomiting
	Constipation
	Abdominal distention
	Confusion, lethargy, coma

BOX 9-6

Calcium

NORMAL VALUE
8.6 to 10 mg/dL

COMMON FOOD SOURCES
Cheese
Collard greens
Milk and soy milk
Rhubarb
Sardines
Spinach
Tofu
Yogurt

14. Prepare for administration of calcitonin (Calcimar) as prescribed to increase incorporation of **calcium** into the bones

XI. HYPOMAGNESEMIA (Table 9-5)

A. Description: A serum **magnesium** level below 1.6 mg/dL (Box 9-7)
B. Interventions
   1. Monitor vital signs
   2. Monitor for dysrhythmias
   3. Monitor for neuromuscular changes
   4. Monitor I&O
   5. Initiate seizure precautions
   6. Administer **magnesium** supplements and monitor laboratory values
   7. Monitor serum **magnesium** levels every 12 to 24 hours when client is receiving **magnesium** by IV
   8. Monitor for reduced deep tendon reflexes suggesting **hypermagnesemia** during administration of **magnesium**
   9. Instruct client to eat food high in **magnesium**

XII. HYPERMAGNESEMIA (see Table 9-5)

A. Description: A serum **magnesium** level that exceeds 2.6 mg/dL (see Box 9-7)
B. Interventions
   1. Monitor vital signs
   2. Monitor for respiratory depression
   3. Monitor for hypotension, bradycardia, and dysrhythmias
   4. Monitor neurological and muscular activity
   5. Monitor level of consciousness
   6. Remove the source of the excess **magnesium**
   7. Monitor laboratory value
   8. Increase renal excretion by forcing fluids or administering loop diuretics as prescribed
   9. Prepare for the administration of **calcium** chloride or **calcium** gluconate if serum levels are more than 7 mEq/L
   10. Instruct clients regarding avoidance of the use of laxatives and antacids containing **magnesium**

XIII. HYPOPHOSPHATEMIA (Table 9-6)

A. Description: A serum **phosphorus** level below 2.7 mg/dL (Box 9-8)
B. Interventions
   1. Monitor vital signs
   2. Monitor respiratory status
   3. Move client carefully
   4. Administer phosphate as prescribed
   5. Check renal system before administering phosphate
   6. Monitor **calcium**, **phosphorus**, **sodium**, and chloride levels

TABLE 9-5

Magnesium Imbalances

Hypomagnesemia	Hypermagnesemia
CAUSES	**CAUSES**
Malnutrition	Overuse of antacids or laxatives containing magnesium
Diarrhea	
Celiac disease	
Crohn's disease	Renal insufficiency and renal failure
Alcoholism	
Prolonged gastric suctioning	Treatment of toxemia of pregnancy with magnesium
Ileostomy or colostomy, intestinal fistulas	
Acute pancreatitis	
Diabetic ketoacidosis	
Eclampsia	
Chemotherapy	
Sepsis	
SIGNS AND SYMPTOMS	**SIGNS AND SYMPTOMS**
Twitching	Hypotension
Paresthesias	Bradycardia
Hyperactive reflexes	Weak pulse
Irritability	Sweating and flushing
Confusion	Respiratory depression
Positive Chvostek's or Trousseau's signs	Loss of deep tendon reflexes
Shallow respirations	Prolonged PR interval, widened QRS complexes
Tetany	
Seizures	
Tachycardia	
Tall T waves depressed ST segment	

BOX 9-7

Magnesium

NORMAL VALUE
1.6 to 2.6 mg/dL

COMMON FOOD SOURCES
Avocado
Canned white tuna fish
Cauliflower
Oatmeal
Green leafy vegetables, such as spinach and broccoli
Yogurt
Milk
Peanut butter
Peas
Pork, beef, chicken
Potatoes
Raisins

TABLE 9-6

Phosphorus Imbalances

Hypophosphatemia	Hyperphosphatemia
CAUSES	**CAUSES**
Decreased nutritional intake and malnutrition	Excessive dietary intake of phosphorus
Use of magnesium-based or aluminum hydroxide–based antacids	Overuse of phosphate-containing laxatives or enemas
Renal failure	Vitamin D intoxication
Hyperparathyroidism	Hypoparathyroidism
Malignancy	Renal insufficiency
Hypercalcemia	Chemotherapy
Alcohol withdrawal	
Diabetic ketoacidosis	
Respiratory alkalosis	
SIGNS AND SYMPTOMS	**SIGNS AND SYMPTOMS**
Confusion	Neuromuscular irritability
Seizures	Muscle weakness
Weakness	Hyperactive reflexes
Decreased deep tendon reflexes	Tetany
Shallow respirations	Positive Chvostek's or Trousseau's sign
Increased bleeding tendency	
Immunosuppression	
Bone pain	

BOX 9-8

Phosphorus

NORMAL VALUE
2.7 to 4.5 mg/dL

COMMON FOOD SOURCES
Fish
Organ meats
Nuts
Pork, beef, chicken
Whole-grain breads and cereals

7. Administer vitamin D
8. Monitor for decreased neuromuscular activity
9. Monitor for **calcium** excess and kidney stones
10. Monitor for hematological changes
11. Decrease intake of **calcium**-rich foods and increase intake of meats and whole grains that contain **phosphorus**
12. Instruct client regarding the use of antacids

XIV. HYPERPHOSPHATEMIA (Table 9-6)
A. Description: A serum **phosphorus** level that exceeds 4.5 mg/dL (see Box 9-8)
B. Interventions
 1. Increase fecal excretion of **phosphorus** by binding **phosphorus** from food in the GI tract (aluminum hydroxide gel)
 2. Monitor laboratory values
 3. Prepare for dialysis if prescribed
 4. Monitor for signs of **hypocalcemia**
 5. Administer **calcium** as prescribed if **hypocalcemia** exists
 6. Monitor for neuromuscular irritability
 7. Monitor for hyperreflexia, tetany, and seizures
 8. Monitor for Trousseau's and Chvostek's signs

9. Instruct clients to avoid phosphate-containing medications, including laxatives and enemas
10. Instruct clients to decrease their intake of foods high in **phosphorus**
11. Instruct clients how to take phosphate-binding medications, emphasizing that these should be taken with meals or immediately after meals

PRACTICE QUESTIONS

1. The registered nurse (RN) tells the licensed practical nurse (LPN) that the physician has prescribed a hypotonic IV solution for a client. Which IV solution would the LPN obtain for administration to the client?
 1. 0.45% saline
 2. 5% dextrose in water
 3. 0% dextrose in water
 4. 5% dextrose in 0.9% saline
2. Intravenous (IV) lactated Ringer's solution is prescribed for a postoperative client. A nursing student is caring for the client, and the nursing instructor asks the student about the tonicity of the prescribed IV solution. The student responds by telling the instructor that the solution is:
 1. Isotonic
 2. Normotonic
 3. Hypotonic
 4. Hypertonic
3. A nurse is reading the physician's progress notes in the client's record and sees that the physician has documented "insensible fluid loss of approximately 800 mL daily." The nurse understands that this type of fluid loss can occur through:
 1. The GI tract
 2. Urinary output
 3. Wound drainage
 4. The skin
4. A nurse is reviewing the health records of assigned clients. The nurse plans care knowing that which client is likely at the lowest risk for the development of third-spacing?
 1. The client with cirrhosis
 2. The client with diabetes mellitus

3. The client with sepsis

4. The client with renal failure

5. A nurse is reviewing the health records of assigned clients. The nurse plans care knowing that which client is at risk for fluid volume deficit?

1. A client with a colostomy

2. A client with cirrhosis

3. A client with congestive heart failure (CHF)

4. A client with decreased kidney function

6. A nurse is caring for a client who has been taking diuretics on a long-term basis. A fluid volume deficit is suspected. Which finding would be noted in the client with this condition?

1. Gurgling respirations

2. Increased blood pressure

3. Decreased hematocrit

4. Increased specific gravity of the urine

7. A nurse is caring for a client with cirrhosis. The nurse notes that the client is dyspneic and crackles are heard on auscultation of the lungs. The nurse suspects fluid volume excess. What additional signs would the nurse expect to note in this client if a fluid volume excess is present?

1. Flat hand and neck veins

2. A weak and thready pulse

3. An increase in blood pressure

4. An increased urine output

8. The nurse is reviewing the health records of assigned clients. The nurse plans care knowing that which client is at risk for a potassium deficit?

1. The client on nasogastric (NG) suction

2. The client with renal disease

3. The client with Addison's disease

4. The client with metabolic acidosis

9. A nurse is instructing a client on how to decrease the intake of magnesium in the diet. The nurse tells the client that which food item contains the least amount of magnesium?

1. Processed drinking water

2. Peanut butter

3. Spinach

4. Broccoli

10. A nurse instructs a client at risk for hypokalemia about the foods high in potassium that should be included in the daily diet. The nurse tells the client that which food provides the least amount of potassium?

1. Spinach

2. Carrots

3. Apricots

4. Apple

11. A nurse reviews a client's electrolyte results and notes a potassium level of 5.5 mEq/L. The nurse understands that a potassium value at this level would be noted in which condition?

1. The client who sustained a traumatic burn

2. The client with Cushing's syndrome

3. The client with colitis

4. The client who has been overusing laxatives

12. A nurse reviews a client's electrolyte results and notes that the potassium level is 5.4 mEq/L. Which of the following would the nurse note on the cardiac monitor as a result of the laboratory value?

1. Narrow, peaked T waves

2. Prominent U wave

3. ST elevation

4. Peaked P wave

13. A nurse prepares to administer sodium polystyrene sulfonate (Kayexalate) to the client. Before administering the medication, the nurse reviews the action of the medication and understands that it:

1. Releases bicarbonate in exchange for primarily sodium ions

2. Releases sodium ions in exchange for primarily bicarbonate ions

3. Releases sodium ions in exchange for primarily potassium ions

4. Releases potassium ions in exchange for primarily sodium ions

14. A nurse reviews electrolyte values and notes a sodium level of 130 mEq/L. The nurse understands that which client is at risk for the development of a sodium value at this level?

1. The client with syndrome of inappropriate secretion of antidiuretic hormone (SIADH)

2. The client with an inadequate daily water intake

3. The client with watery diarrhea

4. The client with diabetes insipidus

15. A nurse is caring for a client with leukemia and notes that the client has poor skin turgor and flat neck and hand veins. The nurse suspects hyponatremia. What additional signs would the nurse expect to note in this client if hyponatremia is present?

1. Dry mucous membranes

2. Postural blood pressure changes

3. Intense thirst

4. Slow bounding pulse

16. A nurse is caring for a client with a diagnosis of hyperthyroidism. Laboratory studies are performed and the serum calcium level is 12.0 mg/dL. Based on this laboratory value, the nurse takes which action?

1. Documents the value in the client's record

2. Places the laboratory result form in the client's record

3. Informs the registered nurse of the laboratory value

4. Reassures the client that the laboratory result is normal

17. A nurse reviews a client's serum sodium level and notes that the level is 150 mEq/L. The physician prescribes dietary instructions for the client based on the sodium level. Which of the following

food items will the nurse instruct the client to avoid?
1. Spinach
2. Squash
3. Processed oat cereals
4. Molasses

18. A nurse reviews the client's serum calcium level and notes that the level is 4.0 mEq/L. The nurse understands that which condition would cause this serum calcium level?
1. Prolonged bed rest
2. Excessive ingestion of vitamin D
3. Renal disease
4. Hyperparathyroidism

19. A nurse is caring for a client with a suspected diagnosis of hypercalcemia. Which of the following signs would be an indication of this diagnosis?
1. Generalized muscle weakness
2. Twitching
3. Hyperactive bowel sounds
4. Positive Trousseau's sign

20. A nurse is instructing a client on how to decrease the intake of calcium in the diet. The nurse tells the client that which food item contains the least amount of calcium?
1. Butter
2. Milk
3. Spinach
4. Collard greens

21. A nurse is caring for a client with hyperparathyroidism and notes that the client's serum calcium level is 13 mg/dL. Which medication would the nurse prepare to administer as prescribed to the client?
1. Calcium gluconate
2. Calcium chloride
3. Calcitonin (Calcimar)
4. Large doses of vitamin D

22. A nurse is instructing a client on how to decrease the intake of potassium in the diet. The nurse tells the client that which food contains the least amount of potassium?
1. Potatoes
2. Apricots
3. Avocado
4. Lettuce

23. The nurse is caring for a client with renal failure. The laboratory results reveal a magnesium level of 3.6 mg/dL. Which of the following signs would the nurse expect to note in the client based on this magnesium level?
1. Twitching
2. Hyperactive reflexes
3. Irritability
4. Loss of deep tendon reflexes

24. The nurse reviews the client's serum phosphorus level and notes that the level is 2.0 mg/dL. The nurse understands that which condition caused this serum phosphorus level?
1. Alcoholism
2. Hypoparathyroidism
3. Chemotherapy
4. Vitamin D intoxication

25. A nurse is instructing a client on how to decrease the intake of phosphorus in the diet. The nurse tells the client that which food item contains the least amount of phosphorus?
1. Oranges
2. Fish
3. Whole-grain bread
4. Almonds

ALTERNATE FORMAT QUESTION: CHART/EXHIBIT

CLIENT'S CHART
Laboratory Test Results
Potassium level of 4.5 mEq/L
Sodium level of 132 mEq/L

A nurse is caring for a client with a nasogastric (NG) tube. NG tube irrigations are prescribed to be performed once every shift. Which solution is the most appropriate to use for the NG irrigation?
1. Tap water
2. Distilled water
3. Sterile water
4. Normal saline

ANSWERS

1. *Answer:* **1**
Rationale: 5% dextrose in water is an isotonic solution. 10% dextrose in water and 5% dextrose in 0.9% saline are hypertonic solutions. 0.45% saline is hypotonic and is probably the only hypotonic solution used in clinical situations. Distilled water is another example of a hypotonic solution. Hypotonic solutions contain a lower concentration of salt or more water than an isotonic solution.
Test-Taking Strategy: Use the process of elimination. Note the similarities in options 2, 3, and 4. All these solutions contain dextrose. Option 1 is different than the others. Review the tonicity of IV solutions if you had difficulty with this question.
Level of Cognitive Ability: Application
Client Needs: Physiological Integrity
Integrated Process: Nursing Process/Implementation
Content Area: Fundamental Skills
Reference: Linton, A., & Maebius, N. (2003). *Introduction to medical-surgical nursing* (3rd ed.). Philadelphia: W.B. Saunders, p. 237.

2. *Answer:* **1**

Rationale: Lactated Ringer's solution is an isotonic solution. Other isotonic solutions include 5% dextrose in water, 0.9% normal saline, and 5% dextrose in 0.225% normal saline. 0.45% normal saline is hypotonic. 10% dextrose in water, 5% dextrose in 0.9% normal saline, and 5% dextrose in 0.45% normal saline are hypertonic solutions.

Test-Taking Strategy: Knowledge regarding the tonicity of the various IV solutions is needed to answer the question. Remember that lactated Ringer's solution is an isotonic solution. Review this information if you had difficulty with this question.

Level of Cognitive Ability: Comprehension
Client Needs: Physiological Integrity
Integrated Process: Teaching/Learning
Content Area: Fundamental Skills
References: Linton, A. & Maebius, N. (2003). *Introduction to medical-surgical nursing* (3rd ed.). Philadelphia: W.B. Saunders, p. 238.
Potter, P. & Perry, A. (2005) *Fundamentals of nursing* (6th ed.). St. Louis: Mosby, p. 1160.

3. *Answer:* **4**

Rationale: Sensible losses are those that the person is aware of, such as through wound drainage, GI tract losses, and urination. Insensible losses may occur without the person's awareness. Insensible losses occur daily through the skin and the lungs.

Test-Taking Strategy: Note that the issue of the question is insensible fluid loss. Use the process of elimination, noting the similarity in options 1, 2, and 3. These types of losses can be measured for accurate output. Fluid loss through the skin cannot be accurately measured, only approximated. If you had difficulty with this question, review the difference between sensible and insensible fluid loss.

Level of Cognitive Ability: Comprehension
Client Needs: Physiological Integrity
Integrated Process: Nursing Process/Data Collection
Content Area: Fundamental Skills
References: Black, J., & Hawks, J. (2005). *Medical-surgical nursing: Clinical management for positive outcomes* (7th ed.). Philadelphia: W.B. Saunders, p. 230.
Linton, A., & Maebius, N. (2003), *Introduction to medical-surgical nursing* (3rd ed.). Philadelphia: W.B. Saunders, pp. 154-159.

4. *Answer:* **2**

Rationale: Fluid that shifts into the interstitial spaces and remains there is referred to as third-space fluid. Common sites for third-spacing include the abdomen, pleural cavity, peritoneal cavity, and pericardial sac. Third-space fluid is physiologically useless because it does not circulate to provide nutrients for the cells. Risk factors include clients with liver or kidney disease, major trauma, burns, sepsis, wound healing or major surgery, malignancy, malabsorption syndrome, malnutrition, and alcoholic or older clients.

Test-Taking Strategy: Note the key words, *lowest risk*. These words indicate a false response question and that you need to select the client at least risk for third-spacing. Eliminate options 1 and 4 first because it is likely that fluid balance disturbances will occur with these conditions. From the remaining options, sepsis is the option that is most acute and therefore is most similar to options 1 and 4. Review the risk factors associated with third-spacing if you had difficulty with this question.

Level of Cognitive Ability: Analysis
Client Needs: Physiological Integrity
Integrated Process: Nursing Process/Planning
Content Area: Fundamental Skills
Reference: Black, J., & Hawks, J. (2005). *Medical-surgical nursing: Clinical management for positive outcomes* (7th ed.). Philadelphia: W.B. Saunders, pp. 213-219.

5. *Answer:* **1**

Rationale: Causes of a fluid volume deficit include vomiting, diarrhea, conditions that cause increased respirations or increased urinary output, insufficient IV fluid replacement, draining fistulas, or an ileostomy or colostomy. A client with cirrhosis, CHF, or decreased kidney function is at risk for fluid volume excess.

Test-Taking Strategy: Read the question carefully, noting that it asks for the client at risk for a deficit. Read each option and think about the fluid imbalance that can occur in each client. The clients presented in options 2, 3, and 4 retain fluid. The only condition that can cause a fluid volume deficit is the condition noted in option 1. If you had difficulty with this question, review the causes of fluid volume deficit.

Level of Cognitive Ability: Analysis
Client Needs: Physiological Integrity
Integrated Process: Nursing Process/Planning
Content Area: Fundamental Skills
Reference: Linton, A., & Maebius, N. (2003). *Introduction to medical-surgical nursing* (3rd ed.). Philadelphia: W.B. Saunders, pp. 158-159, 697.

6. *Answer:* **4**

Rationale: Findings in a client with a fluid volume deficit include increased respirations and heart rate, decreased central venous pressure (CVP), weight loss, poor skin turgor, dry mucous membranes, decreased urine volume, increased specific gravity of the urine, dark-colored and odorous urine, an increased hematocrit, and altered level of consciousness. The signs in options 1, 2, and 3 are seen in a client with fluid volume excess.

Test-Taking Strategy: Use the process of elimination. Eliminate options 1 and 2 first. Gurgling respirations and increased blood pressure are noted in fluid volume excess. Remember that the specific gravity of urine is increased in a client with a fluid volume deficit. If you had difficulty with this question, review the findings noted in fluid volume deficit.

Level of Cognitive Ability: Comprehension
Client Needs: Physiological Integrity
Integrated Process: Nursing Process/Data Collection
Content Area: Fundamental Skills
Reference: Black, J., & Hawks, J. (2005). *Medical-surgical nursing: Clinical management for positive outcomes* (7th ed.). Philadelphia: W.B. Saunders, p. 208.

7. *Answer:* **3**

Rationale: Findings associated with fluid volume excess include cough, dyspnea, crackles, tachypnea, tachycardia, an elevated blood pressure and a bounding pulse, an elevated central venous pressure, weight gain, edema, neck and hand vein distention, altered level of consciousness, and a decreased hematocrit.

Test-Taking Strategy: Use the process of elimination. Note the similarities in options 1, 2, and 4. Each of these signs relates to a decrease in fluid volume. Option 3 reflects an increase. If you had difficulty with this question review the signs noted in fluid volume excess.

Level of Cognitive Ability: Comprehension
Client Needs: Physiological Integrity
Integrated Process: Nursing Process/Data Collection
Content Area: Fundamental Skills
References: Black, J., & Hawks, J. (2005). *Medical-surgical nursing: Clinical management for positive outcomes* (7th ed.). Philadelphia: W.B. Saunders, p. 225.
Linton, A., & Maebius, N. (2003). *Introduction to medical surgical nursing* (3rd ed.). Philadelphia: W.B. Saunders, pp. 159, 730.

8. Answer: 1
Rationale: Potassium-rich gastrointestinal (GI) fluids are lost through GI suction, placing the client at risk for hypokalemia. The client with renal disease, Addison's disease, and metabolic acidosis are at risk for hyperkalemia.

Test-Taking Strategy: Read the question carefully, noting that it asks for the client at risk for hypokalemia. Read each option and think about the electrolyte loss that can occur in each. Option 1 clearly identifies a loss of body fluid. If you had difficulty with this question, review the causes of hypokalemia.

Level of Cognitive Ability: Analysis
Client Needs: Physiological Integrity
Integrated Process: Nursing Process/Planning
Content Area: Fundamental Skills
Reference: Linton, A., & Maebius, N. (2003). *Introduction to medical-surgical nursing* (3rd ed.). Philadelphia: W.B. Saunders, p. 162.

9. Answer: 1
Rationale: Drinking water that has not been processed through a water softener is high in magnesium. Peanut butter, spinach, and broccoli are magnesium-containing foods and should be avoided by the client on a magnesium-restricted diet.

Test-Taking Strategy: Use the process of elimination and note the key words, *least amount.* These words indicate a false response question and that you need to select the item lowest in magnesium. Eliminate options 3 and 4 first because they are similar. Recalling that unprocessed water is high in magnesium will direct you to option 1 from the remaining options. Review the foods that are high in magnesium if you had difficulty with this question.

Level of Cognitive Ability: Application
Client Needs: Health Promotion and Maintenance
Integrated Process: Teaching/Learning
Content Area: Fundamental Skills
Reference: Peckenpaugh, N. (2003). *Nutrition essentials and diet therapy* (9th ed.). Philadelphia: W.B. Saunders, pp. 97, 115.

10. Answer: 4
Rationale: An apple provides approximately 3 mEq of potassium per serving. Spinach and carrots ($^1/_2$ cup cooked) and

four apricots provide approximately 7 mEq of potassium per serving.

Test-Taking Strategy: Use the process of elimination and note the key words, *least amount.* These words indicate a false response question and that you need to select the item lowest in potassium. Recalling the potassium content of the foods identified will direct you to option 4. Review the foods high in potassium if you had difficulty with this question.

Level of Cognitive Ability: Application
Client Needs: Health Promotion and Maintenance
Integrated Process: Teaching/Learning
Content Area: Fundamental Skills
Reference: Peckenpaugh, N. (2003). *Nutrition essentials and diet therapy* (9th ed.). Philadelphia: W.B. Saunders, p. 98.

11. Answer: 1
Rationale: A serum potassium level that exceeds 5.1 mEq/L is indicative of hyperkalemia. Clients who experience cellular shifting of potassium, as in the early stages of massive cell destruction, such as in trauma, burns, sepsis, or with metabolic or respiratory acidosis, are at risk for hyperkalemia. The client with Cushing's syndrome or colitis and the client who has been overusing laxatives are at risk for hypokalemia.

Test-Taking Strategy: Use the process of elimination and eliminate options 3 and 4 first because they are similar and reflect a gastrointestinal loss. From the remaining options, recalling that cell destruction causes potassium shifts will assist in directing you to the correct option. Remember that Cushing's syndrome presents a risk for hypokalemia and that Addison's disease presents a risk for hyperkalemia. Review the causes of hyperkalemia if you had difficulty with this question.

Level of Cognitive Ability: Analysis
Client Needs: Physiological Integrity
Integrated Process: Nursing Process/Data Collection
Content Area: Fundamental Skills
References: Chernecky, C., & Berger, B. (2004). *Laboratory tests and diagnostic procedures* (4th ed.). Philadelphia: W.B. Saunders, p. 889.
Linton, A., & Maebius, N. (2003). *Introduction to medical-surgical nursing* (3rd ed.). Philadelphia: W.B. Saunders, p. 1034.

12. Answer: 1
Rationale: A serum potassium level of 5.4 mEq/L is indicative of hyperkalemia. Cardiac changes include a wide, flat P wave, prolonged PR interval, widened QRS complex, narrow, peaked T waves, and depressed ST segment.

Test-Taking Strategy: From the information in the question, you need to determine that this condition is a hyperkalemic one. From this point, it is necessary to know the cardiac changes that are expected when hyperkalemia exists. Review these cardiac changes if you had difficulty with this question.

Level of Cognitive Ability: Analysis
Client Needs: Physiological Integrity
Integrated Process: Nursing Process/Data Collection
Content Area: Fundamental Skills
Reference: Pagana, K., & Pagana, T. (2003). *Mosby's diagnostic and laboratory test reference* (6th ed.). St. Louis: Mosby, p. 698.

13. *Answer:* **3**

Rationale: Sodium polystyrene sulfonate (Kayexalate) is a cation exchange resin used in the treatment of hyperkalemia. The resin either passes through the intestine or is retained in the colon. It releases sodium ions in exchange for primarily potassium ions. The therapeutic effect occurs 2 to 12 hours after oral administration and longer after rectal administration.

Test-Taking Strategy: Use the process of elimination. Looking at the name of the medication (Kayexalate) closely will assist in recalling the action of the medication. If you had difficulty with this question, review the action of this medication.

Level of Cognitive Ability: Comprehension

Client Needs: Physiological Integrity

Integrated Process: Nursing Process/Planning

Content Area: Pharmacology

Reference: Hodgson, B., & Kizior, R. (2005). *Saunders nursing drug handbook 2005.* Philadelphia: W.B. Saunders, pp. 980-981.

14. *Answer:* **1**

Rationale: Hyponatremia is a serum sodium level below 135 mEq/L. Hyponatremia can result secondary to SIADH. The client with an inadequate daily water intake, watery diarrhea, or diabetes insipidus is at risk for hypernatremia.

Test-Taking Strategy: Knowledge regarding the normal sodium level and the causes of hyponatremia are required to answer the question. Remember that hyponatremia can result secondary to SIADH. Review these causes if you had difficulty with this question.

Level of Cognitive Ability: Analysis

Client Needs: Physiological Integrity

Integrated Process: Nursing Process/Data Collection

Content Area: Fundamental Skills

Reference: Pagana, K., & Pagana, T. (2003). *Mosby's diagnostic and laboratory test reference* (6th ed.). St. Louis: Mosby, p. 814.

15. *Answer:* **2**

Rationale: Postural blood pressure changes occur in the client with hyponatremia. Dry mucous membranes and intense thirst are seen in clients with hypernatremia. A slow, bounding pulse is not indicative of hyponatremia. In hyponatremia, a rapid thready pulse is noted.

Test-Taking Strategy: Use the process of elimination and note the information provided in the question. Eliminate options 1 and 3 first because they are similar (a client with dry mucous membranes is likely to have intense thirst). From the remaining options, it is necessary to recall the signs of hyponatremia. If you have difficulty with this question, review the signs associated with hyponatremia.

Level of Cognitive Ability: Analysis

Client Needs: Physiological Integrity

Integrated Process: Nursing Process/Data Collection

Content Area: Fundamental Skills

Reference: Linton, A., & Maebius, N. (2003). *Introduction to medical-surgical nursing* (3rd ed.). Philadelphia: W.B. Saunders, pp. 160-161.

16. *Answer:* **3**

Rationale: The normal serum calcium level ranges from 8.6 to 10.0 mg/dL. The client is experiencing hypercalcemia and the nurse would inform the registered nurse of the laboratory value.

Because the client is experiencing hypercalcemia, options 1, 2, and 4 are incorrect.

Test-Taking Strategy: Focus on the laboratory value in the question to determine that the client is experiencing hypercalcemia. Also, note that options 1, 2, and 4 are similar and indicate that no action would be taken to report the value. Review the normal calcium level if you had difficulty with this question.

Level of Cognitive Ability: Application

Client Needs: Physiological Integrity

Integrated Process: Nursing Process/Implementation

Content Area: Fundamental Skills

Reference: Malarkey, L., & McMorrow, M. (2005). *Nursing guide to laboratory and diagnostic tests.* Philadelphia: W.B. Saunders, p. 164.

17. *Answer:* **3**

Rationale: The normal serum sodium level is 135 to 145 mEq/L. A serum sodium level of 150 mEq/L is indicative of hypernatremia. Based on this finding, the nurse would instruct the client to avoid foods high in sodium. Spinach and molasses are good food sources of calcium. Squash is high in phosphorus.

Test-Taking Strategy: Note the key word, *avoid*. This word indicates a false response question and that you need to select the food item high in sodium. Recall the normal serum sodium level. After determining that the client has hypernatremia, determining the food to avoid is the issue. Eliminate options 1 and 2 first because these are basically very healthy foods. From the remaining options, note the word "processed" in option 3. Processed foods tend to be higher in sodium content, so this is the food to avoid. Review foods high in sodium content if you had difficulty with this question.

Level of Cognitive Ability: Application

Client Needs: Health Promotion and Maintenance

Integrated Process: Teaching/Learning

Content Area: Fundamental Skills

Reference: Peckenpaugh, N. (2003). *Nutrition essentials and diet therapy* (9th ed.). Philadelphia: W.B. Saunders, p. 156.

18. *Answer:* **1**

Rationale: The normal serum calcium level is 8.6 to 10.0 mg/dL. A client with a serum calcium level of 4.0 mEq/L is experiencing hypocalcemia. Excessive ingestion of vitamin D, renal disease, and hyperparathyroidism are causative factors associated with hypercalcemia. Although immobilization can initially cause hypercalcemia, the long-term effect of prolonged bed rest is hypocalcemia.

Test-Taking Strategy: Knowledge regarding the normal serum calcium level will assist in determining that the client is experiencing hypocalcemia. This should help in eliminating option 2. Recalling the causative factors associated with hypocalcemia is necessary to select the correct option from those remaining. Remember that the long-term effect of prolonged bed rest is hypocalcemia. If you had difficulty with the question, review the causative factors associated with hypocalcemia.

Level of Cognitive Ability: Analysis

Client Needs: Physiological Integrity

Integrated Process: Nursing Process/Data Collection

Content Area: Fundamental Skills

Reference: Pagana, K., & Pagana, T. (2003). *Mosby's diagnostic and laboratory test reference* (6th ed.). St. Louis: Mosby, p. 280.

19. *Answer:* **1**
Rationale: Generalized muscle weakness is seen in hypercalcemia. Options 2, 3, and 4 identify signs of hypocalcemia.
Test-Taking Strategy: Use the process of elimination, noting that options 2, 3, and 4 are similar because they all reflect a hyperactivity of body systems. The option that is different is option 1. Review the signs of hypercalcemia if you had difficulty with this question.
Level of Cognitive Ability: Analysis
Client Needs: Physiological Integrity
Integrated Process: Nursing Process/Data Collection
Content Area: Fundamental Skills
Reference: Phipps, W., Monahan, F., Sands, J., Marek, J., & Neighbors, M. (2003). *Medical-surgical nursing: Health and illness perspectives* (7th ed.). St. Louis: Mosby, p. 257.

20. *Answer:* **1**
Rationale: Butter comes from milk fat and does not contain significant amounts of calcium. Milk, spinach, and collard greens are calcium-containing foods and should be avoided by the client on a calcium-restricted diet.
Test-Taking Strategy: Note the key words, *least amount.* These words indicate a false response question and that you need to select the item lowest in calcium. Option 2 can be easily eliminated first. Eliminate options 3 and 4 next because they are similar. Review the foods high and low in calcium if you had difficulty with this question.
Level of Cognitive Ability: Application
Client Needs: Health Promotion and Maintenance
Integrated Process: Teaching/Learning
Content Area: Fundamental Skills
Reference: Peckenpaugh, N. (2003). *Nutrition essentials and diet therapy* (9th ed.). Philadelphia: W.B. Saunders, p. 97.

21. *Answer:* **3**
Rationale: The normal serum calcium level is 8.6 to 10.0 mg/dL. This client is experiencing hypercalcemia. Calcium gluconate and calcium chloride are medications used in the treatment of tetany, which occurs as a result of acute hypocalcemia. In hypercalcemia, large doses of vitamin D need to be avoided. Calcitonin, a thyroid hormone, decreases the plasma calcium level by inhibiting bone resorption and lowering the serum calcium concentration.
Test-Taking Strategy: Recalling the normal serum calcium level will assist in determining that the client is experiencing hypercalcemia. With this knowledge, you can easily eliminate options 1 and 2, because you would not administer medication that adds calcium to the body. Remembering that excessive vitamin D is a causative factor of hypercalcemia will assist in eliminating option 4. If you had difficulty with this question, review the treatment for hypercalcemia.
Level of Cognitive Ability: Application
Client Needs: Physiological Integrity
Integrated Process: Nursing Process/Planning
Content Area: Pharmacology
Reference: Hodgson, B., & Kizior, R. (2005). *Saunders nursing drug handbook 2005.* Philadelphia: W.B. Saunders, p. 153.

22. *Answer:* **4**
Rationale: Lettuce contains less than 100 mg of potassium. Potatoes, apricots, and avocado are potassium-containing foods and should be avoided by the client on a potassium-restricted diet.
Test-Taking Strategy: Note the key words, *least amount.* These words indicate a false response question and that you need to select the item that is lowest in potassium. Recalling the foods high in potassium will direct you to option 4. If you had difficulty with the question, review these foods.
Level of Cognitive Ability: Application
Client Needs: Health Promotion and Maintenance
Integrated Process: Teaching/Learning
Content Area: Fundamental Skills
Reference: Nix, S. (2005). *Williams' basic nutrition and diet therapy* (12th ed.). St. Louis: Mosby, pp. 137-138.

23. *Answer:* **4**
Rationale: The normal magnesium level is 1.6 to 2.6 mg/dL. A client with a magnesium level of 3.6 mg/dL is experiencing hypermagnesemia. Options 1, 2, and 3 would be noted in a client with hypomagnesemia.
Test-Taking Strategy: Knowledge regarding the normal magnesium level and the associated signs related to an imbalance are helpful in answering the question. Use the process of elimination, noting that options 1, 2, and 3 are similar because they reflect neurological excitability. If you had difficulty with this question, review the signs noted for magnesium imbalance.
Level of Cognitive Ability: Analysis
Client Needs: Physiological Integrity
Integrated Process: Nursing Process/Data Collection
Content Area: Fundamental Skills
Reference: Linton, A., & Maebius, N. (2003), *Introduction to medical-surgical nursing* (3rd ed.). Philadelphia: W.B. Saunders, p. 163.

24. *Answer:* **1**
Rationale: The normal serum phosphorus level is 2.7 to 4.5 mg/dL. The client in this question is experiencing hypophosphatemia. Causative factors relate to decreased nutritional intake and malnutrition. A poor nutritional state is associated with alcoholism. Hypoparathyroidism, chemotherapy, and vitamin D intoxication are causative factors of hyperphosphatemia.
Test-Taking Strategy: Knowledge regarding the normal phosphorus level is required to determine the condition that this client is experiencing. From this point, it is necessary to know the causes of hypophosphatemia. Remember that causative factors relate to decreased nutritional intake and malnutrition. If you had difficulty with this question, review the causative factors associated with hypophosphatemia.
Level of Cognitive Ability: Analysis
Client Needs: Physiological Integrity
Integrated Process: Nursing Process/Data Collection
Content Area: Fundamental Skills
References: Black, J., & Hawks, J. (2005). *Medical-surgical nursing: Clinical management for positive outcomes* (7th ed.). Philadelphia: W.B. Saunders, p. 242.
Pagana, K., & Pagana, T. (2003). *Mosby's diagnostic and laboratory test reference* (6th ed.). St. Louis: Mosby, pp. 672-673.

25. *Answer:* **1**
Rationale: An orange contains the least amount of phosphorus. Foods high in phosphorus include fish, pork, beef, chicken, organ meats, nuts, whole-grain breads, and cereals.

Test-Taking Strategy: Note the key words, *least amount.* These words indicate a false response question and that you need to select the food that contains the least amount of phosphorus. Recalling the foods that are high and low in phosphorus will direct you to option 1. Review these foods if you had difficulty with this question.
Level of Cognitive Ability: Application
Client Needs: Health Promotion and Maintenance
Integrated Process: Teaching/Learning
Content Area: Fundamental Skills
Reference: Nix, S. (2005). *Williams' basic nutrition and diet therapy* (12th ed.). St. Louis: Mosby, pp. 133-134.

ALTERNATE FORMAT QUESTION: CHART/EXHIBIT

Answer: 4
Rationale: A potassium level of 4.5 mEq/L is within normal range. A sodium level of 132 mEq/L is low, indicating hyponatremia. In clients with hyponatremia, normal (isotonic) saline should be used rather than sterile water for GI irrigations.
Test-Taking Strategy: Use the process of elimination. Note that sterile water, distilled water, and tap water are similar. The only option that is different is option 4. If you had difficulty with this question, review the care for the client experiencing hyponatremia.
Level of Cognitive Ability: Application
Client Needs: Physiological Integrity
Integrated Process: Nursing Process/Implementation
Content Area: Fundamental Skills
Reference: Linton, A., & Maebius, N. (2003). *Introduction to medical-surgical nursing* (3rd ed.). Philadelphia: W.B. Saunders, pp. 160-161.

REFERENCES

Black, J., & Hawks, J. (2005). *Medical-surgical nursing: Clinical management for positive outcomes* (7th ed.). Philadelphia: W.B. Saunders.

Chernecky, C., & Berger, B. (2004). *Laboratory tests and diagnostic procedures* (4th ed.). Philadelphia: W.B. Saunders.

Hodgson, B., & Kizior, R. (2005). *Saunders nursing drug handbook 2005.* Philadelphia: W.B. Saunders.

Linton, A., & Maebius, N. (2003). *Introduction to medical-surgical nursing* (3rd ed.). Philadelphia: W.B. Saunders.

Malarkey, L., & McMorrow, M. (2005). *Nursing guide to laboratory and diagnostic tests.* Philadelphia: W.B. Saunders.

Nix, S. (2005). *Williams' basic nursing and diet therapy* (12th ed). St. Louis: Mosby.

Pagana, K., & Pagana, T. (2003). *Mosby's diagnostic and laboratory test reference* (6th ed.). St. Louis: Mosby.

Peckenpaugh, N. (2003). *Nutrition essentials and diet therapy* (9th ed). Philadelphia: W.B. Saunders.

Phipps, W., Monahan, F., Sands, J., Marek, J., & Neighbors, M. (2003). *Medical-surgical nursing: Health and illness perspectives* (7th ed.). St. Louis: Mosby.

Acid-Base Balance

PYRAMID TERMS

Allen's test Test for determining collateral circulation to the hand by evaluating the patency of the radial and ulnar arteries.

metabolic acidosis The total concentration of buffer base is lower than normal, with a relative increase in the H^+ ion concentration. It results from losing buffer bases or retaining too much acid without sufficient base. It occurs in conditions such as renal failure and diabetic ketoacidosis, and from the production of lactic acid or the ingestion of toxins, such as aspirin.

metabolic alkalosis A deficit or loss of H^+ ions or acids or an excess of base (bicarbonate). It results from an accumulation of base or a loss of acid without a comparable loss of base in the body fluids. It is caused by conditions resulting in hypovolemia, the loss of gastric fluid, excessive bicarbonate intake, massive transfusion of whole blood, and hyperaldosteronism.

respiratory acidosis The total concentration of buffer base is lower than normal, with a relatively increasing hydrogen ion (H^+) concentration; thus, a greater number of H^+ ions are circulating in the blood than can be absorbed by the buffer system. It is caused by primary defects in the function of the lungs or by changes in normal respiratory patterns as a result of secondary problems. Any condition that causes an obstruction of the airway or depresses respiratory status can cause respiratory acidosis.

respiratory alkalosis A deficit of carbonic acid (H_2CO_3) or a decrease in H^+ ion concentration; results from an accumulation of base or a loss of acid without a comparable loss of base in the body fluids. It is caused by conditions that cause overstimulation of the respiratory status.

PYRAMID TO SUCCESS

Acid-base imbalance is a content area that is sometimes viewed as complex to understand. It is important to understand the description of each imbalance and then to review the causes of each disorder, correlating the pathophysiology with each cause. From this point, note the signs and symptoms related to each disorder and the treatment associated with the clinical manifestations. Maintenance of a patent airway is a priority. The nurse also needs to monitor vital signs, cardiovascular status, neurological status, intake and output, laboratory values, and arterial blood gas values. Remember, safety and seizure precautions may need to be initiated. The Integrated Processes addressed in this chapter are Clinical Problem-Solving Process (Nursing Process), Caring, Communication and Documentation, and Teaching/Learning.

CLIENT NEEDS
Safe, Effective Care Environment

Accident prevention

Establishment of priorities

Informed consent for invasive procedures, such as obtaining arterial blood gas specimens or treatments, related to the various acid-base imbalances

Medical and surgical asepsis

Providing safety to the client when implementing various treatments for the acid-base disorder

Standard, transmission-based, and other precautions

Health Promotion and Maintenance

Data collection techniques

Disease prevention

Health and wellness

Identifying clients at risk for an acid-base imbalance

Reinforcing instructions to the client and family about the prevention, early detection, and treatment measures for health disorders

Psychosocial Integrity

Emotional support of the client and family

Sensory/perceptual alterations

Support systems

Therapeutic interactions

Physiological Integrity

Administer and monitor medications, IV (intravenous) fluids, and other prescribed therapies

Assist with determining the results from an arterial blood gas study

Assist with obtaining arterial blood gases

Document the expected and unexpected responses to the therapy

Identify clients at risk for an acid-base disturbance

Monitor for changes in status and complications

Provide wound care when blood is obtained for a blood gas determination

Reduce the likelihood that an acid-base disturbance will occur

I. HYDROGEN IONS, ACIDS, AND BASES

A. Hydrogen ions (H^+)
   1. Vital to life
   2. Expressed as pH
   3. pH of body fluid is normally alkaline (between 7.35 and 7.45)

B. Acids
   1. Produced as end products of metabolism
   2. Contain hydrogen ions
   3. Hydrogen ion donors, which means that acids give up H^+ ions to neutralize or decrease the strength of an acid or to form a weaker base
   4. The number of hydrogen ions in body fluid determines whether is acid, alkaline, or neutral

C. Bases
   1. Contain no H^+ ions
   2. Hydrogen ion acceptors
   3. Accept H^+ ions from acids to neutralize or decrease the strength of a base or to form a weaker acid

II. REGULATORY SYSTEMS FOR H^+ CONCENTRATION IN THE BLOOD

A. Buffers
   1. The fastest acting regulatory system
   2. Provide immediate protection against changes in H^+ ion concentration in the extracellular fluid
   3. Serve as a transport mechanism that carries excess H^+ ions to the lungs
   4. Once the primary buffer systems react, they are consumed, and this leaves the body less able to withstand further stress until they are replaced

B. Primary buffer systems in extracellular fluid
   1. Hemoglobin (Hgb) system
      a. In the red blood cells (RBCs)
      b. Maintains acid-base balance by a process called chloride shift
      c. Chloride shifts in and out of the cells in response to the level of oxygen (O_2) in the blood
   2. Plasma proteins system
      a. Functions in conjunction with the liver to vary the amount of H^+ ions in the chemical structure of protein
      b. Plasma proteins have the ability to attract or release H^+ ions
   3. Carbonic acid–bicarbonate system
      a. Maintains a pH of 7.4, with a ratio of 20 parts bicarbonate to 1 part carbonic acid (20:1)
      b. This ratio (20:1) determines H^+ ions concentration of body fluid
      c. Carbonic acid concentration is controlled by the excretion of CO_2 by the lungs; the rate and depth of respiration changes is the response to changes in CO_2
      d. Bicarbonate concentration is controlled by the kidneys, which selectively retain or secrete bicarbonates in response to body needs
   4. Phosphate buffer system
      a. Present in the cells and body fluids
      b. Especially active in the kidneys
      c. Acts like bicarbonate and clears excess H^+

C. Lungs
   1. Body's second defense, which interacts with the buffer system to maintain acid-base balance
   2. In acidosis, the pH goes down and the respiratory rate and depth go up in an attempt to blow off acids; the carbonic acid created by the neutralizing action of bicarbonate can be carried to the lungs, where it is reduced to CO_2 and water (H_2O) and exhaled; thus, H^+ ions are inactivated and excreted
   3. In alkalosis, the pH goes up and the respiratory rate and depth go down; CO_2 is retained, and the carbonic acid concentration increases to neutralize and decrease the strength of excess bicarbonate
   4. The action of the lungs is reversible in controlling an excess or deficit
   5. The lungs can hold H^+ ions until the deficit is corrected or can inactivate H^+ ions, changing them to water molecules to be exhaled as CO_2 and thereby correcting the excess
   6. The lungs can inactivate only H^+ ions carried by carbonic acid (H_2CO_3); excess H^+ ions created by other problems must be excreted by the kidneys

D. Kidneys
   1. The ultimate correction of acid-base disturbances is dependent on the kidneys, even though the renal excretion of acids and alkali occurs more slowly
   2. Compensation requires a few hours to several days; however, it is a more thorough and selective process than that of other regulators
   3. In acidosis, the pH goes down, and excess H^+ ions are secreted into the tubules and combine with buffers for excretion in the urine
   4. In alkalosis, the pH goes up, and bicarbonate ions move into the tubules, combine with sodium, and are excreted in the urine

5. Selective regulation of bicarbonate in the kidneys
   a. The kidneys restore bicarbonate by releasing of H^+ ions and holding on to bicarbonate ions
   b. Extra H^+ ions are excreted in the urine in the form of phosphoric acid
   c. The alteration of certain amino acids in the renal tubules results in a diffusion of ammonia into the kidneys; the ammonia combines with extra H^+ ions and is excreted into the urine

E. Potassium
   1. Plays an exchange role in maintaining acid-base balance
   2. The body changes the potassium (K) level by drawing H^+ ions into the cell or by pushing them out of the cell
   3. In acidosis, the body protects itself from the acid state by moving H^+ ions into the cell; therefore, K moves out to make room for H^+ ions; the K level increases
   4. In alkalosis, the cells release H^+ ions into the blood in an attempt to increase the acidity of the blood and combat alkalinity; the K moves into the cells and the K level decreases

III. RESPIRATORY ACIDOSIS

A. Description: The total concentration of buffer base is lower than normal, with a relatively increasing hydrogen ion (H^+) concentration; thus, a greater number of H^+ ions are circulating in the blood than can be absorbed by the buffer system
B. Causes (Box 10-1)
   1. Due to primary defects in the function of the lungs or by changes in normal respiratory patterns from secondary problems
   2. Remember that any condition that causes an obstruction of the airway or depresses respiratory status can cause **respiratory acidosis**
C. Data collection
   1. In an attempt to compensate, the respiratory rate and depth increase
   2. pH is lower than 7.35 and pCO_2 (partial pressure of CO_2) higher than 45 mm Hg
   3. Headache

BOX 10-1

Causes of Respiratory Acidosis

Asthma
Atelectasis
Brain trauma
Bronchiectasis
Bronchitis
Emphysema
Hypoventilation
Medications
Pulmonary edema

4. Restlessness
5. Mental status changes, such as drowsiness and confusion
6. Visual disturbances
7. Diaphoresis
8. Cyanosis as the hypoxia becomes more acute
9. Hyperkalemia
10. Rapid, irregular pulse
11. Dysrhythmias leading to ventricular fibrillation

D. Interventions
   1. Maintain patent airway
   2. Monitor for signs of respiratory distress
   3. Administer oxygen as prescribed
   4. Place client in semi-Fowler's position unless contraindicated
   5. Encourage and assist the client to turn, cough, and deep breathe
   6. Prepare to administer chest physiotherapy and postural drainage, as prescribed
   7. Encourage hydration to thin secretions unless excess fluid intake is contraindicated
   8. Suction the client as necessary
   9. Monitor electrolyte values
   10. Avoid the use of tranquilizers, narcotics, and hypnotics because they further depress respirations
   11. Administer antibiotics for infection or other medications as prescribed

IV. RESPIRATORY ALKALOSIS

A. Description: A deficit of carbonic acid (H_2CO_3) or a decrease in H^+ ion concentration; results from accumulation of base or loss of acid without comparable loss of base in the body fluids
B. Causes: Conditions that cause overstimulation of the respiratory status (Box 10-2)
C. Data collection
   1. Initially, the hyperventilation and respiratory stimulation cause abnormal rapid and deep respirations (tachypnea); in an attempt to compensate, respiratory rate and depth then decrease
   2. pH is higher than 7.45 and pCO_2 is lower than 35 mm Hg
   3. Headache
   4. Light-headedness, vertigo
   5. Mental status changes

BOX 10-2

Causes of Respiratory Alkalosis

Fever
Hyperventilation
Hypoxia
Hysteria
Overventilation by mechanical ventilators
Pain

6. Paresthesias, such as tingling of the fingers and toes
7. Hypokalemia, hypocalcemia
8. Tetany, convulsions

D. Interventions
1. Maintain a patent airway
2. Provide emotional support and reassurance to the client
3. Encourage appropriate breathing patterns
4. Assist with breathing techniques and breathing aids, as prescribed
   a. Voluntary holding of breath
   b. Rebreathing exhaled CO_2
   c. Rebreathing mask, as prescribed
   d. Carbon dioxide breaths, as prescribed
5. Provide cautious care with ventilator clients so that they are not forced to take breaths too deeply or rapidly
6. Monitor electrolyte values, particularly K and calcium levels
7. Administer medications, as prescribed
8. Prepare to assist with administering calcium gluconate for tetany, as prescribed

V. METABOLIC ACIDOSIS

A. Description: The total concentration of buffer base is lower than normal, with a relative increase in the H^+ ion concentration; occurs as a result of losing buffer bases or retaining too much acid without sufficient base

B. Causes (Box 10-3)
1. Diabetes mellitus–diabetic ketoacidosis: An insufficient supply of insulin causes increased fat metabolism, leading to an excess accumulation of ketones or other acids; bicarbonate then ends up being depleted
2. Renal insufficiency or failure
   a. Increased waste products of protein metabolism are retained
   b. Excessive acids build up, and bicarbonate cannot maintain acid-base balance
3. Insufficient metabolism of carbohydrates: When an insufficient supply of O_2 is available for the proper burning of carbohydrates, glucose, and

---

BOX 10-3

Causes of Metabolic Acidosis

Diabetes mellitus or diabetic ketoacidosis
Excessive ingestion of acetylsalicylic acid (aspirin)
High-fat diet
Insufficient metabolism of carbohydrates
Malnutrition
Renal insufficiency or renal failure
Severe diarrhea

---

water, lactic acid concentration increases and lactic acidosis results
4. Excessive ingestion of acetylsalicylic acid (aspirin): Causes an increase in the H^+ ions concentration
5. Severe diarrhea: Intestinal and pancreatic secretions are normally alkaline; therefore, excessive loss of base leads to acidosis
6. Malnutrition: Improper metabolism of nutrients causes fat catabolism, leading to an excess buildup of ketones and acids
7. High-fat diet: A high intake of fat causes the waste products of fat metabolism to be accumulated much too rapidly, leading to a buildup of ketones and acids

C. Data collection
1. In an attempt to blow off the extra CO_2 and compensate for the acidosis, hyperpnea with Kussmaul's respirations occurs
2. pH lower than 7.35 and HCO_3^- (bicarbonate ion) level lower than 22 mEq/L
3. Headache
4. Nausea, vomiting, diarrhea
5. Fruity-smelling breath as a result of improper fat metabolism
6. Central nervous system depression: mental dullness, drowsiness, stupor, coma
7. Twitching, convulsions
8. Hyperkalemia

D. Interventions
1. Based on the cause of the acidosis
2. Maintain a patent airway
3. Assess level of consciousness (LOC) for central nervous system (CNS) depression
4. Monitor I&O and assist with fluid and electrolyte replacement, as prescribed
5. Initiate safety and seizure precautions
6. Monitor the serum K level closely; when acidosis is being treated, K will move back into the cell and the serum K level will drop

E. Interventions in diabetes mellitus–diabetic ketoacidosis
1. Insulin is given to hasten the movement of serum glucose into the cell, thereby decreasing the concurrent ketosis
2. When glucose is being properly metabolized, the body stops converting fats to glucose
3. Monitor for circulatory collapse caused by polyuria, which can result from the hyperglycemic state, because polyuria or diuresis might lead to extracellular volume deficit

F. Interventions in renal failure
1. In renal failure, dialysis may be used to remove protein and waste products, thereby decreasing the acidosis
2. A diet low in protein and high in calories will decrease the amount of protein waste products; this in turn will lessen the acidosis

VI. METABOLIC ALKALOSIS

A. Description: A deficit of or loss of H^+ or acids, or an excess of base (bicarbonate); results from the accumulation of base or from loss of acid without comparable loss of base in the body fluids

B. Causes (Box 10-4)

C. Data collection

1. In an attempt to compensate, respiratory rate and depth decrease to conserve carbon dioxide (CO_2)
2. Nausea, vomiting, diarrhea
3. Restlessness
4. Numbness and tingling in the extremities
5. Twitching in the extremities
6. Hypokalemia, hypocalcemia
7. Dysrhythmia: tachycardia

D. Interventions

1. Maintain a patent airway
2. Monitor potassium and calcium serum blood levels
3. Institute safety precautions
4. Prepare to administer medications, as prescribed, to promote excretion of bicarbonate by the kidneys
5. Prepare to replace potassium chloride, as prescribed

VII. ARTERIAL BLOOD GASES (Box 10-5)

A. Description: Levels reflect the ability of the lungs to exchange oxygen and carbon dioxide, the effectiveness of the kidneys in balancing retention and elimination of bicarbonate, and the effectiveness of the heart as a pump

B. Obtaining an arterial blood gas specimen

1. Obtain vital signs
2. Perform **Allen's test** to determine the presence of collateral circulation (Box 10-6)
3. Identify factors that might affect the accuracy of the results, such as changes in the O_2 settings on respiratory assistive devices, suctioning within the last 20 minutes, and client activities
4. Assist with the specimen draw by preparing a heparinized syringe
5. Provide emotional support to the client
6. Apply pressure immediately to the puncture site for 5 minutes, and for 10 minutes if the client is taking anticoagulants
7. Appropriately label the specimen and transport on ice to the laboratory
8. Record the client's temperature and the type of supplemental oxygen that the client is receiving on the laboratory form

C. Respiratory imbalances

1. Remember, the respiratory function indicator is the pCO_2
2. In a respiratory imbalance, you will find an opposite relationship between the pH and the pCO_2; in other words, the pH will be up when the pCO_2 is down, or the pH will be down with an elevated pCO_2
3. Remember, the pH is down in an acidotic condition and is elevated in an alkalotic condition
4. Look at the pH and the pCO_2 to determine if the condition is a respiratory problem
5. **Respiratory acidosis**
   a. The pH is down
   b. The pCO_2 is up
6. **Respiratory alkalosis**
   a. The pH is up
   b. The pCO_2 is down

D. Metabolic imbalances

1. Remember, the metabolic function indicator is the bicarbonate ion (HCO_3^-)
2. In a metabolic imbalance, you will find a corresponding relationship between the pH and the HCO_3^-
3. In other words, the pH will be up and the HCO_3^- will be up, or the pH will be down and the HCO_3^- will be down
4. Remember, the pH is down in an acidotic condition and is elevated in an alkalotic condition
5. Look at the pH and the HCO_3^- concentration to determine if the condition is a metabolic problem

---

BOX 10-4

Causes of Metabolic Alkalosis

Diuretics
Excessive vomiting or gastrointestinal suctioning
Hyperaldosteronism
Ingestion of excess sodium bicarbonate
Massive transfusion of whole blood

BOX 10-5

Normal Blood Gas Values

pH = 7.35-7.45
pCO_2 = 35-45 mm Hg
HCO_3^- = 22-27 mEq/L
pO_2 (partial pressure of O_2) = 80-100 mm Hg

BOX 10-6

Performing Allen's Test

Apply direct pressure over the client's ulnar and radial arteries simultaneously
While pressure is applied, ask the client to open and close the hand repeatedly; the hand should blanch
Release pressure from the ulnar artery while compressing the radial artery, and assess the color of the extremity distal to the pressure point
If pinkness fails to return within 6 seconds, the ulnar artery is insufficient, indicating that the radial artery should not be used for obtaining a blood specimen

Analyzing Arterial Blood Gas Results

If you can remember the following pyramid points and steps, you will be able to analyze any blood gas report.

PYRAMID POINTS
In acidosis, the pH is down.
In alkalosis, the pH is up.
The respiratory function indicator is the pco_2 value.
The metabolic function indicator is the HCO_3^- level.

PYRAMID STEPS
Look at the blood gas report.
Pyramid Step 1
Look at the pH. Is it up or down? If it is up, it reflects alkalosis. If it is down, it reflects acidosis.
Pyramid Step 2
Look at the pco_2 level. Is it up or down? If it reflects an opposite relationship to the pH, then you know that the condition is a respiratory imbalance. If it does not reflect an opposite relationship to the pH, then move on to pyramid step 3.
Pyramid Step 3
Look at the HCO_3^- level. Does the HCO_3^- level reflect a corresponding relationship to the pH? If it does, then the condition is a metabolic imbalance.

6. **Metabolic acidosis**
   a. The pH is down
   b. The HCO_3^- is down
7. **Metabolic alkalosis**
   a. The pH is up
   b. The HCO_3^- is up
E. Steps for analyzing arterial blood gas results (Box 10-7)

PRACTICE QUESTIONS

1. A nurse is caring for a client with a diagnosis of chronic obstructive pulmonary disease (COPD). The nurse monitors the client for which acid-base imbalance that most likely occurs in this condition?
   1. Respiratory acidosis
   2. Respiratory alkalosis
   3. Metabolic acidosis
   4. Metabolic alkalosis
2. A licensed practical nurse (LPN) is assigned to care for a client with Guillain-Barré syndrome. The registered nurse (RN) reviews the results of the arterial blood gases with the LPN and tells the LPN that the client is experiencing respiratory acidosis. The LPN would expect to note which of the following on the laboratory result form?
   1. pH 7.40, pco_2 52 mm Hg
   2. pH 7.35, pco_2 40 mm Hg

   3. pH 7.25, pco_2 50 mm Hg
   4. pH 7.50, pco_2 30 mm Hg
3. A nurse is caring for a client with respiratory insufficiency. Arterial blood gas results indicate a pH of 7.50 and a pco_2 of 30 mm Hg, and the nurse is told that the client is experiencing respiratory alkalosis. Which of the following additional laboratory values would the nurse expect to note?
   1. Sodium level, 145 mEq/L
   2. Potassium level, 3.2 mEq/L
   3. Magnesium level, 2.4 mg/dL
   4. Phosphorus level, 4.0 mg/dL
4. The nurse is caring for a client with pneumonia. The nurse is told that the blood gas results indicate a pH of 7.50 and a pco_2 of 30 mm Hg. The nurse determines that these results indicate:
   1. Metabolic acidosis
   2. Metabolic alkalosis
   3. Respiratory alkalosis
   4. Respiratory acidosis
5. A client is scheduled for blood to be drawn from the radial artery for an arterial blood gas (ABG) determination. A nurse assists in performing Allen's test before drawing the blood gas to determine the adequacy of the:
   1. Brachial circulation
   2. Ulnar circulation
   3. Femoral circulation
   4. Carotid circulation
6. A nurse is caring for a client with a nasogastric tube that is attached to low suction. The nurse monitors the client closely for which acid-base disorder that is most likely to occur in this client?
   1. Respiratory acidosis
   2. Respiratory alkalosis
   3. Metabolic acidosis
   4. Metabolic alkalosis
7. A nurse is caring for a client with an ileostomy. The nurse monitors the client closely, understanding that this client is at risk for developing which acid-base disorder?
   1. Respiratory acidosis
   2. Respiratory alkalosis
   3. Metabolic acidosis
   4. Metabolic alkalosis
8. A nurse is caring for a client with diabetic ketoacidosis and documents that the client is experiencing Kussmaul's respirations. Based on this documentation, which of the following did the nurse most likely observe?
   1. Respirations that are abnormally deep, regular, and increased in rate
   2. Respirations that are regular but abnormally slow
   3. Respirations that are labored and increased in depth and rate
   4. Respirations that cease for several seconds
9. A nurse is collecting data from a client with a suspected diagnosis of gastric ulcer. The client tells the

nurse that oral antacids are taken frequently throughout the day. The nurse continues to collect data from the client, understanding that the client is at risk for which acid-base disturbance?

1. Respiratory alkalosis
2. Respiratory acidosis
3. Metabolic acidosis
4. Metabolic alkalosis

10. A nurse is caring for a client with renal failure. The nurse is told that the blood gas results indicate a pH of 7.30 and a HCO_3 of 20 mm Hg, and that the client is experiencing metabolic acidosis. The nurse reviews the laboratory results and expects to note which of the following?

1. Sodium level, 145 mEq/L
2. Magnesium level, 2.6 mg/dL
3. Potassium level, 5.6 mEq/L
4. Phosphorus level, 4.5 mg/dL

ALTERNATE FORMAT QUESTION: PRIORITIZING (ORDERED RESPONSE)

A client is scheduled for an arterial blood gas specimen to be drawn, and the nurse assists with performing Allen's test on the client. Number the steps for performing Allen's test in order of priority. (Number 1 is the first step)

___ Ask the client to open and close the hand repeatedly
___ Apply pressure over the ulnar and radial arteries
___ Assess the color of the extremity distal to the pressure point
___ Release pressure from the ulnar artery
___ Explain the procedure to the client

ANSWERS

1. *Answer:* **1**

Rationale: Respiratory acidosis most often occurs as a result of primary defects in the function of the lungs or changes in normal respiratory patterns from secondary problems. Chronic respiratory acidosis is most commonly caused by COPD. Acute respiratory acidosis also occurs in these clients when superimposed respiratory infection or concurrent respiratory disease increases the work of breathing. Options 2, 3, and 4 are not likely to occur unless other conditions complicate the COPD.

Test-Taking Strategy: Use the process of elimination. Remembering that primary defects in the function of the lungs results in respiratory acidosis will direct you to the correct option. Review the causes of respiratory acidosis if you had difficulty with this question.

Level of Cognitive Ability: Comprehension
Client Needs: Physiological Integrity
Integrated Process: Nursing Process/Data Collection
Content Area: Fundamental Skills
References: Linton, A., & Maebius, N. (2003). *Introduction to medical-surgical nursing* (3rd ed.). Philadelphia: W.B. Saunders, pp. 164, 500.

2. *Answer:* **3**

Rationale: The normal pH is 7.35 to 7.45. The normal pCO_2 is 35 to 45 mm Hg. In respiratory acidosis, the pH is down and the pCO_2 is up.

Test-Taking Strategy: Remember that in a respiratory imbalance you will find an opposite relationship between the pH and pCO_2. Also, remember that the pH is down in an acidotic condition. Options 1 and 4 reflect an elevated pH, which indicates an alkalotic condition. Option 2 reflects a normal blood gas result. Option 3 is the only option that reflects an acidotic condition. Review the interpretation of arterial blood gas results if you had difficulty with this question.

Level of Cognitive Ability: Analysis
Client Needs: Physiological Integrity
Integrated Process: Nursing Process/Data Collection
Content Area: Adult Health/Neurological

Reference: Pagana, K., & Pagana, T. (2003). *Mosby's diagnostic and laboratory test reference* (6th ed.). St. Louis: Mosby, p. 116.

3. *Answer:* **2**

Rationale: Clinical manifestations of respiratory alkalosis include tachypnea, mental status changes, dizziness, pallor around the mouth, spasms of the muscles of the hands, and hypokalemia. Options 1, 3, and 4 identify normal laboratory results.

Test-Taking Strategy: Recalling the clinical manifestations of respiratory alkalosis and the normal laboratory values will assist in answering the question. By the process of elimination, you can then determine that the only abnormal laboratory value is the potassium level. Review the clinical manifestations of respiratory alkalosis if you had difficulty with this question.

Level of Cognitive Ability: Analysis
Client Needs: Physiological Integrity
Integrated Process: Nursing Process/Data Collection
Content Area: Adult Health/Respiratory
References: Black, J., & Hawks, J. (2005). *Medical-surgical nursing: Clinical management for positive outcomes* (7th ed.). Philadelphia: W.B. Saunders, p. 265.
Chernecky, C., & Berger, B. (2004). *Laboratory tests and diagnostic procedures* (4th ed.). Philadelphia: W.B. Saunders, p. 888.

4. *Answer:* **3**

Rationale: The normal pH is 7.35 to 7.45. In a respiratory condition, an opposite relationship will be seen between the pH and the pCO_2. In an alkalotic condition, the pH is up. Clients with pneumonia are at risk for respiratory alkalosis as a result of hypoxia.

Test-Taking Strategy: Remember that, in a respiratory condition, you will find an opposite relationship between the pH and the pCO_2. Therefore, options 1 and 2 can be eliminated. Also, remember that the pH is up in an alkalotic condition. Review the steps related to reading blood gas values if you had difficulty with this question.

Level of Cognitive Ability: Analysis
Client Needs: Physiological Integrity

Integrated Process: Nursing Process/Data Collection
Content Area: Adult Health/Respiratory
Reference: Linton, A., & Maebius, N. (2003). *Introduction to medical-surgical nursing* (3rd ed.). Philadelphia: W.B. Saunders, pp. 165, 481-482.

5. Answer: 2
Rationale: Before radial puncture for obtaining an arterial specimen for ABGs, Allen's test should be performed to determine adequate ulnar circulation. Failure to assess collateral circulation could result in severe ischemic injury to the hand if damage to the radial artery occurs with arterial puncture. Options 1, 3, and 4 are not associated with this test.
Test-Taking Strategy: Use the process of elimination. Note the relationship between the words "radial artery" in the question and option 2. Review this test if you had difficulty with this question.
Level of Cognitive Ability: Analysis
Client Needs: Physiological Integrity
Integrated Process: Nursing Process/Evaluation
Content Area: Adult Health/Cardiovascular
Reference: Chernecky, C., & Berger, B. (2004). *Laboratory tests and diagnostic procedures* (4th ed.). Philadelphia: W.B. Saunders, p. 248.

6. Answer: 4
Rationale: Loss of gastric fluid via nasogastric suction or vomiting causes metabolic alkalosis due to the loss of hydrochloric acid. This results in an alkalotic condition. Options 1, 2, and 3 are incorrect.
Test-Taking Strategy: Remember that hydrochloric acid is lost when the client is on nasogastric suction. This will direct you to the options identifying an alkalotic condition. Because the question addresses a situation other than a respiratory one, the acid-base disorder would be a metabolic condition. If you had difficulty with this question, review the causes of metabolic alkalosis.
Level of Cognitive Ability: Analysis
Client Needs: Physiological Integrity
Integrated Process: Nursing Process/Data Collection
Content Area: Adult Health/Gastrointestinal
References: Black, J., & Hawks, J. (2005). *Medical-surgical nursing: Clinical management for positive outcomes* (7th ed.). Philadelphia: W.B. Saunders, pp. 266-267.
Linton, A., & Maebius, N. (2003). *Introduction to medical-surgical nursing* (3rd ed.). Philadelphia: W.B. Saunders, p. 165.

7. Answer: 3
Rationale: Intestinal secretions high in bicarbonate may be lost through enteric drainage tubes, an ileostomy, or diarrhea. The decreased bicarbonate level creates the actual base deficit of metabolic acidosis. Options 1, 2, and 4 are unlikely to occur in a client with an ileostomy.
Test-Taking Strategy: Note that the client condition described in the question is a client with a gastrointestinal disorder. This will direct you to think about a metabolic disorder. Remembering that intestinal fluids are primarily alkaline will assist in selecting the correct option. When excess bicarbonate is lost, acidosis will result. Review the causes of metabolic acidosis if you had difficulty with this question.

Level of Cognitive Ability: Analysis
Client Needs: Physiological Integrity
Integrated Process: Nursing Process/Data Collection
Content Area: Adult Health/Gastrointestinal
Reference: Linton, A., & Maebius, N. (2003). *Introduction to medical-surgical nursing* (3rd ed.). Philadelphia: W.B. Saunders, p. 165.

8. Answer: 1
Rationale: Kussmaul's respirations are abnormally deep, regular, and increased in rate. In bradypnea, respirations are regular but abnormally slow. In hyperpnea, respirations are labored and increased in depth and rate. In apnea, respirations cease for several seconds.
Test-Taking Strategy: Knowledge regarding the descriptions for alterations in breathing pattern is required to answer the question. Remember, Kussmaul's respirations occur in diabetic ketoacidosis. Review the characteristics of these types of respirations if you had difficulty with this question.
Level of Cognitive Ability: Comprehension
Client Needs: Physiological Integrity
Integrated Process: Nursing Process/Data Collection
Content Area: Fundamental Skills
Reference: Linton, A., & Maebius, N. (2003). *Introduction to medical-surgical nursing* (3rd ed.). Philadelphia: W.B. Saunders, p. 456.

9. Answer: 4
Rationale: Increases in base components occur as a result of oral or parenteral ingestion of bicarbonates, carbonates, acetates, citrates, and lactates. Excessive use of oral antacids containing sodium or calcium bicarbonate can cause a metabolic alkalosis. Options 1, 2, and 3 are incorrect.
Test-Taking Strategy: Remember that antacids contain bicarbonate and that an excess oral intake increases bicarbonate; this will assist in directing you to the correct option. Review the causes of metabolic alkalosis if you had difficulty with the question.
Level of Cognitive Ability: Analysis
Client Needs: Physiological Integrity
Integrated Process: Nursing Process/Data Collection
Content Area: Adult Health/Gastrointestinal
Reference: Linton, A., & Maebius, N. (2003). *Introduction to medical-surgical nursing* (3rd ed.). Philadelphia: W.B. Saunders, p. 165.

10. Answer: 3
Rationale: Clinical manifestations of metabolic acidosis include weakness, malaise, and headache. Hyperkalemia will occur. The pH will be lower than 7.35 and the HCO_3^- ion level lower than 22 mEq/L. Options 1, 2, and 4 identify normal laboratory values, whereas option 3 indicates hyperkalemia.
Test-Taking Strategy: Knowledge regarding the clinical manifestations of metabolic acidosis along with normal laboratory values will assist you in answering the question. By the process of elimination, you can then determine that the only abnormal laboratory value is the potassium level. Review the manifestations of metabolic acidosis if you had difficulty with this question.
Level of Cognitive Ability: Analysis

Client Needs: Physiological Integrity
Integrated Process: Nursing Process/Data Collection
Content Area: Adult Health/Renal
References: Chernecky, C., & Berger, B. (2004). *Laboratory tests and diagnostic procedures* (4th ed.). Philadelphia: W.B. Saunders, p. 245.
Linton, A., & Maebius, N. (2003). *Introduction to medical-surgical nursing* (3rd ed.). Philadelphia: W.B. Saunders, p. 165.

ALTERNATE FORMAT QUESTION: PRIORITIZING (ORDERED RESPONSE)

Answer: 32541

Rationale: Allen's test is performed before obtaining an arterial blood specimen from the radial artery to determine the presence of adequate collateral circulation and the adequacy of the ulnar artery. Failure to determine the presence of adequate collateral circulation could result in severe ischemic injury to the hand if damage to the radial artery occurs with arterial puncture. The nurse would first explain the procedure to the client. To perform the test, the nurse applies direct pressure over the client's ulnar and radial arteries simultaneously.

While pressure is applied, the nurse asks the client to open and close the hand repeatedly; the hand should blanch. The nurse then releases pressure from the ulnar artery while compressing the radial artery and assesses the color of the extremity distal to the pressure point. If pinkness fails to return within 6 seconds, the ulnar artery is insufficient, indicating that the radial artery should not be used for obtaining a blood specimen.

Test-Taking Strategy: Recalling that the procedure needs to be explained to the client will assist in determining the first action. Next, think about the purpose and reason for performing this test and visualize the procedure. This will assist in determining the steps for performing Allen's test. Review this test if you had difficulty with this question.
Level of Cognitive Ability: Application
Client Needs: Physiological Integrity
Integrated Process: Nursing Process/Data Collection
Content Area: Fundamental Skills
Reference: Malarkey, L., & McMorrow, M. (2005). *Nursing guide to laboratory and diagnostic tests.* Philadelphia: W.B. Saunders, p. 105.

REFERENCES

Black, J., & Hawks, J. (2005). *Medical-surgical nursing: Clinical management for positive outcomes* (7th ed.). Philadelphia: W.B. Saunders.
Chernecky, C., & Berger, B. (2004). *Laboratory tests and diagnostic procedures* (4th ed.). Philadelphia: W.B. Saunders.
Linton, A., & Maebius, N. (2003). *Introduction to medical-surgical nursing* (3rd ed.). Philadelphia: W.B. Saunders.

Malarkey, L., & McMorrow, M. (2005). *Nursing guide to laboratory and diagnostic tests.* Philadelphia: W.B. Saunders.
Pagana, K., & Pagana, T. (2003). *Mosby's diagnostic and laboratory test reference* (6th ed.). St. Louis: Mosby.

Laboratory Values

PYRAMID TERMS

capillary puncture Preferred for a peripheral blood smear.

plasma The fluid ground substance; what remains after the cells have been removed from a sample of whole blood.

serum Blood plasma from which clotting agents have been removed.

venipuncture Puncture into a vein to obtain a blood specimen for testing; the antecubital veins are the veins of choice because of ease of access.

▲ PYRAMID TO SUCCESS

This chapter identifies the normal adult values for the most common laboratory tests. If you are familiar with the normal values, you will be able to determine if an abnormality exists when a laboratory value is presented in a question. It is unlikely that a question on NCLEX-PN will simply ask you what a normal value may be. The questions on NCLEX-PN related to laboratory values will require you to identify whether the laboratory value is normal or abnormal, and then you will be required to think about the effects of the laboratory value in terms of the client. Pyramid points focus on knowledge of the normal values for the most common laboratory tests, therapeutic serum medication levels of commonly prescribed medications, and interventions based on the findings. When a question is presented on NCLEX-PN regarding a specific laboratory value, note the disorder presented in the question and the associated body organ that is affected as a result of the disorder. This process will assist you in determining the correct answer. For example, if the question is asking you about the immune status of a client receiving chemotherapy, assessment of laboratory values will focus on the white blood cell count and on the neutrophils, because this client may be at risk for infection. In the client receiving chemotherapy who has a low white blood cell (WBC) count, the plan of care focuses on

the immune system and protecting the client from infection. Implementation focuses on preventive interventions related to infection, perhaps protective isolation measures. Evaluation may focus on maintenance of a normal temperature in the client. Integrated Processes addressed in this chapter are the Clinical Problem-Solving Process (Nursing Process), Caring, Communication and Documentation, and Teaching/Learning. Box 11-1 lists the abbreviations used in laboratory values.

CLIENT NEEDS ▲
Safe, Effective Care Environment

Informed consent for specific procedures

Medical and surgical asepsis when obtaining a specimen

Principles of infection control

Procedures for handling hazardous and infectious materials

Standard, transmission-based, and other precautions

Verifying the identity of the client

BOX 11-1

Pyramid Abbreviations

ABBREVIATION	DESCRIPTION
g/dL	grams per deciliter
mcg/dL	micrograms per deciliter
mg/dL	milligrams per deciliter
mEq/L	milliequivalents per liter
units/L	units per liter
mm/hr	millimeters per hour
IU/L	international units per liter
mcg/mL	micrograms per milliliter
ng/mL	nanograms per milliliter
microunits/mL	microunits per milliliter
mL/kg	milliliters per kilogram

Health Promotion and Maintenance

Client preparation for the laboratory test
Community resources available for the follow up
Importance of follow-up laboratory studies
Post-test procedures
Signs and symptoms that indicate the need to notify the health care provider

Psychosocial Integrity

Communicate purpose of test to client
Communicate with the client regarding laboratory results
Describe specific interventions or home care measures required on the basis of the results
Provide emotional support during testing

Physiological Integrity

Comfort interventions
Determining the need to implement specific actions based on the laboratory results
Monitoring for clinical manifestations associated with an abnormal laboratory value
Monitoring for potential complications related to a test
Normal values for the most common laboratory tests
Reporting significant laboratory values
Therapeutic serum medication levels of commonly prescribed medications

I. ELECTROLYTES (Table 11-1)
A. **Serum** sodium (Na)
  1. Description
    a. A major cation of extracellular fluid
    b. Maintains osmotic pressures and acid-base balance and assists in transmission of nerve impulses
    c. Absorbed from the small intestine and excreted in the urine in amounts dependent on dietary intake
    d. Minimum daily requirement of Na is approximately 15 mEq
  2. Nursing consideration: Drawing blood samples proximal to intravenous (IV) infusion of sodium chloride will falsely elevate results

TABLE 11-1

Normal Adult Electrolyte Values	
Electrolyte	Value (mEq/L)
Sodium	135-145
Potassium	3.5-5.1
Chloride	98-107
Bicarbonate (venous)	22-29

B. **Serum** potassium (K)
  1. Description
    a. A major intracellular cation; regulates cellular water balance, electrical conduction in muscle cells, and acid-base balance
    b. The body obtains K through dietary ingestion, and the kidneys either preserve or excrete K, depending upon cellular need
    c. K levels are used to evaluate cardiac function, renal function, gastrointestinal (GI) function, and the need for IV replacement therapy
  2. Nursing considerations
    a. Use of a tourniquet and clenching and unclenching the hand prior to venous sampling can increase the value
    b. Do not draw blood from an IV infusion site
    c. If the client is receiving K supplementation, note this on the laboratory form
    d. Clients with elevated WBC and platelet counts may have falsely elevated K levels
C. **Serum** chloride
  1. Description
    a. A hydrochloric acid salt that is the most abundant body anion in the extracellular fluid
    b. Functions in counterbalancing cations, such as sodium, and acts as a buffer during oxygen and carbon dioxide exchange in red blood cells
    c. Aids in digestion and maintaining osmotic pressure and water balance
  2. Nursing considerations
    a. Draw blood from an extremity that does not have normal saline infusing into it
    b. Do not allow the client to clench and unclench the hand prior to blood draw
    c. Any condition accompanied by prolonged vomiting, diarrhea, or both will alter levels
D. **Serum** bicarbonate
  1. Description: Part of the bicarbonate-carbonic acid buffering system and mainly responsible for regulating the pH of body fluids
  2. Nursing considerations
    a. Ingestion of acidic or alkaline solutions may cause increased or decreased results, respectively
    b. Prolonged tourniquet application before the blood draw increases **serum** bicarbonate

II. COAGULATION STUDIES
A. Activated partial thromboplastin time (aPTT)
  1. Description
    a. Evaluates how well the coagulation sequence is functioning by measuring the amount of time it takes for recalcified, citrated **plasma** to clot after partial thromboplastin is added to it
    b. Screens for deficiencies and inhibitors of all factors except VII and XIII

c. Most commonly used to monitor heparin therapy and screen for coagulation disorders

2. Value: 20 to 36 seconds, depending on the type of activator used

3. Nursing considerations

   a. If the client is receiving intermittent heparin therapy, draw the blood sample 1 hour prior to the next scheduled dose

   b. Do not draw samples from an arm into which heparin is infusing

   c. Transport specimen to the laboratory immediately

   d. The aPTT should be between 1.5 and 2.5 times normal when the client is receiving heparin therapy; if the value is prolonged, initiate bleeding precautions

B. Prothrombin time (PT) and international normalized ratio (INR)

1. Description

   a. Prothrombin is a vitamin K–dependent glycoprotein, produced by the liver, necessary for firm fibrin clot formation

   b. Each laboratory establishes a normal or control value based on the method used to perform the test (PT)

   c. The PT measures the amount of time it takes for clot formation; used to monitor response to warfarin sodium (Coumadin) therapy or to screen for dysfunction of the extrinsic system resulting from liver disease, vitamin K deficiency, or disseminated intravascular coagulation (DIC)

   d. A PT value within 2 seconds (plus or minus) of the control value is considered normal

   e. The INR standardizes the PT ratio; calculated in the laboratory setting by raising the observed PT ratio to the power of the international sensitivity index specific to the thromboplastin reagent used

   f. The INR measures the effects of oral anticoagulants

2. Values

   a. PT: 9.6 to 11.8 seconds (adult male); 9.5 to 11.3 seconds (adult female)

   b. INR: 2 to 3 for standard warfarin sodium (Coumadin) therapy

   c. INR: 3 to 4.5 for high-dose warfarin sodium (Coumadin) therapy

3. Nursing considerations

   a. Baseline PT should be determined before anticoagulation therapy is started; note the time of collection on laboratory form

   b. Apply direct pressure to the venipuncture site for 3 to 5 minutes if a coagulation defect is present

   c. Concurrent warfarin sodium (Coumadin) therapy with heparin therapy can lengthen the PT for up to 5 hours after dosing

d. Diets high in green leafy vegetables can increase the absorption of vitamin K, which shortens the PT

e. Oral anticoagulation therapy usually maintains the PT at 1.5 to 2 times the laboratory control value

f. PT longer than 30 seconds places the client at risk for hemorrhage

C. Clotting time

1. Description: Measures the time required for the interaction of all factors involved in the clotting process

2. Value: 8 to 15 minutes

3. Nursing considerations

   a. The client should not receive heparin therapy for 3 hours prior to specimen collection because the heparin therapy will affect the results

   b. The test result is prolonged by any anticoagulant therapy, test tube agitation, or high temperature changes that may affect the specimen

D. Platelet count

1. Description

   a. Platelets function in hemostatic plug formation, clot retraction, and coagulation factor activation

   b. Platelets are produced by the bone marrow to function in hemostasis

2. Value: 150,000 to 400,000 cells/μL

3. Nursing considerations

   a. Monitor the venipuncture site for bleeding in clients with known thrombocytopenia

   b. High altitudes, chronic cold weather, and exercise increase platelet counts

   c. Bleeding precautions should be instituted in clients with a low platelet count

III. ERYTHROCYTE STUDIES

A. Erythrocyte sedimentation rate

1. Description

   a. The rate at which erythrocytes settle out of anticoagulated blood in 1 hour

   b. Not diagnostic of any particular disease, but indicates that a disease process is ongoing

2. Value: 0 to 30 mm/hour, depending on age of client

3. Nursing consideration: Fasting is not necessary, but a fatty meal may cause **plasma** alterations

B. Hemoglobin and hematocrit

1. Description

   a. Hemoglobin is the main component of erythrocytes and serves as the vehicle for the transportation of oxygen and carbon dioxide

   b. Hemoglobin determinations are important in identifying anemia

   c. Hematocrit represents red blood cell mass and is an important measurement in the identification of anemia or polycythemia (Table 11-2)

2. Nursing consideration: Fasting is not required

TABLE 11-2

Normal Adult Hemoglobin and Hematocrit Levels

Blood Component	Normal Level
HEMOGLOBIN (g/dL)	
Male	14-16.5
Female	12-15
HEMATOCRIT (%)	
Male	42-52
Female	35-47

TABLE 11-3

Normal Adult Lactate Dehydrogenase Levels

Serum Enzyme/Isoenzyme	Normal Level
Lactate dehydrogenase (LDH)	140-280 U/L
Lactate dehydrogenase isoenzymes (% of LDH level)	
LDH_1	14-26
LDH_2	29-39
LDH_3	20-26
LDH_4	8-16
LDH_5	6-16

C. **Serum** iron
1. Description
   a. Iron is mostly found in hemoglobin
   b. Iron acts as a carrier of oxygen from the lungs to the tissues and indirectly aids in the return of carbon dioxide to the lungs
   c. Aids in diagnosing anemias and hemolytic disorders
2. Values
   a. Male: 65-175 mcg/dL
   b. Female: 50-170 mcg/dL
3. Nursing consideration: Level will be increased if the client has ingested iron prior to the test
D. Red blood cell (RBC) count
1. Description
   a. RBCs function in hemoglobin transport, which results in delivery of oxygen to the body tissues
   b. RBCs are formed by red bone marrow, have a life span of 120 days, and are removed from the blood by the liver, spleen, and bone marrow
   c. Aids in diagnosing anemias and blood dyscrasias
   d. Evaluates the body's ability to produce red blood cells in sufficient numbers
2. Values
   a. Female: 4 to 5.5 million cells/μL
   b. Male: 4.5 to 6.2 million cells/μL
3. Nursing consideration: Fasting is not required

IV. SERUM ENZYMES/CARDIAC MARKERS
A. Creatine kinase (CK)
1. Description
   a. An enzyme found in muscle and brain tissue; reflects tissue catabolism resulting from cell trauma
   b. The test is performed to detect myocardial or skeletal muscle damage or central nervous system damage; normal CK value is 26-174 units/L
   c. Isoenzymes include CK-MB (cardiac), CK-BB (brain), and CK-MM (muscle)
   d. CK-MB is found mainly in cardiac muscle, CK-BB is found mainly in brain tissue, and CK-MM is found mainly in skeletal muscle

2. Values
   a. CK-MB: 0% to 5% of total CK value
   b. CK-MM: 95% to 100% of total CK value
   c. CK-BB: 0% of CK value
3. Nursing considerations
   a. If the test is to evaluate skeletal muscle, instruct the client to avoid strenuous physical activity for 24 hours prior to the test
   b. Instruct the client to avoid ingestion of alcohol for 24 hours prior to the test
   c. Invasive procedures and intramuscular injections may falsely elevate CK levels
B. Lactate dehydrogenase (LDH)
1. Description
   a. The isoenzymes that are particularly affected in acute myocardial infarction are LDH_1 and LDH_2
   b. The LDH level begins to increase approximately 24 hours after myocardial infarction and peaks in 48 to 72 hours; thereafter it returns to normal, usually within 7 to 14 days (Table 11-3)
   c. The presence of an LDH flip (when LDH_1 is higher than LDH_2) is helpful in diagnosing a myocardial infarction
2. Nursing considerations
   a. LDH isoenzymes should be interpreted in view of the clinical findings
   b. Testing should be repeated on 3 consecutive days
C. Troponins
1. Description
   a. Troponin is a regulatory protein found in striated muscle (skeletal and myocardial)
   b. Increased amounts of troponins are released into the bloodstream when an infarction causes damage to the myocardium
   c. Serial measurements are important to compare with baseline test values
2. Values
   a. Troponin I: Lower than 0.6 ng/mL; higher than 1.5 ng/mL is consistent with a myocardial infarction
   b. Troponin T: Higher than 0.1 to 0.2 ng/mL is consistent with a myocardial infarction

3. Nursing consideration: Client does not need to be fasting

V. SERUM GASTROINTESTINAL STUDIES

A. Albumin
1. Description
   a. A main **plasma** protein of blood
   b. Maintains oncotic pressure and transports bilirubin, fatty acids, medications, hormones, and other substances that are insoluble in water
   c. Increased in conditions such as dehydration, diarrhea, and metastatic carcinoma; decreased in conditions such as acute infection, ascites, and alcoholism
   d. The presence of detectable albumin, or protein, in the urine is indicative of abnormal renal function
2. Value: 3.4 to 5 g/dL
3. Nursing considerations: Draw from an extremity that does not have an IV infusing into it

B. Alkaline phosphatase
1. Description
   a. An enzyme normally found in bone, liver, intestine, and placenta
   b. The level rises during periods of bone growth, liver disease, and bile duct obstruction
2. Value: 4.5 to 13 King-Armstrong units/dL
3. Nursing considerations
   a. The client may need to fast 12 hours prior to test
   b. Hepatotoxic medications administered within 12 hours prior to specimen collection can cause false values
   c. Transport the specimen to the laboratory immediately

C. Ammonia
1. Description
   a. A waste product from nitrogen breakdown during protein metabolism
   b. Metabolized by the liver and excreted by the kidneys as urea
   c. Elevated levels resulting from hepatic dysfunction may lead to encephalopathy
   d. Not a reliable indicator of hepatic coma
2. Value: 35 to 65 mcg/dL
3. Nursing considerations
   a. Instruct the client to fast, except for water, and to refrain from smoking for 8 to 10 hours before the test
   b. Place the specimen in ice and transport to the laboratory immediately

D. Amylase
1. Description
   a. An enzyme, produced by the pancreas and salivary glands, that aids in the digestion of complex carbohydrates and is excreted by the kidneys

   b. In acute pancreatitis, the amylase level is greatly increased; the level starts rising 3 to 6 hours after the onset of pain, peaks at about 24 hours, and returns to normal 2 to 3 days after the onset of pain
2. Value: 25 to 151 units/L
3. Nursing considerations
   a. On the laboratory form, list medications that the client has taken for the 24 hours before the test
   b. Note that many medications may cause false-positive or false-negative results
   c. Results are invalidated if the specimen was obtained less than 72 hours after cholecystography with radiopaque dyes

E. Lipase
1. Description
   a. A pancreatic enzyme that changes fats and triglycerides into fatty acids and glycerol
   b. Elevated lipase levels occur in pancreatic disorders; elevations may not occur until 24 to 36 hours after the onset of illness and may remain elevated for up to 14 days
2. Value: 10 to 140 units/L
3. Nursing consideration: Endoscopic retrograde cholangiopancreatography (ERCP) may increase lipase activity

F. Bilirubin
1. Description
   a. Produced by the liver, spleen, and bone marrow; also a by-product of hemoglobin breakdown
   b. Total bilirubin can be broken down into direct bilirubin, which is primarily excreted via the intestinal tract, and indirect bilirubin, which circulates primarily in the bloodstream
   c. Total bilirubin levels rise with any type of jaundice, whereas direct and indirect levels rise depending on the cause of the jaundice
2. Values
   a. Bilirubin, direct: 0 to 0.3 mg/dL
   b. Bilirubin, indirect: 0.1 to 1 mg/dL
   c. Bilirubin, total: Lower than 1.5 mg/dL
3. Nursing considerations
   a. Instruct the client to eat a diet low in yellow foods, such as carrots, yams, yellow beans, and pumpkins, for 3 to 4 days before the blood is drawn
   b. Instruct the client to fast for 4 hours before the blood is drawn
   c. Note that results will be elevated with the ingestion of alcohol or the administration or ingestion of morphine sulfate, theophylline, ascorbic acid, or aspirin
   d. Note that results are invalidated if the client has undergone a radioactive scan within 24 hours prior to the test

G. Lipids
1. Description

a. Blood lipids consist primarily of cholesterol, triglycerides, and phospholipids

b. Lipid assessment includes total cholesterol, high-density lipoprotein (HDL), low-density lipoprotein (LDL), and triglycerides

c. Cholesterol is present in all body tissues and is a major component of LDLs, brain and nerve cells, cell membranes, and some gallbladder stones

d. Triglycerides constitute a major part of very low-density lipoproteins (VLDLs) and a small part of LDLs

e. Triglycerides are synthesized in the liver from fatty acids, protein, and glucose, and are obtained from the diet

f. Increased cholesterol, LDL, and triglyceride levels place the client at risk for coronary artery disease

g. HDLs help protect against the risk of coronary artery disease

2. Values

a. Cholesterol: 140 to 199 mg/dL

b. LDLs: Lower than 130 mg/dL

c. HDLs: 30 to 70 mg/dL

d. Triglycerides: Lower than 200 mg/dL

3. Nursing considerations

a. Oral contraceptives may increase the lipid level

b. Instruct the client to abstain from foods and fluid, except for water, for 12 to 14 hours before the test and from alcohol for 24 hours before the test

c. Instruct the client that the evening meal before the test should be free of high-cholesterol foods

H. Protein

1. Description

a. Reflects the total amount of albumin and globulins in the **serum**

b. Regulates osmotic pressure and comprises coagulation factors for hemostasis, enzymes, hormones, tissue growth and repair, and pH buffers

c. Increased in conditions such as Addison's disease, autoimmune collagen disorders, chronic infection, and Crohn's disease

d. Decreased in conditions such as burns, cirrhosis, edema, and severe hepatic disease

2. Value: 6 to 8 g/dL

3. Nursing considerations

a. Do not draw in an extremity with an IV infusion

b. Instruct the client to avoid a high-fat diet for 8 hours before to the test

I. Uric acid

1. Description

a. Formed as the purines, adenine and guanine; is continuously metabolized during the formation and degradation of DNA and RNA and from the metabolism of dietary purines

b. Elevated amounts deposit in joints and soft tissue and cause gout

c. Conditions of fast cell turnover, as well as slowed renal excretion of uric acid, may cause uricemia

d. Elevated amounts of urinary uric acid form precipitates of urate stones in the kidneys

2. Values

a. Male: 4.5 to 8 mg/dL

b. Female: 2.5 to 6.2 mg/dL

3. Nursing considerations

a. Instruct the client to fast for 8 hours prior to the test

b. Aminophylline, caffeine, and vitamin C may cause falsely elevated results

VI.   GLUCOSE STUDIES

A. Fasting blood glucose

1. Description

a. Glucose is a monosaccharide found in fruits and is formed from the digestion of carbohydrates and the conversion of glycogen by the liver

b. Glucose is the body's main source of cellular energy and is essential for brain and erythrocyte function

c. Fasting blood glucose levels are used to help diagnose diabetes mellitus and hypoglycemia (Table 11-4)

2. Nursing considerations

a. Instruct the client to fast for 8 to 12 hours prior to test

b. Instruct a client with diabetes mellitus to withhold morning insulin or oral hypoglycemic medication until after the blood is drawn

B. Glucose tolerance test (GTT) (see Table 11-4)

1. Description

a. Aids in the diagnosis of diabetes mellitus

b. If the glucose levels peak at higher than normal at 1 to 2 hours after injection or ingestion of glucose and are slower than normal to return

TABLE 11-4

Normal Adult Glucose Values

Point of Measurement	Normal Value (mg/dL)
Glucose, fasting	70-110
Glucose monitoring (capillary blood)	60-110
Glucose tolerance test, oral	
Baseline fasting	70-110
30-minute fasting	110-170
60-minute fasting	120-170
90-minute fasting	100-140
120-minute fasting	70-120
Glucose, 2-hour postprandial	less than 140

to fasting levels, then diabetes mellitus is confirmed

  2. Nursing considerations

    a. Instruct the client to eat a high-carbohydrate (200- to 300-g) diet for 3 days before the test

    b. Instruct the client to avoid alcohol, coffee, and smoking for 36 hours before the test

    c. Instruct the client to fast for 10 to 16 hours before the test

    d. Instruct the client to avoid strenuous exercise for 8 hours before and after the test

    e. Instruct the client with diabetes mellitus to withhold morning insulin or oral hypoglycemic medication

    f. Instruct the client that the test will take 3 to 5 hours; requires intravenous or oral administration of glucose and multiple blood samples

C. Glycosylated hemoglobin

  1. Description

    a. Glycosylated hemoglobin is blood glucose bound to hemoglobin

    b. HbA1c (glycosylated hemoglobin A) is a reflection of how well blood glucose levels have been controlled for up to the prior 4 months

    c. Hyperglycemia in diabetics is usually a cause of an increase in HbA1c

  2. Values

    a. Values are expressed as a percentage of the total hemoglobin

    b. Diabetic with good control: 7.5% or lower

    c. Diabetic with fair control: 7.6% to 8.9%

    d. Diabetic with poor control: 9% or higher

  3. Nursing consideration: Fasting is not required before the test

VII. RENAL FUNCTION STUDIES

A. **Serum** creatinine

  1. Description

    a. Very specific indicator of renal function

    b. Elevated levels indicate a slowing of the glomerular filtration rate

  2. Value: 0.6 to 1.3 mg/dL

  3. Nursing considerations: Instruct the client to avoid excessive exercise for 8 hours and excessive red meat intake for 24 hours before the test

B. Blood urea nitrogen (BUN)

  1. Description

    a. Urea nitrogen is the nitrogen portion of urea, a substance formed in the liver through an enzymatic protein breakdown process

    b. Urea is normally freely filtered through the renal glomeruli, with a small amount reabsorbed in the tubules and the remainder excreted into the urine

    c. Elevated levels indicate a slowing of the glomerular filtration rate

  2. Value: 8 to 25 mg/dL

  3. Nursing considerations: Both creatinine levels and urea nitrogen levels should be analyzed when renal function is evaluated

VIII. ELEMENTS

A. Calcium

  1. Description

    a. Cation that is absorbed into the bloodstream from dietary sources and functions in bone formation, nerve impulse transmission, and contraction of myocardial and skeletal muscles

    b. Aids in blood clotting by converting prothrombin to thrombin

  2. Value: 8.6 to 10 mg/dL

  3. Nursing considerations

    a. Instruct the client to eat a diet with normal calcium levels (800 mg/day) for 3 days before the test

    b. Instruct the client that fasting may be required for 8 hours before the test

B. Magnesium

  1. Description

    a. Used as an index to determine metabolic activity and renal function

    b. Magnesium is needed for the blood-clotting process, regulates neuromuscular activity, acts as a cofactor that modifies the activity of many enzymes, and has an effect on the metabolism of calcium

  2. Value: 1.6 to 2.6 mg/dL

  3. Nursing considerations

    a. Prolonged use of magnesium products will cause increased levels

    b. Long-term total parenteral nutrition therapy or excessive loss of body fluids may cause decreased levels

C. Phosphorus

  1. Description

    a. Important in bone formation, energy storage and release, urinary acid-base buffering, and carbohydrate metabolism

    b. Absorbed from food and excreted by the kidneys

    c. High concentrations of phosphorus are stored in bone and skeletal muscle

  2. Value: 2.7 to 4.5 mg/dL

  3. Nursing consideration: Instruct the client to fast before the test

IX. THYROID STUDIES

A. Description

  1. Performed if a thyroid disorder is suspected

  2. Helpful to differentiate primary thyroid disease from secondary causes and from abnormalities in thyroxine-binding globulin levels

B. Values

1. Thyroid-stimulating hormone (thyrotropin; TSH): 0.2 to 5.4 microunits/mL
2. Throxine (T_4): 5 to 12 mcg/dL
3. Thyroxine, free (FT_4): 0.8 to 2.4 ng/dL
4. Triiodothyronine (T_3): 80 to 230 ng/dL

C. Nursing consideration: Test results may be invalid if client has undergone a radionuclide scan within 7 days before the test

X. WHITE BLOOD CELL (WBC) COUNT

A. Description

1. White blood cells function in the body's immune defense system
2. The WBC count assesses leukocyte distribution

B. Value: 4500 to 11,000 cells/µL (Table 11-5)

C. Nursing considerations

1. A "shift to the left" means that there is an increased number of immature neutrophils in the peripheral blood
2. A low total WBC count with a left shift indicates a recovery from bone marrow depression or an infection of such intensity that the demand for neutrophils in the tissue is greater than the capacity of the bone marrow to release them into the circulation
3. A high total WBC count with a left shift indicates an increased release of neutrophils by the bone marrow in response to an overwhelming infection or inflammation
4. A "shift to the right" means that cells have more than the usual number of nuclear segments; found in liver disease, Down's syndrome, and megaloblastic and pernicious anemia

XI. HEPATITIS TESTS

A. Description

1. Tests include radioimmune assay (RIA), enzyme-linked immunosorbent assay (ELISA), and microparticle enzyme immunoassay (MEIA)
2. Serologic tests for specific hepatitis virus markers assist in defining the specific type of hepatitis

TABLE 11-5

Normal Adult White Blood Cell Differential

Cell Type	Normal Value
Neutrophils	56% or 1800-7800 cells/µL
Bands	3% or 0-700 cells/µL
Eosinophils	2.7% or 0-450 cells/µL
Basophils	0.3% or 0-200 cells/µL
Lymphocytes	34% or 1000-4800 cells/µL
Monocytes	4% or 0-800 cells/µL

B. Values

1. The presence of immunoglobulin M (IgM) antibody to hepatitis A virus (IgM anti-HAV) and total antibody to hepatitis A virus (total anti-HAV) identify the disease
2. Detection of core antigen (HBcAg), envelope antigen (HBeAg), and surface antigen (HBsAg), or their corresponding antibodies, constitutes hepatitis B assessment
3. Hepatitis C is confirmed by the presence of antibodies to hepatitis C (anti-HCV)
4. Serologic hepatitis delta virus (HDV) determination is made by detection of the hepatitis D antigen (HDAg) early in the course of the infection and by detection of anti-HDV antibody in later disease stages
5. Specific serologic tests for hepatitis E virus (HEV) include detection of IgM and IgG antibodies to hepatitis E (anti-HEV)
6. Hepatitis G (HGV) has been found in some blood donors, IV drug users, hemodialysis clients, and clients with hemophilia; however, HGV does not appear to cause significant liver disease

C. Nursing consideration: If the radioimmunoassay technique is being used, the injection of radionuclides within 1 week before the blood test may falsely elevate results

XII. HUMAN IMMUNODEFICIENCY VIRUS (HIV) AND ACQUIRED IMMUNODEFICIENCY SYNDROME (AIDS) TESTING

A. Description

1. Detects HIV, which cause AIDS
2. Tests used to determine the presence of antibodies to HIV include ELISA, Western blot (WB), and immunofluorescence assay (IFA)
3. A single reactive ELISA test by itself cannot be used to diagnose HIV and should be repeated in duplicate with the same blood sample; if the result is repeatedly reactive, follow-up tests using WB or IFA should be done
4. A positive WB or IFA is considered confirmatory for HIV
5. A positive ELISA that fails to be confirmed by WB or IFA should not be considered negative, and repeat testing should take place in 3 to 6 months

B. CD4$^+$ T cell counts

1. Monitors the progression of HIV
2. As the disease progresses, there is usually a decrease in the number of CD4$^+$ T-cell counts and a resultant decrease in immunity
3. Normal CD4$^+$ T-cell count is between 500 and 1600 cells/µL
4. Generally, the immune system remains healthy, with CD4$^+$ T-cell counts greater than 500 cells/µL
5. Immune system problems occur when the CD4$^+$ T-cell cell count is between 200 and 499 cells/µL

6. Severe immune system problems occur when the CD4⁺ T-cell count is lower than 200 cells/μL

C. CD4⁺ to CD8⁺ ratio
1. Monitors the progression of the disease
2. The normal ratio is approximately 2:1
3. In HIV and AIDS, because of the low number of CD4⁺ cells, this ratio is low

D. Viral culture: Involves placing the infected client's blood cells in a culture medium and measuring the amount of reverse transcriptase (RT) activity over a specified period of time

E. Viral load testing: Measures the presence of HIV viral genetic material (ribonucleic acid [RNA]) or other viral protein in the client's blood

F. p24 antigen assay: Quantifies the amount of HIV viral core protein in the client's serum

G. Nursing considerations
1. Maintain issues of confidentiality surrounding HIV and AIDS testing
2. Follow prescribed state regulations and protocols related to reporting positive test results

XIII. URINE TESTS (Table 11-6)

XIV. THERAPEUTIC SERUM MEDICATION LEVELS (Table 11-7)

TABLE 11-6

Normal Adult Values: Urine Tests

Name of Test	Normal Value
Chloride	110-250 mEq/24 hr
Magnesium	7.3-12.2 mg/dL/day
Potassium	25-125 mEq/24 hr
Protein	40-150 mg/24 hr
Sodium	40-220 mEq/24 hr
Uric acid	250-750 mg/24 hr
pH	4.5-7.8
Specific gravity	1.016-1.022

TABLE 11-7

Therapeutic Serum Medication Levels

Medication	Therapeutic Range
Acetaminophen (Tylenol)	10-20 mcg/mL
Carbamazepine (Tegretol)	5-12 mcg/mL
Digoxin (Lanoxin)	0.5-2 ng/mL
Gentamicin (Garamycin)	5-10 mcg/mL
Lithium (Lithobid)	0.5-1.3 mEq/L
Magnesium sulfate	4-7 mg/dL
Phenytoin (Dilantin)	10-20 mcg/mL
Salicylates	100-250 mcg/mL
Theophylline (Aminophylline, Theo-Dur)	10-20 mcg/mL
Tobramycin (Nebcin)	5-10 mcg/mL
Valproic acid (Depakene)	50-100 mcg/mL

PRACTICE QUESTIONS

1. A nurse is reviewing the laboratory results of an adult client with Addison's disease. The nurse determines that the magnesium level is normal if which of the following is noted?
   1. 2 mg/dL
   2. 3 mg/dL
   3. 4 mg/dL
   4. 5 mg/dL

2. A client is suspected of having a myocardial infarction. The nurse would expect elevations in which isoenzyme value reported with the creatine kinase (CK) level?
   1. MM
   2. MB
   3. BB
   4. MK

3. An adult male client has had laboratory work done as part of a routine physical examination. The nurse reviews the client's record and determines that the client may have a mild degree of renal insufficiency if which of the following serum creatinine levels is found?
   1. 0.6 mg/dL
   2. 1.1 mg/dL
   3. 1.9 mg/dL
   4. 3.5 mg/dL

4. A client with a seizure disorder is taking phenytoin (Dilantin). A sample for a serum dilantin level is drawn and the nurse determines that the medication therapy is effective if the laboratory result is:
   1. 3 mcg/mL
   2. 8 mcg/mL
   3. 16 mcg/mL
   4. 24 mcg/mL

5. A client who takes theophylline for chronic obstructive pulmonary disease (COPD) is seen in the urgent care center for respiratory distress. Just before initiating treatment for the respiratory distress, a sample for a theophylline level is drawn. The nurse determines that the client may not be compliant with medication therapy if the result is:
   1. 6 mcg/mL
   2. 11 mcg/mL
   3. 15 mcg/mL
   4. 18 mcg/mL

6. A nurse is told that the laboratory result for the serum digoxin level is 2.4 ng/mL. The nurse plans to do which of the following?
   1. Record the normal value on the client's flow sheet
   2. Administer the next dose of the medication as scheduled
   3. Check the client's last pulse rate
   4. Hold the medication

7. A client with atrial fibrillation who is receiving maintenance therapy of warfarin sodium (Coumadin) has a prothrombin time (PT) of 30 seconds. The nurse

anticipates that which of the following will be prescribed?
1. Holding the next dose of warfarin sodium
2. Administering the next dose of warfarin sodium
3. Increasing the next dose of warfarin sodium
4. Adding a dose of heparin

8. An adult client who has had preadmission testing before surgery has had blood drawn for determination of serum electrolyte levels. The nurse identifies which of the following as an abnormal value?
1. Sodium, 148 mEq/L
2. Potassium, 3.8 mEq/L
3. Chloride, 101 mEq/L
4. Bicarbonate, 26 mEq/L

9. An adult client with a critically high potassium level has received sodium polystyrene sulfonate (Kayexalate). The nurse determines that the medication was most effective if the client's repeat serum potassium level is:
1. 6.2 mEq/L
2. 5.8 mEq/L
3. 5.4 mEq/L
4. 4.9 mEq/L

10. The adult client with a history of cardiac disease is due for a morning dose of furosemide (Lasix). The nurse reviews the client's record and would report which of the following serum potassium levels before administering the dose of furosemide?
1. 3.2 mEq/L
2. 3.8 mEq/L
3. 4.2 mEq/L
4. 4.8 mEq/L

11. A client with diabetes mellitus has a sample for fasting blood glucose drawn. The nurse identifies which of the following results as a critical value?
1. 150 mg/dL
2. 200 mg/dL
3. 220 mg/dL
4. 340 mg/dL

12. An adult client with a history of gastrointestinal bleeding has a platelet count of 300,000 cells/mL. Which of the following actions by the nurse is most appropriate on reading this report?
1. Report the abnormally low count
2. Report the abnormally high count
3. Place the client on bleeding precautions
4. Place the normal report in the client's medical record

13. An adult client with hepatic cirrhosis has been taking a diet with optimal amounts of protein, because neither excess nor deficiency of protein has been helpful. The nurse evaluates the client's status as most satisfactory if the total protein level is which of the following values in the normal range?
1. 0.4 g/dL
2. 3.7 g/dL
3. 6.4 g/dL
4. 9.8 g/dL

14. A client is seen in the urgent care center for complaints of chest pain 3 days ago. Since that time, the client has not been feeling well and fatigues easily. The nurse reviews the results of the laboratory tests and suspects myocardial infarction at the time of chest pain 3 days ago if which of the following isoenzymes for lactic dehydrogenase (LDH) comes back positive?
1. LDH_1
2. LDH_3
3. LDH_4
4. LDH_5

15. An adult client was diagnosed with acute pancreatitis 9 days ago. The nurse interprets that the client is recovering from this episode if the serum lipase level drops to which of the following values, which is just beneath the upper limit of normal?
1. 20 units/L
2. 80 units/L
3. 135 units/L
4. 250 units/L

16. A client arrives in the emergency room complaining of chest pain that began 4 hours ago. A troponin T blood specimen is obtained, and the results indicate a level of 0.6 ng/mL. The nurse interprets that this result indicates:
1. A normal level
2. A level that indicates the presence of possible angina
3. A low value indicating possible gastritis
4. A level that indicates a myocardial infarction

17. An adult female client has a hemoglobin level of 10.8 g/dL. The nurse interprets that this result is most likely due to which of the following factors in the client's history?
1. Chronic obstructive pulmonary disease (COPD)
2. Heart failure
3. Dehydration
4. Iron deficiency anemia

18. An adult male client admitted with dehydration has received fluid volume replacement. The nurse determines that the client has had adequate fluid resuscitation if the client's repeat hematocrit level has decreased to which of the following values in the normal range?
1. 56%
2. 48%
3. 39%
4. 34%

19. A client with diabetes mellitus has a glycosylated hemoglobin A (HbA1c) level of 8%. Based on this test result, the nurse plans to reinforce teaching measures with the client about the need to:
1. Avoid infection
2. Take in adequate fluids
3. Prevent hyperglycemia
4. Prevent hypoglycemia

20. A client has been diagnosed as having syndrome of inappropriate antidiuretic hormone (SIADH) secretion following cranial surgery. The nurse interprets that this complication is not resolving if which of the following urine specific gravity measurements is obtained?
    1. 1.002
    2. 1.016
    3. 1.020
    4. 1.030
21. A nurse is caring for a client with a diagnosis of cancer who is immunosuppressed. The nurse knows that neutropenic precautions will be implemented if the client's white blood cell (WBC) count is:
    1. 2000 cells/μL
    2. 5800 cells/μL
    3. 8400 cells/μL
    4. 11,500 cells/μL
22. A nurse volunteering at the health screening clinic teaches a 22-year-old client that diet and exercise should be used as tools to keep the total cholesterol level under:
    1. 130 mg/dL
    2. 200 mg/dL
    3. 250 mg/dL
    4. 300 mg/dL
23. A client has been admitted for urinary tract infection and dehydration. The nurse determines that the client has received adequate volume replacement if the blood urea nitrogen (BUN) level drops to:
    1. 35 mg/dL
    2. 29 mg/dL
    3. 15 mg/dL
    4. 6 mg/dL
24. A nurse is reviewing the laboratory results of a female adult client suspected of having iron deficiency anemia. The nurse reviews the results knowing that the normal hemoglobin level for this client is:
    1. 10 g/dL
    2. 14 g/dL
    3. 17 g/dL
    4. 19 g/dL
25. A nurse is assigned to a 40-year-old client admitted with chronic pancreatitis. The nurse reviews the client's record and expects to note a serum amylase level that is most similar to which of the following values?
    1. 25 units/L
    2. 100 units/L
    3. 300 units/L
    4. 500 units/L

ALTERNATE FORMAT QUESTION: MULTIPLE RESPONSE

Several laboratory tests are prescribed for a client and the nurse reviews the results of the tests. Select the laboratory tests that are abnormal.

___ White blood cells, 3,000 cells/μL
___ Neutrophils, 1000 cells/μL
___ Thyroid-stimulating hormone (thyrotropin; TSH), 0.4 microunits/mL
___ Phosphorus, 3.6 mg/dL
___ Magnesium, 1.0 mg/dL
___ Calcium, 7.0 mg/dL
___ Blood urea nitrogen, 10 mg/dL
___ Serum creatinine, 1.0 mg/dL

ANSWERS

1. *Answer: 1*
Rationale: The normal magnesium level in an adult client is 1.6 to 2.6 mg/dL. Options 2, 3, and 4 indicate elevated values.
Test-Taking Strategy: Knowledge regarding the normal magnesium level in an adult client is required to answer this question. Remember that the normal magnesium level in an adult client is 1.6 to 2.6 mg/dL. Review this laboratory test if you had difficulty with this question.
Level of Cognitive Ability: Comprehension
Client Needs: Physiological Integrity
Integrated Process: Nursing Process/Data Collection
Content Area: Fundamental Skills
Reference: Chernecky, C., & Berger, B. (2004). *Laboratory tests and diagnostic procedures* (4th ed.). Philadelphia: W.B. Saunders, p. 752.

2. *Answer: 2*
Rationale: CK is a cellular enzyme that can be fractionated into three isoenzymes. The MM band reflects CK from skeletal muscle. The MB band reflects CK from cardiac muscle, which is the level that increases with myocardial infarction. The BB band reflects CK from the brain. There is no MK band.
Test-Taking Strategy: Focus on the key words, *myocardial infarction*. Recalling that the MB band reflects CK from cardiac muscle will direct you to the correct option. Review this information if you had difficulty with this question.
Level of Cognitive Ability: Comprehension
Client Needs: Physiological Integrity
Integrated Process: Nursing Process/Data Collection
Content Area: Fundamental Skills
References: Chernecky, C., & Berger, B. (2004). *Laboratory tests and diagnostic procedures* (4th ed.). Philadelphia: W.B. Saunders, p. 428.
Pagana, K., & Pagana, T. (2003). *Mosby's diagnostic and laboratory test reference* (6th ed.). St. Louis: Mosby, pp. 302, 307.

3. *Answer: 3*
Rationale: The normal serum creatinine level is 0.6 to 1.3 mg/dL. The client with a mild degree of renal insufficiency would

have a slightly elevated level, which would be the value of 1.9 mg/dL. Creatinine levels of 3.5 mg/dL may be associated with acute or chronic renal failure.
Test-Taking Strategy: Note the key word, *mild.* This tells you that the correct option will be an abnormal value, but perhaps not the most abnormal of all the options. Use your knowledge of the normal serum creatinine level to direct you to option 3. Review the normal value of this laboratory test if you had difficulty with this question.
Level of Cognitive Ability: Analysis
Client Needs: Physiological Integrity
Integrated Process: Nursing Process/Data Collection
Content Area: Fundamental Skills
Reference: Pagana, K., & Pagana, T. (2003). *Mosby's diagnostic and laboratory test reference* (6th ed.). St. Louis: Mosby, pp. 308-309.

4. Answer: 3
Rationale: The therapeutic range for serum phenytoin (Dilantin) level is 10 to 20 mcg/mL. If the level is below the therapeutic range, the client may continue to experience seizure activity. If the level is too high, the client could experience phenytoin toxicity.
Test-Taking Strategy: Focus on the issue, that medication therapy is effective. Remember that the therapeutic range for serum phenytoin (Dilantin) level is 10 to 20 mcg/mL. Review this normal range if you had difficulty with this question.
Level of Cognitive Ability: Analysis
Client Needs: Physiological Integrity
Integrated Process: Nursing Process/Evaluation
Content Area: Fundamental Skills
Reference: Black, J., & Hawks, J. (2005). *Medical-surgical nursing: Clinical management for positive outcomes* (7th ed.). Philadelphia: W.B. Saunders, p. 2307.

5. Answer: 1
Rationale: The therapeutic range for the serum theophylline level is 10 to 20 mcg/mL. If the level is below the therapeutic range, the client may experience frequent exacerbations of the disorder. If the level is within the therapeutic range, the client is most likely compliant with medication therapy.
Test-Taking Strategy: Note the key words, *may not be compliant.* Recalling the therapeutic level of theophylline will direct you to option 1. Review this therapeutic range if you had difficulty with this question.
Level of Cognitive Ability: Analysis
Client Needs: Physiological Integrity
Integrated Process: Nursing Process/Evaluation
Content Area: Fundamental Skills
Reference: Hodgson, B., & Kizior, R. (2005). *Saunders nursing drug handbook 2005.* Philadelphia: W.B. Saunders, p. 53.

6. Answer: 4
Rationale: The normal therapeutic range for digoxin is 0.5 to 2 ng/mL. A value of 2.4 ng/mL exceeds the therapeutic range and could be toxic to the client. The nursing action is to hold further doses of digoxin. Option 1 is incorrect because the value is not normal. The next dose should not be administered automatically. Checking the client's pulse is not incorrect but may have limited value. Depending on the time that

has elapsed since the last pulse check, it may be more useful to do a current assessment of the client's status.
Test-Taking Strategy: Recall that the normal therapeutic range for digoxin is 0.5 to 2 ng/mL. Noting that the value is high will direct you to option 4. Review this therapeutic level if you had difficulty with this question.
Level of Cognitive Ability: Application
Client Needs: Physiological Integrity
Integrated Process: Nursing Process/Implementation
Content Area: Fundamental Skills
Reference: Hodgson, B., & Kizior, R. (2005). *Saunders nursing drug handbook 2005.* Philadelphia: W.B. Saunders, p. 326.

7. Answer: 1
Rationale: The normal PT is 9.6 to 11.8 seconds (adult male) and 9.5 to 11.3 seconds (adult female). Because the value stated is extremely high (and perhaps near the critical range), the nurse should anticipate that the client would not receive further doses at this time. If the level were too high, then the antidote (vitamin K) may be prescribed.
Test-Taking Strategy: Note that the PT is 30 seconds. Noting that the PT value is high will direct you to option 1. Review this laboratory value if you had difficulty with this question.
Level of Cognitive Ability: Comprehension
Client Needs: Physiological Integrity
Integrated Process: Nursing Process/Planning
Content Area: Fundamental Skills
Reference: Pagana, K., & Pagana, T. (2003). *Mosby's diagnostic and laboratory test reference* (6th ed.). St. Louis: Mosby, pp. 730-731.

8. Answer: 1
Rationale: The normal serum electrolyte ranges for adults are as follows: sodium, 135 to 145 mEq/L; potassium, 3.5 to 5.1 mEq/L; chloride, 98 to 107 mEq/L; bicarbonate (venous), 22 to 29 mEq/L. The only abnormal value identified is the serum sodium level.
Test-Taking Strategy: Focus on the issue, an abnormal value. Recalling the normal serum electrolyte values will direct you to option 1. Review the normal electrolyte values if you had difficulty with this question.
Level of Cognitive Ability: Comprehension
Client Needs: Physiological Integrity
Integrated Process: Nursing Process/Data Collection
Content Area: Fundamental Skills
Reference: Chernecky, C., & Berger, B. (2004). *Laboratory tests and diagnostic procedures* (4th ed.). Philadelphia: W.B. Saunders, p. 492.

9. Answer: 4
Rationale: The normal serum potassium level in the adult is 3.5 to 5.1 mEq/L. Option 4 is the only option reflecting a value that has dropped down into the normal range.
Test-Taking Strategy: Note the key words, *critically high.* You would expect that this medication is administered to lower the potassium level. Recalling the normal serum potassium level will direct you to option 4. Review this normal level if you had difficulty with this question.
Level of Cognitive Ability: Analysis
Client Needs: Physiological Integrity

Integrated Process: Nursing Process/Evaluation
Content Area: Fundamental Skills
Reference: Chernecky, C., & Berger, B. (2004). *Laboratory tests and diagnostic procedures* (4th ed.). Philadelphia: W.B. Saunders, p. 887.

10. *Answer:* **1**
Rationale: The normal adult serum potassium level is 3.5 to 5.1 mEq/L. Option 1 is the only value that falls below the therapeutic range. Administering furosemide to a client with a low potassium level and a cardiac history could precipitate ventricular dysrhythmias in the client.
Test-Taking Strategy: Use the process of elimination. Recalling the normal serum potassium level will assist you in identifying the value that is not within normal range. This will direct you to option 1. Review the normal adult serum potassium level if you had difficulty with this question.
Level of Cognitive Ability: Comprehension
Client Needs: Physiological Integrity
Integrated Process: Nursing Process/Implementation
Content Area: Fundamental Skills
Reference: Chernecky, C., & Berger, B. (2004). *Laboratory tests and diagnostic procedures* (4th ed.). Philadelphia: W.B. Saunders, p. 887.

11. *Answer:* **4**
Rationale: The normal fasting blood glucose is 70 to 110 mg/dL in the adult client. A critical level is considered to be one that exceeds 300 mg/dL. This makes option 4 the correct option.
Test-Taking Strategy: Use the process of elimination and knowledge of the normal fasting blood glucose level to answer the question. Noting the key words *critical value* will direct you to option 4. Review this laboratory test if you had difficulty with this question.
Level of Cognitive Ability: Comprehension
Client Needs: Physiological Integrity
Integrated Process: Nursing Process/Data Collection
Content Area: Fundamental Skills
Reference: Chernecky, C., & Berger, B. (2004). *Laboratory tests and diagnostic procedures* (4th ed.). Philadelphia: W.B. Saunders, p. 599.

12. *Answer:* **4**
Rationale: A normal platelet count ranges from 150,000 to 400,000 cells/µL. The nurse should place the report containing the normal laboratory value into the client's medical record.
Test-Taking Strategy: Use the process of elimination. Remember that options that are similar are not likely to be correct. With this in mind, eliminate options 1 and 3 first. From the remaining options, recalling the normal range for this laboratory test will direct you to option 4. Review this normal value if you had difficulty with this question.
Level of Cognitive Ability: Application
Client Needs: Physiological Integrity
Integrated Process: Nursing Process/Implementation
Content Area: Fundamental Skills
Reference: Chernecky, C., & Berger, B. (2004). *Laboratory tests and diagnostic procedures* (4th ed.). Philadelphia: W.B. Saunders, p. 879.

13. *Answer:* **3**
Rationale: The normal range for the protein level in the adult client is 6 to 8 g/dL, making option 3 the correct option. Options 1 and 2 indicate low levels. Option 4 indicates an elevated level.
Test-Taking Strategy: Note the key words, *most satisfactory.* Recalling the normal protein level will direct you to option 3. Review this normal level if you had difficulty with this question.
Level of Cognitive Ability: Analysis
Client Needs: Physiological Integrity
Integrated Process: Nursing Process/Evaluation
Content Area: Fundamental Skills
Reference: Chernecky, C., & Berger, B. (2004). *Laboratory tests and diagnostic procedures* (4th ed.). Philadelphia: W.B. Saunders, p. 907.

14. *Answer:* **1**
Rationale: The isoenzymes that are particularly affected in acute myocardial infarction are LDH_1 and LDH_2. The LDH level begins to increase approximately 24 hours after myocardial infarction and peaks in 48 to 72 hours. Thereafter, it returns to normal, usually within 7 to 14 days.
Test-Taking Strategy: Familiarity with the cardiac isoenzymes for LDH is needed to answer this question. Remember that the isoenzymes that are particularly affected with acute myocardial infarction are LDH_1 and LDH_2. Review these enzymes if you had difficulty with this question.
Level of Cognitive Ability: Comprehension
Client Needs: Physiological Integrity
Integrated Process: Nursing Process/Data Collection
Content Area: Fundamental Skills
Reference: Chernecky, C., & Berger, B. (2004). *Laboratory tests and diagnostic procedures* (4th ed.). Philadelphia: W.B. Saunders, p. 710.

15. *Answer:* **3**
Rationale: The normal serum lipase level is 10 to 140 units/L. The client who is recovering from acute pancreatitis usually has elevated lipase levels for approximately 10 days after onset of symptoms. This makes lipase a valuable test in monitoring the client's pancreatic function. Option 3 is the only option that contains a value just beneath the upper limit of normal.
Test-Taking Strategy: Note the key words, *just beneath the upper limit of normal.* Recalling the normal lipase level will direct you to option 3. Review this normal level if you had difficulty with this question.
Level of Cognitive Ability: Comprehension
Client Needs: Physiological Integrity
Integrated Process: Nursing Process/Evaluation
Content Area: Fundamental Skills
Reference: Chernecky, C., & Berger, B. (2004). *Laboratory tests and diagnostic procedures* (4th ed.). Philadelphia: W.B. Saunders, p. 724.

16. *Answer:* **4**
Rationale: Troponin is a regulatory protein found in striated muscle. The troponins function together in the contractile apparatus for striated muscle in skeletal muscle and in the myocardium. Increased amounts of troponins are released into the bloodstream when an infarction causes damage to

the myocardium. A troponin T level that is higher than 0.1 to 0.2 ng/mL is consistent with a myocardial infarction. A normal troponin I level is lower than 0.6 ng/mL, whereas a level higher than 1.5 ng/mL is consistent with a myocardial infarction.

Test-Taking Strategy: Note that the issue of the question relates to the troponin T level. Recalling that a level higher than 0.1 to 0.2 ng/mL is consistent with a myocardial infarction will direct you to option 4. Review this diagnostic test if you are unfamiliar with it.

Level of Cognitive Ability: Analysis
Client Needs: Physiological Integrity
Integrated Process: Nursing Process/Evaluation
Content Area: Adult Health/Cardiovascular
Reference: Malarkey, L., & McMorrow, M. (2005). *Nursing guide to laboratory and diagnostic tests.* Philadelphia: W.B. Saunders, pp. 179-181

17. *Answer: 4*
Rationale: The normal hemoglobin level for an adult female client is 12 to 15 g/dL. Iron deficiency anemia can result in lower hemoglobin levels. Heart failure and COPD may increase the hemoglobin level due to the need by the body for more oxygen-carrying capacity. Dehydration may increase the hemoglobin level by hemoconcentration.
Test-Taking Strategy: Use the process of elimination. Evaluate each condition in the options in terms of whether it is likely to raise or lower the hemoglobin level. This will direct you to option 4. Review the normal hemoglobin level and the causes of a low level if you had difficulty with this question.
Level of Cognitive Ability: Analysis
Client Needs: Physiological Integrity
Integrated Process: Nursing Process/Data Collection
Content Area: Fundamental Skills
Reference: Pagana, K., & Pagana, T. (2003). *Mosby's diagnostic and laboratory test reference* (6th ed.). St. Louis: Mosby, p. 491.

18. *Answer: 2*
Rationale: The normal hematocrit level for an adult male is 42% to 52%. The client who is dehydrated has an elevated level because of hemoconcentration. The client's level may be expected to drift back down to within the normal range once fluid volume has been adequately restored. Thus, option 2 is the only correct choice. Option 1 is too high and options 3 and 4 are low.
Test-Taking Strategy: Use the process of elimination and note the key words, *normal range.* Recalling the normal hematocrit level for an adult male will direct you to option 2. Review this normal value if you had difficulty with this question.
Level of Cognitive Ability: Comprehension
Client Needs: Physiological Integrity
Integrated Process: Nursing Process/Evaluation
Content Area: Fundamental Skills
Reference: Pagana, K., & Pagana, T. (2003). *Mosby's diagnostic and laboratory test reference* (6th ed.). St. Louis: Mosby, pp. 487-489.

19. *Answer: 3*
Rationale: The glycosylated hemoglobin value measures the amount of glucose that has become permanently bound to the red blood cells from circulating glucose. Elevations in

blood glucose levels will cause elevations in the amount of glycosylation. Thus, the test is useful in detecting clients who have periods of hyperglycemia that are undetected in other ways. Values are expressed as a percentage of total hemoglobin and include the following: diabetic with good control of 7.5% or lower; diabetic with fair control of 7.6% to 8.9%; diabetic with poor control of 9% or higher. Elevations indicate continued need for teaching related to prevention of hyperglycemic episodes.
Test-Taking Strategy: Use the process of elimination and focus on the level identified in the question. Recalling the expected values related to this test and their significance will assist in answering correctly. Review this test if you had difficulty with this question.
Level of Cognitive Ability: Application
Client Needs: Health Promotion and Maintenance
Integrated Process: Teaching/Learning
Content Area: Fundamental Skills
Reference: Pagana, K., & Pagana, T. (2003). *Mosby's diagnostic and laboratory test reference* (6th ed.). St. Louis: Mosby, p. 472.

20. *Answer: 4*
Rationale: The normal range for urine specific gravity is from 1.016 to 1.022. Elevations may occur with SIADH, because the kidneys are stimulated to reabsorb water, thus causing unusual concentration of the urine. Option 1 represents a low value, which may be seen in the client with diabetes insipidus. Options 2 and 3 reflect normal values.
Test-Taking Strategy: Use the process of elimination and note the key words, *not resolving.* Recalling the normal values for this test will assist in eliminating options 2 and 3. From the remaining options, recalling the pathophysiology associated with SIADH will direct you to option 4. Review this test if you had difficulty with this question.
Level of Cognitive Ability: Analysis
Client Needs: Physiological Integrity
Integrated Process: Nursing Process/Evaluation
Content Area: Fundamental Skills
Reference: Chernecky, C., & Berger, B. (2004). *Laboratory tests and diagnostic procedures* (4th ed.). Philadelphia: W.B. Saunders, p. 1013.

21. *Answer: 1*
Rationale: The normal WBC count ranges from 4500 to 11,000/μL. The client who is immunosuppressed has a decrease in the number of circulating WBCs. The nurse implements neutropenic precautions when the client's values fall sufficiently below the low-normal level.
Test-Taking Strategy: Knowledge regarding the normal WBC count and the purpose of neutropenic precautions will direct you to option 1. Remember the normal WBC count ranges from 4500 to 11,000/μL. Review this laboratory test if you had difficulty with this question.
Level of Cognitive Ability: Comprehension
Client Needs: Safe, Effective Care Environment
Integrated Process: Nursing Process/Implementation
Content Area: Fundamental Skills
Reference: Chernecky, C., & Berger, B. (2004). *Laboratory tests and diagnostic procedures* (4th ed.). Philadelphia: W.B. Saunders, p. 400.

22. *Answer:* **2**
Rationale: The normal cholesterol level is 140 to 199 mg/dL. The client should be counseled to keep the total cholesterol level under 200 mg/dL. This will aid in prevention of atherosclerosis, which can lead to a number of cardiovascular disorders later in life.
Test-Taking Strategy: Use the process of elimination. Recalling the normal cholesterol level will direct you to option 2. Remember that the normal cholesterol level is 140 to 199 mg/dL. Review this normal level if you had difficulty with this question.
Level of Cognitive Ability: Application
Client Needs: Health Promotion and Maintenance
Integrated Process: Teaching/Learning
Content Area: Fundamental Skills
Reference: Chernecky, C., & Berger, B. (2004). *Laboratory tests and diagnostic procedures* (4th ed.). Philadelphia: W.B. Saunders, p. 369.

23. *Answer:* **3**
Rationale: The normal BUN value for the adult is 8 to 25 mg/dL. Thus, option 3 is correct. Values such as those in options 1 and 2 reflect continued dehydration. Option 4 reflects a lower than normal value, which may occur with fluid overload, among other conditions.
Test-Taking Strategy: Use the process of elimination and note the key words, *adequate volume replacement*. Recalling the normal BUN level will direct you to option 3. Remember that the normal BUN for the adult is 8 to 25 mg/dL. Review this level if you had difficulty with this question.
Level of Cognitive Ability: Comprehension
Client Needs: Physiological Integrity
Integrated Process: Nursing Process/Evaluation
Content Area: Fundamental Skills
Reference: Chernecky, C., & Berger, B. (2004). *Laboratory tests and diagnostic procedures* (4th ed.). Philadelphia: W.B. Saunders, p. 1111.

24. *Answer:* **2**
Rationale: The normal hemoglobin level for an adult female is 12 to 15 g/dL. Option 1 is a low value and would indicate an anemia. Options 3 and 4 are elevated values.
Test-Taking Strategy: Knowledge regarding the normal hemoglobin level will direct you to option 2. Remember that the normal hemoglobin level for an adult female is 12 to 15 g/dL. If you are unfamiliar with this laboratory value, review its normal value.
Level of Cognitive Ability: Comprehension
Client Needs: Physiological Integrity
Integrated Process: Nursing Process/Data Collection

Content Area: Fundamental Skills
Reference: Pagana, K., & Pagana, T. (2003). *Mosby's diagnostic and laboratory test reference* (6th ed.). St. Louis: Mosby, p. 490.

25. *Answer:* **3**
Rationale: The normal serum amylase level is 25 to 151 units/L. In chronic cases of pancreatitis, the rise in serum amylase levels usually does not exceed three times the normal value. In acute pancreatitis, the value may exceed five times the normal value. Therefore, option 3 is correct.
Test-Taking Strategy: Note the key word, *chronic*. Recalling that the normal serum amylase level is 25 to 151 units/L and understanding the effects of chronic pancreatitis on this laboratory value will direct you to option 3. Review these effects if you had difficulty with this question.
Level of Cognitive Ability: Analysis
Client Needs: Physiological Integrity
Integrated Process: Nursing Process/Data Collection
Content Area: Fundamental Skills
Reference: Chernecky, C., & Berger, B. (2004). *Laboratory tests and diagnostic procedures* (4th ed.). Philadelphia: W.B. Saunders, p. 172.

ALTERNATE FORMAT QUESTION: MULTIPLE RESPONSE

Answers:
White blood cells, 3000 cells/μL
Neutrophils, 1000/μL
Magnesium, 1.0 mg/dL
Calcium, 7.0 mg/dL
Rationale: The normal values include the following: white blood cells, 4500 to 11,000/μL; neutrophils, 56% or 1800 to 7800 cells/μL; thyroid-stimulating hormone, 0.2 to 5.4 microunits/mL; phosphorus, 2.7 to 4.5 mg/dL; magnesium, 1.6 to 2.6 mg/dL; calcium, 8.6 to 10.0 mg/dL; blood urea nitrogen, 5 to 20 mg/dL; and serum creatinine, 0.6 to 1.3 mg/dL.
Test-Taking Strategy: Note the key word *abnormal* in the question. Knowledge of the normal laboratory values for these studies will assist in answering this question. Review these normal values if you had difficulty with this question.
Level of Cognitive Ability: Analysis
Client Needs: Physiological Integrity
Integrated Process: Nursing Process/Data Collection
Content Area: Fundamental Skills
Reference: Lewis, S., Heitkemper, M., & Dirksen, S. (2004). *Medical-surgical nursing: Assessment and management of clinical problems* (6th ed.). St. Louis: Mosby, pp. 700, 1034, 1163, 1263-1264.

REFERENCES

Black, J., & Hawks, J. (2005). *Medical-surgical nursing: Clinical management for positive outcomes* (7th ed.). Philadelphia: W.B. Saunders.

Chernecky, C., & Berger, B. (2004). *Laboratory tests and diagnostic procedures* (4th ed.). Philadelphia: W.B. Saunders.

Hodgson, B., & Kizior, R. (2005). *Saunders nursing drug handbook 2005*. Philadelphia: W.B. Saunders.

Lewis, S., Heitkemper, M., & Dirksen, S. (2004). *Medical-surgical nursing: Assessment and management of clinical problems* (6th ed.). St. Louis: Mosby.

Malarkey, L., & McMorrow, M. (2005). *Nursing guide to laboratory and diagnostic tests*. Philadelphia: W.B. Saunders.

National Council of State Boards of Nursing . (2005). *Detailed test plan for the National Council licensure examination for practical/ vocational nurses*. Chicago: Author.

Pagana, K., & Pagana, T. (2003). *Mosby's diagnostic and laboratory test reference* (6th ed.). St. Louis: Mosby.

Nutritional Components of Care

PYRAMID TERMS

absorption   Passage of digested nutrients through the wall of the stomach or small intestine into the blood or lymph system.

digestion   The breakdown of carbohydrates, fats, and proteins into monosaccharides, fatty acids, and amino acids.

enteral nutrition   Administering nutrition with liquefied foods into the gastrointestinal (GI) tract via a tube.

fat emulsion (lipids)   Administered during parenteral nutrition therapy to prevent fatty acid deficiency.

malnutrition   Deficiency of the nutrients required for development and maintenance of the human body.

metabolism   Ongoing chemical process within the body that converts digested nutrients into energy for the functioning of body cells.

nutrients   Include carbohydrates, fats or lipids, proteins, vitamins, minerals, and water. Must be supplied in adequate amounts to provide energy, growth, development, and maintenance of the human body.

parenteral nutrition   The administration of nutrition through a central or peripheral intravenous catheter.

peripheral parenteral nutrition (PPN)   Parenteral nutrition administered through a peripheral vein in an extremity.

total parenteral nutrition (TPN)   Parenteral nutrition administered through a central vein, such as the subclavian vein; also called hyperalimentation, central venous parenteral nutrition, or central parenteral nutrition.

▲ PYRAMID TO SUCCESS

Nutrition is a basic need that must be met for all clients. Nurses must have the knowledge required to educate and care for healthy clients, as well as clients with nutritional needs or disorders requiring alterations in dietary measures. NCLEX-PN will address the dietary measures required for basic needs and for particular body system alterations. When presented with a question related to nutrition, consider the client's diagnosis and the particular requirement or restriction necessary for treatment of the disorder. Pyramid points focus on the common types of therapeutic diets, nutrients contained in food items, enteral feedings, and total parenteral nutrition. Integrated Processes addressed in this chapter include Clinical Problem-Solving Process (Nursing Process), Caring, Communication and Documentation, and Teaching/Learning.

CLIENT NEEDS
Safe, Effective Care Environment

Consultation with members of the health care team
Dietary consultation and referral
Informed consent for invasive procedures
Medical and surgical asepsis
Standard, transmission-based, and other precautions

Health Promotion and Maintenance

Collecting data
Dietary teaching
Disease prevention
Health and wellness
Health promotion programs
Lifestyle choices

Psychosocial Integrity

Coping mechanisms
Cultural preferences related to nutritional patterns and lifestyle choices
Religious and spiritual influences on health

Physiological Integrity

Alteration in body systems
Elimination patterns
Monitoring enteral feedings and the client's ability to tolerate feedings

Monitoring for expected effects of nutritional therapy

Monitoring for potential complications of enteral feedings or total parenteral nutrition

Monitoring laboratory values

Monitoring fluid and electrolyte balance

Monitoring nutritional intake and oral hydration

I. NUTRIENTS

A. Carbohydrates (Box 12-1)
   1. Preferred source of energy
   2. Include sugars, starches, and cellulose, and provide 4 cal/g
   3. Promote normal fat **metabolism,** spare protein, and enhance lower gastrointestinal (GI) function
   4. Major food sources include milk, grains, fruits, and vegetables
   5. Inadequate carbohydrate intake affects **metabolism**
B. Fats (Box 12-2)
   1. Provide a concentrated source and a stored form of energy
   2. Protect internal organs and maintain body temperature
   3. Enhance **absorption** of the fat-soluble vitamins
   4. Provide 9 cal/g
   5. Inadequate fat intake leads to clinical manifestations of sensitivity to cold, skin lesions, increased risk of infection, and amenorrhea in women
   6. Diets high in fat can lead to obesity and increase the risk of cardiovascular disease and some cancers
C. Proteins (Box 12-3)
   1. Made from amino acids, critical to all aspects of growth and development of body tissues, and provide 4 cal/g
   2. Build and repair body tissues, regulate fluid balance, maintain acid-base balance, produce antibodies, provide energy, and produce enzymes and hormones
   3. Essential amino acids (EAAs) are required in the diet because the body cannot manufacture them
   4. High-quality proteins or complete proteins such as eggs, dairy products, meat, fish, and poultry contain adequate amounts of EAAs
   5. Foods that do not contain EAAs in sufficient amounts are lower quality or incomplete proteins
   6. Inadequate protein can cause protein energy **malnutrition** and severe wasting of fat and muscle tissue
D. Vitamins (Box 12-4)
   1. Facilitate **metabolism** of proteins, fats, and carbohydrates; act as catalysts for metabolic functions; promote life and growth processes; and maintain and regulate body functions
   2. Fat-soluble vitamins A, D, E, and K can be stored in the body, so an excess can cause toxicity
   3. The B vitamins and vitamin C are water soluble, are not stored in the body, and can be excreted in the urine
   4. Vitamin K acts as a catalyst for facilitating blood-clotting factors, especially prothrombin
   5. Vitamin C produces collagen, a vital component in wound healing
   6. Vitamin A maintains eyesight and epithelial linings
E. Minerals (Box 12-5)
   1. Components of hormones, cells, tissues, and bones
   2. Act as catalysts for chemical reactions and enhancers of cell function
   3. Almost all foods contain some form of minerals
   4. Deficiency of minerals can occur in chronically ill or hospitalized clients

II. FOOD GUIDE PYRAMID (Figure 12-1)

III. THERAPEUTIC DIETS

A. Clear liquid diet
   1. Indications
      a. Serves a primary function of providing fluids and electrolytes to prevent dehydration

---

BOX 12-1

Carbohydrate Food Sources

GLUCOSE	FRUCTOSE	CELLULOSE	LACTOSE
Grapes	Honey	Bran	Milk
Oranges	Fruits	Apples	
Dates		Beans	
Corn		Cabbage	
Carrots			

SUCROSE	STARCH
Granulated table sugar	Wheat
Molasses	Corn
Apricots	Oats
Peaches	Rye
Plums	Barley
Honeydew and cantaloupe	Potatoes and pasta
Peas and corn	Beets, carrots, and peas

BOX 12-2

Fat Food Sources

SATURATED FATS	MONOUNSATURATED FATS
Beef	Duck and goose
Luncheon meats	Eggs
Hard yellow cheeses	Olive and peanut oils
Butter	

POLYUNSATURATED FATS	CHOLESTEROL
Safflower oil	Animal products
Corn oil	Egg yolks
Sunflower oil	Liver and organ meats

BOX 12-3

Protein Food Sources

Meats
Dairy products
Bread and cereal products
Dried beans

BOX 12-4

Food Sources of Vitamins

WATER-SOLUBLE VITAMINS
Vitamin C (ascorbic acid): Citrus fruits, tomatoes, broccoli, cabbage
Vitamin B_1 (thiamine): Pork and nuts, whole-grain cereals, and legumes
Vitamin B_2 (riboflavin): Milk, lean meats, fish, grains
Niacin: Meats, poultry, fish, beans, peanuts, grains
Vitamin B_6 (pryidoxine): Yeast, corn, meat, poultry, fish
Vitamin B_{12} (cobalamin): Meat, liver
Folic acid: Green, leafy vegetables; liver, beef and fish; legumes; grapefruits and oranges

FAT-SOLUBLE VITAMINS
Vitamin A: Liver, egg yolk, whole milk, green or orange vegetables, fruits
Vitamin D: Fortified milk, fish oils, cereals
Vitamin E: Vegetable oils; green, leafy vegetables; cereals; apricots, apples, and peaches
Vitamin K: Green, leafy vegetables; cauliflower and cabbage

BOX 12-5

Food Sources of Minerals

CALCIUM
Yogurt
Milk
Rhubarb
Collard greens
Cheese
Tofu
Spinach
Broccoli
Green beans
Carrots

Spinach
Bananas
Fish
Oranges
Strawberries
Mushrooms
Carrots
Potatoes
Tomatoes

CHLORIDE
Salt

MAGNESIUM
Green, leafy vegetables
Avocado
Canned white tuna fish
Yogurt
Cooked rolled oats
Milk
Peas
Potatoes
Pork, beef, chicken
Raisins
Peanut butter
Cauliflower

SODIUM
Table salt
Soy sauce
Cured pork
Cottage cheese
American cheese
Milk
Butter
White and whole-wheat bread
Ketchup
Mustard
Bacon
Hot dogs
Lunch meat
Canned food
Processed food
Snack food

PHOSPHORUS
Fish
Pork, beef, chicken
Organ meats
Nuts
Whole-grain breads and cereals

IRON
Liver
Meats
Egg yolk
Dark-green vegetables
Breads and cereals

POTASSIUM
Avocado
Raisins
Pork, beef, veal
Cantaloupe

ZINC
Meats
Eggs
Leafy vegetables
Protein-rich foods

---

b. Initial feeding after complete bowel rest
c. Used initially to feed a malnourished person or a person who has not had any oral intake for some time
d. Bowel preparation for surgery or tests
e. Postsurgical diet
f. Diarrhea
2. Nursing considerations
a. Clear liquid is deficient in energy and most nutrients
b. The body digests and absorbs clear liquids easily
c. Contributes to little or no residue in the GI tract
d. Can be unappetizing and boring
e. Client should not stay on a clear liquid diet for more than a day or two
f. Consists of foods that are relatively transparent to light, and are clear and liquid at room and body temperature
g. Foods include such items as water, bouillon, clear broth, carbonated beverages, gelatin, hard candy, lemonade, Popsicles, and regular or decaffeinated coffee or tea
h. The nurse should limit the amount of caffeine consumed by the client because caffeine can cause an upset stomach and sleeplessness

i. Client may have salt or sugar
j. Dairy products are not allowed
B. Full liquid diet
1. Indication: May be used as a second diet after clear liquids following surgery, or for a client who is unable to chew or swallow
2. Nursing considerations
a. Nutritionally deficient in energy and most nutrients
b. Includes both clear and opaque liquid foods and those that liquefy at body temperature
c. Foods include all clear liquids and such items as plain ice cream, sherbet, breakfast drinks,

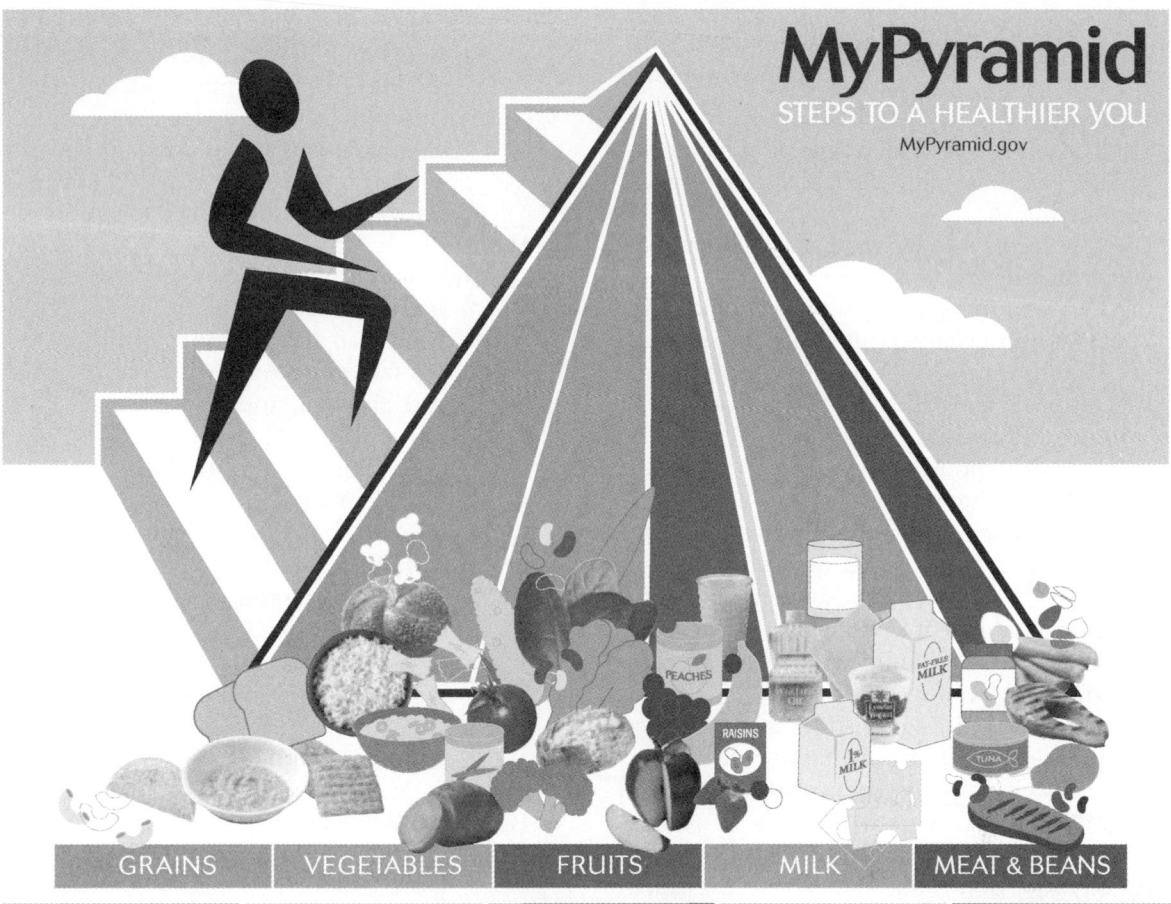

MyPyramid
STEPS TO A HEALTHIER YOU
MyPyramid.gov

GRAINS	VEGETABLES	FRUITS	MILK	MEAT & BEANS
GRAINS Make half your grains whole	**VEGETABLES** Vary your veggies	**FRUITS** Focus on fruits	**MILK** Get your calcium-rich foods	**MEAT & BEANS** Go lean with protein
Eat at least 3 oz. of whole-grain cereals, breads, crackers, rice, or pasta every day 1 oz. is about 1 slice of bread, about 1 cup of breakfast cereal, or ½ cup of cooked rice, cereal, or pasta	Eat more dark-green veggies like broccoli, spinach, and other dark leafy greens Eat more orange vegetables like carrots and sweetpotatoes Eat more dry beans and peas like pinto beans, kidney beans, and lentils	Eat a variety of fruit Choose fresh, frozen, canned, or dried fruit Go easy on fruit juices	Go low-fat or fat-free when you choose milk, yogurt, and other milk products If you don't or can't consume milk, choose lactose-free products or other calcium sources such as fortified foods and beverages	Choose low-fat or lean meats and poultry Bake it, broil it, or grill it Vary your protein routine — choose more fish, beans, peas, nuts, and seeds

For a 2,000-calorie diet, you need the amounts below from each food group. To find the amounts that are right for you, go to MyPyramid.gov.

Eat 6 oz. every day	Eat 2½ cups every day	Eat 2 cups every day	Get 3 cups every day; for kids aged 2 to 8, it's 2	Eat 5½ oz. every day

Find your balance between food and physical activity
- Be sure to stay within your daily calorie needs.
- Be physically active for at least 30 minutes most days of the week.
- About 60 minutes a day of physical activity may be needed to prevent weight gain.
- For sustaining weight loss, at least 60 to 90 minutes a day of physical activity may be required.
- Children and teenagers should be physically active for 60 minutes every day, or most days.

Know the limits on fats, sugars, and salt (sodium)
- Make most of your fat sources from fish, nuts, and vegetable oils.
- Limit solid fats like butter, stick margarine, shortening, and lard, as well as foods that contain these.
- Check the Nutrition Facts label to keep saturated fats, *trans* fats, and sodium low.
- Choose food and beverages low in added sugars. Added sugars contribute calories with few, if any, nutrients.

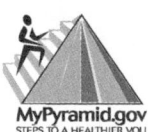

MyPyramid.gov
STEPS TO A HEALTHIER YOU

U.S. Department of Agriculture
Center for Nutrition Policy and Promotion
April 2005
CNPP-15

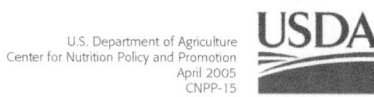

FIG. 12-1   MyPyramid. (From U.S. Department of Agriculture, Center for Nutrition Policy and Promotion. Retrieved April 2005 from www.MyPyramid.gov.)

milk, pudding and custard, soups that are strained, and strained vegetable juices

C. Soft diet
1. Indications
   a. Used in clients with dental problems, poor-fitting dentures, and difficulty chewing or swallowing
   b. Used for clients with ulcerations of the mouth or gums, oral surgery, broken jaw, plastic surgery of head or neck, or dysphasia, or for the stroke client
   c. Therapeutic for clients with impaired digestion and/or absorption as a result of conditions such as ulcerative colitis and Crohn's disease
2. Nursing considerations
   a. Clients with mouth sores should be served foods at cooler temperatures
   b. Clients who have difficulty chewing and swallowing because of reduced flow of saliva can increase salivary flow by sucking on sour candy
   c. Encourage the client to eat a variety of foods
   d. Provide plenty of fluids with meals to ease chewing and swallowing of foods
   e. Sucking fluids through a straw may be easier than drinking them from a cup or glass
   f. All foods and seasonings are permitted; however, liquid, chopped, or puréed foods or regular foods with a soft consistency are tolerated best
   g. Avoid foods that contain nuts or seeds, which can easily become trapped in the mouth and cause discomfort
   h. Raw fruits and vegetables, fried foods, and whole grains are avoided

D. Bland diet
1. Indication: May be prescribed for the client with gastritis, ulcers, reflux esophagitis, or other GI disorders, congestive heart failure (CHF), or myocardial infarction (MI)
2. Nursing considerations
   a. Bland foods are less likely to form gas than food in regular diets
   b. Eliminate foods that stimulate gastric acid secretions
   c. Eliminate foods that are irritating to the gastric mucosa
   d. Foods to be avoided include alcohol, caffeine and caffeine-containing beverages such as cola, cocoa, coffee, and tea, fried foods, hot pepper and spicy foods

E. Low-residue, low-fiber diet
1. Indications
   a. Supplies foods that are least likely to form an obstruction when the intestinal tract is narrowed by inflammation or scarring or when GI motility is slowed
   b. Used for inflammatory bowel disease, partial obstructions of the intestinal tract, enteritis, diarrhea, or other GI disorders

2. Nursing considerations
   a. Foods high in carbohydrates are usually low in residue; include white bread, cereals, and pasta
   b. Foods to be avoided are raw fruits (except bananas), vegetables, seeds, plant fiber, and whole grains
   c. Dairy products are limited to two servings a day

F. High-residue, high-fiber diet
1. Indications
   a. Used in constipation
   b. Used in irritable bowel syndrome, when the primary symptom is alternating constipation and diarrhea, and asymptomatic diverticular disease
   c. Helps regulate blood glucose in clients with diabetes mellitus
   d. Helps control blood cholesterol in clients with heart disease
2. Nursing considerations
   a. Provides 20 to 25 g of dietary fiber daily
   b. Adds volume and weight to the stool and speeds the movement of undigested materials through the intestine
   c. Consists of fruits and vegetables and whole-grain products

G. Fat-controlled diet
1. Indications
   a. Indicated for atherosclerosis, diabetes mellitus, hyperlipidemia, hypertension, myocardial infarction, nephrotic syndrome, and renal failure
   b. Reduces the risk of heart disease
2. Nursing considerations: Limit both the total amounts of fats and polyunsaturated, monounsaturated, and saturated fats and cholesterol

H. High-calorie diet
1. Indications: Severe stress, burns, cancer, human immunodeficiency virus (HIV) infection, acquired immunodeficiency syndrome (AIDS), chronic obstructive pulmonary disease (COPD), respiratory failure, or any other type of debilitating disease
2. Nursing considerations
   a. High-calorie diet should also be high in protein, because the purpose of the diet is to build and/or maintain lean body mass
   b. Add fats to foods whenever possible
   c. Add nuts and dried fruits such as raisins to dessert or cereal if the client can tolerate and eat these foods
   d. Add sugar to food, and provide high-calorie desserts
   e. Encourage snacks between meals, such as milkshakes and instant breakfasts

I. Sodium-restricted diet
1. Indications: Hypertension, CHF, kidney diseases, cardiac diseases, and cirrhosis of the liver
2. Nursing considerations (Box 12-6)

BOX 12-6

Sodium-Free Spices and Flavorings

Allspice	Ginger
Almond extract	Lemon extract
Bay leaves	Maple extract
Caraway seeds	Marjoram
Cinnamon	Mustard powder
Curry powder	Nutmeg
Garlic powder or garlic	

   a. This type of diet consists of 2000 to 4000 mg of sodium daily (mild restriction), 1000 mg of sodium daily (moderate restriction), or 500 mg of sodium daily (strict and seldom prescribed)
   b. Cereals allowed on a sodium-restricted diet include dried or instant cereals, puffed wheat, puffed rice, and shredded wheat
J. Protein-restricted diet
   1. Indications: Acute renal failure, chronic renal disease, cirrhosis of the liver, and hepatic coma
   2. Nursing considerations
      a. Provides enough protein to maintain nutritional status but not an amount that will allow the buildup of waste products from protein metabolism (40 to 60 g of protein daily)
      b. The smaller the amount of protein allowed, the more important it becomes that all protein included in the diet be of high quality
      c. An adequate total energy intake from foods is critical for clients on protein-restricted diets (protein will be used for energy, rather than for protein synthesis)
      d. Special low-protein products, such as pastas, bread, cookies, wafers, and gelatin made with wheat starch, can improve energy intake and add variety to the diet
      e. Carbohydrates in powdered or liquid form can also provide additional energy
      f. Vegetables and fruits contain some protein; for very low-protein diets, these foods must be calculated into the diet
      g. Foods are limited from the milk, meat, bread, and starch exchange
K. High-protein diet
   1. Indications: Tissue building, burns, liver disease, and older clients
   2. Nursing considerations
      a. High-protein diets correct protein loss and assist with tissue repair
      b. Increase foods such as meat, fish, fowl, and dairy products
      c. Client may need protein supplements

L. Low-calcium diet
   1. Indication: May be prescribed to prevent renal calculi in the client at risk for forming calculi composed of calcium
   2. Nursing considerations: Decrease the total intake of calcium to prevent further stone formation; avoid whole grains, milk and dairy products, and green, leafy vegetables
M. High-calcium diet
   1. Indications: Calcium is needed during bone growth and in adulthood to prevent osteoporosis
   2. Nursing considerations
      a. Primary dietary sources of calcium are dairy products (see Chapter 9, Box 9-6) for food items high in calcium)
      b. Clients with lactose intolerance need to incorporate sources of calcium other than dairy products into their dietary patterns regularly
N. Low-purine diet
   1. Indication: Used to treat gout
   2. Nursing considerations
      a. Purine is a precursor for uric acid, which forms stones and crystals
      b. The client needs to avoid consuming fish such as anchovies, herring, mackerel, sardines, and scallops
      c. The client needs to avoid consuming glandular meats, gravies, meat extracts, wild game, goose, and sweetbreads
O. High-iron diet
   1. Indication: Used in anemia
   2. Nursing considerations
      a. Replaces iron deficit from inadequate intake or loss
      b. Includes organ meats, meat, egg yolks, whole-wheat products, leafy vegetables, dried fruit, legumes
P. Diet for diverticular disease
   1. Symptomatic diverticulitis: Fiber is avoided because a high-fiber diet is irritating to the bowel
   2. Asymptomatic diverticular disease: High-fiber diet is consumed to prevent constipation
   3. The client should maintain a liberal fluid intake of 2500 to 3000 mL/day, unless contraindicated
   4. Seeds and nuts should be avoided because they become trapped in the diverticula and cause irritation
   5. Gas-forming foods should be avoided (Box 12-7)
Q. Fluid restriction (Box 12-8)
   1. Indications: Acute renal failure (oliguric phase), chronic renal disease, cirrhosis of the liver, congestive heart failure and other cardiac disorders, and hepatic coma
   2. Nursing considerations: Usually, this diet restricts foods composed largely of water, such as carbonated beverages, coffee, juices, milk, tea, water,

---

BOX 12-7

Gas-Forming Foods

Apples	Figs
Artichokes	Honey
Barley	Melons
Beans	Milk
Bran	Molasses
Broccoli	Nuts
Brussels sprouts	Onions
Cabbage	Radishes
Celery	Soybeans
Cherries	Wheat
Coconuts	Yeast
Eggplant	

BOX 12-8

Measures to Relieve Thirst

Chew gum or suck hard candy
Freeze fluids so that they take longer to consume
Add lemon juice to water to make it more refreshing
Gargle with refrigerated mouthwash

frozen yogurt, gelatin, ice cream, Popsicles, sherbet, soup, cream, and liquid medications

R. Carbohydrate-controlled diet
  1. Indications
     a. Helps maintain normal glucose levels in clients with disorders that cause blood glucose levels to rise or fall abnormally
     b. Used for diabetes mellitus, hypoglycemia, lactose intolerance, galactosemia, dumping syndrome, and obesity
  2. Nursing considerations: Exchange Lists for Meal Planning
     a. The Exchange Lists for Meal Planning, developed by the American Dietetic Association and the American Diabetes Association, is a food guide used to help control diabetes mellitus and manage weight
     b. The Exchange List groups foods according to the amounts of the carbohydrates, fats, and proteins they contain
     c. Major food groups include carbohydrates, meats and meat substitutes, and fats

S. Miscellaneous diets: See Chapter 9, Boxes 9-4, 9-5, 9-7, and 9-8 for foods high in potassium, sodium, magnesium, and phosphorus

---

IV. VEGETARIAN DIETS
A. Types (Box 12-9)
B. Nursing considerations
  1. Ensure that the client eats a sufficient amount of varied foods to meet normal nutrient and energy needs

---

BOX 12-9

Types of Vegetarian Diets

LACTO-OVO VEGETARIANS
Consume plant foods with dairy products and eggs
May consume fish and occasionally poultry

LACTO-VEGETARIANS
Consume plant foods and dairy products, excluding eggs

VEGANS
Follow a strict vegetarian diet and use no animal foods
Food pattern consists entirely of plant foods

  2. Protein consumption can be increased by consuming a variety of vegetable protein sources based on whole grains, legumes, seeds, nuts, and vegetables combined to provide all the essential amino acids
  3. Adequate energy intakes are important to ensure that dietary protein is used for protein synthesis

---

V. ENTERAL NUTRITION
A. Description: Provides liquefied foods into the GI tract via a tube
B. Indications
  1. When the GI tract is functional but oral intake is not feasible
  2. Used for clients with swallowing problems, burns, major trauma, liver failure, or severe **malnutrition**
C. Nursing considerations
  1. Clients with lactose intolerance need to be placed on lactose-free formulas
  2. Refer to Chapter 19 for information regarding the administration of GI tube feedings

---

VI. TOTAL PARENTERAL NUTRITION (TPN)
A. Description
  1. Supplies necessary nutrients via the veins
  2. Supplies carbohydrates in the form of dextrose, fats in special emulsified form, proteins in the form of amino acids, vitamins, minerals, and water
  3. Prevents subcutaneous fat and muscle protein from being catabolized by the body for energy
B. Indications
  1. Clients whose GI tracts are severely dysfunctional or nonfunctional and who cannot process nutrients normally
  2. Clients who can take some oral nutrition, but not enough to meet the body's needs
  3. Clients with multiple GI surgeries, GI trauma, severe intolerance to enteral feedings, or intestinal

BOX 12-10

Complications of Total Parenteral Nutrition

Air embolism
Fluid overload
Hyperglycemia
Infection
Pneumothorax

BOX 12-11

Signs of an Adverse or Allergic Reaction to Lipids

Chills
Fever
Flushing
Diaphoresis
Dyspnea
Cyanosis
Chest and back pain
Nausea and vomiting
Headache
Pressure over the eyes
Thrombophlebitis
Vertigo

obstructions, or in whom the bowel needs to rest for healing

4. Clients with acquired immunodeficiency syndrome (AIDS), cancer, or **malnutrition,** or clients receiving chemotherapy

C. Central parenteral nutrition (CPN)
   1. **TPN** is administered through central venous access when the client requires a larger concentration of carbohydrates (more than 10% glucose)
   2. Subclavian or internal jugular veins are used when **TPN** is a short-term intervention (shorter than 4 weeks)
   3. When **TPN** is anticipated for an extended period (longer than 4 weeks), a more permanent catheter, such as a peripherally inserted central catheter (PICC) line, a tunneled catheter, or an implanted vascular access device, is used

D. Peripheral parenteral nutrition (PPN)
   1. Administered through a peripheral vein
   2. Used for short periods (5 to 7 days) and when the client needs only small concentrations of carbohydrates, fats, and proteins
   3. Used to deliver isotonic or mildly hypertonic solutions; the delivery of highly hypertonic solutions into peripheral veins can cause sclerosis, phlebitis, or swelling

E. Complications of **TPN** (Box 12-10)

F. Precautions
   1. Assist with insertion of catheter; position the client in Trendelenburg position
   2. Ask the client to perform the Valsalva maneuver during insertion to prevent air emboli
   3. When the central line is inserted, placement is confirmed by chest x-ray
   4. **TPN** catheter is not used for blood draws or the administration of other medications or fluids
   5. **TPN** is always delivered via an electronic infusion device
   6. Solutions should be stored under refrigeration
   7. **TPN** solution is changed every 24 hours

G. Nursing interventions
   1. Maintain aseptic technique
   2. Monitor vital signs
   3. Monitor weight and input and output (I&O) daily
   4. Monitor site for redness, swelling, tenderness, or drainage
   5. Monitor blood glucose and urine for glucose and acetone four times daily, or as prescribed
   6. Electrolytes and blood urea nitrogen (BUN) are monitored, as prescribed
   7. Monitor infusion rate hourly
   8. If sepsis is suspected, a blood culture is drawn, and the tip of the catheter is cultured for bacteria
   9. Monitor for signs of fluid overload such as a bounding pulse, jugular vein distention, headache, increased blood pressure, and lung crackles
   10. If the IV tubing becomes disconnected, instruct the client to perform the Valsalva maneuver
   11. Monitor for signs of an air embolus such as confusion, pallor, light-headedness, tachycardia, tachypnea, hypotension, anxiety, and unresponsiveness
   12. Place the client in the left side-lying position with the head lower than the feet if air embolism is suspected, and contact the physician

H. **Lipids (fat emulsion)**
   1. An isotonic solution that can be administered through a peripheral vein
   2. Administered with **TPN** to prevent or correct fatty acid deficiency
   3. Most **fat emulsions** are prepared from soybean oil; the primary components are linoleic, oleic, palmitic, linolenic, and stearic acids
   4. Solution is examined for separation of emulsion into layers or fat globules or for the accumulation of froth; if observed, it is not used and is returned to the pharmacy
   5. Solution is administered slowly; monitor vital signs every 10 minutes, and observe for adverse reactions for the first 30 minutes of the infusion; if signs of an adverse reaction occur, stop the infusion and notify the physician (Box 12-11)

PRACTICE QUESTIONS

1. A low-sodium diet has been prescribed for a client with hypertension. Following diet teaching, which of the following foods, if selected from the menu by the client, would indicate an understanding of this diet?
   1. Tomato soup
   2. Baked turkey
   3. Chicken gumbo soup
   4. Boiled shrimp

2. A nurse is providing dietary instructions to a client with gout. The nurse tells the client to avoid which food item?
   1. Macaroni products
   2. Corn bread
   3. Scallops
   4. Chocolate

3. A clear liquid diet has been prescribed for a client with gastroenteritis. Which item would be most appropriate to offer to the client?
   1. Orange juice
   2. Strained soup
   3. Fat-free broth
   4. Soft custard

4. A client who has recently been started on enteral feedings begins to complain of abdominal cramping, followed by passage of two liquid stools. A nurse notes that the client has abdominal distention as well. The nurse reviews the nutritional content on the label of the can to see if it contains which of the following ingredients?
   1. Maltose
   2. Lactose
   3. Sucrose
   4. Fructose

5. A client has been diagnosed with acute gastroenteritis. Which of the following diets would the nurse anticipate would be prescribed for the client?
   1. High residue
   2. Low residue
   3. High carbohydrate
   4. Low fat

6. A client with heart disease is instructed regarding a low-fat diet. The nurse determines that the client understands the diet if the client states that a food item to avoid is:
   1. Apples
   2. Oranges
   3. Avocado
   4. Cherries

7. A nurse instructs a client to increase the amount of riboflavin in the diet. The nurse instructs the client to select which food item that is high in riboflavin?
   1. Milk
   2. Tomatoes
   3. Citrus fruits
   4. Green, leafy vegetables

8. A nurse instructs a client to increase the amount of thiamine in the diet. The nurse instructs the client to select which food item that is especially high in thiamine?
   1. Chicken
   2. Broccoli
   3. Pork
   4. Milk

9. A nurse caring for a client with a neurological disorder is assisting in planning care to maintain nutritional status. The nurse is concerned about the client's swallowing ability. The nurse avoids including which food item in this client's diet?
   1. Cheese casserole
   2. Scrambled eggs
   3. Mashed potatoes
   4. Spinach

10. A client with a burn injury is transferred to the nursing unit and a regular diet has been prescribed. The nurse encourages the client to eat which dietary items to promote wound healing?
    1. Veal, potatoes, Jell-O, orange juice
    2. Peanut butter and jelly sandwich, cantaloupe, tea
    3. Chicken breast, broccoli, strawberries, milk
    4. Spaghetti with tomato sauce, garlic bread, ginger ale

11. A nurse is assisting a client who has had a cerebrovascular accident (CVA) to eat. The nurse implements which of the following that will best promote independence?
    1. Offer only puréed foods
    2. Sit the client in a high Fowler's position
    3. Place the food tray on the unaffected side
    4. Encourage the client to eat with other clients who have had CVAs

12. A nurse has completed diet teaching for a client on a low-sodium diet to treat hypertension. The nurse determines that further teaching is necessary when the client makes which of these statements?
    1. "This diet will help to lower my blood pressure."
    2. "The reason I need to lower my salt intake is to reduce fluid retention."
    3. "This diet is not a replacement for my antihypertensive medications."
    4. "Fresh foods such as fruits and vegetables are high in sodium."

13. A client is on a diet designed to avoid concentrated sugars. The nurse determines that the client understands the diet plan if which of these diets is selected by the client?
    1. Strawberry yogurt, lettuce salad, coffee
    2. Chicken salad, tomato, Jell-O, instant iced tea
    3. Peanut butter and jelly sandwich, sherbet, cola
    4. Tuna sandwich, lettuce salad, watermelon, herbal tea

14. A nurse is assigned to care for a client receiving enteral feedings. The nurse plans care knowing that which of the following is of highest priority for this client?
    1. Imbalanced nutrition
    2. Risk for aspiration
    3. Risk for deficient fluid volume
    4. Risk for diarrhea

15. A client receiving total parenteral nutrition (TPN) may begin to take small amounts of clear liquids today. The nurse's priority is to collect data regarding which of the following before giving the client anything by mouth?
    1. Client's appetite
    2. Client's weight today
    3. Presence of swallow reflex
    4. Adequate pulse and blood pressure

16. A nurse is preparing to administer a feeding to the client receiving enteral nutrition through a nasogastric tube. The nurse performs which of the following as the priority nursing action?
    1. Measuring intake and output
    2. Weighing the client
    3. Adding blue food coloring to the enteral formula
    4. Determining tube placement

17. A nurse has reinforced discharge teaching with the family of a client who is to have enteral feedings at home. The nurse uses which method of evaluation to best determine the family's competence in performing the feeding procedure?
    1. Return demonstration of the feeding procedure
    2. Selection of appropriate equipment for the feeding procedure
    3. Written testing on the steps of the feeding procedure
    4. Verbal description of the feeding procedure by each member of the family

18. A nurse is asked to assist in preparing a client who will be receiving total parenteral nutrition (TPN) solution via a central line. The nurse plans to obtain which most essential piece of equipment for this procedure?
    1. Electronic infusion pump
    2. Blood glucose meter
    3. Urine test strips
    4. Noninvasive blood pressure monitor

19. A client is receiving nutrition by means of total parenteral nutrition (TPN). The nurse monitors the client for which of the following signs of hyperglycemia, a complication of this therapy?
    1. Nausea, vomiting, and oliguria
    2. Sweating, chills, and abdominal pain
    3. Pallor, weak pulse, and thirst
    4. Increased appetite, thirst, and increased urine output

20. A client receiving total parenteral nutrition (TPN) complains of a headache. The nurse notes that the client has an increased blood pressure and a bounding pulse. The nurse reports the findings knowing that these signs are indicative of which complication of TPN therapy?
    1. Hyperglycemia
    2. Air embolism
    3. Sepsis
    4. Fluid overload

ALTERNATE FORMAT QUESTION: MULTIPLE RESPONSE

A postoperative client has been placed on a clear liquid diet. Select all the items that the client is allowed to consume on this diet.

____ Broth
____ Gelatin
____ Pudding
____ Puréed vegetables
____ Coffee
____ Vegetable juice

ANSWERS

1. *Answer: 2*
Rationale: Regular soup (1 cup) contains 900 mg of sodium. Fresh shellfish (1 oz) contains 50 mg sodium. Poultry (1 oz) contains 25 mg sodium.
Test-Taking Strategy: Use the process of elimination. Eliminate options 1 and 3 first because they are similar. Also, recall that canned foods are high in sodium. From the remaining options, select option 2 over option 4, remembering that shellfish is also high in sodium. Review foods high in sodium if you had difficulty with this question.
Level of Cognitive Ability: Analysis
Client Needs: Health Promotion and Maintenance
Integrated Process: Teaching/Learning
Content Area: Fundamental Skills
References: Nix, S. (2005). *William' basic nutrition and diet therapy* (12th ed.). St. Louis: Mosby, pp. 358-359.
Peckenpaugh, N. (2003). *Nutrition essentials and diet therapy* (9th ed.). Philadelphia: W.B. Saunders, p. 98.

2. *Answer: 3*
Rationale: Scallops should be omitted from the diet of a client who has gout because of the high purine content. The food items identified in options 1, 2, and 4 contain a negligible

purine content and may be consumed by the client with gout.
Test-Taking Strategy: Use the process of elimination and focus on the client's diagnosis. Recalling the food items that are high in purine will direct you to option 3. Review foods high in purine if you had difficulty with this question.
Level of Cognitive Ability: Application
Client Needs: Health Promotion and Maintenance
Integrated Process: Teaching/Learning
Content Area: Fundamental Skills
References: Linton, A., & Maebius, N. (2003), *Introduction to medical-surgical nursing* (3rd ed.). Philadelphia: W.B. Saunders, p. 815.
Nix, S. (2005). *Williams' basic nutrition and diet therapy* (12th ed.). St. Louis: Mosby, pp. 405-406.

3. *Answer:* 3
Rationale: A clear liquid diet consists of foods that are relatively transparent. The food items in options 1, 2, and 4 would be included in a full liquid diet.
Test-Taking Strategy: Remember that a clear liquid diet consists of foods that are relatively transparent. By the process of elimination you should easily select option 3, because this is the only food item that is transparent. Review food items allowed on clear liquid and full liquid diets if you had difficulty with this question.
Level of Cognitive Ability: Application
Client Needs: Physiological Integrity
Integrated Process: Nursing Process/Implementation
Content Area: Fundamental Skills
Reference: Peckenpaugh, N. (2003). *Nutrition essentials and diet therapy* (9th ed.). Philadelphia: W.B. Saunders, p. 54.

4. *Answer:* 2
Rationale: Several tube feeding formulas contain lactose. A client with an unreported history of lactose intolerance would develop symptoms such as these in response to nutritional therapy with these formulas. If the client is diagnosed as lactose intolerant, a lactose-free formula should be prescribed by the physician. This will resolve the client's symptoms and promote adequate nutrition for the client.
Test-Taking Strategy: Focus on the data in the question. The issue is the ability to associate the symptoms experienced by the client with the symptoms of lactose intolerance. If you had difficulty with this question, review the symptoms of lactose intolerance and the nursing considerations related to enteral feedings.
Level of Cognitive Ability: Analysis
Client Needs: Physiological Integrity
Integrated Process: Nursing Process/Data Collection
Content Area: Fundamental Skills
Reference: Perry, A., & Potter, P. (2002), *Clinical nursing skills and techniques* (5th ed.). St. Louis: Mosby, p. 680.

5. *Answer:* 2
Rationale: A low-residue (low-fiber) diet places less strain on the intestines because this type of diet is easier to digest. This diet is prescribed for clients with inflammatory bowel disease, ileostomy, colostomy, partial obstructions of the intestinal tract, acute gastroenteritis, or diarrhea.
Test-Taking Strategy: Note that the diagnosis in the question refers to an inflammation in the colon. With this in mind,

you should easily be directed to option 2, the diet that would place the least strain on the intestinal tract. Review the indications for a low-residue diet if you had difficulty with this question.
Level of Cognitive Ability: Comprehension
Client Needs: Physiological Integrity
Integrated Process: Nursing Process/Planning
Content Area: Fundamental Skills
References: Peckenpaugh, N. (2003). *Nutrition essentials and diet therapy* (9th ed.). Philadelphia: W.B. Saunders, p. 74.
Potter, P., & Perry, A. (2005). *Fundamentals of nursing* (6th ed.). St. Louis: Mosby, p. 1298.

6. *Answer:* 3
Rationale: Fruits and vegetables, except avocado, olives, and coconut, contain minimal amounts of fat.
Test-Taking Strategy: Use the process of elimination and knowledge regarding the fat content of fruits to eliminate options 1 and 2. Recalling that avocado is high in fat content will direct you to option 3 from the remaining options. Review the fruits high in fat if you had difficulty with this question.
Level of Cognitive Ability: Analysis
Client Needs: Health Promotion and Maintenance
Integrated Process: Teaching/Learning
Content Area: Fundamental Skills
Reference: Peckenpaugh, N. (2003). *Nutrition essentials and diet therapy* (9th ed.). Philadelphia: W.B. Saunders, p. 49.

7. *Answer:* 1
Rationale: Food sources of riboflavin include milk, lean meats, fish, and grains. Tomatoes and citrus fruits are high in vitamin C. Green, leafy vegetables are high in folic acid.
Test-Taking Strategy: Knowledge regarding food items high in riboflavin is required to answer this question. Remember that milk is a food source of riboflavin. Review these foods if you had difficulty with this question.
Level of Cognitive Ability: Application
Client Needs: Health Promotion and Maintenance
Integrated Process: Teaching/Learning
Content Area: Fundamental Skills
Reference: Peckenpaugh, N. (2003). *Nutrition essentials and diet therapy* (9th ed.). Philadelphia: W.B. Saunders, p. 94.

8. *Answer:* 3
Rationale: Thiamine is present in a variety of foods of plant and animal origin. Pork products are especially rich in this vitamin. Other good sources include nuts, whole-grain cereals, and legumes. Poultry is high in pyridoxine. Broccoli is high in vitamin C. Milk is high in riboflavin.
Test-Taking Strategy: Knowledge regarding food items high in thiamine is required to answer this question. Remember that pork products are especially rich in this vitamin. Review these foods if you had difficulty with this question.
Level of Cognitive Ability: Application
Client Needs: Health Promotion and Maintenance
Integrated Process: Teaching/Learning
Content Area: Fundamental Skills
Reference: Peckenpaugh, N. (2003). *Nutrition essentials and diet therapy* (9th ed.). Philadelphia: W.B. Saunders, p. 94.

9. *Answer:* **4**
Rationale: Moist pastas, casseroles, egg dishes, and potatoes are usually well tolerated by the client who has difficulty swallowing. Raw vegetables, chunky vegetables such as diced beets, and stringy vegetables such as spinach, corn and peas are foods commonly excluded from the diet of a client who has difficulty swallowing.
Test-Taking Strategy: Note the key words, *swallowing ability* and *avoids.* The word "avoids" indicates a false response question and that you need to select the incorrect food item. Use the process of elimination to select option 4 as the food that would be most difficult to swallow. Review the foods to avoid in a client who has difficulty swallowing if you had difficulty with this question.
Level of Cognitive Ability: Application
Client Needs: Physiological Integrity
Integrated Process: Nursing Process/Implementation
Content Area: Fundamental Skills
References: Nix, S. (2005). *Williams' basic nutrition and diet therapy* (12th ed.). St. Louis: Mosby, pp. 28, 438.
Peckenpaugh, N. (2003). *Nutrition essentials and diet therapy* (9th ed.). Philadelphia: W.B. Saunders, pp. 67-68.

10. *Answer:* **3**
Rationale: Protein and vitamin C are necessary for wound healing. Poultry and milk are good sources of protein. Broccoli and strawberries are good sources of vitamin C. Peanut butter is a source of niacin. Jell-O and jelly have no nutrient value. Spaghetti is a complex carbohydrate.
Test-Taking Strategy: Focus on the issue, promoting wound healing, and recall that protein and vitamin C are necessary for wound healing. Eliminate options 1 and 2 first because jelly and Jell-O have no nutrient value related to healing. From the remaining options, select option 3 over option 4 because of the greater nutrient value in these food items. Review foods high in protein and vitamin C if you had difficulty with this question.
Level of Cognitive Ability: Application
Client Needs: Physiological Integrity
Integrated Process: Nursing Process/Implementation
Content Area: Fundamental Skills
Reference: Peckenpaugh, N. (2003). *Nutrition essentials and diet therapy* (9th ed.). Philadelphia: W.B. Saunders, pp. 34-35.

11. *Answer:* **3**
Rationale: Independence is promoted by allowing the client to have control in a given situation. Placing the tray on the client's unaffected side will facilitate the client's ability to eat. Options 1, 2, and 4 do not offer the client control.
Test-Taking Strategy: Note the key words, *promote independence.* With this issue in mind, by the process of elimination, you should easily be directed to option 3. Review measures related to promoting independence in the client with a CVA if you had difficulty with this question.
Level of Cognitive Ability: Application
Client Needs: Psychosocial Integrity
Integrated Process: Nursing Process/Implementation
Content Area: Fundamental Skills
References: Black, J., & Hawks, J. (2005). *Medical-surgical nursing: Clinical management for positive outcomes* (7th ed.). Philadelphia: W.B. Saunders, pp. 1974-1975.

Linton, A., & Maebius, N. (2003). *Introduction to medical-surgical nursing* (3rd ed.). Philadelphia: W.B. Saunders, p. 426.

12. *Answer:* **4**
Rationale: A low-sodium diet is used as an adjunct to antihypertensive medications for the treatment of hypertension. Sodium retains fluid, which leads to hypertension secondary to increased fluid volume. Fresh foods such as fruits and vegetables are low in sodium.
Test-Taking Strategy: Use the process of elimination noting the key words, *further teaching is necessary.* These words indicate a false response question and that you need to select the incorrect client statement. Eliminate options 1, 2, and 3 because these are accurate statements related to hypertension. Also, remember that fresh foods are low in sodium. Review the purpose of a low-sodium diet if you had difficulty with this question.
Level of Cognitive Ability: Analysis
Client Needs: Health Promotion and Maintenance
Integrated Process: Teaching/Learning
Content Area: Fundamental Skills
References: Nix, S. (2005). *Williams' basic nutrition and diet therapy* (12th ed.). St. Louis: Mosby, pp. 263, 484.
Peckenpaugh, N. (2003). *Nutrition essentials and diet therapy* (9th ed.). Philadelphia: W.B. Saunders, pp. 240-243.

13. *Answer:* **4**
Rationale: Concentrated sugars are found in fruit yogurt, gelatin desserts, prepared drink mixes, jelly, and sherbet.
Test-Taking Strategy: Use the process of elimination. Note that option 4 is the only option that does not identify a prepackaged food item. Review foods containing concentrated sugar if you had difficulty with this question.
Level of Cognitive Ability: Analysis
Client Needs: Health Promotion and Maintenance
Integrated Process: Nursing Process/Evaluation
Content Area: Fundamental Skills
Reference: Peckenpaugh, N. (2003). *Nutrition essentials and diet therapy* (9th ed.). Philadelphia: W.B. Saunders, pp. 34-36.

14. *Answer:* **2**
Rationale: Any condition in which gastrointestinal motility is slowed or esophageal reflux is possible places a client at risk for aspiration. Options 1 and 4 may be appropriate but are not the highest priority. Option 3 is not likely to occur in this client.
Test-Taking Strategy: Note the key words, *highest priority.* Eliminate option 3 first because it is not likely to occur in this client. Next, use the ABCs—airway, breathing, and circulation. Option 2 addresses airway management. Options 1 and 4 are possible problems, but not as high a priority as airway maintenance. Review care of the client receiving enteral feedings if you had difficulty with this question.
Level of Cognitive Ability: Application
Client Needs: Physiological Integrity
Integrated Process: Nursing Process/Planning
Content Area: Fundamental Skills
Reference: Black, J., & Hawks, J. (2005). *Medical-surgical nursing: Clinical management for positive outcomes* (7th ed.). Philadelphia: W.B. Saunders, p. 676.

15. *Answer:* **3**

Rationale: The nurse ensures that the client has intact gag and swallow reflexes. The nurse would also check for the presence of bowel sounds. Pulse, blood pressure, and weight require ongoing monitoring, but are not the most important items, given the wording of the question. The client may be expected to have a poor appetite after being without oral intake for a period of time.

Test-Taking Strategy: Focus on the issue of the question, noting the key word, *priority*. Option 3 is most closely associated with the issue of the question, feeding the client, and addresses prevention of aspiration. Review nursing care measures for the client resuming an oral intake if you had difficulty with this question.

Level of Cognitive Ability: Application
Client Needs: Physiological Integrity
Integrated Process: Nursing Process/Data Collection
Content Area: Fundamental Skills
References: Black, J., & Hawks, J. (2005). *Medical-surgical nursing: Clinical management for positive outcomes* (7th ed.). Philadelphia: W.B. Saunders, p. 675.
deWit, S. (2005). *Fundamental concepts and skills for nursing* (2nd ed.). Philadelphia: W.B. Saunders. p. 483.

16. *Answer:* **4**

Rationale: Initiating a tube feeding before checking tube placement can lead to serious complications, such as aspiration. Options 1 and 2 are part of the total plan of care for a client on enteral feeding. Option 3 may be instituted for a client who has been identified as a high risk for aspiration. Option 4 is the priority nursing action.

Test-Taking Strategy: Use the ABCs—airway, breathing, and circulation—and the clinical problem-solving process (nursing process) to answer the question. Option 4 relates to the risk of aspiration and to data collection. If you had difficulty with this question, review nursing interventions when initiating a tube feeding.

Level of Cognitive Ability: Application
Client Needs: Physiological Integrity
Integrated Process: Nursing Process/Implementation
Content Area: Fundamental Skills
Reference: deWit, S. (2005). *Fundamental concepts and skills for nursing* (2nd ed.). Philadelphia: W.B. Saunders, p. 483.

17. *Answer:* **1**

Rationale: Return demonstration is the most reliable evaluation of procedure performance. Selection of equipment is included in a return demonstration. Written testing is not useful for performance testing of procedures. Verbal description does not allow the nurse to observe the psychomotor skill needed to perform the procedure.

Test-Taking Strategy: Note the similar words in the question and option 1. "Performing" in the question and "demonstration" in the option indicate action. Review basic teaching and learning principles if you had difficulty with this question.

Level of Cognitive Ability: Application
Client Needs: Health Promotion and Maintenance
Integrated Process: Teaching/Learning

Content Area: Fundamental Skills
Reference: Black, J., & Hawks, J. (2005). *Medical-surgical nursing: Clinical management for positive outcomes* (7th ed.). Philadelphia: W.B. Saunders, p. 676.

18. *Answer:* **1**

Rationale: The nurse obtains an electronic infusion pump in preparation for this procedure. It is necessary to use an infusion pump to ensure that the solution does not infuse too rapidly or fall too far behind. Because the client's blood glucose level is monitored every 6 to 8 hours during administration of TPN, a blood glucose meter will also be needed, but this is not the *most essential* item. Urine test strips may be needed to measure glucose. A noninvasive blood pressure cuff is unnecessary for this procedure.

Test-Taking Strategy: Note that the question contains the key words, *most essential*. Use knowledge of principles of TPN administration and the method of administration to eliminate each incorrect option. Review these principles if you had difficulty with this question.

Level of Cognitive Ability: Application
Client Needs: Physiological Integrity
Integrated Process: Nursing Process/Planning
Content Area: Fundamental Skills
References: Christensen, B., & Kockrow, E. (2003). *Foundations of nursing* (4th ed.). St. Louis: Mosby, p. 585.
deWit, S. (2005). *Fundamental concepts and skills for nursing* (2nd ed.). Philadelphia: W.B. Saunders, p. 482.

19. *Answer:* **4**

Rationale: The high glucose concentration in TPN places the client at risk for hyperglycemia. Signs of hyperglycemia include polyuria, polydipsia (thirst), blurred vision, nausea and vomiting, and abdominal pain.

Test-Taking Strategy: Use the process of elimination. Remember that, for an option to be correct, all the parts of that option must be correct. Recalling the signs of hyperglycemia (polyuria, polydipsia, and polyphagia) will direct you to option 4. Review the signs of hyperglycemia if you had difficulty with this question.

Level of Cognitive Ability: Application
Client Needs: Physiological Integrity
Integrated Process: Nursing Process/Data Collection
Content Area: Fundamental Skills
References: Christensen, B., & Kockrow, E. (2003). *Foundations of nursing* (4th ed.). St. Louis: Mosby, p. 537.
Linton, A., & Maebius, N. (2003). *Introduction to medical-surgical nursing* (3rd ed.). Philadelphia: W.B. Saunders, p. 664.

20. *Answer:* **4**

Rationale: The client's signs and symptoms are consistent with fluid overload. The increased intravascular volume increases the blood pressure, while the pulse rate increases as the heart tries to pump the extra fluid volume. A fever would be present in sepsis. Signs and symptoms of an air embolus include confusion, pallor, light-headedness, tachycardia, tachypnea, hypotension, anxiety, and unresponsiveness. Polyuria, polydipsia, and polyphagia are manifestations of hyperglycemia.

Test-Taking Strategy: Use the process of elimination. Focus on the data in the question and recall the complications of TPN and their manifestations. This will direct you to option 4. Review these complications and manifestations if you had difficulty with this question.
Level of Cognitive Ability: Analysis
Client Needs: Physiological Integrity
Integrated Process: Nursing Process/Data Collection
Content Area: Fundamental Skills
References: Christensen, B., & Kockrow, E. (2003). *Foundations of nursing* (4th ed.). St. Louis: Mosby, pp. 536-537.
DeWit, S. (2005). *Fundamental concepts and skills for nursing* (2nd ed.). Philadelphia: W.B. Saunders, p. 487.

ALTERNATE FORMAT QUESTION: MULTIPLE RESPONSE

Answers:
Broth
Gelatin
Coffee

Rationale: A clear liquid diet consists of foods that are relatively transparent to light, and are clear and liquid at room and body temperature. These foods include such items as water, bouillon, clear broth, carbonated beverages, gelatin, hard candy, lemonade, Popsicles, and regular or decaffeinated coffee or tea. The incorrect food items are items that are allowed on a full liquid diet.
Test-Taking Strategy: Focus on the issue, a clear liquid diet. Recalling that a clear liquid diet consists of foods that are relatively transparent to light and are clear will assist in answering the question. Review foods allowed on a clear and full liquid diet if you had difficulty with this question.
Level of Cognitive Ability: Application
Client Needs: Physiological Integrity
Integrated Process: Nursing Process/Implementation
Content Area: Fundamental Skills
Reference: Peckenpaugh, N. (2003). *Nutrition essentials and diet therapy* (9th ed.). Philadelphia: W.B. Saunders, p. 54.

REFERENCES

Black, J., & Hawks, J. (2005). *Medical-surgical nursing: Clinical management for positive outcomes* (7th ed.). Philadelphia: W.B. Saunders.

Christensen, B., & Kockrow, E. (2003). *Foundations of nursing* (4th ed.). St. Louis: Mosby.

deWit, S. (2005). *Fundamental concepts and skills for nursing* (2nd ed.). Philadelphia: W.B. Saunders.

Linton, A., & Maebius, N. (2003), *Introduction to medical-surgical nursing* (3rd ed.). Philadelphia: W.B. Saunders.

National Council of State Boards of Nursing. (2005). *Detailed test plan for the National Council licensure examination for practical/ vocational nurses.* Chicago: Author.

Perry, A., & Potter, P. (2002). *Clinical nursing skills and techniques* (5th ed.). St. Louis: Mosby.

Potter, P., & Perry, A. (2005). *Fundamentals of nursing* (6th ed.). St. Louis: Mosby.

Peckenpaugh, N. (2003). *Nutrition essentials and diet therapy* (9th ed.). Philadelphia: W.B. Saunders.

Nix, S. (2005). *Williams' basic nutrition and diet therapy* (12th ed.). St. Louis: Mosby.

Intravenous Therapy and Blood Administration

PYRAMID TERMS

ABO   A type of antigen system. The ABO type of the donor should be compatible with the recipient's. Type A can match with type A or O; type B can match with type B or O; type O can match only with type O; type AB can match with type A, B, or O.

air embolism   Caused by a bolus of air that enters the vein through an inadequately primed intravenous (IV) line, from a loose connection, or during tubing change or removal of the IV catheter.

fluid (circulatory) overload   A complication resulting from the infusion of blood at a rate too rapid for body size, cardiac status, or clinical condition of the recipient.

compatibility   Determined by two different types of antigen systems, ABO and Rh, present on the membrane surface of the red blood cells (RBCs).

crossmatching   The testing of the donor's blood and the recipient's blood for compatibility.

infiltration   Seepage of IV (intravenous) fluid out of the vein and into the surrounding interstitial spaces.

phlebitis   An inflammation of the vein that can occur from either mechanical or chemical (medication) trauma or a local infection.

Rh factor   A person having the factor is Rh positive; a person lacking the factor is Rh negative.

septicemia   The presence of infective agents or their toxins in the bloodstream. It is a serious infection that must be treated promptly; otherwise, the infection leads to circulatory collapse, profound shock, and death.

transfusion reaction   A hemolytic transfusion reaction is caused by blood type or Rh factor incompatibility. An allergic transfusion reaction is most often seen in clients with a history of allergy. A febrile transfusion reaction most commonly occurs in clients with antibodies directed against the transfused white blood cells (WBCs). A bacterial transfusion reaction occurs after transfusion of contaminated blood products.

◤ PYRAMID TO SUCCESS

The nurse is responsible for monitoring clients receiving parenteral therapies. Pyramid points focus on the safety related to monitoring an infusion rate and monitoring for complications related to the IV. Focus on the signs and symptoms of infiltration, phlebitis, *circulatory overload*, and air embolism and the treatment measures associated with each. Pyramid points also focus on safety related to monitoring a client receiving a blood transfusion and monitoring for complications related to the transfusion. Focus on the signs and symptoms of a transfusion reaction and the immediate interventions if a transfusion reaction occurs. Documentation of expected and unexpected effects of the therapy is also a pyramid point. The primary Integrated Processes addressed in this chapter are Caring, Clinical Problem-Solving Process (Nursing Process), Communication and Documentation, and Teaching/Learning.

CLIENT NEEDS
Safe, Effective Care Environment

Informed consent for therapy
Continuity of care
Close supervision during IV infusion
Error prevention in monitoring IVs
Establishing priorities
Handling hazardous or infectious materials
Asepsis
Standard, transmission-based, and other precautions

Health Promotion and Maintenance

Client teaching about the signs of a transfusion reaction
Lifestyle choices related to the transfusion
Techniques of collecting physical data

Psychosocial Integrity

Identifying coping mechanisms
Support systems for the client

Communication regarding the procedure for IV infusion and blood administration

Religious, spiritual, and cultural considerations related to blood administration

Physiological Integrity

Safe administration of IV and blood transfusion

Monitoring intravenous infusion sites and infusion rates

Monitoring for expected effects

Monitoring for complications

Monitoring laboratory values

Documentation

I. INTRAVENOUS THERAPY (Table 13-1)

A. Used to sustain clients who are unable to take substances orally

B. Replaces water, electrolytes, and nutrients more rapidly than oral administration

C. Provides immediate access to the vascular system for the rapid delivery of specific solutions without the time required for gastrointestinal (GI) tract absorption

D. Provides a vascular route for the administration of medication or blood components

II. INTRAVENOUS DEVICES

A. IV cannulas
1. Steel needles or butterfly set
    a. Used when the infusion time will be short
    b. **Infiltration** is more common with these devices
    c. The butterfly infusion set might commonly be used in children and older clients, whose veins are likely to be small or fragile
2. Plastic cannulas
    a. Used in place of a steel needle or butterfly set when a longer infusion time is expected
    b. Can cause catheter embolism if the tip of the cannula breaks

B. IV gauges
1. The smaller the gauge number, the larger the outside diameter of the cannula
2. The gauge size used depends on the solution to be administered and the diameter of the available vein
3. For rapid emergency fluid administration, blood products, or anesthetics, a large needle such as a 14-, 16-, 18-, or 19-gauge needle is used
4. For standard IV fluid, a 22- or 24-gauge needle is used
5. If the client has very small veins, a 24- to 25-gauge needle is used

C. IV containers (Figure 13-1)
1. Container may be glass or plastic
2. Squeeze the plastic bag to ensure that it is intact and check the glass bottle for any punctures or cracks
3. Do not write on the plastic IV bag with a marking pen because the ink may be absorbed through the plastic into the solution.

TABLE 13-1

Types of Intravenous Solutions

Type	Description
Isotonic	Solutions with the same osmolality as body fluids
Hypotonic	Solutions that are more dilute or have a lower osmolality than body fluids
Hypertonic	Solutions that are more concentrated or have a higher osmolality than body fluids

Solution	Tonicity
0.45% normal saline (½ NS)	Hypotonic
0.9% normal saline (NS)	Isotonic
5% dextrose in water (5% D/W)	Isotonic
5% dextrose in 0.225% saline (5% D/¼ NS)	Isotonic
Lactated Ringer's solution	Isotonic
5% dextrose in lactated Ringer's solution	Hypertonic
5% dextrose in 0.45% saline (5% D/½ NS)	Hypertonic
5% dextrose in 0.9% saline (5% D/NS)	Hypertonic
10% dextrose in water (10% D/W)	Hypertonic

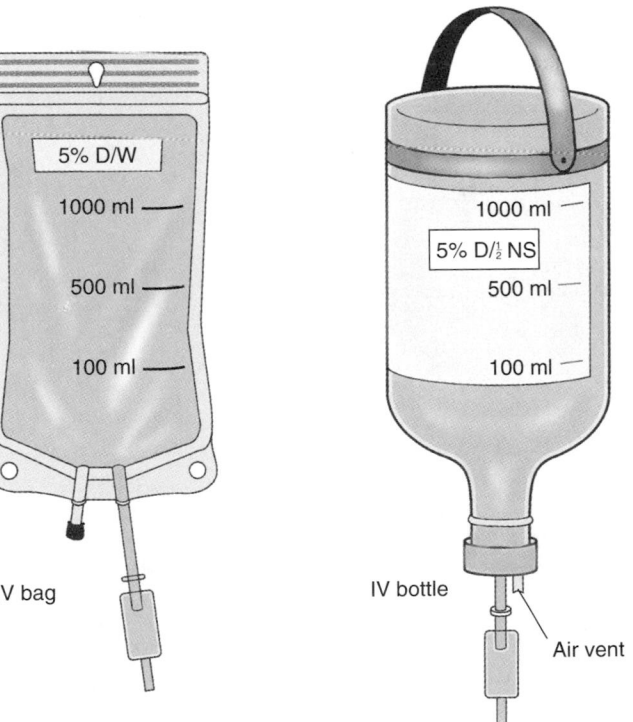

FIG. 13-1 Intravenous containers. (From Kee, J. & Marshall, S. [2004]. *Clinical calculations: With applications to general and specialty areas* [5th ed.]. Philadelphia: W.B. Saunders.)

4. Use a label and a ballpoint pen for marking the bag, placing the label onto the bag

D. Intravenous tubing (Figure 13-2)

1. Contains a spike end for the bag or bottle, a drop chamber, a roller clamp, a Y site, and an adapter end for attachment to the needle
2. Extension tubing may be attached to the IV tubing for children, clients who are restless, or clients who have special mobility needs
3. Vented and nonvented tubing are available
   a. A vent allows air to enter the IV container as the fluid leaves
   b. A vented adapter can be used to add a vent to a nonvented IV tubing system
   c. Use nonvented tubing for flexible containers
   d. Use vented tubing for glass or rigid plastic containers to allow air to enter and displace the fluid as it leaves; fluid will not flow from a rigid IV container unless it is vented

E. Drip chambers (Figure 13-3)

1. Microdrip chamber
   a. Normally, this chamber has a short, vertical, metal piece where the drop forms
   b. Delivers about 60 drops/mL
   c. Read the tubing package to determine how many drops per milliliter are delivered (drop factor)
   d. Used if fluid will be infused at a slow rate (less than 50 mL/hour), if the solution contains medication, and in the pediatric client

2. Macrodrip chamber
   a. Used if the solution is thick or is to infuse rapidly
   b. Drop factor varies from 10 to 20 drops/mL
   c. Read the tubing package to determine how many drops per milliliter are delivered (drop factor)

F. Filters: May be used in IV lines to trap small particles and provide protection by preventing particles from entering the client's veins

G. Needleless systems: Include recessed needles, plastic cannulas, or one-way valves that decrease the exposure to contaminated needles

H. Intermittent infusion sets: Used when intravascular accessibility is desired for intermittent administration of medications or solutions

III. LATEX ALLERGY

A. Ask the client about an allergy to latex
B. IV supplies that may contain latex including IV catheters, IV tubing, IV ports (particularly IV rubber injection ports), rubber stoppers on multidose vials, and adhesive tape
C. Latex-safe IV supplies need to be used for clients with a latex allergy
D. Refer to Chapter 60 for additional information regarding latex allergy

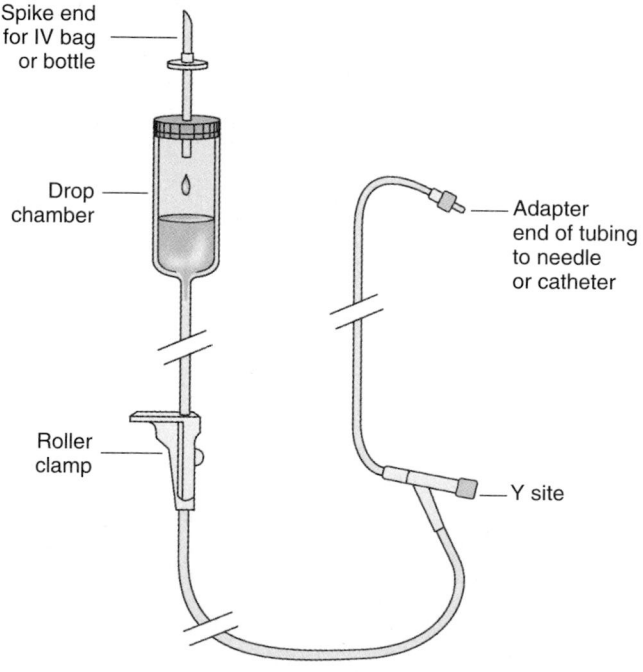

FIG. 13-2 Intravenous tubing. (From Kee, J. & Marshall, S. [2004]. *Clinical calculations: With applications to general and specialty areas* [5th ed.]. Philadelphia: W.B. Saunders.)

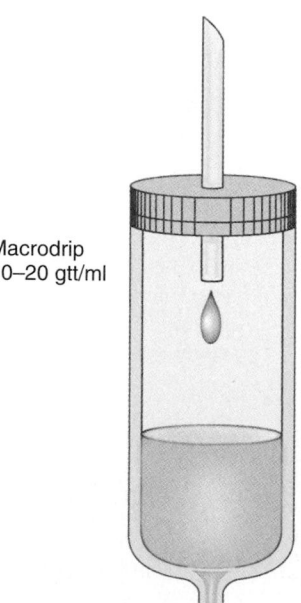
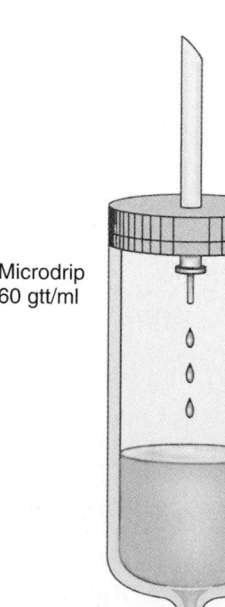

FIG. 13-3 Macrodrip and microdrip sets. (From Kee, J. & Marshall, S. [2004]. *Clinical calculations: With applications to general and specialty areas* [5th ed.]. Philadelphia: W.B. Saunders.)

IV. PERIPHERAL IV SITES

A. The most frequently used sites are the veins of the forearm, because the bones of the forearm act as a natural support and splint

B. Veins in the lower extremities are not suitable because of the risk of thrombus formation and possible pooling in areas of decreased venous return (Box 13-1)

C. Veins in the scalp and feet might be suitable sites for infants

D. Bending the elbow on the arm with an IV may easily obstruct the flow of solution, causing **infiltration**, which could lead to thrombophlebitis

E. Avoid checking the blood pressure on the arm receiving the IV infusion

F. Do not place restraints over the venipuncture site

G. An arm board may be prescribed when the venipuncture site is located in an area of flexion

V. ADMINISTERING IV SOLUTIONS

A. The IV solution should be checked against the physician's orders for the type, amount, percentage of solution, and rate of flow

B. Wash hands thoroughly and use sterile technique when working with an IV

C. When preparing a new solution for administration, clamp the tubing, attach the spike end of the tubing to the IV bag, and then prime the tubing to remove air from the tubing and IV system

D. Change the IV tubing every 24 to 72 hours, depending on agency policy

E. Do not let an IV bag or bottle hang for more than 24 hours

F. Do not allow the IV tubing to touch the floor

G. Change the IV dressing every 72 hours, when the dressing is wet or contaminated, or as specified by the agency policy

H. Label the tubing, dressing, and solution bags clearly, including the date and time when changed

VI. PRECAUTIONS

A. Can cause initial pain and discomfort for the client on insertion

B. Provides a route of entry for microorganisms into the body

---

BOX 13-1

Peripheral Intravenous Sites to Avoid

Edematous extremity
An arm that is weak, traumatized, or paralyzed
The arm on the same side as a mastectomy
An arm that has an arteriovenous fistula or shunt for dialysis
An infected area

C. **Fluid (circulatory) overload** or electrolyte imbalances can occur from an excessive or too-rapid infusion of fluids; an IV infusion should be checked at least once per hour in an adult client

D. Incompatibilities between certain solutions can occur

E. Clients with cardiac, respiratory, renal, or liver diseases, and older and very young clients cannot tolerate an excessive fluid volume; the risk of **fluid (circulatory) overload** exists with these clients

F. A client with congestive heart failure is usually not given a saline solution because this type of fluid encourages the retention of water, and therefore exacerbates heart failure by increasing the fluid overload

G. A client with diabetes mellitus does not typically receive dextrose (glucose) solutions

H. Lactated Ringer's solution contains potassium and should not be administered to clients with renal failure

VII. COMPLICATIONS (Table 13-2)

A. Infection
   1. Description
      a. The entry of microorganisms into the body through the venipuncture site
      b. Venipuncture interrupts the integrity of the skin, the first line of defense against infection
      c. The longer the therapy continues, the greater the risk of infection

TABLE 13-2

Signs of Complications of Intravenous Therapy

Complication	Signs
Phlebitis	Heat, redness, tenderness at site
	Not swollen or hard
	IV infusion sluggish
Thrombophlebitis	Hard and cordlike vein
	Heat, redness, tenderness at site
	IV infusion sluggish
Infiltration	Edema, pain, and coolness at site
	May or may not have a blood return
Catheter embolism	Decrease in blood pressure (BP)
	Pain along vein
	Weak, rapid pulse
	Cyanosis of nail beds
	Loss of consciousness
Fluid overload	Increased BP
	Rapid breathing
	Dyspnea
	Moist cough and crackles
Air embolism	Tachycardia
	Dyspnea
	Cyanosis
	Hypotension
	Decreased level of consciousness

2. At-risk clients
   a. Immunocompromised client from diseases such as cancer or acquired immunodeficiency syndrome (AIDS)
   b. Clients receiving treatments such as chemotherapy that have an altered or lowered white blood cell count
   c. Older clients, because aging alters the effectiveness of the immune system
3. Prevention and interventions
   a. Maintain strict asepsis when caring for the IV site
   b. Monitor vital signs, particularly temperature
   c. Monitor for local inflammation at the IV site
   d. Check fluid containers for cracks, leaks, cloudiness, or other evidence of contamination
   e. Change the tubing and site dressing every 24 to 72 hours according to agency policy
   f. Antimicrobial ointment is used at the IV site
   g. Ensure that the IV solution is not hanging for more than 24 hours
   h. Monitor for systemic infection; this includes malaise, headache, chills, fever, nausea, vomiting, backache, and tachycardia
   i. If infection occurs, the IV is discontinued and the physician is notified; blood cultures may be ordered

B. **Phlebitis** and thrombophlebitis
1. Description
   a. An inflammation of the vein that can occur from mechanical or chemical (medication) trauma or local infection
   b. **Phlebitis** can cause the development of a clot (thrombophlebitis)
2. Prevention and interventions
   a. An IV cannula smaller than the vein is used, and very small veins or veins over an area of flexion are avoided
   b. Anchor the cannula and loop of tubing securely with tape
   c. Use an arm board or splint, as prescribed, if the client is restless or active
   d. If **phlebitis** occurs, the IV device is removed immediately
   e. The physician is notified if **phlebitis** is suspected, and warm, moist compresses are applied if prescribed

C. Infiltration
1. Description
   a. A form of tissue damage also called extravasation
   b. Seepage of the intravenous fluid out of the vein into the surrounding tissues
   c. Occurs when an IV device has become dislodged or perforates the wall of the vein
2. Prevention and interventions
   a. IV sites over an area of flexion are avoided
   b. Anchor the cannula and loop of tubing securely with tape

   c. Use an arm board or splint, as prescribed, if the client is restless or active
   d. Monitor the IV site for pain, edema, or coolness, comparing it with the opposite extremity
   e. Monitor the IV rate for a decrease or a halt in flow
   f. If **infiltration** has occurred, the IV device is removed immediately
   g. Do not rub an infiltrated area, because this can cause the development of a hematoma
   h. If **infiltration** has occurred, the extremity is elevated and compresses are applied (warm or cool, depending on the physician's preference or agency policy) over the affected area

D. Catheter embolism
1. Description: the tip of the catheter breaks off during IV insertion or removal, resulting in the possibility of an embolus
2. Prevention and interventions
   a. Remove the IV catheter carefully and inspect the catheter when removed
   b. If the catheter tip has broken off, the physician is notified; a tourniquet is placed high on the limb of IV site, as prescribed, an x-ray study is obtained, and the client may require surgery to remove catheter pieces

E. **Fluid (circulatory) overload**
1. Description: Results from the administration of fluids too rapidly or in a client at risk for fluid overload
2. Prevention and interventions
   a. Identify clients at risk for fluid overload
   b. Calculate and monitor the drip rate frequently
   c. An infusion controller device may be used for clients at risk for overload
   d. If fluid overload occurs, the physician is notified

F. **Air embolism**
1. Description: A bolus of air enters the vein through an inadequately primed IV line, from a loose connection, or during tubing change or removal of the IV
2. Prevention and interventions
   a. Prime the tubing with fluid before use and monitor for any air bubbles in tubing
   b. Secure all connections
   c. Replace IV fluid before the bag or bottle is empty
   d. If an **air embolism** is suspected, the tubing is clamped, the client is turned on his or her left side, with the head of the bed lowered to trap the air in the right atrium, and the physician is notified

VIII. CENTRAL VENOUS CATHETERS
(Figure 13-4)
A. Description
1. Used to deliver hyperosmolar solutions, measure central venous pressure, and infuse total parenteral

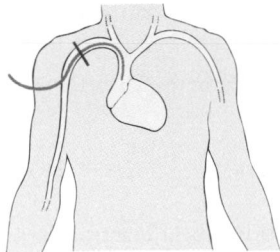

Subclavian catheter site

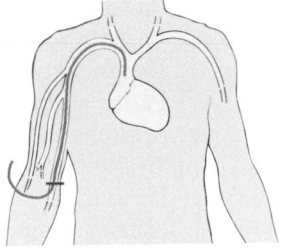

Peripherally inserted
central catheter (PICC)

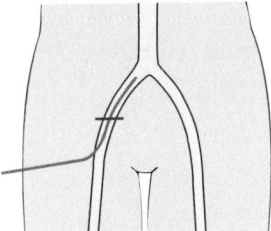

Femoral catheter site

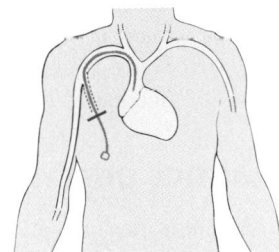

Hickman catheter site

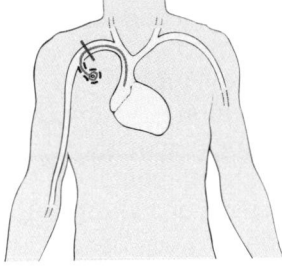

Subclavian catheter
with implantable
vascular access port

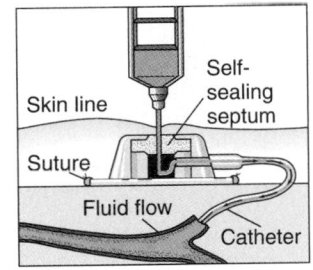

Skin line

Suture

Fluid flow

Self-
sealing
septum

Catheter

Implantable
vascular access port

FIG. 13-4 Central venous access sites and access port. (From Kee, J. & Marshall, S. [2004]. *Clinical calculations: With applications to general and specialty areas* [5th ed.]. Philadelphia: W.B. Saunders.)

nutrition (TPN) and multiple IV infusions or medications
2. Catheter position is determined by x-ray study after insertion
3. May have a single, double, or triple lumen
4. May be inserted peripherally and threaded through the basilic or cephalic vein into the superior vena cava, inserted centrally through the internal jugular or subclavian veins, or surgically tunneled through subcutaneous tissue into the cephalic vein
5. With multilumen catheters, more than one medication can be administered at the same time without incompatibility problems, and there is only one insertion site for care
6. For central line insertion, tubing change, and line removal, place the client in Trendelenburg position (if not contraindicated) or supine position, and instruct the client to perform the Valsalva maneuver to increase pressure in the central veins when the IV system is open

B. Tunneled central venous catheters
1. A more permanent type of catheter, such as the Hickman, Broviac, or Groshong catheter, used for long-term IV therapy
2. May be single or multilumen
3. Inserted in the operating room; the catheter is threaded into the lower part of the vena cava at the entrance of the right atrium
4. The catheter will be fitted with an intermittent infusion device to allow access as needed and to keep the system closed and intact
5. Patency is maintained by flushing with a diluted heparin solution or normal saline solution, depending on the type of catheter and as per agency policy
C. Vascular access ports (implantable ports)
1. Surgically implanted under the skin, such as a Port-a-Cath, Mediport, or Infusaport; used for long-term administration of repeated IV therapy
2. For access, requires palpation and injection through the skin into the self-sealing port with a noncoring needle such as a Huber-point needle
3. Patency is maintained by periodic flushing with a diluted heparin solution, as prescribed per agency policy
D. Peripherally inserted central catheter (PICC) line
1. Used for long-term IV therapy, frequently in the home
2. The basilic vein is usually used, but the median cubital and cephalic veins in the antecubital area can also be used
3. Threaded so that the catheter tip may terminate in either the axillary or subclavian vein or the superior vena cava
4. A small amount of bleeding may occur at the time of insertion and continue for 24 hours, but bleeding thereafter is not expected
5. **Phlebitis** is a common complication
6. Insertion is below the heart level; therefore, **air embolism** is not common

IX. BLOOD ADMINISTRATION

A. Types of blood components
1. Red blood cells (RBCs)
   a. Used to replace erythrocytes
   b. Evaluation of an effective response is based on the resolution of the symptoms of anemia and an increase of the erythrocyte count
2. Whole blood
   a. Rarely used because treatment with a specific blood component is usually prescribed
   b. Used to resolve hypovolemic shock resulting from hemorrhage
   c. Contains RBCs, plasma, and plasma proteins
   d. Evaluation of an effective response is based on the resolution of the symptoms of hypovolemia

3. Platelets
   a. Platelets are used to treat thrombocytopenia and platelet dysfunctions
   b. **Crossmatching** is not required but is usually done (platelet concentrates contain few RBCs)
   c. Evaluation of an effective response is based on improvement in the platelet count
4. Fresh-frozen plasma
   a. Fresh-frozen plasma may be used to provide clotting factors or volume expansion; contains no platelets
   b. **Rh factor** and **ABO compatibility** are required for the transfusion of plasma products
   c. Evaluation of an effective response is assessed by monitoring coagulation studies

B. **Compatibility**
1. To ensure proper identification, client blood samples are drawn and labeled at the bedside; client is asked to state his or her name, which is compared with the identification bracelet
2. The recipient's **ABO** and **Rh factor** are identified
3. An antibody screen is done to determine the presence of antibodies
4. **Crossmatching** testing is done, in which donor RBCs are combined with the recipient's serum and Coombs' serum; **crossmatching** is compatible if no RBC agglutination occurs
5. The universal RBC donor is O negative; the universal recipient is AB positive

C. Interventions
1. The client's temperature is checked before beginning a transfusion; a fever may be a cause for delaying the transfusion; in addition, a fever will mask a possible symptom of an acute transfusion reaction
2. During the transfusion, the client is monitored for signs and symptoms of a **transfusion reaction**; the first 10 to 15 minutes of the transfusion are the most critical, and the nurse must stay with client; if a major **ABO** incompatibility exists or a severe allergic reaction occurs, it is usually evident within the first 50 mL of the transfusion
3. The client is instructed to immediately report anything unusual
4. If a reaction occurs, the transfusion is stopped and the physician is notified; the blood bag and tubing are returned to the blood bank
5. If a reaction occurs, the client is monitored for any life-threatening symptoms and the appropriate blood and urine samples are obtained, as prescribed
6. Document the client's tolerance to the administration of the blood product

D. **Transfusion reactions**
1. Immediate **transfusion reaction**
   a. Chills and diaphoresis
   b. Muscle aches, back pain, or chest pain
   c. Rashes, hives, itching, and swelling
   d. Rapid, thready pulse
   e. Dyspnea, cough, or wheezing
   f. Pallor and cyanosis
   g. Apprehension
   h. Tingling and numbness
   i. Headache
   j. Nausea, vomiting, abdominal cramping, and diarrhea
2. Delayed **transfusion reaction**
   a. Reactions can occur days to years after a transfusion
   b. Signs include fever, mild jaundice, and a decreased hematocrit level

PRACTICE QUESTIONS

1. A client has an order to receive 1000 mL of 5% dextrose in 0.45% sodium chloride. After gathering the appropriate equipment, the nurse takes which of the following actions first before spiking the IV bag with the tubing?
   1. Uncaps the spike portion of the tubing
   2. Uncaps the distal end of the tubing
   3. Closes the roller clamp on the IV tubing
   4. Opens the roller clamp on the IV tubing
2. A nurse is checking the IV dressing of a client with a peripheral intravenous solution infusing. The date on the dressing is 2/9 (February 9). The nurse calculates that the dressing should be changed on which of the following dates?
   1. 2/10
   2. 2/12
   3. 2/14
   4. 2/16
3. A nurse is doing a routine assessment of a client's peripheral IV site. The nurse notes that the site is cool, pale, and swollen and that the IV has stopped running. The nurse determines that which of the following has probably occurred?
   1. Infiltration
   2. Phlebitis
   3. Thrombosis
   4. Infection
4. A nurse is assigned to care for a client with a peripheral IV infusion. The nurse is providing hygiene care to the client and would avoid which of the following while changing the client's hospital gown?
   1. Use a hospital gown with snaps at the sleeves
   2. Put the bag and tubing through the sleeve, followed by the client's arm
   3. Disconnect the IV tubing from the catheter in the vein
   4. Check the IV flow rate immediately after changing the hospital gown
5. A nurse is making a worksheet and is listing the tasks that need to be done on assigned adult clients during

the shift. The nurse writes on the plan to check the IV of an assigned client receiving fluid replacement therapy every:
1. 4 hours
2. 3 hours
3. 2 hours
4. 1 hour

6. A nurse is checking the insertion site of a peripheral intravenous catheter. The nurse notes the site to be reddened, warm, painful, and slightly edematous in the area of the vein proximal to the IV catheter. The nurse interprets that this is most likely due to:
1. Infiltration of the IV line
2. Phlebitis of the vein
3. Hypersensitivity to the IV solution
4. Allergic reaction to the IV catheter material

7. A nurse has been instructed to discontinue an intravenous line. The nurse removes the catheter by withdrawing the catheter while applying pressure to the site with a(n):
1. Alcohol swab
2. Betadine swab
3. Band-Aid
4. Sterile 2 × 2 gauze

8. A nurse is preparing an IV solution and tubing for a client requiring IV fluids. While preparing to prime the tubing, the tubing drops and hits the top of the medication cart. The nurse should plan to do which of the following?
1. Scrub the tubing before attaching it to the IV bag
2. Change the IV tubing
3. Wipe the tubing with Betadine
4. Scrub the tubing with an alcohol swab

9. A client is going to be transfused with a unit of packed red blood cells. The nurse understands that it is necessary to remain with the client for what time period, once the transfusion is started?
1. 5 minutes
2. 15 minutes
3. 30 minutes
4. 45 minutes

10. A nurse is assisting in caring for a client receiving a unit of packed red blood cells. The nurse tells the client that it is most important to report which of the following signs immediately?
1. Mild discomfort at the catheter site
2. Chills, itching, or rash
3. Unusual sleepiness or fatigue
4. Sore throat or ear ache

11. A nurse is assisting in caring for a client who will receive a unit of blood. Just before the infusion, it is most important for the nurse to assess the client's:
1. Skin color
2. Oxygen saturation
3. Vital signs
4. Latest hematocrit level

12. A client receiving a blood transfusion rings the call bell for the nurse. On entering the room, the nurse notes that the client is flushed, dyspneic, and complaining of generalized itching. The nurse interprets that the client is experiencing:
1. Fluid overload
2. Bacteremia
3. Hypovolemic shock
4. Transfusion reaction

13. A client who was receiving a blood transfusion has experienced a transfusion reaction. The nurse sends the blood bag used for the client to which of the following areas?
1. Risk management department
2. Laboratory
3. Pharmacy
4. Blood bank

14. A nurse takes a client's temperature before giving a blood transfusion. The temperature is 100° F orally. The nurse reports the finding to the registered nurse and anticipates that which of the following actions will take place?
1. The transfusion will begin as prescribed
2. The blood will be held and the physician will be notified
3. The transfusion will begin after administering an antihistamine
4. The transfusion will begin after administration of 600 mg of acetaminophen (Tylenol)

15. A nurse is assisting in caring for a client who has received a transfusion of platelets. The nurse evaluates that the client is benefiting most from this therapy if the client exhibits which of the following?
1. Decline of temperature to normal
2. Decrease in oozing from puncture sites and gums
3. Increased hemoglobin level
4. Increased hematocrit level

ALTERNATE FORMAT QUESTION: FILL IN THE BLANK

A nurse is completing a time tape for a 1000-mL IV bag that is scheduled to infuse over 8 hours. The nurse has just placed the 11:00 AM marking at the 500-mL level. The nurse would place the mark for 12:00 noon at which numerical level (mL) on the time tape?

Answer: _____

ANSWERS

1. Answer: 3

Rationale: The nurse should first clamp the tubing to prevent the solution from running freely through the tubing once it is attached to the IV bag. The nurse should next uncap the proximal (spike) portion of the tubing and attach it to the IV bag. Then, the roller clamp is opened slowly and the fluid is allowed to flow through the tubing in a controlled fashion to prevent air from remaining in parts of the tubing.

Test-Taking Strategy: Use the process of elimination and note the key word, *first.* This question tests a specific procedure related to intravenous therapy. Visualize this procedure to answer the question correctly. Review this procedure if you had difficulty with this question.

Level of Cognitive Ability: Application
Client Needs: Physiological Integrity
Integrated Process: Nursing Process/Implementation
Content Area: Fundamental Skills
Reference: Potter, P., & Perry, A. (2005). *Fundamentals of nursing* (6th ed.). St. Louis: Mosby, p. 1184.

2. Answer: 2

Rationale: The IV site dressing should be changed every 48 to 72 hours, which is every 2 to 3 days. With an insertion date of 2/9, the due date for change, depending on agency policy, would be either 2/11 or 2/12. Changing the dressing every 5 to 7 days (options 3 and 4) would place the client at risk for infection. Changing the dressing on a daily basis is not necessary, unless the dressing becomes wet.

Test-Taking Strategy: Use the process of elimination. Recalling that the IV site dressing should be changed every 48 to 72 hours will direct you to option 2. Review the standard accepted guidelines for intravenous site maintenance if you had difficulty with this question.

Level of Cognitive Ability: Application
Client Needs: Physiological Integrity
Integrated Process: Nursing Process/Planning
Content Area: Fundamental Skills
References: Linton, A., & Maebius, N. (2003). *Introduction to medical-surgical nursing* (3rd ed.). Philadelphia: W.B. Saunders, p. 244.
Potter, P., & Perry, A. (2005). *Fundamentals of nursing* (6th ed.). St. Louis: Mosby, pp. 1181, 1187.

3. Answer: 1

Rationale: An infiltrated IV is one that has dislodged from the vein and is lying in subcutaneous tissue. The pallor, coolness, and swelling are the result of IV fluid being deposited into the subcutaneous tissue. When the pressure in the tissues exceeds the pressure in the tubing, the flow of the IV solution will stop. The other three options identify complications that are likely to be accompanied by warmth at the site, not coolness.

Test-Taking Strategy: Focus on the data in the question and note the key word, *cool.* Recalling that coolness occurs at the site of IV infiltration will direct you to option 1. Review the signs of infiltration if you had difficulty with this question.

Level of Cognitive Ability: Analysis
Client Needs: Physiological Integrity
Integrated Process: Nursing Process/Data Collection
Content Area: Fundamental Skills

References: Linton, A., & Maebius, N. (2003). *Introduction to medical-surgical nursing* (3rd ed.). Philadelphia: W.B. Saunders, p. 246.
Potter, P., & Perry, A. (2005). *Fundamentals of nursing* (6th ed.). St. Louis: Mosby, p. 1189.

4. Answer: 3

Rationale: The tubing should not be removed from the IV catheter. With each break in the system, there is an increased chance of introducing bacteria into the system, leading to infection. Options 1 and 2 are appropriate. The flow rate should be checked immediately after changing the hospital gown because the position of the roller clamp may have been affected during the change.

Test-Taking Strategy: Use the process of elimination and note the key word, *avoid.* This word indicates a false response question and that you need to select the incorrect action. Visualize this procedure and use knowledge of the basic principles related to intravenous therapy and asepsis to direct you to option 3. Review these principles if you had difficulty with this question.

Level of Cognitive Ability: Application
Client Needs: Safe, Effective Care Environment
Integrated Process: Nursing Process/Implementation
Content Area: Fundamental Skills
Reference: Potter, P., & Perry, A. (2005) .*Fundamentals of nursing* (6th ed.). St. Louis: Mosby, p. 1181.

5. Answer: 4

Rationale: Safe nursing practice includes monitoring an IV infusion at least once per hour in an adult client. Options 1, 2, and 3 do not provide time frames that are safe or acceptable.

Test-Taking Strategy: Use the process of elimination. To answer this question accurately, it is necessary to be familiar with the specific time frames indicated in this nursing procedure. In questions similar to this one, it is best to select the most frequently occurring time frame. Review the precautions related to administering IV fluid if you had difficulty with this question.

Level of Cognitive Ability: Application
Client Needs: Physiological Integrity
Integrated Process: Communication and Documentation
Content Area: Fundamental Skills
Reference: Linton, A., & Maebius, N. (2003). *Introduction to medical-surgical nursing* (3rd ed.). Philadelphia: W.B. Saunders, p. 242.

6. Answer: 2

Rationale: Phlebitis at an IV site results in discomfort at the site, as well as redness, warmth, and swelling proximal to the IV catheter. The IV catheter should be removed, and a new IV should be inserted at a different site. The remaining options are incorrect.

Test-Taking Strategy: Use the process of elimination. Remember that similar options are not likely to be correct. In this case, options 3 and 4 are similar and are therefore eliminated. Recalling that warmth occurs at the site of phlebitis will direct you to option 2. Review the signs of phlebitis if you had difficulty with this question.

Level of Cognitive Ability: Analysis
Client Needs: Physiological Integrity
Integrated Process: Nursing Process/Data Collection

Content Area: Fundamental Skills
Reference: Linton, A., & Maebius, N. (2003). Introduction to medical-surgical nursing (3rd ed.). Philadelphia: W.B. Saunders, p. 246.

7. Answer: 4
Rationale: A dry sterile dressing, such as a sterile 2 × 2 gauze, is used to apply pressure to the site while the catheter is discontinued and removed. This material is absorbent, sterile, and nonirritating to the site. A Betadine or alcohol swab would irritate the opened puncture site and would not stop the blood flow. A Band-Aid may be used to cover the site once hemostasis has occurred.
Test-Taking Strategy: Use the process of elimination. Visualize this procedure and think about each of the items identified in the options to answer the question. Noting the word "sterile" in option 4 will assist in directing you to this option. Review this procedure if you had difficulty with this question.
Level of Cognitive Ability: Application
Client Needs: Safe, Effective Care Environment
Integrated Process: Nursing Process/Implementation
Content Area: Fundamental Skills
References: Christensen, B., & Kockrow, E. (2003). Foundations of nursing (4th ed.). St. Louis: Mosby, p. 450.
Potter, P., & Perry, A. (2005). Fundamentals of nursing (6th ed.). St. Louis: Mosby, p. 1190.

8. Answer: 2
Rationale: The nurse should change the IV tubing. The tubing has become contaminated and, if used, could result in systemic infection to the client. Wiping or scrubbing the tubing is insufficient to prevent systemic infection.
Test-Taking Strategy: Use knowledge of basic infection control measures and intravenous therapy concepts to answer this question. Note the similarity of options 1, 3, and 4 and eliminate these options. Review aseptic technique and IV therapy if you had difficulty with this question.
Level of Cognitive Ability: Application
Client Needs: Safe, Effective Care Environment
Integrated Process: Nursing Process/Implementation
Content Area: Fundamental Skills
Reference: Potter, P., & Perry, A. (2005). Fundamentals of nursing (6th ed.). St. Louis: Mosby, p. 1180.

9. Answer: 2
Rationale: The nurse must remain with the client for the first 15 minutes of a transfusion, which is usually when a transfusion reaction may occur. This enables the nurse to detect a reaction and intervene quickly. The nurse engages in safe nursing practice by obtaining coverage for the other clients during this time. Options 1, 3, and 4 are incorrect.
Test-Taking Strategy: Use the process of elimination and knowledge regarding blood transfusion procedures to answer this question. Remember, the client must be directly monitored for the first 15 minutes of the transfusion. Review the nursing responsibilities involved in beginning a blood transfusion if you had difficulty with this question.
Level of Cognitive Ability: Application
Client Needs: Physiological Integrity
Integrated Process: Nursing Process/Planning

Content Area: Fundamental Skills
Reference: Potter, P., & Perry, A. (2005). Fundamentals of nursing (6th ed.). St. Louis: Mosby, p. 1191.

10. Answer: 2
Rationale: The client is told to report chills, itching, or rash immediately. These could possibly be signs of a transfusion reaction. Mild discomfort at the catheter site may be indicative of a problem, or could result from the size of the IV catheter required to infuse the blood product. Sleepiness, fatigue, headache, nausea, and vomiting are unrelated to a transfusion reaction.
Test-Taking Strategy: Note the key words, most important and immediately. This tells you that more than one or all the options may be partially or totally correct. Knowing that a transfusion reaction is of greatest concern to the nurse, prioritize and select the option that characterizes this problem. Review the signs of a transfusion reaction if you had difficulty with this question.
Level of Cognitive Ability: Application
Client Needs: Physiological Integrity
Integrated Process: Nursing Process/Implementation
Content Area: Fundamental Skills
Reference: Potter, P., & Perry, A. (2005). Fundamentals of nursing (6th ed.). St. Louis: Mosby, pp. 1190-1192.

11. Answer: 3
Rationale: A change in vital signs may indicate that a transfusion reaction is occurring. The nurse assesses the client's vital signs before the procedure to obtain a baseline, every 15 minutes for the first half-hour after beginning the transfusion, and every half-hour thereafter.
Test-Taking Strategy: Note the key words, just before and most important. This tells you that more than one option may be partially or totally correct. Recalling the signs of a blood transfusion reaction will direct you to option 3. Additionally, vital signs is the umbrella (global) option. Review this procedure if you had difficulty with this question.
Level of Cognitive Ability: Application
Client Needs: Physiological Integrity
Integrated Process: Nursing Process/Data Collection
Content Area: Fundamental Skills
Reference: Potter, P., & Perry, A. (2005). Fundamentals of nursing (6th ed.). St. Louis: Mosby, p. 1191.

12. Answer: 4
Rationale: The signs and symptoms exhibited by the client are consistent with a transfusion reaction. With fluid overload, the client would have crackles in addition to dyspnea. With bacteremia, the client would have a fever, which is not part of the clinical picture presented. There is no correlation between the signs mentioned in the question and hypovolemic shock. The signs identified in the question are indicative of an allergic reaction, which is one type of blood transfusion reaction.
Test-Taking Strategy: Use the process of elimination and focus on the data in the question. Recalling the signs of a transfusion reaction will direct you to option 4. Review the complications of blood administration and the signs of a transfusion reaction if you had difficulty with this question.

Level of Cognitive Ability: Analysis
Client Needs: Physiological Integrity
Integrated Process: Nursing Process/Data Collection
Content Area: Fundamental Skills
Reference: Potter, P., & Perry, A. (2005). *Fundamentals of nursing* (6th ed.). St. Louis: Mosby, p. 1192.

13. *Answer:* **4**
Rationale: The nurse prepares to return the blood transfusion bag containing any remaining blood to the blood bank. This allows the blood bank to complete any follow-up testing procedures needed once a transfusion reaction has been documented. Options 1, 2, and 3 are incorrect.
Test-Taking Strategy: Use the process of elimination. Recalling that blood is obtained from the blood bank will help you to eliminate each of the incorrect options. Review the procedures to follow when a blood transfusion reaction occurs if you had difficulty with this question.
Level of Cognitive Ability: Application
Client Needs: Physiological Integrity
Integrated Process: Nursing Process/Implementation
Content Area: Fundamental Skills
References: Christensen, B., & Kockrow, E. (2003). *Foundations of nursing* (4th ed.). St. Louis: Mosby, p 450.
Potter, P., & Perry, A. (2005). *Fundamentals of nursing* (6th ed.). St. Louis: Mosby, p. 1193.

14. *Answer:* **2**
Rationale: If the client has a temperature equal to or higher than 100° F, the unit of blood should be held until the physician is notified and has the opportunity to give further orders. The other options are incorrect.
Test-Taking Strategy: Use the process of elimination. Eliminate options 1, 3, and 4 because they are similar. Remember that, if the temperature is elevated, the physician needs to be notified before initiating a blood transfusion. Review the procedures related to administering a blood transfusion if you had difficulty with this question.
Level of Cognitive Ability: Application
Client Needs: Physiological Integrity
Integrated Process: Nursing Process/Planning
Content Area: Fundamental Skills

Reference: Christensen, B., & Kockrow, E. (2003). *Foundations of nursing* (4th ed.). St. Louis: Mosby, p. 450.

15. *Answer:* **2**
Rationale: Platelets are necessary for proper blood clotting. The client with insufficient platelets may exhibit frank bleeding or oozing of blood from puncture sites, wounds, and mucous membranes. A temperature would decline to normal after infusion of granulocytes if those transfused cells were then instrumental in fighting infection in the body. Increased hemoglobin and hematocrit levels would be seen when the client has received a transfusion of red blood cells.
Test-Taking Strategy: Use the process of elimination. Recalling that bleeding is a concern when the platelets are low will easily direct you to option 2. Review the action of platelets if you had difficulty with this question.
Level of Cognitive Ability: Analysis
Client Needs: Physiological Integrity
Integrated Process: Nursing Process/Evaluation
Content Area: Fundamental Skills
Reference: Pagana, K., & Pagana, T. (2003). *Mosby's diagnostic and laboratory test reference* (6th ed.). St. Louis: Mosby, p. 680.

ALTERNATE FORMAT QUESTION: FILL IN THE BLANK
Answer: **375**
Rationale: If the IV is scheduled to run over 8 hours, then the hourly rate is 125 mL/hour. Using 500 mL as the reference point, the next hourly marking would be at 375 mL, which is 125 mL less than 500.
Test-Taking Strategy: Use basic principles related to pharmacology mathematics and IV administration to answer this question. If this question was difficult, review the concepts related to marking an IV solution by using a time tape.
Level of Cognitive Ability: Application
Client Needs: Physiological Integrity
Integrated Process: Nursing Process/Implementation
Content Area: Fundamental Skills
Reference: Potter, P., & Perry, A. (2005). *Fundamentals of nursing* (6th ed.). St. Louis: Mosby, p. 1176.

REFERENCES

Christensen, B., & Kockrow, E. (2003). *Foundations of nursing* (4th ed.). St. Louis: Mosby.

Linton, A., & Maebius, N. (2003). *Introduction to medical-surgical nursing* (3rd ed.). Philadelphia: W.B. Saunders.

National Council of State Boards of Nursing. (2005). *Detailed test plan for the National Council licensure examination for practical/vocational nurses.* Chicago: Author.

Pagana, K., & Pagana, T. (2003). *Mosby's diagnostic and laboratory test reference* (6th ed.). St. Louis: Mosby.

Potter, P., & Perry, A. (2005). *Fundamentals of nursing* (6th ed.). St. Louis: Mosby.

Fundamental Skills

Hygiene and Safety

PYRAMID TERMS

chemical restraints Medications given to inhibit a specific behavior or movement.

nosocomial infections Infections acquired in the hospital or other health care facility that were not present or incubating at the time of the client's admission; also referred to as hospital-acquired infections.

physical restraints Devices that are applied to restrict a client's movement.

poison Any substance that impairs health or destroys life when ingested, inhaled, or otherwise absorbed by the body.

standard precautions Guidelines used by all health care providers with all clients to reduce the risk of infection for clients and caregivers.

transmission-based precautions Guidelines that are used in addition to standard precautions; used for specific syndromes that are highly suggestive of infections until a diagnosis is confirmed.

warfare agent May be biological, chemical, or radioactive in nature that can cause mass destruction and fatality.

PYRAMID TO SUCCESS

Safety and Infection Control is a subcategory of the Client Needs component "Safe, Effective Care Environment" of the test plan for NCLEX-PN. Pyramid points focus on maintaining environmental safety, preventing accidents, using restraints, priority nursing actions in the event of a disaster, and biological and chemical warfare agents. Pyramid points also focus on standard and transmission-based precautions and the measures required to handle hazardous or infectious materials. The Integrated Processes addressed in this chapter include Caring, Communication and Documentation, Clinical Problem-Solving Process (Nursing Process), and Teaching/Learning.

CLIENT NEEDS

Safe, Effective Care Environment

Biological and chemical warfare agents
Client rights and informed consent
Disaster planning
Establishing priorities
Guidelines regarding the use of restraints
Handling hazardous and infectious materials
Maintaining precautions to prevent accidents
Standard, transmission-based, and other precautions

Health Promotion and Maintenance

Assisting clients and families to identify environmental hazards in the home
Client and family education regarding accident prevention
Client and family education to prevent the spread of infection
Client and family education regarding measures to be implemented in an emergency or disaster
Home safety measures

Psychosocial Integrity

Cultural and religious lifestyles
Sensory/perceptual alterations
Support systems

Physiological Integrity

Providing comfort and assistance to the client
Assisting the client with activities of daily living (ADLs)
Use of assistive devices to prevent injury

Managing and providing care to clients with infectious diseases

Priority nursing actions in an emergency or disaster

I. HYGIENE

A. Description
1. The activity of providing care or promoting self-care, which includes bathing and grooming
2. Includes care of the skin, hair, nails, mouth, teeth, eyes, ears, nasal cavities, and perineal and genital areas
3. Personal hygiene is the activity of self-care, including bathing and grooming

B. General principles
1. Wash hands and wear gloves
2. Ensure privacy
3. Explain procedures to the client
4. Determine the client's health status and readiness for hygiene procedures
5. Determine the client's routine hygiene practices
6. Use proper body mechanics during bathing and hygiene activities
7. Use time spent with client as an opportunity for communication and teaching
8. Maintain and encourage independence as much as possible

II. ENVIRONMENTAL SAFETY

A. Fire safety (Box 14-1)
1. Keep open spaces free of clutter
2. Clearly mark fire exits
3. Know the locations of all fire alarms, exits, and extinguishers (Table 14-1; Box 14-2)
4. Know the telephone number for reporting fires
5. Know the agency's fire drill and evacuation plan
6. Never use the elevator in the event of a fire
7. Turn off oxygen and appliances in the vicinity of the fire
8. In the event of a fire, if a client is on life support, maintain the client's respiratory status manually with an Ambu bag until the client is moved away from the threat of the fire

9. In the event of a fire, ambulatory clients can be directed to walk by themselves to a safe area, and in some cases may be able to assist moving clients in wheelchairs
10. Bedridden clients are generally moved from the scene of a fire by stretcher, their bed, or wheelchair
11. If a client must be carried from the area of a fire, appropriate transfer techniques need to be used
12. If fire department personnel are at the scene of the fire, they can help evacuate clients

B. Electrical safety
1. Electrical equipment must be maintained in good working order and should be grounded
2. Use a three-pronged electrical cord
3. In a three-pronged electrical cord, the third, longer prong of the cord is the ground; the other two prongs carry the power to the piece of electrical equipment
4. Any electrical equipment that the client brings into the health care facility must be inspected for safety prior to use
5. Check electrical cords and outlets for exposed, frayed, or damaged wires
6. Avoid overloading any circuit
7. Read warning labels on all equipment; never operate unfamiliar equipment
8. Use safety extension cords only when absolutely necessary, and tape them to the floor with electrical tape
9. Never run electrical wiring under carpets
10. Never pull a plug by using the cord; always grasp the plug itself
11. Never use electrical appliances near sinks, bathtubs, or other water sources
12. Always disconnect a plug from the outlet before cleaning equipment or appliances

---

TABLE 14-1

Types of Fire Extinguishers

Type	Class of Fires
A	Wood, cloth, upholstery, paper, rubbish, plastic
B	Flammable liquids or gases, grease, tar, oil-based paint
C	Electrical equipment

BOX 14-1

Priority Actions in the Event of a Fire

Remember the mnemonic **RACE** to set priorities in the event of a fire:

R Rescue: Remove all clients from the vicinity of a fire.
A Alarm: Activate the fire alarm; report a fire before attempting to extinguish it.
C Confine: Close doors and windows when a fire is detected.
E Extinguish: Extinguish the fire, using the appropriate fire extinguisher.

BOX 14-2

Using a Fire Extinguisher

Remember the mnemonic **PASS** to use a fire extinguisher:
P Pull the pin.
A Aim at the base of the fire.
S Squeeze the handles.
S Sweep the fire from side to side.

13. If a client receives an electrical shock, turn off the electricity before touching the client

C. Radiation safety
1. Know the health care agency's protocols and guidelines
2. Label potentially radioactive material
3. To reduce exposure to radiation:
   a. The time spent near the source should be limited
   b. The distance from the source should be as great as possible
   c. A shielding device such as a lead apron should be used
4. Monitor radiation exposure with a film (dosimeter) badge
5. Place the client who has a radiation implant in a private room
6. Never touch dislodged implants

D. Disposal of infectious wastes
1. Handle all infectious materials as a hazard
2. Dispose of waste in designated areas only, using proper containers for disposal
3. Ensure that infectious material is properly labeled
4. Needles should not be recapped, bent, or broken
5. Dispose of all sharps immediately after use in closed, puncture-resistant disposal containers that are leakproof and labeled or color-coded

E. Falls (Box 14-3 lists measures to prevent falls)

F. **Restraints**
1. Protective devices used to limit the physical activity of a client or to immobilize a client or an extremity
2. **Physical restraints**: Restrict client movement through the application of a device
3. **Chemical restraints**: Medications given to inhibit a specific behavior or movement
4. Interventions
   a. When **restraints** are necessary, the physician's orders should state the type of **restraint**, identify specific client behaviors for which **restraints** are to be used, and identify a limited time frame for use
   b. Physician's orders for **restraints** should be renewed within a specific time frame according to agency policy
   c. **Restraints** are not to be ordered PRN (as needed basis)
   d. The reason for the **restraints** should be given to the client and family, and their permission should be sought
   e. **Restraints** should not interfere with any treatments or affect the client's health problem
   f. Use a half-bow or safety knot to secure the device to the bed frame or chair, not to the side rails (provides for quick release)
   g. Ensure that there is enough slack on the straps to allow some movement of the body part
   h. Assess skin integrity and neurovascular and circulatory status every 30 minutes, and remove the **restraint** at least every 2 hours to permit muscle exercise and promote circulation
   i. Continually assess the need for **restraints** (Box 14-4)
5. Alternatives to **restraints**
   a. Orient client and family to surroundings
   b. Explain all procedures and treatments to client and family
   c. Encourage family and friends to stay with the client, and utilize sitters for clients who need supervision
   d. Assign confused and disoriented clients to rooms near the nurses' station
   e. Provide appropriate visual and auditory stimuli to the client, such as a clock, calendar, television, and radio
   f. Place familiar items, such as family pictures, near the client's bedside
   g. Maintain toileting routines
   h. Eliminate bothersome treatments, such as tube feedings, as soon as possible
   i. Evaluate all medications that the client is receiving
   j. Use relaxation techniques with the client
   k. Institute exercise and ambulation schedules as the client's condition allows

---

BOX 14-3

Measures to Prevent Falls

Assess the client's risk for falling.
Ensure that the client at risk for falling is in a room near the nurses' station.
Be alert to clients at risk for falling.
Orient the client to physical surroundings.
Instruct the client to seek assistance when getting up.
Explain use of the call bell system.
Keep the bed in the low position with side rails up, if required.
Lock all beds, wheelchairs, and stretchers.
Keep personal items within reach.
Eliminate clutter and obstacles in the client's room.
Provide adequate lighting.
Reduce bathroom hazards.
Maintain the client's toileting schedule throughout the day.

BOX 14-4

Documentation Points with the Use of a Restraint

Reason for restraint
Method of restraint
Date and time of application of restraint
Duration of use of restraint and client's response
Release from restraint with periodic exercise and circulatory, neurovascular, and skin assessment
Determination of continued need for restraint
Evaluation of client's response

G. Poisons
1. Any substance that impairs health or destroys life when ingested, inhaled, or otherwise absorbed by the body
2. Specific antidotes or treatments are available for only some types of **poisons**
3. The capability of body tissue to recover from a **poison** determines the reversibility of the effect
4. **Poison** can impair the respiratory, circulatory, central nervous, hepatic, gastrointestinal (GI), and renal systems of the body
5. The toddler, the preschooler, and young school-age child must be protected from accidental poisoning
6. In older adults, diminished eyesight and impaired memory may result in accidental ingestion of poisonous substances or an overdose of prescribed medications
7. A **Poison** Control Center phone number should be visible on the telephone in homes with small children; in all cases of suspected poisoning, the number should be called immediately
8. Interventions
   a. Remove any obvious materials from the mouth, eye, or body area immediately
   b. Identify the type and amount of substance ingested
   c. Call the **Poison** Control Center before attempting an intervention
   d. If the victim vomits or vomiting is induced, save the vomitus if requested to do so, and deliver it to the **Poison** Control Center
   e. If instructed by the **Poison** Control Center to take the person to the emergency department, call an ambulance
   f. Vomiting is never induced following ingestion of lye, household cleaners, grease, or petroleum products
   g. Vomiting is never induced in an unconscious victim

III. NOSOCOMIAL INFECTIONS (Box 14-5)
A. Also referred to as hospital-acquired infections
B. Infections acquired in a hospital or other health care facility that were not present or incubating at the time of a client's admission
C. Illness impairs the body's normal defense mechanisms

BOX 14-5

Common Drug-Resistant Nosocomial Infections

Vancomycin-resistant enterococci (VRE)
Methicillin-resistant *Staphylococcus aureus* (MRSA)
Multidrug-resistant (MDR) tuberculosis

D. The hospital environment provides exposure to a variety of virulent organisms that the client has not been exposed to in the past; therefore, the client has not developed resistance to these organisms
E. Infections can be transmitted by health care personnel who fail to practice proper hand washing procedures or fail to change gloves between client contacts
F. Some health care agencies have dispensers mounted at the entrance to each client's room that contain an alcohol-based solution for hand rubs

IV. STANDARD PRECAUTIONS
A. Description
1. Must be practiced with all clients in any setting, regardless of the diagnosis or presumed infectiousness
2. Promotes hand washing and use of gloves, masks, eye protection, and gowns, when appropriate, for client contact
3. These precautions apply to blood, all body fluids, secretions, and excretions, regardless of whether they contain blood, nonintact skin, and mucous membranes
B. Interventions
1. Handle all blood and body fluids from all clients as if they were contaminated
2. Hands are washed between client contacts; after contact with blood, body fluids, secretions, or excretions and after contact with equipment or articles contaminated by them; and immediately after gloves are removed
3. Gloves are worn when blood, body fluids, secretions, excretions, nonintact skin, mucous membranes, or contaminated items are touched; gloves should be removed and hands washed between client care contacts
4. Masks, eye protection, or face shields are worn if client care activities may generate splashes or sprays of blood or body fluid
5. Gowns are worn if soiling of clothing is likely from contact with blood or body fluid; wash hands after removing a gown
6. Client care equipment is properly cleaned and reprocessed, and single-use items are discarded
7. Contaminated linen is placed in leakproof bags and handled to prevent skin and mucous membrane exposure
8. All sharp instruments and needles are discarded in a puncture-resistant container; needles are disposed of uncapped or a mechanical device for recapping is used, if necessary
9. Spills of blood or body fluids are cleaned with a solution of bleach and water (diluted 1:10) or agency-approved disinfectant

10. A private room is unnecessary unless the client's hygiene is unacceptable; the nurse should consult with the infection-control professional

V. TRANSMISSION-BASED PRECAUTIONS
A. Airborne precautions
   1. Diseases
      a. Measles
      b. Chickenpox (varicella)
      c. Disseminated varicella zoster
      d. Tuberculosis (TB)
   2. Barrier protection for airborne precautions
      a. Single room maintained under negative pressure; door kept closed except when someone is entering or exiting the room
      b. Negative airflow pressure in the room, with a minimum of 6 to 12 air exchanges per hour depending on the health care agency
      c. Use of ultraviolet germicide irradiation or high-efficiency particulate air (HEPA) filter in the room
      d. Mask or personal respiratory protection device
      e. Place a mask on the client when the client needs to leave the room; the client leaves the room only if necessary
B. Droplet precautions
   1. Diseases
      a. Adenovirus
      b. Diphtheria (pharyngeal)
      c. Epiglottitis
      d. Influenza
      e. Meningitis
      f. Mumps
      g. Mycoplasma pneumonia or menigococcal pneumonia
      h. Parvovirus B19
      i. Pertussis
      j. Pneumonia
      k. Rubella
      l. Scarlet fever
      m. Sepsis
      n. Streptococcal pharyngitis
   2. Barrier protection
      a. Private room or cohort client
      b. Use of a mask
      c. Place a mask on the client when the client is out of the room; the client leaves the room only if necessary
C. Contact precautions
   1. Diseases
      a. Colonization or infection with a multidrug-resistant organism
      b. Enteric infections such as *Clostridium difficile*
      c. Respiratory infections such as respiratory syncytial virus (RSV)
      d. Wound infections
      e. Skin infections such as cutaneous diphtheria, herpes simplex, impetigo, pediculosis, scabies, *Staphylococcus*, varicella zoster
      f. Eye infection such as conjunctivitis
   2. Barrier protection
      a. Private room or cohort client
      b. Use of gloves and a gown when in contact with the client

VI. DISASTERS
A. Know the agency's disaster plan
B. Internal disasters are those in which the agency is in danger
C. External disasters occur in the community, and victims will be brought to the health care facility for care
D. When the health care agency is notified of a disaster, the nurse would follow the guidelines specified in the agency's disaster plan
E. Refer to Chapter 8 for additional information on disaster planning

VII. BIOLOGICAL WARFARE AGENTS
A. Anthrax
   1. Caused by *Bacillus anthracis* and can be contracted through the digestive system or abrasions in the skin, or inhaled through the lungs
   2. Transmitted by direct contact with bacteria and its spores; spores are dormant encapsulated bacteria that become active when they enter living host (no person-to-person spread) (Box 14-6)
   3. Carried to the lymph nodes and then spreads to the rest of the body by way of the blood and lymph; high levels of toxins lead to shock and death
   4. In the lungs, anthrax can cause buildup of fluid, tissue decay, and death (fatal if untreated)
   5. A blood test is available to detect anthrax (magnifies DNA from the blood sample and matches it to anthrax DNA)
   6. Treated with ciprofloxacin (Cipro), doxycycline, or penicillin
   7. Vaccine has limited availability
B. Smallpox
   1. Transmitted in air droplets and by handling contaminated materials
   2. Highly contagious
   3. Symptoms include fever, back pain, vomiting, malaise, and headache
   4. Papules develop 2 days after symptoms develop and progress to pustular vesicles, which are initially abundant on the face and extremities
   5. A vaccine is available to those at risk for exposure to smallpox

BOX 14-6

Transmission and Symptoms of Anthrax

SKIN

Spores enter the skin through cuts and abrasions and are contracted by handling contaminated animal skin products

Starts with an itchy bump like a mosquito bite that progresses to a small, liquid-filled sac

Sac becomes a painless ulcer with an area of black, dead tissue in the middle

Toxins destroy surrounding tissue

GASTROINTESTINAL SYSTEM

Occurs following ingestion of contaminated undercooked meat

Begins with nausea, loss of appetite, and vomiting

Progresses to severe abdominal pain, vomiting of blood, and severe diarrhea

INHALATION

Caused by the inhalation of bacterial spores, which multiply in the alveoli

Begins with the same symptoms as the flu, including fever, muscle aches, and fatigue

Symptoms suddenly become more severe with the development of breathing problems and shock

Toxins cause hemorrhage and destruction of lung tissue

C. Botulism
1. Serious paralytic illness caused by a nerve toxin that is produced by the bacterium *Clostridium botulinum* (client can die within 24 hours)
2. Spore is found in the soil and can spread through the air or food (improperly canned food) or via a contaminated wound
3. Cannot be spread from person to person
4. Symptoms include abdominal cramps, diarrhea, nausea and vomiting, double vision, blurred vision, drooping eyelids, difficulty swallowing or speaking, dry mouth, and muscle weakness
5. Can progress to paralysis of the arms, legs, trunk, or respiratory muscles (mechanical ventilation is necessary)
6. If diagnosed early, foodborne and wound botulism can be treated with an antitoxin that blocks the action of toxin circulating in the blood
7. Other treatments include induction of vomiting, enemas, and penicillin
8. No available vaccine

D. Plague
1. Caused by *Yersinia pestis*, a bacteria found in rodents and fleas
2. Contracted by being bitten by a rodent or flea carrying the plague bacterium, ingestion of contaminated meat, or handling an animal infected with the bacteria
3. Transmitted by direct person-to-person spread
4. Forms include bubonic (most common), pneumonic, and septicemic (most deadly)
5. Begins with a fever, chest pain, lymph node swelling, and productive cough (hemoptysis)
6. Rapidly progresses to dyspnea, stridor, and cyanosis; death occurs from respiratory failure, shock, and bleeding
7. Antibiotics are only effective if administered immediately; drugs of choice include streptomycin and gentamicin (Garamycin)
8. Vaccine is available

E. Tularemia
1. Infectious disease of animals caused by the bacillus *Francisella tularensis* (also called deerfly fever or rabbit fever)
2. Transmitted by ticks and deerflies or contact with an infected animal
3. Symptoms include fever, headache, ulcerated skin lesion with localized lymph node enlargement, eye infection, gastrointestinal ulceration, and pneumonia
4. Treated with antibiotics
5. Recovery produces life-long immunity (vaccine is available)

F. Hemorrhagic fever
1. Caused by several viruses, including Marburg, Lassa, Junin, and Ebola
2. Virus is carried by rodents and mosquitoes
3. Can be transmitted by direct person-to-person spread via body fluids
4. Symptoms include fever, headache, malaise, conjunctivitis, nausea, vomiting, hypotension, hemorrhage of tissues and organs, and organ failure
5. No known specific treatment is available; treatment is symptomatic

VIII. CHEMICAL AND RADIOACTIVE WARFARE AGENTS

A. Sarin
1. A highly toxic nerve gas that can cause death within minutes of exposure
2. Enters the body through the eyes and skin, and acts by paralyzing the respiratory muscles

B. Phosgene: Colorless gas normally used in chemical manufacturing; if inhaled at high concentrations for a long enough period, leads to severe respiratory distress, pulmonary edema, and death

C. Mustard gas: Yellow to brown in color and has a garlic-like odor that irritates the eyes and causes skin burns and blisters

D. Ionizing radiation
1. Acute radiation poisoning develops after substantial exposure to radiation
2. Can occur from external radiation or internal absorption

3. Symptoms depend on the amount of exposure to the radiation; range from nausea and vomiting, diarrhea, fever, electrolyte imbalances, and neurological and cardiovascular impairment to leukopenia, purpura, hemorrhage, and death

PRACTICE QUESTIONS

1. A nurse enters a client's room and finds that the waste-basket is on fire. The nurse immediately assists the client out of the room. The next nursing action would be to:
   1. Confine the fire by closing the room door
   2. Activate the fire alarm
   3. Call for help
   4. Extinguish the fire

2. A nurse enters the nursing lounge and discovers that a chair is on fire. The nurse activates the alarm, closes the lounge door, and obtains the fire extinguisher to extinguish the fire. The nurse pulls the pin on the fire extinguisher. The next action would be to:
   1. Squeeze the handle on the extinguisher
   2. Aim at the base of the fire
   3. Sweep the fire from side to side with the extinguisher
   4. Sweep the fire from top to bottom with the extinguisher

3. A nurse conducts a home safety assessment with a client preparing for discharge, and the client tells the nurse that a space heater is used to heat the apartment. Which of the following instructions would the nurse provide to the client regarding the use of the space heater?
   1. A space heater should not be used in an apartment
   2. The space heater needs to be placed at least 3 feet from anything that can burn
   3. The space heater should be placed in the hallway at nighttime
   4. The space heater should always be kept at a low setting

4. A nurse is preparing to initiate a tube feeding to a client and the physician has prescribed the use of an electronic food pump. The nurse brings the pump to the bedside to plug the pump cord into the wall and discovers that there is no available outlet in the wall socket. Which of the following would be the appropriate nursing action?
   1. Use an extension cord from the nurse's lounge for the pump plug
   2. Initiate the feeding without the use of a pump
   3. Plug the pump cord into the available outlet above the room sink
   4. Contact the electrical maintenance department for assistance

5. A nurse obtains an order from the physician to restrain a client using a jacket restraint and instructs the nursing assistant to apply the restraint to the client.

Which of the following observations, if made by the nurse, would indicate inappropriate application of the restraint?
   1. A safety knot in the restraint strap
   2. Restraint straps are safely secured to the side rails
   3. The jacket restraint is secure and two fingers can easily slide between the restraint and the client's skin
   4. The jacket restraint strap does not tighten when force is applied against it

6. A nurse is giving a report to the nursing assistant caring for a client who has hand restraints. The nurse instructs the nursing assistant to assess the skin integrity of the restrained hands:
   1. Every 30 minutes
   2. Every 2 hours
   3. Every 3 hours
   4. Every 4 hours

7. A nurse is assisting in planning care for a client with an internal radiation implant. Which of the following is an inappropriate component for the nurse to include in the plan of care?
   1. Placing the client in a semiprivate room at the end of the hallway
   2. Wearing gloves when emptying the client's bedpan
   3. Keeping all linens in the room until the implant is removed
   4. Wearing a lead apron when providing direct care to the client

8. A mother calls a neighborhood nurse and tells the nurse that her 3-year-old child has just ingested liquid furniture polish. The nurse would direct the mother to immediately:
   1. Induce vomiting
   2. Bring the child to the emergency room
   3. Call an ambulance
   4. Call the Poison Control Center

9. An emergency room nurse receives a telephone call and is informed that a tornado has hit a local residential area and numerous casualties have occurred. The victims will be brought to the emergency room. The initial nursing action would be which of the following?
   1. Prepare the triage rooms
   2. Obtain additional supplies from the central supply department
   3. Activate the agency disaster plan
   4. Obtain additional nursing staff to assist in treating the casualties

10. A nurse is caring for a client with a nosocomial infection caused by methicillin-resistant *Staphylococcus aureus* (MRSA) who is on contact precautions. The nurse prepares to provide colostomy care to the client. Which of the following protective items will be required to perform this procedure?
   1. Gloves, gown, and goggles
   2. Gloves and goggles

3. Gloves, gown, and shoe protectors
4. Gloves and a gown

ALTERNATE FORMAT QUESTION: MULTIPLE RESPONSE

A community health nurse is conducting a teaching session about terrorism to members of the community and is discussing information regarding anthrax. The nurse tells those attending that anthrax can be transmitted by which route(s)?

_____ Direct contact with an infected individual
_____ Skin
_____ Gastrointestinal
_____ Inhalation
_____ Sexual contact with an infected individual

ANSWERS

1. *Answer: 2*
Rationale: The order of priority in the event of a fire is to rescue the clients in immediate danger. The next step is to activate the fire alarm. The fire is then confined by closing all doors and, finally, the fire is extinguished.
Test-Taking Strategy: Note the key word, *next*. Remember the mnemonic **RACE** to prioritize in the event of a fire. R = Rescue clients in immediate danger; A = Alarm, sound the alarm; C = Confine the fire by closing all doors; E = Extinguish or evacuate. Review fire safety procedures if you had difficulty with this question.
Level of Cognitive Ability: Application
Client Needs: Safe, Effective Care Environment
Integrated Process: Nursing Process/Implementation
Content Area: Delegating/Prioritizing
Reference: Christensen, B., & Kockrow, E. (2003). *Foundations of nursing* (4th ed.). St. Louis: Mosby. p. 280.

2. *Answer: 2*
Rationale: A fire can be extinguished by smothering it with a blanket or by using a fire extinguisher. To use the extinguisher, the pin is pulled first. The extinguisher should then be aimed at the base of the fire. The handle of the extinguisher is then squeezed and the fire is extinguished by sweeping from side to side to coat the area evenly.
Test-Taking Strategy: Note the key word, *next*. Remember the mnemonic **PASS** to prioritize in the use of a fire extinguisher. P = Pull the pin; A = Aim at the base of the fire; S = Squeeze the handle; S = Sweep from side to side to coat the area evenly. Review the procedures related to the use of a fire extinguisher if you had difficulty with this question.
Level of Cognitive Ability: Application
Client Needs: Safe, Effective Care Environment
Integrated Process: Nursing Process/Implementation
Content Area: Fundamental Skills
Reference: Christensen, B., & Kockrow, E. (2003). *Foundations of nursing* (4th ed.). St. Louis: Mosby. p. 280.

3. *Answer: 2*
Rationale: Space heaters need to be used appropriately because they present a great risk of fire. A space heater needs to be placed at least 3 feet from anything that can burn. Placing a heater in a hallway does not guarantee that it will be 3 feet from anything that can burn. A low setting does not reduce the risk of fire. A space heater can be used in an apartment if there is ample space and safety precautions are followed.
Test-Taking Strategy: Use the process of elimination, keeping in mind the issues related to fire safety. Note that option 2 is the only option that specifically defines a safety measure related to the use of a space heater. Review fire safety prevention measures in the home if you had difficulty with this question.
Level of Cognitive Ability: Application
Client Needs: Safe, Effective Care Environment
Integrated Process: Teaching/Learning
Content Area: Fundamental Skills
Reference: deWit, S. (2005). *Fundamental concepts and skills for nursing.* Philadelphia: W.B. Saunders, pp. 310-311.

4. *Answer: 4*
Rationale: The nurse needs to use hospital resources for assistance. A regular extension cord should not be used because it poses the risk of fire. The use of electrical appliances near a sink also presents a hazard. If the use of a pump is prescribed, the nurse must provide safe means for its use.
Test-Taking Strategy: Use the process of elimination. Eliminate option 2 because the physician has ordered the use of an electronic pump. Recalling safety issues related to electrical hazards will assist in eliminating options 1 and 3. Review electrical safety if you had difficulty with this question.
Level of Cognitive Ability: Application
Client Needs: Safe, Effective Care Environment
Integrated Process: Nursing Process/Implementation
Content Area: Fundamental Skills
Reference: Potter, P., & Perry, A. (2005). *Fundamentals of nursing* (6th ed.). St. Louis: Mosby, pp. 992-993.

5. *Answer: 2*
Rationale: A half-bow or safety knot should be used for applying a restraint because it does not tighten when force is applied against it and it allows quick and easy removal of the restraint in case of an emergency. The restraint strap is secured to the bed frame, never to the side rail, to avoid accidental injury in case the side rail is released. The jacket restraint should be secure, and one to two fingers should easily slide between the restraint and the client's skin.
Test-Taking Strategy: Note the key word, *inappropriate*. This indicates that you are looking for an option that identifies an inaccurate measure related to the application of restraints. The words "secured to the side rails" in option 2 should direct you to this option as an inappropriate action. Review guidelines related to the application of restraints if you had difficulty with this question.
Level of Cognitive Ability: Comprehension
Client Needs: Safe, Effective Care Environment
Integrated Process: Teaching/Learning
Content Area: Fundamental Skills

Reference: Potter, P., & Perry, A. (2005). *Fundamentals of nursing* (6th ed.). St. Louis: Mosby, p. 985.

6. Answer: 1
Rationale: The nurse should instruct the nursing assistant to assess restraints and skin integrity every 30 minutes. Agency guidelines regarding the use of restraints should always be followed.
Test-Taking Strategy: Use the process of elimination. In this situation, it is best to select the option that identifies the most frequent time frame. Review the guidelines related to the use of restraints if you had difficulty with this question.
Level of Cognitive Ability: Application
Client Needs: Safe, Effective Care Environment
Integrated Process: Teaching/Learning
Content Area: Fundamental Skills
Reference: Potter, P., & Perry, A. (2005). *Fundamentals of nursing* (6th ed.). St. Louis: Mosby, p. 987.

7. Answer: 1
Rationale: A private room with a private bath is essential if a client has an internal radiation implant. This is necessary to prevent accidental exposure of radiation to other clients. Options 2, 3, and 4 are accurate interventions for a client with a radiation implant.
Test-Taking Strategy: Use the process of elimination. Note the key word, *inappropriate*. This word indicates a false response question and that you need to select the incorrect action. Option 2 can be eliminated first because this is a component of standard precautions for all clients. Options 3 and 4 can be eliminated next because they directly relate to radiation safety. Review radiation safety principles if you had difficulty with this question.
Level of Cognitive Ability: Application
Client Needs: Safe, Effective Care Environment
Integrated Process: Nursing Process/Planning
Content Area: Fundamental Skills
Reference: Linton, A., & Maebius, N. (2003). *Introduction to medical-surgical nursing* (3rd ed.). Philadelphia: W.B. Saunders, p. 329.

8. Answer: 4
Rationale: If a poisoning occurs, the Poison Control Center should be contacted immediately. Vomiting should not be induced if the victim is unconscious or if the substance ingested is a strong corrosive or petroleum product. Bringing the child to the emergency room or calling an ambulance would not be the initial action, because this would delay treatment. The Poison Control Center may advise the mother to bring the child to the emergency room and, if this is the case, the mother should call an ambulance.
Test-Taking Strategy: Use the process of elimination. Note the key word, *immediately*, in the stem of the question. Eliminate options 2 and 3 because these options will delay treatment. Recalling that vomiting should not be induced if a corrosive substance was ingested will assist in eliminating option 1. Review poison control measures if you had difficulty with this question.
Level of Cognitive Ability: Application
Client Needs: Physiological Integrity

Integrated Process: Nursing Process/Implementation
Content Area: Child Health
Reference: Christensen, B., & Kockrow, E. (2003). *Foundations of nursing* (4th ed.). St. Louis: Mosby, pp. 282-283.

9. Answer: 3
Rationale: In a widespread disaster, many people will be brought to the emergency room for treatment. Although options 1, 2, and 4 may be components of preparing for the casualties, the initial nursing action must be to activate the disaster plan.
Test-Taking Strategy: Note the key word, *initial*. Use the process of elimination in determining the priority action. Note that option 3 is the umbrella (global) option. Review procedures related to management of a disaster if you had difficulty with this question.
Level of Cognitive Ability: Application
Client Needs: Safe, Effective Care Environment
Integrated Process: Nursing Process/Implementation
Content Area: Fundamental Skills
Reference: Christensen, B., & Kockrow, E. (2003). *Foundations of nursing* (4th ed.). St. Louis: Mosby, pp. 280-281.

10. Answer: 1
Rationale: Goggles are worn to protect the mucous membranes of the eye during interventions that may produce splashes of blood, body fluids, secretions, and excretions. In addition, contact precautions require the use of gloves, and a gown should be worn if direct client contact is anticipated. Shoe protectors are not necessary.
Test-Taking Strategy: Note the key words, *contact precautions* and *colostomy*. Use the process of elimination in determining the necessary items required to care for this client. Review this type of precautions if you had difficulty with this question.
Level of Cognitive Ability: Application
Client Needs: Safe, Effective Care Environment
Integrated Process: Nursing Process/Implementation
Content Area: Fundamental Skills
Reference: Christensen, B., & Kockrow, E. (2003). *Foundations of nursing* (4th ed.). St. Louis: Mosby, pp. 247-248.

CRITICAL THINKING: FILL IN THE BLANK
Answers: Skin, Gastrointestinal, Inhalation
Rationale: Anthrax is caused by *Bacillus anthracis* and can be contracted through the digestive system, abrasions in the skin, or inhalation through the lungs. It cannot be spread from person to person.
Test-Taking Strategy: Knowledge regarding the methods of contracting anthrax is needed to answer this question. Remember that it is not spread by person-to-person contact. Review information related to this infection if you had difficulty with this question.
Level of Cognitive Ability: Application
Client Needs: Safe, Effective Care Environment
Integrated Process: Teaching/Learning
Content Area: Fundamental Skills
Reference: Lewis, S., Heitkemper, M., & Dirksen, S. (2004). *Medical-surgical nursing: Assessment and management of clinical problems* (6th ed.). St. Louis: Mosby, p. 1863.

REFERENCES

Christensen, B. & Kockrow, E. (2003). *Foundations of nursing* (4th ed.). St. Louis: Mosby.

deWit, S. (2005). *Fundamental concepts and skills for nursing,* Philadelphia: W.B. Saunders.

Lewis, S., Heitkemper, M., & Dirksen, S. (2004). *Medical-surgical nursing: Assessment and management of clinical problems* (6th ed.). St. Louis: Mosby.

Linton, A. & Maebius, N. (2003). *Introduction to medical-surgical nursing* (3rd ed.). Philadelphia: W.B. Saunders.

National Council of State Boards of Nursing. (2005). *Detailed test plan for the National Council licensure examination for practical/vocational nurses.* Chicago: Author.

Potter, P., & Perry, A. (2005). *Fundamentals of nursing* (6th ed.). St. Louis: Mosby.

Medication and Intravenous Administration

PYRAMID TERMS

conversion   Conversion is the first step in the calculation of a medication problem.

generic name   The common or chemical name of a medication; printed on the label in small letters, usually under the trade name.

milliequivalent(s)   Milliequivalent(s), abbreviated mEq, is an expression of the number of grams of a medication contained in 1 mL of a solution.

parenteral   Parenteral always means injection route. Injections are administered by intravenous, intramuscular, and subcutaneous routes.

percentage solutions   Percentage solutions express the number of grams of a medication per 100 mL of solution.

reconstitution   Powders must be dissolved with a sterile diluent before use, and usually sterile water or normal saline is used. The dissolving procedure is called reconstitution.

ratio solutions   Ratio solutions express the number of grams of a medication per total milliliters of solution.

trade name   Also called the brand name; usually printed on the label in large bold letters.

unit   A measurement of a medication in terms of its action, not its physical weight.

PYRAMID TO SUCCESS

When a medication or intravenous calculation question is presented, a nurse should always use the appropriate formula to solve the problem. Shortcuts should not be used in making these calculations. The problem and the answer should be expressed in the correct units of measure. Be careful with decimal points. It is important to place the decimal points in the correct places, or the answer will be incorrect. When solving a medication calculation problem, the nurse determines whether the answer is within reason and makes sense. In the clinical setting, the nurse should always seek assistance if he or she is unsure of the accuracy of a calculation.

On the NCLEX PN examination, the fill-in-the blank questions may require that you calculate a medication dose or an intravenous flow rate. You will be provided with an optional on-screen calculator for these medication and intravenous problems. Even if you use the calculator to calculate dosages and flow rates, it is important to check the calculation before selecting an option or typing in the answer. Follow the formula, place the decimal points in the correct places, and check the accuracy of the calculation. Remember, practice makes perfect!

The Integrated Processes addressed in this chapter are Caring, the Clinical Problem-Solving Process (Nursing Process), Communication and Documentation, and Teaching/Learning.

CLIENT NEEDS
Safe, Effective Care Environment

Client rights
Error prevention
Handling hazardous or infectious materials
Intravenous fluid and medication calculations
Medical and surgical asepsis
Standard and other precautions

Health Promotion and Maintenance

Collecting physical data
Client teaching regarding prescribed medication(s) or intravenous (IV) therapy
Disease prevention
Lifestyle choices
Physical assessment of client

Psychosocial Integrity

Cultural, religious, and spiritual influences on health
Support systems

Therapeutic interactions
Use of coping mechanisms

Physiological Integrity

Actions of medications and IV therapy
Administration of medications and IV therapy
Adverse effects of and contraindications to medication
or IV therapy
Alterations in body systems
Expected effects of pharmacological therapy
Laboratory values
Unexpected responses to therapy

I. MEDICATION ADMINISTRATION (Box 15-1)

II. DRUG MEASUREMENT SYSTEMS
A. Metric system (Box 15-2)
    1. The basic units of metric measures are meter, liter, and gram
      a. Meter measures length
      b. Liter measures volume
      c. Gram measures weight

BOX 15-1

Medication Administration

Check the medication order.
Ask client about a history of allergies.
Determine the client's current condition and the purpose for the medication or intravenous solution.
Determine the client's understanding regarding the purpose of the prescribed medication or need for IV solution.
Plan to teach the client about the medication and about self-administration at home.
Identify and address concerns (social, cultural, religious) that the client may have about taking the medication.
Determine the need for conversion when preparing a dose of medication for administration to the client.
Check the six rights: right medication, right dose, right client, right route, right time and frequency, and right documentation.
Check vital signs before administering the medication.
Document the administration of the prescribed therapy and client's response to the therapy.

BOX 15-2

Metric System

ABBREVIATIONS/SYMBOLS	EQUIVALENTS
meter: m	1 mg = 1000 mcg or 0.001 g
liter: L	1 g = 1000 mg
gram: g, gm, Gm	1 mL = 0.001 L
milligram: mg	1 kg = 1000 g
microgram: mcg	1 mcg = 0.000001 g
kilogram: kg, Kg	1 mL or 0.001 L
milliliter: mL	1 kg = 2.2 lb

B. Apothecary and household systems (Box 15-3)
    1. The apothecary and household systems are the oldest of the medication measurement systems
    2. The three apothecary measures commonly used are grain, dram, and ounce
      a. Grain, dram, and ounce measure weight
      b. Fluid dram and fluid ounce measure volume
      c. The four household measures commonly used are tablespoon, teaspoon, minim, and drop
C. Additional common drug measures
    1. **Milliequivalent**
      a. Abbreviated mEq
      b. Is an expression of the number of grams of a medication contained in 1 mL of a normal solution
      c. Example: 5 mEq of potassium
    2. **Unit**
      a. Measures a medication in terms of its action, not its physical weight
      b. For example: Penicillin, heparin sodium, insulin are measured in units

III. CONVERSIONS
A. **Conversion** between metric **units** (Box 15-4)
    1. The metric system is a decimal system; therefore, **conversions** between the **units** in this system can be done by either dividing or multiplying by 1000 or by moving the decimal point three places to the right or three places to the left
    2. In the metric system, to convert larger to smaller, multiply by 1000 or move the decimal point three places to the right
    3. In the metric system, to convert smaller to larger, divide by 1000 or move the decimal point three places to the left

BOX 15-3

Apothecary and Household Systems

ABBREVIATIONS	EQUIVALENTS
Apothecary (weight)	gr 1 = 60 mg
grain: gr	gr 5 = 300 mg
dram: dr	gr 15 = 1000 mg or 1 g
ounce: oz	gr 1/150 = 0.4 mg
Household (volume)	1fl oz = 30 mL
minim: min	1 fl dr = 4 mL
quart: qt	1 T = 15 mL or 3 tsp
pint: pt	1 t or tsp = 5 mL
drops: gtt	1 min = 1 gtt
tablespoon: T or tbs	15 min = 1 mL
teaspoon: t or tsp	60 min = 1 fl dr
fluid dram: fl dr	8 dr = 1 fl oz
Household (weight)	1 qt = 1000 mL or 1 L
pounds: lb	1 qt = 2 pt or 32 oz
	1 pt = 16 fl oz
	16 oz = 1 lb
	2.2 lb = 1 kg

B. **Conversion** between apothecary, household, and metric systems
1. **Conversions** between the metric, apothecary, and household systems are equivalent, not *equal*, measures
2. **Conversion** to equivalent measures between systems is necessary when a medication order is written in one system but the medication label is given in another
3. Medications are not always ordered and prepared in the same system of measurement; it is therefore necessary to convert **units** from one system to another
4. **Conversion** is the first step in the calculation of dosages
5. Calculating equivalents between two systems may be done by using the method of ratio and proportion (Box 15-5)

IV. CELSIUS AND FAHRENHEIT TEMPERATURES (Box 15-6)
A. To convert Fahrenheit to Celsius, first subtract 32 and then divide result by 1.8
B. To convert Celsius to Fahrenheit, first multiply by 1.8 and then add 32

V. MEDICATION LABELS
A. A medication label will contain both the **generic name** and the **trade name** of the medication
B. Each medication has only one official name but may have several trade names, each for the exclusive use of the company that manufactures the medication
C. Always check expiration dates on medication labels

VI. MEDICATION ORDERS (Box 15-7)
A. In a medication order, the name of the medication is written first, followed by the dosage, route, and frequency

---

BOX 15-4

Conversion Between Metric Units

PROBLEM 1:
Convert 2 grams (g) to milligrams (mg).
Solution:
Change a larger unit to a smaller unit.
2.000 g = 2000 mg (moving decimal three places to right)

PROBLEM 2:
Convert 250 milliliters (mL) to liters (L).
Solution:
Change a smaller unit to a larger unit.
250 mL = or 0.25 L (moving decimal three places to left)

B. If there are any questions about or inconsistencies in the written order, the person who wrote the order must be contacted immediately, and the order must be verified

VII. ORAL MEDICATIONS
A. Scored tablets contain an indented mark to be used for breakage into partial dosages; when necessary, scored tablets (those marked for division) can be divided into halves or quarters
B. Enteric-coated tablets and sustained-released capsules delay absorption until the medication reaches the small intestine; these medications should not be crushed

---

BOX 15-5

Calculating Equivalents Between Two Systems

Calculating equivalents between two systems may be done by using the method of ratio and proportion.

PROBLEM:
The physician orders nitroglycerin, grain (gr) 1/150. The medication label reads 0.4 milligram (mg) per tablet. The nurse prepares to administer how many tablets to the client?
Solution
gr 1:60 mg = gr 1/150:x mg
$60 \times 1/150 = x$
x = 0.4 mg (1 tablet)

BOX 15-6

Celsius and Fahrenheit Temperature

CONVERTING FAHRENHEIT (F) TO CELSIUS (C)
To convert Fahrenheit to Celsius, subtract 32 and divide result by 1.8.
Formula: C = (F − 32) divided by 1.8

CONVERTING CELSIUS TO FAHRENHEIT
To convert Celsius to Fahrenheit, multiply by 1.8 and add 32.
Formula: $F = 1.8 \times C + 32$

BOX 15-7

Medication Orders

Name of client
Date and time when order is written
Name of medication to be given
Dosage of medication
Medication route
Time and frequency of administration
Signature of person writing the order

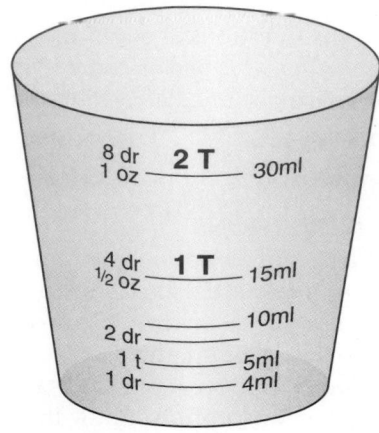

FIG. 15-1 Medicine cup. (From Kee, J., & Marshall, S. [2004]. *Clinical calculations: With applications to general and specialty areas* [5th ed.]. Philadelphia: W.B. Saunders.)

Three-milliliter syringe

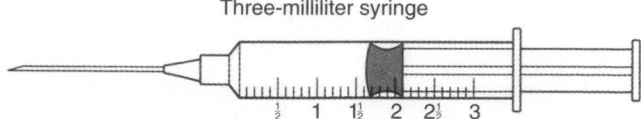

FIG. 15-2 3-mL syringe. (From Kee, J., & Marshall, S. [2004]. *Clinical calculations: With applications to general and specialty areas* [5th ed.]. Philadelphia: W.B. Saunders.)

C. Capsules contain a powered or oily medication in a gelatin cover

D. Oral liquids are supplied in solution form and contain a specific amount of medication in a given amount of solution, as stated on the label

E. The medicine cup (Figure 15-1)
  1. Has a capacity of 30 mL, or 1 ounce
  2. Used for oral liquids
  3. Calibrated to measure teaspoons, tablespoons, and drams
  4. To pour accurately, hold the medication cup at eye level, and then line up the measure that is needed and pour

F. Volumes of less than 5 mL are measured by using a syringe with the needle removed

G. A calibrated dropper is used for giving medicine to children or for adding small amounts of liquid to water or juice; calibrations are in milliliters, cubic centimeters, drops, or minims

VIII. PARENTERAL MEDICATIONS

A. **Parenteral** always means injection route, and **parenteral** medications are administered by intravenous, intramuscular, or subcutaneous routes

B. Parenteral medications are packaged in single-use ampules, in single- and multiple-use rubber-stoppered vials, and in premeasured syringes and cartridges

C. The nurse should not administer more than 3 mL per intramuscular or 1 mL per subcutaneous injection site; larger volumes are difficult for an injection site to absorb and, if prescribed, need to be verified

D. Always question and verify excessively large or small volumes of medication

E. The standard 3-mL syringe is used to measure most injectable medications; it is calibrated in tenths (0.1) of a milliliter (Figure 15-2)

F. The calibrations on a syringe are read from the top black ring on the syringe, not the middle section and not the bottom ring

G. Prefilled medication cartridge (Figure 15-3)
  1. The medication cartridge slips into the cartridge holder, which provides a plunger for injection of the medication
  2. Designed to provide sufficient capacity to allow for the addition of a second medication when combined dosages are prescribed
  3. The prefilled medication cartridge is to be used once and discarded; if a nurse is to give less than the full single dose provided, the nurse needs to discard the extra amount before giving the client the injection, following agency policies and procedures

H. Standard medication doses for adults are to be rounded to the nearest tenth (0.1) of a milliliter and measured on the milliliter scale; for example, 1.25 mL is rounded to 1.3 mL

I. When volumes larger than 3 mL are required, a 5-, 6-, 10-, or 12-mL syringe may be used; these syringes are calibrated in fifths (Figure 15-4)

J. Syringes larger than 12 mL are calibrated in full milliliter measures

K. Tuberculin syringe (Figure 15-5)
  1. Holds a total capacity of 1 mL; used to measure small or critical amounts of medication, such as allergen extract, vaccine, or a child's medication
  2. It is calibrated in hundredths (0.01) of a milliliter, with each one tenth (0.1) marked on the metric scale

L. Insulin syringe (Figure 15-6)
  1. The standard unit-100 insulin syringe is used to measure unit-100 insulin only; it is calibrated for a total of 100 **units**, or 1 mL
  2. Insulin should not be measured in any other type of syringe
  3. When the insulin order states to combine regular and NPH insulin, remember to draw regular insulin first and then draw the NPH insulin

M. Safety needles: Contain shielding devices to reduce the incidence of needlestick injuries (Figure 15-7)

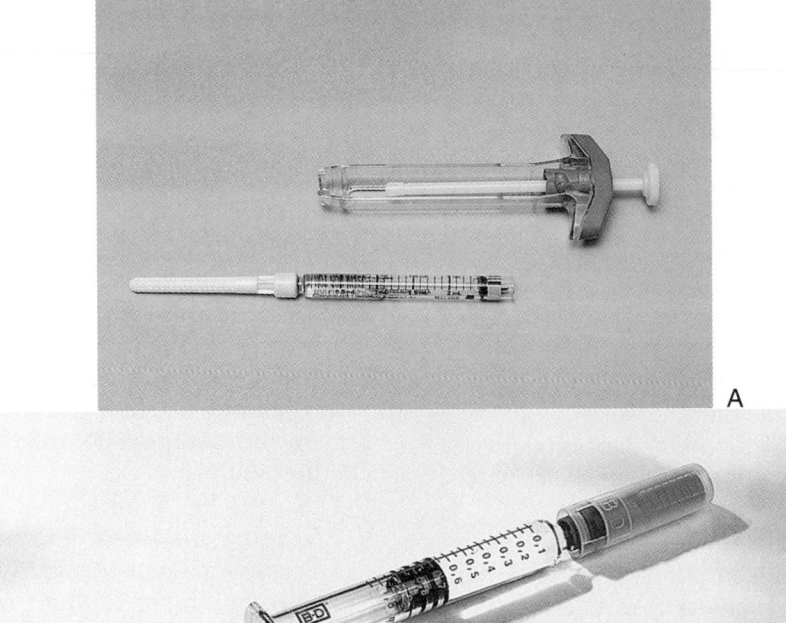

A

B

FIG. 15-3   A, Carpuject syringe and prefilled sterile cartridge with needle. (From Elkin, M., Perry, A., & Potter, P. [2004]. *Nursing interventions and clinical skills,* [3rd ed.]. St. Louis: Mosby); **B,** BD Hypak prefilled syringe. (Courtesy Becton, Dickinson, and Company, Franklin Lakes, NJ.)

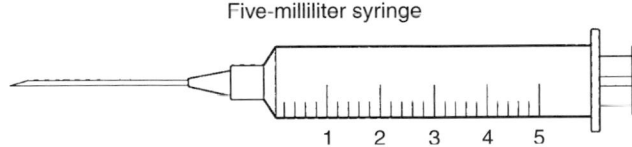

FIG. 15-4   5-mL syringe. (From Kee, J., & Marshall, S. [2004]. *Clinical calculations: With applications to general and specialty areas* [5th ed.]. Philadelphia: W.B. Saunders.)

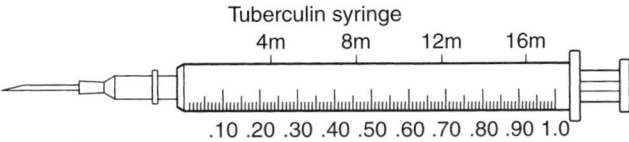

FIG. 15-5   Tuberculin syringe. (From Kee, J., & Marshall, S. [2004]. *Clinical calculations: With applications to general and specialty areas* [5th ed.]. Philadelphia: W.B. Saunders.)

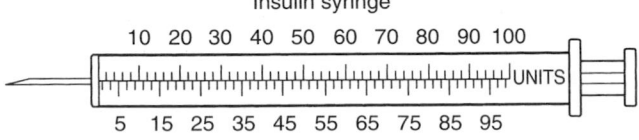

FIG. 15-6   Insulin syringe. (From Kee, J., & Marshall, S. [2004]. *Clinical calculations: With applications to general and specialty areas* [5th ed.]. Philadelphia: W.B. Saunders.)

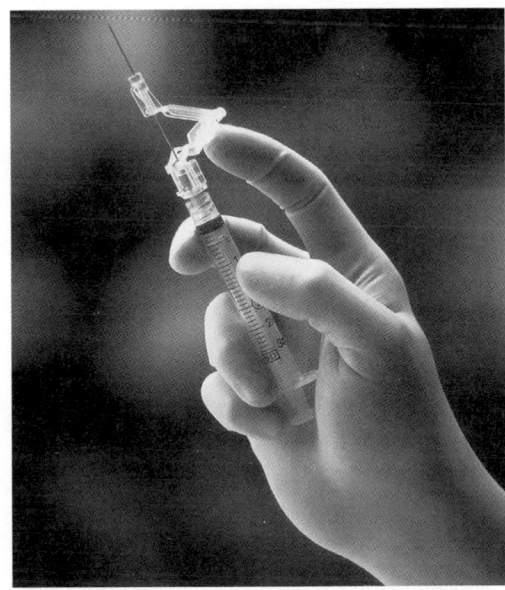

FIG. 15-7   BD SafetyGlide needle. (From Kee, J., & Marshall, S. [2004]. *Clinical calculations: With applications to general and specialty areas* [5th ed.]. Philadelphia: W.B. Saunders. [Courtesy Becton, Dickinson, Franklin Lakes, NJ.])

IX. INJECTABLE MEDICATIONS IN POWDER FORM

A. Some medications become unstable when stored in solution form and are therefore packaged in powder form

B. Powders must be dissolved with a sterile diluent before use; usually sterile water or normal saline is used; the dissolving procedure is called **reconstitution** (Box 15-8)

X. CALCULATING THE CORRECT DOSAGE (Box 15-9)

A. When calculating dosages of oral medications, check the calculation and question an order if the calculation calls for more than three tablets

B. When calculating dosages of **parenteral** medications, check the calculation and question an order if the amount to be given is too large a dose

C. Regardless of the source of an error, if a nurse gives an incorrect dose, he or she is legally responsible for the action

D. Be sure that all measures are in the same system, and that all **units** are in the same size, converting when necessary; carefully consider the reasonable amount of the medication that should be administered

E. Round standard injection doses to tenths and measure in a 3-mL syringe

F. Round small, critical, or children's doses to hundredths and measure in the 1-mL tuberculin syringe

XI. CALCULATING DOSAGES EXPRESSED AS RATIO OR PERCENTAGE

A. **Percentage solutions**
  1. Express the number of grams of the medication per 100 mL of solution
  2. Example: Calcium gluconate 10% = 10 g of pure medication per 100 mL of solution

B. **Ratio solutions**
  1. Express the number of grams of the medication per total milliliters of solution
  2. Example: Epinephrine 1:1000 = 1 g of pure medication per 1000 mL solution

XII. INTRAVENOUS FLOW RATES (Box 15-10)

A. Monitor IVs every 30 minutes for adults and every 15 minutes for children

B. If an IV is running behind schedule, collaborate with the physician to determine the client's ability to tolerate an increased flow rate, particularly clients with cardiac, pulmonary, renal, or neurological conditions

C. The nurse should never increase the rate (speed up) of an IV to catch up if the IV is running behind schedule

D. Whenever a prescribed IV rate is increased, the nurse should assess the client for increased heart rate, increased respirations, or increased lung congestion, which could indicate fluid overload

E. IV fluids are most frequently ordered on the basis of milliliters (mL) per hour to be administered

F. The volume per hour ordered is administered by adjusting the rate at which the IV infuses, which is counted in drops (gtt) per minute

---

BOX 15-8

Reconstitution

When reconstituting the medication, locate the instructions on the label or in the vial package insert, and read and follow the directions carefully.

Instructions will state the volume of diluent to be used and the resulting volume of the reconstituted medication.

Often, the powdered medication adds volume to the solution in addition to the amount of diluent added.

When reconstituting a multiple-dose vial, label the medication vial with the date and time of preparation, your initials, and the date of expiration.

It is also important to label the strength per volume.

The total volume of the prepared solution will always exceed the volume of the diluent added.

BOX 15-9

Formula for Calculating a Medication Dosage

$$\frac{D \text{ (Desired)}}{A \text{ (Available)}} \times Q \text{ (Quantity)} = x$$

D (Desired) = The dosage that the physician ordered

A (Available) = The dosage strength as stated on the medication label

Q (Quantity) = The volume or form in which the dosage strength is available, such as tablets, capsules, or milliliters

---

BOX 15-10

Formulas for Intravenous Calculations

FLOW RATES

$$\frac{\text{Total volume} \times \text{gtt factor}}{\text{Time in minutes}} = \text{gtt/min}$$

INFUSION TIME

$$\frac{\text{Total volume to infuse}}{\text{mL/hour being infused}} = \text{infusion time}$$

NUMBER OF mL/HOUR

$$\frac{\text{Total volume in mL}}{\text{Number of hours}} = \text{number of mL/hour}$$

G. Most flow rate calculations involve changing milliliters per hour into drops per minute

H. IV tubing
1. Calibrated in gtt per milliliter; this calibration is needed for calculating flow rates
2. A standard or macrodrip set is used for routine adult IV administrations; depending on the manufacturer and type of tubing, it requires 10, 15, or 20 gtt to equal 1 mL
3. A minidrip or microdrip set is used when more exact measurements are needed, such as in intensive care units and pediatric units
4. In a minidrip or microdrip set, 60 gtt is equal to 1 mL
5. The calibration, in gtt per mL, is written on the IV tubing package

▲

XIII. ELECTRONIC IV FLOW RATE REGULATORS

A. Controller
1. Works on the same principle of gravity as a regular IV drip, with the rate of flow being maintained by rapid compression and decompression of the IV tubing by the machine
2. The desired flow rate is set on the controller in milliliters per hour
3. Because controllers work by gravity, the height of the solution bag is critical; it must be maintained at a minimum of 36 inches above the controller
4. The nurse should continue to assess the amount of IV solution in the IV container and monitor the controller to ensure proper functioning of the machine

B. Pump
1. A pump is different from a controller in that it physically pumps fluids against resistance
2. Gravity is not a factor in the use of a pump, and the height of the IV solution container is not a critical factor
3. The flow rate on a pump is set in milliliters per hour
4. The nurse should continue to assess the amount of IV solution in the IV container and monitor the pump to ensure proper functioning of the machine

PRACTICE QUESTIONS

The practice questions below are presented in either the multiple-choice format or the fill-in-the-blank format (alternate question format).

1. A physician orders 1000 mL of 0.9% normal saline to run over 12 hours. The drop factor is 15 drops/1 mL. The nurse plans to adjust the flow rate at how many drops per minute?
   1. 15 drops/minute
   2. 17 drops/minute
   3. 21 drops/minute
   4. 23 drops/minute

2. A physician orders an intramuscular dose of 400,000 units of penicillin G benzathine (Bicillin). The label on the 10-mL ampule sent from the pharmacy reads penicillin G benzathine (Bicillin) 300,000 units/mL. The nurse prepares how much medication to administer the correct dose?
   1. 1.3 mL
   2. 13 mL
   3. 1.5 mL
   4. 10 mL

3. A physician orders 3000 mL of 5% dextrose to run over a 24-hour period. The drop factor is 10 drops/1 mL. The nurse plans to adjust the flow rate at how many drops per minute? (Round to the nearest whole number.)

Answer: _____ drops/minute

4. A physician's order reads phenytoin (Dilantin) 0.2 g orally, twice daily. The medication label states 100-mg capsules. How many capsule(s) will the nurse prepare to administer one dose?

Answer: _____ capsule(s)

5. A physician orders 1000 mL of ½%-normal saline to run over 8 hours. The drop factor is 15 drops/1 mL. The nurse plans to adjust the flow rate at how many drops per minute?
   1. 20 drops/minute
   2. 22 drops/minute
   3. 28 drops/minute
   4. 31 drops/minute

6. A physician orders 2000 mL of D5W saline to run over 24 hours. The drop factor is 15 drops/1 mL. The nurse plans to adjust the flow rate at how many drops per minute?
   1. 15 drops/minute
   2. 17 drops/minute
   3. 21 drops/minute
   4. 28 drops/minute

7. A physician's order reads cyanocobalamin (vitamin B12) 100 mcg intramuscular. The medication label reads cyanocobalamin (vitamin B12), 0.5 mg/mL. The nurse administers how many milliters to the client?

Answer: _____ mL

8. A physician orders 3000 mL of 5% dextrose to be administered over a 24-hour period. The nurse prepares to set the infusion rate knowing that how many milliters per hour are to be administered?

Answer: _____ mL

9. A physician's order reads levothyroxine (Synthroid), 150 mcg orally daily. The medication label reads levothyroxine, 0.1 mg/tablet. The nurse prepares to administer how many tablet(s) to the client?
   1. 1 tablet
   2. 1.5 tablets
   3. 2 tablets
   4. 2.5 tablets

10. A physician orders 1000 mL 5% dextrose to run at 125 mL/hour. The nurse calculates the infusion rate knowing that it will take how many hours for 1 L to infuse?

Answer: _____ hours

11. A physician orders one unit of packed red blood cells to infuse over 4 hours. One unit of blood contains 250 mL. The drop factor is 10 drops/1 mL. The registered nurse (RN) asks the licensed practical nurse (LPN) to assist in monitoring the flow rate during the infusion. The LPN monitors the flow rate knowing that how many drops per minute should infuse?
    1. 10 drops
    2. 15 drops
    3. 17 drops
    4. 20 drops

12. A physician's order reads triazolam (Halcion), 125 mcg orally at bedtime daily. The medication bottle is labeled triazolam (Halcion), 0.125-mg tablets. The nurse prepares how many tablet(s) to administer one dose?
    1. 1 tablet
    2. 1.5 tablets
    3. 2 tablets
    4. 2.5 tablets

13. A physician's order reads atenolol (Tenormin), 0.025 g orally daily. The medication bottle reads atenolol (Tenormin), 50 mg-tablets. The nurse prepares how many tablet(s) to administer the dose?
    1. 0.5 tablet
    2. 1 tablet
    3. 2 tablets
    4. 3 tablets

14. A physician's order reads hydromorphone hydrochloride (Dilaudid), 3 mg intramuscular every 4 hours PRN (as needed). The medication label reads hydromorphone hydrochloride (Dilaudid), 4 mg/1 mL. The nurse prepares to administer which of the following to the client?
    1. 1.3 mg
    2. 1.5 mL
    3. 0.8 mL
    4. 4 mg

15. A physician's order reads digoxin (Lanoxin), 0.25 mg PO (orally) daily. The medication label reads digoxin (Lanoxin), 0.125 mg/tablet. The nurse prepares how many tablet(s) to administer the dose?

Answer: _____ tablet(s)

16. A physician's order reads meperidine hydrochloride (Demerol), 80 mg intramuscular PRN (as needed). The medication label reads meperidine hydrochloride (Demerol), 100 mg/mL. The nurse prepares to administer how many millliters to the client?
    1. 100 mL
    2. 1.25 mL
    3. 1 mL
    4. 0.8 mL

17. A physician orders heparin sodium (Liquaemin), 650 units subcutaneous every 12 hours. The medication vial reads heparin sodium (Liquaemin), 1000 units/mL. The nurse prepares how many milliliters to administer one dose? (Round to the nearest tenth.)

Answer: _____ mL

18. A physician orders trimethobenzamide hydrochloride (Tigan), 250 mg intramuscular PRN (as needed). The medication label reads trimethobenzamide hydrochloride (Tigan), 200 mg/2 mL. The nurse plans to prepare how much medication to administer the dose?

Answer: _____ mL

19. A physician orders meperidine hydrochloride (Demerol), 35 mg intramuscular, stat (immediately). The medication label states meperidine hydrochloride (Demerol), 50 mg/mL. The nurse plans to prepare how much medication to administer the dose?
    1. 0.5 mL
    2. 0.6 mL
    3. 0.7 mL
    4. 1 mL

20. A physician orders prochlorperazine (Compazine), 20 mg intramuscular every 4 hours PRN (as needed). The medication label states prochlorperazine (Compazine), 10 mg/mL. The nurse prepares how much medication to administer the dose?
    1. 0.5 mL
    2. 2 mL
    3. 2.5 mL
    4. 2.9 mL

21. A physician orders atropine sulfate, 0.4 mg intramuscular, stat (immediately). The medication label states atropine sulfate, 0.3 mg/0.5 mL. The nurse prepares how much medication to administer the dose? (Round to the nearest tenth.)

Answer: _____ mL

22. A physician orders levodopa (Dopar), 1 g orally twice daily. The medication label states 500-mg tablets. The nurse prepares to administer how many tablets at the evening dose?
    1. 2 tablets
    2. 3 tablets
    3. 4 tablets
    4. 5 tablets

23. A physician orders zidovudine (AZT), 0.2 g orally every 4 hours. The medication label states zidovudine (AZT), 100-mg tablets. The nurse prepares to administer how many tablets for one dose?
    1. 0.5 tablet
    2. 1 tablet

3. 1.5 tablets

4. 2 tablets

24. A physician orders atropine sulfate, gr 1/300, to be administered. The medication label states atropine sulfate, 0.5 mg/0.5 mL. How many milliters will the nurse prepare to administer to the client?

Answer: _____ mL

25. A physician's order states to administer aspirin (acetylsalicylic acid), 650 mg orally for a temperature above 38° C. The medication bottle states aspirin (acetylsalicylic acid), gr 5/tablet. The nurse takes the client's temperature and notes that it is 101° F. The nurse plans to take which of the following actions?

1. Not administer the aspirin at this time

2. Check the client's temperature in 30 minutes

3. Administer 2 aspirin tablets

4. Administer 3 aspirin tablets

ANSWERS

1. *Answer:* 3

Rationale: The prescribed 1000 mL is to be infused over 12 hours. Follow the formula and multiply 1000 mL by 15 (gtt factor). Then, divide the result by 720 minutes (12 hours × 60 minutes). The infusion is to run at 20.8, or 21, drops/minute.

Formula:

$$\frac{\text{Total volume (in mL)} \times \text{drop factor}}{\text{Time in minutes}} = \text{flow rate in drops/minute}$$

$$\frac{1000 \text{ mL} \times 15 \text{ drops}}{720 \text{ minutes}} = \frac{15,000}{720} = 20.8, \text{ or } 21, \text{ drops/minute}$$

Test-Taking Strategy: Follow the formula for calculating an infusion rate for an IV. Be sure to change 12 hours to minutes. After you have performed the calculation, verify your answer using a calculator. Review the formula for calculating infusion rates if you had difficulty with this question.

Level of Cognitive Ability: Application

Client Needs: Physiological Integrity

Integrated Process: Nursing Process/Planning

Content Area: Fundamental Skills

Reference: Kee, J., & Marshall, S. (2004). *Clinical calculations: With applications to general and specialty areas* (5th ed.). Philadelphia: W.B. Saunders, p. 202.

2. *Answer:* 1

Rationale: Follow the formula for dosage calculation.

Formula:

$$\frac{\text{Desired}}{\text{Available}} \times \text{mL} = \text{mL/dose}$$

$$\frac{400,000 \text{ units}}{300,000 \text{ units}} \times 1 \text{ mL} = 1.3 \text{ mL/dose}$$

Test-Taking Strategy: Follow the formula for the calculation of the correct dose. Focus on the key information: 300,000 units/mL. After you have performed the calculation, verify your answer using a calculator. Review medication calculation problems if you had difficulty with this question.

Level of Cognitive Ability: Application

Client Needs: Physiological Integrity

Integrated Process: Nursing Process/Implementation

Content Area: Fundamental Skills

Reference: Christensen, B., & Kockrow, E. (2003). *Foundations of nursing* (4th ed.). St. Louis: Mosby, p. 569.

3. *Answer:* 21

Rationale: The prescribed 3000 mL is to be infused over 24 hours. Follow the formula and multiply 3000 mL by 10 (gtt factor). Then, divide the result by 1440 minutes (24 hours × 60 minutes). The infusion is to run at 20.8, or 21, drops/minute.

Formula:

$$\frac{\text{Total volume (in mL)} \times \text{drop factor}}{\text{Time in minutes}} = \text{flow rate in drops/minute}$$

$$\frac{3000 \text{ mL} \times 10 \text{ drop}}{1440 \text{ minutes}} = \frac{30,000}{1440} = 20.8, \text{ or } 21, \text{ drops/minute}$$

Test-Taking Strategy: Follow the formula for calculating the infusion rate for an IV. Be sure to change 24 hours to minutes. After you have performed the calculation, verify your answer using a calculator and remember to round to the nearest whole number. Review the formula for calculating infusion rates if you had difficulty with this question.

Level of Cognitive Ability: Application

Client Needs: Physiological Integrity

Integrated Process: Nursing Process/Planning

Content Area: Fundamental Skills

Reference: Kee, J., & Marshall, S. (2004). *Clinical calculations: With applications to general and specialty areas* (5th ed.). Philadelphia: W.B. Saunders, p. 202.

4. *Answer:* 2

Rationale: Convert 0.2 g to milligrams. In the metric system, to convert larger to smaller, multiply by 1000 or move the decimal three places to the right. Therefore, 0.2 g = 200 mg.

Formula:

$$\frac{\text{Desired}}{\text{Available}} \times \text{capsules} = \text{capsules per dose}$$

$$\frac{200 \text{ mg}}{100 \text{ mg}} \times 1 \text{ capsule} = 2 \text{ capsules}$$

Test-Taking Strategy: In this medication calculation problem, it is necessary to first convert grams to milligrams. Follow the formula for conversion and read the question carefully. After you have performed the calculation, verify your answer using a calculator. Review medication calculations and conversions if you had difficulty with this question.

Level of Cognitive Ability: Application

Client Needs: Physiological Integrity

Integrated Process: Nursing Process/Implementation

Content Area: Fundamental Skills

Reference: Kee, J., & Marshall, S. (2004). *Clinical calculations: With applications to general and specialty areas* (5th ed.). Philadelphia: W.B. Saunders, p. 116.

5. *Answer:* 4

Rationale: The prescribed 1000 mL is to be infused over 8 hours. Follow the formula and multiply 1000 mL by 15 (gtt factor). Then, divide the result by 480 minutes (8 hours × 60 minutes). The infusion is to run at 31.2, or 31, drops/minute.

Formula:

$$\frac{\text{Total volume in mL} \times \text{drop factor}}{\text{Time in minutes}} = \text{flow rate in drops/minute}$$

$$\frac{1000 \text{ mL} \times 15 \text{ drops}}{480 \text{ minutes}} = \frac{15{,}000}{480} = 31.2, \text{ or } 31, \text{ drops/minute}$$

Test-Taking Strategy: Follow the formula for calculating the infusion rate for an IV. Be sure to change 8 hours to minutes. After you have performed the calculation, verify your answer using a calculator. Review the formula for calculating infusion rates if you had difficulty with this question.

Level of Cognitive Ability: Application
Client Needs: Physiological Integrity
Integrated Process: Nursing Process/Planning
Content Area: Fundamental Skills
Reference: Kee, J., & Marshall, S. (2004). *Clinical calculations: With applications to general and specialty areas* (5th ed.). Philadelphia: W.B. Saunders, p. 202.

6. **Answer: 3**
Rationale: The prescribed 2000 mL is to be infused over 24 hours. Follow the formula and multiply 2000 mL by 15 (gtt factor). Then, divide the result by 1440 minutes (24 hours × 60 minutes). The infusion is to run at 20.8, or 21, drops/minute.

Formula:

$$\frac{\text{Total volume (in mL)} \times \text{drop factor}}{\text{Time in minutes}} = \text{flow rate in drops/minute}$$

$$\frac{2000 \text{ mL} \times 15 \text{ drops}}{1440 \text{ minutes}} = \frac{30{,}000}{1440} = 20.8, \text{ or } 21, \text{ drops/minute}$$

Test-Taking Strategy: Follow the formula for calculating the infusion rate for an IV. Be sure to change 24 hours to minutes. After you have performed the calculation, verify your answer using a calculator. Review the formula for calculating infusion rates if you had difficulty with this question.

Level of Cognitive Ability: Application
Client Needs: Physiological Integrity
Integrated Process: Nursing Process/Planning
Content Area: Fundamental Skills
Reference: Kee, J., & Marshall, S. (2004). *Clinical calculations: With applications to general and specialty areas* (5th ed.). Philadelphia: W.B. Saunders, p. 202.

7. **Answer: 0.2**
Rationale: Convert 100 mcg to milligrams. In the metric system, to convert smaller to larger, divide by 1000 or move the decimal three places to the left. Therefore, 100 mcg = 0.1 mg.

Formula:

$$\frac{\text{Desired}}{\text{Available}} \times \text{mL} = \text{mL/dose}$$

$$\frac{0.1 \text{ mg}}{0.5 \text{ mg}} \times 1 \text{ mL} = \frac{0.1}{0.5} = 0.2 \text{ mL}$$

Test-Taking Strategy: In this medication calculation problem, it is necessary to first convert micrograms to milligrams. Follow the formula for conversion and read the question carefully. Focus on the key information, 0.5 mg/mL. After you have performed the calculation, verify your answer using a calculator. Review medication calculations and conversions if you had difficulty with this question.

Level of Cognitive Ability: Application
Client Needs: Physiological Integrity
Integrated Process: Nursing Process/Implementation
Content Area: Fundamental Skills
Reference: Kee, J., & Marshall, S. (2004). *Clinical calculations: With applications to general and specialty areas* (5th ed.). Philadelphia: W.B. Saunders, p. 116.

8. **Answer: 125**
Rationale: To determine how many milliters per hour are to be administered, simply divide the total prescribed amount of IV solution by the prescribed time period for infusion.

Formula:

$$\frac{\text{Total volume in mL}}{\text{Number of hours}} = \text{amount of mL/hour}$$

$$\frac{3000 \text{ mL}}{24 \text{ hours}} = 125 \text{ mL/hour}$$

Test-Taking Strategy: Focus on the issue of the question, mL per hour. Follow the formula and, after you have performed the calculation, verify your answer using a calculator. Review the formula for determining the amount of milliters to infuse per hour if you had difficulty with this question.

Level of Cognitive Ability: Application
Client Needs: Physiological Integrity
Integrated Process: Nursing Process/Planning
Content Area: Fundamental Skills
Reference: Kee, J., & Marshall, S. (2004). *Clinical calculations: With applications to general and specialty areas* (5th ed.). Philadelphia: W.B. Saunders, p. 202.

9. **Answer: 2**
Rationale: Convert 150 mcg to milligrams. In the metric system, to convert smaller to larger, divide by 1000 or move the decimal three places to the left. Therefore, 150 mcg = 0.15 mg.

Formula:

$$\frac{\text{Desired}}{\text{Available}} \times \text{tablet(s)} = \text{tablet(s)/dose}$$

$$\frac{0.15 \text{ mg}}{0.1 \text{ mg}} \times 1 \text{ tablet} = 1.5 \text{ tablets}$$

Test-Taking Strategy: In this medication calculation problem, it is necessary to first convert micrograms to milligrams. Follow the formula and, after you have performed the calculation, verify your answer using a calculator. Review medication calculations and conversions if you had difficulty with this question.

Level of Cognitive Ability: Application
Client Needs: Physiological Integrity
Integrated Process: Nursing Process/Planning
Content Area: Fundamental Skills
Reference: Kee, J., & Marshall, S. (2004). *Clinical calculations: With applications to general and specialty areas* (5th ed.). Philadelphia: W.B. Saunders, p. 202.

10. **Answer: 8**
Rationale: To determine how many hours it will take for 1 L to infuse, first recall that 1 L is equal to 1000 mL. Next, divide the 1000 mL by the amount being delivered in 1 hour.

Formula:

$$\frac{\text{Total volume in mL}}{\text{mL/hour}} = \text{infusion time in hours}$$

$$\frac{1000 \text{ mL}}{125 \text{ mL}} = 8 \text{ hours}$$

Test-Taking Strategy: Focus on the issue of the question—how many hours for 1 L to infuse. Follow the formula and, after you have performed the calculation, verify your answer using a calculator. Review the formula for determining the infusion time if you had difficulty with this question.
Level of Cognitive Ability: Application
Client Needs: Physiological Integrity
Integrated Process: Nursing Process/Implementation
Content Area: Fundamental Skills
Reference: Asperheim, M. (2005). *Introduction to pharmacology* (10th ed.). Philadelphia: Elsevier/Saunders, p. 38.

11. *Answer:* **1**
Rationale: The prescribed 250 mL is to be infused over 4 hours. Follow the formula and multiply 250 mL by 10 (gtt factor). Then, divide the result by 240 minutes (4 hours × 60 minutes). The infusion is to run at 10.4, or 10, drops/minute.
Formula:
$$\frac{\text{Total volume (in mL)} \times \text{drop factor}}{\text{Time in minutes}} = \text{flow rate in drops/minute}$$
$$\frac{250 \text{ mL} \times 10 \text{ drops}}{240 \text{ minutes}} = \frac{2500}{240} = 10.4, \text{ or } 10, \text{ drops/minute}$$
Test-Taking Strategy: Follow the formula for calculating the infusion rate for an IV. Be sure to change 4 hours to minutes. After you have performed the calculation, verify your answer using a calculator. Review the formula for calculating infusion rates if you had difficulty with this question.
Level of Cognitive Ability: Application
Client Needs: Physiological Integrity
Integrated Process: Nursing Process/Implementation
Content Area: Fundamental Skills
Reference: Kee, J., & Marshall, S. (2004). *Clinical calculations: With applications to general and specialty areas* (5th ed.). Philadelphia: W.B. Saunders, p. 202.

12. *Answer:* **1**
Rationale: Convert 125 mcg to milligrams. In the metric system, to convert smaller to larger, divide by 1000 or move the decimal three places to the left. Therefore, 125 mcg = 0.125 mg. One tablet is administered.
Test-Taking Strategy: In this medication calculation problem, it is necessary to first convert mcg to mg. Follow the formula for conversion and, after you have performed the calculation, verify your answer using a calculator. Review medication calculations and conversions if you had difficulty with this question.
Level of Cognitive Ability: Application
Client Needs: Physiological Integrity
Integrated Process: Nursing Process/Planning
Content Area: Fundamental Skills
Reference: Kee, J., & Marshall, S. (2004). *Clinical calculations: With applications to general and specialty areas* (5th ed.). Philadelphia: W.B. Saunders, pp. 22-23.

13. *Answer:* **1**
Rationale: Convert 0.025 g to milligrams. In the metric system, to convert larger to smaller, multiply by 1000 or move the decimal three places to the right. Therefore, 0.025 g = 25.0 mg.

Formula:
$$\frac{\text{Desired}}{\text{Available}} \times \text{tablet} = \text{number of tablets/dose}$$
$$\frac{25.0 \text{ mg}}{50 \text{ mg}} \times 1 \text{ tablet} = 0.5 \text{ tablet}$$
Test-Taking Strategy: In this medication calculation problem, it is necessary to first convert grams to milligrams. Follow the formula for conversion and, after you have performed the calculation, verify your answer using a calculator. Review medication calculations and conversions if you had difficulty with this question.
Level of Cognitive Ability: Application
Client Needs: Physiological Integrity
Integrated Process: Nursing Process/Planning
Content Area: Fundamental Skills
Reference: Kee, J., & Marshall, S. (2004). *Clinical calculations: With applications to general and specialty areas* (5th ed.). Philadelphia: W.B. Saunders, pp. 22-23.

14. *Answer:* **3**
Rationale: Follow the formula for dosage calculation.
Formula:
$$\frac{\text{Desired}}{\text{Available}} \times \text{mL} = \text{mL/dose} \quad \frac{3 \text{ mg}}{4 \text{ mg}} \times 1 \text{ mL} = 0.75, \text{ or } 0.8, \text{ mL}$$
Test-Taking Strategy: Follow the formula for the calculation of the correct dose. Focus on the key information: 4 mg/1 mL. After you have performed the calculation, verify your answer using a calculator. Review medication calculations if you had difficulty with this question.
Level of Cognitive Ability: Application
Client Needs: Physiological Integrity
Integrated Process: Nursing Process/Planning
Content Area: Fundamental Skills
Reference: Kee, J., & Marshall, S. (2004). *Clinical calculations: With applications to general and specialty areas* (5th ed.). Philadelphia: W.B. Saunders, p. 116.

15. *Answer:* **2**
Rationale: Follow the formula for dosage calculation.
Formula:
$$\frac{\text{Desired}}{\text{Available}} \times \text{tablet} = \text{number of tablets per dose}$$
$$\frac{0.25 \text{ mg}}{0.125 \text{ mg}} \times 1 \text{ tablet} = 2 \text{ tablets}$$
Test-Taking Strategy: Follow the formula for the calculation of the correct dose. Focus on the key information: 0.125 mg/tablet. After you have performed the calculation, verify your answer using a calculator. Review medication calculations if you had difficulty with this question.
Level of Cognitive Ability: Application
Client Needs: Physiological Integrity
Integrated Process: Nursing Process/Planning
Content Area: Fundamental Skills
Reference: Kee, J., & Marshall, S. (2004). *Clinical calculations: With applications to general and specialty areas* (5th ed.). Philadelphia: W.B. Saunders, p. 116.

16. *Answer:* **4**
Rationale: Follow the formula for dosage calculation.

Formula:

$$\frac{Desired}{Available} \times mL = mL/dose$$

$$\frac{80\ mg}{100\ mg} \times 1\ mL = 0.8\ mL$$

Test-Taking Strategy: Follow the formula for the calculation of the correct dose. Focus on the key information: 100 mg/mL. After you have performed the calculation, verify your answer using a calculator. Review medication calculations if you had difficulty with this question.
Level of Cognitive Ability: Application
Client Needs: Physiological Integrity
Integrated Process: Nursing Process/Planning
Content Area: Fundamental Skills
Reference: Kee, J., & Marshall, S. (2004). *Clinical calculations: With applications to general and specialty areas* (5th ed.). Philadelphia: W.B. Saunders, p. 116.

17. *Answer:* **0.7**
Rationale: Follow the formula for dosage calculation.
Formula:

$$\frac{Desired}{Available} \times mL = mL/dose$$

$$\frac{650\ units}{1000\ units} \times 1\ mL = 0.65,\ or\ 0.7,\ mL$$

Test-Taking Strategy: Follow the formula for the calculation of the correct dose. Focus on the key information: 1000 units/mL. After you have performed the calculation, verify your answer using a calculator and remember to round to the nearest tenth. Review medication calculations if you had difficulty with this question.
Level of Cognitive Ability: Application
Client Needs: Physiological Integrity
Integrated Process: Nursing Process/Planning
Content Area: Fundamental Skills
Reference: Kee, J., & Marshall, S. (2004). *Clinical calculations: With applications to general and specialty areas* (5th ed.). Philadelphia: W.B. Saunders, p. 116.

18. *Answer:* **2.5**
Rationale: Follow the formula for dosage calculation.
Formula:

$$\frac{Desired}{Available} \times mL = mL/dose$$

$$\frac{250\ mg}{200\ mg} \times 2\ mL = 2.5\ mL$$

Test-Taking Strategy: Follow the formula for the calculation of the correct dose. Focus on the key information: 200 mg/2 mL. After you have performed the calculation, verify your answer using a calculator. Review medication calculations if you had difficulty with this question.
Level of Cognitive Ability: Application
Client Needs: Physiological Integrity
Integrated Process: Nursing Process/Planning
Content Area: Fundamental Skills
Reference: Kee, J., & Marshall, S. (2004). *Clinical calculations: With applications to general and specialty areas* (5th ed.). Philadelphia: W.B. Saunders, p. 116.

19. *Answer:* **3**
Rationale: Follow the formula for dosage calculations.
Formula:

$$\frac{Desired}{Available} \times mL = mL/dose$$

$$\frac{35\ mg}{50\ mg} \times 1\ mL = 0.7\ mL$$

Test-Taking Strategy: Follow the formula for the calculation of the correct dose. Focus on the key information: 50 mg/mL. After you have performed the calculation, verify your answer using a calculator. Review medication calculations if you had difficulty with this question.
Level of Cognitive Ability: Application
Client Needs: Physiological Integrity
Integrated Process: Nursing Process/Planning
Content Area: Fundamental Skills
Reference: Kee, J., & Marshall, S. (2004). *Clinical calculations: With applications to general and specialty areas* (5th ed.). Philadelphia: W.B. Saunders, p. 116.

20. *Answer:* **2**
Rationale: Follow the formula for dosage calculation.
Formula:

$$\frac{Desired}{Available} \times mL = mL/dose$$

$$\frac{20\ mg}{10\ mg} \times 1\ mL = 2\ mL$$

Test-Taking Strategy: Follow the formula for the calculation of the correct dose. Focus on the key information: 10 mg/mL. After you have performed the calculation, verify your answer using a calculator. Review medication calculations if you had difficulty with this question.
Level of Cognitive Ability: Application
Client Needs: Physiological Integrity
Integrated Process: Nursing Process/Planning
Content Area: Fundamental Skills
Reference: Kee, J., & Marshall, S. (2004). *Clinical calculations: With applications to general and specialty areas* (5th ed.). Philadelphia: W.B. Saunders, p. 116.

21. *Answer:* **0.7**
Rationale: Follow the formula for dosage calculation.
Formula:

$$\frac{Desired}{Available} \times mL = mL/dose$$

$$\frac{0.4\ mg}{0.3\ mg} \times 0.5\ mL = 0.66,\ or\ 0.7,\ mL$$

Test-Taking Strategy: Follow the formula for the calculation of the correct dose. Focus on the key information: 0.3 mg/0.5 mL. After you have performed the calculation, verify your answer using a calculator and remember to round to the nearest tenth. Review medication calculations if you had difficulty with this question.
Level of Cognitive Ability: Application
Client Needs: Physiological Integrity
Integrated Process: Nursing Process/Planning
Content Area: Fundamental Skills

Reference: Kee, J., & Marshall, S. (2004). *Clinical calculations: With applications to general and specialty areas* (5th ed.). Philadelphia: W.B. Saunders, p. 116.

22. Answer: 1
Rationale: Convert 1 g to milligrams. In the metric system, to convert larger to smaller, multiply by 1000 or move the decimal three places to the right. Therefore, 1 g = 1000 mg.
Formula:

$$\frac{Desired}{Available} \times tablet = number\ of\ tablets\ per\ dose$$

$$\frac{1000\ mg}{500\ mg} \times 1\ tablet = 2\ tablets$$

Test-Taking Strategy: In this medication calculation problem, it is necessary to first convert grams to milligrams. Follow the formula for conversion and read the question carefully. After you have performed the calculation, verify your answer using a calculator. Review medication calculations and conversions if you had difficulty with this question.
Level of Cognitive Ability: Application
Client Needs: Physiological Integrity
Integrated Process: Nursing Process/Planning
Content Area: Fundamental Skills
Reference: Kee, J., & Marshall, S. (2004). *Clinical calculations: With applications to general and specialty areas* (5th ed.). Philadelphia: W.B. Saunders, pp. 22-23.

23. Answer: 4
Rationale: Convert 0.2 g to mg. In the metric system, to convert larger to smaller, multiply by 1000 or move the decimal three places to the right. Therefore, 0.2 g = 200 mg.
Formula:

$$\frac{Desired}{Available} \times tablet = number\ of\ tablets/dose$$

$$\frac{200\ mg}{100\ mg} \times 1\ tablet = 2\ tablets$$

Test-Taking Strategy: In this medication calculation problem, it is necessary to first convert grams to milligrams. Follow the formula for conversion and read the question carefully. After you have performed the calculation, verify your answer using a calculator. Review medication calculations and conversions if you had difficulty with this question.
Level of Cognitive Ability: Application
Client Needs: Physiological Integrity
Integrated Process: Nursing Process/Planning
Content Area: Fundamental Skills
Reference: Kee, J., & Marshall, S. (2004). *Clinical calculations: With applications to general and specialty areas* (5th ed.). Philadelphia: W.B. Saunders, pp. 22-23.

24. Answer: 0.2
Rationale: Convert gr 1/300 to milligrams using ratio and proportion. Then, use the dosage calculation formula.
Ratio and Proportion:
gr 1:60 mg = gr 1/300:x mg
60 × 1/300 = x
x = 0.2 mg

Formula:

$$\frac{Desired}{Available} \times mL = mL/dose$$

$$\frac{0.2\ mg}{0.5\ mg} \times 0.5\ mL = 0.2\ mL$$

Test-Taking Strategy: In this medication calculation problem, it is necessary to first convert grains to milligrams. Follow the formula for conversion and read the question carefully. Focus on the issue: 0.5 mg/0.5 mL. After you have performed the calculation, verify your answer using a calculator. Review medication calculations and conversions if you had difficulty with this question.
Level of Cognitive Ability: Application
Client Needs: Physiological Integrity
Integrated Process: Nursing Process/Planning
Content Area: Fundamental Skills
Reference: Kee, J., & Marshall, S. (2004). *Clinical calculations: With applications to general and specialty areas* (5th ed.). Philadelphia: W.B. Saunders, pp. 9, 22-23.

25. Answer: 3
Rationale: Calculation of this problem requires more than one step. Convert Fahrenheit to Celsius, convert milligrams to grains, and then calculate the dose to be administered.
Step 1: Convert Fahrenheit to Celsius
Formula: To convert Fahrenheit to Celsius, subtract 32 and divide the result by 1.8:
C = (101 − 32) divided by 1.8; C = (69) divided by 1.8; C = 38.3°
Step 2: Convert milligrams to grains
gr 1:60 mg = x gr:650 mg
60x = 650
x = gr 10.8
Step 3: Dosage calculation

$$\frac{Desired}{Available} \times tablet = number\ of\ tablets/dose$$

$$\frac{gr\ 10.8}{gr\ 5} \times 1\ tablet = 2.16,\ or\ 2,\ tablets$$

Test-Taking Strategy: Focus on what the question is asking you to determine. In this medication calculation problem, it is necessary to first convert Fahrenheit to Celsius, and then you need to convert milligrams to grains. Follow the formula for conversion and read the question carefully. After you have performed the calculation, verify your answer using a calculator. Review these formulas if you had difficulty with this question.
Level of Cognitive Ability: Application
Client Needs: Physiological Integrity
Integrated Process: Nursing Process/Planning
Content Area: Fundamental Skills
References: Asperheim, M. (2005). *Introduction to pharmacology* (10th ed.). Philadelphia: Elsevier/Saunders, p. 13.
Kee, J., & Marshall, S. (2004). *Clinical calculations: With applications to general and specialty areas* (5th ed.). Philadelphia: W.B. Saunders, pp. 9, 22-23.

REFERENCES

Asperheim, M. (2005). *Introduction to pharmacology* (10th ed.). Philadelphia: Elsevier/Saunders.

Christensen, B., & Kockrow, E. (2003). *Foundations of nursing* (4th ed). St. Louis: Mosby.

Kee, J., & Marshall, S. (2004). *Clinical calculations: With applications to general and specialty areas* (5th ed.). Philadelphia: W.B. Saunders.

National Council of State Boards of Nursing. (2005). *Detailed test plan for the National Council licensure examination for practical/vocational nurses.* Chicago: Author.

Basic Life Support

PYRAMID TERMS

automated external defibrillator (AED) Converts ventricular fibrillation into a perfusing rhythm and allows for early defibrillation by first responders.

basic life support (BLS) Providing oxygen to the brain, heart and other vital organs until help arrives.

cardiopulmonary resuscitation (CPR) An interchangeable term for basic life support.

head tilt–chin lift Preferred method to open a victim's airway.

Heimlich maneuver Method to relieve a foreign body airway obstruction (FBAO).

jaw thrust maneuver Method used to open a victim's airway if a neck injury is suspected.

▲ PYRAMID TO SUCCESS

The Pyramid to Success focuses on the emergency measures related to performing basic life support. Focus on the points related to the breath and compression ratio with one-person and two-person adult CPR and with CPR in the infant and the child. Pyramid points focus on airway management in CPR and on performing the Heimlich maneuver to relieve a foreign body airway obstruction (FBAO). Focus on the correct hand placements for cardiac compressions and on the differences between the adult, the child, and the infant. Remember, before initiating CPR, determining unresponsiveness is the initial action. Remember the ABCDs—airway, breathing, circulation, and difibrillation or definitive treatment—when performing CPR. The Integrated Processes addressed in this chapter include Caring, the Clinical Problem-Solving Process (Nursing Process), Communication and Documentation, and Teaching/Learning.

▲ CLIENT NEEDS
Safe, Effective Care Environment

Advance directives regarding the client's documented requests

Advocacy regarding the client's wishes
Client rights
Establishing priorities
Ethical and legal responsibilities
Standard, transmission-based, and other precautions

Health Promotion and Maintenance

Health promotion programs
Teaching significant others to perform CPR and the Heimlich maneuver
Techniques of data collection

Psychosocial Integrity

Cultural diversity
End-of-life issues
Emotional support to significant others
Grief and loss
Religious and spiritual influences
Therapeutic communications

Physiological Integrity

Administration of emergency medications and intravenous lines
Alterations in cardiopulmonary system
Handling medical emergencies
Performing CPR or the Heimlich maneuver
Use of special equipment
Documentation of response to BLS measures

I. **BASIC LIFE SUPPORT (BLS)** (Box 16-1)
A. Providing oxygen to the brain, heart, and other vital organs until help arrives
B. Also known as **cardiopulmonary resuscitation (CPR)**

BOX 16-1

ABCDs of Basic Life Support (BLS)

A: Airway
B: Breathing
C: Circulation
D: Defibrillation or definitive treatment
Each step of the ABCDs of BLS begins with assessment!

II. ADULT BLS

A. Description: An adult can be defined as a person who is 8 years of age or older

B. Airway
1. Remember that data collection is the first step of the nursing process; assessing a victim of sudden illness or accident for unconsciousness is the initial action; assess for 5 to 10 seconds
2. Gently shake the victim's shoulders and ask "Are you OK?"; be alert to the potential for a head or neck injury
3. Activate emergency medical service(s) (EMS): "phone first" for children 8 years of age or older and for adults; "phone last" for children younger than 8 years old
4. Place the victim in a supine position on a firm, flat surface (logroll the victim, using spine precautions)
   a. One-person rescue: The rescuer is positioned on his or her knees, perpendicular to the victim's sternum and facing the victim
   b. Two-person rescue: One rescuer faces the victim, kneeling perpendicular to the victim's head; the second rescuer moves to the opposite side and faces the victim, kneeling perpendicular to the victim's sternum
   c. The rescuers apply gloves and a face shield, if available
5. Open the airway
6. The **head tilt–chin lift** is the preferred method for opening the airway; if there is a neck injury, the **jaw thrust maneuver** is used to open the airway (Figure 16-1)
7. Look for any foreign material, liquids, or solids in the victim's mouth; wipe out any foreign material with a hooked index or middle finger

C. Breathing
1. Assess breathing, maintaining an open airway
2. The rescuer places his or her ear over the victim's nose and mouth and looks for the chest to rise and fall, listens for air moving in and out of the lungs, and feels for the flow of air
3. Breathing victim
   a. Place the victim on his or her side if no cervical trauma is suspected; logroll the victim onto his or her side as a unit (without twisting) to help

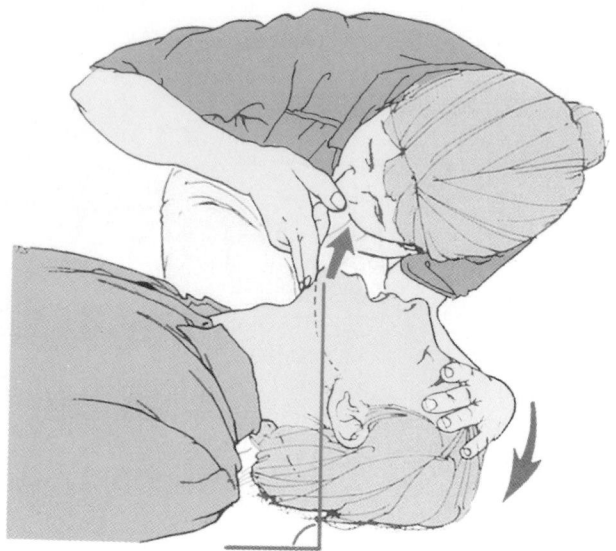

FIG. 16-1 Head tilt–chin lift maneuver. (From Christensen, B., & Kockrow, E. [2003]. *Foundations of nursing* [4th ed.]. St. Louis: Mosby.)

maintain an open airway and decrease the risk of aspiration
   b. If trauma or injury is suspected, the victim should not be moved
4. Nonbreathing victim
   a. Maintain the **head tilt–chin lift**; pinch the nostrils closed, and give two, slow full ventilations (breaths) of 2 seconds per breath (use resuscitation bag or face shield if available, ensuring an adequate air seal); allow victim to exhale between breaths
   b. Give 10 to 12 ventilations per minute
   c. If unsuccessful at giving the breath or ventilation, reposition the victim's head and try again (improper chin and head positions is the most common cause of difficulty in ventilating the victim)
   d. If still unsuccessful, check the victim's mouth for a foreign body or for loose dentures (remove dentures only if they interfere with the mouth seal), clear the airway, and try to ventilate again
   e. Be alert to gastric distention when giving ventilations
5. Mouth to nose: Recommended when it is impossible to ventilate through the victim's mouth, the mouth cannot be opened, the mouth is seriously injured, or a tight mouth-to-mouth seal is difficult to achieve
6. Mouth to stoma: Used for the victim who has had a laryngectomy or has a temporary tracheostomy; to be effective, an adequate seal over the victim's mouth and nose is necessary

D. Circulation
1. Assess circulation; always check for the absence of a pulse before beginning chest compressions on the victim
2. Maintain an open airway and palpate for a carotid pulse for 5 to 10 seconds
3. If there is a pulse, continue to give 10 to 12 ventilations per minute
4. Recheck the pulse after 1 minute; if there is no pulse, start chest compressions

E. Chest compressions
1. Hand placement (Figure 16-2)
   a. Correct hand placement for chest compressions is crucial
   b. Hand placement is on the lower half of the sternum
   c. With the hand closest to the victim's feet, locate the lower margin of the rib cage
   d. Move the fingertips along the margin to the notch where the ribs meet the sternum
   e. Place the middle finger on the notch and the index finger next to the middle finger
   f. Place the heel of the opposite hand next to the index finger, and place the other hand on top (Figure 16-3)
2. Complications of chest compressions
   a. Laceration of internal organs
   b. Punctured lungs
   c. Fractured ribs or sternum

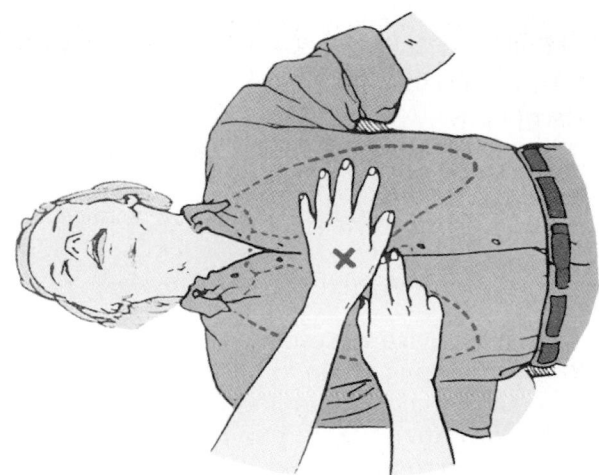

FIG. 16-2 Position for hand placement for external cardiac compressions. (From Christensen, B., & Kockrow, E. [2003]. *Foundations of nursing* [4th ed.]. St. Louis: Mosby.)

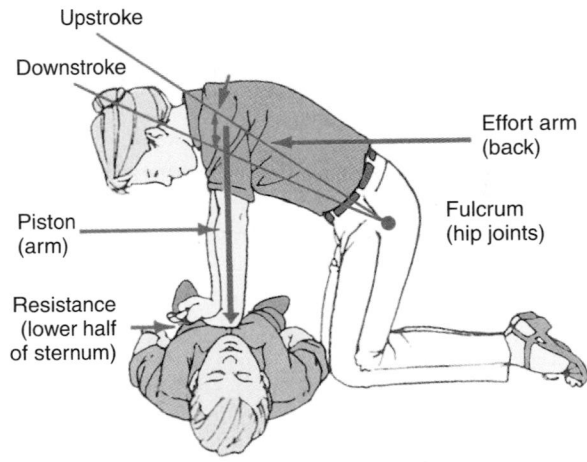

FIG. 16-3 Positioning for proper compression techniques. (From Christensen, B., & Kockrow, E. [2003]. *Foundations of nursing* (4th ed.). St. Louis: Mosby.)

III. ADULT ONE-PERSON BLS

A. The ratio is 15:2; that is, 15 compressions at a rate of 100 per minute and at a depth of 1.5 to 2 inches, and 2 ventilations at 2 seconds per breath
B. Perform four complete cycles and then reassess the victim
C. Check the carotid pulse after the first four cycles of CPR and every few minutes thereafter; if no pulse is felt, continue CPR

IV. ADULT TWO-PERSON BLS

A. The ratio is 15:2, the same as adult one-person BLS
B. One person is at the victim's side performing chest compressions; one person is at the victim's head, maintaining an open airway, monitoring the carotid pulse, and doing the rescue breathing
C. When the second rescuer arrives at the scene, he or she must identify himself or herself and tell the first rescuer that he or she knows two-person CPR
D. The second rescuer then activates EMS, if this has not been done, and then returns to the scene to help
E. The second rescuer can perform one-person CPR if the first rescuer is fatigued; or, the first rescuer finishes 15 compressions, gives 2 ventilations,

moves to the head, opens the airway, and checks the carotid pulse
F. If there is no pulse, the first rescuer announces, "No pulse, continue CPR"
G. The second rescuer locates the landmark for chest compressions
H. The two rescuers begin CPR at a ratio of 15 compressions to 2 ventilations
I. At the end of 1 minute, the ventilator checks for a pulse and checks for breathing; if there is none, the ventilator says, "No pulse, continue CPR"
J. When the compressor becomes tired, the compressor should change positions with minimal interruption of chest compressions
K. The rescuer ventilating the victim assumes responsibility for monitoring for signs of circulation and breathing

V. PEDIATRIC DIFFERENCES

A. Description
1. A child is defined as a person between 1 and 8 years of age
2. An infant is defined as a person younger than 1 year of age

B. Airway: Assess unresponsiveness

C. Breathing
1. Breathing victim: Keep the airway open
2. Nonbreathing victim
   a. Give 2 ventilations at 1 to 1.5 seconds per breath
   b. With the infant, provide ventilations by mouth to mouth and nose
   c. With the older child, provide ventilations by mouth to mouth
   d. With the infant or the child, give 20 ventilations per minute
   e. Activate EMS as soon as possible

D. Circulation
1. Assess circulation
2. If the victim is older than 1 year, assess circulation via the carotid pulse
3. If the victim is younger than 1 year, assess circulation via the brachial pulse
4. The ratio is 5 compressions to 1 ventilation
5. Reassess every few minutes
6. Infant chest compressions
   a. Visualize an imaginary line between the nipples (intermammary line) over the breastbone (sternum).
   b. The index finger of the hand farthest from the infant's head is placed just under the intermammary line, where it intersects the sternum
   c. The area of compression is one fingerwidth below this intersection, at the middle and ring fingers
   d. With the use of two or three fingers, the breastbone is compressed 0.5 to 1 inch at least 100 times per minute
   e. Two-thumb encircling hands technique is the preferred two-rescuer technique
7. Chest compressions for a child
   a. The location for hand placement is the same as for an adult
   b. Depress the chest 1 to 1.5 inches at 100 times per minute with the heel of one hand

VI. FOREIGN BODY AIRWAY OBSTRUCTION

A. Conscious adult
1. Ask the victim, "Are you choking?" (the victim will not be able to speak or cough if he or she is choking)
2. If the victim's airway is partially obstructed, a crowing sound is heard; encourage the victim to cough

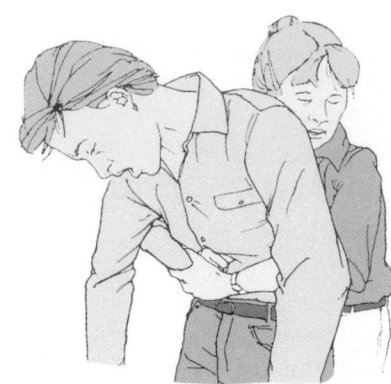

FIG. 16-4 Heimlich maneuver. (From Christensen, B., & Kockrow, E. [2003]. *Foundations of nursing* [4th ed.]. St. Louis: Mosby.)

BOX 16-2

Heimlich Maneuver

Stand behind the victim.
Place arms around the victim's waist.
Make a fist.
Place the thumb side of the fist just above the umbilicus (belly button) and well below the xiphoid process.
Perform five quick in-and-up thrusts (between the umbilicus and the xiphoid process).
Use chest thrusts for the markedly obese or for the advanced pregnancy victim.

---

3. Relieve the obstruction by the **Heimlich maneuver** (Figure 16-4; Box 16-2)
4. Continue abdominal thrusts until the object is dislodged or the victim becomes unconscious

B. Unconscious adult
1. Assess unconsciousness
2. Call for help; activate EMS as soon as possible
3. Perform tongue-jaw lift technique; finger sweep to remove the object
4. Open the airway
5. Attempt ventilation
6. Reposition the head if unsuccessful; reattempt ventilation
7. Relieve the obstruction by the **Heimlich maneuver** with five thrusts; then finger sweep the mouth
8. To perform the **Heimlich maneuver**, straddle the victim's thighs, place the heel of one hand on top of the other between the umbilicus and xiphoid process, and give five thrusts in and up with the heel of the bottom hand
9. Reattempt ventilation
10. Repeat the sequence of tongue-jaw lift, finger sweep, breaths, and **Heimlich maneuver** until successful

11. Be sure to assess the victim's pulse and respirations
12. Perform **CPR** if required

C. Choking child or infant

1. Choking is suspected in infants and children experiencing acute respiratory distress associated with coughing, gagging, or stridor (high-pitched noisy breathing)

2. Allow the victim to continue to cough if the cough is forceful

3. If the cough is ineffective or the victim develops increased respiratory difficulty accompanied by a high-pitched noise while inhaling, help is needed

4. Conscious child

   a. Assess for obstruction by asking the child, "Are you choking?"

   b. Relieve the obstruction by the **Heimlich maneuver** until the obstruction is dislodged or the child becomes unconscious

5. Unconscious child

   a. Assess unconsciousness

   b. Open the airway by the tongue-jaw lift technique

   c. Check for breathing and look for a foreign object

   d. Attempt ventilation

   e. If unsuccessful, reposition the head; reattempt ventilation

   f. Relieve the obstruction by using the **Heimlich maneuver,** giving five abdominal thrusts, and finger sweep the mouth only if the object is seen

   g. Assess airway for foreign object and reattempt ventilation

   h. Repeat the sequence

   i. Assess pulse and respirations and perform **CPR** if required

6. Conscious infant

   a. Assess for obstruction and note breathing problems

   b. Relieve the obstruction by five back blows and five chest thrusts

   c. Straddle the infant over the arm, place the infant's head lower than the trunk, and support the head firmly, holding the jaw

   d. Give five back blows with the heel of the hand between the shoulder blades (Figure 16-5)

   e. Turn the infant; place the head lower than the trunk

   f. Give five chest thrusts at the same location as for chest compressions

   g. Check for the object and remove if seen

   h. Blind finger sweeps are avoided in infants and small children, because the object may be pushed back farther into the airway, causing further obstruction

   i. Continue until the object is removed or the infant becomes unconscious

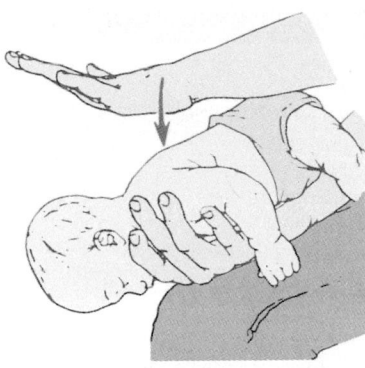

FIG. 16-5 Clearing airway obstruction in an infant. (From Christensen, B., & Kockrow, E. [2003]. *Foundations of nursing* [4th ed.]. St. Louis: Mosby.)

7. Unconscious infant

   a. Assess unconsciousness by gentle taps

   b. Open the airway by the tongue-jaw lift

   c. Check for breathing and look for a foreign object

   d. Attempt ventilation

   e. Reposition the head if unsuccessful; reattempt ventilation

   f. Relieve the obstruction by five back blows and five chest thrusts

   g. Finger sweep the mouth only if the object is seen

   h. Reattempt ventilation and repeat the sequence

   i. Activate EMS after 1 minute of unresponsiveness

   j. Perform **CPR** if required

VII. PREGNANT OR OBESE VICTIM

A. **Heimlich maneuver** and relieving a foreign body airway obstruction

1. Place arms under the victim's axilla and across the chest

2. Place the thumb side of a clenched fist against the middle of the sternum, and place the other hand over the fist

3. Perform backward chest thrusts until the foreign body is expelled or until the victim becomes unconscious

4. If the victim is pregnant and becomes unconscious, place her on her back; a wedge, such as a pillow or rolled blanket, should be placed under her right abdominal flank and hip to displace the uterus to the left side of the abdomen

5. If unable to ventilate, position the hands as for chest compressions and deliver chest thrusts firmly to remove the obstruction

B. Defibrillation in the pregnant client: If defibrillation is needed, place the paddles one rib interspace higher than usual, because the heart is displaced slightly by the enlarged uterus

BOX 16 3

Pyramid Points

Do not interrupt CPR for more than 5 seconds!

STOP CPR ONLY IF:
Pulse and respiration return
EMS assistance arrives
Administering AED
Physician declares the victim deceased

ADDITIONAL PYRAMID POINT
In a non–health care setting, another indication to stop CPR would be that the rescuer was exhausted and physically unable to continue to perform CPR.

VIII. AUTOMATED EXTERNAL DEFIBRILLATOR (AED)

A. Description
1. Used to convert ventricular fibrillation into a perfusing rhythm
2. Differentiates nonventricular fibrillation rhythms and allows for early defibrillation by first responders
3. Use of an **AED** is not recommended on a child who is younger than 8 years of age or a child who weighs less than 25 kg

B. Interventions
1. Attach **AED** leads to the victim
2. Turn on the **AED** and push the button to activate the analyzer
3. Follow instructions given for the **AED,** usually "assess," "stand back," "shock," and "reassess"
4. Evaluate for return of the pulse, and if the victim is pulseless, repeat defibrillation as directed up to three times; if defibrillation is still ineffective, perform **CPR** for 1 minute, and then deliver another series of three shocks (Box 16-3)

PRACTICE QUESTIONS

1. A nurse on the day shift walks into a client's room and finds the client unresponsive. The client is not breathing and does not have a pulse, and the nurse immediately calls out for help. The next nursing action is which of the following?
   1. Ventilate with a mouth-to-mask device
   2. Start chest compressions
   3. Give the client oxygen
   4. Open the airway
2. A nurse is performing cardiopulmonary resuscitation (CPR) on an adult client. When performing chest compressions, the nurse understands that correct hand placement is located over the:
   1. Lower third of the sternum
   2. Upper half of the sternum
   3. Upper third of the sternum
   4. Lower half of the sternum
3. A nurse witnesses a neighbor's husband sustain a fall from the roof of his house. The nurse rushes to the victim and determines the need to open the airway. The nurse opens the airway in this victim by using which appropriate method?
   1. Head tilt–chin lift
   2. Flexed position
   3. Modified head tilt–chin lift
   4. Jaw thrust maneuver
4. A nurse is preparing to attempt to relieve an airway obstruction in a 3-year-old conscious child. The nurse performs this maneuver by placing the hands between the:
   1. Umbilicus and the groin
   2. Groin and the abdomen
   3. Umbilicus and the xiphoid process
   4. Lower abdomen and the chest
5. A nurse is performing basic life support (BLS) on a 7-year-old child. The nurse delivers how many breaths per minute to the child?
   1. 12
   2. 16
   3. 18
   4. 20
6. A nurse is performing cardiopulmonary resuscitation (CPR) on an infant. When performing chest compressions, the nurse understands that the compression rate is at least:
   1. 60 times per minute
   2. 80 times per minute
   3. 100 times per minute
   4. 160 times per minute
7. A nursing instructor teaches a group of students about basic life support (BLS). The instructor asks a student to identify the most appropriate location to assess the pulse of an infant under 1 year of age. Which of the following, if stated by the student, would indicate that the student understands the appropriate procedure?
   1. Brachial
   2. Carotid
   3. Popliteal
   4. Radial
8. A nurse is teaching cardiopulmonary resuscitation (CPR) to a group of community members. The nurse asks a member of the group to describe the reason why blind finger sweeps are avoided in infants. The nurse determines that the person understands this reason if the person makes which statement?
   1. "The object may be forced back farther into the throat."
   2. "The mouth is too small to see the object."
   3. "The object may have been swallowed."
   4. "The infant may bite down on the finger"
9. A nurse is performing cardiopulmonary resuscitation (CPR) on an adult client. The nurse understands that,

when chest compressions are performed, the sternum should be depressed:

1. $\frac{1}{2}$ to $\frac{3}{4}$ inch
2. $\frac{3}{4}$ to 1 inch
3. $1\frac{1}{2}$ to 2 inches
4. $2\frac{1}{2}$ to 3 inches

10. A nursing instructor asks a nursing student to describe the procedure for performing the Heimlich maneuver on an unconscious pregnant woman at 8 months' gestation. The student describes the procedure correctly if the student states that which of the following should be done?

   1. Perform abdominal thrusts until the object is dislodged
   2. Place the hands in the pelvis to perform the thrusts
   3. Place a rolled blanket under the right abdominal flank and hip area
   4. Perform left lateral abdominal thrusts until the object is dislodged

ALTERNATE FORMAT QUESTION: PRIORITIZING (ORDERED RESPONSE)

A nursing student is asked to describe the correct steps for performing adult cardiopulmonary resuscitation (CPR). Number in order of priority the steps of adult CPR.

___ Check for a pulse at the carotid artery
___ Perform chest compressions
___ Determine breathlessness
___ Initiate breathing
___ Open the client's airway
___ Determine unconsciousness by shaking the client and asking, "Are you OK?"

ANSWERS

1. *Answer:* **4**
Reference: The next nursing action would be to open the airway. Ventilation cannot be initiated unless the airway is opened. Chest compressions are started after the airway is opened and ventilation is initiated. Oxygen may be helpful at some point, but the airway is opened first.
Test-Taking Strategy: Visualize the steps of basic life support to answer the question. Recalling the ABCDs—airway, breathing, circulation, defibrillation or definitive treatment—will assist in directing you to option 4. Review the steps of BLS if you had difficulty with this question.
Level of Cognitive Ability: Application
Client Needs: Physiological Integrity
Integrated Process: Nursing Process/Implementation
Content Area: Delegating/Prioritizing
Reference: Christensen, B., & Kockrow, E. (2003). *Foundations of nursing* (4th ed.). St. Louis: Mosby, pp. 462, 616.

2. *Answer:* **4**
Rationale: Proper hand placement for chest compressions is determined by locating the notch where the rib margin meets the sternum, and placing the middle finger on this notch and the index finger next to it. Then, the heel of the opposite hand is placed on the lower half of the sternum, close to the index finger. The first hand is removed and placed on top of the hand on the sternum, and chest compressions are begun. This location is the lower half of the sternum.
Test-Taking Strategy: Use the process of elimination. Eliminate options 2 and 3 first because these locations would be ineffective. From the remaining options, visualizing the procedure and considering the anatomical location of the heart will direct you to option 4. If you had difficulty with this question, review the landmarks for chest compressions.
Level of Cognitive Ability: Application
Client Needs: Physiological Integrity
Integrated Process: Nursing Process/Implementation
Content Area: Adult Health/Cardiovascular

Reference: Christensen, B., & Kockrow, E. (2003). *Foundations of nursing* (4th ed.). St. Louis: Mosby, p. 616.

3. *Answer:* **4**
Rationale: If a neck injury is suspected, the jaw thrust maneuver is used to open the airway. The head tilt–chin lift produces hyperextension of the neck and could cause complications if a neck injury is present. A flexed position is an inappropriate position for opening the airway.
Test-Taking Strategy: Use the process of elimination. Eliminate options 1 and 3 first because they are similar. Next, eliminate option 2, because this position would not open the airway. If you had difficulty with this question, review the appropriate methods to open an airway.
Level of Cognitive Ability: Application
Client Needs: Physiological Integrity
Integrated Process: Nursing Process/Implementation
Content Area: Adult Health/Neurological
Reference: Christensen, B., & Kockrow, E. (2003). *Foundations of nursing* (4th ed.). St. Louis: Mosby, pp. 614-615.

4. *Answer:* **3**
Rationale: To perform the Heimlich maneuver on a child, the rescuer stands behind the victim and places the arms directly under the victim's axillae and around the victim. The thumb side of one fist is placed against the victim's abdomen in the midline, slightly above the umbilicus and well below the tip of the xiphoid process. The fist is grasped with the other hand, and up to five thrusts are delivered. Care must be taken not to touch the xiphoid process or the lower margins of the rib cage, because force applied to these structures may damage internal organs.
Test-Taking Strategy: Use the process of elimination, noting the age of the child. Eliminate options 1 and 2 first because they are similar. From the remaining options, considering the anatomical location and the effect of the maneuver in dislodging an obstruction will direct you to option 3. If you had difficulty with this question, review the correct hand placement for the Heimlich maneuver.

Level of Cognitive Ability: Application
Client Needs: Physiological Integrity
Integrated Process: Nursing Process/Implementation
Content Area: Child Health
Reference: Linton, A., & Maebius, N. (2003) *Introduction to medical-surgical nursing* (3rd ed.). Philadelphia: W.B. Saunders, p. 192.

5. *Answer:* **4**
Rationale: In a child between the ages of 1 and 8 years, 20 breaths per minute are delivered. Options 1, 2, and 3 are incorrect.
Test-Taking Strategy: Use the process of elimination and note the age of the child. Recalling the normal respiratory rate in a child of this age will assist in directing you to option 4. If you had difficulty with this question, review BLS for a child.
Level of Cognitive Ability: Application
Client Needs: Physiological Integrity
Integrated Process: Nursing Process/Implementation
Content Area: Child Health
Reference: Christensen, B., & Kockrow, E. (2003). *Foundations of nursing* (4th ed.). St. Louis: Mosby, p. 615.

6. *Answer:* **3**
Rationale: In an infant, the rate of chest compressions is at least 100 times per minute. Options 1 and 2 identify rates that are too low, and option 4 identifies a rate that is too high.
Test-Taking Strategy: Use the process of elimination, considering the normal heart rate of an infant. Eliminate options 1 and 2 because of the low rates identified in the options. Eliminate option 4 because this rate would be much too rapid for an infant. If you had difficulty with this question, review CPR for an infant.
Level of Cognitive Ability: Application
Client Needs: Physiological Integrity
Integrated Process: Nursing Process/Implementation
Content Area: Child Health
Reference: Christensen, B., & Kockrow, E. (2003). *Foundations of nursing* (4th ed.). St. Louis: Mosby, p. 618.

7. *Answer:* **1**
Rationale: To assess a pulse in an infant (under 1 year of age), the pulse should be checked at the brachial artery. The infant's relatively short, fat neck makes palpation of the carotid artery difficult. The popliteal and radial pulses are also difficult to palpate in an infant.
Test-Taking Strategy: Use the process of elimination and knowledge regarding circulatory assessment in an infant. Considering the body structure of an infant will assist in directing you to option 1. Review cardiac assessment and BLS for an infant if you had difficulty with this question.
Level of Cognitive Ability: Comprehension
Client Needs: Physiological Integrity
Integrated Process: Teaching/Learning
Content Area: Child Health
Reference: Christensen, B., & Kockrow, E. (2003). *Foundations of nursing* (4th ed.). St. Louis: Mosby, p. 618.

8. *Answer:* **1**
Rationale: Blind finger sweeps are not recommended for infants and children because of the risk of forcing the object

farther down into the airway. Options 2, 3, and 4 are not directly related to the issue of the question.
Test-Taking Strategy: Use the ABCDs—airway, breathing, circulation, and defibrillation or definitive treatment—to answer this question. Option 1 addresses the concern of airway patency. If you had difficulty with this question, review obstructed airway management for an infant or a child.
Level of Cognitive Ability: Analysis
Client Needs: Physiological Integrity
Integrated Process: Teaching/Learning
Content Area: Child Health
Reference: James, S., Ashwill, J., & Droske, S. (2002). *Nursing care of children: Principles and practice* (2nd ed.). Philadelphia: W.B. Saunders, p. 280.

9. *Answer:* **3**
Rationale: When performing CPR on an adult client, the sternum should be depressed 1.5 to 2 inches. Options 1 and 2 identify compression depths that would be ineffective in an adult. Option 4 identifies a depth that could cause injury to the client.
Test-Taking Strategy: Note the key word, *adult*, in the question. Consider the normal body structure of an adult to assist in answering the question. If you had difficulty with this question, review the procedure for performing adult BLS.
Level of Cognitive Ability: Application
Client Needs: Physiological Integrity
Integrated Process: Nursing Process/Implementation
Content Area: Adult Health/Cardiovascular
Reference: Christensen, B., & Kockrow, E. (2003). *Foundations of nursing* (4th ed.). St. Louis: Mosby, p. 616.

10. *Answer:* **3**
Rationale: To perform the Heimlich maneuver on an unconscious woman in an advanced stage of pregnancy, the woman is placed on her back. A wedge, such as a pillow or rolled blanket, should be placed under the right abdominal flank and hip to displace the uterus to the left side of the abdomen. Options 1, 2, and 4 are incorrect and can cause harm to the woman and the fetus.
Test-Taking Strategy: Use the process of elimination and note that the client is an unconscious pregnant woman at 8 months' gestation. Recall the concepts associated with hypotension and vena cava syndrome to assist in directing you to option 3. Review the principles associated with performing the Heimlich maneuver on a pregnant woman if you had difficulty with this question.
Level of Cognitive Ability: Analysis
Client Needs: Physiological Integrity
Integrated Process: Nursing Process/Evaluation
Content Area: Maternity/Antepartum
References: Lowdermilk, D., & Perry, A. (2004). *Maternity and woman's health care* (8th ed.). St. Louis: Mosby, p. 918.
Potter, P., & Perry, A. (2005). *Fundamentals of nursing* (6th ed.). St. Louis: Mosby, p. 414.

ALTERNATE FORMAT QUESTION: PRIORITIZING (ORDERED RESPONSE)

Answer: 563421
Rationale: The first step in CPR is to determine that the client is unconscious as opposed to being intoxicated, sleeping,

or hearing impaired. Once unconsciousness had been determined, use the ABCDs—airway, breathing, and circulation, and defibrillation or, definitive treatment—and the steps of the nursing process (clinical problem-solving process) to determine the correct order of action. The nurse would not initiate breathing or perform cardiac compressions unless the client were breathless or lacked a pulse, respectively. Breathlessness is determined before initiating breathing. Then, pulselessness is determined before initiating cardiac compressions.

Test-Taking Strategy: Use the ABCDs—airway, breathing, and circulation, and defibrillation or definitive treatment. This will assist in determining the steps of CPR. Review these steps if you had difficulty with this question.
Level of Cognitive Ability: Application
Client Needs: Physiological Integrity
Integrated Process: Nursing Process/Implementation
Content Area: Delegating/Prioritizing
Reference: Christensen, B., & Kockrow, E. (2003). *Foundations of nursing* (4th ed.). St. Louis: Mosby, pp. 462, 616.

REFERENCES

American Heart Association. (2001). *Basic life support for health care providers.* Dallas: Author.

American Heart Association and International Liaison Committee on Resuscitation. (2000). *Guidelines 2000 for cardiopulmonary resuscitation and emergency cardiovascular care.* Dallas: Author.

Christensen, B., & Kockrow, E. (2003). *Foundations of nursing* (4th ed.). St. Louis: Mosby.

James, S., Ashwill, J., & Droske, S. (2002). *Nursing care of children: Principles and practice* (2nd ed.). Philadelphia: W.B. Saunders.

Linton, A., & Maebius, N. (2003). *Introduction to medical-surgical nursing* (3rd ed.). Philadelphia: W.B. Saunders.

Lowdermilk, D., & Perry, A. (2004). *Maternity and woman's health care* (8th ed.). St. Louis: Mosby.

National Council of State Boards of Nursing. (2005). *Detailed test plan for the National Council licensure examination for practical/vocational nurses.* Chicago: Author.

Potter, P., & Perry, A. (2005). *Fundamentals of nursing* (6th ed.). St. Louis: Mosby.

Perioperative Nursing Care

PYRAMID TERMS

atelectasis   A collapsed or airless state of the lung that may be the result of airway obstruction because of accumulated secretions or failure of the client to deep breathe. It is a common postoperative complication and usually occurs 1 to 2 days after surgery.

extended postoperative stage   The period of at least 1 to 4 days after surgery.

immediate postoperative stage   The period of 1 to 4 hours after surgery.

intermediate postoperative stage   The period of 4 to 24 hours after surgery.

wound dehiscence   An opening of the wound edges.

wound evisceration   Protrusion of internal organs through an opening in wound edges.

◢ PYRAMID TO SUCCESS

Pyramid points focus on reinforcing instructions to the client and family or significant other in the preoperative stage, preparing the client for the operative procedure, and ensuring that prescribed preoperative procedures have been performed, and that the results of the procedures are within expected range and are documented. In the postoperative stage, pyramid points focus on monitoring for surgical complications and on the implementation of initial nursing measures if a complication arises. Pyramid points also focus on preparing the client for discharge, reinforcing instructions related to the prescribed treatments, and identifying the need for home care support services. The Integrated Processes addressed in this chapter include Caring, Communication and Documentation, the Clinical Problem-Solving Process (Nursing Process), and Teaching/Learning.

◢ CLIENT NEEDS
Safe, Effective Care Environment

Advance directives
Client rights

Establishing priorities
Informed consent for the surgical procedure
Informing the client of the surgical process
Providing safety to the medicated client
Suggesting appropriate home care and other support services
Surgical asepsis
Standard precautions

Health Promotion and Maintenance

Expected body image changes
Reinforcing instructions related to the prescribed discharge plan
Preventing complications
Promoting lifestyle choices
Techniques of data collection

Psychosocial Integrity

Assisting the client to develop coping methods
Promoting an environment that will allow the client to express concerns
Support systems
Therapeutic interactions
Unexpected body image changes

Physiological Integrity

Initiating nursing interventions when surgical complications arise
Monitoring for surgical complications
Monitoring for unexpected responses to treatments and procedures
Monitoring for wound infection
Providing respiratory care
Providing basic care and comfort
Safe administration of preoperative and postoperative medications

I. PREOPERATIVE CARE

A. Obtaining informed consent

1. The surgeon is responsible for obtaining the consent for surgery
2. No sedation should be administered to the client before signing the consent
3. Minors may need a parent or legal guardian to sign the consent form
4. Older clients may need a legal guardian to sign the consent form
5. The nurse may witness the client signing the preoperative consent, but the nurse must be sure that the client has understood the surgeon's explanation of the surgery
6. The nurse needs to document the witnessing of the signing of the operative consent after the client acknowledges understanding the procedure

B. Nutrition

1. Check the physician's orders regarding the NPO (nothing by mouth) status before surgery
2. Solid foods and liquids are generally withheld for 6 to 8 hours before general anesthesia and for 3 hours before surgery with local anesthesia to avoid aspiration
3. Monitor intravenous (IV) fluids, if prescribed
4. Note that total parenteral nutrition (TPN) may be prescribed for clients who are malnourished, have protein or metabolic deficiencies, or cannot ingest foods

C. Elimination

1. If the client is to have intestinal or abdominal surgery, an enema, laxative, or both may be prescribed the night before surgery
2. The client should void immediately before surgery
3. Prepare to insert a Foley catheter, if prescribed
4. If there is a Foley catheter in place, it should be emptied immediately before surgery and the amount and quality of urine output documented

D. Surgical site

1. Prepare to clean the surgical site with a mild antiseptic soap the night before surgery, as prescribed
2. Prepare to shave the operative site, as prescribed
3. Hair should be shaved only if it will interfere with the surgical procedure and only if prescribed

E. Reinforcing preoperative instructions

1. Inform the client about what to expect after surgery
2. Inform the client to notify the nurse if he or she experiences any postoperative pain and that pain medication will be prescribed to be given as the client requests
3. Instruct the client to use the noninvasive pain relief techniques before the pain occurs and as soon as the pain is noticed
4. Reinforce instructions about the use of a client-controlled analgesia pump if its use is prescribed

---

BOX 17-1

Preoperative Instructions

DEEP BREATHING AND COUGHING EXERCISES

Instruct the client that a sitting position provides the best lung expansion for coughing and deep breathing exercises.

Instruct the client to breathe deeply three times, inhaling through the nostrils and exhaling slowly through pursed lips.

Instruct the client that the third breath should be held for 3 seconds; then the client should cough deeply three times

The client should perform this exercise every 2 hours.

INCENTIVE SPIROMETRY

Instruct the client to assume a sitting or upright position.

Instruct the client to place the mouth tightly around the mouthpiece.

Instruct the client to inhale slowly to raise and maintain the flow rate indicator between the 600 and 900 marks.

Instruct the client to hold his or her breath for 5 seconds, and then to exhale through pursed lips.

Instruct the client to repeat this process 10 times every hour.

LEG AND FOOT EXERCISES

Gastrocnemius (calf) pumping: Instruct the client to move both ankles by pointing the toes up and then down.

Quadriceps (thigh) setting: Instruct the client to press the back of the knees against the bed, and then to relax the knees; this contracts and relaxes the thigh and calf muscles to prevent thrombus formation.

Foot circles: Instruct the client to rotate each foot in a circle.

Hip and knee movements: Instruct the client to flex the knee and thigh and straighten the leg, and to hold the position for 5 seconds before lowering (not performed if the client is having abdominal surgery or if the client has a back problem).

SPLINTING THE INCISION

If the surgical incision is abdominal or thoracic, instruct the client to place a pillow, or one hand with the other hand on top, over the incisional area.

During deep breathing and coughing, the client presses gently against the incisional area to splint or support it.

---

5. Inform the client that requesting a narcotic after surgery will not make the client a drug addict
6. The client should be instructed not to smoke for at least 24 hours before surgery
7. Instruct the client in deep breathing and coughing techniques, the use of incentive spirometry, and the importance of performing the techniques after surgery to prevent the development of pneumonia and **atelectasis** (Box 17-1; Figure 17-1)
8. Instruct the client in leg and foot exercises to prevent venous stasis of blood and facilitate venous blood return (Figure 17-2; see Box 17-1)
9. Instruct the client how to splint an incision and to turn and reposition (Figure 17-3; see Box 17-1)

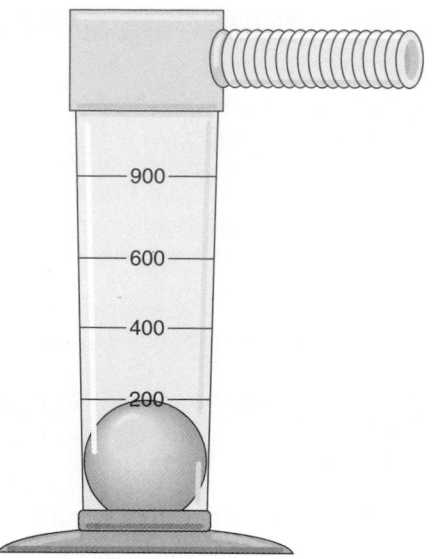

FIG. 17-1 Incentive spirometer. (From Phipps, W., Monahan, F., Sands, J., Marek, J., & Neighbors, M. [2003]. *Medical-surgical nursing: Health and illness perspectives* [7th ed.]. St. Louis: Mosby.)

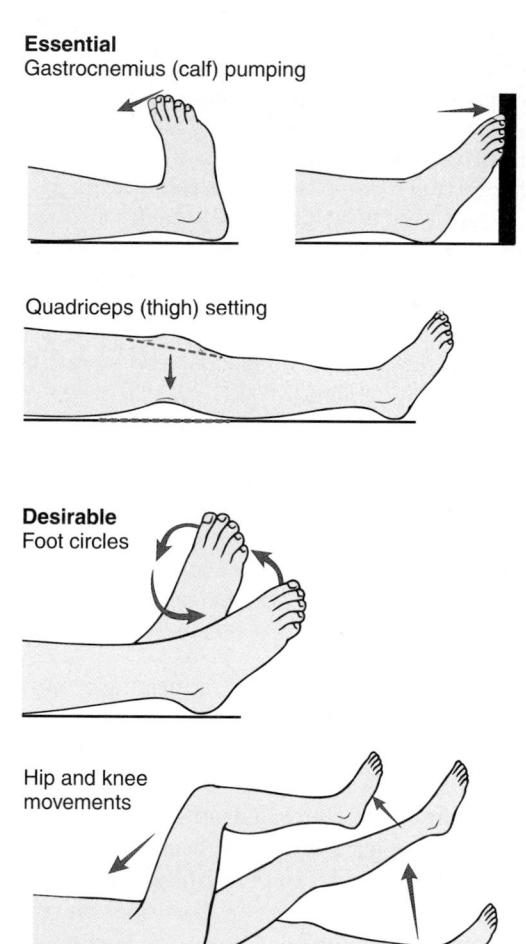

FIG. 17-2 Postoperative leg exercises. (From Lewis, S., Heitkemper, M., & Dirksen, S. [2004]. *Medical-surgical nursing: Assessment and management of clinical problems* [6th ed.]. St. Louis: Mosby.)

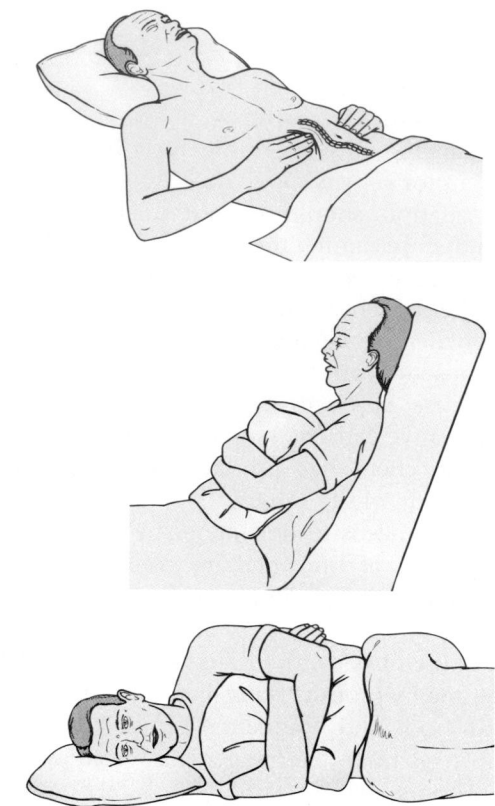

FIG. 17-3 Techniques for splinting wound when coughing. (From Lewis, S., Heitkemper, M., & Dirksen, S. [2004]. *Medical-surgical nursing: Assessment and management of clinical problems* [6th ed.]. St. Louis: Mosby.)

10. Inform the client of any invasive devices that may be needed after surgery, such as tubes, drains, Foley catheter, or intravenous lines
11. Inform the client not to pull on any of the invasive devices, because they will be removed as soon as possible

F. Psychosocial preparation
   1. Be alert to the client's anxiety level
   2. Ask the client about questions or concerns he or she may have regarding surgery
   3. Allow time for privacy for the client to prepare psychologically for surgery
   4. Provide support and assistance as needed

G. Preoperative checklist
   1. Ensure that the client has an identification bracelet on
   2. Check for client allergies (refer to Chapter 60 for information on latex allergy)
   3. Review the preoperative check list to be sure that each item is addressed before the client is transported to surgery
   4. Ensure that consent forms have been signed for the operative procedure, anesthesia, any blood transfusions, disposal of a limb, or surgical sterilization procedures

5. Ensure that a history and physical examination was completed and documented in the client's record

6. Ensure that consultations prescribed were completed and documented in the client's record

7. Ensure that the prescribed laboratory test results are documented in the client's record

8. Ensure that electrocardiography (ECG) and chest radiography reports are noted in the client's record

9. Ensure that blood type and screen, or type and crossmatch, are noted in the client's record

10. Document that the client has voided before surgery

11. Remove jewelry, makeup, dentures, hairpins, nail polish, glasses, and any prosthesis

12. Document that valuables were given to the client's family members or locked in the hospital safe

13. Document that the prescribed preoperative medication was given (Box 17-2)

14. Monitor and document the client's vital signs

15. Document the last time the client ate or drank

H. Preoperative medications

1. Prepare to administer preoperative medications as prescribed, or to be administered on call to the operating room immediately before the surgery

2. Instruct the client that he or she will feel drowsy after the medications are given

3. After administering the preoperative medications, keep the client in bed, with the side rails up

4. Place the call bell next to the client; instruct the client not to get out of bed and to call for assistance if needed

I. Arrival at the operating room

1. When the client arrives to the operating room, the operating room nurse will verify the identification bracelet with the client's verbal response and will review the client's chart

2. The operating room nurse will confirm the operative procedure and site to be operated on

3. The client's chart will be checked for completeness

4. The client's chart will be reviewed for consent forms, history and physical examination, and allergic reaction information

5. The physician's orders will be reviewed and their completion verified

6. The IV line may be initiated at this time, if prescribed

7. The anesthesia team will administer the prescribed anesthesia

II. POSTOPERATIVE CARE

A. **Immediate postoperative stage**

1. Description: the period of 1 to 4 hours after surgery

2. Respiratory system

BOX 17-2

Substances That Can Affect the Surgical Client

ANTIBIOTICS
Potentiate the action of anesthetic agents.

ANTICHOLINERGICS
Medications with anticholinergic effects increase the potential for confusion.

ANTICOAGULANTS
These alter normal clotting factors and increase the risk of hemorrhaging.
Aspirin (acetylsalicylic acid, ASA) and nonsteroidal anti-inflammatory drugs (NSAIDs) are commonly used medications that can alter clotting mechanisms.
These medications should be discontinued at least 48 hours before surgery.

ANTICONVULSANTS
Long-term use of certain anticonvulsants can alter the metabolism of anesthetic agents.

ANTIDEPRESSANTS
These may lower the blood pressure during anesthesia.

ANTIDYSRHYTHMICS
These reduce cardiac contractility and impair cardiac conduction during anesthesia.

ANTIHYPERTENSIVES
These can interact with anesthetic agents and cause bradycardia, hypotension, and impaired circulation.

CORTICOSTEROIDS
These cause adrenal atrophy and reduce the body's ability to withstand stress.
Before and during surgery, dosages may be temporarily increased.

DIURETICS
These potentiate electrolyte imbalances after surgery.

HERBAL SUBSTANCES
These can interact with anesthesia and cause a variety of adverse effects. These substances may need to be stopped at a specific point of time before surgery. During the preoperative period, the client needs to be asked if he or she is taking a herbal substance.

INSULIN
The need for insulin after surgery in a diabetic either may be reduced because the client's nutritional intake is decreased or may be increased because of the stress response and IV administration of glucose solutions.

a. Monitor vital signs

b. Monitor airway patency and adequate ventilation, because prolonged mechanical ventilation during anesthesia may affect postoperative lung function

c. Remember that extubated clients who are lethargic may not be able to maintain an airway

d. Monitor for secretions and remove by suctioning if the client is unable to clear the airway by coughing

e. Observe chest movement for symmetry and the use of accessory muscles

f. Monitor oxygen administration, if prescribed

g. Monitor pulse oximetry, as prescribed

h. Encourage coughing and deep breathing exercises as soon as possible

i. Note the rate, depth, and quality of respirations: the respiratory rate should be more than 10 and less than 30 breaths per minute

j. Monitor the client for signs of **atelectasis,** pneumonia, and pulmonary embolism

3. Cardiovascular system

a. Check the client's color

b. Observe capillary refill, mucous membranes, and sclera

c. Check peripheral pulses and for peripheral edema

d. Monitor for bleeding

e. Check pulse for rate and rhythm; a bounding pulse may indicate hypertension, fluid overload, or anxiety

f. Monitor for signs of hypertension and hypotension

g. Monitor for cardiac irregularities

h. Check for Homan's sign, particularly in clients in the lithotomy position during surgery, because these clients may be predisposed to developing deep vein thrombosis

4. Musculoskeletal system

a. Check the client for moving extremities

b. Check the physician's orders regarding client positioning or restrictions

c. Unless contraindicated, place the client in a low Fowler's position after surgery to increase the size of the thorax

d. Avoid positioning the client in a supine position until pharyngeal reflexes have returned

e. If the client is comatose or semicomatose, position on his or her side unless contraindicated

5. Neurological system

a. Check level of consciousness

b. Closely monitor the client who may be drowsy or unconscious

c. Periodic frequent attempts to awaken the client should continue until the client awakens

d. Orient the client to the environment

e. Speak in a soft tone and filter out extraneous noises in the environment

f. Maintain body temperature and prevent heat loss by providing the client with warm blankets and raising the room temperature, as necessary

6. Temperature control

a. Monitor temperature

b. Monitor for signs of hypothermia that may result from anesthesia, a cool operating room, and exposure of the skin and internal organs during surgery

c. Apply warm blankets and continue oxygen, as prescribed, if the client is shivering

7. Integumentary system

a. Check surgical site, drains, and wound dressings

b. Monitor for and document any drainage or bleeding from the surgical site

c. Check skin for redness, abrasions, or breakdown that may have resulted from surgical positioning

8. Fluid and electrolyte balance

a. Monitor IV administration as prescribed

b. Accurately record input and output (I&O)

9. Gastrointestinal system

a. Monitor for nausea and vomiting

b. Maintain patency of nasogastric tube, if present, as prescribed

c. Monitor for abdominal distention

d. Monitor for return of bowel sounds

10. Renal system

a. Check bladder for distention

b. Monitor color, quantity, and quality of urine output if a Foley catheter is present

c. Expect the client to void 6 to 8 hours after the surgical procedure, depending on the type of anesthesia administered

11. Pain management

a. Check for pain

b. Note the type of anesthetic used and preoperative medication that the client received, and note if the client received any pain medications in the postanesthesia period

c. Ask the client to rate the degree of pain on a scale of 1 to 10, with 10 being the most severe

d. Monitor such objective data as facial expressions, body gestures, pulse rate, blood pressure, and respirations

e. Inquire about the effectiveness of the last pain medication

f. If a narcotic has been prescribed, during the initial administration, check the client every 30 minutes for respiratory rate and pain relief

g. Use noninvasive measures to relieve postoperative pain including distraction, comfort measures, positioning, back rubs, and providing a quiet and restful environment

h. Document effectiveness of pain medication

B. **Intermediate postoperative stage**

1. Description

a. The period of 4 to 24 hours after surgery

b. Nursing care implemented during the **immediate postoperative stage** is continued

2. Respiratory system: Encourage coughing and deep breathing

3. Cardiovascular system: Encourage the use of antiembolism stockings, if prescribed, to promote venous return, strengthen muscle tone, and prevent pooling of secretions in the lungs

4. Musculoskeletal system
   a. Before ambulation, instruct the client to sit at the edge of the bed with the feet supported
   b. If client is unable to walk, turn the client every 1 to 2 hours

5. Neurological system: Check level of consciousness

6. Integumentary system
   a. Monitor wound for signs of infection
   b. Maintain a dry and intact dressing
   c. Reinforce with a sterile dressing if necessary and notify the primary health care provider if bleeding occurs from the site
   d. Change dressings as prescribed, noting the amount of bleeding or drainage, odor, and intactness of sutures or staples
   e. Use an abdominal binder for obese and debilitated individuals to prevent rupture of the incision (Figure 17-4)
   f. Drains should be patent, and there should be minimal bleeding or drainage
   g. Prepare to assist with the removal of drains as prescribed by the physician when the drainage amount becomes insignificant

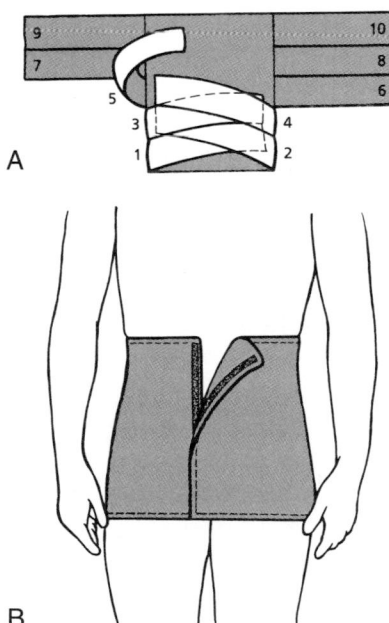

FIG. 17-4 Abdominal binders. **A,** Binder with flaps that wrap over each other; **B,** binder with Velcro. (From Perry, P., & Potter, A. [2002]. *Clinical nursing skills and techniques* [5th ed.]. St. Louis: Mosby.)

7. Gastrointestinal system
   a. Turn the unconscious client to a side-lying position if vomiting occurs, and have suctioning equipment available and ready to use
   b. Administer frequent mouth care
   c. Maintain the NPO (nothing by mouth) status until the gag reflex and peristalsis return
   d. Assess for bowel sounds in all four quadrants
   e. When oral fluids are permitted, start with ice chips and water
   f. Ensure that the client advances to clear liquids and then to a regular diet, as prescribed
   g. Monitor the client for flatus and encourage ambulation, as prescribed

8. Renal system
   a. Monitor urinary output (should be greater than 30 mL/hour)
   b. If the client does not have a Foley catheter, client is expected to void within 6 to 8 hours after the surgical procedure; ensure that the amount is at least 200 mL

9. Pain management: Continue with data collection and interventions, as during the **immediate postoperative stage**

C. **Extended postoperative stage**
   1. Description: The period of at least 1 to 4 days after the surgical procedure
   2. Interventions
      a. Continue to check and observe the client's body systems during this stage
      b. Monitor for signs of infection such as redness, swelling, and tenderness at the surgical site, fever, and leukocytosis
      c. Encourage active range of motion every 2 hours
      d. Continue to encourage ambulation that will promote peristalsis and the passage of fluid and flatus
      e. Increase ambulation every day to increase muscle strength
      f. Encourage the client to perform as many activities of daily living as possible
      g. Instruct the client to eat foods that are high in protein and vitamin C content to promote wound healing

III. PNEUMONIA AND ATELECTASIS
(Figure 17-5; Box 17-3)

A. Description
   1. Pneumonia, an inflammation of the alveoli caused by infectious process, may develop 3 to 5 days after the surgical procedure because of infection, aspiration, or immobility
   2. **Atelectasis**, a collapse of the alveoli with retained mucous secretions, is the most common postoperative complication and usually occurs 1 to 2 days after the surgical procedure

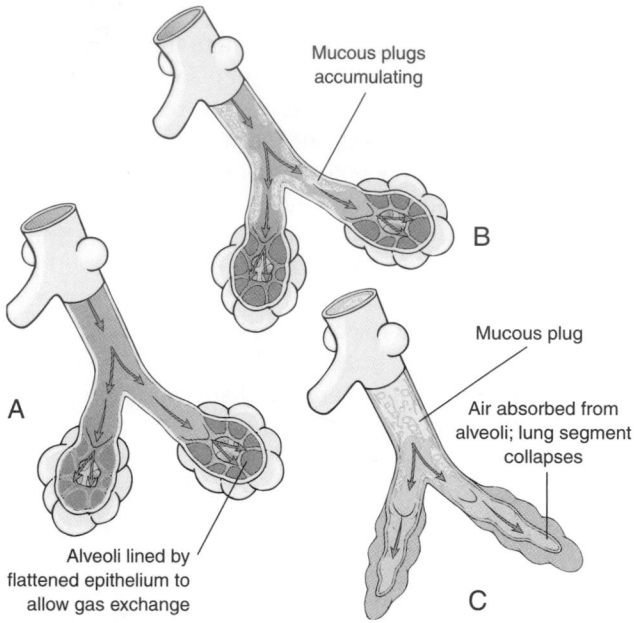

FIG. 17-5 Postoperative atelectasis. **A,** Normal bronchiole and alveoli. **B,** Mucous plug in bronchiole. **C,** Collapse of alveoli due to atelectasis following absorption of air. (Lewis, S., Heitkemper, M., & Dirksen, S. [2004]. *Medical-surgical nursing: Assessment and management of clinical problems* [6th ed.]. St. Louis: Mosby.)

BOX 17-3

Postoperative Complications

Constipation
Hemorrhage
Hypoxia
Paralytic ileus
Pneumonia and atelectasis
Pulmonary embolism
Shock
Thrombophlebitis
Urinary retention
Wound dehiscence
Wound evisceration
Wound infection

*The licensed practical vocational nurse always notifies the RN and/or physician if signs of complications are noted.

B. Data collection
  1. Dyspnea and increased respiratory rate
  2. Elevated temperature
  3. Productive cough and chest pain
  4. Crackles over involved lung area
C. Interventions
  1. Monitor temperature
  2. Encourage ambulation
  3. Reposition the client every 1 to 2 hours
  4. Encourage the client to use incentive spirometer, and to cough and deep breathe
  5. Check lung sounds and suction to clear secretions if the client is unable to cough
  6. Encourage fluid intake

IV. HYPOXIA (see Box 17-3)
A. Description: An inadequate concentration of oxygen in arterial blood
B. Data collection
  1. Restlessness
  2. Dyspnea
  3. Increased heart rate and blood pressure
  4. Diaphoresis
  5. Cyanosis
C. Interventions
  1. Monitor for signs of hypoxia and eliminate cause of hypoxia
  2. Monitor pulse oximetry
  3. Administer oxygen as prescribed
  4. Encourage coughing and deep breathing and use of incentive spirometry
  5. Turn and reposition client frequently

V. PULMONARY EMBOLISM (see Box 17-3)
A. Description: An embolus blocking the pulmonary artery and disrupting blood flow to one or more lobes of the lung
B. Data collection
  1. Dyspnea
  2. Sudden sharp chest or upper abdominal pain
  3. Increased heart rate and a decrease in blood pressure
  4. Cyanosis
C. Interventions
  1. Notify the registered nurse and/or physician immediately
  2. Monitor vital signs

VI. HEMORRHAGE (see Box 17-3)
A. Description: Loss of a large amount of blood externally or internally in a short period of time
B. Data collection
  1. Restlessness
  2. Weak, rapid pulse and hypotension
  3. Cool, clammy skin
  4. Tachypnea
  5. Reduced urine output
C. Interventions
  1. Apply pressure to the site of bleeding
  2. Notify the registered nurse and/or physician immediately

VII. SHOCK (see Box 17-3)
A. Description: Loss of circulatory fluid volume that is usually caused by hemorrhage
B. Data collection: Similar to data collection findings in hemorrhage
C. Interventions

1. If shock develops, elevate the legs
2. If the client has had spinal anesthesia, do not elevate the legs any higher than placing them on the pillow; otherwise, diaphragm muscles could be impaired
3. Notify the registered nurse and/or physician immediately

VIII. THROMBOPHLEBITIS (see Box 17-3)

A. Description
  1. Inflammation of a vein, often accompanied by clot formation
  2. Veins in the legs are most commonly affected
B. Data collection
  1. Aching or cramping leg pain
  2. Vein inflammation; vein feels hard and cordlike and is tender to touch
  3. Elevated temperature
  4. Positive Homan's sign
C. Interventions
  1. Monitor legs for swelling, inflammation, cyanosis, pain, tenderness, and venous distention
  2. Elevate the extremity 30 degrees without allowing any pressure on the popliteal area
  3. Encourage the use of antiembolism stockings, as prescribed, removing them twice a day to wash and inspect the legs
  4. Use intermittent pulsatile compression device as prescribed (Figure 17-6)
  5. Perform passive range of motion every 2 hours if the client is on bed rest
  7. Do not allow the client's to dangle the legs
  8. Instruct the client not to sit in one position for an extended period of time
  9. Heparin sodium or warfarin (Coumadin) may be prescribed

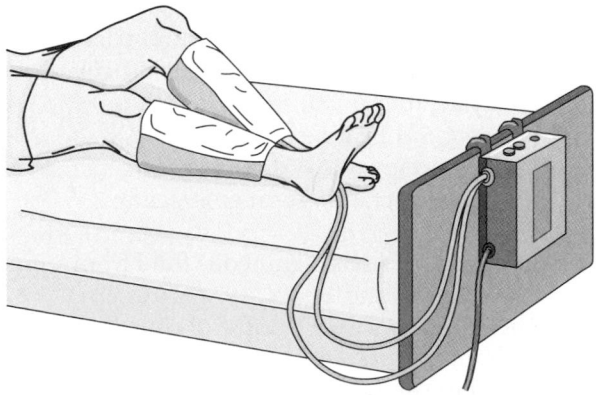

FIG. 17-6 Intermittent pulsatile compression device. (From Phipps, W., Monahan, F., Sands, J., Marek, J. & Neighbors, M. [2003]. *Medical-surgical nursing: Health and illness perspectives* [7th ed.]. St. Louis: Mosby.)

IX. URINARY RETENTION (see Box 17-3)

A. Description
  1. Involuntary accumulation of urine in the bladder from loss of muscle tone
  2. Occurs as a result of the effects of anesthetics and narcotic analgesics
  3. Appears 6 to 8 hours after surgery
B. Data collection
  1. Restlessness and diaphoresis
  2. Lower abdominal pain
  3. Inability to void and a distended bladder
  4. Elevated blood pressure
  5. On percussion, the bladder sounds like a drum
C. Interventions
  1. Monitor for voiding and check for distended bladder
  2. Encourage fluid intake unless contraindicated
  3. Assist the client to void by helping to stand
  4. Provide privacy
  5. Pour warm water over the perineum or allow the client to hear running water to promote voiding
  6. Catheterize the client as prescribed after all non-invasive techniques have been attempted

X. CONSTIPATION (see Box 17-3)

A. Description
  1. Abnormal infrequent passage of stool
  2. When the client resumes a solid diet after surgery, failure to pass stool within 48 hours is a cause for concern
B. Data collection
  1. Abdominal distention
  2. Absence of bowel movements
  3. Anorexia, headache, and nausea
C. Interventions
  1. Check bowel sounds
  2. Encourage fluid intake up to 3000 mL/day unless contraindicated
  3. Encourage early ambulation
  4. Encourage consumption of fiber foods unless contraindicated
  5. Administer stool softeners and laxatives as prescribed
  6. Provide privacy and adequate time for bowel elimination

XI. PARALYTIC ILEUS (see Box 17-3)

A. Description
  1. Failure of appropriate forward movement of bowel contents
  2. May occur as a result of anesthetic medications or manipulation of the bowel during the surgical procedure

B. Data collection
   1. Postoperative nausea and vomiting
   2. Abdominal distention
   3. Absence of bowel sounds, bowel movement, or flatus
C. Interventions
   1. Maintain NPO status until bowel sounds return
   2. Maintain patency of nasogastric (NG) tube if in place
   3. Encourage ambulation
   4. Monitor IV fluids as prescribed
   5. Administer medications as prescribed to increase gastrointestinal (GI) motility and secretions
   6. If ileus occurs, it is first treated nonsurgically by bowel decompression by insertion of an NG tube attached to intermittent to constant suction

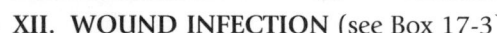

XII. WOUND INFECTION (see Box 17-3)

A. Description
   1. Caused by poor aseptic technique or a contaminated wound before surgical exploration
   2. Usually occurs 3 to 6 days after surgery
   3. Purulent material may exit from the drains or separated wound edges
B. Data collection
   1. Fever and chills
   2. Warm, tender, painful, and inflamed incision site
   3. Edematous skin at incision and tight skin sutures
   4. Elevated white blood cell count
C. Interventions
   1. Monitor temperature
   2. Monitor incision site for approximation of suture line, edema, or bleeding, and signs of infection (REEDA: *r*edness, *e*rythema, *e*cchymosis, *d*rainage, *a*pproximation of the wound edges)
   3. Maintain patency of drains, and keep drain and tubes away from incision line
   4. Monitor drains, and assess drainage amount, color, and consistency
   5. Change dressing, as prescribed
   6. Administer antibiotics, as prescribed

XIII. WOUND DEHISCENCE (Figure 17-7; see Box 17-3)

A. Description
   1. Separation of the wound edges at the suture line
   2. Usually occurs 6 to 8 days after surgery
B. Data collection
   1. Increased drainage
   2. Opened wound edges
   3. Appearance of underlying tissues through the wound
C. Interventions
   1. Notify the registered nurse and/or physician immediately

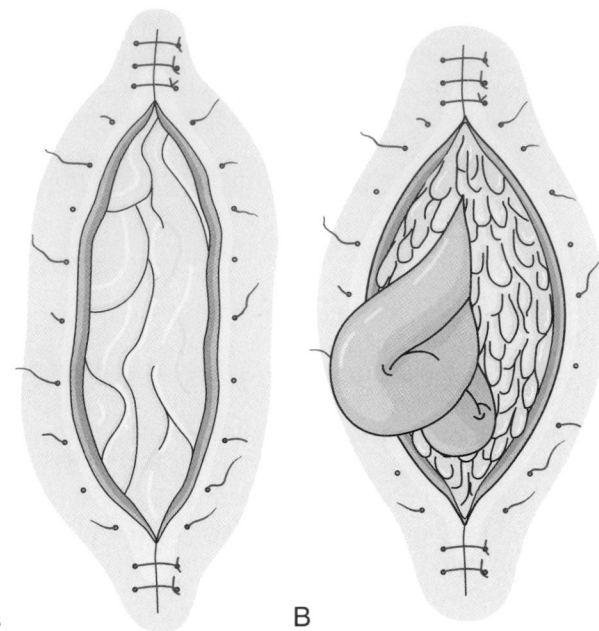

A **B**

FIG. 17-7 **A,** Wound dehiscence and **B,** wound evisceration. (From Phipps, W., Monahan, F., Sands, J., Marek, J. & Neighbors, M. [2003]. *Medical-surgical nursing: Health and illness perspectives* [7th ed.]. St. Louis: Mosby.)

   2. Place the client in low Fowler's position with knees bent to prevent abdominal tension on abdominal wounds
   3. Cover the wound with a sterile normal saline dressing
   4. Prevent wound infection
   5. Administer antiemetics, as prescribed, to prevent vomiting and further strain on the incision
   6. Instruct the client to splint the incision when coughing

XIV. WOUND EVISCERATION (see Box 17-3 and Figure 17-7)

A. Description
   1. Protrusion of the internal organs and tissues through an opening in the wound edges
   2. Most common among obese clients, clients who have had abdominal surgery, or those who have poor wound-healing ability
   3. Usually occurs 6 to 8 days after surgery
   4. **Wound evisceration** is an emergency
B. Data collection
   1. Discharge of serosanguineous fluid from a previously dry wound
   2. The appearance of loops of bowel or other abdominal contents through the wound
   3. The client may report feeling a popping sensation after coughing or turning
C. Interventions
   1. Notify the registered nurse and/or physician immediately

2. Place the client in a low Fowler's position with the knees bent to prevent abdominal tension
3. Cover the wound with a sterile normal saline dressing
4. Prevent wound infection
5. Administer antiemetics, as prescribed, to prevent vomiting and further strain on the incision
6. Instruct the client to splint the incision when coughing

XV. AMBULATORY SURGERY

A. Criteria for client discharge
1. Is alert and oriented
2. Has voided
3. Has no respiratory distress
4. Is able to ambulate, swallow, and cough
5. Has minimal pain
6. Is not vomiting
7. Has minimal, if any, bleeding from incision site
8. A responsible adult is available to drive the client home
9. The surgeon has signed a release form

B. Reinforcing discharge instructions (Box 17-4)
1. Should be performed before the date of the scheduled procedure
2. Provide written instructions to the client and family regarding the specifics of care
3. Instruct the client and family about postoperative complications that can occur
4. Suggest appropriate resources for home care support
5. Instruct the client not to drive for 24 hours if he or she has had a general anesthetic
6. Inform the client to call the surgeon, ambulatory center, or emergency department if postoperative problems occur
7. Instruct the client to keep follow-up appointments with the surgeon

PRACTICE QUESTIONS

1. A nurse is reviewing the laboratory results of a client scheduled for surgery. Which of these laboratory results would indicate to the nurse that the surgery might be postponed?
   1. Sodium, 140 mEq/L
   2. Hemoglobin, 9.2 g/dL
   3. Platelets, 200,000/mm^3
   4. Serum creatinine, 0.9 mg/dL
2. A nurse is assisting in developing a plan of care for a client scheduled for surgery. The nurse would include which of the following activities in the nursing care plan for the client on the day of surgery?
   1. Have the client void immediately before surgery
   2. Report immediately any slight increase in blood pressure or pulse

---

BOX 17-4

Reinforcing Discharge Instructions

Determine the client's readiness to learn, educational level, and desire to change or modify lifestyle.

Determine the need for resources needed for home care.

Demonstrate care to the incision and how to change the dressing.

Instruct the client to cover the incision with plastic if showering is allowed.

Be sure the client is provided with a 48-hour supply of dressings for home use.

Instruct the client on the importance of returning to the physician's office for follow-up.

Instruct the client that sutures are usually removed in the physician's office 7 to 10 days after surgery.

Inform the client that staples are removed 7 to 14 days after surgery and that the skin may become slightly reddened when they are ready to be removed.

Steri-Strips may be applied to provide extra support after the sutures are removed.

Instruct the client on the use of medications, their purpose, doses, administration, and side effects.

Instruct the client on diet and to drink 6 to 8 glasses of liquid a day.

Instruct the client on activity levels and to resume normal activities gradually.

Instruct the client to avoid lifting for 6 weeks if a major surgical procedure was performed.

Instruct the client with an abdominal incision not to lift anything weighing 10 lb or more and not to engage in any activities that involve pushing or pulling.

Clients usually can return to work in 6 to 8 weeks, as prescribed by the physician.

Instruct the client on the signs and symptoms of complications and when to call a physician.

---

   3. Verify that the client has not eaten for the last 24 hours
   4. Avoid oral hygiene and rinsing with mouthwash

3. Emergency surgery is scheduled for a client with a bowel obstruction. The licensed practical nurse (LPN) tells the registered nurse (RN) that he or she is unable to obtain informed consent from the client because the client has received narcotic analgesics and is very sedated. The LPN understands that which of the following is the appropriate action?
   1. Performing the surgery without an informed consent
   2. Calling the family and telling them that they must come to the hospital immediately to sign the informed consent
   3. Obtaining a telephone consent from the family member and ensuring that the oral consent is witnessed by two persons
   4. Having the client sign the consent form because this is an emergency situation

4. A nurse is caring for a client scheduled for surgery. The client is concerned about the surgical procedure.

To alleviate the client's fears and misconceptions about surgery, the nurse should:

1. Provide explanations about the procedures involved in the planned surgery
2. Explain all nursing care and possible discomfort that may result
3. Tell the client that preoperative fear is normal
4. Ask the client to discuss information known about the planned surgery

5. A nurse is reinforcing instructions to a client regarding the use of the incentive spirometer. Which of the following statements, if made by the client, would indicate that the client does not clearly understand the procedure?
   1. "My lips should cover the mouthpiece completely."
   2. "I should inhale slowly to maintain a constant flow through the unit."
   3. "After maximum inspiration, I should hold my breath for 2 to 3 seconds, and then exhale slowly."
   4. "I can use the incentive spirometer in any position to achieve optimal lung expansion."

6. A nurse is collecting data from a client who is scheduled for surgery in 1 week in the ambulatory care surgical center. The nurse notes that the client has a history of arthritis and has been taking acetylsalicylic acid (ASA, aspirin). The nurse reports the information to the physician and anticipates that the physician will prescribe which of the following?
   1. Continue to take the aspirin as prescribed
   2. Decrease the dose of the aspirin to half of what is normally taken
   3. Discontinue the aspirin immediately
   4. Discontinue the aspirin 48 hours before the scheduled surgery

7. A nurse preparing a client for surgery reviews the client's medication record. The client is to be NPO after midnight. Which of the following medications, if noted on the client's record, would the nurse question?
   1. Cyclobenzaprine (Flexeril)
   2. Fentanyl (Duragesic)
   3. Allopurinol (Zyloprim)
   4. Prednisone (Deltasone)

8. A nurse obtains the vital signs on a postoperative client who just returned to the nursing unit. The client's blood pressure (BP) is 100/60 mm Hg, pulse is 90 beats per minute, and respiration rate is 20 breaths per minute. Based on these findings, which of the following nursing actions should be performed?
   1. Cover the client with a warm blanket
   2. Shake gently to arouse
   3. Continue to monitor the vital signs
   4. Call the registered nurse (RN) immediately

9. A client arrives to the surgical nursing unit after surgery. The initial nursing action is to check the:
   1. Dressing for bleeding
   2. Tubes or drains for patency
   3. Patency of the airway
   4. Vital signs to compare with preoperative measurements

10. A nurse is monitoring an adult client for postoperative complications. Which of the following would be most indicative of a potential postoperative complication that requires further observation?
    1. Urinary output of 20 mL/hour
    2. Temperature of 37.6°C (99.6°F)
    3. Serous drainage on the surgical dressing
    4. Blood pressure of 100/70 mm Hg

11. A nurse monitors the postoperative client frequently for the presence of secretions in the lungs, knowing that accumulated secretions can lead to:
    1. Pulmonary edema
    2. Pneumonia
    3. Fluid imbalance
    4. Carbon dioxide retention

12. A nurse is caring for a postoperative client who has a drain inserted into the surgical wound. Which of the following nursing actions would be inappropriate in the care of the drain?
    1. Maintain aseptic technique when emptying
    2. Observe for bright red bloody drainage
    3. Check the drain for patency
    4. Secure the drain by curling or folding it and taping it firmly to the body

13. A nurse checks the client's surgical incision for signs of infection. Which of the following would be indicative of a potential infection?
    1. The presence of serous drainage
    2. Temperature of 98.8°F (37.1°C)
    3. Client complains of feeling cold
    4. The presence of purulent drainage

14. A nurse is checking a client's surgical incision and notes an increase in the amount of drainage, a separation of the incision line, and the appearance of underlying tissue. Which of the following is the initial action?
    1. Clean the wound using aseptic technique, and apply a sterile dry dressing
    2. Apply a sterile dressing soaked with normal saline to the wound
    3. Leave the incision open to the air to assist in drying the drainage
    4. Cover the wound with a Betadine-soaked dressing

15. A nurse monitors a postoperative client for signs of complications. Which of the following would the nurse determine to be indicative of a sign of a potential complication?
    1. Faint bowel sounds heard in all four quadrants
    2. A negative Homan's sign
    3. A blood pressure of 120/70 mm Hg with a pulse of 90 beats per minute
    4. Increasing restlessness

ALTERNATE FORMAT QUESTION: MULTIPLE RESPONSE

A client who had abdominal surgery complains of feeling as though "something gave way" in the incisional site. The nurse removes the dressing and notes the presence of a loop of bowel protruding through the incision. Select all nursing interventions that the nurse would take.

___ Place the client in a supine position without a pillow under the head
___ Instruct the client to remain quiet
___ Place a sterile saline dressing and ice packs over the wound
___ Notify the registered nurse
___ Prepare the client for wound closure

ANSWERS

1. Answer: 2
Rationale: Routine screening tests include a complete blood cell count, serum electrolyte analysis, coagulation studies, and serum creatinine tests. The complete blood count includes the hemoglobin analysis. All these values are within normal range, except the hemoglobin. If a client has a low hemoglobin level, the surgery may be postponed.
Test-Taking Strategy: Use the process of elimination. Recalling the normal values for serum sodium, hemoglobin, platelets, and creatinine will direct you to option 2. This is the only abnormal value. Review these normal laboratory values if you had difficulty with this question.
Level of Cognitive Ability: Analysis
Client Needs: Physiological Integrity
Integrated Process: Nursing Process/Data Collection
Content Area: Fundamental Skills
References: Pagana, K., & Pagana, T. (2003). *Mosby's diagnostic and laboratory test reference* (6th ed.). St. Louis: Mosby, p. 490.
Potter, P., & Perry, A. (2005). *Fundamentals of nursing* (6th ed.). St. Louis: Mosby, p. 1606.

2. Answer: 1
Rationale: The nurse would assist the client to void immediately before surgery so that the bladder will be empty. A slight increase in blood pressure and pulse is common during the preoperative period and is generally the result of anxiety. The client usually has a restriction of food and fluids for 8 hours prior to surgery instead of 24 hours. Oral hygiene is allowed, but the client should not swallow any water.
Test-Taking Strategy: Use the process of elimination and read each option carefully. Eliminate option 2 because of the words "immediately" and "slight." Eliminate option 3, knowing that the client should be NPO for 8 hours prior to surgery. There is no useful reason for option 4; in fact, oral hygiene may make the client feel more comfortable. Review general preoperative care if you had difficulty with this question.
Level of Cognitive Ability: Application
Client Needs: Physiological Integrity
Integrated Process: Nursing Process/Planning
Content Area: Fundamental Skills
Reference: Potter, P., & Perry, A. (2005), *Fundamentals of nursing* (6th ed.). St. Louis: Mosby, pp. 1606, 1609.

3. Answer: 3
Rationale: Every effort must be made to obtain permission from a responsible family member to perform surgery if the client is unable to sign the consent form. A telephone consent must be witnessed by two persons who hear the family member's oral consent. The two witnesses then sign the consent and document the name of the family member, noting that an oral consent was obtained. In emergencies, the client may be unable to sign and family members may not be available. In this type of a situation, the physician is legally permitted to perform surgery without consent. Consent is not informed if it is obtained from the client who is confused, unconscious, mentally incompetent, or under the influence of sedatives.
Test-Taking Strategy: Use the process of elimination. Note the key word, *appropriate*. Eliminate options 1 and 4 first because they are inappropriate. From the remaining options, select option 3 because it is legally acceptable to obtain telephone permission from a family member if two persons witness it. Review the issues related to informed consent if you had difficulty with this question.
Level of Cognitive Ability: Comprehension
Client Needs: Safe, Effective Care Environment
Integrated Process: Nursing Process/Implementation
Content Area: Fundamental Skills
References: Linton, A., & Maebius, N. (2003). *Introduction to medical-surgical nursing* (3rd ed.). Philadelphia: W.B. Saunders, p. 212.
Potter, P., & Perry, A. (2005). *Fundamentals of nursing* (6th ed.). St. Louis: Mosby, p. 416.

4. Answer: 4
Rationale: Explanations should begin with the information that the client knows. Option 3 is a block to communication. Options 1 and 2 may produce additional anxiety in the client.
Test-Taking Strategy: Use the process of elimination. Remember always to focus on the client's feelings first. This will direct you to option 4. Additionally, option 4 is the only option that addresses data collection, the first step of the nursing process. Review the psychosocial aspects related to the preoperative client if you had difficulty with this question.
Level of Cognitive Ability: Application
Client Needs: Psychosocial Integrity
Integrated Process: Caring
Content Area: Fundamental Skills
Reference: Potter, P., & Perry, A. (2005). *Fundamentals of nursing* (6th ed.). St. Louis: Mosby, p. 1604.

5. Answer: 4
Rationale: For optimal lung expansion with the incentive spirometer, the client should assume the semi-Fowler's or high Fowler's position. The mouthpiece should be covered completely while the client inhales slowly, with a constant

flow through the unit. The client's breath should be held for 2 to 3 seconds before exhaling slowly.
Test-Taking Strategy: Use the process of elimination and note the key words, *does not clearly understand.* Remember that, for optimal lung expansion, the head should be elevated to decrease the pressure of the internal organs on the diaphragm and to increase the expansion of the diaphragm. If you had difficulty with this question, review the correct procedure related to the use of an incentive spirometer.
Level of Cognitive Ability: Analysis
Client Needs: Physiological Integrity
Integrated Process: Nursing Process/Evaluation
Content Area: Fundamental Skills
Reference: Potter, P., & Perry, A. (2005). *Fundamentals of nursing* (6th ed.). St. Louis: Mosby, p. 1614.

6. *Answer:* 4
Rationale: Anticoagulants alter normal clotting factors and increase the risk of hemorrhage. Aspirin has properties that can alter the clotting mechanism and should be discontinued at least 48 hours before surgery.
Test-Taking Strategy: Use the process of elimination. Remembering that aspirin has properties that can alter normal clotting factors and that it should be discontinued at least 48 hours before surgery will assist in directing you to option 4. Review the medications that affect the preoperative client if you had difficulty with this question.
Level of Cognitive Ability: Application
Client Needs: Physiological Integrity
Integrated Process: Nursing Process/Planning
Content Area: Fundamental Skills
Reference: Potter, P., & Perry, A. (2005). *Fundamentals of nursing* (6th ed.). St. Louis: Mosby, p. 1602.

7. *Answer:* 4
Rationale: Prednisone is a corticosteroid that can cause adrenal atrophy, which reduces the body's ability to withstand stress. Before and during surgery, dosages may be temporarily increased. Cyclobenzaprine is a skeletal muscle relaxant. Fentanyl is an opioid analgesic. Allopurinol is an antigout medication.
Test-Taking Strategy: Use the process of elimination and knowledge regarding the medications that may have special implications for the surgical client to answer this question. Review these medications if you had difficulty with this question.
Level of Cognitive Ability: Application
Client Needs: Physiological Integrity
Integrated Process: Nursing Process/Implementation
Content Area: Fundamental Skills
Reference: Potter, P., & Perry, A. (2005). *Fundamentals of nursing* (6th ed.). St. Louis: Mosby, p. 1602.

8. *Answer:* 3
Rationale: A slightly lower than normal BP and an increased pulse rate are common after surgery. Warm blankets are applied to maintain the client's body temperature. Level of consciousness can be determined by checking the client's response to light touch and verbal stimuli, rather than by shaking the client. There is no reason to contact the RN immediately.

Test-Taking Strategy: Focus on the data in the question. Noting that the vital signs are within normal limits will direct you to option 3. Review expected postoperative findings if you had difficulty with this question.
Level of Cognitive Ability: Application
Client Needs: Physiological Integrity
Integrated Process: Nursing Process/Implementation
Content Area: Fundamental Skills
Reference: Potter, P., & Perry, A. (2005). *Fundamentals of nursing* (6th ed.). St. Louis: Mosby, pp. 1631-1632.

9. *Answer:* 3
Rationale: If the airway is not patent, immediate measures must be taken for the survival of the client. After checking the client's airway, the nurse would next check the client's vital signs and then check the dressing and tubes and drains.
Test-Taking Strategy: Use the ABCs—airway, breathing, and circulation. Airway patency is the first action to be taken. Options 1, 2, and 4 are all nursing actions that should be performed after a patent airway has been established. Review care to the postoperative client if you had difficulty with this question.
Level of Cognitive Ability: Application
Client Needs: Physiological Integrity
Integrated Process: Nursing Process/Implementation
Content Area: Delegating/Prioritizing
Reference: Potter, P., & Perry, A. (2005). *Fundamentals of nursing* (6th ed.). St. Louis: Mosby, p. 1632.

10. *Answer:* 1
Rationale: Urine output is maintained at a minimum of at least 30 mL/hour for an adult. An output of less than 30 mL/hour for each of two consecutive hours should be reported to the physician. A temperature above 37.7°C (100°F) or below 36.1°C (97°F) and a falling systolic blood pressure under 90 mm Hg are to be reported. The client's preoperative or baseline blood pressure is used to make informed postoperative comparisons. Moderate or light serous drainage from the surgical site is considered normal.
Test-Taking Strategy: Knowledge of the normal ranges for temperature, blood pressure, urinary output, and wound drainage is necessary to determine the correct option. Through the process of elimination, you can determine that the urinary output is the only observation that is not within the normal range. Review expected postoperative findings if you had difficulty with this question.
Level of Cognitive Ability: Analysis
Client Needs: Physiological Integrity
Integrated Process: Nursing Process/Data Collection
Content Area: Fundamental Skills
Reference: Potter, P., & Perry, A. (2005). *Fundamentals of nursing* (6th ed.). St. Louis: Mosby, pp. 1637-1640.

11. *Answer:* 2
Rationale: The most common postoperative respiratory problems are atelectasis, pneumonia, and pulmonary emboli. Pneumonia is the inflammation of lung tissue that causes productive cough, dyspnea, and crackles. Pulmonary edema usually results from left-sided heart failure and can be caused

by medications, fluid overload, and smoke inhalation. Carbon dioxide retention results from the inability to exhale carbon dioxide in conditions such as chronic obstructive pulmonary disease. Fluid imbalance can be a deficit or excess related to fluid loss or overload.

Test-Taking Strategy: Use the process of elimination and note the key words, *presence of secretions in the lungs.* Focusing on the issue of the question, the postoperative client, will direct you to option 2. Options 1, 3, and 4 most commonly occur with other conditions. Review postoperative complications if you had difficulty with this question.

Level of Cognitive Ability: Application
Client Needs: Physiological Integrity
Integrated Process: Nursing Process/Data Collection
Content Area: Fundamental Skills
Reference: Potter, P., & Perry, A. (2005). *Fundamentals of nursing* (6th ed.). St. Louis: Mosby, p. 1636.

12. *Answer: 4*
Rationale: Aseptic technique must be used when emptying the drainage container or changing the dressing to avoid contamination of the wound. Usually, drainage from the wound is pale, red, and watery. Active bleeding will be bright red in color. The drain should be checked for patency to provide an exit for the fluid or blood to promote healing. The nurse needs to ensure that drainage flows freely and that there are no kinks in the drains. Curling or folding the drain prevents the flow of the drainage.

Test-Taking Strategy: Use the process of elimination and note the key word, *inappropriate.* Remember that the nurse needs to ensure that drainage flows freely from a drain. Review care of the surgical client with a drain if you had difficulty with this question.

Level of Cognitive Ability: Application
Client Needs: Physiological Integrity
Integrated Process: Nursing Process/Implementation
Content Area: Fundamental Skills
Reference: Potter, P., & Perry, A. (2005). *Fundamentals of nursing* (6th ed.). St. Louis: Mosby, pp. 1640-1641.

13. *Answer: 4*
Rationale: Signs and symptoms of a wound infection include warm, red, and tender skin around the incision. The client may have fever and chills. Purulent material may exit from drains or from separated wound edges. It may be caused by poor aseptic technique and a contaminated wound before surgical exploration. It appears 3 to 6 days after surgery. Serous drainage is not indicative of a wound infection. A temperature of 98.8° F is not an abnormal finding in a postoperative client. Complaining of feeling cold is not indicative of an infection, although chills along with a fever are signs of an infection.

Test-Taking Strategy: Use the process of elimination. Noting the word "purulent" in option 4 will direct you to this option. Review the signs of a wound infection if you had difficulty with this question.

Level of Cognitive Ability: Comprehension
Client Needs: Physiological Integrity
Integrated Process: Nursing Process/Data Collection
Content Area: Fundamental Skills

References: Christensen, B., & Kockrow, E. (2003). *Foundations of nursing* (4th ed.). St. Louis: Mosby, p. 414.
Potter, P., & Perry, A. (2005). *Fundamentals of nursing* (6th ed.). St. Louis: Mosby, p. 1640.

14. *Answer: 2*
Rationale: Wound dehiscence is the separation of wound edges at the suture line. Signs and symptoms include increased drainage and the appearance of underlying tissues. It usually occurs as a complication 6 to 8 days after surgery. The client should be instructed to remain quiet and to avoid coughing or straining. The client should be positioned to prevent further stress on the wound. Sterile dressings soaked with sterile normal saline should be used to cover the wound. The physician needs to be notified.

Test-Taking Strategy: Use the process of elimination. Eliminate option 3 first because this action would expose the open wound and underlying tissues to infection. Eliminate options 1 and 4 next. A dry dressing and a dressing soaked with Betadine will irritate the exposed body tissues. Review emergency care when dehiscence or evisceration occurs if you had difficulty with this question.

Level of Cognitive Ability: Application
Client Needs: Physiological Integrity
Integrated Process: Nursing Process/Implementation
Content Area: Fundamental Skills
Reference: Christensen, B., & Kockrow, E. (2003). *Foundations of nursing* (4th ed.). St. Louis: Mosby, pp. 419-420.

15. *Answer: 4*
Rationale: Increasing restlessness noted in a client is a sign that requires continuous and close monitoring, because it could be a potential indication of a complication such as hemorrhage or shock. Faint bowel sounds heard in all four quadrants is a normal occurrence. A negative Homan's sign is also normal. A positive Homan's sign, however, may be indicative of thrombophlebitis. A blood pressure of 120/70 mm Hg with a pulse of 90 beats per minute is a relatively normal sign.

Test-Taking Strategy: Use the process of elimination. Eliminate options 1, 2, and 3 because these are normal expected findings. Review the normal expected postoperative findings if you had difficulty with this question.

Level of Cognitive Ability: Analysis
Client Needs: Physiological Integrity
Integrated Process: Nursing Process/Data Collection
Content Area: Fundamental Skills
Reference: Potter, P., & Perry, A. (2005). *Fundamentals of nursing* (6th ed.). St. Louis: Mosby, p. 1636.

ALTERNATE FORMAT QUESTION: MULTIPLE RESPONSE

Answers:
Instruct the client to remain quiet
Notify the registered nurse
Prepare the client for wound closure
Rationale: Wound dehiscence is the separation of the wound edges. Wound evisceration is protrusion of the internal organs through an incision. If wound dehiscence or evisceration occurs, the registered nurse is notified and then contacts the

surgeon immediately. The client is placed in a low Fowler's position, kept quiet, and instructed not to cough. Protruding organs are covered with a warm, sterile saline dressing. The treatment for evisceration is immediate wound closure under local or general anesthesia.

Test-Taking Strategy: Focus on the information in the question to determine that the client is experiencing wound evisceration. Visualizing this occurrence will assist in determining that the client would not be placed supine and that ice packs would not be placed on the incision. Review this surgical complication if you had difficulty with this question.

Level of Cognitive Ability: Application
Client Needs: Physiological Integrity
Integrated Process: Nursing Process/Implementation
Content Area: Fundamental Skills
References: Christensen, B., & Kockrow, E. (2003). *Foundations of nursing* (4th ed.). St. Louis: Mosby, pp. 419-420.
Phipps, W., Monahan, F., Sands, J., Marek, J., & Neighbors, M. (2003). *Medical-surgical nursing: Health and illness perspectives* (7th ed.). St. Louis: Mosby, p. 452.

REFERENCES

Christensen, B., & Kockrow, E. (2003). *Foundations of nursing* (4th ed.). St. Louis: Mosby.

Linton, A., & Maebius, N. (2003). *Introduction to medical-surgical nursing* (3rd ed.). Philadelphia: W.B. Saunders.

National Council of State Boards of Nursing. (2005). *Detailed test plan for the National Council licensure examination for practical/ vocational nurses.* Chicago: Author.

Pagana, K., & Pagana, T. (2003). *Mosby's diagnostic and laboratory test reference* (6th ed.). St. Louis: Mosby.

Phipps, W., Monahan, F., Sands, J., Marek, J., & Neighbors, M. (2003). *Medical-surgical nursing: Health and illness perspectives* (7th ed.). St. Louis: Mosby.

Potter, P., & Perry, A. (2005). *Fundamentals of nursing* (6th ed.). St. Louis: Mosby.

Positioning Clients

PYRAMID TERMS

Fowler's position   The client is supine and the head of the bed is elevated to 45 to 60 degrees.

high Fowler's position   The client is supine and the head of the bed is elevated to 90 degrees.

lateral (side-lying) position   The client is lying on the side, and the head and shoulders are aligned with the hips and the spine, parallel to the edge of the mattress. The head, neck, and upper arm are supported by a pillow. The lower shoulder is pulled forward slightly and, along with the elbow, flexed at 90 degrees. The legs are flexed or extended. A pillow is placed to support the back.

lithotomy position   The client is lying on the back with the hips and knees flexed at right angles and the feet in stirrups.

prone position   The client is lying on the abdomen, with the head turned to the side.

reverse Trendelenburg position   The bed is tilted so that the client's foot of the bed is down.

semi-Fowler's position (low Fowler's)   The client is supine, and the head of the bed is elevated approximately 30 degrees.

Sims' position   The client is lying on the side, with the body turned prone at 45 degrees. The lower leg is extended, with the upper leg flexed at the hip and knee at a 45- to 90-degree angle.

supine position   The client is lying on the back. The head and shoulders are usually slightly elevated with a small pillow. The arms and legs are extended, and the legs are slightly abducted.

Trendelenburg's position   The bed is tilted so that the head of the client's bed is down. This position is contraindicated in clients with head injuries, increased intracranial pressure, spinal cord injuries, and certain respiratory disorders.

▲ PYRAMID TO SUCCESS

Nursing responsibilities include positioning clients in a safe and appropriate manner to provide safety and comfort. Knowledge regarding the client's position required for a certain procedure or condition is expected.

It is the nurse's responsibility to reduce the likelihood and prevent the development of complications related to an existing condition, prescribed treatment, or medical or surgical procedure. It is imperative that the nurse review the physician's orders after treatments or procedures and take note of instructions regarding positioning and mobility (Figures 18-1, 18-2, and 18-3).

Fowler's position

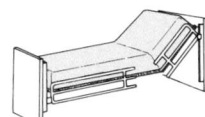

Semi-Fowler's position

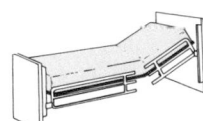

Trendelenburg's position

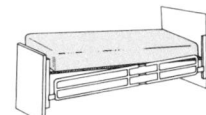

Reverse Trendelenburg's position

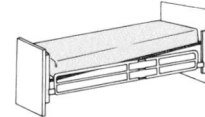

Flat position

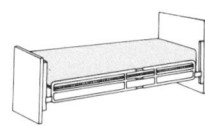

FIG. 18-1   Common bed positions. (From Potter, P., & Perry, A. [2001]. *Fundamentals of nursing* [5th ed.]. St. Louis: Mosby.)

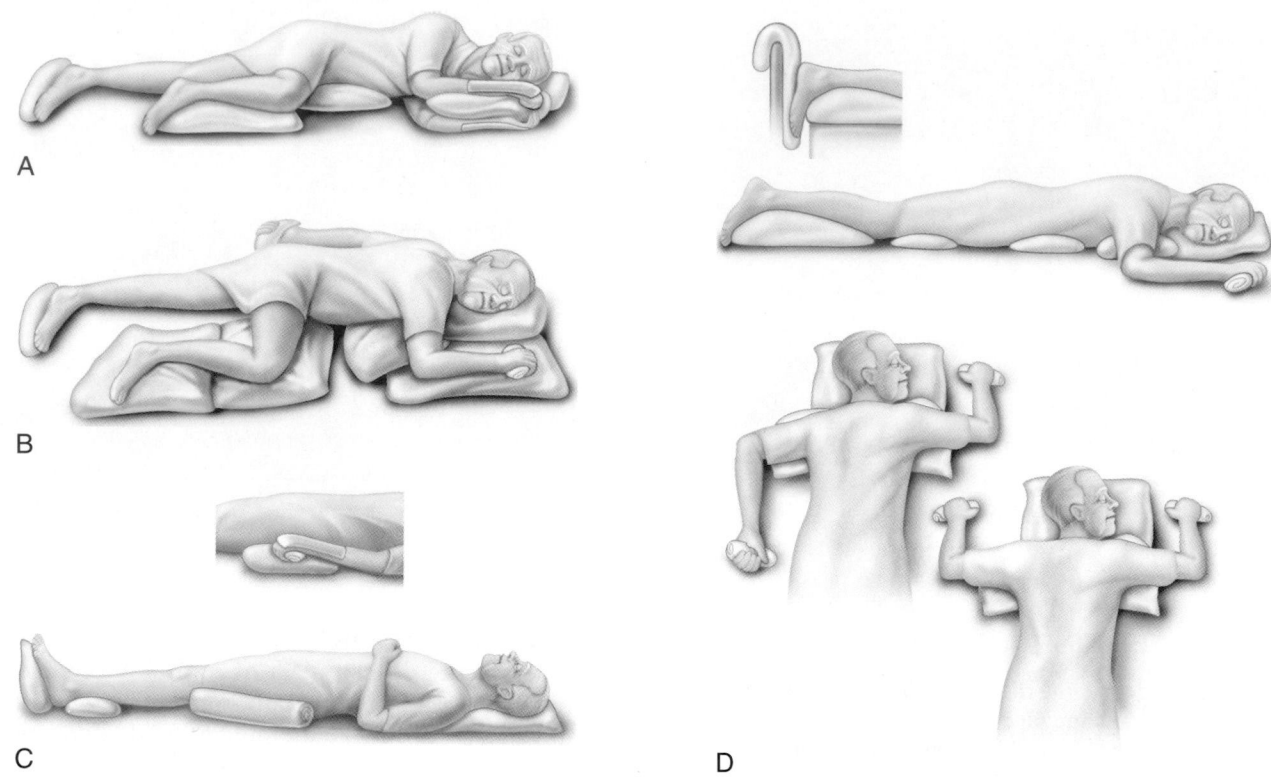

FIG. 18-2 A, Lateral (side-lying) position; **B,** semiprone (Sims') position; **C,** supine position; and **D,** prone position. (From Harkreader, H., & Hogan, M.A. [2004]. *Fundamentals of nursing: Caring and clinical judgment* [2nd ed.]. Philadelphia: W.B. Saunders.)

The Integrated Processes addressed in this chapter include Caring, Communication and Documentation, the Clinical Problem-Solving Process (Nursing Process), and Teaching/Learning.

▲ CLIENT NEEDS
Safe, Effective Care Environment

Accident and injury prevention
Appropriate positioning
Environmental and personal safety
Informed consent
Priority establishment
Protective measures
Safe use of equipment

Health Promotion and Maintenance

Information regarding the need for prescribed therapies
Techniques of data collection

Psychosocial Integrity

Assisting the client to use coping mechanisms
Keeping the family informed of client progress
Providing support to the client
Therapeutic communications

Physiological Integrity

Comfort measures for rest and sleep
Immobility
Preventing complications
Providing nutrition and oral intake
Providing personal hygiene as needed
Use of assistive devices

I. GUIDELINES FOR POSITIONING
A. Position in a safe and appropriate manner to provide safety and comfort
B. Review the physician's orders, especially after treatments or procedures, and take note of instructions regarding positioning and mobility
C. Select a position that will prevent the development of complications related to an existing condition, prescribed treatment, or medical or surgical procedure

II. POSITIONS TO ENSURE SAFETY AND COMFORT
A. Integumentary system
  1. Autograft: After surgery, the site is immobilized for approximately 3 to 7 days to provide the time

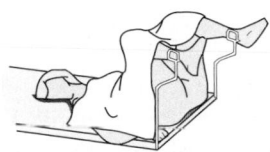

FIG. 18-3 Lithotomy position. (From Potter, P., & Perry, A. [2005]. *Fundamentals of nursing* [6th ed.]. St. Louis: Mosby.)

needed for the graft to adhere and attach to the wound bed

2. Burns of the face and head: Elevate the head of the bed to prevent or reduce facial, head, and tracheal edema
3. Circumferential burns of the extremities: Elevate the extremities above the level of the heart to prevent or reduce dependent edema
4. Skin graft: Elevate and immobilize the graft site to prevent movement and shearing of the graft and disruption of tissue; avoid weight bearing

B. Reproductive system
1. Mastectomy
   a. Position the client with the head of the bed elevated at least 30 degrees (see Figure 18-1; **semi-Fowler's position**), with the affected arm elevated on a pillow to promote lymphatic fluid return after the removal of axillary lymph nodes
   b. Turn the client only to the back and unaffected side
2. Perineal and vaginal procedures: Place the client in the **lithotomy position** (see Figure 18-3)

C. Endocrine system
1. Hypophysectomy: Elevate the head of the bed to prevent increased intracranial pressure
2. Thyroidectomy
   a. Place in **semi-Fowler's position** to reduce swelling and edema in the neck area
   b. Sandbags or pillows may be used to support the client's head or neck

D. Gastrointestinal system
1. Hemorrhoidectomy: Assist the client to a **lateral (side-lying) position** to prevent pain and bleeding
2. Gastroesophageal reflux disease: **Reverse Trendelenburg's position** may be prescribed to promote gastric emptying and prevent esophageal reflux
3. Liver biopsy
   a. During procedure
      (1) Position client **supine,** with the right side of the upper abdomen exposed
      (2) The client's right arm is raised and extended over the left shoulder behind the head
      (3) The liver is located on the right side, and this position provides for maximal exposure of the right intercostal space
   b. After procedure
      (1) Assist the client into a right **lateral (side-lying) position**
      (2) Place a small pillow or folded towel under the puncture site for at least 3 hours to provide pressure to the site and prevent bleeding
4. Nasogastric tube
   a. Insertion
      (1) Position the client in **high Fowler's position**, with the head tilted forward
      (2) This position will help close the trachea and open the esophagus
   b. Irrigations and tube feedings
      (1) Elevate the head of the bed 30 degrees **(semi-Fowler's position)** to prevent aspiration
      (2) Maintain head elevation for 1 hour after an intermittent feeding
      (3) Head of the bed should remain elevated for continuous feedings
5. Rectal enemas or irrigations: Place client in left **Sims' position** to allow the solution to flow by gravity in the natural direction of the colon
6. Sengstaken-Blakemore and Minnesota tubes: Maintain elevation of the head of the bed to increase lung expansion and reduce portal blood flow, permitting effective compression of the esophageal varices

E. Respiratory system
1. Chronic obstructive pulmonary disease: In advanced disease, place in a sitting position, leaning forward, with the client's arms over several pillows or on an overbed table; this position will help the client to breathe easier
2. Laryngectomy (radical neck dissection): Place the client in **semi-Fowler's** or **Fowler's position** to maintain a patent airway and minimize edema
3. Bronchoscopy postprocedure: Place the client in a **semi-Fowler's position** to prevent choking or aspiration resulting from an impaired ability to swallow
4. Postural drainage: the lung segment to be drained should be in the uppermost position; **Trendelenburg's position** may be used
5. Thoracentesis
   a. During procedure: To facilitate removal of fluid from the chest wall, position the client sitting on the edge of the bed and leaning over the bedside table, with the feet supported on a stool, or lying in bed on the unaffected side with the head of the bed elevated approximately 45 degrees **(Fowler's position)**
   b. After procedure: Assist the client to a position of comfort

6. Thoracotomy: Check physician's orders regarding positioning

F. Cardiovascular system

1. Abdominal aneurysm resection
   a. After surgery, limit elevation of the head of the bed to 45 degrees (**Fowler's position**) to avoid flexion of the graft
   b. The client may be turned from side to side

2. Amputation of the lower extremity
   a. During the first 24 hours after amputation, elevate the foot of the bed to reduce edema (the stump is supported with pillows but not elevated because of the risk of flexion contractures)
   b. Consult with the physician, and then position the client **prone** twice a day for a 20- to 30-minute period to stretch muscles and prevent flexion contractures of the hip

3. Arterial vascular grafting of an extremity
   a. To promote graft patency after the procedure, bed rest is usually maintained for approximately 24 hours, and the affected extremity is kept straight
   b. Limit movement and avoid flexion of the hip and knee

4. Cardiac catheterization
   a. If the femoral artery was used, the client is maintained on bed rest for approximately 3 to 4 hours; the client may turn from side to side
   b. The affected extremity is kept straight and the head elevated no more than 30 degrees, until hemostasis is adequately achieved

5. Congestive heart failure and pulmonary edema: Position the client upright (**high Fowler's position**), preferably with the legs dangling over the side of the bed, to decrease venous return and lung congestion

6. Peripheral arterial disease
   a. Obtain the physician's order for positioning
   b. Because swelling can prevent arterial blood flow, clients may be advised to elevate their feet at rest, but they should not raise their legs above the level of the heart because extreme elevation slows arterial blood flow; some clients may be advised to maintain a slightly dependent position to promote perfusion

7. Deep vein thrombosis
   a. If the extremity is red, edematous, and painful, and traditional heparin therapy is initiated, bed rest with leg elevation may be prescribed for the client
   b. Clients receiving low-molecular-weight heparin (LMWH) can usually be out of bed after 24 hours, if pain level permits

8. Varicose veins: Leg elevation above heart level is usually prescribed; the client is also advised to minimize prolonged sitting or standing during daily activities

9. Venous leg ulcers: Leg elevation is usually prescribed

G. Sensory system

1. Cataract surgery: Postoperatively, elevate the head of the bed (**semi-Fowler's** to **Fowler's position**) and position the client on the back or nonoperative side to prevent development of edema at the operative site

2. Retinal detachment
   a. If the detachment is large, bed rest and bilateral eye patching may be prescribed to minimize eye movement and prevent extension of the detachment
   b. Restrictions in activity and positioning following repair of the detachment depend on the physician's preference and surgical procedure performed
   c. If a gas bubble has been injected into the eye to flatten the retina and reinforce the repair, the client may have to be positioned so that the gas rises in the eye and presses against the repair (usually face down or angled toward the unoperative side)

H. Neurological system

1. Autonomic dysreflexia: Elevate the head of the bed to a **high Fowler's position** to help with adequate ventilation and prevention of hypertensive stroke

2. Cerebral aneurysm: Bed rest is maintained, with the head of the bed elevated 30 to 45 degrees (**semi-Fowler's** to **Fowler's position**) to prevent pressure on the aneurysm site

3. Cerebral angiography
   a. Maintain bed rest for 12 to 24 hours as prescribed
   b. The extremity into which the contrast medium was injected is kept straight and immobilized for approximately 8 hours

4. Cerebrovascular accident (CVA)
   a. In clients with hemorrhagic strokes, the head of the bed is usually elevated to 30 degrees to reduce intracranial pressure and facilitate venous drainage
   b. For clients with ischemic strokes, the head of the bed is usually kept flat
   c. Maintain the head in a midline, neutral position to facilitate venous drainage from the head
   d. Avoid extreme hip and neck flexion; extreme hip flexion may increase intrathoracic pressure, whereas extreme neck flexion prohibits venous drainage from the brain

5. Craniotomy
   a. The client should *not* be positioned on the site that was operated on, especially if the bone flap has been removed, because the brain has no bony covering over the affected site

b. Elevate the head of the bed 30 to 45 degrees (**semi-Fowler's** to **Fowler's position**) and maintain the head in a midline, neutral position to facilitate venous drainage from the head

c. Avoid extreme hip and neck flexion

6. Laminectomy
   a. Logroll the client
   b. When the client is out of bed, the client's back is kept straight (the client is placed in a straight-backed chair) with the feet resting comfortably on the floor

7. Increased intracranial pressure
   a. Elevate the head of the bed 30 to 45 degrees (**semi-Fowler's** to **Fowler's position**) and maintain the head in a midline, neutral position to facilitate venous drainage from the head
   b. Avoid extreme hip and neck flexion

8. Lumbar puncture
   a. During procedure: Assist the client to the **lateral (side-lying) position**, with the back bowed at the edge of the examining table, the knees flexed up to the abdomen, and the head bent so that the chin is resting on the chest
   b. After procedure: Place the client in the **supine position** for 4 to 12 hours as prescribed

9. Myelogram postprocedure
   a. If water-soluble dye is used, the head of the bed should be elevated 30 to 60 degrees for approximately 12 hours to keep the dye from irritating the cerebral meninges
   b. If an oil-based dye is used, a **supine position** is maintained for several hours after the dye is removed to prevent leakage of cerebrospinal fluid

10. Spinal cord injury
    a. Immobilize the client on a spinal backboard, with the head in a neutral position, to prevent incomplete injury from becoming complete
    b. Prevent head flexion, rotation, or extension; the head is immobilized with a firm, padded cervical collar
    c. Logroll the client; no part of the body should be twisted or turned, nor should the client be allowed to assume a sitting position

I. Musculoskeletal system
   1. Total hip replacement
      a. Positioning depends on the surgical techniques used, the method of implantation, and the prosthesis
      b. Avoid extreme internal and external rotation

c. Avoid adduction; side-lying on the operative side is not allowed (unless specifically prescribed by the physician)

d. Maintain abduction when the client is in a supine position or positioned on the unoperative side

e. Place a pillow between the client's legs to maintain abduction; instruct the client not to cross the legs

f. Check the physician's orders regarding elevation of the head of the bed; flexion is usually limited to 60 degrees during the first postoperative week and then 90 degrees for 2 to 3 months thereafter

PRACTICE QUESTIONS

1. A client returns to the nursing unit after an above-the-knee amputation of the right leg. The nurse positions the client:
   1. With the stump flat on the bed
   2. With the foot of the bed elevated
   3. In reverse Trendelenburg's position
   4. Prone

2. A nurse is assigned to assist in caring for a client who has had an autograft placed on the lower extremity. The nurse plans to:
   1. Maintain the surgical extremity in a flat position
   2. Keep the surgical extremity covered with a blanket
   3. Maintain the client in a prone position
   4. Elevate and immobilize the surgical extremity

3. A nurse is assigned to assist in caring for a client after cardiac catheterization. The nurse plans to maintain bed rest with:
   1. Head elevation at 45 degrees
   2. Head elevation no greater than 30 degrees
   3. Bathroom privileges only
   4. In high Fowler's position

4. A nurse is reinforcing home care instructions to a client and family regarding care after right eye cataract removal. Which of the following statements, if made by the client, would indicate an understanding of the instructions?
   1. "I will not sleep on my right side."
   2. "I will not sleep on my left side."
   3. "I will take aspirin if I have any pain."
   4. "I will not wear my glasses until my physician says it is OK."

5. After a liver biopsy, the nurse places the client in which of the following positions?
   1. Supine
   2. Prone
   3. A left side-lying position with a small pillow or folded towel under the puncture site
   4. A right side-lying position with a small pillow or folded towel under the puncture site

6. A nurse is administering a cleansing enema to a client with a fecal impaction. Before administering the enema, the nurse assists the client to which of the following positions?
    1. On the left side of the body, with the head of the bed elevated 45 degrees
    2. On the right side of the body, with the head of the bed elevated 45 degrees
    3. Left Sims' position
    4. Right Sims' position
7. A client is being prepared for a thoracentesis. The nurse assigned to care for the client assists the client to which of the following positions for the procedure?
    1. Lying in bed on the affected side, with the head of the bed elevated 45 degrees
    2. Lying in bed on the unaffected side, with the head of the bed elevated 45 degrees
    3. Prone, with the head turned to the side supported by a pillow
    4. Sims' position, with the head of the bed flat
8. A nurse is assisting to insert a nasogastric tube into a client. The nurse places the client in which position for insertion?
    1. High Fowler's position
    2. Supine, with the head flat
    3. Right side
    4. Low Fowler's position

9. A client is diagnosed with thrombophlebitis. The nurse tells the client that which of the following is necessary?
    1. Bed rest, with the affected extremity in a dependent position
    2. Bed rest, with bathroom privileges only
    3. Bed rest, keeping the affected extremity flat
    4. Bed rest, with elevation of the affected extremity
10. A nurse is assisting in caring for a client after a craniotomy. The nurse plans to position the client:
    1. Prone
    2. Supine
    3. Semi-Fowler's position
    4. Dorsal recumbent

ALTERNATE FORMAT QUESTION: FILL IN THE BLANK

A nurse is caring for a client with congestive heart failure. The client suddenly becomes anxious and restless, has a sudden onset of breathlessness, and becomes cyanotic. The nurse suspects pulmonary edema and immediately places the client in what position?

Answer: _____

ANSWERS

1. *Answer: 2*
Rationale: During the first 24 hours after amputation, the nurse elevates the foot of bed (but not the stump itself) to reduce edema. After the first 24 hours, the bed is kept flat to prevent hip flexion contractures. The physician's postoperative orders regarding positioning are always followed.
Test-Taking Strategy: Note the key words, *returns to the nursing unit after.* Recalling that edema is a concern after surgery will direct you to option 2. Review postoperative positioning after amputation if you had difficulty with this question.
Level of Cognitive Ability: Application
Client Needs: Physiological Integrity
Integrated Process: Nursing Process/Implementation
Content Area: Fundamental Skills
Reference: Linton, A., & Maebius, N. (2003). *Introduction to medical-surgical nursing* (3rd ed.). Philadelphia: W.B. Saunders, p. 847.

2. *Answer: 4*
Rationale: Autografts placed over joints or on lower extremities are often elevated and immobilized after surgery for 3 to 7 days. This period of immobilization allows the autograft time to adhere and attach to the wound bed. Options 1, 2, and 3 are incorrect positions.
Test-Taking Strategy: Use the process of elimination. Options 2 and 3 can be eliminated first because both a blanket and a prone position can easily disrupt a graft. From the

remaining options, note that option 4 specifically addresses immobilization of the extremity. Review care after an autograft if you had difficulty with this question.
Level of Cognitive Ability: Application
Client Needs: Physiological Integrity
Integrated Process: Nursing Process/Planning
Content Area: Fundamental Skills
References: Lewis, S., Heitkemper, M., & Dirksen, S. (2004). *Medical-surgical nursing: Assessment and management of clinical problems* (6th ed.). St. Louis: Mosby, p. 534.
Phipps, W., Monahan, F., Sands, J., Marek, J., & Neighbors, M. (2003). *Medical-surgical nursing: Health and illness perspectives* (7th ed.). St. Louis: Mosby, pp. 2000-2001.

3. *Answer: 2*
Rationale: After cardiac catheterization, the extremity into which the catheter was inserted is kept straight for the time period as prescribed. The client may turn from side to side. The head of the bed is not elevated higher than 30 degrees to keep the affected leg straight at the groin and prevent arterial occlusion. Bathroom privileges are not allowed in the immediate post catheterization period. In high Fowler's position, the head of the bed is elevated 90 degrees.
Test-Taking Strategy: Use the process of elimination. Recalling that a concern after this procedure is bleeding and arterial occlusion will direct you to option 2. Review care to the client after cardiac catheterization if you had difficulty with this question.
Level of Cognitive Ability: Application

Client Needs: Physiological Integrity
Integrated Process: Nursing Process/Planning
Content Area: Fundamental Skills
References: Linton, A., & Maebius, N. (2003). *Introduction to medical-surgical nursing* (3rd ed.). Philadelphia: W.B. Saunders, p. 564.
Phipps, W., Monahan, F., Sands, J., Marek, J., & Neighbors, M. (2003). *Medical-surgical nursing: Health and illness perspectives* (7th ed.). St. Louis: Mosby, p. 640.

4. *Answer:* **1**
Rationale: After cataract surgery, the client should not sleep on the side of the body that was operated on. Clients should be instructed not to take aspirin or medications containing aspirin. Acetaminophen (Tylenol) can be taken as needed for pain. Clients may wear their glasses.
Test-Taking Strategy: Use the process of elimination. If you can remember to instruct clients to stay off the operative side, this will assist you with answering questions related to cataract surgery. Review care after this type of surgery if you had difficulty with this question.
Level of Cognitive Ability: Comprehension
Client Needs: Health Promotion and Maintenance
Integrated Process: Nursing Process/Evaluation
Content Area: Fundamental Skills
Reference: Linton, A., & Maebius, N. (2003). *Introduction to medical-surgical nursing* (3rd ed.). Philadelphia: W.B. Saunders, pp. 1065-1066.

5. *Answer:* **4**
Rationale: After a liver biopsy, the client is assisted to assume a right side-lying position with a small pillow or folded towel under the puncture site for at least 3 hours. Options 1, 2, and 3 are incorrect positions.
Test-Taking Strategy: Knowledge regarding the anatomy of the body will assist in answering this question. Remember that the liver is on the right side of the body, and that the application of pressure on the right side will minimize the escape of blood or bile through the puncture site. Review care after a liver biopsy if you had difficulty with this question.
Level of Cognitive Ability: Application
Client Needs: Physiological Integrity
Integrated Process: Nursing Process/Implementation
Content Area: Fundamental Skills
References: Linton, A., & Maebius, N. (2003). *Introduction to medical-surgical nursing* (3rd ed.). Philadelphia: W.B. Saunders, p. 720.
Pagana, K., & Pagana, T. (2003). *Mosby's diagnostic and laboratory test reference* (6th ed.). St. Louis: Mosby, p. 659.

6. *Answer:* **3**
Rationale: When administering an enema, the client is placed in a left Sims' position so that the enema solution can flow by gravity in the natural direction of the colon. The head of the bed is not elevated.
Test-Taking Strategy: Recalling the anatomy of the bowel will assist in eliminating options 2 and 4. Option 1 can be eliminated next because the head of the bed should be flat during enema administration. Review the procedure for enema administration if you had difficulty with this question.

Level of Cognitive Ability: Application
Client Needs: Physiological Integrity
Integrated Process: Nursing Process/Implementation
Content Area: Fundamental Skills
Reference: Christensen, B., & Kockrow, E. (2003). *Foundations of nursing* (4th ed.). St. Louis: Mosby, p. 486.

7. *Answer:* **2**
Rationale: To facilitate removal of fluid from the chest wall, the client is positioned sitting on the edge of bed, leaning over the bedside table, with the feet supported on a stool, or lying in bed on the unaffected side with the head of the bed elevated 45 degrees (Fowler's position). Options 1, 3, and 4 are incorrect.
Test-Taking Strategy: Visualize this procedure. Option 1 can be eliminated because, if the client were lying on the affected side, it would be very difficult to perform the procedure. Option 4 can be eliminated because the Sims' position is primarily used for rectal enemas or irrigations. In the prone position, the client is lying on the abdomen, which is not an appropriate position for this procedure. Review this procedure if you had difficulty with this question.
Level of Cognitive Ability: Application
Client Needs: Physiological Integrity
Integrated Process: Nursing Process/Implementation
Content Area: Fundamental Skills
References: Chernecky, C., & Berger, B. (2004). *Laboratory tests and diagnostic procedures* (4th ed.). Philadelphia: W.B. Saunders, p. 1043.
Linton, A., & Maebius, N. (2003). *Introduction to medical-surgical nursing* (3rd ed.). Philadelphia: W.B. Saunders, p. 466.

8. *Answer:* **1**
Rationale: During insertion of a nasogastric tube, the client is placed in a sitting or high Fowler's position to reduce the risk of pulmonary aspiration if the client should vomit. Options 2, 3, and 4 will not facilitate insertion of the tube or prevent aspiration.
Test-Taking Strategy: Use the process of elimination. Recalling that a concern with insertion of a nasogastric tube is pulmonary aspiration will direct you to option 1. Review the procedure for inserting a nasogastric tube if you had difficulty with this question.
Level of Cognitive Ability: Application
Client Needs: Physiological Integrity
Integrated Process: Nursing Process/Implementation
Content Area: Fundamental Skills
Reference: Perry, A., & Potter, P. (2002). *Clinical nursing skills and techniques* (5th ed.). St. Louis: Mosby, p. 660.

9. *Answer:* **4**
Rationale: Elevation of the affected leg facilitates blood flow by the force of gravity and also decreases venous pressure, which in turn relieves edema and pain. The foot of the bed is elevated and bed rest is indicated to prevent emboli and to prevent pressure fluctuations in the venous system that occur with walking. The positions in options 1, 2, and 3 are incorrect.
Test-Taking Strategy: Use the process of elimination. Recalling the pathophysiology related to the venous system will assist

in directing you to option 4. Review care to the client with thrombophlebitis if you had difficulty with this question.
Level of Cognitive Ability: Application
Client Needs: Physiological Integrity
Integrated Process: Nursing Process/Implementation
Content Area: Fundamental Skills
References: Linton, A., & Maebius, N. (2003). *Introduction to medical-surgical nursing* (3rd ed.). Philadelphia: W.B. Saunders, p. 633.
Phipps, W., Monahan, F., Sands, J., Marek, J., & Neighbors, M. (2003). *Medical-surgical nursing: Health and illness perspectives* (7th ed.). St. Louis: Mosby, p. 797.

10. *Answer:* **3**
Rationale: After craniotomy, the head of the bed is elevated 30 to 45 degrees (semi-Fowler's to Fowler's position), and the client's head is maintained in a midline, neutral position to facilitate venous drainage. Options 1, 2, and 4 are incorrect positions.
Test-Taking Strategy: Focus on the surgical procedure. Recalling that a goal of care after this surgery is to facilitate venous drainage will direct you to option 3. Review care to the client after craniotomy if you had difficulty with this question.
Level of Cognitive Ability: Application
Client Needs: Physiological Integrity
Integrated Process: Nursing Process/Planning

Content Area: Fundamental Skills
Reference: Linton, A., & Maebius, N. (2003). *Introduction to medical-surgical nursing* (3rd ed.). Philadelphia: W.B. Saunders, p. 382.

ALTERNATE FORMAT QUESTION: FILL IN THE BLANK
Answer: High Fowler's position
Rationale: Positioning the client upright (high Fowler's position), with the legs dangling over the side of the bed, has an immediate effect of decreasing venous return and decreasing lung congestion.
Test-Taking Strategy: Think about the physiological effects of pulmonary edema. Recall that the lung congestion that occurs in this disorder results in severe hypoxemia. This will help in determining the optimal position for the client. Review care of the client who develops pulmonary edema if you had difficulty with this question.
Level of Cognitive Ability: Application
Client Needs: Physiological Integrity
Integrated Process: Nursing Process/Implementation
Content Area: Fundamental Skills
Reference: Ignatavicius, D., & Workman, M. (2002). *Medical surgical nursing: Critical thinking for collaborative care* (4th ed.). Philadelphia: W.B. Saunders, p. 710.

REFERENCES

Chernecky, C., & Berger, B. (2004). *Laboratory tests and diagnostic procedures* (4th ed.). Philadelphia: W.B. Saunders.

Christensen, B., & Kockrow, E. (2003). *Foundations of nursing* (4th ed.). St. Louis: Mosby.

Ignatavicius, D., & Workman, M. (2002). *Medical surgical nursing: Critical thinking for collaborative care* (4th ed.). Philadelphia: W.B. Saunders.

Lewis, S., Heitkemper, M., & Dirksen, S. (2004). *Medical-surgical nursing: Assessment and management of clinical problems* (6th ed.). St. Louis: Mosby.

Linton, A., & Maebius, N. (2003). *Introduction to medical-surgical nursing* (3rd ed.). Philadelphia: W.B. Saunders.

National Council of State Boards of Nursing. (2005). *Detailed test plan for the National Council licensure examination for practical/vocational nurses.* Chicago: Author.

Pagana, K., & Pagana, T. (2003). *Mosby's diagnostic and laboratory test reference* (6th ed.). St. Louis: Mosby.

Perry, A., & Potter, P. (2002). *Clinical nursing skills and techniques* (5th ed.). St. Louis: Mosby.

Phipps, W., Monahan, F., Sands, J., Marek, J., & Neighbors, M. (2003). *Medical-surgical nursing: Health and illness perspectives* (7th ed.). St. Louis: Mosby.

Care of a Client with a Tube

PYRAMID TERMS

chest tube Returns negative pressure to the intrapleural space; used to remove abnormal accumulations of air and fluids from the plural space.

endotracheal tube Used to maintain a patent airway and is indicated when the client needs mechanical ventilation.

gastrointestinal (GI) intubation Insertion of a tube into the stomach or intestine.

intestinal tube Passed nasally and designed to enter the small intestine through the pyloric sphincter because of the weight of a small bag of mercury at the end of the tube; used to decompress the bowel or to remove intestinal contents.

Miller-Abbott tube A double-lumen tube passed nasally into the small intestine; used to decompress the bowel or to remove intestinal contents.

Sengstaken-Blakemore Tube A triple-lumen gastric tube with an inflatable esophageal balloon, an inflatable gastric balloon, and a gastric aspiration lumen; used as a treatment modality for the client with esophageal varices.

Tracheostomy Artificial opening created into the trachea to establish an airway.

◢ PYRAMID TO SUCCESS

The Pyramid to Success focuses on the common types of tubes used in the clinical setting. The NCLEX-PN examination is likely to address content areas related to the appropriate care of certain tubes and the immediate interventions required if a complication arises. Focus on the specific data collection points related to the specific type of tube. Review procedures for verifying correct placement of a tube and procedures for administering medications or feedings through a tube, if appropriate. Pyramid points also focus on interventions associated with complications or emergencies that may occur. The Integrated Processes addressed in this chapter include Caring, Clinical Problem-Solving Process (Nursing Process), Communication and Documentation, and Teaching/ Learning.

CLIENT NEEDS
Safe, Effective Care Environment

Advance directives
Advocacy related to client's concerns
Asepsis in administering care
Client rights
Consultations and referrals as prescribed
Establishing priorities
Handling infectious materials
Informed consent for invasive procedure
Standard precautions

Health Promotion and Maintenance

Client and family instructions regarding care at home
Disease prevention
Lifestyle choices
Techniques of collecting physical data

Psychosocial Integrity

Home care services
Situational role changes
Support systems
Therapeutic interactions
Unexpected body image changes

Physiological Integrity

Administering medications through a gastrointestinal (GI) tube
Assisting with emergency interventions for complications
Diagnostic tests to confirm accurate placement of tube
Laboratory values
Measures to ensure basic care and comfort
Nutrition and hydration
Potential complications associated with the tube

I. NASOGASTRIC (NG) TUBES (Figure 19-1)

A. Description
1. Short tubes used to intubate the stomach
2. Inserted from the nose to the stomach

B. Types of tubes (Figure 19-2)
1. Levine
   a. Single-lumen nasogastric tube
   b. Used to remove gastric contents via intermittent suction, or to provide tube feedings
2. Salem sump
   a. Double-lumen nasogastric tube with an air vent (pigtail)
   b. Used for decompression with continuous suction
   c. Air vent is not to be clamped and is to be kept above the level of the stomach
   d. If leakage occurs through the air vent, instill 30 mL of air into the air vent and irrigate the main lumen with normal saline (NS)

C. Determining placement
1. Note that the most reliable method to determine placement is by x-ray study, which should be performed after initial placement
2. Determine tube placement every 4 hours and before administering feedings or medications
3. Determine tube placement by aspirating gastric contents and measuring the pH, which should be 4 or lower (pH values higher than 6 indicate intestinal placement)
4. Inserting 5 to 10 mL of air into the NG tube and listening for the rush of air over the stomach with a stethoscope is an alternative method for determining placement, but is not as reliable as an x-ray study or checking gastric pH

D. Checking residual
1. Check residual volumes every 4 hours, before each feeding, or before giving medications
2. Aspirate all stomach contents (residual) and measure amount
3. Reinstill residual feeding to prevent excessive fluid and electrolyte losses unless the residual volume appears abnormal
4. Usually, if the residual is less than 100, the feeding is administered (physician's orders and agency policy are followed)

E. Irrigating
1. Perform irrigation every 4 hours to check the patency of the tube
2. Check placement before irrigating
3. Gently instill 30 to 50 mL water or normal saline (depending on agency policy) with an irrigation syringe
4. Pull back on the syringe plunger to withdraw the fluid to check patency; repeat if the tube remains sluggish

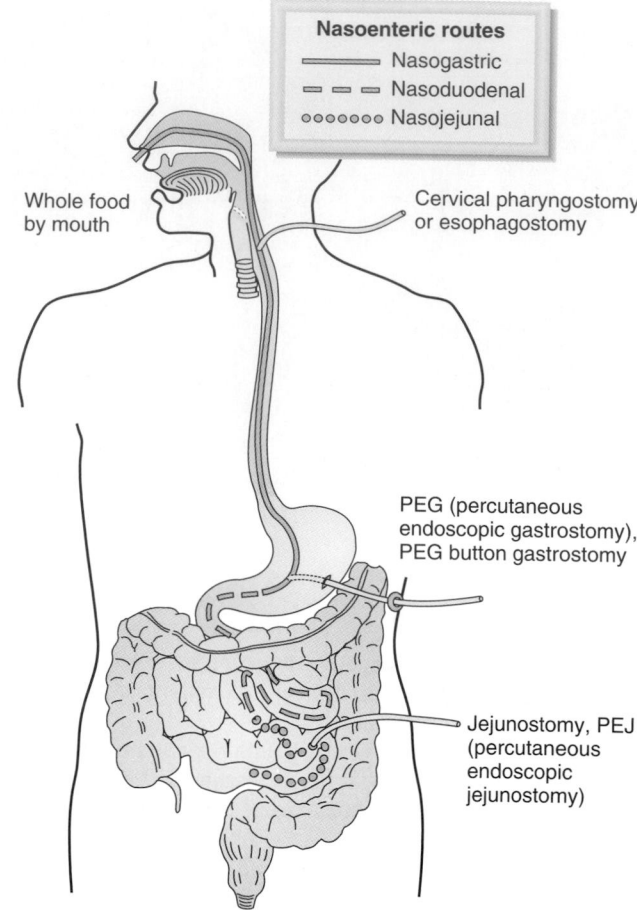

FIG. 19-1 Diagram of the placement of enteral feeding tubes. (From Linton, A., & Maebius, N. [2003]. *Introduction to medical-surgical nursing* (3rd ed.). Philadelphia: W.B. Saunders.)

F. Removal of an NG tube: Ask the client to take a deep breath and hold; remove the tube slowly and evenly over the course of 3 to 6 seconds (coil the tube around the hand as it is being removed)

II. GI TUBE FEEDINGS

A. Tubes
1. Nasogastric: Nose to stomach
2. Gastrostomy: Stomach
3. Jejunostomy: Jejunum

B. Types of administration
1. Intermittent (bolus)
   a. Resembles normal meal feeding patterns
   b. Approximately 300 to 400 mL of formula is administered over a 30- to 60-minute period every 3 to 6 hours
2. Continuous
   a. Administered continuously for 24 hours
   b. An infusion pump regulates the flow
3. Cyclical
   a. Administered either in the daytime or nighttime for 8 to 16 hours

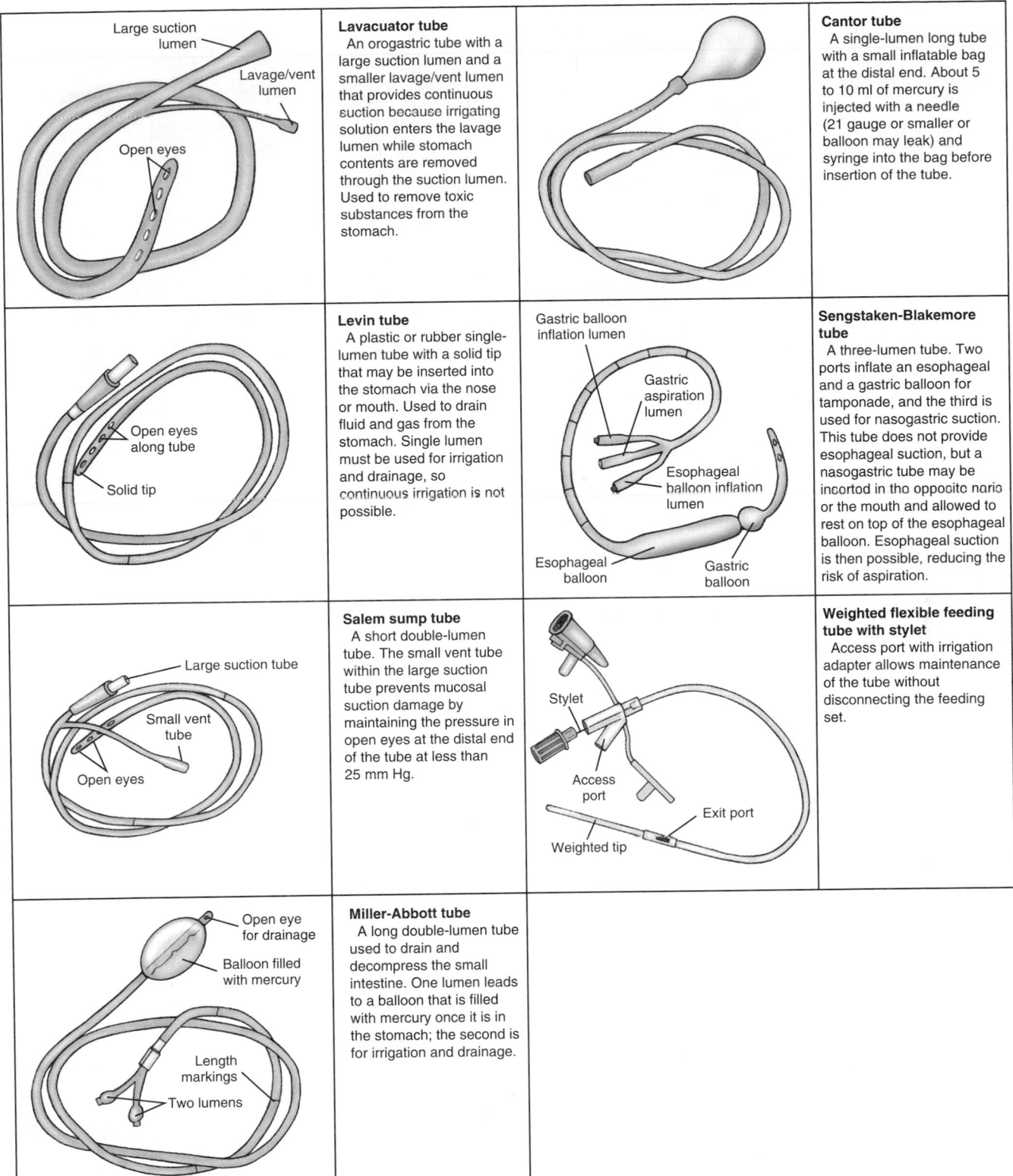

Lavacuator tube
An orogastric tube with a large suction lumen and a smaller lavage/vent lumen that provides continuous suction because irrigating solution enters the lavage lumen while stomach contents are removed through the suction lumen. Used to remove toxic substances from the stomach.

Cantor tube
A single-lumen long tube with a small inflatable bag at the distal end. About 5 to 10 ml of mercury is injected with a needle (21 gauge or smaller or balloon may leak) and syringe into the bag before insertion of the tube.

Levin tube
A plastic or rubber single-lumen tube with a solid tip that may be inserted into the stomach via the nose or mouth. Used to drain fluid and gas from the stomach. Single lumen must be used for irrigation and drainage, so continuous irrigation is not possible.

Sengstaken-Blakemore tube
A three-lumen tube. Two ports inflate an esophageal and a gastric balloon for tamponade, and the third is used for nasogastric suction. This tube does not provide esophageal suction, but a nasogastric tube may be inserted in the opposite naris or the mouth and allowed to rest on top of the esophageal balloon. Esophageal suction is then possible, reducing the risk of aspiration.

Salem sump tube
A short double-lumen tube. The small vent tube within the large suction tube prevents mucosal suction damage by maintaining the pressure in open eyes at the distal end of the tube at less than 25 mm Hg.

Weighted flexible feeding tube with stylet
Access port with irrigation adapter allows maintenance of the tube without disconnecting the feeding set.

Miller-Abbott tube
A long double-lumen tube used to drain and decompress the small intestine. One lumen leads to a balloon that is filled with mercury once it is in the stomach; the second is for irrigation and drainage.

FIG. 19-2 Examples of tubes used in the digestive tract. (From Linton, A., & Maebius, N. [2003]. *Introduction to medical-surgical nursing* [3rd ed.]. Philadelphia: W.B. Saunders.)

b. An infusion pump regulates the flow

c. Feedings at night allow for more freedom during the day

C. Administering feedings

1. If feedings are prescribed, x-ray confirmation should be done before initiating feedings after insertion of the tube

2. Position the client in high Fowler's; also position on the right side if comatose

3. Warm feeding to room temperature to prevent diarrhea and cramps

4. Aspirate all stomach contents (residual), measure amount, and return contents to the stomach to prevent electrolyte imbalances (unless residual appears abnormal)

5. Check physician's orders and agency policy regarding residual amounts; usually, if the residual is less than 100 mL, the feeding is administered; large-volume aspirates indicate delayed gastric emptying and place the client at risk for aspiration

6. Check tube placement by aspirating gastric contents and measuring the pH (should be 4 or lower)

7. Check bowel sounds; feeding is held and the physician is notified if bowel sounds are absent

8. Use a feeding pump for continuous or cyclic feedings

9. For an intermittent (bolus) feeding, leave the client in a high Fowler's position for 30 minutes after feeding

10. For a continuous feeding, keep the client in a semi-Fowler's position at all times (30 to 45 degrees)

D. Precautions

1. Change feeding container and tubing every 24 hours

2. Do not hang more solution than will be required for a 4-hour period to prevent bacterial growth

3. Check the expiration date on the formula before administering

4. Shake the formula well before inserting it into the feeding bag

5. Always check placement of the tube before feeding

6. Always check bowel sounds, and do not administer any feedings if bowel sounds are absent

7. Add a drop of methylene blue to the feeding, particularly with clients who have endotracheal or tracheal tubes; suspect tracheoesophageal fistula when blue gastric contents appear in tracheal excretion; if this is noted, notify the registered nurse and physician immediately

8. Administer the feeding at the prescribed rate, or via gravity flow (intermittent bolus feedings) with a 60-mL syringe with the plunger removed (Figure 19-3)

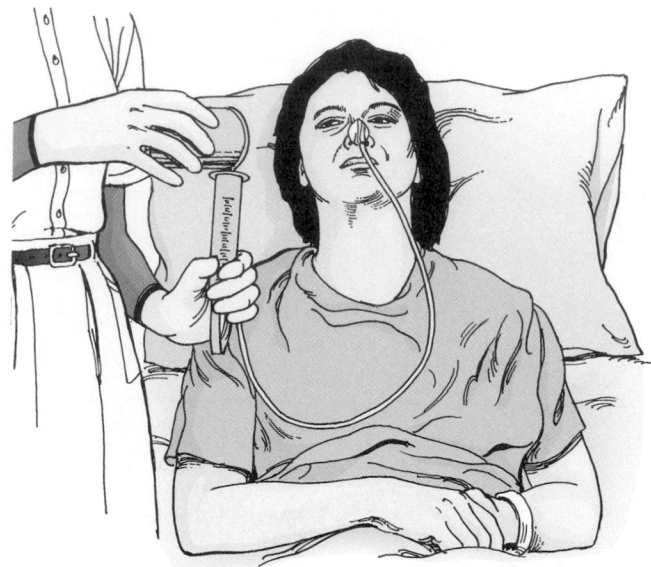

FIG. 19-3 Intermittent feeding. (From Perry A., & Potter P. [2002]. *Clinical nursing skills and nursing techniques.* St. Louis: Mosby.)

9. Gently flush with 30 to 50 mL water or normal saline (depending on agency policy) with an irrigation syringe after feeding

III. MEDICATIONS VIA NASOGASTRIC OR GASTROSTOMY TUBE

A. Crush medications or use elixir forms of medications

B. Ensure that the medication ordered can be crushed or that the capsule can be opened

C. Dissolve crushed medication or capsule contents in 5 to 10 mL of water

D. Check placement and residual before instilling medications

E. Draw up the medication into a catheter tip syringe, clear excess air, and insert the medication into the tube

F. Flush with 30 to 50 mL of water or NS (depending on agency policy)

G. Clamp the tube for 30 to 60 minutes (depending on the medication and agency policy)

IV. INTESTINAL TUBES (Figure 19-4)

A. Description

1. Passed nasally into the small intestine

2. Used to decompress the bowel or to remove intestinal contents

3. Designed to enter the small intestine through the pyloric sphincter because of the weight of a small bag of mercury at the end

B. Types of tubes (see Figure 19-2)

1. Cantor or Harris

2. **Miller-Abbott tube**

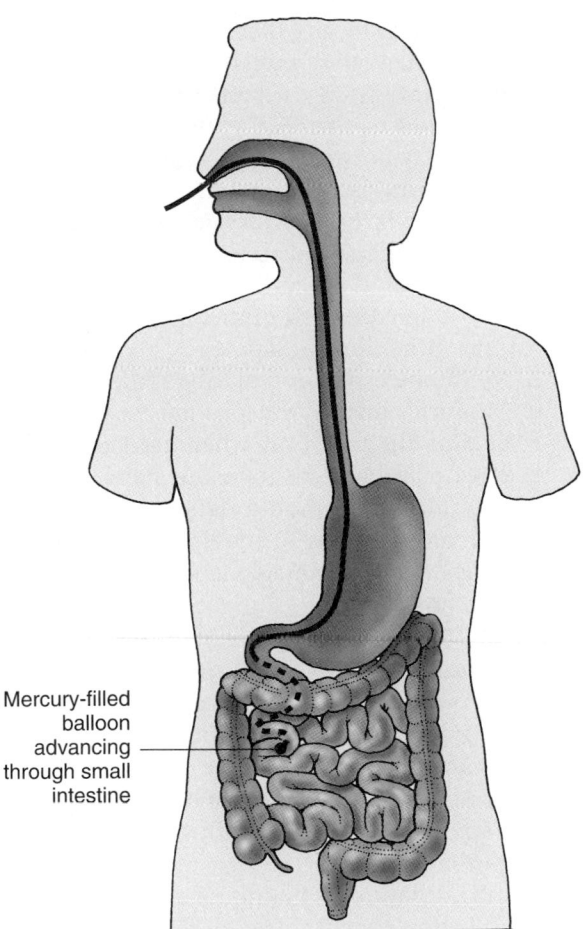

Mercury-filled
balloon
advancing
through small
intestine

FIG. 19-4   A nasoenteric tube. (From Linton, A., &
Maebius, N. [2003]. *Introduction to medical-surgical
nursing* (3rd ed.). Philadelphia: W.B. Saunders.)

C. Interventions
  1. Position the client on the right side to facilitate passage of the mercury bag within the tube through the pylorus of the stomach and into the small intestine
  2. Do not secure the tube to the client's face with tape until it has reached final placement (may take several hours) in the intestines
  3. An x-ray study is performed to verify desired placement
  4. Monitor drainage from the tube
  5. If the tube becomes blocked, the registered nurse and physician is notified; a small amount of air injected into the lumen may be prescribed to clear the tube
  6. Check the abdomen and measure abdominal girth
  7. When the tube is removed, dispose of the mercury in the appropriate manner as per agency policy

V. ESOPHAGEAL AND GASTRIC TUBES
A. Description
  1. Used to apply pressure against esophageal veins to control bleeding

  2. Not used if the client has ulceration or necrosis of the esophagus or has had previous esophageal surgery
B. **Sengstaken-Blakemore tube** (see Figure 19-2)
  1. Triple-lumen gastric tube with an inflatable esophageal balloon, an inflatable gastric balloon, and a gastric aspiration lumen
  2. The gastric balloon applies pressure at the cardioesophageal junction to compress gastric varices directly and to decrease blood flow to esophageal varices; traction is applied to maintain the gastric balloon in place
  3. The esophageal balloon directly compresses esophageal varices
  4. An x-ray study of the upper abdomen and chest confirms placement
  5. Gastric contents are aspirated by gastric lavage or intermittent suction via the gastric aspiration port
  6. With the **Sengstaken-Blakemore tube**, a nasogastric tube is also inserted into the opposite nares to collect secretions that accumulate above the esophageal balloon
C. Interventions
  1. The patency and integrity of all balloons are checked before insertion, and each lumen is labeled
  2. The client is placed in an upright or Fowler's position for insertion
  3. Prepare the client for an x-ray study immediately after insertion to verify placement
  4. Maintain head elevation once the tube is in place
  5. The balloon ports are double-clamped to prevent air leaks
  6. Scissors are kept at the bedside at all times
  7. The client is monitored for respiratory distress; if it occurs, notify the registered nurse immediately; the tubes will be cut to deflate the balloons
  8. Monitor for increased bloody drainage that may indicate persistent bleeding
  9. Monitor for signs of esophageal rupture that include a drop in blood pressure, increased heart rate, back and upper abdominal pain (esophageal rupture is an emergency and must be reported immediately)

VI. URINARY AND RENAL TUBES
A. Routine urinary catheter care
  1. Use gloves and wash the perineal area with warm soapy water
  2. With the nondominant hand, pull back the labia or foreskin to expose the meatus (in the adult male, return the foreskin to its normal position)
  3. Clean along the catheter with soap and water
  4. Anchor the catheter to the thigh
  5. Maintain the catheter bag below the level of the bladder
B. Ureteral and nephrostomy tubes
  1. Never clamp the tubes

2. Maintain patency
3. Monitor output closely; urine output of less than 30 mL/hour or a lack of output for more than 15 minutes should be reported immediately

VII. RESPIRATORY SYSTEM TUBES

A. Endotracheal tubes (Figure 19-5)
   1. Description
      a. Used to maintain a patent airway
      b. Indicated when the client needs mechanical ventilation
      c. If the client requires an artificial airway for longer than 10 to 14 days, a **tracheostomy** may be created to avoid mucosal and vocal cord damage that can be caused by the **endotracheal tube**
   2. Orotracheal
      a. Inserted through the mouth; allows use of a larger diameter tube and reduces the work of breathing
      b. Indicated when the client has a nasal obstruction or a predisposition to epistaxis
      c. Uncomfortable and can be manipulated by the tongue, causing airway obstruction; an oral airway may be needed to prevent the client from biting on the tube
   3. Nasotracheal
      a. Inserted through the nose and allows use of a smaller sized tube, which increases resistance and increases the client's work of breathing
      b. Discouraged in clients with bleeding disorders
      c. More comfortable for the client, and the client is unable to manipulate the tube with tongue
   4. Interventions
      a. Placement is confirmed by chest x-ray study (correct placement is 1 to 2 cm above the

carina) and by auscultating both sides of chest while manually ventilating with a resuscitation (Ambu) bag; if breath sounds and chest wall movement are absent on the left side, the tube may be in the right main stem bronchus
      b. If the tube is in the stomach, louder breath sounds will be heard over the stomach than over the chest, and abdominal distention will be present
      c. The tube is secured immediately after intubation with adhesive tape
      d. Monitor the position of tube at the lip or nose
      e. Monitor skin and mucous membranes
      f. Suction the tube only when needed
      g. The oral tube needs to be moved to the opposite side of the mouth daily to prevent pressure and necrosis of the lip and mouth area, prevent nerve damage, and facilitate inspection and cleaning of the mouth; moving the tube to the opposite side of the mouth should be done by two health care providers
      h. To prevent dislodgment, prevent pulling or tugging on the tube; suction, and coughing or speaking attempts by the client place extra stress on the tube and can cause dislodgment
      i. Keep a resuscitation (Ambu) bag at bedside at all times
      j. Cuff inflation is maintained to create a seal and allow for complete mechanical control of respiration
   5. Extubation
      a. Hyperoxygenate the client and suction the **endotracheal tube** and the oral cavity
      b. Place the client in semi-Fowler's position
      c. The cuff is deflated; have the client inhale and, at peak inspiration, the tube is removed and the airway is suctioned through the tube as it is pulled out
      d. After removal, instruct the client to cough and deep breathe to assist in removing accumulated secretions in the throat
      e. Apply oxygen therapy as prescribed
      f. Monitor for respiratory difficulty; contact the registered nurse and physician if respiratory difficulty occurs
      g. Inform the client that hoarseness or a sore throat is normal and that he or she should limit talking if it occurs

B. **Tracheostomy**
   1. Description
      a. A tracheotomy is a surgical incision into the trachea for the purpose of establishing an airway
      b. A **tracheostomy** is the stoma or opening that results from the tracheotomy
      c. The **tracheostomy** can be temporary or permanent

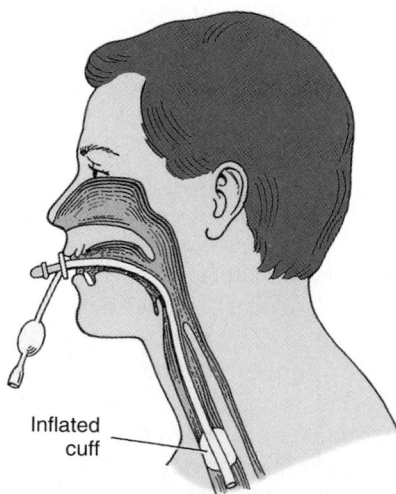

Inflated cuff

FIG. 19-5 Endotracheal tube with inflated cuff. (From Perry A., & Potter P. [2002]. *Clinical nursing skills and nursing techniques.* St. Louis: Mosby.)

2. Single-cannula tube: Has an outer but no inner cannula; used for client with a thick neck or client in whom a standard tube will not enter the trachea
3. Cuffed tube: Has an outer and inner cannula, obturator, and cuff
4. Cuffless tube
   a. Has an outer cannula, an open and plugged inner cannula, and obturator
   b. Used over the long term for evaluating the client's ability to breathe through the upper airway and for the client no longer at risk for aspiration
5. Fenestrated tube (Figure 19-6)
   a. Has an opening along the posterior wall of the outer cannula
   b. When the tube is capped, the client can breathe through the upper airway and can speak
   c. The cuff is always deflated before capping the tube
6. Foam-cuffed tube
   a. Cuff is larger than the standard cuffed tube
   b. Filled with foam, which may apply less pressure to the tracheal mucosa
7. Metal tube
   a. Has an outer and inner cannula and can be reused after sterilization
   b. Does not have a cuff and is most often used after a permanent tracheostomy or laryngectomy
8. Interventions
   a. Monitor respirations and for bilateral breath sounds
   b. Monitor pulse oximetry
   c. Encourage coughing and deep breathing
   d. Maintain a semi- to high Fowler's position
   e. Monitor for bleeding, difficulty breathing, and crepitus, which are indications of hemorrhage, pneumothorax, and subcutaneous emphysema
   f. Provide respiratory treatments, as prescribed
   g. Suction as needed; hyperoxygenate the client before suction
   h. If the client is allowed to eat, sit the client up for meals and ensure that the cuff is inflated (if the tube is not capped) for meals and for 1 hour after meals
   i. Assess the stoma and secretions for blood or purulent drainage
   j. Follow the physician's orders and agency policy for cleaning the **tracheostomy** site and inner cannula; usually, half-strength hydrogen peroxide is used
   k. Administer humidified oxygen as prescribed because the normal humidification process is bypassed in a client with a **tracheostomy**
   l. Obtain assistance in changing **tracheostomy** ties; after placing the new ties, cut and remove the old ties holding the tracheostomy tube in place (Figure 19-7)
   m. Never insert a decannulation plug into a **tracheostomy** tube until the cuff is deflated and the inner cannula is removed; prior insertion prevents airflow to the client
   n. Keep a resuscitation (Ambu) bag, obturator, clamps, and tracheotomy set at the bedside
9. Complications of a **tracheostomy** (Box 19-1)
   a. Tube obstruction
   b. Tube dislodgment
   c. Tracheomalacia
   d. Tracheal stenosis
   e. Tracheoesophageal fistula
   f. Trachea–innominate artery fistula

VIII. CHEST TUBE DRAINAGE SYSTEM
   (Figures 19-8 and 19-9)
A. Description
   1. Returns negative pressure to the intrapleural space

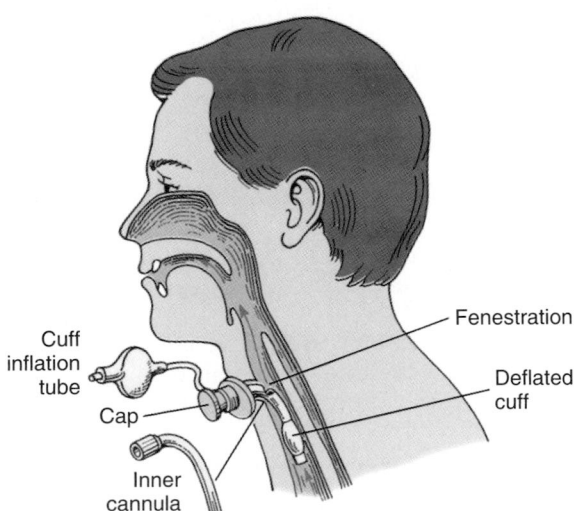

FIG. 19-6 Tracheostomy tube (fenestrated). (From Perry A., & Potter P. [2002]. *Clinical nursing skills and nursing techniques.* St. Louis: Mosby.)

Cuff inflation tube
Cap
Inner cannula
Fenestration
Deflated cuff

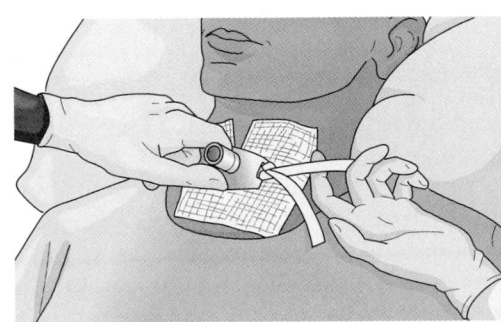

FIG. 19-7 Tracheostomy ties properly placed. (From Perry A., & Potter P. [2002]. *Clinical nursing skills and nursing techniques.* St. Louis: Mosby.)

BOX 19-1

Complications of a Tracheostomy

TUBE OBSTRUCTION
Data Collection
Difficulty in breathing
Noisy respirations
Difficulty in inserting the suction catheter
Thick, dry secretions
Unexplained peak pressures if client is on a mechanical
    ventilator
Prevention and Interventions
Assist the client to cough and deep breathe.
Provide humidification and suctioning.
Clean the inner cannula regularly.
Physician repositions or replaces the tube if obstruction
    occurs as a result of cuff prolapse over the end of the
    tube.

TUBE DISLODGMENT
Prevention and Interventions
Secure the tube in place.
Minimize manipulation and traction on the tube.
Ensure that the client does not pull on the tube.
Ensure that a tracheostomy tube of the same type and
    size is at the client's bedside.
Be familiar with institutional policy regarding replace-
    ment of a tracheostomy tube as a nursing procedure.
During the first 72 hours following surgical
placement of the tracheostomy:
The nurse manually ventilates the client by using a
    manual resuscitation (Ambu) bag while another nurse
    calls the resuscitation team for help.
After 72 hours following surgical placement of the
tracheostomy:
Extend the client's neck and open the tissues of the
    stoma to secure the airway.
Grasp the retention sutures (if they are present) to
    spread the opening.
Use a tracheal dilator (curved clamp) to hold the stoma
    open.
Prepare to assist in inserting the tracheostomy tube;
    place obturator into tracheostomy tube, replace the
    tube, and remove the obturator.
Maintain ventilation by resuscitation (Ambu) bag.
Check airflow and check for bilateral breath sounds.
If unable to secure an airway, call the resuscitation team
    and the anesthesiologist.

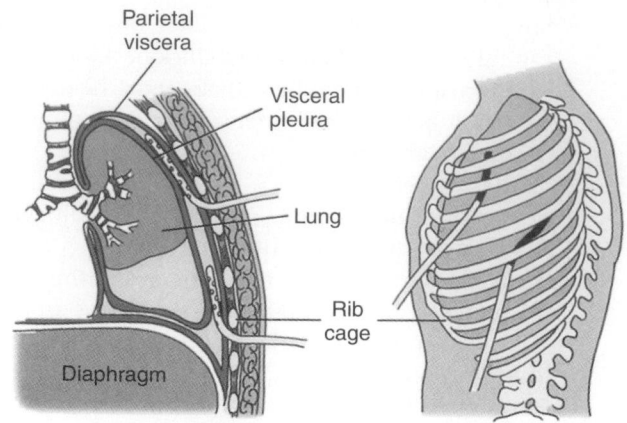

FIG. 19-8   Diagram of sites for chest tube placement. (From Perry A., & Potter P. [2002]. *Clinical nursing skills and nursing techniques.* St. Louis: Mosby.)

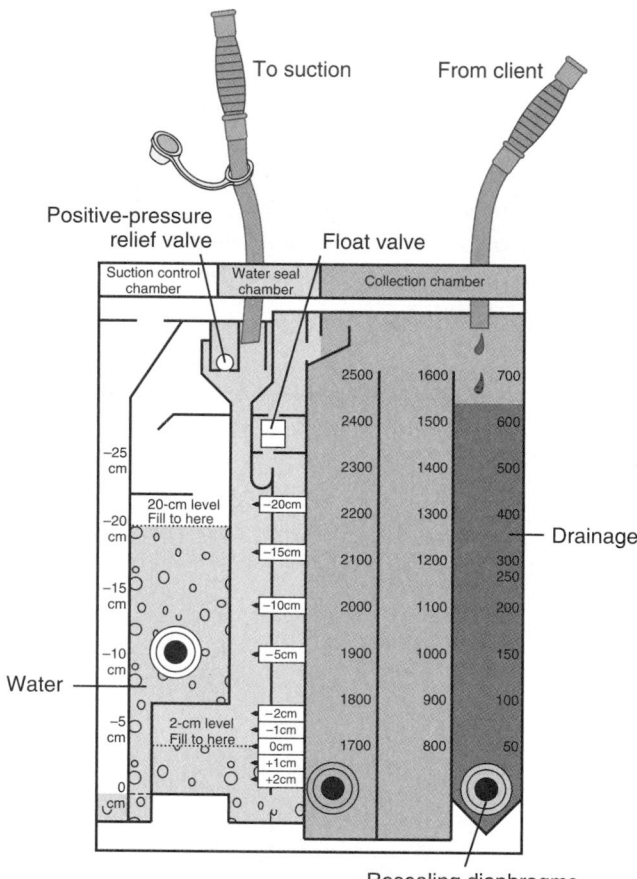

FIG. 19-9   A commonly used disposable chest drainage system combines the three bottles into a single device. (Courtesy Teleflex Medical, Fall River, MA.)

   2. Used to remove abnormal accumulations of air
      and fluid from the plural space
B. Collection chamber
   1. Where the **chest tube** from the client connects to
      the system
   2. Drainage from the tube drains into and collects
      in a series of calibrated columns in this chamber
C. Water seal chamber
   1. The tip of the tube is underwater, allowing fluid
      and air to drain from the pleural space and
      preventing air from entering the pleural space

   2. Water oscillates (moves up as the client inhales
      and moves down as the client exhales)
   3. Continuous bubbling indicates an air leak in the
      chest tube system

D. Suction control chamber
1. Provides suction, which can be controlled to provide negative pressure to the chest
2. This chamber is filled with various levels of water to achieve the desired level of suction; without this control, lung tissue could be sucked into the **chest tube**
3. Gentle bubbling in this chamber indicates that there is suction; does not indicate that air is escaping from the pleural space

E. Dry suction system
1. Because this is a dry suction system, absence of bubbling is noted in the suction control chamber
2. A knob on the collection device is used to set the prescribed amount of suction; then the wall suction source dial is turned until a small orange floater valve appears in the window on the device (when the orange floater valve is in the window, the correct amount of suction has been applied)

F. Interventions
1. Collection chamber
   a. Monitor drainage; the physician is notified if drainage is greater than 100 mL/hour, or if drainage becomes bright red or increases suddenly
   b. Mark the **chest tube** drainage in the collection chamber at 1- to 4-hour intervals, using a piece of tape
2. Water seal chamber
   a. Monitor for fluctuation of the fluid level in the water seal chamber
   b. Fluctuation in the water seal chamber stops if the tube is obstructed, if a dependent loop exists, if the suction is not working properly, or if the lung has re-expanded
   c. If the client has a known pneumothorax, intermittent bubbling in the water seal chamber is expected as air is drained from the chest, but continuous bubbling indicates an air leak in the system
   d. Notify the registered nurse and physician if there is continuous bubbling in the water seal chamber
3. Suction control chamber: Gentle bubbling should be noted in the suction control chamber (vigorous bubbling indicates an air leak, and the registered nurse and physician should be notified)
4. An occlusive sterile dressing is maintained at the insertion site
5. A chest radiograph assesses the position of the tube and determines whether the lung has re-expanded
6. Monitor respiratory status and listen to lung sounds
7. Monitor for signs of extended pneumothroax or hemothorax
8. Keep the drainage system below the level of the chest and the tubes free of kinks, dependent loops, or other obstructions
9. Ensure that all connections are secure
10. Encourage coughing and deep breathing
11. Change the client's position frequently to promote drainage and ventilation
12. Stripping or milking a **chest tube** is not done unless specifically ordered by a physician and if agency policy allows
13. Keep a clamp and a sterile occlusive dressing at the bedside at all times
14. A **chest tube** is never clamped without a written order from the physician; also, determine agency policy for clamping **chest tubes**
15. If the drainage system cracks or breaks, insert the chest tube into a bottle of sterile water; the cracked or broken system is removed and replaced with a new system
16. If the **chest tube** is accidentally pulled out of the chest, pinch the skin opening together, apply an occlusive sterile dressing, cover the dressing with overlapping pieces of 2-inch tape, and notify the registered nurse and the physician immediately
17. When the **chest tube** is removed, the client is asked to take a deep breath and hold it, and the tube is removed; a dry sterile dressing, petroleum gauze dressing, or Telfa dressing (depending on the physician's preference) is taped in place after removal of the **chest tube**
18. Depending on the physician's preference, when the **chest tube** is removed, the client may be asked to take a deep breath, exhale, and bear down (Valsalva's maneuver)

PRACTICE QUESTIONS

1. A registered nurse is preparing to insert a nasogastric (NG) tube in a client and asks the licensed practical nurse (LPN) to obtain supplies needed for the procedure. Which of the following supplies, if obtained by the LPN, indicates a need for education regarding this procedure?
   1. $^1/_2$-inch tape
   2. Oil-soluble lubricant
   3. A straw
   4. 50-mL catheter tip syringe

2. A nurse is checking for correct placement of a nasogastric (NG) tube. The nurse aspirates the stomach contents and checks the contents for pH. Which of the following pH values indicates correct placement of the tube?
   1. pH of 7.5
   2. pH of 7.35
   3. pH of 7.0
   4. pH of 4.0

3. A licensed practical nurse (LPN) is preparing to assist the registered nurse (RN) in removing a nasogastric (NG) tube from the client. The LPN would plan to instruct the client to do which of the following?

1. To perform a Valsalva maneuver
2. To take and hold a deep breath
3. To exhale
4. To inhale and exhale quickly

4. A nurse is preparing to administer medication through a nasogastric (NG) tube that is connected to suction. Which of the following indicates the accurate procedure related to the medication administration?
   1. Aspirate the NG tube after medication administration to maintain patency
   2. Position the client supine to assist in medication absorption
   3. Clamp the NG tube for 30 minutes after administration of the medication
   4. Change the suction setting to low intermittent suction for 30 minutes after medication administration

5. A nurse assists a physician with the insertion of a Miller-Abbott tube. After insertion of the tube, the nurse would assist the client to which of the following positions?
   1. On the right side
   2. On the left side
   3. Prone
   4. Left lateral Sims' position

6. A nurse is assigned to assist in caring for a client with esophageal varices who has a Sengstaken-Blakemore tube inserted. The nurse checks the client's room to ensure that which of the following priority items is at the bedside?
   1. An irrigation set
   2. A pair of scissors
   3. A Kelly clamp
   4. An obturator

7. A nurse is inserting an indwelling urinary catheter into the urethra of a male client. As the nurse inflates the balloon, the client complains of discomfort. The appropriate nursing action is to:
   1. Remove the syringe from the balloon; discomfort is normal and temporary
   2. Aspirate the fluid, advance the catheter farther, and reinflate the balloon
   3. Aspirate the fluid, withdraw the catheter slightly, and reinflate the balloon
   4. Aspirate the fluid, remove the catheter, and reinsert a new catheter

8. A nurse is inserting an indwelling urinary catheter into a male client. As the catheter is inserted into the urethra, urine begins to flow into the tubing. At this point, the nurse:
   1. Immediately inflates the balloon
   2. Withdraws the catheter approximately 1 inch and inflates the balloon
   3. Inserts the catheter until resistance is met and inflates the balloon
   4. Inserts the catheter 2.5 to 5 cm and inflates the balloon

9. A nurse is assigned to assist in caring for a client who has a chest tube. The nurse notes fluctuation of the fluid level in the water seal chamber. Based on this observation, which of the following actions would be appropriate?
   1. Empty the drainage
   2. Encourage the client to deep breathe
   3. Continue to monitor, because this is an expected finding
   4. Encourage the client to hold his or her breath periodically

10. A nurse is assigned to assist the physician with the removal of a chest tube. The nurse instructs the client to do which of the following during removal of the chest tube?
    1. Stay very still
    2. Inhale and exhale quickly
    3. Exhale slowly
    4. Perform the Valsalva maneuver

11. A nurse is preparing to change the neck ties on a tracheostomy tube. To perform this procedure, the nurse would plan to:
    1. Remove the old ties, clean the site, and then apply the new ties
    2. Obtain a second health care team member to assist
    3. Call the physician for assistance in changing the ties
    4. Call the respiratory therapy department for assistance in changing the ties

12. A nurse is preparing to begin a continuous tube feeding on a client with a nasogastric tube. The nurse positions the client:
    1. Supine
    2. Supine on the right side
    3. With the head elevated 15 degrees
    4. With the head elevated 45 degrees

13. A nurse is preparing to administer an intermittent tube feeding to a client with a nasogastric tube. The nurse checks the residual and obtains an amount of 200 mL. The nurse would:
    1. Administer the feeding
    2. Flush the tubing with 30 mL of water
    3. Hold the feeding
    4. Elevate the head of the bed to 90 degrees and administer the feeding

14. A nurse is preparing to administer a continuous tube feeding to a client with a nasogastric tube. The physician has prescribed an amount of 100 mL/hour. The nurse plans to fill the feeding bag with:
    1. 400 mL of formula
    2. 600 mL of formula
    3. 800 mL of formula
    4. Enough formula to last for 8 hours

15. A nurse is preparing to suction a client through a tracheostomy tube. The nurse avoids which of the following when performing this procedure?

1. Moistening the catheter tip in sterile saline solution before suctioning
2. Preoxygenating the client before suctioning
3. Introducing the catheter into the tracheostomy tube using a sterile gloved hand
4. Placing suction on the catheter while introducing the catheter into the tracheostomy tube

16. A nurse is suctioning a client through a tracheostomy tube. The nurse plans to apply suction during the withdrawal of the catheter for a period of time no greater than:
   1. 10 seconds
   2. 25 seconds
   3. 30 seconds
   4. 35 seconds

17. A nurse is told that an assigned client will have a fenestrated tracheostomy tube inserted. The nurse prepares the client for the procedure knowing that this type of tube:
   1. Is necessary for mechanical ventilation
   2. Enables the client to speak
   3. Prevents air from being inhaled through the tracheostomy opening
   4. Prevents the client from speaking

18. A nurse is told that an assigned client will have the chest tubes removed. In preparation for the procedure, the nurse plans to:
   1. Clamp the chest tubes
   2. Disconnect the drainage system
   3. Empty the drainage system
   4. Administer pain medication 30 minutes before the procedure

19. A nurse is assisting in caring for a client with a chest tube. The nurse understands that which of the following is an incorrect action in the care of the client?
   1. Be sure all connections remain airtight
   2. Be sure all connections are taped
   3. Pin the tubing to the bed clothes
   4. Do not allow the tubing to become kinked or obstructed by the weight of the client

20. A nurse is assigned to care for a client who has a chest tube. The nurse is told to monitor the client for subcutaneous emphysema. The nurse monitors the client for this complication by:
   1. Monitoring respirations hourly
   2. Palpating for leakage of air into the subcutaneous tissues
   3. Monitoring for pain
   4. Checking the blood pressure every 2 hours

ALTERNATE FORMAT QUESTION: MULTIPLE RESPONSE

A nurse is assisting in monitoring the functioning of a chest tube drainage system in a client who just returned from the recovery room following a thoracotomy with wedge resection. Select all expected findings.

___ Excessive bubbling in the water seal chamber
___ Vigorous bubbling in the suction control chamber
___ Fluctuation of water in the tube in the water seal chamber during inhalation and exhalation
___ 50 mL of drainage in the drainage collection chamber
___ An occlusive dressing is in place over the chest tube insertion site
___ The drainage system is maintained below the client's chest

ANSWERS

1. *Answer:* 2
Rationale: Water-soluble lubricant is used to lubricate 3 inches of the tube at the insertion end. An oil lubricant is not used because, if the tube accidentally enters the bronchus, pneumonia can develop. Half-inch tape is used to secure the tube after correct placement is verified. A 50-mL catheter tip syringe is used to aspirate gastric contents to confirm placement. The client will be asked to take a sip of water through a straw to help with the passage of the tube.
Test-Taking Strategy: Note the key words, *indicates a need for education*, in the stem of the question. Remember that water-soluble lubricant must be used to lubricate the tube. Review this procedure if you had difficulty with this question.
Level of Cognitive Ability: Comprehension
Client Needs: Physiological Integrity
Integrated Process: Teaching/Learning
Content Area: Fundamental Skills
Reference: Christensen, B., & Kockrow, E. (2003). *Foundations of nursing* (4th ed.). St. Louis: Mosby, p. 478.

2. *Answer:* 4
Rationale: If the NG tube is in the stomach, the pH of the contents will be acidic. Option 1 indicates an alkaline pH. Option 2 indicates a neutral pH. Option 3 indicates a slightly acidic pH.
Test-Taking Strategy: Use the process of elimination. Recalling that gastric contents are acidic will easily direct you to option 4. Review the procedure for checking NG tube placement if you had difficulty with this question.
Level of Cognitive Ability: Comprehension
Client Needs: Physiological Integrity
Integrated Process: Nursing Process/Evaluation
Content Area: Fundamental Skills
Reference: Christensen, B., & Kockrow, E. (2003). *Foundations of nursing* (4th ed.). St. Louis: Mosby, p. 479.

3. *Answer:* 2
Rationale: When the nurse removes an NG tube, the client is instructed to take and hold a deep breath. This will close the epiglottis and the airway will be temporarily obstructed during the tube removal. This allows for easy withdrawal of

the tube through the esophagus into the nose. The nurse removes the tube with one very smooth continuous pull. Options 1, 3, and 4 are incorrect.
Test-Taking Strategy: Use the process of elimination and focus on the issue, removing an NG tube. Visualize the procedure as a guide considering what each client action identified in the options would produce. Review the procedure for removing an NG tube if you had difficulty with this question.
Level of Cognitive Ability: Application
Client Needs: Physiological Integrity
Integrated Process: Nursing Process/Implementation
Content Area: Fundamental Skills
Reference: Christensen, B., & Kockrow, E. (2003). *Foundations of nursing* (4th ed.). St. Louis: Mosby, p. 483.

4. *Answer: 3*
Rationale: If a client has an NG tube connected to suction, the nurse should wait up to 30 minutes before reconnecting the tube to the suction apparatus to allow adequate time for medication absorption. Aspirating the NG tube will remove the medication just administered. Low intermittent suction will also remove the medication just administered. The client should not be placed in the supine position because of the risk for aspiration.
Test-Taking Strategy: Use the process of elimination. Eliminate options 1 and 4 first because these actions are similar and will produce the same effect. Recalling that the client should not be placed in a supine position will assist in eliminating option 2. Review the procedure for administering medications through an NG tube if you had difficulty with this question.
Level of Cognitive Ability: Application
Client Needs: Physiological Integrity
Integrated Process: Nursing Process/Implementation
Content Area: Fundamental Skills
References: Potter, P., & Perry, A. (2005). *Fundamentals of nursing* (6th ed.). St. Louis: Mosby, p. 464.
Phipps, W., Monahan, F., Sands, J., Marek, J., & Neighbors, M. (2003). *Medical-surgical nursing: Health and illness perspectives* (7th ed.). St. Louis: Mosby, p. 1058.

5. *Answer: 1*
Rationale: A Miller-Abbott tube is an intestinal tube that has a double lumen, one for a mercury balloon and the other for suction or drainage. After insertion of the tube, the tube is allowed to advance for several hours. The client is positioned on the right side to facilitate passage through the pylorus of the stomach and into the small intestine. Options 2, 3, and 4 are incorrect.
Test-Taking Strategy: Use the process of elimination. Eliminate options 2 and 4 because they are similar. From the remaining options, recalling the purpose of this tube and the anatomy of the body will assist in directing you to option 1. Review care of the client with a Miller-Abbott tube if you had difficulty with this question.
Level of Cognitive Ability: Application
Client Needs: Physiological Integrity
Integrated Process: Nursing Process/Implementation
Content Area: Fundamental Skills
Reference: Lewis, S., Heitkemper, M., & Dirksen, S. (2004). *Medical-surgical nursing: Assessment and management of clinical problems* (6th ed.). St. Louis: Mosby, p. 1081.

6. *Answer: 2*
Rationale: When the client has a Sengstaken-Blakemore tube, a pair of scissors must be kept at the client's bedside at all times. The client needs to be observed for sudden respiratory distress that occurs if the gastric balloon ruptures and the entire tube moves upward. If this occurs, the registered nurse (RN) is notified immediately and the balloon lumens will be cut. An obturator and a Kelly clamp are kept at the bedside of a client with a tracheostomy. An irrigation set may be kept at the bedside, but is not the priority item.
Test-Taking Strategy: Use knowledge regarding the structure, function, and placement of a Sengstaken-Blakemore tube to answer this question. Note the key word, *priority*, in the stem of the question. This should assist in eliminating options 1, 3, and 4. Review care of a client with a Sengstaken-Blakemore tube if you had difficulty with this question.
Level of Cognitive Ability: Application
Client Needs: Safe, Effective Care Environment
Integrated Process: Nursing Process/Implementation
Content Area: Fundamental Skills
Reference: Black, J., & Hawks, J. (2005). *Medical-surgical nursing: Clinical management for positive outcomes* (7th ed.). Philadelphia: W.B. Saunders, p. 1345.

7. *Answer: 2*
Rationale: If the balloon is malpositioned in the urethra, inflating the balloon could produce trauma, and pain will occur. If pain occurs, the fluid should be aspirated and the catheter inserted a little farther to provide sufficient space to inflate the balloon. The catheter's balloon is behind the opening at the insertion tip. Inserting the catheter the extra distance will ensure that the balloon is inflated inside the bladder and not in the urethra. There is no need to remove the catheter and reinsert a new one. Pain when the balloon is inflated is not normal or temporary.
Test-Taking Strategy: Visualize the procedure to answer the question. Option 1 can be eliminated, because discomfort is neither normal nor temporary when caused by the balloon being inflated. It is not necessary to remove the catheter and reinsert a new catheter. Option 3 will not properly position the balloon in the bladder for safe balloon inflation. Review the procedure for inserting a urinary catheter if you had difficulty with this question.
Level of Cognitive Ability: Application
Client Needs: Physiological Integrity
Integrated Process: Nursing Process/Implementation
Content Area: Fundamental Skills
Reference: Christensen, B., & Kockrow, E. (2003). *Foundations of nursing* (4th ed). St. Louis: Mosby, p. 467.

8. *Answer: 4*
Rationale: The catheter's balloon is behind the opening at the insertion tip. The catheter is inserted 2.5 to 5 cm after urine begins to flow to provide sufficient space to inflate the balloon. Inserting the catheter the extra distance will ensure that the balloon is inflated inside the bladder and not in the urethra. Inflating the balloon in the urethra could produce trauma.
Test-Taking Strategy: Visualize the proper procedure for inserting an indwelling urinary catheter to assist you in answering this question. Note the key words, *urine begins to flow*. Options 2 and 3 can easily be eliminated. Eliminate option 1 next

because of the word "immediately." Review the procedure for bladder catheterization if you had difficulty with this question.
Level of Cognitive Ability: Application
Client Needs: Physiological Integrity
Integrated Process: Nursing Process/Implementation
Content Area: Fundamental Skills
References: Christensen, B., & Kockrow, E. (2003). *Foundations of nursing* (4th ed.). St. Louis: Mosby, p. 467.
Potter, P., & Perry, A. (2005). *Fundamentals of nursing* (6th ed.). St. Louis: Mosby, p. 1355.

9. *Answer: 3*
Rationale: The presence of fluctuation of the fluid level in the water seal chamber indicates a patent drainage system. With normal breathing, the water level rises with inspiration and falls with expiration. The apparatus and all connections must remain airtight at all times and the drainage is never emptied. Encouraging the client to deep breathe is unrelated to this observation. The client is not told to hold his or her breath.
Test-Taking Strategy: Focusing on the issue of the question, fluctuation of the fluid level in the water seal chamber, will assist in eliminating options 1, 2, and 4. Review expected and unexpected findings when caring for a client with a chest tube if you had difficulty with this question.
Level of Cognitive Ability: Application
Client Needs: Physiological Integrity
Integrated Process: Nursing Process/Implementation
Content Area: Fundamental Skills
References: Linton, A., & Maebius, N. (2003). *Introduction to medical-surgical nursing* (3rd ed.). Philadelphia: W.B. Saunders, pp. 473-474.
Potter, P., & Perry, A. (2005). *Fundamentals of nursing* (6th ed.). St. Louis: Mosby, p. 1120.

10. *Answer: 4*
Rationale: When the chest tube is removed, the client is asked to perform the Valsalva maneuver (take a deep breath, exhale, and bear down), the tube is quickly withdrawn, and an airtight dressing is taped in place. An alternative instruction is to ask the client to take a deep breath and hold the breath while the tube is removed. Options 1, 2, and 3 are incorrect client instructions.
Test-Taking Strategy: Use the process of elimination. Visualize the procedure and the client instructions in each option as you answer the question. This will direct you to option 4. If you had difficulty with this question, review the procedure for removal of a chest tube.
Level of Cognitive Ability: Application
Client Needs: Physiological Integrity
Integrated Process: Nursing Process/Implementation
Content Area: Fundamental Skills
References: Lewis, S., Heitkemper, M., & Dirksen, S. (2004). *Medical-surgical nursing: Assessment and management of clinical problems* (6th ed.). St. Louis: Mosby, p. 625.
Potter, P., & Perry, A. (2005). *Fundamentals of nursing* (6th ed.). St. Louis: Mosby, p. 403.

11. *Answer: 2*
Rationale: It is best to have two people help change the ties at the tracheostomy. The movement of the tube can easily cause the client to cough and expel the tube from the stoma. Removing the old ties, cleaning the site, and then applying the new ties is not appropriate because, if the client coughs, the tube could be expelled. This procedure is a nursing procedure; therefore, it is not appropriate to call the physician. The respiratory therapist can assist in changing the ties, but it is not necessary to specifically call the therapist for the procedure.
Test-Taking Strategy: Visualize this procedure. Eliminate option 1 knowing that this action can create a risk of the tube being expelled if the client coughs. Eliminate option 3 next knowing that this is a nursing procedure. For the remaining options, select option 2 because it is the umbrella (global) option. Review care of the client with a tracheostomy if you had difficulty with this question.
Level of Cognitive Ability: Application
Client Needs: Safe, Effective Care Environment
Integrated Process: Nursing Process/Planning
Content Area: Fundamental Skills
References: Christensen, B., & Kockrow, E. (2003). *Foundations of nursing* (4th ed). St. Louis: Mosby, p. 459.
Potter, P., & Perry, A. (2005). *Fundamentals of nursing* (6th ed.). St. Louis: Mosby, p. 382.

12. *Answer: 4*
Rationale: When a tube feeding is administered, the client is placed in a high Fowler's position for a bolus feeding and in semi-Fowler's (30 to 45 degrees) to allow gravity to help the flow of formula, prevent reflux, and prevent aspiration. Options 1, 2, and 3 are inappropriate positions during a tube feeding.
Test-Taking Strategy: Use the process of elimination. Eliminate options 1 and 2 first because they are similar. Recalling the risks associated with administering a tube feeding will easily direct you to option 4. Review the procedure for administering tube feedings if you had difficulty with this question.
Level of Cognitive Ability: Application
Client Needs: Physiological Integrity
Integrated Process: Nursing Process/Implementation
Content Area: Fundamental Skills
References: Christensen, B., & Kockrow, E. (2003). *Foundations of nursing* (4th ed). St. Louis: Mosby, p. 533.
Potter, P., & Perry, A. (2005). *Fundamentals of nursing* (6th ed.). St. Louis: Mosby, p. 658.

13. *Answer: 3*
Rationale: When 200 mL of residual formula is obtained, the feeding is held and the physician is notified because it is an indication that the feeding is not being absorbed. Usually, if the residual is less than 100 mL, the feeding is administered; large-volume aspirates indicate delayed gastric emptying and place the client at risk for aspiration. Always check the physician's orders and agency policy regarding residual amounts. Elevating the head of the bed to 90 degrees and flushing the tubing are not appropriate actions.
Test-Taking Strategy: Use the process of elimination. Eliminate options 1 and 4 first because they are similar. Recalling that the feeding is held when more that 100 mL of residual is obtained will direct you to option 3. Review this procedure if you had difficulty with this question.
Level of Cognitive Ability: Application

Client Needs: Physiological Integrity
Integrated Process: Nursing Process/Implementation
Content Area: Fundamental Skills
Reference: Christensen, B., & Kockrow, E. (2003). *Foundations of nursing* (4th ed). St. Louis: Mosby, p. 534.

14. *Answer:* 1
Rationale: Feeding can be hung at room temperature for a period of 4 hours. If 100 mL/hour is prescribed, the nurse would fill the feeding bag with a maximum amount of 400 mL. Feeding hung longer than 4 hours at room temperature creates the risk of bacterial invasion in the formula.
Test-Taking Strategy: Use the process of elimination. Eliminate options 3 and 4 first because they are similar. From the remaining options, recalling that feeding can be hung at room temperature for 4 hours will direct you to option 1. Review the procedure for administering tube feedings if you had difficulty with this question.
Level of Cognitive Ability: Application
Client Needs: Safe, Effective Care Environment
Integrated Process: Nursing Process/Planning
Content Area: Fundamental Skills
References: Christensen, B., & Kockrow, E. (2003). *Foundations of nursing* (4th ed.). St. Louis: Mosby, p. 534.
Potter, P., & Perry, A. (2005). *Fundamentals of nursing* (6th ed.). St. Louis: Mosby, p. 1306.

15. *Answer:* 4
Rationale: Suction is not placed on the catheter when the catheter is introduced into the tracheostomy tube. Suction draws out oxygen and, placing suction on the catheter at this time, could traumatize tracheal tissue. Options 1, 2, and 3 are appropriate components of the plan of care for suctioning.
Test-Taking Strategy: Note the key word, *avoids*. This word indicates a false response question and that you need to select the incorrect nursing action. Visualize the procedure, recalling the risks associated with this procedure. Review the procedure for suctioning if you had difficulty with this question.
Level of Cognitive Ability: Application
Client Needs: Physiological Integrity
Integrated Process: Nursing Process/Implementation
Content Area: Fundamental Skills
References: Lewis, S., Heitkemper, M., & Dirksen, S. (2004). *Medical-surgical nursing: Assessment and management of clinical problems* (6th ed.). St. Louis: Mosby, p. 579.
Potter, P., & Perry, A. (2005). *Fundamentals of nursing* (6th ed.). St. Louis: Mosby, pp. 1103-1104.

16. *Answer:* 1
Rationale: During suctioning, the nurse would apply suction during the withdrawal of the catheter for a period of 5 to 10 seconds. Suction applied longer than this can cause hypoxia in the client.
Test-Taking Strategy: Visualize this procedure and recall the complications associated with suctioning. Note the key words, *no greater than*. It is best to select the option that identifies the least amount of time. Review the procedure for suctioning if you had difficulty with this question.
Level of Cognitive Ability: Application
Client Needs: Physiological Integrity

Integrated Process: Nursing Process/Planning
Content Area: Adult Health/Respiratory
Reference: Christensen, B., & Kockrow, E. (2003). *Foundations of nursing* (4th ed.). St. Louis: Mosby, p. 458.

17. *Answer:* 2
Rationale: Fenestrated tubes have a small opening in the outer cannula that allows some air to escape through the larynx. This type of tube enables the client to speak. Options 1, 3, and 4 are incorrect regarding this type of tube.
Test-Taking Strategy: Knowledge regarding the design and purpose of a fenestrated tracheostomy tube will direct you to option 2. Review the purpose of a fenestrated tube if you had difficulty with this question.
Level of Cognitive Ability: Comprehension
Client Needs: Physiological Integrity
Integrated Process: Nursing Process/Planning
Content Area: Fundamental Skills
References: Lewis, S., Heitkemper, M., & Dirksen, S. (2004). *Medical-surgical nursing: Assessment and management of clinical problems* (6th ed.). St. Louis: Mosby, p. 577.
Phipps, W., Monahan, F., Sands, J., Marek, J., & Neighbors, M. (2003). *Medical-surgical nursing: Health and illness perspectives* (7th ed.). St. Louis: Mosby, p. 516.

18. *Answer:* 4
Rationale: Removal of chest tubes can be uncomfortable for a client. The nurse should medicate the client 30 to 60 minutes before the chest tube is removed. Options 1, 2, and 3 are inappropriate actions and would not be performed by the nurse.
Test-Taking Strategy: Use the process of elimination and Maslow's Hierarchy of Needs theory to answer the question. Option 4 is the only client-centered nursing action, and this option addresses physiological integrity. Review care of the client in preparation for chest tube removal if you had difficulty with this question.
Level of Cognitive Ability: Application
Client Needs: Physiological Integrity
Integrated Process: Nursing Process/Implementation
Content Area: Fundamental Skills
References: Lewis, S., Heitkemper, M., & Dirksen, S. (2004). *Medical-surgical nursing: Assessment and management of clinical problems* (6th ed.). St. Louis: Mosby, p. 625.
Potter, P., & Perry, A. (2005). *Fundamentals of nursing* (6th ed.). St. Louis: Mosby, p. 403.

19. *Answer:* 3
Rationale: Chest tube tubing is never pinned to bed clothing because it presents the risk of accidental dislodgment of the tube when the client moves. Options 1, 2, and 4 are appropriate interventions in the plan of care for a client with a chest tube.
Test-Taking Strategy: Note the key word, *incorrect*, in the stem of the question. This word indicates a false response question and that you need to select the incorrect action. Use the process of elimination, recalling the complications associated with a chest tube. Review care of the client with a chest tube if you had difficulty with this question.
Level of Cognitive Ability: Application

Client Needs: Physiological Integrity
Integrated Process: Nursing Process/Implementation
Content Area: Fundamental Skills
Reference: Potter, P., & Perry, A. (2005). *Fundamentals of nursing* (6th ed.). St. Louis: Mosby, pp. 1118-1119.

20. **Answer: 2**
Rationale: Subcutaneous emphysema is also known as crepitus. It presents as a "puffed-up" appearance caused by leakage of air into the subcutaneous tissues. It is monitored by palpating and feels like bubble wrap when palpated. Although options 1, 3, and 4 may be a component of the plan of care for a client with a chest tube, these actions will not identify subcutaneous emphysema.
Test-Taking Strategy: Use the process of elimination. Note the similarity between the words "subcutaneous emphysema" in the question and "subcutaneous tissues" in the correct option. Review this complication if you had difficulty with this question.
Level of Cognitive Ability: Application
Client Needs: Physiological Integrity
Integrated Process: Nursing Process/Data Collection
Content Area: Fundamental Skills
Reference: Black, J., & Hawks, J. (2005). *Medical-surgical nursing: Clinical management for positive outcomes* (7th ed.). Philadelphia: W.B. Saunders, p. 1780.

ALTERNATE FORMAT QUESTION: MULTIPLE RESPONSE

Answers:
Fluctuation of water in the tube in the water seal chamber during inhalation and exhalation
50 mL of drainage in the drainage collection chamber
An occlusive dressing is in place over the chest tube insertion site
The drainage system is maintained below the client's chest

Rationale: The bubbling of water in the water seal chamber indicates air drainage from the client. This is usually seen when intrathoracic pressure is greater than atmospheric pressure and may occur during exhalation, coughing, or sneezing. Excessive bubbling in the water seal chamber may indicate an air leak, an unexpected finding. Fluctuation of water in the tube in the water seal chamber during inhalation and exhalation is expected. An absence of fluctuation may indicate that the chest tube is obstructed or that the lung has re-expanded and that no more air is leaking into the pleural space. Gentle (not vigorous) bubbling should be noted in the suction control chamber. A total of 50 mL of drainage is not excessive in a client returning to the nursing unit from the recovery room. Drainage that is more than 100 mL/hour is considered excessive and requires physician notification. The chest tube insertion site is covered with an occlusive (airtight) dressing to prevent air from entering the pleural space. Positioning the drainage system below the client's chest allows gravity to drain the pleural space.
Test-Taking Strategy: Thinking about the physiology associated with the functioning of a chest tube drainage system will help in answering this question. The words "excessive bubbling" and "vigorous bubbling" will assist in eliminating these findings. Review care of the client with a chest tube drainage system if you had difficulty with this question.
Level of Cognitive Ability: Analysis
Client Needs: Physiological Integrity
Integrated Process: Nursing Process/Data Collection
Content Area: Adult Health/Respiratory
References: Linton, A., & Maebius, N. (2003). *Introduction to medical-surgical nursing* (3rd ed.). Philadelphia: W.B. Saunders, pp. 473-474.
Potter, P., & Perry, A. (2005). *Fundamentals of nursing* (6th ed.). St. Louis: Mosby, p. 1120.

REFERENCES

Black, J., & Hawks, J. (2005). *Medical-surgical nursing: Clinical management for positive outcomes* (7th ed.). Philadelphia: W.B. Saunders.

Christensen, B., & Kockrow, E. (2003). *Foundations of nursing* (4th ed.). St. Louis: Mosby.

Lewis, S., Heitkemper, M., & Dirksen, S. (2004). *Medical-surgical nursing: Assessment and management of clinical problems* (6th ed.). St. Louis: Mosby.

Linton, A., & Maebius, N. (2003). *Introduction to medical-surgical nursing* (3rd ed.). Philadelphia: W.B. Saunders.

National Council of State Boards of Nursing. (2005). *Detailed test plan for the National Council licensure examination for practical/vocational nurses.* Chicago: Author.

Phipps, W., Monahan, F., Sands, J., Marek, J., & Neighbors, M. (2003). *Medical-surgical nursing: Health and illness perspectives* (7th ed.). St. Louis: Mosby.

Potter, P., & Perry, A. (2005). *Fundamentals of nursing* (6th ed.). St. Louis: Mosby.

Maternity Nursing

PYRAMID TERMS

amniotic fluid   Fluid that surrounds and protects the fetus; 800 to 1200 mL by the end of pregnancy. The fetus floats in the amniotic fluid, which serves as a cushion against injury from sudden blows or movements and helps maintain a constant body temperature for the fetus. The fetus voids into the amniotic fluid and also drinks and breathes the fluid.

ballottement   Rebounding of the fetus against the examiner's finger on palpation. When the cervix is tapped, the fetus floats upward in the amniotic fluid. A rebound is felt by the examiner when the fetus falls back.

Chadwick's sign   Bluish coloration of the mucous membranes of cervix, vagina, and vulva that occurs at about 6 weeks of pregnancy and is a probable sign of pregnancy.

delivery   Actual event of birth; the expulsion or extraction of the neonate and fetal membranes at birth.

fertilization   Takes place when sperm and ovum unite; occurs within 12 hours of ovulation and within 2 to 3 days of insemination, the average duration of viability for the ovum and sperm.

Goodell's sign   Softening of the cervix; occurs at the beginning of the second month of gestation and is a probable sign of pregnancy.

gravida   A pregnant woman; called gravida I (primigravida) during the first pregnancy, gravida II during the second, and so on.

Hegar's sign   Compressibility and softening of the lower uterine segment; occurs at about week 6 of gestation; a probable sign of pregnancy.

implantation   Zygote propels toward the uterus and implants in the uterine wall 6 to 8 days after ovulation.

infant   A baby born alive; also, from 28 days of age until the first birthday.

labor   Coordinated sequence of involuntary uterine contractions resulting in effacement and dilation of cervix, followed by expulsion of the products of conception.

lochia   Discharge from the uterus that consists of blood from the vessels of the placental site and debris from the decidua; lasts for 2 to 3 weeks after delivery.

Nagele's rule   Determines the estimated date of confinement (EDC) and works on the premise that the woman has a 28-day menstrual cycle. Add 7 days to the first day of last menstrual period (LMP). Subtract 3 months and add 1 year. Alternatively, add 7 days to the last menstrual period and count forward 9 months.

neonate   A human offspring from the time of birth to the 28th day of life; also called a newborn.

newborn   A human offspring from the time of birth to the 28th day of life; also called a neonate.

parity   The number of pregnancies that have been carried to viability.

placenta   The organ that provides for the exchange of nutrients and waste products between the fetus and mother and produces hormones to maintain pregnancy; develops by the third month of gestation; also called afterbirth.

quickening   First perception of fetal movement appearing usually in the 16th to 18th week of pregnancy.

PYRAMID TO SUCCESS

The Pyramid to Success focuses on the physiological and psychosocial aspects related to the experience of pregnancy. Pyramid points begin with instructing the pregnant client in measures that will promote a healthy environment for both the mother and fetus. Focus on the importance of antenatal follow-up care, nutrition, and the interventions for common discomforts that occur during pregnancy. Review the purpose of the commonly prescribed diagnostic tests and procedures in the antenatal period. Focus on disorders that can occur during pregnancy, particularly pregnancy-induced hypertension (PIH) and diabetes. Review the labor and delivery process and the immediate interventions when the mother or fetal status is compromised, such as prolapsed cord or altered fetal heart rate. Review fetal effects resulting from the mother with acquired immunodeficiency syndrome or the substance abuse mother. Focus on the normal expectations of the postpartum period and the complications that can occur. Pyramid points also focus on the normal physical assessment findings in the newborn and the early identification of disorders in the newborn. The Integrated Processes addressed in this unit include Caring, Clinical Problem-Solving Process (Nursing Process), Communication and Documentation, and Teaching/Learning.

▲ CLIENT NEEDS

Safe, Effective Care Environment

Asepsis
Confidentiality
Consultations with other members of the health care team
Continuity of care
Establishing priorities
Handling infectious materials
Informed consent for procedures
Parent rights
Standard, transmission-based, and other precautions when delivering care

Health Promotion and Maintenance

Antenatal, intrapartum, and postpartum care
Birthing and parenting issues
Expected body image changes
Family interaction patterns
Family planning
Growth and development and health care screening
Health and wellness
Lifestyle choices
Reproduction and human sexuality
Techniques of data collection

Psychosocial Integrity

Communication
Coping mechanisms
Cultural, spiritual, and religious influences regarding birth and motherhood
Role changes
Support systems

Physiological Integrity

Alterations in body systems
Commonly prescribed diagnostic tests and procedures
Interventions for unexpected events during the pregnancy
Labor and delivery process
Normal expectations during pregnancy
Nutrition
Physiological changes that occur during pregnancy
Risk identification during pregnancy

REFERENCES

Christensen, B., & Kockrow, E. (2003). *Foundations of nursing* (4th ed.). St. Louis: Mosby.
deWit, S. (2005). *Fundamental concepts and skills for nursing* (2nd ed.). Philadelphia: W.B. Saunders.
Leifer, G. (2005). *Maternity nursing* (9th ed.). Philadelphia: W.B. Saunders.
McKinney, E., James, S., Murray, S., & Ashwill, J. (2005). *Maternal-child nursing* (2nd ed.). St. Louis: Mosby.
Morrison-Valfre, M. (2005). *Foundations of mental health care* (3rd ed.). St. Louis: Mosby.
Murray, S., McKinney, E., & Gorrie, T. (2002). *Foundations of maternal-newborn nursing* (3rd ed.). Philadelphia: W.B. Saunders.
National Council of State Boards of Nursing. (2005). *Detailed test plan for the National Council licensure examination for practical/vocational nurses.* Chicago: Author.
Nix, S. (2005). *Williams basic nutrition and diet therapy* (11th ed.). St. Louis: Mosby.
Price, D., & Gwin, J. (2005). *Thompson's pediatric nursing* (9th ed.). Philadelphia: W.B. Saunders.

Female Reproductive System

I. ORGANS

A. Ovaries
1. Form and expel ova
2. Secrete estrogen and progesterone

B. Fallopian tubes
1. Muscular tubes (oviducts) approximate to the ovaries and connect to the uterus
2. Propel the ova from the ovaries to the uterus

C. Uterus
1. Organ (muscular, pear-shaped cavity) in which the fetus develops
2. Organ from which menstruation occurs

D. Cervix
1. Internal os opens into the body of the uterine cavity
2. Cervical canal is located between the internal os and external os
3. External os opens into the vagina

E. Vagina
1. Mucous membrane–lined channel through the muscles of the pelvic floor
2. Known as the birth canal
3. Passage between the cervical os and the external environment
   a. Passageway for fetus
   b. Passageway for menstrual blood

II. MENSTRUAL CYCLE (Table 20-1)

A. Ovarian hormones
1. Include follicle-stimulating hormone (FSH) and luteinizing hormone (LH)
2. Released by the anterior pituitary gland
3. Produce changes in the ovaries
4. Secretion of ovarian hormones leads to changes in the endometrium
5. Menstrual cycle: The regularly recurring physiological changes in the endometrium that culminate in its shedding; may vary in duration, with average of approximately 28 days

B. Ovarian changes
1. Preovulatory phase
2. Luteal phase

C. Uterine changes
1. Menstrual phase
2. Proliferative phase
3. Secretory phase

III. FEMALE PELVIS AND MEASUREMENTS

A. True pelvis
1. Lies below pelvic brim
2. Consists of the pelvic inlet, mid pelvis, and pelvic outlet

B. False pelvis
1. Shallow portion above the pelvic brim
2. Supports the abdominal viscera

C. Types of pelvis (Figure 20-1)
1. Gynecoid
   a. Normal female pelvis
   b. Transversely rounded or blunt
   c. Most favorable for successful labor and birth
2. Android
   a. Wedge-shaped or angulated
   b. Seen in males
   c. Not favorable for labor
   d. Narrow pelvic planes can cause slow descent and midpelvis arrest
3. Anthropoid
   a. Oval shape
   b. The outlet is adequate, with a normal or moderately narrow pubic arch
4. Platypelloid
   a. Flat shape with an oval inlet
   b. Transverse diameter is wide but anteroposterior diameter is short, making the outlet inadequate

TABLE 20-1

Menstrual Cycle

OVARIAN CHANGES

Pre-Ovulatory Phase	Luteal Phase
The hypothalamus releases gonadotropin-releasing hormone (GnRH) through the portal system to the anterior pituitary system	Begins with ovulation.
	Body temperature drops and then rises by 0.5°F to 1°F around the time of ovulation.
Secretion of FSH by the anterior lobe of the pituitary gland stimulates growth of follicles.	Corpus luteum is formed from follicle cells that remain in the ovary following ovulation.
Most follicles die, leaving one to mature into a large graafian follicle.	Corpus luteum secretes estrogen and progesterone during remaining 14 days of cycle.
	Corpus luteum degenerates if the ovum is not fertilized, and secretion of estrogen and progesterone declines.
Estrogen produced by the follicle stimulates increased secretions of LH by the anterior lobe of the pituitary gland.	Estrogen and progesterone inhibit secretions of FSH and LH.
The follicle ruptures and releases an ovum into the peritoneal cavity.	Once corpus luteum degenerates, pituitary secretion of estrogen and progesterone decreases and ovarian cycle begins again.

UTERINE CHANGES

Menstrual Phase	Proliferative Phase	Secretory Phase
Consists of 4 to 6 days of bleeding as endometrium breaks down owing to the decreased amount of estrogen and progesterone.	Estrogen stimulates proliferation and growth of endometrium.	Lasts about 12 days
	Lasts about 9 days.	Follows ovulation.
	As estrogen increases, it suppresses secretion of FSH and increases the secretion of LH.	Initiated in response to the increase of LH.
FSH rises, enabling the beginning of a new cycle.		Graafian follicle replaced by corpus luteum.
	LH stimulates ovulation and development of the corpus luteum.	Corpus luteum secretes progesterone and estrogen.
	Ovulation occurs between day 12 and day 16.	Progesterone prepares endometrium for pregnancy should a fertilized ovum be implanted.
	Estrogen is high and progesterone is low.	

D. Pelvic inlet diameters
   1. Anteroposterior diameters
      a. Diagonal conjugate: Distance from the lower margin of the symphysis pubis to the sacral promontory
      b. True conjugate or conjugate vera: Distance from the upper margin of the symphysis pubis to the sacral promontory
      c. Obstetric conjugate: Smallest front-to-back distance through which the fetal head must pass in moving through the pelvic inlet
   2. Transverse diameter: Largest of the pelvic inlet diameters; located at right angles to the true conjugate
   3. Oblique (diagonal) diameter: Not clinically measurable
   4. Posterior sagittal diameter: Distance from the point where the anteroposterior and transverse diameters cross each other to the middle of the sacral promontory

E. Pelvic midplane diameters
   1. Transverse diameter (interspinous diameter)
   2. Midplane normally is the largest plane, with greatest diameter
F. Pelvic outlet diameters
   1. Transverse (intertuberous)
   2. Outlet presents the smallest plane of the pelvic canal

IV. FERTILIZATION AND IMPLANTATION
A. **Fertilization**
   1. Occurs in the upper region of the fallopian tubes
   2. Occurs within 12 hours of ovulation and within 2 to 3 days of insemination, the average duration of viability for the ovum and sperm
   3. Takes place when sperm and ovum unite
   4. Once fertilized, the membrane of the ovum undergoes changes that prevent the entry of other sperm

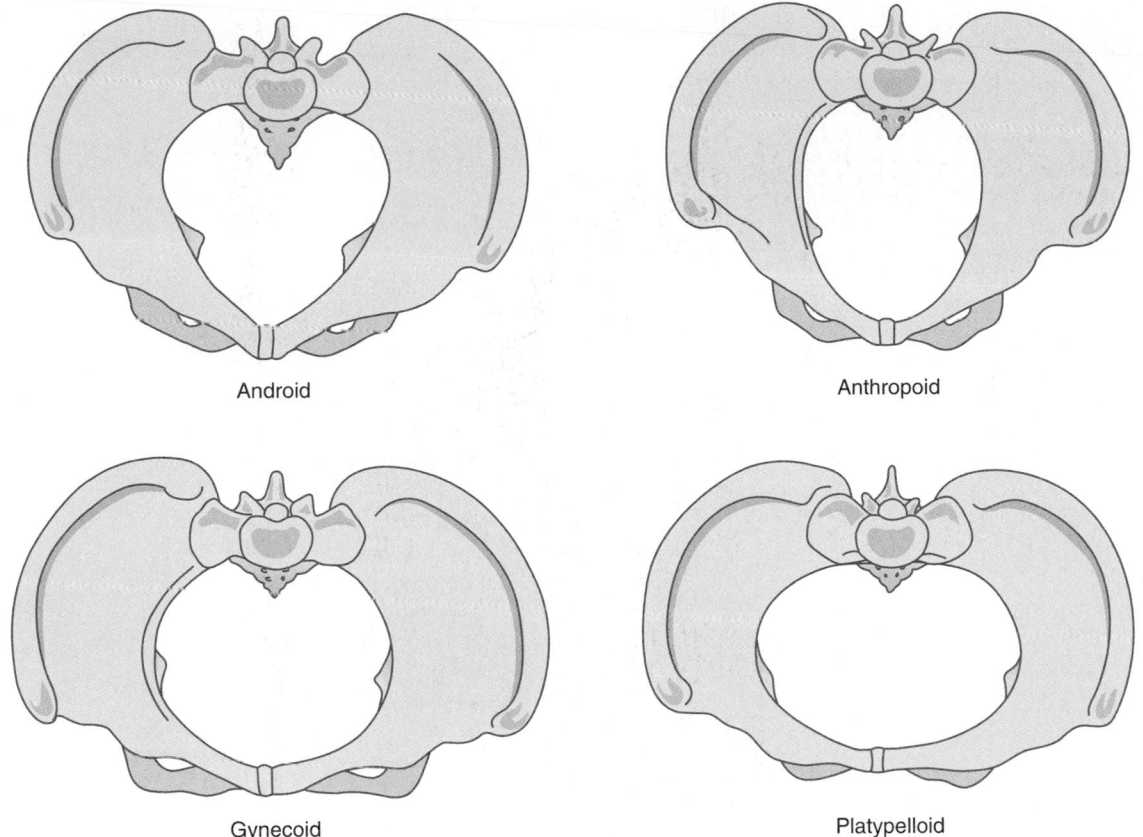

Android

Anthropoid

Gynecoid

Platypelloid

FIG. 20-1 Types of pelves. (From Matteson, P. [2001]. *Women's health during the childbearing years: A community-based approach.* St. Louis: Mosby.)

5. Each reproductive cell carries 23 chromosomes
6. Sperm carry an X and Y chromosome, egg carries an XX chromosome; XY: male, XX: female

B. Implantation
   1. Zygote is propelled toward the uterus
   2. Implants 6 to 8 days after ovulation
   3. Blastocyst secretes chorionic gonadotropin to ensure that the corpus luteum remains viable; secretes estrogen and progesterone for the first 2 to 3 months of gestation

V. FETAL DEVELOPMENT (Table 20-2)

A. Pre-embryonic period: First 2 weeks after conception
B. Embryonic stage: Beginning of the third week through the eighth week after conception
C. Fetal period: Beginning of the ninth week after conception and ending with birth

VI. FETAL ENVIRONMENT

A. Amnion
   1. Encloses the amniotic cavity
   2. Inner membrane that forms about the second week of embryonic development
   3. Forms a fluid-filled sac that surrounds the embryo and later the fetus

B. Chorion
   1. Outer membrane
   2. Becomes vascularized and forms the fetal part of the **placenta**

C. **Amniotic fluid**
   1. Consists of 800 to 1200 mL by the end of pregnancy
   2. Surrounds, cushions, and protects the fetus and allows for fetal movement
   3. Maintains body temperature of the fetus
   4. Consists largely of fetal urine and is therefore a measure of fetal kidney function
   5. The fetus drinks, swallows, and urinates the **amniotic fluid** and breathes the **amniotic fluid** into its lungs

D. **Placenta**
   1. Provides for exchange of nutrients and waste products between fetus and mother
   2. Develops by the third month
   3. Dependent on maternal circulation
   4. Produces hormones to maintain pregnancy; assumes full responsibility for the production of these hormones by the 12th week of gestation
   5. Large particles such as bacteria cannot pass through the **placenta**
   6. In addition to nutrients, drugs, antibodies, and viruses can pass through the **placenta**

TABLE 20-2

Fetal Development

Embryonic Stage	Fetal Period
WEEK 1 Free-floating blastocyst	**WEEK 16** Active movements are present Fetal skin is transparent Lanugo hair begins to develop Skeletal ossification occurs Sex of fetus can be determined at this time
WEEK 2 TO 3 Two mm in length Groove formed along middle of back Beginning of blood circulation Heart tubular in shape	**WEEK 20** 19 cm in length 465 g in weight Lanugo covers the entire body Fetus has nails Muscles developed Enamel and dentin depositing Heartbeat detected by fetoscope
WEEK 5 4 to 6 mm in length 0.4 g in weight Double heart chambers visible Heart beginning to beat Limb buds	**WEEK 24** 28 cm in length 780 g in weight Hair on head well formed Skin reddish and wrinkled Reflex hand grasp Vernix caseosa covers entire body Has ability to hear
WEEK 8 3 cm in length 2 g in weight Eyelids begin to fuse Circulatory system through umbilical cord well established Every organ system present	**WEEK 28** 38 cm in length 1200 g in weight Limbs are well flexed Brain develops rapidly Eyelids open and close Lungs sufficiently developed to provide gas exchange (lecithin forming) If born, neonate can breathe at this time
WEEK 12 8 cm in length 45 g in weight Face well formed Limbs long and slender Kidneys begin to form urine Spontaneous movements occur Heart tones detected by electronic devices between 10 and 12 weeks Sex visually recognizable	**WEEK 32** 40 cm in length 2000 g (5.5 lb) in weight Bones are fully developed Subcutaneous fat collected L/S (lecithin/sphingomyelin) ratio switching to 1.2:1
	WEEK 36 42 to 48 cm length 2500 g in weight Skin pink, body rounded Less wrinkled Lanugo disappearing L/S (lecithin/sphingomyelin) ratio to 2:1 or higher
	WEEK 40 48 to 52 cm in length 3000 to 3600 g in weight Skin pinkish and smooth Lanugo present in upper arms and shoulders Vernix caseosa decreases Fingernails extend beyond fingertips Sole (plantar) creases down to heel Testes in scrotum Labia majora well developed

7. In the third trimester, transfer of maternal immunoglobulin provides fetus passive immunity to certain diseases for the first few months after birth
8. By week 8, genetic testing can be done

VII. FETAL CIRCULATION

A. Umbilical cord
1. Contains two arteries and one vein
2. Arteries carry deoxygenated blood and waste products from the fetus
3. The vein carries oxygenated blood and provides oxygen and nutrients to the fetus

B. Fetal heart rate
1. Depends on gestational age: 160 to 170 beats per minute in the first trimester, but slows with fetal growth to 120 to 160 beats per minute near or at term
2. Approximately twice the maternal heart rate

C. Fetal circulation bypass
1. Present because of nonfunctioning lungs
2. Bypasses must close after birth to allow blood to flow through the lungs and the liver
3. Ductus arteriosus connects the pulmonary artery to aorta, bypassing the lungs
4. Ductus venosus connects the umbilical vein and inferior vena cava, bypassing the liver
5. Foramen ovale is the opening between the right and left atria of heart, bypassing the lungs

PRACTICE QUESTIONS

1. A pregnant client asks the nurse about the hormone that causes milk production. The nurse tells the client that the primary hormone that stimulates the secretion of milk is:
   1. Testosterone
   2. Oxytocin
   3. Prolactin
   4. Progesterone

2. A licensed practical nurse (LPN) is assisting a high school nurse in conducting a session with female adolescents regarding the menstrual cycle. The LPN tells the adolescents that the normal duration of the menstrual cycle is about:
   1. 14 days
   2. 28 days
   3. 30 days
   4. 45 days

3. A maternity nursing instructor asks a nursing student to identify the hormones that are produced by the ovaries. Which of the following, if identified by the student, indicates an understanding of the hormones produced by this endocrine gland?
   1. Estrogen and progesterone
   2. Follicle-stimulating hormone (FSH)

   3. Luteinizing hormone (LH)
   4. Oxytoxin

4. A nurse-midwife is conducting a session on the process of fertilization with a group of nursing students. The nurse-midwife asks a student to identify the structure where fertilization of an ovum takes place. Which of the following, if identified by the student, indicates an understanding of this process?
   1. Fallopian tube
   2. Fundus of the uterus
   3. In the ovary
   4. In the corpus of the uterus

5. A nursing student is conducting a clinical conference regarding the hormones that are related to pregnancy. The instructor asks the student about the function of progesterone. Which of the following responses, if made by the student, indicates an understanding of the function of this hormone?
   1. "It softens the muscles and joints of the pelvis."
   2. "It is the primary hormone of milk production."
   3. "It increases during pregnancy to stimulate the basal metabolic rate."
   4. "It maintains the uterine lining for implantation and relaxes all smooth muscle, including the uterus."

6. A nurse is reinforcing teaching to a pregnant woman about the physiological effects and hormone changes that occur in pregnancy. The woman asks the nurse about the purpose of estrogen. The nurse bases the response on which of the following purposes of estrogen?
   1. It maintains the uterine lining for implantation
   2. It stimulates metabolism of glucose and converts the glucose to fat
   3. It prevents the involution of the corpus luteum and maintains the production of progesterone until the placenta is formed
   4. It stimulates uterine development to provide an environment for the fetus and stimulates the breasts to prepare for lactation

7. A maternity nurse is describing the ovarian cycle to a group of nursing students. The instructor asks a nursing student to identify the phases of the cycle. Which phase, if stated by the nursing student, indicates a need to further research this area?
   1. Follicular phase
   2. Ovulatory phase
   3. Luteal phase
   4. Proliferative phase

8. A nursing student is asked to describe the size of the uterus in a nonpregnant client. Which of the following responses, if made by the student, indicates an understanding of the anatomy of this structure?
   1. "The uterus weighs about 2 ounces."
   2. "The uterus weighs about 2.2 pounds."

3. "The uterus has a capacity of about 50 milliliters."
4. "The uterus is round in shape and weighs approximately 1000 grams."

9. A nurse is collecting data from a pregnant client. The client asks the nurse about the purpose of the fallopian tubes. The nurse responds to the client, knowing that the fallopian tubes:
   1. Secrete estrogen and progesterone
   2. Are the organ of copulation
   3. Are where the fetus develops
   4. Are where fertilization occurs

10. A nursing student is assigned to care for an adolescent female client in the health care clinic. The instructor reviews the menstrual cycle with the student. The instructor determines that the student understands the process of secretion of the follicle-stimulating hormone (FSH) and the luteinizing hormone (LH) if the student states:
    1. "FSH and LH are released from the anterior pituitary gland."
    2. "FSH and LH are secreted by the corpus luteum of the ovary."
    3. "FSH and LH are secreted by the adrenal glands."
    4. "FSH and LH stimulate the formation of milk during pregnancy."

11. A nurse working in a prenatal clinic reviews a client's chart and notes that the physician documents that the client has a gynecoid pelvis. Based on this documentation, the nurse understands that this type of pelvis is:
    1. Not favorable for labor
    2. Seen in 25% of women
    3. A wide pelvis with a short diameter
    4. The most favorable for labor and birth

12. A client asks the nurse about the purpose of the placenta. The nurse plans to respond to the client, knowing that the placenta:
    1. Prevents antibodies and viruses from passing to the fetus
    2. Cushions and protects the fetus
    3. Provides an exchange of nutrients and waste products between the mother and fetus
    4. Maintains the body temperature of the fetus

13. A nurse is describing the process of fetal circulation to a client during a prenatal visit. The nurse tells the client that fetal circulation consists of:
    1. Two umbilical veins and one umbilical artery
    2. Two umbilical arteries and one umbilical vein
    3. Arteries carrying oxygenated blood to the fetus
    4. Veins carrying deoxygenated blood to the fetus

14. A nursing student is assigned to a client in labor. The nursing instructor asks the student to describe fetal circulation, specifically the ductus venosus. The instructor determines that the student understands the structure of the ductus venosus if the student states that it:
    1. Connects the pulmonary artery to the aorta
    2. Is an opening between the right and left atria
    3. Connects the umbilical artery to the inferior vena cava
    4. Connects the umbilical vein to the inferior vena cava

15. During the prenatal visit, the nurse checks the fetal heart rate (FHR) of a client in the third trimester of pregnancy. The nurse determines that the FHR is normal if which of the following heart rates is noted?
    1. 80 beats per minute
    2. 100 beats per minute
    3. 150 beats per minute
    4. 180 beats per minute

ALTERNATE FORMAT QUESTION: FILL IN THE BLANK

A client who has just been told that she is pregnant asks a clinic nurse when the fetus's heart will be developed and beating. The nurse tells the client that the fetal heart is beating at what gestational week?

Answer: _____

ANSWERS

1. *Answer: 3*
Rationale: Prolactin stimulates the secretion of milk, called lactogenesis. Oxytocin stimulates contractions during birth and stimulates postpartum contractions to compress uterine vessels and control bleeding. Testosterone is produced by the adrenal glands in the female and induces the growth of pubic and axillary hair at puberty. Progesterone stimulates the secretions of the endometrial glands and causes the endometrial vessels to become dilated and tortuous in preparation for possible embryo implantation.
Test-Taking Strategy: Use the process of elimination. Note the relationship between "secretion of milk" in the question and the hormone "prolactin" in the correct option. Review the functions of the various hormones of the reproductive system if you had difficulty with this question.

Level of Cognitive Ability: Application
Client Needs: Physiological Integrity
Integrated Process: Teaching/Learning
Content Area: Maternity/Antepartum
Reference: Leifer, G. (2005). *Maternity nursing* (9th ed.). Philadelphia: W.B. Saunders, pp. 198, 348.

2. *Answer: 2*
Rationale: The normal duration of the menstrual cycle is about 28 days, although it may range from 20 to 45 days. The first day of the menstrual period is counted as day 1 of the woman's cycle. Options 1, 3, and 4 are incorrect.
Test-Taking Strategy: Recalling the duration of the menstrual cycle will direct you to the correct option. Note the key words, *normal duration,* in the question. This will assist in eliminating

options 1, 3, and 4. Review the physiology related to the menstrual cycle if you had difficulty with this question.
Level of Cognitive Ability: Application
Client Needs: Physiological Integrity
Integrated Process: Teaching/Learning
Content Area: Maternity/Antepartum
Reference: Leifer, G. (2005). *Maternity nursing* (9th ed.). Philadelphia: W.B. Saunders, p. 15.

3. *Answer:* **1**
Rationale: The ovaries are the endocrine glands that produce estrogen and progesterone. FSH and LH are produced by the anterior pituitary gland. Oxytoxin is produced by the posterior pituitary gland and stimulates the uterus to produce contractions during birth.
Test-Taking Strategy: Recalling the various hormones and the production and secretion of the hormones will direct you to the correct option. Review this information if you had difficulty with this question.
Level of Cognitive Ability: Comprehension
Client Needs: Physiological Integrity
Integrated Process: Teaching/Learning
Content Area: Maternity/Antepartum
Reference: Leifer, G. (2005). *Maternity nursing* (9th ed.). Philadelphia: W.B. Saunders, p. 12.

4. *Answer:* **1**
Rationale: Fallopian tubes, also called oviducts, are 8 to 14 cm long and are quite narrow. The fallopian tubes are a pathway for the ovum between the ovary and the uterus. Fertilization occurs in the fallopian tube. Options 2, 3, and 4 are incorrect.
Test-Taking Strategy: Recalling the process of fertilization and the area in which fertilization occurs will direct you to the correct option. Review this information if you had difficulty with this question.
Level of Cognitive Ability: Comprehension
Client Needs: Physiological Integrity
Integrated Process: Teaching/Learning
Content Area: Maternity/Antepartum
Reference: Leifer, G. (2005). *Maternity nursing* (9th ed.). Philadelphia: W.B. Saunders, pp. 22, 25.

5. *Answer:* **4**
Rationale: Progesterone maintains the uterine lining for implantation and relaxes all smooth muscle, including the uterus. Relaxin is the hormone that softens the muscles and joints of the pelvis. Thyroxine increases during pregnancy to stimulate basal metabolic rates, and prolactin is the primary hormone of milk production.
Test-Taking Strategy: Recalling the function of the various hormones related to pregnancy will direct you to the correct option. Review the functions of these hormones if you had difficulty with this question.
Level of Cognitive Ability: Comprehension
Client Needs: Physiological integrity
Integrated Process: Teaching/Learning
Content Area: Maternity/Antepartum
Reference: Leifer, G. (2005). *Maternity nursing* (9th ed.). Philadelphia: W.B. Saunders, p. 12.

6. *Answer:* **4**
Rationale: Estrogen stimulates uterine development to provide an environment for the fetus and stimulates the breasts to prepare for lactation. Progesterone maintains the uterine lining for implantation and relaxes all smooth muscle. Human placental lactogen stimulates the metabolism of glucose and converts the glucose to fat. Human chorionic gonadotropin prevents involution of the corpus luteum and maintains the production of progesterone until the placenta is formed.
Test-Taking Strategy: Recalling the functions of various hormones related to pregnancy will direct you to the correct option. Review these various hormones if you had difficulty with this question.
Level of Cognitive Ability: Application
Client Needs: Physiological Integrity
Integrated Process: Teaching/Learning
Content Area: Maternity/Antepartum
Reference: McKinney, E., James, S., Murray, S., & Ashwill, J. (2005). *Maternal-child nursing* (2nd ed.). St. Louis: Elsevier, p. 258.

7. *Answer:* **4**
Rationale: The ovarian cycle consists of three phases: follicular, ovulatory, and luteal. The proliferative phase is a phase of the endometrial cycle.
Test-Taking Strategy: Note the key words, *indicates a need to further research.* These words indicate a false response question and that you need to select the incorrect student statement. Recalling the ovarian cycle and the phases included in the cycle will direct you to option 4. Review the ovarian cycle if you had difficulty with this question.
Level of Cognitive Ability: Comprehension
Client Needs: Physiological Integrity
Integrated Process: Teaching/Learning
Content Area: Maternity/Antepartum
Reference: Leifer, G. (2005). *Maternity nursing* (9th ed.). Philadelphia: W.B. Saunders, p. 15.

8. *Answer:* **1**
Rationale: Before conception, the uterus is a small pear-shaped organ contained entirely in the pelvic cavity. Before pregnancy, the uterus weighs approximately 60 g (2 oz) and has a capacity of about 10 mL ($^1/_3$ oz). At the end of pregnancy, the uterus weighs approximately 1000 g (2.2 lb) and has a sufficient capacity for the fetus, placenta, and amniotic fluid.
Test-Taking Strategy: Use the process of elimination. Note the key word, *nonpregnant,* and visualize each of the items identified in the options to assist in directing you to the correct option. Review the anatomy of the uterus if you had difficulty with this question.
Level of Cognitive Ability: Comprehension
Client Needs: Physiological Integrity
Integrated Process: Teaching/Learning
Content Area: Maternity/Antepartum
Reference: Leifer, G. (2005). *Maternity nursing* (9th ed.). Philadelphia: W.B. Saunders, p. 12.

9. *Answer:* **4**
Rationale: Each fallopian tube is a hollow muscular tube that transports a mature oocyte for final maturation and fertilization.

Fertilization typically occurs near the boundary between the ampulla and isthmus of the tube. Estrogen is a hormone produced by the ovarian follicles, corpus luteum, adrenal cortex, and placenta during pregnancy. Progesterone is a hormone secreted by the corpus luteum of the ovary, adrenal glands, and placenta during pregnancy. The vagina is the organ of copulation, and the fetus develops in the uterus.
Test-Taking Strategy: Recalling the anatomy and physiology of the female reproductive system will direct you to the correct option. Review this information if you had difficulty with this question.
Level of Cognitive Ability: Comprehension
Client Needs: Physiological Integrity
Integrated Process: Nursing Process/Implementation
Content Area: Maternity/Antepartum
Reference: Leifer, G. (2005). *Maternity nursing* (9th ed.). Philadelphia: W.B. Saunders, p. 12.

10. *Answer:* **1**
Rationale: FSH and LH are released from the anterior pituitary gland to stimulate follicular growth and development, growth of the graafian follicle, and the production of progesterone. Options 2, 3, and 4 are incorrect.
Test-Taking Strategy: Use the process of elimination. Option 4 can be eliminated because the case of the question does not address pregnancy. From this point, use your knowledge related to the menstrual cycle to select the correct option. Review the menstrual cycle if you had difficulty with this question.
Level of Cognitive Ability: Comprehension
Client Needs: Physiological Integrity
Integrated Process: Teaching/Learning
Content Area: Maternity/Antepartum
References: Leifer, G. (2005). *Maternity nursing* (9th ed.). Philadelphia: W.B. Saunders, pp. 15-16.
McKinney, E., James, S., Murray, S., & Ashwill, J. (2005). *Maternal-child nursing* (2nd ed.). St. Louis: Elsevier, pp. 224-226.

11. *Answer:* **4**
Rationale: A gynecoid pelvis is a normal female pelvis and is the most favorable for successful labor and birth. An android pelvis would not be favorable for labor because of the narrow pelvic planes. An anthropoid pelvis has an outlet that is adequate, with a normal or moderately narrow pubic arch. The platypelloid pelvis has a wide transverse diameter, but the anteroposterior diameter is short, making the outlet inadequate.
Test-Taking Strategy: Knowledge regarding pelvic types is required to answer this question. Remember that the gynecoid pelvis is the normal female pelvis. Review pelvic types if you had difficulty with this question.
Level of Cognitive Ability: Comprehension
Client Needs: Physiological Integrity
Integrated Process: Nursing Process/Data Collection
Content Area: Maternity/Antepartum
Reference: Leifer, G. (2005). *Maternity nursing* (9th ed.). Philadelphia: W.B. Saunders, p. 14.

12. *Answer:* **3**
Rationale: The placenta provides an exchange of nutrients and waste products between the mother and fetus. The amniotic

fluid surrounds, cushions, and protects the fetus and maintains the body temperature of the fetus.
Test-Taking Strategy: Knowledge regarding the purpose of the placenta and amniotic fluid is required to answer this question. Remember that the placenta provides nutrients. Review the structure and function of the placenta and amniotic fluid if you had difficulty with this question.
Level of Cognitive Ability: Comprehension
Client Needs: Physiological Integrity
Integrated Process: Nursing Process/Planning
Content Area: Maternity/Antepartum
Reference: Leifer, G. (2005). *Maternity nursing* (9th ed.). Philadelphia: W.B. Saunders, p. 24.

13. *Answer:* **2**
Rationale: Blood pumped by the fetus's heart leaves the fetus through two umbilical arteries. Once oxygenated, the blood is then returned by one umbilical vein. Arteries carry deoxygenated blood and waste products from the fetus and veins carry oxygenated blood and provide oxygen and nutrients to the fetus.
Test-Taking Strategy: Knowledge regarding fetal circulation is required to answer this question. Remember that there are three umbilical vessels within an umbilical cord (two arteries and one vein). Review fetal circulation if you had difficulty with this question.
Level of Cognitive Ability: Application
Client Needs: Physiological Integrity
Integrated Process: Nursing Process/Implementation
Content Area: Maternity/Antepartum
References: Leifer, G. (2005). *Maternity nursing* (9th ed.). Philadelphia: W.B. Saunders, p. 27.
Murray, S., McKinney, E., & Gorrie, T. (2002). *Foundations of maternal-newborn nursing* (3rd ed.). Philadelphia: W.B. Saunders, pp. 114, 334.

14. *Answer:* **4**
Rationale: The ductus venosus connects the umbilical vein to the inferior vena cava. The foramen ovale is a temporary opening between the right and left atria. The ductus arteriosus joins the aorta and the pulmonary artery.
Test-Taking Strategy: Knowledge regarding fetal circulation is required to answer this question. Remember that the ductus venosus connects the umbilical vein to the inferior vena cava. Review fetal circulation if you had difficulty with this question.
Level of Cognitive Ability: Comprehension
Client Needs: Physiological Integrity
Integrated Process: Teaching/Learning
Content Area: Maternity/Antepartum
Reference: Leifer, G. (2005). *Maternity nursing* (9th ed.). Philadelphia: W.B. Saunders, p. 27.

15. *Answer:* **3**
Rationale: Fetal heart rate depends on gestational age. It normally is 160 to 170 beats per minute in the first trimester, but slows with fetal growth to 110 or 120 (low end) to 160 (high end) beats per minute near or at term.
Test-Taking Strategy: Knowledge regarding normal fetal heart rate is required to answer this question. Noting the key words, *third trimester*, will direct you to option 3. Review fetal heart rate if you had difficulty with this question.

Level of Cognitive Ability: Comprehension
Client Needs: Physiological Integrity
Integrated Process: Nursing Process/Data Collection
Content Area: Maternity
Reference: Leifer, G. (2005). *Maternity nursing* (9th ed.). Philadelphia: W.B. Saunders, p. 78.

ALTERNATE FORMAT QUESTION: FILL IN THE BLANK

Answer: **5**
Rationale: The fetal heart is beating and has developed four chambers by gestational week 5.

Test-Taking Strategy: Recalling the weekly development of the fetus will assist in answering this question. Review fetal development in relation to the fetal heart beat if you had difficulty with this question.
Level of Cognitive Ability: Application
Client Needs: Physiological Integrity
Integrated Process: Teaching/Learning
Content Area: Maternity/Antepartum
Reference: Murray, S., McKinney, E., & Gorrie, T. (2002). *Foundations of maternal-newborn nursing* (3rd ed.). Philadelphia: W.B. Saunders, p. 106.

REFERENCES

Leifer, G. (2005). *Maternity nursing* (9th ed.). Philadelphia: W.B. Saunders.

Matteson, P. (2001). *Women's health during the childbearing years: A community-based approach.* St. Louis: Mosby.

McKinney, E., James, S., Murray, S., & Ashwill, J. (2005). *Maternal-child nursing* (2nd ed.). St. Louis: Elsevier.

Murray, S., McKinney, E., & Gorrie, T. (2002). *Foundations of maternal-newborn nursing* (3rd ed.). Philadelphia: W.B. Saunders.

Obstetrical Assessment

I. GESTATION

A. Estimated date of confinement (EDC) or estimated date of delivery (EDD)

B. Lasts approximately 280 days

C. **Nagele's rule** for estimating EDC (Box 21-1)

1. For **Nagele's rule** to be accurate, the woman must have a regular 28-day menstrual cycle

2. Add 7 days to the first day of the last menstrual period (LMP), subtract 3 months, and then add 1 year to that date; alternatively, add 7 days to the date of the last menstrual period and count forward 9 months

II. GRAVIDITY AND PARITY

A. Gravidity

1. **Gravida** refers to a pregnant woman

2. Gravidity refers to the number of pregnancies

3. Nulligravida is a woman who has never been pregnant

4. Primigravida is a woman who is pregnant for the first time

5. Multigravida is a woman in at least her second pregnancy

BOX 21-1

Nagele's Rule for Determining Estimated Date of Confinement (EDC)

First day of LMP: September 11, 2007
Add 7 days: September 18, 2007
Subtract 3 months: June 18, 2007
Add 1 year: June 18, 2008
EDC: June 18, 2008

B. Parity

1. **Parity** is the number of births (not the number of fetuses, e.g., twins) past 20 weeks' gestation, whether or not the fetus was born alive

2. Nullipara is a woman who has not had a birth at more than 20 weeks' gestation

3. Primipara is a woman who has had one birth after the 20th week of gestation

4. Multipara is a woman who has had two or more pregnancies resulting in viable offspring

C. Use of GTPAL: Pregnancy outcomes can be described with the GTPAL acronym (Box 21-2)

1. **G** = gravidity = number of pregnancies

2. **T** = term births = number born at term (40 weeks)

3. **P** = preterm births = number born before 40 weeks' gestation

4. **A** = abortions or miscarriages = number of abortions/miscarriages (included in gravida if

---

BOX 21-2

GTPAL Acronym

G = gravidity
T = term births
P = preterm births
A = abortions/miscarriages
L = live births

Example: A woman is pregnant for the fourth time. She had one elective abortion in the first trimester, a daughter who was born at 40 weeks' gestation, and a son who was born at 36 weeks' gestation. Therefore, she is gravida (G) 4, para 2, and term (T) 1 (the daughter born at 40 weeks); preterm (P) = 1 (the son born at 36 weeks); abortion (A) = 1 (the abortion is counted in the gravida but is not included in the para because it occurred before 20 weeks); live births (L) = 2.
GTPAL = 4, 1, 1, 1, 2

---

before 20 weeks' gestation; included in para if past 20 weeks' gestation)

    5. **L** = live births = number of live births or living children

---

III. PREGNANCY SIGNS

A. Presumptive signs
1. Amenorrhea
2. Nausea and vomiting
3. Increased size and increased feeling of fullness in breasts
4. Pronounced nipples
5. Urinary frequency
6. **Quickening:** First perception of fetal movement; may occur as early as the 14th to 16th week of gestation
7. Fatigue
8. Discoloration and thickening of vaginal mucosa

B. Probable signs
1. Uterine enlargement
2. **Hegar's sign:** Softening of the uterus that occurs at about week 6
3. **Goodell's sign:** Softening of the cervix that occurs at the beginning of the second month
4. **Chadwick's sign:** Bluish coloration of the mucous membranes of cervix, vagina, and vulva that occurs about week 6
5. **Ballottement:** Rebounding of the fetus against the examiner's fingers on palpation
6. Braxton Hicks contractions
7. Positive pregnancy test measuring level of human chorionic gonadotropin (hCG)

C. Positive signs
1. Fetal heart rate detected by electronic device (Doppler transducer) at 10 to 12 weeks and by nonelectronic device (fetoscope) at 20 weeks of gestation
2. Active fetal movements palpable by examiner
3. Outline of fetus via radiography or ultrasound

IV. FUNDAL HEIGHT (Box 21-3)

A. Measured to evaluate gestational age of fetus
B. During the second and third trimesters (weeks 18 to 30), fundal height in centimeters approximately equals the fetus's age in weeks plus or minus 2 cm

---

BOX 21-3

Measuring Fundal Height

1. Place the client in a supine position.
2. Place the end of the tape measure at the level of the symphysis pubis.
3. Stretch the tape to the top of the uterine fundus.
4. Note and record measurement.

C. At 16 weeks, the fundus can be found halfway between the symphysis pubis and the umbilicus
D. At 20 to 22 weeks, the fundus is at the umbilicus
E. At 36 weeks, the fundus is at the xiphoid process

V. MATERNAL RISK FACTORS

A. German measles (rubella)
1. The risks of maternal and fetal or congenital infection are related to the trimester of placental infection
2. Maternal infection during the first 8 weeks of gestation carries the highest rate of maternal and fetal infection

B. Sexually transmitted diseases
1. Syphilis
    a. May cross the **placenta**
    b. Usually leads to spontaneous abortions
    c. Increases the incidence of mental subnormality and physical deformities in the fetus
2. Genital herpes
    a. May cross **placenta**
    b. Fetus contaminated after membranes rupture or with vaginal **delivery**
3. Gonorrhea
    a. The fetus is contaminated at the time of **delivery**
    b. May result in postpartum infection of the **neonate**
    c. Risks to the **neonate** include ophthalmia neonatorum, pneumonia, sepsis

C. Human immunodeficiency virus (HIV)
1. The virus is transmitted through blood, blood products, and other bodily fluids such as urine, semen, and vaginal fluid
2. Repeated exposure to HIV during pregnancy through unsafe sex practices or intravenous drug use can increase the risk of transmission to the fetus

D. Substance abuse
1. Many substances cross the **placenta**; therefore, no drugs, including over-the-counter medications, should be taken unless prescribed by the physician
2. Substances commonly abused include alcohol, cocaine, crack, marijuana, amphetamines, barbiturates, and heroin
3. Substance abuse threatens normal fetal growth and successful term completion of the pregnancy
4. Substance abuse places the pregnancy at risk for fetal growth retardation, abruptio placentae, and fetal bradycardia
5. Physical signs of drug abuse may include dilated or contracted pupils, fatigue, track (needle) marks, skin abscesses, inflamed nasal mucosa, and inappropriate behavior by the mother
6. Consumption of alcohol during pregnancy may lead to fetal alcohol syndrome; can cause jitteriness, physical abnormalities, congenital anomalies, and growth deficits

7. Smoking leads to low birth weights, higher incidence of birth defects, and stillbirths

E. Adolescent pregnancy

1. Factors that result in adolescent pregnancy include the early onset of menarche, changing sexual behaviors in this age-group, problems with family development, poverty, and the lack of knowledge of reproduction and birth control

2. Major concerns related to adolescent pregnancy include poor nutritional status, emotional and behavioral difficulties, lack of support systems, increased risk of stillbirth, low-birth-weight newborn infants, fetal mortality, cephalopelvic disproportion, and increased risks of maternal complications such as hypertension, anemia, prolonged labor, and infections

PRACTICE QUESTIONS

1. A client arrives at the prenatal clinic for the first prenatal assessment. The client tells the nurse that the first day of her last menstrual period was September 19, 2007. Using Nagele's rule, the nurse determines the estimated date of confinement as:
   1. July 26, 2008
   2. June 12, 2008
   3. June 26, 2008
   4. July 12, 2008

2. A nurse is collecting data during an admission assessment of a client who is pregnant with twins. The client has a healthy 5-year-old child who was delivered at 38 weeks, and tells the nurse that she does not have a history of any type of abortion or fetal demise. The nurse would document the GTPAL for this client as:
   1. G = 3, T = 2, P = 0, A = 0, L = 1
   2. G = 2, T = 0, P = 1, A = 0, L = 1
   3. G = 1, T = 1, P = 1, A = 0, L = 1
   4. G = 2, T = 0, P = 0, A = 0, L = 1

3. A nurse is collecting data during an admission assessment on a client who is pregnant with twins. The client also has a 5-year-old child. The nurse would document which gravida and para status on this client?
   1. Gravida III, para II
   2. Gravida II, para II
   3. Gravida I, para I
   4. Gravida II, para I

4. A primipara is being evaluated in the clinic during her second trimester of pregnancy. Which of the following would indicate an abnormal physical finding necessitating further testing?
   1. Consistent increase in fundal height
   2. Fetal heart rate of 180 beats per minute
   3. Braxton Hicks contractions
   4. Quickening

5. A nurse is providing instructions to a pregnant client with genital herpes about the measures that need to be implemented to protect the fetus. The nurse tells the client that:
   1. Daily administration of acyclovir (Zovirax) is necessary during the entire pregnancy
   2. Total abstinence from sexual intercourse is necessary during the entire pregnancy
   3. Sitz baths need to be taken every 4 hours while awake if vaginal lesions are present
   4. A cesarean section will be necessary if vaginal lesions are present at the time of labor

6. A nurse is collecting data on a pregnant client who is at 28 weeks' gestation. The nurse measures the fundal height in centimeters and expects the findings to be which of the following?
   1. 22 cm
   2. 28 cm
   3. 36 cm
   4. 40 cm

7. A pregnant client is seen in the health care clinic for a regular prenatal visit. The client tells the nurse that she is experiencing irregular contractions. The nurse determines that the client is experiencing Braxton Hicks contractions. Based on this finding, which nursing action is appropriate?
   1. Instruct the client to maintain bed rest for the remainder of the pregnancy
   2. Instruct the client that these are common and may occur throughout the pregnancy
   3. Contact the physician
   4. Call the maternity unit and inform them that the client will be admitted in a prelabor condition

8. A nurse is reviewing the record of a client who has just been told that a pregnancy test is positive. The physician has documented the presence of Goodell's sign. The nurse determines that this sign is indicative of:
   1. A softening of the cervix
   2. soft blowing sound that corresponds to the maternal pulse while auscultating the uterus
   3. The presence of human chorionic gonadotropin (hCG) in the urine
   4. The presence of fetal movement

9. A nursing instructor asks a nursing student to describe the process of quickening. Which of the following statements, if made by the student, indicates an understanding of this term?
   1. "It is the irregular, painless contractions that occur throughout pregnancy."
   2. "It is the soft blowing sound that can be heard when the uterus is auscultated."
   3. "It is the fetal movement that is felt by the mother."
   4. "It is the thinning of the lower uterine segment."

10. A pregnant client asks the nurse in the clinic when she will be able to start feeling the fetus move.

The nurse responds by telling the mother that fetal movements will be noted between:
1. 6 and 8 weeks' gestation
2. 8 and 10 weeks' gestation
3. 10 and 12 weeks' gestation
4. 14 and 16 weeks' gestation

ALTERNATE FORMAT QUESTION: MULTIPLE RESPONSE

A nurse is assisting in performing an assessment on a client who suspects that she is pregnant and is checking the client for probable signs of pregnancy. Select all probable signs of pregnancy.

____ Uterine enlargement
____ Fetal heart rate detected by a nonelectronic device
____ Outline of fetus via radiography or ultrasound
____ Chadwick's sign
____ Braxton Hicks contractions
____ Ballottement

ANSWERS

1. Answer: 3
Rationale: Accurate use of Nagele's rule requires that the woman have a regular 28-day menstrual cycle. Add 7 days to the first day of the last menstrual period (LMP), subtract 3 months, and then add 1 year to that date. First day of the LMP: September 19, 2007; add 7 days: September 26, 2007; subtract 3 months: June 26, 2007; add 1 year: June 26, 2008.
Test-Taking Strategy: Knowledge regarding the use of Nagele's rule is required to answer this question. Read all of the options carefully, noting the dates and years in the options, before selecting an answer. Review Nagele's rule if you had difficulty with this question.
Level of Cognitive Ability: Comprehension
Client Needs: Physiological Integrity
Integrated Process: Nursing Process/Data Collection
Content Area: Maternity/Antepartum
Reference: Leifer, G. (2005). *Maternity nursing* (9th ed.). Philadelphia: W.B. Saunders, p. 34.

2. Answer: 2
Rationale: Pregnancy outcomes can be described with the GTPAL acronym: G = gravidity = number of pregnancies; T = term births = number born at term (40 weeks); P = preterm births = number born before 40 weeks' gestation; A = abortions/miscarriages = number of abortions/miscarriages (included in gravida if before 20 weeks' gestation; included in para if past 20 weeks' gestation); L = live births = number of live births or living children. Therefore, a woman who is pregnant with twins and has a child has a gravida of 2. Because the child was delivered at 38 weeks, the number of preterm births is 1 and number of term births is 0. The number of abortions is 0 and number of live births is 1.
Test-Taking Strategy: Knowledge and understanding of the GTPAL acronym will direct you to option 2. If you had difficulty answering this question, review this method of describing pregnancy outcomes.
Level of Cognitive Ability: Application
Client Needs: Health Promotion and Maintenance
Integrated Process: Nursing Process/Data Collection
Content Area: Maternity/Antepartum
Reference: Wong, D., Perry, S., & Hockenberry, M. (2002). *Maternal child nursing care* (2nd ed.). St. Louis:Mosby, p. 168.

3. Answer: 4
Rationale: Gravida is a term that refers to a woman who is or has been pregnant, regardless of the duration of the pregnancy. Para is a term that means the number of births past 20 weeks' gestation. Parity does not reflect the number of fetuses or infants. Option 1, 2, and 3 are incorrect based on the above definition.
Test-Taking Strategy: Knowledge of the terms *gravida* and *para* is necessary to answer this question correctly. Review the description of these terms if you had difficulty with this question.
Level of Cognitive Ability: Application
Client Needs: Physiological Integrity
Integrated Process: Communication and Documentation
Content Area: Maternity/Antepartum
Reference: Leifer, G. (2005). *Maternity nursing* (9th ed.). Philadelphia: W.B. Saunders, pp. 33-34.

4. Answer: 2
Rationale: The fetal heart rate depends on gestational age. It is 160 to 170 beats per minute in the first trimester and slows with fetal growth to approximately 110 or 120 to 160 beats per minute. Options 1, 3, and 4 are normal expected findings.
Test-Taking Strategy: Use the process of elimination. Note the key words, *indicates an abnormal physical finding*. Recalling the normal fetal heart rate will direct you to option 2. Review normal assessment findings in pregnancy if you had difficulty with this question.
Level of Cognitive Ability: Comprehension
Client Needs: Physiological Integrity
Integrated Process: Nursing Process/Data Collection
Content Area: Maternity/Antepartum
Reference: Leifer, G. (2005). *Maternity nursing* (9th ed.). Philadelphia: W.B. Saunders, p. 78.

5. Answer: 4
Rationale: For women with active lesions, either recurrent or primary at the time of labor, delivery should be by cesarean section to prevent the fetus from being in contact with the genital herpes. The safety of acyclovir has not been established during pregnancy and should be used only when a life-threatening infection is present. Clients should be advised to abstain from sexual contact while the lesions are present. If this is an initial infection, they should continue to abstain

until they become culture-negative, because prolonged viral shedding may occur in such cases. Keeping the genital area clean and dry will promote healing.
Test-Taking Strategy: Use the process of elimination. Eliminate options 1 and 2 first because of the absolute word "entire" in these options. From the remaining options, recalling that the lesions should be kept clean and dry to promote healing will assist in eliminating option 3. If you had difficulty with this question, review the content related to genital herpes as a maternal risk factor.
Level of Cognitive Ability: Application
Client Needs: Safe, Effective Care Environment
Integrated Process: Teaching/Learning
Content Area: Maternity/Antepartum
Reference: Leifer, G. (2005). *Maternity nursing* (9th ed.). Philadelphia: W.B. Saunders, p. 338.

6. *Answer: 2*
Rationale: During the second and third trimesters (weeks 18 to 30), fundal height in centimeters approximately equals the fetus's age in weeks plus or minus 2 cm. At 16 weeks, the fundus can be located halfway between the symphysis pubis and the umbilicus. At 20 to 22 weeks, the fundus is at the umbilicus and, at 36 weeks, the fundus is at the xiphoid process.
Test-Taking Strategy: Use the process of elimination. Remember that during the second and third trimesters (weeks 18 to 30), fundal height in centimeters approximately equals the fetus's age in weeks plus or minus 2 cm. If you are unfamiliar with this data collection technique, review this content area.
Level of Cognitive Ability: Comprehension
Client Needs: Health Promotion and Maintenance
Integrated Process: Nursing Process/Data Collection
Content Area: Maternity/Antepartum
References: Leifer, G. (2005). *Maternity nursing* (9th ed.). Philadelphia: W.B. Saunders, p. 192.
Murray, S., McKinney, E., & Gorrie, T. (2002). *Foundations of maternal-newborn nursing* (3rd ed.). Philadelphia: W.B. Saunders, p. 425.

7. *Answer: 2*
Rationale: Braxton Hicks contractions are irregular, painless contractions that may occur intermittently throughout pregnancy. Because Braxton Hicks contractions may occur and are normal in some pregnant women during pregnancy, options 1, 3, and 4 are unnecessary and inappropriate actions.
Test-Taking Strategy: Use the process of elimination. Options 3 and 4 are similar and can be eliminated first. From the remaining options, knowing that Braxton Hicks contractions are common and can occur throughout pregnancy will assist in directing you to option 2. If you had difficulty with this question, review the physiology associated with Braxton Hicks contractions.
Level of Cognitive Ability: Application
Client Needs: Health Promotion and Maintenance
Integrated Process: Teaching/Learning
Content Area: Maternity/Antepartum
Reference: Leifer, G. (2005). *Maternity nursing* (9th ed.). Philadelphia: W.B. Saunders, p. 83.

8. *Answer: 1*
Rationale: In the early weeks of pregnancy, the cervix becomes softer as a result of pelvic vasoconstriction, which causes Goodell's sign. Cervical softening is noted by the examiner during pelvic examination. A soft blowing sound that corresponds to the maternal pulse may be auscultated over the uterus and is due to blood circulation through the placenta. hCG is noted in maternal urine in a positive urine pregnancy test. Goodell's sign does not indicate the presence of fetal movement.
Test-Taking Strategy: Use the process of elimination and knowledge regarding the physiological findings in Goodell's sign to answer this question. Remember that Goodell's sign refers to a softening of the cervix. If you had difficulty with this question, review the changes in the cervix that occur during pregnancy.
Level of Cognitive Ability: Comprehension
Client Needs: Health Promotion and Maintenance
Integrated Process: Nursing Process/Data Collection
Content Area: Maternity/Antepartum
Reference: McKinney, E., James, S., Murray, S., & Ashwill, J. (2005). *Maternal-child nursing* (2nd ed.). St. Louis: Elsevier, p. 264.

9. *Answer: 3*
Rationale: Quickening is fetal movement and may occur as early as the 14th to 16th week of gestation, when the expectant mother first notices subtle fetal movements that gradually increase in intensity. A soft blowing sound that corresponds to the maternal pulse may be auscultated over the uterus, which is known as uterine souffle. This sound is due to the blood circulation to the placenta and corresponds to the maternal pulse. Braxton Hicks contractions are irregular, painless contractions that may occur throughout pregnancy. A thinning of the lower uterine segment occurs about the sixth week of pregnancy and is called Hegar's sign.
Test-Taking Strategy: Use the process of elimination and knowledge regarding the term *quickening* to answer this question. Remember that quickening is fetal movement. If you are unfamiliar with this sign associated with pregnancy, review this content area.
Level of Cognitive Ability: Comprehension
Client Needs: Health Promotion and Maintenance
Integrated Process: Teaching/Learning
Content Area: Maternity/Antepartum
References: Leifer, G. (2005). *Maternity nursing* (9th ed.). Philadelphia: W.B. Saunders, p. 386.
Murray, S., McKinney, E., & Gorrie, T. (2002). *Foundations of maternal-newborn nursing* (3rd ed.). Philadelphia: W.B. Saunders, p. 163.

10. *Answer: 4*
Rationale: Quickening is fetal movement and may occur as early as the 14th to 16th week of gestation. The expectant mother first notices subtle fetal movements during this time, which gradually increase in intensity. Options 1, 2, and 3 are incorrect.
Test-Taking Strategy: Use the process of elimination and knowledge regarding the occurrence of quickening. In this situation, it is best to select the option that indicates the greatest

length of gestational time. Review the process of quickening if you had difficulty with this question.

Level of Cognitive Ability: Application
Client Needs: Health Promotion and Maintenance
Integrated Process: Teaching/Learning
Content Area: Maternity/Antepartum
Reference: Murray, S., McKinney, E., & Gorrie, T. (2002). *Foundations of maternal-newborn nursing* (3rd ed.). Philadelphia: W.B. Saunders, p. 147.

ALTERNATE FORMAT QUESTION: MULTIPLE RESPONSE

Answers:
Uterine enlargement
Chadwick's sign
Braxton Hicks contractions
Ballottement
Rationale: The probable signs of pregnancy include uterine enlargement, Hegar's sign (softening and thinning of the lower uterine segment that occurs at about week 6), Goodell's sign (softening of the cervix that occurs at the beginning of the second month), Chadwick's sign (bluish coloration of the mucous membranes of the cervix, vagina, and vulva that occurs about week 6), ballottement (rebounding of the fetus against the examiner's fingers on palpation), Braxton Hicks contractions, and a positive pregnancy test measuring for human chorionic gonadotropin (hCG). Positive signs of pregnancy include fetal heart rate detected by an electronic device (Doppler transducer) at 8 to 12 weeks and by a nonelectronic device (fetoscope) at 20 weeks' gestation, active fetal movements palpable by the examiner, and an outline of the fetus via radiography or ultrasound.

Test-Taking Strategy: Focusing on the issue, probable signs of pregnancy, will assist in answering this question. Remember that detection of the fetal heart rate and an outline of the fetus via radiography or ultrasound are positive signs of pregnancy. Review the probable signs of pregnancy if you had difficulty with this question.

Level of Cognitive Ability: Analysis
Client Needs: Health Promotion and Maintenance
Integrated Process: Nursing Process/Data Collection
Content Area: Maternity/Antepartum
Reference: Murray, S., McKinney, E., & Gorrie, T. (2002). *Foundations of maternal-newborn nursing* (3rd ed.). Philadelphia: W.B. Saunders, p. 132.

REFERENCES

Leifer, G. (2005). *Maternity nursing* (9th ed.). Philadelphia: W.B. Saunders.

McKinney, E., James, S., Murray, S., & Ashwill, J. (2005). *Maternal-child nursing* (2nd ed.). St. Louis: Elsevier.

Murray, S., McKinney, E., & Gorrie, T. (2002). *Foundations of maternal-newborn nursing* (3rd ed.). Philadelphia: W.B. Saunders.

Wong, D., Perry, S., & Hockenberry, M. (2002). *Maternal child nursing care* (2nd ed.). St. Louis: Mosby.

Prenatal Period and Risk Conditions

I. PHYSIOLOGICAL MATERNAL CHANGES

A. Cardiovascular system
  1. Circulating blood volume increases
  2. Heart is elevated upward and to the left because of displacement of the diaphragm as the uterus enlarges
  3. Pulse may increase about 10 beats per minute; blood pressure may decline in the second trimester
  4. Physiological anemia may occur; iron requirements are increased
  5. Sodium and water retention may occur

B. Respiratory system
  1. Oxygen consumption increases
  2. Diaphragm is elevated as a result of the enlarged uterus
  3. Respiratory rate remains unchanged
  4. Shortness of breath may be experienced

C. Gastrointestinal (GI) system
  1. Nausea and vomiting may occur as a result of the secretion of human chorionic gonadotropin (hCG), which subsides by the third month
  2. Constipation resulting from decreased GI motility or pressure of the uterus
  3. Poor appetite, flatulence, and heartburn resulting from decreased GI motility and slow emptying of the stomach
  4. Alterations in taste and smell may occur
  5. Hemorrhoids resulting from increased venous pressure

D. Renal system
  1. Frequency of urination occurs in the first and third trimester as a result of pressure of the enlarging uterus on the bladder
  2. Decreased bladder tone is caused by hormonal changes
  3. Decreased bladder capacity is present
  4. Renal function increases
  5. Renal threshold for glucose may be reduced

E. Endocrine system: basal metabolic rate rises

F. Reproductive system
  1. Uterus
    a. Uterus enlarges from 60 to 1000 g
    b. Irregular contractions occur
  2. Cervix
    a. Becomes shorter, more elastic, and larger in diameter
    b. Endocervical glands secrete a thick mucus plug, which is expelled from the canal when dilation begins
    c. Increased vascularization causes a softening and blue-purple discoloration (Chadwick's sign)
  3. Ovaries: Cease ovum production
  4. Vagina
    a. Hypertrophy and thickening of muscle occurs
    b. Increase in vaginal secretions occurs; secretions are usually thick, white, and acidic
  5. Breast
    a. Breast size increases
    b. Nipples become more pronounced and areola becomes darker
    c. Colostrum may appear from the breast

G. Skin
  1. A dark streak down the midline of the abdomen may appear (linea nigra)
  2. Chloasma (mask of pregnancy), a blotchy brownish hyperpigmentation, may occur over the forehead, cheeks, and nose
  3. Reddish purple stretch marks (striae) may occur on the abdomen, breasts, thighs, and upper arms

H. Skeletal system: Postural changes occur as the increased weight of the uterus causes a forward pull of the bony pelvis

I. Metabolism
1. Metabolic function increases
2. Body weight increases
3. Water retention is increased, which can contribute to weight gain

II. PSYCHOLOGICAL MATERNAL CHANGES

A. Ambivalence
1. Occurs early in pregnancy, even when the pregnancy is planned
2. Mother may experience dependence-independence conflict and ambivalence related to role changes
3. Father may experience ambivalence related to new role he is assuming, increased financial responsibilities, and sharing wife's attention with the child

B. Acceptance: Factors that may be related to acceptance of the pregnancy are the woman's readiness for the experience and her identification with the motherhood role

C. Emotional lability
1. May be manifested by frequency in the change of emotional states or extremes in emotional states
2. These emotional changes are common, but the mother may believe that these changes are abnormal

D. Body image changes: Changes in a woman's perception of her image during pregnancy occur gradually and may be either positive or negative

E. Relationship with the fetus
1. The woman may daydream to prepare for motherhood and think about the maternal qualities she would like to possess
2. The woman first accepts the biological fact that she is pregnant
3. The woman next accepts the growing fetus as distinct from herself and a person to nurture
4. Finally, the woman prepares realistically for the birth and parenting of the child

III. DISCOMFORTS OF PREGNANCY

A. Nausea and vomiting
1. Occur in the first trimester
2. Caused by elevated human chorionic gonadotropin (hCG) levels and changes in carbohydrate metabolism
3. Interventions
   a. Eating dry crackers before arising
   b. Avoiding brushing teeth immediately after arising
   c. Eating small, frequent, low-fat meals during the day
   d. Drinking liquids between meals rather than at meals
   e. Avoiding fried foods and spicy foods

f. Acupressure (some types may require a prescription)
g. Herbal remedies, only if approved by a physician or nurse-midwife

B. Syncope
1. Usually occurs in the first trimester; supine hypotension occurs, particularly in the second and third trimesters
2. May be hormonally triggered or caused by increased blood volume, anemia, fatigue, sudden position changes, or lying supine
3. Interventions
   a. Sitting with the feet elevated
   b. Changing positions slowly
   c. Changing the position to the lateral recumbent to relieve the pressure of the uterus on the inferior vena cava

C. Urinary urgency and frequency
1. Usually occurs in first and third trimesters
2. Caused by pressure of the uterus on the bladder
3. Interventions
   a. Drinking 2 quarts of fluid during the day
   b. Limiting fluid intake in the evening
   c. Voiding at regular intervals
   d. Sleeping on the side at night
   e. Wearing perineal pads, if necessary
   f. Performing Kegel's exercises

D. Breast tenderness
1. Can occur from the first through the third trimesters
2. Caused by increased levels of estrogen and progesterone
3. Interventions
   a. Encouraging the use of a supportive bra with nonelastic straps
   b. Avoiding the use of soap on the nipples and areola area to prevent drying

E. Increased vaginal discharge
1. Can occur from the first through the third trimesters
2. Caused by hyperplasia of vaginal mucosa and increased mucus production
3. Interventions
   a. Wearing cotton underwear
   b. Avoiding douching
   c. Using proper cleansing and hygiene techniques
   d. Advising the client to consult the physician or nurse-midwife if infection is suspected

F. Nasal stuffiness
1. Occurs during the first through the third trimesters
2. Occurs because of increased estrogen that causes swelling of the nasal tissues and dryness
3. Interventions
   a. Encouraging the use of humidifier
   b. Avoiding the use of nasal sprays or antihistamines

G. Fatigue
1. Occurs usually in the first and third trimesters
2. Is usually due to hormonal changes
3. Interventions
   a. Arranging frequent rest periods throughout the day
   b. Using correct body mechanics
   c. Engaging in regular exercise
   d. Performing muscle relaxation and strengthening exercises for the legs and hip joints
   e. Avoiding eating and drinking foods containing stimulants throughout pregnancy

H. Heartburn
1. Occurs in the second and third trimesters
2. Results from increased progesterone levels, decreased GI motility and esophageal reflux, and displacement of the stomach by the enlarging uterus
3. Interventions
   a. Eating small, frequent meals, and avoiding fatty and spicy food
   b. Sitting upright for 30 minutes after a meal
   c. Drinking milk between meals
   d. Performing tailor-sitting exercises
   e. Taking antacids only if recommended by the physician or nurse-midwife

I. Ankle edema
1. Usually occurs in the second and third trimesters
2. Occurs because of vasodilation, venous stasis, and increased venous pressure below the uterus
3. Interventions
   a. Elevating the legs during the day
   b. Sleeping on the left side
   c. Wearing supportive stockings
   d. Avoiding sitting or standing in one position for long periods

J. Varicose veins
1. Usually occur in the second and third trimesters
2. Occur because of weakening walls of the veins or valves and venous congestion
3. Interventions
   a. Wearing support hose
   b. Elevating the feet when sitting
   c. Lying with the feet and hips elevated
   d. Avoiding long periods of standing or sitting
   e. Moving about while standing to improve circulation
   f. Avoiding leg crossing
   g. Avoiding constricting articles of clothing

K. Headaches
1. Usually occur in the second and third trimesters
2. Occur as a result of changes in blood volume and vascular tone
3. Interventions
   a. Changing position slowly
   b. Applying a cool cloth to the forehead

   c. Eating a small snack
   d. Using acetaminophen (Tylenol) only if prescribed by the physician or nurse-midwife

L. Hemorrhoids
1. Usually occur in the second and third trimesters
2. Occur because of increased venous pressure and/or constipation
3. Interventions
   a. Soaking in a warm sitz bath
   b. Sitting on a soft pillow
   c. Eating high-fiber foods and avoiding constipation
   d. Drinking sufficient fluids
   e. Increasing exercise, such as walking
   f. Applying ointments, suppositories, or compresses as prescribed by the physician or nurse-midwife

M. Constipation
1. Usually occurs in the second and third trimesters
2. Occurs because of decreased intestinal motility, displacement of the intestines, and taking iron supplements
3. Interventions
   a. Eating high-fiber foods
   b. Drinking sufficient fluids
   c. Exercising regularly
   d. Laxatives and enemas are avoided unless their use is approved by the physician or nurse-midwife

N. Backache
1. Usually occurs in the second and third trimesters
2. Occurs from an exaggerated lumbosacral curve because of the enlarged uterus
3. Interventions
   a. Encouraging rest
   b. Using correct body mechanics and improving posture
   c. Wearing low-heeled shoes
   d. Performing pelvic rocking and abdominal breathing exercises
   e. Sleeping on a firm mattress

O. Leg cramps
1. Usually occur in the second and third trimesters
2. Occur because of an altered calcium-phosphorus balance and pressure of the uterus on nerves, or from fatigue
3. Interventions
   a. Getting regular exercise, especially walking
   b. Dorsiflexing the foot of the affected leg
   c. Increasing calcium intake

P. Shortness of breath
1. Can occur in the second and third trimesters
2. Occurs as a result of pressure on the diaphragm
3. Interventions
   a. Allowing frequent rest periods and avoiding overexertion
   b. Sleeping with the head elevated or on the side
   c. Performing tailor-sitting exercises

IV. LABORATORY TESTS (Box 22-1)

A. Blood type and Rh factor
  1. ABO typing is performed to determine the woman's blood type
  2. Rh typing is done to determine the presence or absence of Rh antigen (Rh positive or Rh negative)
  3. If the client is Rh negative and has a negative antibody screen, the client will need repeat antibody screens and should receive Rh immune globulin at 28 weeks' gestation

B. Rubella titer
  1. If the client has a negative titer, indicating susceptibility to the rubella virus, the client should receive the appropriate immunization postpartum
  2. The client must be using effective birth control at the time of the immunization; must be counseled not to become pregnant for 3 months following immunization and to avoid contact with anyone who is immunocompromised
  3. If the rubella vaccine is administered at the same time as Rh immune globulin, it may not be effective

C. Hemoglobin and hematocrit levels
  1. Hemoglobin and hematocrit levels will drop during gestation as a result of increased plasma volume
  2. An increase in the hematocrit level may indicate the development of pregnancy-induced hypertension (PIH)
  3. A decrease in the hemoglobin level below 10 g/dL or a decrease in the hematocrit level below 30 g/dL indicates anemia

D. Papanicolaou (Pap) smear: Done during the initial prenatal examination to screen for cervical neoplasia

E. Sexually transmitted diseases (Table 22-1)

F. Sickle cell screening
  1. Indicated for clients at risk for sickle cell disease
  2. A positive test result may indicate a need for further screening

G. Tuberculin skin test
  1. The health care provider may prefer to perform this skin test after **delivery**
  2. A positive skin test indicates the need for a chest radiograph (using an abdominal lead shield) to rule out active disease; in a pregnant client, a chest radiograph will not be performed until after 20 weeks' gestation (after fetal organs are formed)
  3. Converters to positive may be referred for treatment with medication following **delivery**

H. Hepatitis B surface antigens
  1. Recommended for all women because of the prevalence of the disease in the general population
  2. Vaccination for hepatitis B antigen may be specifically indicated for:
     a. Health care workers
     b. Clients born in Asia, Africa, Haiti, or the Pacific islands
     c. Clients with previously undiagnosed jaundice or chronic liver disease
     d. IV drug abusers
     e. Clients with tattoos
     f. Clients with histories of blood transfusions
     g. Clients with histories of multiple episodes of sexually transmitted diseases
     h. Clients who have been previously rejected as blood donors
     i. Clients with histories of dialysis or renal transplantation
     j. Clients from households having hepatitis B–infected members or hemodialysis clients

I. Urinalysis and urine culture
  1. A urine specimen for glucose and protein determinations should be obtained at every prenatal visit
  2. Glycosuria is a common result of decreased renal threshold that occurs during pregnancy
  3. If glycosuria persists, this may indicate diabetes

BOX 22-1

Prenatal Visits

Every 4 weeks from 28 to 32 weeks
Every 2 weeks from 32 to 36 weeks
Every week from 36 to 40 weeks

TABLE 22-1

Monitoring for Sexually Transmitted Diseases

Disease	Laboratory Test
Gonorrhea	A culture is done during the initial prenatal examination to screen for gonorrhea. The culture may be repeated during the third trimester in high-risk clients.
Syphilis	A culture is done during the initial prenatal examination to screen for syphilis. The culture may be repeated during the third trimester in high-risk clients.
Herpesvirus infection	A culture is indicated for clients with a positive history or those with active lesions. Performed to determine the route of delivery. Weekly cultures may be done at the 35th or 36th week of pregnancy until delivery.
Chlamydia	A culture is indicated if the client is in a high-risk group or if infants from previous pregnancies have developed neonatal conjunctivitis or pneumonia.

4. White blood cells in the urine may indicate infection
5. Ketonuria may result from insufficient food intake or vomiting
6. Levels of 2+ to 4+ protein in the urine may indicate infection or pregnancy-induced hypertension (PIH)

V. DIAGNOSTIC TESTS

A. Ultrasonography
  1. Outlines and identifies fetal and maternal structures
  2. Helps confirm gestational age and estimated date of **delivery**
  3. May be done abdominally or transvaginally during pregnancy
  4. Interventions
    a. If the abdominal ultrasound is being performed, the woman may need to drink water to fill the bladder before the procedure to obtain a better image of the fetus
    b. If the transvaginal ultrasound is being performed, a lubricated probe is inserted into the vagina
    c. Inform the client that the test presents no known risks to the client or the fetus

B. Alpha-fetoprotein (AFP) screening
  1. Assesses the quantity of fetal serum proteins; if elevated, is associated with open neural tube and abdominal wall defects
  2. Can detect spina bifida and Down syndrome
  3. Interventions
    a. Explain that the level is determined by a single maternal blood sample drawn at 15 to 18 weeks' gestation
    b. If the level is elevated and the gestation is less than 18 weeks, a second sample is drawn
    c. Ultrasonography is performed if AFP level is elevated to rule out fetal abnormalities or multiple gestation

C. Chorionic villus sampling (CVS)
  1. The physician aspirates a small sample of chorionic villus tissue at 8 to 12 weeks' gestation
  2. Test is performed to detect genetic abnormalities
  3. Interventions
    a. Obtain informed consent
    b. Instruct the client to drink water to fill the bladder before the procedure to aid in positioning the uterus for catheter insertion
    c. Instruct the client to report bleeding, infection, or leakage of fluid at insertion site after the procedure
    d. Rh-negative women may be given Rho (D) immune globulin (RhoGAM) because CVS increases the risk of Rh sensitization

D. Kick counts (fetal movement counting)
  1. Mother sits quietly or lies down on her left side and counts fetal kicks for a period of time, as instructed
  2. Instruct the client to notify the physician or nurse-midwife if there are fewer than 10 kicks in a 12-hour period or as instructed by the physician or nurse-midwife

E. Amniocentesis
  1. Aspiration of **amniotic fluid** done from 13th to 14th week of pregnancy and thereafter
  2. Performed to determine genetic disorders, metabolic defects, and fetal lung maturity
  3. Risks
    a. Maternal hemorrhage
    b. Infection
    c. Rh isoimmunization
    d. Abruptio placentae
    e. **Amniotic fluid** emboli
    f. Premature rupture of the membranes
  4. Interventions
    a. Obtain informed consent
    b. Instruct the client to empty the bladder before the procedure
    c. Prepare the client for ultrasonography, which is performed to locate the **placenta**
    d. Obtain baseline vital signs and fetal heart rate (FHR), and monitor every 15 minutes
    e. Position the client supine
    f. Instruct the client that if chills, fever, leakage of fluid at the needle insertion site, decreased fetal movement, or uterine contractions occur, she is to notify the physician or nurse-midwife

F. Fern test
  1. A microscopic slide test to determine the presence of **amniotic fluid** leakage
  2. By use of sterile technique, a specimen is obtained from the external os of the cervix and vaginal pool and examined on a slide under a microscope
  3. A fernlike pattern occurring from the salts of **amniotic fluid** indicates the presence of **amniotic fluid**
  4. Interventions
    a. Place the client in the dorsal lithotomy position
    b. Instruct the client to cough; this causes the fluid to leak from the uterus if the membranes are ruptured

G. Nitrazine test
  1. A Nitrazine test strip is used to detect the presence of **amniotic fluid** in vaginal secretions
  2. Vaginal secretions have a pH of 4.5 to 5.5 and do not affect the yellow color of the Nitrazine strip or swab
  3. **Amniotic fluid** has a pH of 7.0 to 7.5 and turns the yellow Nitrazine strip or swab a blue color

4. Interventions
   a. Place the client in the dorsal lithotomy position
   b. Touch the test tape to the fluid
   c. Assess the test tape for a blue-green, blue-gray, or deep blue color, which indicates that the membranes are probably ruptured
H. Nonstress test (Box 22-2)
I. Contraction stress test (Box 22-3)

VI. NUTRITION
A. General guidelines
   1. The average expected weight gain during pregnancy is 25 to 35 pounds for women with a normal prepregnancy weight
   2. An increase of about 300 calories per day is needed during pregnancy
   3. Calorie needs are greater in the last two trimesters than in the first

4. An increase of about 500 calories per day is needed during lactation
5. Encourage a diet high in folic acid, with folic acid supplements
6. A diet rich in folic acid is necessary for all women of childbearing age to prevent neural tube defect in the fetus during the first trimester of pregnancy
7. Drink at least 8 to 10 (8-oz) glasses of fluid each day, of which 4 to 6 glasses are water
8. Sodium is not restricted unless specifically ordered by the physician or nurse-midwife
B. Vegetarianism (Box 22-4)
   1. Ensure that the client eats a sufficient amount of varied foods to meet normal nutrient and energy needs
   2. Protein consumption can be increased by consuming a variety of vegetable protein sources based on whole grains, legumes, seeds, nuts,

---

BOX 22-2

Nonstress Test (NST)

DESCRIPTION
Performed to assess placental function and oxygenation
Determines fetal well-being
Evaluates fetal heart rate (FHR) in response to fetal movement

INTERVENTIONS
An external ultrasound transducer and tocodynamometer (toco) are applied to the mother, and a tracing of at least 20 minutes' duration is obtained so that the FHR and the uterine activity can be observed.
Obtain baseline blood pressure (BP) and monitor BP frequently.
Position mother in the left lateral position to avoid vena cava compression.
The mother may be asked to press a button every time she feels fetal movement; the monitor records a mark at each point of fetal movement, which is used as a reference point to assess FHR response.

RESULTS
Reactive Nonstress Test (Normal, Negative)
Indicates a healthy fetus
Two or more FHR accelerations of at least 15 beats per minute, lasting at least 15 seconds from the beginning of the acceleration to the end, in association with fetal movement, during a 20-minute period
Nonreactive Nonstress Test (Abnormal)
No accelerations or accelerations of less than 15 beats per minute or lasting less than 15 seconds in duration for a 40-minute observation
Unsatisfactory
Cannot be interpreted because of the poor quality of the FHR tracing

---

BOX 22-3

Contraction Stress Test

DESCRIPTION
Assesses placental oxygenation and function
Determines fetal ability to tolerate labor and determines fetal well-being
Fetus is exposed to the stressor of contractions to assess the adequacy of placental perfusion under simulated labor conditions
Performed if the nonstress test is abnormal

INTERVENTIONS
The external fetal monitor is applied to the mother, and a 20- to 30-minute baseline strip is recorded.
The uterus is stimulated to contract, either by the administration of a dilute dose of oxytocin (Pitocin) or by having the mother use nipple stimulation, until three palpable contractions with a duration of 40 seconds or more in a 10-minute period have been achieved.
Frequent maternal BP readings are done, and the mother is monitored closely while increasing doses of oxytocin are given.

RESULTS
Negative Contraction Stress Test
No late or variable decelerations of the FHR
Positive Contraction Stress Test (Abnormal)
Late or variable decelerations of the FHR, with 50% or more of the contractions in the absence of hyperstimulation of the uterus
Equivocal
Contains decelerations but with less than 50% of the contractions, or uterine activity shows a hyperstimulated uterus
Unsatisfactory
Adequate uterine contractions cannot be achieved, or the FHR tracing not of sufficient quality for adequate interpretation

and vegetables combined to provide all essential amino acids

3. Adequate energy intakes are important to ensure that dietary protein is used for protein synthesis

C. Lactose intolerance

1. Lactose consumed by an individual with a lactose intolerance can cause abdominal distention, discomfort, nausea, vomiting, cramps, and loose stools

2. Clients experiencing lactose intolerance need to incorporate sources of calcium other than dairy products regularly into their dietary patterns

3. Milk may be tolerated in cooked form, such as in custards or fermented dairy products

4. Cheese and yogurt are sometimes tolerated

5. Lactase, an enzyme, may be prescribed and is taken before ingesting milk or milk products

6. Lactase-treated milk or lactose-free products are also available commercially

D. Pica

1. Definition: Eating nonfood substances such as dirt, clay, starch, and freezer frost

2. The cause is unknown; cultural values, such as beliefs regarding a material's effect on the mother or fetus, may make pica a common practice

3. Iron deficiency anemia may occur as a result of pica

E. Cultural considerations: Refer to Chapter 6 for information on cultural considerations in nutrition

VII. ABORTION

A. Description: A pregnancy that ends before 20 weeks' gestation, either spontaneously or electively

B. Data collection

1. Spontaneous vaginal bleeding

2. Passage of clots and tissue through vagina

3. Low uterine cramping and contractions

4. Hemorrhage and shock can occur

C. Interventions

1. Maintain bed rest

2. Monitor vital signs

3. Monitor cramping and bleeding

4. Count perineal pads to evaluate blood loss and save expelled tissues and clots

5. Maintain intravenous (IV) fluids as prescribed; monitor for signs of shock

6. Prepare client for dilatation and curettage as prescribed for incomplete abortion

7. Rh immune globulin is given to appropriate Rho(D)-negative woman

VIII. ACQUIRED IMMUNODEFICIENCY SYNDROME (AIDS)

A. Description

1. The human immunodeficiency virus (HIV) is the a causative factor in the development of AIDS

2. Women infected with HIV virus may first demonstrate symptoms at the time of pregnancy or possibly develop life-threatening infections, because normal pregnancy involves some suppression of the maternal immune system

3. Zidovudine (AZT) is recommended for the prevention of maternal-fetal HIV transmission and is administered orally beginning after 14 weeks' gestation, intravenously during **labor**, and in the form of syrup to the **neonate** after birth for 6 weeks

B. Transmission

1. Sexual exposure to genital secretions of an infected person

---

BOX 22-4

Types of Vegetarian Diets

LACTO-OVO VEGETARIANS
Consume plant foods with dairy products and eggs
May consume fish and occasionally poultry

LACTO-VEGETARIANS
Consume plant foods and dairy products excluding eggs

VEGANS
Follow a strict vegetarian diet and consume no animal foods
Food pattern consists entirely of plant foods

BOX 22-5

Stages of AIDS

STAGE 1
Fever
Myalgia
Lymphadenopathy
Headache

STAGE 2
Active but asymptomatic; may remain so for years
May experience an outbreak of herpes zoster (shingles)
May experience a transient thrombocytopenia

STAGE 3
Symptomatic
Evidence of immune dysfunction
All body systems can present with signs of immune dysfunction
Integumentary and gynecological problems are common

STAGE 4
Advanced HIV infection
Vulnerable to common bacterial infections
Development of opportunistic infections
Serious immune compromise

2. Parenteral exposure to infected blood and tissue
3. Perinatal exposure of an infant to infected maternal secretions through birth process or breast-feeding

C. Risks to the mother: The mother with HIV is managed as high risk because she is vulnerable to infections

D. Diagnosis (Box 22-5)
1. Tests used to determine the presence of antibodies to HIV include enzyme-linked immunosorbent assay (ELISA), Western blot (WB), and indirect fluorescent antibody (IFA)
2. A single reactive ELISA test result by itself cannot be used to diagnose HIV and should be repeated in duplicate with the same blood sample; if the result is repeatedly reactive, follow-up tests using WB or IFA should be done
3. A positive WB or IFA is considered confirmatory for HIV
4. A positive ELISA that fails to be confirmed by WB or IFA should not be considered negative; repeat testing should take place in 3 to 6 months
5. Refer to Chapter 11 for additional laboratory tests

E. Interventions
1. Prenatal period
   a. Prevention of opportunistic infections
   b. Avoid procedures that increase the risk of perinatal transmission, such as amniocentesis and fetal scalp sampling
2. Intrapartum period
   a. If the fetus has not been exposed to HIV in utero, the highest risk exists during **delivery** through the birth canal
   b. Avoid the use of scalp electrodes
   c. Avoid episiotomy to decrease the amount of maternal blood in and around the birth canal
   d. Avoid the administration of oxytocin (Pitocin), because oxytocin contractions can be strong, inducing vaginal tears or necessitating the need for an episiotomy
   e. Place heavy absorbent pads under the mother's hips to absorb **amniotic fluid** and maternal blood
   f. Minimize the **neonate's** exposure to maternal blood and body fluids; promptly remove the **neonate** from the mother's blood following **delivery**
   g. Suction the **infant** promptly
   h. Prepare to administer zidovudine (AZT) intravenously, as prescribed to the mother during **labor** and **delivery**
3. Postpartum period
   a. Monitor for signs of infection
   b. Place the mother in protective isolation if the mother is immunosuppressed
   c. Restrict breast-feeding
   d. Instruct the mother to monitor for signs of infection and report any signs if they occur

F. The **neonate** and HIV
1. Description
   a. **Neonates** born to HIV-positive clients may test positive because the mother's positive antibodies may persist for as long as 18 months after birth; all **neonates** acquire maternal antibody to HIV infection, but not all acquire infection
   b. The use of antiviral medication, reduction of **neonate** exposure to maternal blood and body fluids, and early identification of HIV in pregnancy reduce the risk of transmission to the **neonate**
2. Interventions
   a. Bathe **neonate** carefully before any invasive procedure, such as the administration of vitamin K, heel sticks, or venipunctures; the umbilical cord stump is cleaned meticulously every day until healed
   b. **Neonate** can room with mother
   c. Prepare to administer zidovudine (AZT) to the **newborn infant** as prescribed for the first 6 weeks of life
   d. All HIV-exposed **newborn infants** should be treated with medication to prevent infection by *Pneumocystis jiroveci* (formerly known as *P. carinii*)
   e. Note that an HIV culture is recommended at age 1 month and after 4 months of age; **infants** at risk for HIV infection should be seen by the physician at birth and at 1 week, 2 weeks, 1 month, 2 months, and 4 months of life
   f. **Infants** at risk for HIV infection need to receive all recommended immunizations at the regular schedule; no live-virus vaccines should be administered
   g. The **neonate** may be asymptomatic for the first several years of life and needs to be monitored for early signs of immunodeficiency

IX. ANEMIA

A. Description
1. Condition that can develop as a result of iron deficiency
2. Anemia predisposes the client to postpartum infection and hemorrhage

B. Data collection
1. Fatigue
2. Headache
3. Pallor
4. Tachycardia
5. Hemoglobin value usually below 10 g/dL and hematocrit value usually below 30%

C. Interventions
1. Monitor hemoglobin and hematocrit levels every 2 weeks

2. Administer and instruct the client about iron and folic acid supplements
3. Instruct the client to take iron with a source of vitamin C and to avoid taking iron with tea
4. Instruct the client to eat foods high in iron, folic acid, and protein
5. Teach the client to monitor for signs and symptoms of infection
6. Prepare to administer injectable iron; may be prescribed for severe anemia
7. Prepare to administer transfusions if prescribed for severe anemia
8. Prepare for the administration of oxytoxic medications in the postpartum period to prevent hemorrhage

X. CARDIAC DISEASE

A. Description: Inability to cope with the added plasma volume and increased cardiac output
B. Data collection
   1. Cough
   2. Dyspnea and fatigue
   3. Palpitations and tachycardia
   4. Peripheral edema
   5. Angina-type pain
   6. Signs of pulmonary edema
   7. Signs of respiratory infection
C. Interventions
   1. Monitor vital signs, fetal heart rate (FHR), and condition of fetus
   2. Plan activities and stress the need for sufficient rest
   3. Encourage adequate nutrition to prevent anemia
   4. Maintain bed rest for the client as prescribed during the last weeks of pregnancy
   5. During **labor**
      a. Monitor vital signs frequently
      b. Place the client on a cardiac monitor and on an external fetal monitor
      c. Maintain bed rest, with mother lying on her side and her head and shoulders elevated
      d. Administer oxygen as prescribed
      e. Monitor for signs of heart failure

XI. CHRONIC HYPERTENSION

A. Description
   1. Hypertension that occurs before pregnancy, is diagnosed before the 20th week of gestation, or is diagnosed for the first time during pregnancy and persists beyond the 42nd day postpartum
   2. The condition predisposes the client to pregnancy-induced hypertension (PIH)
   3. Can cause **abruptio placentae** and intrauterine growth retardation
B. Data collection
   1. Headaches

2. Visual changes
3. Elevated blood pressure, usually 140/90 mm Hg or higher
4. Delayed fetal growth

C. Interventions
   1. Monitor blood pressure
   2. Monitor fetal activity and fetal growth
   3. Encourage frequent rest periods, instructing the client to lie in the left lateral position
   4. Administer antihypertensive medications as prescribed for diastolic pressures higher than 100 mm Hg
   5. Monitor intake and output (I&O)
   6. Evaluate renal function through prescribed studies such as blood urea nitrogen (BUN), serum creatinine, and 24-hour urine levels to determine creatinine clearance and protein

XII. DIABETES MELLITUS

A. Description
   1. Pregnancy places demands on carbohydrate metabolism and causes insulin requirements to change
   2. Premature **delivery** is more frequent
   3. The **newborn infant** of a diabetic mother may be large in size but will have functions related to gestational age rather than size
   4. The **newborn infant** of a diabetic mother is subject to hypoglycemia, hyperbilirubinemia, respiratory distress syndrome, hypocalcemia, and congenital anomalies
   5. Stillborn and neonatal mortality rates are higher in pregnancies of diabetic women
B. Type 1 diabetes mellitus
   1. Maternal glucose crosses the **placenta** but insulin does not
   2. The fetus produces its own insulin and pulls glucose from the mother, which predisposes the mother to hypoglycemic reactions
   3. During the first trimester, maternal insulin needs decrease
   4. During the second and third trimesters, increases in **placental** hormones cause an insulin-resistant state, requiring an increase in the client's insulin dose
   5. After **placental delivery, placental** hormone levels drop abruptly and insulin requirements decrease
C. Gestational diabetes mellitus
   1. Occurs in pregnancy (during the second or third trimester) in clients not previously diagnosed as diabetic; occurs when the pancreas cannot respond to the demand for more insulin
   2. Pregnant women should be screened for gestational diabetes between 24 and 28 weeks of pregnancy
   3. An oral glucose tolerance test (OGTT) will be performed to confirm gestational diabetes mellitus

4. Oral hypoglycemic agents are never used during pregnancy
5. Frequently can be treated by diet alone; however, insulin may be needed for some clients
6. Most gestational diabetics convert to normal after **delivery**; however, these individuals have an increased risk of developing diabetes mellitus in their lifetimes

D. Predisposing conditions to gestational diabetes
1. Over age 35
2. Obesity
3. Multiple gestation
4. Family history of diabetes mellitus

E. Data collection
1. Excessive thirst
2. Hunger
3. Weight loss
4. Blurred vision
5. Frequent urination
6. Recurrent urinary tract infections and vaginal yeast infections
7. Glycosuria and ketonuria
8. Signs of pregnancy-induced hypertension
9. Polyhydramnios
10. Fetus may be large for gestational age

F. Interventions
1. Include diet, insulin (if diet cannot control blood glucose levels), exercise, and blood glucose determinations to maintain blood glucose levels between 65 and 130 mg/dL
2. Observe for signs of hyperglycemia, glycosuria and ketonuria, and hypoglycemia
3. Monitor weight
4. Increase calorie intake as prescribed, with adequate insulin therapy, so that glucose will move into the cells
5. Assess for signs of maternal complications such as preeclampsia (hypertension, proteinuria, and edema)
6. Monitor for signs of infection
7. Instruct the client to report burning and pain on urination, vaginal discharge or itching, or any other signs of infection to the health care provider
8. Assess fetal status and monitor for signs fetal compromise

G. Interventions during **labor**
1. Monitor fetal status continuously for signs of distress and, if noted, prepare the client for immediate cesarean section
2. Carefully regulate insulin and provide IV glucose as prescribed, because **labor** depletes glycogen

H. Interventions during the postpartum period
1. Observe client closely for a hypoglycemic reaction, because a precipitous drop in insulin requirements normally occurs (the client may not require insulin for the first 24 hours)

2. Reregulate insulin needs as prescribed after the first day, according to blood glucose testing
3. Assess dietary needs on the basis of blood glucose and insulin requirements
4. Monitor for signs of infection or postpartum hemorrhage

XIII. DISSEMINATED INTRAVASCULAR COAGULATION (DIC)

A. Description
1. Condition in the mother's body that result in an exaggerated clotting process, which increases the formation of clots in the microcirculation
2. The rapid and extensive formation of clots results in bleeding and the potential vascular occlusion of organs from thromboembolus formation

B. Predisposing conditions (Box 22-6)

C. Data collection
1. Uncontrolled bleeding
2. Bruising, purpura, petechiae, and ecchymosis
3. Hematuria, hematemesis, or vaginal bleeding
4. Signs of shock
5. Decreased fibrinogen level, platelet count, and hematocrit level
6. Increased prothrombin time (PT) and partial thromboplastin time (PTT), clotting time, and fibrin degradation products

D. Interventions
1. Remove the underlying cause
2. Monitor vital signs; assess for bleeding and signs of shock
3. Prepare for oxygen therapy, volume replacement, blood component therapy, and possibly heparin therapy
4. Monitor for complications associated with fluid and blood replacement and heparin therapy
5. Monitor urine output and maintain at 30 mL/hour (renal failure is a complication of DIC)

XIV. ECTOPIC PREGNANCY

A. Description: Pregnancy that occurs in a site other than a uterine site, with **implantation** usually occurring in the fallopian tubes

---

BOX 22-6

Predisposing Conditions for Disseminated Intravascular Coagulation (DIC)

Abruptio placentae
Intrauterine fetal death
Amniotic fluid embolism
Pregnancy-induced hypertension
Liver disease
Sepsis

B. Data collection
   1. Missed period
   2. Abdominal pain
   3. Vaginal spotting to bleeding that is dark red or brown
   4. Rupture: Increased pain, referred shoulder pain, signs of shock
C. Interventions
   1. Obtain assessment data and vital signs
   2. Monitor bleeding and initiate measures to prevent rupture and shock
   3. Methotrexate (a folic acid antagonist) may be prescribed to inhibit cell division in the developing embryo
   4. Prepare the client for laparotomy and removal of the pregnancy and tube, if necessary, or repair of the tube
   5. Administer antibiotics; Rh immune globulin is given to appropriate Rho(D)-negative women

XV. ENDOMETRITIS

A. Description
   1. Infection of the lining of the uterus after **delivery;** caused by bacteria that invade the uterus at the **placental** site
   2. The infection may spread and involve the entire endometrium and cause peritonitis, pelvic thrombophlebitis, or cellulitis
B. Data collection
   1. Chills and fever
   2. Increased pulse
   3. Decreased appetite
   4. Headache
   5. Backache
   6. Prolonged, severe afterpains
   7. Tender, large uterus
   8. Foul odor to **lochia** or reddish-brown **lochia**
   9. Ileus
   10. Elevated white blood cell count
C. Interventions
   1. Monitor vital signs
   2. Place the mother in Fowler's position to facilitate drainage of **lochia**
   3. Provide a private room for the mother
   4. Inform the mother that it is not necessary to isolate the **newborn infant** from the mother
   5. Instruct the mother in proper handwashing techniques
   6. Initiate wound and skin precautions, as necessary
   7. Monitor I&O and encourage fluid intake
   8. IV antibiotics may be prescribed
   9. Administer comfort measures, such as back rubs and positioning changes, and pain medications, as prescribed
   10. Oxytoxic medications may be prescribed to improve uterine tone

XVI. FETAL DEATH IN UTERO (FDIU)

A. Description
   1. Death of a fetus after the 20th week of gestation and before birth
   2. DIC can develop if the dead fetus is retained in the uterus for 3 to 4 weeks or more
B. Data collection
   1. Absence of fetal movement
   2. Absence of fetal heart tones
   3. Maternal weight loss
   4. Lack of fetal growth or decrease in fundal height
   5. Lack of cardiac activity and other characteristics suggestive of fetal death noted on the ultrasound
C. Interventions
   1. Prepare for **delivery** of the fetus
   2. Support the client's decision about **labor**, birth, and the postpartum period
   3. Facilitate the grieving process
   4. Allow parents to hold the **infant** after birth
   5. Allow parents to name the **infant**
   6. Accept such behaviors as anger and hostility from parents
   7. Refer parents to an appropriate support group

XVII. HEPATITIS B

A. Description
   1. The risks of prematurity, low birth weight, and neonatal death increases if the mother has hepatitis B infection
   2. It is transmitted through blood, saliva, vaginal secretions, semen, breast milk, and across the placental barrier
B. Interventions
   1. Minimize the risk for intrapartum ascending infections (limit the number of vaginal examinations)
   2. Remove maternal blood from the **neonate** immediately after birth
   3. Suction the **neonate** immediately after birth
   4. Bathe the **neonate** prior to any invasive procedures
   5. Clean and dry the face and eyes of the neonate before instilling eye prophylaxis
   6. Infection of the neonate can be prevented by the administration of hepatitis B immune globulin and hepatitis B vaccine soon after birth
   7. Discourage the mother from kissing the **neonate** until the **neonate** has received the vaccine
   8. Support breast-feeding after neonatal treatment; breast-feeding is not contraindicated if the neonate has been vaccinated
   9. Inform the mother that the hepatitis B vaccine will be administered to the **neonate,** and that the second dose will be administered at 1 month; the third dose is administered at 6 months

XVIII. HEMATOMA

A. Description
  1. Occurs following the escape of blood into the tissues of the reproductive sac after the **delivery**
  2. Predisposing conditions include operative **delivery** with forceps or injury to a blood vessel

B. Data collection (Box 22-7)

C. Interventions
  1. Monitor vital signs
  2. Monitor client for abnormal pain, especially when forceps **delivery** has occurred
  3. Apply ice to the hematoma site
  4. Administer analgesics as prescribed
  5. Monitor I&O
  6. Encourage fluids and voiding; prepare for urinary catheterization if client is unable to void
  7. Prepare to administer blood replacements as prescribed
  8. Monitor for signs of infection, such as increased temperature, pulse rate, and white blood cell (WBC) count
  9. Administer antibiotics as prescribed, because infection is common following hematoma formation
  10. Prepare for incision and evacuation of hematoma, if necessary

XIX. HYDATIDIFORM MOLE

A. Description
  1. Developmental anomaly of the **placenta** that changes chorionic villi into a mass of clear vesicles
  2. Presents as an edematous grapelike cluster that may be nonmalignant or may develop into choriocarcinoma

B. Data collection
  1. Fetal heart rate not detectable
  2. Vaginal bleeding, which usually occurs by week 12, is bright red or dark brown in color; may be slight, profuse, or intermittent
  3. Symptoms of PIH, such as an elevated blood pressure, edema, and proteinuria, may be present before week 20

BOX 22-7

Hematoma: Data Collection Findings

Abnormal, severe pain
Pressure in perineal area
Palpable, sensitive tumor in perineal area, with discolored skin
Inability to void
Decreased hemoglobin and hematocrit levels
Signs of shock, such as pallor, tachycardia, and hypotension, if significant blood loss has occurred

---

  4. Fundal height is greater than expected for date
  5. Elevated human chorionic gonadotropin (hCG) levels
  6. Ultrasound shows a characteristic snowstorm pattern

C. Interventions
  1. Prepare mother for uterine evacuation (before evacuation, diagnostic tests are done to detect metastatic disease)
  2. Evacuation of the mole is done by vacuum aspiration; oxytocin (Pitocin) is administered after evacuation to contract the uterus
  3. Tissue is sent to the laboratory for evaluation; follow-up is important to detect changes suggestive of malignancy
  4. Monitor for postprocedure hemorrhage and infection
  5. hCG levels are monitored every 1 to 2 weeks until normal prepregnancy levels are attained; the levels are then checked every 1 to 2 months for 1 year
  6. Instruct parents regarding birth control measures so that pregnancy can be prevented during the 1-year follow-up

XX. HYPEREMESIS GRAVIDARUM

A. Description: Intractable nausea and vomiting that persists beyond the first trimester and causes disturbances in nutrition, electrolytes, and fluid balance

B. Data collection
  1. Nausea most pronounced on arising; however, can occur at other times during the day
  2. Persistent vomiting and weight loss
  3. Signs of dehydration and electrolyte imbalances

C. Interventions
  1. Measures to alleviate nausea, including medication therapy, are initiated; if unsuccessful, and weight loss and electrolyte imbalances occur, administration of intravenous fluid and electrolyte replacement or total parenteral nutrition may be necessary
  2. Monitor vital signs, I&O, weight, and calorie count
  3. Monitor laboratory data and for signs of dehydration and electrolyte imbalances
  4. Monitor urine for ketones
  5. Monitor fetal heart rate, fetal activity, and fetal growth
  6. Encourage intake of small portions of food (low-fat, easily digestible carbohydrates, such as cereals, rice, and pasta)
  7. Liquids should be taken between meals to avoid distending the stomach and triggering vomiting
  8. Encourage the client to sit upright after meals

XXI. INCOMPETENT CERVIX

A. Description
   1. Premature dilation of cervix, which occurs in the 4th or 5th month of pregnancy
   2. Associated with cervical trauma as a result of a previous surgery or birth
   3. Treatment is surgical

B. Data collection
   1. Vaginal bleeding
   2. Fetal membranes visible through the cervix

C. Interventions
   1. Provide bed rest, hydration, and tocolysis, as prescribed, to inhibit uterine contractions
   2. Prepare for cervical cerclage (at 10 to 14 weeks' gestation), in which a band of fascia or nonabsorbable ribbon is placed around the cervix beneath the mucosa to constrict the internal os of the cervix
   3. Following cervical cerclage, the woman is told to refrain from intercourse and avoid prolonged standing and heavy lifting
   4. The cervical cerclage is removed at 37 weeks' gestation or left in place and a cesarean delivery performed; if removed, cerclage must be repeated with each successive pregnancy
   5. Following the procedure, monitor for contractions, rupture of the membranes, and signs of infection
   6. Instruct the woman to report any postprocedure vaginal bleeding or increased uterine contractions immediately to the health care provider

XXII. INFECTIONS

A. Toxoplasmosis
   1. Caused by infection with the protozoan intracellular parasite *Toxoplasma gondii*
   2. Produces a rash and symptoms of acute, flulike infection in the mother
   3. Transmitted to the mother through raw meat or handling cat litter of infected cats
   4. Organism is transmitted to the fetus across the **placenta**
   5. Can cause spontaneous abortion

B. Rubella (German measles)
   1. Extremely teratogenic in the first trimester
   2. Organism is transmitted to the fetus across the **placenta**
   3. Causes congenital defects of the eyes, heart, ears, and brain
   4. If not immune (titer of 1:8 or less), the mother should be vaccinated in the postpartum period; she must then wait at least 3 months before becoming pregnant

C. Cytomegalovirus (CMV)
   1. Produces mononucleosis-like symptoms in the mother
   2. Organism is transmitted across the **placenta** to the fetus, or the fetus may be infected through the birth canal
   3. May be asymptomatic at birth; causes fetal death, mental retardation, blindness, deafness, and/or seizures
   4. Antiviral therapy may be prescribed

D. Genital herpes
   1. Affects the external genitalia, vagina, and cervix
   2. Causes draining, painful vesicles
   3. Virus is usually transmitted to the fetus during birth through the infected vagina or via an ascending infection after rupture of the membranes
   4. No vaginal examinations are done in the presence of active vaginal herpetic lesions
   5. Can cause death or severe neurological impairment in the newborn
   6. **Delivery** of the fetus is usually by cesarean section if active lesions are present in the vagina; **delivery** may be performed vaginally if the lesions are in the anal, perineal, or inner thigh area (strict precautions are necessary to protect the fetus during **delivery**)
   7. Maintain contact precautions

XXIII. MULTIPLE GESTATION

A. Description: Results from double ovulation (fraternal or dizygotic) or splitting of the fertilized egg (identical or monozygotic)

B. Data collection
   1. Excessive fetal activity
   2. Uterus large for gestational age
   3. Palpation of three or four large fetal parts in the uterus
   4. Auscultation of more than one fetal heart rate
   5. Excessive weight gain

C. Interventions
   1. Monitor vital signs
   2. Monitor fetal heart rates, fetal activity, and fetal growth
   3. Monitor for cervical changes
   4. Prepare client for ultrasound, as prescribed
   5. Monitor for anemia; administer supplemental vitamins as prescribed
   6. Monitor for preterm **labor** and treat preterm **labor** promptly
   7. Prepare for cesarean section for abnormal presentations
   8. Prepare to administer oxytoxic medications after **delivery** to prevent postpartum hemorrhage from uterine overdistention

XXIV. PREGNANCY-INDUCED HYPERTENSION (PIH)

A. Description
   1. Also known as gestational hypertension; an acute hypertensive state that develops after the 20th week of gestation

2. The condition may be mild or severe and can progress to seizures (eclampsia) (Box 22-8)
3. The classic signs of preeclampsia are hypertension, generalized edema, and proteinuria

B. Predisposing conditions
1. Primigravida
2. Age younger than 19 years or older than 40 years
3. Chronic renal disease
4. Chronic hypertension
5. Diabetes mellitus
6. Rh incompatibility
7. History of or family history of PIH

C. Complications of PIH
1. Abruptio placentae
2. DIC
3. Thrombocytopenia
4. **Placental** insufficiency
5. Intrauterine fetal death

D. Mild preeclampsia
1. Data collection
   a. Elevated blood pressure (usually 15 to 30 mm Hg above baseline)
   b. Weight gain of 1 lb or more per week in the last trimester
   c. Mild, generalized edema
   d. Proteinuria of 1+ to 2+
2. Interventions
   a. Provide bed rest and place the client in left lateral position
   b. Monitor blood pressure and weight
   c. Monitor neurological status, because changes can indicate cerebral hypoxia or impending seizure
   d. Monitor deep tendon reflexes and for the presence of clonus, because hyperreflexia indicates increased central nervous system irritability (Box 22-9)
   e. Provide adequate fluids
   f. Monitor I&O; a urinary output of 30 mL/hour indicates adequate renal perfusion
   g. Increase dietary protein and carbohydrates, with no added salt
   h. Administer medications as prescribed to lower the blood pressure; blood pressure should not be lowered drastically, because **placenta** perfusion can be compromised

E. Severe preeclampsia
1. Data collection
   a. Severe hypertension, (systolic blood pressure of at least 160 mm Hg or a diastolic blood pressure of at least 110 mm Hg)
   b. Massive, generalized edema and weight gain
   c. Proteinuria greater than 3+ to 4+
   d. Oliguria—urine output less than 400 to 500 mL/24 hours
   e. Cerebral or visual disturbances such as altered level of consciousness, headache, or blurred vision

---

BOX 22-9

Checking Reflexes

BICEPS REFLEX
Position your thumb over the client's biceps tendon, supporting the client's elbow with the palm of the hand.
Strike a downward blow over the thumb with the percussion hammer.
Normal Response
Flexion of the arm at the elbow.

PATELLAR REFLEX
Position the client with legs dangling over the edge of the examining table or lying on her back, with the legs slightly flexed.
Strike the patellar tendon just below the kneecap with the percussion hammer.
Normal Response
Extension or kicking out of leg.

CLONUS REFLEX
Position the client with the legs dangling over the edge of the examining table.
Support the leg with one hand and sharply dorsiflex the client's foot with the other hand.
Maintain the dorsiflexed position for a few seconds; then release the foot.
Normal Response (Negative Clonus Response)
Foot will remain steady in the dorsiflexed position.
No rhythmic oscillations or jerking of the foot will be felt.
When released, the foot will drop to a plantarflexed position, with no oscillations.
Abnormal Response (Positive Clonus Response)
Rhythmic oscillations when the foot is dorsiflexed.
Similar oscillations will be noted when the foot drops to the plantarflexed position.

GRADING THE RESPONSE
0 = reflex absent
1+ = reflex present but hypoactive
2+ = normal reflex
3+ = hyperactive reflex
4+ = hyperactive reflex with clonus present

BOX 22-8

Signs of Worsening Pregnancy-Induced Hypertension (PIH) or Impending Seizures

Blood pressure, 160/110 mm Hg or higher
Epigastric pain
Decreased urinary output
Visual changes
Headache
Excessive proteinuria

f. Epigastric pain, nausea and vomiting

g. Hepatic, pulmonary, or cardiac involvement

h. Thrombocytopenia

i. **HELLP** syndrome: Laboratory diagnosis for severe preeclampsia characterized by hemolysis (H), elevated liver enzymes (EL), and low platelet count (LP)

2. Interventions

a. Maintain client on bed rest

b. Prepare for the administration of magnesium sulfate (use a controlled infusion device), as prescribed, to prevent seizures; may be continued for 24 to 48 hours postpartum

c. Monitor for signs of magnesium toxicity, including flushing, sweating, hypotension, depressed deep tendon reflexes, and central nervous system depression including respiratory depression; keep antidote (calcium gluconate) at the client's bedside

d. Administer antihypertensives as prescribed

e. Prepare for the induction of **labor**

F. Eclampsia

1. Data collection: Characterized by generalized seizures (Box 22-10)

2. Interventions

a. Maintain a patent airway and administer oxygen

b. Protect the client from injury

c. Monitor fetal heart rate and contractions

d. Prepare for the administration of medications to control the seizures (magnesium sulfate may be prescribed)

e. Prepare for **delivery** of the fetus after stabilization of the client

XXV. SEXUALLY TRANSMITTED DISEASES (STDs)

A. Chlamydia

1. Description

a. Common, sexually transmitted pathogen associated with an increased risk for premature births, stillborns, neonatal conjunctivitis, and **newborn** chlamydial pneumonia

---

BOX 22-10

Eclampsia

Seizure typically begins with twitching around the mouth.

The body then becomes rigid in a state of tonic muscular contractions, which last 15 to 20 seconds.

The facial muscles, and then all body muscles, alternatively contract and relax in rapid succession (clonic phase; may last about 1 minute).

Respiration is halted during the seizure because the diaphragm tends to remain fixed (breathing resumes shortly after the seizure).

---

b. In the nonpregnant state, can cause salpingitis, pelvic abscesses, chronic pelvic pain, and infertility

c. Diagnostic test is positive culture for *Chlamydia trachomatis*

2. Data collection

a. Usually asymptomatic

b. Bleeding between periods or after coitus

c. Mucoid or purulent cervical discharge

d. Dysuria

e. In the **newborn**, conjunctivitis and pneumonia

3. Interventions

a. Screen the client to determine whether client is at high risk; instruct the client in the importance of rescreening, because reinfection can occur as the client nears term

b. Instruct the client about the prescribed medication for treatment

c. Instruct the mother about medication for the **neonate**, if prescribed

d. Administer appropriate eye prophylaxis to the **neonate**

e. Monitor neonate for signs and symptoms of pneumonia, if at risk

f. Ensure that the sexual partner is treated

B. Syphilis

1. Description

a. Chronic infectious disease caused by the organism *Treponema pallidum*

b. Transmission is by intimate physical contact with syphilitic lesions, which are usually found on the skin or mucous membranes of the mouth and genitals

c. Infection may cause abortion or premature **labor**; passed to the fetus after the fourth month of pregnancy as congenital syphilis

2. Data collection (Box 22-11)

3. Interventions

a. Obtain a serum sample to test for syphilis on the first prenatal visit; prepare to repeat the test at 36 weeks' gestation, because the disease may be acquired after the initial visit

b. If positive, treatment is necessary with an antibiotic, such as penicillin

c. Instruct the client that treatment of her partner is necessary if infection is present

C. Gonorrhea

1. Description

a. Infection caused by *Neisseria gonorrhoeae*, which causes inflammation of the mucous membranes of the genital and urinary tracts

b. Transmission of organism is by sexual intercourse

c. Infection may be transmitted to the **newborn's** eyes during **delivery**, causing blindness (ophthalmia neonatorum)

BOX 22-11

Stages of Syphilis

PRIMARY STAGE
Most infectious stage
Appearance of ulcerative, painless lesions produced by spirochetes at the point of entry into the body

SECONDARY STAGE
Highly infectious stage
Lesions appear about 3 weeks after the primary stage; may occur anywhere on the skin and mucous membranes
Generalized lymphadenopathy occurs

TERTIARY STAGE
Spirochetes enter internal organs and cause permanent damage; symptoms may occur 10 to 30 years following occurrence of an untreated primary lesion
Invades the CNS, causing meningitis, ataxia, general paresis, and progressive mental deterioration
Affects the aortic valve and aorta

2. Data collection
   a. Female: Usually asymptomatic; vaginal discharge, urinary frequency, and pain possible
   b. Male: Fever, painful urination, pelvic pain, epididymitis with pain, tenderness, and swelling
3. Interventions
   a. Obtain culture for gonorrhea on the first prenatal visit; prepare to repeat culture, because infection may occur during pregnancy
   b. Administer prophylactic antibiotics to the **newborn infant's** eyes as prescribed
   c. Instruct client that treatment of her partner is necessary if infection occurs
D. Condylomata acuminata (venereal warts)
   1. Description
      a. Caused by human papillomavirus (HPV); affects the cervix, urethra, anus, penis, and scrotum
      b. Transmitted through sexual contact
   2. Data collection
      a. Small to large wartlike growths on genitals
      b. Cervical cell changes may be noted because HPV is associated with cervical malignancies
   3. Interventions
      a. Lesions are removed by the use of cytotoxic agents, cryotherapy, electrocautery, and laser
      b. Encourage yearly Papanicolaou (Pap) smear
      c. Avoid sexual contact until the lesions are healed (condoms are used to reduce transmission)

XXVI. TUBERCULOSIS (TB)

A. Description
   1. A highly communicable disease caused by *Mycobacterium tuberculosis*
   2. Transmitted by the airborne route

3. A multidrug-resistant strain of TB (MDR-TB) can exist as a result of improper compliance or noncompliance with treatment programs and the development of mutations in the tubercle bacilli
B. Transmission
   1. Transplacental transmission is rare
   2. Can occur during birth through aspiration of infected **amniotic** fluid
   3. **Neonate** can become infected from contact with infected individuals
C. Risk to mother: Active disease during pregnancy has been associated with an increase in hypertensive disorders of pregnancy
D. Diagnosis
   1. If a chest radiograph is required for the mother, it is obtained *only* after 20 weeks' gestation, and a lead shield for the abdomen is required
   2. TB skin testing is safe during pregnancy
E. Data collection
   1. Maternal
      a. May be asymptomatic
      b. Fever and chills
      c. Night sweats
      d. Weight loss
      e. Fatigue
      f. Cough, hemoptysis, or green or yellow sputum
      g. Dyspnea
      h. Pleural pain
   2. **Neonate**
      a. Fever
      b. Lethargy
      c. Poor feeding
      d. Failure to thrive
      e. Respiratory distress
      f. Hepatosplenomegaly
      g. Meningitis
      h. Disease may spread to all major organs
F. Interventions
   1. Pregnant client
      a. Administration of isoniazid (INH), pyrazinamide, and rifampin (Rifadin) daily for 9 months; ethambutol (Myambutol) is added if medication resistance is probable
      b. Pyridoxine (vitamin B_6) should be administered along with INH to pregnant women to prevent fetal neurotoxicity caused by the INH
      c. Encourage breast-feeding only if the mother is noninfectious
   2. **Newborn infant**
      a. Management focuses on preventing disease and treating early infection
      b. The infant is skin tested at birth and may be placed on INH therapy; the skin test is repeated in 3 to 4 months and INH may be stopped if the skin test results remain negative
      c. If the skin test result is positive, the infant should receive INH for at least 6 months

d. If the mother's sputum is free of organisms, the infant does not need to be isolated from the mother while in the hospital

PRACTICE QUESTIONS

1. A client is in her second trimester of pregnancy. She complains of frequent low back pain and ankle edema at the end of the day. The nurse recommends which measure to help relieve both discomforts?
   1. Lie on the floor with the legs elevated onto a couch or padded chair, with the hips and knees at a right angle
   2. Lie on the left side with the feet dorsiflexed
   3. Soak the feet in hot water after performing 10 pelvic tilt exercises
   4. Lie on the right side with the feet elevated on pillow and a heating pad on the back

2. A client beginning week 30 of gestation comes to the clinic for a routine visit. Which of the following observations by the nurse indicates a need for teaching?
   1. The client is wearing panty hose
   2. The client is wearing shoes with arch supports
   3. The client is wearing nonslip shoes
   4. The client is wearing knee-high hose

3. The plan of care for a pregnant teen should include teaching regarding which of the following concerning dental care?
   1. Use toothpaste with baking soda to decrease plaque buildup
   2. Avoid the use of local anesthetics during dental work
   3. Expect to lose at least one tooth because of calcium and phosphorus leaving the teeth to nourish the fetus
   4. Tell the dentist office staff that she is pregnant

4. A pregnant woman complains of being awakened frequently by leg cramps. The nurse reinforces instructions to the client's partner and tells the partner to:
   1. Dorsiflex the client's foot while flexing the knee
   2. Dorsiflex the client's foot while extending the knee
   3. Plantarflex the client's foot while flexing the knee
   4. Plantarflex the client's foot while extending the knee

5. A nurse is providing instructions to a pregnant client with heartburn regarding measures that will alleviate the discomfort. The nurse instructs the client to:
   1. Lie down for 30 minutes after eating
   2. Drink decaffeinated coffee and tea
   3. Substitute salt in cooking for other spices
   4. Eliminate between-meal snacks

6. A nurse is reinforcing instructions to a pregnant woman who is complaining of low back pain. The nurse instructs the woman:
   1. To wear an abdominal support
   2. In the technique of pelvic tilt
   3. To relax abdominal muscles when standing
   4. To wear at least a 2-inch heel on her shoes

7. A client at 28 weeks' gestation is Rh negative and Coombs' antibody negative. The nurse determines that the client understands what the nurse has taught her about Rh sensitization when the client states:
   1. "I know I can never have another child."
   2. "I will have to have an injection once a month until the baby is born."
   3. "I will tell the nurse at the hospital that I had RhoGAM during pregnancy."
   4. "I am glad I won't have to have these shots if I have another child."

8. While assisting with the measurement of fundal height, the client (36 weeks' gestation) states that she is feeling lightheaded. Based on the nurse's knowledge of pregnancy, the nurse determines that this is most likely due to:
   1. Emotional instability
   2. Compression of the vena cava
   3. A full bladder
   4. Insufficient iron intake

9. A nurse is providing information to a pregnant woman about food items high in folic acid. Which of the following midafternoon snacks would be recommended to supply folic acid?
   1. One medium banana
   2. Nuts and green, leafy vegetables
   3. 1 cup milk with two graham crackers
   4. 1 cup yogurt

10. A contraction stress test is scheduled for a client. The woman asks the nurse about the test. The most accurate description of the test includes which of the following?
    1. "Small amounts of oxytocin (Pitocin) are administered during internal fetal monitoring to stimulate uterine contractions."
    2. "An internal fetal monitor is attached and you will walk on a treadmill until contractions begin."
    3. "The uterus is stimulated to contract by either small amounts of oxytocin (Pitocin) or by nipple stimulation."
    4. "Uterine contractions are stimulated by Leopold's maneuvers."

11. A client at 38 weeks of pregnancy is admitted to the birthing center in early labor. The client is carrying twins, and one of the fetuses is a breech presentation. The nurse assists in planning care for the client and identifies which of the following as the lowest priority in the care of this client?
    1. Attach electronic fetal monitoring
    2. Prepare the client for a possible cesarean section
    3. Measure fundal height
    4. Gather equipment for starting an IV

12. A stillborn was delivered in the birthing suite a few hours ago. After the birth, the family has remained together, holding and touching the baby. Which statement by the nurse would further assist the family in their initial period of grief?
    1. "Don't worry, there is nothing you could do to prevent this from happening."
    2. "We need to take the baby from you now so that you can get some sleep."
    3. "What have you named your lovely baby?"
    4. "We will see to it that you have an early discharge so that you don't have to be reminded of this experience."

13. A nurse is collecting data from a prenatal client. The nurse determines that which of the following places the client in the high-risk category for contracting human immunodeficiency virus (HIV)?
    1. Living in an area where HIV infections are minimal
    2. A history of IV drug use in the past year
    3. A history of one sexual partner within the past 10 years
    4. A spouse who is heterosexual and who has had only one sexual partner in the past 10 years

14. A perinatal client is admitted to the obstetric unit during an exacerbation of a heart condition. When planning for the nutritional requirements of the client, the nurse would consult with the dietitian to ensure which of the following?
    1. A low-calorie diet to ensure absence of weight gain
    2. A diet low in fluids and fiber to decrease blood volume
    3. A diet high in fluids and fiber to decrease constipation
    4. Unlimited sodium intake to increase circulating blood volume

15. A perinatal client is at risk for toxoplasmosis. The nurse would teach the client which of the following to prevent exposure to this disease?
    1. Wash hands only before meals
    2. Eat raw meats
    3. Avoid exposure to litter boxes used by cats
    4. Use topical corticosteroid treatments prophylactically

16. A nurse caring for a client with abruptio placentae is monitoring the client for signs of disseminated intravascular coagulopathy (DIC). The nurse would suspect DIC if he or she observes:
    1. Pain and swelling of the calf of one leg
    2. Rapid clotting times
    3. Laboratory values indicating increased platelets
    4. Petechiae, oozing from injection sites, and hematuria

17. A nurse has a teaching session with a malnourished client regarding iron supplementation to prevent anemia during pregnancy. Which of the following statements, if made by the client, would indicate successful learning?
    1. "The iron is needed for the red blood cells."
    2. "Meat does not provide iron and should be avoided."
    3. "Iron supplements will give me diarrhea."
    4. "My body has all the iron it needs and I don't need to take supplements."

18. During a prenatal visit, a nurse is explaining dietary management to a client with diabetes mellitus. The nurse determines that the teaching has been effective when the client states:
    1. "I can eat more sweets now because I need more calories."
    2. "I need more fat in my diet so the baby can gain enough weight."
    3. "I need to eat a high-protein, low-carbohydrate diet now to control my blood glucose."
    4. "I need to increase the fiber in my diet to control my blood glucose and prevent constipation."

19. A nurse is assigned to assist in caring for a client at risk for eclampsia. When a client progresses from preeclampsia to eclampsia, the nurse's first action should be to:
    1. Prepare for the administration of IV magnesium sulfate
    2. Check the blood pressure and fetal heart tones
    3. Clear and maintain an open airway
    4. Administer oxygen by face mask

20. A nurse is doing a 48-hour postpartum check on a client with mild pregnancy-induced hypertension (PIH). Which of the following data indicate that the PIH is not resolving?
    1. Blood pressure reading has returned to the prenatal baseline
    2. Urinary output has increased
    3. The client complains of a headache and blurred vision
    4. There is no evidence of dependent edema

ALTERNATE FORMAT QUESTIONS: FILL IN THE BLANK

A nurse is monitoring a pregnant client with pregnancy-induced hypertension who is at risk for preeclampsia. The nurse checks the client for which three classic signs of preeclampsia?

Answer:_____

ANSWERS

1. Answer: 1

Rationale: The position described in option 1 will produce the posture of the pelvic tilt while countering gravity as the force that leads to edema of the lower extremities. Although the other options might seem useful, options 3 and 4 identify heat, which should be prescribed by the physician. Option 2 will not relieve back pain and ankle edema.

Test-Taking Strategy: Use the process of elimination. Focus on the issue of the question, back pain and ankle edema. Eliminate options 3 and 4 because the application of heat needs to be prescribed by the physician. From the remaining options, focus on the issue, which will direct you to option 1. Review measures that will reduce these discomforts if you had difficulty with this question.

Level of Cognitive Ability: Application
Client Needs: Physiological Integrity
Integrated Process: Nursing Process/Implementation
Content Area: Maternity/Antepartum
Reference: Leifer, G. (2005). *Maternity nursing* (9th ed.). Philadelphia: W.B. Saunders, p. 55.

2. Answer: 4

Rationale: Varicose veins often develop in the lower extremities during pregnancy. Any constricting clothing, such as knee-high hose, impedes venous return from the lower legs and thus places the client at higher risk for developing varicosities. Clients should be encouraged to wear support (panty) hose. Flat, nonslip shoes with proper support are important to help the pregnant woman maintain proper posture and balance and minimize fall risks.

Test-Taking Strategy: Note the key words, *need for teaching.* Use the process of elimination, seeking the option that will cause complications. Recalling that knee-high hose impedes venous return from the lower legs will direct you to option 4. Review these measures if you had difficulty with this question.

Level of Cognitive Ability: Comprehension
Client Needs: Health Promotion and Maintenance
Integrated Process: Nursing Process/Data collection
Content Area: Maternity/Antepartum
Reference: Leifer, G. (2005). *Maternity nursing* (9th ed.). Philadelphia: W.B. Saunders, pp. 195-196.

3. Answer: 4

Rationale: Baking soda may irritate the gums, which are more likely to bleed because of hormonal changes of pregnancy. Local anesthetics for minor dental work should not have adverse effects on the fetus. Option 3 is inaccurate information. The dental staff needs to know about the pregnancy so that care is taken during examinations and x-ray studies are avoided.

Test-Taking Strategy: Use the process of elimination. Focus on the safety of the unseen client (fetus). Option 4 is the umbrella (global) option. Review client teaching points related to pregnancy if you had difficulty with this question.

Level of Cognitive Ability: Application
Client Needs: Safe, Effective Care Environment
Integrated Process: Nursing Process/Planning
Content Area: Maternity/Antepartum
Reference: Leifer, G. (2005). *Maternity nursing* (9th ed.). Philadelphia: W.B. Saunders, p. 51.

4. Answer: 2

Rationale: Leg cramps often occur when the pregnant woman stretches her leg and plantarflexes her foot. Dorsiflexion of the foot while extending the knee stretches the gastrocnemius muscle, prevents the muscle from contracting, and halts the cramping.

Test-Taking Strategy: Use the process of elimination. Knowledge regarding the actions that will alleviate muscle cramps will assist you in answering the question. Visualize each of the descriptions in the options to help direct you to the correct option. Review these measures if you had difficulty with this question.

Level of Cognitive Ability: Application
Client Needs: Health Promotion and Maintenance
Integrated Process: Teaching/Learning
Content Area: Maternity/Antepartum
Reference: Leifer, G. (2005). *Maternity nursing* (9th ed.). Philadelphia: W.B. Saunders, p. 51.

5. Answer: 2

Rationale: Lying down after meals is likely to lead to reflux of stomach contents. Spices tend to trigger heartburn. Salt leads to the retention of fluid. Eating smaller, more frequent portions is preferable to eating three large meals to control heartburn. Caffeine, like spices, may cause heartburn.

Test-Taking Strategy: Use the process of elimination, recalling those items that cause heartburn. This will direct you to option 2. Review measures to alleviate heartburn if you had difficulty with this question.

Level of Cognitive Ability: Application
Client Needs: Health Promotion and Maintenance
Integrated Process: Teaching/Learning
Content Area: Maternity/Antepartum
Reference: Murray, S., McKinney, E., & Gorrie, T. (2002). *Foundations of maternal-newborn nursing* (3rd ed.). Philadelphia: W.B. Saunders, p. 148.

6. Answer: 2

Rationale: Pelvic tilt exercises decrease strain to the muscles of the abdomen and lower back caused by the added weight of the abdomen and the shift in the center of gravity. An abdominal support should be worn only if recommended by the physician. Relaxing abdominal muscles will add to the problem. Wearing 2-inch heels on shoes will add to the strain on the muscles and exaggerate the shift in the center of gravity.

Test-Taking Strategy: Focus on the issue and use the process of elimination. Visualize each of the instructions in the options and think about its effect on relieving low back pain. Review the measures to relieve low back pain in the pregnant client if you had difficulty with this question.

Level of Cognitive Ability: Application
Client Needs: Physiological Integrity
Integrated Process: Teaching/Learning
Content Area: Maternity/Antepartum
Reference: Leifer, G. (2005). *Maternity nursing* (9th ed.). Philadelphia: W.B. Saunders, p. 55.

7. Answer: 3

Rationale: As described in the question, it is accepted practice to administer RhoGAM to a woman at 28 weeks of gestation,

with a second injection within 72 hours of delivery. This prevents sensitization, which could jeopardize a future pregnancy. For subsequent pregnancies or abortions, the injections must be repeated, because the immunity is passive. Options 1, 2, and 4 are inaccurate information.
Test-Taking Strategy: Note the key words, *that the client understands.* Recalling the guidelines regarding the administration of RhoGAM will direct you to option 3. Review Rh sensitization if you had difficulty with this question.
Level of Cognitive Ability: Comprehension
Client Needs: Physiological Integrity
Integrated Process: Nursing Process/Evaluation
Content Area: Maternity/Antepartum
References: Leifer, G. (2005). *Maternity nursing* (9th ed.). Philadelphia: W.B. Saunders, p. 278.

8. Answer: 2
Rationale: Compression of the inferior vena cava and aorta by the uterus may cause supine hypotension syndrome in pregnancy. Having the woman turn onto her left side or elevating the left buttock during fundal height measurement will prevent or correct the problem. Options 1, 3, and 4 are not the cause of the client's problem described in the question.
Test-Taking Strategy: Focus on the data in the question and recall the complications associated with pregnancy. Use the ABCs—airway, breathing, and circulation—to direct you to option 2. Review vena cava syndrome if you had difficulty with this question.
Level of Cognitive Ability: Comprehension
Client Needs: Physiological Integrity
Integrated Process: Nursing Process/Data collection
Content Area: Maternity/Antepartum
Reference: Leifer, G. (2005). *Maternity nursing* (9th ed.). Philadelphia: W.B. Saunders, p. 39.

9. Answer: 2
Rationale: Folic acid is needed during pregnancy for healthy cell growth and repair. A pregnant woman should have at least four daily servings of foods rich in folic acid. The food items in option 2 contain folic acid. Bananas provide potassium. Milk and yogurt supply calcium.
Test-Taking Strategy: Knowledge regarding food sources high in folic acid is required to answer the question. Remembering that green, leafy vegetables are high in folic acid will direct you to option 2. Review the foods high in folic acid if you had difficulty with this question.
Level of Cognitive Ability: Application
Client Needs: Physiological Integrity
Integrated Process: Nursing Process/Implementation
Content Area: Maternity/Antepartum
Reference: Leifer, G. (2005). *Maternity nursing* (9th ed.). Philadelphia: W.B. Saunders, p. 62.

10. Answer: 3
Rationale: A contraction stress test assesses placental oxygenation and function, determines fetal ability to tolerate labor, determines fetal well-being, and is performed if the nonstress test result is abnormal. In this test, the fetus is exposed to the stressor of contractions to assess the adequacy of placental perfusion under simulated labor conditions. An external fetal monitor is applied to the mother and a 20- to 30-minute baseline strip is recorded. The uterus is stimulated to contract, either by the administration of a dilute dose of oxytocin (Pitocin) or by having the mother use nipple stimulation, until three palpable contractions with a duration of 40 seconds or more in a 10-minute period have occurred. Frequent maternal blood pressure readings are done and the client is monitored closely while increasing doses of oxytocin are given.
Test-Taking Strategy: Knowledge regarding the contraction stress test is required to answer the question. Remember that, in both the nonstress test and the contraction stress test, external monitoring is performed. Review this test if you had difficulty with this question.
Level of Cognitive Ability: Application
Client Needs: Physiological Integrity
Integrated Process: Nursing Process/Implementation
Content Area: Maternity/Antepartum
Reference: Leifer, G. (2005). *Maternity nursing* (9th ed.). Philadelphia: W.B. Saunders, p. 70.

11. Answer: 3
Rationale: Option 3 is a low priority because fundal height should be measured at each antepartal clinic visit and not as a priority of care in the intrapartum period. Options 1, 2, and 4 are all high priorities. The twins should be monitored by dual electronic fetal monitoring and, in so doing, any signs of distress need to be reported. Many physicians choose to perform a cesarean birth if either of the twins is breech. The mother should have an IV in place in case fluid or blood replacement is required.
Test-Taking Strategy: Note the key words, *lowest priority.* Use Maslow's Hierarchy of Needs theory and the ABCs—airway, breathing, and circulation—to prioritize and direct you to option 3. Review care to the pregnant client with a breech presentation if you had difficulty with this question.
Level of Cognitive Ability: Application
Client Needs: Physiological Integrity
Integrated Process: Nursing Process/Planning
Content Area: Delegating/Prioritizing
Reference: Leifer, G. (2005). *Maternity nursing* (9th ed.). Philadelphia: W.B. Saunders, p. 241.

12. Answer: 3
Rationale: Nurses should explore measures that assist the family to create memories of an infant so that the existence of the child is confirmed and the parents can complete the grieving process. Option 3 meets this goal and also demonstrates a caring and empathetic response. Options 1, 2, and 4 are blocks to communication and devalue parents' feelings.
Test-Taking Strategy: Use therapeutic communication techniques and always focus on the client's feelings first. Option 3 demonstrates a caring and empathetic response by the nurse and addresses the grieving process. Review the grief process if you had difficulty with this question.
Level of Cognitive Ability: Application
Client Needs: Psychosocial Integrity
Integrated Process: Caring
Content Area: Maternity/Postpartum
References: Lowdermilk, D., & Perry, A. (2004). *Maternity and woman's health care* (8th ed.). St. Louis: Mosby, pp. 1152-1153.

Wong, D., & Hockenberry, M. (2003). *Nursing care of infants and children* (7th ed.). St. Louis: Mosby, p. 370.

13. Answer: 2

Rationale: HIV is transmitted by intimate sexual contact and by the exchange of body fluids, exposure to infected blood, and the transmission from an infected woman to her fetus. Women who fall into the high-risk category for HIV infection include those with persistent and recurrent sexually transmitted diseases or a history of multiple sexual partners and those who use or have used IV drugs. Options 1, 3, and 4 are not situations that contribute to contracting HIV infection.

Test-Taking Strategy: Knowledge regarding risk factors for HIV infection is necessary to answer the question. Use the process of elimination, recalling that IV drug use places the client at high risk for contracting the disease. Review these risk factors if you had difficulty with this question.

Level of Cognitive Ability: Comprehension
Client Needs: Health Promotion and Maintenance
Integrated Process: Nursing Process/Data collection
Content Area: Maternity/Antepartum
Reference: Leifer, G. (2005). *Maternity nursing* (9th ed.). Philadelphia: W.B. Saunders, p. 339.

14. Answer: 3

Rationale: Constipation causes the client to use the Valsalva maneuver. This causes blood to rush to the heart and overload the cardiac system. Absence of weight gain is not recommended during pregnancy. Diets low in fluid and fiber cause a decrease in blood volume, which in turn deprives the fetus of nutrients. Too much sodium could cause an overload to the circulating blood volume and contribute to the cardiac condition.

Test-Taking Strategy: Use the process of elimination and try to relate the situation to something with which you are familiar. Look for options that would apply to any heart condition and think about the needs of a pregnant client. Then, use the process of elimination. Review dietary measures for the client with cardiac disease if you had difficulty with question.

Level of Cognitive Ability: Application
Client Needs: Physiological Integrity
Integrated Process: Nursing Process/Planning
Content Area: Maternity/Antepartum
Reference: Leifer, G. (2005). *Maternity nursing* (9th ed.). Philadelphia: W.B. Saunders, pp. 225-226.

15. Answer: 3

Rationale: Infected house cats transmit toxoplasmosis through feces. Handling litter boxes can transmit the disease to the maternity client. Meats that are undercooked can harbor microorganisms that can cause infection. Hands should be washed throughout the day when items that could be contaminated are handled. Topical corticosteroid treatment is not the pharmacological treatment of choice for toxoplasmosis.

Test-Taking Strategy: Use the process of elimination. Eliminate option 1 because of the absolute word "only." Option 2 also represents an extreme statement and should be eliminated. From the remaining options, recalling the causes and treatment for toxoplasmosis will direct you to option 3. Review the causes of toxoplasmosis if you had difficulty with this question.

Level of Cognitive Ability: Application
Client Needs: Health Promotion and Maintenance
Integrated Process: Teaching/Learning
Content Area: Maternity/Antepartum
Reference: Leifer, G. (2005). *Maternity nursing* (9th ed.). Philadelphia: W.B. Saunders, p. 388.

16. Answer: 4

Rationale: DIC is a state of diffuse clotting in which clotting factors are consumed. This leads to widespread bleeding. Platelet counts are decreased because they are consumed by the process, coagulation studies show no clot formation (and clotting times are thus prolonged), and fibrin plugs may clog the microvasculature diffusely, rather than in an isolated area.

Test-Taking Strategy: Use the process of elimination. Eliminate option 1 based on the knowledge that DIC is a widespread problem, not a localized one. Eliminate options 2 and 3 next because they are similar. Review the signs related to DIC if you had difficulty with this question.

Level of Cognitive Ability: Comprehension
Client Needs: Physiological Integrity
Integrated Process: Nursing Process/Data collection
Content Area: Maternity/Antepartum
Reference: Leifer, G. (2005). *Maternity nursing* (9th ed.). Philadelphia: W.B. Saunders, pp. 287-288.

17. Answer: 1

Rationale: A nutritional supplement commonly needed during pregnancy is iron. Anemia of pregnancy is primarily caused by iron deficiency. Iron supplements usually cause constipation. Meats are an excellent source of iron. Iron for the fetus comes from the maternal serum.

Test-Taking Strategy: Use the process of elimination. Note the key word, *malnourished*. Eliminate options 2 and 4 because of the absolute terminology "not" and "all." Knowledge regarding the effects of iron supplements would assist in eliminating option 3. Review the relationship of nutrition to anemia if you had difficulty with this question.

Level of Cognitive Ability: Comprehension
Client Needs: Physiological Integrity
Integrated Process: Teaching/Learning
Content Area: Maternity/Antepartum
Reference: Leifer, G. (2005). *Maternity nursing* (9th ed.). Philadelphia: W.B. Saunders, pp. 225-226.

18. Answer: 4

Rationale: An increase in calories is needed during pregnancy, but concentrated sugars should be avoided because they may cause hyperglycemia. The fat intake should be 20% to 30% of the total calories. The client with diabetes needs about 50% to 60% of the diet from carbohydrates and about 12% to 20% from protein. High-fiber foods will control blood glucose levels and prevent constipation.

Test-Taking Strategy: Note the key words, *teaching has been effective*. Use the process of elimination and knowledge regarding diabetes mellitus and diet therapy to direct you to the correct option. Review these components of the diabetic diet if you had difficulty with this question.

Level of Cognitive Ability: Comprehension

Client Needs: Health Promotion and Maintenance
Integrated Process: Nursing Process/Evaluation
Content Area: Maternity/Antepartum
References: Leifer, G. (2005). *Maternity nursing* (9th ed.).
Philadelphia: W.B. Saunders, pp. 228-229.
Lowdermilk, D., & Perry, A. (2003). *Maternity nursing* (6th ed.).
St. Louis: Mosby, p. 854.

19. *Answer:* **3**
Rationale: The first action is to maintain an open airway and prevent injuries to the client. Options 1, 2, and 4 may be components of care but are not the first action.
Test-Taking Strategy: Note the key word, *first.* Use the ABCs—airway, breathing, and circulation—to answer the question. Airway is the first priority. Review care of the client with eclampsia if you had difficulty with this question.
Level of Cognitive Ability: Application
Client Needs: Physiological Integrity
Integrated Process: Nursing Process/Implementation
Content Area: Delegating/Prioritizing
Reference: Lowdermilk, D., & Perry, A. (2004). *Maternity and woman's health care* (8th ed.). St. Louis: Mosby, p. 854.

20. *Answer:* **3**
Rationale: Options 1, 2, and 4 are all signs that the PIH is being resolved. Option 3 is a symptom of worsening of the PIH.

Test-Taking Strategy: Note the key words, *not resolving.* Recalling the signs of worsening PIH will direct you to the correct option. Review these signs if you had difficulty with this question.
Level of Cognitive Ability: Analysis
Client Needs: Physiological Integrity
Integrated Process: Nursing Process/Evaluation
Content Area: Maternity/Antepartum
Reference: Leifer, G. (2005). *Maternity nursing* (9th ed.).
Philadelphia: W.B. Saunders, p. 223.

ALTERNATE FORMAT QUESTION:
FILL IN THE BLANK

Answer: Hypertension, generalized edema, and proteinuria
Rationale: The three classic signs of preeclampsia are hypertension, generalized edema, and proteinuria.
Test-Taking Strategy: It is necessary to know the classic signs of preeclampsia to answer this question. If you had difficulty with this question, review preeclampsia and learn these signs.
Level of Cognitive Ability: Application
Client Needs: Physiological Integrity
Integrated Process: Nursing Process/Data collection
Content Area: Maternity/Antepartum
Reference: Wong, D., Perry, S. & Hockenberry, M. (2002). *Maternal child nursing care* (2nd ed.). St. Louis: Mosby, p. 277.

REFERENCES

Leifer, G. (2005). *Maternity nursing* (9th ed.). Philadelphia: W.B. Saunders.
Lowdermilk, D., & Perry, A. (2004). *Maternity and woman's health care* (8th ed.) St. Louis: Mosby.

Murray, S., McKinney, E., & Gorrie, T. (2002). *Foundations of maternal-newborn nursing* (3rd ed.). Philadelphia: W.B. Saunders.
Wong, D., Perry, S., & Hockenberry, M. (2002). *Maternal child nursing care* (2nd ed.). St. Louis: Mosby.

Labor and Delivery and Associated Complications

I. THE PROCESS OF LABOR: "THE 4 P's" (Box 23-1)

A. Description
   1. Labor: Coordinated sequence of involuntary uterine contractions
   2. **Delivery:** Actual event of birth
B. Four major factors (four P's) interact during normal childbirth; all four P's are interrelated
C. Powers: Uterine contractions
   1. The forces acting to expel the fetus
   2. Effacement: Shortening and thinning of the cervix during the first stage of **labor**
   3. Dilation: Enlargement of cervical os and cervical canal during first stage
   4. Pushing efforts of mother during second stage
D. Passageway: Composed of the mother's rigid bony pelvis and the soft tissues of the cervix, pelvic floor, vagina, and introitus
E. Passenger: The fetus
F. Psyche: Mother may experience anxiety or fear
G. Attitude
   1. The relationship of the fetal body parts to one another
   2. Normal intrauterine attitude is flexion, in which the fetal back is rounded, the head is forward on the chest, and the arms and legs are folded in against the body
H. Lie
   1. Relationship of the spine of the fetus to the spine of the mother
   2. Longitudinal or vertical
      a. Fetal spine is parallel to the mother's spine
      b. Fetus is either cephalic or breech presentation
   3. Transverse or horizontal
      a. Fetal spine is at a right angle, or perpendicular, to the mother's spine
      b. Presenting part is the shoulder
      c. **Delivery** by cesarean section
   4. Oblique
      a. Fetal spine is at a slight angle from a true horizontal lie
      b. **Delivery** is by cesarean section if uncorrectable
I. Presentation
   1. Presenting part: Portion of the fetus that enters the pelvis first
   2. Cephalic
      a. The most common presentation
      b. Fetal head presents first
   3. Breech
      a. Buttocks present first
      b. **Delivery** by cesarean section may be required, although it is often possible to deliver vaginally
   4. Shoulder
      a. Fetus is in a transverse lie, or the arm, back, abdomen, or side could present
      b. If the fetus does not spontaneously rotate or if it is not possible to turn the fetus manually, a cesarean section may be performed
J. Position: Relationship of assigned area of the presenting part or landmark to the maternal pelvis (Box 23-2)
K. Station
   1. The measurement of the progress of descent in centimeters above or below the midplane from the presenting part to the ischial spine
   2. Station 0: at ischial spine
   3. Minus station: above ischial spine
   4. Plus station: below ischial spine

II. MECHANISMS OF LABOR (Box 23-3)

A. Data collection
   1. Lightening or dropping: Fetus descends into the pelvis about 2 weeks prior to **delivery** for a primipara; the fetus may engage into the pelvis after **labor** commences for a multipara

BOX 23-1

Four P's

Powers
Passageway
Passenger
Psyche

BOX 23-2

Fetal Positions

ROA : Right occiput anterior
LOA: Left occiput anterior
ROP: Right occiput posterior
LOP: Left occiput posterior
ROT: Right occiput transverse
LOT: Left occiput transverse
RMA: Right mentum anterior
LMA: Left mentum anterior
RMP: Right mentum posterior
LSA: Left sacrum anterior
LSP: Left sacrum posterior

2. Braxton Hicks contractions increase
3. Show
4. Vaginal mucosa congested and vaginal mucus increases
5. Brownish or blood-tinged cervical mucus passed
6. Cervix ripens, becomes soft, partly effaced, and may begin to dilate
7. Sudden burst of energy
8. Loss of 1 to 3 pounds from water loss resulting from fluid shifts produced by the changes in progesterone and estrogen levels
9. Spontaneous rupture of membranes
B. True **labor** (Box 23-4)
    1. Contractions increase in duration and intensity with a change in activity
    2. Cervical dilation and effacement are progressive
C. False labor (see Box 23-4)
    1. Exaggeration of normal contractions
    2. Does not produce dilation, effacement, or descent
    3. Contractions are irregular without progression
    4. Walking has no effect on contractions and often relieves false **labor**

III. LEOPOLD'S MANEUVERS
A. Description: To determine position, presentation, and engagement
B. Preparation
    1. Ask the mother to empty the bladder
    2. Warm hands and apply them to the mother's abdomen with firm and gentle pressure
C. First maneuver
    1. Determines which part of the fetus is in the fundus

BOX 23-3

Mechanisms of Labor

ENGAGEMENT
Mechanism by which the fetus nestles into the pelvis
Also termed lightening or dropping

DESCENT
The process that the fetal head undergoes as it begins its journey through the pelvis
A continuous process from the time of engagement until birth; assessed by the measurement called station

FLEXION
Process of the fetal head's nodding forward toward the fetal chest

INTERNAL ROTATION
Internal rotation of the fetus; most commonly from the occiput transverse position, assumed at engagement into the pelvis, to the occiput anterior position while continuously descending

EXTENSION
Enables the head to emerge when the fetus is in a cephalic position
Begins after the head crowns
Is complete when the head passes under the symphysis pubis and occiput, and the anterior fontanel, brow, face, and chin pass over the sacrum and coccyx and are over the perineum

RESTITUTION
Realignment of the fetal head with the body after the head emerges

EXTERNAL ROTATION
The shoulders externally rotate after the head emerges and restitution occurs, so that the shoulders are in the anteroposterior diameter of the pelvis

EXPULSION
The birth of the entire body

2. Place palms on each side of the upper abdomen and palpate around the fundus
3. If the head is in the fundus, one feels a hard, round, movable object
4. The buttocks will feel soft, have an irregular shape, and are more difficult to move
D. Second maneuver
    1. Move hands downward over each side of the abdomen, applying firm, even pressure
    2. The fetus's back, which is a smooth, hard surface, should be felt on one side of the abdomen
    3. Irregular knobs and lumps, which may be the hands, feet, elbows, and knees, will be felt on the opposite side of the abdomen

BOX 23-4

True Labor and False Labor

TRUE LABOR
Contractions increase in duration and intensity with a change in activity
Cervical dilation and effacement are progressive

FALSE LABOR
Does not produce dilation, effacement, or descent
Contractions are irregular without progression
Walking has no effect on contractions and often relieves false labor
Example: A woman has been sleeping and wakes up with contractions. If she gets up and moves around and her contractions become stronger and closer together, this is true labor. If the contractions go away, this is false labor.

E. Third maneuver
  1. Confirms fetal position
  2. Place hand above the symphysis pubis
  3. Bring thumb and fingers together and grasp the part of fetus between them (may be either the head or the buttocks)
F. Fourth maneuver
  1. Used in the late stage of pregnancy to determine how far the fetus has descended into the pelvic inlet
  2. Place hands on the sides of the lower abdomen, close to the midline
  3. Slide hands downward and press inward
  4. If it has been determined that the buttocks are in the fundus, then feel for the head
  5. If the head cannot be felt, it has probably descended

IV. BREATHING TECHNIQUES (Box 23-5)
A. Provide a focus during contractions, interfering with pain sensory transmission
B. Begin with simple breathing patterns and progress to more complex ones, as needed
C. Promote relaxation and oxygenation

V. FETAL MONITORING
A. Description
  1. Displays fetal heart rate (FHR)
  2. Monitors the uterine activity, frequency, duration, and intensity of contractions
  3. Monitors the FHR in relation to maternal contractions
  4. Baseline FHR is measured between contractions; the normal FHR at term is 120 to 160 beats per minute
B. External fetal monitoring
  1. Noninvasive and performed by the use of a toco-transducer or Doppler ultrasonic transducer

BOX 23-5

Breathing Techniques

FIRST-STAGE BREATHING
Cleansing Breath
Each contraction begins and ends with a deep inspiration and expiration
Slow-Paced Breathing
A slow deep breathing that promotes relaxation
Used as long as possible during labor
Modified-Paced Breathing
Used when slow-paced breathing is no longer effective
Shallow, fast breathing
Pattern-Paced Breathing
Sometimes called pant-blow
After a certain number of breaths (modified-paced breathing), the woman exhales with a slight emphasis or blow, and then begins the modified-paced breathing again
Breathing to Prevent Pushing
The woman blows repeatedly using short puffs when the urge to push is strong

SECOND-STAGE BREATHING
Traditional Pushing
The woman takes one or more cleansing breaths at the beginning of a contraction and then holds her breath, pushing as hard as she can for as long as possible
She then quickly exhales, takes another breath, and pushes again, repeating the process until the contraction is over
Other Pushing Methods
Exhalation of small amounts of air through an open glottis during pushing
The woman may push in short bursts only when the urge is very strong instead of using prolonged expulsive efforts

  2. Leopold's maneuvers are performed to determine on which side the fetal back is located, and the ultrasound transducer is placed over this area (fasten with a belt)
  3. The tocotransducer is placed the over the fundus of the uterus where contractions feel the strongest (fasten with a belt)
  4. Allow the client to assume a comfortable position, avoiding vena cava compression
C. Internal fetal monitoring
  1. Invasive and requires rupturing of the membranes and attaching an electrode to the presenting part of the fetus
  2. Mother must be dilated 2 to 3 cm to perform internal monitoring
D. Periodic patterns in the FHR
  1. Fetal bradycardia and tachycardia
    a. Bradycardia: FHR is less than 120 beats per minute for 10 minutes or more
    b. Tachycardia: FHR is greater than 160 beats per minute for 10 minutes or more

c. Change position of the mother and administer oxygen

d. The physician is notified

2. Variability

a. Irregular fluctuations in the baseline FHR of 2 cycles per minute or more

b. Decreased variability can result from fetal hypoxemia, acidosis, or certain medications

c. A temporary decrease in variability can occur when the fetus is in a sleep state (sleep states do not usually last longer than 30 minutes)

3. Accelerations

a. Brief, temporary increases in the FHR of at least 15 beats above the baseline, lasting at least 15 seconds

b. Usually a reassuring sign, reflecting a responsive, nonacidotic fetus

c. Usually occur with fetal movement

d. May occur with uterine contractions, vaginal examinations, or mild cord compression or when the fetus is in a breech presentation

4. Early decelerations

a. Decrease in FHR below baseline

b. Occur during contractions as the fetal head is pressed against the woman's pelvis or soft tissues, such as the cervix, and return to the baseline FHR by the end of the contraction

c. Not associated with fetal compromise and requires no intervention

5. Late decelerations

a. A nonreassuring pattern that reflects impaired **placental** exchange or uteroplacental insufficiency

b. Interventions include improving **placental** blood flow and fetal oxygenation

6. Variable decelerations

a. Caused by conditions that restrict flow through the umbilical cord (cord compression)

b. Significant when the FHR repeatedly decreases to less than 70 beats per minute and persists at that level for at least 60 seconds before returning to the baseline

7. Hypertonic uterine activity

a. Checking uterine activity includes frequency, duration, intensity of the contractions, and uterine resting tone

b. The uterus should relax between contractions for 60 seconds or longer

c. In hypertonic uterine activity, reduced uterine blood flow and decreased fetal oxygen supply occurs

8. Interventions for nonreassuring (altered) patterns (Box 23-6)

a. The registered nurse and physician are notified

b. Identify the cause (check for cord prolapse)

c. Change the mother's position (avoid the supine position for patterns associated with cord compression)

BOX 23-6

Nonreassuring Patterns

Tachycardia
Bradycardia
Decreased or absent variability
Late decelerations
Variable decelerations falling to less than 70 beats per minutes for longer than 60 seconds
Prolonged decelerations
Hypertonic uterine activity

---

d. Administer oxygen by face mask at 8 to 10 L/minute

e. Oxytocin (Pitocin) if infusing is discontinued, as prescribed

f. Intravenous fluids are increased, as prescribed

g. Prepare to obtain a fetal scalp pH monitor to determine a blood pH value

h. Prepare to initiate continuous electronic fetal monitoring with internal devices if not contraindicated

i. Prepare for cesarean **delivery** if necessary

VI. STAGES OF LABOR

A. Stage 1, latent phase

1. Data collection

a. Cervical dilation of 1 to 4 cm

b. Uterine contractions every 15 to 30 minutes, 15 to 30 seconds in duration, and of mild intensity

c. Mother talkative and eager to be in **labor**

2. Interventions

a. Encourage mother and partner to participate in care

b. Assist with comfort measures, changes of position, and ambulation

c. Keep mother and partner informed of progress

d. Offer fluids and ice chips

e. Encourage voiding every 1 to 2 hours

B. Stage 1, active phase

1. Data collection

a. Cervical dilation of 4 to 7 cm

b. Uterine contractions every 3 to 5 minutes, 30 to 60 seconds in duration, and of moderate intensity

c. Mother may experience feelings of helplessness

d. Mother becomes restless and anxious as contractions become stronger

2. Interventions

a. Encourage maintenance of effective breathing patterns

b. Provide a quiet environment

c. Keep mother and partner informed of progress

d. Promote comfort with back rubs, sacral pressure, pillow support, and position changes

e. Instruct partner in effleurage

f. Offer fluids and ice chips and ointment for dry lips

g. Encourage voiding every 1 to 2 hours

C. Stage 1, transition phase

1. Data collection

a. Cervical dilation of 8 to 10 cm

b. Uterine contractions every 2 to 3 minutes, 45 to 90 seconds in duration, and of strong intensity

c. Mother becomes tired, is restless and irritable, and feels out of control

2. Interventions

a. Encourage rest between contractions

b. Wake mother at beginning of contraction so she can begin breathing pattern

c. Keep mother and partner informed of progress

d. Provide privacy

e. Offer fluids and ice chips and ointment for dry lips

f. Encourage voiding every 1 to 2 hours

D. Interventions throughout stage 1

a. Monitor maternal vital signs

b. Monitor FHR via ultrasound, Doppler, fetoscope, or electronic fetal monitor

c. Assess FHR before, during, and after a contraction, noting that the normal FHR is 120 to 160 beats per minute

d. Monitor uterine contractions by palpation or monitor, determining frequency, duration, and intensity

e. Assist with monitoring the status of cervical dilation and effacement

f. Assist with monitoring fetal station presentation and position by Leopold's maneuvers

g. Assist with pelvic examinations and prepare for a fern test

h. Check the color of the **amniotic fluid** if the membranes have ruptured, because meconium-stained fluid can indicate fetal distress

E. Stage 2

1. Data collection

a. Cervical dilation is complete

b. Progress of **labor** is measured by descent of fetal head through the birth canal (change in fetal station)

c. Uterine contractions occur every 2 to 3 minutes, lasting 60 to 75 seconds, and the intensity is strong

d. Increase in bloody show occurs

e. Mother feels urge to bear down; assist mother in pushing efforts

2. Interventions

a. Monitor maternal vital signs

b. Check the FHR before, during, and after a contraction, noting that normal fetal heart rate is 120 to 160 beats per minute

c. Monitor uterine contractions by palpation or monitor, determining frequency, duration, and intensity

d. Provide mother with encouragement and praise and provide for rest between contractions

e. Keep mother and partner informed of progress

f. Maintain privacy

g. Provide ice chips and ointment for dry lips

h. Assist mother into a position that promotes comfort and assists pushing efforts, such as lithotomy, semisitting, kneeling, side-lying, or squatting

i. Monitor for signs of approaching birth, such as perineal bulging or visualization of the fetal head

j. Prepare for birth

F. Stage 3

1. Data collection

a. Contractions occur until **placenta** is born

b. **Placental** separation and expulsion occur

c. Birth of **placenta** occurs 5 to 30 minutes after birth of the baby

d. Schultze's mechanism: Center portion of **placenta** separates first, and its shiny fetal surface emerges from the vagina

e. Duncan's mechanism: Margin of **placenta** separates, and the dull, red, rough maternal surface emerges from the vagina first

2. Interventions

a. Monitor maternal vital signs and uterine status

b. Following birth of **placenta**, uterine fundus remains firm and is located 2 fingerbreadths below the umbilicus

c. Examine **placenta** for cotyledons and membranes to verify that it is intact

d. Monitor mother for shivering and provide warmth

e. Promote parental-neonatal attachment

G. Stage 4

1. Description: The period of time from 1 to 4 hours after **delivery**

2. Data collection

a. Blood pressure returns to prelabor level

b. Pulse is slightly lower than during **labor**

c. Fundus remains contracted, in the midline, 1 to 2 fingerbreadths below the umbilicus

d. **Lochia** is moderate or scant and is red

3. Interventions

a. Maternal assessments are performed every 15 minutes for 1 hour, every 30 minutes for 1 hour, and hourly for 2 hours

b. Provide warm blankets

c. Apply ice packs to the perineum

d. Massage the uterus if needed and teach the mother to massage the uterus

e. Provide breast-feeding support as needed

f. Refer to Chapter 25 for information on caring for the **newborn**

VII. ANESTHESIA

A. Local anesthesia
1. Used for blocking pain during episiotomy
2. Administered just before the birth of baby
3. No effect on the fetus

B. Pudendal block
1. Administered just before the birth of the baby
2. Injection site at pudendal nerve through a transvaginal route
3. Blocks perineal area for episiotomy
4. Effect lasts about 30 minutes
5. No effect on contractions or fetus

C. Lumbar epidural block
1. Injection site in epidural space at L3-L4
2. Administered after **labor** is established or just before a scheduled cesarean birth
3. Relieves pain from contractions and numbs vagina and perineum
4. May cause hypotension
5. Does not cause headache because the dura mater is not penetrated
6. Monitor maternal blood pressure
7. Maintain the mother in side-lying position or place a rolled blanket beneath the right hip to displace the uterus from the vena cava
8. Intravenous fluids are administered, as prescribed
9. Increase fluids as prescribed if hypotension occurs

D. Subarachnoid (spinal) block
1. Injection site in spinal subarachnoid space at L3-L5
2. Administered just before birth
3. Relieves uterine and perineal pain and numbs vagina, perineum, and lower extremities
4. May cause maternal hypotension
5. May cause postpartum headache
6. The mother must lie flat 8 to 12 hours following spinal injection
7. Intravenous fluids are administered as prescribed
8. Increase fluids as prescribed if hypotension occurs

E. General anesthesia
1. May be used for some surgical interventions
2. The mother is not awake
3. Presents a danger of respiratory depression and vomiting

VIII. OBSTETRICAL PROCEDURES

A. Bishop score (Table 23-1)
1. Used to determine maternal readiness for **labor**
2. Evaluates cervical status and fetal position
3. Indicated before the induction of **labor**
4. The five factors are assigned a score of 0 to 3, and the total score is calculated
5. A score of 6 or more indicates a readiness for **labor** induction

TABLE 23-1

Factors of the Bishop Score

SCORE	0	1	2	3
Dilation of cervix (cm)	0	1-2	3-4	≥5
Effacement of cervix (%)	0-30	40-50	60-70	≥80
Consistency of cervix	Firm	Medium	Soft	
Position of cervix	Posterior	Midposition	Anterior	
Station of presenting part	−3	−2	−1	+1, +2

B. Induction
1. A deliberate initiation of uterine contractions that stimulates **labor**
2. Elective induction may be accomplished by oxytocin (Pitocin) infusion
3. Baseline tracing of uterine contractions and FHR is obtained
4. Intravenous dosage of oxytocin may be increased as prescribed only after assessing contractions, FHR, and maternal blood pressure and pulse
5. The rate of oxytocin is not increased once the desired contraction pattern is obtained (contraction frequency of 2 to 3 minutes, lasting 60 seconds)
6. Oxytocin infusion is discontinued as prescribed if contraction frequency is less than every 2 minutes or duration is more than 90 seconds, or if fetal distress is noted

C. Amniotomy
1. Artificial rupture of membranes (AROM); performed by the physician to stimulate **labor**
2. Performed if the fetus is at "0" or "+" station
3. Increases risk of prolapsed cord and infection
4. Monitor FHR before and after AROM
5. Record time of AROM, FHR, and characteristics of fluid
6. Meconium-stained **amniotic fluid** may be associated with fetal distress
7. Bloody **amniotic fluid** may indicate abruptio placentae or fetal trauma
8. An unpleasant odor to **amniotic fluid** is associated with infection
9. Polyhydramnios is associated with maternal diabetes and certain congenital disorders
10. Oligohydramnios is associated with intrauterine growth retriction (IUGR) and congenital disorders
11. Expect more variable decelerations after rupture of the membranes as a result of cord compression during contractions
12. Limit client activity after AROM, if prescribed

▲ D. External version
  1. External manipulation of the fetus from an abnormal position into a normal presentation
  2. Indicated for an abnormal presentation that exists after the 34th week
  3. Monitor vital signs
  4. If the mother is Rh-negative, ensure that Rh immune globulin was given at 28 weeks' gestation
  5. Prepare for nonstress test to evaluate fetal well-being
  6. Intravenous fluids and tocolytic therapy may be administered to relax the uterus and permit easier manipulation of fetus
  7. Ultrasound is used during the procedure to evaluate fetal position and **placental** placement and guide direction of the fetus
  8. Abdominal wall is manipulated to direct fetus into a cephalic presentation if possible
  9. Monitor blood pressure to identify vena cava compression
  10. Monitor for unusual pain
  11. Following the procedure
     a. Perform nonstress test to evaluate fetal well-being
     b. Monitor for uterine activity, bleeding, ruptured membranes, and decreased fetal activity
     c. With Rh-negative clients, a Kleihauer-Betke test is performed as prescribed to detect the presence and amount of fetal blood in the maternal circulation and to identify clients who need additional Rh immune globulin

▲ E. Episiotomy
  1. Incision made into the perineum to enlarge vaginal outlet and facilitate **delivery**
  2. Check episiotomy site
  3. Institute measures to relieve pain
  4. Provide ice pack during the first 24 hours
  5. Instruct the client in the use of sitz baths
  6. Apply analgesic spray or ointment as prescribed
  7. Provide perineal care, using clean technique
  8. Instruct the client in the proper care of the incision
  9. Instruct the client to dry the perineal area from front to back and to blot the area rather than wipe it
  10. Instruct the client to shower rather than bathe in a tub
  11. Apply a peripad without touching the inside surface of the pad
  12. Report any bleeding or discharge to the physician

▲ F. Forceps **delivery**
  1. Two double-crossed, spoonlike articulated blades used to assist in the **delivery** of the fetal head
  2. Reassure the mother and explain the need for forceps
  3. Monitor mother and fetus during **delivery**

  4. Check **neonate** and mother after **delivery** for any possible injury
  5. Assist with repair of any lacerations

G. Vacuum extraction ▲
  1. A caplike suction device is applied to the fetal head to facilitate extraction
  2. Suction is used to assist in **delivery** of the fetal head
  3. Traction is applied during uterine contractions until descent of the fetal head is achieved
  4. The suction device should not be kept in place any longer than 25 minutes
  5. Monitor FHR every 5 minutes if external fetal monitoring is not used
  6. Check the **newborn infant** at birth and monitor throughout the postpartum period for signs of cerebral trauma
  7. Monitor for developing cephalhematoma
  8. Caput succedaneum is normal and will resolve in 24 hours

H. Cesarean **delivery** ▲
  1. **Delivery** of the fetus usually through a transabdominal, low-segment incision of the uterus
  2. Preoperative
     a. If planned, prepare the mother and partner
     b. If an emergency, quickly explain the need and procedure to the mother and partner
     c. Obtain informed consent
     d. Make sure that the preoperative diagnostic tests are done, including testing for the Rh factor
     e. Prepare the mother for insertion of an IV line and a Foley catheter
     f. Prepare the abdomen, as prescribed
     g. Monitor the mother and fetus continuously for signs of **labor**
     h. Provide emotional support
     i. Administer preoperative medications as prescribed
  3. Postoperative
     a. Monitor vital signs
     b. Provide pain relief
     c. Encourage turning, coughing, and deep breathing
     d. Encourage ambulation
     e. Monitor for signs of infection and bleeding
     f. Burning and pain on urination may indicate a bladder infection
     g. A tender uterus and foul-smelling **lochia** may indicate endometritis
     h. A productive cough or chills may indicate pneumonia
     i. A positive Homans' sign, pain, or edema of extremity may indicate thrombophlebitis

IX. DYSTOCIA
A. Description
  1. Difficult **labor** that is prolonged or more painful

2. Occurs because of problems caused by uterine contractions, the fetus, or the bones and tissues of the maternal pelvis
3. Contractions may be hypotonic or hypertonic
4. Fetus may be excessively large, malpositioned, or in an abnormal presentation
5. Can result in maternal dehydration, infection, fetal injury or death

B. Data collection
1. Excessive abdominal pain
2. Abnormal contraction pattern
3. Fetal distress
4. Maternal or fetal tachycardia
5. Lack of progress in **labor**

C. Interventions
1. Check fetal heart rate (FHR); monitor for fetal distress
2. Monitor uterine contractions
3. Monitor maternal temperature and heart rate
4. Assist with pelvic examination, measurements, ultrasound, and other procedures
5. Prophylactic antibiotics may be prescribed to prevent infection
6. Intravenous fluids may be prescribed
7. Monitor intake and output (I&O)
8. Monitor for dehydration
9. Instruct the mother in breathing techniques and relaxation exercises
10. Fetal monitoring is needed if oxytocin (Pitocin) is prescribed
11. Monitor color of **amniotic** fluid
12. Provide rest and comfort as with a normal **delivery**, such as back rubs and position changes
13. Assess mother's fatigue and pain and administer sedatives and pain medications as prescribed
14. Monitor for prolapse of the cord after rupture of the membranes

X. PROLAPSED CORD

A. Description: The umbilical cord is displaced, either between the presenting part and the amnion or protruding through the cervix, causing compression of the cord and compromising fetal circulation

B. Data collection
1. A feeling that something is coming through the vagina
2. Umbilical cord is seen or palpated
3. FHR is irregular and slow
4. Fetal heart monitor will show variable deceleration or bradycardia after rupture of the membranes
5. If fetal hypoxia is severe, violent fetal activity may occur and then cease

C. Interventions (Box 23-7)

BOX 23-7

Interventions: Cord Prolapse

Relieve cord pressure immediately.
Reposition mother; turn on her side or her hips may be elevated to shift the fetal presenting part toward her diaphragm.
Elevate the fetal presenting part that is lying on the cord by applying finger pressure with a sterile gloved hand.
Do not attempt to push the cord into the uterus.
Monitor FHR.
Monitor fetus for hypoxia.
Administer oxygen by face mask to the mother, as prescribed.
Prepare for emergency cesarean birth.

XI. PRECIPITOUS LABOR AND DELIVERY

A. Description: **Labor** lasts less than 3 hours
B. Interventions
1. Stay with the mother at all times
2. Provide emotional support and keep the mother calm
3. Encourage the mother to pant between contractions
4. Prepare for rupturing membranes when head crowns if they are not already ruptured
5. Do not try to keep fetus from being delivered
6. If delivery is necessary before the arrival of the health care provider
   a. Apply gentle pressure to fetal head upward toward the vagina to prevent damage to the fetal head and vaginal lacerations
   b. Support the infant's body during delivery
   c. Deliver the infant between contractions, checking for the cord around the neck
   d. Restitution is used to deliver the posterior shoulder
   e. Gentle downward pressure is used to move the anterior shoulder under the pubic symphysis
   f. Clear the **infant's** mouth
7. Dry and cover the infant to keep the body warm
8. Allow the **placenta** to separate naturally
9. Place the **infant** on the mother's abdomen or breast to induce uterine contractions

XII. PRETERM LABOR

A. Description
1. **Labor** occurring after the 20th week but before the 37th week
2. Contractions occur more frequently than every 10 minutes, last 30 seconds or longer, and persist
3. May be associated with infection

B. Data collection
   1. Uterine contractions (painful or painless)
   2. Abdominal cramping (may be accompanied by diarrhea)
   3. Low back pain
   4. Pelvic pressure or heaviness
   5. Change in the character and amount of usual discharge; may be thicker or thinner, bloody, brown or colorless, and may be odorous
   6. Rupture of amniotic membranes
C. Interventions
   1. Focus is on stopping the labor: identify and treat infection, restrict activity, and ensure hydration
   2. Maintain bed rest and a lateral position
   3. Monitor fetal status
   4. Administer fluids
   5. Medications may be prescribed to suppress labor (Box 23-8)

BOX 23-8

Medications Used In Preterm Labor

Magnesium sulfate
Terbutaline (Brethine)
Nifedipine (Procardia)
Indomethacin (Indocin)

XIII. RUPTURE OF UTERUS

A. Description
   1. Complete or incomplete separation of the uterine tissue as a result of a tear in the wall of the uterus from the stress of **labor**
   2. Complete: A direct communication between the uterine and peritoneal cavities
   3. Incomplete: A rupture into the peritoneum covering the uterus (but not into the peritoneal cavity)
   4. Manifestations vary with the degree of rupture
B. Data collection
   1. Abdominal pain or tenderness
   2. Chest pain
   3. Contractions may stop or fail to progress
   4. Rigid abdomen
   5. Absent fetal heart rate
   6. Signs of maternal shock
   7. Fetus palpated outside the uterus (complete rupture)
C. Interventions
   1. Monitor for and assist in treating signs of shock (oxygen, intravenous [IV] fluids, and blood products may be prescribed)
   2. Prepare the client for cesarean section or hysterotomy with hysterectomy
   3. Provide emotional support for the client and partner

XIV. PLACENTA PREVIA

A. Description
   1. Improperly implanted **placenta** in the lower uterine segment near or over the internal cervical os
   2. Total: The internal os is entirely covered by the **placenta** when the cervix is fully dilated
   3. Partial: Incomplete coverage of the internal os

   4. Marginal: Only an edge of the **placenta** extends to the internal os but may extend onto the os during dilation of the cervix during **labor**
   5. Low-lying **placenta**: The **placenta** is implanted in the lower uterine segment but does not reach the os
   6. Management depends on the classification of the previa and gestational age of the fetus
B. Data collection
   1. Sudden onset of painless, bright red vaginal bleeding in the last half of pregnancy
   2. Soft, relaxed, nontender uterus
   3. Fundal height may be greater than expected for gestational age
C. Interventions
   1. Monitor maternal vital signs, fetal heart rate, and fetal activity
   2. Prepare for ultrasound to confirm diagnosis
   3. Vaginal examination or any other action that would stimulate uterine activity is avoided
   4. Maintain bed rest in a left lateral position
   5. Monitor amount of bleeding (treat signs of shock)
   6. IV fluids, blood products, or tocolytic medications may be prescribed
   7. If bleeding is heavy, a cesarean section may be performed
   8. Prepare to administer Rh immune globulin if the mother is Rh-negative and has not been given the injection at 28 weeks' gestation

XV. ABRUPTIO PLACENTAE

A. Description: Premature separation of the **placenta** from the uterine wall after the 20th week of gestation and before the fetus is delivered
B. Data collection
   1. Painful vaginal bleeding (dark red)
   2. Uterine tenderness
   3. Uterine rigidity
   4. Severe abdominal pain
   5. Signs of fetal distress
   6. Signs of maternal shock if bleeding is excessive
C. Interventions
   1. Monitor maternal vital signs and fetal heart rate
   2. Monitor for excessive vaginal bleeding, abdominal pain, and increase in fundal height

3. Maintain bed rest; oxygen, IV fluids, and blood products may be prescribed
4. Monitor and report any uterine activity
5. Prepare for the delivery of the fetus as quickly as possible, with vaginal delivery preferable if the fetus is healthy and stable and the presenting part is in the pelvis; emergency cesarean section is performed if the fetus is alive but shows signs of distress
6. Monitor for signs of disseminated intravascular coagulation (DIC) in the postpartum period
7. Prepare to administer Rh immune globulin

XVI. UTERINE INVERSION

A. Description
   1. Uterus completely or partly turns inside out
   2. Usually occurs during delivery or after delivery of the placenta
B. Data collection
   1. A depression in the fundal area of the uterus is noted
   2. Interior of the uterus may be seen through the cervix or protruding through the vagina
   3. Severe pain
   4. Hemorrhage
   5. Signs of shock
C. Interventions
   1. Monitor for hemorrhage, signs of shock, and treat shock
   2. Prepare the client for a return of the uterus to the correct position via the vagina; if unsuccessful, laparotomy with replacement is done

XVII. AMNIOTIC FLUID EMBOLISM

A. Description
   1. The escape of amniotic fluid into the maternal circulation
   2. The debris containing amniotic fluid deposits in the pulmonary arterioles and is usually fatal to the mother
B. Data collection
   1. Abrupt onset of respiratory distress and chest pain
   2. Cyanosis
   3. Seizures
   4. Heart failure and pulmonary edema
   5. Fetal bradycardia and distress if delivery has not occurred at the time of the embolism
C. Interventions
   1. Institute emergency measures to maintain life

2. Administer oxygen at 8 to 10 L/minute by face mask or resuscitation bag delivering 100% oxygen, as prescribed
3. Prepare the client for intubation and mechanical ventilation
4. Position the woman on her side
5. IV fluids, blood products, and medications may be prescribed to correct coagulation failure
6. Monitor fetal status
7. Prepare for emergency delivery once the woman is stabilized
8. Provide emotional support to the woman, partner, and family

XVIII. SUPINE HYPOTENSIVE SYNDROME
   (Figure 23-1)

A. Description
   1. Occurs when the venous return to the heart is impaired by the weight of the uterus
   2. Results in partial occlusion of the vena cava and descending aorta and in reduced cardiac return, cardiac output, and blood pressure
B. Data collection
   1. Faintness, lightheadedness, dizziness
   2. Hypotension
   3. Fetal distress
C. Interventions
   1. Position the client in a lateral recumbent position to shift the weight of the fetus off the inferior vena cava
   2. Monitor vital signs and fetal heart rate

XIX. FETAL DISTRESS

A. Data collection
   1. Fetal heart rate below 120 or above 160 beats per minute
   2. Meconium-stained amniotic fluid
   3. Fetal hyperactivity
   4. Progressive decrease in baseline variability
   5. Severe variable decelerations
   6. Late decelerations
B. Interventions
   1. Place the mother in a lateral position; elevate her legs
   2. Administer oxygen at 8 to 10 L/minute via face mask, as prescribed
   3. Oxytocin (Pitocin) if infusing is discontinued, as prescribed
   4. Monitor maternal and fetal status
   5. Prepare for emergency cesarean section

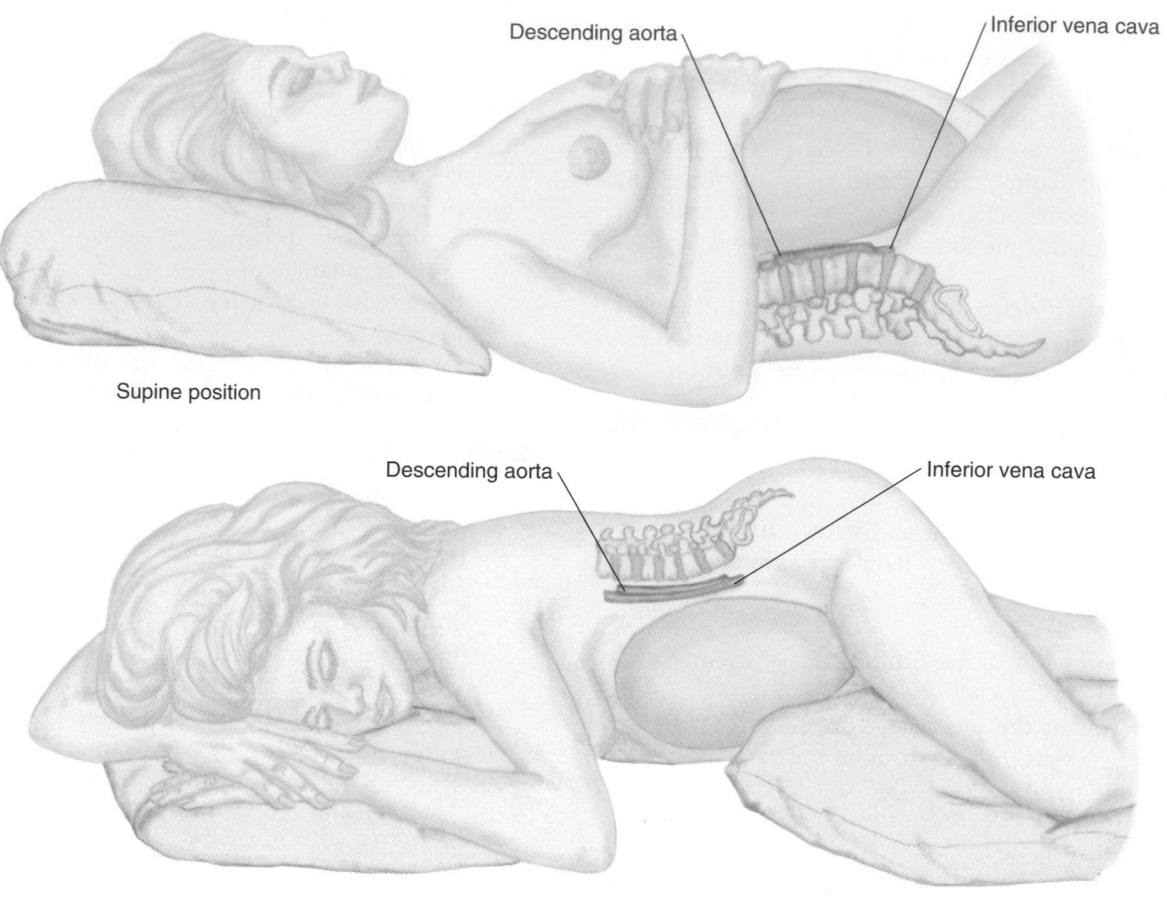

Descending aorta

Inferior vena cava

Supine position

Descending aorta

Inferior vena cava

Right lateral position

FIG. 23-1 Supine hypotensive syndrome. (From Murray, S., McKinney, E., & Gorrie, T. [2002]. *Foundations of maternal-newborn nursing* [3rd ed.]. Philadelphia: W.B. Saunders.)

PRACTICE QUESTIONS

1. The nurse is assigned to assist in caring for a client admitted to the labor unit. The client is 9 cm dilated and is experiencing precipitous labor. A priority nursing action is to:
   1. Prepare for an oxytocin infusion
   2. Keep the client in a side-lying position
   3. Prepare the client for an epidural anesthesia
   4. Encourage the client to start pushing with the contractions

2. A client is admitted to the labor suite complaining of painless vaginal bleeding. The nurse assists with the examination of the client knowing that a routine labor procedure contraindicated with this client's situation is:
   1. Leopold maneuvers
   2. External electronic fetal heart rate monitoring
   3. A manual pelvic examination
   4. Hemoglobin and hematocrit evaluation

3. A nurse is assigned to assist in caring for a client with abruptio placentae who is experiencing vaginal bleeding. The nurse collects data from the client knowing that abruptio placentae is accompanied by which additional finding?
   1. Abdomen soft on palpation
   2. No complaints of abdominal pain
   3. Lack of uterine irritability or tetanic contractions
   4. Uterine tenderness on palpation

4. A nurse is assigned to work in the delivery room and is assisting in caring for a client who has just delivered a newborn infant. The nurse is monitoring for signs of placental separation knowing that which of the following indicates that the placenta has separated?
   1. Shortening of the umbilical cord
   2. Decrease in blood loss from the introitus
   3. Change in the uterine contour
   4. Sudden sharp abdominal pain

5. A nurse is assisting in caring for a client with abruptio placenta. While caring for the client, the nurse notes that the client begins to develop signs of shock. The nurse would first:
   1. Turn the client onto her side
   2. Monitor the maternal pulse

3. Monitor urinary output
4. Monitor the maternal blood pressure

6. A client being prepared for a cesarean delivery is brought to the delivery room. To maintain optimal perfusion of oxygenated blood to the fetus, the nurse places the client in the:
   1. Trendelenburg position
   2. Semi-Fowler's position
   3. Supine position with a wedge under the right hip
   4. Prone position

7. A nurse is asked to assist the primary health care provider in performing Leopold maneuvers on a client. Which nursing intervention should be implemented before this procedure is performed?
   1. Locate fetal heart tones
   2. Have the client drink 8 ounces of water
   3. Warm the sonogram gel
   4. Have the client empty her bladder

8. A woman in active labor has contractions every 2 to 3 minutes lasting 45 seconds. The fetal heart rate between contraction is 100 beats per minute. Based on these findings, the priority nursing intervention is to:
   1. Notify the registered nurse (RN) immediately
   2. Encourage relaxation and breathing techniques between contractions
   3. Continue monitoring labor and fetal heart rate
   4. Monitor maternal vital signs

9. A nurse is assigned to assist in caring for a client being admitted to the birthing center in early labor. On admission, the nurse would initially:
   1. Check pelvic adequacy
   2. Administer an analgesic
   3. Estimate fetal size
   4. Determine maternal and fetal vital signs

10. Leopold's maneuvers will be performed on a pregnant client. The client asks the nurse about this procedure. The nurse responds knowing that this procedure:
    1. Determines the "lie" and "attitude" of the fetus
    2. Is a systemic method for palpating the fetus through the maternal back
    3. Is a systemic method for palpating the fetus through the maternal abdominal wall
    4. Measures the height of the maternal fundus

11. A nurse is assigned to care for a client who is in early labor. When collecting data from the client it is most important for the nurse to first determine which of the following?
    1. Intensity of contractions
    2. Frequency of contractions
    3. Baseline fetal heart rate
    4. Maternal blood pressure

12. A nurse is caring for a client in labor. The nurse rechecks the client's blood pressure and notes that it has dropped. To decrease the incidence of supine hypotension, the nurse should encourage the client to remain in which position?
    1. Left lateral
    2. Semi-Fowler's
    3. Squatting
    4. Tailor sitting

13. After a precipitous delivery, a nurse notes that the new mother is passive and only touches her newborn infant briefly with her fingertips. The nurse would do which of the following to help the woman process what has happened?
    1. Encourage the mother to breast-feed soon after birth
    2. Tell the mother that it is important to hold the newborn infant
    3. Document a complete account of the mother's reaction on the birth record
    4. Support the mother in her reaction to the newborn infant

14. A primigravida's membranes rupture spontaneously. The nurse's first action is to:
    1. Monitor contraction pattern
    2. Determine the fetal heart rate
    3. Note the amount, color, and odor of the amniotic fluid
    4. Prepare for immediate delivery

15. After a client vaginally delivers a viable newborn, the nurse observes the umbilical cord lengthen and a spurt of blood from the vagina. The nurse recognizes these findings as signs of:
    1. Abruptio placentae
    2. Placenta previa
    3. Placental separation
    4. Uterine atony

ALTERNATE FORMAT QUESTION: MULTIPLE RESPONSE

A nurse is collecting data on a client diagnosed with placenta previa. Select all findings that the nurse would expect to note.

_____ Bright red vaginal bleeding
_____ Uterine rigidity
_____ Soft, relaxed, nontender uterus
_____ Uterine tenderness
_____ Severe abdominal pain
_____ Fundal height may be greater than expected for gestational age

ANSWERS

1. Answer: 2
Rationale: Priority care of this client includes promotion of fetal oxygenation. Precipitous labor progresses quickly with frequent contractions and short periods of relaxation between contractions. This does not allow for maximal reperfusion of the placenta with oxygenated blood. A side-lying position can assist in blood flow to the uterus by preventing vena cava and abdominal aorta compression. Further stimulation with oxytocin is contraindicated. There may not be enough time to administer an epidural anesthesia before a delivery with such quick progression. Pushing with contractions is not indicated, especially with this type of labor. Controlled delivery of the fetus is essential to prevent maternal and fetal injury.
Test-Taking Strategy: Note the key words, *precipitous* and *priority*. Use the ABCs—airway, breathing, and circulation—and include the baby's needs as well as the mother's needs. Option 2 will promote fetal oxygenation. Review care of the client with precipitous labor if you had difficulty with this question.
Level of Cognitive Ability: Application
Client Needs: Physiological Integrity
Integrated Process: Nursing Process/Implementation
Content Area: Maternity/Intrapartum
Reference: McKinney, E., James, S., Murray, S., & Ashwill, J. (2005). *Maternal-child nursing* (2nd ed.). St. Louis: Elsevier, p. 679.

2. Answer: 3
Rationale: Painless vaginal bleeding is a sign of a possible placenta previa. Digital examination of the cervix can lead to maternal and fetal hemorrhage. Leopold's maneuver can reveal a nonengaged presenting part or malpresentation, both of which often accompany placenta previa because of the placenta filling the lower uterine segment. Hemoglobin and hematocrit values help estimate the amount of blood loss. Electronic fetal monitoring (external) is crucial in evaluating the status of the fetus, who is at risk for severe hypoxia. Options 1, 2, and 4 are procedures that would not place the client at further risk.
Test-Taking Strategy: Use the process of elimination and note the key word, *contraindicated*. Option 3 is the only procedure that is invasive to the pregnancy and endangers the physiological safety of the client and fetus. Review care of the client with placenta previa if you had difficulty with this question.
Level of Cognitive Ability: Analysis
Client Needs: Physiological Integrity
Integrated Process: Nursing Process/Data collection
Content Area: Maternity/Intrapartum
Reference: Leifer, G. (2005). *Maternity nursing* (9th ed.). Philadelphia: W.B. Saunders, p. 216.

3. Answer: 4
Rationale: Vaginal bleeding in a pregnant client most often is caused by placenta previa or a placental abruption. Uterine tenderness accompanies abruptio placentae, especially with a central abruption and trapped blood behind the placenta. The abdomen will feel hard and boardlike on palpation as the blood penetrates the myometrium and causes uterine irritability. A sustained tetanic contraction can occur if the client is in labor and the uterine muscle cannot relax.

Test-Taking Strategy: Note the issue of the question, abruptio placentae. It can be easy to confuse a placenta previa and abruption. Remember, the difference involves the presence of uterine pain and tenderness with an abruptio placentae as opposed to painless bleeding with a placenta previa. Options 1, 2, and 3 describe the absence of a sign or symptom of abruptio placentae, whereas option 4 is the only one that describes the presence of one. Review the signs of abruptio placentae if you had difficulty with this question.
Level of Cognitive Ability: Comprehension
Client Needs: Physiological Integrity
Integrated Process: Nursing Process/Data collection
Content Area: Maternity/Intrapartum
Reference: Leifer, G. (2005). *Maternity nursing* (9th ed.). Philadelphia: W.B. Saunders, p. 218.

4. Answer: 3
Rationale: Signs of placental separation include lengthening of the umbilical cord, a sudden gush of dark blood from the introitus, a firmly contracted uterus, and the uterus changing from a discoid to globular shape. The client may experience vaginal fullness, but not sudden and sharp abdominal pain.
Test-Taking Strategy: Use the process of elimination. Thinking about what one would expect to occur when the placenta separates will assist in eliminating options 1 and 2. Option 4 is eliminated because of the words "sudden, sharp." Review the signs of placental separation if you had difficulty with this question.
Level of Cognitive Ability: Comprehension
Client Needs: Physiological Integrity
Integrated Process: Nursing Process/Data collection
Content Area: Maternity/Intrapartum
Reference: Leifer, G. (2005). *Maternity nursing* (9th ed.). Philadelphia: W.B. Saunders, pp. 128, 386.

5. Answer: 1
Rationale: With a client in shock, the nurse would want to increase perfusion to the placenta. A simple way to do this, requiring no equipment, would be to turn the mother on her side. This would increase blood flow to the placenta by relieving pressure from the gravid uterus on the great vessels. The nurse would immediately contact the registered nurse would then contact the physician. The other options would follow quickly.
Test-Taking Strategy: Note the key word, *first*. Eliminate options 2 and 4 because they are similar. Recalling that positioning will affect the status of blood flow will assist in directing you to option 1 from the remaining options. Review care of the client in shock if you had difficulty with this question.
Level of Cognitive Ability: Application
Client Needs: Physiological Integrity
Integrated Process: Nursing Process/Implementation
Content Area: Delegating/Prioritizing
Reference: McKinney, E., James, S., Murray, S., & Ashwill, J. (2005). *Maternal-child nursing* (2nd ed.). St. Louis: Elsevier, p. 629.

6. Answer: 3
Rationale: Vena cava and descending aorta compression by the pregnant uterus impede blood return from the lower trunk and extremities, therefore decreasing cardiac return, cardiac

output, and blood flow to the uterus and subsequently to the fetus. The best position to prevent this would be side-lying, with the uterus displaced off the abdominal vessels. Positioning for abdominal surgery necessitates a supine position; however, a wedge placed under the right hip provides displacement of the uterus. The Trendelenburg position places pressure from the pregnant uterus on the diaphragm and lungs, decreasing respiratory capacity and oxygenation. A semi-Fowler's or prone position is not practical for this type of abdominal surgery.
Test-Taking Strategy: Note the key words, *maintain optimal perfusion.* Use the process of elimination and visualize each of the positions and their effect on the fetus. Review client positioning if you had difficulty with this question.
Level of Cognitive Ability: Application
Client Needs: Physiological Integrity
Integrated Process: Nursing Process/Implementation
Content Area: Maternity/Intrapartum
Reference: McKinney, E., James, S., Murray, S., & Ashwill, J. (2005). *Maternal-child nursing* (2nd ed.). St. Louis: Elsevier, p. 456.

7. Answer: 4
Rationale: An empty bladder contributes to a woman's comfort during the examination. Drinking water to fill the bladder and warming sonogram gel may be performed prior to a sonogram (ultrasound). Often, Leopold's maneuvers are performed to aid the examiner in locating the fetal heart tones.
Test-Taking Strategy: Use the process of elimination. Eliminate option 1 because Leopold's maneuvers are often used to help locate fetal heart tones. Eliminate options 2 and 3 because sonogram gel is used for an ultrasound and not during Leopold's maneuvers. Also, a client is requested to have a full bladder before ultrasonography. Review the preparation of a client for this procedure if you had difficulty with this question.
Level of Cognitive Ability: Application
Client Needs: Physiological Integrity
Integrated Process: Nursing Process/Implementation
Content Area: Maternity/Intrapartum
Reference: McKinney, E., James, S., Murray, S., & Ashwill, J. (2005). *Maternal-child nursing* (2nd ed.). St. Louis: Elsevier, p. 366.

8. Answer: 1
Rationale: Fetal bradycardia between contractions may indicate the need for immediate medical management. The nurse would immediately contact the RN, who in turn would contact the physician. Options 2, 3, and 4 will delay necessary and immediate interventions.
Test-Taking Strategy: Use the ABCs—airway, breathing, and circulation. Note that the woman is in active labor and that the fetal heart rate is below normal. It is imperative that the circulation in the fetus be restored to normal limits. Review care of the client in active labor if you had difficulty with this question.
Level of Cognitive Ability: Application
Client Needs: Physiological Integrity
Integrated Process: Nursing Process/Implementation
Content Area: Maternity/Intrapartum
Reference: Lowdermilk, D. & Perry, A. (2004). *Maternity and woman's health care* (8th ed.). St. Louis: Mosby, p. 525.

9. Answer: 4
Rationale: To evaluate a woman's physical well-being, the temperature, pulse, respirations, and blood pressure, as well as the fetal heartbeat, are checked. Option 2 is incorrect because it would be too premature for an analgesic. Medication given too early tends to slow or stop labor contractions. Options 1 and 3 are incorrect. These assessments should be done by the physician or a nurse midwife during prenatal visits.
Test-Taking Strategy: Note the key word, *initially.* Use the ABCs—airway, breathing, and circulation. This will direct you to option 4. Remember, measuring vital signs is the priority. Review care of the client in labor if you had difficulty with this question.
Level of Cognitive Ability: Application
Client Needs: Physiological Integrity
Integrated Process: Nursing Process/Implementation
Content Area: Maternity/Intrapartum
References: Leifer, G. (2005). *Maternity nursing* (9th ed.). Philadelphia: W.B. Saunders, pp. 104-105.
Lowdermilk, D., & Perry, A. (2004). *Maternity and woman's health care* (8th ed.). St. Louis: Mosby, p. 556.

10. Answer: 3
Rationale: Leopold's maneuvers comprise a systemic method for palpating the fetus through the maternal abdominal wall. Options 1, 2, and 4 are incorrect.
Test-Taking Strategy: Knowledge of the purpose and procedure for Leopold's maneuvers is required to answer this question. Visualizing this procedure will assist in directing you to option 3. Review Leopold's maneuvers if you had difficulty with this question.
Level of Cognitive Ability: Comprehension
Client Needs: Physiological Integrity
Integrated Process: Nursing Process/Implementation
Content Area: Maternity/Intrapartum
Reference: Lowdermilk, D. & Perry, A. (2004). *Maternity and woman's health care* (8th ed.). St. Louis: Mosby, p. 562.

11. Answer: 3
Rationale: The nurse should first determine the baseline fetal heart rate. Although options 1, 2, and 4 are a component of the data collection process, the fetal heart rate is the priority.
Test-Taking Strategy: Note the key word, *first.* Use the ABCs when selecting an answer. Remember the order of priority of airway, breathing, and circulation. Fetal heart rate reflects the ABCs. Review care of the client in labor if you had difficulty with this question.
Level of Cognitive Ability: Application
Client Needs: Physiological Integrity
Integrated Process: Nursing Process/Implementation
Content Area: Delegating/Prioritizing
Reference: Leifer, G. (2005). *Maternity nursing* (9th ed.). Philadelphia: W.B. Saunders, p. 105.

12. Answer: 1
Rationale: Pressure from the enlarged uterus and the aorta and vena cava when the woman is supine can result in hypotension. This can be relieved by having the woman lie on her left side. Options 2, 3, and 4 are incorrect.

Test-Taking Strategy: Use the process of elimination and knowledge of the anatomy of the pregnant uterus and the physiological response caused by pressure on the large abdominal vessels. Note that options 2, 3, and 4 are all similar in that the client is upright. Review nursing measures when the pregnant client becomes hypotensive if you had difficulty with this question.
Level of Cognitive Ability: Application
Client Needs: Physiological Integrity
Integrated Process: Nursing Process/Implementation
Content Area: Maternity/Intrapartum
References: Leifer, G. (2005). *Maternity nursing* (9th ed.). Philadelphia: W.B. Saunders, p. 49.
Lowdermilk, D., & Perry, A. (2004). *Maternity and woman's health care* (8th ed.). St. Louis: Mosby, p. 357.

13. *Answer: 4*
Rationale: Women who have experienced precipitous labor and delivery often describe feelings of disbelief that their labor has progressed so rapidly. To assist the woman in understanding what has happened, it is best to support the mother in her reaction to the newborn infant. Options 1, 2, and 3 do not acknowledge the mother's feelings.
Test-Taking Strategy: Use therapeutic communication techniques. Option 4 is the only option that acknowledges the mother's feelings. If you had difficulty with this question, review these techniques and care of the mother following a precipitous birth.
Level of Cognitive Ability: Application
Client Needs: Psychosocial Integrity
Integrated Process: Caring
Content Area: Maternity/Intrapartum
Reference: Lowdermilk, D., & Perry, S. (2003). *Maternity nursing* (6th ed.). St. Louis: Mosby, p. 666.

14. *Answer: 2*
Rationale: When the membranes rupture, the nurse immediately assesses the fetal heart rate to detect changes associated with prolapse or compression of the umbilical cord. Monitoring the contraction pattern and noting the amount, color, and odor of the amniotic fluid may be performed, but would not be the first action. There is no information in the question that indicates the necessity to prepare the client for immediate delivery.
Test-Taking Strategy: Note the key word, *first.* Use the ABCs—airway, breathing, and circulation. Fetal heart rate is associated with fetal breathing and circulation. Review the initial nursing interventions when the membranes rupture if you had difficulty with this question.
Level of Cognitive Ability: Application
Client Needs: Physiological Integrity
Integrated Process: Nursing Process/Implementation
Content Area: Maternity/Intrapartum

References: Leifer, G. (2005). *Maternity nursing* (9th ed.). Philadelphia: W.B. Saunders, p. 83.
Lowdermilk, D., & Perry, A. (2004). *Maternity and woman's health care* (8th ed.). St. Louis: Mosby, p. 567.

15. *Answer: 3*
Rationale: As the placenta separates, it settles downward into the lower uterine segment, the umbilical cord lengthens, and a sudden trickle or spurt of blood appears. The clinical manifestations identified in the question are not related to options 1, 2, and 4.
Test-Taking Strategy: Use the process of elimination. Note the similarity between options 1, 2, and 4 in that they represent complications associated with pregnancy. Option 3 indicates a normal finding following vaginal delivery of the newborn. Review this stage of labor if you had difficulty with this question.
Level of Cognitive Ability: Comprehension
Client Needs: Physiological Integrity
Integrated Process: Nursing Process/Data collection
Content Area: Maternity/Intrapartum
Reference: Leifer, G. (2005). *Maternity nursing* (9th ed.). Philadelphia: W.B. Saunders, p. 126.

ALTERNATE FORMAT QUESTION: MULTIPLE RESPONSE

Answers:
Bright red vaginal bleeding
Soft, relaxed, nontender uterus
Fundal height may be greater than expected for gestational age
Rationale: Painless bright red vaginal bleeding in the second or third trimester of pregnancy is a sign of placenta previa. The client will have a soft, relaxed, nontender uterus and fundal height may be greater than expected for gestational age. In abruptio placentae, severe abdominal pain is present. Uterine tenderness accompanies placental abruption. Additionally, in abruptio placentae, the abdomen will feel hard and boardlike on palpation as the blood penetrates the myometrium and causes uterine irritability.
Test-Taking Strategy: Remember that the difference between placenta previa and abruptio placentae involves the presence of uterine pain and tenderness with an abruption, as opposed to painless bleeding with a previa. Review the signs of placenta previa and abruptio placentae if you had difficulty with this question.
Level of Cognitive Ability: Analysis
Client Needs: Physiological Integrity
Integrated Process: Nursing Process/Data collection
Content Area: Maternity/Intrapartum
Reference: Murray, S., McKinney, E., & Gorrie, T., (2002). *Foundations of maternal-newborn nursing* (3rd ed.). Philadelphia: W.B. Saunders, p. 353.

REFERENCES

Leifer, G. (2005). *Maternity nursing* (9th ed.). Philadelphia: W.B. Saunders.

Lowdermilk, D., & Perry, S. (2003). *Maternity nursing* (6th ed.) St. Louis: Mosby,

Lowdermilk, D., & Perry, A. (2004). *Maternity and woman's health care* (8th ed.). St. Louis: Mosby.

McKinney, E., James, S., Murray, S., & Ashwill, J. (2005). *Maternal-child nursing* (2nd ed.). St. Louis: Elsevier.

The Postpartum Period and Associated Complications

I. POSTPARTUM

A. Description: Period when the reproductive tract returns to the normal, nonpregnant state

B. Postpartum period: Starts immediately after **delivery** and is usually completed by week 6 after **delivery**

II. PHYSIOLOGICAL MATERNAL CHANGES

A. Involution (Figure 24-1)
   1. Description
      a. The rapid decrease in the size of the uterus as it returns to the nonpregnant state
      b. Clients who breast-feed may experience a more rapid involution
   2. Data collection
      a. Weight of the uterus decreases from 2 lb to 2 oz in 6 weeks
      b. Fundus steadily descends into pelvis; the fundal height decreases about one finger-breadth (1 cm) per day
      c. By 10 days postpartum, the uterus cannot be palpated abdominally
      d. A flaccid fundus indicates uterine atony and should be massaged until firm
      e. A tender fundus indicates an infection

B. Lochia (Figure 24-2)
   1. Description: Discharge from the uterus that consists of blood from vessels of the **placental** site and debris from the decidua
   2. Data collection
      a. Rubra: Bright red discharge that occurs from **delivery** day to day 3 postpartum
      b. Serosa: Brownish-pink discharge that occurs from days 4 to 10 postpartum
      c. Alba: White discharge that occurs from days 10 to 14 postpartum
      d. Normally, the discharge smells like normal menstrual flow
      e. Discharge decreases daily in amount
      f. Discharge increases with ambulation
      g. Weigh the perineal pad before and after use and identify the amount of time between pad changes to determine the amount of **lochial** flow most accurately

C. Cervix: Cervical involution occurs; after 1 week, the muscle begins to regenerate

D. Vagina: Vaginal distention decreases, although muscle tone is never restored completely to the pregravid state

E. Ovarian function and menstruation
   1. Ovarian function depends on the rapidity with which pituitary function is restored
   2. Menstrual flow resumes within 8 weeks in non–breast-feeding mothers
   3. Menstrual flow usually resumes within 3 to 4 months in breast-feeding mothers
   4. Breast-feeding mothers may experience amenor-rhea during the entire period of lactation
   5. A woman may ovulate without menstruating, so breast-feeding should not be considered a form of birth control

F. Breasts
   1. A decrease of estrogen and progesterone levels after **delivery** stimulates increased prolactin levels, which promote breast milk production
   2. Breasts become distended with milk on the third day
   3. Engorgement occurs in 48 to 72 hours in non–breast-feeding mothers; breast-feeding will relieve engorgement

G. Urinary tract
   1. May have urinary retention because of loss of elasticity and tone and loss of sensation in the

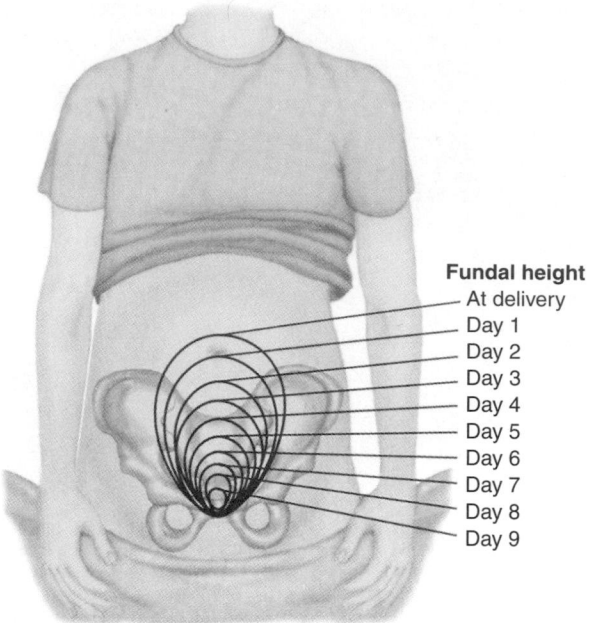

Fundal height
- At delivery
- Day 1
- Day 2
- Day 3
- Day 4
- Day 5
- Day 6
- Day 7
- Day 8
- Day 9

FIG. 24-1 Involution of the uterus. (From Murray, S., McKinney, E., & Gorrie, T. [2002]. *Foundations of maternal-newborn nursing* [3rd ed.]. Philadelphia: W.B. Saunders.)

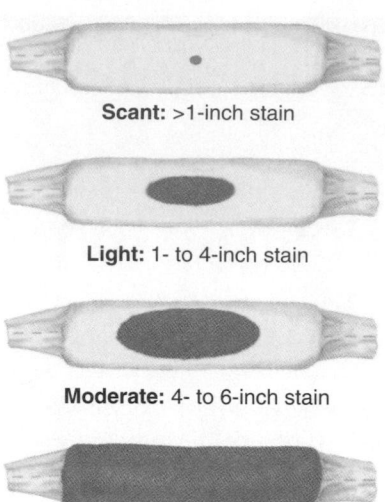

Scant: >1-inch stain

Light: 1- to 4-inch stain

Moderate: 4- to 6-inch stain

Large: Saturated in 1 hour

FIG. 24-2 Guidelines for assessing the amount of lochia on the perineal pad. (From Murray, S., McKinney, E., & Gorrie, T. [2002]. *Foundations of maternal-newborn nursing* [3rd ed.]. Philadelphia: W.B. Saunders.)

bladder from trauma, medications, anesthesia, and lack of privacy
2. Diuresis usually begins within the first 12 hours after **delivery**

H. Gastrointestinal tract
1. Women are usually very hungry after **delivery**
2. Constipation can occur
3. Hemorrhoids are common

I. Vital signs
1. Temperature may be elevated during the first 24 hours because of dehydration
2. Bradycardia is common during the first week, with a range of 50 to 70 beats per minute
3. Blood pressure remains unchanged

III. POSTPARTUM INTERVENTIONS

A. Data collection
1. Monitor vital signs
2. Monitor height, consistency, and location of the fundus
3. Monitor color, amount, and odor of **lochia**
4. Check breasts for engorgement
5. Monitor perineum for swelling or discoloration; check episiotomy for healing
6. Check incisions or dressings of cesarean birth client
7. Monitor input and output (I&O)
8. Monitor bowel status
9. Encourage frequent voiding
10. Encourage ambulation
11. Rh$_o$(D) immune globulin (RhoGAM) is prescribed to be administered within 72 hours postpartum to the Rh-negative client who has given birth to an Rh-positive **neonate**
12. Monitor parent-**newborn** bonding
13. Monitor emotional status (Box 24-1)

B. Client teaching
1. Demonstrate **newborn** care skills, as necessary
2. Provide the opportunity for the mother to bathe the **newborn**
3. Instruct on feeding technique
4. Instruct the mother to avoid heavy lifting for at least 3 weeks
5. Instruct the mother to plan at least one rest period per day
6. Instruct the mother that contraception should begin after **delivery** or with the initiation of intercourse
7. Instruct the mother on the importance of follow-up care, which should be scheduled at 4 to 6 weeks postpartum
8. Instruct the mother to report immediately any signs of chills, fever, increased **lochia**, or depressed feelings to the physician

IV. POSTPARTUM DISCOMFORTS

A. Afterbirth pains
1. Occur because of contractions of the uterus
2. Are more common in multiparas, breast-feeding mothers, clients treated with oxytocin (Pitocin), and clients who had an overdistended uterus during pregnancy, such as with carrying twins

BOX 24-1

Rubin's Postpartum Phases of Regeneration

TAKING-IN PHASE: FIRST 3 DAYS

Mother focuses on her own primary needs, such as sleep and food

Important for the nurse to listen and to help the mother interpret the events of delivery to make them more meaningful

Not an optimum time to teach the mother about baby care

TAKING-HOLD PHASE: DAYS 3 TO 10

More in control of independence

Begins to assume the tasks of mothering

An optimum time to teach the mother about baby care

LETTING-GO PHASE

Mother may feel deep loss over separation of the baby from her body and may grieve over the loss

Mother may be caught in a dependent-independent role, wanting to feel safe and secure yet wanting to make decisions

Teenage mothers need special consideration because of the conflict taking place within them as part of adolescence

B. Perineal discomfort
   1. Apply ice packs to the perineum as prescribed during the first 24 hours to reduce swelling
   2. After the first 24 hours, apply warmth by sitz baths as prescribed
C. Episiotomy
   1. Instruct the client to administer perineal care after each voiding
   2. Encourage the use of analgesic spray, as prescribed
   3. Administer analgesics as prescribed if comfort measures are unsuccessful
D. Breast discomfort from engorgement
   1. Encourage wearing a support bra at all times, even while sleeping
   2. Encourage the use of ice packs if the client is not breast-feeding
   3. Encourage the use of warm soaks before feeding for the breast-feeding mother
   4. Administer analgesics as prescribed if comfort measures are unsuccessful
E. Postpartum blues
   1. The condition may be caused by physiological or emotional stress
   2. The mother may feel upset and depressed at times
   3. Verbalization should be encouraged
   4. If unresolved, postpartum blues may progress to postpartum depression

V. NUTRITION

A. Discuss caloric intake for breast-feeding and non–breast-feeding mothers

B. Nutritional needs depend on prepregnancy weight, ideal weight for height, and whether the mother is breast-feeding

C. If the mother is breast-feeding, calorie needs increase by approximately 200 to 500 cal/day, and the mother may require increased fluids and the continuance of prenatal vitamins and minerals

VI. BREAST-FEEDING

A. Interventions
   1. Put the baby to the mother's breast as soon as the mother's and baby's conditions are stable (on **delivery** table if possible)
   2. Stay with the mother each time she nurses until she feels secure and confident with the baby and her feelings
   3. Assess LATCH (L = latch achieved by infant; A = audible swallowing; T = type of nipple; C = comfort of mother; H = help given to mother with nursing)
   4. Uterine cramping may occur the first day after **delivery** while the mother is nursing, when oxytocin simulation causes the uterus to contract
   5. Use general hygiene and wash the breasts once daily
   6. If engorgement occurs, have the mother breast-feed frequently, apply warm packs before feeding, apply ice packs after feedings, and massage the breasts
   7. Do not use soap on the breasts, because it tends to remove natural oils, which increases the chance of cracked nipples
   8. If cracked nipples develop, expose the nipples to air for 10 to 20 minutes after feeding, rotate the position of the baby for each feeding, and be sure that the baby is latched on to the areola, not just the nipple
   9. Bra should be well-fitted and supporting
   10. Breasts may leak between feedings or during coitus; place breast pad in bra
   11. Calories should be increased by 200 to 500 cal/day, and the diet should include additional fluids; prenatal vitamins should be taken as prescribed
   12. Baby's stools will be light yellow, seedy, watery, and frequent
   13. Medications should be avoided unless prescribed
   14. Gas-producing foods and caffeine should be avoided
   15. Hormonal contraceptives may cause a decrease in the milk supply and are best avoided during the first 6 weeks after birth
   16. Oral contraceptives containing estrogen are not recommended for breast-feeding mothers; progestin-only birth control pills are less likely to interfere with the milk supply

17. Baby will develop his or her own feeding schedule
B. Breast-feeding procedure for mother (Box 24-2)
C. Engorgement
   1. Breast-feed frequently
   2. Apply warm packs before feeding
   3. Apply ice packs between feedings
D. Cracked nipples
   1. Expose nipples to air for 10 to 20 minutes after feeding
   2. Rotate the position of the baby for each feeding
   3. Be sure that the baby is latched on to the areola, not just the nipple

VII. CYSTITIS

A. Description: Infection of the bladder
B. Data collection
   1. Burning and pain on urination
   2. Lower abdominal pain
   3. Increased frequency of urination
   4. Fever
   5. Proteinuria, hematuria, bacteriuria, and white blood cells (WBCs) in the urine
C. Interventions
   1. Palpate the bladder for distention
   2. Palpate the fundus for position
   3. Obtain a urine specimen for culture and sensitivity, if prescribed
   4. Institute measures to assist the client to void
   5. Encourage frequent and complete emptying of the bladder
   6. Encourage fluids to 3000 mL/day
   7. Administer antibiotics as prescribed after the urine culture is obtained

---

BOX 24-2

Breast-Feeding Procedure for Mother

Wash the hands and assume a comfortable position.
Start with the breast that the last feeding ended with.
Brush the newborn infant's lower lip with the nipple.
Tickle the lips to have the infant open the mouth wide.
Guide the nipple and surrounding areola into the infant's mouth.
After the baby has nursed, release suction by depressing the infant's chin or inserting a clean finger into the infant's mouth.
Burp the infant after the first breast.
Repeat the procedure on the second breast until the infant stops nursing.
Burp the infant again.
Instruct the mother to listen for audible sucking and swallowing.

---

8. Instruct the client in the methods of prevention and treatment of cystitis

VIII. HEMATOMA

A. Description
   1. Localized collection of blood into the tissues of the reproductive sac after the **delivery**
   2. Predisposing conditions include operative **delivery** with forceps or injury to a blood vessel
   3. Can be a life-threatening condition
B. Data collection
   1. Abnormal severe pain
   2. Pressure in the perineal area
   3. Sensitive, bulging mass in the perineal area with discolored skin
   4. Inability to void
   5. Decreased hemoglobin and hematocrit (H&H) levels
   6. Signs of shock, such as pallor, tachycardia, and hypotension, if significant blood loss has occurred
C. Interventions
   1. Monitor vital signs
   2. Monitor the client for abnormal pain, especially when forceps **delivery** has occurred
   3. Place ice to the hematoma site
   4. Administer analgesics and antibiotics as prescribed
   5. Monitor I&O; encourage fluids
   6. Prepare for urinary catheterization if the client is unable to void
   7. Monitor for signs of infection, such as increased temperature, pulse rate, and WBC count
   8. Prepare the client for incision and evacuation of hematoma if necessary

IX. HEMORRHAGE

A. Description: Bleeding of 500 mL or more after **delivery**
B. Data collection
   1. Early
      a. Hemorrhage occurs during the first 24 hours after **delivery**
      b. Caused by uterine atony, lacerations, or inversion of uterus
   2. Late
      a. Hemorrhage occurs later than the first 24 hours after **delivery**
      b. Caused by retained **placental** fragments
C. Interventions
   1. Massage fundus, with care not to overmassage
   2. Physician or health care provider is notified if hemorrhage occurs; monitor vital signs and fundus every 5 to 15 minutes
   3. Monitor and estimate blood loss by pad count
   4. Maintain asepsis because hemorrhage predisposes to infection
   5. Administer fluids as prescribed and monitor I&O

6. Monitor level of consciousness
7. Oxytocin (Pitocin) may be administered
8. Hemoglobin and hematocrit levels are monitored; blood transfusions may be administered

X. INFECTION

A. Description: Any infection of the reproductive organs that occurs within 28 days of **delivery** or abortion
B. Data collection
   1. Fever and chills
   2. Pelvic discomfort or pain
   3. Vaginal discharge
   4. Elevated white blood cell count
C. Interventions
   1. Monitor vital signs and temperature every 2 to 4 hours
   2. Make the mother as comfortable as possible; position for comfort and to promote drainage
   3. Keep the mother warmed if chilled
   4. Isolate the baby from the mother only if the mother can infect the baby
   5. Provide a nutritious high-calorie, high-protein diet
   6. Encourage fluids to 3000 to 4000 mL/day, if not contraindicated
   7. Encourage frequent voiding; monitor I&O
   8. Monitor culture results if cultures were prescribed
   9. Administer antibiotics as prescribed

XI. MASTITIS

A. Description
   1. Inflammation of the breast as a result of infection
   2. Primarily seen in breast-feeding mothers 2 to 3 weeks after **delivery** but may occur at any time during lactation
B. Data collection
   1. Localized heat and swelling
   2. Pain
   3. Elevated temperature
   4. Complaints of flulike symptoms
C. Interventions
   1. Instruct the mother in good hand washing and breast hygiene techniques
   2. Apply heat or cold to site as prescribed
   3. Maintain lactation in breast-feeding mothers
   4. Encourage manual expression of breast milk or use of breast pump every 4 hours
   5. Encourage the mother to support the breasts with a supportive bra
   6. Administer analgesics or antibiotics as prescribed

XII. PULMONARY EMBOLISM

A. Description: Passage of thrombus, often originating in one of the uterine or other pelvic veins, into the lungs, where it disrupts the circulation of blood

B. Data collection
   1. Dyspnea, tachypnea, and tachycardia
   2. Congested cough
   3. Hemoptysis
   4. Pleuritic chest pain
   5. Feeling of impending doom
C. Interventions
   1. Administer oxygen, as prescribed
   2. Position the client with the head of the bed elevated to promote comfort
   3. Monitor vital signs frequently
   4. Frequently monitor respiratory rate
   5. Monitor for signs of respiratory distress and for signs of hypoxemia, such as tachypnea, tachycardia, restlessness, cool and clammy skin, cyanosis, and the use of accessory muscles
   6. Intravenous fluids may be prescribed
   7. Anticoagulants may be prescribed

XIII. SUBINVOLUTION

A. Description: Incomplete involution or failure of the uterus to return to its normal size and condition
B. Data collection
   1. Uterine pain on palpation
   2. Uterus is larger than expected
   3. Greater than normal vaginal bleeding
C. Interventions
   1. Monitor vital signs
   2. Monitor uterus and fundus and for vaginal bleeding
   3. Elevate the legs to promote venous return
   4. Encourage frequent voiding
   5. Hemoglobin and hematocrit are monitored
   6. Methylergonovine maleate (Methergine) may be prescribed

XIV. THROMBOPHLEBITIS

A. Description
   1. A condition in which a clot forms in a vessel wall as a result of inflammation of the vessel wall
   2. A partial obstruction of the vessel can occur
   3. Increased blood-clotting factors in the postpartum period place the client at risk
B. Types
   1. Superficial thrombophlebitis
   2. Femoral thrombophlebitis
   3. Pelvic thrombophlebitis
C. Data collection (Box 24-3)
D. Interventions
   1. Assess lower extremities for edema, tenderness, varices, and increased skin temperature
   2. Evaluate legs for Homans' sign by extending the legs with the knees slightly flexed and dorsiflexing the foot
   3. Maintain bed rest

BOX 24-3

Data Collection: Types of Thrombophlebitis

SUPERFICIAL
Tenderness and pain in the affected lower extremity
Warm and pinkish-red color over thrombus area
Palpable thrombus that feels bumpy and hard

FEMORAL
Chills and fever
Malaise
Pain, stiffness, and swelling of the affected leg
Shiny, white skin over the affected area
Positive Homans' sign
Diminished peripheral pulses

PELVIC
Severe chills
Dramatic body temperature changes
Occurrence of pulmonary embolism may be the first sign

BOX 24-4

Client Teaching for Thrombophlebitis

Avoid pressure behind the knees.
Avoid prolonged sitting.
Avoid constrictive clothing.
Avoid crossing the legs.
Never massage the leg.
Know how to apply support hose if prescribed.
Understand the importance of anticoagulant therapy if prescribed.
Understand the importance of follow-up with the health care provider.

4. Elevate the affected leg
5. Apply a bed cradle and keep bedclothes off the affected leg
6. Never massage the leg
7. Monitor for manifestations of pulmonary embolism
8. Superficial thrombophlebitis
   a. Provide rest
   b. Apply hot packs to the affected site as prescribed
   c. Apply elastic stockings
   d. Administer analgesics as prescribed
9. Femoral thrombophlebitis
   a. Provide bed rest
   b. Elevate the affected leg
   c. Apply moist heat continuously to affected area if prescribed to alleviate discomfort
   d. Administer analgesics, as prescribed
   e. Administer antibiotics, if prescribed
   f. Intravenous heparin sodium may be prescribed to prevent further thrombus formation

10. Pelvic thrombophlebitis
    a. Provide bed rest
    b. Administer analgesics as prescribed
    c. Administer antibiotics if prescribed
    d. Intravenous heparin sodium may be prescribed to prevent further thrombus formation
D. Client teaching (Box 24-4)

PRACTICE QUESTIONS

1. A nurse palpates the fundus and checks the character of the lochia of a postpartum client in the fourth stage of labor. The nurse expects the lochia to be:
   1. White
   2. Pink
   3. Serosanguineous
   4. Red

2. After episiotomy and delivery of a newborn, the nurse performs a perineal check on the mother. The nurse notes a trickle of bright red blood coming from the perineum. The nurse checks the fundus and notes that it is firm. The nurse determines that:
   1. This is a normal expectation after episiotomy
   2. The perineal assessment should be performed more frequently
   3. The bright red bleeding is abnormal and should be reported
   4. The mother should be allowed bathroom privileges only

3. A nurse is assigned to care for a client in the postpartum period. The client asks the nurse what the term *involution* means. The nurse responds to the client, knowing that involution is:
   1. A progressive descent of the uterus into the pelvic cavity occurring approximately 1 cm/day
   2. The gradual reversal of the uterine muscle into the abdominal cavity
   3. The descent of the uterus into the pelvic cavity occurring at a rate of 2 cm/day
   4. The inverted uterus returning to normal

4. A mother is breast-feeding her newborn baby and experiences breast engorgement. The nurse encourages the mother to do which of the following measures to provide comfort for the engorgement?
   1. Breast-feed only during the daytime hours
   2. Apply cold compresses to the breast before feeding
   3. Massage the breasts before feeding to stimulate let-down
   4. Avoid the use of a bra while the breasts are engorged

5. A nurse is assisting in developing a plan of care for a client in the fourth stage of labor. Which of the following problems is most likely to occur during this stage?
   1. Pain because of the process of labor or birth
   2. Anxiety related to childbirth

3. Fatigue resulting from physical exertion during labor
4. Urinary retention caused by the loss of sensation to void and rapid bladder filling

6. After delivery, a nurse checks the height of the uterine fundus. The nurse expects that the position of the fundus would most likely be noted:
   1. At the level of the umbilicus
   2. Above the level of the umbilicus
   3. One fingerbreadth above the symphysis pubis
   4. To the right of the abdomen

7. A nurse is caring for a postpartum client. Four hours postpartum, the client's temperature is 102° F (38.9° C). The appropriate nursing action would be to:
   1. Continue to monitor the temperature
   2. Notify the registered nurse, who will then contact the physician
   3. Apply cool packs to the abdomen
   4. Remove the blanket from the client's bed

8. A nurse is assigned to care for a client in the immediate postpartum period who received epidural anesthesia for delivery, and the nurse monitors the client for complications. Which of the following would most likely indicate a hematoma?
   1. Complaints of a tearing sensation
   2. Complaints of lower abdominal discomfort
   3. Changes in vital signs
   4. Signs of heavy bruising

9. A nurse is assisting in planning care for the postpartum woman who has small vulvar hematomas. To assist in reducing the swelling, the nurse should:
   1. Check the vital signs every 4 hours
   2. Prepare a heat pack for application to the area
   3. Measure the fundal height every 4 hours
   4. Prepare an ice pack for application to the area

10. A client received epidural anesthesia during labor and had a forceps delivery after pushing for 2 hours. At 6 hours postpartum, the client's systolic blood pressure (BP) drops 20 points, the diastolic BP drops 10 points, and the pulse is 120 beats per minute. The client is very anxious and restless. The nurse is told that the client has a vulvar hematoma. Based on this diagnosis, the nurse would plan to:
    1. Monitor fundal height
    2. Apply perineal pressure
    3. Prepare the client for surgery
    4. Reassure the client

11. A nurse is assigned to care for a client after cesarean section. To prevent thrombophlebitis, the nurse encourages the woman to:
    1. Ambulate frequently
    2. Apply warm, moist packs to the legs
    3. Remain on bed rest with the legs elevated
    4. Wear support stockings

12. A postpartum client has developed thrombophlebitis. The nurse knows that the affected extremity should be elevated by:
    1. Elevating it on two pillows
    2. Elevating the foot of the bed only
    3. Placing the bed in reverse Trendelenburg position
    4. Placing the bed in Trendelenburg position

13. A nurse is caring for a postpartum client with a diagnosis of thrombophlebitis. The client suddenly complains of chest pain and dyspnea. The nurse would initially check:
    1. Level of consciousness (LOC)
    2. Fundal height
    3. Presence of Homans' sign
    4. Vital signs

14. A nurse suspects that a client has a pulmonary embolism. The most important nursing action is to:
    1. Administer oxygen by face mask, as prescribed
    2. Elevate the head of the bed
    3. Increase the intravenous flow rate
    4. Monitor vital signs

15. A nurse notes that the 4-hour postpartum client has cool, clammy skin, and is restless and excessively thirsty. The nurse immediately notifies the registered nurse and then:
    1. Encourages ambulation
    2. Checks vital signs
    3. Begins fundal massage
    4. Encourages the client to drink fluids

16. A new mother attempting breast-feeding for the first time has developed mastitis. She states, "My breasts look terrible and I think that I will stop breast-feeding." The nurse plans care, knowing that the client's statement relates to:
    1. Body image
    2. Newborn nutrition
    3. Feelings of inadequacy
    4. Infection

17. Breast-feeding instructions for the postpartum mother should include avoidance of soaps on the nipples, frequent changing of breast pads, intermittent exposure of nipples to air, and hand washing before handling the breast and before breast-feeding. The nurse understands that these measures are specific to the prevention of:
    1. Engorgement
    2. Newborn colic
    3. "Let-down" reflex
    4. Mastitis

18. The new breast-feeding mother is being discharged from the hospital after being treated for mastitis. The nurse knows that the mother needs further teaching when the mother states:
    1. "I need to change my breast pads when they are wet."
    2. "I will wash my breasts gently with plain water."

3. "My left breast is sore, so I will offer only my right breast frequently for breast-feeding."

4. "When my breasts feel engorged, I will use an ice pack for the pain."

19. A postpartum client with a pulmonary embolism was separated from her newborn infant for 2 days. Which observation by the nurse indicates a potential client need?

   1. The client nurses her newborn infant in the side-lying position
   2. The client needs the head of the bed elevated for comfort
   3. The newborn infant prefers the bottle over breast milk
   4. The client turns herself from side to side

20. A nurse is assisting in caring for a postpartum client experiencing uterine hemorrhage. In planning to meet the psychosocial needs of the client, the nurse would:

   1. Keep the client and her family members informed of progress

   2. Monitor vital signs every 2 hours
   3. Maintain strict bed rest
   4. Perform firm fundal massage every 2 hours

ALTERNATE FORMAT QUESTION: MULTIPLE RESPONSE

A nurse is preparing a list of self-care instructions for a postpartum client who was diagnosed with mastitis. Select all instructions that would be included on the list.

___ Take the prescribed antibiotics until the soreness subsides

___ Wear a supportive bra

___ Avoid decompression of the breasts by breast-feeding or breast pump

___ Rest during the acute phase

___ Continue to breast-feed if the breasts are not too sore

ANSWERS

1. **Answer: 4**
Rationale: The color of the lochia during the fourth stage of labor is bright red. This may last from 1 to 3 days. The color of the lochia then changes to a pinkish brown that lasts 4 to 10 days. Finally, the lochia changes to a creamy white color that lasts approximately 10 to 14 days.
Test-Taking Strategy: Focus on the key words, *fourth stage of labor.* This will direct you to option 4. Review postpartum expected findings if you had difficulty with this question.
Level of Cognitive Ability: Comprehension
Client Needs: Physiological Integrity
Integrated Process: Nursing Process/Data Collection
Content Area: Maternity/Postpartum
Reference: Leifer, G. (2005). *Maternity nursing* (9th ed.). Philadelphia: W.B. Saunders, p. 193.

2. **Answer: 3**
Rationale: Lochial flow should be distinguished from bleeding originating from a laceration or episiotomy, which is usually brighter red than lochia and presents as a continuous trickle of bleeding, even though the fundus of the uterus is firm. This bright red bleeding is abnormal and needs to be reported.
Test-Taking Strategy: Note the key words, *bright red.* This should be an indication that the flow is not normal. Review lochial flow and complications associated with episiotomy if you had difficulty with this question.
Level of Cognitive Ability: Analysis
Client Needs: Physiological Integrity
Integrated Process: Nursing Process/Data Collection
Content Area: Maternity/Postpartum
Reference: Leifer, G. (2005). *Maternity nursing* (9th ed.). Philadelphia: W.B. Saunders, p. 204.

3. **Answer: 1**
Rationale: Involution is a progressive descent of the uterus into the pelvic cavity. After birth, descent occurs approximately one fingerbreadth, or approximately 1 cm/day.
Test-Taking Strategy: Use knowlege of medical terminology to help you in defining the word "involution." This will assist in directing you to the correct option. Review the process of involution if you had difficulty with this question.
Level of Cognitive Ability: Comprehension
Client Needs: Physiological Integrity
Integrated Process: Nursing Process/Implementation
Content Area: Maternity/Postpartum
References: Leifer, G. (2005). *Maternity nursing* (9th ed.). Philadelphia: W.B. Saunders, p. 384.
McKinney, E., James, S., Murray, S., & Ashwill, J. (2005). *Maternal-child nursing* (2nd ed.). St. Louis: Elsevier, p. 465.

4. **Answer: 3**
Rationale: Comfort measures for breast engorement include massaging the breasts before feeding to stimulate let-down, wearing a supportive well-fitting bra at all times, taking a warm shower or applying warm compresses just before feeding, and alternating breasts during feeding.
Test-Taking Strategy: Use the process of elimination to answer the question. Eliminate option 1 because of the absolute word "only." From the remaining options, recalling the self-care measures to promote comfort to the mother with breast engorgement will assist in directing you to option 3. Review these measures if you had difficulty with this question.
Level of Cognitive Ability: Application
Client Needs: Health Promotion and Maintenance
Integrated Process: Nursing Process/Implementation
Content Area: Maternity/Postpartum

References: Leifer, G. (2005). *Maternity nursing* (9th ed.). Philadelphia: W.B. Saunders, p. 185.
McKinney, E., James, S., Murray, S., & Ashwill, J. (2005). *Maternal-child nursing* (2nd ed.). St. Louis: Elsevier, pp. 587-588.

5. *Answer: 4*
Rationale: The fourth stage of labor is the first hour postpartum, when the woman's body begins to readjust and relax. Options 1 and 2 relate to the first stage of labor. Option 3 relates to the second stage of labor. Option 4 is related to the third and fourth stages of labor.
Test-Taking Strategy: Use the process of elimination. Focus on the key words, *fourth stage of labor*. Remembering that the fourth stage of labor is the last stage will direct you toward the correct option. Review the stages of labor if you had difficulty with this question.
Level of Cognitive Ability: Comprehension
Client Needs: Physiological Integrity
Integrated Process: Nursing Process/Planning
Content Area: Maternity/Postpartum
Reference: Leifer, G. (2005). *Maternity nursing* (9th ed.). Philadelphia: W.B. Saunders, p. 92.

6. *Answer: 1*
Rationale: Immediately after delivery, the uterine fundus should be at the level of the umbilicus or 1 to 3 fingerbreadths below it and in the midline of the abdomen. If the fundus is above the umbilicus, this may indicate that there are blood clots in the uterus that need to be expelled by fundal massage. If the fundus is noted to the right of the abdomen, it may indicate a full bladder.
Test-Taking Strategy: Note the key words, *after delivery*. Remember that, immediately after delivery, the uterine fundus should be at the level of the umbilicus or one to three fingerbreadths below it and in the midline of the abdomen. Review expected postdelivery findings if you had difficulty with this question.
Level of Cognitive Ability: Comprehension
Client Needs: Physiological Integrity
Integrated Process: Nursing Process/Data Collection
Content Area: Maternity/Postpartum
References: Leifer, G. (2005). *Maternity nursing* (9th ed.). Philadelphia: W.B. Saunders, p. 192.
Lowdermilk, D., & Perry, A. (2004). *Maternity and woman's health care* (8th ed.). St. Louis: Mosby, p. 619.

7. *Answer: 2*
Rationale: In the postpartum period, the mother's temperature may be elevated during the first 24 hours as a result of dehydration. However, if the temperature is more than 2° F above normal, this may indicate infection, and the physician will need to be notified.
Test-Taking Strategy: Use the process of elimination. Focus on the key words, *4 hours* and *102° F*. Noting that the temperature is extreme compared with the normal temperature will direct you to option 2. Review the expected findings in the postpartum period if you had difficulty with this question.
Level of Cognitive Ability: Application
Client Needs: Physiological Integrity

Integrated Process: Nursing Process/Implementation
Content Area: Maternity/Postpartum
Reference: Leifer, G. (2005). *Maternity nursing* (9th ed.). Philadelphia: W.B. Saunders, pp. 208, 292.

8. *Answer: 3*
Rationale: Changes in vital signs indicate hypovolemia in the anesthetized postpartum woman with vulvar hematoma. Options 1 and 2 are inaccurate for a client who is anesthetized. Heavy bruising may be noted, but vital sign changes are most likely to indicate the presence of a hematoma.
Test-Taking Strategy: Use the process of elimination. Eliminate options 1 and 2 first. Because the woman is anesthetized, she cannot feel pain or lower abdominal discomfort. Option 4 (heavy bruising) may be visualized, but vital sign changes indicate hematoma caused by blood collection in the perineal tissues. Review the signs of a hematoma if you had difficulty with this question.
Level of Cognitive Ability: Analysis
Client Needs: Physiological Integrity
Integrated Process: Nursing Process/Data Collection
Content Area: Maternity/Postpartum
References: Leifer, G. (2005). *Maternity nursing* (9th ed.). Philadelphia: W.B. Saunders, p. 287.
Lowdermilk, D., & Perry, A. (2004). *Maternity and woman's health care* (8th ed.). St. Louis: Mosby, p. 1038.

9. *Answer: 4*
Rationale: Application of ice will reduce swelling caused by hematoma formation in the vulvar area. Options 1, 2, and 3 will not reduce the swelling.
Test-Taking Strategy: Use the process of elimination. Focus on the issue of the question, "reducing the swelling." This will assist in eliminating options 1 and 3. Recalling the principles related to heat and cold will direct you to option 4 from the remaining options. Review nursing care of the client with a hematoma if you had difficulty with this question.
Level of Cognitive Ability: Application
Client Needs: Physiological Integrity
Integrated Process: Nursing Process/Implementation
Content Area: Maternity/Postpartum
Reference: Leifer, G. (2005). *Maternity nursing* (9th ed.). Philadelphia: W.B. Saunders, p. 287.

10. *Answer: 3*
Rationale: The information provided in the question indicates that the client is experiencing blood loss. Surgery would be indicated for this complication to stop the bleeding. Options 1, 2, and 4 would not assist in controlling the bleeding in this emergency situation.
Test-Taking Strategy: Focus on the information provided in the question. Note that the signs and symptoms in the question indicates the presence of bleeding. This should direct you to option 3. Review nursing interventions related to vulvar hematomas if you had difficulty with this question.
Level of Cognitive Ability: Analysis
Client Needs: Physiological Integrity
Integrated Process: Nursing Process/Planning
Content Area: Maternity/Postpartum

Reference: Lowdermilk, D., & Perry, A. (2004). *Maternity and woman's health care* (8th ed.). St. Louis: Mosby, pp. 1040-1041.

11. Answer: 1
Rationale: Stasis is believed to be a major predisposing factor in the development of thrombophlebitis. Because cesarean delivery poses a risk factor, the client should ambulate early and frequently to promote circulation and prevent stasis. Options 2, 3, and 4 are implemented if thrombophlebitis occurs.
Test-Taking Strategy: Focus on the issue of the question, prevention of thrombophlebitis. Options 2, 3, and 4 are implemented if thrombophlebitis occurs. Ambulating frequently (option 1) is a preventive measure. Review content related to the prevention of thrombophlebitis in the postoperative period if you had difficulty with this question.
Level of Cognitive Ability: Application
Client Needs: Physiological Integrity
Integrated Process: Nursing Process/Implementation
Content Area: Maternity/Postpartum
Reference: Leifer, G. (2005). *Maternity nursing* (9th ed.). Philadelphia: W.B. Saunders, p. 291.

12. Answer: 4
Rationale: Placing the bed in Trendelenburg position rather than flexing the leg at the hip promotes venous drainage. The reverse Trendelenburg position will not aid in promoting venous return. Elevating the extremity by using a pillow or elevating the foot of the bed will cause flexion at the hip, thus impeding venous drainage.
Test-Taking Strategy: Focus on the issue of the question and use the process of elimination. Eliminate option 2 first because of the absolute word "only." From the remaining options, recalling that flexion at the hip area restricts venous flow will direct you to option 4. Review these concepts if you had difficulty answering this question.
Level of Cognitive Ability: Comprehension
Client Needs: Physiological Integrity
Integrated Process: Nursing Process/Implementation
Content Area: Maternity/Postpartum
Reference: Lowdermilk, D., & Perry, A. (2004). *Maternity and woman's health care* (8th ed.). St. Louis: Mosby, p. 1046.

13. Answer: 4
Rationale: Pulmonary embolism is a complication of thrombophlebitis. Vital signs will be one of the first changes to occur with pulmonary embolism as pulmonary blood flow is compromised. LOC may change as the condition worsens and would indicate hypoxia. Homans' sign is an indicator of thrombophlebitis. Fundal height is unrelated to the issue of the question.
Test-Taking Strategy: Note the key word, *initially.* Use the ABCs—airway, breathing, and circulation—to assist in directing you to option 4. Review the complications of thrombophlebitis if you had difficulty with this question.
Level of Cognitive Ability: Application
Client Needs: Physiological Integrity
Integrated Process: Nursing Process/Data Collection
Content Area: Maternity/Postpartum
Reference: Lowdermilk, D., & Perry, A. (2004). *Maternity and woman's health care* (8th ed.). St. Louis: Mosby, p. 1046.

14. Answer: 1
Rationale: Because pulmonary circulation is compromised in the presence of an embolus, cardiorespiratory support is initiated by oxygen administration. Options 2 and 4 may be a component of the plan of care but are not the most important action. The nurse would not increase the IV rate without a physician's order to do so.
Test-Taking Strategy: Note the key words, *most important,* and use the ABCs—airway, breathing, and circulation. This will direct you to option 1. Review care of the client in the event of a pulmonary embolism if you had difficulty with this question.
Level of Cognitive Ability: Application
Client Needs: Physiological Integrity
Integrated Process: Nursing Process/Implementation
Content Area: Maternity/Postpartum
Reference: Leifer, G. (2005). *Maternity nursing* (9th ed.). Philadelphia: W.B. Saunders, p. 291.

15. Answer: 2
Rationale: Symptoms of hypovolemia include cool, clammy, pale skin, feelings of anxiety, restlessness, and thirst. The nurse would check the vital signs. The nurse would not ambulate the client or encourage fluids until specific orders are given to do so. There is no information in the question to indicate the need for fundal massage.
Test-Taking Strategy: Focus on the symptoms in the question. Use the ABCs—airway, breathing, and circulation—to assist in directing you to option 2. Review nursing care for the client with hypovolemia if you had difficulty with this question.
Level of Cognitive Ability: Application
Client Needs: Physiological Integrity
Integrated Process: Nursing Process/Implementation
Content Area: Maternity/Postpartum
Reference: Leifer, G. (2005). *Maternity nursing* (9th ed.). Philadelphia: W.B. Saunders, p. 287.

16. Answer: 1
Rationale: Inflammation and engorgement are symptoms of mastitis that may alter the new breast-feeding mother's body image. The client's statement does not relate to a problem with newborn nutrition, inadequacy, or infection.
Test-Taking Strategy: Focus on the information in the question and use the process of elimination. Noting the key words, *My breasts look terrible,* will direct you to option 1. Review the psychosocial issues related to mastitis if you had difficulty with this question.
Level of Cognitive Ability: Comprehension
Client Needs: Psychosocial Integrity
Integrated Process: Nursing Process/Planning
Content Area: Maternity/Postpartum
Reference: Leifer, G. (2005). *Maternity nursing* (9th ed.). Philadelphia: W.B. Saunders, pp. 41, 293.

17. Answer: 4
Rationale: Mastitis is an infection frequently associated with a break in the skin surface of the nipple. The measures described in the question are personal hygiene measures to help prevent mastitis. The data in the question is unrelated to options 1, 2, and 3.

Test-Taking Strategy: Use the process of elimination and knowledge of the cause and prevention of mastitis to answer this question. Focusing on the data in the question will assist in directing you to option 4. Review the preventive measures for mastitis if you had difficulty with this question.
Level of Cognitive Ability: Comprehension
Client Needs: Health Promotion and Maintenance
Integrated Process: Teaching/Learning
Content Area: Maternity/Postpartum
Reference: Leifer, G. (2005). *Maternity nursing* (9th ed.). Philadelphia: W.B. Saunders, p. 294.

18. *Answer:* **3**
Rationale: Failure to nurse equally on both sides will decrease the flow of milk through the breast, causing engorgement of the breast that has been offered less frequently. Options 1, 2, and 4 are appropriate measures.
Test-Taking Strategy: Note the key words, *needs further teaching.* These words indicate a false response question and that you need to select the incorrect client statement. Use knowledge regarding the treatment for mastitis and the process of elimination to select the correct option. Review the concepts related to breast-feeding and mastitis if you had difficulty with this question.
Level of Cognitive Ability: Comprehension
Client Needs: Health Promotion and Maintenance
Integrated Process: Nursing Process/Evaluation
Content Area: Maternity/Postpartum
Reference: Leifer, G. (2005). *Maternity nursing* (9th ed.). Philadelphia: W.B. Saunders, p. 294.

19. *Answer:* **3**
Rationale: Breast-feeding will be compromised and the newborn infant may begin to prefer the bottle over the breast if the mother and newborn are separated for an extended period. When the mother's condition is stable after being separated, reestablishing breast-feeding should be a nursing priority. Options 1, 2, and 4 do not indicate the need for intervention.
Test-Taking Strategy: Use the process of elimination, focusing on the key words, *separated from her newborn infant for 2 days.* This should easily direct you to option 3. Review the concepts related to maternal-infant bonding if you had difficulty with this question.
Level of Cognitive Ability: Comprehension
Client Needs: Psychosocial Integrity
Integrated Process: Nursing Process/Evaluation
Content Area: Maternity/Postpartum
Reference: Leifer, G. (2003). *Introduction to maternity and pediatric nursing* (4th ed.). Philadelphia: W.B. Saunders, pp. 153, 223.

20. *Answer:* **1**
Rationale: Keeping the client and her family informed of her condition will help minimize fear and apprehension. Options 2, 3, and 4 identify physiological interventions.
Test-Taking Strategy: Use the process of elimination. Focus on the key words, *meet the psychosocial needs.* Option 1 is the only option that addresses psychosocial needs. Review the interventions that will meet the psychosocial needs of a client if you had difficulty with this question.
Level of Cognitive Ability: Application
Client Needs: Psychosocial Integrity
Integrated Process: Nursing Process/Implementation
Content Area: Maternity/Postpartum
Reference: Lowdermilk, D., & Perry, A. (2004). *Maternity and woman's health care* (8th ed.). St. Louis: Mosby, p. 44.

ALTERNATE FORMAT QUESTION: MULTIPLE RESPONSE

Answers:
Wear a supportive bra
Rest during the acute phase
Continue to breast-feed if the breasts are not too sore
Rationale: Mastitis is an infection of the lactating breast. Client instructions include resting during the acute phase, maintaining a fluid intake of at least 3000 mL/day, and analgesics to relieve discomfort. Antibiotics may be prescribed and are taken until the complete prescribed course is finished. Antibiotics are not stopped when the soreness subsides. Additional supportive measures include the use of moist heat or ice packs and wearing a supportive bra. Continued decompression of the breast by breast-feeding or breast pump is important to empty the breast and prevent the formation of an abscess.
Test-Taking Strategy: Think about the pathophysiology associated with mastitis. Recalling that supportive measures include rest, moist heat or ice packs, antibiotics, analgesics, breast support, and decompression of the breasts will assist in answering the question. Review the measures to treat mastitis if you had difficulty with this question.
Level of Cognitive Ability: Application
Client Needs: Physiological Integrity
Integrated Process: Teaching/Learning
Content Area: Maternity/Postpartum
Reference: Murray, S., McKinney, E., & Gorrie, T. (2002). *Foundations of maternal-newborn nursing* (3rd ed.). Philadelphia: W.B. Saunders, pp. 792-793.

REFERENCES

Leifer, G. (2003). *Introduction to maternity and pediatric nursing* (4th ed.). Philadelphia: W.B. Saunders.
Leifer, G. (2005). *Maternity nursing* (9th ed.). Philadelphia: W.B. Saunders.
Lowdermilk, D., & Perry, A. (2004). *Maternity and woman's health care* (8th ed.). St. Louis: Mosby.
McKinney, E., James, S., Murray, S., & Ashwill, J. (2005). *Maternal-child nursing* (2nd ed.). St. Louis: Elsevier.
Murray, S., McKinney, E., & Gorrie, T. (2002). *Foundations of maternal-newborn nursing* (3rd ed.). Philadelphia: W.B. Saunders.

Care of the Newborn

I. INITIAL CARE OF THE NEWBORN
A. Data collection
   1. Observe or assist with initiation of respirations
   2. Check Apgar score
   3. Note characteristics of cry
   4. Monitor for nasal flaring, grunting, retractions, abnormal respirations
   5. Obtain vital signs
   6. Observe **newborn** for signs of hypothermia or hyperthermia
   7. Check for gross anomalies
B. Interventions
   1. Suction mouth, then nares, with bulb syringe
   2. Dry **newborn** and stimulate crying by rubbing
   3. Maintain temperature stability; wrap **newborn** in warm blankets and place a stockinette cap on **newborn's** head
   4. Keep **newborn** with mother to facilitate bonding
   5. Place **newborn** at mother's breast if breast-feeding is planned, or place on mother's abdomen
   6. Place **newborn** in warmer
   7. Position **newborn** on side, on abdomen or in modified Trendelenburg position to facilitate drainage of mucus

   8. Ensure **newborn's** proper identification
   9. Footprint **newborn** and fingerprint mother on identification sheet, per agency policies and procedures
   10. Place matching identification bracelets on mother and **newborn**
C. Apgar scoring system
   1. Determine and record Apgar score at 1 minute and at 5 minutes
   2. Assess each of five items to be scored, and assign value of 0 (very poor) to 2 (excellent) for each item
   3. Add the points to determine the **newborn's** total score
   4. Five vital indicators (Table 25-1)
   5. Interventions: Apgar score (Table 25-2)

II. INITIAL PHYSICAL EXAMINATION
A. General guidelines
   1. Keep **newborn** warm during the examination
   2. Begin with general observations; then first perform assessments that are least disturbing to the **newborn**

TABLE 25-1

Five Vital Indicators of Apgar Scoring

Indicator	0 Points	1 Point	2 Points
Heart rate	Absent	Less than 100/minute	More than 100/minute
Respiratory rate	Absent	Slow, irregular weak cry	Good vigorous cry
Muscle tone	Flaccid, limp	Minimal flexion of extremities	Good flexion, active motion
Reflex irritability	No response	Minimal response (grimace) to suction or gentle slap on soles	Responds promptly with a cry or active movement
Skin color	Pallor or cyanosis	Body skin normal, extremities blue	Body and extremity skin color normal

3. Initiate nursing interventions for abnormal findings
4. Document all abnormal findings
B. Vital signs
  1. Heart rate: 100 to 170 beats per minute (apical); check for a full minute because of irregularities after birth
  2. Respirations: 30 to 80 breaths per minute; check for a full minute
  3. Axillary temperature: 96.8° to 99° F
  4. Blood pressure: 73/55 mm Hg
C. Body measurements
  1. Length: 45 to 55 cm (18 to 22 inches)
  2. Weight: 2500 to 4300 g (5.5 to 9.5 pounds)
  3. Head circumference: 33 to 35.5 cm (13 to 14 inches)
  4. Chest circumference: 30 to 33 cm (12 to 13 inches); should be equal to or 2 to 3 cm less than the head circumference
D. Head
  1. 25% of the body length (cephalocaudal development)
  2. Bones of the skull are not fused
  3. Palpable sutures (connective tissue between the skull bones)
  4. Fontanels: Unossified membranous tissue at the junction of the sutures (Table 25-3)
  5. Molding: Asymmetry of the head as a result of pressure in the birth canal; disappears in about 72 hours
  6. Masses from birth trauma
    a. Caput succedaneum: Edema of the soft tissue over bone (crosses over suture line); subsides within a few days
    b. Cephalhematoma: Swelling caused by bleeding into an area between the bone and its periosteum (does not cross over suture line); usually absorbed within 6 weeks with no treatment
  7. Head lag
    a. Common when pulling **newborn** to a sitting position
    b. When prone, **newborn** should be able to lift the head slightly and turn the head from side to side
E. Eyes
  1. Slate gray (light skin) or brown-gray (dark skin)
  2. Symmetrical and clear
  3. Pupils equal, round, react to light by accommodation
  4. Blink reflex present
  5. Eyes cross because of weak extraocular muscles
  6. Able to track and fixate momentarily
  7. Red reflex present
  8. Eyelids often edematous as a result of pressure during the birth process and the effects of eye medication
F. Ears
  1. Symmetrical
  2. Firm cartilage with recoil
  3. Pinna should be on or above line drawn from canthus of eye
  4. Low-set ears associated with Down syndrome
G. Nose
  1. Flat, broad, in center of face
  2. Obligatory nose breathing
  3. Occasional sneezing to remove obstructions
H. Mouth
  1. Pink, moist gums
  2. Soft and hard palates intact
  3. Epstein's pearls (small, white cysts) may be present on hard palate
  4. Uvula in midline
  5. Tongue moves freely, is symmetrical, has short frenulum
  6. Sucking and crying movements symmetrical
  7. Able to swallow
  8. Gag reflex present
I. Neck
  1. Short and thick
  2. Head held in midline
  3. Trachea on midline
  4. Good range of motion (ROM) and is able to flex and extend
J. Chest
  1. Appears circular because anteroposterior and lateral diameters are about equal
  2. Respirations appear diaphragmatic
  3. Bronchial sounds heard on auscultation

TABLE 25-2

Apgar Score Interventions

Score	Intervention
8 to 10	No intervention except support the infant's spontaneous efforts
4 to 7	Gently stimulate
	Rub infant's back
	Administer oxygen to infant
0 to 3	Infant requires resuscitation

TABLE 25-3

Fontanels

Fontanel	Characteristics	Closure
Anterior	Soft, flat, diamond-shaped, 3 to 4 cm wide by 2 to 3 cm long	Closes between 12 and 18 months of age
Posterior	Triangular, 0.5 to 1 cm wide	Closes between birth and 2 to 3 months of age
	Located between occipital and parietal bones	

4. Nipples prominent and often edematous
5. Milky secretion (witch's milk) common
6. Breast tissue present
7. Clavicles need to be palpated to check for fractures

K. Skin
1. Pinkish-red (light-skinned **newborn**) to pinkish-brown or pinkish-yellow (dark-skinned **newborn**)
2. Vernix caseosa
3. Lanugo
4. Milia
5. Dry, peeling skin
6. Dark red color common in premature **newborns**
7. Cyanosis common with hypothermia, infection, and hypoglycemia, and with cardiac, respiratory, or neurological abnormalities
8. Acrocyanosis (peripheral cyanosis) is normal in the first few hours after birth and if the infant becomes cold; results from poor perfusion of blood to the periphery of the body
9. Check for ecchymosis and petechiae resulting from the trauma of birth
10. Check skin turgor over the abdomen to determine hydration status
11. Observe for forceps marks
12. Harlequin sign
   a. Deep pink or red color develops over one side of the **newborn's** body while the other side remains pale or of normal color
   b. May indicate shunting of blood with a cardiac problem or may indicate sepsis
13. Birthmarks (Table 25-4)

L. Abdomen
1. Umbilical cord
   a. Three vessels, two arteries and one vein, in cord; if fewer than three vessels are noted, notify the physician
   b. Small, thin cord may be associated with poor fetal growth
   c. Check for intact cord, and ensure that clamp is secured
   d. Cord should be clamped for at least the first 24 hours after birth; clamp can be removed when the cord is dried and occluded
   e. Note any bleeding or drainage from the cord
   f. Triple dye or alcohol may be applied for initial cord care because it minimizes microorganisms and promotes drying; use a cotton-tipped applicator to paint the dye, once on the cord and once on 1 inch of surrounding skin
   g. Application of alcohol to the cord should be done with each diaper change and at least two or three times a day to minimize microorganisms and promote drying
   h. If symptoms of infection such as moistness, oozing, discharge, and a reddened base occur, antibiotic treatment is prescribed

TABLE 25-4

Birthmarks

Birthmark	Characteristics
Telangiectatic nevi (stork bites)	Pale pink or red, flat, dilated capillaries
	On eyelids, nose, lower occipital bone, and nape of neck
	Blanch easily
	More noticeable during crying periods
	Disappear by age 2 years
Nevus flammeus (port-wine stain)	Capillary angioma directly below epidermis
	Nonelevated, sharply demarcated, red to purple, dense areas of capillaries
	Commonly appears on face
	Does not fade with time
	May require surgery in the future
Nevus vasculosus (strawberry mark)	Capillary hemangioma
	Raised, clearly delineated, dark red, with a rough surface
	Common in head region
	Disappears by age 7 to 9 years
Mongolian spots	Bluish black pigmentation
	On lumbar dorsal area and buttocks
	Gradually fade during first and second years of life
	Common in Asians and dark-skinned individuals

2. Gastrointestinal
   a. Monitor cord for meconium staining
   b. Check for umbilical hernia
   c. Note abdominal depression associated with diaphragmatic hernia
   d. Check for abdominal distension associated with obstruction, mass, or sepsis
   e. Monitor bowel sounds, which should occur within 1 to 2 hours after birth
3. Anus
   a. Anal opening patent
   b. First-stool meconium should pass within first 24 hours

M. Genitals
1. Female
   a. Labia edematous, clitoris enlarged
   b. Smegma present (thick, white mucous discharge)
   c. Pseudomenstruation possible (blood-tinged mucus)
   d. Hymen tag may be visible
   e. First voiding should occur within 24 hours
2. Male
   a. Prepuce (foreskin) covers glans penis
   b. Scrotum edematous
   c. Meatus at tip of penis
   d. Testes descended but may retract with cold
   e. Check for hernia or hydrocele
   f. First voiding should occur within 24 hours

N. Spine
1. Straight
2. Posture flexed
3. Supports head momentarily when prone
4. Arms and legs flexed
5. Chin flexed on upper chest
6. Sporadic movements that are well coordinated
7. A degree of hypotonicity or hypertonicity is indicative of central nervous system (CNS) damage

O. Extremities
1. Flexed
2. Full ROM; movements symmetrical
3. Fists clenched
4. Should be 10 fingers and 10 toes, all separate
5. Legs bowed
6. Major gluteal folds even
7. Creases on soles of feet
8. Check for fractures (especially clavicle) or dislocations (hip)
9. Check for hip dysplasia; when thighs are rotated outward, no clicks should be heard
10. Pulses palpable (radial, brachial, femoral)
11. Slight tremors are common but could be a sign of hypoglycemia or drug withdrawal

III. BODY SYSTEMS

A. Cardiovascular system
1. Keep **newborn** warm
2. Take apical heart rate for 1 full minute
3. Listen for murmurs
4. Palpate pulses
5. Check for cyanosis; blanch skin on trunk and extremities to assess circulation
6. Observe for cardiac distress when **newborn** is feeding

B. Respiratory system
1. Position **newborn** on side
2. Suction as necessary: use a bulb syringe for upper airway suctioning (compress bulb before insertion) and a French catheter for deeper suctioning
3. Observe for respiratory distress and hypoxemia
   a. Nasal flaring
   b. Increasingly severe retractions
   c. Grunting
   d. Cyanosis
   e. Bradycardia and periods of apnea lasting longer than 15 seconds
4. Administer oxygen via hood if necessary and as prescribed

C. Hepatic system
1. Normal or physiological jaundice appears after the first 24 hours in full-term **neonates** and after the first 48 hours in premature **neonates**; jaundice occurring prior to this time (pathological jaundice) may indicate early hemolysis of red blood cells (RBCs) and must be reported to the physician
2. Physiological jaundice peaks about the fifth day of life (indirect bilirubin levels: 6 to 7 mg/dL)
3. Monitor serum bilirubin levels
4. Feed early to stimulate intestinal activity and to keep the bilirubin level low
5. Prevent chilling, because hypothermia can cause acidosis, which interferes with bilirubin conjugation and excretion
6. The newborn's liver stores iron that was passed from the mother for 5 to 6 months
7. Glycogen storage occurs in the liver
8. **Neonate** is at risk for hemorrhagic disorders; coagulation factors synthesized in the liver are dependent on vitamin K, which is not synthesized until intestinal bacteria are present
9. Handle **neonate** carefully and monitor for any bruising or bleeding episodes
10. Watch for meconium stool and subsequent stools
11. Administer one dose of vitamin K (Aqua-MEPHYTON), usually 0.5 to 1.0 mg intramuscular as prescribed, to the **neonate** in the lateral aspect of the middle third of the vastus lateralis muscle, to prevent hemorrhagic disorders
12. Check **newborn's** hemoglobin and blood glucose levels

D. Renal system
1. The immature kidneys cannot concentrate urine
2. A weight loss of 5% to 15% during the first week of life occurs as a result of voiding and limited intake
3. Weigh **newborn** daily
4. Monitor intake and output (I&O); weigh diapers if necessary
5. Measure specific gravity of urine if necessary
6. Monitor for signs of dehydration (dry mucous membranes, sunken eyeballs, poor skin turgor, sunken fontanels)

E. Immune system
1. Passive immunity via the **placenta** (immunoglobulin G, IgG)
2. Passive immunity from colostrum (immunoglobulin A, IgA)
3. Elevations in IgM indicate infection in utero
4. Use aseptic technique when caring for the **newborn**
5. Observe standard precautions when handling the **newborn**
6. Ensure meticulous hand washing
7. Ensure that infection-free staff members care for the **newborn**
8. Monitor **newborn's** temperature
9. Observe for any cracks or openings in the skin
10. Administer eye medication within 1 hour after birth to prevent ophthalmia neonatorum

a. Eye prophylaxis may be delayed until an hour or so after birth so that eye contact and parent-**infant** attachment and bonding are facilitated

b. Erythromycin (0.5%) and tetracycline (1%) ophthalmic ointment or drops are both bacteriostatic and bactericidal; provide prophylaxis against infection by *Neisseria gonorrhoeae* and *Chlamydia trachomatis*

c. Silver nitrate (1%) solution may be prescribed, but its use is minimal because it does not protect against chlamydial infection and can cause chemical conjunctivitis

11. Provide cord care

a. Umbilical clamp can be removed after 24 hours

b. Teach mother how to perform cord care

c. Keep the cord clean and dry; wash with soap and water at least two or three times a day

d. Keep diaper from covering cord; fold diaper below cord

e. Monitor cord for odor, swelling, or discharge

f. Sponge bathe the **newborn** until the cord falls off (within 2 weeks)

12. Provide circumcision care

a. Apply petroleum jelly gauze to the penis, except when a Plastibell is used

b. Remove petroleum jelly gauze, if applied, after first voiding following circumcision

c. Observe for swelling, infection, or bleeding from the circumcision site

d. Teach mother care of circumcision site

e. Cleanse the penis after each voiding by squeezing warm water over the penis

f. A milky covering over the glans penis is normal and should not be disrupted

g. Monitor for urinary retention

▲ F. Metabolic system and gastrointestinal system

1. **Newborns** can digest simple carbohydrates but cannot digest fats because of the lack of lipase

2. Proteins may be only partially broken down, so they may serve as antigens and provoke an allergic reaction

3. The **newborn** has a small stomach capacity (about 90 mL) with rapid intestinal peristalsis (bowel emptying time is 2.5 to 3 hours)

4. Breast-feeding can usually begin immediately after birth; bottle-fed **newborns** may be offered a few milliliters of sterile water or 5% dextrose 1 to 4 hours after birth prior to a feeding with formula

5. Observe feeding reflexes, such as rooting, sucking, and swallowing

6. Assist mother with breast-feeding or formula feeding

7. Burp **newborn** during and after feeding

8. Monitor for regurgitation or vomiting

9. Position **newborn** on right side after feeding

10. Observe for normal stool and the passage of meconium

a. Meconium stool, which is greenish-black with a thick, sticky, tarlike consistency, is usually passed within the first 24 hours of life

b. Transitional stool, the second type of stool excreted by the **newborn**, is greenish-brown and of looser consistency than meconium

c. Seedy, yellow stools are noted in breast-fed **newborns**; pale yellow to light brown stools in formula-fed **newborns**

11. **Newborn**: Screening test is performed (includes the test for phenylketonuria, PKU) before discharge after sufficient protein intake occurs; the **newborn** should be on formula or breast milk for 24 hours before screening

G. Neurological system

1. **Newborn** head size is proportionally larger than that of adults because of cephalocaudal development

2. Myelinization of nerve fibers is incomplete, so primitive reflexes are present

3. Fontanels are open to allow for brain growth

4. Check for an abnormal head size and a bulging or depressed anterior fontanel

5. Measure and graph head circumference in relation to chest circumference and length

6. Monitor **newborn's** movements, noting symmetry, posture, and abnormal movements

7. Observe for jitteriness, marked tremors, and seizures

8. Test **newborn's** reflexes

9. Monitor for lethargy

10. Monitor pitch of cry

H. Thermal regulatory system

1. **Newborns** do not shiver to produce heat

2. **Newborns** have brown fat deposits, which produce heat

3. Heat is dissipated through vasodilation

4. Prevent heat loss resulting from evaporation by keeping **newborn** dry and well-wrapped with a blanket

5. Prevent heat loss resulting from radiation by keeping **newborn** away from cold objects and outside walls

6. Prevent heat loss resulting from convection by shielding the **newborn** from drafts

7. Prevent heat loss resulting from conduction by performing all treatments on a warm, padded surface

8. Keep temperature in room warm

9. Take **newborn's** axillary temperature every hour for the first 4 hours of life, every 4 hours for the remainder of the first 24 hours, and then every shift

I. Reflexes

1. Sucking and rooting

a. Touch the **newborn's** lip, cheek, or corner of the mouth with a nipple

b. **Newborn** turns head toward the nipple, opens the mouth, takes hold of the nipple, and sucks

c. Rooting reflex usually disappears after 3 to 4 months but may persist for up to 1 year

2. Swallowing reflex
   a. Occurs spontaneously after sucking and obtaining fluids
   b. **Newborn** swallows in coordination with sucking without gagging, coughing, or vomiting

3. Tonic neck or fencing
   a. While the **newborn** is falling asleep or sleeping, gently and quickly turn the head to one side
   b. As the **newborn** faces the left side, the left arm and leg extend outward while the right arm and leg flex
   c. When the head is turned to the right side, the right arm and leg extend outward while the left arm and leg flex
   d. Usually disappears within 3 to 4 months

4. Palmar-plantar grasp
   a. Place a finger in the palm of the **newborn's** hand; then place a finger at the base of the toes
   b. The **newborn's** fingers curl around the examiner's fingers, and the **newborn's** toes curl downward
   c. Palmar response lessens within 3 to 4 months
   d. Plantar response lessens within 8 months

5. Moro reflex
   a. Hold the **newborn** in a semisitting position; then, allow the head and trunk to fall backward to at least a 30-degree angle
   b. The **newborn** symmetrically abducts and extends the arms
   c. The **newborn** fans the fingers out and forms a C with the thumb and the forefinger
   d. The **newborn** adducts the arms to an embracing position and returns to a relaxed flexion state
   e. Present at birth; a complete response may occur up to 8 weeks
   f. A body jerk motion occurs from 8 to 18 weeks
   g. No response may be noted by 6 months as long as neurological maturation has not been delayed
   h. A persistent response lasting more than 6 months may indicate the occurrence of brain damage during pregnancy

6. Startle reflex
   a. The response is best elicited if the **newborn** is at least 24 hours old
   b. The examiner makes a loud noise or claps hands to elicit the response
   c. The **newborn's** arms adduct while the elbows flex
   d. The hands stay clenched
   e. The reflex should disappear within 4 months

7. Pull to sit
   a. Pull the **newborn** up from the wrist while the **newborn** is in the prone position

b. The head will lag until the **newborn** is in an upright position; then the head will be level with the chest and shoulders momentarily before falling forward

c. The head will then lift for a few minutes

d. The response depends on the **newborn's** general muscle tone and condition as well as maturity level

8. Babinski sign—plantar reflex
   a. Beginning at the heel of the foot, gently stroke upward along the lateral aspect of the sole; then the examiner moves the finger along the ball of the foot
   b. The **newborn's** toes hyperextend while the big toe dorsiflexes
   c. Reflex disappears after the **newborn** is 1 year old
   d. Absence of this reflex indicates the need for a neurological examination

9. Stepping or walking
   a. Hold the **newborn** in a vertical position, allowing one foot to touch a table surface
   b. The **newborn** simulates walking, alternately flexing and extending the feet
   c. The reflex is usually present for 3 to 4 months

10. Crawling
    a. Place the **newborn** on the abdomen
    b. The **newborn** begins making crawling movements with the arms and legs
    c. The reflex usually disappears after about 6 weeks

IV. PARENT TEACHING

A. Formula feeding
   1. Teach sterilization techniques if the water supply is from an area where the purification process of the water is questionable
   2. Remind the mother not to heat the bottle of formula in a microwave oven
   3. Inform the mother that formula is a sufficient diet for the first 4 to 6 months
   4. Determine the mother's ability to burp the **newborn**

B. Breast-feeding
   1. Monitor the **newborn's** ability to attach to the mother's breast and suck
   2. Teach the mother about engorgement
   3. Teach the mother how to pump her breasts and how to store breast milk properly
   4. Inform the mother that breast milk is a sufficient and superior diet for the first 4 to 6 months
   5. Give the mother the phone numbers of local organizations that offer support to breast-feeding mothers

C. Bathing
   1. Bathe the **newborn** in a warm room before feeding
   2. Have all equipment for bathing available
   3. Use a mild soap (not on the face)

4. Proceed from the cleanest area to the dirtiest
5. Clean eyes from the inner canthus outward
6. Special care should be taken to clean under the folds of the neck, underarms, groin, and genitals
7. Make bath time enjoyable for both the **newborn** and the mother

D. Clothing
1. Determine diaper and clothing needs for the **newborn** with the mother
2. Instruct the mother that the **newborn's** head should be covered in cold weather to prevent heat loss
3. Instruct the mother to layer the **newborn's** clothing in cooler weather

E. Cord care: Refer to cord care under Body Systems
F. Circumcision: Refer to circumcision care under Body Systems
G. Uncircumcised **newborn**
1. Inform the mother that the foreskin and glans are two similar layers of cells that separate from each other, and that the separation process is normally complete between 3 and 5 years of age
2. Instruct the mother not to pull back the foreskin but to allow for the natural separation to occur
3. Inform the mother that, as the process of separation occurs, sterile sloughed cells build up between the layers of the foreskin and the glans; when retraction occurs, daily gentle washing of the glans with soap and water is sufficient to maintain adequate cleanliness

V. PRETERM NEWBORN

A. Description
1. A **neonate** born before 37 weeks' gestation
2. The primary concern relates to immaturity of all body systems

B. Data collection
1. Respirations irregular with periods of apnea
2. Body temperature is below normal
3. **Newborn** has poor suck and swallow reflexes
4. Bowel sounds are diminished
5. Increased or decreased urinary output
6. Extremities are thin, with minimal creasing on soles and palms
7. **Newborn** extends extremities and does not maintain flexion
8. Lanugo, on skin and in the hair on the **newborn's** head, is present in woolly patches
9. Skin is thin, with visible blood vessels and minimal subcutaneous fat pads
10. Skin may appear jaundiced
11. Testes are undescended in boys
12. Labia are narrow in girls

C. Interventions
1. Monitor vital signs every 2 to 4 hours
2. Maintain cardiopulmonary function

3. Administer oxygen and humidification, as prescribed
4. Monitor input and output (I&O) and electrolyte balance
5. Monitor weight daily
6. Maintain **newborn** in a warming device
7. Position every 1 to 2 hours, and handle **newborn** carefully
8. Avoid exposure to infections
9. Provide **newborn** with appropriate stimulation, such as touch

VI. POST-TERM NEWBORN

A. Description: A **neonate** born after 42 weeks' gestation
B. Data collection
1. Hypoglycemia
2. Parchment-like skin (dry and cracked) without lanugo
3. Fingernails long and extended over ends of fingers
4. Profuse scalp hair
5. Body is long and thin
6. Extremities show wasting of fat and muscle
7. Meconium staining may be present on nails and umbilical cord

C. Interventions
1. Provide normal **newborn** care
2. Monitor for hypoglycemia
3. Maintain **newborn's** temperature
4. Monitor for meconium aspiration

VII. SMALL FOR GESTATIONAL AGE

A. Description: A **neonate** who is plotted at or below the 10th percentile on the intrauterine growth curve
B. Data collection
1. Fetal distress
2. Gestational age and physical maturity
3. Lowered or elevated body temperature
4. Physical abnormalities
5. Hypoglycemia
6. Signs of polycythemia
   a. Ruddy appearance
   b. Cyanosis
   c. Jaundice
7. Signs of infection
8. Signs of aspiration of meconium

C. Interventions
1. Maintain airway
2. Maintain body temperature
3. Observe for signs of respiratory distress
4. Monitor for infection and initiate measures to prevent sepsis
5. Monitor blood glucose levels and for signs of hypoglycemia

6. Initiate early feedings and monitor for signs of aspiration
7. Provide stimulation, such as touch and cuddling

VIII. LARGE FOR GESTATIONAL AGE

A. Description: A **neonate** who is plotted at or above the 90th percentile on the intrauterine growth curve
B. Data collection
1. Gestational age
2. Birth trauma or injury
3. Respiratory distress
4. Hypoglycemia
C. Interventions
1. Monitor vital signs
2. Monitor blood glucose levels and for signs of hypoglycemia
3. Initiate early feedings
4. Monitor for infection and initiate measures to prevent sepsis
5. Provide stimulation, such as touch and cuddling

IX. RESPIRATORY DISTRESS SYNDROME (RDS)

A. Description: A serious lung disorder caused by immaturity and inability to produce surfactant, resulting in hypoxia and acidosis
B. Data collection
1. Tachypnea
2. Flaring nares
3. Expiratory grunting
4. Retractions
5. Decreased breath sounds
6. Apnea
7. Pallor and cyanosis
8. Hypothermia
9. Poor muscle tone
C. Interventions
1. Monitor color, respiratory rate, and degree of effort in breathing
2. Support respirations as prescribed
3. Monitor arterial blood gases (ABGs) and oxygen saturation levels (ABGs from umbilical artery)
4. Monitor ABGs so that oxygen administered to the **newborn** is at the lowest possible concentration necessary to maintain adequate arterial oxygenation
5. Schedule any premature **newborn** who has been given oxygen support for an eye examination before discharge to check for retinal damage
6. Suction every 2 hours, or more often as necessary
7. Position **newborn** on side or back, with neck slightly extended
8. Prepare to administer surfactant replacement therapy (instilled into the endotracheal tube)
9. Administer respiratory therapy (percussion and vibration) as prescribed; use padded small plastic cup or small oxygen mask for percussion; use padded electric toothbrush for vibration
10. Provide nutrition
11. Support bonding
12. Prepare parents for short- to long-term period of oxygen dependency, if necessary
13. Encourage mother to pump breasts for future breast-feeding if she so desires
14. Encourage as much parental participation in **newborn's** care as condition allows

---

X. HYPERBILIRUBINEMIA

A. Description
1. At any serum bilirubin level, the appearance of jaundice during the first day of life indicates a pathological process
2. Evaluation is indicated when serum bilirubin levels are over 12 mg/dL in the term **newborn**
3. Therapy is aimed at preventing kernicterus, which results in permanent neurological damage resulting from the deposition of bilirubin in the brain cells
B. Data collection
1. Jaundice
2. Elevated serum bilirubin levels
3. Enlarged liver
4. Poor muscle tone
5. Lethargy
6. Poor sucking reflex
C. Interventions
1. Monitor for the presence of jaundice
a. Examine the **newborn's** skin color in natural light
b. Press finger over a bony prominence or tip of the **newborn's** nose to press out capillary blood from the tissues
c. Note that jaundice starts at the head first, spreads to the chest, then the abdomen, then the arms and legs, followed by the hands and feet, which are the last to be jaundiced
2. Keep **newborn** well hydrated to maintain blood volume
3. Facilitate early, frequent feeding to hasten passage of meconium and encourage excretion of bilirubin
4. Report to the physician any signs of jaundice in the first 24 hours and any abnormal signs and symptoms
5. Prepare for phototherapy, and monitor the **newborn** closely during the treatment
D. Phototherapy
1. Description
a. Use of intense fluorescent lights to reduce serum bilirubin levels in the **newborn**
b. Injury from treatment, such as eye damage, dehydration, or sensory deprivation, can occur

2. Interventions
   a. Expose as much of the **newborn's** skin as possible
   b. Cover the genital area, and monitor genital area for skin irritation or breakdown
   c. Cover the **newborn's** eyes with eye shields or patches; make sure eyelids are closed when shields or patches are applied
   d. Remove the shields or patches at least once per shift to inspect the eyes for infection or irritation and to allow eye contact
   e. Measure the quantity of light every 8 hours
   f. Monitor skin temperature closely
   g. Increase fluids to compensate for water loss
   h. Expect loose green stools and green urine
   i. Monitor the **newborn's** skin color, with the fluorescent light turned off, every 4 to 8 hours
   j. Monitor the skin for bronze baby syndrome, a grayish-brown discoloration of the skin
   k. Reposition **newborn** every 2 hours
   l. Provide stimulation
   m. After treatment, continue monitoring for signs of hyperbilirubinemia, because rebound elevations are normal after therapy is discontinued

XI. ERYTHROBLASTOSIS FETALIS

A. Description
   1. Destruction of red blood cells (RBCs) that results from an antigen-antibody reaction
   2. Characterized by hemolytic anemia or hyperbilirubinemia
   3. Exchange of fetal and maternal blood takes place primarily when the **placenta** separates at birth
   4. Rh antigens from the baby's blood enter the maternal bloodstream
   5. The mother produces anti-Rh antibodies against the fetal blood cells
   6. Antibodies are harmless to the mother but attach to the erythrocytes in the fetus and cause hemolysis
   7. Sensitization is rare with the first pregnancy
   8. ABO incompatibility is usually less severe

B. Data collection
   1. Anemia
   2. Jaundice that develops rapidly after birth and before 24 hours
   3. Edema

C. Interventions
   1. Administer Rh$_o$(D) immune globulin (RhoGAM) to the mother during the first 72 hours after **delivery** if the Rh-negative mother delivers an Rh-positive fetus but remains unsensitized
   2. Assist with exchange transfusion after birth or intrauterine transfusion, as prescribed
   3. The baby's blood is replaced with Rh-negative blood to stop the destruction of the baby's red blood cells; the Rh-negative blood is gradually replaced with the baby's own blood
   4. Reassure the mother that the **newborn** will suffer no untoward effects from the condition

XII. SEPSIS

A. Description: Generalized infection resulting from the presence of bacteria in the blood
B. Data collection
   1. Pallor
   2. Tachypnea, tachycardia
   3. Poor feeding
   4. Abdominal distention
   5. Temperature instability
C. Interventions
   1. Monitor for periods of apnea or irregular respirations
   2. If apnea is present, stimulate by gently rubbing chest or foot
   3. Administer oxygen, as prescribed
   4. Monitor vital signs
   5. Maintain warmth in an Isolette
   6. Provide isolation as necessary
   7. Monitor for a fever
   8. Monitor I&O and obtain daily weight
   9. Monitor for diarrhea
   10. Monitor feeding and sucking reflex, which may be poor
   11. Monitor for jaundice
   12. Monitor for irritability and lethargy
   13. Administer antibiotics as prescribed and observe carefully for toxicity, because a **newborn's** liver and kidneys are immature

XIII. TORCH SYNDROME

A. Description
   1. Refers to infections of the fetus or **newborn**
   2. Caused by one of the following (**TORCH**)
      a. **T**oxoplasmosis
      b. **O**ther infections
      c. **R**ubella
      d. **C**ytomegalovirus
      e. **H**erpes
B. Infections (Table 25-5)

XIV. SYPHILIS

A. Description
   1. Sexually transmitted disease
   2. Congenital syphilis can result in premature **delivery**, skin lesions, abnormal skeletal development
   3. The organism *Treponema pallidum*, a spirochete, can cross the **placenta** throughout pregnancy and infect the fetus, usually after 18 weeks' gestation

TABLE 25-5

Infections Included in TORCH Syndrome

Infection	Characteristics
Toxoplasmosis	Protozoan infection
	Produces no serious effects in the mother
	Can be transmitted to the fetus
	Can result in severe physical and developmental abnormalities
	Common carriers include cat feces and raw beef
Other infections	Syphilis
Rubella	Systemic viral infection
	Causes congenital rubella syndrome, which includes congenital heart disease, cataracts, growth retardation, and pneumonia if the mother becomes infected during the first trimester
	Deafness and some learning disabilities can occur if the mother becomes infected during the first trimester
Cytomegalovirus	A viral infection that persists in the body indefinitely, with periods of reactivation without symptoms
	Can infect the fetus or infant during delivery or after birth through breast milk, blood transfusions, or contact with infected secretions
	May cause microcephaly, blindness, deafness, and mental and motor retardation
Herpes simplex	Sexually transmitted disease caused by a virus
	Periods of reactivation
	Neonate is commonly infected during delivery by direct contact with lesions in the genital tract
	Can cause neurological impairment or death

4. Risks include preterm birth, stillbirth, and low birth weight
5. Congenital effects are irreversible and may include central nervous system damage and hearing loss

B. Data collection
 1. Hepatosplenomegaly
 2. Joint swelling
 3. Palmar rash
 4. Anemia
 5. Jaundice
 6. Snuffles (syphilitic rhinitis)
 7. Ascites
 8. Pneumonitis
 9. Cerebrospinal fluid changes

C. Interventions
 1. Monitor **newborn** for signs of syphilis
 2. Monitor for palmar rash and snuffles
 3. Prepare **newborn** for serological testing if prescribed
 4. Administer antibiotic therapy, as prescribed
 5. Use standard precautions and drainage and secretion precautions with suspected congenital syphilis
 6. Wear gloves when handling **neonate** until antibiotic therapy has been administered for 24 hours
 7. Provide psychological support to the mother, and provide instructions regarding follow-up care of the **newborn**

XV. ADDICTED NEWBORN

A. Description: **Newborn** who has become passively addicted to drugs that have passed through the **placenta**

B. Addicting drugs
 1. Heroin
    a. **Newborn** may appear normal at birth, with a low birth weight
    b. Withdrawal occurs within 12 to 24 hours and may last 5 to 7 days
 2. Methadone
    a. Withdrawal occurs within 1 to 2 days to 1 week or more, is most evident at 48 to 72 hours, and may last 6 days to 8 weeks
    b. **Newborn** appears very ill
    c. May develop jaundice as a result of prematurity
 3. Cocaine
    a. Causes decreased interactive behavior
    b. Feeding problems are present
    c. Irregular sleep patterns and diarrhea occur

C. Data collection
 1. Irritability
 2. Tremors
 3. Hyperactivity and hypertonicity
 4. Respiratory distress
 5. Vomiting
 6. High-pitched cry
 7. Sneezing
 8. Fever
 9. Diarrhea
 10. Excessive sweating
 11. Poor feeding
 12. Extreme sucking of fists
 13. Convulsions

D. Interventions
 1. Monitor respiratory and cardiac status frequently
 2. Monitor temperature and vital signs
 3. Hold **newborn** firm and close to the body during feeding and when giving care
 4. Initiate seizure precautions (pad sides of crib)
 5. Provide small frequent feedings and allow a longer period for feeding
 6. Monitor I&O
 7. Administer IV hydration if prescribed
 8. Protect **neonate's** skin from injury, which can be caused by the constant rubbing from hyperactive jitters

9. Swaddle **newborn**

10. Place **newborn** in a quiet room and reduce stimulation

11. Allow mother to ventilate feelings of anxiety and guilt

12. Refer mother for treatment of substance abuse problem

XVI. FETAL ALCOHOL SYNDROME

A. Description
1. Caused by maternal alcohol use during pregnancy
2. Most serious cause of teratogenesis
3. Causes mental and physical retardation

B. Data collection
1. Facial changes
   a. Short palpebral fissures
   b. Hypoplastic philtrum
   c. Short, upturned nose
   d. Flat midface
   e. Thin upper lip
   f. Low nasal bridge
2. Abnormal palmar creases
3. Respiratory distress (apnea, cyanosis)
4. Congenital heart disorders
5. Irritability, hypersensitivity to stimuli
6. Tremors
7. Poor feeding
8. Seizures

C. Interventions
1. Monitor for respiratory distress
2. Position **newborn** on side to facilitate drainage of secretions
3. Keep resuscitation equipment at the bedside
4. Monitor for hypoglycemia
5. Check suck and swallow reflex
6. Administer small feedings and burp well
7. Suction as necessary
8. Monitor I&O
9. Monitor weight and head circumference
10. Decrease environmental stimuli

XVII. NEWBORN WITH ACQUIRED IMMUNODEFICIENCY SYNDROME (AIDS)

A. Description
1. The fetus of a human immunodeficiency virus (HIV) antibody–positive woman should be monitored closely throughout the pregnancy
2. Serial ultrasound screenings should be done during pregnancy to identify intrauterine growth restriction
3. Weekly nonstress testing after 32 weeks' gestation and biophysical profiles may be necessary during pregnancy
4. **Neonates** born to HIV-positive clients may test positive because the mother's positive anti-

bodies may persist for as long as 18 months after birth

5. The use of antiviral medication, the reduction of **neonate** exposure to maternal blood and body fluids, and the early identification of HIV in pregnancy reduce the risk of transmission to the **newborn**

6. All **neonates** born to HIV-positive mothers acquire maternal antibody to HIV infection, but not all acquire the infection

7. The **neonate** may be asymptomatic for the first several years of life

B. Transmission
1. Across **placental** barrier
2. During **labor** and **delivery**
3. Breast milk

C. Data collection
1. May have no outward signs for the first several months of life
2. Signs of immune deficiency
3. Hepatomegaly
4. Splenomegaly
5. Lymphadenopathy
6. Impairment in growth and development

D. Interventions
1. Cleanse **newborn's** skin carefully before any invasive procedure, such as the administration of vitamin K, heel sticks, or venipunctures
2. Circumcisions are not done on **newborns** with HIV-positive mothers until the **newborn's** status is determined
3. **Newborn** can room with mother
4. All HIV-exposed **newborns** should be treated with medication to prevent infection by *Pneumocystis jiroveci* (formerly known as *Pneumocystis carinii*)
5. Zidovudine (AZT) may be administered as prescribed for the first 6 weeks of life
6. Monitor for early signs of immune deficiency, such as enlarged spleen or liver, lymphadenopathy, and impairment in growth and development
7. **Newborns** at risk for HIV infection should be seen by the physician at birth and at 1 week, 2 weeks, 1 month, and 2 months of life
8. Inform the mother that an HIV culture is recommended at age 1 month and after 4 months of age

E. Immunizations
1. **Newborns** at risk for HIV infection need to receive all recommended immunizations at the regular schedule
2. Immunizations with live vaccines, such as measles-mumps-rubella (MMR), should not be done until the **newborn's, infant's,** or child's HIV status is confirmed
3. If a child is infected, live vaccine will not be given

XVIII. NEWBORN OF DIABETIC MOTHER

A. Description
   1. **Neonate** born to an insulin-dependent or gestational diabetic mother
   2. High incidence of hypoglycemia, hyperbilirubinemia, respiratory distress syndrome, hypocalcemia, and congenital anomalies

B. Data collection
   1. Excessive size and weight as a result of excess fat and glycogen in tissues
   2. Edema or puffiness in the face and cheeks
   3. Signs of hypoglycemia, such as twitching, difficulty in feeding, lethargy, apnea, seizures, and cyanosis
   4. Hyperbilirubinemia
   5. Signs of respiratory distress, such as tachypnea, cyanosis, retractions, grunting, and nasal flaring

C. Interventions
   1. Monitor for signs of respiratory distress
   2. Monitor bilirubin and blood glucose levels
   3. Monitor weight
   4. Feed the infant soon after birth with glucose in water, breast milk, or formula, as prescribed
   5. Administer IV glucose to treat hypoglycemia if necessary and as prescribed
   6. Monitor for edema
   7. Monitor for apnea, tremors, and seizures

XIX. HYPOGLYCEMIA

A. Description
   1. Abnormally low level of glucose in the blood (lower than 30 mg/dL in the first 72 hours or below 45 mg/dL after the first 3 days of life)
   2. Normal blood glucose level is 40 to 60 mg/dL in a 1-day-old **neonate** and 50 to 90 mg/dL in a **neonate** older than 1 day

B. Data collection
   1. Increased respiratory rate
   2. Twitching, nervousness, or tremors
   3. Unstable temperature
   4. Cyanosis

C. Interventions
   1. Prevent low blood glucose through early feedings
   2. Administer glucose orally or by IV as prescribed
   3. Monitor blood glucose levels as prescribed
   4. Monitor for feeding problems
   5. Monitor for apneic periods
   6. Monitor for shrill or intermittent cries
   7. Evaluate lethargy and poor muscle tone

PRACTICE QUESTIONS

1. A nurse is reinforcing measures regarding the care of the newborn with a mother. To bathe a newborn, a mother should be taught to:
   1. Start with the dirtiest area first
   2. Begin with the eyes and face
   3. Begin with the feet and work upward
   4. Only wash the diaper area, because this is the only part of the baby that gets soiled

2. Following birth, the nurse prevents hypothermia due to evaporation in the newborn by:
   1. Warming the crib pad
   2. Turning on the overhead radiant warmer
   3. Closing the doors to the room
   4. Drying the baby with a warm blanket

3. A nurse is planning to teach cord care to a new mother. The nurse plans to tell the mother that:
   1. Cord care is done only at birth to control bleeding
   2. Alcohol is the only agent used to clean the cord
   3. The process of keeping the cord clean and dry will decrease bacterial growth
   4. It takes 21 days for the cord to dry up and fall off

4. A male neonate has just been circumcised. The nurse would expect the surgical site to appear:
   1. Pink, without drainage
   2. Reddened, with a small amount of bloody drainage
   3. Reddened, with a large amount of bloody drainage that requires a dressing change every 30 minutes
   4. Reddened, with a small amount of yellow exudate on the glans

5. The parents of a male neonate who is not circumcised request information on how to clean the newborn's penis. The nurse makes which response to the parents?
   1. "Retract the foreskin and cleanse the glans when bathing the neonate."
   2. "Avoid retracting the foreskin to cleanse the glans because this may cause adhesions."
   3. "Retract the foreskin no farther than it will easily go and replace it over the glans after cleaning."
   4. "Retract the foreskin and cleanse with every diaper change."

6. Preterm newborns are at the risk for developing respiratory distress syndrome (RDS). The nurse monitors for the clinical signs associated with RDS, knowing that these signs include:
   1. Hypotension and bradycardia
   2. Tachypnea and retractions
   3. Acrocyanosis and grunting
   4. The presence of a barrel chest with acrocyanosis

7. A nurse notes hypotonia, irritability, and a poor sucking reflex in a full-term newborn infant upon admission to the nursery. The nurse suspects fetal alcohol syndrome (FAS) and is aware that which of the following additional signs would be consistent with FAS?
   1. Head circumference appropriate for gestational age
   2. Birth weight of 6 pounds 14 ounces
   3. Length of 19 inches
   4. Abnormal palmar creases

8. A pregnant human immunodeficiency virus (HIV)–positive woman delivers a baby. The nurse provides guidance to help the client make decisions regarding newborn care. The nurse determines that additional guidance is needed if the woman states that she will:
   1. Be sure to wash her hands before and following bathroom use
   2. Be sure to wash her hands before feeding the newborn
   3. Breast-feed, especially for the first 6 weeks postpartum
   4. Administer the prescribed antiviral medication to the newborn for the first 6 weeks after delivery

9. A pregnant woman has a positive history of genital herpes, but has not had lesions during this pregnancy. The nurse plans to provide which of the following information to the client?
   1. "You will be isolated from your newborn following delivery."
   2. "You will be evaluated at the time of delivery for herpetic genital tract lesions; if present, a cesarean delivery will be needed."
   3. "There is little risk to your neonate during this pregnancy, birth, and following delivery."
   4. "Vaginal deliveries can reduce neonatal infection risks, even if you have an active lesion at birth."

10. A nurse administers erythromycin ointment (0.5%) to the newborn's eyes, and the mother asks the nurse why this is done. The nurse tells the client that this is routinely done to:
    1. Minimize the spread of microorganisms to the neonate from invasive procedures during labor
    2. Protect the neonate's eyes from possible infections acquired while hospitalized
    3. Prevent ophthalmia neonatorum from occurring after delivery to a neonate born to a woman with an untreated gonococcal infection
    4. Prevent cataracts in the neonate born to a woman who is susceptible to rubella

11. A client asks the nurse why her newborn baby needs an injection of vitamin K. The nurse makes which statement to the client?
    1. "Your newborn needs vitamin K to develop immunity."
    2. "The vitamin K will protect your newborn from becoming jaundiced."
    3. "Newborns are deficient in vitamin K. This injection prevents your baby from abnormal bleeding."
    4. "Newborns have sterile bowels and the vitamin K will colonize the bowel with the necessary bacteria."

12. A nurse is assigned to assist in caring for a neonate born to a mother with acquired immunodeficiency syndrome (AIDS). The nurse understands that which of the following should be included in the plan of care?
    1. Instruct breast-feeding mothers regarding treatment of their nipples with an antifungal cream
    2. Monitor the neonate's vital signs routinely
    3. Maintain standard precautions at all times while caring for the neonate
    4. Initiate referral to evaluate for blindness, deafness, learning, or behavioral problems in the neonate

13. A nurse in the newborn nursery receives a telephone call to prepare for the admission of a 43-week-gestation newborn infant with Apgar scores of 1 and 4. In planning for admission of this infant, the nurse's highest priority should be to:
    1. Connect the resuscitation bag to the oxygen outlet
    2. Turn on the apnea and cardiorespiratory monitor
    3. Set up the intravenous line with 5% dextrose in water
    4. Set up the radiant warmer control temperature at 36.5° C (97.6° F)

14. A nurse is caring for a post-term neonate immediately after admission to the nursery. The priority nursing action would be to monitor:
    1. Urinary output
    2. Total bilirubin levels
    3. Blood glucose levels
    4. Hemoglobin and hematocrit

15. A nurse is reinforcing instructions to a new mother about cord care and how to monitor for infection. The nurse tells the mother that which of the following is a sign of infection?
    1. A darkened drying stump
    2. A moist cord with discharge
    3. A purple stump that shows pinkness around the base
    4. A purple stump that shows some moistness at the base

ALTERNATE FORMAT QUESTION: MULTIPLE RESPONSE

Select all interventions for a newborn receiving phototherapy.
___ Expose all of the newborn's skin
___ Cover the newborn's eyes with eye shields or patches
___ Monitor skin temperature closely
___ Decrease fluid intake
___ Monitor the skin for bronze baby syndrome, a grayish-brown discoloration of the skin
___ Reposition newborn every 2 hours
___ Avoid stimulation

ANSWERS

1. Answer: 2

Rationale: Bathing should start at the eyes and face, usually the cleanest area. Next, the external ear and behind the ears are cleansed. The newborn's neck should be washed because formula, lint, or breast milk will often accumulate in the folds of the neck. Hands and arms are then washed. The baby's legs are washed, and the diaper area is washed last.

Test-Taking Strategy: Use the basic techniques of bathing a client to answer the question. Remember, when bathing an adult or baby, start with the cleanest part of the body and proceed to the dirtiest part. Options 1, 3, and 4 are incorrect. Review the techniques for bathing a newborn if you had difficulty with this question.

Level of Cognitive Ability: Application
Client Needs: Health Promotion and Maintenance
Integrated Process: Nursing Process/Implementation
Content Area: Maternity/Postpartum
Reference: Leifer, G. (2003). *Introduction to maternity and pediatric nursing* (4th ed.). Philadelphia: W.B. Saunders, p. 295.

2. Answer: 4

Rationale: Evaporation occurs when moisture from the newborn's wet body surface dissipates heat along with moisture. By keeping the newborn dry (by drying the wet newborn at birth), evaporation is prevented. Conduction occurs when the newborn is on a cold surface, such as a cold pad or mattress. Convection occurs as air moves across the newborn's skin from an open door and heat is transferred to the air. Radiation occurs when heat from the newborn radiates to a colder surface.

Test-Taking Strategy: Recalling the methods of preventing heat loss in a newborn and focusing on the issue, evaporation, will direct you to option 4. Review these methods of heat loss if you had difficulty with this question.

Level of Cognitive Ability: Application
Client Needs: Physiological Integrity
Integrated Process: Nursing Process/Implementation
Content Area: Maternity/Postpartum
Reference: Leifer, G. (2003). *Introduction to maternity and pediatric nursing* (4th ed.). Philadelphia: W.B. Saunders, p. 135.

3. Answer: 3

Rationale: The cord should be kept clean and dry to decrease bacterial growth. This includes keeping the diaper folded below the cord to keep urine away from the cord. The cord should be cleansed two to three times a day. It usually falls off within 7 to 14 days. Agents other than alcohol may be used to clean the cord.

Test-Taking Strategy: Use the process of elimination. Eliminate options 1 and 2, noting the absolute word "only." Also, recall that cord care is required until the cord dries up and falls off and that agents other than alcohol may be used on the cord. Option 4 is incorrect because the cord should fall off between 7 and 14 days after birth. Review the concepts of cord care if you had difficulty answering the question.

Level of Cognitive Ability: Comprehension
Client Needs: Physiological Integrity
Integrated Process: Teaching/Learning
Content Area: Maternity/Postpartum

Reference: Leifer, G. (2005). *Maternity nursing* (9th ed.). Philadelphia: W.B. Saunders, pp. 154, 156.

4. Answer: 2

Rationale: The glans penis is normally dark red. Following circumcision, a small amount of bloody drainage is expected. During the normal healing process, the glans become covered with a yellow exudate. If excessive bleeding is noted from the circumcision, the nurse applies gentle pressure to the site of bleeding with a sterile gauze pad. If bleeding is not controlled, the physician is notified because a blood vessel may need to be ligated.

Test-Taking Strategy: Use the process of elimination and focus on the issue, an expected appearance. Remember, a small amount of bloody drainage is expected. Review the expected findings following circumcision if you had difficulty with this question.

Level of Cognitive Ability: Comprehension
Client Needs: Physiological Integrity
Integrated Process: Nursing Process/Data collection
Content Area: Maternity/Postpartum
References: Leifer, G. (2005). *Maternity nursing* (9th ed.). Philadelphia: W.B. Saunders, pp. 167-168.
Leifer, G. (2003). *Introduction to maternity and pediatric nursing* (4th ed.). Philadelphia: W.B. Saunders, p. 291.

5. Answer: 2

Rationale: In newborn males, the prepuce is continuous with the epidermis of the glans and is nonretractable. Forced retraction may cause adhesions to develop. Separation should be allowed to occur naturally, which will take place between 3 years and 5 years of age. Most foreskins are retractable by 3 years of age and should be pushed back gently for cleaning once a week.

Test-Taking Strategy: Use the process of elimination, and note the similarities between options 1, 3, and 4. Options 1, 3, and 4 are incorrect because retracting the foreskin is not recommended in an uncircumcised male. Option 2 is the only different option, stating that retraction of the foreskin is avoided. Review care to the neonate who is uncircumcised if you had difficulty with this question.

Level of Cognitive Ability: Application
Client Needs: Physiological Integrity
Integrated Process: Teaching/Learning
Content Area: Maternity/Postpartum
Reference: Leifer, G. (2003). *Introduction to maternity and pediatric nursing* (4th ed.). Philadelphia: W.B. Saunders, p. 291.

6. Answer: 2

Rationale: The newborn infant with respiratory distress syndrome may present with clinical signs of cyanosis, tachypnea or apnea, nasal flaring, chest wall retractions, or audible grunts. Acrocyanosis is a bluish discoloration of the hands and feet, associated with immature peripheral circulation, and is not uncommon in the first few hours of life. Options 1, 3, and 4 do not indicate clinical signs of RDS.

Test-Taking Strategy: Use the process of elimination. Recalling that acrocyanosis may be a normal sign in a newborn infant will assist in eliminating options 3 and 4. From the remaining

options, it is necessary to be familiar with the signs of respiratory distress syndrome. Also, note the relationship between the diagnosis and the signs noted in option 2. If you had difficulty with this question, review the signs of RDS.
Level of Cognitive Ability: Analysis
Client Needs: Physiological Integrity
Integrated Process: Nursing Process/Data collection
Content Area: Maternity/Postpartum
Reference: Leifer, G. (2003). *Introduction to maternity and pediatric nursing* (4th ed.). Philadelphia: W.B. Saunders, p. 309.

7. *Answer:* **4**
Rationale: Features of newborn infants diagnosed with FAS include craniofacial abnormalities, intrauterine growth retardation (IUGR), cardiac abnormalities, abnormal palmar creases, and respiratory distress. Options 1, 2, and 3 are normal findings in the full-term newborn infant.
Test-Taking Strategy: Use the process of elimination and knowledge regarding normal findings in the full-term newborn infant to answer this question. Note that options 1, 2, and 3 are similar and represent normal findings in the full-term newborn infant. If you had difficulty with this question, review the content related to normal newborn infant findings and FAS.
Level of Cognitive Ability: Analysis
Client Needs: Physiological Integrity
Integrated Process: Nursing Process/Data collection
Content Area: Maternity/Postpartum
References: Lowdermilk, D., & Perry, S. (2003). *Maternity nursing* (6th ed.). St. Louis: Mosby, p. 758.
Murray, S., McKinney, E., & Gorrie, T. (2002). *Foundations of maternal-newborn nursing* (3rd ed.). Philadelphia: W.B. Saunders, p. 638.

8. *Answer:* **3**
Rationale: The mode of perinatal transmission of HIV to the fetus or neonate of an HIV-positive woman can occur during the antenatal, intrapartal, or postpartum periods. HIV transmission can occur during breast-feeding; thus, HIV-positive clients are encouraged to bottle feed their neonates. Antiviral medications will be prescribed for the neonate for the first 6 weeks of life. The principles related to hand washing need to be taught to the mother.
Test-Taking Strategy: Use the process of elimination and note the key words, *additional guidance is needed*. These words indicate a false response question and that you need to select the incorrect client statement. Options 1 and 2 can be eliminated first because they are similar. From the remaining options, recalling the modes of transmission of HIV from the mother to the newborn will direct you to option 3. Review these modes of transmission if you had difficulty with this question.
Level of Cognitive Ability: Application
Clients Needs: Safe, Effective Care Environment
Integrated Process: Teaching/Learning
Content Area: Maternity/Postpartum
Reference: Leifer, G. (2003). *Introduction to maternity and pediatric nursing* (4th ed.). Philadelphia: W.B. Saunders, p. 110.

9. *Answer:* **2**
Rationale: If herpetic genital lesions are present at the time of delivery, a cesarean delivery will be necessary to reduce the risk of infecting the neonate. In the absence of herpetic genital lesions, a vaginal delivery may be indicated unless there are other reasons for performing a cesarean delivery. Maternal isolation is not necessary, but potentially exposed neonates should be cultured on the day of delivery.
Test-Taking Strategy: Use the process of elimination. Focusing on the issue of the question, a positive history of genital herpes and recalling the risks to the neonate will direct you to option 2. Review the methods of transmission of genital herpes to the neonate if you had difficulty with this question.
Level of Cognitive Ability: Application
Clients Needs: Safe, Effective Care Environment
Integrated Process: Nursing Process/Implementation
Content Area: Maternity/Antepartum
Reference: Leifer, G. (2003). *Introduction to maternity and pediatric nursing* (4th ed.). Philadelphia: W.B. Saunders, p. 109.

10. *Answer:* **3**
Rationale: Erythromycin ophthalmic ointment (Ilotycin ophthalmic) 0.5% is used as a prophylactic treatment of ophthalmia neonatorum, which is caused by the bacteria *Neisseria gonorrhoeae*. Preventive treatment of gonorrhea is required by law. Options 1, 2, and 4 are not the purposes of administering this medication to the newborn infant.
Test-Taking Strategy: Use the process of elimination and knowledge of the purpose of administering erythromycin ophthalmic ointment to the newborn infant. Remember that erythromycin ophthalmic ointment (Ilotycin ophthalmic) 0.5% is used as a prophylactic treatment of ophthalmia neonatorum in newborns. If you had difficulty with this question, review initial care of the newborn infant.
Level of Cognitive Ability: Application
Clients Needs: Safe, Effective Care Environment
Integrated Process: Nursing Process/Implementation
Content Area: Maternity/Postpartum
Reference: Leifer, G. (2003). *Introduction to maternity and pediatric nursing* (4th ed.). Philadelphia: W.B. Saunders, pp. 153-154.

11. *Answer:* **3**
Rationale: Vitamin K is necessary for the body to synthesize coagulation factors. Vitamin K is administered to the newborn infant to prevent abnormal bleeding. It promotes liver formation of the clotting factors II, VII, IX, and X. Newborn infants are vitamin K deficient because the bowel does not have the bacteria necessary for synthesizing fat-soluble vitamin K. The normal flora in the intestinal tract produces vitamin K. The newborn infant's bowel does not support the normal production of vitamin K until bacteria adequately colonize it. The bowel becomes colonized by bacteria as food is ingested. Vitamin K does not promote the development of immunity or prevent the infant from becoming jaundiced.
Test-Taking Strategy: Use the process of elimination. Because jaundice and immunity are not related to the action of vitamin K, eliminate options 1 and 2. From the remaining options, recall the action of vitamin K to direct you to option 3.

If you had difficulty with this question, review the purpose of vitamin K injection.
Level of Cognitive Ability: Application
Client's Needs: Psychological Integrity
Integrated Process: Nursing Process/Implementation
Content Area: Maternity/Postpartum
Reference: Leifer, G. (2003). *Introduction to maternity and pediatric nursing* (4th ed.). Philadelphia: W.B. Saunders, p. 153.

12. *Answer:* 3
Rationale: The neonate born of a mother with AIDS must be cared for with strict attention to standard precautions. This prevents the transmission of the infection from the neonate, if infected, to others, and prevents the transmission of other infectious agents to the possibly immunocompromised neonate. A mother with AIDS should not breast-feed. Options 2 and 4 are not specifically associated with the care of a potentially AIDS infected neonate.
Test-Taking Strategy: Use the process of elimination and knowledge regarding care to a neonate infant born to a woman with AIDS. Eliminate options 2 and 4 first because they are not specifically associated with the care of a potentially infected neonate. Recalling that AIDS-infected mothers should not breast-feed will direct you to option 3 from the remaining options. Review care to a neonate born to a woman with AIDS if you had difficulty with this question.
Level of Cognitive Ability: Application
Client Needs: Safe, Effective Care Environment
Integrated Process: Nursing Process/Planning
Content Area: Maternity/Postpartum
Reference: Leifer, G. (2003). *Introduction to maternity and pediatric nursing* (4th ed.). Philadelphia: W.B. Saunders, p. 759.

13. *Answer:* 1
Rationale: The highest priority on admission to the nursery for a newborn with low Apgar scores is airway support, which would involve preparing respiratory resuscitation equipment. The remaining options are also important, although they are of somewhat lower priority. The newborn infant will be placed on a cardiorespiratory monitor. Setting up an IV with 5% dextrose in water would provide circulatory support. The radiant warmer will provide an external heat source, which is necessary to prevent further respiratory distress.
Test-Taking Strategy: Use the process of elimination and note the key words, *highest priority*. This question asks you to prioritize care based on information about a newborn infant's condition. Use the ABCs—airway, breathing, and circulation. A method of planning for airway support is to have the resuscitation bag connected to an oxygen source. Review care of the newborn infant with low Apgar scores if you had difficulty with this question.
Level of Cognitive Ability: Application
Client Needs: Physiological Integrity
Integrated Process: Nursing Process/Planning
Content Area: Delegating/Prioritizing
Reference: Leifer, G. (2003). *Introduction to maternity and pediatric nursing* (4th ed.). Philadelphia: W.B. Saunders, pp. 153, 288.

14. *Answer:* 3
Rationale: The most common metabolic complication in the post-term newborn is hypoglycemia, which can produce central nervous system abnormalities and mental retardation if not corrected immediately. Urinary output, although important, is not the highest priority action. Hemoglobin and hematocrit levels are monitored because the post-term neonate exhibits polycythemia, although this also does not require immediate attention. The polycythemia contributes to increased bilirubin levels, usually beginning on the second day after delivery.
Test-Taking Strategy: Use the process of elimination, and note the key word, *priority*. Recalling that hypoglycemia is a primary concern in the post-term newborn will direct you to option 3. Review the post-term newborn content if you had difficulty with this question.
Level of Cognitive Ability: Application
Client Needs: Physiological Integrity
Integrated Process: Nursing Process/Data collection
Content Area: Delegating/Prioritizing
Reference: Leifer, G. (2003). *Introduction to maternity and pediatric nursing* (4th ed.). Philadelphia: W.B. Saunders, p. 728.

15. *Answer:* 2
Rationale: Signs of infection at the umbilical cord are moistness, oozing, discharge, and a reddened base. If signs of infection occur, the health care provider is notified. Antibiotic treatment may be necessary.
Test-Taking Strategy: Use the process of elimination. Options 1 and 3 identify normal signs and are eliminated first. From the remaining options, noting the word "discharge" in option 2 will direct you to this option. Review the signs and symptoms of infection if you had difficulty with this question.
Level of Cognitive Ability: Application
Client Needs: Health Promotion and Maintenance
Integrated Process: Teaching/Learning
Content Area: Maternity/Postpartum
Reference: Leifer, G. (2003). *Introduction to maternity and pediatric nursing* (4th ed.). Philadelphia: W.B. Saunders, p. 221.

ALTERNATE FORMAT QUESTION: MULTIPLE RESPONSE

Answers:
Cover the newborn's eyes with eye shields or patches
Monitor skin temperature closely
Monitor the skin for bronze baby syndrome, a grayish-brown discoloration of the skin
Reposition newborn every 2 hours
Rationale: Phototherapy is the use of intense fluorescent lights to reduce serum bilirubin levels in the newborn. Injury from treatment, such as eye damage, dehydration, or sensory deprivation, can occur. Interventions include exposing as much of the newborn's skin as possible; however, the genital area is covered and the nurse monitors the genital area for skin irritation or breakdown. The newborn's eyes are also covered with eye shields or patches, ensuring that the eyelids are closed when shields or patches are applied. The shields or patches are removed at least once per shift to inspect the

eyes for infection or irritation and to allow eye contact. The nurse measures the quantity of light every 8 hours, monitors skin temperature closely, and increases fluids to compensate for water loss. The newborn will have loose green stools and green-colored urine. The newborn's skin color is monitored every 4 to 8 hours with the fluorescent light turned off, and is monitored for bronze baby syndrome, a grayish-brown discoloration of the skin. The newborn is repositioned every 2 hours and stimulation is provided. After treatment, the newborn is monitored for signs of hyperbilirubinemia, because rebound elevations are normal after therapy is discontinued.

Test-Taking Strategy: Focus on the issue, phototherapy. Recalling that injury from treatment, such as eye damage, dehydration, or sensory deprivation can occur will assist in determining the correct interventions. Review the interventions for the newborn receiving phototherapy if you had difficulty with this question.
Level of Cognitive Ability: Application
Client Needs: Safe, Effective Care Environment
Integrated Process: Nursing Process/Implementation
Content Area: Maternity/Postpartum
Reference: Lowdermilk, D., & Perry, S. (2003). *Maternity nursing* (6th ed.). St. Louis: Mosby, pp. 497-498.

REFERENCES

Leifer, G. (2003). *Introduction to maternity and pediatric nursing* (4th ed.). Philadelphia: W.B. Saunders.
Leifer, G. (2005). *Maternity nursing* (9th ed.). Philadelphia: W.B. Saunders.

Lowdermilk, D., & Perry, S. (2003). *Maternity nursing.* (6th ed.). St. Louis: Mosby.
Murray, S., McKinney, E., & Gorrie, T. (2002). *Foundations of maternal-newborn nursing* (3rd ed.). Philadelphia: W.B. Saunders.

Maternity and Newborn Medications

I. OXYTOCIC MEDICATION: OXYTOCIN (PITOCIN)

A. Description
1. Stimulates the smooth muscle of the uterus and induces contraction of the myocardium
2. Promotes milk let-down
3. Routes of administration include intranasal, intramuscular (IM), and intravenous (IV)
4. Minimal cervical change is usually noted until the active phase of **labor** is achieved

B. Uses
1. Induces or augments **labor**
2. Controls postpartum bleeding
3. Promotes milk let-down and facilitates breastfeeding (intranasal route)
4. Induces or completes an abortion

C. Adverse reactions and contraindications
1. Rare, but may include allergies, dysrhythmias, changes in blood pressure (BP), uterine rupture, and water intoxication; intranasal administration may cause nasal vasoconstriction
2. May produce uterine hypertonicity resulting in fetal or maternal injury
3. High doses may cause hypotension, with rebound hypertension
4. Postpartum hemorrhage can occur because the uterus may become atonic when the medication wears off
5. Should not be used in a client who cannot deliver vaginally or in a client with hypertonic uterine contractions

D. Interventions
1. Monitor maternal vital signs (every 15 minutes), especially the blood pressure (BP) and heart rate, weight, intake and output (I&O), level of consciousness (LOC), and lung sounds
2. Monitor frequency, duration, force of contractions, and resting uterine tone every 15 minutes

3. Monitor fetal heart rate (FHR) every 15 minutes; notify the registered nurse if significant changes occur; an internal fetal scalp electrode should be used if possible
4. Administered by IV infusion via an infusion monitoring device (Y setup or stopcock used, with normal saline in the primary line); dose administered is carefully monitored
5. Do not leave the client unattended while the oxytocin is infusing
6. Administer oxygen if prescribed
7. Monitor for hypertonic contractions
8. The medication is stopped if uterine hyperstimulation or a nonreassuring FHR occurs; if these occur, notify the registered nurse, turn the client on her side, and administer oxygen via face mask
9. Notify the registered nurse if uterine hyperstimulation or nonreassuring FHR occurs
10. Monitor for signs of water intoxication
11. Have emergency equipment available
12. Keep the family informed of the client's progress

II. ERGOT ALKALOIDS (Box 26-1)

A. Description
1. Directly stimulate uterine muscle and increase the force and frequency of contractions
2. Produce a firm tetanic contraction of the uterus
3. Produce arterial vasoconstriction; can cause vasospasm of the coronary arteries

---

BOX 26-1

Ergot Alkaloids

Ergonovine (Ergotrate)
Methylergonovine (Methergine)

---

4. Not administered before delivery of the **placenta**
5. May be administered by the oral or intramuscular route; may be administered by the IV route undiluted in an emergency

B. Uses
   1. Postpartum hemorrhage
   2. Postabortal hemorrhage resulting from atony or involution

C. Adverse reactions and contraindications
   1. Nausea
   2. Uterine cramping
   3. Can cause bradycardia, dysrhythmias, myocardial infarction, and severe hypertension
   4. High doses are associated with peripheral vasospasm or vasoconstriction, angina, miosis, confusion, respiratory depression, seizures, or unconsciousness; uterine tetany can occur
   5. Contraindicated during pregnancy
   6. Contraindicated in clients with significant cardiovascular disease, peripheral vascular disease, hypertension, eclampsia, or preeclampsia

D. Interventions
   1. Monitor maternal vital signs, weight, I&O, LOC, and lung sounds
   2. Monitor the BP closely; the medication produces vasoconstriction, and if a rise in BP is noted, withhold the medication and notify the registered nurse
   3. Monitor uterine contractions (frequency, strength, and duration)
   4. Assess for chest pain, headache, shortness of breath, itching, pale or cold hands or feet, nausea, diarrhea, or dizziness
   5. Notify the registered nurse if chest pain occurs
   6. Assess the extremities for color, warmth, movement, and pain
   7. Assess vaginal bleeding
   8. Administer analgesics as prescribed; may be required because the medication produces painful uterine contractions

III. PROSTAGLANDINS (Box 26-2)

A. Description
   1. Potent stimulators of the myometrium
   2. Dinoprostone is administered as a gel or suppository directly into the vagina
   3. Carboprost can be administered by deep intramuscular injection

---

BOX 26-2

Prostaglandins

Carboprost (Hemabate)
Dinoprostone (Cervidil)

B. Uses
   1. Abortifacient
   2. Induce abortion during the second trimester, when the uterus is resistant to oxytocin
   3. Dinoprostone is also used to soften and promote dilation of the cervix to facilitate vaginal **delivery**

C. Adverse reactions and contraindications
   1. Significant gastrointestinal side effects, including diarrhea, nausea, vomiting, and stomach cramps
   2. Fever, chills, and flushing
   3. Anaphylaxis, dysrhythmias, bronchoconstriction, chest pain, hypertension, and peripheral vasoconstriction
   4. Contraindicated in clients with significant cardiovascular disease or those with a history of asthma or pulmonary disease
   5. High doses can cause uterine cramping and tetany

D. Interventions
   1. Monitor maternal vital signs, especially the BP and heart rate, weight, I&O, LOC, and lung sounds
   2. Monitor frequency, duration, force of uterine contractions, and resting uterine tone frequently; palpate the fundus
   3. Monitor vaginal bleeding
   4. Remain with the client for 30 minutes after administration to monitor for anaphylaxis; signs include shortness of breath or difficulty breathing, tachycardia, hives, tightness in the chest, and swelling of the face
   5. Maintain client in a supine position for 30 minutes following administration of the medication
   6. Keep side rails up; have a suction machine at the bedside
   7. Administer antidiarrheal and antiemetic medications as prescribed

IV. MAGNESIUM SULFATE

A. Description
   1. Central nervous system (CNS) depressant and anticonvulsant
   2. Causes smooth muscle relaxation
   3. Antidote: Calcium gluconate

B. Uses
   1. Prevent and control seizures in preeclamptic and eclamptic clients
   2. Treat preterm **labor**

C. Adverse reactions and contraindications
   1. Can cause reduced respiratory rate, decreased reflexes, flushing, hypotension, and decreased heart rate
   2. Continuous IV infusion increases the risk of magnesium toxicity in the **neonate**
   3. IV administration should not be used for 2 hours preceding **delivery**

4. Magnesium sulfate is continued for the first 12 to 24 hours postpartum if used for preeclampsia
5. High doses can cause loss of deep tendon reflexes, heart block, respiratory paralysis, and cardiac arrest
6. Contraindicated in the client with heart block, myocardial damage, or renal failure
7. Used with caution in the client with severe renal impairment

D. Interventions
1. Monitor maternal vital signs, especially respirations, every 30 to 60 minutes
2. Notify the registered nurse if respirations are less than 12/minute, indicating respiratory depression
3. Monitor renal function and cardiac function closely
4. Monitor magnesium levels, because the target range is 4 to 7 mEq/L; if a rise in the magnesium level occurs, the health care provider is notified
5. Administered by IV infusion via an infusion monitoring device
6. Keep calcium gluconate on hand in case of magnesium sulfate overdose, because calcium gluconate antagonizes the effect of magnesium sulfate
7. Deep tendon reflexes are monitored hourly for signs of developing toxicity
8. The patellar reflex is tested before administering repeat parenteral doses (used as an indicator of CNS depression; suppressed reflex may be a sign of impending respiratory arrest)
9. Patellar reflex must be present and respiratory rate must be greater than 16 breaths per minute before each parenteral dose
10. Monitor I&O hourly; output should be maintained at 30 mL/hour because the medication is eliminated through the kidneys

V. MEPERIDINE HYDROCHLORIDE (DEMEROL)
A. Description
1. Narcotic analgesic
2. Administered by the intramuscular or IV route
3. Antidote: Naloxone (Narcan)
B. Use: Relieves moderate to severe pain associated with **labor**
C. Adverse reactions and contraindications
1. Dizziness, nausea, vomiting, sedation, decreased BP, decreased respirations, diaphoresis, flushed face, decreased urination
2. May be administered with promethazine (Phenergan) to prevent nausea
3. High doses may result in respiratory depression, skeletal muscle flaccidity, cold, clammy skin, cyanosis, extreme somnolence progressing to convulsions, stupor, and coma

4. Used cautiously in clients delivering preterm **infants**
5. Not administered in early **labor** because it may slow the **labor** process
6. Not administered in advanced **labor** (within 1 hour of **delivery**) if the **neonate** is to be delivered before the medication has been adequately removed from the fetal circulation (may cause respiratory depression)
7. Regular use of opiates during pregnancy may produce withdrawal symptoms in the **neonate** (e.g., irritability, excessive crying, tremors, hyperactive reflexes, fever, vomiting, diarrhea, yawning, sneezing, seizures)

D. Interventions
1. Monitor vital signs, particularly respiratory status; if respirations are 12/minute or less frequent, withhold medication and notify the registered nurse
2. Monitor for BP changes (hypotension); maintain in a recumbent position
3. Have antidote available

VI. Rh$_0$(D) IMMUNE GLOBULIN (RhoGAM)
A. Description
1. Prevention of anti-Rh (D) antibody formation is most successful if the medication is administered twice, at 28 weeks' gestation and again within 72 hours after **delivery**
2. Should also be administered within 72 hours after potential or actual exposure to Rh-positive blood; must be given with each subsequent exposure or potential exposure to Rh-positive blood
3. Of no benefit once the client has developed a positive antibody titer to the Rh antigen
B. Use: Prevents isoimmunization in Rh-negative clients who are exposed or potentially exposed to Rh-positive red blood cells by transfusion, termination of pregnancy, amniocentesis, chorionic villus sampling (CVS), abdominal trauma, or bleeding during pregnancy or the birth process
C. Adverse reactions and contraindications
1. Elevated temperature
2. Tenderness at the injection site
3. Contraindicated for Rh-positive women
4. Contraindicated in clients with a history of systemic allergic reactions to preparations containing human immunoglobulins
5. Not administered to a **newborn infant**
D. Interventions
1. Administer to mother by intramuscular injection at 28 weeks' gestation and within 72 hours after **delivery**
2. Never administered by the IV route
3. Monitor for temperature elevation
4. Monitor injection site for tenderness

VII. BETAMETHASONE (CELESTONE)

A. Description
1. Corticosteroid
2. Increases production of surfactant

B. Use: For client in preterm **labor** between 28 and 32 weeks whose **labor** can be inhibited for 48 hours without jeopardizing mother or fetus

C. Adverse reactions and contraindications
1. Decreases mother's resistance to infection
2. Breast-feeding is contraindicated during medication administration

D. Interventions
1. Monitor maternal vital signs
2. Monitor mother for signs of infection
3. White blood cell count is monitored

VIII. LUNG SURFACTANTS (Box 26-3)

A. Description
1. Replenish surfactant and restore surface activity to the lungs
2. Administered by the intratracheal route

B. Use: Prevent or treat respiratory distress syndrome (hyaline membrane disease) in premature **infants**

C. Adverse reactions and contraindications
1. Side effects include transient bradycardia and oxygen desaturation
2. Administered with caution in those at risk for circulatory overload

D. Interventions
1. The medication is instilled through a catheter inserted into **infant's** endotracheal tube; avoid suctioning for at least 2 hours after administration
2. Monitor for bradycardia and decreased oxygen saturation during administration
3. Check lung sounds for moist breath sounds

IX. EYE PROPHYLAXIS FOR THE NEONATE

A. Description
1. Erythromycin (0.5% Ilotycin) and tetracycline (1%) ophthalmic ointment or drops are both bacteriostatic and bactericidal; provide prophylaxis against infection by *Neisseria gonorrhoeae* and *Chlamydia trachomatis*
2. Silver nitrate (1%) solution may be prescribed, but its use is minimal because it does not protect against chlamydial infection and can cause chemical conjunctivitis

---

BOX 26-3

Lung Surfactants

Beractant (Survanta)
Colfosceril palmitate (Exosurf)

---

3. Preventive treatment of gonorrhea is required by law

B. Use: As a prophylactic measure to protect against infection by *Neisseria gonorrhoeae* and *Chlamydia trachomatis*

C. Adverse reaction: Silver nitrate (1%) solution can cause chemical conjunctivitis

D. Interventions
1. Cleanse the **neonate's** eyes before instilling drops or ointment
2. Instill into each of the **neonate's** conjunctival sacs within 1 hour after **delivery**; eye prophylaxis may be delayed until an hour or so after birth so that eye contact and parent-**infant** attachment and bonding are facilitated
3. Do not flush the eyes after instillation

X. VITAMIN K (AquaMEPHYTON)

A. Description
1. Necessary for aiding in the production of active prothrombin
2. **Newborns** are deficient in vitamin K for the first 5 to 8 days of life because of the lack of intestinal flora necessary to absorb vitamin K

B. Use: For prophylaxis and to treat hemorrhagic disease of the **newborn**

C. Adverse reaction: Can cause hyperbilirubinemia in the **newborn**

D. Interventions
1. Protect the medication from light
2. Administer during the early neonatal period
3. Administer in the vastus lateralis muscle of the thigh
4. Monitor for bruising at the injection site and for bleeding from the cord
5. Monitor for jaundice and monitor bilirubin level because the medication can cause hyperbilirubinemia in the **newborn**

PRACTICE QUESTIONS

1. Epidural analgesia is administered to a woman for pain relief following a cesarean birth. The nurse assisting in caring for the woman ensures that which medication is readily available if respiratory depression occurs?
   1. Betamethasone (Celestone)
   2. Morphine sulfate
   3. Meperidine hydrochloride (Demerol)
   4. Naloxone (Narcan)

2. Rh$_o$(D) immune globulin (RhoGAM) is prescribed for a woman following delivery of a newborn infant and the nurse provides information to the woman about the purpose of the medication. The nurse determines that the woman understands the purpose of the medication if the woman states that it

will protect her next baby from which of the following?

1. Being affected by Rh incompatibility
2. Having Rh-positive blood
3. Developing a rubella infection
4. Developing physiological jaundice

3. Methylergonovine (Methergine) is prescribed for a postpartum woman to treat postpartum hemorrhage. The nurse assisting in caring for the woman collects data regarding which priority item before administration of the medication?

1. Amount of lochia
2. Blood pressure
3. Deep tendon reflexes
4. Uterine tone

4. A nurse is assisting with the administration of beractant (Survanta) to a premature infant who has respiratory distress syndrome (hyaline membrane disease). The nurse understands that the medication will be administered by which of the following routes?

1. Subcutaneous
2. Intratracheal
3. Intramuscular
4. Intradermal

5. A nurse is assisting in caring for a client who is receiving pitocin (Oxytocin) for the induction of labor. The nurse notifies the registered nurse if which of the following is noted in the client?

1. Drowsiness
2. Fatigue
3. Fetal heart rate of 140 beats per minute
4. Uterine hyperstimulation

6. A pregnant client is receiving magnesium sulfate for the management of preeclampsia. The nurse assisting in caring for the client identifies that the client has developed an unwanted outcome if which of the following is noted?

1. Presence of deep tendon reflexes
2. Serum magnesium level of 6 mEq/L
3. Proteinuria of 3+
4. Respirations of 10 breaths per minute

7. A woman with preeclampsia is receiving magnesium sulfate. The nurse assisting in caring for the client determines that the magnesium sulfate therapy is effective if:

1. Ankle clonus is noted
2. The blood pressure decreases
3. Seizures do not occur
4. Scotomas are present

8. Methylergonovine (Methergine) is prescribed for a client with postpartum hemorrhage. The nurse

assisting in caring for the client notifies the registered nurse if which of the following conditions were documented in the client's medical history?

1. Peripheral vascular disease
2. Hypothyroidism
3. Hypotension
4. Diabetes mellitus

9. Vitamin K (AquaMEPHYTON) is prescribed for the neonate. The nurse prepares the medication and selects which muscle site to administer the medication?

1. Deltoid
2. Tricep
3. Vastus lateralis
4. Bicep

10. A nursing instructor asks a nursing student to describe the procedure for administering erythromycin (0.5% Ilotycin) ointment to the eyes of the neonate. The instructor determines that the student needs to further research this procedure if the student states:

1. "I will cleanse the neonate's eyes before instilling ointment."
2. "I will flush the eyes after instilling the ointment."
3. "I will instill the eye ointment into each of the neonate's conjunctival sacs within 1 hour after birth."
4. "Administration of the eye ointment may be delayed until an hour or so after birth so that eye contact and parent-infant attachment and bonding can occur."

ALTERNATE FORMAT QUESTION: MULTIPLE RESPONSE

A nurse is caring for a pregnant client with severe preeclampsia who is receiving IV magnesium sulfate. Select all nursing interventions that apply in the care of the client.

____ Monitor maternal vital signs every 2 hours
____ Notify the registered nurse if respirations are less than 18/minute
____ Monitor renal function and cardiac function closely
____ Keep calcium gluconate on hand in case of a magnesium sulfate overdose
____ Deep tendon reflexes are monitored hourly
____ Monitor I&O hourly
____ Notify the registered nurse if urinary output is less than 30 mL/hour

ANSWERS

1. *Answer:* 4

Rationale: Narcotics are used for epidural analgesia. An adverse reaction of epidural analgesia is a delayed respiratory depression. Naloxone (Narcan) is a narcotic antagonist, which reverses the effects of narcotics and is given for respiratory depression. Morphine sulfate and meperidine hydrochloride are narcotics. Celestone is a corticosteroid administered to enhance fetal lung maturity.

Test-Taking Strategy: Use the process of elimination focusing on the issue of the question, the antidote for respiratory depression. Eliminate options 2 and 3 first, knowing that these medications are narcotics. Next, eliminate option 1, knowing that this medication is a corticosteroid. Review the purpose and actions of these medications if you had difficulty with this question.

Level of Cognitive Ability: Application
Client Needs: Physiological Integrity
Integrated Process: Nursing Process/Implementation
Content Area: Maternity/Postpartum
Reference: Hodgson, B., & Kizior, R. (2005). *Saunders nursing drug handbook 2005*. Philadelphia: W.B. Saunders, pp. 748-749.

2. *Answer:* 1

Rationale: Rh incompatibility can occur when an Rh-negative mother becomes sensitized to the Rh antigen. Sensitization may develop when an Rh-negative woman becomes pregnant with a fetus who is Rh positive. During pregnancy and at delivery, some of the baby's Rh-positive blood can enter the maternal circulation, causing the woman's immune system to form antibodies against Rh-positive blood. Administration of Rh$_o$(D) immune globulin (RhoGAM) prevents the woman from developing antibodies against Rh-positive blood by providing passive antibody protection against the Rh antigen.

Test-Taking Strategy: Use the process of elimination. Options 3 and 4 can be easily eliminated first because they are unrelated to the medication. From the remaining options, note the relationship between the name of the medication, Rh$_o$(D) immune globulin, and the word "incompatibility" in the correct option. Review the purpose of this medication if you had difficulty with this question.

Level of Cognitive Ability: Comprehension
Client Needs: Health Promotion and Maintenance
Integrated Process: Nursing Process/Evaluation
Content Area: Maternity/Postpartum
Reference: McKinney, E., James, S., Murray, S., & Ashwill, J. (2005). *Maternal-child nursing* (2nd ed.). St. Louis: Elsevier, p. 643.

3. *Answer:* 2

Rationale: Methylergonovine, an ergot alkaloid, is an agent that is used to prevent or control postpartum hemorrhage by contracting the uterus. It causes continuous uterine contractions and may elevate the blood pressure. A priority assessment before the administration of the medication is to check the blood pressure. The physician should be notified if hypertension is present. Although options 1, 3, and 4 may be a component of the postpartum data collection, option 2, blood pressure, is specifically related to the administration of this medication.

Test-Taking Strategy: Use the process of elimination. Eliminate options 1 and 4 first because they are similar and relate to one another. From the remaining options, use the ABCs—airway, breathing, and circulation. Blood pressure is a method of checking circulation. Review the adverse effects of this medication if you had difficulty with this question.

Level of Cognitive Ability: Application
Client Needs: Physiological Integrity
Integrated Process: Nursing Process/Data Collection
Content Area: Maternity/Postpartum
Reference: Hodgson, B., & Kizior, R. (2005). *Saunders nursing drug handbook 2005*. Philadelphia: W.B. Saunders, p. 694.

4. *Answer:* 2

Rationale: Respiratory distress is common in premature neonates and may be due to lung immaturity as a result of surfactant deficiency. The mainstay of treatment is the administration of exogenous surfactant. It is administered by the intratracheal route. Options 1, 3, and 4 are not routes of administration for this medication.

Test-Taking Strategy: Use the process of elimination. Note the relationship between the diagnosis, "respiratory distress syndrome," and the correct option, "intratracheal." Review this medication if you had difficulty with this question.

Level of Cognitive Ability: Comprehension
Client Needs: Physiological Integrity
Integrated Process: Nursing Process/Planning
Content Area: Maternity/Postpartum
Reference: Hodgson, B., & Kizior, R. (2005). *Saunders nursing drug handbook 2005*. Philadelphia: W.B. Saunders, p. 117.

5. *Answer:* 4

Rationale: Pitocin stimulates uterine contractions and is a common pharmacological method used to induce labor. An adverse reaction associated with administration of the medication is hyperstimulation of uterine contractions. Therefore, pitocin infusion must be stopped when there are any signs of uterine hyperstimulation. Drowsiness and fatigue may be due to the labor experience. The normal fetal heart rate is approximately 120 to 160 beats per minute.

Test-Taking Strategy: Use the process of elimination focusing on the issue, an adverse reaction to pitocin. Options 1 and 2 can be eliminated first because they are similar. From the remaining options, recalling the normal fetal heart rate will assist in eliminating option 3. Review the nursing responsibilities associated with this medication if you had difficulty with this question.

Level of Cognitive Ability: Application
Client Need: Physiological Integrity
Integrated Process: Nursing Process/Implementation
Content Area: Maternity/Intrapartum
Reference: Hodgson, B., & Kizior, R. (2005). *Saunders nursing drug handbook 2005*. Philadelphia: W.B. Saunders, p. 818.

6. *Answer:* 4

Rationale: Magnesium toxicity can occur from magnesium sulfate therapy. Signs of magnesium sulfate toxicity relate to central nervous system (CNS) depressant effects of the medication and include respiratory depression, loss of deep tendon reflexes, sudden drop in fetal heart rate and/or maternal heart rate and blood pressure. Therapeutic serum levels of magnesium are 4 to 7 mEq/L. Proteinuria of 3+ is likely to be noted in a client with preeclampsia.

Test-Taking Strategy: Use the process of elimination and eliminate option 1 first, because it is a normal finding. Next, eliminate option 2, knowing that the therapeutic serum level of magnesium is between 4 and 7 mEq/L. From the remaining options, recalling that proteinuria of 3+ would be noted in a client with preeclampsia will direct you to the correct option. Review the adverse effects of magnesium sulfate if you had difficulty with this question.

Level of Cognitive Ability: Analysis
Client Needs: Physiological Integrity
Integrated Process: Nursing Process/Data Collection
Content Area: Pharmacology
Reference: Hodgson, B., & Kizior, R. (2005). *Saunders nursing drug handbook 2005.* Philadelphia: W.B. Saunders, p. 661.

7. *Answer:* 3

Rationale: For a client with preeclampsia, the goal of care is directed at preventing eclampsia (seizures). Magnesium sulfate is an anticonvulsant; it is not an antihypertensive agent. Although a decrease in blood pressure may be noted initially, this effect is usually transient. Ankle clonus indicates hyperreflexia and may precede the onset of eclampsia. Scotomas are areas of complete or partial blindness. Visual disturbances, such as scotomas, often precede an eclamptic seizure.

Test-Taking Strategy: Use the process of elimination, and note the key words, *therapy is effective.* Knowing that magnesium sulfate is an anticonvulsant will direct you to option 3. Review this medication if you had difficulty with this question.

Level of Cognitive Ability: Analysis
Client Needs: Physiological Integrity
Integrated Process: Nursing Process/Evaluation
Content Area: Pharmacology
Reference: Hodgson, B., & Kizior, R. (2005). *Saunders nursing drug handbook 2005.* Philadelphia: W.B. Saunders, p. 659.

8. *Answer:* 1

Rationale: Methylergonovine is an ergot alkaloid used for postpartum hemorrhage. Ergot alkaloids are avoided in clients with significant cardiovascular disease, peripheral disease, hypertension, eclampsia, or preeclampsia. These conditions are worsened by the vasoconstrictive effects of the ergot alkaloids. Options 2, 3, and 4 are not contraindications related to the use of ergot alkaloids.

Test-Taking Strategy: Use the process of elimination. Recalling that ergot alkaloids produce vasoconstriction will direct you to option 1. Review the effects of this medication and the associated contraindications if you had difficulty with this question.

Level of Cognitive Ability: Analysis
Client Needs: Safe, Effective Care Environment
Integrated Process: Nursing Process/Implementation
Content Area: Maternity/Postpartum
Reference: Hodgson, B., & Kizior, R. (2005). *Saunders nursing drug handbook 2005.* Philadelphia: W.B. Saunders, p. 693.

9. *Answer:* 3

Rationale: Newborns are deficient in vitamin K for the first 5 to 8 days of life because of the lack of intestinal flora necessary to absorb vitamin K. Vitamin K is administered to the neonate to aid in the production of active prothrombin and to prevent hemorrhagic disease. It is administered in the vastus lateralis muscle. The vastus lateralis is the largest muscle mass in infants and small children (younger than 3 years of age) and has few major nerves and blood vessels. Options 1, 2, and 4 are incorrect administration sites.

Test-Taking Strategy: Use the process of elimination. Visualize the procedure for administering an injection to a neonate to assist in directing you to option 3. Review this procedure if you had difficulty with this question.

Level of Cognitive Ability: Application
Client Needs: Physiological Integrity
Integrated Process: Nursing Process/Implementation
Content Area: Maternity/Postpartum
References: Hodgson, B., & Kizior, R. (2005). *Saunders nursing drug handbook 2005.* Philadelphia: W.B. Saunders, p. 1119.
Leifer, G. (2005). *Maternity nursing* (9th ed.). Philadelphia: W.B. Saunders, p. 157.
Price, D., & Gwin, J. (2005). *Thompson's pediatric nursing* (9th ed.). Philadelphia: W.B. Saunders. p. 366.

10. *Answer:* 2

Rationale: Eye prophylaxis protects the neonate against *Neisseria gonorrhoeae* and *Chlamydia trachomatis* infection. The eyes are not flushed after instilling the medication because the flush will wash away the administered medication. Options 1, 3, and 4 are correct statements regarding the procedure for administering eye medication to the neonate.

Test-Taking Strategy: Use the process of elimination noting the key words, *needs to further research.* Eliminate options 3 and 4 first because they are similar. From the remaining options, visualize the effect of each. This will direct you to option 2. Review the procedure for administering eye medication to the neonate if you had difficulty with this question.

Level of Cognitive Ability: Analysis
Client Needs: Safe, Effective Care Environment
Integrated Process: Teaching/Learning
Content Area: Maternity/Postpartum
Reference: McKinney, E., James, S., Murray, S., & Ashwill, J. (2005). *Maternal-child nursing* (2nd ed.). St. Louis: Elsevier, p. 555.

ALTERNATE FORMAT QUESTION: MULTIPLE RESPONSE

Answers:
Monitor renal function and cardiac function closely
Keep calcium gluconate on hand in case of a magnesium sulfate overdose
Deep tendon reflexes are monitored hourly
Monitor I&O hourly
Notify the registered nurse if urinary output is less than 30 mL/hour
Rationale: Magnesium sulfate is a central nervous system (CNS) depressant and anticonvulsant used to prevent and control seizures in preeclamptic and eclamptic clients and to treat preterm labor. When caring for a client receiving

magnesium sulfate, the nurse would monitor maternal vital signs, especially respirations, every 30 to 60 minutes and notify the registered nurse if respirations are less than 12/minute, because this would indicate respiratory depression. Calcium gluconate is kept on hand in case of a magnesium sulfate overdose, because calcium gluconate antagonizes the effect of magnesium sulfate. Deep tendon reflexes are monitored hourly for signs of developing toxicity, and the patellar reflex is tested before administering repeat parenteral doses (used as an indicator of CNS depression; suppressed reflex may be a sign of impending respiratory arrest). The patellar reflex must be present and the respiratory rate must be more than 16 breaths/minute before each parenteral dose. Cardiac and renal function is monitored closely. The urine output should be maintained at 30 mL/hour because the medication is eliminated through the kidneys.

Test-Taking Strategy: Recalling that magnesium sulfate is a central nervous system (CNS) depressant and anticonvulsant and recalling the guidelines for its administration will assist in answering this question. If you are unfamiliar with the guidelines for the administration of this medication, review this content.

Level of Cognitive Ability: Application
Client Needs: Physiological Integrity
Integrated Process: Nursing Process/Implementation
Content Area: Maternity/Intrapartum
Reference: Hodgson, B., & Kizior, R. (2005). *Saunders nursing drug handbook 2005.* Philadelphia: W.B. Saunders, p. 659.

REFERENCES

Hodgson, B., & Kizior, R. (2005). *Saunders nursing drug handbook 2005.* Philadelphia: W.B. Saunders.

Leifer, G. (2005). *Maternity nursing* (9th ed.). Philadelphia: W.B. Saunders.

McKinney, E., James, S., Murray, S., & Ashwill, J. (2005). *Maternal-child nursing* (2nd ed.). St. Louis: Elsevier.

Price, D., & Gwin, J. (2005). *Thompson's pediatric nursing* (9th ed.). Philadelphia: W.B. Saunders.

Growth and Development across the Life Span

PYRAMID TERMS

abuse The willful infliction of pain, injury, or mental anguish; unreasonable confinement or willful deprivation of services, including medical care. Abuse can include failure to prevent injury, verbal assaults, the demand to perform demeaning tasks, theft, or mismanagement of personal belongings.

accommodation The ability to change a schema (an individual's cognitive structure or framework of thought) in order to introduce new ideas, objects, or experiences.

aging The biopsychosocial process of change occurring between birth and death.

assimilation The ability to incorporate new ideas, objects, and experiences into the framework of one's thoughts.

conscious Includes all experiences that are within an individual's awareness and that the individual can control.

dementia Organic syndrome identified by gradual and progressive deterioration in intellectual functioning. Long- and short-term memory loss occur with impairment in judgment, abstract thinking, problem-solving ability, and behavior; results in a self-care deficit. The most common type of dementia is Alzheimer's disease.

depression A functional disorder of mood that is not linked with aging. The depression may be precipitated by losses related to aging. Depression can be manifested by cognitive impairment or may be the cause of a decline in mental status. Depression can be identified by feelings of sadness, hopelessness, and worthlessness, and a decreased interest in activities.

ego One's "sense of self"; provides such functions as problem solving, mobilization of defense mechanisms, reality testing, and the capability of functioning independently; the mediator between the id and the superego.

exploitation Illegal or improper use of the individual's resources.

gerontology The study of the process of aging.

id Source of all primitive drives and instincts; thought of as the reservoir of all psychic energy.

neglect The lack of providing services necessary for physical or mental health.

schema Refers to an individual's cognitive structure or framework of thought.

schemata Categories that an individual forms in his or her mind to organize and understand the world.

self-neglect The person chooses to avoid medical care or other services that could improve optimal function. Unless declared legally incompetent, an individual has the right to refuse care.

subconscious Often called the preconscious; includes experiences, thoughts, feelings, or desires that might not be in immediate awareness but can be recalled to consciousness; helps repress unpleasant thoughts or feelings.

superego Represents the moral component of personality; includes internalizing the values, ideals, and moral standards of society.

unconscious Includes memories, feelings, thoughts, or wishes that are repressed and that are not available to the conscious mind.

PYRAMID TO SUCCESS

Normal growth and development proceed in an orderly, systematic, and predictable pattern, which provides a basis for identifying an individual's abilities. Understanding the path of growth and development across the life span assists the nurse in identifying appropriate and expected human behavior. The Pyramid to Success focuses on Sigmund Freud's Theory of Psychosexual Development, Jean Piaget's Theory of Cognitive Development, Erik Erikson's Psychosocial Theory, and Lawrence Kohlberg's Theory of Moral Development. Growth and development concepts focus on the aging process, and on physical characteristics, nutritional behaviors, skills, play, and specific safety measures relevant to a particular age group that will ensure a safe and hazard-free environment. If an age is identified in a question presented on the NCLEX-PN examination, note the age and think about the associated growth and developmental concepts. The Integrated Processes addressed in this unit include Caring, Clinical Problem-Solving Process (Nursing Process), Communication and Documentation, and Teaching/Learning.

▲ **CLIENT NEEDS**
Safe, Effective Care Environment

Accident prevention
Advocacy
Client rights
Confidentiality
Consultation with members of the health care team
Establishing priorities
Ethical practice
Legal responsibilities
Referrals
Respect for client and family needs on the basis of their preferences

Health Promotion and Maintenance

Aging process
Client and family teaching
Developmental stages and transition
Expected body image changes
Family planning and family systems
Growth and development
Health and wellness
Health care beliefs and preferences
Lifestyle choices

Psychosocial Integrity

Abuse and neglect
Adjustment to potential deterioration in physical and mental health and well-being in the older client
Changes and adjustment in role function in the older client (threat to independent functioning)
Coping mechanisms
Grief and loss issues with the older client

Loss of quantity and quality of relationships with the older client
Sensory and perceptual alterations
Support systems
Use of resources for the client and family

Physiological Integrity

Alterations in body systems and the related risks from the aging process
Basic care and comfort needs
Health care preferences
Interventions compatible with client's age, cultural, religious, and health care beliefs, education level, and language.
Practices or restrictions related to procedures and treatments
Providing care using a nonjudgmental approach
Safe medication administration

REFERENCES

Christensen, B., & Kockrow, E. (2003). *Foundations of nursing* (4th ed.). St. Louis: Mosby.

Linton, A., & Maebius, N. (2003). *Introduction to medical-surgical nursing* (3rd ed.). Philadelphia: W.B. Saunders.

Lowdermilk, D., & Perry, S. (2003). *Maternity nursing* (6th ed.) St. Louis: Mosby.

McKinney, E., James, S., Murray, S., & Ashwill, J. (2005). *Maternal-child nursing* (2nd ed.). St. Louis: Elsevier.

National Council of State Boards of Nursing. (2005). *Detailed test plan for the National council licensure examination for practical/vocational nurses.* Chicago: Author.

Potter, P., & Perry, A. (2005). *Fundamentals of nursing* (6th ed.). St. Louis: Mosby.

Price, D., & Gwin, J. (2005). *Thompson's pediatric nursing* (9th ed.). Philadelphia: W.B. Saunders.

Wold, G. (2004). *Basic geriatric nursing* (3rd ed.). St. Louis: Mosby.

Theories of Growth and Development

I. PSYCHOSOCIAL DEVELOPMENT AND ERIK ERIKSON

A. The theory
1. Describes the human life cycle as a series of eight **ego** developmental stages from birth to death
2. Each stage presents a psychosocial crisis, the goal of which is to integrate physical, maturation, and societal demands
3. Focuses on psychosocial tasks that are accomplished throughout the life cycle
4. The **ego** is separate and liberated from the **id**, developing across the course of the complete life cycle
5. **Ego** development is influenced by family, social, and developmental factors

B. Psychosocial development
1. A lifelong series of conflicts affected by social and cultural factors
2. Each conflict must be resolved for the child or adult to progress emotionally
3. Unsuccessful resolution leaves the individual emotionally handicapped

C. Stages of psychosocial development (Table 27-1)

II. COGNITIVE DEVELOPMENT AND JEAN PIAGET

A. The theory
1. Defines cognitive acts as ways in which the mind organizes and adapts to its environment
2. **Schema:** Refers to an individual's cognitive structure or framework of thought
3. **Schemata**
   a. Categories that an individual forms in his or her mind to organize and understand the world
   b. A young child has only a few **schemata** with which to understand the world, and gradually these are increased

c. Adults use a wide variety of **schemata** to understand the world
4. **Assimilation**
   a. The ability to incorporate new ideas, objects, and experiences into the framework of one's thoughts
   b. The growing child will perceive and give meaning to new information according to what is already known and understood
5. **Accommodation**
   a. The ability to change a **schema** in order to introduce new ideas, objects, or experiences
   b. Changes the mental structure so that new experiences can be added

B. Stages of cognitive development
1. Sensorimotor stage
   a. 0 to 2 years
   b. Development proceeds from reflex activity to imagining and solving problems through the senses and movement
2. Preoperational stage
   a. 2 to 7 years
   b. Learning to think in terms of past, present, and future
   c. The child moves from knowing the world through sensation and movement to prelogical thinking and finding solutions to problems
3. Concrete operational
   a. 7 to 11 years
   b. Able to classify, order, and sort facts
   c. The child moves from prelogical thought to solving concrete problems through logic
4. Formal operations
   a. 11 years to adulthood
   b. Able to think abstractly and logically
   c. Logical thinking is expanded to include solving abstract and concrete problems

TABLE 27-1

Erik Erikson's Stages of Psychosocial Development

Age	Psychosocial Crisis	Task
Infancy (0-18 months)	Trust vs. mistrust	Attachment to the mother

Resolution of Crisis
Trust in people; faith and hope about the environment and the future
Unsuccessful Resolution of Crisis
General difficulties relating to people effectively; suspicion; trust-fear conflict, fear of the future

Age	Psychosocial Crisis	Task
Early childhood (18 months to 3 years)	Autonomy vs. shame and doubt	Gaining some basic control over self and environment

Resolution of Crisis
Sense of self-control and adequacy; will power
Unsuccessful Resolution of Crisis
Independence-fear conflict; severe feelings of self-doubt

Age	Psychosocial Crisis	Task
Late childhood (3-6 years)	Initiative vs. guilt	Becoming purposeful and directive

Resolution of Crisis
Ability to initiate one's own activities; sense of purpose
Unsuccessful Resolution of Crisis
Aggression-fear conflict; sense of inadequacy or guilt

Age	Psychosocial Crisis	Task
School age (6-12 years)	Industry vs. inferiority	Developing social, physical, and school skills

Resolution of Crisis
Competence; ability to learn and work
Unsuccessful Resolution of Crisis
Sense of inferiority; difficulty learning and working

Age	Psychosocial Crisis	Task
Adolescence (12-20 years)	Identity vs. role confusion	Developing sense of identity

Resolution of Crisis
Sense of personal identity
Unsuccessful Resolution of Crisis
Confusion about who one is; identity submerged in relationships or group memberships

Age	Psychosocial Crisis	Task
Early adulthood (20-35 years)	Intimacy vs. isolation	Establishing intimate bonds of love and friendship

Resolution of Crisis
Ability to love deeply and commit oneself
Unsuccessful Resolution of Crisis
Emotional isolation, egocentricity

Age	Psychosocial Crisis	Task
Middle adulthood (35-65 years)	Generativity vs. stagnation	Fulfilling life goals that involve family, career, and society

Resolution of Crisis
Ability to give and care for others
Unsuccessful Resolution of Crisis
Self-absorption; inability to grow as a person

Age	Psychosocial Crisis	Task
Later (65 years to death)	Integrity vs. despair	Looking back over one's life and accepting its meaning

Resolution of Crisis
Sense of integrity and fulfillment
Unsuccessful Resolution of Crisis
Dissatisfaction with life

Modified from Varcarolis, E.M. (2002). *Foundations of psychiatric mental health nursing* (4th ed.). Philadelphia: W.B. Saunders, p. 30.

III. MORAL DEVELOPMENT AND LAWRENCE KOHLBERG

A. Moral development
1. A complicated process involving the acceptance of the values and rules of society in a way that shapes behavior
2. Classified into a series of levels and behaviors

B. Levels of moral development (Box 27-1)

IV. PSYCHOSEXUAL DEVELOPMENT AND SIGMUND FREUD

A. Components of the theory (Box 27-2)
1. Levels of awareness
2. Agencies of the mind (**id, ego, superego**)
3. Concept of anxiety and defense mechanisms
4. Psychosexual stages of development

B. Levels of awareness

BOX 27-1

Moral Development and Lawrence Kohlberg

LEVEL ONE: PRECONVENTIONAL

Stage 0 (0-2 years)

The infant has no awareness of right or wrong.

Stage 1 (2-3 years)

At this stage, children cannot reason as mature members of society.

Children view the world in a selfish way, with no real understanding of right or wrong.

The child obeys rules and demonstrates acceptable behavior to avoid punishment and displeasing those who are in power, and because he or she fears punishment from a superior force, such as a parent.

A toddler typically is at the first substage of the preconventional stage, involving punishment and obedience orientation, in which the toddler makes judgments on the basis of avoiding punishment or obtaining a reward.

Physical punishment and withholding privileges tend to give the toddler a negative view of morals.

Withdrawing love and affection as punishment leads to feelings of guilt in the toddler.

Appropriate discipline includes providing simple explanations why certain behaviors are unacceptable, praising appropriate behavior, and using distractions when the toddler is headed for danger.

Stage 2 (4-7 years)

The child conforms to rules to obtain rewards or have favors returned.

The child's moral standards are those of others, and the child's observes them to avoid punishment or obtain rewards.

A preschooler is in the preconventional stage of moral development.

In this stage, conscience emerges and the emphasis is on external control.

LEVEL TWO: CONVENTIONAL

The child conforms to rules to please others.

The child has increased awareness of others' feelings.

A concern for social order begins to emerge.

A child views good behavior as that which those in authority will approve.

If the behavior is not acceptable, the child feels guilty.

Stage 3 (7-10 years)

Conformity occurs to avoid disapproval or dislike by others.

This stage involves living up to what is expected by individuals close to the child or what individuals generally expect of others in their roles as son, brother, friend, and so on.

Being good is important and is interpreted as having good motives and showing concern about others.

It also means maintaining mutual relationships, such as trust, loyalty, respect, and gratitude.

Stage 4 (10-12 years)

The child has more concern with society as a whole.

Emphasis is on obeying laws to maintain social order.

Moral reasoning develops as the child shifts the focus of living to society.

The school-age child is at the conventional level of the role conformity stage and has an increased desire to please others.

The child observes and to some extent internalizes the standards of others.

The child wants to be considered "good" by those individuals whose opinions matter to him or her.

LEVEL THREE: POSTCONVENTIONAL

The individual focuses on individual rights and principles of conscience.

The focus is a concern regarding what is best for all.

Stage 5 (12 years and older)

The adolescent is aware that people hold a variety of values and opinions and that most values and rules are relative to the group.

The adolescent in this stage gives as well as takes, and does not expect to get something without paying for it.

Stage 6

Conformity is based on universal principles of justice and occurs to avoid self-condemnation.

This stage involves following self-chosen ethical principles.

The development of the postconventional level of morality occurs in the adolescent at about age 13 years, marked by the development of an individual conscience and a defined set of moral values.

The adolescent can now acknowledge a conflict between two socially accepted standards and try to decide between them.

Control of conduct is now internal, both in standards observed and in reasoning about right and wrong.

BOX 27-2

Psychosexual Development and Sigmund Freud: Components of the Theory

Levels of awareness
Agencies of the mind (id, ego, superego)
Concept of anxiety and defense mechanisms
Psychosexual stages of development

1. **Conscious** level of awareness
   a. The **conscious** mind is logical and is regulated by the Reality Principle
   b. Includes all experiences that are within an individual's awareness and that the individual is able to control
   c. Includes all information that is easily remembered and immediately available to an individual
2. Preconscious level of awareness
   a. Called the **subconscious**
   b. Includes experiences, thoughts, feelings, or desires that might not be in immediate awareness but can be recalled to consciousness
   c. The **subconscious** can help repress unpleasant thoughts or feelings and can examine and censor certain wishes and thinking
3. **Unconscious** level of awareness
   a. The **unconscious** is not logical and is governed by the Pleasure Principle, which refers to seeking immediate tension reduction
   b. Memories, feelings, thoughts, or wishes are repressed and are not available to the **conscious** mind
   c. These repressed memories, thoughts, or feelings, if made prematurely **conscious,** can cause anxiety
C. Agencies of the mind
   1. **Id, ego,** and **superego**
      a. The three systems of personality
      b. The psychological processes that follow different operating principles
      c. In a mature and well-adjusted personality, they work together as a team under the leadership of the ego
   2. The **id**
      a. Source of all drives
      b. Is present at birth
      c. Includes genetic inheritance, reflexes, capacities to respond, instincts, basic drives, needs, and wishes that motivate an individual
      d. It operates according to the Pleasure Principle
      e. The **id** does not tolerate uncomfortable states and seeks to discharge tension and return to a more comfortable, constant level of energy
      f. The **id** acts immediately in an impulsive, irrational way, pays no attention to the consequences of its actions, and therefore often behaves in ways harmful to self and others

   g. The "primary" process is a psychological activity in which the **id** attempts to reduce tension
   h. The "primary" process can include hallucinating or forming an image of the object that will satisfy its needs and remove the tension
   i. The "primary" process by itself is not capable of reducing tension; therefore, a "secondary" psychological process must develop if the individual is to survive; when this occurs, the structure of the second system of the personality, the **ego,** begins to take form
3. The **ego**
   a. The functions of the **ego** include reality testing and problem solving
   b. Begins its development during the fourth or fifth month of life
   c. The **ego** emerges out of the **id** and acts as an intermediary between the **id** and the external world
   d. Emerges because the needs, wishes, and demands of the **id** require appropriate exchanges with the outside world of reality
   e. Distinguishes between things in the mind and things in the external world
   f. Reality testing is a function of the **ego,** and the **ego** uses realistic thinking
   g. The **ego** follows the Reality Principle and operates by means of the "secondary" process—that is, realistic thinking
   h. The aim of the Reality Principle is to satisfy the **id's** impulses in the external world with an object that is suitable; the Reality Principle determines whether an experience is true or false and whether it has external existence or not
   i. The **ego** devises a plan and tests the plan by some kind of action to see if it will work
4. The **superego**
   a. A necessary part of socialization that develops during the phallic stage of 3 to 6 years of age
   b. It develops from the interactions with one's parents during the extended period of childhood dependency
   c. It includes the internalization of the values, ideals, and moral standards of society
   d. The child internalizes the moral standards of parents and society
   e. The **superego** consists of the **conscience** and the **ego** ideal
   f. The **conscience** refers to the capacity for self-evaluation and criticism
   g. When moral codes are violated, the **conscience** punishes the individual by instilling guilt
   h. What parents approve of, and what they reward the child for doing, become incorporated as the **ego** ideal by the mechanism of introjection

---

BOX 27-3

Freud's Psychosexual Stages of Development

ORAL STAGE (0-1 YEARS)

During this stage, the infant is concerned with his or her own gratification.

The infant is all id, operating on the Pleasure Principle and striving for immediate gratification of needs.

When the infant experiences gratification of basic needs, a sense of trust and security begins.

The ego begins to emerge as the infant begins to see self as separate from the mother; this marks the beginning of the development of a sense of self.

ANAL STAGE (1-3 YEARS)

Toilet training occurs during this period, and the child gains pleasure both from the elimination of the feces and from their retention.

The conflict of this stage is between demands from society and parents and the sensations of pleasure associated with the anus.

The child begins to gain a sense of control over instinctive drives and learns to delay immediate gratification to gain a future goal.

PHALLIC STAGE (3-6 YEARS)

The child experiences both pleasurable and conflicting feelings associated with the genital organs.

The pleasures of masturbation and the fantasy life of children set the stage for the Oedipus complex.

The child's unconscious sexual attraction to and wish to possess the parent of the opposite sex, the hostility and desire to remove the parent of the same sex, and the subsequent guilt for these wishes comprise the conflict the child faces.

The conflict is resolved when the child identifies with the parent of the same sex.

The emergence of the superego is both the solution to and the result of these intense impulses.

LATENCY STAGE (6-12 YEARS)

During this stage, there is a tapering off of conscious biological and sexual urges.

The sexual impulses are channeled and elevated into a more culturally accepted level of activity.

Growth of ego functions and the ability to care about and relate to others outside the home are the tasks of this stage of development.

GENITAL STAGE (12 YEARS AND BEYOND)

This emerges at adolescence with the onset of puberty, when the genital organs mature.

The individual gains gratification from his or her own body.

During this stage, the individual develops satisfying sexual and emotional relationships with members of the opposite sex.

The individual plans life goals and gains a strong sense of personal identity.

---

     i. The **superego** strives for perfection rather than pleasure and represents the ideal rather than the real

     j. Living up to one's **ego** ideal results in the individual feeling proud and increases self-esteem

D. Anxiety and defense mechanisms

    1. The **ego** develops defenses or defense mechanisms to fight off anxiety

    2. Defense mechanisms operate on an **unconscious** level, except for suppression, so the individual is not aware of their operation

    3. Defense mechanisms deny, falsify, or distort reality to make it less threatening

    4. An individual cannot survive without defense mechanisms; however, if they become too extreme in distorting reality, then interference in healthy adjustment and personal growth may occur

E. Psychosexual stages of development (Box 27-3)

    1. Human development proceeds through a series of stages from infancy to adulthood

    2. Each stage is characterized by the inborn tendency of all individuals to reduce tension and seek pleasure

    3. Each stage is associated with a particular conflict that must be resolved before the child can move successfully to the next stage

    4. Experiences during the early stages determine an individual's adjustment patterns and the personality traits that the individual has as an adult

PRACTICE QUESTIONS

1. A nurse is reinforcing instructions to a new mother regarding the psychosocial development of the infant. Using Erikson's psychosocial development theory, the nurse would instruct the mother to:

  1. Allow the infant to signal a need

  2. Anticipate all of the needs of the infant

  3. Avoid the infant during the first 10 minutes of crying

  4. Attend to the infant immediately when crying

2. A mother of a 3-year-old tells the nurse that the child is constantly rebelling and having temper tantrums. The appropriate instruction to the mother is to:

  1. Punish the child every time the child says "no," to change the behavior

  2. Allow the behavior, because this is normal at this age period

  3. Set limits on the child's behavior

  4. Ignore the child when this behavior occurs

3. A nurse employed in long-term care facility is caring for a 70-year-old woman. The client reminisces about

past life experiences in a positive way. The nurse interprets this behavior as:

1. A normal psychosocial response
2. Requiring a psychiatric consultation
3. A mental status alteration
4. A sensory deficit requiring social activities

4. A mother of an 8-year-old child tells the nurse that she is concerned about the child because the child seems to be more attentive to friends than anything else. The appropriate nursing response would be which of the following?

1. "You need to be concerned."
2. "You need to monitor the child's behavior closely."
3. "At this age, the child is developing his or her own personality."
4. "You need to provide more praise to the child to stop this behavior."

5. A mother of a 4-year-old child tells the nurse that she is concerned because the child has been masturbating. The appropriate response by the nurse is which of the following?

1. "The child is very young to begin this behavior and should be brought to the mental health clinic."
2. "This is not normal behavior and the child should be brought to the mental health clinic."
3. "This is a normal behavior at this age."
4. "Children usually begin this behavior at age 8 years."

6. A nursing instructor asks a nursing student to present a clinical conference to peers regarding Freud's psychosexual stages of development, specifically the anal stage. The nursing student prepares for the conference knowing that which of the following appropriately relates to this stage of development?

1. This stage is associated with toilet training
2. This stage is associated with pleasurable and conflicting feelings about the genital organs
3. This stage is characterized by a tapering off of conscious biological and sexual urges
4. This stage is characterized by the gratification of self

7. A mother of a 5-year-old child tells the nurse that the child scolds the floor or table if the child hurts herself on the object. According to Piaget's theory of cognitive development, this behavior is identified as:

1. Object permanence
2. Egocentric speech

3. Animism
4. Global organization

8. A nursing instructor asks a nursing student to describe the formal operations stage of Piaget's cognitive developmental theory. The appropriate response by the nursing student is:

1. "The child has the ability to think abstractly."
2. "The child develops logical thought patterns."
3. "The child has difficulty separating fantasy from reality."
4. "The child begins to understand the environment."

9. According to Kohlberg's theory of moral development, in the preconventional level, moral development is thought to be motivated by which of the following?

1. The parents' behavior
2. Peer pressure
3. Social pressures
4. Punishment and reward

10. A nursing instructor asks a nursing student about Kohlberg's theory of moral development. The instructor determines that the student needs to further research this theory if the student states that a component of the theory includes which of the following?

1. Moral development progresses in relationship to cognitive development
2. Individuals move through all six stages in a sequential fashion
3. It provides a framework for understanding how individuals determine a moral code to guide their behavior
4. A person's ability to make moral judgments develops over a period of time

ALTERNATE FORMAT QUESTION: PRIORITIZING (ORDERED RESPONSE)

Freud's psychosocial stages of human development proceed through a series of stages from infancy to adulthood. List the stages in order, as they proceed from infancy to adulthood. (Number 1 would indicate the stage that occurs at infancy.)

___ Latency stage
___ Anal stage
___ Oral stage
___ Phallic stage
___ Genital stage

ANSWERS

1. *Answer*: 1

Rationale: According to Erikson, the caregiver should not try to anticipate the infant's needs at all times but must allow the infant to signal needs. If an infant is not allowed to signal a need, he or she will not learn how to control the environment. Erikson believed that a delayed or prolonged response to an infant's signal would inhibit the development of trust and lead to mistrust of others.

Test-Taking Strategy: Use the process of elimination. Eliminate options 3 and 4 first because of the words "avoid" and "immediately." Additionally, option 2 can be eliminated because of the absolute word "all." Review Erikson's psychosocial development theory if you had difficulty with this question.

Level of Cognitive Ability: Application

Client Needs: Psychosocial Integrity

Integrated Process: Teaching/Learning

Content Area: Child Health

References: Leifer, G., & Hartston, H. (2004). *Growth and development.* Philadelphia: Elsevier, pp. 54-55.

McKinney, E., James, S., Murray, S., & Ashwill, J. (2005). *Maternal-child nursing* (2nd ed.). St. Louis: Elsevier, p. 59.

2. *Answer*: 3

Rationale: According to Erikson, the child focuses on independence between ages 1 and 3 years. Gaining independence often means that the child has to rebel against the parents' wishes. Saying things like "no" or "mine" and having temper tantrums are common during this period of development. Being consistent and setting limits on the child's behavior are necessary elements.

Test-Taking Strategy: Use the process of elimination. Options 2 and 4 can be eliminated first because they are similar. Eliminate option 1 next because this action is likely to produce a negative response during this normal developmental pattern. Review psychosocial development of the toddler according to Erikson if you had difficulty with this question.

Level of Cognitive Ability: Application

Client Needs: Psychosocial Integrity

Integrated Process: Nursing Process/Implementation

Content Area: Child Health

Reference: Leifer, G. (2003). *Introduction to maternity and pediatric nursing* (4th ed.). Philadelphia: W.B. Saunders, pp. 364-365.

3. *Answer*: 1

Rationale: According to Erikson, the later years are 65 years of age to death. The adult reminisces about past life experiences, viewing them in a positive way. The adult needs to feel good about accomplishments, see successes in life, and feel that he or she has made a contribution to society.

Test-Taking Strategy: Use knowledge regarding Erikson's theory of psychosocial development of late adulthood to answer the question. Note the similarity in options 2, 3, and 4. This will direct you to option 1. Review psychosocial development if you had difficulty with this question.

Level of Cognitive Ability: Comprehension

Client Needs: Psychosocial Integrity

Integrated Process: Nursing Process/Data Collection

Content Area: Fundamental Skills

Reference: Leifer, G., & Hartston, H. (2004). *Growth and development.* Philadelphia: Elsevier, p. 55.

4. *Answer*: 3

Rationale: According to Erikson, during ages 7 to 12 years, the child begins to move for support toward peers and friends and away from the parents. The child also begins to develop special interests that reflect his or her own developing personality instead of the parents.

Test-Taking Strategy: Use Erikson's psychosocial development theory related to school-age children to assist in eliminating options 1 and 2. Eliminate option 4 next because, although praising the child for accomplishments is important at this age, the behavior that the child is exhibiting is normal. Review Erikson's psychosocial development theory if you had difficulty with this question.

Level of Cognitive Ability: Application

Client Needs: Psychosocial Integrity

Integrated Process: Caring

Content Area: Child Health

Reference: Leifer, G. (2003). *Introduction to maternity and pediatric nursing* (4th ed.). Philadelphia: W.B. Saunders, p. 364.

5. *Answer*: 3

Rationale: According to Freud's psychosexual stages of development, the child is in the phallic stage between the ages of 3 and 6 years. At this time, the child devotes much energy to examining his or her genitalia, masturbating, and expressing interest in sexual concerns.

Test-Taking Strategy: Use the process of elimination. Eliminate options 1 and 2 because they are similar. From the remaining options, use Freud's psychosexual stages of development to direct you to option 3. If you had difficulty with this question, review Freud's psychosocial stages of development.

Level of Cognitive Ability: Application

Client Needs: Psychosocial Integrity

Integrated Process: Nursing Process/Implementation

Content Area: Child Health

Reference: Leifer, G. (2003). *Introduction to maternity and pediatric nursing* (4th ed.). Philadelphia: W.B. Saunders, pp. 364, 426.

6. *Answer*: 1

Rationale: Generally, toilet training occurs during this period. According to Freud, the child gains pleasure both from the elimination of feces and from their retention. Option 2 relates to the phallic stage. Option 3 relates to the latency period. Option 4 relates to the oral stage.

Test-Taking Strategy: Use the process of elimination. Note the relationship between the words "anal" in the question and "toilet training" in the correct option. If you had difficulty with this question, review Freud's psychosocial stages of development.

Level of Cognitive Ability: Comprehension

Client Needs: Psychosocial Integrity

Integrated Process: Nursing Process/Planning

Content Area: Child Health

Reference: McKinney, E., James, S., Murray, S., & Ashwill, J. (2005). *Maternal-child nursing* (2nd ed.). St. Louis: Elsevier, pp. 59-60, 122-123.

7. *Answer:* **3**

Rationale: Animism means that all inanimate objects are given living meaning. Object permanence, the realization that something out of sight still exists, occurs in the later stages of the sensorimotor stage of development. Egocentric speech occurs when the child talks just for fun and cannot see another's point of view. Global organization means that if any part of an object or situation changes, the whole thing has changed. Options 2 and 4 occur during the preoperational stage.

Test-Taking Strategy: Use the process of elimination. Make a relationship with the behavior identified in the question and the correct option. This will direct you to option 3. If you had difficulty with this question, review the concepts of Piaget's theory of cognitive development.

Level of Cognitive Ability: Comprehension
Client Needs: Psychosocial Integrity
Integrated Process: Nursing Process/Data Collection
Content Area: Child Health
Reference: Leifer, G. (2003). *Introduction to maternity and pediatric nursing* (4th ed.). Philadelphia: W.B. Saunders, p. 423.

8. *Answer:* **1**

Rationale: In the formal operation stage, the child has the ability the think abstractly and solve problems. Option 2 identifies the concrete operations stage. Option 3 identifies the preoperational stage. Option 4 identifies the sensorimotor stage.

Test-Taking Strategy: Knowledge regarding the characteristics of Piaget's cognitive developmental theory is required to answer this question. Remember, in the formal operation stage, the child has the ability to think abstractly and solve problems. If you had difficulty with this question, review these concepts.

Level of Cognitive Ability: Comprehension
Client Needs: Psychosocial Integrity
Integrated Process: Teaching/Learning
Content Area: Child Health
Reference: Leifer, G. (2003). *Introduction to maternity and pediatric nursing* (4th ed.). Philadelphia: W.B. Saunders, p. 364.

9. *Answer:* **4**

Rationale: In the preconventional stage, morals are thought to be motivated by punishment and reward. If the child is obedient and is not punished, then he or she is being moral. The child sees actions as either good or bad. If the child's actions are good, the child is praised. If the child's actions are bad, the child is punished.

Test-Taking Strategy: Use the process of elimination. Eliminate options 2 and 3 because they are similar. Knowledge that the preconventional stage occurs between the ages of 2 and 7 years will assist in directing you to option 4. If you had difficulty with this question, review Kohlberg's theory of moral development.

Level of Cognitive Ability: Comprehension
Client Needs: Psychosocial Integrity
Integrated Process: Nursing Process/Data Collection
Content Area: Child Health
Reference: Leifer, G. (2003). *Introduction to maternity and pediatric nursing* (4th ed.). Philadelphia: W.B. Saunders, p. 364.

10. *Answer:* **2**

Rationale: Kohlberg's theory states that individuals move through the six stages of development in a sequential fashion but that not everyone reaches stages 5 and 6 in their development of personal morality. Options 1, 3, and 4 are correct statements regarding Kohlberg's theory.

Test-Taking Strategy: Note the key words, *needs to further research.* These words indicate a false response question and that you need to select the incorrect statement. Also, note the absolute word "all" in option 2. If you had difficulty with this question, review Kohlberg's theory.

Level of Cognitive Ability: Comprehension
Client Needs: Psychosocial Integrity
Integrated Process: Teaching/Learning
Content Area: Fundamental Skills
Reference: Leifer, G. (2003). *Introduction to maternity and pediatric nursing* (4th ed.). Philadelphia: W.B. Saunders, p. 364.

ALTERNATE FORMAT QUESTION: PRIORITIZING (ORDERED RESPONSE)

Answer: 42135

Rationale: According to Freud, human development proceeds through a series of stages from infancy to adulthood. Each stage is characterized by the inborn tendency of all individuals to reduce tension and seek pleasure and is associated with a particular conflict that must be resolved before the child can move successfully to the next stage. Experiences during the early stages determine an individual's adjustment patterns and the personality traits that the individual has as an adult. The oral stage occurs in infancy from 0 to 1 years of age; the anal stage, 1 to 3 years of age; the phallic stage, 3 to 6 years of age; latency stage, 6 to 12 years of age; and the genital stage, 12 years of age and beyond.

Test-Taking Strategy: Knowledge regarding Freud's psychosocial stages of development is needed to answer this question. Review these stages if you had difficulty with this question.

Level of Cognitive Ability: Comprehension
Client Needs: Psychosocial Integrity
Integrated Process: Nursing Process/Implementation
Content Area: Child Health
References: Leifer, G., & Hartston, H. (2004). *Growth and development*, Philadelphia: Elsevier, pp. 54-55.
McKinney, E., James, S., Murray, S., & Ashwill, J. (2005). *Maternal-child nursing* (2nd ed.). St. Louis: Elsevier, p. 59.

REFERENCES

Leifer, G. (2003). *Introduction to maternity and pediatric nursing* (4th ed.). Philadelphia: W.B. Saunders.

Leifer, G., & Hartston, H. (2004). *Growth and development.* Philadelphia: Elsevier.

McKinney, E., James, S., Murray, S., & Ashwill, J. (2005). *Maternal-child nursing* (2nd ed.). St. Louis: Elsevier.

Varcarolis, E.M. (2002). *Foundations of psychiatric mental health nursing* (4th ed.). Philadelphia: W.B. Saunders.

Developmental Stages

I. THE HOSPITALIZED INFANT AND TODDLER

A. Separation anxiety
1. Protest
   a. Cries, screams, searches for a parent; avoids and rejects contact with strangers
   b. Verbal attack on others
   c. Physical fighting; kicks, fights, hits, pinches
2. Despair
   a. Withdrawn, depressed, uninterested in the environment
   b. Loss of newly learned skills
3. Detachment
   a. Is uncommon; sometimes called denial
   b. Superficially, the toddler appears to have adjusted to the loss
   c. During this phase, the toddler again becomes more interested in the environment, plays with others, and seems to form new relationships; this behavior is a form of resignation and is not a sign of contentment
   d. The toddler detaches from the parents in an effort to escape the emotional pain of desiring the parent's presence
   e. The toddler copes by forming shallow relationships with others, becoming increasingly self-centered, and attaching primary importance to material objects
   f. This is the most serious phase because reversal of the potential adverse effects is less likely to occur once detachment is established; in most situations, the temporary separation imposed by hospitalization does not cause such prolonged parental absence that the toddler enters into detachment

B. Fear of injury and pain: Affected by previous experiences, separation from parents, and preparation for the experience

C. Loss of control
1. Hospitalization with its own set of rituals and routines can severely disrupt the life of a toddler
2. The lack of control is often exhibited in behaviors related to feeding, toileting, playing, and bedtime
3. The toddler may demonstrate regression

D. Interventions
1. Provide swaddling and soft talking to the infant
2. Provide opportunities for sucking and oral stimulation for the infant using a pacifier if the infant is not to receive anything by mouth
3. Provide stimulation, if appropriate, for the infant, using objects of contrasting colors and textures
4. Provide routines and rituals as close as possible to what the toddler is used to at home
5. Provide as many choices to the toddler as possible to provide some control
6. Approach the toddler with a positive attitude
7. Allow the toddler to express feelings of protest
8. Encourage the toddler to talk about parents or others in their lives
9. Accept regressive behavior without ridiculing the toddler
10. Provide the toddler with favorite and comforting objects
11. Allow the toddler as much mobility as possible
12. Anticipate temper tantrums from the toddler, and maintain a safe environment for physical acting out
13. Employ pain-reduction techniques as appropriate

II. THE HOSPITALIZED PRESCHOOLER

A. Separation anxiety
1. Generally less obvious and less serious than in the toddler
2. As stress increases, the preschooler's ability to separate from the parents decreases

3. Protest
   a. Less direct and aggressive than the toddler
   b. May displace feelings onto others
4. Despair
   a. Similar to the toddler
   b. Quietly withdrawn, depressed, uninterested in the environment
   c. Loss of newly learned skills
   d. The preschooler becomes generally uncooperative, refusing to eat or take medication
   e. The preschooler repeatedly asks when the parents will be visiting
5. Detachment: Similar to the toddler

B. Fear of injury and pain
   1. The preschooler has a general lack of understanding of body integrity
   2. Fears invasive procedures and mutilation
   3. Imagines things to be much worse than they are
   4. Preschoolers believe that they are ill because of something they did or thought

▲ C. Loss of control
   1. Likes familiar routines and rituals and may show regression if not allowed to maintain some control
   2. Has attained a good deal of independence and self-care at home and may expect that to continue in the hospital

▲ D. Interventions
   1. Provide a safe and secure environment
   2. Take time for communication
   3. Allow the preschooler to express anger
   4. Acknowledge fears and anxieties
   5. Accept regressive behavior; assist the preschooler in moving from regressive to appropriate behaviors according to age
   6. Encourage rooming-in or leave favorite toy
   7. Allow mobility, and provide play and diversional activities
   8. Place the preschooler with other children of the same age if possible
   9. Encourage the preschooler to be independent
   10. Explain procedures simply, on the preschooler's level
   ▲ 11. Avoid intrusive procedures when possible
   ▲ 12. Allow wearing of underpants

▲ **III. THE HOSPITALIZED SCHOOL-AGE CHILD**
A. Separation anxiety
   1. Accustomed to periods of separation from the parents, but as stressors are added, the separation becomes more difficult
   2. More concerned with missing school and the fear that their friends will forget them
   3. Usually do not see the stage of behavior of protest, despair, and detachment with school-age children
B. Fear of injury and pain
   1. Fear bodily injury and pain

2. Fear of illness itself, disability, death, and intrusive procedures in genital areas
3. Uncomfortable with any type of sexual examination
4. Groans or whines, holds rigidly still, communicates about pain

C. Loss of control
   1. Is usually highly social, independent, and involved with activities
   2. Seeks information and asks relevant questions about tests and procedures and the illness
   3. Associates his or her actions with the cause of the illness
   4. May feel helpless and dependent if physical limitations occur

D. Interventions
   1. Encourage rooming-in
   2. Focus on the school-age child's abilities and needs
   3. Encourage the school-age child to become involved with his or her own care
   4. Accept regression but encourage independence
   5. Provide choices to the school-age child
   6. Allow expression of feelings both verbally and nonverbally
   7. Acknowledge fears and concerns and allow for discussion
   8. Explain all procedures, using body diagrams or outlines
   9. Provide privacy
   10. Avoid intrusive procedures if possible
   11. Allow the school-age child to wear underpants
   12. Involve the school-age child in activities appropriate to developmental level and illness
   13. Encourage the school-age child to contact friends
   14. Provide for educational needs
   15. Employ appropriate interventions to relieve pain

IV. THE HOSPITALIZED ADOLESCENT
A. Separation anxiety
   1. Not sure whether they want their parents with them when they are hospitalized
   2. Separation from friends is a source of anxiety
   3. Become upset if friends go on with their lives, excluding them
B. Fear of injury and pain
   1. Fear of being different from others and their peers
   2. May give the impression that they are not afraid even though they are terrified
   3. Become guarded when any areas related to sexual development are examined
C. Loss of control
   1. Behaviors exhibited include anger, withdrawal, and uncooperativeness
   2. Seek help and then reject it
D. Interventions
   1. Encourage questions about appearance and effects of the illness on the future

2. Explore feelings about the hospital and the significance the illness might have for relationships
3. Encourage to wear own clothes and perform normal grooming
4. Allow favorite foods to be brought in to the hospital if possible
5. Provide privacy
6. Use body diagrams to prepare for procedures
7. Introduce to other adolescents in the nursing unit
8. Encourage maintaining contact with peer groups
9. Provide for educational needs
10. Identify formation of future plans
11. Help develop positive coping mechanisms

V. COMMUNICATION APPROACHES

A. General guidelines
   1. Allow the child to feel comfortable with the nurse
   2. Communicate through the use of objects
   3. Allow the child to express fears and concerns
   4. Speak clearly and in a quiet, unhurried voice
   5. Offer choices when possible
   6. Be honest with the child
   7. Set limits with the child as appropriate
B. Infant
   1. Infants respond to nonverbal communication behaviors of adults, such as holding, rocking, patting, and touching
   2. Use a slow approach and allow the infant to get to know the nurse
   3. Use a calm, soft, soothing voice
   4. Be responsive to cries
   5. Talk and read to infants
   6. Allow security objects such as blankets and pacifiers if the infant has them
C. Toddler
   1. Approach toddler cautiously
   2. Remember that toddlers accept verbal communications of others literally
   3. Learn the toddler's words for common items and use them in conversations
   4. Use short, concrete terms
   5. Prepare the toddler for procedures immediately before the event
   6. Repeat explanations and descriptions
   7. Use play for demonstrations
   8. Use visual aids such as picture books, puppets, and dolls
   9. Allow the toddler to handle the equipment or instruments; explain what the equipment or instrument does and how it feels
   10. Encourage the use of comfort objects
D. Preschooler
   1. Seek opportunities to offer choices
   2. Speak in simple sentences
   3. Be concise and limit the length of explanations
   4. Allow asking questions

5. Describe procedures as they are about to be performed
6. Use play to explain procedures and activities
7. Allow handling the equipment or instruments, which will ease fear and help answer questions
E. School-age child
   1. Establish limits
   2. Provide reassurance to help in alleviating fears and anxieties
   3. Engage in conversations that encourage thinking
   4. Use medical play techniques
   5. Use photographs, books, dolls, and videos to explain procedures
   6. Explain in clear terms
   7. Allow time for composure and privacy
F. Adolescent
   1. Remember that the adolescent may be preoccupied with body image
   2. Encourage and support independence
   3. Provide privacy
   4. Use photographs, books, and videos to explain procedures
   5. Engage in conversations about adolescent's interests
   6. Avoid becoming too abstract, too detailed, and too technical
   7. Avoid responding to less than desirable social behaviors by prying, confrontation, or judgmental attitudes

VI. DEVELOPMENTAL CHARACTERISTICS

A. Infant
   1. Physical
      a. Height increases by $3/4$ inch per month
      b. Weight is doubled at 5 to 6 months and tripled at 12 months
      c. At birth, head circumference is 2 to 3 cm greater than chest circumference
      d. By 1 to 2 years of age, head circumference and chest circumference are equal
      e. Anterior fontanel (soft and flat in a normal infant) closes at 12 to 18 months
      f. Posterior fontanel (soft and flat in a normal infant) closes by 2 to 3 months
      g. Ten upper and 10 lower deciduous teeth by $2^1/_2$ years of age
      h. Lower central incisors present by 6 to 8 months
      i. Sleeps most of the time
   2. Vital signs (Box 28-1)
   3. Nutrition
      a. The infant may breast-feed or bottle-feed, depending on the mother's choice
      b. Iron stores from birth are depleted by 4 months
      c. Human milk is the best food for infants under 6 months of age
      d. Infants should remain on human milk or iron-fortified formula for the first year of life

e. Whole milk should not be introduced to infants until after 1 year of age

f. Skim and low-fat milk should not be given, because the essential fatty acids are inadequate and the solute concentration of protein and electrolytes is too high

g. Fluoride supplementation may be needed at about 6 months of age, depending on the infant's intake of fluoridated tap water

h. Solid foods are introduced at 5 to 6 months of age; introduce solid foods one at a time, usually at intervals of 4 to 5 days, to identify food allergens

i. Sequence of introduction of solid foods is as follows: rice cereal; fruits and vegetables, starting with yellow and then green; meats; and then egg yolks, avoiding egg whites (introduce egg whites toward the end of the first year); cheese may be used as a substitute for meat and as a finger food

j. Avoid solid foods that place the infant at risk for choking, such as nuts, foods with seeds, raisins, popcorn, grapes, pieces of a hot dog

k. Avoid microwaving baby bottles and baby food

l. Never mix food and/or medications with formula

m. Avoid adding honey to formula, water, or other fluid to prevent botulism

n. Offer fruit juice from a cup (12 to 13 months) rather than a bottle to prevent nursing (bottle-mouth) caries

4. Skills (Box 28-2)
5. Play
   a. Solitary
   b. Birth to 3 months: Verbal, visual, and tactile stimuli
   c. 4 to 6 months: Initiates actions and recognizes new experiences
   d. 6 to 12 months: Aware of self, imitates, repeats pleasurable actions
   e. Enjoys soft stuffed animals, crib mobiles with contrasting colors, squeeze toys, rattles, musical toys, water toys during the bath, large picture books, and push toys after he or she begins to walk

---

BOX 28-1

Vital Signs: Newborn and 1-Year-Old Infant

NEWBORN
Temperature: Axillary, 97.7° to 99.5° F
Apical rate: 120-160 beats per minute (100 sleeping, 180 crying)
Respirations: 30-60 (average, 40 breaths per minute)
Blood pressure (BP): 73/55 mm Hg

1-YEAR-OLD INFANT
Temperature: Axillary, 96.8° to 99° F
Apical rate: 90 to 130 beats per minute
Respirations: 20 to 40 breaths per minute
BP: 90/56 mm Hg

BOX 28-2

Infant Skills

2-3 MONTHS
Smiles
Turns head side to side
Cries
Follows objects
Holds head in midline

4-5 MONTHS
Grasps objects
Switches objects from hands
Rolls over for the first time
Enjoys social interaction
Begins to show memory
Aware of unfamiliar surroundings

6-7 MONTHS
Creeps
Sits with support
Imitates
Exhibits fear of strangers
Holds arms out
Frequent mood swings
Waves bye-bye

8-9 MONTHS
Sits steadily unsupported
Crawls
May stand while holding on
Begin to stand without help

10-11 MONTHS
Can change from prone to sitting position
Walks while holding onto furniture
Stands securely
Entertains self for periods of time

12-13 MONTHS
Walks with one hand held
Can take a few steps without falling

14-15 MONTHS
Walks alone
Can crawl up stairs
Shows emotions such as anger and affection
Will explore away from mother in familiar surroundings

6. Safety
   a. Baby-proof home
   b. Infants who weigh up to 20 pounds should be restrained in a car seat (convertible restraint) in a semireclined, rear-facing position
   c. Rear-facing infant seats (convertible restraint) are not placed in the front seats of cars equipped with an air bag on the passenger side; the child could be seriously injured if the air bag is released, because rear-facing infant seats extend closer to the dashboard
   d. Guard infant when on bed or changing table
   e. Use gates to protect infant from stairs
   f. Never vigorously shake an infant
   g. Be sure that bath water is not hot; do not leave infant unattended in bath
   h. Do not hold infant while drinking or working near hot liquids
   i. Cool vaporizers should be used instead of steam vaporizers to prevent burn injuries
   j. Avoid offering food that is round and similar to the size of the airway to prevent choking
   k. Be sure toys have no small pieces
   l. Hanging toys or mobiles over the crib should be well out of reach to prevent strangulation
   m. Avoid placing large toys in the crib because an older infant may use them as steps to climb
   n. Cribs should be positioned away from curtains and blind cords
   o. Cover electrical outlets
   p. Remove hazardous objects from low, reachable places
   q. Remove chemicals, medications, poisons, and plants from infant's reach
   r. Keep the poison control number available
   s. The mother is instructed to contact the poison control center immediately in the event of a poisoning

B. Toddler
   1. Physical
      a. Height and weight increase in a steplike fashion, reflecting growth spurts and lags
      b. Head circumference increases about 1 inch between ages 1 and 2 years; thereafter, head circumference increases about $\frac{1}{2}$ inch per year until age 5 years
      c. Anterior fontanel closes between ages 12 and 18 months
      d. Weight gain is slower than in infancy; by age 2 years, the average weight is 27 pounds
      e. Normal height changes include a growth of about 3 inches per year; the average height of the toddler is 34 inches at age 2 years
      f. Lordosis (pot belly) is evident
      g. The toddler should see a dentist soon after the first teeth erupt, usually around 1 year of age;

fluoride supplements may be necessary if the water is not fluoridated
   h. A toddler should never be allowed to fall asleep with a bottle containing milk, juice, soda pop, or sweetened water because of the risk of nursing (bottle-mouth) caries
   i. Typically sleeps through the night; has one daytime nap, and discontinues the daytime nap at about age 3
   j. A consistent bedtime ritual helps prepare the toddler for sleep
   k. Security objects at bedtime may assist in sleep
   2. Vital signs (Box 28-3)
   3. Nutrition
      a. Most toddlers prefer to feed themselves
      b. The toddler generally does best by eating several small nutritious meals each day rather than three large meals
      c. Offer a limited number of foods at any one time
      d. Offer finger foods and avoid concentrated sweets and empty calories
      e. At risk for aspiration of small foods that are not easily chewed, such as nuts, foods with seeds, raisins, popcorn, grapes, pieces of a hot dog
      f. Physiological anorexia is normal, because of the alternating periods of fast and slow growth
      g. Sit the toddler in a high chair at the family table for meals
      h. Allow sufficient time to eat, but remove food when toddler begins playing with it
      i. The toddler drinks well from a cup held with both hands
      j. Avoid using food as a reward or punishment
   4. Skills
      a. The toddler begins to walks with one hand held by age 12 to 13 months
      b. Runs by age 2 years; walks backward and hops on one foot by age 3 years
      c. The toddler usually cannot alternate feet when climbing stairs
      d. The toddler begins to master fine motor skills for building, undressing, and drawing lines
      e. The young toddler often uses "no," even when he or she means "yes," to assert independence
      f. Begins to use short sentences and has a vocabulary of about 300 words by age 2 years
      g. Tends to ask many "why" questions

BOX 28-3

Toddler's Vital Signs

Temperature: Axillary, 97.5° to 98.6° F
Apical rate: 80 to 120 beats per minute
Respirations: 20 to 30 breaths per minute
Blood pressure: Average, 92/55 mm Hg

5. Bowel and bladder control
   a. Signs that a toddler is ready for toilet training (Box 28-4)
   b. Bowel control develops before bladder control
   c. By age 3 years, the toddler achieves fairly good bowel and bladder control
   d. The toddler may stay dry during the day, but may need a diaper at night until about age 4 years
6. Play
   a. The major socializing mechanism is parallel play, and therapeutic play can begin at this age
   b. Has a short attention span, causing the toddler to change toys often
   c. Explores body parts of self and others
   d. Typical toys include push-pull toys, blocks, sand, finger paints and bubbles, large balls, crayons, trucks and dolls, containers, Play-Doh, toy telephones, cloth books, wooden puzzles
7. Safety
   a. Toddlers are eager to explore the world around them
   b. The toddler should be supervised at play
   c. The toddler can be placed in an upright forward-facing position in a car seat (convertible restraint); the transition point for switching to a forward-facing position is defined by the manufacturer of the car seat but is generally at a body weight of at least 9 kg (20 pounds) and 1 year of age
   d. Convertible car safety seats are used until the child weighs at least 40 pounds
   e. Lock car doors
   f. Use back burners on the stove to prepare a meal, and turn pot handles inward and toward the middle of the stove
   g. Keep dangling cords from small appliances away from the toddler
   h. Place inaccessible locks on windows and doors, and keep furniture away from windows
   i. Secure screens on all windows
   j. Place gates at stairways
   k. Do not allow the toddler to sleep or play in an upper bunk bed
   l. Never leave the toddler alone near a bathtub, pail of water, swimming pool, or any other body of water
   m. Keep toilet lids closed
   n. Keep all medicines, poisons, household plants, and toxic products high and locked out of reach
   o. Keep the poison control number available
   p. The mother is instructed to contact the poison control center immediately in the event of a poisoning
C. Preschooler
   1. Physical
      a. Grows 2½ to 3 inches per year
      b. Average height is 37 inches at age 3, 40½ inches at age 4, and 43 inches at age 5
      c. Gains 5 pounds per year; average weight of 32 pounds at age 5
      d. Requires about 12 hours of sleep each day
      e. A security object and a nightlight help with sleeping
      f. At the beginning of the preschool period, the eruption of the deciduous (primary) teeth is complete
      g. Regular dental care is essential, and the preschooler requires assistance with brushing and flossing of teeth; fluoride supplements may be necessary if the water is not fluoridated
   2. Vital signs (Box 28-5)
   3. Nutrition
      a. Exhibits food fads and strong taste preferences
      b. By 5 years old, tends to focus on social aspects of eating, table conversations, manners, and willingness to try new foods
   4. Skills
      a. Has good posture
      b. Develops fine motor coordination
      c. Can hop, skip, and run more smoothly
      d. Athletic abilities begin to develop
      e. Demonstrates increased skills in balancing
      f. Alternates feet when climbing stairs
      g. Can tie shoelaces
      h. May talk continuously and ask many "why" questions
      i. Vocabulary increases to about 900 words by age 3 and 2100 words by age 5
      j. By age 3, usually talks in three- or four-word sentences and speaks in short phrases

---

BOX 28-4

Signs of Readiness for Toilet Training

Able to stay dry for 2 hours
Waking dry from a nap
Able to sit, squat, and walk
Able to remove clothing
Recognizes urge to defecate or urinate
Expresses willingness to please parent
Able to sit on toilet for 5 to 10 minutes without fussing or getting off

---

BOX 28-5

Preschooler's Vital Signs

Temperature: Axillary, 97.5° to 98.6° F
Apical rate: 70 to 110 beats per minute
Respirations: 16 to 22 breaths per minute
Blood pressure: Average, 95/57 mm Hg

k. By age 4, uses five- or six-word sentences and, by age 5, speaks in longer sentences that contain all parts of speech

l. Can be readily understood by others and can clearly understand what others are saying

5. Bowel and bladder control
    a. By age 4, the preschooler has daytime control of bowel and bladder but may experience bed-wetting accidents at night
    b. By age 5, the preschooler achieves both bowel and bladder control, although accidents may occur in stressful situations

6. Play
    a. Cooperative
    b. Imaginary playmates
    c. Likes to build and create things, and play is simple and imaginative
    d. Understands sharing and is able to interact with peers
    e. Requires regular socialization with age mates
    f. Play activities include a large space for running and jumping
    g. Likes dress-up clothes, paints, paper, and crayons for creative expressions
    h. Swimming and sports aid with growth and development
    i. Puzzles and toys aid with fine motor development

7. Safety
    a. Preschoolers are active and inquisitive
    b. Because of their magical thinking, they may believe that daring feats seen in cartoons are possible and they may attempt them
    c. Can learn simple safety practices because they can follow simple and verbal directions and their attention span is lengthened
    d. Once the child has outgrown the convertible restraint car safety seat (weighs more than 40 pounds), the preschooler should be placed and restrained in a booster seat (until the preschooler weighs at least 60 pounds, is 8 years old, or his or her head is higher than the vehicle's back seat)
    e. A universal child safety seat system (UCSSS) for automobiles provides a uniform anchorage in the rear seat of the vehicle for child safety seats; seat belts are not needed to anchor child safety seats
    f. Teach the preschooler basic safety rules to ensure safety when playing in a playground near swings and ladders
    g. Never allow the preschooler to play with matches or lighters
    h. The preschooler should be taught what to do in the event of a fire or if clothes catch fire; fire drills should be practiced with preschooler

i. Guns should be stored unloaded and secured under lock and key; the preschooler should be taught to leave an area immediately if a gun is seen, and to tell an adult

j. The preschooler should be taught never to point a toy gun at another person

k. Teach the preschooler that, if another person touches his or her body in an inappropriate way, to tell an adult

l. Teach the preschooler to avoid speaking to strangers and never to accept a ride, toys, or gifts from a stranger

m. Teach the preschooler his or her full name, address, parents' names, and telephone number

n. Teach the preschooler how to dial 911 in an emergency situation

o. Keep the poison control number available

p. The mother is instructed to contact the poison control center immediately in the event of a poisoning

D. School-age child
1. Physical
    a. Girls usually grow faster than boys
    b. Growth of about 2 inches per year between ages 6 and 12
    c. Height ranges from 45 inches at age 6 to 59 inches at age 12
    d. Weight gain of $4^1/_2$ to $6^1/_2$ pounds per year
    e. Average weight of 46 pounds at age 6 and 88 pounds at age 12
    f. The first permanent (secondary) teeth erupt around age 6, and deciduous teeth are gradually lost
    g. Regular dentist visits are necessary, and the school-age child needs to be supervised with brushing and flossing teeth; fluoride supplements may be necessary if the water is not fluoridated
    h. For school-age children with primary and permanent dentition, the best toothbrush is one with soft nylon bristles and an overall length of about 6 inches
    i. Sleep requirements range from 10 to 12 hours a night

2. Vital signs (Box 28-6)
3. Nutrition
    a. Increased growth needs
    b. Balanced diet from foods in MyPyramid (see Figure 12-1)
    c. May still be a picky eater, but willing to try new foods
4. Skills
    a. Refinement of fine motor skills
    b. Continued development of gross motor skills
    c. Increase in strength and endurance
5. Play
    a. Play is more competitive

BOX 28-6

School-age Child's Vital Signs

Temperature: Oral, 97.5° to 98.6° F
Apical rate: 60 to 100 beats per minute
Respirations: 16 to 20 breaths per minute
Blood pressure: Average, 107/64 mm Hg

BOX 28-7

Adolescent's Vital Signs

Temperature: Oral, 97.5° to 98.6° F
Apical rate: 55 to 90 beats per minute
Respirations: 12 to 20 breaths per minute
Blood pressure: Average, 121/70 mm Hg

b. Rules and rituals are important aspects of play and games
c. Enjoys drawing, collecting items, dolls, pets, guessing games, board games, listening to the radio, TV, reading, and videos and computer games
d. Participates in team sports
e. Participates in secret clubs, peer group activities, scout organizations

6. Safety
   a. Experiences less fear in play activities and frequently imitates real life by using tools and household items
   b. Car safety belts should be worn low on the hips; the shoulder belt is used only if it does not cross over the child's neck and face
   c. Major causes of injuries include bicycles, skateboards, and team sports as the child increases motor abilities and independence
   d. Children should always wear a helmet when riding a bike or using inline skates or skateboards
   e. Teach the school-age child water safety rules
   f. Instruct the school-age child to avoid teasing or playing roughly with animals
   g. Never allow the school-age child to play with matches or lighters
   h. The school-age child should be taught what to do in the event of a fire or if clothes catch fire; fire drills should be practiced with the school-age child
   i. Guns should be stored unloaded and secured under lock and key; the school-age child should be taught to leave an area immediately if a gun is seen, and to tell an adult
   j. Teach the school-age child that, if another person touches his or her body in an inappropriate way, to tell an adult
   k. Teach the school-age child to avoid speaking to strangers and never to accept a ride, toys, or gifts from a stranger
   l. Teach the school-age child traffic safety rules
   m. Teach the school-age child how to dial 911 in an emergency situation
   n. Keep the poison control number available
   o. The mother is instructed to contact the poison control center immediately in the event of a poisoning

E. Adolescent
   1. Physical
      a. Puberty: The maturational, hormonal, and growth process that occurs when the reproductive organs begin to function and the secondary sex characteristics develop
      b. Body mass increases to adult size
      c. Sebaceous and sweat glands become active and fully functional
      d. Body hair distribution occurs
      e. Increase in height, weight, breast development, and pelvic girth in girls
      f. Menstrual periods occur about $2^{1}/_{2}$ years after the onset of puberty
      g. In boys, an increase in height, weight, muscle mass, and penis and testicle size occurs
      h. Voice deepens in boys
      i. Normal weight gain during puberty: Girls gain 15 to 55 pounds and boys gain 15 to 65 pounds
      j. Careful brushing and care of the teeth are important, and many adolescents need to wear braces
      k. Sleep patterns include a tendency to stay up late; therefore, in an attempt to catch up on missed sleep, adolescents sleep late whenever possible; an overall average of 8 hours per night is recommended
   2. Vital signs (Box 28-7)
   3. Nutrition
      a. Teaching about the food guide MyPyramid is important (see Figure 12-1)
      b. Typically eat whenever they have a break in activities
      c. Calcium, zinc, iron, folic acid, and protein are especially important nutritional needs
      d. Tend to snack on empty calories
      e. Body image is very important
   4. Skills
      a. Gross and fine motor skills are well developed
      b. Strength and endurance increase
   5. Play
      a. Games and athletics are the most common forms of play
      b. Competition and strict rules are important
      c. Enjoy activities such as sports, videos, movies, reading, parties, dancing, hobbies,

computer games, music, and experimenting, such as with makeup, hairstyles, tattoos, and piercings

    d. Friends are important and adolescents like to gather in small groups

6. Safety

    a. Risk takers

    b. Have a natural urge to experiment and be independent

    c. Instruct in the dangers related to drugs, alcohol, cigarettes, caffeine, and suntanning

    d. Help to recognize that there are choices when difficult or potentially dangerous situations arise

    e. Advocate the use of seat belts

    f. Instruct in the consequences of injuries that motor vehicle crashes can cause

    g. Instruct in water safety and emphasize that they should enter the water feet first, as opposed to diving, especially when the depth of the water is unknown

    h. Instruct about the dangers associated with guns, violence, and gangs

    i. Instruct about the complications associated with body piercing, tattooing, and suntanning

    j. Discuss issues such as date rape, sexual relationships, and the transmission of sexually transmitted diseases (STDs)

F. Early adulthood

  1. Description: Period between the late teens and mid- to late 30s

  2. Physical changes

    a. Has completed physical growth by the age of 20

    b. Quite active

    c. Severe illnesses are less common than in older age groups

    d. Tend to ignore physical symptoms and postpone seeking health care

    e. Lifestyle habits such as smoking, stress, lack of exercise, poor personal hygiene, and family history of disease increase the risk of future illness

  3. Cognitive changes

    a. Rational thinking habits

    b. Conceptual, problem-solving, and motor skills increase

    c. Identifying preferred occupational areas

  4. Psychosocial changes

    a. Separate from their families of origin

    b. Give much attention to occupational and social pursuits to improve socioeconomic status

    c. Making decisions regarding career, marriage, and parenthood

    d. Need to adapt to new situations

  5. Sexuality

    a. Have the emotional maturity to develop mature sexual relationships

    b. At risk for sexually transmitted diseases

G. Middle adulthood

  1. Description: Period between the mid- to late 30s and the mid-60s

  2. Physical changes

    a. Occur between 40 and 65 years of age

    b. Individual becomes aware that changes in reproductive and physical abilities signify the beginning of another stage in life

    c. Menopause occurs in women and climacteric occurs in men

    d. Often, physiological changes have an impact on self-concept and body image

    e. Physiological concerns include stress, level of wellness, and the formation of positive health habits

  3. Cognitive changes

    a. May be interested in learning new skills

    b. May become involved in educational or vocational programs for entering the job market or for changing careers

  4. Psychosocial changes

    a. May include expected events, such as children moving away from home (postparental family stage), or unexpected events such as death of a close friend

    b. Time and financial demands decrease as children move away from home and the couple faces redefining their relationship

    c. May become grandparents

    d. Achieving generativity

  5. Sexuality

    a. Many couples renew their relationships and find increased marital and sexual satisfaction

    b. The onset of menopause and climacteric may affect sexual health

    c. Stress, health, and medications can affect sexuality

PRACTICE QUESTIONS

1. The parents of a 2-year-old arrive at the hospital to visit the child. The child is in the play room and ignores the parents during the visit. This 2-year-old behavior indicates:

  1. The child is withdrawn

  2. The child is more interested in playing with other children

  3. The child has adjusted to the hospitalized setting

  4. A normal pattern

2. The most appropriate toy to provide to a 3-year-old child is which of the following?

  1. A farm set

  2. A golf set

  3. A puzzle

  4. A wagon

3. A nurse reinforces instructions to the parents of a newborn infant regarding car travel and safety seats.

Which of the following is the correct information related to the safety of the infant?

1. Restrain in a car seat in the front seat in a semi-reclined, rear-facing position
2. Restrain in a car seat in the front seat in a semi-reclined, face-forward position
3. Restrain in a car seat in the back seat in a semi-reclined, rear-facing position
4. Restrain in a car seat in the back seat in a semi-reclined, face-forward position

4. A nurse is assigned to monitor a 3-month-old infant for increased intracranial pressure. On palpation of the fontanels, the nurse notes that the anterior fontanel has not closed and is soft and flat. Which of the following actions should the nurse take?
   1. Elevate the head of the bed to 90 degrees
   2. Notify the registered nurse (RN)
   3. Increase oral fluids
   4. Document the findings

5. A nurse is caring for a 5-year-old child who has been placed in traction following a fracture to the femur. Which of the following is the most appropriate activity for this child?
   1. Large picture books
   2. A radio
   3. A sports video
   4. Finger paints

6. The mother of a 16-year-old child tells the nurse that she is concerned because the child sleeps until noon every weekend, and whenever the child has a day off from school. The appropriate nursing response is which of the following?
   1. "The child should have a blood test to check for anemia."
   2. "Adolescents love to sleep late in the morning."
   3. "The child shouldn't be staying up so late at night."
   4. "If the child eats properly, that shouldn't be happening."

7. A 16-year-old child is admitted to the hospital for acute appendicitis and an appendectomy is performed. Which of the following interventions is most appropriate to facilitate normal growth and development?
   1. Allow the family to bring in favorite computer games
   2. Encourage the parents to room in with the child
   3. Encourage the child to rest and read
   4. Allow the child to participate in activities with other individuals in the same age group when the condition permits

8. A 2-year-old child is treated in the emergency room for a burn to the chest and abdomen. The child sustained the burn from grabbing a cup of hot coffee that was left on the kitchen counter. The nurse reinforces safety principles with the parents before discharge. Which statement, if made by the parents, indicates an understanding of the measures to provide safety in the home?
   1. "I guess my children need to understand what the word 'hot' means."
   2. "We will install a safety gate as soon as we get home so the children can't get into the kitchen."
   3. "We will be sure that the children stay in their rooms when we work in the kitchen."
   4. "We will be sure not to leave hot liquids unattended."

9. A mother of a 4-year-old child expresses concern because her hospitalized child has started sucking his thumb. The mother states that this behavior began 2 days after hospital admission. The most appropriate nursing response is which of the following?
   1. "A 4-year-old is too old for this type of behavior."
   2. "Your child is acting like a baby."
   3. "The doctor will need to notified."
   4. "It is best to ignore the behavior."

10. The mother of a toddler asks the nurse when it is safe to place the car safety seat in a face-forward position. The best nursing response is which of the following?
    1. Once the toddler weigh 20 pounds
    2. The seat should not be placed in a face-forward position unless there are safety locks in the car
    3. The seat should never be placed in a face-forward position because of the risk of the child unbuckling the harness
    4. When the toddler weighs 40 pounds

ALTERNATE FORMAT QUESTION: MULTIPLE RESPONSE

Select the interventions appropriate for the care of an infant.

___ Provide swaddling
___ Talk in a loud voice
___ Hang mobiles with black and white contrast designs
___ Allow the infant to cry for at least 10 minutes before responding
___ Caress infant while bathing and during diaper changes

ANSWERS

1. Answer: 4
Rationale: The toddler is particularly vulnerable to separation. A toddler often shows anger at being left by ignoring the parent or by pretending to be more interested in play than in going home. Parents of hospitalized toddlers are frequently distressed by such behavior. The toddler normally engages in parallel play and plays alongside, but not with, other children. Options 1, 2, and 3 are incorrect.
Test-Taking Strategy: Use concepts of growth and development. Option 3 can be easily eliminated first. There is no information in the question to support option 1. From the remaining options, knowledge regarding separation anxiety in the toddler will direct you to option 4. Review these concepts if you had difficulty with this question.
Level of Cognitive Ability: Comprehension
Client Needs: Psychosocial Integrity
Integrated Process: Nursing Process/Data Collection
Content Area: Child Health
Reference: Price, D., & Gwin, J. (2005). *Thompson's pediatric nursing* (9th ed.). Philadelphia: W.B. Saunders, pp. 169, 171.

2. Answer: 4
Rationale: Toys for the toddler must be strong, safe, and too large to swallow or place in the ear or nose. Toddlers need supervision at all times. Push-pull toys, large balls, coloring with large crayons, trucks, and dolls are some appropriate toys. A farm set and a golf set may contain items that the child could swallow. A puzzle with large pieces only may be appropriate.
Test-Taking Strategy: Use the process of elimination. Options 1 and 2 can be easily eliminated because they contain items that could be swallowed by the child. From the remaining options, the most appropriate toy is a wagon. Remember that large and strong toys are safest for the toddler. Review the safety measures for the toddler if you had difficulty with this question.
Level of Cognitive Ability: Comprehension
Client Needs: Safe, Effective Care Environment
Integrated Process: Nursing Process/Implementation
Content Area: Child Health
Reference: Price, D., & Gwin, J. (2005). *Thompson's pediatric nursing* (9th ed.). Philadelphia: W.B. Saunders, pp. 178-179.

3. Answer: 3
Rationale: The infant should be placed in a car safety seat restraint in the back seat of the car, in a rear-facing position, until the infant weighs 20 pounds. The infant should never be placed in a forward-facing position or in the front seat.
Test-Taking Strategy: Visualize each of the descriptions in the options with a focus of safety in mind. Use the process of elimination. Eliminate options 1 and 2 because of the words "front seat." Next, eliminate option 4 because of the words "face-forward." If you had difficulty with this question, review the car safety measures for the infant.
Level of Cognitive Ability: Application
Client Needs: Health Promotion and Maintenance
Integrated Process: Teaching/Learning
Content Area: Child Health
Reference: Leifer, G. (2003). *Introduction to maternity and pediatric nursing* (4th ed.). Philadelphia: W.B. Saunders, p. 402.

4. Answer: 4
Rationale: The anterior fontanel is diamond-shaped and located on the top of the head. It should be soft and flat in a normal infant, and it normally closes by 12 to 18 months of age. The posterior fontanel closes by 2 to 3 months of age. Therefore, because the findings are normal, the nurse would document the findings.
Test-Taking Strategy: Use the process of elimination. Note the key words, *soft and flat.* This should provide you with the clue that this is a normal finding. A bulging or tense fontanel may result from crying or increased intracranial pressure. Review normal findings in the infant if you had difficulty with this question.
Level of Cognitive Ability: Application
Client Needs: Physiological Integrity
Integrated Process: Nursing Process/Implementation
Content Area: Child Health
References: Leifer, G. (2003). *Introduction to maternity and pediatric nursing* (4th ed.). Philadelphia: W.B. Saunders, pp. 284-285.
Price, D., & Gwin, J. (2005). *Thompson's pediatric nursing* (9th ed.). Philadelphia: W.B. Saunders, p. 49.

5. Answer: 4
Rationale: In the preschooler, play is simple and imaginative, and includes activities such as dressing up, finger paints, clay, pasting, and simple board and card games. Large picture books are most appropriate for the infant. A radio and sports video are most appropriate for the adolescent.
Test-Taking Strategy: Note the age of the child and think about the age-related activity that would be most appropriate. Eliminate options 2 and 3, knowing that they are most appropriate for the adolescent. From the remaining options, the word "large" in option 1 should provide you with the clue that this activity would be more appropriate for a child younger than age 5. Review the appropriate activities for a preschooler if you had difficulty with this question.
Level of Cognitive Ability: Application
Client Needs: Psychosocial Integrity
Integrated Process: Nursing Process/Implementation
Content Area: Child Health
Reference: Price, D., & Gwin, J. (2005). *Thompson's pediatric nursing* (9th ed.). Philadelphia: W.B. Saunders, p. 222.

6. Answer: 2
Rationale: Sleep patterns in the adolescent vary according to individual need. Adolescents love to sleep late in the morning but they should be encouraged to be responsible for waking themselves, particularly in time to get ready for school. Options 1, 3, and 4 are incorrect.
Test-Taking Strategy: Use the process of elimination. Options 3 and 4 can be eliminated first because they are inappropriate responses. From the remaining options, there is no indication that a physiological alteration is present; therefore, option 2 is most appropriate. Review adolescent sleep patterns if you had difficulty with this question.
Level of Cognitive Ability: Application
Client Needs: Physiological Integrity
Integrated Process: Nursing Process/Implementation
Content Area: Child Health

Reference: Price, D., & Gwin, J. (2005). *Thompson's pediatric nursing* (9th ed.). Philadelphia: W.B. Saunders, 320.

7. *Answer:* **4**
Rationale: Adolescents often are not sure whether they want their parents with them when they are hospitalized. Because of the importance of the peer group, separation from friends is a source of anxiety. Ideally, the peer group will support their ill friend. Options 1, 2, and 3 isolate the child from the peer group.
Test-Taking Strategy: Consider the psychosocial needs of the adolescent when answering the question. Options 1, 2, and 3 are similar in that they isolate the child from their own peer group. Review the psychosocial needs of the adolescent if you had difficulty with this question.
Level of Cognitive Ability: Application
Client Needs: Psychosocial Integrity
Integrated Process: Nursing Process/Implementation
Content Area: Child Health
Reference: Price, D., & Gwin, J. (2005). *Thompson's pediatric nursing* (9th ed.). Philadelphia: W.B. Saunders, 314.

8. *Answer:* **4**
Rationale: Toddlers, with their increased mobility and developing of motor skills, can reach hot water, open fires, or hot objects placed on counters and stoves above their eye level. Parents should be encouraged to remain in the kitchen when preparing a meal and reminded to use the back burners on the stove; pot handles should be turned inward and toward the middle of the stove. Hot liquids should never be left unattended, and the toddler should always be supervised. Options 1, 2, and 3 do not reflect an adequate understanding of the principles of safety.
Test-Taking Strategy: Use the process of elimination. Option 1 can be easily eliminated. Option 2 and 3 are similar in that they isolate the child from the environment. Review safety principles for the toddler if you had difficulty with question.
Level of Cognitive Ability: Comprehension
Client Needs: Safe, Effective Care Environment
Integrated Process: Nursing Process/Evaluation
Content Area: Child Health
Reference: Price, D., & Gwin, J. (2005). *Thompson's pediatric nursing* (9th ed.). Philadelphia: W.B. Saunders, p. 181.

9. *Answer:* **4**
Rationale: In the hospitalized preschooler, it is best to accept regression if it occurs. Regression is most often due to the stress of the hospitalization. Parents may be overly concerned about regression and should be told that their child may continue the behavior at home. There is no need to call the physician. Options 1 and 2 are inappropriate.
Test-Taking Strategy: Use the process of elimination. Options 1, 2, and 3 will cause additional stress and concern in the parent. Review the psychosocial issues related to the hospitalized preschool child if you had difficulty with this question.
Level of Cognitive Ability: Application

Client Needs: Psychosocial Integrity
Integrated Process: Nursing Process/Implementation
Content Area: Child Health
Reference: Price, D., & Gwin, J. (2005). *Thompson's pediatric nursing* (9th ed.). Philadelphia: W.B. Saunders, p. 217.

10. *Answer:* **1**
Rationale: The transition point for switching to the forward-facing position is defined by the manufacturer of the car safety seat, but is generally at a body weight of 9 kg (20 pounds). The car safety seat should be used until the child weighs at least 40 pounds, regardless of age. Options 2, 3, and 4 are incorrect.
Test-Taking Strategy: Use the process of elimination and focus on the issue of the question. Eliminate options 2 and 3 first because of the absolute words "not" and "never." From the remaining options, use knowledge regarding car safety and the toddler to answer the question. Review these safety principles if you had difficulty with this question.
Level of Cognitive Ability: Application
Client Needs: Safe, Effective Care Environment
Integrated Process: Nursing Process/Implementation
Content Area: Child Health
Reference: Price, D., & Gwin, J. (2005). *Thompson's pediatric nursing* (9th ed.). Philadelphia: W.B. Saunders, p. 181.

ALTERNATE FORMAT QUESTION: MULTIPLE RESPONSE

Answers:
Provide swaddling
Hang mobiles with black and white contrast designs
Caress infant while bathing and during diaper changes
Rationale: Holding, caressing, and swaddling provides warmth and tactile stimulation for the infant. To provide auditory stimulation, the nurse should talk to the infant in a soft voice and should instruct the mother to do so also. Additional interventions include playing a music box, radio, or television, or having a ticking clock or metronome nearby. Hanging a bright shiny object within 20 to 25 cm of the infant's face and in midline, and hanging mobiles with contrasting colors, such as blank and white, provides visual stimulation. Crying is an infant's way of communicating; therefore, the nurse would respond to the infant's crying. The mother is taught to do so also.
Test-Taking Strategy: Focus on the issue, care of the infant. Noting the word "loud" and the words "at least 10 minutes before responding" will assist in eliminating these interventions. Review the guidelines related to the care of an infant if you had difficulty with this question.
Level of Cognitive Ability: Application
Client Needs: Psychosocial Integrity
Integrated Process: Nursing Process/Implementation
Content Area: Child Health
Reference: Lowdermilk, D., & Perry, S. (2003). *Maternity nursing* (6th ed.). St. Louis: Mosby, pp. 430, 433.

REFERENCES

Leifer, G. (2003). *Introduction to maternity and pediatric nursing* (4th ed.). Philadelphia: W.B. Saunders.

Leifer, G. (2005). *Maternity nursing* (9th ed.). Philadelphia: W.B. Saunders.

Lowdermilk, D., & Perry, S. (2003). *Maternity nursing* (6th ed.). St. Louis: Mosby.

Price, D., & Gwin, J. (2005). *Thompson's pediatric nursing* (9th ed.). Philadelphia: W.B. Saunders.

Care of the Older Client

I. PHYSIOLOGICAL CHANGES

A. Integumentary system
1. Loss of pigment in hair and skin
2. Wrinkling of the skin
3. Thinning of the epidermis and easy bruising and tearing of the skin
4. Decreased skin turgor, elasticity, and subcutaneous fat
5. Increased nail thickness and decreased nail growth
6. Decreased perspiration
7. Dry, itchy, scaly skin
8. Seborrheic dermatitis and keratosis formation

B. Neurological system
1. Slowed reflexes
2. Slight tremors and difficulty with fine motor movement
3. Loss of balance
4. Experience an increased incidence of awakening after sleep onset
5. Increased susceptibility to hypothermia and hyperthermia
6. Short-term memory may decline
7. Long-term memory usually maintained

C. Musculoskeletal system
1. Muscle mass and strength decrease and muscles atrophy
2. Decreased mobility, range of motion, flexibility, coordination, and stability
3. Change of gait, with shortened step and wider base
4. Posture and stature changes causing a decrease in height
5. Increased brittleness of the bones
6. Joint capsule components deteriorate
7. Kyphosis of the dorsal spine

D. Cardiovascular system
1. Diminished energy and endurance, with lowered tolerance to exercise
2. Decreased compliance of the heart muscle, and heart valves become thicker and more rigid
3. Decreased cardiac output and decreased efficiency of blood return to the heart
4. Decreased resting heart rate
5. Weak peripheral pulses
6. Increased blood pressure but susceptible to postural hypotension

E. Respiratory system
1. Decreased stretch and compliance of the chest wall
2. Decreased strength and function of respiratory muscles
3. Decreased size and number of alveoli
4. Increased rate of respirations, generally 16 to 25 breaths per minute
5. Decreased depth of respirations and oxygen intake
6. Decreased ability to cough and expectorate sputum

F. Hematological system
1. Hemoglobin and hematocrit levels average toward the low end of normal
2. Prone to increased blood clotting

G. Immune system
1. Lymphocyte counts tend to be low
2. Decreased resistance to infection and disease

H. Gastrointestinal system
1. Decreased need for calories
2. Decreased appetite, thirst, and oral intake
3. Decreased lean body weight
4. Digestive disturbances
5. Decreased stomach-emptying time
6. Decreased absorption of carbohydrates, proteins, fats, and vitamins

7. Increased tendency toward constipation
8. Increased susceptibility for dehydration
9. Tooth loss
10. Difficulty in chewing and swallowing food
  I. Endocrine system
  1. Decreased secretion of hormones, with specific changes related to each hormone function
  2. Decreased metabolic rate
  3. Decreased glucose tolerance with resistance to insulin in peripheral tissues
  J. Renal system
  1. Decreased kidney size, function, and ability to concentrate urine
  2. Decreased glomerular filtration rate
  3. Decreased capacity of the bladder
  4. Increased residual urine and increased incidence of infection and incontinence
  5. Impaired medication excretion
  K. Reproductive system
  1. Decreased testosterone production and decreased size of testes
  2. Changes in the prostate gland leading to urinary problems
  3. Decreased secretion of hormones with the cessation of menses
  4. Vaginal changes, including decreased muscle tone and lubrication
  5. Impotence or sexual dysfunction for both sexes; sexual function varies and depends on general physical condition, mental health status, and medications
  L. Special senses
  1. Decreased visual acuity
  2. Decreased accommodation in eyes, requiring increased adjustment time to changes in light
  3. Decreased peripheral vision and increased sensitivity to glare
  4. Presbyopia and cataract formation
  5. Possible loss of hearing ability; low-pitched tones are more easily heard
  6. Inability to discern taste of food
  7. Decreased smell acuity
  8. Changes in touch sensation
  9. Decreased pain awareness

II. PSYCHOSOCIAL CONCERNS

A. Adjustment to deterioration in physical and mental health and well-being
B. Threat to independent functioning and fear of becoming a burden to loved ones
C. Adjustment to retirement and loss of income
D. Loss of skills and competencies developed early in life
E. Coping with changes in role function and social life
F. Diminished quantity and quality of relationships and coping with loss

G. Dependence on governmental and social systems
H. Access to social support systems
I. Costs of health care and medications

III. MENTAL HEALTH CONCERNS (Box 29-1)

A. Isolation: Client is alone and desires contact with others, but is unable to make that contact
B. Grief: Reaction to the client's perception of loss, including physical, psychological, social, and spiritual aspects
C. **Depression:** The increased dependency that older adults may experience can lead to hopelessness, helplessness, a lowered sense of self-control, and decreased self-esteem and self worth; these changes can interfere with daily functioning and lead to depression
D. Suicide: All suicide threats from an older client should be taken seriously

IV. PAIN

A. Description
  1. Pain can occur from numerous causes and most often occurs from degenerative changes in the musculoskeletal system
  2. The failure to alleviate pain in the older client can lead to functional limitations affecting their ability to function independently
B. Data collection
  1. Agitation
  2. Moaning
  3. Crying
  4. Restlessness
  5. Verbal reporting of pain
C. Interventions
  1. Monitor the client for signs of pain
  2. Identify the pattern of pain
  3. Identify the precipitating factor(s) for the pain
  4. Monitor the impact of the pain on activities of daily living
  5. Provide pain relief through measures such as distraction, relaxation, massage, biofeedback
  6. Administer pain medication as prescribed and instruct the client in their use
  7. Evaluate the effects of pain-reducing measures

BOX 29-1

Mental Health Concerns

Isolation
Grief
Depression
Suicide

V. MEDICATIONS

A. Major problems with prescriptive medications include adverse affects, medication interactions, medication errors, noncompliance, and the cost

B. Determine the use of over-the-counter medications

C. Keep the use of medications to a minimum

D. Medication dosages are normally prescribed at one third to one half of normal adult doses

E. Closely monitor for adverse effects and response to therapy because of the increased risk for medication toxicity

F. Note that a common sign of an adverse reaction in the older client in an acute change in mental status

G. Assess for medication interactions in client taking multiple medications

H. Advise the client to use one pharmacy and notify the consulting physicians of the medications taken

I. Administration of medications

1. Place the client in a sitting position when administering medication
2. Check for mouth dryness, because medication may stick and dissolve in mouth
3. Administer liquid preparations if the client has difficulty swallowing tablets
4. Crush tablets if necessary and give with textured food (nectar, applesauce) if not contraindicated
5. Do not crush enteric-coated tablets and do not open capsules
6. If administering a suppository, do not insert suppository immediately after removing from the refrigerator
7. A suppository may take longer to dissolve because of decreased body core temperature
8. When administering parenteral medication, monitor the site, because it may ooze medication or bleed as a result of decreased tissue elasticity
9. Do not use an immobile limb for administering parenteral medication
10. Monitor client compliance with taking prescribed medications
11. Monitor for safety in correctly taking medications
12. Use a medication cassette to facilitate proper administration of medication

VI. ABUSE OF THE OLDER ADULT

A. Involves physical, emotional, or sexual **abuse**; can also involve **neglect** or economic exploitation

B. Individuals at most risk include those who are dependent because of their immobility or altered mental status

C. Factors that contribute to **abuse** and **neglect** include long-standing family violence, caregiver stress, and the individual's increasing dependence on others

D. Victims may attempt to dismiss injuries as accidental, and abusers may prevent victims from receiving proper medical care to avoid discovery

E. Victims are often socially isolated by their abusers

F. For additional information on **abuse** of the older client, refer to Chapter 75

PRACTICE QUESTIONS

1. The nurse is assigned to care for an older client with hearing loss. The nurse plans care, knowing that older clients:
   1. Are often distracted
   2. Respond to low-pitched tones
   3. Have middle-ear changes
   4. Develop moist cerumen production

2. An older male client is admitted to the hospital with a diagnosis of malnutrition. The nurse is told that blood will be drawn to determine whether the client has a protein deficiency. Which of the following laboratory data indicates that the client is experiencing a protein deficiency?
   1. Creatinine, 0.6 mg/dL
   2. Transferrin, 90 mg/dL
   3. Calcium, 10 mg/dL
   4. Sodium, 138 mEq/L

3. The nurse is attending an educational session and the topic is abuse of the older client. The nurse understands that which client is most characteristic of a victim of abuse?
   1. A 90-year-old woman with advanced Parkinson's disease
   2. A 68-year-old man with newly diagnosed cataracts
   3. A 70-year-old woman with early diagnosed Lyme disease
   4. A 75-year-old man with moderate hypertension

4. An older female client confides to the visiting nurse that she is afraid she will fall while going to the bathroom at night. Which suggestion, if made by the nurse, indicates that the nurse understands the visual changes affecting the older client?
   1. "Use a bell to call your daughter if you need to get up."
   2. "Keep a red light on in the bathroom at night."
   3. "Use a commode in your bedroom at night."
   4. "Limit your fluid intake during the day."

5. A nurse is assigned to care for an older client. To reduce the risk of aspiration during meals, the nurse positions the client:
   1. Upright in a chair
   2. On the left side in bed
   3. In low Fowler's position, with the legs elevated
   4. On the right side in bed

6. The nurse who volunteers at a senior citizens' center is planning activities for the members who attend

the center. Which activity would best promote health and maintenance for these senior citizens?

1. Gardening every day for an hour
2. Cycling three times a week for 20 minutes
3. Sculpting once a week for 40 minutes
4. Walking three to five times a week for 30 minutes

7. The nurse is working with older clients in a long-term care facility. Which of the following activities performed by the nurse fosters reminiscence among these clients?

1. Displaying calendars and clocks
2. Encouraging client participation in pottery class
3. Setting up pet therapy sessions
4. Having story-telling hours

8. The nurse is performing an environmental assessment in the home of an older client. Which of the following, if observed by the nurse, requires immediate attention?

1. An operable smoke detector
2. A prefilled medication cassette
3. Unsecured scatter rugs
4. Clear exit passageways

9. The nurse is teaching an older client about measures to prevent constipation. Which statement, if made by the client, indicates that further teaching about bowel elimination is necessary?

1. "I drink six to eight glasses of water per day."
2. "I walk 1 to 2 miles per day."
3. "I need to decrease fiber in my diet."
4. "I have a bowel movement every other day."

10. The nurse is providing information to nursing assistants regarding caring for the older adult. The nurse tells the nursing assistants that which of the following situations portrays ageism?

1. Accepting differences among older adults
2. Allowing older adults to make decisions
3. Informing the older adult of their rights
4. Advising older adults to forego aggressive treatment

11. The nurse is providing medication instructions to an older client who is taking digoxin (Lanoxin) on a daily basis. The nurse bears in mind that which age-related body changes could place the client at risk for digitalis toxicity?

1. Decreased cough efficiency and decreased vital capacity
2. Decreased lean body mass and decreased glomerular filtration rate
3. Decreased salivation and decreased gastrointestinal motility
4. Decreased muscle strength and loss of bone density

12. The nurse employed in a long-term care facility is caring for an older male client. Which of the following nursing actions would contribute to encouraging autonomy in the client?

1. Scheduling his barber appointments
2. Allowing him to choose social activities
3. Decorating his room
4. Planning his meals

13. The nurse assigned to care for an older client places an extra blanket in the client's room. The nurse understands that the older client is less able to regulate hot and cold body changes because of alterations in the activity of the:

1. Parotid glands
2. Thymus gland
3. Pineal gland
4. Sweat glands

14. The nurse is caring for an older female client whose husband died 6 months ago. Which behavior, by the client, indicates ineffective coping?

1. Visiting her husband's grave once a month
2. Participating in a senior citizens program
3. Looking at old snapshots of her family
4. Neglecting her personal grooming

15. The nurse is preparing to communicate with an older client who is hearing-impaired. The most appropriate initial nursing action is to:

1. Stand in front of the client
2. Exaggerate lip movements
3. Obtain a sign language interpreter
4. Pantomime and write the client notes

16. The nurse is collecting data from an older client who is having difficulty sleeping at night. Which statement, if made by the client, indicates that teaching about promoting sleep is necessary?

1. "I drink hot chocolate before bedtime."
2. "I have stopped smoking cigars."
3. "I swim three times a week."
4. "I read for 40 minutes before bedtime."

17. The nurse observes that an older male client is confined by his daughter-in-law to his room. When the nurse suggests that he walk to the den and join the family, he says, "I'm in everyone's way, and my son needs me to stay here." The most important action for the nurse to take is to:

1. Suggest to the client and daughter-in-law that they consider a nursing home for the client
2. Suggest appropriate resources to the client and daughter-in-law, such as respite care and a senior citizens' center
3. Say nothing, because it is best for the nurse to remain neutral and wait to be asked for help
4. Say to the son, "Confining your father to his room is inhuman."

18. The nurse is collecting data from an older adult client. Which of the following indicates a potential complication associated with the skin of this client?

1. Wrinkling
2. Thinning and loss of elasticity in the skin
3. Deepening of expression lines
4. Crusting

19. The nurse provides medication instructions to an older hypertensive client who is taking lisinopril (Prinivil, Zestril) 20 mg orally daily. Which statement, if made by the client, indicates that further teaching is necessary?
    1. "I take the pill after breakfast each day."
    2. "I need to change my position slowly."
    3. "If I get a bad headache, I should call my doctor immediately."
    4. "I can skip a dose once a week."
20. The nurse is caring for an older client who is on bed rest. The nurse plans which intervention to prevent respiratory complications?
    1. Monitoring vital signs every shift
    2. Decreasing oral fluid intake
    3. Changing the client's position every 2 hours
    4. Instructing the client to bear down every hour and hold his or her breath

ALTERNATE FORMAT QUESTION: MULTIPLE RESPONSE

Select all the normal age-related physiological changes.
___ Decline in visual acuity
___ Decreased respiratory rate
___ Increased heart rate
___ Increased susceptibility to urinary tract infections
___ Decline in long-term memory
___ Increased incidence of awakening after sleep onset

ANSWERS

1. *Answer:* **2**
Rationale: Presbycusis refers to the age-related, irreversible, degenerative changes of the inner ear leading to decreased hearing acuity. As a result of these changes, the older client has a decreased response to high-frequency sounds. Low-pitched tones of voice are more easily heard and interpreted by the older client. Options 1, 3, and 4 are not accurate.
Test-Taking Strategy: Use the process of elimination. Recalling that the client with a hearing loss responds to low-pitched tones will direct you to option 2. If you had difficulty with this question, review the characteristics associated with presbycusis and hearing loss.
Level of Cognitive Ability: Application
Client Needs: Physiological Integrity
Integrated Process: Nursing Process/Planning
Content Area: Adult Health/Ear
Reference: Wold, G. (2004). *Basic geriatric nursing* (3rd ed.). St. Louis: Mosby, pp. 52-53, 133.

2. *Answer:* **2**
Rationale: Serum transferrin is an iron transport protein that can be measured directly or calculated as an indirect measurement of total iron-binding capacity. It is a more sensitive indicator of protein status than albumin. When the serum transferrin level is less than 100 mg/dL, the level of visceral protein depletion is severe. Options 1, 3, and 4 identify normal laboratory values.
Test-Taking Strategy: Use the process of elimination. Note the key word, *protein.* The only option that refers to the analysis of protein is option 2. Additionally, eliminate options 1, 3, and 4, because these are normal laboratory values. Review these laboratory values if you had difficulty with this question.
Level of Cognitive Ability: Analysis
Client Needs: Physiological Integrity
Integrated Process: Nursing Process/Data Collection
Content Area: Fundamental Skills
Reference: Chernecky, C., & Berger, B. (2004). *Laboratory tests and diagnostic procedures* (4th ed.). Philadelphia: W.B. Saunders, pp. 1082-1083.

3. *Answer:* **1**
Rationale: Elder abuse is widespread and occurs among all subgroups of the population. It includes physical and psychological abuse, misuse of property, and violation of rights. The typical abuse victim is a woman of advanced age with few social contacts and at least one physical or mental impairment that limits her ability to perform activities of daily living. In addition, the client usually lives alone or with the abuser, and depends on the abuser for care.
Test-Taking Strategy: Use the process of elimination. Read each option carefully and identify the client who is most defenseless as the result of the disease process. If you had difficulty with this question, review content related to elder abuse.
Level of Cognitive Ability: Comprehension
Client Needs: Psychosocial Integrity
Integrated Process: Nursing Process/Implementation
Content Area: Mental Health
Reference: O'Neill, P. (2002). *Caring for the older adult.* Philadelphia: W.B. Saunders, p. 255.

4. *Answer:* **2**
Rationale: Because it takes longer to adapt to changes from dark to light and vice versa, older people are at greater risk of falls and injuries. Any place where there is a sudden change from dark to light or from light to dark can be dangerous. Getting up during the night is hazardous for an older client. Eyes adapt to the dark by using the rod receptors, which are sensitive to short blue-green wavelengths. Red wavelengths are longer and are perceived by the cones. Thus, a red light in the bathroom at night allows for adequate vision to function in the dark without the need for adaptation.
Test-Taking Strategy: Use the process of elimination focusing on the issue. Eliminate options 1 and 3 because they do not meet the client's need for independence. Additionally, there is no information in the question indicating that the client lives with the daughter. Option 4 is incorrect because the older client needs to be encouraged to drink at least 2 L of fluid a day to prevent dehydration. Review the physiological changes in the eye that occur with aging if you had difficulty with this question.
Level of Cognitive Ability: Comprehension
Client Needs: Physiological Integrity

Integrated Process: Nursing Process/Implementation
Content Area: Adult Health/Eye
Reference: Wold, G. (2004). *Basic geriatric nursing* (3rd ed.). St. Louis: Mosby, pp. 124, 138.

5. *Answer:* 1

Rationale: It is preferable to get clients out of bed and sitting in a chair for meals. This position facilitates chewing and swallowing and prevents the reflux of stomach contents and aspiration. Options 2, 3, and 4 do not identify positions that will reduce the risk of aspiration.
Test-Taking Strategy: Use the process of elimination. Focus on the issue of the question, "reduce the risk of aspiration." This should direct you to option 1. Review the measures that will prevent aspiration if you had difficulty with this question.
Level of Cognitive Ability: Application
Client Needs: Safe, Effective Care Environment
Integrated Process: Nursing Process/Implementation
Content Area: Fundamental Skills
Reference: Wold, G. (2004). *Basic geriatric nursing* (3rd ed.). St. Louis: Mosby, p. 218.

6. *Answer:* 4

Rationale: Exercise and activity are essential for health promotion and maintenance in the older adult and to achieve an optimal level of functioning. Approximately half of the physical deterioration of the older client is caused by disuse rather than by the aging process or disease. One of the best exercises for an older adult is walking, progressing to 30-minute sessions three to five times each week. Swimming and dancing are also beneficial.
Test-Taking Strategy: Use the process of elimination, noting the key word, *best*. Options 1, 2, and 3, although possible, are not the best activities. Remember, walking is one of the best forms of exercise. Review this content if you had difficulty with this question.
Level of Cognitive Ability: Application
Client Needs: Health Promotion and Maintenance
Integrated Process: Nursing Process/Planning
Content Area: Fundamental Skills
Reference: Wold, G. (2004). *Basic geriatric nursing* (3rd ed.). St. Louis: Mosby, pp. 63-64, 263.

7. *Answer:* 4

Rationale: Clients who like to retell stories or past events need to be provided the opportunity to do so. This phenomenon is called life review or reminiscence. In a sense, it is a way for the elder client to relive and restructure life experiences, and is a part of achieving ego identity. Option 1 indicates reality orientation techniques. Options 2 and 3 indicate socialization and physical activity.
Test-Taking Strategy: Use the process of elimination. Focusing on the key word, *reminiscence*, and recalling its definition will direct you to option 4. Review this form of activity if you had difficulty with this question.
Level of Cognitive Ability: Application
Client Needs: Psychosocial Integrity
Integrated Process: Caring
Content Area: Mental Health

Reference: Wold, G. (2004). *Basic geriatric nursing* (3rd ed.). St. Louis: Mosby, pp. 155-156.

8. *Answer:* 3

Rationale: Trauma to the older client in the home may be caused by a variety of factors. Some of these factors include an unsteady gait, the presence of unsecured scatter rugs, cluttered passageways, inoperable smoke detectors, or a history of previous falls.
Test-Taking Strategy: Use the process of elimination. Note the key words, *requires immediate attention*. Focusing on the issue and looking for the item that identifies an unsafe condition will direct you to option 3. Review the components of an environmental assessment if you had difficulty with this question.
Level of Cognitive Ability: Comprehension
Client Needs: Safe, Effective Care Environment
Integrated Process: Nursing Process/Data Collection
Content Area: Fundamental Skills
Reference: Wold, G. (2004). *Basic geriatric nursing* (3rd ed.). St. Louis: Mosby, p. 124.

9. *Answer:* 3

Rationale: Adequate dietary fiber is an important factor in aiding bowel function. Dietary fiber increases fecal weight and water content and accelerates the transit of fecal mass through the gastrointestinal tract. The retention of water by the fiber has the ability to soften stools and promote regularity. Fluid intake and exercise also facilitate bowel elimination.
Test-Taking Strategy: Note the key words, *further teaching about bowel elimination is necessary*. These words indicate a false response question and that you need to select the incorrect client statement. Use the process of elimination and basic principles related to preventing constipation. If you had difficulty with this question, review these basic principles.
Level of Cognitive Ability: Comprehension
Client Needs: Physiological Integrity
Integrated Process: Teaching/Learning
Content Area: Fundamental Skills
Reference: Wold, G. (2004). *Basic geriatric nursing* (3rd ed.). St. Louis: Mosby, p. 244.

10. *Answer:* 4

Rationale: Ageism is a form of prejudice, in which older adults are stereotyped by characteristics found in only a few members of their group. Fundamental to ageism is the view that older people are different from "me" and will remain different from "me." Therefore, they are portrayed as not experiencing the same desires, needs, and concerns. Options 1, 2, and 3 identify supportive roles that the nurse engages in when dealing with the older adult. Option 4 suggests that the older adult is not worthy of aggressive treatment and demonstrates ageism.
Test-Taking Strategy: Use the process of elimination and focus on the issue, ageism. Recalling the definition of ageism will direct you to option 4. Review this concept if you had difficulty with this question.
Level of Cognitive Ability: Comprehension
Client Needs: Health Promotion and Maintenance
Integrated Process: Caring
Content Area: Fundamental Skills

Reference: Wold, G. (2004). *Basic geriatric nursing* (3rd ed.). St. Louis: Mosby, pp. 5-7, 152.

11. *Answer: 2*

Rationale: The older client is at risk for medication toxicity because of decreased lean body mass and age-associated decreased glomerular filtration rate. Although options 1, 3, and 4 identify age-related changes that occur in the older client, they are not specifically associated with this risk.

Test-Taking Strategy: Use the process of elimination and focus on the issue, an age-related body change that could place the client at risk for medication toxicity. Note that option 2 is the only option that addresses renal excretion. If you had difficulty with this question, review the physiological changes associated with aging.

Level of Cognitive Ability: Comprehension
Client Needs: Physiological Integrity
Integrated Process: Teaching/Learning
Content Area: Fundamental Skills
Reference: Wold, G. (2004). *Basic geriatric nursing* (3rd ed.). St. Louis: Mosby, pp. 94-97.

12. *Answer: 2*

Rationale: Autonomy is the personal freedom to direct one's own life as long as it does not impinge on the rights of others. An autonomous person is capable of rational thought. This individual can identify problems, search for alternatives, and choose solutions that allow continued personal freedom as long as the rights and property of others are not harmed. Loss of autonomy, and therefore independence, is a very real fear among older clients. Option 2 is the only option that allows the client to be a decision-maker.

Test-Taking Strategy: Use the process of elimination focusing on the issue, encouraging autonomy. Recalling the definition of autonomy will direct you to the correct option. Remember, to promote independence in clients, it is essential to give the client choices. Review the concept of autonomy if you had difficulty with this question.

Level of Cognitive Ability: Application
Client Needs: Safe, Effective Care Environment
Integrated Process: Caring
Content Area: Fundamental Skills
Reference: Linton, A., & Maebius, N. (2003) *Introduction to medical-surgical nursing* (3rd ed.). Philadelphia: W.B. Saunders, p. 21.

13. *Answer: 4*

Rationale: Functions of the skin include protection, sensory reception, homeostasis, and temperature regulation. The skin helps regulate the body temperature in two ways, by dilation and constriction of blood vessels and by the activity of the sweat glands. As aging progresses, alterations in sweat gland activity make the glands less effective in temperature regulation, so the aging person is less able to regulate hot and cold body changes. The parotid glands are responsible for the drainage of saliva, which plays an important role in digestion. The pineal gland is a major site of melatonin biosynthesis. The thymus gland plays an immunological role throughout life.

Test-Taking Strategy: Use the process of elimination and focus on the issue, temperature regulation. Recalling the function of the skin and that the sweat glands control temperature regulation will direct you to the correct option. Review the age-related changes that occur in the older client if you had difficulty with this question.

Level of Cognitive Ability: Comprehension
Client Needs: Physiological Integrity
Integrated Process: Nursing Process/Implementation
Content Area: Fundamental Skills
Reference: Linton, A., & Maebius, N. (2003) *Introduction to medical-surgical nursing* (3rd ed.). Philadelphia: W.B. Saunders, p. 1012.

14. *Answer: 4*

Rationale: Coping mechanisms are behaviors used to decreased stress and anxiety. In response to a death, ineffective coping is manifested by an extreme behavior that in some instances may be harmful to the individual, physically and/or psychologically. Option 4 is indicative of a behavior that identifies an ineffective coping behavior in the grieving process.

Test-Taking Strategy: Use the process of elimination and note the issue, an ineffective coping behavior. Eliminate options 1, 2, and 3 because they are similar and are positive activities that the individual is engaging in to get on with her life. Review coping mechanisms in response to grief and loss if you had difficulty with this question.

Level of Cognitive Ability: Analysis
Client Needs: Mental Health
Integrated Process: Nursing Process/Data Collection
Content Area: Fundamental Skills
Reference: Wold, G. (2004). *Basic geriatric nursing* (3rd ed.). St. Louis: Mosby, pp. 172-175.

15. *Answer: 1*

Rationale: The nurse would ensure that the hearing-impaired client can see the nurse when speaking by providing adequate lighting and by standing in front of the client. The nurse should enunciate words clearly but not exaggerate lip movements. If the client is profoundly hearing-impaired and uses signing, a sign language interpreter should be obtained. If a client cannot understand by reading lips, the nurse would try using gestures, pantomiming, or writing notes.

Test-Taking Strategy: Note the key words, *initial nursing action*. To communicate effectively with a hearing impaired client, the nurse first makes sure that the client can see her or him. If you had difficulty with this question, review the nursing interventions for the hearing-impaired client.

Level of Cognitive Ability: Application
Client Needs: Health Promotion and Maintenance
Integrated Process: Nursing Process/Implementation
Content Area: Fundamental Skills
Reference: Wold, G. (2004). *Basic geriatric nursing* (3rd ed.). St. Louis: Mosby, p. 136.

16. *Answer: 1*

Rationale: Many nonpharmacological sleep aids can be used to influence sleep. The client should avoid caffeinated beverages and stimulants, such as tea, cola, and chocolate, and foods containing tyrosine, such as cheddar cheese. The client should exercise regularly, because exercise promotes sleep by burning off tension that accumulates during the day.

A 20- to 30-minute walk, swim, or bicycle ride three time a week is helpful. Smoking and alcohol should be avoided. The client should avoid large meals, peanuts, beans, fruit and raw vegetables that produce gas, and snacks high in fat that are difficult to digest.

Test-Taking Strategy: Focus on the issue, that teaching is necessary. Options 2, 3, and 4 are positive statements indicating that the client understands the methods of promoting sleep. Review the factors that can interfere with sleep if you had difficulty with this question.

Level of Cognitive Ability: Comprehension
Client Needs: Physiological Integrity
Integrated Process: Teaching/Learning
Content Area: Fundamental Skills
Reference: Wold, G. (2004). *Basic geriatric nursing* (3rd ed.). St. Louis: Mosby, pp. 279-281.

17. *Answer:* 2
Rationale: Assisting clients and families to become aware of available community support systems is a role and responsibility of the nurse. Option 1 suggests committing the client to a nursing home and is a premature action on the nurse's part. Although the data provided tell the nurse that this client requires nursing care, the nurse does not know the extent of nursing care. Observing that the client has begun to be confined to his room makes it necessary for the nurse to intervene legally and ethically, so option 3 is not appropriate and is passive in terms of advocacy. Option 4 is incorrect and judgmental.

Test-Taking Strategy: Use the process of elimination. Note the key words, *most important action*. Using principles related to the ethical and legal responsibility of the nurse and knowledge of the nurse's role will direct you to option 2. Review these principles if you had difficulty with this question.

Level of Cognitive Ability: Application
Client Needs: Health Promotion and Maintenance
Integrated Process: Nursing Process/Implementation
Content Area: Fundamental Skills
Reference: Wold, G. (2004). *Basic geriatric nursing* (3rd ed.). St. Louis: Mosby, pp. 16-17, 78.

18. *Answer:* 4
Rationale: The normal physiological changes that occur in the skin of older adults include thinning of the skin, loss of elasticity, deepening of expression lines, and wrinkling. Crusting noted on the skin would indicate a potential complication.

Test-Taking Strategy: Use the process of elimination and note the key words, *potential complication*. Recall the normal physiological changes that occur in the aging process to direct you to option 4. Review these age-related skin changes if you had difficulty with this question.

Level of Cognitive Ability: Comprehension
Client Needs: Physiological Integrity
Integrated Process: Nursing Process/Data Collection
Content Area: Fundamental Skills
Reference: Wold, G. (2004). *Basic geriatric nursing* (3rd ed.). St. Louis: Mosby, pp. 26-27, 223.

19. *Answer:* 4
Rationale: Lisinopril is an antihypertensive, angiotensin-converting enzyme inhibitor (ACE inhibitor). The usual dosage range is 20 to 40 mg/day. Adverse effects include headache, dizziness, fatigue, orthostatic hypotension, tachycardia, and angioedema. Specific client teaching points include taking one pill a day, not stopping the medication without consulting the physician, and monitoring for side effects and adverse reactions. The client should notify the physician if side effects occur.

Test-Taking Strategy: Use the process of elimination. Note the key words, *further teaching is necessary*. Basic principles related to the administration of prescribed medications will direct you to option 4. If you had difficulty with this question, review teaching points related to medication administration.

Level of Cognitive Ability: Analysis
Client Needs: Physiological Integrity
Integrated Process: Teaching/Learning
Content Area: Pharmacology
Reference: Skidmore-Roth, L. (2005). *Mosby's drug guide for nurses* (6th ed.). St. Louis: Mosby, p. 504.

20. *Answer:* 3
Rationale: Frequent position changes help mobilize lung secretions and prevent pooling. This is the only intervention identified in the options that will prevent respiratory complications. The nurse should assess the client's vital signs every 4 hours to identify an elevated temperature, which may suggest infection. The nurse would encourage fluid intake to thin secretions and thus enable the client to expectorate more easily. It is important to encourage coughing and deep breathing to mobilize lung secretions. The client should be instructed to avoid the Valsalva maneuver or any activity involving holding the breath.

Test-Taking Strategy: Use the process of elimination. Note the key words, *prevent respiratory complications*. Changing the position of the immobilized client every 2 hours will help prevent pooling of lung secretions. The other options do not assist the client to improve ventilatory efforts or prevent respiratory complications. Review nursing interventions to prevent respiratory complications in the client who is immobilized if you had difficulty with this question.

Level of Cognitive Ability: Application
Client Needs: Physiological Integrity
Integrated Process: Nursing Process/Planning
Content Area: Fundamental Skills
Reference: Linton, A., & Maebius, N. (2003) *Introduction to medical-surgical nursing* (3rd ed.). Philadelphia: W.B. Saunders, pp. 269-270.

ALTERNATE FORMAT QUESTION: MULTIPLE RESPONSE

Answers:
Decline in visual acuity
Increased susceptibility to urinary tract infections
Increased incidence of awakening after sleep onset
Rationale: Anatomic changes to the eye affect the individual's visual ability, leading to potential problems with activities of daily living. Light adaptation and visual fields are reduced.

Respiratory rates are generally higher in older adults, ranging from 16 to 25 breaths per minute. Heart rate decreases and heart valves thicken. Age-related changes that affect the urinary tract increase an older client's susceptibility to urinary tract infections. Short-term memory may decline with age but long-term memory is usually maintained. Change in sleep patterns is a consistent, age-related change. Older persons experience an increased incidence of awakening after sleep onset.

Test-Taking Strategy: Knowledge regarding the normal age-related changes is needed to answer this question. Read each characteristic carefully and think about the physiological changes that occur with aging to select the correct items. Review the normal age-related changes if you had difficulty with this question.
Level of Cognitive Ability: Comprehension
Client Needs: Health Promotion and Maintenance
Integrated Process: Nursing Process/Data Collection
Content Area: Fundamental Skills
Reference: Wold, G. (2004). *Basic geriatric nursing* (3rd ed.). St. Louis: Mosby, pp. 26-27, 223.

REFERENCES

Chernecky, C., & Berger, B. (2004). *Laboratory tests and diagnostic procedures* (4th ed.). Philadelphia: W.B. Saunders.

Linton, A., & Maebius, N. (2003). *Introduction to medical-surgical nursing* (3rd ed.). Philadelphia: W.B. Saunders.

O'Neill, P. (2002). *Caring for the older adult.* Philadelphia: W.B. Saunders.

Skidmore-Roth, L. (2005) *Mosby's drug guide for nurses* (6th ed.). St. Louis: Mosby.

Wold, G. (2004). *Basic geriatric nursing* (3rd ed.). St. Louis: Mosby.

Pediatric Nursing

PYRAMID TERMS

abuse   Nonaccidental physical injury or the nonaccidental act of omission by a parent or person responsible for the care of a child.

active immunity   The protection, which can last months, years, or even a lifetime, that forms in response to exposure to antigens in nature or vaccines.

atresia   Congenital absence or closure of a body orifice.

attenuated vaccines   Vaccines derived from microorganisms or viruses whose virulence has been weakened as a result of passage through another host.

cephalocaudal   Characterized by growth and development that proceeds from head to toe.

chronological age   Age in years.

developmental age   Age based on functional behavior and ability to adapt to the environment. It does not necessarily correspond to chronological age.

encopresis   Fecal incontinence after the age of 4 years.

functional age   The age equivalent at which a child is actually able to perform specific self-care or related tasks.

growth   Measurable physical and physiological changes that occur over time.

growth spurts   Brief periods of rapid increase in growth rate.

hereditary   Involving the transmission of genetic characteristics from parent to offspring.

inactivated vaccines   Vaccines that contain killed microorganisms.

intelligence   What an individual can do relative to learning, thinking, and problem solving.

learning   Behavior changes that occur as a result of both maturation and experience with the environment.

nasal flaring   A serious sign of air hunger; a widening of the nares to enable an infant or child to take in more oxygen.

passive immunity   Antibody transfer from a person with active immunity to a person who does not have that antibody.

puberty   The period of time during which the adolescent experiences a growth spurt, develops secondary sex characteristics, and achieves reproductive maturity.

regression   Behavior that is more appropriate to an earlier stage of development and is often used to cope with stress or anxiety.

regurgitation   An abnormal backward flow of body fluid.

retractions   An abnormal movement of the chest walls during inspiration.

separation anxiety   Distress and apprehension caused by being removed from parents, home, or familiar surroundings.

shunt   Tube or device implanted in the body to redirect a body fluid from one cavity or vessel to another

stenosis   The narrowing or constriction of an opening.

stridor   A shrill harsh sound heard during inspiration or expiration, or both, that is produced by the flow of air through a narrowed segment of the respiratory tract.

wheezing   High-pitched musical whistles heard with or without a stethoscope.

PYRAMID TO SUCCESS

Pyramid points focus on growth and development, safety and the age-appropriate measures to ensure a safe and hazard-free environment for the child, and acute disorders that can occur in children. Focus on specific feeding techniques, positioning techniques, and interventions that will provide and maintain adequate airway, breathing, and circulation patterns in the child. On the NCLEX-PN examination, be alert to the age of the child if the age is presented in a question. The Integrated Processes addressed in this unit include Caring, the Clinical Problem-Solving Process (Nursing Process), Communication and Documentation, and Teaching/Learning.

CLIENT NEEDS
Safe, Effective Care Environment

Accident prevention

Confidentiality

Continuity of care

Environmental and personal safety related to the developmental age of the child

Establishing priorities

Informed consent in regard to minors

Parent and child rights

Protection of the child and other contacts to prevent illness

Protective measures

Spread and control of infectious agents, particularly with regard to communicable diseases

Health Promotion and Maintenance

Developmental stages
Disease prevention
Family systems
Health promotion programs
Immunizations and communicable diseases
Instructions to the child and parents regarding care at home

Psychosocial Integrity

Child abuse and neglect
Communication
Cultural, religious, and spiritual differences
End-of-life issues
Family and support systems
Grief and loss
Play

Physiological Integrity

Age-appropriate normal body structure and function
Comfort measures
Elimination
Illness management
Infectious diseases
Intrusive procedures

Medical emergencies
Medication administration
Nutrition
Potential for alterations in body systems
Responses to therapies
Rest and sleep
Surgical procedures and health alterations

REFERENCES

Christensen, B., & Kockrow, E. (2003). *Foundations of nursing* (4th ed.). St. Louis: Mosby.

deWit, S. (2005). *Fundamental concepts and skills for nursing* (2nd ed.). Philadelphia: W.B. Saunders.

Leifer, G. (2003). *Introduction to maternity and pediatric nursing* (4th ed.). Philadelphia: W.B. Saunders.

Malarkey, L., & McMorrow, M. (2005). *Nursing guide to laboratory and diagnostic tests.* Philadelphia: W.B. Saunders.

National Council of State Boards of Nursing. (2005). *Detailed test plan for the National Council licensure examination for practical/vocational nurses.* Chicago: Author.

Potter, P., & Perry, A. (2005). *Fundamentals of nursing* (6th ed.). St. Louis: Mosby.

Price, D., & Gwin, J. (2005). *Thompson's pediatric nursing* (9th ed.). Philadelphia: W.B. Saunders.

Skidmore-Roth, L. (2005). *Mosby's drug guide for nurses* (6th ed.). St. Louis: Mosby.

Stuart, G., & Laraia, M. (2005). *Principles and practice of psychiatric nursing* (8th ed.). St. Louis: Mosby.

Wong, D., & Hockenberry, M. (2003). *Nursing care of infants and children* (7th ed.). St. Louis: Mosby.

Neurological, Cognitive, and Psychosocial Disorders

I. HEAD INJURY

A. Description

1. The pathological result of any mechanical force to the skull, scalp, meninges, or brain
2. Manifestations depend on the type of injury and the subsequent amount of increased intracranial pressure (ICP)

B. Data collection (ICP)

1. Early signs
   a. Headache
   b. Visual disturbances, diplopia
   c. Nausea and vomiting
   d. Dizziness or vertigo
   e. Slight change in vital signs
   f. Change in pupillary response and equality
   g. Sunsetting eyes
   h. Slight change in level of consciousness (LOC)
   i. Infant: Bulging fontanel, wide sutures, increased head circumference, dilated scalp veins, high-pitched cry

2. Late signs
   a. Significant decrease in LOC
   b. Cushing's triad: Increased systolic blood pressure and widened pulse pressure, bradycardia, irregular respirations
   c. Decorticate posturing: Adduction of the arms at the shoulders, the arms being flexed on the chest with the wrists flexed and the hands fisted, and the lower extremities being extended and adducted; seen with severe dysfunction of the cerebral cortex (Figure 30-1)
   d. Decerebrate posturing: Rigid extension and pronation of the arms and the legs; a sign of dysfunction at the level of the midbrain (see Figure 30-1)
   e. Fixed and dilated pupils

C. Interventions

1. Monitor the airway

2. Check for injuries; immobilize the neck if a cervical injury is suspected
3. Monitor vital signs and neurological function
4. Monitor for decreased responsiveness to pain (a significant sign of altered LOC)
5. Initiate seizure precautions
6. Maintain an NPO status or provide clear liquids if prescribed, until it is determined that vomiting will not occur
7. Administer oxygen and intravenous (IV) fluids as prescribed
8. Monitor IV fluids carefully to avoid aggravating any cerebral edema and to minimize the possibility of overhydration

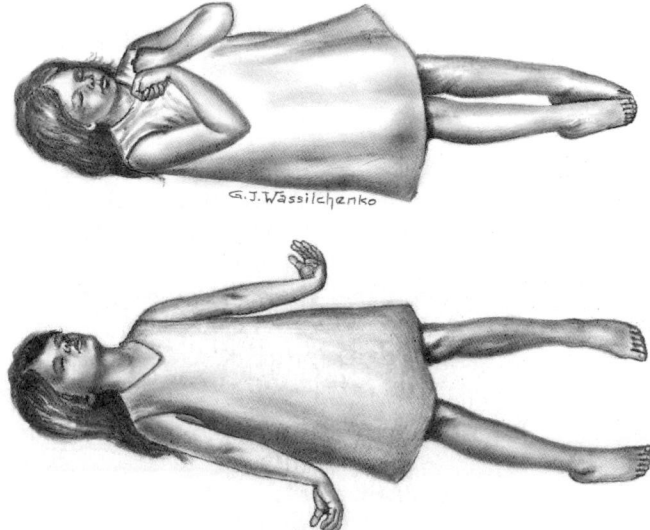

G.J.Wassilchenko

FIG. 30-1 Decorticate posturing (*top*) and decerebrate posturing (*bottom*). (From Hockenberry, M. [2003]. *Nursing care of infants and children* [7th ed.]. St. Louis: Mosby.)

9. Elevate the head of the bed 15 to 30 degrees if not contraindicated

10. Position so that the head is maintained midline to facilitate venous drainage and avoid jugular vein compression; turning side to side is contraindicated because of the risk of jugular vein compression

11. Check wound dressings for the presence of drainage and monitor for nose or ear drainage, which could indicate leakage of cerebrospinal fluid (CSF); drainage that is positive indicates leakage of CSF from a skull fracture

12. Administer tepid sponge baths or place on a hypothermia blanket if hyperthermia occurs

13. Suctioning through the nares is contraindicated because of the high risk of a secondary infection and the probability of the catheter entering the brain through a fracture

14. As prescribed, administer acetaminophen (Tylenol) for headache, anticonvulsants for seizures, antibiotics if a laceration is present, and tetanus toxoid as appropriate

15. Sedating medications are withheld during the acute phase of the injury

16. Monitor for signs of brainstem involvement (Box 30-1)

17. Epidural hematoma: Monitor for asymmetrical pupils (one dilated, unreactive pupil in a comatose child is a neurosurgical emergency that may require evacuation of the hematoma)

▲

II. HYDROCEPHALUS

A. Description
   1. An imbalance of CSF absorption or production, caused by malformations, tumors, hemorrhage, infections, or trauma
   2. Results in head enlargement and increased ICP
B. Types (Box 30-2)
C. Data collection
   1. Infant
      a. Increased head circumference
      b. Bones of the head are thin and widely separated and produce a cracked-pot sound (Macewen's sign) on percussion
      c. Anterior fontanel tense, bulging, and non-pulsating
      d. Scalp veins dilated
      e. Frontal bossing
      f. Sunsetting eyes
   2. Child
      a. Behavior changes such as irritability and lethargy
      b. Headache on awakening
      c. Nausea and vomiting
      d. Ataxia
      e. Nystagmus
   3. Late signs: A high, shrill cry and seizure activities
D. Surgical interventions
   1. The goal of surgical treatment is to prevent further CSF accumulation by bypassing the blockage and draining the fluid from the ventricles to a location where it may be reabsorbed
   2. Ventriculoperitoneal **shunt** (VP **shunt**): CSF drains into the peritoneal cavity from the lateral ventricle (Figure 30-2)
   3. Atrioventricular **shunt** (AV **shunt**): CSF drains into the right atrium of the heart from the lateral ventricle, bypassing the obstruction (used in older children and in children with abdominal pathology)
E. Interventions postoperatively
   1. Monitor vital signs and neurological signs
   2. Position on the unoperated side to prevent ▲ pressure on the **shunt** valve
   3. The child is kept flat as prescribed to avoid rapid ▲ reduction of intracranial fluid
   4. Observe for increased ICP; if increased ICP occurs, ▲ elevate the head of the bed to 15 to 30 degrees to enhance gravity flow through the **shunt**
   5. Monitor for signs of infection and check dressings for drainage
   6. Measure head circumference
   7. Monitor input and output (I&O)
   8. Provide comfort measures; administer medications as prescribed, which may include diuretics, antibiotics, or anticonvulsants
   9. Instruct parents in how to recognize **shunt** infection or malfunction
   10. In a toddler, headache and a lack of appetite are the earliest common signs of **shunt** malfunction

---

BOX 30-1

Signs of Brainstem Involvement

Deep, rapid, or intermittent and gasping respirations
Wide fluctuations or noticeable slowing of the pulse
Widening pulse pressure or extreme fluctuations in blood pressure

---

BOX 30-2

Types of Hydrocephalus

COMMUNICATING
Occurs as a result of impaired absorption within the subarachnoid space
No interference of CSF within the ventricular system

NONCOMMUNICATING
Obstruction of CSF flow within the ventricular system

III. SPINA BIFIDA

A. Description
1. Central nervous system (CNS) defect that occurs as a result of neural tube failure to close during embryonic development
2. Associated deficits include sensory motor disturbance, dislocated hips, clubfoot, and hydrocephalus
3. Defect closure is usually done during infancy

B. Types
1. Spina bifida occulta
   a. Posterior vertebral arches fail to close in the lumbosacral area
   b. Spinal cord remains intact and usually is not visible
   c. Meninges are not exposed on the skin surface
   d. Neurological deficits are not usually present
2. Spina bifida cystica
   a. Protrusion of the spinal cord and/or its meninges
   b. Results in incomplete closure of the vertebral and neural tubes, resulting in a saclike protrusion in the lumbar or sacral area, with varying degrees of nervous tissue involvement
   c. Can include meningocele, myelomeningocele, lipomeningocele, and lipomeningomyelocele
3. Meningocele
   a. Protrusion involves meninges and a saclike cyst that contains CSF in the midline of the back, usually in the lumbosacral area

b. No involvement of the spinal cord
c. Neurological deficits are usually not present
4. Myelomeningocele
   a. Protrusion of meninges, CSF, nerve roots, and a portion of the spinal cord
   b. The sac (defect) is covered by a thin membrane that is prone to leakage or rupture
   c. Neurological deficits are evident

C. Data collection
1. Depends on the spinal cord involvement
2. Visible spinal defect
3. Flaccid paralysis of the legs
4. Altered bladder and bowel function
5. Hip and joint deformities

D. Interventions
1. Evaluate the sac and measure the lesion
2. Perform neurological assessment
3. Monitor for increased ICP, which might indicate developing hydrocephalus
4. Measure head circumference; assess the anterior fontanel for fullness
5. Protect the sac; cover with a sterile, moist (normal saline), nonadherent dressing to maintain the moisture of the sac and contents, and change the dressing every 2 to 4 hours, as prescribed
6. Place in a prone position to minimize tension on the sac and the risk of trauma; the head is turned to one side for feeding
7. Change the dressing covering the sac whenever soiled, because of the risk of infection; diapering may be contraindicated until the defect has been repaired

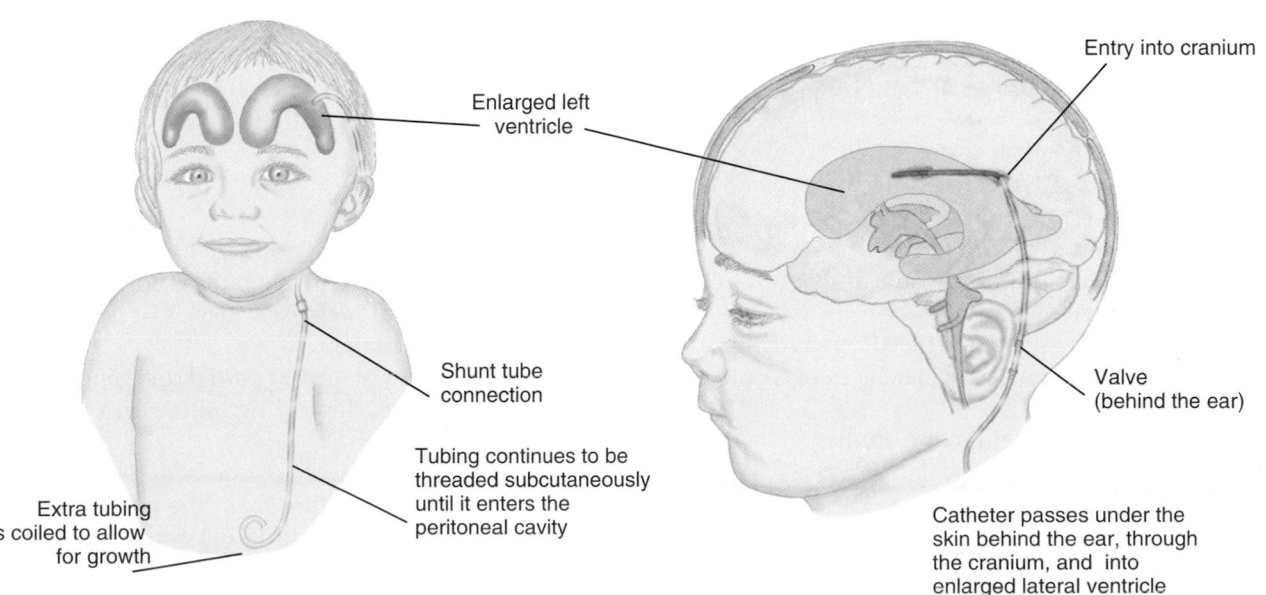

FIG. 30-2 Ventriculoperitoneal shunt. (From McKinney, E., James, S., Murray, S., & Ashwill, J. [2005]. *Maternal-child nursing* [2nd ed.]. St. Louis: W.B. Saunders.)

8. Use aseptic technique to prevent infection
9. Check the sac for redness, clear or purulent drainage, abrasions, irritation, and signs of infection
10. Early signs of infection include elevated temperature (axillary), irritability, lethargy, and nuchal rigidity
11. Monitor for physical impairments such as hip and joint deformities
12. Prepare the child and family for surgery
13. Antibiotics may be prescribed to prevent infection
14. In the child, anticholinergics may be prescribed to improve urinary continence, laxatives to achieve bowel continence, and antispasmodics to control bladder spasms

IV. REYE'S SYNDROME
A. Description
  1. Acute encephalopathy that follows a viral illness; characterized pathologically by cerebral edema and fatty changes in the liver
  2. The exact cause is not clear
  3. It is recommended that aspirin not be administered to children with varicella or influenza because of its association with Reye's syndrome
  4. Acetaminophen (Tylenol) is considered the medication of choice for pediatric clients
  5. The goal of treatment is to maintain effective cerebral perfusion and control increasing ICP
B. Data collection
  1. History of systemic viral illness 4 to 7 days before the onset of symptoms
  2. Malaise
  3. Nausea and vomiting
  4. Progressive neurological deterioration
C. Interventions
  1. Monitor neurological status
  2. Monitor for altered level of consciousness and signs of increased ICP
  3. Monitor I&O
  4. Provide rest and decrease stimulation in the environment
  5. Monitor for signs of bleeding and signs of impaired coagulation, such as a prolonged bleeding time
  6. Monitor liver and function studies

V. MENINGITIS
A. Description
  1. An infectious process of the CNS caused by bacteria and viruses that may be acquired as a primary disease or as a result of compli-

cations of neurosurgery, trauma, infection of the sinus or ears, or systemic infections
  2. Diagnosis is made by testing CSF obtained by lumbar puncture, which shows increased pressure, cloudy CSF, high protein, and low glucose
  3. Meningococcal meningitis occurs in epidemic form and is the only type readily transmitted by droplet infection from nasopharyngeal secretions
  4. Viral meningitis is associated with viruses such as mumps, paramyxovirus, herpes virus, and enterovirus
B. Data collection
  1. Signs and symptoms vary, depending on the type, the age of the child, and the duration of the preceding illness; there is no one classic sign or symptom
  2. Fever, chills
  3. Vomiting, diarrhea
  4. Poor feeding or anorexia
  5. Nuchal rigidity
  6. Poor or high-pitched cry
  7. Altered level of consciousness, such as lethargy or irritability
  8. Bulging anterior fontanel in the infant
  9. Kernig's sign and Brudzinski's sign in children and adolescents
  10. Muscle or joint pain
  11. Petechial or purpuric rashes (meningococcal infection)
C. Interventions
  1. Provide isolation and maintain for at least 24 hours after antibiotics are initiated
  2. Administer antibiotics as prescribed
  3. Perform neurological assessment
  4. Monitor for personality changes and irritability
  5. Monitor I&O
  6. Monitor nutritional status
  7. Determine close contacts of the child with meningitis, because the contacts will need prophylactic treatment

VI. SEIZURE DISORDERS
A. Description
  1. Sudden, transient alterations in brain function resulting from excessive levels of electrical activity in the brain
  2. Classified as either partial or generalized, or unclassified, depending on the area of the brain involved
B. Data collection
  1. Obtain information from the parents about the time of onset, precipitating events, and behavior before and after the seizure
  2. Determine the child's history related to seizures
C. Seizure precautions (Box 30-3)
D. Interventions (Box 30-4)

BOX 30-3

Seizure Precautions

Raise the side rails when the child is sleeping or resting.
Pad the side rails and other hard objects.
Place a waterproof mattress or pad on the bed or crib.
Instruct the child to wear or carry medical identification.
Instruct the child in precautions to take during potentially hazardous activities.
Instruct the child to swim with a companion.
Instruct the child to use a protective helmet and padding during bicycle riding, skateboarding, and inline skating.
Alert caregivers to the need for any special precautions.

BOX 30-4

Emergency Treatment for Seizures

Ensure airway patency.
Time the seizure episode.
If the child is standing or sitting, ease the child down to the floor; place in a side-lying position.
Place a pillow or folded blanket under the child's head; if no bedding is available, place your hands under the child's head or place the child's head in your lap.
Loosen restrictive clothing.
Remove eyeglasses from the child if present.
Clear area of any hazards or hard objects.
Allow seizure to proceed and end without interference.
If vomiting occurs, turn child to one side as a unit.
Do not restrain the child, place anything in the child's mouth, or give any food or liquids to the child.
Prepare to administer medications as prescribed.
Remain with the child until the child fully recovers.
Observe for incontinence, which may have occurred during the seizure.
Document the occurrence.

VII. CEREBRAL PALSY (CP)

A. Description
1. Disorder characterized by impaired movement and posture resulting from an abnormality in the extrapyramidal or pyramidal motor system
2. The most common clinical type is spastic CP, which represents an upper motor neuron type of muscle weakness

B. Data collection
1. Extreme irritability and crying
2. Feeding difficulties
3. Stiff and rigid arms or legs
4. Delayed gross development
5. Abnormal motor performance
6. Alterations of muscle tone
7. Abnormal posturing, such as opisthotonos (exaggerated arching of the back)
8. Persistence of primitive infantile reflexes

C. Interventions
1. The goal of management is early recognition and intervention to maximize the child's abilities
2. A multidisciplinary team approach is implemented to meet the many needs of the child
3. Therapeutic management includes physical therapy, occupational therapy, speech therapy, education, and recreation
4. Assess the child's developmental level and **intelligence**
5. Encourage early intervention and participation in school programs
6. Prepare for using mobilizing devices to help prevent or reduce deformities
7. Encourage communication and interaction with the child on his or her developmental level rather than **chronological age** level
8. Provide a safe environment, such as by removing sharp objects, using a protective helmet if the child falls frequently, and implementing seizure precautions if necessary
9. Provide safe, appropriate toys for age and developmental level
10. Position upright after meals
11. Administer medications as prescribed to decrease spasticity
12. Surgical interventions are reserved for the child who does not respond to more conservative measures or for the child whose spasticity causes progressive deformity

VIII. MENTAL RETARDATION

A. Description
1. Subaverage general intellectual functioning along with a deficit in adaptation in behavior
2. Down syndrome is a congenital condition that results in moderate to severe retardation and has been linked to an extra group G chromosome, chromosome 21 (trisomy 21)

B. Data collection
1. Deficits in cognitive skills and level of adaptive functioning
2. Delays in fine and gross motor skills
3. Speech delays
4. Decreased spontaneous activity
5. Nonresponsiveness
6. Irritability
7. Poor eye contact during feeding

C. Interventions
1. Medical strategies are focused at correcting structural deformities and treating associated behaviors
2. Implement community and educational services, using a multidisciplinary approach
3. Promote care skills as much as possible
4. Assist with communication and socialization skills

5. Facilitate appropriate playtime
6. Initiate safety precautions as necessary
7. Assist the family with decisions regarding care
8. Provide information regarding support services and community agencies

IX. AUTISM

A. Description
1. A severe mental disorder beginning in infancy or toddlerhood
2. Apparent to the parents before the age of 3
3. Characterized by impairment in reciprocal social interaction and in verbal and nonverbal communication
4. The cause is unknown and the prognosis may be poor
5. Diagnosis is established on the basis of symptoms and through the use of specialized autism assessment tools
6. Also called infantile autism

B. Data collection
1. Disturbance in the rate and appearance of physical, social, and language skills
2. Abnormal responses of body sensations
3. Abnormal ways of relating to people, objects, and events; the child is self-absorbed and unable to relate to others
4. There are no delusions, hallucinations, or incoherence, and the facies is intelligent and responsive
5. The child may play happily alone for hours, but have temper tantrums if interrupted
6. Language disturbance often includes repetition of previously heard speech and reversal of the pronouns "I" and "you"
7. If the child can talk, he or she uses speech not for communication but to repeat words or phrases meaninglessly
8. The child may develop an unusual attachment to a significant object and may display frequent rocking, spinning, twirling, or other bizarre behaviors

C. Interventions
1. Determine the child's routines, habits, and preferences, and maintain consistency as much as possible
2. Determine the specific ways in which the child communicates
3. Facilitate communication through the use of picture boards
4. Evaluate the child for safety
5. Implement safety precautions as necessary for self-injurious behaviors such as head banging
6. Monitor for stress and anxiety
7. Avoid placing demands on the child
8. Initiate referrals to special programs as required
9. Provide support to parents

X. ATTENTION-DEFICIT HYPERACTIVITY DISORDER (ADHD)

A. Description
1. A developmental disorder characterized by developmentally inappropriate degrees of inattention, overactivity, and impulsivity
2. One of the most common reasons for referral of children to mental health services
3. Childhood problems include lowered intellectual development, some minor physical abnormalities, sleeping disturbances, behavioral or emotional disorders, and difficulty in social relationships
4. Diagnosis is established on the basis of self-reports, parent and teacher reports, and psychological assessments

B. Data collection
1. Fidgets with hands or feet or squirms in the seat
2. Easily distracted with external or internal stimuli
3. Difficulty with following through on instructions
4. Poor attention span
5. Shifts from one uncompleted activity to another
6. Talks excessively
7. Interrupts or intrudes on others
8. Engages in physically dangerous activities without considering the possible consequences

C. Interventions
1. Provide environmental and physical safety measures
2. Enhance capabilities and self-esteem
3. Encourage support groups for parents
4. Administer prescribed medication; some commonly prescribed medications include methylphenidate hydrochloride (Ritalin), pemoline (Cylert), and dextroamphetamine sulfate (Dexadrine)
5. Instruct the child and parents regarding medication administration
6. Inform the child and parents that positive effects of the medication may be seen within 1 to 2 weeks if taken as prescribed

XI. TOURETTE'S DISORDER

A. Description: Appears between ages 2 and 15 and is characterized by recurrent involuntary and rapid movements affecting various parts of the body, accompanied by vocal noises such as barks, grunts, or profanities

B. Interventions
1. Establish a trusting one-to-one relationship
2. Protect the child from harm by providing a helmet or protective padding
3. Allow the child to have a favorite toy or other object

4. Provide positive reinforcement for appropriate behaviors
5. Maintain eye contact
6. Assess suicide potential
7. Remove dangerous objects from the environment
8. Set limits on socially inappropriate or manipulative behaviors
9. Encourage the child to confront tension and frustration before they emerge as inappropriate behaviors
10. Provide noncompetitive group situations

XII. CHILD ABUSE

A. Description: Involves emotional or physical **abuse** or neglect, as well as sexual exploitation or molestation by caretakers or other individuals
B. Data collection
1. Physical **abuse**
a. Unexplained bruises, burns, or fractures
b. Bald spots on the scalp
c. Apprehensive child
d. Extreme aggressiveness or withdrawal
e. Fear of parents
f. Lack of crying when approached by a stranger
2. Physical neglect
a. Inadequate weight gain
b. Poor hygiene
c. Consistent hunger
d. Inconsistent school attendance
e. Constant fatigue
f. Reports of lack of child supervision
g. Delinquency
3. Emotional **abuse**
a. Speech disorders
b. Habit disorders such as sucking, biting, and rocking
c. Psychoneurotic reactions
d. **Learning** disorders
e. Suicide attempts
4. Sexual **abuse**
a. Difficulty walking or sitting
b. Torn, stained, or bloody underclothing
c. Pain, swelling, or itching of the genitals
d. Bruises, bleeding, or lacerations in the genital or anal area
e. Unwillingness to change clothes or unwillingness to participate in gym activities
f. Poor peer relations
5. Shaken baby syndrome
a. Can cause intracranial hemorrhage leading to cerebral edema and death
b. Full bulging fontanelles and a head circumference greater than expected would be noted
C. Interventions
1. Support the child during a thorough physical assessment

2. Assess injuries
3. Report case of suspected **abuse**
4. Place the child in an environment that is safe, thereby preventing further injury
5. Document in an objective manner information related to the suspected **abuse**
6. Assess parents' strengths and weaknesses, normal coping mechanisms, and presence or absence of support systems
7. Assist the family in identifying stressors, support systems, and resources
8. Refer the family to appropriate support groups

PRACTICE QUESTIONS

1. A nurse is assisting in collecting data on a 6-month-old infant with a diagnosis of hydrocephalus. The nurse checks for the major symptom associated with hydrocephalus by doing which of the following?
   1. Testing the urine for protein
   2. Taking the apical pulse
   3. Palpating the anterior fontanel
   4. Taking the blood pressure

2. A mother arrives at the emergency room with her 5-year-old child and states that the child fell off a bunk bed. A head injury is suspected, and the nurse checks the child for signs of increased intracranial pressure (ICP). Which of the following is a late sign of increased ICP?
   1. Bulging fontanel
   2. Altered level of consciousness
   3. Nausea
   4. Widening pulse pressure

3. A nurse is caring for a child with Reye's syndrome. The nurse understands that the major symptom associated with Reye's syndrome is:
   1. Persistent vomiting
   2. Protein in the urine
   3. A history of a staphylococcus infection
   4. Symptoms of hyperglycemia

4. A child is diagnosed with Reye's syndrome. The nurse assists in preparing a nursing care plan for this child and suggests which of the following?
   1. Providing a quiet atmosphere with dimmed lights
   2. Checking for hearing loss
   3. Monitoring output
   4. Changing body position every 2 hours

5. Which of the following, if noted by the nurse, would indicate a potential complication associated with a tonic-clonic seizure?
   1. Blood on the pillow
   2. Blanched toenails
   3. Migraine headaches
   4. High-pitched cry

6. A nurse plans for a safe environment when caring for an infant at risk for a seizure. In the plan of care, the

seizure precautions would include placing which of the following items at the bedside?
1. A suction apparatus and an airway
2. Oxygen with a tracheotomy set
3. Emergency cart
4. Airway and a tracheotomy set

7. A nurse is reinforcing instructions with an adolescent with a history of seizures, who is on an anticonvulsant medication. Which of the following statements, if made by the adolescent, indicates an understanding of the instructions?
1. "I will never be able to drive a car."
2. "My anticonvulsant medication will clear up my skin."
3. "I can't drink alcohol while I am taking my medication."
4. "If I forget my morning medication, I can take two pills at bedtime."

8. A nurse is collecting data on a child admitted to the hospital with a diagnosis of seizures. The nurse checks for causes of the seizure activity by:
1. Testing the child's urine for specific gravity
2. Obtaining a family history of psychiatric illness
3. Obtaining a history regarding factors that might precipitate seizure activity
4. Asking the child what happens during a seizure

9. A nurse is caring for a child recently diagnosed with cerebral palsy. The parents of the child ask the nurse about the disorder. The nurse bases the response to the parents on the understanding that cerebral palsy is:
1. A chronic disability characterized by a difficulty in controlling the muscles
2. An infectious disease of the central nervous system
3. An inflammation of the brain as a result of a viral illness
4. A congenital condition that results in moderate to severe retardation

10. A nurse is caring for a child with cerebral palsy. The primary goal to be included in the plan of care is to:
1. Eliminate the cause of the disease
2. Prevent the occurrence of emotional disturbances
3. Maximize the child's assets and minimize the limitations caused by the disease
4. Improve muscle control and coordination

11. A nurse is assigned to care for an 8-year-old child with a basilar skull fracture. Which of the following physician orders written in the child's medical record would the nurse question?
1. Restrict fluid intake
2. Keep an intravenous (IV) line patent
3. Insert an indwelling urinary catheter
4. Suction via the nasotracheal route PRN

12. A lumbar puncture is performed on a child suspected of having bacterial meningitis and cerebrospinal fluid (CSF) is obtained for analysis. The nurse understands that which of the following results would verify the diagnosis?
1. Cloudy CSF with low protein and low glucose levels
2. Cloudy CSF with high protein and low glucose levels
3. Clear CSF with high protein and low glucose levels
4. Decreased pressure and cloudy CSF with high protein level

13. A nurse is caring for a child with meningococcal meningitis. Based on the mode of transmission of this infection, which of the following would be included in the plan of care?
1. No precautions are required as long as antibiotics have been started
2. Maintain enteric precautions
3. Maintain isolation precautions for at least 24 hours after the initiation of antibiotics
4. Maintain neutropenic precautions

14. A nurse is observing a child diagnosed with autism. The nurse knows that the primary characteristic(s) of autism include which of the following?
1. Consistent imitation of others actions
2. Normal social play
3. Lack of social interaction and awareness
4. Normal verbal but abnormal nonverbal communication

15. An emergency room nurse is collecting data on a child suspected of being sexually abused. Which of the following data would most likely indicate this suspicion?
1. Poor hygiene
2. Bald spots on the scalp
3. Fear of the parents
4. Swelling of the genitals

ALTERNATE FORMAT QUESTION: MULTIPLE RESPONSE

A nurse is developing a plan of care for a child who is at risk for seizures. Select all interventions that apply if the child has a seizure.

___ Place the child in a prone position
___ Restrain the child
___ Time the seizure
___ Insert a padded tongue blade into the child's mouth
___ Stay with the child
___ Move furniture away from the child

ANSWERS

1. Answer: 3

Rationale: An elevated or bulging anterior fontanel indicates an increase in cerebrospinal fluid collection in the cerebral ventricle. Proteinuria, apical pulse, and blood pressure changes are not specifically associated with increasing cerebrospinal fluid in the brain tissue.

Test-Taking Strategy: Use the principles associated with excessive fluid buildup in the cranial cavity and note the age of the infant. Additionally, correlate "hydrocephalus" in the question, with "anterior fontanel" in option 3. Review the symptoms associated with hydrocephalus if you had difficulty with this question.

Level of Cognitive Ability: Application
Client Needs: Physiological Integrity
Integrated Process: Nursing Process/Data Collection
Content Area: Child Health
Reference: Price, D., & Gwin, J. (2005). *Thompson's pediatric nursing* (9th ed.). Philadelphia: W.B. Saunders, p. 105.

2. Answer: 4

Rationale: Late signs of increased ICP include tachycardia leading to bradycardia, apnea, systolic hypertension, widening pulse pressure, and posturing. A bulging fontanel is a sign of increased ICP in an infant. Nausea and altered level of consciousness are signs of increased ICP in a child. Options 1, 2, and 3 are not late signs.

Test-Taking Strategy: Note the age of the child and that the question asks for the "late" sign. Option 1 can be eliminated because the fontanels are closed in a child. Knowledge of the early and late signs will direct you to the correct option from those remaining. Review these signs if you had difficulty with this question.

Level of Cognitive Ability: Comprehension
Client Needs: Physiological Integrity
Integrated Process: Nursing Process/Data Collection
Content Area: Child Health
Reference: Leifer, G. (2003). *Introduction to maternity and pediatric nursing* (4th ed.). Philadelphia: W.B. Saunders, pp. 560-562.

3. Answer: 1

Rationale: Persistent vomiting is a major symptom associated with intracranial pressure. Options 2, 3, and 4 are incorrect. Protein is not present in the urine. Reye's syndrome is related to a history of viral infections, and hypoglycemia is a symptom of this disease.

Test-Taking Strategy: Note the key words, *major symptom.* Recalling that increased ICP is an associated characteristic will direct you to option 1. Review the symptoms of Reye's syndrome and the signs of increased ICP if you had difficulty with this question.

Level of Cognitive Ability: Comprehension
Client Needs: Physiological Integrity
Integrated Process: Nursing Process/Data Collection
Content Area: Child Health
Reference: Price, D., & Gwin, J. (2005). *Thompson's pediatric nursing* (9th ed.). Philadelphia: W.B. Saunders, p. 304.

4. Answer: 1

Rationale: The major elements of care are to maintain effective cerebral perfusion and control intracranial pressure. Decreasing stimuli in the environment would decrease the stress on the cerebral tissue and neuron responses. Cerebral edema is a progressive part of this disease process. Hearing loss and output are not affected. Changing the body position every 2 hours would not affect the cerebral edema and intracranial pressure directly. The child should be in a head-elevated position to decrease the progression of the cerebral edema and promote drainage of cerebrospinal fluid.

Test-Taking Strategy: Focus on the pathophysiology associated with Reye's syndrome to answer the question. Recalling the effects of environmental stimuli, the responses of the brain cells to stimuli, and how cerebral edema can result will direct you to option 1. Review the symptoms of Reye's syndrome and the signs of increased ICP if you had difficulty with this question.

Level of Cognitive Ability: Application
Client Needs: Physiological Integrity
Integrated Process: Nursing Process/Planning
Content Area: Child Health
References: Leifer, G. (2003). *Introduction to maternity and pediatric nursing* (4th ed.). Philadelphia: W.B. Saunders, p. 545.
Price, D., & Gwin, J. (2005). *Thompson's pediatric nursing* (9th ed.). Philadelphia: W.B. Saunders, p. 304.

5. Answer: 1

Rationale: The complications associated with seizures include airway compromise, extremity and teeth injuries, and tongue lacerations. Night seizures can cause the child to bite down on the tongue. Cyanosis can occur during the tonic-clonic part of the seizure activity, but blanching does not occur. Migraine headaches are not common in children with seizures. Seizures do not cause a high-pitched cry, unless a tumor or intracranial pressure is the cause of the seizure diagnosis.

Test-Taking Strategy: Use knowledge of tonic-clonic activity and the involuntary tightening of all the body muscles that occurs during seizure activity when answering this question. Recall that the tongue can get easily caught by the child's teeth when the seizure activity occurs. This causes injury, swelling, and bleeding of the tongue tissue. Review the complications associated with seizures if you had difficulty with this question.

Level of Cognitive Ability: Comprehension
Client Needs: Physiological Integrity
Integrated Process: Nursing Process/Data Collection
Content Area: Child Health
Reference: Price, D., & Gwin, J. (2005). *Thompson's pediatric nursing* (9th ed.). Philadelphia: W.B. Saunders, p. 241.

6. Answer: 1

Rationale: Seizures cause tightening of all body muscles followed by tremors. Obstructive airway and increased oral secretions are the major complications during and following the seizure. Options 2 and 4 are incorrect because inserting a tracheostomy is not done. Suctioning is helpful to prevent choking and cyanosis. Option 3 is incorrect, because an emergency cart would not be left at the bedside, but would be available in the treatment room or on the nursing unit.

Test-Taking Strategy: Use the process of elimination. Recalling that seizures produce excessive oral secretions and airway obstruction will direct you to option 1. Review the plan of

care associated with seizure precautions if you had difficulty with this question.
Level of Cognitive Ability: Application
Client Needs: Safe, Effective Care Environment
Integrated Process: Nursing Process/Planning
Content Area: Child Health
References: Leifer, G. (2005). *Maternity nursing* (9th ed.). Philadelphia: W.B. Saunders, p. 553.
Wong, D., & Hockenberry, M. (2003). *Nursing care of infants and children* (7th ed.). St. Louis: Mosby, pp. 1693-1694.

7. **Answer: 3**
Rationale: Alcohol will lower the seizure threshold and should be avoided. Adolescents can obtain a driver's license, in most states, when they are seizure-free for 1 year. Anticonvulsants cause acne and oily skin; therefore, a dermatologist may need to be consulted. If an anticonvulsant medication is missed, the physician should be notified.
Test-Taking Strategy: Use the process of elimination and note the key words, *indicates an understanding.* Using general principles related to medication instructions will direct you to option 3. Review teaching points related to anticonvulsants if you had difficulty with this question.
Level of Cognitive Ability: Comprehension
Client Needs: Physiological Integrity
Integrated Process: Nursing Process/Evaluation
Content Area: Pharmacology
Reference: Price, D., & Gwin, J. (2005). *Thompson's pediatric nursing* (9th ed.). Philadelphia: W.B. Saunders, p. 243.

8. **Answer: 3**
Rationale: Fever and infections increase the body's metabolic rate. This can cause seizure activity in children under the age of 5 years old. Dehydration and electrolyte imbalance can also contribute to the occurrence of a seizure. Falls can cause head injury, which would increase intracranial pressure or cerebral edema. Some medications could cause seizures. Specific gravity would not be a reliable test because it varies, depending on the existing condition. Psychiatric illness has no impact on seizure occurrence or cause. Children do not remember what happened during the seizure itself.
Test-Taking Strategy: Use the process of elimination and focus on the issue, the cause of the seizure activity. Note the relationship between the issue and option 3. Review the precipitating factors associated with seizures if you had difficulty with this question.
Level of Cognitive Ability: Application
Client Needs: Physiological Integrity
Integrated Process: Nursing Process/Data Collection
Content Area: Child Health
Reference: Price, D., & Gwin, J. (2005). *Thompson's pediatric nursing* (9th ed.). Philadelphia: W.B. Saunders, p. 239.

9. **Answer: 1**
Rationale: Cerebral palsy is a chronic disability characterized by difficulty in controlling the muscles as a result of an abnormality in the extrapyramidal or pyramidal motor system. Meningitis is an infectious process of the central nervous system. Encephalitis is an inflammation of the brain that occurs as a result of viral illness or central nervous

system infection. Down syndrome is an example of a congenital condition that results in moderate to severe retardation.
Test-Taking Strategy: Use the process of elimination. Eliminate options 2 and 3 first noting that they are similar. From the remaining options, noting the relationship between "palsy" in the question and "muscles" in option 1 will direct you to this option. Review the characteristics associated with cerebral palsy if you had difficulty with this question.
Level of Cognitive Ability: Comprehension
Client Needs: Physiological Integrity
Integrated Process: Nursing Process/Implementation
Content Area: Child Health
Reference: Price, D., & Gwin, J. (2005). *Thompson's pediatric nursing* (9th ed.). Philadelphia: W.B. Saunders, p. 199.

10. **Answer: 3**
Rationale: The goal of managing the child with cerebral palsy is early recognition and intervention to maximize the child's abilities. The cause of the disease cannot be eliminated. It is best to minimize emotional disturbances, if possible, but not to prevent them, because it is healthy for the child to express emotions. Improvement of muscle control and coordination is a component of the plan, but the primary goal is to maximize the child's assets and minimize the limitations caused by the disease.
Test-Taking Strategy: Use the process of elimination. Eliminate options 1 and 2 first because the cause of the disease cannot be eliminated nor can emotional disturbances be prevented. From the remaining options, identify the option that is the umbrella or most global option, which is option 3. Review the goals of care for the child with cerebral palsy if you had difficulty with this question.
Level of Cognitive Ability: Application
Client Needs: Psychosocial Integrity
Integrated Process: Nursing Process/Planning
Content Area: Child Health
Reference: Price, D., & Gwin, J. (2005). *Thompson's pediatric nursing* (9th ed.). Philadelphia: W.B. Saunders, pp. 199-201.

11. **Answer: 4**
Rationale: Nasotracheal suctioning is contraindicated in a child with a basilar skull fracture. Because of the nature of the injury, the suction catheter may be introduced into the brain. The child may need a urinary catheter for accurate monitoring of I&O. Fluids are restricted to prevent fluid overload. An IV line is maintained to administer fluids or medications if necessary.
Test-Taking Strategy: Use the process of elimination and note the key words, *would the nurse question.* Note that options 1, 2, and 3 are similar in that they all address the issue of fluid intake or output. Review care to the child with this type of skull fracture if you had difficulty with this question.
Level of Cognitive Ability: Analysis
Client Needs: Safe, Effective Care Environment
Integrated Process: Nursing Process/Implementation
Content Area: Child Health
References: Leifer, G. (2003). *Introduction to maternity and pediatric nursing* (4th ed.). Philadelphia: W.B. Saunders, pp. 562-563.

Price, D., & Gwin, J. (2005). *Thompson's pediatric nursing* (9th ed.). Philadelphia: W.B. Saunders, pp. 202-203.

12. Answer: 2
Rationale: A diagnosis of meningitis is made by testing CSF obtained by lumbar puncture. In the case of bacterial meningitis, findings usually include increased pressure, cloudy CSF, high protein level, and low glucose level.
Test-Taking Strategy: Use the process of elimination and knowledge regarding the diagnostic findings in meningitis. Eliminate options 3 and 4 first because clear CSF and decreased pressure are not likely to be found if an infectious process such as meningitis is suspected. From this point, recalling that a high protein level indicates a possible diagnosis of meningitis will direct you to option 2. Review the findings in meningitis if you had difficulty with this question.
Level of Cognitive Ability: Comprehension
Client Needs: Physiological Integrity
Integrated Process: Nursing Process/Data Collection
Content Area: Child Health
References: Chernecky, C., & Berger, B. (2004). *Laboratory tests and diagnostic procedures* (4th ed.). Philadelphia: W.B. Saunders, p. 741.
Leifer, G. (2005). *Maternity nursing* (9th ed.). Philadelphia: W.B. Saunders, pp. 507, 546.
Price, D., & Gwin, J. (2005). *Thompson's pediatric nursing* (9th ed.). Philadelphia: W.B. Saunders, p. 361.

13. Answer: 3
Rationale: Meningococcal meningitis is transmitted primarily by droplet infection. Isolation is begun and maintained for at least 24 hours after antibiotics are given. Options 1, 2, and 4 are incorrect.
Test-Taking Strategy: Use the process of elimination, eliminating options 2 and 4 first. Both enteric and neutropenic precautions are unrelated to the mode of transmission of meningococcal meningitis. Recalling that it takes approximately 24 hours for antibiotics to reach a therapeutic blood level will assist in directing you to option 3 from the remaining options. Review the mode of transmission of meningococcal meningitis if you had difficulty with this question.
Level of Cognitive Ability: Application
Client Needs: Safe, Effective Care Environment
Integrated Process: Nursing Process/Planning
Content Area: Child Health
References: Leifer, G. (2005). *Maternity nursing* (9th ed.). Philadelphia: W.B. Saunders, p. 549.
Price, D., & Gwin, J. (2005). *Thompson's pediatric nursing* (9th ed.). Philadelphia: W.B. Saunders, p. 159.

14. Answer: 3
Rationale: Autism is a severe developmental disorder that begins in infancy or toddlerhood. The primary characteristic is lack of social interaction and awareness. Social behaviors in autism include lack of or abnormal imitation of others actions, and the lack of or abnormal social play. Additional characteristics include lack of or impaired verbal communication and markedly abnormal nonverbal communication.
Test-Taking Strategy: Use the process of elimination. Eliminate options 2 and 4 first because they address

normal behaviors. From the remaining options, recalling that the autistic child lacks social interaction and awareness will direct you to option 3. Review the characteristics associated with autism if you had difficulty with this question.
Level of Cognitive Ability: Comprehension
Client Needs: Psychosocial Integrity
Integrated Process: Nursing Process/Data Collection
Content Area: Child Health
Reference: Price, D., & Gwin, J. (2005). *Thompson's pediatric nursing* (9th ed.). Philadelphia: W.B. Saunders, p. 205.

15. Answer: 4
Rationale: The most likely findings in sexual abuse include difficulty walking or sitting, torn, stained, or bloody underclothing, pain, swelling, or itching of the genitals, and bruises, bleeding, or lacerations in the genital or anal area. Poor hygiene may be indicative of physical neglect. Bald spots on the scalp and fear of the parents are most likely associated with physical abuse.
Test-Taking Strategy: Use the process of elimination. Note the key words, *sexually abused*. The only option that specifically addresses a finding related to sexual abuse is option 4. Review the findings in a child suspected of abuse if you had difficulty with this question.
Level of Cognitive Ability: Comprehension
Client Needs: Physiological Integrity
Integrated Process: Nursing Process/Data Collection
Content Area: Child Health
Reference: Price, D., & Gwin, J. (2005). *Thompson's pediatric nursing* (9th ed.). Philadelphia: W.B. Saunders, p. 165.

ALTERNATE FORMAT QUESTION: MULTIPLE RESPONSE

Answers:
Time the seizure
Stay with the child
Move furniture away from the child
Rationale: During a seizure, the child is placed on his or her side in a lateral position. Positioning on the side will prevent aspiration because saliva will drain out the corner of the child's mouth. The child is not restrained because this could cause injury to the child. The nurse would loosen clothing around the child's neck and ensure a patent airway. Nothing is placed into the child's mouth during a seizure because this action may cause injury to the child's mouth, gums, or teeth. The nurse would stay with the child to reduce the risk of injury and allow for observation and timing of the seizure.
Test-Taking Strategy: Visualize this clinical situation. Recalling that airway patency and safety is the priority will assist in determining the appropriate interventions. Review care to the child experiencing a seizure if you had difficulty with this question.
Level of Cognitive Ability: Application
Client Needs: Physiological Integrity
Integrated Process: Nursing Process/Implementation
Content Area: Child Health
References: James, S., Ashwill, J., & Droske, S. (2002). *Nursing care of children: Principles and practice* (2nd ed.). Philadelphia: W.B. Saunders, p. 973.
Price, D., & Gwin, J. (2005). *Thompson's pediatric nursing* (9th ed.). Philadelphia: W.B. Saunders, p. 241.

REFERENCES

Chernecky, C., & Berger, B. (2004). *Laboratory tests and diagnostic procedures* (4th ed.). Philadelphia: W.B. Saunders.

James, S., Ashwill, J., & Droske, S. (2002). *Nursing care of children: Principles and practice* (2nd ed.). Philadelphia; W.B. Saunders.

Leifer, G. (2003). *Introduction to maternity and pediatric nursing* (4th ed.). Philadelphia: W.B. Saunders.

Leifer, G. (2005). *Introduction to maternity and pediatric nursing* (4th ed.). Philadelphia: W.B. Saunders.

Price, D., & Gwin, J. (2005). *Thompson's pediatric nursing* (9th ed.). Philadelphia: W.B. Saunders.

Wong, D., & Hockenberry, M. (2003). *Nursing care of infants and children* (7th ed.). St. Louis: Mosby.

Eye, Ear, Throat, and Respiratory Disorders

I. STRABISMUS

A. Description
1. Called "squint" or "lazy eye"
2. A condition in which the eyes are not aligned because of lack of coordination of the extraocular muscles
3. Most often results from muscle imbalance or paralysis of extraocular muscles, but may also result from conditions such as a brain tumor, myasthenia gravis, or infection
4. Normal in the young infant, but should not be present after about age 4 months

B. Data collection
1. Amblyopia if not treated early
2. Permanent loss of vision if not treated early
3. Loss of binocular vision
4. Impairment of depth perception
5. Frequent headaches
6. Squints or tilts head to see

C. Interventions
1. Corrective lenses as indicated
2. Instruct the parents regarding patching (occlusion therapy) of the "good" eye to strengthen the weak eye
3. Prepare for botulinum toxin (Botox) injection into the eye muscle, which produces temporary paralysis and allows muscles opposite the paralyzed muscle to straighten the eye
4. Inform the parents that the injection of botulinum toxin wears off in about 2 months and, if successful, correction will occur
5. Prepare for surgery to realign the weak muscles as prescribed if nonsurgical interventions are unsuccessful
6. Instruct the parents about the need for follow-up visits

II. CONJUNCTIVITIS

A. Description
1. Also known as "pinkeye"
2. Inflammation of the conjunctiva
3. Usually caused by allergy, infection, or trauma
4. Bacterial or viral conjunctivitis is extremely contagious
5. Chlamydial conjunctivitis is rare in older children and, if diagnosed in a child who is not sexually active, the child should be assessed for possible sexual **abuse**

B. Data collection
1. Itching, burning, or scratchy eyelids
2. Redness
3. Edema
4. Discharge

C. Interventions
1. Instruct in infection control measures such as good hand washing and not sharing towels and washcloths
2. Administer antibiotic or antiviral eyedrops or ointment as prescribed if infection is present
3. Administer antihistamines as prescribed if an allergy is present
4. Instruct the child and parents in the administration of the prescribed medications
5. Instruct the parents that the child should be kept home from school or day care until antibiotic eyedrops have been administered for 24 hours
6. Instruct in the use of cool compresses to lessen irritation and in wearing dark glasses for photophobia
7. Instruct the child to avoid rubbing the eye to prevent injury
8. Instruct the child who is wearing contact lenses to discontinue wearing them and to obtain new lenses to eliminate the chance of reinfection

9. Instruct the adolescent that eye makeup should be discarded and replaced

III. OTITIS MEDIA

A. Description
   1. Infection of the middle ear occurring as a result of a blocked eustachian tube, which prevents normal drainage
   2. Otitis media is a common complication of an acute respiratory infection
   3. Infants and children are more prone to otitis media because their eustachian tubes are shorter, wider, and straighter

B. Data collection
   1. Fever
   2. Irritability and restlessness
   3. Loss of appetite
   4. Rolling of head from side to side
   5. Pulling on or rubbing the ear
   6. Earache or pain
   7. Signs of hearing loss
   8. Purulent ear drainage
   9. Red, opaque, bulging, or retracting tympanic membrane

C. Interventions
   1. Encourage fluids
   2. Teach the parents to feed infants in upright position
   3. Instruct the child to avoid chewing during the acute period because chewing increases pain
   4. Provide local heat, and have the child lie with the affected ear down
   5. Instruct the parents in the appropriate procedure to clean drainage from the ear with sterile cotton swabs
   6. Instruct the parents in the administration of analgesics or antipyretics such as acetaminophen (Tylenol) to decrease fever and pain
   7. Instruct the parents in the administration of prescribed antibiotics, emphasizing that the 10- to 14-day period is necessary to eradicate positive organisms
   8. Instruct the parents that screening for hearing loss may be necessary
   9. Instruct the parents about the procedure for administering ear medications (Box 31-1)

BOX 31-1

Administering Ear Medications

In a child younger than age 3 years, pull the pinna down and back.
In a child older than 3 years, pull the pinna up and back.

D. Myringotomy
   1. Description: Insertion of tympanoplasty tubes into the middle ear to equalize pressure and keep the ear aerated
   2. Interventions postoperatively
      a. Instruct the parents and child to keep the ears dry
      b. Earplugs should be worn during bathing, shampooing, and swimming
      c. Diving and submerging under water are not allowed

IV. TONSILLECTOMY AND ADENOIDECTOMY

A. Description
   1. Tonsillitis refers to inflammation and infection of the tonsils
   2. Adenoiditis refers to inflammation and infection of the adenoids

B. Data collection
   1. Persistent or recurrent sore throat
   2. Enlarged bright red tonsils that may be covered with white exudate
   3. Difficulty in swallowing
   4. Mouth breathing and an unpleasant mouth odor
   5. Fever
   6. Cough
   7. Enlarged adenoids may cause nasal quality of speech, mouth breathing, hearing difficulty, snoring, or obstructive sleep apnea

C. Interventions preoperatively
   1. Monitor for signs of active infection
   2. Monitor bleeding and clotting studies because the throat is very vascular
   3. Prepare the child for a sore throat postoperatively, and inform the child that he or she will need to drink liquids
   4. Check for any loose teeth to decrease the risk of aspiration during surgery

D. Interventions postoperatively
   1. Position prone or side-lying to facilitate drainage
   2. Have suction equipment available, but do not suction unless there is an airway obstruction
   3. Monitor for signs of hemorrhage (frequent swallowing may be indicative of hemorrhage); if hemorrhage occurs, turn the child to the side and notify the physician
   4. Discourage coughing or clearing the throat
   5. Provide clear, cool, noncitrus and noncarbonated fluids
   6. Avoid milk products initially because they will coat the throat
   7. Avoid red liquids, which will simulate the appearance of blood if the child vomits
   8. Do not give the child any straws, forks, or sharp objects that can be put into the mouth
   9. Administer acetaminophen (Tylenol) for sore throat as prescribed

10. Instruct the parents to notify the physician if bleeding, a persistent earache, or fever occurs
11. Instruct the parents to keep the child away from crowds until healing has occurred

V. EPIGLOTTITIS
A. Description
   1. A bacterial form of croup
   2. An inflammation of the epiglottis, which may be caused by *Haemophilus influenzae* type B or *Streptococcus pneumoniae*
   3. Occurs most frequently in children 2 to 5 years of age
   4. The onset is abrupt, and the condition occurs most often in the winter
   5. Considered an emergency situation
B. Data collection
   1. High fever
   2. Sore, red, and inflamed throat
   3. Absence of spontaneous cough
   4. Drooling
   5. Difficulty in swallowing
   6. Muffled voice
   7. Inspiratory **stridor**
   8. Agitation
   9. Tripod positioning; while supporting the body with the hands and arms, the child thrusts the chin forward and opens the mouth in an attempt to widen the airway
C. Interventions
   1. Maintain a patent airway
   2. Check respiratory status and breath sounds, noting **nasal flaring,** the use of accessory muscles, and the presence of **stridor**
   3. Check temperature by the axillary route, not the oral route
   4. To prevent spasm of epiglottis and airway occlusion, *no* attempts should be made to visualize the posterior pharynx or to obtain a throat culture
   5. Prepare the child for lateral neck films to confirm the diagnosis
   6. Maintain nothing by mouth (NPO) status
   7. Do not leave the child unattended
   8. Do not force the child to lie down
   9. Do not restrain the child
   10. Administer intravenous (IV) fluids and antibiotics, as prescribed
   11. Administer analgesics and antipyretics (acetaminophen [Tylenol]) to reduce fever and throat pain, as prescribed
   12. Provide cool mist oxygen therapy, as prescribed
   13. Provide high humidification to cool the airway and decrease swelling
   14. Have resuscitation equipment available, and prepare for enotracheal intubation or tracheotomy for severe respiratory distress
   15. Ensure that the child is up to date with immunization schedule, including *Haemophilus influenzae* type b (Hib) conjugate vaccine

VI. LARYNGOTRACHEOBRONCHITIS (LTB)
A. Description
   1. Inflammation of larynx, trachea, and bronchi
   2. Most common type of croup; may be viral or bacterial
   3. Has a gradual onset and may be preceded by an upper respiratory infection
B. Data collection
   1. Fever, low-grade fever to high fever
   2. Irritability and restlessness
   3. Hoarse voice
   4. Seal bark and brassy cough
   5. Inspiratory **stridor** and suprasternal **retractions**
   6. Use of accessory muscles for breathing
   7. Crackles and **wheezing** on lung auscultation
   8. Anorexia, nausea, and vomiting
   9. Signs of anoxia and carbon dioxide retention
   10. Cyanosis
C. Interventions
   1. Maintain a patent airway
   2. Monitor respiratory status, checking for **nasal flaring,** sternal **retraction,** and inspiratory **stridor**
   3. Monitor for pallor or cyanosis
   4. Elevate the head of the bed and provide bed rest
   5. Provide humidified oxygen via cool mist tent for the hospitalized child
   6. Instruct the parents to use a cool air vaporizer or humidifier at home; other measures include having the child breathe in the cool night air or the air from an open freezer, or taking the child to a cool basement or garage
   7. Provide and encourage fluid intake; IVs may be prescribed to maintain hydration status if the child is unable to take oral fluids
   8. Administer acetaminophen (Tylenol) as prescribed to reduce fever
   9. Avoid cough syrups and cold medicines, which may dry and thicken secretions
   10. Administer bronchodilators if prescribed to relax smooth muscle and relieve **stridor**
   11. Administer corticosteroids if prescribed for the anti-inflammatory effect
   12. Administer nebulized epinephrine (racemic epinephrine) as prescribed for children with severe disease, **stridor** at rest, **retractions,** or difficulty breathing
   13. Administer antibiotics as prescribed, noting that they are not indicated unless a bacterial infection is present
   14. Have resuscitation equipment available

VII. BRONCHITIS

A. Description: Infection of the major bronchi; may be referred to as tracheobronchitis

B. Data collection
1. Fever
2. Dry, hacking, and nonproductive cough that is worse at night and becomes productive in 2 to 3 days

C. Interventions
1. Monitor for respiratory distress
2. Provide cool, humidified air
3. Monitor for signs of dehydration, such as a sunken fontanel, poor skin turgor, and decreased and concentrated urinary output
4. Increased fluid intake
5. Administer acetaminophen (Tylenol) for fever as prescribed

VIII. BRONCHIOLITIS–RESPIRATORY SYNCYTIAL VIRUS (RSV)

A. Description
1. An inflammation of the bronchioles that causes a thick production of mucus, which occludes bronchiole tubes and small bronchi
2. RSV is a common cause of bronchiolitis
3. RSV, although not airborne, is highly communicable and is usually transferred by the hands

B. Data collection
1. Upper respiratory infection (URI) symptoms such as rhinorrhea and low-grade fever
2. Lethargy, poor feeding, and irritability in infants
3. Tachypnea
4. Increased difficulty in breathing
5. **Nasal flaring** and retractions
6. Expiratory wheeze and grunt
7. Diminished breath sounds

C. Interventions
1. Maintain a patent airway
2. Position the child at a 30- to 40-degree angle with the neck slightly extended to maintain an open airway and decrease pressure on the diaphragm
3. Provide cool, humidified oxygen
4. Encourage fluids; IV fluids may be necessary until the acute stage has passed
5. Monitor for signs of dehydration

D. The child with RSV
1. Isolate in a single room or place in a room with another RSV child
2. Maintain good hand washing procedures
3. Ensure that nurses caring for these children do not care for other high-risk children
4. Wear gowns when soiling of clothing may occur during care
5. Administer ribavirin (Virazole), an antiviral respiratory medication, if prescribed (Box 31-2)
6. Prepare for the administration of respiratory syncytial virus immune globulin (RSV-IG IV or RespiGam or palivizumab [synagis] (Box 31-3)

IX. PNEUMONIA

A. Description (Box 31-4)
1. Inflammation of the alveoli caused by a virus, mycoplasmal agent, bacteria, or aspiration of foreign substances
2. The causative agent is usually introduced into the lungs through inhalation or from the bloodstream
3. Viral pneumonia occurs more frequently than bacterial pneumonia and is often associated with a viral upper respiratory infection (URI)
4. Primary atypical pneumonia (*Mycoplasma pneumoniae*) is the most common cause of pneumonia in children between the ages of 5 and 12 years; occurs primarily in the fall and winter months, and is more prevalent in crowded living conditions
5. Bacterial pneumonia is often a serious infection; hospitalization is indicated when pleural effusion or empyema accompanies the disease, and is mandatory for children with staphylococcal pneumonia

---

BOX 31-2

Administering Ribavirin (Virazole)

Ribavarin is administered via aerosol by hood, tent, or mask or through ventilator tubing.
Pregnant health care providers should not care for a child receiving ribavirin.
The nurse wearing contact lenses should wear goggles when coming in contact with ribavirin, because the mist may dissolve soft lenses.

BOX 31-3

Respiratory Syncytial Virus Immune Globulin

Used prophylactically to prevent RSV in high-risk infants
Not administered to infants or children with congenital heart disease (CHD) or with cyanotic CHD

BOX 31-4

Types of Pneumonia

Viral pneumonia
Primary atypical pneumonia (*Mycoplasma pneumoniae*)
Bacterial pneumonia
Aspiration pneumonia

6. Aspiration pneumonia occurs when food, secretions, liquids, or other materials enter the lung and cause inflammation and a chemical pneumonitis; classic symptoms include an increasing cough or fever with foul-smelling sputum, deteriorating results on chest x-rays, and other signs of airway involvement

B. Viral pneumonia
   1. Data collection
      a. Mild fever, slight cough, and malaise, to high fever, severe cough, and prostration
      b. Nonproductive or productive cough of small amounts of whitish sputum
      c. Wheezes or fine crackles
   2. Interventions
      a. Administer oxygen with cool mist as prescribed
      b. Increase fluid intake
      c. Administer antipyretics for fever as prescribed
      d. Administer chest physiotherapy and postural drainage as prescribed
      e. Antimicrobial therapy is reserved for children in whom the presence of infection is demonstrated by cultures

C. Primary atypical pneumonia
   1. Data collection
      a. Fever, chills, anorexia, headache, malaise, and muscle pain
      b. Rhinitis, sore throat, and dry, hacking cough
      c. Cough is nonproductive initially, then produces seromucoid sputum, which becomes mucopurulent or blood-streaked
   2. Interventions: Symptomatic

D. Bacterial pneumonia
   1. Data collection
      a. Acute onset, fever, toxic appearance
      b. Infant: Irritability, lethargy, poor feeding; abrupt fever (may be accompanied by seizures); respiratory distress (air hunger, tachypnea, and circumoral cyanosis)
      c. Older child: Headache, chills, abdominal pain, chest pain, meningeal symptoms (meningism)
      d. Hacking, nonproductive cough
      e. Diminished breath sounds or scattered crackles
      f. As the infection resolves, coarse crackles and **wheezing** are heard; cough becomes productive with purulent sputum
   2. Interventions
      a. Antimicrobial therapy is initiated as soon as the diagnosis is suspected
      b. Administer oxygen (via hood, mist tent, or nasal cannula) for respiratory distress as prescribed
      c. Place the child in a mist tent, as prescribed; cool humidification moistens the airways and assists in temperature reduction
      d. Suction the infant to maintain a patent airway if the infant is unable to handle secretions

e. Administer chest physiotherapy and postural drainage every 4 hours, as prescribed
f. Promote bed rest to conserve energy
g. Encourage the child to lie on the affected side (if pneumonia is unilateral) to splint the chest and reduce the discomfort caused by pleural rubbing
h. Provide liberal fluid intake (administer cautiously to prevent aspiration); IV fluids may be necessary
i. Administer antipyretics for fever as prescribed; monitor temperature frequently because of the risk for febrile seizures
j. Institute isolation precautions with pneumococcal or staphylococcal pneumonia (according to agency policy)
k. Administer antitussives as prescribed before rest times and meals if the cough is disturbing
l. Continuous closed chest drainage may be instituted if purulent fluid is present (usually noted in staphylococcal infections)
m. Fluid accumulation in the pleural cavity may be removed by thoracentesis; thoracentesis also provides a means for obtaining fluid for culture and for instilling antibiotics directly into the pleural cavity

X. TUBERCULOSIS (TB)

A. Description
   1. A contagious disease caused by *Mycobacterium tuberculosis,* an acid-fast bacillus
   2. Multidrug-resistant strains of *Mycobacterium tuberculosis* occur because of client or family noncompliance with therapeutic regimens
   3. The route of transmission of *Mycobacterium tuberculosis* is through inhalation of droplets from an individual with active TB
   4. Most children are infected by a family member or by another individual with whom they have frequent contact, such as a babysitter

B. Data collection
   1. May be asymptomatic or develop symptoms such as malaise, fever, cough, weight loss, anorexia, and lymphadenopathy
   2. Specific symptoms related to the site of infection, such as the lungs, brain, or bone, may be present

C. Mantoux test (Box 31-5)
   1. Will produce a positive reaction 2 to 10 weeks after the initial infection
   2. Determines whether the child has been infected and has developed a sensitivity to the protein of the tubercle bacillus; a positive reaction does not confirm the presence of active disease
   3. Once the child reacts positively, the child will always react positively; a positive reaction in a

Mantoux Test Results

Induration measuring 15 mm or more is considered to be a positive reaction in children 4 years of age or older who do not have any risk factors.

Induration measuring 10 mm or more is considered to be a positive reaction in children younger than 4 years of age and in those with chronic illness or at high risk for exposure to TB.

Induration measuring 5 mm or more is considered to be positive for those in the highest risk groups, such as children with immunosuppressive conditions or human immunodeficiency virus (HIV) infection.

previously negative test indicates that the child has been infected since the last test

4. TB testing should not be done at the same time as measles immunization; viral interference from the measles vaccine may cause a false-negative reaction

▲ D. Sputum culture

1. A definitive diagnosis is made by demonstrating the presence of mycobacteria in a culture
2. Because an infant or young child often swallows sputum rather than expectorates, gastric washings (aspiration of lavaged contents from the fasting stomach) may be done to obtain a specimen; specimen is obtained in the early morning, before breakfast

▲ E. Interventions

1. Medications
   a. Include isoniazid (INH), rifampin (Rifadin), and pyrazinamide
   b. A 9-month course of INH may be prescribed to prevent a latent infection from progressing to clinically active TB and to prevent initial infection in children in high-risk situations; a 12-month course may be prescribed for the HIV-infected child
   c. Recommendation for the child with clinically active TB may include INH, rifampin, and pyrazinamide daily for 2 months, and then INH and rifampin twice weekly for 4 months
2. Place children with infectious disease on airborne precautions until medications have been initiated, sputum cultures demonstrate a diminished number of organisms, and cough is improving
3. Wear a mask if the child is coughing and does not reliably cover his or her mouth
4. Maintain airborne precautions with family members until they are demonstrated not to have infectious TB
5. Stress the importance of adequate rest and adequate diet

6. Instruct the child and family in measures to prevent transmission of TB

▲

XI. ASTHMA

A. Description
1. Chronic inflammatory disease of the airways
2. Is commonly caused by physical and chemical irritants such as foods, pollens, dust mites, cockroaches, smoke, animal dander, temperature changes, respiratory infection, activity, and stress
3. The allergic reaction in the airways can cause an immediate reaction, with obstruction occurring, and can precipitate a late bronchial obstructive reaction several hours after the initial exposure
4. A common symptom is coughing in the absence of respiratory infection, especially at night
5. Status asthmaticus ▲
   a. Child displays respiratory distress despite vigorous treatment measures
   b. A medical emergency that can result in respiratory failure and death if left untreated

B. Data collection ▲
1. Episodes of **wheezing**, breathlessness, dyspnea, chest tightness, and cough, particularly at night and/or in the early morning
2. Itching localized at the front of the neck or over the upper part of the back
3. Exacerbations are episodes of progressively worsening shortness of breath, cough, **wheezing**, chest tightness, decreases in expiratory airflow because of bronchospasm, mucosal edema, and mucus plugging; air is trapped behind occluded or narrow airways, and hypoxemia can occur
4. Asthmatic episode ▲
   a. Begins with irritability, restlessness, headache, feeling tired, or chest tightness
   b. Respiratory symptoms include a hacking, irritable, nonproductive cough caused by bronchial edema
   c. Accumulated secretions stimulate the cough, and the cough becomes rattling and productive of frothy, clear, gelatinous sputum
   d. Child may be pale or flushed, and the lips may have a deep, dark red color that may progress to cyanosis observed in the nail beds and skin, especially around the mouth
   e. Restlessness, apprehension, and diaphoresis occur
   f. Younger children assume the tripod sitting ▲ position; older children sit upright with the shoulders in a hunched-over position, with the hands on the bed or a chair, and arms braced to facilitate the use of accessory muscles of breathing (child refuses to lie down)
   g. Child speaks in short, broken phrases

h. Retractions

i. Hyperresonance on percussion of the chest

j. Breath sounds are coarse and loud, with crackles, coarse rhonchi, and inspiratory and expiratory **wheezing**; expiration is prolonged

5. Exercise-induced bronchospasm (EIB): Cough, shortness of breath, chest pain or tightness, **wheezing**, and endurance problems during exercise

6. Severe spasm or obstruction: Breath sounds and crackles may become inaudible, and the cough is ineffective (represents a lack of air movement)

7. Ventilatory failure and asphyxia: Shortness of breath, with air movement in the chest restricted to the point of absent breath sounds accompanied by a sudden rise in the respiratory rate

C. Interventions: Acute episode (Box 31-6)

D. Medications

1. Quick-relief (rescue) medications: To treat symptoms and exacerbations (Box 31-7)

2. Long-term control (preventer) medications: To achieve and maintain control of inflammation (Box 31-8)

3. Nebulizer, metered-dose inhaler (MDI), or peak expiratory flow meters (PEFMs)

a. Used to deliver many of the medications used to treat asthma

b. If the child has difficulty using the MDI, medication can be administered by nebulization (medication is mixed with saline and then nebulized with compressed air by a machine)

E. Chest physiotherapy (CPT)

1. Includes breathing exercises and physical training

2. Not recommended during an acute exacerbation

F. Allergen control

1. Prevents and reduces exposure to airborne and environmental allergens

2. Skin testing to identify allergens; immunotherapy (hyposensitization) is not recommended for allergens that can be eliminated effectively

G. Home care measures

1. Instruct in measures to eliminate allergens

2. Avoid extremes of environmental temperature; in cold temperatures, instruct the child to breathe through the nose, not the mouth, and to cover the nose and mouth with a scarf

3. Avoid exposure to individuals with a viral respiratory infection

4. Instruct the child in how to recognize early symptoms of an asthma attack

5. Instruct the child in the administration of medications, as prescribed

6. Instruct the child in the use of a nebulizer, MDI, or PEFM

7. Instruct the child about the importance of home monitoring of peak expiratory flow rate; decrease in rate may be indicative of impending infection or exacerbation

---

BOX 31-6

Interventions in the Event of an Acute Asthma Attack

Assess airway patency.

Administer humidified oxygen by nasal prongs or face-mask.

Administer quick-relief (rescue) medications.

Continuously monitor respiratory status, pulse oximetry, and color; be alert to decreased wheezing or a silent chest, which may signal the inability to move air.

Initiate an IV line, and prepare to correct dehydration, acidosis, or electrolyte imbalances.

Prepare the child for a chest x-ray.

Prepare to obtain blood samples for determining arterial blood gases and serum electrolytes.

BOX 31-7

Quick-Relief (Rescue) Medications

Short-acting β_2 agonists

Anticholinergics (for relief of acute bronchospasm)

Systemic corticosteroids (for anti-inflammatory action to treat reversible airflow obstruction)

BOX 31-8

Long-term Control (Preventer Medications)

Corticosteroids

Antiallergic agents

Nonsteroidal anti-inflammatory drugs

Long-acting β_2 agonists

Leukotriene modifiers to prevent bronchospasm and inflammatory cell infiltration

Long-acting bronchodilators

Nebulizer, metered-dose inhaler (MDI), or peak expiratory flow meters (PEFMs)

---

8. Instruct the child in the cleaning of devices used for inhaled medications (oral candidiasis can occur with the use of aerosolized steroids)

9. Encourage adequate rest, sleep, and a well-balanced diet

10. Instruct the child in the importance of adequate fluid intake to liquefy secretions

11. Assist in developing an exercise program

12. Instruct the child in the procedure for respiratory treatments and exercises, as prescribed

13. Encourage the child to cough effectively

14. Encourage the parents to keep immunizations up to date; annual influenza vaccinations are recommended

15. Inform other health care providers and school personnel of the asthma condition

16. Allow the child to take control of self-care measures on the basis of age appropriateness

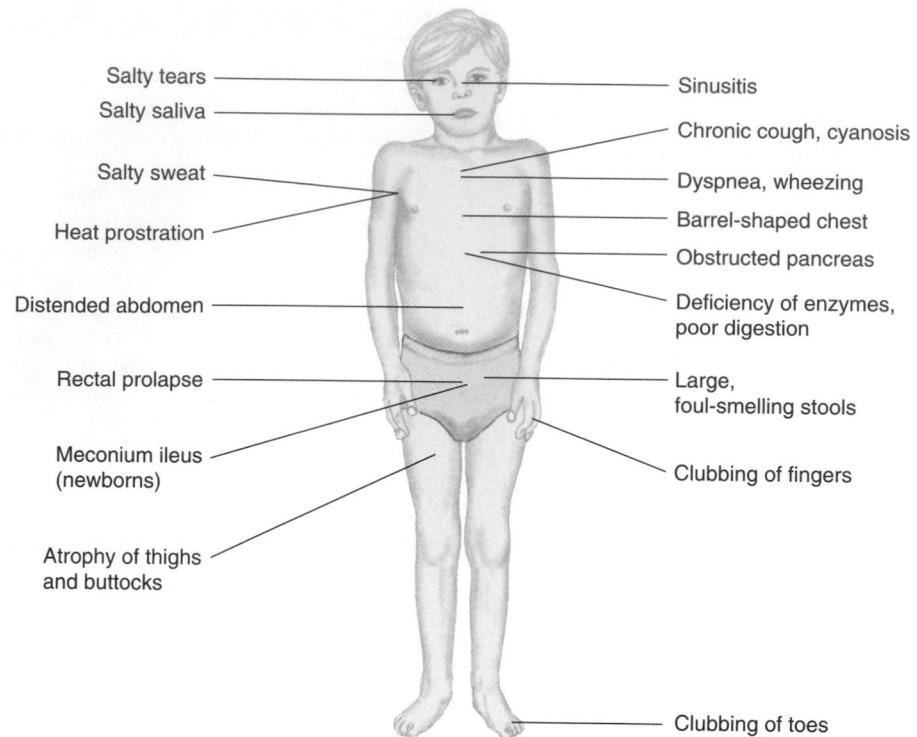

Salty tears
Salty saliva
Salty sweat
Heat prostration
Distended abdomen
Rectal prolapse
Meconium ileus
(newborns)
Atrophy of thighs
and buttocks

Sinusitis
Chronic cough, cyanosis
Dyspnea, wheezing
Barrel-shaped chest
Obstructed pancreas
Deficiency of enzymes,
poor digestion
Large,
foul-smelling stools
Clubbing of fingers
Clubbing of toes

FIG. 31-1 Manifestations of cystic fibrosis. (From Price, D., & Gwin, J. [2005]. *Thompson's pediatric nursing* [9th ed.]. Philadelphia: W.B. Saunders.)

XII. CYSTIC FIBROSIS (CF) (Figure 31-1)

A. Description

1. A chronic multisystem disorder (autosomal recessive trait disorder) characterized by exocrine gland dysfunction
2. The mucus produced by the exocrine glands is abnormally thick, causing obstruction of the small passageways of the affected organs
3. The most common symptoms are pancreatic enzyme deficiency caused by duct blockage, progressive chronic lung disease associated with infection, and sweat gland dysfunction resulting in increased sodium and chloride sweat concentrations
4. An increase in sodium and chloride in both sweat and saliva forms the basis for the most reliable diagnostic test, the sweat chloride test

B. Respiratory system

1. Symptoms are produced by the stagnation of mucus in the airway, leading to bacterial colonization and destruction of lung tissue
2. Emphysema and atelectasis occur as the airways become increasingly obstructed
3. Chronic hypoxemia causes contraction and hypertrophy of the muscle fibers in pulmonary arteries and arterioles, leading to pulmonary hypertension and eventual cor pulmonale

4. Pneumothorax from ruptured bullae and hemoptysis from erosion of the bronchial wall through an artery occur as the disease progresses
5. **Wheezing** and dry nonproductive cough
6. Dyspnea
7. Cyanosis
8. Clubbing of the fingers and toes (Figure 31-2)
9. Repeated episodes of bronchitis and pneumonia

C. Gastrointestinal system

1. Meconium ileus in the neonate
2. Intestinal obstruction (distal intestinal obstructive syndrome) caused by thick intestinal secretions; signs include pain, abdominal distention, nausea, and vomiting
3. Steatorrhea (frothy, foul-smelling stools)
4. Deficiency of the fat-soluble vitamins A, D, E, and K, which causes easy bruising and anemia
5. Malnutrition and failure to thrive; demonstration of hypoalbuminemia from diminished absorption of protein, resulting in generalized edema
6. Rectal prolapse can occur as a result of the large, bulky stools, and lack of the supportive fat pads around the rectum

D. Integumentary system

1. Abnormally high concentrations of sodium and chloride in sweat
2. Parents report that the infant tastes "salty" when kissed

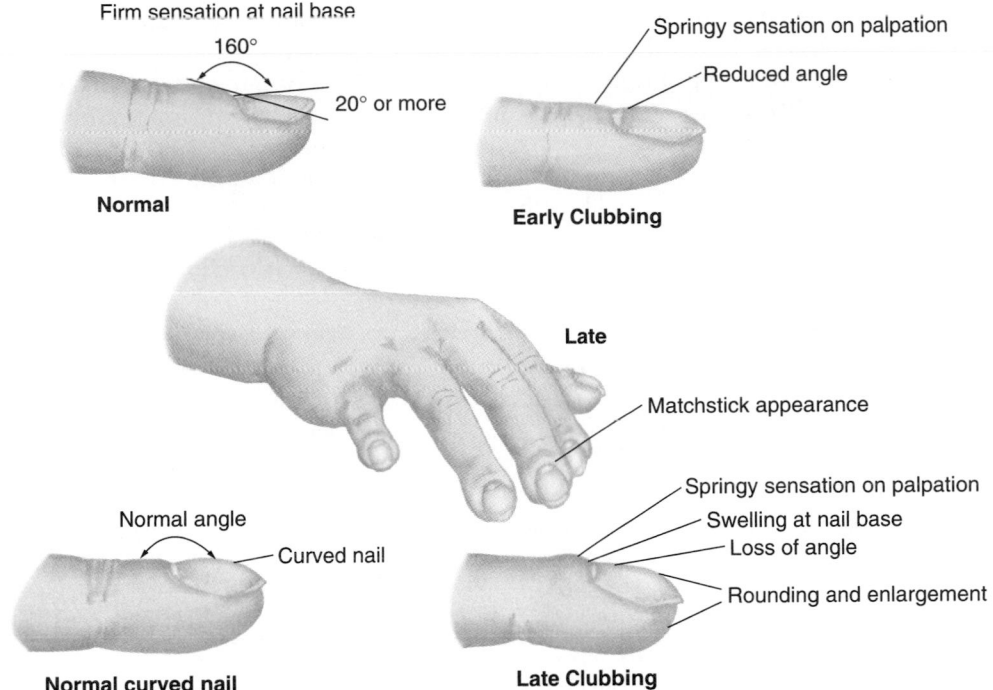

FIG. 31-2 Clubbing of fingers. (From McKinney, E., James, S., Murray, S., & Ashwill, J. [2005]. *Maternal-child nursing* [2nd ed.]. St. Louis: W.B. Saunders.)

3. Dehydration and electrolyte imbalances, especially during hyperthermic conditions

E. Reproductive system
   1. Delayed **puberty** in females
   2. Fertility can be inhibited by highly viscous cervical secretions, which act as a plug and block sperm entry
   3. Males are usually sterile, caused by the blockage of the vas deferens by abnormal secretions or by failure of normal development of duct structures

F. Diagnostic tests
   1. Quantitative sweat chloride test (Box 31-9)
   2. Chest x-ray: Reveals atelectasis and obstructive emphysema
   3. Pulmonary function tests: Provide evidence of abnormal small airway function
   4. Stool fat and/or enzyme analysis: A 72-hour stool sample is collected to check the fat and/or enzyme (trypsin) content (food intake is recorded during the collection)

G. Interventions
   1. Respiratory system
      a. Goals of treatment include preventing and treating pulmonary infection by improving aeration, removing secretions, and administering antimicrobial medications
      b. Chest physiotherapy (percussion and postural drainage) on awakening and in the evening (more frequently during pulmonary infection)
      c. Chest physiotherapy (CPT) should not be performed before or immediately after a meal

---

BOX 31-9

Quantitative Sweat Chloride Test

The production of sweat is stimulated (pilocarpine iontophoresis), the sweat is collected, and the sweat electrolytes are measured (a minimum of 50 mg of sweat is needed).

Normally, sweat chloride concentration is lower than 40 mEq/L.

A chloride concentration higher than 60 mEq/L is a positive test result.

Chloride concentrations of 40 to 60 mEq/L are highly suggestive of CF and require a repeat test.

---

      d. Bronchodilator medication by aerosol to open the bronchi for easier expectoration (administered before the CPT, when the child has reactive airway disease or is **wheezing**)
      e. Use of a Flutter Mucus Clearance Device (a small, hand-held plastic pipe with a stainless steel ball on the inside) that facilitates removal of mucus; store away from small children because if the device separates, the steel ball poses a choking hazard
      f. Use of a ThAIRapy vest device, which provides high-frequency chest wall oscillations to help loosen secretions
      g. Administration of recombinant human deoxyribonuclease (DNase), known generically as dornase alfa (Pulmozyme), which decreases the viscosity of mucus

h. Instruct the parents not to give cough suppressants, because they will inhibit expectoration of secretions and promote infection

i. Teach the child forced expiratory technique (huffing) to mobilize secretions

j. Develop a physical exercise program with the aim of establishing a good habitual breathing pattern

k. Administer antibiotics as prescribed, which may be prescribed prophylactically or when pulmonary symptoms develop

l. Aerosolized antibiotics may be prescribed and are administered after CPT is performed, or IV antibiotics may be prescribed and administered at home through a central venous access device

m. Administer oxygen as prescribed during acute episodes; monitor closely for oxygen narcosis

n. Monitor for hemoptysis; more than 300 mL in 24 hours for the older child (less for a younger child) needs to be treated immediately

o. Hemoptysis may be controlled by bed rest, cough suppressants, antibiotics, and vitamin K; if hemoptysis persists, the site of bleeding may be cauterized or embolized

p. Lung transplantation is a final therapeutic option for the end-stage child

2. Gastrointestinal system

a. The goal of treatment for pancreatic insufficiency is to replace pancreatic enzymes; administered with meals and snacks (or within 30 minutes of eating meals and snacks) to ensure that digestive enzymes are mixed with food in the duodenum

b. The amount of pancreatic enzymes administered is adjusted to achieve normal **growth** and a decrease in the number of stools to two or three per day

c. Enteric-coated pancreatic enzymes should not be crushed or chewed

d. Pancreatic enzymes should not be given if the child is NPO

e. Encourage a well-balanced, high-protein, high-calorie diet; multivitamins and vitamins A, D, E, and K are also administered

f. Monitor weight and monitor for failure to thrive

g. Monitor for constipation and intestinal obstruction

h. Supplement the child's diet with salt during extremely hot weather or if the child has a fever; include fluids such as Gatorade or Exceed, which provide an adequate supply of electrolytes

H. Home care

1. Instruct the parents about the prescribed treatment measures and their importance

2. Instruct the parents to be sure immunizations are up to date

3. Inform the parents that the child should be vaccinated yearly for pneumococcus and influenza

4. Inform the parents about the Cystic Fibrosis Foundation

XIII. SUDDEN INFANT DEATH SYNDROME (SIDS)

A. Description

1. Unexpected death of an apparently healthy infant under age 1 year for which a thorough autopsy fails to demonstrate an adequate cause of death

2. The cause is not known; may be related to a brainstem abnormality in the neurologic regulation of cardiorespiratory control

3. Time of year: Most frequent during winter months

4. Time of death: Usually occurs during sleep

5. Age: Most frequently occurs from 2 to 4 months of life

6. Sex and race

a. Incidence higher in males

b. Incidence higher in Native Americans, African Americans, and Hispanics

7. Sleep risk habits

a. Prone position

b. Use of soft bedding

c. Overheating (thermal stress)

d. Possibly, sleeping with an adult

B. Appearance when found

1. Apneic, blue, lifeless

2. Frothy blood-tinged fluid in the nose and mouth

3. May be found in any position but is typically found in a disheveled bed, with blankets over the head, and huddled in a corner

4. May be clutching bedding

5. Diaper may be wet and full of stool

C. Prevention

1. Infants should be placed in the supine position for sleep

2. Soft moldable mattresses and bedding, such as pillows or quilts, should not be used under the infant for bedding

3. Stuffed animals should be removed from the crib while the infant is sleeping

4. Discourage bed sharing (sleeping with an adult)

5. Avoid overheating during sleep

PRACTICE QUESTIONS

1. A day care nurse is observing a 2-year-old child and suspects that the child may have strabismus. Which of the following observations might be indicative of this condition?

1. The child consistently tilts his or her head to see

2. The child consistently turns his or her head to see

3. The child does not respond when spoken to

4. The child has difficulty hearing

2. A nurse has provided instructions to a mother of a child diagnosed with bacterial conjunctivitis. Which of the following, if stated by the mother, would indicate a need for further instructions?

1. "I need to wash my hands frequently."

2. "I need to clean the eye as prescribed."

3. "I need to give the eyedrops as prescribed."

4. "It is OK to share towels and washcloths."

3. A nurse provides instructions to parents regarding the methods that will decrease the risk of recurrent otitis media in infants. Which of the following would the nurse include in the instructions?

1. Feed the infant in an upright position

2. Allow the infant to have a bottle during nap time

3. Maintain bottle-feeding as long as possible

4. Discontinue breast-feeding as soon as possible

4. A nurse is assigned to care for a child following myringotomy with insertion of tympanostomy tubes. The nurse notes a small amount of reddish drainage from the child's ear following the surgery. Based on this finding, the nurse takes which action?

1. Notifies the registered nurse (RN) immediately

2. Changes the ear tubes so that they do not become blocked

3. Documents the findings

4. Checks the ear drainage for the presence of cerebrospinal fluid (CSF)

5. A nurse prepares a teaching plan regarding the administration of eardrops for the parents of a 2-year-old child. Which of the following would be included in the plan?

1. Pull the ear up and back before instilling the eardrops

2. Wear gloves when administering the eardrops

3. Hold the child in a sitting position when administering the eardrops

4. Pull the earlobe down and back before instilling the eardrops

6. A child is scheduled for a tonsillectomy. Which of the following would present the highest risk of aspiration during surgery?

1. Difficulty swallowing

2. The presence of loose teeth

3. Bleeding during surgery

4. Exudate in the throat area

7. The appropriate child position following a tonsillectomy is which of the following?

1. Supine

2. Trendelenburg

3. Side-lying

4. High Fowler's

8. Following tonsillectomy, the child begins to vomit bright red blood. The initial nursing action would be to:

1. Administer the prescribed antiemetic

2. Turn the child to the side

3. Notify the registered nurse (RN)

4. Maintain an NPO status

9. Following tonsillectomy, which of the following fluid or food items would be appropriate to offer to the child?

1. Cool cherry Kool-Aid

2. Vanilla pudding

3. Cold ginger ale

4. Jell-O

10. A nurse is reinforcing instructions to the mother of an 8-year-old child who had a tonsillectomy. The mother tells the nurse that the child loves tacos and asks when the child can safely eat one. The nurse makes which response to the mother?

1. "In 1 week."

2. "In 3 weeks."

3. "Two days following surgery."

4. "When the physician says it's OK."

11. A nurse reinforces instructions to the mother of a child with croup about the measures to take if an acute spasmodic episode occurs. Which statement by the mother indicates a need for further instruction?

1. "I will place a steam vaporizer in my child's room."

2. "I will place my child in a closed bathroom and allow my child to inhale steam from the running water."

3. "I will place a cool mist humidifier in my child's room."

4. "I will take my child out into the cool, humid night air."

12. A nurse reinforces instructions to the mother of a child hospitalized with croup. Which of the following statements, if made by the mother, would indicate a need for further instruction?

1. "I will give my child cough syrup if a cough develops."

2. "I will be sure that my child drinks at least two to four glasses of fluids every day."

3. "I will give acetaminophen (Tylenol) if my child develops a fever."

4. "Sips of warm fluid will help if my child develops a croup attack."

13. A nurse working in the emergency room is caring for a child diagnosed with epiglottitis. Indications that the child may be experiencing airway obstruction include which of the following?

1. Child leans backward, supporting self with the hands and arms

2. A low-grade fever and complaints of a sore throat

3. Child leans forward, with the chin thrust out

4. Nasal flaring and bradycardia

14. A nurse is caring for a hospitalized infant with bronchiolitis. Diagnostic tests have confirmed respiratory syncytial virus (RSV). Based on this finding,

which of the following would be the appropriate nursing action?

1. Plan to move the infant to another room with another RSV child
2. Leave the infant in the present room because RSV is not contagious
3. Wear a mask when caring for the child
4. Initiate strict enteric precautions

15. A child is brought to the emergency room for treatment of an acute asthma attack. The nurse prepares to administer which of the following medications first?
    1. A leukotriene modifier
    2. A nonsteroidal anti-inflammatory
    3. Oral corticosteroids
    4. Albuterol (Proventil HFA, Ventolin)

16. A nursing student is asked to discuss sudden infant death syndrome (SIDS) at the clinical conference being held at the end of the clinical day. The student plans to include which of the following in the discussion during the conference?
    1. SIDS usually occurs during sleep and is more common in premature infants
    2. SIDS usually occurs during sleep and is more common in girls
    3. SIDS usually occurs during sleep and most frequently occurs between 8 and 10 months of age
    4. SIDS usually occurs during sleep and is more common in high-birth-weight infants

17. A nurse is instructing a mother of a child with cystic fibrosis (CF) about the appropriate dietary measures. Which diet will be included in the instructions?
    1. Low-calorie, low-fat diet
    2. High-calorie, high-protein diet
    3. High-calorie, low-protein diet
    4. Low-calorie, restricted fat diet

18. A nurse prepares to administer a pancreatic enzyme powder to the child with cystic fibrosis (CF). Which of the following food items will the nurse mix with the medication?
    1. Applesauce
    2. Tapioca
    3. Mashed potatoes
    4. Hot oatmeal

19. A nurse reviews the results of a Mantoux test performed on a 3-year-old child. The results indicate an area of induration measuring 10 mm. The nurse would interpret these results as:
    1. Negative
    2. Positive
    3. Inconclusive
    4. Definitive, requiring a repeat test

20. Isoniazid (INH) is prescribed for a 2-year-old child with a positive Mantoux test. The mother of the child asks the nurse how long the child will need to take the medication. The appropriate response is:
    1. Six months
    2. Nine months
    3. Fifteen months
    4. Eighteen months

ALTERNATE FORMAT QUESTION: MULTIPLE RESPONSE

A nurse is preparing for the admission of an infant with a diagnosis of bronchiolitis caused by the respiratory syncytial virus (RSV). Select all interventions that would be included in the plan of care.

_____ Place the infant in a private room

_____ Position the infant side-lying, with the head lower than the chest

_____ Place the infant in a room near the nurses' station

_____ Place the child in a tent that delivers warm humidified air

_____ Wear a mask at all times when in contact with the infant

ANSWERS

1. *Answer:* **1**

Rationale: The nurse may suspect strabismus in a child when the child complains of frequent headaches, squints, or tilts the head to see. Options 2, 3, and 4 are not indicative of this condition.

Test-Taking Strategy: Use the process of elimination. Begin by eliminating option 3 and 4 because they are similar and refer to hearing. From the remaining options, recalling the signs of this condition will assist in directing you to option 1. Review these signs if you had difficulty with this question.

Level of Cognitive Ability: Comprehension
Client Needs: Physiological Integrity
Integrated Process: Nursing Process/Data Collection
Content Area: Child Health
Reference: Leifer, G. (2003). *Introduction to maternity and pediatric nursing* (4th ed.). Philadelphia: W.B. Saunders, p. 541.

2. *Answer:* **4**

Rationale: Bacterial conjunctivitis is highly contagious and infection control measures should be taught. These include frequent hand washing and not sharing towels and washcloths. Options 2 and 3 are correct treatment measures.

Test-Taking Strategy: Note the key words, *indicates a need for further instruction.* These words indicate a false response question and that you need to select the incorrect client statement. Recalling that bacterial conjunctivitis is highly contagious will direct you to option 4. Review infection control measures for bacterial conjunctivitis if you had difficulty with this question.
Level of Cognitive Ability: Comprehension
Client Needs: Health Promotion and Maintenance
Integrated Process: Teaching/Learning
Content Area: Child Health
Reference: Leifer, G. (2003). *Introduction to maternity and pediatric nursing* (4th ed.). Philadelphia: W.B. Saunders, p. 541.

3. *Answer:* **1**
Rationale: To decrease the risk of recurrent otitis media, parents should be encouraged to breast-feed during infancy, discontinue bottle-feeding as soon as possible, feed the infant in an upright position, and not to give the infant a bottle in bed. Parents should be told not to smoke in the child's presence, because passive smoking increases the incidence of otitis media.
Test-Taking Strategy: Use the process of elimination. Option 2 can be eliminated first, recalling the principles related to bottle-feeding. Recalling that breast-feeding offers some protection by providing maternal antibodies will assist in eliminating options 3 and 4. Review measures that will assist in preventing otitis media if you had difficulty with this question.
Level of Cognitive Ability: Application
Client Needs: Health Promotion and Maintenance
Integrated Process: Nursing Process/Implementation
Content Area: Child Health
Reference: Wong, D., & Hockenberry, M. (2003). *Nursing care of infants and children* (7th ed.). St. Louis: Mosby, p. 1360.

4. *Answer:* **3**
Rationale: Following myringotomy with insertion of tympanostomy tubes, the child is monitored for ear drainage. A small amount of reddish drainage is normal for the first few days after surgery. Any heavy bleeding or bleeding that occurs after 3 days should be reported. The nurse would document the findings. Options 1, 2, and 4 are not necessary.
Test-Taking Strategy: Use the process of elimination. Note the key words, *small amount.* Considering both the anatomical location of the surgery and these key words will direct you to the correct option. Review postoperative findings following this type of surgery if you had difficulty with this question.
Level of Cognitive Ability: Application
Client Needs: Physiological Integrity
Integrated Process: Nursing Process/Implementation
Content Area: Child Health
Reference: McKinney, E., James, S., Murray, S., & Ashwill, J. (2005). *Maternal-child nursing* (2nd ed.). St. Louis: Elsevier, p. 1199.

5. *Answer:* **4**
Rationale: To administer eardrops in a child younger than age 3 years, the ear should be pulled down and back. In children older than 3 years, the ear is pulled up and back. Gloves do not need to be worn by the parents, but hand washing before

and after the procedure needs to be performed. The child needs to be in a side-lying position with the affected ear facing upward to facilitate the flow of medication down the ear canal by gravity.
Test-Taking Strategy: Use the process of elimination. Visualizing this procedure will assist in eliminating options 2 and 3 first. From the remaining options, recalling the anatomy of the child's ear canal will direct you to option 4. Review this procedure if you had difficulty with this question.
Level of Cognitive Ability: Application
Client Needs: Health Promotion and Maintenance
Integrated Process: Nursing Process/Planning
Content Area: Child Health
Reference: Price, D., & Gwin, J. (2005). *Thompson's pediatric nursing* (9th ed.). Philadelphia: W.B. Saunders, p. 365.

6. *Answer:* **2**
Rationale: In the preoperative period, the child should be observed for the presence of loose teeth to decrease the risk of aspiration during surgery. Options 1 and 4 are incorrect. Bleeding during surgery will be controlled via packing and suction as needed.
Test-Taking Strategy: The issue of the question relates to aspiration. Note the key words, *highest risk.* Options 1 and 4 can be eliminated because they are similar. Recalling that the tonsillar area is vascular, anticipation of bleeding during surgery is expected and would be controlled. Review preoperative assessment procedures related to tonsillectomy if you had difficulty with this question.
Level of Cognitive Ability: Comprehension
Client Needs: Physiological Integrity
Integrated Process: Nursing Process/Data Collection
Content Area: Child Health
References: Leifer, G. (2005). *Maternity nursing* (9th ed.). Philadelphia: W.B. Saunders, p. 599.
Price, D., & Gwin, J. (2005). *Thompson's pediatric nursing* (9th ed.). Philadelphia: W.B. Saunders, p. 236.

7. *Answer:* **3**
Rationale: The child should be placed in a prone or side-lying position following tonsillectomy to facilitate drainage. Options 1, 2, and 4 will not achieve this goal.
Test-Taking Strategy: Visualize each of the positions described in the options. Keeping in mind that the goal is to facilitate drainage will direct you to option 3. Review positioning procedures following tonsillectomy if you had difficulty with this question.
Level of Cognitive Ability: Application
Client Needs: Physiological Integrity
Integrated Process: Nursing Process/Implementation
Content Area: Child Health
Reference: Price, D., & Gwin, J. (2005). *Thompson's pediatric nursing* (9th ed.). Philadelphia: W.B. Saunders, p. 237.

8. *Answer:* **2**
Rationale: Following tonsillectomy, if bleeding occurs, the child is turned to the side and the RN is notified, who will then contact the physician. An NPO status would be maintained and an antiemetic may be prescribed; however, the initial nursing action would be to turn the child to the side.

Test-Taking Strategy: Note the key word, *initial*. Although all the options may be appropriate, to maintain physiological integrity, the initial action is to turn the child to the side. Review care to the child following tonsillectomy if you had difficulty with this question.
Level of Cognitive Ability: Application
Client Needs: Physiological Integrity
Integrated Process: Nursing Process/Implementation
Content Area: Child Health
References: Leifer, G. (2003). *Introduction to maternity and pediatric nursing* (4th ed.). Philadelphia: W.B. Saunders, p. 599. Wong, D., & Hockenberry, M. (2003). *Nursing care of infants and children* (7th ed.). St. Louis: Mosby, p. 1374.

9. **Answer: 4**
Rationale: Following tonsillectomy, clear, cool liquids should be administered. Citrus, carbonated, and extremely hot or cold liquids need to be avoided because they may irritate the throat. Red liquids need to be avoided because they give the appearance of blood if the child vomits. Milk and milk products (pudding) are avoided because they coat the throat and cause the child to clear the throat, thus increasing the risk of bleeding.
Test-Taking Strategy: Use the process of elimination. Remember, avoiding foods and fluids that may irritate or cause bleeding is the concern. This will assist in eliminating options 2 and 3. The word "cherry" in option 1 should be the clue that this is not an appropriate food item. Review dietary measures following tonsillectomy if you had difficulty with this question.
Level of Cognitive Ability: Application
Client Needs: Physiological Integrity
Integrated Process: Nursing Process/Implementation
Content Area: Child Health
Reference: Leifer, G. (2003). *Introduction to maternity and pediatric nursing* (4th ed.). Philadelphia: W.B. Saunders, p. 599.

10. **Answer: 2**
Rationale: Rough, scratchy foods or spicy foods are to be avoided for 3 weeks. Citrus juices, which irritate the throat, need to be avoided for 10 days. Red liquids are avoided because they will give the appearance of blood if the child vomits. A full liquid diet is allowed on the second postoperative day and soft foods are allowed as the child tolerates them.
Test-Taking Strategy: Use the process of elimination and knowledge regarding the specific instructions related to food and fluids following tonsillectomy to answer this question. Eliminate option 4 because it places the mother's question on hold and is not a therapeutic response. From the remaining options, focus on the issue, when the child can safely eat a taco, and select option 2 because it is the longest period following surgery. Review dietary instructions following tonsillectomy if you had difficulty with this question.
Level of Cognitive Ability: Application
Client Needs: Health Promotion and Maintenance
Integrated Process: Nursing Process/Implementation
Content Area: Child Health
References: Leifer, G. (2003). *Introduction to maternity and pediatric nursing* (4th ed.). Philadelphia: W.B. Saunders, p. 599.

Price, D., & Gwin, J. (2005). *Thompson's pediatric nursing* (9th ed.). Philadelphia: W.B. Saunders, p. 237.

11. **Answer: 1**
Rationale: Steam from warm running water in a closed bathroom and cool mist from a bedside humidifier are effective in reducing mucosal edema. Cool mist humidifiers are recommended over steam vaporizers, which present a danger of scald burns. Taking the child out into the cool humid night air may also relieve mucosal swelling. Remember, however, that a cold mist may precipitate bronchospasm.
Test-Taking Strategy: Note the key words, *need for further instructions*, and focus on the issue, to reduce mucosal edema and to provide a safe environment. Option 1 is the option that would provide an unsafe environment for the child. Review management of acute spasmodic croup if you had difficulty with this question.
Level of Cognitive Ability: Comprehension
Client Needs: Safe, Effective Care Environment
Integrated Process: Teaching/Learning
Content Area: Child Health
Reference: Leifer, G. (2003). *Introduction to maternity and pediatric nursing* (4th ed.). Philadelphia: W.B. Saunders, p. 595.

12. **Answer: 1**
Rationale: Cough syrups and cold medicines are not to be given because they may dry and thicken secretions. Adequate hydration of 500 to 1000 mL of fluids daily is important in thinning secretions. Acetaminophen is used if a fever develops. Sips of warm fluids during a croup attack help relax the vocal cords and thin mucus.
Test-Taking Strategy: Note the key words, *a need for further instruction*. These words indicate a false response question and that you need to select the incorrect client statement. Knowledge of the pathophysiology related to croup will assist in eliminating options 2 and 3 first. Recalling that warm fluids can relax membranes and thin secretions will assist in directing you to option 1 from the remaining options. Review the effects of cough medicines if you had difficulty with this question.
Level of Cognitive Ability: Comprehension
Client Needs: Physiological Integrity
Integrated Process: Teaching/Learning
Content Area: Child Health
Reference: Wong, D., & Hockenberry, M. (2003). *Nursing care of infants and children* (7th ed.). St. Louis: Mosby, p. 1397.

13. **Answer: 3**
Rationale: Clinical manifestations suggestive of airway obstruction include tripod positioning (leaning forward supported by the hands and arms, chin thrust out, mouth open), nasal flaring, tachycardia, a high fever, and sore throat.
Test-Taking Strategy: Use the process of elimination. Eliminate option 4 first, because tachycardia rather than bradycardia will occur in a child experiencing respiratory distress. Eliminate option 2 next, knowing that a high fever occurs with epiglottitis. From the remaining options, visualize the descriptions in each, and determine which position would best assist a child experiencing respiratory distress. Review tripod position if you had difficulty with this question.

Level of Cognitive Ability: Comprehension
Client Needs: Physiological Integrity
Integrated Process: Nursing Process/Data Collection
Content Area: Child Health
References: Leifer, G. (2003). *Introduction to maternity and pediatric nursing* (4th ed.). Philadelphia: W.B. Saunders, p. 596. Price, D., & Gwin, J. (2005). *Thompson's pediatric nursing* (9th ed.). Philadelphia: W.B. Saunders, p. 190.

14. Answer: 1
Rationale: RSV is a highly communicable disorder. It is not transmitted via the airborne route. It is usually transferred by the hands, and meticulous hand washing is necessary to decrease the spread of organisms. The infant with RSV is isolated in a single room or placed in a room with another RSV child. Enteric precautions are not necessary; however, the nurse should wear a gown when soiling of clothing may occur.
Test-Taking Strategy: Knowledge regarding the transmission of RSV will direct you to option 1. Remember, RSV is usually transferred by the hands and meticulous hand washing is necessary to decrease the spread of organisms. Review care of the child with RSV if you had difficulty with this question.
Level of Cognitive Ability: Application
Client Needs: Safe, Effective Care Environment
Integrated Process: Nursing Process/Implementation
Content Area: Child Health
Reference: Price, D., & Gwin, J. (2005). *Thompson's pediatric nursing* (9th ed.). Philadelphia: W.B. Saunders, p. 143.

15. Answer: 4
Rationale: In treating an acute asthma attack, a short acting β_2 agonist such as albuterol will be given to produce bronchodilation. Options 1, 2, and 3 are long-term control (preventer) medications.
Test-Taking Strategy: Use the process of elimination and note the key words *acute asthma attack* and *first*. Recalling that asthma is a reversible obstructive airway disease should assist in directing you to option 4. It would seem logical that the first action would be to dilate the bronchi. Review the treatment for an acute asthma attack if you had difficulty with this question.
Level of Cognitive Ability: Application
Client Needs: Physiological Integrity
Integrated Process: Nursing Process/Planning
Content Area: Child Health
References: Leifer, G. (2003). *Introduction to maternity and pediatric nursing* (4th ed.). Philadelphia: W.B. Saunders, p. 604. Price, D., & Gwin, J. (2005). *Thompson's pediatric nursing* (9th ed.). Philadelphia: W.B. Saunders, p. 291.

16. Answer: 1
Rationale: SIDS usually occurs during sleep. It most frequently occurs between the second and fourth months of life. It is more common in boys, low-birth-weight infants, and premature infants.
Test-Taking Strategy: Use the process of elimination and knowledge regarding the characteristics related to the causes and incidence of SIDS. Review this information if you are unfamiliar with it.

Level of Cognitive Ability: Application
Client Needs: Health Promotion and Maintenance
Integrated Process: Teaching/Learning
Content Area: Child Health
Reference: Price, D., & Gwin, J. (2005). *Thompson's pediatric nursing* (9th ed.). Philadelphia: W.B. Saunders, p. 161.

17. Answer: 2
Rationale: Children with CF are managed with a high-calorie, high-protein diet. Pancreatic enzyme replacement therapy is undertaken, and fat-soluble vitamin supplements are administered. Fats are not restricted unless steatorrhea cannot be controlled by increased pancreatic enzymes.
Test-Taking Strategy: Use the process of elimination. Eliminate options 1 and 4 first because of the words "low-calorie." From the remaining options, recalling the appropriate diet in the child with CF will direct you to option 2. Review the treatment measures in CF if you had difficulty with this question.
Level of Cognitive Ability: Application
Client Needs: Physiological Integrity
Integrated Process: Nursing Process/Implementation
Content Area: Child Health
Reference: Price, D., & Gwin, J. (2005). *Thompson's pediatric nursing* (9th ed.). Philadelphia: W.B. Saunders, p. 146.

18. Answer: 1
Rationale: Pancreatic enzyme powders are not to be mixed with hot foods or foods containing tapioca or other starches. Enzyme powder should be mixed with nonfat, nonprotein foods such as applesauce. Pancreatic enzymes are inactivated by heat and are partially degraded by gastric acids.
Test-Taking Strategy: Use the process of elimination. Eliminate option 4 first because of the word "hot" and option 2 because of the probable warm temperature of mashed potatoes. From the remaining options, recalling that enzyme powder should be mixed with nonfat, nonprotein foods will direct you to option 1. Review the procedure for administering pancreatic enzyme powder if you had difficulty with this question.
Level of Cognitive Ability: Application
Client Needs: Physiological Integrity
Integrated Process: Nursing Process/Implementation
Content Area: Child Health
Reference: Leifer, G. (2003). *Introduction to maternity and pediatric nursing* (4th ed.). Philadelphia: W.B. Saunders, p. 611.

19. Answer: 2
Rationale: An induration measuring 10 mm or more is considered to be a positive result in children younger that 4 years of age and in those with chronic illness or high risk for environmental exposure to tuberculosis. A reaction of 5 mm or more is considered to be a positive result for those in the highest risk groups.
Test-Taking Strategy: Use the process of elimination and knowledge regarding a positive Mantoux test in children to answer this question. Option 4 can be easily eliminated first. Note the child's age in the question to determine the correct option from the remaining three. Review analysis of a Mantoux test in children if you had difficulty with this question.

Level of Cognitive Ability: Analysis
Client Needs: Physiological Integrity
Integrated Process: Nursing Process/Data Collection
Content Area: Child Health
Reference: deWit, S. (2005) *Fundamental concepts and skills for nursing.* Philadelphia: W.B. Saunders, p. 679.

20. *Answer: 2*
Rationale: INH is given to prevent TB infection from progressing to active disease. A chest x-ray film is obtained prior to initiation of preventative therapy. In infants and children, the recommended duration of INH therapy is 9 months. For children with human immunodeficiency virus infection, a minimum of 12 months is recommended.
Test-Taking Strategy: Knowledge regarding treatment with INH in a 2-year-old child is required to answer this question. Remember, in infants and children, the recommended duration of INH therapy is 9 months. Review the recommended treatment plans for a child with TB if you had difficulty with this question.
Level of Cognitive Ability: Application
Client Needs: Health Promotion and Maintenance
Integrated Process: Nursing Process/Implementation
Content Area: Child Health
Reference: Price, D., & Gwin, J. (2005). *Thompson's pediatric nursing* (9th ed.). Philadelphia: W.B. Saunders, p. 86.

ALTERNATE FORMAT QUESTION: MULTIPLE RESPONSE

Answers:
Place the infant in a private room
Place the infant in a room near the nurses' station

Rationale: The infant with RSV should be isolated in a private room or in a room with another infant with RSV infection. The infant should be placed in a room near the nurses' station for easy observation. The infant should be positioned with the head and chest at a 30- to 40-degree angle and the neck slightly extended to maintain an open airway and decrease pressure on the diaphragm. Cool, humidified oxygen is delivered to relieve dyspnea, hypoxemia, and insensible water loss from tachypnea. Contact precautions (wearing gloves and a gown) reduces nosocomial transmission of RSV.
Test-Taking Strategy: Recalling the mode of transmission of RSV will assist in determining that the infant needs to be placed in a private room or in a room with another infant with RSV infection, and that contact precautions need to be maintained. Recalling the need to maintain a patent airway (edema and the accumulation of mucus obstruct the bronchioles) will assist in determining that the infant needs to be observed closely, that the infant's head should be elevated, and that the infant should receive cool, humidified oxygen. Review care of the child with bronchiolitis and RSV if you had difficulty with this question.
Level of Cognitive Ability: Application
Client Needs: Physiological Integrity
Integrated Process: Nursing Process/Planning
Content Area: Child Health
References: James, S., Ashwill, J., & Droske, S. (2002). *Nursing care of children: Principles and practice* (2nd ed.). Philadelphia; W.B. Saunders, pp. 647-648.
Price, D., & Gwin, J. (2005). *Thompson's pediatric nursing* (9th ed.). Philadelphia: W.B. Saunders, p. 143.

REFERENCES

American Lung Association. Web site: http://www.lungusa.org
American SIDS Institute. Web site: http://www.sids.org
Asthma and Allergy Foundation of America. Web site: http://www.aafa.org
Cystic Fibrosis Foundation of America. Web site: http://www.CFF.org
deWit, S. (2005). *Fundamental concepts and skills for nursing* (2nd ed.). Philadelphia: W.B. Saunders.
James, S., Ashwill, J., & Droske, S. (2002). *Nursing care of children: Principles and practice* (2nd ed.). Philadelphia; W.B. Saunders.

Leifer, G. (2003). *Introduction to maternity and pediatric nursing* (4th ed.). Philadelphia: W.B. Saunders.
McKinney, E., James, S., Murray, S., & Ashwill, J. (2005). *Maternal-child nursing* (2nd ed.). St. Louis: W.B. Saunders.
Price, D., & Gwin, J. (2005). *Thompson's pediatric nursing* (9th ed.). Philadelphia: W.B. Saunders.
Wong, D., & Hockenberry, M. (2003). *Nursing care of infants and children* (7th ed.). St. Louis: Mosby.

Cardiovascular Disorders

I. CONGESTIVE HEART FAILURE (CHF)

A. Description

1. Inability of the heart to pump sufficiently to meet the metabolic needs of the body
2. In infants and children, inadequate cardiac output is most commonly caused by congenital heart defects that produce an excessive volume or pressure load on the myocardium
3. In infants and children, a combination of both left-sided and right-sided heart failure is usually present
4. The goals of treatment are to improve cardiac function, remove accumulated fluid and sodium, decrease cardiac demands, improve tissue oxygenation, and decrease oxygen consumption

B. Data collection of early signs

1. Tachycardia, especially during rest and slight exertion
2. Tachypnea
3. Profuse scalp sweating, especially in infants
4. Fatigue and irritability
5. Sudden weight gain
6. Respiratory distress

C. Interventions

1. Monitor vital signs closely and for the early signs of CHF
2. Monitor for respiratory distress (count respirations for 1 full minute)
3. Monitor apical pulse (count pulse for 1 full minute) and monitor for dysrhythmias
4. Monitor temperature for hyperthermia and for other signs of infection, particularly respiratory infection
5. Monitor input and output (I&O); weigh diapers
6. Monitor daily weight to assess for fluid retention; a weight gain of 0.5 kg (1 pound) in 1 day is a result of the accumulation of fluid
7. Monitor for facial or peripheral edema, auscultate lung sounds, and report abnormal findings
8. Elevate the head of the bed (semi-Fowler's position)
9. Maintain a neutral thermal environment to prevent cold stress in infants
10. Provide rest; decrease environmental stimuli
11. Administer cool, humidified oxygen as prescribed; use an oxygen hood for young infants and a nasal cannula or face tent for older infants and children
12. Organize nursing activities to allow for uninterrupted sleep
13. Maintain adequate nutritional status
14. Feed when hungry and soon after awakening (crying exhausts the limited energy supply), accommodating the infant's sleep and wake patterns; the infant should be well rested before feeding
15. Provide small, frequent feedings, which will be less tiring
16. Administer sedation as prescribed during the acute stage to promote rest
17. Administer digoxin (Lanoxin), as prescribed; monitor digoxin levels and for signs of digoxin toxicity, especially bradycardia and vomiting
18. Count the apical heart rate for 1 minute before administering digoxin
19. Check regarding parameters for withholding digoxin; generally, digoxin is withheld if the pulse is below 90 to 110 beats per minute in infants and young children or below 70 beats per minute in older children
20. Note that infants rarely receive more than 1 mL (50 mcg, or 0.05 mg) of digoxin (Lanoxin) in one dose

21. Angiotensin-converting enzyme (ACE) inhibitors such as captopril (Capoten) or enalapril (Vasotec) may be prescribed
22. Monitor for hypotension, renal dysfunction, and cough when ACE inhibitors are administered
23. Administer diuretics as prescribed; monitor for hypokalemia with furosemide (Lasix) and with thiazide diuretics
24. Administer potassium supplements and provide dietary sources of potassium, as prescribed
25. Monitor serum electrolytes, particularly the potassium level
26. Restrict fluid as prescribed in the acute stage; monitor for dehydration
27. Check the physician's orders regarding sodium restriction; note that most infant formulas have slightly more sodium than breast milk
28. Instruct the parents regarding the diagnosis and administration of medications (Box 32-1)
29. Instruct the parents in cardiopulmonary resuscitation (CPR)

II. DEFECTS WITH INCREASED PULMONARY BLOOD FLOW (Box 32-2)

A. Description
   1. Intracardiac communications along the septum or an abnormal connection between the great arteries allows blood to flow from the high-pressure left side of the heart to the low-pressure right side of the heart
   2. The infant typically demonstrates signs and symptoms of CHF

BOX 32-1

Home Care Instructions for Administering Digoxin

Administer as prescribed.
Administer 1 hour before or 2 hours after feedings.
Use a calendar to mark off the dose administered.
Do not mix the medication with foods or fluid.
If a dose is missed and more than 4 hours has elapsed, withhold the dose and give the next dose at the scheduled time; if less than 4 hours has elapsed, administer the missed dose.
If the child vomits, do not administer a second dose.
If more than two consecutive doses have been missed, notify the physician; do not increase or double the dose for missed doses.
If the child has teeth, give water after the medication; if possible, brush the child's teeth to prevent tooth decay from the sweetened liquid.
If the child becomes ill, notify the physician.
Keep the medication in a locked cabinet.
Call the poison control center immediately if accidental overdose occurs.

B. Atrial septal defect (ASD)
   1. Abnormal opening between the atria that causes an increased flow of oxygenated blood into the right side of the heart
   2. Right atrial and ventricular enlargement occur
   3. Infant may be asymptomatic or may develop CHF
   4. Nonsurgical treatment: May be closed by using devices during a cardiac catheterization
   5. Surgical treatment: Open repair with cardiopulmonary bypass is usually performed before school age

C. Ventricular septal defect (VSD)
   1. Abnormal opening between the right and left ventricles
   2. Many VSDs close spontaneously during the first year of life in children having small or moderate defects
   3. A characteristic murmur is present; CHF is common
   4. Nonsurgical treatment: Device closure during cardiac catheterization may be possible
   5. Surgical treatment: Open repair with cardiopulmonary bypass

D. Atrioventricular canal (AVC) defect
   1. Incomplete fusion of the endocardial cushions
   2. Most common cardiac defect in Down syndrome
   3. A characteristic murmur is present
   4. The infant usually has mild to moderate CHF; mild cyanosis increases with crying
   5. Surgical treatment: Can include either pulmonary artery banding for infants with severe symptoms (palliative) or complete repair via cardiopulmonary bypass

E. Patent ductus arteriosus (PDA)
   1. Failure of the fetal ductus arteriosus (artery connecting the aorta and the pulmonary artery) to close within the first weeks of life
   2. A characteristic machine-like murmur is present; asymptomatic or may show signs of CHF
   3. A widened pulse pressure and bounding pulses are present
   4. Medical management: Indomethacin (prostaglandin inhibitor) may be administered to close a patent ductus in premature infants and some newborns
   5. Other therapy: Use of coils to occlude the PDA during cardiac catheterization or may require surgical management

---

BOX 32-2

Defects with Increased Pulmonary Blood Flow

Atrial septal defect (ASD)
Ventricular septal defect (VSD)
Atrioventricular canal (AVC) defect
Patent ductus arteriosus (PDA)

III. OBSTRUCTIVE DEFECTS (Box 32-3)

A. Description
1. Blood exiting the heart meets an area of anatomic narrowing (**stenosis**), causing obstruction to blood flow
2. The location of narrowing is usually near the valve of the obstructive defect
3. Infants and children exhibit signs of CHF
4. Children with mild obstruction may be asymptomatic

B. Coarctation of the aorta (COA)
1. Localized narrowing near the insertion of the ductus arteriosus
2. Collateral circulation develops during fetal life to maintain flow from the ascending to the descending aorta
3. Signs of CHF in infants
4. High blood pressure and bounding pulses in the arms, weak or absent femoral pulses, and cool lower extremities may be present
5. Children may experience headaches, dizziness, fainting, and epistaxis resulting from hypertension
6. Treatment: Balloon angioplasty in children; however, restenosis can occur or surgical treatment may be necessary

C. Aortic **stenosis** (AS)
1. Narrowing or stricture of the aortic valve, causing resistance to blood flow in the left ventricle, decreased cardiac output, left ventricular hypertrophy, and pulmonary vascular congestion
2. A characteristic murmur is present
3. Infants with severe defects demonstrate signs of decreased cardiac output with faint pulses, hypotension, tachycardia, and poor feeding
4. Children show signs of exercise intolerance, chest pain, and dizziness when standing for long periods
5. Treatment: Balloon angioplasty during cardiac catheterization to dilate the narrowed valve, or surgery may be necessary

D. Pulmonary **stenosis** (PS)
1. Narrowing at the entrance to the pulmonary artery
2. Resistance to blood flow causes right ventricular hypertrophy and decreased pulmonary blood flow; the right ventricle may be hypoplastic
3. Pulmonary **atresia** is the extreme form of PS—total fusion of the commissures and no blood flows to the lungs
4. A characteristic murmur is present
5. May be asymptomatic; mild cyanosis or CHF occurs
6. Newborns with severe narrowing will be cyanotic
7. If PS is severe, CHF occurs
8. Treatment: Balloon angioplasty during cardiac catheterization to dilate the narrowed valve, or surgery may be necessary

IV. DEFECTS WITH DECREASED PULMONARY BLOOD FLOW (Box 32-4)

A. Description
1. Obstructed pulmonary blood flow and an anatomic defect (ASD or VSD) between the right and left sides of the heart
2. Pressure on the right side of the heart increases, exceeding left-sided pressure, which allows desaturated blood to **shunt** right to left; this causes desaturation in the left side of the heart and in the systemic circulation
3. Typically, hypoxemia and cyanosis appear

B. Tetralogy of Fallot (TOF)
1. Includes four defects: VSD, PS, overriding aorta, and right ventricular hypertrophy
2. If pulmonary vascular resistance is higher than systemic resistance, the **shunt** is from right to left; if systemic resistance is higher than pulmonary resistance, the **shunt** is left to right
3. Infants
   a. May be acutely cyanotic at birth or may have mild cyanosis that progresses over the first year of life as the pulmonic **stenosis** worsens
   b. A characteristic murmur is present
   c. Acute episodes of cyanosis and hypoxia (hypercyanotic spells), called blue spells or tet spells, occur when the infant's oxygen requirements exceed the blood supply (usually during crying or after feeding)
4. Children: With increasing cyanosis, there may be clubbing of the fingers, squatting, and poor **growth**
5. Surgical treatment may include a palliative **shunt** or complete repair

C. Tricuspid **atresia**
1. Failure of the tricuspid valve to develop
2. There is no communication from the right atrium to the right ventricle

---

BOX 32-3

Obstructive Defects

Coarctation of the aorta (COA)
Aortic stenosis (AS)
Pulmonary stenosis (PS)

BOX 32-4

Defects with Decreased Pulmonary Blood Flow

Tetralogy of Fallot (TOF)
Tricuspid atresia

3. Blood flows through an ASD or a patent foramen ovale to the left side of the heart and through a VSD to the right ventricle and out to the lungs
4. Often associated with pulmonic **stenosis** and transposition of the great arteries
5. Complete mixing of unoxygenated and oxygenated blood in the left side of the heart, resulting in systemic desaturation, pulmonary obstruction, and decreased pulmonary blood flow
6. Cyanosis, tachycardia, and dyspnea are seen in the newborn
7. Older children exhibit signs of chronic hypoxemia and clubbing
8. Surgical treatment is necessary; for the neonate whose pulmonary blood flow depends on the patency of the ductus arteriosus, a continuous infusion of prostaglandin E$_1$ is initiated until surgery

V. MIXED DEFECTS (Box 32-5)
A. Description
1. Fully saturated systemic blood flow mixes with the desaturated blood flow, causing a desaturation of the systemic blood flow
2. Pulmonary congestion occurs and cardiac output decreases
3. Signs of CHF; symptoms depend on the degree of desaturation
B. Transposition of the great arteries (TGA) or transposition of the great vessels (TGV)
1. The pulmonary artery leaves the left ventricle, and the aorta exits from the right ventricle
2. No communication between the systemic and pulmonary circulations
3. Infants with minimal communication are severely cyanotic and depressed at birth
4. Infants with large septal defects or a patent ductus arteriosus may be less severely cyanotic but may have symptoms of CHF
5. Cardiomegaly is evident a few weeks after birth
6. Treatment includes balloon atrial septostomy during cardiac catheterization, or surgery may be required
C. Total anomalous pulmonary venous connection (TAPVC)
1. Failure of the pulmonary veins to join the left atrium

BOX 32-5

Mixed Defects

Transposition of the great arteries (TGA) or transposition of the great vessels (TGV)
Total anomalous pulmonary venous connection (TAPVC)
Truncus arteriosus (TA)
Hypoplastic left heart syndrome (HLHS)

---

2. Results in mixed blood being returned to the right atrium and shunted from the right to the left through an ASD
3. The right side of the heart hypertrophies, whereas the left side of the heart may remain small
4. CHF develops
5. Cyanosis worsens with pulmonary vein obstruction; once obstruction occurs, the infant's condition deteriorates rapidly
6. Surgical treatment is necessary
D. Truncus arteriosus (TA)
1. Failure of normal septation and division of the embryonic bulbar trunk into the pulmonary artery and the aorta, resulting in a single vessel that overrides both ventricles
2. Blood from both ventricles mixes in the common great artery, causing desaturation and hypoxemia
3. A characteristic murmur is present
4. The infant exhibits moderate to severe CHF and variable cyanosis, poor **growth**, and activity intolerance
5. Surgical treatment is necessary
E. Hypoplastic left heart syndrome (HLHS)
1. Underdevelopment of the left side of the heart, resulting in a hypoplastic left ventricle and aortic **atresia**
2. Mild cyanosis and signs of CHF occur until the ductus arteriosus closes; then, progressive deterioration with cyanosis and decreased cardiac output occurs, leading to cardiovascular collapse
3. Fatal in the first few months of life without intervention
4. Surgical treatment is necessary

VI. INTERVENTIONS: CARDIOVASCULAR DEFECTS
A. Monitor for signs of a defect in the infant or child
B. Monitor vital signs closely
C. Monitor respiratory status for the presence of **nasal flaring** and use of accessory muscles; the physician is notified if any changes occur
D. Breath sounds are auscultated for crackles, wheezes, or rhonchi
E. If respiratory effort is increased, place the child in reverse Trendelenburg position (elevate head and upper body) to decrease the work of breathing
F. Administer humidified oxygen as prescribed
G. Endotracheal tube and ventilator care may be necessary; restrain the hands of an intubated child
H. Monitor for hypercyanotic spells (Box 32-6)
I. Monitor for signs of CHF, such as fluid retention in the eyes, hands, feet, and chest
J. Monitor peripheral pulses
K. Monitor I&O and notify the physician if a decrease in urine output occurs
L. Monitor urine output, weighing diapers as necessary

M. Obtain daily weight

N. Maintain fluid restriction if prescribed

O. Provide adequate nutrition (high calorie requirements) as prescribed

P. Administer medications, as prescribed

Q. Keep child as stress-free as possible; plan interventions to allow maximal rest for the child

R. Prepare parents and child, if appropriate, for surgery

S. Allow parents and child to verbalize feelings and concerns regarding disorder

T. Familiarize parents and child with hospital procedures and equipment

VII. CARDIAC SURGERY

A. Postoperative interventions

1. Monitor vital signs frequently

2. Monitor temperature; the physician is notified if a fever occurs

3. Monitor for signs of sepsis, such as fever, chills, diaphoresis, lethargy, and altered levels of consciousness

4. Maintain aseptic technique

5. Assist with monitoring lines, tubes, or catheters that are in place and remove promptly as prescribed when no longer needed to prevent infection

6. Monitor for signs of discomfort, such as irritability, changes in heart rate, respiratory rate, and blood pressure, and inability to sleep

7. Administer pain medications as prescribed, noting effectiveness

8. Administer antibiotics and antipyretics, as prescribed

9. Encourage rest periods

10. Facilitate parent-child contact as soon as possible

B. Postoperative home care (Box 32-7)

VIII. RHEUMATIC FEVER

A. Description

1. An inflammatory autoimmune disease that affects the connective tissues of the heart, joints, subcutaneous tissues, and/or blood vessels of the central nervous system (CNS)

2. The most serious complication is rheumatic heart disease, which affects the cardiac valves

---

BOX 32-6

Treatment for Hypercyanotic Spells

Place the infant in a knee-chest position.
Administer 100% oxygen by face mask.
Administer morphine sulfate, as prescribed.
Administer IV fluids, as prescribed.

---

3. Presents 2 to 6 weeks following an untreated or partially treated group A beta-hemolytic streptococcal infection of the upper respiratory tract

4. Jones criteria are utilized in determining the diagnosis

B. Data collection (Figure 32-1)

1. Fever: Low-grade fever that spikes in the late afternoon

2. Elevated antistreptolysin O titer

3. Elevated sedimentation rate

4. Elevated C-reactive protein

5. Aschoff bodies (lesions): Found in the heart, blood vessels, brain, and serous surfaces of the joints and pleura

C. Interventions

1. Monitor vital signs

2. Control joint pain and inflammation with massage and alternating hot and cold applications, as prescribed

3. Provide bed rest during acute febrile phase

4. Limit physical exercise in the child with carditis

5. Administer antibiotics (penicillin) as prescribed

6. Administer salicylates and anti-inflammatory agents as prescribed (should not be instituted before the diagnosis is confirmed, because these medications mask polyarthritis)

7. Initiate seizure precautions if the child is experiencing chorea

---

BOX 32-7

Home Care After Cardiac Surgery

Omit play outside for several weeks.
Avoid activities in which the child could fall, such as bike riding, for 2 to 4 weeks.
Avoid crowds for 2 weeks after discharge.
Follow a no-salt added diet if prescribed.
Do not add any new foods to the infant's eating schedule.
Do not place creams, lotions, or powders on the incision until completely healed.
The child may return to school the third week after discharge, starting with half-days.
The child should have no physical education for 2 months.
Instruct the parents to discipline the child normally.
Instruct the parents about the importance of the 2-week follow-up.
Avoid immunizations, invasive procedures, and dental visits for 2 months.
Advise the parents regarding the importance of a dental visit every 6 months after age 3 years and to inform the dentist of the cardiac problem so that antibiotics can be prescribed, if necessary.
Instruct the parents to call the physician when coughing, tachypnea, cyanosis, vomiting, diarrhea, anorexia, pain, fever, or any swelling, redness, or drainage occurs at the site of the incision.

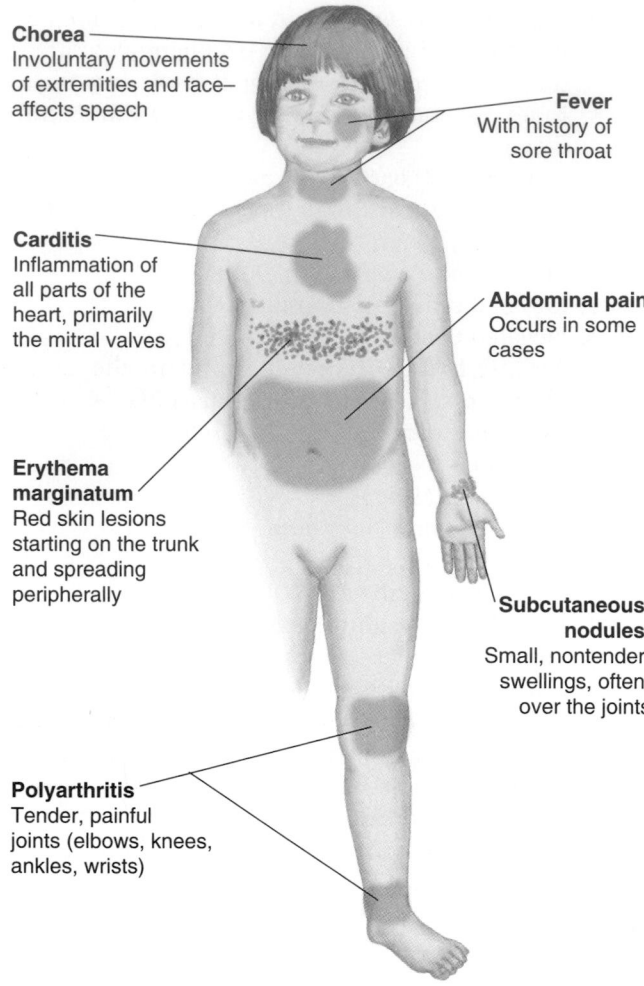

Chorea
Involuntary movements of extremities and face—affects speech

Fever
With history of sore throat

Carditis
Inflammation of all parts of the heart, primarily the mitral valves

Abdominal pain
Occurs in some cases

Erythema marginatum
Red skin lesions starting on the trunk and spreading peripherally

Subcutaneous nodules
Small, nontender swellings, often over the joints

Polyarthritis
Tender, painful joints (elbows, knees, ankles, wrists)

FIG. 32-1 Clinical manifestations of rheumatic fever. (From McKinney, E., James, S., Murray, S., & Ashwill, J. [2005]. *Maternal-child nursing* [2nd ed.]. St. Louis: W.B. Saunders.)

8. Instruct the parents about the importance of follow-up and the need for antibiotic prophylaxis for dental work, infection, and invasive procedures
9. Advise the child to inform the parents if anyone in school develops a streptococcal throat infection

IX. KAWASAKI DISEASE

A. Description
 1. Known as mucocutaneous lymph node syndrome; an acute systemic inflammatory illness
 2. The cause is unknown but may be associated with an infection by an organism or toxin
 3. Cardiac involvement is the most serious complication; aneurysms can develop
B. Data collection
 1. Acute stage

   a. Fever
   b. Conjunctival hyperemia
   c. Red throat
   d. Swollen hands, rash, and enlargement of the cervical lymph nodes
 2. Subacute stage
   a. Cracking lips and fissures
   b. Desquamation of the skin on the tips of the fingers and toes
   c. Joint pain
   d. Cardiac manifestations
   e. Thrombocytosis
 3. Convalescent stage: Child appears normal but signs of inflammation may be present
C. Interventions
 1. Monitor temperature frequently
 2. Monitor heart sounds and rhythm
 3. Monitor extremities for edema, redness, and desquamation
 4. Examine eyes for conjunctivitis
 5. Monitor mucous membranes for inflammation
 6. Monitor dietary and fluid intake (I&O)
 7. Administer soft foods and liquids that are neither too hot nor too cold
 8. Weigh daily
 9. Provide passive range-of-motion exercises to facilitate joint movement
 10. Administer acetylsalicylic acid (aspirin) as prescribed for its antipyretic and antiplatelet effects
 11. IV immune globulin (IVIG) may be prescribed to reduce the duration of fever and the incidence of coronary artery lesions and aneurysms
 12. Instruct the parents in the administration of prescribed medications, the need to monitor for bleeding, and the need for follow-up to monitor for cardiac complications

PRACTICE QUESTIONS

1. A nurse caring for an infant with congenital heart disease is monitoring the infant closely for signs of congestive heart failure (CHF). The nurse monitors the infant closely for which early sign of CHF?
 1. Cough
 2. Tachycardia
 3. Slow and shallow breathing
 4. Pallor
2. A physician has prescribed oxygen as needed (PRN) for the child with congestive heart failure (CHF). In which of the following situations does the nurse administer the oxygen to the child?
 1. During feeding
 2. When the mother is holding the child
 3. When changing the child's diapers
 4. When drawing blood for measurement of electrolyte levels

3. An infant with congestive heart failure (CHF) is receiving diuretic therapy and the nurse is closely monitoring the intake and output (I&O). Which is the best method for the nurse to use to monitor the urine output?
   1. Inserting a Foley catheter
   2. Weighing the diapers
   3. Comparing intake with output
   4. Measuring the amount of water added to formula

4. A nurse is monitoring the daily weight of an infant with congestive heart failure (CHF). Which of the following alerts the nurse to suspect fluid accumulation and the need to notify the registered nurse?
   1. Bradypnea
   2. Diaphoresis
   3. Decreased blood pressure (BP)
   4. A weight gain of 1 pound in 1 day

5. A nurse provides home care instructions to the parents of a child with congestive heart failure (CHF) regarding the procedure for the administration of digoxin (Lanoxin). Which statement, if made by a parent, indicates the need for further instruction?
   1. "If my child vomits after medication administration, I will repeat the dose."
   2. "I will take my child's pulse before administering the medication."
   3. "I will not mix the medication with food."
   4. "If more than one dose is missed, I will call the physician."

6. A nurse is assigned to care for an infant with a diagnosis of tricuspid atresia. The nurse plans care, knowing that in this disorder:
   1. There is no communication from the systemic and pulmonary circulations
   2. Frequent episodes of hypercyanotic spells occur
   3. There is no communication from the right atrium to the right ventricle
   4. A single vessel overrides both ventricles

7. Prostaglandin E₁ is prescribed for a child with transposition of the great arteries. The mother of the child asks the nurse why the child needs the medication. The nurse tells the mother that the medication:
   1. Maintains an adequate hormone level
   2. Maintains the position of the great arteries
   3. Provides adequate oxygen saturation and maintains cardiac output
   4. Prevents hypercyanotic (tet) spells

8. A nurse reviews the record of a child just seen by the physician. The physician has documented a diagnosis of suspected aortic stenosis. The nurse expects to note documentation of which clinical manifestation specifically found in this disorder?
   1. Hyperactivity
   2. Exercise intolerance
   3. Pallor
   4. Gastrointestinal disturbances

9. A nurse has reinforced home care instructions to the mother of a child who is being discharged following cardiac surgery. Which statement made by the mother indicates a need for further instructions?
   1. "Large crowds of people need to be avoided for at least 2 weeks following surgery."
   2. "I can apply lotion or powder to the incision if it is itchy."
   3. "A balance of rest and exercise is important."
   4. "Activities where the child could fall need to be avoided for 2 to 4 weeks."

10. A nurse is reviewing the physician's orders for a child who was just admitted to the hospital with a diagnosis of Kawasaki disease. The nurse expects to note an order for which of the following as part of the treatment plan?
    1. Morphine sulfate
    2. Immune globulin
    3. Heparin infusion
    4. Digoxin (Lanoxin)

11. A nurse is told that a child with rheumatic fever (RF) will be arriving to the nursing unit for admission. On admission, the nurse prepares to ask the mother which question to elicit information specific to the development of RF?
    1. "Did the child have a sore throat or an unexplained fever within the last 2 months?"
    2. "Has the child had any nausea or vomiting?"
    3. "Has the child complained of headaches?"
    4. "Has the child complained of back pain?"

12. Acetylsalicylic acid (Aspirin) is prescribed for the child with rheumatic fever. The nurse would question this order if the child had documented evidence of which of the following?
    1. A viral infection
    2. Joint pain
    3. Facial edema
    4. Arthralgia

13. A nurse is caring for a child with a suspected diagnosis of rheumatic fever (RF). The nurse reviews the laboratory results, knowing that which laboratory study would assist in confirming the diagnosis of RF?
    1. White blood cell count
    2. Red blood cell count
    3. Immunoglobulin
    4. Antistreptolysin O titer

14. A nurse is caring for a child with a diagnosis of Kawasaki disease. The mother of the child asks the nurse about the disorder. The nurse tells the mother that:
    1. It is an acquired cell-mediated immunodeficiency disorder
    2. It is an inflammatory autoimmune disease that affects the connective tissue of the heart, joints, and subcutaneous tissues

3. It is a chronic multisystem autoimmune disease characterized by the inflammation of connective tissue
4. Is also called mucocutaneous lymph node syndrome and is a febrile generalized vasculitis of unknown cause

15. A nurse assists in admitting a child with a diagnosis of acute stage Kawasaki disease. On data collection, the nurse expects to note which clinical manifestation of the acute stage of the disease?
    1. Conjunctival hyperemia
    2. Cracked lips
    3. Desquamation of the skin
    4. A normal appearance

ALTERNATE FORMAT QUESTION: MULTIPLE RESPONSE

A nurse is caring for an infant with a diagnosis of tetralogy of Fallot. The infant suddenly becomes cyanotic, and the nurse recognizes that the infant is experiencing a hypercyanotic spell. Select the interventions that the nurse takes.
____ Place the infant in a prone position
____ Notify the registered nurse
____ Prepare to administer 100% oxygen by face mask
____ Call a code blue
____ Prepare to administer morphine sulfate

ANSWERS

1. *Answer: 2*
Rationale: The early signs of CHF include tachycardia, tachypnea, profuse scalp sweating, fatigue and irritability, sudden weight gain, and respiratory distress. A cough may occur in CHF as a result of mucosal swelling and irritation, but it is not an early sign. Pallor may be noted in the infant with CHF, but is also not an early sign.
Test-Taking Strategy: Use the process of elimination and note the key word, *early*. Think about the physiology and the effects on the heart when fluid overload occurs. These concepts will assist in directing you to option 2. If you had difficulty with this question, review the early signs of CHF in an infant.
Level of Cognitive Ability: Application
Client Needs: Physiological Integrity
Integrated Process: Nursing Process/Data Collection
Content Area: Child Health
Reference: Price, D., & Gwin, J. (2005). *Thompson's pediatric nursing* (9th ed.). Philadelphia: W.B. Saunders, p. 87.

2. *Answer: 4*
Rationale: Oxygen administration may be ordered for stressful periods, especially during bouts of crying or invasive procedures. Drawing blood is an invasive procedure that would likely cause the child to cry.
Test-Taking Strategy: Use the process of elimination. Read the options and recall the situations that would place stress and an increased workload on the heart. This concept should direct you to option 4. Review care of the child with CHF if you had difficulty with this question.
Level of Cognitive Ability: Application
Client Needs: Physiological Integrity
Integrated Process: Nursing Process/Implementation
Content Area: Child Health
Reference: Price, D., & Gwin, J. (2005). *Thompson's pediatric nursing* (9th ed.). Philadelphia: W.B. Saunders, p. 94.

3. *Answer: 2*
Rationale: The best method to monitor urine output in an infant on diuretic therapy is to weigh the diapers. Comparing intake with output would not provide an accurate measure of urine output. Measuring the amount of water added to formula is unrelated to the amount of output. Although Foley catheter drainage is most accurate in determining output, it is not the best method, and places the infant at risk for infection.
Test-Taking Strategy: Use the process of elimination. Eliminate options 3 and 4 first because they will not provide an indication of urine output. From the remaining options, note the word "best" in the stem of the question. This will direct you to option 2. Review care of the infant receiving diuretic therapy if you had difficulty with this question.
Level of Cognitive Ability: Application
Client Needs: Physiological Integrity
Integrated Process: Nursing Process/Data Collection
Content Area: Child Health
Reference: Price, D., & Gwin, J. (2005). *Thompson's pediatric nursing* (9th ed.). Philadelphia: W.B. Saunders, p. 94.

4. *Answer: 4*
Rationale: A weight gain of 0.5 kg (1 pound) in 1 day is due to the accumulation of fluid. The nurse should monitor urine output, monitor for evidence of facial or peripheral edema, check the lung sounds, and report the weight gain. Tachypnea and an increased BP would occur with fluid accumulation. Diaphoresis is a sign of CHF but is not specific to fluid accumulation, and usually occurs with exertional activities.
Test-Taking Strategy: Use the process of elimination and focus on the issue, fluid accumulation. Note the relationship between "fluid accumulation" in the question and "weight gain" in the correct option. Review the indications of fluid accumulation in an infant with CHF if you had difficulty with this question.
Level of Cognitive Ability: Comprehension
Client Needs: Physiological Integrity
Integrated Process: Nursing Process/Data Collection
Content Area: Child Health
Reference: Price, D., & Gwin, J. (2005). *Thompson's pediatric nursing* (9th ed.). Philadelphia: W.B. Saunders, p. 94.

5. *Answer: 1*
Rationale: The parents need to be instructed that if the child vomits after the digoxin is administered, they are not to repeat

the dose. Options 2, 3, and 4 are accurate instructions regarding the administration of this medication. Additionally, the parents should be instructed that, if a dose is missed and it is not noticed until 4 hours later, the dose should not be administered.

Test-Taking Strategy: Note the key words, *need for further instruction.* These words indicate a false response question and that you need to select the incorrect client statement. General knowledge regarding digoxin administration will assist in eliminating option 2. Principles related to administering medications to children will assist in eliminating option 3. From the remaining options, select option 1 over option 4 because, if the child vomits, it would be difficult to determine if the medication was also vomited or absorbed by the body. Review home care instructions regarding the administration of digoxin if you had difficulty with this question.

Level of Cognitive Ability: Comprehension
Client Needs: Health Promotion and Maintenance
Integrated Process: Teaching/Learning
Content Area: Child Health
Reference: Leifer, G. (2003). *Introduction to maternity and pediatric nursing* (4th ed.). Philadelphia: W.B. Saunders, p. 624.

6. Answer: 3
Rationale: In tricuspid atresia, there is no communication from the right atrium to the right ventricle. Option 1 describes transposition of the great arteries. Frequent episodes of hypercyanotic spells occur in tetralogy of Fallot. Option 4 describes truncus arteriosus.

Test-Taking Strategy: Use the process of elimination. Note the relationship between "tricuspid atresia" and the description in option 3. Recalling that the tricuspid valve is located between the right atrium and the right ventricle will direct you to this option. Review the characteristics of tricuspid atresia if you had difficulty with this question.

Level of Cognitive Ability: Comprehension
Client Needs: Physiological Integrity
Integrated Process: Nursing Process/Planning
Content Area: Child Health
Reference: Wong, D., & Hockenberry, M. (2003). *Nursing care of infants and children* (7th ed.). St. Louis: Mosby, p. 1497.

7. Answer: 3
Rationale: A child with transposition of the great arteries may receive prostaglandin E$_1$ temporarily to increase blood mixing if systemic and pulmonary mixing are inadequate to maintain adequate cardiac output. Options 1, 2, and 4 are incorrect. Additionally, tet spells occur in tetralogy of Fallot.

Test-Taking Strategy: Use the ABCs—airway, breathing, and circulation—to answer the question. Option 3 addresses circulation. Review the purpose of this medication in this condition if you had difficulty with this question.

Level of Cognitive Ability: Application
Client Needs: Physiological Integrity
Integrated Process: Nursing Process/Implementation
Content Area: Child Health

Reference: Wong, D., & Hockenberry, M. (2003). *Nursing care of infants and children* (7th ed.). St. Louis: Mosby, p. 1499.

8. Answer: 2
Rationale: The child with aortic stenosis shows signs of exercise intolerance, chest pain, and dizziness when standing for long periods. Pallor may be noted, but is not specific to this type of disorder alone. Options 1 and 4 are not related to this disorder.

Test-Taking Strategy: Use the process of elimination focusing on the disorder. Options 1 and 4 can be eliminated first because they are not associated with a cardiac disorder. From the remaining options, noting the word "specifically" in the stem of the question will direct you to option 2. Review the manifestations associated with aortic stenosis if you had difficulty with this question.

Level of Cognitive Ability: Comprehension
Client Needs: Physiological Integrity
Integrated Process: Nursing Process/Data Collection
Content Area: Child Health
Reference: Wong, D., & Hockenberry, M. (2003). *Nursing care of infants and children* (7th ed.). St. Louis: Mosby, p. 1495.

9. Answer: 2
Rationale: The mother should be instructed that lotions and powders should not be applied to the incision site. Options 1, 3, and 4 are accurate instructions regarding home care following cardiac surgery.

Test-Taking Strategy: Note the key words, *indicates a need for further instructions.* These words indicate a false response question and that you need to select the incorrect client statement. Using general principles related to postoperative incisional site care will direct you to option 2. Review home care instructions following cardiac surgery if you had difficulty with this question.

Level of Cognitive Ability: Comprehension
Client Needs: Health Promotion and Maintenance
Integrated Process: Teaching/Learning
Content Area: Child Health
Reference: Price, D., & Gwin, J. (2005). *Thompson's pediatric nursing* (9th ed.). Philadelphia: W.B. Saunders, p. 95.

10. Answer: 2
Rationale: Intravenous immune globulin (IVIG) is administered to the child with Kawasaki disease to decrease the incidence of coronary artery lesions and aneurysms and to decrease fever and inflammation. Options 1, 3, and 4 are not components of the treatment plan for this disease.

Test-Taking Strategy: Use the process of elimination. Remember that the pharmacological treatment for this disease is acetylsalicylic acid (aspirin) and IVIG. If you had difficulty with this question, review the treatment plan for the child with Kawasaki disease.

Level of Cognitive Ability: Analysis
Client Needs: Physiological Integrity
Integrated Process: Nursing Process/Planning
Content Area: Child Health
Reference: Leifer, G. (2003). *Introduction to maternity and pediatric nursing* (4th ed.). Philadelphia: W.B. Saunders, p. 629.

11. Answer: 1

Rationale: RF characteristically presents 2 to 6 weeks following an untreated or partially treated group A beta-hemolytic streptococcal infection of the upper respiratory tract. Initially, the nurse determines if the child has had a sore throat or an unexplained fever within the past 2 months. Options 2, 3, and 4 are unrelated RF.

Test-Taking Strategy: Use the process of elimination. Note the similarity between rheumatic "fever" in the question and the word "fever" in the correct option. If you had difficulty with this question, review the etiology related to RF.

Level of Cognitive Ability: Application

Client Needs: Physiological Integrity

Integrated Process: Nursing Process/Data Collection

Content Area: Child Health

Reference: Leifer, G. (2003). *Introduction to maternity & pediatric nursing* (4th ed.). Philadelphia: W.B. Saunders, p. 626.

12. Answer: 1

Rationale: Anti-inflammatory agents, including aspirin, may be prescribed for the child with RF. Aspirin should not be given to a child who has chickenpox or other viral infections such as the flu. Options 2 and 4 are clinical manifestations of RF. Facial edema may be associated with the development of a cardiac complication.

Test-Taking Strategy: Use the process of elimination. Options 2 and 4 can be eliminated because they are similar. Recalling that facial edema may indicate a cardiac complication will assist in eliminating this option. Review the contraindications related to the use of aspirin if you had difficulty with this question.

Level of Cognitive Ability: Application

Client Needs: Safe, Effective Care Environment

Integrated Process: Nursing Process/Implementation

Content Area: Child Health

References: Leifer, G. (2003). *Introduction to maternity and pediatric nursing* (4th ed.). Philadelphia: W.B. Saunders, p. 626.
Price, D., & Gwin, J. (2005). *Thompson's pediatric nursing* (9th ed.). Philadelphia: W.B. Saunders, p. 298.

13. Answer: 4

Rationale: A diagnosis of RF is confirmed by the presence of two major manifestations or one major and two minor manifestations from the Jones criteria. Additionally, evidence of a recent streptococcal infection is confirmed by a positive anti-streptolysin O titer, streptozyme, or an anti-DNase B assay. Options 1, 2, and 3 will not assist in confirming the diagnosis of RF.

Test-Taking Strategy: Use the process of elimination. Recalling that RF is characteristically associated with streptococcal infection will direct you to option 4. If you had difficulty with this question, review the tests used to confirm RF.

Level of Cognitive Ability: Comprehension

Client Needs: Physiological Integrity

Integrated Process: Nursing Process/Data Collection

Content Area: Child Health

Reference: Price, D., & Gwin, J. (2005). *Thompson's pediatric nursing* (9th ed.). Philadelphia: W.B. Saunders, p. 297.

14. Answer: 4

Rationale: Kawasaki disease, also called mucocutaneous lymph node syndrome, is a febrile generalized vasculitis of unknown etiology. Option 1 describes human immunodeficiency virus (HIV) infection. Option 2 describes rheumatic fever. Option 3 describes systemic lupus erythematosus.

Test-Taking Strategy: Knowledge regarding the description of Kawasaki disease is required to answer this question. Remember, Kawasaki disease is a febrile generalized vasculitis of unknown etiology. Review the characteristics of this disorder if you are unfamiliar with it.

Level of Cognitive Ability: Application

Client Needs: Physiological Integrity

Integrated Process: Nursing Process/Implementation

Content Area: Child Health

Reference: Leifer, G. (2003). *Introduction to maternity and pediatric nursing* (4th ed.). Philadelphia: W.B. Saunders, p. 628.

15. Answer: 1

Rationale: In the acute stage, the child presents with fever, conjunctival hyperemia, a red throat, swollen hands, a rash, and enlargement of the cervical lymph nodes. In the subacute stage, cracking lips and fissures, desquamation of the skin on the tips of the fingers and toes, joint pain, cardiac manifestations, and thrombocytosis occur. In the convalescent stage, the child appears normal, but signs of inflammation may be present.

Test-Taking Strategy: Use the process of elimination. Noting the key words, *acute stage*, in the question will assist in directing you to option 1. Review the clinical manifestations associated with each stage of Kawasaki disease if you had difficulty with this question.

Level of Cognitive Ability: Comprehension

Client Needs: Physiological Integrity

Integrated Process: Nursing Process/Data Collection

Content Area: Child Health

Reference: Leifer, G. (2003). *Introduction to maternity and pediatric nursing* (4th ed.). Philadelphia: W.B. Saunders, p. 628.

ALTERNATE FORMAT QUESTION: MULTIPLE RESPONSE

Answers:

Notify the registered nurse

Prepare to administer 100% oxygen by face mask

Prepare to administer morphine sulfate

Rationale: Hypercyanotic episodes often occur in infants with tetralogy of Fallot and may occur in infants whose heart defect includes obstruction to pulmonary blood flow and communication between the ventricles. If a hypercyanotic episode occurs, the infant is placed in a knee-chest position immediately. The registered nurse is then notified, who will then contact the physician. The knee-chest position improves systemic arterial oxygen saturation by decreasing venous return, so that smaller amounts of highly saturated blood reach the heart. Toddlers and children squat to get into this position and relieve chronic hypoxia. There is no reason to call a code blue unless respirations cease. Additional interventions include administering 100% oxygen

by face mask, morphine sulfate, and intravenous fluids, as prescribed.
Test-Taking Strategy: Focus on the infant's diagnosis. Review the nursing interventions when a hypercyanotic episode occurs in an infant if you had difficulty with this question.
Level of Cognitive Ability: Application

Client Needs: Physiological Integrity
Integrated Process: Nursing Process/Implementation
Content Area: Child Health
Reference: Wong, D., & Hockenberry, M. (2003). *Nursing care of infants and children* (7th ed.). St. Louis: Mosby, p. 1488.

REFERENCES

Leifer, G. (2003). *Introduction to maternity and pediatric nursing* (4th ed.). Philadelphia: W.B. Saunders.

Price, D., & Gwin, J. (2005). *Thompson's pediatric nursing* (9th ed.). Philadelphia: W.B. Saunders.

Wong, D., & Hockenberry, M. (2003). *Nursing care of infants and children* (7th ed.). St. Louis: Mosby.

CHAPTER 33

Metabolic, Endocrine, and Gastrointestinal Disorders

I. FEVER

A. Description
1. An abnormal body temperature elevation
2. A child's temperature can vary depending on activity, emotional stress, the type of clothing the child is wearing, and the temperature of the environment
3. Data collection findings associated with the fever provide important indications of the seriousness of the fever

B. Data collection
1. Temperature elevation
2. Flushed skin
3. Diaphoresis
4. Chills
5. Restlessness or lethargy

C. Interventions
1. Monitor vital signs
2. Administer a sponge bath with lukewarm water for 20 to 30 minutes
3. Administer antipyretics such as acetaminophen (Tylenol), as prescribed
4. Do not administer aspirin (acetylsalicylic acid, ASA), because of the risk of Reye's syndrome
5. Retake the temperature 30 to 60 minutes after the antipyretic is administered
6. Provide adequate fluid intake as tolerated and as prescribed
7. Monitor for dehydration and fluid and electrolyte imbalance
8. Instruct the parents in how to take the child's temperature, how to safely medicate the child, and when it is necessary to call the physician

II. VOMITING

A. Description
1. The major concerns when a child is vomiting are the risk of dehydration, the loss of fluid and electrolytes, and the development of metabolic alkalosis
2. Additional concerns include aspiration, atelectasis, and the development of pneumonia

B. Data collection
1. Signs of aspiration
2. Character of vomitus
3. Pain and abdominal cramping
4. Dehydration
5. Fluid and electrolyte imbalances
6. Metabolic alkalosis

C. Interventions
1. Maintain a patent airway
2. Position the child on side to prevent aspiration
3. Monitor vital signs
4. Monitor the character, amount, and frequency of vomiting
5. Note the force of the vomiting, because projectile vomiting is indicative of pyloric **stenosis** or increased intracranial pressure
6. Monitor intake and output (I&O) and for signs of dehydration
7. Monitor electrolyte levels
8. Provide oral rehydration therapy as tolerated and as prescribed; start feeding slowly, with small amounts of fluid at frequent intervals
9. Monitor for diarrhea or abdominal pain
10. Inform the parents to contact the physician when signs of dehydration, blood in vomitus, forceful vomiting, or abdominal pain is present

III. DIARRHEA

A. Description: The major concerns when a child is having diarrhea are the risk of dehydration, the loss of fluid and electrolytes, and the development of metabolic acidosis

B. Data collection

1. Character of stools
2. Pain and abdominal cramping
3. Dehydration
4. Fluid and electrolyte imbalances
5. Metabolic acidosis

C. Interventions
1. Monitor vital signs
2. Monitor the character, amount, and frequency of diarrhea
3. Monitor skin integrity
4. Monitor I&O and for signs of dehydration
5. Monitor electrolyte levels
6. For mild to moderate dehydration, prepare to provide oral rehydration therapy; avoid carbonated beverages and those containing high amounts of sugar
7. For severe dehydration, prepare to maintain NPO status to place the bowel at rest and provide fluid and electrolyte replacement by intravenous fluids as prescribed; if potassium is prescribed intravenously, monitor urine output
8. Prepare to reintroduce a normal diet once rehydration is achieved
9. Provide enteric isolation as required
10. Instruct the parents in good hand washing technique

IV. DEHYDRATION (Box 33-1)

A. Description
1. Dehydration is a common fluid and electrolyte imbalance in infants and children
2. Infants and children are more vulnerable to fluid volume deficit because a greater amount of their body water is in the extracellular fluid compartment
3. In infants and children, the organs that conserve water are immature, placing them at risk for fluid volume deficit
4. The causes can include decreased fluid intake, diaphoresis, vomiting, diarrhea, diabetic ketoacidosis, and extensive burns or other serious injuries

---

BOX 33-1

Types of Dehydration

ISOTONIC DEHYDRATION
Electrolyte and water deficits occur in approximately balanced proportions.

HYPERTONIC DEHYDRATION
Water loss exceeds electrolyte loss.

HYPOTONIC DEHYDRATION
Electrolyte loss exceeds water loss.

B. Data collection
1. Tachycardia
2. Dry skin and mucous membranes
3. Sunken eyeballs and fontanels
4. Decreased urine output and increased urine specific gravity
5. Changes in level of consciousness and responses to stimuli
6. Signs of circulatory failure, such as coolness and mottling of the extremities
7. Loss of skin elasticity and turgor
8. Delayed capillary filling time
9. Weight loss
10. Decreased blood pressure
11. Thirst
12. Absence of tears

C. Interventions
1. Monitor vital signs
2. Monitor for signs of dehydration
3. Monitor weight and monitor for weight changes, including fluid gains and losses
4. Monitor I&O and urine for specific gravity
5. Monitor level of consciousness
6. Monitor skin turgor and mucous membranes for dryness
7. Provide oral rehydration therapy with solutions, as prescribed, if the child is able to take fluids orally
8. Intravenous fluids and electrolyte replacements may be prescribed if the child is unable to take sufficient fluids orally
9. Introduce a regular diet as prescribed when the child is rehydrated
10. Provide instructions to the parents about the types and amounts of fluid to encourage, the signs of dehydration, and the indications of the need to notify the physician

V. PHENYLKETONURIA (PKU)

A. Description
1. Genetic disorder that results in central nervous system (CNS) damage from toxic levels of phenylalanine in the blood
2. An autosomal recessive disorder
3. PKU is characterized by blood phenylalanine levels higher than 8 mg/dL (normal level is lower than 2 mg/dL 2 to 5 days after birth)
4. All 50 states require routine screening of all newborn infants for PKU

B. Data collection
1. In all children
   a. Digestive problems and vomiting
   b. Seizures
   c. Musty or mousy odor of the urine
   d. Mental retardation
2. In older children

a. Eczema
b. Hypertonia
c. Hypopigmentation of the hair, skin, and irises
d. Hyperactive behavior

C. Interventions
1. Screening of newborn infants for PKU: the infant should have begun formula or breast milk feeding before specimen collection
2. If initial screening is positive, a repeat test is performed and further diagnostic evaluation is required to verify the diagnosis
3. Infants are rescreened by 14 days of age if the initial screening was done before 48 hours of age
4. If PKU is diagnosed:
   a. Phenylalanine intake is restricted; high-protein foods (meats and dairy products) and a aspartame are avoided because they contain large amounts of phenylalanine
   b. Monitor physical, neurological, and intellectual development
   c. Stress the importance of follow-up treatment
   d. Encourage the parents to express feelings about the diagnosis and the risk of PKU in future children

VI. TYPE 1 DIABETES MELLITUS

A. Description
1. Type 1 diabetes mellitus is also known as insulin-dependent diabetes mellitus; most children with diabetes mellitus have type 1
2. Type 1 diabetes mellitus is caused by the partial or complete lack of secretory capacity of the beta cells of the pancreas, resulting in insulin deficiency
3. Complete insulin deficiency requires the use of exogenous insulin to promote appropriate glucose use and to prevent complications related to elevated blood glucose levels, such as hyperglycemia, diabetic ketoacidosis, and death
4. Diagnosis is based on the presence of classic symptoms and on an elevated blood glucose level (normal blood glucose level is 70 to 110 mg/dL)

B. Data collection
1. Polyuria, polydipsia, polyphagia
2. Hyperglycemia
3. Weight loss
4. Unexplained fatigue or lethargy
5. Headaches
6. Stomachaches
7. Occasional enuresis in a previously toilet-trained child
8. Vaginitis in adolescent girls (caused by *Candida*, which thrives in hyperglycemic tissues)
9. Fruity odor to breath
10. Dehydration
11. Blurred vision
12. Slow wound healing
13. Changes in level of consciousness (LOC)

C. Long-term effects
1. Failure to grow at a normal rate
2. Delayed maturation
3. Recurrent infections
4. Neuropathy
5. Cardiovascular disease
6. Retinal microvascular disease
7. Renal microvascular disease

D. Complications
1. Hypoglycemia
2. Hyperglycemia
3. Diabetic ketoacidosis
4. Coma
5. Hypokalemia
6. Hyperkalemia
7. Microvascular changes
8. Cardiovascular changes

E. Diet
1. Total number of calories is individualized on the basis of the child's age and **growth** expectations
2. As prescribed by the physician, the child may be instructed to follow the food exchange from the American Diabetic Association diet or the dietary guidelines for Americans (MyPyramid Food Guide; see Figure 12-1) issued by the U.S. Departments of Agriculture and Health and Human Services
3. Dietary intake should include three meals per day, eaten at consistent intervals, plus a midafternoon carbohydrate snack and a bedtime snack high in protein; a consistent intake of carbohydrates at each meal and snack is needed
4. Instruct the child and the parents that the child should carry candy with him or her at all times
5. Incorporate the diet into individual child's needs, likes and dislikes, lifestyle, and cultural and socioeconomic patterns
6. Allow the child to participate in making food choices to provide a sense of control

F. Exercise
1. Instruct the child in dietary adjustments when exercising
2. Extra food needs to be consumed for increased activity, usually 10 to 15 g of carbohydrate for every 30 to 45 minutes of activity
3. Instruct the child to monitor blood glucose prior to exercising
4. Plan an appropriate exercise regimen with the child, incorporating the developmental stage

G. Insulin
1. Diluted insulin may be required for some infants to provide small enough doses to avoid hypoglycemia; diluted insulin should be clearly labeled to avoid dosage errors
2. Laboratory evaluation of glycosylated hemoglobin should be performed every 3 months

3. Illness, infection, and stress increase the need for insulin, and insulin should not be withheld during illness, infection, or stress, because hyperglycemia and ketoacidosis can result

4. When the child is NPO for a special procedure, verify with the physician the need to withhold the morning insulin and when food, fluids, and insulin are to be given

5. Instruct the child and parents in the administration of the insulin

6. Instruct the child and parents to recognize symptoms of hypoglycemia and hyperglycemia

7. Instruct the parents in the administration of intramuscular or subcutaneous glucagon if the child has a hypoglycemic reaction and is unable to consume sugar-containing items orally

8. Instruct the child and parents always to have a spare bottle of insulin available

9. Advise the parents to obtain a Medic-Alert bracelet indicating the type and daily insulin dosage prescribed for the child

H. Blood glucose monitoring
1. Results provide information needed to maintain good glycemic control
2. More accurate than urine testing
3. Requires that the child prick himself or herself several times a day, as prescribed
4. Instruct the child and parents in the proper procedure for obtaining the blood glucose level
5. Inform the child and parents that the procedure must be done precisely to obtain accurate results
6. Stress the importance of hand washing before and after performing the procedure to prevent infection
7. Stress the importance of following the manufacturer's instructions for the blood glucose monitoring device
8. Instruct the child and parents to calibrate the monitor as instructed by the manufacturer
9. Instruct the child and parents to check the expiration date on the test strips used for blood glucose monitoring
10. Instruct the child and parents that, if the blood glucose results do not seem reasonable, reread the instructions, reassess technique, check the expiration date of the test strips, and perform the procedure again to verify results

I. Urine testing
1. Instruct the parents and child in the procedure for testing urine for ketones and glucose
2. Teach the child that the second voided urine specimen is most accurate
3. The presence of ketones may indicate impending ketoacidosis
4. Urine glucose testing is not recommended as the only means of monitoring control in the child taking insulin, because it is a less reliable indicator as compared with blood glucose monitoring

J. Hypoglycemia
1. Description
a. A blood glucose level below 70 mg/dL
b. Occurs as a result of too much insulin, not enough food, or excessive activity
2. Interventions (Boxes 33-2 and 33-3)

K. Hyperglycemia
1. Description: Elevated blood glucose level over 200 mg/dL
2. Interventions (Box 33-4)
3. Sick Day Rules (Box 33-5)

L. Diabetic ketoacidosis (DKA)
1. Description
a. A complication of diabetes mellitus that develops when a severe insulin deficiency occurs
b. DKA is a life-threatening condition
c. Hyperglycemia that progresses to metabolic acidosis occurs
d. It develops over a period of several hours to days
e. The blood glucose level is higher than 300 mg/dL and urine and serum ketones are positive
2. Interventions
a. Restore circulating volume and protect against cerebral, coronary, or renal hypoperfusion

---

BOX 33-2

Interventions for Hypoglycemia

If possible, confirm with a blood glucose reading.

Administer glucose immediately; the rapid-releasing sugar is followed by a complex carbohydrate and protein, such as a slice of bread or a peanut butter cracker.

Give an extra snack if the next meal is not planned for more than 30 minutes or if activity is planned.

If the child becomes unconscious, squeeze cake frosting or glucose paste onto the gums and retest the blood glucose level if the child does not improve within 15 to 20 minutes; if the reading remains low, administer additional sugar.

If the child remains unconscious, it may be necessary to administer glucagon.

In the hospital setting, prepare to administer IV dextrose.

BOX 33-3

Food Items to Treat Hypoglycemia

$1/2$ cup of orange juice or a sugar-sweetened carbonated beverage

One small box of raisins

Three or four hard candies such as Life Savers

Two to four sugar cubes

One candy bar

1 tsp honey

Two or three glucose tablets

Interventions for Hyperglycemia

Instruct the parents to notify the physician when:
Blood glucose results are greater than the targeted range (usually 200 mg/dL).
Moderate or high ketonuria is present.
The child is unable to take food or fluids.
Illness persists.

BOX 33-5

Sick Day Rules for the Diabetic Child

Always give insulin even if the child does not have an appetite, or contact the physician for specific instructions.
Test blood glucose levels at least every 4 hours.
Test for urinary ketones with each voiding.
Notify the physician if moderate or large amounts of urinary ketones are present.
Follow the child's usual meal plan.
Encourage consumption of calorie-free liquids to aid in clearing ketones.
Encourage rest, especially if urinary ketones are present.
Notify the physician if vomiting, fruity odor to the breath, deep rapid respirations, decreasing level of consciousness, or persistent hyperglycemia occurs.

b. Dehydration is corrected with intravenous (IV) infusions of 0.9% or 0.45% saline, as prescribed
c. Hyperglycemia is corrected with IV regular insulin administration as prescribed
d. Monitor vital signs, urine output, and mental status closely
e. Correct acidosis and electrolyte imbalances
f. Administer oxygen, as prescribed
g. Monitor blood glucose level frequently
h. Monitor potassium level closely because, when the child receives insulin to lower the blood glucose level, the serum potassium level will decrease as the acidosis improves, and potassium replacement may be required
i. Monitor the child closely for signs of fluid overload
j. IV dextrose is added as prescribed when the blood glucose reaches an appropriate level
k. Treat the cause of hyperglycemia

VII. CLEFT LIP AND CLEFT PALATE (Figure 33-1)
A. Description
    1. A congenital anomaly that occurs as a result of failure of soft tissue or bony structure to fuse during embryonic development

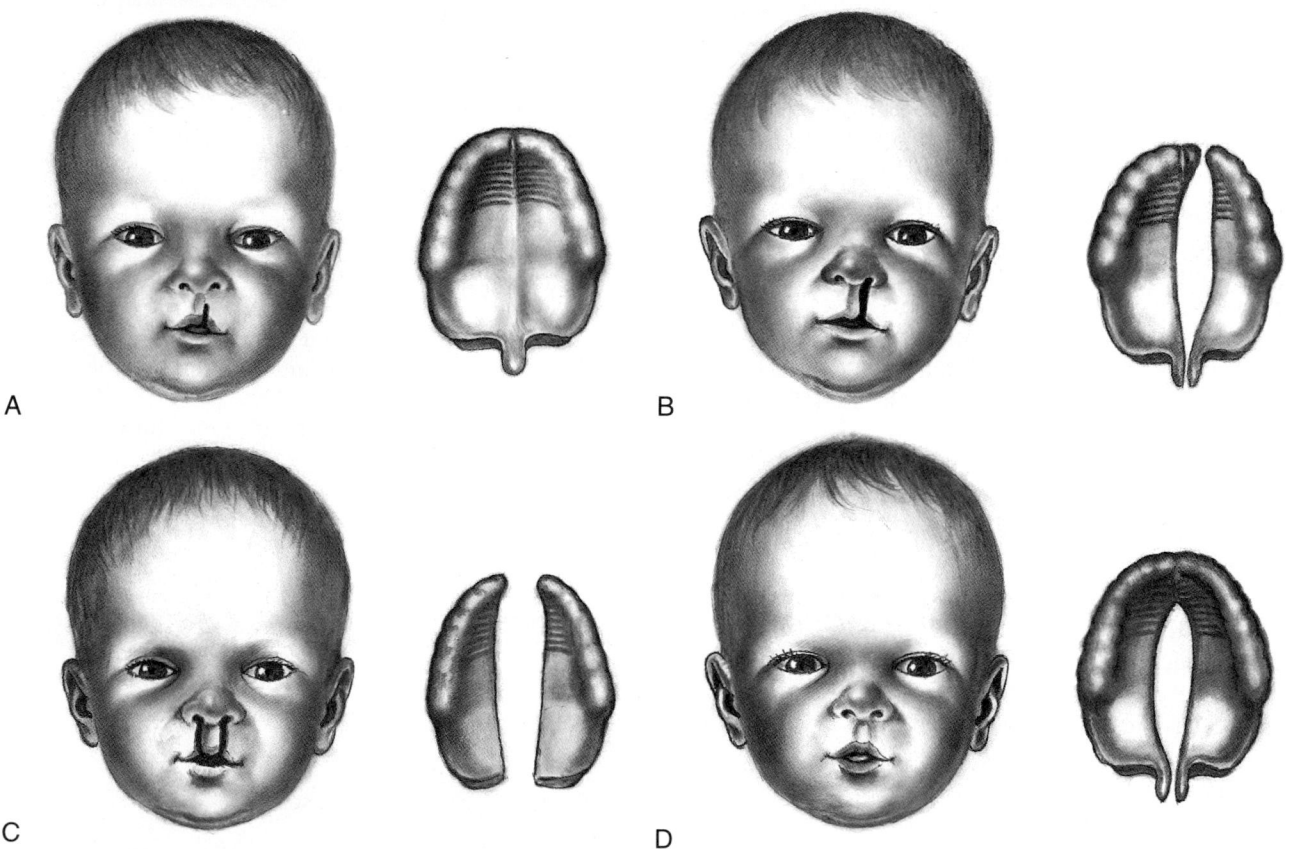

FIG. 33-1 Cleft lip and cleft palate. **A,** Notch in vermelion border; **B,** unilateral cleft lip and cleft palate; **C,** bilateral cleft lip and cleft palate; **D,** cleft palate. (From Wong, D., & Hockenberry, M. [2003]. *Nursing care of infants and children* [7th ed.]. St. Louis: Mosby.)

2. Involves abnormal openings in the lip or palate that may occur unilaterally or bilaterally and are readily apparent at birth
3. Causes include genetic, **hereditary**, and environmental factors; exposure to radiation or rubella virus; chromosome abnormalities; and teratogenic factors
4. Closure of cleft lip defect precedes that of the palate and is performed usually during the first weeks of life
5. Cleft palate repair is performed sometime between 12 and 18 months of age to allow for the palatal changes that take place with normal **growth**; a cleft palate is closed before the child develops faulty speech habits

B. Data collection
1. Cleft lip can range from a slight notch to a complete separation from the floor of the nose
2. Cleft palate can include nasal distortion, midline or bilateral cleft, and variable extension from the uvula and soft and hard palate

C. Interventions
1. Check the ability to suck, swallow, handle normal secretions, and breathe without distress
2. Monitor fluid and calorie intake daily and monitor weight
3. Modify feeding techniques; plan to use specialized feeding techniques, obturators, and special nipples and feeders
4. Hold the child in an upright position and direct the formula to the side and back of the mouth to prevent aspiration; feed small amounts gradually and burp frequently
5. Position on side after feeding
6. Keep suction equipment and bulb syringe at bedside
7. Encourage breast-feeding, if appropriate
8. Teach the parents special feeding or suctioning techniques
9. Teach the parents the **ESSR** (*e*nlarge, *s*timulate sucking, *s*wallow, *r*est) method of feeding (Box 33-6)
10. Encourage the parents to describe their feelings related to the deformity

D. Postoperative interventions
1. Cleft lip repair
   a. A lip protector device may be taped securely to the cheeks to prevent trauma to the suture line

---

BOX 33-6

ESSR Method of Feeding

Enlarge the nipple.
Stimulate the suck reflex.
Swallow.
Rest to allow the child to finish swallowing what has been placed in the mouth.

---

   b. Position the child on the side lateral to the repair or on the back; avoid the prone position to prevent rubbing of the surgical site on the mattress
   c. After feeding, cleanse the suture line of formula or serosanguineous drainage with a cotton-tipped swab dipped in saline; apply antibiotic ointment if prescribed
2. Cleft palate repair
   a. Child is allowed to lie on the abdomen
   b. Feedings are resumed by bottle, breast, or cup
   c. Oral packing may be secured to the palate (removed in 2 to 3 days)
   d. Do not allow the child to brush his or her teeth
   e. Instruct the parents to avoid offering hard food items to the child, such as toast or cookies
3. Soft elbow or jacket restraints may be used (check agency policies and procedures) to keep the child from touching the repair site; remove restraints at least every 2 hours to assess skin integrity and allow for exercising the arms
4. Avoid contact with sharp objects near the surgical site
5. Avoid the use of oral suction or placing objects in the mouth such as a tongue depressor, thermometer, straw, spoon, fork, or pacifier
6. Provide analgesics for pain
7. Instruct the parents in feeding techniques and in the care of the surgical site
8. Instruct the parents to monitor for signs of infection at the surgical site, such as redness, swelling, or drainage
9. Encourage the parents to hold the child
10. Assist with initiating appropriate referrals for speech impairment or language-based **learning** difficulties

---

VIII. ESOPHAGEAL ATRESIA AND TRACHEOESOPHAGEAL FISTULA (TEF)
(Figure 33-2)

A. Description
1. The esophagus terminates before it reaches the stomach and/or a fistula is present that forms an unnatural connection with the trachea
2. The condition causes oral intake to enter the lungs or a large amount of air to enter the stomach, and choking, coughing, and severe abdominal distention can occur
3. Aspiration pneumonia and severe respiratory distress will develop, and death will occur without surgical intervention
4. Treatment includes maintenance of a patent airway, prevention of pneumonia, gastric or blind pouch decompression, supportive therapy, and surgical repair

B. Data collection
  1. Frothy saliva in the mouth and nose, and drooling
  2. Coughing, choking during feedings, and unexplained cyanosis (3C's)
  3. **Regurgitation** and vomiting
  4. Abdominal distention
  5. Inability to pass a small-gauge (such as a No. 5 French) orogastric feeding tube via the mouth into the stomach

▲ C. Preoperative interventions
  1. Infant may be placed in an incubator or radiant warmer, and humidified oxygen is administered (intubation and mechanical ventilation may be necessary if respiratory distress occurs)
  2. Maintain an NPO status
  3. Maintain IV fluids, as prescribed
  4. Suction accumulated secretions from the mouth and pharynx
  5. A double-lumen catheter is placed into the upper esophageal pouch and attached to intermittent or continuous low suction to keep the pouch empty of secretions; it is irrigated with normal saline as prescribed to prevent clogging
  6. Maintain in an upright position to facilitate drainage and to prevent aspiration of gastric secretions
  7. A gastrostomy tube may be placed and is left open so that air entering the stomach through the fistula can escape, minimizing the danger of **regurgitation**
  8. Administer broad-spectrum antibiotics as prescribed, because of the high risk for aspiration pneumonia

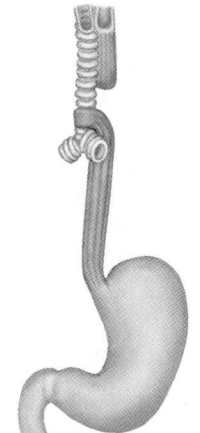

Esophageal atresia
with distal TEF

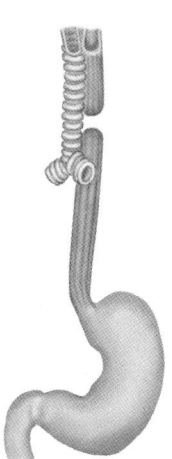

Esophageal atresia
without fistula

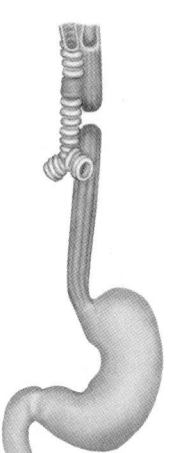

Proximal esophageal fistula with
trachea; distal segment has no
communication

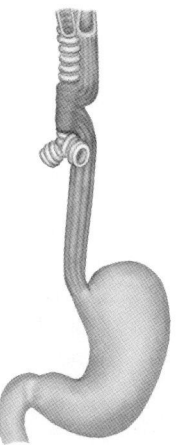

Proximal and distal esophageal
fistulas with trachea

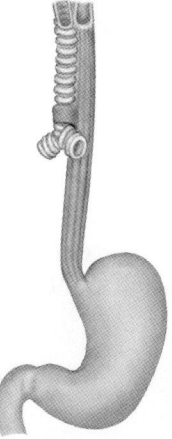

TEF without atresia
(also called "H type")

FIG. 33-2 Esophageal atresia and tracheoesophageal fistula (TEF). (From McKinney, E., James, S., Murray, S., & Ashwill, J. [2005]. *Maternal-child nursing* [2nd ed.]. St. Louis: W.B. Saunders.)

D. Postoperative interventions
1. Monitor respiratory status
2. Maintain IV fluids, antibiotics, and parenteral nutrition, as prescribed
3. Monitor I&O and weight daily
4. Inspect surgical site
5. Provide care to the chest tube if in place
6. Monitor for signs of pain
7. Monitor for dehydration and possible fluid overload
8. Monitor for anastomotic leaks as evidenced by purulent chest drainage, increased temperature, and an increased white blood cell count
9. The double-lumen catheter is attached to low suction
10. If a gastrostomy tube is present, it is attached to gravity drainage until the infant can tolerate feedings (usually the fifth to seventh day postoperatively)
11. Before oral feedings and removal of the chest tube, a barium swallow is performed to verify the integrity of the esophageal anastomosis
12. Before feeding, the gastrostomy tube is elevated and secured above the level of the stomach to allow gastric secretions to pass to the duodenum and swallowed air to escape through the open gastrostomy tube
13. Feedings through the gastrostomy tube may be prescribed until the anastomosis is healed
14. Oral feedings are begun with sterile water, followed by frequent small feedings of formula
15. The gastrostomy tube may be removed prior to discharge or may be maintained for supplemental feedings at home
16. If the infant is awaiting esophageal replacement, a cervical esophagostomy may be performed
17. Check the cervical esophagostomy site for redness, breakdown, or exudate (continued discharge or saliva can cause skin breakdown); remove drainage frequently and apply a protective ointment, a barrier dressing, and/or a collection device
18. If the infant is awaiting esophageal replacement, non-nutritive sucking is provided by a pacifier; infants who remain NPO for extended periods and have not received oral stimulation frequently may have difficulty eating by mouth after surgery and may develop oral hypersensitivity and food aversion
19. Reinforce instructions to the parents in the techniques of suctioning, gastrostomy tube care and feedings, and skin site care as appropriate
20. Instruct parents to identify behaviors that indicate the need for suctioning, signs of respiratory distress, and signs of a constricted esophagus (poor feeding, dysphagia, drooling, or regurgitated undigested food)

IX. GASTROESOPHAGEAL REFLUX (GER)

A. Description
1. Backflow of gastric contents into the esophagus as a result of relaxation or incompetence of the lower esophageal or cardiac sphincter
2. Complications include esophagitis, esophageal strictures, aspiration of gastric contents, and aspiration pneumonia
3. Most infants with GER have a mild problem that improves in about 1 year and requires only medical therapy
4. Treatment (Box 33-7)

B. Data collection
1. Passive **regurgitation** or emesis
2. Poor weight gain
3. Hematemesis and melena
4. Irritability
5. Heartburn (in older children)
6. Anemia from blood loss

C. Interventions
1. Monitor amount and characteristics of emesis
2. Monitor the relation of vomiting to the times of feedings and infant activity
3. Monitor breath sounds before and after feedings
4. Place suction equipment at the bedside
5. Monitor I&O
6. Monitor for signs and symptoms of dehydration
7. Maintain IV fluids, as prescribed

D. Positioning: Place in either the flat prone position or the head-elevated prone position following feedings and at night

E. Diet
1. Provide small, frequent feedings to decrease the amount of **regurgitation;** nasogastric tube feedings are indicated if severe **regurgitation** and poor **growth** are present
2. For infants, thicken formula by adding 1 tbsp of rice cereal per 6 ounces of formula and cross-cut the nipple; monitor for coughing during feeding
3. Breast-feeding may continue, and the mother may provide more frequent feeding times or express milk for thickening with rice cereal
4. Burp the infant frequently when feeding and handle the infant minimally after feedings
5. For toddlers, feed solids first, followed by liquids
6. The parents are instructed to avoid feeding the child fatty foods, chocolate, tomato products,

---

BOX 33-7

Treatment for Gastroesophageal Reflux

Diet
Positioning
Medications
Surgery: Performed when severe complications occur

carbonated liquids, fruit juices, citrus products, and spicy foods

7. Avoid vigorous play after feeding and avoid feeding just before bedtime

F. Medications

1. Administer antacids and histamine receptor antagonists as prescribed to reduce the amount of acid present in gastric secretions and to prevent esophagitis

2. Administer prokinetic agents to accelerate gastric emptying and decrease reflux

3. Administer acetaminophen (Tylenol) as prescribed to relieve reflux pain

G. Surgery

1. If surgery is prescribed, it will require a procedure known as fundoplication, in which a wrap to the stomach fundus is made around the distal esophagus (restores the competence of the lower esophageal sphincter)

2. A gastrostomy may be performed at the same time as the fundoplication for decompression of the stomach postoperatively

3. Fundoplication may be combined with pyloroplasty in children with gastroesophageal reflux who also have delayed gastric emptying

4. Postoperative care is similar to that for other types of abdominal surgery

5. Instruct parents about potential postoperative problems, such as bloating symptoms or discomfort after consuming large, solid meals

X. HYPERTROPHIC PYLORIC STENOSIS (Figure 33-3)

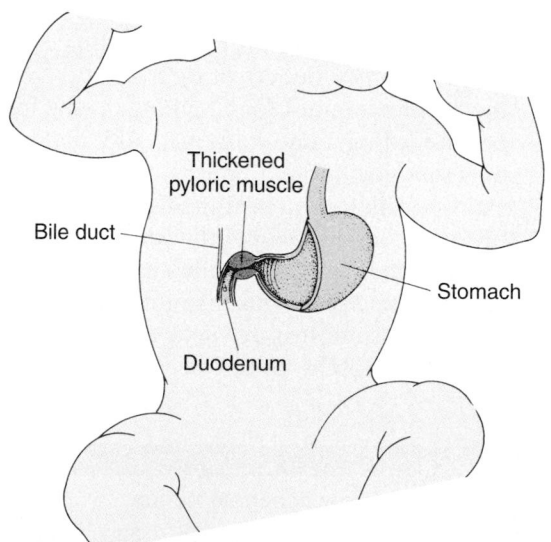

FIG. 33-3 Hypertrophic pyloric stenosis. (From Leifer, G. [2003]. *Introduction to maternity and pediatric nursing* [4th ed.]. Philadelphia: W.B. Saunders.)

A. Description

1. Hypertrophy of the circular muscles of the pylorus causes narrowing of the pyloric canal between the stomach and the duodenum

2. Usually develops in the first few weeks of life, causing projectile vomiting, dehydration, metabolic alkalosis, and failure to thrive

B. Data collection

1. Vomiting that progresses from mild **regurgitation** to forceful and projectile and usually occurs after a feeding

2. Vomitus contains gastric contents such as milk or formula; may contain mucus, may be blood-tinged, and does not usually contain bile

3. Hunger and irritability

4. Peristaltic waves visible from left to right across the epigastrium during or immediately following a feeding

5. Olive-shaped mass in the epigastrium just right of the umbilicus

6. Dehydration and malnutrition

7. Electrolyte imbalances

8. Metabolic alkalosis

C. Interventions

1. Monitor vital signs

2. Monitor I&O and weight

3. Monitor for signs of dehydration and electrolyte imbalances

4. Prepare the child and parents for pyloromyotomy if prescribed

D. Pyloromyotomy

1. Description: An incision through the muscle fibers of the pylorus; may be performed by laparoscopy

2. Interventions preoperatively

a. Monitor hydration status by daily weights, I&O, and urine for specific gravity

b. Correct fluid and electrolyte imbalances; IV fluids may be prescribed for rehydration

c. Maintain NPO status

d. Monitor the number and character of stools

e. Maintain patency of the nasogastric (NG) tube placed for stomach decompression

3. Postoperative interventions

a. Monitor I&O

b. Maintain IV fluids until the infant is taking and retaining adequate amounts by mouth

c. Begin small, frequent feedings of glucose, water, or electrolyte solution 4 to 6 hours postoperatively, as prescribed; advance the diet to formula 24 hours postoperatively, as prescribed

d. Gradually increase amount and interval between feedings until a full feeding schedule is reinstated, usually by 48 hours postoperatively

e. Feed the infant slowly, burping frequently; handle the infant minimally after feedings

f. Monitor for abdominal distention

g. Monitor the surgical wound and for signs of infection

h. Instruct the parents about wound care and feeding

XI. LACTOSE INTOLERANCE

A. Description: Inability to tolerate lactose as a result of an absence or deficiency of lactase, an enzyme found in the secretions of the small intestine that is required for the digestion of lactose

B. Data collection (Box 33-8)

C. Interventions

1. Eliminate the offending dairy product or administer an enzyme replacement

2. Provide information to parents about enzyme tablets (Lactaid, Lactrase, Dairy Ease) that predigest the lactose in milk or supplement the body's own lactase

3. In infants, soy-based formula can be substituted for cow's milk formula or human milk

4. Provide calcium and vitamin D supplements to prevent deficiency

5. Limit milk consumption to one glass at a time

6. If milk is consumed, drink with other foods rather than alone

7. Encourage consumption of hard cheese, cottage cheese, or yogurt (contains inactive lactase enzyme) instead of drinking milk

8. Encourage consumption of small amounts of dairy foods daily to help colonic bacteria adapt to ingested lactose

9. Instruct parents about the importance of calcium and vitamin D supplements

10. Instruct parents about the foods that contain lactose, including hidden sources

XII. CELIAC DISEASE

A. Description

1. Also known as gluten enteropathy or tropical sprue

2. Intolerance to gluten, the protein component of wheat, barley, rye, and oats

3. It results in the accumulation of the amino acid glutamine, which is toxic to intestinal mucosal cells

4. Intestinal villi atrophy occurs, which affects absorption of ingested nutrients

5. Symptoms of the disorder occur most often between the ages of 1 and 5 years; there is usually an interval of several months between the introduction of gluten in the diet and the onset of symptoms

6. Strict dietary avoidance of gluten minimizes the risk of developing malignant lymphoma of the small intestine and other gastrointestinal (GI) malignancies

B. Data collection

1. Acute or insidious diarrhea; stools are watery and pale with an offensive odor

2. Anorexia

3. Abdominal pain and distention

4. Muscle wasting, particularly in the buttocks and extremities

5. Vomiting

6. Anemia

7. Irritability

C. Celiac crisis (Box 33-9)

D. Interventions

1. Gluten-free diet and substituting corn, rice, and millet as grain sources

2. Lifelong elimination of gluten sources such as wheat, rye, oats, and barley

3. Mineral and vitamin supplements, including iron, folic acid, and fat-soluble supplements A, D, E, and K

4. Teach the parents about a gluten-free diet and to read food labels carefully for hidden sources of gluten (Box 33-10)

BOX 33-9

Celiac Crisis

Precipitated by infection, fasting, and ingestion of gluten
Can lead to electrolyte imbalance, rapid dehydration, and severe acidosis
Causes profuse watery diarrhea and vomiting

BOX 33-10

Basics of a Gluten-Free Diet

FOODS ALLOWED
Meat such as beef, pork, and poultry; fish; eggs, milk and dairy products; vegetables, fruits; grains, rice, corn, gluten-free wheat flour, puffed rice, cornflakes, cornmeal, precooked gluten-free cereals

FOODS PROHIBITED
Commercially prepared ice cream; malted milk; prepared puddings; grains, including anything made from wheat, rye, oats, or barley, such as breads, rolls, cookies, cakes, crackers, cereal, spaghetti, macaroni noodles, beer, and ale

---

BOX 33-8

Data Collection Findings: Lactose Intolerance

Symptoms occur after the ingestion of milk products
Diarrhea
Abdominal distention
Crampy, abdominal pain
Excessive flatus

5. Instruct the parents in the measures to prevent celiac crisis
6. Inform the parents about the Celiac Sprue Association/United States of America

XIII. APPENDICITIS

A. Description
   1. Inflammation of the appendix
   2. When the appendix becomes inflamed or infected, perforation may occur within a matter of hours, leading to peritonitis and sepsis
   3. Treatment is surgical removal of the appendix before perforation occurs
B. Data collection
   1. Pain in periumbilical area that descends to the right lower quadrant
   2. Abdominal pain that is most intense at McBurney's point
   3. Referred pain indicating the presence of peritoneal irritation
   4. Rebound tenderness and abdominal rigidity
   5. Elevated white blood cell (WBC) count
   6. Side-lying position with abdominal guarding (legs flexed)
   7. Difficulty walking and pain in the right hip
   8. Low-grade fever
   9. Anorexia, nausea, and vomiting after the pain develops
   10. Diarrhea
C. Peritonitis
   1. Data collection
      a. Results from a perforated appendix
      b. Increased fever
      c. Sudden relief of pain after the perforation; then, a subsequent increase in pain accompanied by right guarding of the abdomen occurs
      d. Progressive abdominal distention
      e. Tachycardia and tachypnea
      f. Pallor
      g. Chills
      h. Restlessness and irritability
D. Appendectomy
   1. Description: Surgical removal of the appendix
   2. Preoperative interventions
      a. Maintain NPO status
      b. IV fluids and electrolytes may be prescribed to prevent dehydration and correct electrolyte imbalances
      c. Monitor for signs of ruptured appendix and peritonitis
      d. Antibiotics may be prescribed
      e. Monitor for changes in the level of pain
      f. Monitor bowel sounds
      g. Position in right side-lying or low to semi-Fowler's position to promote comfort

h. Apply ice packs to the abdomen for 20 to 30 minutes every hour if prescribed
      i. Avoid the application of heat to the abdomen
      j. Avoid the administration of laxatives or enemas
   3. Postoperative interventions
      a. Monitor temperature for signs of infection
      b. Maintain NPO status until bowel function has returned; advance diet gradually as tolerated and as prescribed when bowel sounds return
      c. Monitor incision for signs of infection, such as redness, swelling, drainage, and pain
      d. If perforation of the appendix had occurred, expect a drain (Penrose drain) to be inserted or the incision may be left open to heal from the inside out
      e. Expect that drainage from the drain may be profuse for the first 12 hours
      f. Position the client in right side-lying or low to semi-Fowler's position with legs flexed to facilitate drainage
      g. Change the dressing as prescribed, and record type and amount of drainage
      h. Perform wound irrigations if prescribed
      i. Maintain NG tube suction and patency of tube if present
      j. Administer antibiotics and analgesics, as prescribed

XIV. HIRSCHSPRUNG'S DISEASE (Figure 33-4)

A. Description
   1. A congenital anomaly also known as congenital aganglionosis or megacolon
   2. Occurs as the result of an absence of ganglion cells in the rectum and upward in the colon

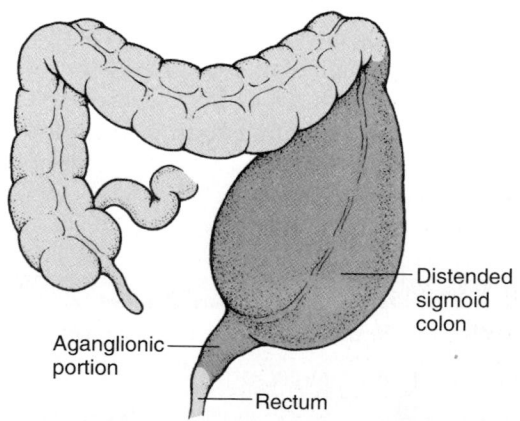

Distended sigmoid colon

Aganglionic portion

Rectum

FIG. 33-4   Hirschsprung's disease. (From Leifer, G. [2003]. *Introduction to maternity and pediatric nursing* [4th ed.]. Philadelphia: W.B. Saunders.)

3. Results in mechanical obstruction from inadequate motility in an intestinal segment
4. May be a familial congenital defect or may be associated with other anomalies, such as Down syndrome and genital urinary abnormalities
5. A rectal biopsy demonstrates histologic evidence of the absence of ganglionic cells
6. The most serious complication is enterocolitis; signs include fever, severe prostration, GI bleeding, and explosive watery diarrhea
7. Treatment for mild or moderate disease is based on relieving the chronic constipation with stool softeners and rectal irrigations; however, most children require surgery
8. Treatment for moderate to severe disease involves a two-step surgical procedure
9. Initially, in the neonatal period, the obstruction is relieved by a temporary colostomy to relieve obstruction and allow the normally innervated, dilated bowel to return to its normal size
10. A complete surgical repair is performed, when the child weighs approximately 9 kg (20 pounds), via a pull-through procedure to excise portions of the bowel; at this time, the colostomy is closed

B. Data collection
  1. Newborn infants
    a. Failure to pass meconium stool
    b. Refusal to suck
    c. Abdominal distention
    d. Bile-stained vomitus
  2. Children
    a. Failure to gain weight and delayed **growth**
    b. Abdominal distention
    c. Vomiting
    d. Constipation alternating with diarrhea
    e. Ribbon-like and foul-smelling stools

C. Nonsurgical interventions
  1. Dietary management
  2. Stool softeners
  3. Daily rectal irrigations with normal saline to promote adequate elimination and prevent obstruction

D. Surgical management: Preoperative interventions
  1. Monitor bowel function and administer bowel preparation as prescribed
  2. Maintain NPO status
  3. Monitor hydration and fluid and electrolyte status; IV fluids may be prescribed for hydration
  4. Antibiotics may be prescribed to clear the bowel of bacteria
  5. Monitor I&O and weight
  6. Measure abdominal girth
  7. Avoid rectal temperatures
  8. Monitor for respiratory distress associated with abdominal distention

E. Postoperative interventions
  1. Monitor vital signs, avoiding rectal temperatures

2. Measure abdominal girth
3. Check the surgical site for redness, swelling, and drainage
4. Check the stoma for bleeding or skin breakdown (stoma should be pink and moist)
5. Check anal area for the presence of stool, redness, or discharge
6. Maintain NPO status until bowel sounds return or flatus is passed; bowel sounds usually return within 48 to 72 hours
7. Maintain the NG tube to allow intermittent suction until peristalsis returns
8. Maintain the IV until the child tolerates appropriate oral intake; begin the diet with clear liquids, advancing to regular as tolerated and as prescribed
9. Monitor for dehydration and fluid overload
10. Monitor I&O and weight
11. Monitor pain level and provide comfort measures as required
12. Provide the parents with instructions regarding colostomy care and skin care
13. Teach the parents about the appropriate diet and the need for adequate fluid intake

XV. INTUSSUSCEPTION (Figure 33-5)

A. Description
  1. Telescoping of one portion of the bowel into another portion

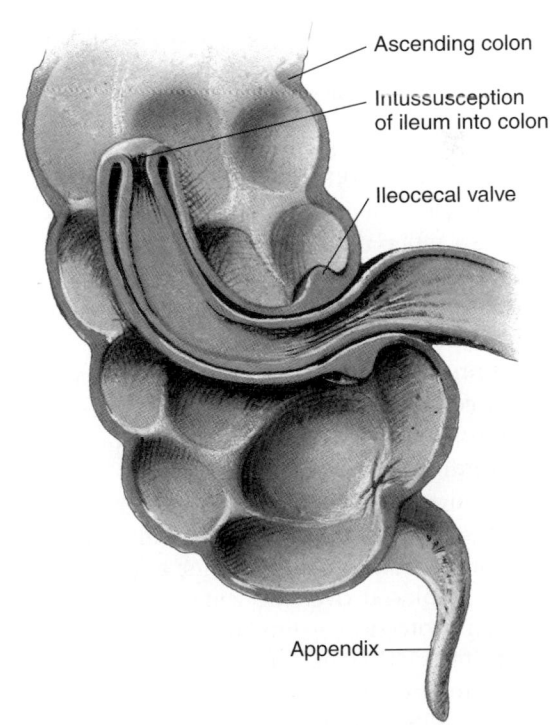

FIG. 33-5 Intussusception. (From Leifer, G. [2003]. *Introduction to maternity and pediatric nursing* [4th ed.]. Philadelphia: W.B. Saunders.)

2. Results in an obstruction to the passage of intestinal contents

B. Data collection
   1. Colicky abdominal pain that causes the child to scream and draw his or her knees to the abdomen
   2. Vomiting of gastric contents
   3. Bile-stained fecal emesis
   4. Currant jelly–like stools containing blood and mucus
   5. Hypoactive or hyperactive bowel sounds
   6. Tender distended abdomen, possibly with a palpable sausage-shaped mass in the upper right quadrant

C. Interventions
   1. Monitor for signs of perforation and shock as evidenced by fever, increased heart rate, changes in level of consciousness (LOC) or blood pressure, and respiratory distress, and report immediately
   2. Prepare for hydrostatic reduction if prescribed (not performed if signs of perforation or shock occur)
      a. Antibiotics, IV fluids, and NG decompression may be prescribed
      b. Monitor for the passage of normal, brown stool, which indicates that the intussusception has reduced itself
   3. After hydrostatic reduction:
      a. Monitor for the return of normal bowel sounds, the passage of barium, and the characteristics of stool
      b. Administer clear fluids and advance the diet gradually as prescribed
   4. If surgery is required, postoperative care is similar to that following any abdominal surgery

XVI. ABDOMINAL WALL DEFECTS
A. Omphalocele
   1. Occurs when there is a herniation of the abdominal contents through the umbilical ring (hernia of the umbilical cord), usually with an intact peritoneal sac
   2. The protrusion is covered by a translucent sac that may contain bowel or other abdominal organs
   3. Rupture of the sac results in evisceration of the abdominal contents
   4. Immediately after birth, the sac is covered with sterile gauze soaked in normal saline to prevent drying of abdominal contents; a layer of plastic wrap is placed over the gauze to provide additional protection against heat and moisture loss
   5. Monitor vital signs every 2 to 4 hours, particularly temperature, because the infant can lose heat through the sac
   6. Preoperatively: Maintain NPO status, IV fluids will be prescribed to maintain hydration and electrolyte balance; monitor for signs of infection,

and handle the infant carefully to prevent rupture of the sac
   7. Postoperatively: Control pain, prevent infection, maintain fluid and electrolyte balance, and ensure adequate nutrition

B. Gastroschisis
   1. Occurs when the herniation of the intestine is lateral to the umbilical ring
   2. There is no membrane covering the exposed bowel
   3. The exposed bowel is loosely covered in saline-soaked pads, and the abdomen is wrapped in a plastic drape; wrapping around the exposed bowel is contraindicated because if the exposed bowel expands, wrapping could cause pressure and necrosis
   4. Preoperatively: Care is similar to that for omphalocele; surgery is performed within several hours after birth because there is no membrane covering the sac
   5. Postoperatively: Most infants have a prolonged ileus and require mechanical ventilation and parenteral nutrition; otherwise, care is similar to that for omphalocele

XVII. UMBILICAL HERNIA, INGUINAL HERNIA, OR HYDROCELE
A. Description
   1. A hernia is a protrusion of the bowel through an abnormal opening in the abdominal wall
   2. In children, a hernia most commonly occurs at the umbilicus and through the inguinal canal
   3. A hydrocele is the presence of abdominal fluid in the scrotal sac

B. Data collection
   1. Umbilical hernia: Soft swelling or protrusion around the umbilicus that is usually reducible with the finger
   2. Inguinal hernia
      a. Painless inguinal swelling that is reducible
      b. Swelling may disappear during periods of rest and is most noticeable when the infant cries or coughs
   3. Incarcerated hernia
      a. The descended portion of bowel becomes tightly caught in the hernial sac, compromising blood supply
      b. A medical emergency requiring surgical repair
      c. Irritability
      d. Tenderness at site
      e. Anorexia
      f. Abdominal distention
      g. Difficulty defecating
      h. May lead to complete intestinal obstruction and gangrene
   4. Noncommunicating hydrocele

a. Occurs when residual peritoneal fluid is trapped with no communication to the peritoneal cavity

b. Usually disappears by age 1 year

5. Communicating hydrocele

a. Associated with a hernia that remains open from the scrotum to the abdominal cavity

b. Data collection findings include a bulge in the inguinal area or the scrotum that increases with crying or straining and decreases when the child is at rest

C. Postoperative interventions (hernia)

1. Monitor vital signs
2. Monitor for wound infection
3. Monitor for redness or drainage
4. Monitor I&O and hydration status
5. Advance the diet as tolerated and as prescribed
6. Administer analgesics, as prescribed

D. Postoperative interventions (hydrocele)

1. Provide ice bags and a scrotal support to relieve pain and swelling
2. Instruct the child and parents to avoid tub bathing until the incision heals
3. Instruct the child and parents to avoid strenuous physical activities

XVIII. CONSTIPATION AND ENCOPRESIS

A. Description

1. Constipation is the infrequent and difficult passage of dry, hard stools
2. **Encopresis** is fecal incontinence, and children often complain that soiling is involuntary and occurs without warning
3. If the child does not have a neurological or anatomic disorder, **encopresis** is usually the result of fecal impaction and an enlarged rectum caused by chronic constipation

B. Data collection

1. Constipation

a. Abdominal pain and cramping without distention
b. Palpable movable fecal masses
c. Normal or decreased bowel sounds
d. Malaise and headache
e. Anorexia, nausea, and vomiting

2. **Encopresis**

a. Evidence of soiling of clothing
b. Scratching or rubbing of anal area
c. Fecal odor
d. Social withdrawal

C. Interventions

1. Simple constipation may resolve by using only dietary changes or methods to change the habit of retention
2. Severe **encopresis** may require that interventions be continued over a period of 3 to 6 months

3. Overcoming withholding

a. Administer enemas as prescribed until the impaction is cleared
b. Monitor for hypernatremia or hyperphosphatemia when administering repeated enemas
c. Administer stool softener or laxative as prescribed
d. Administer mineral oil, 30 to 75 mL twice daily, as prescribed; administer chilled or mixed with cold drinks to disguise the taste

4. Dietary changes

a. Increase water and fiber intake
b. Decrease sugar and milk intake
c. Plan to administer fat-soluble vitamins during the use of mineral oil because the oil can interfere with vitamin absorption in the small intestine

5. Changing the retention habit: Have the child sit on the toilet for 5 to 10 minutes approximately 20 to 30 minutes after breakfast and dinner to assist with defecation

XIX. IRRITABLE BOWEL SYNDROME

A. Description

1. Occurs as a result of increased motility, which can lead to spasm and pain
2. The diagnosis is based on the elimination of pathology
3. It is a self-limiting, intermittent problem with no definitive treatment
4. Stress and emotional factors may contribute to its occurrence

B. Data collection

1. Diffuse abdominal pain unrelated to meals or activity
2. Alternating constipation and diarrhea with the presence of undigested food and mucus in the stool

C. Interventions

1. Reassure the parents that the problem is self-limiting and intermittent and will resolve
2. Encourage the maintenance of a healthy, well-balanced, moderate-fiber diet
3. Encourage health promotion activities such as exercise and school activities
4. Inform the parents of psychosocial resources if required

XX. IMPERFORATE ANUS

A. Description: Incomplete development or absence of the anus in its normal position in the perineum

B. Data collection (Box 33-11)

C. Preoperative interventions

1. Determine patency of the anus

BOX 33-11

Data Collection Findings: Imperforate Anus

Failure to pass meconium stool
Absence or stenosis of the anal rectal canal
Presence of an anal membrane
External fistula to the perineum

---

2. Monitor for the presence of stool in the urine and vagina and report immediately

D. Postoperative interventions
   1. Monitor the skin for signs of infection
   2. Position side-lying with legs flexed or in a prone position to keep the hips elevated to reduce edema and pressure on the surgical site
   3. Keep the anal surgical incision clean and dry, and monitor for redness, swelling, or drainage
   4. Maintain NPO status and NG tube if in place
   5. Maintain IV fluids until gastrointestinal (GI) motility returns
   6. Provide colostomy care if prescribed
   7. A fresh colostomy stoma will be red and edematous, but this should decrease with time
   8. Instruct the parents to perform anal dilation if prescribed to achieve and maintain bowel patency
   9. Instruct the parents to use only dilators supplied by the physician and a water-soluble lubricant, and to insert the dilator no more than 1 to 2 cm into the anus to prevent damage to the mucosa

XXI. HEPATITIS

A. This section contains specific information regarding hepatitis as it relates to infants and children; refer to Chapters 22 and 46 for additional information on hepatitis

B. Description: An acute or chronic inflammation of the liver that may be caused by a virus, a medication reaction, or another disease process

C. Hepatitis A (HAV)
   1. Highest incidence occurs among preschool or school-age children under 15 years of age
   2. Many affected children are asymptomatic, but mild nausea, vomiting, and diarrhea may occur
   3. Infected children who are asymptomatic can still spread HAV to others

D. Hepatitis B (HBV)
   1. Most HBV in children is acquired perinatally
   2. Newborn infants are at risk if the mother is infected with HBV or was a carrier of HBV during pregnancy
   3. Possible routes of maternal-fetal (infant) transmission include leakage of the virus across the placenta late in pregnancy or during labor, ingestion of amniotic fluid or maternal blood, and breast-feeding, especially if the mother has cracked nipples

4. The severity in the infant varies from no liver disease to fulminant (severe, acute course) or chronic, active disease
5. In children and adolescents, HBV occurs in specific high-risk groups, including:
   a. Children with hemophilia or other disorders who have received multiple blood transfusions
   b. Children or adolescents involved in drug abuse
   c. Institutionalized children
   d. Preschool children in endemic areas
   e. Children who might be involved with heterosexual activity or sexual activity with homosexual males
6. HBV infection can cause a carrier state and lead to eventual cirrhosis or hepatocellular carcinoma in adulthood

E. Hepatitis C (HCV)
   1. Transmission is primarily by the parenteral route
   2. Some children may be asymptomatic, but HCV often becomes a chronic condition and can cause cirrhosis and hepatocellular carcinoma

F. Hepatitis D (HDV)
   1. Occurs in children already infected with HBV
   2. Both acute and chronic forms tend to be more severe than HBV and can lead to cirrhosis

G. Hepatitis E (HEV)
   1. Uncommon in children
   2. Is not a chronic condition, does not cause chronic liver disease, and has no carrier state

H. Hepatitis G
   1. Bloodborne and similar to HCV
   2. High-risk groups include transfusion recipients, IV drug users, and individuals infected with HCV
   3. Individuals are often asymptomatic, and most infections are chronic

I. Data collection (Box 33-12)

J. Diagnostic evaluation: Refer to Chapter 11 for laboratory studies used to diagnose hepatitis

K. Prevention
   1. Proper hand washing and standard precautions can prevent the spread of viral hepatitis
   2. Prophylactic use of standard immune globulin (IG) to prevent HAV in situations of preexposure (such as anticipated travel to areas where HAV is prevalent) or within 2 weeks of exposure
   3. Hepatitis B immune globulin (HBIG) is effective in preventing infection following one-time exposures, such as accidental needle punctures or other contact of contaminated material with mucous membranes; should be given to newborns whose mothers are positive for HBsAg (hepatitis B surface antigen); should be given within 72 hours of exposure
   4. Hepatitis A vaccine is recommended for children 2 years and older who reside in communities with high endemic rates and for preexposure prophylaxis

BOX 33-12

Data Collection Findings: Hepatitis

PRODROMAL OR ANICTERIC PHASE

Lasts 5 to 7 days

Absence of jaundice

Anorexia, malaise, lethargy, easy fatigability

Fever (especially in adolescents)

Nausea and vomiting

Epigastric or right upper quadrant abdominal pain

Arthralgia and skin rashes (more likely with HBV)

Hepatomegaly

ICTERIC PHASE

Jaundice, which is best assessed in the sclera, nail beds, and mucous membranes

Dark urine and pale stools

Pruritus

5. Hepatitis B vaccine: Refer to Chapter 38 for immunization schedule

L. Interventions

1. Strict hand washing
2. Hospitalization is required in the event of coagulopathy or fulminant hepatitis
3. Standard precautions are followed during hospitalization
4. Hospitalized child is not usually isolated in a separate room unless he or she is fecally incontinent and items are likely to become contaminated with feces
5. Children are discouraged from sharing toys
6. Instruct child and parents in good hand washing techniques
7. Instruct the parents to thoroughly disinfect diaper-changing surfaces using $^1/_4$ cup bleach in 1 gallon of water
8. Maintain comfort and provide adequate rest and sleep
9. Provide a low-fat, balanced diet
10. Provide enteric precautions for at least 1 week after the onset of jaundice with HAV
11. Inform the parents that, because hepatitis A is not infectious within 1 week after the onset of jaundice, the child may return to school at that time if he or she feels well enough
12. Inform the parents that jaundice may get worse before it resolves
13. Caution parents about administering any medications to the child (liver is unable to detoxify and excrete medications)
14. Instruct the parents in the signs indicating a worsening of the child's condition, such as changes in the neurological status, bleeding, and fluid retention

XXII. INGESTION OF POISONS

A. Lead poisoning

1. Description: Excessive accumulation of lead in the blood
2. Causes
   a. The pathway for exposure may be food, air, or water
   b. Dust and soil contaminated with lead may be a source of exposure
   c. Lead enters the child's body through ingestion or inhalation, or through placental transmission to an unborn child when the mother is exposed; the most common route is ingestion either from hand-to-mouth behavior from contaminated objects or from eating loose paint chips that contain lead
   d. When lead enters the body, it affects the erythrocytes, bones and teeth, and organs and tissues, including the brain and nervous system; the most serious consequences are the effects on the central nervous system
3. Universal screening
   a. Recommended in high-risk areas at the age of 1 to 2 years; children at high risk should be screened earlier
   b. Any child between the ages of 3 and 6 years who has not been screened should be tested
4. Targeted screening
   a. Acceptable in low-risk areas
   b. At the age of 1 to 2 years (or a child between the ages of 3 and 6 years who has not been screened) may be targeted for screening if determined to be at risk
5. Blood lead level (BLL) test: Used for screening and diagnosis (Table 33-1)
6. Erythrocyte protoporphyrin (EP) test
   a. An indicator of anemia
   b. Normal value for a child is 35 mcg/100 mL of whole blood or lower
7. Chelation therapy
   a. Removes lead from the circulating blood and from some organs and tissues
   b. Does not counteract any effects of the lead
   c. Medications: Dimercaprol (BAL in Oil); calcium disodium edetate (CaNa$_2$EDTA); succimer (Chemet)
   d. Dimercaprol (BAL in Oil) is contraindicated in children with an allergy to peanuts because the medication is prepared in a peanut oil solution
   e. Ensure adequate urinary output before administering medications
   f. Provide adequate hydration and monitor kidney function for nephrotoxicity when medication is given, because the medication is excreted via the kidneys

TABLE 33-1

Blood Lead Level (BLL) Test

Level	Intervention
Lower than 10 mcg/dL	Reassess or rescreen in 1 year; sooner if exposure status changes
10 to 14 mcg/dL	Provide family lead education, follow-up testing, and social service referral if necessary
15 to 19 mcg/dL	Provide family lead education, follow-up testing, and social service referral if necessary; on follow-up testing, initiate actions for BLL level of 20 to 44 mcg/dL
20 to 44 mcg/dL	BLL level higher than 20 mcg/dL is considered acute; provide coordination of care, clinical management, including treatment, environmental investigation, and lead hazard control (the child must not remain in a lead-hazardous environment if resolution is necessary)
70 mcg/dL or higher	Medical treatment is immediately provided, including coordination of care, clinical management, environmental investigation, and lead-hazard control

g. Follow-up lead levels to monitor progress are essential

h. Provide instructions to parents about safety from lead hazards, medication administration, and the need for follow-up

i. Confirm that the child will be discharged to home without lead hazards

B. Acetaminophen (Tylenol) poisoning
   1. Description
      a. Seriousness of ingestion is determined by the amount ingested and the length of time before intervention
      b. Toxic dose is 150 mg/kg or higher in children
   2. Data collection
      a. First 2 to 4 hours: Malaise, nausea, vomiting, sweating, pallor, weakness
      b. Latent period: 24 to 36 hours; child improves
      c. Hepatic involvement: May last up to 7 days and be permanent; right upper quadrant pain, jaundice, confusion, stupor, elevated liver enzymes and bilirubin, prolonged prothrombin time (PT)
   3. Interventions
      a. Administer antidote: N-acetylcysteine (NAC)
      b. Dilute antidote in juice or soda because of its offensive odor
      c. Loading dose is followed by maintenance doses

C. Acetylsalicylic acid (aspirin, ASA) poisoning
   1. Description
      a. May be caused by acute ingestion or chronic ingestion
      b. Acute: Severe toxicity occurs with 300 to 500 mg/kg
      c. Chronic: More than 100 mg/kg/day for 2 days or more; can be more serious than acute ingestion
   2. Data collection
      a. GI effects: Nausea, vomiting, and thirst from dehydration
      b. CNS effects: Hyperpnea, confusion, tinnitus, convulsions, coma, respiratory failure, circulatory collapse

c. Renal effects: Oliguria

d. Hematopoietic effects: Bleeding tendencies

e. Metabolic effects: Diaphoresis, dehydration, fever, hyponatremia, hypokalemia, dehydration, hypoglycemia

3. Interventions
   a. To induce vomiting, the physician may prescribe syrup of ipecac, or gastric lavage may be performed
   b. Activated charcoal may be prescribed to decrease absorption of salicylate (important in early ASA toxicity)
   c. IVs, sodium bicarbonate, electrolytes, or volume expanders may be prescribed
   d. Vitamin K may be given for bleeding tendencies, as prescribed
   e. Glucose may be prescribed to treat hypoglycemia
   f. Prepare the child for dialysis as prescribed if the child is unresponsive to the therapy

PRACTICE QUESTIONS

1. A nurse is caring for an 18-month-old child who has been vomiting. The appropriate position in which to place the child during naps and sleep time is:
   1. Side-lying position
   2. Prone with the face turned to the side
   3. Supine
   4. Prone with the head elevated

2. A nurse is monitoring for signs of dehydration in a 1-year-old child who has been hospitalized for diarrhea and prepares to take the child's temperature. Which method of temperature measurement would be avoided?
   1. Tympanic
   2. Axillary
   3. Rectal
   4. Electronic

3. An infant returns to the nursing unit following a surgical repair of a cleft lip located on the right side of the lip. The best position to place this infant at this time is:
   1. On the right side
   2. On the left side
   3. Prone
   4. Supine

4. A nurse reviews the record of an infant seen in the clinic. The nurse notes that a diagnosis of esophageal atresia with tracheoesophageal fistula (TEF) is suspected. The nurse expects to note which most likely clinical manifestation of this condition documented in the record?
   1. Severe projectile vomiting
   2. Coughing at nighttime
   3. Choking with feedings
   4. Incessant crying

5. A nurse is reviewing the record of a child with a diagnosis of pyloric stenosis. Which data would the nurse expect to note documented in the child's record?
   1. Vomiting large amounts of bile
   2. Watery diarrhea
   3. Increased urine output
   4. Projectile vomiting

6. A nurse reinforces instructions to the mother about dietary measures for a 5-year-old child with lactose intolerance. The nurse tells the mother that which of the following supplements will be required due to the necessity of lactose avoidance in the diet?
   1. Zinc
   2. Protein
   3. Calcium
   4. Fats

7. A nurse reinforces home care instructions to the parents of a child with celiac disease. Which of the following food items would the nurse advise the parents to include in the child's diet?
   1. Rice
   2. Rye toast
   3. Oatmeal
   4. Wheat bread

8. A nurse is caring for a child who is scheduled for an appendectomy. When the nurse reviews the physician's preoperative orders, which of the following would be questioned?
   1. Maintain IV fluids as prescribed
   2. Maintain NPO status
   3. Administer a Fleet enema
   4. Administer preoperative medication on call to the operating room

9. A nurse reviews the record of a 3-week-old infant and notes that the physician has documented a diagnosis of suspected Hirschsprung's disease. The nurse understands that which of the following symptoms led the mother to seek health care for the infant?
   1. Diarrhea

   2. Projectile vomiting
   3. Regurgitation of feedings
   4. Foul-smelling ribbon-like stools

10. A nurse is caring for a child with a diagnosis of intussusception. Which of the following symptoms would the nurse expect to note in this child?
    1. Blood and mucus in the stools
    2. Profuse projectile vomiting
    3. Watery diarrhea
    4. Ribbon-like stools

11. A child with a diagnosis of umbilical hernia has been scheduled for surgical repair in 2 weeks. The nurse reinforces instructions to the parents about the signs of possible hernial strangulation. The nurse tells the parents that which of the following signs would require physician notification by the parents?
    1. Fever
    2. Diarrhea
    3. Constipation
    4. Vomiting

12. A nurse reinforces home care instructions to the parents of a child with hepatitis regarding care of the child and the prevention of transmission of the virus. Which statement by a parent indicates a need for further instruction?
    1. "Frequent hand washing is important."
    2. "I need to clean contaminated household surfaces with bleach."
    3. "I need to provide a well-balanced, high-fat diet to my child."
    4. "Diapers should not be changed near any surfaces used to prepare food."

13. A child is hospitalized with a diagnosis of lead poisoning. The nurse assisting in caring for the child would prepare to assist in administering which of the following medications?
    1. Activated charcoal
    2. Sodium bicarbonate
    3. Ipecac syrup
    4. Dimercaprol (BAL in Oil)

14. An emergency nurse is caring for a child brought to the emergency room following the ingestion of approximately one half-bottle of acetylsalicylic acid (aspirin). The nurse anticipates that the most likely initial treatment will be:
    1. The administration of syrup of ipecac
    2. The administration of sodium bicarbonate
    3. The administration of vitamin K
    4. Dialysis

15. A licensed practical nurse (LPN) asks a nursing assistant to gather supplies in preparation for administering a tepid bath to a child with a fever. The LPN intervenes if the nursing assistant obtains which unnecessary item(s)?
    1. Washcloths and towels
    2. A bottle of alcohol

3. Toys
4. Lightweight pajamas

16. A cooling blanket is prescribed for a child with a fever. The nurse prepares to use the cooling blanket and avoids which of the following?
    1. Placing the cooling blanket on the bed and covering it with a sheet
    2. Checking the skin condition of the child before, during, and after the use of the cooling blanket
    3. Keeping the child uncovered to assist in reducing the fever
    4. Keeping the child dry while on the cooling blanket to prevent the risk of frostbite

17. A nursing instructor asks a nursing student about phenylketonuria (PKU). Which statement, if made by the student, indicates an understanding of this disorder?
    1. "PKU is an autosomal dominant disorder."
    2. "Treatment includes dietary restriction of tyramine."
    3. "All 50 states require routine screening of all newborns for PKU."
    4. "PKU primarily affects the gastrointestinal system."

18. A school-age child with type 1 diabetes mellitus has soccer practice three afternoons a week. The nurse reinforces instructions regarding how to prevent hypoglycemia during practice. The nurse tells the child to:
    1. Take half the amount of prescribed insulin on practice days
    2. Eat twice the amount normally eaten at lunchtime
    3. Take the prescribed insulin at noontime rather than in the morning
    4. Drink $1/2$ cup of orange juice before soccer practice

19. The nurse is reinforcing instructions to an adolescent with type 1 diabetes mellitus regarding insulin administration and rotation sites. Which statement, if made by the adolescent, would indicate an understanding of the instructions?
    1. "I need to use one major site for the morning injection and another major site for the evening injection for 2 to 3 weeks before changing major sites."
    2. "I need to use a different site for each insulin injection."
    3. "I need to use the same site for 1 month before rotating to another site."
    4. "I should use only my stomach and my thighs for injections."

20. A mother of a 6-year-old with type 1 diabetes mellitus calls the clinic nurse and tells the nurse that the child has been sick. The mother reports that she checked the child's urine and it showed positive ketones. Which of the following would the nurse instruct the mother to do?
    1. Come to the clinic immediately
    2. Hold the next dose of insulin
    3. Administer an additional dose of regular insulin
    4. Encourage the child to drink calorie-free liquids

ALTERNATE FORMAT QUESTION: MULTIPLE RESPONSE

Select all interventions for a child with type 1 diabetes mellitus who has a blood glucose level of 60 mg/dL.
___ Give the child a teaspoon of honey
___ Prepare to administer glucagon subcutaneously if unconsciousness occurs
___ Encourage the child to ambulate
___ Administer regular insulin

ANSWERS

1. *Answer:* **1**
Rationale: The vomiting child should be placed in an upright or side-lying position to prevent aspiration. Options 2, 3, and 4 will place the child at risk for aspiration if vomiting occurs. *Test-Taking Strategy:* Use the process of elimination. Eliminate options 2 and 4 first because they are similar. Additionally, these positions would place the child at risk for aspiration if vomiting occurred. Visualize the remaining two positions. Option 3 is also inappropriate and would cause aspiration. Review appropriate positioning for the child who has been vomiting if you had difficulty with this question.
Level of Cognitive Ability: Application

Client Needs: Physiological Integrity
Integrated Process: Nursing Process/Implementation
Content Area: Child Health
Reference: Price, D., & Gwin, J. (2005). *Thompson's pediatric nursing* (9th ed.). Philadelphia: W.B. Saunders, pp. 156-157.

2. *Answer:* **3**
Rationale: Rectal temperature measurements should be avoided if diarrhea is present. Use of a rectal thermometer can stimulate peristalsis and cause more diarrhea. Axillary and tympanic measurements of temperature would be acceptable. Most measurements are done via electronic devices.

Test-Taking Strategy: Use the process of elimination and note the key word, *avoided.* Eliminate option 4 first because most methods of temperature measurement are done using an electronic device. Next, note the diagnosis stated in the question. This should direct you to option 3. Review interventions for the child with diarrhea if you had difficulty with this question.
Level of Cognitive Ability: Application
Client Needs: Physiological Integrity
Integrated Process: Nursing Process/Implementation
Content Area: Child Health
Reference: McKinney, E., James, S., Murray, S., & Ashwill, J. (2005). *Maternal-child nursing* (2nd ed.). St. Louis: Elsevier, p. 1093.

3. Answer: 2
Rationale: Following cleft lip repair, the infant should be positioned on the side lateral to the repair to prevent contact of the suture lines with the bed linens. It is best to place the infant on the left side rather than supine immediately after surgery to prevent the risk of aspiration if the infant vomits.
Test-Taking Strategy: Use the process of elimination. Consider the anatomical location of the surgical site and the key words, *right side.* You should easily be directed to the correct option using these concepts. Review postoperative positioning techniques if you had difficulty with this question.
Level of Cognitive Ability: Application
Client Needs: Physiological Integrity
Integrated Process: Nursing Process/Implementation
Content Area: Child Health
Reference: Leifer, G. (2003). *Introduction to maternity and pediatric nursing* (4th ed.). Philadelphia: W.B. Saunders, p. 658.

4. Answer: 3
Rationale: Any child who exhibits the "3 C's," coughing and choking during feedings, and unexplained cyanosis, should be suspected of TEF. Options 1, 2, and 4 are not specifically associated with TEF.
Test-Taking Strategy: Use the process of elimination focusing on the diagnosis. Recalling the "3 C's" associated with this disorder will assist in directing you to the correct option. Review the clinical manifestations associated with this disorder if you had difficulty with this question
Level of Cognitive Ability: Comprehension
Client Needs: Physiological Integrity
Integrated Process: Nursing Process/Data Collection
Content Area: Child Health
Reference: Leifer, G. (2003). *Introduction to maternity and pediatric nursing* (4th ed.). Philadelphia: W.B. Saunders, p. 658.

5. Answer: 4
Rationale: Clinical manifestations of pyloric stenosis include projectile, nonbilious vomiting, irritability, hunger and crying, constipation, and signs of dehydration including a decrease in urine output.
Test-Taking Strategy: Use the process of elimination. Considering the anatomical location of this disorder and its potential effects will assist in eliminating options 2 and 3. Recalling that a major clinical manifestation is projectile,

nonbilious vomiting will assist in directing you to option 4. Review these clinical manifestations if you had difficulty with this question.
Level of Cognitive Ability: Comprehension
Client Needs: Physiological Integrity
Integrated Process: Nursing Process/Data Collection
Content Area: Child Health
Reference: Price, D., & Gwin, J. (2005). *Thompson's pediatric nursing* (9th ed.). Philadelphia: W.B. Saunders, pp. 152-153.

6. Answer: 3
Rationale: Lactose intolerance is the inability to tolerate lactose, the sugar found in dairy products. Removing milk from the diet can provide relief from symptoms. Additional dietary changes may be required to provide adequate sources of calcium and, if the child is an infant, protein and calories.
Test-Taking Strategy: Knowledge that lactose is the sugar found in dairy products will easily direct you to option 3, because dairy products contain high sources of calcium. Review the dietary management for lactose intolerance if you had difficulty with this question.
Level of Cognitive Ability: Application
Client Needs: Health Promotion and Maintenance
Integrated Process: Nursing Process/Implementation
Content Area: Child Health
Reference: Wong, D., & Hockenberry, M. (2003). *Nursing care of infants and children* (7th ed.). St. Louis: Mosby, p. 571.

7. Answer: 1
Rationale: Dietary management is the main stay of treatment in celiac disease. All wheat, rye, barley, and oats should be eliminated from the diet and replaced with corn and rice. Vitamin supplements, especially fat-soluble vitamins and folate, may be needed in the early period of treatment to correct deficiencies. These restrictions are likely to be lifelong, although small amounts of grains may be tolerated after the ulcerations have healed.
Test-Taking Strategy: Use the process of elimination and knowledge regarding the dietary management in celiac disease to answer this question. Recalling that corn and rice are substitute food replacements in this disease will direct you to option 1. Review the dietary management of this disorder if you had difficulty with this question.
Level of Cognitive Ability: Application
Client Needs: Health Promotion and Maintenance
Integrated Process: Teaching/Learning
Content Area: Child Health
Reference: Price, D., & Gwin, J. (2005). *Thompson's pediatric nursing* (9th ed.). Philadelphia: W.B. Saunders, p. 238.

8. Answer: 3
Rationale: In the preoperative period, enemas or laxatives should not be administered. No heat should be applied to the abdomen because this may increase the chance of perforation secondary to vasodilation. IV fluids would be started and the child would be NPO. Prescribed preoperative medications most likely would be administered on call to the operating room.
Test-Taking Strategy: Use the process of elimination. Consider the anatomical location and the concern of rupture in

this disorder. Options 1, 2, and 4 are standard preoperative measures. Option 3 would place the child at risk for a perforated appendix. Review preoperative care in the child with appendicitis if you had difficulty with this question.
Level of Cognitive Ability: Analysis
Client Needs: Physiological Integrity
Integrated Process: Nursing Process/Implementation
Content Area: Child Health
Reference: Price, D., & Gwin, J. (2005). *Thompson's pediatric nursing* (9th ed.). Philadelphia: W.B. Saunders, p. 299.

9. *Answer: 4*
Rationale: Chronic constipation beginning in the first month of life resulting in foul-smelling ribbon-like or pellet-like stools is a clinical manifestation of this disorder. Delayed passage or absence of meconium stool in the neonatal period is the cardinal sign. Bowel obstruction, especially in the neonatal period, abdominal pain and distention, and failure to thrive are also clinical manifestations. Options 1, 2, and 3 are incorrect.
Test-Taking Strategy: Knowledge regarding the clinical manifestations associated with Hirschsprung's disease is required to answer this question. Remember that foul-smelling ribbon-like or pellet-like stools is a clinical manifestation of this disorder. Review these manifestations if you had difficulty with this question.
Level of Cognitive Ability: Comprehension
Client Needs: Physiological Integrity
Integrated Process: Nursing Process/Data Collection
Content Area: Child Health
Reference: Price, D., & Gwin, J. (2005). *Thompson's pediatric nursing* (9th ed.). Philadelphia: W.B. Saunders, p. 156.

10. *Answer: 1*
Rationale: The child with intussusception classically presents with severe abdominal pain that is crampy and intermittent, causing the child to draw in his or her knees to the chest. Vomiting may be present but it is not projectile. Bright red blood and mucus are passed through the rectum and is commonly described as currant jelly–like stools. Ribbon-like stools are not a manifestation of this disorder.
Test-Taking Strategy: Knowledge related to the clinical manifestations associated with intussusception is required to answer this question. Recalling that a classic manifestation is currant jelly–like stools will assist in directing you to option 1. Review this disorder if you had difficulty with this question.
Level of Cognitive Ability: Comprehension
Client Needs: Physiological Integrity
Integrated Process: Nursing Process/Data Collection
Content Area: Child Health
Reference: Price, D., & Gwin, J. (2005). *Thompson's pediatric nursing* (9th ed.). Philadelphia: W.B. Saunders, p. 154.

11. *Answer: 4*
Rationale: The parents of a child with an umbilical hernia need to be instructed about the signs of strangulation. These signs include vomiting, pain, and irreducible mass at the umbilicus. The parents should be instructed to contact the physician immediately if strangulation is suspected.

Test-Taking Strategy: Use the definition of the word "strangulation" to help answer this question. This will assist in eliminating options 1 and 2. From the remaining options, knowledge regarding the signs of strangulation will assist in answering the question. Review the signs of strangulation if you had difficulty with this question.
Level of Cognitive Ability: Application
Client Needs: Health Promotion and Maintenance
Integrated Process: Teaching/Learning
Content Area: Child Health
Reference: Price, D., & Gwin, J. (2005). *Thompson's pediatric nursing* (9th ed.). Philadelphia: W.B. Saunders, p. 152.

12. *Answer: 3*
Rationale: The child with hepatitis should consume a well-balanced, low-fat diet to allow the liver to rest. Options 1, 2, and 4 are components of the home care instructions to the family of a child with hepatitis.
Test-Taking Strategy: Note the key words, *need for further instruction.* These words indicate a false response question and that you need to select the incorrect client statement. Options 1, 2, and 4 can be eliminated by using the basic principles related to standard precautions. Review home care instructions to the parents of a child with hepatitis if you had difficulty with this question.
Level of Cognitive Ability: Comprehension
Client Needs: Safe, Effective Care Environment
Integrated Process: Teaching/Learning
Content Area: Child Health
Reference: Leifer, G. (2005). *Maternity nursing* (9th ed.). Philadelphia: W.B. Saunders, p. 663.

13. *Answer: 4*
Rationale: Dimercaprol (BAL in Oil) is a chelating agent that is administered to remove lead from the circulating blood and from some tissues and organs for excretion in the urine. Sodium bicarbonate may be used in salicylate poisoning. Ipecac syrup is used in poisonings to induce vomiting. Activated charcoal is used to decrease absorption in certain poisoning situations.
Test-Taking Strategy: Knowledge regarding the treatment related to lead poisoning is required to answer this question. Remember that dimercaprol (BAL in Oil) is a chelating agent that is administered to remove lead from the circulating blood and from some tissues and organs for excretion in the urine. Review this treatment if you are unfamiliar with it.
Level of Cognitive Ability: Application
Client Needs: Physiological Integrity
Integrated Process: Nursing Process/Planning
Content Area: Child Health
References: Leifer, G. (2005). *Maternity nursing* (9th ed.). Philadelphia: W.B. Saunders, p. 681.
Price, D., & Gwin, J. (2005). *Thompson's pediatric nursing* (9th ed.). Philadelphia: W.B. Saunders, p. 208.

14. *Answer: 1*
Rationale: Initial treatment of salicylate overdose includes inducing vomiting with syrup of ipecac or gastric lavage. Activated charcoal may be administered to decrease absorption. IV fluids and sodium bicarbonate may be administered

to enhance excretion but would not be the initial treatment. Dialysis is used in extreme cases if the child is unresponsive to therapy. Vitamin K is the antidote for warfarin (Coumadin) overdose.

Test-Taking Strategy: Note the key word, *initial* in the stem of the question. This key word and knowledge regarding the treatment for aspirin overdose will assist in directing you to option 1. Remember, initial treatment of salicylate overdose includes inducing vomiting with syrup of Ipecac, or gastric lavage. Review the treatment for this overdose if you had difficulty with this question.

Level of Cognitive Ability: Comprehension
Client Needs: Physiological Integrity
Integrated Process: Nursing Process/Planning
Content Area: Child Health
Reference: Wong, D., & Hockenberry, M. (2003). *Nursing care of infants and children* (7th ed.). St. Louis: Mosby, pp. 671-672.

15. *Answer: 2*
Rationale: Alcohol should never be used for bathing the child with a fever because it can cause rapid cooling, peripheral vasoconstriction, and chilling, thus elevating the temperature further. Washcloths can be used to squeeze water over the child's body. Towels are used to dry the child. Toys, especially water toys, can be used to provide distraction during the bath. Lightweight clothing should be placed on the child after the child is dried.

Test-Taking Strategy: Use the process of elimination. Note the key word, *intervenes*. This word indicates a false response question and that you need to select the incorrect item. Options 1 and 4 can be easily eliminated first. From the remaining options, select option 2 because of the harmful effects of alcohol and the effect of potentially elevating the temperature. Review the procedure for administering a tepid bath if you had difficulty with this question.

Level of Cognitive Ability: Application
Client Needs: Physiological Integrity
Integrated Process: Nursing Process/Implementation
Content Area: Leadership/Management
Reference: Price, D., & Gwin, J. (2005). *Thompson's pediatric nursing* (9th ed.). Philadelphia: W.B. Saunders, p. 357.

16. *Answer: 3*
Rationale: While on a cooling blanket, the child should be covered lightly to maintain privacy and reduce shivering. Options 1, 2, and 4 are important interventions to prevent shivering, frostbite, and skin breakdown.

Test-Taking Strategy: Note the key word, *avoids*. This word indicates a false response question and that you need to select the incorrect intervention. Knowledge regarding the physiological response associated with fever will direct you to option 3. Review the procedure associated with the use of a cooling blanket if you had difficulty with this question.

Level of Cognitive Ability: Application
Client Needs: Physiological Integrity
Integrated Process: Nursing Process/Implementation
Content Area: Child Health
References: McKinney, E., James, S., Murray, S., & Ashwill, J. (2005). *Maternal-child nursing* (2nd ed.). St. Louis: Elsevier, pp. 945-946.

Wong, D., & Hockenberry, M. (2003). *Nursing care of infants and children* (7th ed.). St. Louis: Mosby, pp. 1130-1131.

17. *Answer: 3*
Rationale: PKU is an autosomal recessive disorder. Treatment includes dietary restriction of phenylalanine intake. PKU is a genetic disorder that results in central nervous system (CNS) damage from toxic levels of phenylalanine in the blood. Option 3 is accurate.

Test-Taking Strategy: Use the process of elimination. Recalling that PKU is a recessive disorder will assist in eliminating option 1. Reading option 2 carefully will direct you to eliminate this option because tyramine is restricted in clients on monoamine oxidase inhibitors, not in PKU. Recalling that PKU affects the CNS will direct you to option 3 from the remaining options. Review the characteristics associated with this disorder if you had difficulty with this question.

Level of Cognitive Ability: Comprehension
Client Needs: Physiological Integrity
Integrated Process: Teaching/Learning
Content Area: Child Health
Reference: Leifer, G. (2003). *Introduction to maternity and pediatric nursing* (4th ed.). Philadelphia: W.B. Saunders, p. 334.

18. *Answer: 4*
Rationale: An extra snack of 10 to 15 g of carbohydrate eaten before activities and for every 30 to 45 minutes of activity will prevent hypoglycemia. One-half cup of orange juice will provide the needed carbohydrate. The child or parents should not be instructed to adjust the amount or time of insulin administration. Meal amounts should not be doubled.

Test-Taking Strategy: Use the process of elimination. Options 1 and 3 can be eliminated first because insulin dosages and times should not be adjusted. From the remaining options, recalling the manifestations and treatment associated with hypoglycemia will direct you to option 4. Review the treatment to prevent hypoglycemia if you had difficulty with this question.

Level of Cognitive Ability: Application
Client Needs: Health Promotion and Maintenance
Integrated Process: Teaching/Learning
Content Area: Child Health
Reference: Price, D., & Gwin, J. (2005). *Thompson's pediatric nursing* (9th ed.). Philadelphia: W.B. Saunders, p. 285.

19. *Answer: 1*
Rationale: To help decrease variations in absorption from day to day, the child should use one location within a major site for the morning injection. The child should then rotate to another site for the evening injection, and a third site for the bedtime injection. The child should follow this pattern for a period of 2 to 3 weeks before changing major sites.

Test-Taking Strategy: Use the process of elimination. Eliminate option 4 first because of the word "only." From the remaining options, it is necessary to know the physiology associated with absorption of insulin. Review insulin administration if you had difficulty with this question.

Level of Cognitive Ability: Analysis
Client Needs: Physiological Integrity

Integrated Process: Nursing Process/Evaluation
Content Area: Child Health
Reference: Price, D., & Gwin, J. (2005). *Thompson's pediatric nursing* (9th ed.). Philadelphia: W.B. Saunders, pp. 282-284.

20. *Answer:* 4
Rationale: When the child is sick, the mother should test for urinary ketones with each voiding. If ketones are present, liquids are essential to aid in clearing. The child should be encouraged to drink calorie-free liquids. It is not necessary to bring the child to the clinic immediately. Insulin doses should not be adjusted or changed.
Test-Taking Strategy: Use the process of elimination. Eliminate options 2 and 3 first because insulin doses should not be adjusted or changed. From the remaining options, note the words "positive ketones." This finding does not require immediate physician referral. Review home care instructions for the sick diabetic child if you had difficulty with this question.
Level of Cognitive Ability: Application
Client Needs: Health Promotion and Maintenance
Integrated Process: Nursing Process/Implementation
Content Area: Child Health
Reference: McKinney, E., James, S., Murray, S., & Ashwill, J. (2005). *Maternal-child nursing* (2nd ed.). St. Louis: Elsevier, p. 1478.

ALTERNATE FORMAT QUESTION: MULTIPLE RESPONSE

Answers:
Give the child a teaspoon of honey
Prepare to administer glucagon subcutaneously if unconsciousness occurs

Rationale: Hypoglycemia is defined as a blood glucose level below 70 mg/dL. It occurs as a result of too much insulin, not enough food, or excessive activity. If possible, the nurse should confirm with a blood glucose reading. Oral glucose is administered immediately; the rapid-releasing sugar is followed by a complex carbohydrate and protein, such as a slice of bread or a peanut butter cracker. An extra snack is given if the next meal is not planned for more than 30 minutes or if activity is planned. If the child becomes unconscious, cake frosting or glucose paste is squeezed onto the gums and the blood glucose level is retested if the child does not improve within 15 to 20 minutes; if the reading remains low, additional sugar is administered. If the child remains unconscious, it may be necessary to administer glucagon and the nurse should be prepared for this intervention. In the hospital setting, the nurse should be prepared to administer IV dextrose. Encouraging the child to ambulate and administering regular insulin will result in a lowered blood glucose level.
Test-Taking Strategy: Focus on the information in the question. Recalling that a blood glucose level of 60 mg/dL indicates hypoglycemia will assist in determining the correct interventions. Review the interventions for hypoglycemia if you had difficulty with this question.
Level of Cognitive Ability: Application
Client Needs: Physiological Integrity
Integrated Process: Nursing Process/Implementation
Content Area: Child Health
Reference: Price, D., & Gwin, J. (2005). *Thompson's pediatric nursing* (9th ed.). Philadelphia: W.B. Saunders, p. 285.

REFERENCES

Leifer, G. (2003). *Introduction to maternity and pediatric nursing* (4th ed.). Philadelphia: W.B. Saunders.
McKinney, E., James, S., Murray, S., & Ashwill, J. (2005). *Maternal-child nursing* (2nd ed.). St. Louis: W.B. Saunders.
Price, D., & Gwin, J. (2005). *Thompson's pediatric nursing* (9th ed.). Philadelphia: W.B. Saunders.
Wong, D., & Hockenberry, M. (2003). *Nursing care of infants and children* (7th ed.). St. Louis: Mosby.

Renal and Urinary Disorders

I. GLOMERULONEPHRITIS

A. Description
1. A term that includes a variety of disorders, most of which are caused by an immunological reaction
2. It results in proliferative and inflammatory changes within the glomerular structure
3. Destruction, inflammation, and sclerosis of the glomeruli of both kidneys occur
4. Inflammation of the glomeruli results from an antigen-antibody reaction produced by an infection elsewhere in the body
5. Loss of kidney function develops

B. Causes
1. Immunological diseases
2. Autoimmune diseases
3. Streptococcal infection, group A beta-hemolytic
4. History of pharyngitis or tonsillitis 2 to 3 weeks prior to symptoms

C. Types (Box 34-1)

D. Data collection
1. Periorbital and facial edema that is more prominent in the morning
2. Anorexia
3. Decreased urinary output
4. Cloudy, smoky brown colored urine
5. Pallor, irritability, lethargy
6. In the older child: Headaches, abdominal or flank pain, dysuria
7. Hypertension
8. Proteinuria that produces a persistent and excessive foam in the urine
9. Azotemia
10. Increased blood urea nitrogen (BUN) and creatinine levels
11. Increased antistreptolysin O titer (used to diagnose disorders caused by streptococcal infections)

E. Interventions
1. Monitor vital signs, weight, intake and output (I&O), and characteristics of urine
2. Limit activity; provide safety measures
3. Nutrition
   a. Restrictions depend on the stage and severity of the disease, especially the extent of the edema
   b. In uncomplicated cases, a regular diet is permitted but sodium is restricted to no added salt to foods
   c. Moderate sodium restriction is prescribed for the child with hypertension or edema
   d. Foods high in potassium are restricted during periods of oliguria
   e. Protein is restricted if the child has severe azotemia resulting from prolonged oliguria
4. Monitor for complications (renal failure, hypertensive encephalopathy, pulmonary edema, and heart failure)
5. Administer diuretics (if significant edema and fluid overload are present), antihypertensives (for hypertension), and antibiotics (to the child with evidence of persistent streptococcal infections), as prescribed
6. Initiate seizure precautions and administer anticonvulsants as prescribed for seizures associated with hypertensive encephalopathy
7. Instruct the parents to report signs of bloody urine, headache, or edema

---

BOX 34-1

Types of Glomerulonephritis

Acute: Occurs 2 to 3 weeks after a streptococcal infection
Chronic: Can occur after the acute phase or slowly over time

8. Instruct the parents that the child needs to obtain treatment for infections, specifically sore throats and upper respiratory infections

II. NEPHROTIC SYNDROME

A. Description
   1. A kidney disorder characterized by massive proteinuria, hypoalbuminemia, and edema
   2. The primary objective of therapeutic management is to reduce the excretion of urinary protein and maintain protein-free urine

B. Data collection (Box 34-2)

C. Interventions
   1. Monitor vital signs, I&O, and daily weights
   2. Monitor urine for specific gravity and albumin
   3. Monitor for edema
   4. Nutrition: A regular diet without added salt is prescribed if the child is in remission; sodium is restricted during periods of massive edema
   5. Corticosteroid therapy: Prescribed as soon as the diagnosis has been determined (monitor child closely for signs of infection)
   6. Immunosuppressant therapy may be prescribed to reduce the relapse rate and induce long-term remission; may be administered in conjunction with the corticosteroid
   7. Diuretics may be prescribed to reduce edema
   8. Plasma expanders such as salt-poor human albumin may be prescribed for the severely edematous child
   9. Instruct the parents about testing the urine for albumin, medication administration, side effects of medications, and general care of the child
   10. Instruct the parents regarding the signs of infection and the need to avoid contact with other children who may be infectious

III. CRYPTORCHIDISM

A. Description: Occurs when one or both testes fail to descend through the inguinal canal into the scrotal sac

B. Data collection: Testes not palpable or easily guided into the scrotum

C. Interventions

BOX 34-2

Findings in Nephrotic Syndrome

Child gains weight
Periorbital and facial edema most prominent in the morning
Leg, ankle, labial or scrotal edema occurs
Decreased urine output; urine is dark and frothy
Abdominal swelling
Blood pressure is normal or slightly decreased

---

1. Monitor during the first 12 months of life to determine if spontaneous descent occurs
2. After age 1, medical or surgical treatment may be instituted
3. Human chorionic gonadotropin (hCG), a pituitary hormone that stimulates the production of testosterone, may be prescribed
4. Surgical correction, if needed, is done by orchiopexy before the child's second birthday (preferably between 1 and 2 years of age) if the testes do not descend spontaneously
5. Monitor for bleeding and infection postoperatively
6. Instruct the parents in postoperative home care measures, including preventing infection, pain control, and activity restrictions
7. Provide an opportunity for parental counseling if the parents are concerned about the future fertility of the child

IV. EPISPADIAS AND HYPOSPADIAS (Figure 34-1)

A. Description: Congenital defects involving abnormal placement of the urethral orifice of the penis

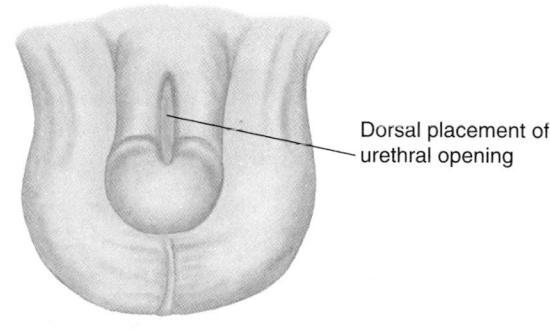

Dorsal placement of urethral opening

Epispadias

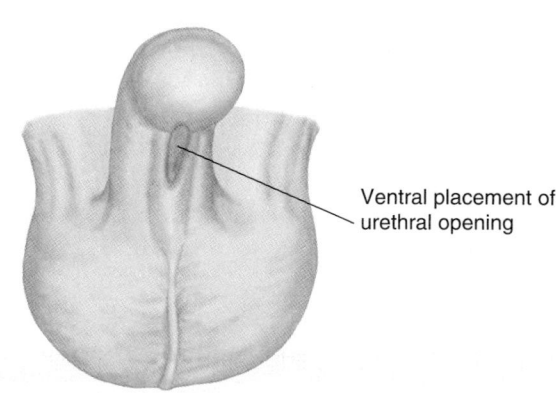

Ventral placement of urethral opening

Hypospadias

FIG. 34-1 Epispadias and hypospadias. (From McKinney, E., James, S., Murray, S., & Ashwill, J. [2005]. *Maternal-child nursing* [2nd ed.]. St. Louis: W.B. Saunders.)

B. Data collection
1. Epispadias: Urethral orifice located on the dorsal surface of the penis; often occurs with exstrophy of the bladder
2. Hypospadias: Urethral orifice located below the glans penis, along the ventral surface

C. Surgical interventions
1. Done before the age of toilet training, preferably between 16 and 18 months of age
2. The child should not be circumcised because the foreskin may be used in surgical reconstruction

D. Postoperative interventions
1. The child will have a pressure dressing and may have some type of urinary diversion or a urinary stent (used to maintain patency of the urethral opening) while healing of the meatus occurs
2. Monitor vital signs
3. Encourage fluid intake to maintain adequate urine output and to maintain patency of the stent
4. Monitor I&O and the urine for cloudiness or a foul odor
5. Notify the registered nurse if there is no urinary drainage for 1 hour, because this may indicate kinks in the system or obstruction by sediment
6. Provide pain medication (acetaminophen [Tylenol]) or medication to relieve bladder spasms (anticholinergic), as prescribed
7. Administer antibiotics, as prescribed
8. Instruct the parents in the care of the urinary diversion or stent if present
9. Instruct the parents to avoid giving the child a tub bath until the stent, if present, is removed
10. Instruct the parents about fluid intake, medication administration, the signs and symptoms of infection, and the need for physician follow-up for dressing removal approximately 4 days after surgery

V. BLADDER EXSTROPHY

A. Description
1. A congenital anomaly characterized by extrusion of the urinary bladder to the outside of the body through a defect in the lower abdominal wall
2. The cause is unknown
3. Treatment requires surgical management and occurs in a series of staged reconstructions
4. Initial surgery for closure of the abdominal defect should occur within the first few days of life
5. The goal of subsequent operations is to reconstruct the bladder and genitalia and enable the child to achieve urinary continence

B. Data collection
1. Exposed bladder mucosa
2. Widened symphysis pubis
3. Defects of the external genitalia

C. Interventions
1. Monitor urinary output
2. Monitor for signs of urinary tract or wound infection
3. Maintain the integrity of the exposed bladder mucosa
4. Prevent the bladder tissue from drying, while allowing the drainage of urine, until surgical closure is performed
   a. The bladder is covered with sterile, nonadherent, clear plastic wrap or a sterile thin film dressing without adhesive
   b. Petroleum jelly is avoided because it tends to dry out, adhere to the bladder mucosa, and damage the delicate tissues when the dressing is removed
5. Monitor laboratory values and urinalysis to assess for renal function
6. Administer antibiotics as prescribed
7. Provide emotional support to the parents, and encourage verbalization of their fears and concerns

VI. ENURESIS

A. Description
1. Refers to a condition in which the child is unable to control bladder function even though the child has reached an age at which control of voiding is expected
2. By age 5, most children are aware of bladder fullness and are able to control voiding

B. Primary nocturnal enuresis
1. Bed-wetting in a child who has never been dry for extended periods
2. Common in children, and most children will eventually outgrow bed-wetting without therapeutic intervention
3. The child is not able to sense a full bladder and does not awaken to void
4. The child may have delayed maturation of the central nervous system (CNS)

C. Secondary or acquired enuresis
1. The onset of wetting after a period of established urinary continence
2. May occur during nighttime sleep (nocturnal), only during the waking hours (diurnal), or during both times of the day
3. The child may complain of dysuria, urgency, or frequency
4. The child should be assessed for urinary tract infections

D. Data collection
1. Normal voiding pattern
2. History of bed-wetting with no extended period of dryness in a child older than age 5 years

E. Interventions
   1. Obtain urinalysis and urine culture as prescribed to rule out infection or existing disorder
   2. Assist the family with identifying a treatment plan that will best fit their needs
   3. Limit fluid intake at night, and encourage the child to void just before going to bed
   4. Involve the child in caring for the wet sheets and changing the bed to assist the child to take ownership of the problem
   5. Provide reward systems as appropriate for the child
   6. Incorporate behavioral conditioning techniques
   7. Encourage follow-up to determine the effectiveness of the treatment

PRACTICE QUESTIONS

1. A nurse is reviewing the health record of a child recently diagnosed with glomerulonephritis. Which finding noted in the child's record is associated with the diagnosis of glomerulonephritis?
   1. Streptococcal throat infection 2 weeks prior to diagnosis
   2. Child fell off a bike onto the handlebars
   3. Nausea and vomiting for the last 24 hours
   4. Urticaria and itching for 1 week prior to diagnosis

2. A nurse is assigned to care for a child suspected of having glomerulonephritis. The nurse reviews the child's record and notes that which finding is associated with the diagnosis of glomerulonephritis?
   1. Low blood urea nitrogen (BUN) level
   2. Hypotension
   3. Low urinary specific gravity
   4. Red-brown urine

3. A nurse is assisting in developing a plan of care for a 7-year-old child diagnosed with acute glomerulonephritis. The nurse includes which intervention in the plan of care?
   1. Encourage limited activity and provide safety measures
   2. Catheterize the child to strictly monitor intake and output
   3. Force intake of oral fluids to prevent hypovolemic shock
   4. Encourage classmates to visit and to keep the child informed of school events

4. A nurse is assisting in performing an admission assessment on a 2-year-old child who has been diagnosed with nephrotic syndrome. The nurse collects data knowing that a common characteristic associated with nephrotic syndrome is:
   1. Generalized edema
   2. Frank, bright red blood in the urine
   3. Increased urinary output
   4. Hypotension

5. A 7-year-old child is seen in the clinic and the primary health care provider documents a diagnosis of primary nocturnal enuresis. The mother asks the nurse about the diagnosis. The nurse bases the response of the fact that primary nocturnal enuresis:
   1. Requires surgical intervention to improve the problem
   2. Is caused by a psychiatric problem
   3. Is common and most children will outgrow bed-wetting without therapeutic intervention
   4. Does not respond to treatment

6. A nurse is caring for an 8-month-old infant. A urinalysis has been ordered and the nurse plans to collect the specimen. The nurse implements which appropriate method to collect the specimen?
   1. Catheterizes the infant, using a No. 5 French Foley
   2. Obtains the specimen from the diaper, using a syringe, after the infant voids
   3. Attaches a urinary collection device to the infant's perineum
   4. Monitors the urinary patterns and prepares to collect the specimen into a cup when the infant voids

7. The child with cryptorchidism is being discharged following orchiopexy, which was performed on an outpatient basis. The nurse informs the parents about which priority care measure?
   1. Administering anticholinergics
   2. Measuring intake and output
   3. Applying cold, wet compresses to the surgical site
   4. Preventing infection at the surgical site

8. A nurse is reinforcing discharge instructions to the mother of a 2-year-old child who has had an orchiopexy to correct cyptorchidism. Which of the following statements, if made by the mother of the child, indicates that further teaching is necessary?
   1. "I'll check his temperature."
   2. "I'll let him decide when to return to his play activities."
   3. "I'll give him medication so he'll be comfortable."
   4. "I'll check his voiding to be sure there are no problems."

9. A nurse collects a urine specimen preoperatively from a child with epispadias who is scheduled for surgical repair. The nurse reviews the child's record for the laboratory results of the urine test and would most likely expect to note which of the following?
   1. Hematuria
   2. Proteinuria
   3. Bacteriuria
   4. Glucosuria

10. A 1-year-old child with hypospadias is scheduled for surgery to correct this condition. A nurse is asked to assist in preparing a plan of care for this child and makes suggestions, knowing that this surgery is taking place at a time when:
    1. Fears of separation and mutilation are great
    2. Sibling rivalry will cause regression to occur
    3. Embarrassment of voiding irregularities is common
    4. Concern over size and function of the penis is present

11. An 18-month-old child is being discharged following surgical repair of hypospadias. Which post-operative nursing care measure should the nurse stress to the parents as they prepare to take this child home?
    1. Encourage toilet training to ensure that flow of urine is normal
    2. Restrict fluid intake to reduce urinary output for the first few days
    3. Avoid tub baths until the stent has been removed
    4. Leave the diapers off to allow the site to heal

12. A nurse is reviewing the treatment plan with the parents of a newborn infant with hypospadias. Which statement by the parents indicates their understanding of the plan?
    1. "Circumcision has been delayed to save tissue for surgical repair."
    2. "Catheterization will be necessary if my infant does not void."
    3. "Caution should be used when straddling my infant on a hip."
    4. "Vital signs should be taken daily to check for bladder infection."

13. The parents of a newborn have been told that their child was born with bladder exstrophy, and the parents ask the nurse about this condition. The nurse bases the response on knowledge that this condition is:
    1. Caused by the use of medications taken by the mother during pregnancy
    2. A hereditary disorder that occurs in every other generation
    3. A condition in which the urinary bladder is abnormally located in the pelvic cavity
    4. An extrusion of the urinary bladder to the outside of the body through a defect in the lower abdominal wall

14. The nurse assists in preparing a plan of care for the infant with bladder exstrophy. The nurse identifies which of the following nursing diagnoses as the priority for the infant?
    1. Alteration in elimination
    2. Impaired tissue integrity
    3. Parental knowledge deficit
    4. Potential for infection

15. A nurse is caring for an infant with a diagnosis of bladder exstrophy. To protect the exposed bladder tissue, the nurse plans to:
    1. Cover the bladder with petroleum jelly gauze
    2. Keep the bladder tissue dry by covering it with dry sterile gauze
    3. Cover the bladder with a nonadhering plastic wrap
    4. Apply sterile distilled water dressings over the bladder mucosa

ALTERNATE FORMAT QUESTION: MULTIPLE RESPONSE

A child is admitted to the hospital with a probable diagnosis of nephrotic syndrome. Select the data collection finding that the nurse would expect to note in the child.

___ Reports of weight loss
___ Edema around the eyes
___ Increased urine output
___ Elevated blood pressure
___ Dark frothy urine

ANSWERS

1. *Answer: 1*
Rationale: Group A beta-hemolytic streptococcal infection is a cause of glomerulonephritis. Often, the child becomes ill with streptococcal infection of the upper respiratory tract and then develops symptoms of acute poststreptococcal glomerulonephritis after an interval of 1 to 2 weeks. The data in options 2, 3, and 4 are unrelated to a diagnosis of glomerulonephritis.
Test-Taking Strategy: Use knowledge regarding the causes of glomerulonephritis and the process of elimination to answer the question. Option 2 relates to a kidney injury. Options 3 and 4 are not related to the diagnosis of glomerulonephritis. Review the causes of glomerulonephritis if you had difficulty with this question.
Level of Cognitive Ability: Comprehension
Client Needs: Physiological Integrity
Integrated Process: Nursing Process/Data Collection
Content Area: Child Health
Reference: Price, D., & Gwin, J. (2005). *Thompson's pediatric nursing* (9th ed.). Philadelphia: W.B. Saunders, p. 245.

2. *Answer:* **4**

Rationale: Gross hematuria resulting in dark, smoky, cola-colored or red-brown urine is a classic symptom of glomerulonephritis. Hypertension is also common. BUN levels may be elevated. A mid to high urinary specific gravity is associated with glomerulonephritis.

Test-Taking Strategy: Use the process of elimination. Eliminate options 2 and 3 first because hypertension and a high specific gravity is most likely to occur in this kidney disorder. Recalling that BUN levels elevate will assist in directing you to option 4 from the remaining options. If you had difficulty with this question, review the clinical manifestations associated with glomerulonephritis.

Level of Cognitive Ability: Comprehension
Client Needs: Physiological Integrity
Integrated Process: Nursing Process/Data Collection
Content Area: Child Health
Reference: Price, D., & Gwin, J. (2005). *Thompson's pediatric nursing* (9th ed.). Philadelphia: W.B. Saunders, p. 245.

3. *Answer:* **1**

Rationale: Activity is limited and most children, because of fatigue, voluntarily restrict their activities during the active phase of the disease. Catheterization may cause a risk of infection. Fluids should not be forced. Visitors should be limited to allow for adequate rest.

Test-Taking Strategy: Use the process of elimination. Eliminate option 4 because rest is the priority over socialization. Eliminate option 2 next. Although monitoring I&O is essential, the risk of infection could occur with catheterization. From the remaining options, eliminate option 3 because of the words "force fluids." Review the appropriate nursing interventions for the child with glomerulonephritis if you had difficulty with this question.

Level of Cognitive Ability: Application
Client Needs: Physiological Integrity
Integrated Process: Nursing Process/Planning
Content Area: Child Health
Reference: Price, D., & Gwin, J. (2005). *Thompson's pediatric nursing* (9th ed.). Philadelphia: W.B. Saunders, p. 246.

4. *Answer:* **1**

Rationale: Nephrotic syndrome is defined as massive proteinuria, hypoalbuminemia, and edema. Urine is dark, foamy, and frothy, but microscopic hematuria may be present; frank bright red blood in the urine does not occur. Urine output is decreased and the blood pressure is normal or slightly decreased.

Test-Taking Strategy: Use the process of elimination. Eliminate option 3 first, because urine output is most likely to be decreased in a renal disorder. From the remaining options, associate edema with nephrotic syndrome because this will be helpful to you if you encounter a similar question. If you had difficulty with this question, review the characteristics of nephrotic syndrome.

Level of Cognitive Ability: Comprehension
Client Needs: Physiological Integrity
Integrated Process: Nursing Process/Data Collection
Content Area: Child Health
Reference: Price, D., & Gwin, J. (2005). *Thompson's pediatric nursing* (9th ed.). Philadelphia: W.B. Saunders, p. 247.

5. *Answer:* **3**

Rationale: Primary nocturnal enuresis occurs in a child that has never been dry at night for extended periods. It is common in children and most children will eventually outgrow bed-wetting without therapeutic intervention. The child is not able to sense a full bladder and does not awaken to void. The child may have delayed maturation of the central nervous system (CNS). It is not caused by a psychiatric problem.

Test-Taking Strategy: Use the process of elimination. Note the relationship between the words "enuresis" in the question and "bed-wetting" in the correct option. If you had difficulty with this question, review the characteristics associated with enuresis.

Level of Cognitive Ability: Application
Client Needs: Physiological Integrity
Integrated Process: Nursing Process/Implementation
Content Area: Child Health
Reference: Leifer, G. (2005). *Maternity nursing* (9th ed.). Philadelphia: W.B. Saunders, p. 431.

6. *Answer:* **3**

Rationale: Although many methods have been used to collect urine from an infant, the most reliable method is the urine collection device. This device is a plastic bag that has an opening lined with adhesive so that it may be attached to the perineum. Urine for certain tests, such as specific gravity, may be obtained from a diaper. Urinary catheterization is not to be done unless specifically prescribed, because of the risk of infection. It is not reasonable to monitor urinary patterns and attempt to collect the specimen in a cup when the infant voids.

Test-Taking Strategy: Use the process of elimination. Eliminate option 4, because this is unrealistic. Eliminate option 1, because catheterization is not prescribed and the risk of infection exists with this procedure. Eliminate option 2 because only certain tests can be done on the urine in a diaper. Review the procedure for collecting urine specimens from an infant if you had difficulty with this question.

Level of Cognitive Ability: Application
Client Needs: Physiological Integrity
Integrated Process: Nursing Process/Implementation
Content Area: Child Health
Reference: Price, D., & Gwin, J. (2005). *Thompson's pediatric nursing* (9th ed.). Philadelphia: W.B. Saunders, pp. 357-358.

7. *Answer:* **4**

Rationale: The most common complications associated with orchiopexy are bleeding and infection. The parents are instructed in postoperative home care measures, including preventing infection, pain control, and activity restrictions. Anticholinergics are prescribed for the relief of bladder spasms and are not necessary following orchiopexy. Measurement of intake and output is not required. Cold wet compresses are not prescribed. Additionally, the moisture from a wet compress presents a potential for infection.

Test-Taking Strategy: Note the key word, *priority*, in the stem of the question. Use Maslow's Hierarchy of Needs theory to answer the question. Of the options presented, the potential for infection is the physiological priority. Review home care

instructions following orchiopexy if you had difficulty with this question.
Level of Cognitive Ability: Application
Client Needs: Health Promotion and Maintenance
Integrated Process: Teaching/Learning
Content Area: Child Health
Reference: Leifer, G. (2005). *Maternity nursing* (9th ed.). Philadelphia: W.B. Saunders, pp. 688, 697.

8. Answer: 2
Rationale: All vigorous activities should be restricted for 2 weeks following surgery to promote healing and prevent injury. This will prevent dislodging of the suture, which is internal. Normally, 2-year-olds will want to be very active; therefore, allowing the child to decide when to return to his play activities may prevent healing and cause injury. The parents should be taught to monitor the temperature, provide analgesics as needed, and monitor the urine output.
Test-Taking Strategy: Note the key words, *further teaching is necessary*. These words indicate a false response question and that you need to select the incorrect client statement. Option 1 is an important action in order to recognize signs of infection. Option 3 is appropriate to keep pain to a minimum. Option 4 monitors voiding pattern, which is also important following this type of surgery. If you had difficulty with this question, review the discharge instructions following surgical correction of cryptorchidism.
Level of Cognitive Ability: Comprehension
Client Needs: Health Promotion and Maintenance
Integrated Process: Teaching/Learning
Content Area: Child Health
Reference: McKinney, E., James, S., Murray, S., & Ashwill, J. (2005). *Maternal-child nursing* (2nd ed.). St. Louis: W.B. Saunders, p. 1171.

9. Answer: 3
Rationale: Epispadias is a congenital defect involving abnormal placement of the urethral orifice of the penis. The urethral opening is located anywhere on the dorsum of the penis. This anatomical characteristic leads to the easy access of bacterial entry into the urine. Options 1, 2, and 4 are not characteristically noted in this condition.
Test-Taking Strategy: Use knowledge regarding the anatomical characteristic of epispadias and the process of elimination to answer the question. Options 1, 2, and 4 do not relate to the potential for infection, which can be present in the condition of epispadias. If you had difficulty with this question, review the diagnostic findings associated with epispadias.
Level of Cognitive Ability: Comprehension
Client Needs: Physiological Integrity
Integrated Process: Nursing Process/Data Collection
Content Area: Child Health
Reference: Wong, D., & Hockenberry, M. (2003). *Nursing care of infants and children* (7th ed.). St. Louis: Mosby, p. 483.

10. Answer: 1
Rationale: At the age of 1 year, a child's fears of separation and mutilation are great, because the child is facing the developmental task of trusting others. As the child gets older,

fears about virility and reproductive ability may surface. The question does not provide enough data to determine that siblings exist. Options 3 and 4 may be issues if the child were older.
Test-Taking Strategy: Focus on the age of the child and use knowledge regarding the stages of growth and development to answer the question. Review the stages of growth and development if you had difficulty with this question.
Level of Cognitive Ability: Application
Client Needs: Health Promotion and Maintenance
Integrated Process: Nursing Process/Planning
Content Area: Child Health
Reference: Leifer, G. (2003). *Introduction to maternity and pediatric nursing* (4th ed.). Philadelphia: W.B. Saunders, pp. 687-688.

11. Answer: 3
Rationale: Following hypospadias repair, the parents are instructed to avoid giving the child a tub bath until the stent has been removed to prevent infection. Diapers are placed on the child to prevent contamination of the surgical site. Fluids should be encouraged to maintain hydration. Toilet training should not be an issue during this stressful period.
Test-Taking Strategy: Use the process of elimination. Option 1 is eliminated first, because toilet training should not be initiated during times of stress, such as following surgery. Option 2 is inappropriate, because fluids should be encouraged rather than restricted. Eliminate option 4, because this action can cause contamination of the surgical site. If you had difficulty with this question, review the postoperative care following surgical repair of hypospadias.
Level of Cognitive Ability: Application
Client Needs: Health Promotion and Maintenance
Integrated Process: Teaching/Learning
Content Area: Child Health
References: Price, D., & Gwin, J. (2005). *Thompson's pediatric nursing* (9th ed.). Philadelphia: W.B. Saunders, p. 161.
Wong, D., & Hockenberry, M. (2003). *Nursing care of infants and children* (7th ed.). St. Louis: Mosby, p. 482.

12. Answer: 1
Rationale: Hypospadias is a congenital defect involving abnormal placement of the urethral orifice of the penis. In hypospadias, the urethral orifice is located below the glans penis along the ventral surface. The infant should not be circumcised because the dorsal foreskin tissue will be used for surgical repair of the hypospadias. Options 2, 3, and 4 are unrelated to this disorder.
Test-Taking Strategy: Use the process of elimination. Note the key words, *indicates their understanding*. Recalling that hypospadias is a congenital defect involving abnormal placement of the urethral orifice of the penis will direct you to option 1. Review the treatment plan related to the repair of the hypospadias if you had difficulty with this question.
Level of Cognitive Ability: Comprehension
Client Needs: Health Promotion and Maintenance
Integrated Process: Nursing Process/Evaluation
Content Area: Child Health
Reference: Price, D., & Gwin, J. (2005). *Thompson's pediatric nursing* (9th ed.). Philadelphia: W.B. Saunders, p. 161.

13. *Answer:* **4**

Rationale: Bladder exstrophy is a congenital anomaly characterized by the extrusion of the urinary bladder to the outside of the body through a defect in the lower abdominal wall. The cause in not known, and there is a higher incidence males. Options 1, 2, and 3 are not characteristics of this disorder.

Test Taking Strategy: Use the process of elimination. If you are unfamiliar with this condition, note the relationship of *ex*-strophy in the name of the disorder to the word *ex*-trusion in the correct option. This should remind you that this condition is located external to the body. If you had difficulty with this question, review the characteristics of bladder exstrophy.

Level of Cognitive Ability: Comprehension
Client Needs: Physiological Integrity
Integrated Process: Nursing Process/Implementation
Content Area: Child Health
Reference: Wong, D., & Hockenberry, M. (2003). *Nursing care of infants and children* (7th ed.). St. Louis: Mosby, p. 483.

14. *Answer:* **2**

Rationale: In bladder exstrophy, the bladder is exposed and external to the body. The highest priority is impaired tissue integrity related to the exposed bladder mucosa. Although the infant needs to be monitored for elimination patterns and kidney function, this is not the priority concern for this condition. Parental knowledge deficit related to the diagnosis and treatment of the condition will need to be addressed, but again is not the priority. Although infection related to the anatomically located defect is an appropriate nursing diagnosis, it is a potential problem and not an actual one.

Test-Taking Strategy: Use the process of elimination. Eliminate option 4 first because this addresses a potential problem rather than an actual one. Eliminate option 3 next because physiological needs take precedence over psychosocial needs. From the remaining options, knowledge that the bladder mucosa is exposed in this condition should direct you to the correct option. Review this disorder if you had difficulty with this question.

Level of Cognitive Ability: Analysis
Client Needs: Physiological Integrity
Integrated Process: Nursing Process/Planning
Content Area: Child Health
Reference: Wong, D., & Hockenberry, M. (2003). *Nursing care of infants and children* (7th ed.). St. Louis: Mosby, p. 483.

15. *Answer:* **3**

Rationale: In this disorder, care must be taken to protect the exposed bladder tissue from drying while allowing the drainage of urine. This is best accomplished by covering the bladder with a nonadhering plastic wrap. The use of petroleum jelly gauze should be avoided because this type of dressing can dry out, adhere to the mucosa, and damage the delicate tissue when removed. Dry sterile dressings and dressings soaked in solutions (that can dry out) also damage the mucosa when removed.

Test-Taking Strategy: Use the process of elimination. Also, note the key word, *nonadherent*, in the correct option. If you had difficulty with this question, review care of the infant with bladder exstrophy.

Level of Cognitive Ability: Application
Client Needs: Physiological Integrity
Integrated Process: Nursing Process/Planning
Content Area: Child Health
Reference: Wong, D., & Hockenberry, M. (2003). *Nursing care of infants and children* (7th ed.). St. Louis: Mosby, p. 484.

ALTERNATE FORMAT QUESTION: MULTIPLE RESPONSE

Answers:

Edema around the eyes
Dark frothy urine

Rationale: Nephrotic syndrome is a kidney disorder characterized by massive proteinuria, hypoalbuminemia, and edema. The urine output is decreased, and the urine is dark and frothy in appearance. The child gains weight and periorbital edema, facial edema, and edema in the legs, ankles, labia or scrotum occur. The blood pressure is normal or slightly decreased.

Test-Taking Strategy: Focus on the diagnosis of the child and think about the definition of nephrotic syndrome. Remember that this disorder is characterized by massive proteinuria, hypoalbuminemia, and edema. Review the clinical manifestations associated with nephrotic syndrome if you had difficulty with this question.

Level of Cognitive Ability: Comprehension
Client Needs: Physiological Integrity
Integrated Process: Nursing Process/Data Collection
Content Area: Child Health
Reference: Price, D., & Gwin, J. (2005). *Thompson's pediatric nursing* (9th ed.). Philadelphia: W.B. Saunders, p. 247.

REFERENCES

Leifer, G. (2005). *Maternity nursing* (9th ed.). Philadelphia: W.B. Saunders.

McKinney, E., James, S., Murray, S., & Ashwill, J. (2005). *Maternal-child nursing* (2nd ed.). St. Louis: W.B. Saunders.

Price, D., & Gwin, J. (2005). *Thompson's pediatric nursing* (9th ed.). Philadelphia: W.B. Saunders.

Wong, D., & Hockenberry, M. (2003). *Nursing care of infants and children* (7th ed.). St. Louis: Mosby.

Integumentary Disorders

I. ECZEMA (ATOPIC DERMATITIS)

A. Description
1. A superficial inflammatory process involving primarily the epidermis
2. The major goals of management are to relieve pruritus, hydrate the skin, reduce inflammation, and prevent or control secondary infections

B. Forms of eczema (Box 35-1)

C. Data collection
1. Redness
2. Itching
3. Minute papules and vesicles
4. Weeping, oozing, and crusting of lesions

D. Interventions
1. Avoid exposure to skin irritants such as soaps, detergents, fabric softeners, diaper wipes, and powder
2. Improve skin hydration
3. Apply cool, wet compresses to soothe the skin
4. Administer antihistamines and topical corticosteroids as prescribed; corticosteroids are applied in a thin layer and are rubbed into the area thoroughly
5. Prevent or minimize scratching; keep the nails short and clean, and place gloves or cotton socks over the hands
6. Eliminate conditions that increase itching, such as heat, woolen clothes or blankets, rough fabrics, or furry stuffed animals
7. Instruct the parents to wash clothing in a mild detergent and rinse thoroughly; putting the clothes through a second complete wash cycle without detergent will minimize the amount of residue remaining on the fabric
8. Instruct the parents in the measures to prevent skin infections
9. Instruct the parents to monitor the lesions for signs of infection (honey-colored crusts with surrounding erythema)

BOX 35-1

Forms of Eczema

INFANTILE
Usually begins at 2 to 6 months of age and generally undergoes spontaneous remission by 3 years of age

CHILDHOOD
May follow the infantile form and occurs at 2 to 3 years of age

PREADOLESCENT AND ADOLESCENT
Begins at about 12 years of age and may continue into the early adult years, or indefinitely

---

II. IMPETIGO

A. Description
1. A highly contagious, bacterial infection of the skin caused by beta-hemolytic streptococci, *Staphylococcus aureus*, or both
2. The most common sites of infection are the face, around the mouth, the hands, the neck, and the extremities
3. The lesions begin as a vesicle or pustule that is surrounded by edema and redness, usually at a site that has been injured; this progresses to an exudative and crusting stage
4. After the crusting of the lesions, the initially serous vesicular fluid becomes cloudy, and the vesicle ruptures, leaving a honey-colored crust covering an ulcerated base

B. Data collection
1. Lesions
2. Pruritus

3. Burning
4. Secondary lymph node involvement
C. Interventions
   1. Contact isolation; use standard precautions and implement agency-specific isolation procedures for the hospitalized child
   2. Allow lesions to dry by air exposure
   3. Assist the child with daily bathing with antibacterial soap, such as pHisoHex, as prescribed
   4. Apply warm compresses to lesions 2 or 3 times per day, as prescribed, to remove crusts and to allow for healing
   5. Apply and instruct the parents in the use of antibiotic ointments; the infection is communicable for 48 hours after antibiotic ointment treatment is begun
   6. Administer oral antibiotics, which may be prescribed if there is no response to topical antibiotic treatment
   7. Apply and instruct the parents in the use of emollients, as prescribed, to prevent skin cracking
   8. Instruct the parents in the methods to prevent the spread of the infection, especially careful hand washing
   9. Inform the parents that the child needs to use separate towels, linens, and dishes
   10. Inform the parents that all linens and clothing should be washed separately with detergent in hot water

III. PEDICULOSIS CAPITIS (LICE)
A. Description
   1. An infestation of the hair and scalp with lice
   2. The most common sites of involvement are the occipital area, behind the ears at the nape of the neck, and occasionally the eyebrows and eyelashes
   3. The female louse lays her eggs (nits) on the hair shaft, close to the scalp; the incubation period is 8 to 10 days
   4. Head lice live and reproduce only on humans and are transmitted by direct and indirect contact, such as sharing of brushes, hats, towels, and bedding
   5. All contacts of the infested child should be examined
B. Data collection (Box 35-2)
C. Interventions
   1. Use of a pediculicide shampoo; the hair is towel-dried, the nits are removed with a fine-toothed comb, and the treatment is repeated in 7 days
   2. Use of permethrin (Nix) rinse
      a. Apply to washed and towel-dried hair, leave in place for 10 minutes, and then rinse
      b. After rinsing, towel-dry the hair and remove the nits with a fine-toothed comb

---

BOX 35-2

Data Collection Findings: Pediculosis Capitis

Intense pruritus is present.
Adult lice are difficult to see and appear as small gray specks; they may crawl very fast.
Nits are visible and firmly attached to the hair shaft near the scalp; they appear as tiny silver or gray specks resembling dandruff.

---

      c. The hair should not be shampooed for 24 hours following treatment
   3. Instruct the parents in the use of shampoo and rinse, as prescribed
   4. Instruct the parents that bedding and clothing used by the child should be changed daily, laundered in hot water with detergent, and dried in a hot dryer for 20 minutes
   5. Instruct the parents that nonessential bedding and clothing can be stored in a tightly sealed bag for 10 to 14 days and then washed
   6. Instruct the parents to seal toys that cannot be washed or dry cleaned in a plastic bag for 2 weeks
   7. Instruct the parents that hairbrushes or combs should be discarded or soaked in hot water (54.4° C [130° F]) for 15 minutes
   8. Instruct the parents that furniture and carpets need to be vacuumed frequently
   9. Teach the child not to share clothing, headwear, or brushes and combs

IV. SCABIES
A. Description (see Chapter 40 for additional information related to scabies)
   1. A parasitic skin disorder caused by an infestation of *Sarcoptes scabiei* (itch mite)
   2. Is endemic among schoolchildren and institutionalized populations as a result of close personal contact
   3. Incubation period
      a. Female mite burrows into epidermis, lays eggs, and dies in the burrow after 4 to 5 weeks
      b. The eggs hatch in 3 to 5 days, and larvae migrate to the skin to mature and complete their life cycle
   4. Infectious period: During the course of the infestation
   5. Transmission: By close personal contact with infected person
B. Data collection (Box 35-3)
C. Interventions
   1. Topical application of a scabicide such as lindane cream (Kwell, Scabene), crotamiton (Eurax), or permethrin 5% (Elimite)
   2. Lindane cream (Kwell, Scabene) should not be used in children younger than age 2 because of the risk of neurotoxicity and seizures

Data Collection Findings: Scabies

Intense pruritus, especially at night
Burrows (fine, grayish-red lines that may be difficult to see) on the skin

3. Instruct the parents in the application of the scabicide
   a. Application should be preceded by a warm soap-and-water bath
   b. Skin must be cool and dry before the application of the lotion
   c. Lotion is left in place for 8 to 14 hours before it is washed off
4. When permethrin 5% (Elimite) is used, the cream is thoroughly and gently massaged into all skin surfaces (not just the areas that have the rash) from the head to the soles of the feet; care should be taken to avoid contact with the eyes
5. Household members and contacts of the infected child need to be treated at the same time
6. Instruct the parents about the importance of frequent hand washing
7. Instruct the parents that all clothing, bedding, and pillowcases used by the child need to be changed daily, washed in hot water with detergent, dried in a hot dryer, and ironed before reuse
8. Instruct the parents that nonwashable toys and other items should be sealed in plastic bags for 4 days

V. TINEA (RINGWORM)

A. Description
   1. Known as tinea capitis (scalp), tinea corporis (body), tinea pedis (feet)
   2. A fungal infection spread by direct contact
B. Data collection
   1. Papules and dry scales
   2. Itching
C. Interventions
   1. Provide meticulous skin care
   2. Apply antifungal ointments as prescribed
   3. Administer oral antifungal medications as prescribed

VI. THE BURNED CHILD

A. Pediatric differences (see Chapter 40 for additional information related to burns)
   1. Very young children who have been severely burned have a higher mortality rate than older children and adults with comparable burns

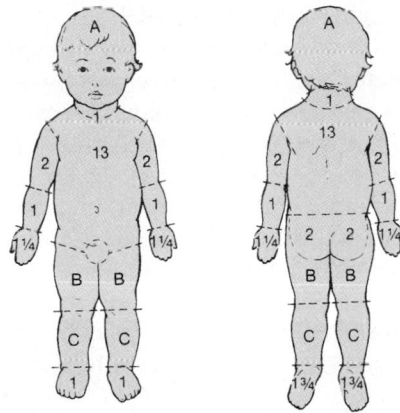

RELATIVE PERCENTAGES OF AREAS AFFECTED BY GROWTH

AREA	BIRTH	AGE 1 YR	AGE 5 YR
A = ½ of head	9½	8½	6½
B = ½ of one thigh	2¾	3¼	4
C = ½ of one leg	2½	2½	2¾

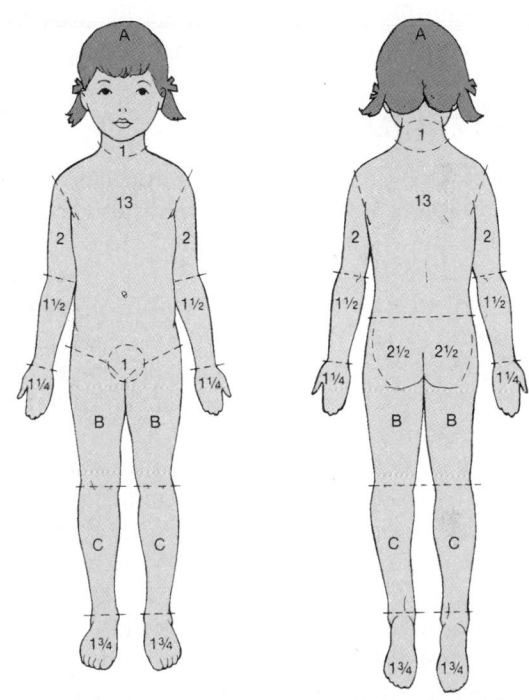

RELATIVE PERCENTAGES OF AREAS AFFECTED BY GROWTH

AREA	AGE 10 YR	AGE 15 YR	ADULT
A = ½ of head	5½	4½	3½
B = ½ of one thigh	4½	4½	4¾
C = ½ of one leg	3	3¼	3½

FIG. 35-1 Estimation of burn distribution in children. (From Wong, D., & Hockenberry, M. [2003]. *Nursing care of infants and children* [7th ed.]. St. Louis: Mosby.)

2. Lower burn temperatures and shorter exposure to heat can cause a more severe burn in a child than in an adult because a child's skin is thinner
3. Severely burned children are at increased risk for fluid and heat loss, dehydration, and metabolic acidosis than an adult

4. The higher proportion of body fluid to mass in children increases the risk of cardiovascular problems
5. Burns involving more than 10% of total body surface area (TBSA) require some form of fluid resuscitation
6. Infants and children are at increased risk for protein and calorie deficiency because they have smaller muscle mass and less body fat than adults
7. Scarring is more severe in a child
8. An immature immune system presents an increased risk of infection for infants and young children
9. A delay in **growth** may occur following a burn

B. Extent of burn injury
1. The rule of nines, used for an adult with a burn injury, gives an inaccurate estimate because of the differences in body proportion between children and adults
2. A modified rule of nines may be used for the pediatric population (Figure 35-1)

PRACTICE QUESTIONS

1. Corticream is prescribed by the physician for a child with atopic dermatitis (eczema) and the nurse instructs the mother how to apply the cream. The nurse tells the mother to:
   1. Avoid cleansing the area before applying the cream
   2. Apply the cream over the entire body
   3. Apply a thin layer of cream and rub into the area thoroughly
   4. Apply a thick layer of cream in affected areas only

2. A nurse assists in providing an instructional session to parents regarding impetigo. Which statement by a parent indicates a need for further instruction?
   1. "It is most common in humid weather."
   2. "It begins in an area of broken skin, such as an insect bite."
   3. "It is extremely contagious."
   4. "Lesions are most often located on the arms and chest."

3. A nurse provides instructions to the mother of a child with impetigo regarding the application of antibiotic ointment and the mother asks the nurse when the child can return to school. The nurse tells the mother that the child can return to school:
   1. Twenty-four hours after using antibiotic ointment
   2. Forty-eight hours after using antibiotic ointment
   3. One week after using antibiotic ointment
   4. Ten days after using antibiotic ointment

4. A nurse provides instructions regarding the use of permethrin 1% (Nix) to the parents of a child diagnosed with pediculosis (head lice). Which statement by a parent indicates a need for further instruction?

   1. "The medication can be obtained over the counter in a local pharmacy."
   2. "The medication is applied to the hair after shampooing and left on for 24 hours."
   3. "The medication is applied to the hair after shampooing, left on for 10 minutes, and then rinsed out."
   4. "The hair should not be shampooed for 24 hours following treatment."

5. A nurse prepares a list of home care instructions for the parents of schoolchildren diagnosed with pediculosis (head lice). Which of the following is included in the list?
   1. Use antilice sprays on all bedding and furniture
   2. Take all bedding and linens to the cleaners to be dry cleaned
   3. Boil combs and brushes in hot water for 2 hours
   4. Vacuum floors, play areas, and furniture to remove any hairs that might carry live nits

6. A mother of a 3-year-old child tells the nurse that the child has been continuously scratching the skin and has developed a rash. The nurse inspects the child and suspects the presence of scabies if which of the following is observed?
   1. Clusters of fluid-filled vesicles
   2. Fine grayish-red lines
   3. Purple-colored lesions
   4. Thick, honey-colored crusts

7. Permethrin 5% (Elimite) is prescribed for a 4-year-old child with a diagnosis of scabies. The nurse instructs the mother regarding the use of this treatment and tells the mother to:
   1. Apply the lotion in the hair and on the face and entire body
   2. Apply the lotion and leave it on for 4 hours
   3. Apply the lotion to cool dry skin at least $1/2$ hour after bathing
   4. The child should wear no clothing while the lotion is in place

8. A 2-year-old child is admitted to the burn unit with partial- and full-thickness burns over 35% of the body. The nurse assisting in caring for the child plans care, understanding that the priority nursing intervention is:
   1. Sedating the child with morphine sulfate
   2. Restricting intravenous (IV) fluids
   3. Inserting a nasogastric tube
   4. Inserting a Foley catheter

9. Griseofulvin (Fulvicin, Grisactin) is prescribed for a child with tinea capitis and the nurse provides instructions to the mother regarding administration of the medication. Which statement by the mother indicates a need for further instructions?
   1. "I need to administer the medication 2 hours before meals."
   2. "I need to shake the oral suspension before preparing the dose."

3. "I need to continue the therapy as long as it is prescribed."
4. "I need to keep my child out of the sun."

10. A nurse is providing home care instructions to an adolescent who has been diagnosed with tinea pedis. Which statement by the adolescent indicates a need for further instruction?
    1. "I need to dry my feet carefully, especially between the toes."
    2. "I need to wear clean socks."
    3. "I need to wear shoes that are well ventilated."
    4. "I should wear plastic shoes as much as possible."

ALTERNATE FORMAT QUESTION: FILL IN THE BLANK

An 8-year-old child has sustained a burn injury to the posterior thorax and both buttocks. According to the modified rule of nines for the pediatric population, what percent of the child's body was burned? (Refer to the chart in Figure 35-1 for assistance in answering the question)

Answer: _____

ANSWERS

1. *Answer: 3*
Rationale: Corticream is a topical corticosteroid. It should be applied sparingly and rubbed into the area thoroughly. The affected area should be cleansed gently before application. It should not be applied over extensive areas. Systemic absorption is more likely to occur with extensive application.
Test-Taking Strategy: Use the process of elimination. Eliminate options 1 because it does not make sense to avoid cleansing an affected area. Eliminate option 2 because cream should be applied only to the area that is affected. Eliminate option 4 because of the words "thick" and "only." Review the procedure for application of this cream if you had difficulty with this question.
Level of Cognitive Ability: Application
Client Needs: Health Promotion and Maintenance
Integrated Process: Teaching/Learning
Content Area: Child Health
Reference: Skidmore-Roth, L. (2005). *Mosby's drug guide for nurses* (6th ed.). St. Louis: Mosby, p. 999.

2. *Answer: 4*
Rationale: Impetigo is most common during hot, humid summer months. It begins in an area of broken skin, such as an insect bite. It may be caused by *Staphylococcus aureus*, group A beta-hemolytic streptococci, or a combination of these bacteria. It is extremely contagious. Lesions are usually located around the mouth and nose, but may be present on the extremities.
Test-Taking Strategy: Use the process of elimination and note the key words, *indicates a need for further instruction*. These words indicate a false response question and that you need to select the incorrect client statement. Recalling that the lesions are most commonly located around the mouth and nose will direct you to option 4. Review this disorder if you had difficulty with this question.
Level of Cognitive Ability: Comprehension
Client Needs: Health Promotion and Maintenance
Integrated Process: Teaching/Learning
Content Area: Child Health
Reference: Price, D., & Gwin, J. (2005). *Thompson's pediatric nursing* (9th ed.). Philadelphia: W.B. Saunders, p. 133.

3. *Answer: 2*
Rationale: The child should not attend school for 24 to 48 hours after the initiation of systemic antibiotics or 48 hours after using antibiotic ointment. The school should be notified of the diagnosis. Therefore, options 1, 3, and 4 are incorrect.
Test-Taking Strategy: Use knowledge related to the administration of antibiotics to answer the question. Eliminate options 3 and 4 first because the time frames are closely related and rather lengthy. Note the key word, *ointment*, in the question; this should assist in directing you to option 2. Review the treatment measures for impetigo if you had difficulty with this question.
Level of Cognitive Ability: Application
Client Needs: Safe, Effective Care Environment
Integrated Process: Nursing Process/Implementation
Content Area: Child Health
Reference: McKinney, E., James, S., Murray, S., & Ashwill, J. (2005). *Maternal-child nursing* (2nd ed.). St. Louis: Elsevier, p. 366.

4. *Answer: 2*
Rationale: Permethrin 1% is an over-the-counter antilice product that kills both lice and eggs with one application and has residual activity for 10 days. It is applied to the hair after shampooing and left for 10 minutes before rinsing out. The hair should not be shampooed for 24 hours after the treatment.
Test-Taking Strategy: Use the process of elimination and note the key words, *need for further instruction*. These words indicate a false response question and that you need to select the incorrect client statement. Recalling the treatment for the use of this medication will direct you to option 2. Review this treatment if you had difficulty with this question.
Level of Cognitive Ability: Comprehension
Client Needs: Safe, Effective Care Environment
Integrated Process: Teaching/Learning
Content Area: Child Health
Reference: Leifer, G. (2003). *Introduction to maternity and pediatric nursing* (4th ed.). Philadelphia: W.B. Saunders, p. 712.

5. *Answer: 4*
Rationale: Antilice sprays are unnecessary. Additionally, they should never be used on a child. Bedding and linens

should be washed with hot water and dried on a hot setting. Items that cannot be washed should be dry cleaned or sealed in plastic bags in a warm place for 3 weeks. Combs and brushes should be boiled or soaked in antilice shampoo or hot water for 15 minutes. Thorough home cleaning is necessary to remove any remaining lice or nits.
Test-Taking Strategy: Use the process of elimination. Eliminate option 1, knowing that antilice sprays should not be used. Knowing that bedding and linens can be washed will eliminate option 2. The time for boiling in option 3 is rather lengthy; therefore, eliminate this option. Review home care instructions regarding pediculosis if you had difficulty with this question.
Level of Cognitive Ability: Application
Client Needs: Safe, Effective Care Environment
Integrated Process: Nursing Process/Implementation
Content Area: Child Health
Reference: Price, D., & Gwin, J. (2005). *Thompson's pediatric nursing* (9th ed.). Philadelphia: W.B. Saunders, p. 279.

6. **Answer: 2**
Rationale: Scabies appears as burrows or fine, grayish, lines. They may be difficult to see if they are obscured by excoriation and inflammation. Clusters of fluid-filled vesicles are seen in herpesvirus. Thick, honey-colored crusts are characteristic of impetigo. Purple-colored lesions may be indicative of various disorders, including systemic conditions.
Test-Taking Strategy: Use the process of elimination. Recalling that scabies infestation produces burrows will assist in directing you to option 2. Review the characteristics of scabies if you had difficulty with this question.
Level of Cognitive Ability: Comprehension
Client Needs: Physiological Integrity
Integrated Process: Nursing Process/Data Collection
Content Area: Child Health
References: Leifer, G. (2003). *Introduction to maternity and pediatric nursing* (4th ed.). Philadelphia: W.B. Saunders, p. 713.
Wong, D., & Hockenberry, M. (2003). *Nursing care of infants and children* (7th ed.). St. Louis: Mosby, p. 760.

7. **Answer: 3**
Rationale: Permethrin is applied from the neck downward, making sure that the soles of the feet, behind the ears, and under the toenails and fingernails are covered. The lotion should be kept on for 8 to 14 hours, and then the child should be given a bath. The lotion should not be applied for at least 30 minutes after bathing and should be applied only to cool, dry skin. The child should be clothed during treatment.
Test-Taking Strategy: Use the process of elimination. Reading options 1 and 4 carefully will assist in eliminating these options. From the remaining options, recalling the treatment time for this medication will assist in directing you to option 3. Review this treatment if you had difficulty with this question.
Level of Cognitive Ability: Application
Client Needs: Health Promotion and Maintenance
Integrated Process: Teaching/Learning
Content Area: Child Health

Reference: Wong, D., & Hockenberry, M. (2003). *Nursing care of infants and children* (7th ed.). St. Louis: Mosby, p. 161.

8. **Answer: 4**
Rationale: A Foley catheter is inserted into the child's bladder so that urine output can be accurately measured on an hourly basis. Although pain medication may be required, the child should not be sedated. IV fluids are not restricted and are administered at a rate sufficient to maintain adequate tissue perfusion. A nasogastric tube may or may not be required but would not be the priority intervention.
Test-Taking Strategy: Use the process of elimination and note the key word, *priority*. Option 1 can be eliminated first, because the child should not be sedated. Eliminate option 2 next, knowing that fluid resuscitation is an important component of therapy to prevent burn shock. From the remaining options, recalling that urine output reflects adequate tissue perfusion will direct you to option 4. Review the treatment of burns if you had difficulty with this question.
Level of Cognitive Ability: Application
Client Needs: Physiological Integrity
Integrated Process: Nursing Process/Planning
Content Area: Child Health
Reference: Price, D., & Gwin, J. (2005). *Thompson's pediatric nursing* (9th ed.). Philadelphia: W.B. Saunders, p. 228.

9. **Answer: 1**
Rationale: Griseofulvin is given with or after meals to avoid gastrointestinal (GI) irritation and increase absorption. Oral suspensions should be shaken well. Parents are instructed to continue therapy as prescribed and not to miss a dose. Exposure to the sun is avoided during treatment.
Test-Taking Strategy: Use the process of elimination and note the key words, *need for further instructions*. These words indicate a false response question and that you need to select the incorrect client statement. Recalling that this medication causes GI irritation will direct you to option 1. Review this medication if you had difficulty with this question.
Level of Cognitive Ability: Analysis
Client Needs: Health Promotion and Maintenance
Integrated Process: Teaching/Learning
Content Area: Child Health
References: Skidmore-Roth, L. (2005). *Mosby's drug guide for nurses* (6th ed.). St. Louis: Mosby, p. 936.
Wong, D., & Hockenberry, M. (2003). *Nursing care of infants and children* (7th ed.). St. Louis: Mosby, p. 760.

10. **Answer: 4**
Rationale: Plastic shoes retain heat and should be avoided because this condition is aggravated by heat and moisture. Options 1, 2, and 3 are appropriate measures to treat this condition.
Test-Taking Strategy: Use the process of elimination. Note the key words, *need for further instruction*. These words indicate a false response question and that you need to select the incorrect client statement. Recalling that heat and moisture aggravate the condition will direct you to option 4. Review the measures to treat tinea pedis if you had difficulty with this question.
Level of Cognitive Ability: Comprehension

Client Needs: Health Promotion and Maintenance
Integrated Process: Teaching/Learning
Content Area: Child Health
Reference: Leifer, G. (2003). *Introduction to maternity and pediatric nursing* (4th ed.). Philadelphia: W.B. Saunders, p. 711.

ALTERNATE FORMAT QUESTION: FILL IN THE BLANK

Answer: 18
Rationale: A modified rule of nines is used for the pediatric population. For an older child, the posterior thorax equals 13% and each buttock equals 2.5% (both buttocks equal 5%). Therefore the total extent of the burn injury equals 18%.

Test-Taking Strategy: Focus on the age of the child and use the chart to assist in answering this question. Review the procedures for estimating the distribution of burns in children if you had difficulty with this question.
Level of Cognitive Ability: Analysis
Client Needs: Physiological Integrity
Integrated Process: Nursing Process/Data Collection
Content Area: Child Health
Reference: Wong, D., & Hockenberry, M. (2003). *Nursing care of infants and children* (7th ed.). St. Louis: Mosby, p. 1228.

REFERENCES

Leifer, G. (2003). *Introduction to maternity and pediatric nursing* (4th ed.). Philadelphia: W.B. Saunders.

McKinney, E., James, S., Murray, S., & Ashwill, J. (2005). *Maternal-child nursing* (2nd ed.). St. Louis: W.B. Saunders.

Price, D., & Gwin, J. (2005). *Thompson's pediatric nursing* (9th ed.). Philadelphia: W.B. Saunders.

Skidmore-Roth, L. (2005). *Mosby's drug guide for nurses* (6th ed.). St. Louis: Mosby.

Wong, D., & Hockenberry, M. (2003). *Nursing care of infants and children* (7th ed.). St. Louis: Mosby.

Musculoskeletal Disorders

I. DYSPLASIA OF THE HIP

A. Description
1. A condition in which the head of the femur is improperly seated in the acetabulum, or hip socket, of the pelvis
2. Can range from very mild to severely dislocated
3. Can be congenital or develop after birth

B. Data collection (Figure 36-1)
1. Neonates: Laxity of the ligaments around the hip, which allows the femoral head to be displaced from the acetabulum on manipulation
2. Infants beyond the newborn period
   a. Asymmetry of the gluteal and thigh skinfolds when the child is placed prone and the legs are extended against the examining table
   b. Limited range of motion (ROM) in the affected hip
   c. Asymmetrical abduction of the affected hip when the child is placed supine with the knees and hips flexed
   d. Apparent short femur on the affected side
3. Positive Barlow or Ortolani maneuver
4. The walking child: minimal to pronounced variations in gait with lurching toward the affected side; positive Trendelenburg sign

C. Interventions
1. In the neonatal period, splinting of the hips with Pavlik harness to maintain flexion and abduction and external rotation (Figure 36-2)
2. Following the neonatal period, traction and/or surgery to release muscles and tendons

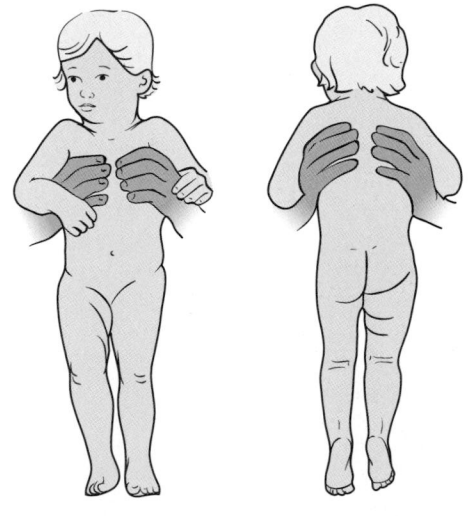 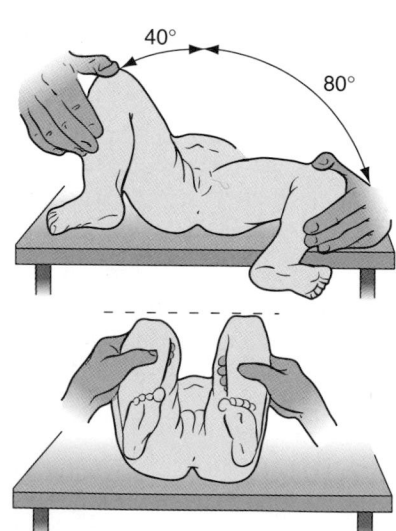

FIG. 36-1 Dysplasia of the hip. (From Price, D., & Gwin, J. [2005]. *Thompson's pediatric nursing* [9th ed.]. Philadelphia: W.B. Saunders.)

3. Following surgery, positioning and immobilization in a spica cast until healing is achieved; then an abduction splint is used
4. Operative reduction may be required in the older child
5. Instruct parents regarding proper care of a Pavlik harness or spica cast

II. CONGENITAL CLUBFOOT (Figure 36-3)

A. Description
   1. A congenital malformation of the lower extremities
   2. The defect may be unilateral or bilateral
   3. Defects are rigid and cannot be manipulated into a neutral position
   4. Long-term interval follow-up is required until the child reaches skeletal maturity
B. Data collection: The foot is plantar flexed with an inverted heel and adducted forefoot
C. Interventions
   1. Treatment begins as soon after birth as possible
   2. Serial manipulation and casting are performed weekly, and if correction is not achieved in 3 to 6 months, surgery is indicated
   3. Monitor for pain
   4. Monitor neurovascular status of the toes
   5. Instruct parents in cast care and the signs of neurovascular impairment that require physician notification

III. SCOLIOSIS

A. Description
   1. A lateral curvature of the spine

2. Surgical and nonsurgical interventions are employed, and the type of treatment depends on the degree of curvature, the age of the child, and the amount of **growth** that is anticipated
3. Long-term monitoring is essential to detect any progression of the curve
B. Data collection
   1. Visible curve fails to straighten when the child bends forward and hangs arms down toward feet
   2. Hips, ribs, and shoulders are asymmetrical
   3. Apparent leg length discrepancy
C. Interventions
   1. Monitor progression of the curvature
   2. Prepare the child and parents for the use of a brace if prescribed
   3. Prepare the child and parents for surgery (spinal fusion; placement of internal instrumentation rods) if prescribed
D. Braces
   1. Usually worn from 16 to 23 hours a day
   2. Inspect the skin for signs of redness or breakdown
   3. Keep the skin clean and dry, avoiding lotions and powders
   4. Advise the child to wear soft, nonirritating clothing under the brace
   5. Instruct in prescribed exercises
   6. Encourage verbalization about body image
E. Postoperative interventions (spinal fusion)
   1. Maintain proper alignment; avoid twisting movements
   2. Logroll the child when turning to maintain alignment
   3. Monitor extremities for neurovascular status
   4. Encourage coughing and deep breathing and use of incentive spirometry

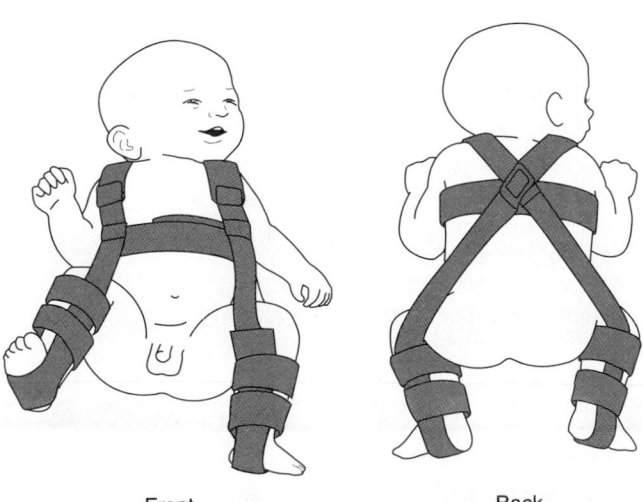

Front   Back

FIG. 36-2 Child in Pavlik harness. (From Wong, D., & Hockenberry, M. [2003]. *Nursing care of infants and children* [7th ed.]. St. Louis: Mosby.)

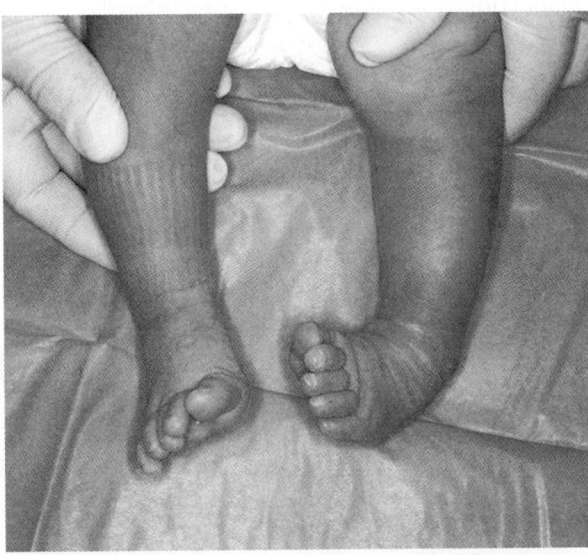

FIG. 36-3 Clubfoot. (From Leifer, G. [2003]. *Introduction to maternity and pediatric nursing* [4th ed.]. Philadelphia: W.B. Saunders.)

5. Monitor pain level and administer prescribed analgesics
6. Monitor for incontinence
7. Monitor for superior mesenteric artery syndrome disorder, caused by mechanical changes in the position of the child's abdominal contents during surgery, and the physician is notified if it occurs; symptoms include emesis and abdominal distention similar to that which occurs with intestinal obstruction or paralytic ileus
8. Instruct in activity restrictions
9. Instruct the child to roll from a side-lying position to a sitting position, and assist with ambulation
10. Prepare the child for the use of a molded plastic jacket to provide external stability of the spine when resuming activities

IV. JUVENILE RHEUMATOID ARTHRITIS (JRA)

A. Description
1. An inflammatory disease affecting the joints; occurs most often in girls
2. The cause is unknown
3. Iridocyclitis (inflammation of the iris and ciliary body) can occur
4. Treatment of JRA is supportive and directed toward preserving joint function, controlling inflammation, minimizing deformity, and reducing the impact that the disease may have on the development of the child
5. Therapy includes medications, physical and occupational therapies, and child and family education
6. Surgical intervention may be implemented when the child has problems with joint contractures and unequal **growth** of extremities

B. Data collection (Box 36-1)

C. Interventions
1. Facilitate social and emotional development
2. Instruct the parents and child in the administration of medications (Box 36-2)
3. Instruct the parent regarding the signs of aspirin toxicity; aspirin is stopped if signs of toxicity occur, and the physician is notified

4. Assist the child with ROM exercises and instruct in prescribed exercises
5. Encourage normal performance of activities of daily living (ADLs)
6. Instruct the parents and child in the use of hot or cold packs, splinting, and positioning the affected joint in a neutral position during painful episodes
7. Encourage and support prescribed physical and occupational therapy
8. Instruct in the importance of preventive eye care and reporting visual disturbances
9. Assess the child's perception regarding the chronic illness

V. FRACTURES

A. Description
1. A break in the continuity of the bone as a result of trauma, twisting, or bone decalcification
2. Fractures in children usually result from increased mobility and inadequate or immature motor and cognitive skills
3. Fractures in children may result from trauma or bone diseases
4. Fractures in infancy are generally rare and warrant further investigation to rule out the possibility of child abuse

B. Data collection
1. Pain or tenderness over the involved area
2. Loss of function
3. Obvious deformity
4. Crepitation
5. Ecchymosis
6. Edema
7. Muscle spasm

C. Initial care of a fracture (Box 36-3)

BOX 36-1

Data Collection Findings: Juvenile Rheumatoid Arthritis

Stiffness, swelling, and limited motion in the affected joints
Affected joints are warm to touch
Morning stiffness present on arising in the morning and after inactivity
Affected joints may be painful and tender

BOX 36-2

Medications Used in Juvenile Rheumatoid Arthritis

Acetylsalicylic acid (aspirin, ASA)
Nonsteroidal anti-inflammatory drugs (NSAIDs)
Slower acting antirheumatic drugs (SAARDs)
Cytotoxic medications
Corticosteroids
Immunological modulators

BOX 36-3

Initial Care of a Fracture

Assess the extent of injury and immobilize the affected extremity.
If a compound fracture exists, splint the extremity and cover the wound with a sterile dressing.

D. Interventions
  1. Reduction
     a. Restoring the bone to proper alignment
     b. Closed reduction: Accomplished by manual alignment of the fragments, followed by immobilization
     c. Open reduction: Requires the surgical insertion of internal fixation devices, such as rods, wires, or pins, that help maintain alignment while healing occurs
  2. Retention: The application of traction or a cast to maintain alignment until healing occurs
E. Traction
  1. Russell skin traction
     a. Used to stabilize a fractured femur before surgery
     b. Similar to Buck's traction but provides a double pull with the use of a knee sling
     c. Traction pulls at the knee and the foot
  2. Balanced suspension
     a. Used with skin or skeletal traction
     b. Used to approximate fractures of the femur, tibia, or fibula
     c. Produced by a counterforce other than the child
     d. Types include Thomas ring splint with Pearson attachment, Steinmann pin, Kirschner wires
     e. Protect the skin from breakdown
     f. Provide pin care if pins are used with the skeletal traction
  3. 90-degree–90-degree traction
     a. The lower leg is supported by a boot cast or a calf sling
     b. A skeletal Steinmann pin or Kirschner wire is placed in the distal fragment of the femur, resulting in a 90-degree angle at both the hip and the knee
  4. Interventions
     a. Maintain correct amount of weight as ordered
     b. Ensure that weights hang freely
     c. Check ropes for fraying, and be sure that they are placed appropriately on the pulleys
     d. Monitor neurovascular status of involved extremity
     e. Monitor for signs and symptoms of immobilization: Constipation, skin breakdown, disuse syndrome of unaffected extremities
     f. Provide therapeutic and diversional play
F. Casts
  1. Description
     a. Made of plaster or fiberglass to provide immobilization of bone(s) and joints after a fracture or injury
     b. Fractures of the hip or the knee may require a spica cast
  2. Interventions
     a. Examine the cast for pressure areas
     b. Monitor the extremity for circulatory impairment, such as pain, swelling, discoloration, tingling, numbness, coolness, or diminished pulse
     c. Notify the physician if circulatory impairment occurs
     d. Prepare for bivalving or cutting the cast if circulatory impairment occurs
     e. Instruct the child not to stick objects down the cast
     f. Teach the child to keep the cast clean and dry
     g. Instruct the child in isometric exercises to prevent muscle atrophy

PRACTICE QUESTIONS

1. A nurse is assisting a physician during the examination of an infant with hip dysplasia and the physician performs the Ortolani maneuver. The nurse understands that this maneuver is performed to:
   1. Push the unstable femoral head out of the acetabulum
   2. Reduce the dislocated femoral head back into the acetabulum
   3. Determine the extent of range of motion
   4. Check for asymmetry on the affected side

2. A 6-month-old infant is seen in the clinic and is diagnosed with unilateral hip dysplasia. The nurse reviews the health care record and understands that which of the following findings is not associated with this condition?
   1. An apparent short femur on the affected side
   2. Limited range of motion in the affected hip
   3. Adduction of the affected hip when placed supine with the knees and hips flexed
   4. Asymmetry of the gluteal skin folds when the infant is placed prone and the legs are extended against the examining table

3. A nurse reinforces instructions to the parents of an infant with hip dysplasia regarding care of the Pavlik harness. The nurse tells the parents that the:
   1. Harness must be worn 12 hours a day
   2. Harness must be removed for diaper changes and for feeding
   3. Harness is removed to check the skin and for bathing
   4. Infant should never be moved when out of the harness

4. A nurse provides information to the mother of a 2-week-old infant diagnosed with clubfoot at the time of birth. Which statement by the mother indicates a need for further instruction regarding this disorder?
   1. "I need to bring my child back to the clinic in 1 month for a new cast."
   2. "Treatment needs to be started as soon as possible."
   3. "I need to come to the clinic every week with my child for the casting."

4. "I realize my child will require follow-up care until full grown."

5. A nurse is assigned to care for a child following spinal fusion for the treatment of scoliosis. The child complains of abdominal discomfort and begins to have episodes of vomiting. On further data collection, the nurse notes abdominal distention. The nurse takes which action?
   1. Administers an antiemetic
   2. Places the child in a side-lying Sims' position
   3. Notifies the registered nurse (RN)
   4. Increases the IV fluids

6. A nurse is providing instructions to the parents of a child with scoliosis regarding the use of a brace. Which statement by a parent indicates a need for further instruction?
   1. "I will apply lotion under the brace to prevent skin breakdown."
   2. "I need to avoid applying powder under the brace because it will cake."
   3. "I need to have my child wear a soft fabric under the brace."
   4. "I need to encourage my child to perform prescribed exercises."

7. The mother of a child with juvenile rheumatoid arthritis (JRA) calls the nurse because the child is experiencing a painful exacerbation of the disease. The mother asks the nurse if the child should perform range-of-motion (ROM) exercises at this time. The nurse makes which response to the mother?
   1. "The ROM exercises must be performed every day."
   2. "Avoid all exercise during painful periods."
   3. "Administer additional pain medication before performing ROM exercises."
   4. "Have the child perform simple isometric exercises during this time."

8. A 4-year-old child sustains a fall at home and is brought to the emergency room by the mother. Following x-ray, it has been determined that the child has a fractured arm and a plaster cast is applied. The nurse provides instructions to the mother regarding cast care for the child. Which statement by the mother indicates a need for further instructions?
   1. "The cast may feel warm as the cast dries."
   2. "If the cast becomes wet, a blow drier set on the cool setting may be used to dry the cast."
   3. "A small amount of white shoe polish can touch up a soiled white cast."
   4. "I can use lotion or powder around the cast edges to relieve itching."

9. A nurse is assigned to care for a child with a spica cast. The nurse avoids which of the following when caring for the child?
   1. Checking neurovascular status of the extremities

2. Observing for nonverbal signs of pain
3. Placing the child on a stretcher and bringing the child to the playroom
4. Using pillows to elevate the head and shoulders

10. A child with a fractured femur is placed in Buck's skin traction. The nurse plans care knowing that this type of traction:
    1. Requires frequent pin care
    2. Places the child at risk for infection
    3. Is a type of skin traction that pulls the hip and leg into extension
    4. Uses skeletal traction and weights to provide a counterforce

11. A nurse is preparing to perform a neurovascular check for tissue perfusion in the child with an arm cast. Which of the following is the priority in performing this procedure?
    1. Taking the blood pressure
    2. Taking the temperature
    3. Checking the apical heart rate
    4. Checking the peripheral pulse in the affected arm

12. A nurse is checking the capillary refill in a child with a cast applied to the left arm. The nurse compresses the nail bed of a finger and it returns to its original color in 2 seconds. Based on this finding, the nurse would:
    1. Notify the registered nurse (RN)
    2. Document the findings
    3. Prepare the child for bivalving the cast
    4. Elevate the extremity and recheck the capillary refill immediately

13. A nurse is performing a neurovascular check on a child with a cast applied to the lower leg. The child complains of tingling in the toes distal to the fracture site. The nurse would:
    1. Ambulate the child with crutches
    2. Elevate the extremity
    3. Document the findings
    4. Notify the registered nurse (RN)

14. A nurse is assigned to care for a child in skeletal traction. The nurse avoids which of the following when caring for the child?
    1. Keeping the weights hanging freely
    2. Placing the bed linen on the traction ropes
    3. Ensuring that the ropes are in the pulleys
    4. Ensuring that the weights are out of the child's reach

15. The nurse is reinforcing information to the mother of a child about a synthetic cast that has been applied to the child for the treatment of a clubfoot. Which of the following information will the nurse provide to the mother?
    1. The cast takes 24 hours to dry
    2. The cast is heavier than a plaster cast
    3. The cast is stronger than a plaster cast
    4. The cast allows for greater mobility than a plaster cast

ALTERNATE FORMAT QUESTION: MULTIPLE RESPONSE

A nurse prepares a list of home care instructions for the parents of a child who has a plaster cast applied to the left forearm. Select all instructions that would be included on the list.

___ Keep small toys and sharp objects away from the cast

___ Use fingertips to lift the cast while it is drying

___ Use a padded ruler or another padded object to scratch the skin under the cast if it itches

___ Contact the physician if the child complains of numbness or tingling in the extremity

___ Elevate the extremity on pillows for the first 24 to 48 hours after casting to prevent swelling

ANSWERS

1. *Answer:* 2

Rationale: In the Barlow maneuver, the examiner pushes the unstable femoral head out of the acetabulum. In the Ortolani maneuver, the examiner reduces the dislocated femoral head back into the acetabulum. A positive effect of the Ortolani maneuver is a palpable clink on entry or exit of the femoral head over the acetabular ring. Options 3 and 4 are data collection techniques for identification of the clinical manifestations of hip dysplasia but do not describe the Ortolani maneuver.

Test-Taking Strategy: Use the process of elimination. Eliminate options 3 and 4 first because they are data collection techniques. From the remaining options, it is necessary to know the purpose of the Ortolani maneuver. Review the purpose of these maneuvers if you had difficulty with this question.

Level of Cognitive Ability: Comprehension

Client Needs: Physiological Integrity

Integrated Process: Nursing Process/Implementation

Content Area: Child Health

References: Leifer, G. (2003). *Introduction to maternity and pediatric nursing* (4th ed.). Philadelphia: W.B. Saunders, p. 33. Price, D., & Gwin, J. (2005). *Thompson's pediatric nursing* (9th ed.). Philadelphia: W.B. Saunders, p. 101.

2. *Answer:* 3

Rationale: Asymmetrical abduction of the affected hip, when placed supine with the knees and hips flexed, would be a finding in hip dysplasia in infants beyond the newborn period. Options 1, 2, and 4 are accurate assessment findings in this disorder.

Test-Taking Strategy: Use the process of elimination and note the key words, *not associated*. This indicates a false response question and that you need to select the incorrect finding. Visualize each of the findings described in the options to assist in directing you to option 3. Review the findings in hip dysplasia if you had difficulty with this question.

Level of Cognitive Ability: Comprehension

Client Needs: Physiological Integrity

Integrated Process: Nursing Process/Data collection

Content Area: Child Health

Reference: Price, D., & Gwin, J. (2005). *Thompson's pediatric nursing* (9th ed.). Philadelphia: W.B. Saunders, p. 101.

3. *Answer:* 3

Rationale: The harness should be worn 23 hours a day and should be removed only to check the skin and for bathing. The hips and buttocks should be supported carefully when the infant is out of the harness. The harness does not need to be removed for diaper changes or feedings.

Test-Taking Strategy: Visualize this harness. This will assist in eliminating options 2 and 4. Select option 3 over option 1, because the time frame in option 1 is rather short. Also, note the absolute word "must" in options 1 and 2 and "never" in option 4. Review home care instruction regarding this harness if you had difficulty with this question.

Level of Cognitive Ability: Application

Client Needs: Health Promotion and Maintenance

Integrated Process: Teaching/Learning

Content Area: Child Health

Reference: Leifer, G. (2003). *Introduction to maternity and pediatric nursing* (4th ed.). Philadelphia: W.B. Saunders, p. 332.

4. *Answer:* 1

Rationale: Treatment for clubfoot is started as soon as possible after birth. Serial manipulation and casting are performed at least weekly. If sufficient correction is not achieved in 3 to 6 months, surgery is usually indicated. Because clubfoot can recur, all children with clubfoot require long-term interval follow-up until they reach skeletal maturity to ensure an optimal outcome.

Test-Taking Strategy: Use the process of elimination and focus on the issue, the treatment plan for clubfoot. Note the key words, *indicates a need for further instruction*, to assist in eliminating options 2 and 4. Recalling that serial manipulations and casting are required weekly will assist in directing you to option 1 from the remaining options. Review these treatment procedures if you had difficulty with this question.

Level of Cognitive Ability: Comprehension

Client Needs: Physiological Integrity

Integrated Process: Teaching/Learning

Content Area: Child Health

Reference: Price, D., & Gwin, J. (2005). *Thompson's pediatric nursing* (9th ed.). Philadelphia: W.B. Saunders, p. 320.

5. *Answer:* 3

Rationale: A complication following surgical treatment of scoliosis is superior mesenteric artery syndrome. This disorder is caused by mechanical changes in the position of the child's abdominal contents, resulting from lengthening of the child's body. It results in a syndrome of emesis and abdominal distention similar to that which occurs with intestinal obstruction or paralytic ileus. Postoperative vomiting in children with body casts or those who have undergone spinal fusion warrants attention because of the possibility of superior mesenteric artery syndrome.

Test-Taking Strategy: Use the process of elimination. Eliminate option 4 first, because it should not be implemented without a prescribed order. Eliminate option 2 next, because this child requires logrolling and the Sims' position may cause injury following surgery. From the remaining options, note the signs and symptoms in the question. These should alert you that the RN needs to be notified. Review superior mesenteric artery syndrome if you had difficulty with this question.
Level of Cognitive Ability: Application
Client Needs: Physiological Integrity
Integrated Process: Nursing Process/Implementation
Content Area: Child Health
References: McKinney, E., James, S., Murray, S., & Ashwill, J. (2005). *Maternal-child nursing* (2nd ed.). St. Louis: W.B. Saunders, p. 1402.
Price, D., & Gwin, J. (2005). *Thompson's pediatric nursing* (9th ed.). Philadelphia: W.B. Saunders, p. 333.

6. *Answer:* **1**
Rationale: Both the use of lotions or powders should be avoided because they can become sticky or cake under the brace, causing irritation. Options 2, 3, and 4 are appropriate statements regarding care of a child with a brace.
Test-Taking Strategy: Use the process of elimination and note the key words, *need for further instructions.* These words indicate a false response question and that you need to select the incorrect client statement. Recalling that lotions and powders need to be avoided will assist in directing you to option 1. Review home care instructions regarding the care of a child in a brace if you had difficulty with this question.
Level of Cognitive Ability: Comprehension
Client Needs: Health Promotion and Maintenance
Integrated Process: Teaching/Learning
Content Area: Child Health
Reference: Price, D., & Gwin, J. (2005). *Thompson's pediatric nursing* (9th ed.). Philadelphia: W.B. Saunders, pp. 331-332.

7. *Answer:* **4**
Rationale: During painful episodes, hot or cold packs, splinting, and positioning the affected joint in a neutral position help reduce the pain. Although resting the extremity is appropriate, it is important to begin simple isometric or tensing exercises as soon as the child is able. These exercises do not involve joint movement.
Test-Taking Strategy: Use the process of elimination. Eliminate options 1, 2, and 3 because of the words "must," "all," and "additional" in each of these options. Review pain management and care during exacerbations if you had difficulty with this question.
Level of Cognitive Ability: Application
Client Needs: Physiological Integrity
Integrated Process: Nursing Process/Implementation
Content Area: Child Health
Reference: Leifer, G. (2003). *Introduction to maternity and pediatric nursing* (4th ed.). Philadelphia: W.B. Saunders, p. 581.

8. *Answer:* **4**
Rationale: The mother needs to be instructed not to use lotion or powders on the skin around the cast edges or inside the cast. Lotions or powders can become sticky or caked

and cause skin irritation. Options 1, 2, and 3 are appropriate instructions.
Test-Taking Strategy: Use the process of elimination and note the key words, *indicates a need for further instructions.* These words indicate a false response question and that you need to select the incorrect client statement. Recalling the principles related to routine cast care should direct you to option 4. Review home care instructions regarding cast care if you had difficulty with this question.
Level of Cognitive Ability: Comprehension
Client Needs: Health Promotion and Maintenance
Integrated Process: Teaching/Learning
Content Area: Child Health
Reference: Wong, D., & Hockenberry, M. (2003). *Nursing care of infants and children* (7th ed.). St. Louis: Mosby, p. 1786.

9. *Answer:* **4**
Rationale: Pillows should not be used to elevate the head or shoulders of a child in a body cast because the pillows will thrust the child's chest against the cast and cause discomfort and respiratory difficulty. Neurovascular checks are a critical component of care to ensure that the cast is not causing circulatory compromise. The nurse should observe for nonverbal signs of pain and should ask the older child if pain is experienced. A ride on a stretcher to the playroom or around the hospital provides changes of position and scenery.
Test-Taking Strategy: Use the process of elimination and note the key word, *avoids.* This word indicates a false response question and that you need to select the incorrect intervention. Visualize this type of cast to direct you to option 4. Review care of the child with a spica cast if you had difficulty with this question.
Level of Cognitive Ability: Application
Client Needs: Physiological Integrity
Integrated Process: Nursing Process/Implementation
Content Area: Child Health
Reference: Leifer, G. (2003). *Introduction to maternity and pediatric nursing* (4th ed.). Philadelphia: W.B. Saunders, p. 332.

10. *Answer:* **3**
Rationale: Buck's skin traction is a type of skin traction used in fractures of the femur and in hip and knee contractures. It pulls the hip and leg into extension. Countertraction is applied by the child's body. Options 1, 2, and 4 describe skeletal traction.
Test-Taking Strategy: Use the process of elimination. Noting the key word, *skin,* in the question will assist in directing you to option 3. Review the purpose of Buck's traction if you had difficulty with this question.
Level of Cognitive Ability: Comprehension
Client Needs: Physiological Integrity
Integrated Process: Nursing Process/Planning
Content Area: Child Health
Reference: Leifer, G. (2003). *Introduction to maternity and pediatric nursing* (4th ed.). Philadelphia: W.B. Saunders, p. 570.

11. *Answer:* **4**
Rationale: The neurovascular check for tissue perfusion is performed on the toes or fingers distal to an injury or cast and includes peripheral pulse, color, capillary refill time,

warmth, motion, and sensation. Options 1, 2, and 3 may be components of care but are not the priority in this situation.
Test-Taking Strategy: Use the process of elimination and note the key word, *priority*. Option 4 is the only option that addresses a neurovascular check. Review the components of a neurovascular check if you had difficulty with this question.
Level of Cognitive Ability: Application
Client Needs: Physiological Integrity
Integrated Process: Nursing Process/Data Collection
Content Area: Delegating/Prioritizing
Reference: Leifer, G. (2003). *Introduction to maternity and pediatric nursing* (4th ed.). Philadelphia: W.B. Saunders, p. 573.

12. *Answer:* **2**
Rationale: When checking capillary refill, the nurse would expect to note that a compressed nail bed will return to its original color in less than 3 seconds. Options 1, 3, and 4 are unnecessary actions.
Test-Taking Strategy: Focus on the data in the question. Recalling the normal finding when checking the capillary refill will direct you to option 2. Review this data collection technique if you had difficulty with this question.
Level of Cognitive Ability: Application
Client Needs: Physiological Integrity
Integrated Process: Nursing Process/Implementation
Content Area: Child Health
Reference: Leifer, G. (2003). *Introduction to maternity and pediatric nursing* (4th ed.). Philadelphia: W.B. Saunders, p. 574.

13. *Answer:* **4**
Rationale: Reduced sensation to touch or complaints of numbness or tingling at a site distal to a fracture may indicate poor tissue perfusion. This finding should be reported to the RN. Options 1, 2, and 3 are inappropriate and would delay the required and immediate interventions.
Test-Taking Strategy: Use the process of elimination and recall the signs of circulatory compromise. Noting the child's complaint will assist in directing you to option 4. Review the complications associated with a cast if you had difficulty with this question.
Level of Cognitive Ability: Application
Client Needs: Physiological Integrity
Integrated Process: Nursing Process/Implementation
Content Area: Child Health
Reference: deWit, S. (2005). *Fundamental concepts and skills for nursing.* Philadelphia: W.B. Saunders, p. 798.

14. *Answer:* **2**
Rationale: Bed linens should not be placed on the traction ropes because of the risk of disrupting the traction apparatus. Options 1, 3, and 4 are appropriate measures when caring for a child in skeletal traction.
Test-Taking Strategy: Note the key word, *avoids*. This word indicates a false response question and that you need to select the incorrect intervention. Use the process of elimination and knowledge regarding the care to the child in traction

to assist in directing you to option 2. Review these nursing measures if you had difficulty with this question.
Level of Cognitive Ability: Application
Client Needs: Physiological Integrity
Integrated Process: Nursing Process/Implementation
Content Area: Child Health
Reference: Leifer, G. (2003). *Introduction to maternity and pediatric nursing* (4th ed.). Philadelphia: W.B. Saunders, p. 570.

15. *Answer:* **4**
Rationale: Synthetic casts dry quickly (in less than 30 minutes) and are lighter than plaster casts. Synthetic casts allow for greater mobility than a plaster cast. However, synthetic casts are not as strong as plaster casts and are more expensive.
Test-Taking Strategy: Use the process of elimination and note the key word, *synthetic*. Recalling the differences between a plaster and a synthetic cast will assist in directing you to option 4. Review these differences if you had difficulty with this question.
Level of Cognitive Ability: Application
Client Needs: Health Promotion and Maintenance
Integrated Process: Nursing Process/Implementation
Content Area: Child Health
Reference: Leifer, G. (2003). *Introduction to maternity and pediatric nursing* (4th ed.). Philadelphia: W.B. Saunders, pp. 329-330.

ALTERNATE FORMAT QUESTION: MULTIPLE RESPONSE

Answers:
Keep small toys and sharp objects away from the cast
Contact the physician if the child complains of numbness or tingling in the extremity
Elevate the extremity on pillows for the first 24 to 48 hours after casting to prevent swelling
Rationale: While the cast is drying, the palms of the hands are used to lift the cast. If the fingertips are used, indentations in the cast could occur and cause pressure on the underlying skin. Small toys and sharp objects are kept away from the cast and no objects (including padded objects) are placed inside the cast because of the risk of altered skin integrity. The extremity is elevated to prevent swelling, and the physician is notified immediately if any signs of neurovascular impairment develop.
Test-Taking Strategy: Use of the ABCs—airway, breathing, and circulation—and recalling the general principles related to care of a child with a cast will assist in answering the question. Review these general principles if you had difficulty with this question.
Level of Cognitive Ability: Application
Client Needs: Health Promotion and Maintenance
Integrated Process: Teaching/Learning
Content Area: Child Health
References: deWit, S. (2005). *Fundamental concepts and skills for nursing.* Philadelphia: W.B. Saunders, p. 798.
Leifer, G. (2003). *Introduction to maternity and pediatric nursing* (4th ed.). Philadelphia: W.B. Saunders, p. 574.

REFERENCES

deWit, S. (2005). *Fundamental concepts and skills for nursing.* Philadelphia: W.B. Saunders.

Leifer, G. (2003). *Introduction to maternity and pediatric nursing* (4th ed.). Philadelphia: W.B. Saunders.

McKinney, E., James, S., Murray, S., & Ashwill, J. (2005). *Maternal-child nursing* (2nd ed.). St. Louis: W.B. Saunders.

Price, D., & Gwin, J. (2005). *Thompson's pediatric nursing* (9th ed.). Philadelphia: W.B. Saunders.

Wong, D., & Hockenberry, M. (2003). *Nursing care of infants and children* (7th ed.). St. Louis: Mosby.

Hematological and Oncological Disorders

I. SICKLE CELL DISEASE (SCD)

A. Description

1. A group of diseases collectively termed *hemoglobinopathies*, in which hemoglobin (hemoglobin A [HgbA]) is partly or completely replaced by abnormal sickle hemoglobin (HgbS)

2. Caused by the inheritance of a gene for a structurally abnormal portion of the hemoglobin (Hgb) chain

3. HgbS is sensitive to changes in the oxygen content of the red blood cell (RBC)

4. Insufficient oxygen causes the cells to assume a sickle shape, and the cells become rigid and clumped together, obstructing capillary blood flow

5. Situations that precipitate sickling include fever and emotional or physical stress; any condition that increases the body's need for oxygen or alters the transport of oxygen can result in sickle cell crisis

6. Risk factors include having parents heterozygous for HgbS or being African American

7. The sickling response is reversible under conditions of adequate oxygenation and hydration; after repeated sickling, the cell becomes permanently sickled

8. The clinical manifestations are primarily the result of obstruction caused by sickled RBCs and increased RBC destruction

9. Sickle cell crises are acute exacerbations of the disease, which vary markedly in severity and frequency; these include vaso-occlusive crisis, splenic sequestration, and aplastic crisis

10. Care focuses on the prevention (preventing exposure to infection and maintaining normal hydration) and treatment (oxygen, hydration, pain management, and bed rest) of the crisis

B. Sickle cell crisis: Data collection (Box 37-1)

C. Interventions

1. Maintain adequate hydration and blood flow with intravenous (IV) normal saline as prescribed and with oral fluids

2. Administer oxygen as prescribed to increase tissue perfusion; blood transfusions may also be prescribed

3. Administer analgesics as prescribed (around the clock); administration of meperidine (Demerol) is avoided because of the risk of normeperidine-induced seizures

4. Assist the child to assume a comfortable position so that the child keeps the extremities extended to promote venous return; elevate the head of the bed no more than 30 degrees, avoid putting strain on painful joints, and do not raise the knee gatch of the bed

---

BOX 37-1

Sickle Cell Crisis

VASO-OCCLUSIVE CRISIS
Most common type of crisis
Caused by stasis of blood with clumping of the cells in the microcirculation, ischemia, and infarction
Signs include fever, pain, and tissue engorgement

SPLENIC SEQUESTRATION
Life-threatening crisis caused by the pooling of blood in the spleen
Signs include profound anemia, hypovolemia, and shock

APLASTIC CRISIS
Caused by the diminished production and increased destruction of red blood cells (RBCs) triggered by viral infection or the depletion of folic acid
Signs include profound anemia and pallor

5. Encourage consumption of a high-calorie, high-protein diet with folic acid supplementation
6. Administer antibiotics as prescribed to prevent infection
7. Monitor for signs of increasing anemia and shock (mental status changes, pallor, vital sign changes)
8. Instruct the child and parents about the early signs and symptoms of crisis and the measures to prevent crisis
9. Inform the parents about the **hereditary** aspects of the disorder

II. IRON DEFICIENCY ANEMIA

A. Description
1. Iron stores are depleted, resulting in a decreased supply of iron for the manufacture of hemoglobin in RBCs
2. Commonly results from blood loss, increased metabolic demands, syndromes of gastrointestinal (GI) malabsorption, and dietary inadequacy

B. Data collection
1. Pallor
2. Weakness and fatigue
3. Irritability

C. Interventions
1. Increase the oral intake of iron
2. Instruct the child and parents in food choices that are high in iron (Box 37-2)
3. Administer iron supplements as prescribed
4. Teach how to administer the iron supplements
   a. Give between meals for maximum absorption
   b. Give with a multivitamin or fruit juice because vitamin C increases absorption
   c. Do not give with milk or antacids because these decrease absorption
5. Teach the child and parents that liquid iron preparation stains the teeth and should be taken through a straw
6. Instruct the child and parents about the side effects of iron supplements (black stools, constipation, and foul aftertaste)

III. APLASTIC ANEMIA

A. Description
1. A deficiency of circulating erythrocytes resulting from the arrested development of RBCs within the bone marrow
2. There are several possible causes, including chronic exposure to myelotoxic agents, viruses, infection, autoimmune disorders, and allergic states
3. The definitive diagnosis is determined by bone marrow aspiration (demonstrates conversion of red bone marrow to fatty red bone marrow)
4. Therapeutic management focuses on restoring function to the bone marrow and involves immunosuppressive therapy and bone marrow transplantation (treatment of choice if a suitable donor exists)

B. Data collection
1. Pancytopenia (a deficiency of erythrocytes, leukocytes, and thrombocytes)
2. Petechiae, purpura, bleeding, pallor, weakness, tachycardia, and fatigue

C. Interventions
1. Prepare the child for bone marrow transplantation, if planned
2. Immunosuppressive medications: Antilymphocyte globulin (ALG) or antithymocyte globulin (ATG) may be prescribed to suppress the autoimmune response
3. Colony-stimulating factors may be prescribed to enhance bone marrow production
4. Corticosteroids and cyclosporine (Sandimmune) may be prescribed
5. Blood transfusions may be prescribed
6. Advise the parents to obtain a Medic-Alert bracelet for the child

IV. HEMOPHILIA

A. Description (Box 37-3)
1. An X-linked recessive trait
2. Males inherit hemophilia from their mothers, and females inherit the carrier status from their fathers
3. Some females who are carriers have an increased tendency to bleed and, although it is rare, females can have hemophilia if their fathers

---

BOX 37-2

Iron-Rich Foods

Breads and cereals
Egg yolks
Dark green leafy vegetables
Kidney beans
Liver
Meats
Raisins

BOX 37-3

Hemophilia

HEMOPHILIA A (CLASSIC HEMOPHILIA)
Results from a deficiency of factor VIII

HEMOPHILIA B (CHRISTMAS DISEASE)
Results from a deficiency of factor IX

have the disorder and their mothers are carriers of the genetic disorder

4. The primary treatment is replacement of the missing clotting factor; products used are factor VIII concentrate and desmopressin (DDAVP; 1-desamino-8-D-arginine vasopressin)

B. Data collection
1. Abnormal bleeding in response to trauma or surgery
2. Joint bleeding causing pain, tenderness, swelling, and limited range of motion
3. Tendency to bruise easily
4. Prolonged partial thromboplastin time (PTT)
5. Bleeding time, prothrombin time (PT), and platelet count are normal

C. Interventions
1. Monitor for bleeding and maintain bleeding precautions
2. Factor VIII concentrate or desmopressin (DDAVP) may be prescribed
3. Monitor for joint pain; immobilize the affected extremity if joint pain occurs
4. Monitor neurological status (child is at risk for intracranial hemorrhage)
5. Monitor urine for hematuria
6. Control bleeding by immobilization, elevation, and the application of ice; in addition, apply pressure (15 minutes) for superficial bleeding
7. Instruct the child and parents about the signs of internal bleeding
8. Instruct the parents in how to control the bleeding
9. Instruct the parents regarding activities for the child, emphasizing the avoidance of contact sports
10. Instruct the child to wear protective devices such as helmets, knee, and elbow pads when participating in sports such as bicycling and skating
11. Instruct the parents to obtain a Medic-Alert bracelet for the child

V. β-THALASSEMIA MAJOR

A. Description
1. An autosomal recessive disorder
2. Also called Cooley's anemia; includes a group of disorders characterized by the reduced production of a globin chain in the synthesis of hemoglobin
3. The incidence is highest in individuals of Mediterranean descent
4. Treatment is supportive; goal of therapy is to maintain normal hemoglobin levels by the administration of blood transfusions
5. Bone marrow transplantation may be offered as an alternative therapy
6. A splenectomy may be performed in a child with severe splenomegaly who demonstrate increased transfusion requirements (assists in relieving abdominal pressure and may increase the life span of supplemental red blood cells)

B. Data collection
1. Frontal bossing
2. Maxillary prominence
3. Wide-set eyes with a flattened nose
4. Greenish-yellow skin tone
5. Hepatosplenomegaly
6. Severe anemia
7. Microcytic, hypochromic RBCs

C. Interventions
1. Blood transfusions may be prescribed
2. Monitor for iron overload and administer chelation therapy with deferoxamine (Desferal), as prescribed, to treat iron overload and to prevent organ damage from the elevated levels of iron caused by the multiple transfusion therapy
3. If the child has had a splenectomy, instruct the parents to report any signs of infection because of the risk of sepsis
4. Provide genetic counseling

VI. LEUKEMIA (Table 37-1)

A. Description
1. Malignant exacerbation in the number of leukocytes, usually at an immature stage, in the bone marrow
2. Affects the bone marrow, causing anemia from decreased erythrocytes, infection from neutropenia, and bleeding from decreased platelet production
3. The cause is unknown and appears to involve gene damage of cells, leading to the transformation of cells from a normal state to a malignant state
4. Risk factors include genetic, viral, immunological, and environmental factors and exposure to radiation, chemicals, and medications
5. Acute lymphocytic leukemia (ALL) is the most frequent type of cancer in children; peak onset is age 2 to 6 years
6. More common in boys than girls after 1 year of age
7. Treatment involves the use of chemotherapeutic agents with or without cranial radiation

TABLE 37-1

Classification of Leukemia

Acute Lymphocytic Leukemia (ALL)	Acute Myelogenous Leukemia (AML)
Mostly lymphoblasts present in bone marrow	Mostly myeloblasts present in bone marrow
Age of onset is younger than 15 years	Age of onset is between 15 and 39 years

8. The phases of treatment include the following: induction, which achieves a complete remission or disappearance of leukemic cells; intensification or consolidation therapy, which further decreases the tumor burden; central nervous system prophylactic therapy, which prevents leukemic cells from invading the central nervous system; and maintenance, which serves to maintain the remission phase

9. Bone marrow transplantation (BMT) may also be performed to treat some children with leukemia

B. Data collection

1. Infiltration of the bone marrow causes fever, pallor, fatigue, anorexia, hemorrhage (usually petechiae), and bone and joint pain; pathological fractures can occur as a result of bone marrow invasion with leukemic cells

2. Signs of infection as a result of neutropenia

3. Hepatosplenomegaly, lymphadenopathy

4. Normal, elevated, or low white blood cell (WBC) count

5. Decreased hemoglobin and hematocrit levels

6. Decreased platelet count

7. Positive bone marrow biopsy identifying leukemic blast (immature) phase cells

8. Signs of increased intracranial pressure, such as severe headache, vomiting, papilledema, irritability, lethargy, and eventually coma, as a result of central nervous system involvement

9. Signs of cranial nerve (cranial nerve VII, or the facial nerve, is most commonly affected) or spinal nerve involvement; clinical manifestations relate to the area involved

10. Clinical manifestations that indicate the invasion of leukemic cells to the kidneys, testes, prostate, ovaries, gastrointestinal (GI) tract, and lungs

C. Infection (Box 37-4)

1. A major cause of death in the immunosuppressed child

2. Can occur through autocontamination or cross contamination

3. Most common sites of infection are the skin (any break in the skin is a potential site of infection), respiratory tract, and GI tract

D. Bleeding (Box 37-5)

1. Children with platelet counts below 20,000/mm³ may need a platelet transfusion

2. For children with severe blood loss, packed red blood cells may be prescribed

E. Fatigue and nutrition

1. Assist the child in selecting a well-balanced diet

2. Provide small meals that require little chewing

3. Assist the child in self-care and mobility activities

4. Allow adequate rest periods during care

5. Do not perform activities unless they are essential

F. Chemotherapy

1. Monitor for severe bone marrow suppression; during the period of greatest bone marrow

---

BOX 37-4

Protecting the Child from Infection

Initiate protective isolation procedures.

Maintain frequent and thorough hand washing.

Maintain the child in a private room and a room with high-efficiency particulate air (HEPA) filtration or laminar airflow system, if possible.

Be sure that the child's room is cleaned daily.

Use strict aseptic technique for all nursing procedures.

Limit the number of caregivers entering the child's room, and ensure that anyone entering the child's room is wearing a mask.

Keep supplies for the child separate from supplies for other children.

Reduce exposure to environmental organisms by eliminating raw fruits and vegetables and fresh flowers, and by not leaving standing water in the child's room.

Assist the child with daily bathing, using antimicrobial soap.

Assist the child to perform oral hygiene frequently.

Monitor for signs and symptoms of infection.

Monitor temperature, pulse, and blood pressure.

Change wound dressings daily and inspect wounds for redness, swelling, or drainage.

Monitor urine for color and cloudiness.

Monitor the skin and oral mucous membranes for signs of infection.

Check lung sounds.

Encourage the child to cough and deep breathe.

Monitor the white blood cell and the neutrophil count.

The physician is notified if signs of infection are present; prepare to obtain specimens for culture of open lesions, urine, and sputum.

Initiate a bowel program to prevent constipation and rectal trauma.

Avoid invasive procedures such as injections, rectal temperatures, and urinary catheterization.

Administer antibiotic, antifungal, and antiviral medication, as prescribed.

Administer granulocyte colony-stimulating factor (GCSF), as prescribed.

Instruct the parents to keep the child away from crowds and those with infections.

Instruct the parents that the child should not receive immunization with a live virus.

Keep any child with chickenpox or any child who has been exposed to the virus away from the child with leukemia.

Instruct the parents to inform the teacher that they should be notified immediately if a case of chickenpox occurs in another child at school.

---

suppression (the nadir), blood counts will be extremely low

2. Monitor for infection and bleeding

3. Protect the child from life-threatening infections

4. Monitor for nausea, vomiting, and diarrhea

5. Administer antiemetics as prescribed

6. Monitor for signs of dehydration

BOX 37-5

Protecting the Child from Bleeding

Examine the child for signs and symptoms of bleeding.

Handle the child gently.

Measure abdominal girth, which can indicate internal hemorrhage.

Instruct the child to use a soft toothbrush and to avoid dental floss.

Provide soft foods that are cool to warm in temperature.

Avoid injections if possible, to prevent trauma to the skin and bleeding.

Apply firm and gentle pressure to a needlestick site for at least 10 minutes.

Pad side rails and sharp corners of the bed and furniture.

Discourage the child from engaging in activities involving the use of sharp objects.

Instruct the child to avoid constrictive or tight clothing.

Use caution when taking the blood pressure to prevent skin injury.

Instruct the child to avoid blowing his or her nose.

Avoid rectal suppositories, enemas, and rectal thermometers.

Examine all body fluids and excrement for the presence of blood.

Count the number of pads or tampons used if the female adolescent is menstruating.

Instruct the child in the signs and symptoms of bleeding.

Instruct the parents to avoid administering nonsteroidal anti-inflammatory drugs (NSAIDs) and products that contain aspirin to the child.

---

7. Monitor for signs of hemorrhagic cystitis
8. Monitor for signs of peripheral neuropathy
9. Check oral mucous membranes for mucositis; administer frequent mouth rinses (normal saline with or without sodium bicarbonate solution) to promote healing if mucositis occurs
10. Instruct the parents in signs and symptoms to monitor after chemotherapy and when to notify the physician
11. Inform the parents that hair loss may occur from chemotherapy (hair will regrow in 3 to 6 months and may be a slightly different color or texture)
12. Instruct the parents about the care of a central venous access device as necessary
13. Listen to the child and family, and encourage them to verbalize their feelings and express their concerns
14. Introduce the family to other families of children with cancer
15. Consult social services and chaplains as necessary

VII. HODGKIN'S DISEASE (Box 37-6)

A. Description
   1. A malignancy of the lymph nodes that originates in a single lymph node or a single chain of nodes

---

BOX 37-6

Staging of Hodgkin's Disease

STAGE I

Involvement of a single lymph node region or only one extralymphatic organ or site such as the liver, kidneys, lungs, or intestines

STAGE II

Involvement of two or more lymph node regions on the same side of the diaphragm or one additional extralymphatic organ or site on the same side of the diaphragm

STAGE III

Involvement of lymph node regions on both sides of the diaphragm or one extralymphatic organ or site or spleen or both

STAGE IV

Diffuse or disseminated involvement of one or more extralymphatic organs with or without associated lymph node involvement

---

2. It predictably metastasizes to nonnodal or extralymphatic sites, especially the spleen, liver, bone marrow, lungs, and mediastinum
3. Characterized by the presence of the Reed-Sternberg cell in the lymph nodes
4. Possible causes include viral infections and previous exposure to alkalating chemical agents
5. The prognosis is dependent on the stage of disease; the prognosis is excellent in children with localized disease
6. The primary treatment modalities are radiation and chemotherapy; each may be used alone or in combination, depending on the clinical staging of the disease
7. BMT may be a consideration in treating Hodgkin's disease

B. Data collection
   1. Painless enlargement of lymph nodes
   2. Enlarged, firm, nontender, movable nodes in the supraclavicular area; in children, the "sentinel" node located near the left clavicle may be the first enlarged node
   3. Nonproductive cough as a result of mediastinal lymphadenopathy
   4. Abdominal pain as a result of enlarged retroperitoneal nodes
   5. Advanced lymph node and extralymphatic involvement may cause systemic symptoms such as low-grade and/or intermittent fever, anorexia, nausea, weight loss, night sweats, and pruritus
   6. Positive biopsy of lymph node (presence of Reed-Sternberg cell) and positive bone marrow biopsy
   7. Computed tomography (CT) scan of the liver, spleen, and bone marrow to detect metastasis

C. Interventions
1. For stages 1 and 2 without mediastinal node involvement, the treatment of choice is extensive external radiation of the involved lymph node regions
2. With more extensive disease, radiation in combination with multiagent chemotherapy is used
3. Monitor for drug-induced pancytopenia, which increases the risk for infection, bleeding, and anemia
4. Monitor for signs of infection and bleeding
5. Protect the child from infection
6. Provide a safe, hazard-free environment
7. Monitor for side effects related to chemotherapy or radiation; the most common complication of radiation to the neck area is hypothyroidism
8. Monitor for nausea and vomiting; administer antiemetics, as prescribed
9. Monitor for skin irritation and breakdown as a result of radiation therapy

VIII. NEPHROBLASTOMA (WILMS' TUMOR)

A. Description
1. A tumor of the kidney that may present unilaterally and localized or bilaterally, sometimes with metastasis to other organs
2. The peak incidence is at 3 years of age
3. Associated with a genetic inheritance and with several congenital anomalies
4. Therapeutic management includes a combined treatment of surgery (partial to total nephrectomy) and chemotherapy with or without radiation, depending on the clinical stage and histologic pattern

B. Data collection
1. Swelling or mass within the abdomen (mass is characteristically firm, nontender, confined to one side, and deep within the flank)
2. Abdominal pain
3. Urinary retention and/or hematuria
4. Anemia (secondary to hemorrhage within the tumor)
5. Pallor, anorexia, lethargy (occurs as a result of anemia)
6. Hypertension (caused by secretion of excess amounts of renin by the tumor)
7. Weight loss and fever
8. Symptoms of lung involvement, such as dyspnea, shortness of breath, and pain in the chest, if metastasis has occurred

C. Preoperative interventions
1. Monitor vital signs, particularly blood pressure
2. Place a sign at the bedside: "Do Not Palpate Abdomen"
3. Avoid palpation of the abdomen
4. Measure abdominal girth

D. Postoperative interventions
1. Monitor temperature and blood pressure closely
2. Monitor for signs of hemorrhage and infection
3. Monitor input and output (I&O) and urine output closely
4. Monitor for abdominal distention, bowel sounds, and other signs of gastrointestinal (GI) activity because of the risk for intestinal obstruction

IX. NEUROBLASTOMA

A. Description
1. An embryonal tumor found in children that arises from the neural crest
2. The primary site is in the abdomen because the tumor arises from the adrenal gland or from the retroperitoneal sympathetic chain; may also occur in the head, neck, chest, or pelvis
3. Most presenting signs are caused by the tumor compressing adjacent normal tissue and organs
4. Diagnostic evaluation is aimed at locating the primary site of the tumor
5. The prognosis is poor because of the frequency of invasiveness of the tumor and because, in most cases, diagnosis is not made until after metastasis has occurred
6. Therapeutic management
   a. Surgery to remove as much of the tumor as possible and to obtain samples for biopsy; in stages I and II, complete surgical removal of the tumor is the treatment of choice
   b. Surgery is usually limited to biopsy in stages III and IV because of the extensive metastasis
   c. Radiation is commonly used with stage III disease and provides palliation for metastatic lesions in bones, lungs, liver, or brain
   d. Chemotherapy is the mainstay of treatment for extensive local or disseminated disease

B. Data collection
1. Firm, nontender, irregular mass in the abdomen that crosses the midline
2. Urinary frequency or retention from compression of the kidney, ureter, or bladder
3. Lymphadenopathy, especially in the cervical and supraclavicular area
4. Bone pain if skeletal involvement occurs
5. Supraorbital ecchymosis, periorbital edema, and exophthalmos as a result of invasion of retrobulbar soft tissue
6. Pallor, weakness, irritability, anorexia, weight loss
7. Signs of respiratory impairment (thoracic lesion)
8. Signs of neurological impairment (intracranial lesion)
9. Paralysis from compression of the spinal cord

C. Preoperative interventions
1. Monitor for signs and symptoms related to the location of the tumor

2. Provide emotional support to the child and parents

D. Postoperative interventions
   1. Monitor for postoperative complications related to the location (organ) of the surgery
   2. Monitor for complications related to chemotherapy or radiation if prescribed
   3. Provide support to the parents and encourage them to express their feelings; many parents suffer from guilt for not having recognized signs in the child earlier
   4. Refer the parents to appropriate community services

X. OSTEOGENIC SARCOMA

A. Description
   1. The most common bone cancer in children
   2. Usually found in the metaphysis of long bones, especially in the lower extremities, with most tumors occurring in the femur
   3. Peak age of incidence is between 10 and 25 years
   4. Symptoms in the earliest stage are almost always attributed to extremity injury or normal growing pains
   5. Treatment may include surgical resection by limb salvage to remove affected tissue or amputation
   6. Chemotherapy plays a vital role in treatment and may be employed both before and after surgery

B. Data collection
   1. Localized pain at the affected site (may be severe or dull) that may be attributed to trauma or the vague complaint of "growing pains"; pain is often relieved by a flexed position
   2. Palpable mass
   3. Limping if weight-bearing limb is affected
   4. Progressively limited range of motion; child curtails physical activity
   5. Child may be unable to hold heavy objects
   6. Pathological fractures at the tumor site

C. Interventions
   1. Prepare the child and family for prescribed treatment modalities, which may include surgical resection by limb salvage to remove affected tissue, amputation, and chemotherapy
   2. Provide honesty and support for the child and family
   3. Prepare for prosthetic fitting as necessary
   4. Assist the child in dealing with problems of self-image

XI. BRAIN TUMORS

A. Description
   1. An infratentorial (below the tentorium cerebelli) tumor is located in the posterior third of the brain (primarily in the cerebellum or brainstem) and accounts for the frequency of symptoms resulting from increased intracranial pressure (ICP)
   2. A supratentorial tumor is located within the anterior two thirds of the brain, mainly the cerebrum
   3. The signs and symptoms of a brain tumor depend on its anatomical location and size and to some extent on the age of the child
   4. Therapeutic management includes surgery, radiation, and chemotherapy; the treatment of choice is total removal of the tumor without residual neurological damage

B. Data collection
   1. Headache that is worse on awakening and improves during the day
   2. Vomiting that is unrelated to feeding or eating
   3. Ataxia
   4. Seizures
   5. Behavioral changes
   6. Clumsiness; awkward gait or difficulty walking
   7. Diplopia
   8. Facial weakness

C. Preoperative interventions
   1. Monitor neurological status
   2. Institute safety measures
   3. Monitor weight and nutritional status
   4. Initiate seizure precautions
   5. The child's head will be shaved (provide a favorite cap or hat for the child)
   6. Prepare the child as much as possible; tell the child that he or she will wake up with a large head dressing

D. Postoperative interventions
   1. Monitor neurological and motor function and level of consciousness (LOC)
   2. Monitor temperature closely, which may be elevated because of hypothalamus or brainstem involvement during surgery; maintain a cooling blanket by the bedside
   3. Monitor for signs of respiratory infection
   4. Monitor for signs of meningitis (opisthotonos, Kernig and Brudzinski signs)
   5. Monitor for signs of increased ICP or hemorrhage (check the back of the head dressing for posterior pooling of blood)
   6. Monitor pupillary response; sluggish, dilated, or unequal pupils are reported immediately because they may indicate increased ICP and potential brainstem herniation
   7. Monitor for colorless drainage on the dressing or from the ears or nose, which indicates cerebrospinal fluid (CSF) and should be reported immediately
   8. Check the physician's order for positioning, including the degree of neck flexion (Box 37-7)
   9. Monitor IV fluids closely

BOX 37-7

Positioning Following Craniotomy

Check the physician's order for positioning, including the degree of neck flexion.

If a large tumor was removed, the child is not placed on the operative side because the brain may suddenly shift to that cavity.

In an infratentorial procedure, the child is usually positioned flat and on either side.

In a supratentorial procedure, the head is usually elevated above the heart level to facilitate CSF drainage and to decrease excessive blood flow to the brain to prevent hemorrhage.

Never place the child in the Trendelenburg position because it increases ICP and the risk of hemorrhage.

10. Promote measures that prevent vomiting (vomiting increases ICP and the risk for incisional rupture)
11. Provide a quiet environment
12. Administer analgesics, as prescribed
13. Provide emotional support to the child and parents, and promote maximum functioning in the child

PRACTICE QUESTIONS

1. A pediatric nursing instructor asks a nursing student to describe the cause of the clinical manifestations that occur in sickle cell disease. Which of the following is the correct response by the nursing student?
   1. "Sickled cells increase the blood flow through the body and cause a great deal of pain."
   2. "The sickled cells mix with the unsickled cells and cause the immune system to become depressed."
   3. "Bone marrow depression occurs because of the development of sickled cells."
   4. "Sickled cells are unable to flow easily through the microvasculature and their clumping obstructs blood flow."

2. A child suspected of having sickle cell disease (SCD) is seen in a clinic, and laboratory studies are performed. A nurse checks the laboratory results, knowing that which of the following would be increased in this disease?
   1. Platelet count
   2. Hematocrit level
   3. Reticulocyte count
   4. Hemoglobin level

3. A nurse instructs the mother of a child with sickle cell disease regarding the precipitating factors related to pain crisis. Which of the following, if identified by the mother as a precipitating factor, indicates the need for further instructions?
   1. Infection
   2. Trauma

3. Fluid overload
4. Stress

4. Oral iron supplements are prescribed for the 6-year-old child with iron deficiency anemia. The nurse instructs the mother to administer the iron with which best food item?
   1. Water
   2. Milk
   3. Apple juice
   4. Orange juice

5. A nurse caring for a child with aplastic anemia reviews the laboratory results and notes a white blood cell (WBC) count of $6000/\mu L$ and a platelet count of $27,000/mm^3$. Which nursing intervention will the nurse suggest to incorporate into the plan of care?
   1. Maintain strict isolation precautions
   2. Encourage naps
   3. Encourage a diet high in iron
   4. Encourage quiet play activities

6. A nurse reinforces instructions regarding home care to the parents of a 3-year-old child hospitalized with hemophilia. Which statement by a parent indicates a need for further instructions?
   1. "I will supervise my child closely."
   2. "I will pad corners of the furniture."
   3. "I will remove household items that can easily fall over."
   4. "I will avoid immunizations being administered and dental hygiene treatments for my child."

7. A nurse is reinforcing home care instructions to the mother of a 10-year-old child with hemophilia. Which activity would the nurse suggest that the child could safely participate in with peers?
   1. Basketball
   2. Swimming
   3. Soccer
   4. Field hockey

8. A nursing student is presenting a clinical conference and discusses the causative factors related to β-thalassemia. The student informs the group that the child at greatest risk of developing this disorder is:
   1. A child whose intake of iron is extremely poor
   2. A child breast-fed by a mother with chronic anemia
   3. A child of Mediterranean descent
   4. A child of Mexican descent

9. A nurse reinforces instructions to the parents of a child with leukemia regarding measures related to monitoring for infection. Which statement by the parents indicates a need for further instructions?
   1. "I need to use proper hand washing techniques."
   2. "I need to take a rectal temperature daily on my child."
   3. "I need to inspect my child's skin daily for redness."
   4. "I need to inspect my child's mouth daily for lesions."

10. A 6-year-old child with leukemia is hospitalized and is receiving chemotherapy. Laboratory results indicate that the child is neutropenic and protective isolation procedures are initiated. The grandmother of the child visits and brings a fresh bouquet of flowers picked from her garden and asks the nurse for a vase for the flowers. The nurse makes which appropriate response to the grandmother?
    1. "I have a vase in the utility room and I will get it for you."
    2. "The flowers from your garden are beautiful, but should not be placed in the child's room at this time."
    3. "I will get the vase and wash it well before you put the flowers in it."
    4. "When you bring the flowers into the room, place them on the bedside stand as far away from the child as possible."

11. A nurse is reviewing the health record of a 10-year-old child suspected of having Hodgkin's disease. Which of the following would the nurse expect to note documented in the record that is most characteristic of this disease?
    1. Painful, enlarged inguinal lymph nodes
    2. Fever and malaise
    3. Painless, firm, and movable adenopathy in the cervical area
    4. Anorexia and weight loss

12. A 4-year-old child is hospitalized with a suspected diagnosis of Wilms' tumor. The nurse assists in developing a plan of care and suggests avoiding which of the following?
    1. Palpating the abdomen for a mass
    2. Checking the urine for the presence of hematuria
    3. Monitoring the temperature for the presence of fever
    4. Monitoring the blood pressure for the presence of hypertension

13. A nursing instructor asks a student nurse to describe osteogenic sarcoma. Which statement by the student indicates the need to further research the disease?
    1. "The symptoms of the disease in the early stage are almost always attributed to normal growing pains."
    2. "The femur is the most common site of this sarcoma."
    3. "Limping, if a weight-bearing limb is affected, is a clinical manifestation."
    4. "The child does not experience pain at the primary tumor site."

14. A 13-year-old child is diagnosed with osteogenic sarcoma of the femur. Following a course of chemotherapy, it has been decided that leg amputation is necessary. Following the amputation, the child becomes very frightened because of aching and cramping felt in the missing limb. The nurse makes which statement to assist in alleviating the child's fear?
    1. "This aching and cramping is normal and temporary and will subside."
    2. "This always occurs after the surgery and we will teach you ways to deal with it."
    3. "The pain medication that I give you will take these feelings away."
    4. "This pain is not real pain and relaxation exercises will help it go away."

15. A nurse is monitoring for bleeding in a child following surgery for removal of a brain tumor. The nurse checks the head dressing for the presence of blood and notes a colorless drainage on the back of the dressing. The nurse takes which appropriate action?
    1. Circles the area of drainage and continues to monitor
    2. Reinforces the dressing
    3. Notifies the registered nurse (RN)
    4. Documents the findings and continue to monitor

ALTERNATE FORMAT QUESTION: MULTIPLE RESPONSE

A nurse is reviewing a physician's orders for a child with sickle cell anemia who was admitted to the hospital for the treatment of vaso-occlusive crisis. Select the orders that the nurse would expect to note written in the client's chart.

___ Increase oral fluid intake
___ Intravenous (IV) fluids of normal saline at 50 mL/hour
___ Administer oxygen at 2 L/minute
___ Elevate the head of the bed 60 degrees at all times
___ Administer meperidine (Demerol) 25 mg intramuscular for pain

ANSWERS

1. *Answer:* **4**
Rationale: All the clinical manifestations of sickle cell disease are a result of the sickled cells being unable to flow easily through the microvasculature, and their clumping obstructs blood flow. With reoxygenation, most of the sickled red blood cells resume their normal shape. Options 1, 2, and 3 are inaccurate.
Test-Taking Strategy: Use the process of elimination. Recalling that sickled cells clump will assist in directing you to the correct option. Review the pathophysiology associated with sickle cell disease if you had difficulty with this question.

Level of Cognitive Ability: Comprehension
Client Needs: Physiological Integrity
Integrated Process: Teaching/Learning
Content Area: Child Health
Reference: Price, D., & Gwin, J. (2005). *Thompson's pediatric nursing* (9th ed.). Philadelphia: W.B. Saunders, p. 138.

2. Answer: 3
Rationale: A diagnosis is established on the basis of a complete blood count, examination for sickled red blood cells (RBCs) in the peripheral smear, and hemoglobin electrophoresis. Laboratory studies will show decreased hemoglobin and hematocrit levels and a decreased platelet count, an increased reticulocyte count, and the presence of nucleated red blood cells. Increased reticulocyte counts occur in children with SCD because the life span of their sickled RBCs is shortened.
Test-Taking Strategy: Use the process of elimination. Recalling that the life span of the sickled RBCs is shortened in SCD and noting the relationship between this concept and the reticulocytes will direct you to the correct option. Review the laboratory tests that are diagnostic for this disorder if you had difficulty with this question.
Level of Cognitive Ability: Analysis
Client Needs: Physiological Integrity
Integrated Process: Nursing Process/Data Collection
Content Area: Child Health
Reference: James, S., Ashwill, J., & Droske, S. (2002). *Nursing care of children: Principles and practice* (2nd ed.). Philadelphia: W.B. Saunders, p. 747.

3. Answer: 3
Rationale: Pain crisis may be precipitated by infection, dehydration, hypoxia, trauma, or general stress. The mother of a child with sickle cell disease should encourage fluid intake of 1.5 to 2 times the daily requirement to prevent dehydration.
Test-Taking Strategy: Note the key words, *need for further instructions*. These words indicate a false response question and that you need to select the incorrect item. Recalling that fluids is a main component of treatment in sickle cell disease to prevent dehydration and pain crisis will direct you to option 3. Review the precipitating factors of pain crisis if you had difficulty with this question.
Level of Cognitive Ability: Comprehension
Client Needs: Health Promotion and Maintenance
Integrated Process: Teaching/Learning
Content Area: Child Health
Reference: Price, D., & Gwin, J. (2005). *Thompson's pediatric nursing* (9th ed.). Philadelphia: W.B. Saunders, p. 140.

4. Answer: 4
Rationale: Vitamin C increases the absorption of iron by the body. The mother should be instructed to administer the medication with a citrus fruit or juice high in vitamin C.
Test-Taking Strategy: Use the process of elimination. Recalling that vitamin C increases the absorption of iron will assist in eliminating options 1 and 2. From the remaining options, select option 4, because this food item contains the highest amount of vitamin C. Review the procedure for administering oral iron if you had difficulty with this question.

Level of Cognitive Ability: Application
Client Needs: Health Promotion and Maintenance
Integrated Process: Teaching/Learning
Content Area: Pharmacology
Reference: Price, D., & Gwin, J. (2005). *Thompson's pediatric nursing* (9th ed.). Philadelphia: W.B. Saunders, p. 137.

5. Answer: 4
Rationale: Precautionary measures to prevent bleeding should be taken when a child has a low platelet count. These include no injections, no rectal temperatures, use of a soft toothbrush, and abstinence from contact sports or activities that could cause an injury. Strict isolation would be required if the WBC count were low. Options 2 and 3 are unrelated to the risk of bleeding.
Test-Taking Strategy: Use the process of elimination. Note that the WBC count is normal and that the platelet count is low. Recall that a low platelet count places the client at risk for bleeding. This will assist in eliminating options 1, 2, and 3. Review normal WBC and platelet counts if you had difficulty with this question.
Level of Cognitive Ability: Analysis
Client Needs: Physiological Integrity
Integrated Process: Nursing Process/Planning
Content Area: Child Health
References: McKinney, E., James, S., Murray, S., & Ashwill, J. (2005). *Maternal-child nursing* (2nd ed.). St. Louis: Elsevier, pp. 1324-1325.
Wong, D., & Hockenberry, M. (2003). *Nursing care of infants and children* (7th ed.). St. Louis: Mosby, p. 1565.

6. Answer: 4
Rationale: The nurse needs to stress the importance of immunizations, dental hygiene, and routine well-child care. Options 1, 2, and 3 are appropriate statements. The parents are also provided instructions regarding measures to take in the event of blunt trauma, especially trauma involving the joints, and are instructed to apply prolonged pressure to superficial wounds until the bleeding has stopped.
Test-Taking Strategy: Use the process of elimination and note the key words, *need for further instructions*. These words indicate a false response question and that you need to select the incorrect client statement. Recalling that bleeding is a concern in this disorder will assist in eliminating options 1, 2, and 3 because they include measures of protection and safety for the child. Review home care measures for the child with hemophilia if you had difficulty with this question.
Level of Cognitive Ability: Comprehension
Client Needs: Health Promotion and Maintenance
Integrated Process: Teaching/Learning
Content Area: Child Health
Reference: Price, D., & Gwin, J. (2005). *Thompson's pediatric nursing* (9th ed.). Philadelphia: W.B. Saunders, p. 235.

7. Answer: 2
Rationale: Children with hemophilia need to avoid contact sports and need to take precautions, such as wearing elbow and knee pads and helmets, when participating in other sports. The safest activity that will prevent injury is swimming.

Test-Taking Strategy: Note the key word, *safely.* Recalling that bleeding is a major concern in this condition will assist in directing you to option 2. Also, note that the activities in options 1, 3, and 4 present the potential for injury. Review home care instructions for the child with hemophilia if you had difficulty with this question.
Level of Cognitive Ability: Application
Client Needs: Health Promotion and Maintenance
Integrated Process: Teaching/Learning
Content Area: Child Health
Reference: Price, D., & Gwin, J. (2005). *Thompson's pediatric nursing* (9th ed.). Philadelphia: W.B. Saunders, p. 235.

8. *Answer:* 3
Rationale: β-Thalassemia is an autosomal recessive disorder. This disorder is found primarily in individuals of Mediterranean descent. The disease has also been reported in Asian and African populations.
Test-Taking Strategy: Knowledge regarding the causative factors associated with this disorder is required to answer this question. Remember that this disorder is found primarily in individuals of Mediterranean descent. Review this disorder if you had difficulty with this question.
Level of Cognitive Ability: Comprehension
Client Needs: Physiological Integrity
Integrated Process: Teaching/Learning
Content Area: Child Health
Reference: Leifer, G. (2003). *Introduction to maternity and pediatric nursing* (4th ed.). Philadelphia: W.B. Saunders, p. 638.

9. *Answer:* 2
Rationale: The risk of injury to fragile mucous membranes is so great in the child with leukemia that only oral, axillary, or tympanic temperatures should be taken. Rectal abscesses can easily occur in damaged rectal tissue. No rectal temperatures should be taken. Additionally, oral temperatures should be avoided if the child has oral ulcers. Options 1, 3, and 4 are appropriate teaching measures.
Test-Taking Strategy: Use the process of elimination and note the key words, *need for further instructions.* These words indicate a false response question and that you need to select the incorrect client statement. Options 1 and 3 can be easily eliminated first. From the remaining options, note the word "rectal" in option 2. Recalling that rectal temperatures should be avoided will direct you to this option. Review home care instructions related to infection in the leukemic child if you had difficulty with this question.
Level of Cognitive Ability: Comprehension
Client Needs: Safe, Effective Care Environment
Integrated Process: Teaching/Learning
Content Area: Child Health
Reference: Leifer, G. (2003). *Introduction to maternity and pediatric nursing* (4th ed.). Philadelphia: W.B. Saunders, p. 644.

10. *Answer:* 2
Rationale: For the hospitalized neutropenic child, flowers or plants should not be kept in the room because standing water and damp soil harbor *Aspergillus* and *Pseudomonas* organisms, to which these children are very susceptible.

Additionally, fruits and vegetables that are not peeled before being eaten harbor molds and should be avoided until the white blood cell count rises.
Test-Taking Strategy: Use the process of elimination and knowledge regarding protective isolation procedures for a neutropenic child. Note that options 1 and 3 are similar and should be eliminated first. From the remaining options, select option 2, because this nursing response maintains the procedure required. Review protective isolation procedures for the neutropenic child if you had difficulty with this question.
Level of Cognitive Ability: Application
Client Needs: Safe, Effective Care Environment
Integrated Process: Communication and Documentation
Content Area: Child Health
Reference: McKinney, E., James, S., Murray, S., & Ashwill, J. (2005). *Maternal-child nursing* (2nd ed.). St. Louis: Elsevier, pp. 1339-1340.

11. *Answer:* 3
Rationale: Clinical manifestations specifically associated with Hodgkin's disease include painless, firm, and movable adenopathy in the cervical and supraclavicular areas. Hepatosplenomegaly is also noted. Although anorexia, weight loss, fever, and malaise are associated with Hodgkin's disease, these manifestations are seen in many disorders.
Test-Taking Strategy: Note the key words, *most characteristic.* Eliminate options 2 and 4 first because these symptoms are general and vague. Recalling that painless adenopathy is associated with Hodgkin's disease will direct you to option 3. Review the clinical manifestations related to Hodgkin's disease if you had difficulty with this question.
Level of Cognitive Ability: Comprehension
Client Needs: Physiological Integrity
Integrated Process: Nursing Process/Data Collection
Content Area: Child Health
Reference: Price, D., & Gwin, J. (2005). *Thompson's pediatric nursing* (9th ed.). Philadelphia: W.B. Saunders, p. 325.

12. *Answer:* 1
Rationale: A Wilms' tumor is a tumor of the kidney. If Wilms' tumor is suspected, the mass should not be palpated. Excessive manipulation can cause seeding of the tumor and cause the spread of the cancerous cells. Fever, hematuria, and hypertension are clinical manifestations associated with Wilms' tumor.
Test-Taking Strategy: Use the process of elimination and note the key word, *avoiding.* This word indicates a false response question and that you need to select the incorrect intervention. Knowledge that this tumor is located in the kidney will assist in eliminating options 2, 3, and 4 because of the relationship of these options to renal function. Review nursing interventions for the child with Wilms' tumor if you had difficulty with this question.
Level of Cognitive Ability: Application
Client Needs: Physiological Integrity
Integrated Process: Nursing Process/Planning
Content Area: Child Health
Reference: Price, D., & Gwin, J. (2005). *Thompson's pediatric nursing* (9th ed.). Philadelphia: W.B. Saunders, p. 205.

13. *Answer: 4*

Rationale: A clinical manifestation of osteogenic sarcoma is progressive, insidious, intermittent pain at the tumor site. By the time these children receive medical attention, they may be in considerable pain from the tumor. Options 1, 2, and 3 are accurate regarding osteogenic sarcoma.

Test-Taking Strategy: Note the key words, *need to further research.* Recalling that osteogenic sarcoma is a malignant tumor of the bone will direct you to option 4. Review the clinical manifestations associated with osteogenic sarcoma if you had difficulty with this question.

Level of Cognitive Ability: Comprehension

Client Needs: Physiological Integrity

Integrated Process: Teaching/Learning

Content Area: Child Health

References: Leifer, G. (2003). *Introduction to maternity and pediatric nursing* (4th ed.). Philadelphia: W.B. Saunders, p. 580.

Wong, D., & Hockenberry, M. (2003). *Nursing care of infants and children* (7th ed.). St. Louis: Mosby, p. 1627.

14. *Answer: 1*

Rationale: Following amputation, phantom limb pain is a temporary condition that some children may experience. This sensation of aching or cramping in the missing limb is most distressing to the child. The child needs to be reassured that the condition is normal and only temporary.

Test-Taking Strategy: Use the process of elimination and therapeutic communication techniques to answer this question. Note that the issue of the question relates to alleviating the child's fear. Option 1 is the only option that will alleviate fear. Options 2, 3, and 4 infer that this pain may be permanent. Also, option 2 contains the absolute word "always." Review care of the child following amputation if you had difficulty with this question.

Level of Cognitive Ability: Application

Client Needs: Psychosocial Integrity

Integrated Process: Communication and Documentation

Content Area: Child Health

References: Leifer, G. (2003). *Introduction to maternity and pediatric nursing* (4th ed.). Philadelphia: W.B. Saunders, p. 580.

Wong, D., & Hockenberry, M. (2003). *Nursing care of infants and children* (7th ed.). St. Louis: Mosby, p. 1628.

15. *Answer: 3*

Rationale: Colorless drainage on the dressing would indicate the presence of cerebrospinal fluid and should be reported to the RN immediately. The RN would then contact the physician. Options 1, 2, and 4 delay required immediate interventions.

Test-Taking Strategy: Use the process of elimination. Note the key words, *colorless drainage.* This should quickly alert you to the possibility of the presence of cerebrospinal fluid. Therefore, eliminate options 1, 2, and 4. Review care of the child with a brain tumor if you had difficulty with this question.

Level of Cognitive Ability: Application

Client Needs: Physiological Integrity

Integrated Process: Nursing Process/Implementation

Content Area: Child Health

Reference: Wong, D., & Hockenberry, M. (2003). *Nursing care of infants and children* (7th ed.). St. Louis: Mosby, p. 1623.

ALTERNATE FORMAT QUESTION: MULTIPLE RESPONSE

Answers:

Increase oral fluid intake

Intravenous (IV) fluids of normal saline at 50 mL/hour

Administer oxygen at 2 L/minute

Rationale: Vaso-occlusive crisis is caused by stasis of blood, with clumping of the cells in the microcirculation, ischemia, and infarction. Signs include fever, pain, and tissue engorgement. Increased fluids and oxygen are used to treat vaso-occlusive crisis. Although analgesics are prescribed, meperidine (Demerol) is not recommended for the child with sickle cell disease because of the risk for normeperidine-induced seizures. Normeperidine, a metabolite of meperidine, is a central nervous system stimulant that produces anxiety, tremors, myoclonus, and generalized seizures when it accumulates with repetitive dosing. The head of the bed is elevated no more than 30 degrees to prevent flexion of joints and strain on painful areas.

Test-Taking Strategy: Focus on the pathophysiology associated with vaso-occlusive crisis. Recall that this type of crisis is caused by stasis of blood, with clumping of the cells in the microcirculation, ischemia, and infarction. This will assist in identifying the expected physician's orders. Review care of the child with sickle cell disease experiencing a crisis if you had difficulty with this question.

Level of Cognitive Ability: Analysis

Client Needs: Physiological Integrity

Integrated Process: Nursing Process/Planning

Content Area: Child Health

Reference: Price, D., & Gwin, J. (2005). *Thompson's pediatric nursing* (9th ed.). Philadelphia: W.B. Saunders, pp. 138; 140.

REFERENCES

Agency for Health Care Research and Quality. Web site: http://www.ahcpr.gov.

American Cancer Society. Web site: http://www.cancer.org.

Cooley's Anemia Foundation. Web site: http://www.thalassemia.org.

James, S., Ashwill, J., & Droske, S. (2002). *Nursing care of children: Principles and practice* (2nd ed.). Philadelphia: W.B. Saunders.

Leifer, G. (2003). *Introduction to maternity and pediatric nursing* (4th ed.). Philadelphia: W.B. Saunders.

McKinney, E., James, S., Murray, S., & Ashwill, J. (2005). *Maternal-child nursing* (2nd ed.). St. Louis: Elsevier.

National Brain Tumor Foundation. Web site: http://www.braintumor.org.

Price, D., & Gwin, J. (2005). *Thompson's pediatric nursing* (9th ed.). Philadelphia: W.B. Saunders.

Wong, D., & Hockenberry, M. (2003). *Nursing care of infants and children* (7th ed.). St. Louis: Mosby.

Communicable Diseases and Acquired Immunodeficiency Syndrome

I. RUBEOLA (MEASLES)

A. Description
  1. Agent: Virus
  2. Incubation period: 10 to 20 days
  3. Communicable period: From 4 days before to 5 days after the rash appears; mainly during prodromal (catarrhal) stage
  4. Source: Respiratory tract secretions, blood, or urine of infected person
  5. Transmission: Airborne or direct contact with infectious droplets

B. Data collection
  1. Fever
  2. Malaise
  3. Coryza and cough
  4. Rash appears as red, discrete maculopapules that blanch easily with pressure and gradually turn a brownish color (lasts 6 to 7 days); rash begins behind the ears and spreads downward to the feet
  5. Koplik spots: small, red spots with a bluish-white center and a red base; located on the mucosa and last 3 days

C. Interventions
  1. Respiratory precautions if the child is hospitalized
  2. Restrict to quiet activities and bed rest
  3. Use a cool mist vaporizer for cough and coryza
  4. Dim lights if photophobia is present
  5. Administer antipyretics for fever

II. ROSEOLA (EXANTHEMA SUBITUM)

A. Description
  1. Agent: Human herpesvirus type 6 (HHV-6)
  2. Incubation period: 5 to 15 days
  3. Communicable period: Unknown but thought to extend from the febrile stage to when the rash first appears
  4. Source: Unknown
  5. Transmission: Unknown

B. Data collection
  1. Fever for 3 to 5 days followed by a rash (rose-pink maculas that blanch with pressure)
  2. The rash appears 2 to 3 days after the onset of fever and lasts 1 to 2 days

C. Interventions: Supportive

III. RUBELLA (GERMAN MEASLES)

A. Description
  1. Agent: Rubella virus
  2. Incubation period: 14 to 21 days
  3. Communicable period: 7 days before to approximately 5 days after the rash appears
  4. Source: Nasopharyngeal secretions; virus is also present in blood, stool, and urine
  5. Transmission
    a. Airborne or direct contact with infectious droplets
    b. Indirectly via articles freshly contaminated with nasopharyngeal secretions, feces, or urine
    c. Transplacental

B. Data collection
  1. Low-grade fever
  2. Malaise
  3. Pinkish-red maculopapular rash that begins on the face and spreads to the entire body
  4. Petechial spots may occur on the soft palate

C. Interventions
  1. Supportive treatment
  2. Isolate the infected child from pregnant women

IV. MUMPS

A. Description
  1. Agent: Paramyxovirus

2. Incubation period: 14 to 21 days
3. Communicable period: Immediately before and after the swelling begins
4. Source: Saliva of infected person and possibly urine
5. Transmission
   a. Direct contact with infected person
   b. Droplet spread from infected person
B. Data collection
   1. Fever
   2. Headache and malaise
   3. Anorexia
   4. Earache aggravated by chewing, followed by parotid glandular swelling
C. Interventions
   1. Respiratory precautions
   2. Bed rest until the parotid glandular swelling subsides
   3. Avoid foods that require chewing
   4. Apply hot or cold compresses as prescribed to the neck
   5. To relieve orchitis, apply warmth and local support with tight-fitting underpants

V. CHICKENPOX (VARICELLA)

A. Description
   1. Agent: Varicella zoster virus (VZV)
   2. Incubation period: 13 to 17 days
   3. Communicable period: 1 to 2 days before the onset of the rash to 6 days after the first crop of vesicles, when crusts have formed
   4. Source: Respiratory tract secretions of infected person; skin lesions
   5. Transmission: Direct contact, droplet (airborne) spread, and contact with contaminated objects
B. Data collection
   1. Slight fever, malaise, and anorexia followed by a macular rash that first appears on the trunk and scalp and moves to the extremities
   2. Lesions become pustules, begin to dry, and develop a crust
   3. Lesions may appear on the mucous membranes of the mouth, the genital area, and the rectal area
C. Interventions
   1. In the hospital setting, strict isolation (contact and airborne precautions)
   2. In the home setting, isolate the infected child until the vesicles have dried; isolate high-risk children from the infected child

VI. PERTUSSIS (WHOOPING COUGH)

A. Description
   1. Agent: *Bordetella pertussis*
   2. Incubation period: 5 to 21 days (usually 10 days)

3. Communicable period: Greatest during the catarrhal stage
4. Source: Discharge from the respiratory tract of the infected person
5. Transmission: Direct contact or droplet spread from infected person; indirect contact with freshly contaminated articles
B. Data collection: Symptoms of respiratory infection followed by increased severity of cough
C. Interventions
   1. Isolation during the catarrhal stage; if the child is hospitalized, institute respiratory precautions
   2. Administer antimicrobial therapy, as prescribed
   3. Administer pertussis immune globulin, as prescribed
   4. Reduce environmental factors that promote paroxysms of coughing, such as dust, smoke, and sudden changes in temperature
   5. Encourage fluid intake
   6. Provide high humidity with the use of a humidifier or tent

VII. DIPHTHERIA

A. Description
   1. Agent: *Corynebacterium diphtheriae*
   2. Incubation period: 2 to 5 days
   3. Communicable period: Variable; until virulent bacilli are no longer present (three negative cultures), usually 2 weeks but as long as 4 weeks
   4. Source: Discharge from the mucous membranes of the nose and nasopharynx, skin, and other lesions of the infected person
   5. Transmission: Direct contact with infected person, carrier, or contaminated articles
B. Data collection
   1. Low-grade fever, malaise, sore throat
   2. Foul-smelling, mucopurulent nasal discharge
   3. Gray membrane on the tonsils and pharynx
   4. Lymphadenitis (neck edema)
C. Interventions
   1. Strict isolation of the hospitalized child
   2. Administer antitoxin as prescribed (preceded by a skin or conjunctival test to rule out sensitivity to horse serum)
   3. Bed rest
   4. Administer antibiotics as prescribed

VIII. POLIOMYELITIS

A. Description
   1. Agent: Enteroviruses
   2. Incubation period: 7 to 14 days
   3. Communicable period: Not exactly known; the virus is present in the throat and feces shortly after infection and persists for approximately 1 week in the throat and 4 to 6 weeks in the feces

4. Source: Oropharyngeal secretions and feces of the infected person
5. Transmission: Direct contact with infected person; fecal-oral and oropharyngeal routes

B. Data collection
1. Fever, malaise, anorexia, nausea, headache, sore throat
2. Abdominal pain followed by soreness and stiffness of the trunk, neck, and limbs that progresses to flaccid paralysis

C. Interventions
1. Enteric precautions
2. Supportive treatment
3. Bed rest
4. Monitor for respiratory paralysis
5. Physical therapy

IX. SCARLET FEVER

A. Description
1. Agent: Group A beta-hemolytic streptococci
2. Incubation period: 1 to 7 days
3. Communicable period: During the incubation period and clinical illness, approximately 10 days; during the first 2 weeks of the carrier stage, although may persist for months
4. Source: Nasopharyngeal secretions of infected person and carriers
5. Transmission: Direct contact with infected person or droplet spread; indirectly by contact with contaminated articles, ingestion of contaminated milk or other contaminated foods

B. Data collection
1. Abrupt high fever, vomiting, headache, malaise, abdominal pain
2. A red, fine papular rash in the axilla, groin, and neck that spreads to cover the entire body
3. The rash blanches with pressure except in areas of deep creases and folds of the joints (Pastia's sign)
4. The tongue is coated and papillae become red and swollen (white strawberry tongue); by the fourth to fifth day the white coat sloughs off, leaving prominent papillae (red strawberry tongue)
5. Tonsils are edematous and covered with a gray-white exudate
6. Pharynx is edematous and beefy red

C. Interventions
1. Respiratory precautions until 24 hours after the initiation of treatment
2. Supportive therapy
3. Bed rest
4. Encourage fluid intake
5. Administer antibiotics as prescribed

X. ERYTHEMA INFECTIOSUM (FIFTH DISEASE)

A. Description

1. Agent: Human parvovirus B19 (HPV)
2. Incubation period: 4 to 14 days; may be as long as 20 days
3. Communicable period: Uncertain but before the onset of symptoms in most children
4. Source: Infected person
5. Transmission: Unknown; possibly respiratory secretions and blood

B. Data collection
1. Fever, myalgia, lethargy, nausea, vomiting, abdominal pain
2. Stages of the rash
   a. Erythema of the face (slapped face appearance), chiefly on the cheeks; disappears by 1 to 4 days
   b. Approximately 1 day after the rash appears on the face, maculopapular red spots appear, symmetrically distributed in the extremities; rash progresses from proximal to distal surfaces and may last a week or more
   c. Rash subsides but may reappear if the skin becomes irritated or traumatized by such factors as sun, heat, cold, or friction

C. Interventions
1. Respiratory isolation of the hospitalized child
2. Pregnant women should not be in contact with or care for the infected person
3. Supportive
4. Administer antipyretics, analgesics, and antiinflammatory medications, as prescribed

XI. INFECTIOUS MONONUCLEOSIS

A. Description
1. Agent: Epstein-Barr (EB) virus
2. Incubation period: 4 to 6 weeks
3. Communicable period: Unknown; the virus is shed before the onset of the disease until 6 months or longer after recovery
4. Source: Oral secretions
5. Transmission: Direct intimate contact, infected blood

B. Data collection
1. Fever, sore throat, malaise, headache, fatigue, nausea, abdominal pain
2. Lymphadenopathy and hepatosplenomegaly

C. Interventions
1. Supportive
2. Monitor for signs of splenic rupture, which include abdominal pain, left upper quadrant pain, and left shoulder pain

XII. ROCKY MOUNTAIN SPOTTED FEVER

A. Description
1. Agent: *Rickettsia rickettsii*
2. Incubation period: 2 to 14 days

3. Source: Tick; mammal source—wild rodents, dogs

4. Transmission: Bite of infected tick

B. Data collection

1. Fever, malaise, anorexia, vomiting, headache, myalgia

2. Maculopapular or petechial rash primarily on the extremities (ankles and wrists) but may spread to other areas, characteristically on the palms and soles

C. Interventions

1. Vigorous supportive care

2. Administer antibiotics as prescribed

3. Teaching regarding protection from tick bites

XIII. ENTEROBIASIS (PINWORM)

A. Description

1. Agent: *Enterobius vermicularis*

2. Source

a. Universally present in temperate climatic zones

b. Eggs are ingested or inhaled (eggs float in the air), hatch in the upper intestine, mature in 2 to 8 weeks, and migrate to the cecal area; females then mate, migrate out the anus, and lay eggs

3. Transmission

a. Favored in crowded conditions

b. Ingestion or inhalation of eggs

c. Hands to mouth or fecal-oral route

d. Contaminated items (pinworm eggs persist in the environment for 2 to 3 weeks)

B. Infectious: Intense perianal itching, irritability, restlessness, poor sleep, bed-wetting, distractibility, short attention span; in females, the worm may migrate to the vagina and urethra and cause infection

C. Interventions

1. Identify the worms

a. Use a flashlight to inspect the anal area 2 to 3 hours after the child is asleep

b. Tape test: Transparent, sticky tape is used to obtain a specimen from the child's perianal area; specimen is collected in the morning as soon as the child awakens and before a bowel movement or a bath

2. Enteric precautions

3. Anthelmintic medications (all household members are treated); course of medication is repeated in 2 weeks following the first course to prevent reinfection

4. Teach home care measures to prevent reinfection

XIV. IMMUNIZATIONS

A. Guidelines

1. In the United States, the recommended age for beginning primary immunizations of infants is at birth

2. Children born prematurely should receive the full dose of each vaccine at the appropriate chronological age

3. Children who began primary immunizations at the recommended age, but have failed to receive all of the doses, do not need to begin the series again but instead receive only the missed doses

4. If it is suspected that the parent will not bring the child to the pediatrician or health care clinic for follow-up immunizations according to the optimal immunization schedule, any of the recommended vaccines can be administered simultaneously

B. General contraindications (Box 38-1)

C. Guidelines for administration (Box 38-2)

BOX 38-1

General Contraindications to Immunizations

Moderate or severe illnesses with or without a fever

Anaphylactic reaction to a previously administered vaccine or a substance in the vaccine

Live virus vaccines generally not administered to anyone with a compromised immune system

---

BOX 38-2

Guidelines for Vaccine Administration

Follow manufacturer's recommendations for route of administration, storage, and reconstitution of the vaccine.

If refrigeration is necessary, store on a center shelf and not in the door; frequent temperature increases from opening the refrigerator door can alter the vaccine's potency.

For protection against light, wrap the vial in aluminum foil.

A vaccine information statement needs to be given to the parents or individual and informed consent for administration needs to be obtained.

Check expiration date on vaccine bottle.

Parenteral vaccines are given in separate syringes in different injection sites.

Vaccines administered intramuscularly are given in the vastus lateralis muscle (best site) in newborns and in the deltoid for older infants and children (dorsogluteal site is avoided).

Maintain immunization record; document day, month, and year of administration; manufacturer and lot number of vaccine; name, address, title of person administering vaccine; site and route of administration.

A Vaccine Adverse Event Report (VAERS form) needs to be filed and the health department needs to be notified if an adverse reaction to an immunization occurs.

XV. RECOMMENDED IMMUNIZATIONS: CHILD AND ADOLESCENT (Box 38-3)

A. Hepatitis B vaccine
1. Protects against hepatitis B
2. The first dose of hepatitis B vaccine should be administered soon after birth and before hospital discharge; the first dose may also be given by age 2 years if the infant's mother is hepatitis B surface antigen (HBsAg)–negative
3. Only monovalent hepatitis B vaccine can be used for the birth dose and monovalent or combination vaccine containing hepatitis B may be used to complete the series
4. The second dose is administered at least 4 weeks after the first dose (except for combination vaccines, which cannot be administered before age 6 weeks)
5. The last dose in the vaccination series should not be administered before age 6 months
6. All children from birth through 18 years of age need three doses of hepatitis B vaccine if they have not already received them
7. Administered intramuscularly in the vastus lateralis muscle in newborns and in the deltoid for older infants and children (dorsogluteal site is avoided)
8. Contraindication: Anaphylactic reaction to common baker's yeast
9. HBsAg-positive mothers
   a. Infant should receive hepatitis B vaccine and hepatitis B immune globulin (HBIG) within 12 hours of birth at two different injection sites
   b. The second dose is recommended at age 1 to 2 months

BOX 38-3

Recommended Childhood and Adolescent Immunizations

AGE	VACCINE(S)
Birth	Hepatitis B
1 month	Hepatitis B
2 months	IPV, DTaP, Hib, PCV
4 months	DTaP, Hib, IPV, PCV
6 months	DTaP, Hib, hepatitis B, IPV, PCV
12-15 months	Hib, MMR, PCV
12-18 months	Varicella zoster
15-18 months	DTaP
4-6 years	DTaP, IPV, MMR
11-12 years	MMR (if not administered at 4-6 years), Td

DTaP, Diphtheria, tetanus, acellular pertussis; *Hib,* Haemophilus influenzae; *IPV,* inactivated polio vaccine; *MMR,* measles, mumps, rubella; *Td,* tetanus, diphtheria; *PCV,* pneumococcal vaccine.

c. The last dose should not be administered before age 6 months
d. Infant should be tested for HBsAg and anti-HBs antibodies at 9 to 15 months of age
10. Mother whose HBsAg status is unknown
    a. Infant should receive the first dose of hepatitis B vaccine series within 12 hours of birth
    b. Maternal blood should be drawn as soon as possible to determine the mother's HBsAg status
    c. If the HBsAg test is positive, the infant should receive HBIG as soon as possible (no later than age 1 week)
    d. The second dose is recommended at age 1 to 2 months
    e. The last dose should not be administered before age 6 months

B. Diphtheria, tetanus, acellular pertussis (DTaP), and tetanus and diphtheria (Td) toxoids
1. Protects against diphtheria, tetanus, and pertussis
2. DTaP is administered at 2 months, 4 months, 6 months, between 15 and 18 months, and between 4 and 6 years of age
3. The fourth dose of DTaP can be given at 12 months of age if 6 months have elapsed since the previous dose and if the child might not return for follow-up by 18 months of age
4. Td is given at 11 to 12 years of age if at least 5 years have passed since the last dose of Td-containing vaccine
5. Subsequent routine Td boosters are recommended every 10 years
6. Contraindication: Encephalopathy within 7 days of administration of previous dose of DTaP

C. *Haemophilus influenzae* type b (Hib) conjugate vaccine
1. Protects against a number of serious infections caused by *Haemophilus influenzae* type b, such as bacterial meningitis, epiglottitis, bacterial pneumonia, septic arthritis, and sepsis
2. Hib is administered at 2 months, 4 months, 6 months, and between 12 and 15 months of age
3. Depending on the brand of Hib vaccine used for the first and second doses, a dose at 6 months of age may not be needed
4. DTap-Hib combination products should not be used for primary immunization in infants ages 2, 4, or 6 months, but can be used as boosters following any Hib vaccine
5. Hib vaccines are administered by intramuscular injection and given at a separate site from any concurrent vaccinations
6. Contraindication: None identified

D. Inactivated poliovirus vaccine (IPV)
1. Protects against polio
2. IPV is administered at 2 months, 4 months, 6 months, and between 4 and 6 years of age

3. The third dose of IPV may be administered between 6 and 18 months of age
4. Contraindication: Anaphylactic reaction to neomycin or streptomycin

E. Measles, mumps, rubella vaccine (MMR)
1. Protects against measles, mumps, and rubella (German measles)
2. The first dose of MMR is administered between 12 and 15 months of age; the second dose is administered at 4 to 6 years of age (the second dose may be administered during any visit as long as at least 4 weeks have elapsed since the first dose, and as long as both doses have been administered beginning at or after age 12 months)
3. If the second dose was not given by 4 to 6 years of age, it should be given at the next scheduled pediatrician or health care clinic visit
4. Those who have not previously received the second dose should complete the schedule by the 11- to 12-year-old pediatrician or health care clinic visit
5. MMR contains minute amounts of neomycin; measles and mumps vaccines, which are grown on chick embryo tissue cultures, are not believed to contain significant amounts of egg cross-reacting proteins
6. Contraindications
   a. Pregnancy
   b. Known altered immunodeficiency
   c. Allergy to contents of immunization (prior to the administration of MMR vaccine, assess for a known history of allergy to neomycin or related antibiotics)
   d. Presence of recently acquired passive immunity through blood transfusions, immunoglobulin, or maternal antibodies (MMR should be postponed for a minimum of 3 months after passive immunization with immunoglobulins or blood transfusions, except washed blood cells, which do not interfere with the immune response)

F. Varicella zoster vaccine
1. Protects against chickenpox
2. Varicella zoster vaccine is administered between 12 and 18 months of age
3. Susceptible children 13 years of age and older (who have not had chickenpox or have not been previously vaccinated) need two doses given at least 4 weeks apart
4. Administered by subcutaneously injection
5. The vaccine should be kept frozen and used within 30 minutes of reconstitution to ensure viral potency
6. Contraindications
   a. Pregnancy
   b. Immunocompromised individuals
   c. Children receiving corticosteroids

G. Pneumococcal vaccine
1. A heptavalent pneumococcal conjugate vaccine (PCV) is recommended for all children 2 to 23 months of age
2. Can be given concurrently with other childhood vaccines at 2, 4, 6, and 12 to 15 months of age
3. Additionally, a single dose is recommended for certain children 24 to 59 months of age
4. Pneumococcal polysaccharide vaccine (PPV) is recommended in addition to PCV for children in certain high-risk groups

XVI. REACTIONS TO A VACCINE

A. Local reactions
1. Tenderness, erythema, and swelling at the injection site
2. Low-grade fever
3. Behavioral changes such as drowsiness, unusual crying, eating less

B. Minimizing local reactions
1. Select a needle of adequate length (1 inch in infants) to deposit the antigen deep into the muscle mass
2. Inject into the vastus lateralis muscle or ventrogluteal muscle; the deltoid may be used in children 18 months of age or older
3. Use an air bubble to clear the needle after injecting the vaccine

C. Anaphylactic reactions
1. The goals of treatment are to provide ventilation, restore adequate circulation, and prevent further exposure to the antigen
2. For a mild reaction with no evidence of respiratory distress or cardiovascular compromise: subcutaneous injection of an antihistamine such as diphenhydramine (Benadryl) and epinephrine (Adrenalin) will be prescribed
3. For moderate or severe distress: Establish an airway; cardiopulmonary resuscitation is initiated if not breathing; a head-elevated position is maintained; epinephrine, fluids, and vasopressor medications may be prescribed; monitor vital signs and urine output

XVII. VACCINES FOR SELECTED POPULATIONS

A. Hepatitis A vaccine
1. Recommended for children and adolescents in selected states and regions (communities with high-infection rates), and for certain high-risk groups
2. Given by the intramuscular route in the deltoid muscle

B. Influenza vaccine
1. Recommended annually for children from age 6 months with certain risk factors such as but

not limited to asthma, sickle cell disease, human immunodeficiency infection, diabetes mellitus, and household members of persons in groups at high risk

2. Recommended annually for adult groups at high risk
   a. Anyone 50 years of age or older
   b. Adults of any age with a chronic cardiac or pulmonary disease or chronic metabolic disease
   c. Residents of long-term care facilities
   d. Immunocompromised adults
   e. Women who will be in the second or third trimester of pregnancy during influenza season
   f. Health care workers
3. Usually administered by intramuscular injection; intranasal administration of influenza vaccine (FluMist) may be recommended for selected persons
4. Contraindicated in persons with anaphylactic hypersensitivity to eggs

C. Pneumococcal vaccine
   1. Recommended (one dose) for persons 65 years of age or older and those with chronic cardiovascular disease, chronic pulmonary disease, or diabetes mellitus
   2. Revaccination is advised if the individual was less than 65 years of age at the time of vaccination
   3. In immunocompromised persons, an initial vaccination is recommended, followed by revaccination every 5 years

D. Meningococcal vaccine
   1. Recommended for persons with medical indications, such as adults with terminal complement component deficiencies or anatomical or functional asplenia, or persons traveling to countries where the disease is hyperendemic or epidemic (revaccination at 3 to 5 years may be indicated for persons at high risk for infection)
   2. College freshman should be counseled about meningococcal disease so that they can make an informed decision about receiving the vaccine
   3. Administered by subcutaneous injection

E. Smallpox vaccine
   1. Protects people who work with smallpox or related viruses in laboratories
   2. The vaccinia virus is the "live virus" used in the smallpox vaccine; it is a "pox"-type virus related to smallpox
   3. The vaccine does not contain the smallpox virus and cannot cause smallpox
   4. Recommendations for use (Box 38-4)
   5. Getting the vaccine before exposure will most likely prevent smallpox

---

BOX 38-4

Recommendations for Smallpox Vaccine

ROUTINE NONEMERGENCY USE

Laboratory workers who handle cultures or animals contaminated with vaccinia or other related viruses such as monkeypox, cowpox, variola

Public health, hospital, and other personnel, generally 18 to 65 years of age, who may have to respond to a smallpox case or outbreak

EMERGENCY USE (SMALLPOX OUTBREAK)

Anyone directly exposed to smallpox virus: should get one dose of the vaccine as soon as possible after exposure

Anyone at risk of exposure to smallpox virus: may need to get one dose of the vaccine when the risk occurs or becomes known

---

6. Getting the vaccine within 3 days after exposure will help prevent the disease or make it less severe
7. Getting the vaccine within a week after exposure can also make the disease less severe
8. Protection from infection lasts 3 to 5 years, and protection from severe illness and death can last 10 years or more
9. Vaccinated persons may need to be revaccinated after 3 to 10 years, depending on risk
10. Site should be checked at about 7 days after vaccination to make sure that the vaccine is working (a successful vaccination is characterized by a pustular lesion or an area of definite induration or congestion surrounding a central lesion, which might be a scab or ulcer)
11. Expected reactions
    a. Formation of a blister and then a scar
    b. Swelling and tenderness of the lymph nodes lasting 2 to 4 weeks after the blister has healed, itching at the site, fatigue, mild fever, headache, or muscle aches
12. Adverse reactions
    a. Mild to moderate reactions: Mild rash, lasting 2 to 4 days, fever over 100° F (37.7° C), blisters on the body
    b. Moderate to severe problems: Eye infection (spread of the vaccine to the eye), rash on entire body
    c. Potentially life-threatening problems: Severe rash that can lead to scarring, encephalitis that can lead to permanent brain damage and death, severe progressive infection that can lead to death
    d. Can cause heart inflammation (myocarditis, pericarditis, myopericarditis)
13. Contraindications (Box 38-5)
14. Care of the vaccination site (Box 38-6)

BOX 38-5

Contraindications to Smallpox Vaccine

Anyone who has eczema or atopic dermatitis, or a past history of either condition

Anyone with a skin condition that causes breaks in the skin: should wait until the condition clears up

Anyone whose immune system is weakened

Pregnancy (women should avoid getting pregnant for 4 weeks after getting smallpox vaccine)

Breast-feeding mothers

Individuals who live with or have close physical contact with someone with a skin condition, a compromised immune system, who is pregnant, or younger than 1 year of age should not get the smallpox vaccine because it poses a risk to that person

Not recommended for anyone under 18 years of age

History of anaphylaxis reaction to polymyxin B, streptomycin, chlortetracycline, neomycin, or a previous dose of smallpox vaccine

Persons using steroid drops in their eyes

Persons who are moderately or severely ill at the time of vaccination: should usually wait until they recover before getting the vaccine

BOX 38-6

Care of the Vaccination Site

A scab will form in the spot where the vaccination was administered; this scab should be left alone so that the vaccinia virus in the vaccine doesn't spread to other parts of the body.

Hands need to be washed frequently and whenever the site is touched or the bandage is changed (the eyes or any other body part should not be touched after changing the bandage or touching the vaccination site).

The site is loosely covered with a gauze bandage; health care workers may need additional measures, such as placing a semipermeable dressing over the gauze bandage.

Gauze bandage is covered with a waterproof bandage while bathing.

Clothing is worn over the vaccination site as an extra precaution.

Used bandages are discarded in a plastic zip bag (the scab is discarded in the same manner).

Avoid sharing towels, and launder items that have touched the vaccination site.

Avoid scratching or putting ointment on the vaccination site.

XVIII. ACQUIRED IMMUNODEFICIENCY SYNDROME (AIDS)

A. Description
  1. A disorder caused by the human immunodeficiency virus (HIV); characterized by a generalized dysfunction of the immune system

  2. Both the cellular and the humoral immunity are compromised
  3. Horizontal transmission of HIV occurs through intimate sexual contact or parenteral exposure to blood or body fluids containing visible blood
  4. Vertical (perinatal) transmission occurs when an HIV-infected pregnant woman passes the infection to her infant
  5. The most common opportunistic infection of children infected with HIV is *Pneumocystis jiroveci* pneumonia (formerly known as *Pneumocystis carinii* pneumonia, PCP); it occurs most frequently between 3 and 6 months of age, when HIV status may be indeterminate
  6. The goals of therapy include slowing the growth of the virus, preventing and treating opportunistic viruses, and providing nutritional support and symptomatic treatment

B. Data collection
  1. During neonatal period
    a. Lymphadenopathy
    b. Hepatosplenomegaly
    c. *Pneumocystis jiroveci* pneumonia (formerly known as *Pneumocystis carinii* pneumonia, PCP)
    d. Progressive encephalopathy
    e. Microcephaly
  2. Infants
    a. Failure to thrive
    b. Diarrhea
    c. Developmental delays
    d. Oral candidiasis
    e. Hepatosplenomegaly
    f. Chronic cough and lymphoid interstitial pneumonia (LIP)
    g. Chronic otitis media
  3. Children and adolescents
    a. Malaise and fatigue
    b. Night sweats
    c. Weight loss
    d. Diarrhea
    e. Fever
    f. **Regression** of developmental milestones
    g. Generalized lymphadenopathy
    h. Nephropathy
    i. *Pneumocystis jiroveci pneumonia* and LIP
    j. Encephalopathy

C. Diagnostic tests (Box 38-7)
  1. Enzyme-linked immunosorbent assay (ELISA)
    a. ELISA determines the response of antibodies to the HIV virus
    b. Useful in children older than 18 months of age
  2. Western blot
    a. Confirms the presence of HIV antibodies
    b. Useful in children older than 18 months of age
    c. A positive HIV antibody test in children younger than 18 months of age indicates only

---

BOX 38-7

Diagnostic and Evaluative Tests

CD4$^+$
Enzyme-linked immunosorbent assay (ELISA)
p24 antigen detection
Polymerase chain reaction (PCR)
Virus culture
Western blot

---

that the mother is infected; other diagnostic tests will be used, including virus culture, polymerase chain reaction (PCR) for detection of proviral DNA, and p24 antigen detection, which is HIV-specific

3. p24 antigen
   a. Used to detect HIV antigen in children younger than 18 months of age
   b. Test can be useful at any age
   c. Only a positive result is significant
   d. Two or more positive results are diagnostic for HIV infection
4. CD4$^+$: Used to assess a child's immune status, risk for disease progression, and the need for prophylaxis against pneumonia after 1 year of age

XIX. CARE OF THE CHILD WITH HIV/AIDS

A. Prophylaxis
   1. Provide prophylaxis as prescribed against pneumonia during the first year of life to the infant born to an HIV-infected woman; after 1 year of age, the need for prophylaxis is determined by the presence of severe immunosuppression or a history of *pneumocystis jiroveci* pneumonia
   2. Provide continued prophylaxis through 12 months of age for children diagnosed with HIV
   3. For HIV-infected children older than 12 months, continued prophylaxis is based on CD4$^+$ counts and whether pneumonia has previously occurred
B. Antiretroviral therapy: Goal is to suppress viral replication to preserve immune function and to delay disease progression
C. Highly active antiretroviral therapy (HAART)
   1. Combination therapy that usually includes two nucleoside analogues, which target viral replication during the reverse transcription phase, and a protease inhibitor, which targets viral replication at a different phase
   2. Usually prescribed for an HIV-infected infant or child who exhibits clinical signs of infection or whose immune status in depressed, or for an HIV-infected infant younger than 1 year of age when the diagnosis is confirmed
D. Parent instructions
   1. Frequent hand washing

2. Monitor for fever, malaise, fatigue, weight loss, vomiting and diarrhea, altered activity level, and oral lesions; notify the physician if these occur
3. Monitor signs and symptoms of opportunistic infections
4. Administer antiretroviral medications, as prescribed
5. The child should avoid exposure to other illnesses
6. Keep immunizations up to date
7. Keep the child home when sick
8. Avoid kissing the child on the mouth
9. Monitor weight
10. Provide a high-calorie and high-protein diet
11. Avoid sharing eating utensils
12. Wash eating utensils in the dishwasher
13. Cover unused food and formula, and refrigerate
14. Discard unused refrigerated formula and food after 24 hours
15. Wear gloves for care, especially when in contact with body fluids and changing diapers
16. Change diapers frequently, away from food areas
17. Fold soiled disposable diapers inward, close with tabs, and dispose in a tightly covered plastic-lined container
18. Dispose of trash daily
19. Cover sandboxes when not in use to create a barrier to germs
20. Clean up spills with bleach solution (10:1 ratio of water to bleach)
E. Immunizations
   1. Immunizations against common childhood illnesses are recommended for all children exposed to or infected with HIV
   2. The varicella (chickenpox) vaccine is avoided
   3. Pneumococcal and influenza vaccines are administered
   4. Measles, mumps, rubella (MMR) vaccine is administered if the child is not severely immunocompromised (the child receiving IV gamma globulin prophylaxis may not respond to the MMR vaccine)

PRACTICE QUESTIONS

1. A child with rubeola (measles) is being admitted to the hospital. In preparing for the admission of the child, the nurse plans to institute which precaution for this child?
   1. Contact
   2. Enteric
   3. Respiratory
   4. Protective
2. Several children have contracted rubeola (measles) in a local school and the school nurse conducts

a teaching session for the mothers of the school-children. Which statement made by a mother indicates a need for further teaching regarding this communicable disease?

1. "Respiratory symptoms such as a very runny nose, cough, and fever occur before the development of a rash."
2. "Small blue-white spots with a red base may appear in the mouth."
3. "The rash usually begins behind the ears and spreads downward toward the feet."
4. "The communicable period ranges from 10 days before the onset of symptoms to 15 days after the rash appears."

3. A mother of a 15-month-old child brings the child to the clinic and reports that the child has a fever and has developed a rash on the neck and trunk. Roseola is diagnosed, and the mother is concerned that her other children will contract the disease. The nurse provides which instruction to the mother regarding prevention of transmission of the disease?

1. The disease is transmitted through the urine and feces, so the other children should use a separate bathroom
2. Disease transmission is unknown
3. The disease is transmitted through the respiratory tract, so the child should be isolated from the other children as much as possible
4. The disease is transmitted by contact with body fluids, so any items contaminated with body fluids need to discarded in a separate receptacle

4. The nurse provides instructions regarding respiratory precautions to the mother of a child with mumps. The mother asks the nurse about the length of time required for the respiratory precautions. The nurse tells the mother that:

1. Respiratory isolation in not necessary
2. Mumps is not transmitted by the respiratory system
3. Respiratory precautions are indicated during the period of communicability
4. Respiratory precautions are indicated for 18 days following the onset of parotid swelling

5. The mother brings her 6-year-old child to the clinic because the child has developed a rash on the trunk and on the scalp. The mother reports that the child has had a low-grade fever, has not felt like eating, and has been generally tired. The child is diagnosed with chickenpox, and the mother inquires about the communicable period associated with chickenpox. The nurse plans to base the response on which of the following?

1. The communicable period is unknown
2. The communicable period is 1 to 2 days before the onset of the rash to 6 days after the onset and crusting of lesions

3. The communicable period is 10 days before the onset of symptoms to 15 days after the rash appears
4. The communicable period ranges from 2 weeks or less up to several months

6. The nurse reinforces home care instructions to the parents of a child hospitalized with pertussis who is in the convalescent stage and is being prepared for discharge. Which statement by the parents indicates a need for further instructions?

1. "We need to maintain respiratory precautions and a quiet environment for at least 2 weeks."
2. "Coughing spells may be triggered by dust or smoke."
3. "We need to encourage an adequate fluid intake."
4. "Good hand washing techniques must be instituted to prevent spreading the disease to others."

7. A 6-month-old infant receives a DTaP (diphtheria, tetanus, and acellular pertussis) immunization at the well-baby clinic. The mother returns home and calls the clinic to report that the infant has developed swelling and redness at the site of injection. The nurse tells the mother to:

1. Leave the injection site alone because this always occurs
2. Bring the infant back to the clinic
3. Apply an ice pack to the injection site
4. Monitor the infant for a fever

8. A child is diagnosed with scarlet fever. The nurse collects data on the child, knowing that which of the following is a clinical manifestation associated with this disease?

1. Pastia's sign
2. Foul smelling mucopurulent nasal drainage
3. Gray membrane on the tonsils and pharynx
4. Abdominal pain and flaccid paralysis

9. A child is diagnosed with infectious mononucleosis, and the nurse reinforces home care instructions to the parents about the care of the child. The nurse tells the parents to:

1. Maintain the child on bed rest for 2 weeks
2. Maintain respiratory precautions for 1 week
3. Notify the physician if the child develops a fever
4. Notify the physician if the child develops abdominal pain or left shoulder pain occurs

10. The mother of a preschooler who attends day care calls the nurse and tells the nurse that the child is constantly itching the perianal area and that the area is irritated. The nurse suspects the possibility of pinworm infection (enterobiasis). The nurse instructs the mother to obtain a rectal specimen by the tape test and to obtain the specimen:

1. When the child is put to bed
2. After toileting
3. After bathing
4. In the morning when the child awakens

11. A nursing student is assigned to help administer immunizations to children in a clinic. The nursing instructor asks the student about the contraindications to receiving an immunization. The student responds correctly by telling the instructor that a contraindication for receiving an immunization is if a child has:
    1. A cold
    2. Otitis media
    3. Mild diarrhea
    4. A severe febrile illness

12. A mother with human immunodeficiency virus (HIV) infection brings her 10-month-old infant to the clinic for a routine checkup. The physician has documented that the infant is asymptomatic for HIV infection. After the checkup, the mother tells the nurse that she is so pleased that the infant will not get HIV. The nurse makes which response to the mother?
    1. "I am so pleased also that everything has turned out fine."
    2. "Everything looks great, but be sure that you return with your infant next month for the scheduled visit."
    3. "Most children infected with HIV develop symptoms within the first 9 months of life, and some become symptomatic some time before the age of 3 years."
    4. "Since symptoms have not developed, it is unlikely that the infant will develop HIV infection."

13. The clinic nurse prepares to administer an MMR (measles, mumps, rubella) vaccine to a 5-year-old child. The nurse administers this vaccine:
    1. Intramuscularly in the anterolateral aspect of the thigh
    2. Intramuscularly in the deltoid muscle
    3. Subcutaneously in the outer aspect of the upper arm
    4. Subcutaneously in the gluteal muscle

14. A child is scheduled to receive an MMR (measles, mumps, rubella) vaccine. The nurse preparing to administer the vaccine reviews the child's record and questions the order if which of the following is documented in the child's record?
    1. A local reaction at the site of a previous MMR vaccine injection
    2. A history of an anaphylactoid reaction to neomycin
    3. A history of frequent respiratory infections
    4. Recent recovery from a cold

15. A mother brings her 4-month-old infant to the well baby clinic for immunizations. The nurse would prepare to administer which of the following immunizations to this infant?
    1. DTaP (diphtheria, tetanus, acellular pertussis), MMR (measles, mumps, rubella), IPV (inactivated poliovirus vaccine)
    2. MMR, Hib (*Haemophilus influenzae* type b), DTaP
    3. DTaP, Hib, IPV, pneumococcal vaccine (PCV)
    4. Varicella and hepatitis B vaccines

ALTERNATE FORMAT QUESTION: MULTIPLE RESPONSE

Select the home care instructions that the nurse would provide to the mother of a child with acquired immunodeficiency syndrome (AIDS).

____ Frequent hand washing is important
____ Fever, malaise, fatigue, weight loss, vomiting and diarrhea are expected to occur and do not require special intervention
____ The child should avoid exposure to other illnesses
____ The child's immunization schedule will need revision
____ Kissing the child on the mouth will never transmit the virus
____ Clean up body fluid spills with bleach solution (10:1 ratio of water to bleach)

ANSWERS

1. *Answer: 3*
Rationale: Rubeola is transmitted via airborne particles or direct contact with infectious droplets. Respiratory precautions are required and a mask is worn by those in contact with the child. Gowns and gloves are not indicated. Articles that are contaminated should be bagged and labeled. Options 1, 2, and 4 are not indicated in rubeola.
Test-Taking Strategy: Use the process of elimination. Recalling that rubeola is transmitted via the airborne route will direct you to option 3. Review the route of transmission and therapeutic management of rubeola if you had difficulty with this question.
Level of Cognitive Ability: Application
Client Needs: Safe, Effective Care Environment
Integrated Process: Nursing Process/Planning
Content Area: Child Health
References: McKinney, E., James, S., Murray, S., & Ashwill, J. (2005). *Maternal-child nursing* (2nd ed.). St. Louis: Elsevier, p. 1020.

Wong, D., & Hockenberry, M. (2003). *Nursing care of infants and children* (7th ed.). St. Louis: Mosby, p. 655.

2. Answer: 4
Rationale: The communicable period for rubeola ranges from 4 days before to 5 days after the rash appears, mainly during the prodromal (catarrhal) stage. Options 1, 2, and 3 are accurate descriptions of rubeola. The small blue-white spots found in this communicable disease are called Koplik spots. Option 4, the incorrect option, describes the incubation period for rubella, not rubeola.
Test-Taking Strategy: Note the key words, *need for further teaching*. These words indicate a false response question and that you need to select the incorrect client statement. Remember that the communicable period for rubeola ranges from 4 days before to 5 days after the rash appears. Review the clinical manifestations associated with rubeola if you had difficulty with this question.
Level of Cognitive Ability: Comprehension
Client Needs: Health Promotion and Maintenance
Integrated Process: Teaching/Learning
Content Area: Child Health
Reference: Price, D., & Gwin, J. (2005). *Thompson's pediatric nursing* (9th ed.). Philadelphia: W.B. Saunders, p. 254.

3. Answer: 2
Rationale: The method of transmission of roseola is unknown. Options 1, 3, and 4 are not correct transmission routes of roseola.
Test-Taking Strategy: Use the process of elimination. Eliminate options 1 and 4 first because they are similar. From the remaining options, recall that the method of transmission of roseola is unknown. Review the characteristics of roseola if you had difficulty with this question.
Level of Cognitive Ability: Application
Client Needs: Safe, Effective Care Environment
Integrated Process: Teaching/Learning
Content Area: Child Health
Reference: Price, D., & Gwin, J. (2005). *Thompson's pediatric nursing* (9th ed.). Philadelphia: W.B. Saunders, p. 254.

4. Answer: 3
Rationale: Mumps is transmitted via direct contact or droplet spread from an infected person and possibly by contact with urine. Respiratory precautions are indicated during the period of communicability. Options 1, 2, and 4 are incorrect.
Test-Taking Strategy: Use the process of elimination. Options 1 and 2 can be eliminated first because they are similar. From the remaining options, select option 3, because it is the umbrella (global option), and addresses communicability. Also, the time frame indicated in option 4 seems rather lengthy. Review the infectious period related to mumps if you had difficulty with this question.
Level of Cognitive Ability: Application
Client Needs: Safe, Effective Care Environment
Integrated Process: Teaching/Learning
Content Area: Child Health
References: Price, D., & Gwin, J. (2005). *Thompson's pediatric nursing* (9th ed.). Philadelphia: W.B. Saunders, p. 255.

Wong, D., & Hockenberry, M. (2003). *Nursing care of infants and children* (7th ed.). St. Louis: Mosby, p. 657.

5. Answer: 2
Rationale: The communicable period for chickenpox is 1 to 2 days before the onset of the rash to 6 days after the onset and crusting of lesions. In roseola, the communicable period is unknown. Option 3 describes rubella. Option 4 describes diphtheria.
Test-Taking Strategy: Use the process of elimination. Option 1 can be easily eliminated first. Eliminate options 3 and 4 next because the time frames in these two options seem rather lengthy and are similar. If you had difficulty with this question, review the communicable period for chickenpox.
Level of Cognitive Ability: Application
Client Needs: Safe, Effective Care Environment
Integrated Process: Teaching/Learning
Content Area: Child Health
Reference: Price, D., & Gwin, J. (2005). *Thompson's pediatric nursing* (9th ed.). Philadelphia: W.B. Saunders, p. 250.

6. Answer: 1
Rationale: Pertussis is transmitted by direct contact or respiratory droplets from coughing. The communicable period occurs primarily during the catarrhal stage. Respiratory precautions are not required during the convalescent phase. Options 2, 3, and 4 are components of home care instructions.
Test-Taking Strategy: Note the key words, *convalescent* and *need for further instructions*. These words indicate a false response question and that you need to select the incorrect statement. Options 3 and 4 can be easily eliminated because they are general interventions associated with convalescence. Knowing that coughing spells are associated with pertussis will assist in directing you to option 1 from the remaining options. Additionally, a 2-week period of respiratory precautions is not required. If you had difficulty with this question, review home care instructions for the child with pertussis.
Level of Cognitive Ability: Comprehension
Client Needs: Health Promotion and Maintenance
Integrated Process: Teaching/Learning
Content Area: Child Health
Reference: Leifer, G. (2003). *Introduction to maternity and pediatric nursing* (4th ed.). Philadelphia: W.B. Saunders, p. 744.

7. Answer: 3
Rationale: Occasionally, tenderness, redness, or swelling may occur at the site of the injection. This can be relieved with ice packs for the first 24 hours, followed by warm compresses if the inflammation persists. It is not necessary to bring the infant back to the clinic. Option 4 may be an appropriate intervention but is not specific to the issue of the question.
Test-Taking Strategy: Use the process of elimination. Eliminate option 1 first because of the absolute word "always." Option 4 can be eliminated next because it does not relate specifically to the issue of the question, and then eliminate option 2 as an unnecessary intervention. Review interventions following immunizations and injections if you had difficulty with this question.

Level of Cognitive Ability: Application
Client Needs: Health Promotion and Maintenance
Integrated Process: Nursing Process/Implementation
Content Area: Child Health
Reference: Wong, D., & Hockenberry, M. (2003). *Nursing care of infants and children* (7th ed.). St. Louis: Mosby, pp. 534-535.

8. Answer: 1
Rationale: Pastia's sign describes a rash seen in scarlet fever that will blanch with pressure, except in areas of deep creases and the folds of joints. The tongue is initially coated with a white furry covering with red projecting papillae (white strawberry tongue). By the fourth to fifth day, the white strawberry tongue sloughs off, leaving a red swollen tongue (strawberry tongue). The pharynx is edematous and beefy red in color. Options 2 and 3 are characteristics of diphtheria. Option 4 is associated with poliomyelitis.
Test-Taking Strategy: Focus on the issue, the clinical manifestation associated with scarlet fever. Remember that Pastia's sign describes the rash noted in scarlet fever. Review the clinical manifestations associated with scarlet fever if you had difficulty with this question.
Level of Cognitive Ability: Analysis
Client Needs: Physiological Integrity
Integrated Process: Nursing Process/Data Collection
Content Area: Child Health
Reference: Leifer, G. (2003). *Introduction to maternity and pediatric nursing* (4th ed.). Philadelphia: W.B. Saunders, p. 746.

9. Answer: 4
Rationale: The parents need to be instructed to notify the physician if abdominal pain, especially in the left upper quadrant, or left shoulder pain occurs, because this may indicate splenic rupture. Children with enlarged spleens are also instructed to avoid contact sports until splenomegaly resolves. Bed rest is not necessary, and children usually self-limit their activity. Respiratory precautions are not required, although transmission can occur via direct intimate contact or contact with infected blood. Fever is treated with acetaminophen (Tylenol).
Test-Taking Strategy: Use the process of elimination and knowledge regarding the organs affected in mononucleosis. Options 1 and 2 can be eliminated first because they are unnecessary interventions in this disease. From the remaining options, knowledge that splenic rupture is a concern will direct you to option 4. Review the complications associated with mononucleosis if you had difficulty with this question.
Level of Cognitive Ability: Application
Client Needs: Physiological Integrity
Integrated Process: Teaching/Learning
Content Area: Child Health
Reference: Price, D., & Gwin, J. (2005). *Thompson's pediatric nursing* (9th ed.). Philadelphia: W.B. Saunders, p. 325.

10. Answer: 4
Rationale: Diagnosis is confirmed by direct visualization of the worms. Parents can view the sleeping child's anus with a flashlight. The worm is white, thin, about ½-inch long,

and moves. A simple technique, the tape test, is used to capture worms and eggs. Transparent tape is lightly touched to the anus and then applied to a slide for examination. The best specimens are obtained as the child awakens, before toileting or bathing.
Test-Taking Strategy: Use the process of elimination. Thinking about the test and the purpose of the test (to obtain a specimen that contains worms and eggs) will direct you to option 4. Review the procedure for this test if you are unfamiliar with it.
Level of Cognitive Ability: Application
Client Needs: Physiological Integrity
Integrated Process: Nursing Process/Implementation
Content Area: Child Health
Reference: Price, D., & Gwin, J. (2005). *Thompson's pediatric nursing* (9th ed.). Philadelphia: W.B. Saunders, p. 192.

11. Answer: 4
Rationale: A severe febrile illness is a reason to delay immunization, but only until the child has recovered from the acute stage of the illness. Minor illnesses such as a cold, otitis media, or mild diarrhea are not contraindications to immunization.
Test-Taking Strategy: Use the process of elimination focusing on the issue of the question, a contraindication to receiving an immunization. Noting the word "severe" in option 4 will direct you to this option. If you had difficulty with this question, review the contraindications associated with immunizations.
Level of Cognitive Ability: Comprehension
Client Needs: Physiological Integrity
Integrated Process: Teaching/Learning
Content Area: Child Health
Reference: Price, D., & Gwin, J. (2005). *Thompson's pediatric nursing* (9th ed.). Philadelphia: W.B. Saunders, p. 122.

12. Answer: 3
Rationale: Most children infected with HIV develop symptoms within the first 9 months of life. The remainder of these infected children become symptomatic sometime before the age of 3 years. Children, with their immature immune systems, have a much shorter incubation period than adults. Options 1, 2, and 4 are incorrect.
Test-Taking Strategy: Use the process of elimination. Eliminate options 1, 2, and 4 because they are similar in content. Option 3 is the only option that provides specific and accurate data regarding HIV infection in the infant. Review assessment findings associated with HIV infection if you had difficulty with this question.
Level of Cognitive Ability: Application
Client Needs: Psychosocial Integrity
Integrated Process: Nursing Process/Implementation
Content Area: Child Health
Reference: James, S., Ashwill, J., & Droske, S. (2002). *Nursing care of children: Principles and practice* (2nd ed.). Philadelphia; W.B. Saunders, p. 488.

13. Answer: 3
Rationale: MMR vaccine is administered subcutaneously in the outer aspect of the upper arm. The gluteal muscle is most

often used for intramuscular injections. MMR vaccine is not administered by the intramuscular route.

Test-Taking Strategy: Use the process of elimination. Recalling that MMR vaccine is administered subcutaneously will assist in eliminating options 1 and 2. From the remaining options, recalling that the gluteal muscle is most often used for intramuscular injections will assist in directing you to option 3. Review the procedures related to the administration of MMR vaccine if you had difficulty with this question.

Level of Cognitive Ability: Application
Client Needs: Physiological Integrity
Integrated Process: Nursing Process/Implementation
Content Area: Child Health
Reference: Price, D., & Gwin, J. (2005). *Thompson's pediatric nursing* (9th ed.). Philadelphia: W.B. Saunders, p. 123.

14. Answer: 2
Rationale: MMR vaccine contains minute amounts of neomycin. A history of an anaphylactoid reaction to neomycin is considered a contraindication to the MMR vaccine. The general contraindication to all immunizations is a severe febrile illness. The presence of minor illnesses such as a common cold is not a contraindication. Additionally, a history of frequent respiratory infections is not a contraindication to receiving a vaccine. A local reaction to an immunization is treated with ice packs for the first 24 hours after injection, followed by warm compresses if the inflammation persists.

Test-Taking Strategy: Use the process of elimination. Recalling that a general contraindication to all immunizations is a severe febrile illness will assist in eliminating options 3 and 4. From the remaining options, note that option 1 identifies a local reaction. This will direct you to option 2, the systemic reaction, and a potential life-threatening condition. Review the contraindications to receiving immunizations if you had difficulty with this question.

Level of Cognitive Ability: Analysis
Client Needs: Physiological Integrity
Integrated Process: Nursing Process/Implementation
Content Area: Child Health
Reference: Schulte, E., Price, D., & Gwin, J. (2001). *Thompson's pediatric nursing* (8th ed.). Philadelphia: W.B. Saunders, pp. 386-387.

15. Answer: 3
Rationale: DTaP, Hib, IPV, and PCV are administered at 4 months of age. DTaP is administered at 2 months, 4 months, 6 months, between 12 and 18 months, and between 4 and 6 years of age. Hib is administered at 2 months, 4 months, 6 months, and between 12 and 15 months of age. IPV is administered at 2 months, 4 months, 6 months, and between 4 to 6 years of age. The first dose of MMR is administered between 12 and 15 months of age; the second dose is administered at 4 to 6 years of age (if the second dose was not given by 4 to 6 years of age, it should be given at the next visit). The first dose of hepatitis B vaccine is administered between the birth and 2 months, the second dose is administered between 1 and 4 months, and the third dose is administered between 6 and 18 months of age. Varicella zoster vaccine is administered between 12 and 18 months of age. PCV is administered at 2,4,6, and between 12 and 15 months of age.

Test-Taking Strategy: Knowledge regarding the immunization schedule for infants and children is required to answer this question. Noting the age of the infant in the question will assist in directing you to option 3. Learn the immunization schedule if you are unfamiliar with it.

Level of Cognitive Ability: Application
Client Needs: Health Promotion and Maintenance
Integrated Process: Nursing Process/Planning
Content Area: Child Health
References: Centers for Disease Control and Prevention. (2005). *Recommended childhood and adolescent immunization schedule.* Atlanta: CDC. Retrieved April 29, 2005, from http://www.cdc.gov/nip.

ALTERNATE FORMAT QUESTION: MULTIPLE RESPONSE

Answers:
Frequent hand washing is important
The child should avoid exposure to other illnesses
Clean up body fluid spills with bleach solution (10:1 ratio of water to bleach)

Rationale: AIDS is a disorder caused by the human immunodeficiency virus (HIV) and is characterized by a generalized dysfunction of the immune system. Both cellular and humoral immunity are compromised. Horizontal transmission of HIV occurs through intimate sexual contact or parenteral exposure to blood or body fluids containing visible blood. Vertical (perinatal) transmission occurs when an HIV-infected pregnant woman passes the infection to her infant. Home care instructions include the following: frequent hand washing; monitoring for fever, malaise, fatigue, weight loss, vomiting and diarrhea, altered activity level, and oral lesions, and notifying the physician if these occur; monitoring for signs and symptoms of opportunistic infections; administering antiretroviral medications as prescribed; avoiding exposure to other illnesses; keeping immunizations up to date; avoiding kissing the child on the mouth; monitoring weight and providing a high-calorie and high-protein diet; and washing eating utensils in the dishwasher and avoiding sharing of eating utensils. Gloves are worn for care, especially when in contact with body fluids and changing diapers (diapers are changed frequently and away from food areas) and soiled disposable diapers are folded inward, tabbed, and disposed of in a tightly covered plastic-lined container. Any body fluid spills are cleaned with a bleach solution (10:1 ratio of water to bleach).

Test-Taking Strategy: Focus on the issue, care of the child with AIDS. Recalling that this disorder is characterized by a generalized dysfunction of the immune system and recalling the modes of transmission of the virus will assist in selecting the home care instructions. Review these instructions if you had difficulty with this question.

Level of Cognitive Ability: Application
Client Needs: Safe, Effective Care Environment
Integrated Process: Teaching/Learning
Content Area: Child Health
Reference: James, S., Ashwill, J., & Droske, S. (2002). *Nursing care of children: Principles and practice* (2nd ed.). Philadelphia; W.B. Saunders, p. 489.

REFERENCES

American Academy of Family Physicians. Web site: http://www.aafp.org.

American Academy of Pediatrics. Web site: http://www.aap.org.

Centers for Disease Control and Prevention. (2005). *Recommended childhood and adolescent immunization schedule.* Atlanta: CDC. Retrieved April 29, 2005 from http://www.cdc.gov/nip.

Centers for Disease Control and Prevention. (2004). *Smallpox prevaccination information packet.* Atlanta: CDC. Retrieved January 16, 2004 from http://www.bt.cdc.gov/agent/smallpox/basics/index.asp.

Immunization Action Coalition. Web site: http://www.immunize.org.

James, S., Ashwill, J., & Droske, S. (2002). *Nursing care of children: Principles and practice* (2nd ed.). Philadelphia; W.B. Saunders.

Leifer, G. (2003). *Introduction to maternity and pediatric nursing* (4th ed.). Philadelphia: W.B. Saunders.

McKinney, E., James, S., Murray, S., & Ashwill, J. (2005). *Maternal-child nursing* (2nd ed.). St. Louis: Elsevier.

Price, D., & Gwin, J. (2005). *Thompson's pediatric nursing* (9th ed.). Philadelphia: W.B. Saunders.

Schulte, E., Price, D., & Gwin, J. (2001). *Thompson's pediatric nursing* (8th ed.). Philadelphia: W.B. Saunders.

U.S. Department of Health and Human Services. (2003). *Smallpox vaccine: What you need to know.* Atlanta: Centers for Disease Control and Prevention, National Immunization Program, pp. 1-2.

Wong, D., & Hockenberry, M. (2003). *Nursing care of infants and children* (7th ed.). St. Louis: Mosby.

Pediatric Medication Administration

I. MEDICATIONS AND THE PEDIATRIC CLIENT

A. Pediatric clients are smaller than an adult and their medications have to be adapted to their size and age

B. Neonates and premature infants have immature body systems

C. The absorption, distribution, metabolism, and excretion of medications differ substantially, and the pediatric client will react more quickly to medication than an adult (Figure 39-1)

D. Medication reactions are not as predictable in a pediatric client as they are in an adult

II. ADMINISTERING ORAL MEDICATIONS

A. Most oral pediatric medications are in liquid or suspension form, because children usually cannot swallow a tablet

B. Solutions may be measured by using an oral syringe; if an oral syringe is not available, hypodermic syringes without the needle can be used for dosage measurement

C. When volumes are extremely small, oral liquids are measured by using a calibrated medication dropper

D. Medications in suspension settle to the bottom of the bottle between uses, and thorough mixing is required prior to pouring of the medication

▲ E. Suspensions must be administered immediately after measurement to prevent settling and administration of an incomplete dose

▲ F. Administer oral medications with the child sitting in an upright position, and with the head elevated, to prevent aspiration if the child cries or resists

▲ G. Never pinch the infant or child's nostrils when administering medication

▲ H. Do not place medication into a baby's bottle

I. Draw the required dose of an unpleasant medication into a small syringe, and place the syringe into the side and toward the back of the infant's mouth; administer the medication slowly, allowing the infant to swallow

J. Place the small child sideways on the adult's lap; the child's closest arm should be placed under the adult's arm and behind the adult's back; cradle the child's head, hold the child's hand, and administer the medication slowly with a plastic spoon or small plastic cup

K. Mix liquid medications with less than 1 ounce of fluid to disguise the taste if necessary

L. If a tablet or capsule has been administered, check the child's mouth to ensure that it has been swallowed; if swallowing is a problem, some tablets can be crushed and given in small amounts of pureed food or flavored syrup (enteric-coated tablets, timed-release tablets, and capsules cannot be crushed)

III. ADMINISTERING PARENTERAL MEDICATIONS

A. Subcutaneous and intramuscularly administered medications

1. Medications most often given via the subcutaneous route are insulin and most immunizations

2. Any site with sufficient subcutaneous tissue may be used for subcutaneous injections; common sites include the central third of the lateral aspect of the upper arm, the abdomen, and the center third of the anterior thigh

3. The safe use of all injection sites is based on normal muscle development and the size of the child; the preferred site for intramuscular injections in infants is the vastus lateralis (Figure 39-2)

4. Usually not more than 0.5 mL (infant) to 2.0 mL (child) is injected per intramuscular or

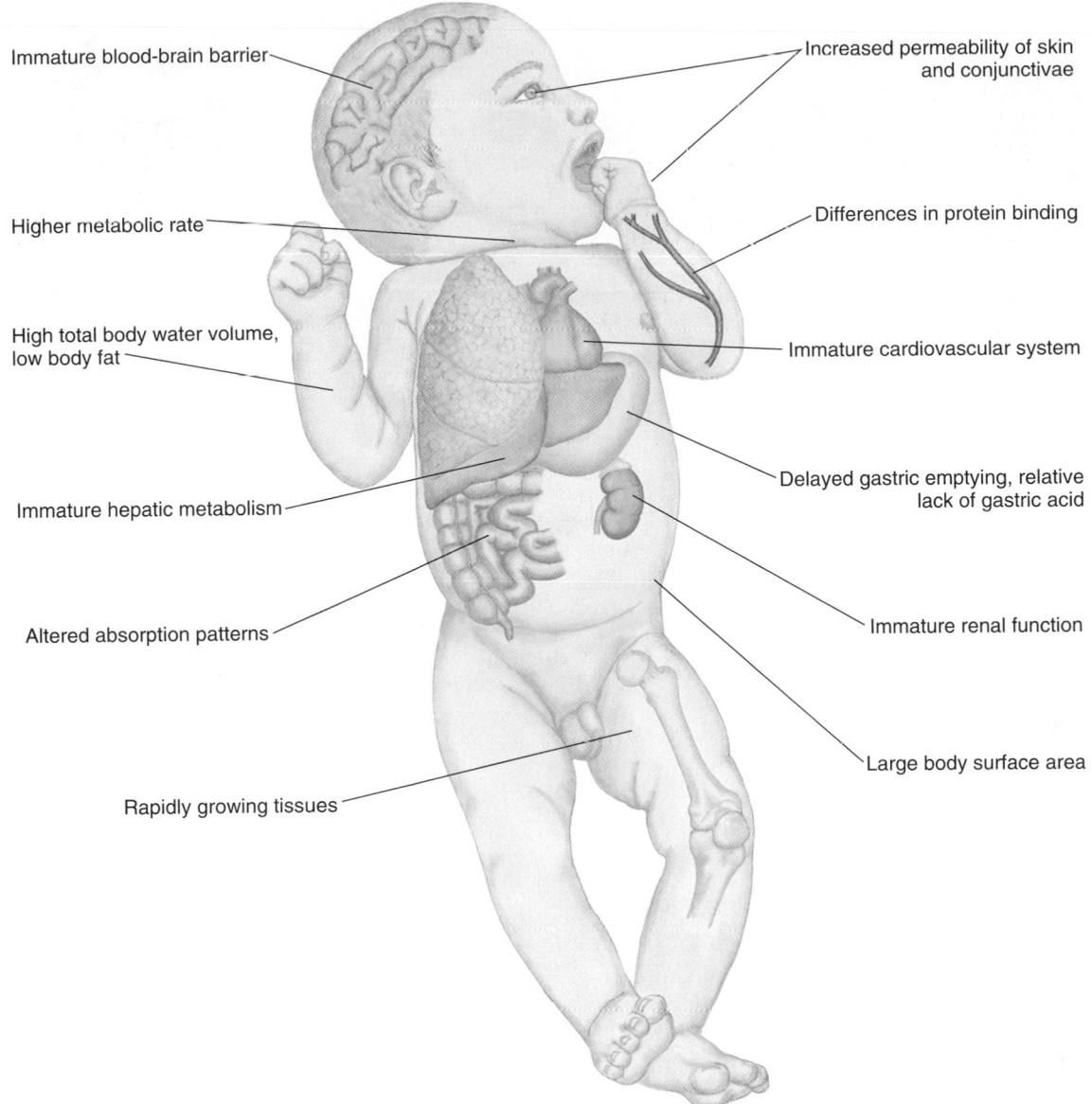

Immature blood-brain barrier

Increased permeability of skin and conjunctivae

Higher metabolic rate

Differences in protein binding

High total body water volume, low body fat

Immature cardiovascular system

Immature hepatic metabolism

Delayed gastric emptying, relative lack of gastric acid

Altered absorption patterns

Immature renal function

Large body surface area

Rapidly growing tissues

FIG. 39-1 Some factors affecting drug disposition in children. (From Price, D., & Gwin, J. [2005]. *Thompson's pediatric nursing* [9th ed.]. Philadelphia: W.B. Saunders.)

subcutaneous site; the site of injection is rotated if frequent injections are necessary

5. For pediatric clients, the usual needle length is $\frac{1}{2}$ to 1 inch and needle gauge is 22 to 25

6. Needle length can also be estimated by grasping the muscle for injection between the thumb and forefinger; half the resulting distance between thumb and forefinger would be the needle length

7. Pediatric dosages for subcutaneous and intramuscular administration are calculated to the nearest hundredth and measured by using a tuberculin (TB) syringe

8. For the toddler or preschooler, place an adhesive bandage or decorated Band-Aid over the puncture site

B. Monitoring intravenous (IV) medications

1. When an infant or child is receiving an IV medication, the IV site needs to be assessed for signs of infiltration and inflammation immediately before, during, and after completion of administration of each medication (Box 39-1)

2. Signs of infiltration or inflammation need to be reported

IV. **CALCULATION OF MEDICATION DOSAGE BY BODY WEIGHT**

A. Conversion of body weight (Box 39-2)

B. Calculating daily dosages

1. Abbreviations (Box 39-3)

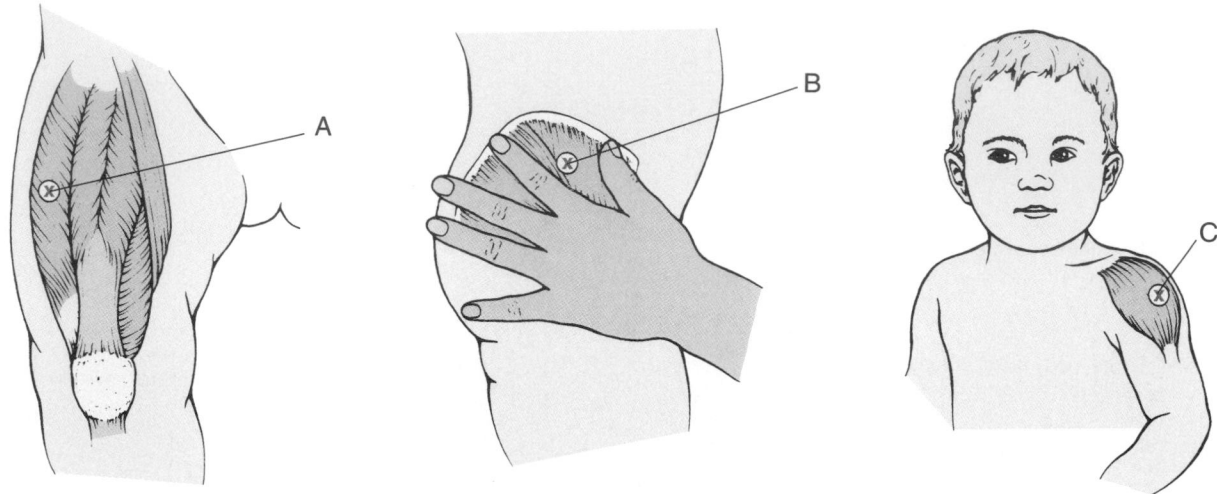

FIG. 39-2 Appropriate sites for intramuscular injections in children. **A,** Vastus lateralis. **B,** Ventrogluteal. **C,** Deltoid. (From Leifer, G. [2003]. *Introduction to maternity and pediatric nursing* [4th ed.]. Philadelphia: W.B. Saunders.)

2. Dosages are expressed in terms of mg/kg/day, mg/lb/day, or mg/kg/dose
3. The total daily dosage is usually administered in divided (more than one) doses per day
4. Express the child's body weight in kilograms or pounds to correlate with the dosage specifications
5. Calculate the total daily dosage
6. Divide the total daily dosage by the number of doses to be administered in 1 day

V. CALCULATION OF BODY SURFACE AREA (BSA)

A. The body surface area is determined by comparing body weight and height with averages or norms on a graph called a nomogram
B. Not all children are the same size at the same age; therefore, the nomogram chart is used to determine the BSA of a child
C. Look at the nomogram chart (Figure 39-3), and note that the height is on the left-hand side of the chart and the weight is on the right-hand side
D. Place a ruler on the chart
E. Line up the left side of the ruler on the height and the right side of the ruler on the weight; read the BSA at the point where the straight edge of the ruler intersects the surface area (SA) column
F. The estimated SA is given in square meters (m^2)
G. See Box 39-4 for an example

VI. CALCULATION BASED ON BSA

A. When dosage recommendations for children specify mg, mcg, or unit per m^2, calculating the dosage is simple multiplication (Box 39-5)
B. When dosages are specified only for adults, a formula is used to calculate a child's dosage from the adult dosage (Box 39-6)

BOX 39-1

Intravenous Site: Signs of Inflammation and Infiltration

Inflammation: Redness, heat, swelling, and tenderness
Infiltration: Swelling, coolness, pain, and lack of blood return

---

BOX 39-2

Conversion of Body Weight

POUNDS (lb) TO KILOGRAMS (kg)
1 kg = 2.2 lb
To convert from pounds to kilograms, divide by 2.2. Kilograms are expressed to the nearest tenth.

KILOGRAMS (kg) TO POUNDS (lb)
1 kg = 2.2 lb
To convert from kilograms to pounds, multiply by 2.2. Pounds are expressed to the nearest tenth.

BOX 39-3

Abbreviations

gr = grain(s)
g = gram(s)
mcg = microgram(s)
mg = milligram(s)
kg = kilogram(s)
lb = pound(s)
mL = milliliter(s)
BSA = body surface area
SA = surface area
m^2 = square meters

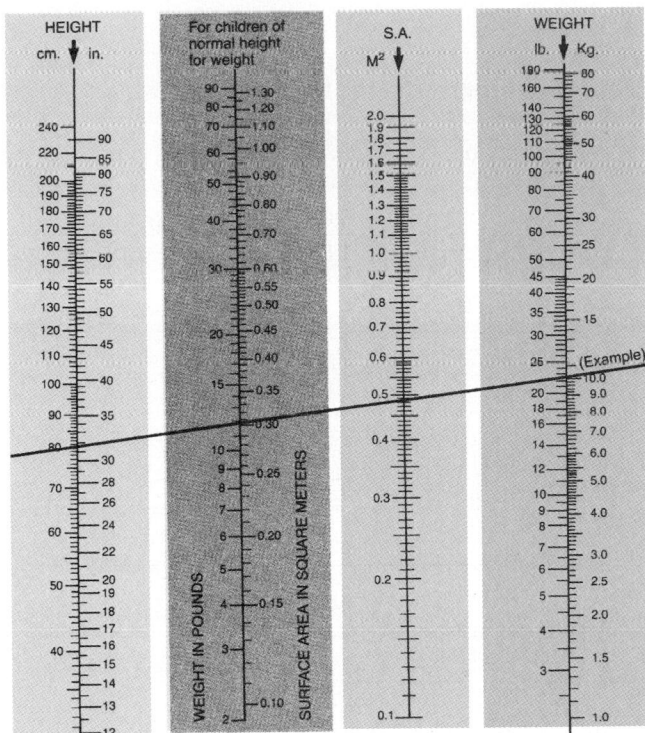

FIG. 39-3 Nomogram chart for estimating body surface area. (From Price, D., & Gwin, J. [2005]. *Thompson's pediatric nursing* [9th ed.]. Philadelphia: W.B. Saunders.)

PRACTICE QUESTIONS

1. Penicillin V (Pen-Veek), 250 mg orally every 8 hours, is prescribed for a child with a respiratory infection. The child's weight is 45 pounds. The safe pediatric dosage is 25 to 50 mg/kg/day. The nurse determines that:
   1. The dose is too low
   2. The dose is too high
   3. The dose is within the safe dosage range
   4. There is not enough information to determine the safe dose

2. A physician has prescribed phenobarbital sodium (Luminal Sodium), 25 mg orally twice daily, for a child with febrile seizures. The medication label reads "phenobarbital sodium, 20 mg/5 mL." The nurse has determined that the dose prescribed is a safe dose for the child. The nurse administers how many milliliters per dose to the child?
   1. 2 mL
   2. 4.5 mL
   3. 6.25 mL
   4. 7 mL

3. Cloxacillin (Tegopen), 100 mg orally every 8 hours, is prescribed for a child with an elevated temperature who is suspected of having a respiratory tract infection. The child weighs 17 pounds. The safe pediatric dosage is 50 mg/kg/day. The nurse determines that:
   1. The dose is too low

BOX 39-4

How to Use the Nomogram

Example: Use the nomogram and calculate the body surface area (BSA) for a child whose height is 58 inches and weight is 12 kg.

Look at the nomogram chart and note that the height is on the left-hand side of the chart and the weight is on the right-hand side

Place a ruler on the chart and line up the left side of the ruler on the height and the right side of the ruler on the weight. Read the BSA at the point where the straight edge of the ruler intersects the surface area (SA) column.

The estimated SA is given in square meters (m^2).

Answer: BSA = 0.66 m^2

BOX 39-5

Calculating Medication Dosage

When dosage recommendations for children specify mg, mcg, or unit/m^2, calculating the dosage is simple multiplication.

Example: The dosage recommendation is 4 mg/m^2. The child has a body surface area (BSA) of 1.1 m^2. What is the dosage to be administered?

Answer: 1.1 × 4 mg = 4.4 mg

BOX 39-6

Calculating a Child's Dosage from the Adult Dosage

When dosages are specified only for adults, a formula is used to calculate a child's dosage from the adult dosage

Example: A physician has prescribed an antibiotic for a child. The average adult dose is 250 mg. The child has a body surface area (BSA) of 0.41 m^2. What is the dose for the child?

Answer: 59.24 mg

Formula:

$$\frac{\text{BSA of child } (m^2)}{1.73 \ m^2} \times \text{adult dose} = \text{child's dose}$$

$$\frac{0.41}{1.73} \times 250 \text{ mg} = 59.24 \text{ mg}$$

   2. The dose is too high
   3. The dose is within the safe dosage range
   4. There is not enough information to determine the safe dose

4. Sulfisoxazole (Gantrisin), 1.0 g orally four times daily, is prescribed for an adolescent with a urinary tract infection. The medication label reads "500-mg tablets." The nurse has determined that the dose prescribed is safe. The nurse administers how many tablets per dose to the adolescent?
   1. 0.5 tablet

   2. 1 tablet
   3. 2 tablets
   4. 3 tablets

5. Diphenhydramine hydrochloride (Benadryl), 25 mg orally every 6 hours, is prescribed for a child with an allergic reaction. The child weighs 25 kg. The safe pediatric dosage is 5 mg/kg/day. The nurse determines that:
   1. The dose is too low
   2. The dose is too high
   3. The dose is within the safe dosage range
   4. There is not enough information to determine the safe dose

6. Penicillin G procaine (Wycillin), 1,000,000 units intramuscular, is prescribed for an adolescent with an infection. The medication label reads "1,200,000 units/2 mL." The nurse has determined that the dose prescribed is safe. The nurse administers how many milliliters per dose to the adolescent?
   1. 0.8 mL
   2. 1.2 mL
   3. 1.44 mL
   4. 1.66 mL

7. Morphine sulfate, 2.5 mg, is prescribed for a child with cancer. The safe pediatric dose is 0.05 to 0.1 mg/kg/dose. The child weighs 50 kg. The nurse determines that:
   1. The dose is too low
   2. The dose is too high
   3. The dose is within the safe dosage range
   4. There is not enough information to determine the safe dosage range

8. Morphine sulfate, 2.5 mg subcutaneously, is prescribed for a child postoperatively. The medication label reads "$^1/_{15}$ grains/mL." The nurse has determined that the dose is safe. The nurse administers how many milliliters to the child?

   1. 0.62 mL
   2. 0.82 mL
   3. 1.35 mL
   4. 1.62 mL

9. A physician's order reads "ampicillin (Omnipen), 125 mg intramuscular every 6 hours." The medication label reads "1 gram and reconstitute with 7.4 mL of bacteriostatic water." The nurse draws up how many milliliters to administer one dose?
   1. 0.54 mL
   2. 0.92 mL
   3. 1.1 mL
   4. 7.4 mL

10. A pediatric client with ventricular septal defect repair is placed on a maintenance dosage of digoxin (Lanoxin) elixir. The safe dosage is 0.03 mg/kg/day, and the client's weight is 7.2 kg. The physician orders the digoxin to be given twice daily. The nurse prepares how much digoxin to administer to the client at each dose?
   1. 0.1 mg
   2. 0.37 mg
   3. 0.5 mg
   4. 2.5 mg

ALTERNATE FORMAT QUESTION: FILL IN THE BLANK

Atropine sulfate, 0.2 mg intramuscular, is prescribed for a child preoperatively. The medication label reads "0.4 mg per mL." The nurse has determined that the dose prescribed is safe. The nurse prepares to administer how many milliliters to the child?

Answer: _____

ANSWERS

1. *Answer: 3*
Rationale: Convert pounds to kilograms by dividing by 2.2.
Pounds to kilograms:

$$45 \text{ lb divided by } 2.2 \text{ lb/kg} = 20.45 \text{ kg}$$

Dosage parameters:

$$25 \text{ mg/kg/day} \times 20.45 \text{ kg} = 511.25 \text{ mg/day}$$
$$50 \text{ mg/kg/day} \times 20.45 \text{ kg} = 1022.5 \text{ mg/day}$$

Dose frequency:

$$250 \text{ mg} \times 3 \text{ doses (every 8 hours)} = 750 \text{ mg/day}$$

The dose is within the safe dosage range.
Test-Taking Strategy: Identify the key components of the question and what the question is asking. In this case, the question asks for the safe dosage range for medication. Change pounds to kilograms. Calculate the dosage parameters using the safe dose range identified in the question and the child's weight in kilograms. Use a calculator to verify the answer and remember to determine the total daily dosage before selecting an option.

Review pediatric medication calculations if you had difficulty with this question.
Level of Cognitive Ability: Analysis
Client Needs: Physiological Integrity
Integrated Process: Nursing Process/Planning
Content Area: Child Health
Reference: Kee, J., & Marshall, S. (2004). *Clinical calculations: With applications to general and specialty areas* (5th ed.). Philadelphia: W.B. Saunders, pp. 234-236.

2. *Answer: 3*
Rationale: Use the medication calculation formula.
Formula:

$$\frac{\text{Desired}}{\text{Available}} \times \text{volume} = \frac{25 \text{ mg}}{20 \text{ mg}} \times 5 \text{ mL} = 6.25 \text{ mL/dose}$$

Test-Taking Strategy: Identify the key components of the question and what the question is asking. In this case, the question asks for milliliters per dose. Use the formula to determine the

correct dosage and use a calculator to verify the answer. Review pediatric medication calculations if you had difficulty with this question.
Level of Cognitive Ability: Application
Client Needs: Physiological Integrity
Integrated Process: Nursing Process/Implementation
Content Area: Child Health
Reference: Kee, J., & Marshall, S. (2004). *Clinical calculations: With applications to general and specialty areas* (5th ed.). Philadelphia: W.B. Saunders, p. 134.

3. *Answer:* 3
Rationale: Convert pounds to kilograms by dividing by 2.2.
Pounds to kilograms:
$$17 \text{ lb divided by } 2.2 \text{ lb/kg} = 7.72 \text{ kg}$$
Safe dose parameter:
$$50 \text{ mg/kg/day} \times 7.72 \text{ kg} = 386 \text{ mg/day}$$
Dosage frequency:
$$100 \text{ mg} \times 3 \text{ doses (every 8 hours)} = 300 \text{ mg/day}$$
The dose is within the safe dosage range.
Test-Taking Strategy: Identify the key components of the question and what the question is asking. In this case, the question asks for the safe dose of the medication. Change pounds to kilograms. Calculate the dosage using the safe dose identified in the question and the child's weight in kilograms. Use a calculator to verify the answer, and remember to determine the total daily dosage prior to selecting an option. Review pediatric medication calculations if you had difficulty with this question.
Level of Cognitive Ability: Analysis
Client Needs: Physiological Integrity
Integrated Process: Nursing Process/Planning
Content Area: Child Health
Reference: Kee, J., & Marshall, S. (2004). *Clinical calculations: With applications to general and specialty areas* (5th ed.). Philadelphia: W.B. Saunders, pp. 234-236.

4. *Answer:* 3
Rationale: Change grams to milligrams, knowing that 1000 mg = 1 g. When converting from grams to milligrams (larger to smaller), move the decimal point three places to the right. Therefore, 1.0 g = 1000 mg. Then, use the medication calculation formula.
Formula:

$$\frac{\text{Desired}}{\text{Available}} \times \text{tablet} = \frac{1000 \text{ mg}}{500 \text{ mg}} \times 1 \text{ tablet} = 2 \text{ tablets}$$

Test-Taking Strategy: Identify the key components of the question and what the question is asking. In this case, the question asks for tablets per dose. Change grams to milligrams first. Then, use the formula to determine the correct dosage. Remember to verify the answer using a calculator. Review pediatric medication calculations if you had difficulty with this question.
Level of Cognitive Ability: Application
Client Needs: Physiological Integrity
Integrated Process: Nursing Process/Implementation
Content Area: Child Health
References: Asperheim, M. (2005). *Introduction to pharmacology* (10th ed.). Philadelphia: W.B. Saunders, p. 15.

Kee, J., & Marshall, S. (2004). *Clinical calculations: With applications to general and specialty areas* (5th ed.). Philadelphia: W.B. Saunders, p. 22.

5. *Answer:* 3
Rationale: Use the formula for calculating a safe dosage range.
Safe dose parameter:
$$5 \text{ mg/kg/day} \times 25 \text{ kg} = 125 \text{ mg/day}$$
Dosage frequency:
$$25 \text{ mg} \times 4 \text{ doses (every 6 hours)} = 100 \text{ mg/day}$$
The dose is within the safe dosage range.
Test-Taking Strategy: Identify the key components of the question and what the question is asking. In this case, the question asks for the safe dose of the medication. Calculate the dosage parameters using the safe dose identified in the question and the child's weight in kilograms. Use a calculator to verify the answer, and remember to determine the total daily dosage prior to selecting an option. Review pediatric medication calculations if you had difficulty with this question.
Level of Cognitive Ability: Analysis
Client Needs: Physiological Integrity
Integrated Process: Nursing Process/Planning
Content Area: Child Health
Reference: Kee, J., & Marshall, S. (2004). *Clinical calculations: With applications to general and specialty areas* (5th ed.). Philadelphia: W.B. Saunders, pp. 234-236.

6. *Answer:* 4
Rationale: Use the medication calculation formula.
Formula:

$$\frac{\text{Desired}}{\text{Available}} \times \text{volume} = \frac{1,000,000}{1,200,000} \times 2 \text{ mL} = 1.66 \text{ mL/dose}$$

Test-Taking Strategy: Identify the key components of the question and what the question is asking. In this case, the question asks for milliters per dose. Use the formula to determine the correct dose, and verify the answer with a calculator. Review pediatric medication calculations if you had difficulty with this question.
Level of Cognitive Ability: Application
Client Needs: Physiological Integrity
Integrated Process: Nursing Process/Implementation
Content Area: Child Health
Reference: Kee, J., & Marshall, S. (2004). *Clinical calculations: With applications to general and specialty areas* (5th ed.). Philadelphia: W.B. Saunders, p. 80.

7. *Answer:* 3
Rationale: Use the formula for calculating a safe dosage range.
Dosage parameters:
$$0.05 \text{ mg/kg/dose} \times 50 \text{ kg} = 2.5 \text{ mg/dose}$$
$$0.1 \text{ mg/kg/dose} \times 50 \text{ kg} = 5 \text{ mg/dose}$$
The dose is within the safe dosage range.
Test-Taking Strategy: Identify the key components of the question and what the question is asking. In this case, the question asks for the safe dosage range of the medication. Calculate the dosage parameters, using the safe dosage range identified in the question and the child's weight in kilograms. Verify the answer using a calculator. Review pediatric medication calculations if you had difficulty with this question.
Level of Cognitive Ability: Analysis

Client Needs: Physiological Integrity
Integrated Process: Nursing Process/Planning
Content Area: Child Health
Reference: Kee, J., & Marshall, S. (2004). *Clinical calculations: With applications to general and specialty areas* (5th ed.). Philadelphia: W.B. Saunders, pp. 234-236.

8. *Answer:* **1**

Rationale: Convert grains (gr) to milligrams (mg) and then use the medication calculation formula.

$$1 \text{ gr} = 60 \text{ mg}$$
$$^1/_{15} \text{ gr} \times 60 \text{ mg} = 4 \text{ mg}$$

Formula:

$$\frac{\text{Desired}}{\text{Available}} \times \text{volume} \times \frac{2.5 \text{ mg}}{4 \text{ mg}} \times 1 \text{ mL} = 0.62 \text{ mL}$$

Test-Taking Strategy: Identify the key components of the question and what the question is asking. In this case, the question asks for milliliters per dose. Begin by converting grains to milligrams. Then, use the formula to determine the correct dose, and verify the answer using a calculator. Review pediatric medication calculations if you had difficulty with this question.
Level of Cognitive Ability: Application
Client Needs: Physiological Integrity
Integrated Process: Nursing Process/Implementation
Content Area: Child Health
Reference: Kee, J., & Marshall, S. (2004). *Clinical calculations: With applications to general and specialty areas* (5th ed.). Philadelphia: W.B. Saunders, p. 80.

9. *Answer:* **2**

Rationale: Convert grams to milligrams. In the metric system, to convert larger to smaller, multiply by 1000 or move the decimal three places to the right. Then, use the medication calculation formula:

$$1 \text{ g} = 1000 \text{ mg}$$

Formula:

$$\frac{\text{Desired}}{\text{Available}} \times \text{volume} = \frac{125 \text{ g}}{1000 \text{ mg}} \times 7.4 \text{ mL} = 0.925 \text{ mL per dose}$$

Test-Taking Strategy: Identify the key components of the question and what the question is asking. In this case, the question asks for milliliters per dose. Convert grams to milligrams first. Next, use the formula to determine the correct dosage, knowing that 1000 mg = 7.4 mL. Verify the answer using a calculator. Review pediatric medication calculations if you had difficulty with this question.
Level of Cognitive Ability: Application
Client Needs: Physiological Integrity

Integrated Process: Nursing Process/Implementation
Content Area: Fundamental Skills
References: Asperheim, M. (2005). *Introduction to pharmacology* (10th ed.). Philadelphia: Elsevier/Saunders, p. 15.
Kee, J., & Marshall, S. (2004). *Clinical calculations: With applications to general and specialty areas* (5th ed.). Philadelphia: W.B. Saunders, p. 22.

10. *Answer:* **1**

Rationale: Calculate the dosage by weight first; therefore, 0.03 mg/day × 7.2 kg = 0.21 mg/day. Next, note that the physician orders digoxin twice daily; therefore, two doses in 24 hours will be administered; 0.21 mg/day divided by 2 doses = 0.1 mg for each dose.
Test-Taking Strategy: Identify the key components of the question and what the question is asking. Read the question carefully, noting the key words, *twice daily* and *each dose*. Calculate the dosage by weight first and then determine the milligrams per each dose. Verify the answer using a calculator. Review pediatric medication calculations if you had difficulty with this question.
Level of Cognitive Ability: Application
Client Needs: Physiological Integrity
Integrated Process: Nursing Process/Implementation
Content Area: Child Health
Reference: Kee, J., & Marshall, S. (2004). *Clinical calculations: With applications to general and specialty areas* (5th ed.). Philadelphia: W.B. Saunders, pp. 234-236.

ALTERNATE FORMAT QUESTION: FILL IN THE BLANK

Answer: 0.5

Rationale: Use the formula for calculating medication dosage.
Formula:

$$\frac{\text{Desired}}{\text{Available}} \times \text{volume} = \frac{0.2 \text{ mg}}{0.4 \text{ mg}} \times 1 \text{ mL} = 0.5 \text{ mL}$$

Test-Taking Strategy: Identify what the question is asking. In this case, the question asks for the milliliters to be administered. Use the formula to determine the correct dose and use a calculator to verify your answer. Review this formula if you had difficulty with this question.
Level of Cognitive Ability: Application
Client Needs: Physiological Integrity
Integrated Process: Nursing Process/Implementation
Content Area: Child Health
Reference: Kee, J., & Marshall, S. (2004). *Clinical calculations: With applications to general and specialty areas* (5th ed.). Philadelphia: W.B. Saunders, pp. 22-23.

REFERENCES

Asperheim, M. (2005). *Introduction to pharmacology* (10th ed.). Philadelphia: W.B. Saunders.

Christensen, B., & Kockrow, E. (2003). *Foundations of nursing* (4th ed.). St. Louis: Mosby.

Hodgson, B., & Kizior, R. (2005). *Saunders nursing drug handbook 2004.* Philadelphia: W.B. Saunders.

Joint Commission on Accreditation of Healthcare Organizations. *2004 national patient safety goals* (2004). Oakbrook Terrrace, IL: JCAHO. Web site: http://www.jcaho.org/accredited+organizations/patient+safety/04+npsg/04_faqs.htm.

Kee, J., & Marshall, S. (2004). *Clinical calculations: With applications to general and specialty areas* (5th ed.). Philadelphia: W.B. Saunders.

The Adult Client with an Integumentary Disorder

PYRAMID TERMS

burns Cell destruction of the layers of the skin and the resultant depletion of fluid and electrolytes.

carbon monoxide poisoning Carbon monoxide is a colorless, odorless, and tasteless gas that has an affinity for hemoglobin 200 times greater than that of oxygen. Oxygen molecules are displaced and carbon monoxide reversibly binds to hemoglobin to form carboxyhemoglobin. Tissue hypoxia occurs.

chemical burns Caused by tissue contact with strong acids, alkalis, or organic compounds. Systemic toxicity from cutaneous absorption can occur.

decubitus Localized areas of skin breakdown that occurs as a result of poor circulation to the area; also called a pressure ulcer.

deep full-thickness burn Similar to a fourth-degree burn. Involves injury to the muscle and bone. Injured area appears black. Edema is absent.

electrical burns Caused by heat generated from electrical energy as it passes through the body; results in internal tissue damage.

full-thickness burn Similar to a third-degree burn. The injured area appears deep red, black, white, or brown. The injured surface appears dry. Tissue disruption is noted with fat exposed. The skin is edematous.

herpes zoster (shingles) An acute viral infection of the nerve structure caused by varicella-zoster. Herpes zoster is contagious to individuals who have not had chickenpox.

Kaposi's sarcoma Skin lesions that occur in individuals with a compromised immune system.

Lyme disease An infection acquired from a tick bite. Ticks live in wooded areas and survive by attaching to a host.

partial-thickness superficial burn Similar to a second-degree burn. A mottled red base and broken epidermis with a wet shiny and weeping surface are present. Large blisters cover an extensive area. The skin is edematous and painful.

skin cancer A malignant lesion of the skin that may or may not metastasize. Causes include chronic friction and irritation to a skin area and exposure to ultraviolet rays. Diagnosis is confirmed by a skin biopsy that is positive for cancer cells.

smoke inhalation injury Results when the victim is trapped in an enclosed, smoke-filled space.

superficial-thickness burn Similar to a first-degree burn. Mild to severe erythema is noted and the skin blanches with pressure.

thermal burns Caused by exposure to flames, hot liquids, steam, or hot objects.

PYRAMID TO SUCCESS

The Pyramid to Success focuses on the concept that the integumentary system provides the first line of defense against infections. Focus on the protective measures necessary to prevent infection. Pyramid points address the risk factors related to the development of integumentary disorders, the preventive measures related to skin cancer, and the content related to Kaposi's sarcoma and Lyme disease. Focus on the emergency measures related to a client with a burn, fluid resuscitation, monitoring for complications, and skin grafting. Psychosocial issues relate to the body image disturbances that can occur as a result of the integumentary disorder. The Integrated Processes addressed in this unit include Caring, the Clinical Problem-Solving Process (Nursing Process), Communication and Documentation, and Teaching/Learning.

CLIENT NEEDS
Safe, Effective Care Environment

Confidentiality related to the disorder
Consultation with members of the health care team
Establishing priorities
Handling infectious materials

Informed consent for treatments and procedures
Medical and surgical asepsis
Referrals
Standard and other precautions

Health Promotion and Maintenance

Disease prevention measures
Health promotion programs
Health screening
Instructions to the client regarding care of the integumentary disorder
Data collection related to the integumentary system

Psychosocial Integrity

Coping mechanisms
End-of-life issues
Situational role changes
Unexpected body image changes
Use of support systems

Physiological Integrity

Adequate nutrition for healing
Alteration in body systems
Basic care and comfort
Expected effects of treatments
Fluid and electrolyte imbalances

Monitoring for complications
Monitoring laboratory values
Providing emergency care

REFERENCES

Black, J., & Hawks, J., (2005). *Medical-surgical nursing: Clinical management for positive outcomes* (7th ed.). Philadelphia: W.B. Saunders.

Chernecky, C., & Berger, B. (2004). *Laboratory tests and diagnostic procedures* (4th ed.). Philadelphia: W.B. Saunders.

Christensen, B., & Kockrow, E. (2003). *Foundations of nursing* (4th ed.). St. Louis: Mosby.

DeWit, S. (2005). *Fundamental concepts and skills for nursing* (2nd ed.). Philadelphia: W.B. Saunders.

Ignatavicius, D., & Workman, M. (2002). *Medical surgical nursing: Critical thinking for collaborative care* (4th ed.). Philadelphia: W.B. Saunders.

Jarvis, C. (2004). *Physical examination and health assessment* (4th ed.). Philadelphia: W.B. Saunders, pp. 542-543.

Lewis, S., Heitkemper, M., & Dirksen, S. (2004). *Medical-surgical nursing: Assessment and management of clinical problems* (6th ed.). St. Louis: Mosby.

Linton, A., & Maebius, N. (2003). *Introduction to medical-surgical nursing* (3rd ed.). Philadelphia: W.B. Saunders.

National Council of State Boards of Nursing. (2005). *Detailed test plan for the National Council licensure examination for practical/vocational nurses.* Chicago: Author.

Pagana, K., & Pagana, T. (2003). *Mosby's diagnostic and laboratory test reference* (6th ed.). St. Louis: Mosby.

Phipps, W., Monahan, F., Sands, J., Marek, J., & Neighbors, M. (2003). *Medical-surgical nursing: Health and illness perspectives* (7th ed.). St. Louis: Mosby.

Thompson, J., McFarland, G., Hirsch, J., & Tucker, S. (2002). *Mosby's clinical nursing* (5th ed.). St. Louis: Mosby.

Integumentary System

I. ANATOMY AND PHYSIOLOGY

A. The skin is the largest sensory organ of the body, with a surface area of 15 to 20 square feet and a weight of about 9 pounds

B. Functions
1. First line of defense against infections
2. Protects underlying tissues and organs from injury
3. Receives stimuli from the external environment; detects touch, pressure, pain, and temperature stimuli and relays that information to the nervous system
4. Maintains normal body temperature
5. Excretes salts, water, and organic wastes
6. Protects the body from excessive water loss
7. Synthesizes vitamin D_3, which converts to calcitriol for normal calcium metabolism
8. Stores nutrients

C. Layers
1. Epidermis
2. Dermis
3. Hypodermis (subcutaneous fat)

D. Epidermal appendages
1. Nails
2. Hair
3. Glands
   a. Sebaceous
   b. Sweat

E. Normal bacterial flora
1. Types of normal bacterial flora
   a. Gram-positive and gram-negative staphylococci
   b. Pseudomonas
   c. Streptococcus
2. Organisms are shed with normal exfoliation
3. A pH of 4.2 to 5.6 halts the growth of bacteria

II. RISK FACTORS FOR INTEGUMENTARY DISORDERS

A. Exposure to chemical and environmental pollutants
B. Exposure to radiation
C. Exposure to the sun
D. Lack of personal hygiene habits
E. Use of cosmetics and harsh soaps
F. Medications, such as long-term corticosteroid and/or anticoagulant therapy
G. Nutritional deficiencies
H. Moderate to severe emotional stress
I. Infection, with injured areas as the potential entry points for infection
J. Changes associated with developmental stages and aging

III. PSYCHOSOCIAL IMPACT

A. Change in body image and decreased self-esteem
B. Social isolation and fear of rejection (from embarrassment about changes in skin appearance)
C. Restrictions in physical activity
D. Pain
E. Disruption or loss of employment
F. Cost of medications, hospitalizations, and follow-up care, including dressing supplies

IV. DIAGNOSTIC TESTS

A. Skin biopsy
1. Description
   a. Obtaining a small piece of skin tissue for histopathologic study
   b. Methods include punch, excisional, incisional, and shave

2. Preprocedure interventions
   a. Obtain informed consent
   b. Cleanse site as prescribed
3. Postprocedure interventions
   a. Place specimen when obtained by physician in the appropriate container, and send to pathology laboratory for analysis
   b. Use surgically aseptic technique for biopsy site dressings
   c. Check the biopsy site for bleeding and infection

B. Skin cultures
   1. Description
      a. Noninvasive procedure
      b. A small skin culture sample is obtained, using a sterile applicator and appropriate type of culture tube (bacterial versus viral)
      c. Viral culture is placed immediately on ice
      d. Sample is sent to laboratory to identify existing organism
   2. Preprocedure intervention: Obtain skin culture samples before instituting antibiotic therapy
   3. Postprocedure intervention: Send skin culture sample to the laboratory

C. Wood's light examination
   1. Description: Skin is viewed under ultraviolet light through a special glass (Wood's glass) to identify superficial infections of the skin
   2. Preprocedure intervention: Darken room prior to the examination
   3. Postprocedure intervention: Assist the client during adjustment from the darkened room

D. Skin testing
   1. Description
      a. The administration of an allergen onto the skin's surface or into the dermis
      b. Administered by patch, scratch, or intradermal technique
   2. Preprocedure interventions
      a. Discontinue systemic corticosteroids or antihistamine therapy 5 days prior to the test, as prescribed
      b. Obtain informed consent
      c. Have resuscitation equipment available if a scratch test is performed, because it may induce an anaphylactic reaction
   3. Postprocedure interventions
      a. Instruct the client to keep skin testing area dry
      b. Instruct the client to avoid activities that may produce sweating if a patch test was performed (if the patch loosens or falls off it should not be reapplied)
      c. Record the site, date, and time of the test
      d. Record the date and time for follow-up site reading
      e. Inspect the site for erythema, papules, vesicles, edema, and induration

f. Provide the client with a list of potential allergens, if identified

V. SKIN DISORDERS
A. Skin cancer
   1. Description
      a. A malignant lesion of the skin, which may or may not metastasize
      b. Causes include chronic friction and irritation to a skin area and exposure to ultraviolet rays
      c. Diagnosis is confirmed by a skin biopsy that is positive for cancer cells
   2. Types
      a. Basal cell: The most common type, arising from the basal cells contained in the epidermis
      b. Squamous cell: The second most common type of **skin cancer** in whites; it is a tumor of the epidermal keratinocytes and can infiltrate surrounding structures, metastasize to lymph nodes, and be subsequently fatal
      c. Malignant melanoma: Cancer of the melanocytes that can metastasize to the brain, lungs, bone, liver, and skin, and is ultimately fatal
   3. Data collection (Box 40-1)
      a. Change in color, size, or shape of pre-existing lesion
      b. Pruritus
      c. Local soreness
   4. Interventions
      a. Instruct the client regarding preventative measures
      b. Instruct the client to monitor for lesions that do not heal or that change characteristics
      c. Instruct the client to have moles or lesions removed that are subject to chronic irritation
      d. Instruct the client to avoid contact with chemical irritants
      e. Instruct the client to wear layered clothing and use sunscreen with an appropriate skin protection factor (SPF) when outdoors
      f. Instruct the client to avoid sun exposure between 11 AM and 3 PM
      g. Assist with surgical excision of the lesion as prescribed

---

BOX 40-1

Appearance of Skin Cancer Lesions

A waxy nodule
An irregular, circular, bordered lesion with hues of tan, black, or blue
A small, red, nodular lesion
An oozing, bleeding, crusting lesion

B. Contact dermatitis
   1. Description: An inflammatory response of the skin that produces skin changes after contact with a specific antigen
   2. Data collection
      a. Pruritus and burning
      b. Edema
      c. Erythema at the point of contact
      d. Signs of infection
      e. Vesicles with drainage
   3. Interventions
      a. Elevation of the extremity to reduce edema
      b. Application of cool, wet dressings and tepid baths, as prescribed
      c. Maintain a cool environment
      d. Protect the affected area from trauma
      e. Prevent scratching and rubbing of the affected area
      f. Assist with skin testing, as prescribed, to determine allergen(s)
      g. Instruct the client to avoid contact with the allergen when determined
      h. Instruct the client to avoid harsh soaps
      i. Instruct the client to avoid using heating pads or blankets
      j. Administer antibiotic for infection, antipruritic or antihistamine for itching, and/or corticosteroids for inflammation, as prescribed
C. Poison ivy, poison oak, and poison sumac
   1. Description: A dermatitis that develops from contact with urushiol from poison ivy, oak, or sumac plants
   2. Data collection
      a. Papulovesicular lesions
      b. Severe itching
   3. Interventions
      a. Cleanse the skin of the plant oils
      b. Apply cool, wet dressings with Burow's solution as prescribed to relieve the itching
      c. Apply lotion or topical corticosteroids, as prescribed
      d. Administer oral corticosteroids as prescribed for severe reaction
D. Lyme disease
   1. Description
      a. An infection caused by the spirochete *Borrelia burgdorferi*, acquired from a tick bite
      b. Ticks live in wooded areas and survive by attaching to a host
   2. Data collection (Box 40-2)
   3. Interventions
      a. Gently remove the tick with tweezers, wash skin with antiseptic, and dispose of tick by flushing it down the toilet
      b. Obtain a blood test 4 to 6 weeks after a bite to detect the presence of the disease (testing before this time is not reliable)

      c. Instruct the client in the administration of antibiotics as prescribed if the disease is confirmed
      d. Instruct the client to avoid areas that contain ticks, such as wooded grassy areas, especially in the summer months
      e. Instruct the client to wear long-sleeved tops, long pants, closed shoes, and hats while outside
      f. Instruct the client to spray the body with tick repellent before going outside
      g. Instruct the client to examine the body when returning inside
E. Erysipelas and cellulitis
   1. Description
      a. Erysipelas is an acute, superficial, rapidly spreading inflammation of the dermis and lymphatics, caused by group A beta-hemolytic streptococcus, that enters the tissue via an abrasion, bite, trauma, or wound
      b. Cellulitis is a skin infection into the deeper dermis and subcutaneous fat; causative organism is usually *Streptococcus pyogenes*
   2. Data collection
      a. Pain
      b. Itching
      c. Swelling
      d. Redness and warmth
   3. Interventions
      a. Promote rest
      b. Apply warm compresses as prescribed (usually twice a day) to promote circulation and to decrease discomfort, erythema, and edema
      c. Administer antibiotics as prescribed for infection following a culture of the area

---

BOX 40-2

Stages of Lyme Disease

FIRST STAGE
Symptoms can occur several days to months following the bite.
A small red pimple develops that spreads into a ring-shaped rash.
The rash may be large or small, or may not occur at all.
Flulike symptoms occur, such as headache, stiff neck, muscle aches, and fatigue.

SECOND STAGE
This occurs several weeks following the bite.
Joint pain develops.
Neurological complications are seen.
Symptoms of heart disease are present.

THIRD STAGE
Large joints become involved.
Arthritis progresses.

d. Clean skin daily with an antibacterial soap, as prescribed

F. Psoriasis
  1. Description
     a. A chronic, noninfectious skin inflammation involving keratin synthesis that results in psoriatic patches
     b. Various forms exist, with psoriasis vulgaris being the most common
     c. Possible causes of the disorder include stress, trauma, infection, and changes in climate
     d. The disorder may also be exacerbated by the use of certain medications
     e. Koebner phenomenon is the development of psoriatic lesions at a site of injury, such as a scratched or sunburned area
  2. Data collection
     a. Pruritus
     b. Shedding, silvery, white scales on a raised, reddened, round plaque; usually affects the scalp, knees, elbows, extensor surfaces of arms and legs, and sacral regions
     c. A yellow discoloration, pitting, and a thickening of nails, if they are affected
     d. Joint inflammation with psoriatic arthritis
  3. Interventions
     a. Administer daily soaks and tepid, wet compresses, to the affected areas to remove scales; oils or coal tar preparations are added to the bath water
     b. Assist the client to remove the scales during the soak, using a soft washcloth and gentle, circular motions; emollient cream or salicylic acid is applied to affected areas after the bath to continue to soften thick scales
  4. Topical pharmacological therapy
     a. Includes tar preparations, anthralin, salicylic acid, and corticosteroids; vitamin D preparation, calcipotriene (Dovonex), and a retinoid compound, tazarotene (Tazorac) suppress epidermopoiesis and cause sloughing of the rapidly growing epidermal cells
     b. Occlusive dressings may be applied following application of the corticosteroid to increase its effectiveness
     c. Use plastic wrap or bags as the occlusive dressing, and use rubber gloves on the client's hands, plastic bags on the feet, and a shower cap on the head, if affected; a plastic vinyl jogging suit may be used for the client being treated at home
  5. Intralesional therapy: Involves the administration of injections of triamcinolone acetonide (Aristocort, Kenalog) into highly visible or isolated patches of psoriasis that are resistant to other forms of therapy
  6. Systemic therapy
     a. Systemic medications may be prescribed to treat extensive psoriasis that does not respond to other forms of therapy
     b. Prescribed medications may include methotrexate and hydroxyurea (Hydrea)
  7. Photochemotherapy
     a. A combination of psoralens and ultraviolet A (PUVA) light therapy (decreases cellular proliferation)
     b. The client takes a photosensitizing medication (8-methoxypsoralen) and is subsequently exposed to long-wave ultraviolet light
  8. Client education
     a. Instruct the client not to scratch the affected areas and to keep the skin lubricated to minimize itching
     b. Monitor for and instruct the client to recognize the signs and symptoms of infection
     c. Instruct the client to wear light cotton clothing over affected areas
     d. Instruct the client regarding prescribed treatments and medications and to avoid over-the-counter medications
     e. Assist the client to identify ways to reduce stress

G. **Kaposi's sarcoma**
  1. Description: Skin lesions that occur primarily in individuals with a compromised immune system
  2. Data collection
     a. Slow-growing tumors that appear as raised, oblong, purplish, reddish-brown lesions; may be tender or nontender
     b. Organ involvement includes the lymph nodes, airways or lungs, or any part of the gastrointestinal tract from the mouth to anus
  3. Interventions
     a. Maintain standard precautions
     b. Provide protective isolation if the immune system is depressed
     c. Prepare the client for radiation therapy or chemotherapy, as prescribed
     d. Administer immunotherapy, as prescribed, to stabilize the immune system

H. **Herpes zoster (shingles)**
  1. Description
     a. An acute viral infection of the dorsal nerve root ganglion, caused by the varicella-zoster virus
     b. Can be caused by reactivation of the varicella-zoster virus or exposure to varicella-zoster, or can occur during any immunocompromised state
     c. Diagnosis is determined by visual examination, skin cultures, and skin stains that identify the organism and by an antinuclear antibody (ANA) blood test that will produce a positive result
     d. A culture provides the definitive diagnosis

e. **Herpes zoster** is contagious to individuals who have not had chickenpox
2. Data collection
   a. Unilaterally clustered skin vesicles along peripheral sensory nerves on the trunk, thorax, or face
   b. Fever
   c. Burning and neuralgia
   d. Pruritus
   e. Paresthesia
3. Interventions
   a. Isolate the client, because exudate from the lesions contain the virus (maintain standard and other precautions, such as contact precautions)
   b. Monitor neurovascular status and seventh cranial nerve function
   c. Monitor for signs and symptoms of infection
   d. Keep blisters intact if formed
   e. Assist the client with acetic acid compresses, cool, wet compresses, and/or tepid baths as prescribed
   f. Prepare to assist physician with a nerve block using lidocaine (Xylocaine), if prescribed
   g. Administer antiviral agents, analgesics, antianxiety agents, antipruritics, and corticosteroids, as prescribed
   h. Use an air mattress and a bed cradle on the client's bed and keep environment cool; warmth and touch aggravate pain
   i. Prevent the client from scratching and rubbing the affected area
   j. Instruct the client to wear light-weight, loose cotton clothing and to avoid wool and synthetic clothing
I. Paronychia
   1. Description: An infection of the tissue around the nail plate that most commonly occurs in middle-aged women and in the client with diabetes mellitus
   2. Data collection
      a. Redness and swelling around the nail bed
      b. Soreness at the nail bed
   3. Interventions
      a. Monitor temperature
      b. Monitor for infection around the nails
      c. Monitor for cellulitis in the affected area
      d. Assist the client with warm soaks, as prescribed
      e. Prepare to assist with incision and drainage of infected area, if prescribed
      f. Administer antibiotic or fungicidal ointments, as prescribed
J. Impetigo: See Chapter 35 for information on this disorder
K. Boils
   1. Description
      a. A deep bacterial inflammation of a hair follicle caused by staphylococcus

b. Commonly occur on the face, neck, arms, legs, and groin
2. Data collection
   a. Redness on skin
   b. Tender and painful furuncle
   c. Skin swelling at the site
   d. A yellow or white center in the furuncle
3. Interventions
   a. Instruct the client in good hand washing technique to prevent the spread of infection
   b. Apply hot moist compresses until drainage occurs
   c. Assist the physician in incision and drainage, which relieves pain and allows the escape of purulent drainage
   d. Instruct the client in daily cleanliness, the use of separate bath linens, and in the administration of antibiotics if prescribed
L. Frostbite
   1. Description
      a. Damage to tissues and blood vessels as a result of prolonged exposure to cold
      b. Fingers, toes, nose, and ears are often affected
   2. Data collection
      a. Numbness
      b. Paresthesia
      c. Pallor
      d. Severe pain, swelling, erythema, and blistering occur once the client is in a warm environment
      e. Necrosis and gangrene may develop in severe cases
   3. Interventions
      a. Handle the tissues gently
      b. Rewarm the affected part rapidly and continuously with a warm water bath (90° to 107° F; 32.2° to 41.6° C) for 15 to 20 minutes or until skin flushing occurs
      c. Avoid slow thawing, interrupted periods of warmth, or massage (may result in further tissue damage)
      d. Do not debride blisters
      e. Leave area exposed initially for continued assessment; then, apply bulky dressings as prescribed to permit drainage and provide protection
M. Scabies
   1. Description
      a. A parasitic skin disorder caused by an infestation of the *Sarcoptes scabiei* (itch mite)
      b. Is endemic among schoolchildren and institutionalized populations because of close personal contact
      c. Risk factors include close personal contact with an infected person or contaminated article
      d. There is usually a 1-month delay between the initial infestation and onset of pruritus in the host

2. Data collection
   a. Erythematous papules and pustules
   b. Threadlike, brownish, linear burrows up to 1 cm long
   c. Secondary lesions consist of vesicles, crusts, reddish-brown nodules, and excoriations
   d. Intense pruritus that worsens at night
3. Interventions
   a. Administer antihistamines or topical steroids to relieve itching as prescribed
   b. Apply topical antiscabies creams or lotions such as lindane (Kwell, Scabene), crotamiton (Eurax), or permethrin 5% (Elimite) as prescribed
   c. Lindane (Kwell, Scabene) should not be used in children younger than age 2 because of the risk of neurotoxicity and seizures
   d. Instruct the client to apply the antiscabies preparation thinly to the entire skin from the neck down (face and scalp are not affected in scabies) and to leave on for 12 to 24 hours, as prescribed
   e. Instruct the client to apply antiscabies preparations to dry skin, because moist skin increases absorption and the potential for central nervous system side effects, such as seizures
   f. Following treatment with antiscabies preparations, instruct the client to remove the medication by thoroughly washing with soap and water
   g. All family members and close contacts should be treated simultaneously
   h. Instruct the client that all bedding and clothing should be washed in very hot water and dried on the hot drier cycle or dry cleaned (mites can survive up to 36 hours on linen)
N. Acne vulgaris
   1. Description
      a. A common, self-limiting, multifactorial disorder
      b. Requires active treatment for control until it spontaneously resolves
      c. Types of lesions include comedones (open and closed), pustules, papules, and nodules
      d. The exact cause is unknown, but may include androgenic influence on sebaceous glands, increased sebum production, and proliferation of *Propionibacterium acnes* (whose enzymes reduce lipids to irritating fatty acids)
      e. Exacerbations coincide with the menstrual cycle from hormonal activity
      f. Heat, humidity, and excessive perspiration have a role in increased acne
   2. Data collection
      a. Closed comedones: Whiteheads and noninflamed lesions that develop as a follicle and enlarge with the retention of horny cells
      b. Open comedones: Blackheads that result from continuing accumulation of horny cells and sebum, which dilate the follicles

   c. Pustules and papules result as the inflammatory process progresses
   d. Nodules result from total disintegration of a comedone and subsequent collapse of the follicle
   e. Deep scarring can result from nodules
3. Interventions
   a. Instruct the client in the administration (provide written instructions) of topical or oral antibiotics as prescribed
   b. Instruct the client in the use of isotretinoin (Accutane) or other medications if prescribed to inhibit sebum production and reduce sebaceous gland size
   c. Instruct the client about the adverse effects of isotretinoin (Accutane), which include cheilitis (lip inflammation), skin dryness, elevated triglycerides, and eye discomfort
   d. Instruct the client to stop taking vitamin A supplements during treatment with isotretinoin (Accutane)
   e. Inform the client that improvement may not be apparent for 4 to 6 weeks
   f. Instruct the client in appropriate skin-cleansing methods, with emphasis on not scrubbing the face and using only the agreed-on topical agents
   g. Instruct the client not to squeeze, prick, or pick at lesions
   h. Instruct the client to use products labeled noncomedogenic and cosmetics that are water-based and to avoid contact with excessively oil-based products
   i. Instruct the client on the importance of follow-up treatment
O. **Decubitus**
   1. Description
      a. An impairment of skin integrity
      b. Localized areas of necrosis of the skin and subcutaneous tissue caused by pressure
      c. Prevention of skin breakdown is a major role of the nurse, particularly in caring for the bedridden or immobile client
   2. Risk factors
      a. Malnutrition
      b. Incontinence
      c. Immobility
      d. Skin shearing
      e. Decreased sensory perception
   3. Data collection (Box 40-3)
   4. Interventions
      a. Institute measures to prevent **decubitus**
      b. Monitor the nutritional status of the client
      c. Provide adequate nutritional intake to promote tissue integrity
      d. Monitor for an alteration in skin integrity
      e. Relieve or remove pressure on the skin

BOX 40-3
Stages of Decubiti

STAGE 1
A reddened area that returns to normal skin color after 15 to 20 minutes of pressure relief, such as turning the client to another position
The skin is intact.
The area is red and does not blanche with external pressure.

STAGE 2
The area has the top layer of skin missing.
The ulcer usually is shallow with a pink to red base, and a white or yellow eschar may be present.

STAGE 3
Deep ulcers extend into the dermis and subcutaneous tissues.
White, gray, or yellow eschar usually is present at the bottom of the ulcer, and the ulcer crater may have a lip or edge.
Purulent drainage is common.

STAGE 4
Deep ulcers extend into muscle and bone.
Brown or black eschar is present.
Purulent drainage is common.

BOX 40-4
Methods to Estimate Extent of Burn Injury

RULE OF NINES: ADULT
Head and neck: 9%
Anterior trunk: 18%
Posterior trunk: 18%
Arms (9% each): 18%
Legs (18% each): 36%
Perineum: 1%

LUND AND BROWDER METHOD
Modifies percentages for body segments according to age
Provides a more accurate estimate of the burn size
Uses a diagram of the body divided into sections, with the representative percentage of the total body surface area for ages older than 1 year
Should be reevaluated after initial wound debridement

f. Turn and reposition the immobile client every 2 hours, or more frequently if necessary
g. Ambulate the client
h. Provide active and passive exercises every 8 hours
i. Keep the skin clean and dry and the sheets wrinkle-free
j. Apply moisture barrier as prescribed to protect the skin
k. Use assistive devices to prevent pressure, such as alternating air pressure mattress or sheepskin padding
l. Apply medications or dressings to the wound as prescribed

VI. BURN INJURIES

A. Description: Cell destruction of the layers of the skin and the resultant depletion of fluid and electrolytes

B. **Burn** size
1. Small **burns**: The body's response to injury is localized to the injured area
2. Large or extensive **burns**
   a. Consists of 25% or more of the total body surface area (TBSA)
   b. The body's response to the injury is systemic
   c. Affects all of the major systems of the body

C. Estimating the extent of injury (Box 40-4; Figure 40-1)

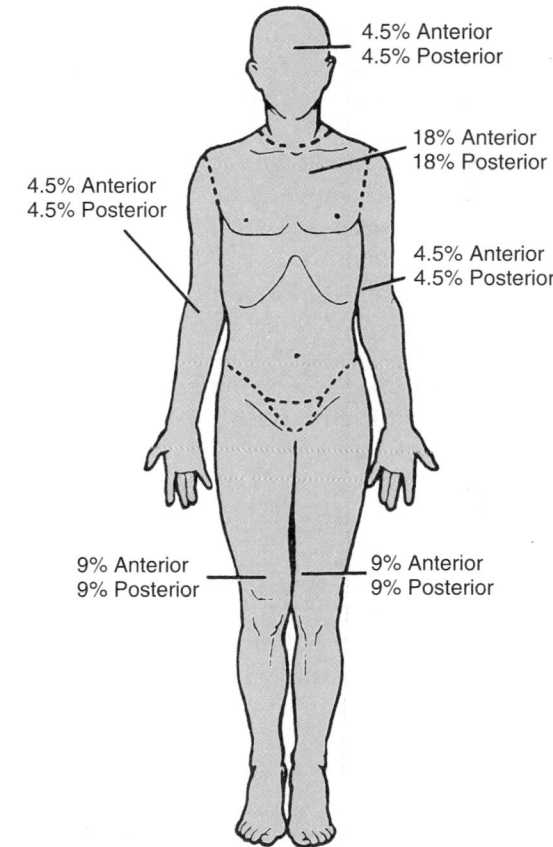

FIG. 40-1 Rule of Nines for estimating burn percentage. (From Ignatavicius, D., & Workman, M. [2002]. *Medical surgical nursing: Critical thinking for collaborative care* [4th ed.]. Philadelphia: W.B. Saunders.)

D. **Burn** depth
1. **Superficial-thickness burn** (similar to first-degree **burn**)
   a. Mild to severe erythema (pink to red), no blisters

b. Skin blanches with pressure
c. Painful, tingling
d. Pain is eased by cooling
e. Discomfort lasts about 48 hours; healing occurs in about 3 to 7 days
f. Skin grafts are not required

2. **Partial-thickness superficial burn** (similar to second-degree **burn**)
   a. Large blisters covering an extensive area
   b. Edema
   c. Mottled red base and broken epidermis, with a wet, shiny, and weeping surface
   d. Painful
   e. Injured area is sensitive to cold air
   f. Superficial partial thickness **burn** heals in 2 to 3 weeks
   g. Deep partial-thickness **burn** heals in 3 to 6 weeks
   h. Grafts may be used if the healing process is prolonged

3. **Full-thickness burn** (similar to third-degree **burn**)
   a. Deep red, black, white, yellow, or brown area
   b. Injured surface appears dry
   c. Edema
   d. Tissue disruption with fat exposed
   e. Little or no pain
   f. Spontaneous healing will not occur
   g. Requires removal of eschar and split- or full-thickness skin grafting
   h. Scarring and wound contractures are likely to develop without preventive measures
   i. Healing takes weeks to months

4. **Deep full-thickness burn** (similar to fourth-degree **burn**)
   a. Involves injury to the muscle and bone
   b. Injured area appears black
   c. Edema is absent
   d. Pain is absent
   e. No blisters
   f. Eschar is hard and inelastic
   g. Healing time takes weeks to months
   h. Grafts are required

E. Age and general health
   1. Mortality rates are higher for children younger than 4 years of age, particularly in the 0- to 1-year age-group, and for clients older than 65 years
   2. Debilitating disorders, such as cardiac, respiratory, endocrine, and renal disorders, negatively influence the client's response to injury and treatment
   3. Mortality rate is higher when the client has a pre-existing disorder at the time of the **burn** injury

▲ F. **Burn** location
   1. **Burns** of the head, neck, and chest are associated with pulmonary complications
   2. **Burns** of the face are associated with corneal abrasion

3. **Burns** of the ear are associated with auricular chondritis
4. Hands and joints require intensive therapy to prevent disability
5. The perineal area is prone to autocontamination by urine and feces
6. Circumferential **burns** of the extremities can produce a tourniquet-like effect and lead to vascular compromise (compartment syndrome)
7. Circumferential thorax **burns** lead to inadequate chest wall expansion and pulmonary insufficiency

G. Types of **burns**
   1. **Thermal burns**: Caused by exposure to flames, hot liquids, steam, or hot objects
   2. **Chemical burns**
      a. Caused by tissue contact with strong acids, alkalis, or organic compounds
      b. Systemic toxicity from cutaneous absorption can occur
   3. **Electrical burns**
      a. Caused by heat generated by an electrical energy as it passes through the body
      b. Results in internal tissue damage
      c. Cutaneous **burns** cause muscle and soft tissue damage that may be extensive, particularly in high-voltage electrical injuries
      d. The voltage, type of current, contact site, and duration of contact are important to identify
      e. Alternating current is more dangerous than direct current because it is associated with cardiopulmonary arrest, ventricular fibrillation, tetanic muscle contractions, and long bone or vertebral fractures
   4. **Radiation burns**: Caused by exposure to ultraviolet light, x-rays, or a radioactive source

VII. INHALATION INJURIES

A. **Smoke inhalation injury**
   1. Description: Results when the victim is trapped in an enclosed, hot, smoke-filled space
   2. Data collection
      a. Facial burns
      b. Erythema
      c. Swelling of oropharynx and nasopharynx
      d. Singed nasal hairs
      e. Flaring nostrils
      f. Stridor, wheezing, and dyspnea
      g. Hoarse voice
      h. Sooty (carbonaceous) sputum and cough
      i. Agitation and anxiety
      j. Tachycardia

B. **Carbon monoxide** poisoning
   1. Description
      a. **Carbon monoxide** is a colorless, odorless, and tasteless gas that has an affinity for hemoglobin 200 times greater than that of oxygen

b. Oxygen molecules are displaced and **carbon monoxide** reversibly binds to hemoglobin to form carboxyhemoglobin

c. Tissue hypoxia occurs

2. Data collection (Table 40-1)

C. Smoke poisoning

1. Description

a. Caused by the inhalation of the by-products of combustion

b. A localized inflammatory reaction occurs, causing a decrease in bronchial ciliary action and a decrease in surfactant

2. Data collection

a. Mucosal edema in the airways

b. Wheezing on auscultation

c. After several hours, sloughing of the tracheobronchial epithelium may occur, and hemorrhagic bronchitis may develop

d. Adult respiratory distress syndrome (ARDS) can result

D. Direct thermal heat injury

1. Description

a. Can occur to the lower airways by the inhalation of steam or explosive gases or the aspiration of scalding liquids

b. Can occur to the upper airways, which appear erythematous and edematous, with mucosal blisters and ulcerations

c. Mucosal edema can lead to upper airway obstruction, especially during the first 24 to 48 hours

d. All clients with head or neck **burns** should be monitored closely for the development of airway obstruction and are immediately considered for endotracheal intubation if obstruction occurs

2. Data collection

a. Erythema and edema of the upper airways

b. Mucosal blisters and ulcerations

VIII. MANAGEMENT OF THE BURN INJURY
(Box 40-5)

A. Emergent phase

1. Description

a. Begins at the time of injury and ends with the restoration of capillary permeability (fluid resuscitation), usually at 48 to 72 hours following the injury; includes prehospital and emergency room care

b. The primary goal is to prevent hypovolemic shock and preserve vital organ functioning

2. Prehospital care

a. Begins at the scene of the accident and ends when emergency care is obtained

b. Remove the victim from the source of the **burn**

c. Remove the source of heat

d. Assess airway, breathing, and circulation

BOX 40-5

Phases of Management of the Burn Injury

EMERGENT PHASE

Begins at time of injury; ends with the restoration of capillary permeability, usually at 48-72 hours following the injury

Primary goal is to prevent hypovolemic shock and preserve vital organ functioning

Includes prehospital care and emergency room care

RESUSCITATIVE PHASE

Begins with the initiation of fluids; ends when capillary integrity returns to near-normal levels and large fluid shifts have decreased

Amount of fluid administered is based on the client's weight and extent of injury

Most fluid replacement formulas are calculated from time of injury and not from time of arrival at the hospital

Goal is to prevent shock by maintaining adequate circulating blood volume and maintaining vital organ perfusion

ACUTE PHASE

Begins when the client is hemodynamically stable, capillary permeability is restored, and diuresis has begun

Usually begins 48-72 hours after time of injury

Emphasis during this phase is placed on restorative therapy; phase continues until wound closure is achieved

Focus is on infection control, wound care, wound closure, nutritional support, pain management, and physical therapy

REHABILITATIVE PHASE

Final phase of burn care

Overlaps the acute care phase and goes well beyond hospitalization

Goals of this phase designed so that client can gain independence and achieve maximal function

---

TABLE 40-1

Carbon Monoxide Poisoning

Blood Level (%)	Clinical Manifestation
1-10	Impaired visual activity
11-20	Flushing
21-30	Nausea
	Impaired dexterity
31-40	Vomiting
	Dizziness
	Syncope
41-50	Tachypnea
	Tachycardia
Higher than 50	Coma and death

e. Assess for associated trauma

f. Conserve body heat

g. Cover **burns** with sterile or clean cloths

h. Remove constricting jewelry and clothing

i. The need for intravenous fluids is assessed

j. Transport to emergency room

▲ 3. Emergency room care: Continuation of care administered at the scene of the injury

4. Major **burns**

a. Evaluate the degree and extent of the **burn** and treat life-threatening conditions

b. Ensure a patent airway and administer 100% oxygen as prescribed if the **burn** occurred in an enclosed area

c. Monitor for respiratory distress and the need for intubation

d. Check oropharynx for blisters and erythema

e. Arterial blood gases (ABGs) and carboxyhemoglobin levels will be monitored

f. For an inhalation injury, administer 100% oxygen via a tight-fitting, nonrebreather face mask as prescribed until carboxyhemoglobin levels fall below 15%

g. A peripheral intravenous (IV) access line is initiated to nonburned skin proximal to any extremity **burn**, or prepare for the insertion of a central venous pressure line, as prescribed

h. Monitor for hypovolemia and prepare to administer IV fluids to maintain fluid balance

i. Monitor vital signs closely

j. Insert a Foley catheter as prescribed, and maintain urine output at 30 to 50 mL/hour

k. Maintain NPO status

l. A nasogastric (NG) tube is inserted as prescribed to prevent paralytic ileus, to prevent vomiting, and to reduce the risk of aspiration

m. Administer tetanus prophylaxis, as prescribed

n. Pain medication is administered as prescribed by the IV route

o. Prepare the client for an escharotomy or fasciotomy, as prescribed

5. Minor **burns**

a. Instruct the client in the use of oral analgesics, as prescribed

b. Administer tetanus prophylaxis, as prescribed

c. Administer wound care as prescribed, which may include cleansing, debriding loose tissue, and removing any damaging agents, followed by the application of topical antimicrobial cream and a sterile dressing

d. Instruct the client in follow-up care, including active range-of-motion exercises and wound care

▲ B. Resuscitative phase

1. Description

a. Begins with the initiation of fluids; ends when capillary integrity returns to near-normal levels and large fluid shifts have decreased

b. The amount of fluid administered is based on client's weight and extent of injury

c. Most fluid replacement formulas are calculated from the time of injury, not from the time of arrival at the hospital

d. The goal is to prevent shock by maintaining adequate circulating blood volume and maintaining vital organ perfusion

2. Fluid resuscitation

a. The amount of fluid administered depends on how much intravenous fluid per hour is required to maintain a urinary output of 30 to 50 mL/hour

b. Successful fluid resuscitation is evaluated by stable vital signs, an adequate urine output, palpable peripheral pulses, and clear sensorium

c. Urinary output is the most common and most sensitive noninvasive assessment parameter for cardiac output and tissue perfusion

d. If the hemoglobin and hematocrit levels decrease or if the urinary output exceeds 50 mL/hour, the rate of IV fluid administration may be decreased

3. Interventions

a. Monitor for tracheal or laryngeal edema and administer respiratory treatments as prescribed

b. Monitor pulse oximetry and prepare for measurement of ABGs and carboxyhemoglobin (COHB) levels if inhalation injury is suspected

c. Elevate the head of the bed to 30 degrees or more for **burns** of the face and head

d. Initiate electrocardiography (ECG) monitoring

e. Monitor temperature and assess for infection

f. Initiate protective isolation techniques; maintain strict hand washing, use sterile sheets and linens when caring for the client, and use gloves, cap, masks, shoe covers, scrub clothes, and plastic aprons

g. Shave or cut body hair around wound margins

h. Monitor daily weights, expecting a weight gain of 15 to 20 pounds in the first 72 hours

i. Monitor gastric output and pH levels and for gastric discomfort and bleeding, indicating a stress ulcer

j. Administer antacids, H$_2$-receptor antagonists, and antiulcer medications such as sucralfate (Carafate), as prescribed

k. Auscultate bowel sounds for ileus and monitor for abdominal distention and gastrointestinal (GI) dysfunction

l. Monitor stools for occult blood

m. Obtain urine specimen for myoglobin and hemoglobin levels

n. Monitor IV fluids and hourly intake and output (I&O) to determine the adequacy of fluid replacement therapy; notify the registered nurse if urine output is lower than 30 or higher than 50 mL per hour

o. Elevate circumferential **burns** of the extremities on pillows above the level of heart to reduce dependent edema if no obvious fractures are present

p. Monitor pulses and capillary refill of the affected extremities and assess perfusion of the distal extremity with a circumferential **burn**

q. Prepare for chest and other x-rays to rule out fractures or associated trauma

r. Keep the room temperature warm

s. Place the client on an air-fluidized bed and use a bed cradle to keep sheets off the client's skin

4. Pain management

a. Morphine sulfate or meperidine (Demerol) is administered as prescribed by the IV route

b. Intramuscular or subcutaneous routes are avoided because absorption through the soft tissue is unreliable when hypovolemia and large fluid shifts are occurring

c. Administering medication by the oral route is avoided because of the possibility of GI dysfunction

d. Ensure that the client is medicated before painful procedures

5. Nutrition

a. Essential to promote wound healing and prevent infection

b. The basal metabolic rate (BMR) is 40 to 100 times higher than normal

c. Maintain nothing by mouth (NPO) status until the bowel sounds are heard; then, advance to clear liquids, as prescribed

d. Nutrition may be provided via enteral tube feeding, peripheral parenteral nutrition, or total parenteral nutrition

e. Provide a diet high in protein, carbohydrates, fats, and vitamins

f. Monitor calorie intake

6. Escharotomy

a. A lengthwise incision is made through the **burn** eschar to relieve constriction and pressure and to improve circulation

b. Performed for circulatory compromise due to circumferential **burns**

c. Performed at the bedside without anesthesia because nerve endings have been destroyed by the **burn** injury

d. Escharotomy can be performed on the thorax to improve ventilation

e. Following the escharotomy, monitor pulses, color, movement, and sensation of affected extremity, and control any bleeding with pressure

f. Pack incision gently with fine mesh gauze for 24 hours after escharotomy, as prescribed

g. Apply topical antimicrobial agents to the area as prescribed following the procedure

7. Fasciotomy

a. An incision is made extending through the subcutaneous tissue and fascia

b. The procedure is performed if adequate tissue perfusion does not return following an escharotomy

c. Performed in the operating room with the client under general anesthesia

d. Following the procedure, monitor pulses, color, movement, and sensation of affected extremity, and control any bleeding with pressure

e. Apply topical antimicrobial agents and dressings to the area as prescribed following the procedure

C. Acute phase

1. Description

a. Begins when the client is hemodynamically stable, capillary permeability is restored, and diuresis has begun

b. Usually begins 48 to 72 hours after the time of injury

c. Emphasis during this phase is placed on restorative therapy, and the phase continues until wound closure is achieved

d. The focus is on infection control, wound care, wound closure, nutritional support, pain management, and physical therapy

2. Interventions

a. Continue with protective isolation techniques

b. Provide wound care as prescribed and prepare for wound closure

c. Provide pain management

d. Provide adequate nutrition, as prescribed

e. Prepare client for rehabilitation

D. Wound care (Table 40-2)

1. Description: The cleansing, debridement, and dressing of the **burn** wounds

2. Hydrotherapy

a. Wounds are cleansed by immersion, showering, or spraying

b. Hydrotherapy occurs for 30 minutes or less to prevent increased sodium loss through the **burn** wound, heat loss, pain, and stress

c. Client should be premedicated before the procedure

d. Hydrotherapy is generally not used for clients who are hemodynamically unstable or those with new skin grafts

e. Care is taken to minimize bleeding and maintain body temperature during the procedure

f. If hydrotherapy is not used, wounds are washed and rinsed in bed before the application of antimicrobial agents

TABLE 40-2

Open versus Closed Method of Wound Care

Method	Advantages	Disadvantages
OPEN Antimicrobial cream is applied, and wound is left open to the air without a dressing Antimicrobial cream is applied every 12 hours	Visualization of the wound Easier mobility and joint range of motion Simplicity in wound care	Increased chance of hypothermia from exposure
CLOSED Gauze dressings are carefully wrapped from the distal to the proximal area of the extremity to ensure circulation is not compromised No two burn surfaces should be allowed to touch: touching can promote webbing of digits and poor cosmetic outcome Dressings are changed every 8-12 hours	Decreases evaporative fluid and heat loss Aids in debridement	Mobility limitations Prevents effective range-of-motion exercises Wound assessment is limited

3. Debridement (Box 40-6)
   a. Removal of eschar to prevent bacterial proliferation under the eschar and to promote wound healing
   b. Debridement may be mechanical, enzymatic, or surgical
   c. Deep partial- or **deep full-thickness burns:** Wound is cleansed and debrided; topical antimicrobial agents are applied once or twice daily

E. Wound closure
   1. Description
      a. Prevents infection and loss of fluid
      b. Promotes healing
      c. Prevents contractures
      d. Performed between days 5 and 21, depending on the extent of the **burn**
   2. Temporary wound coverings (Box 40-7)
   3. Autografting (Box 40-8)
      a. Permanent wound coverage
      b. Surgical removal of a thin layer of the client's own unburned skin, which is then applied to the excised **burn** wound
      c. Performed in the operating room under anesthesia
      d. Monitor for bleeding following the graft, because bleeding beneath an autograft can prevent adherence
      e. Small amounts of blood or serum can be removed by gently rolling the fluid from the center of the graft to the periphery with a sterile gauze pad, where it can be absorbed
      f. For large accumulations of blood, the physician will aspirate the blood using a small-gauge needle and syringe
      g. Autografts are immobilized following surgery for 3 to 7 days to allow time to adhere and attach to the wound bed

BOX 40-6

Debridement

MECHANICAL
Use of scissors and forceps to lift and trim away loose eschar
Wet to dry or wet to wet dressing changes
Painful procedure

ENZYMATIC
Application of prepared proteolytic and fibrinolytic topical enzymes that digest necrotic tissue, which facilitates eschar removal
Requires a moist environment to be effective; enzymes are applied directly to the burn wound
Pain and bleeding are major problems

SURGICAL
Excision of eschar and coverage of wound
Tangential
Very thin layers of eschar shaved until viable tissue is reached
Fascial
Used for very deep burns and for removal of burn tissue and underlying fat down to the fascia

      h. Position for immobilization and elevation of the graft site to prevent movement and shearing of the graft
   4. Care of the graft site
      a. Elevate and immobilize graft site
      b. Keep site free from pressure
      c. Avoid weight-bearing
      d. When graft takes, roll a cotton-tipped applicator over the graft to remove exudate, because exudate can lead to infection and prevent graft adherence

BOX 40-7

Temporary Wound Coverings

BIOLOGICAL

Amnion

Amniotic membranes from human placenta

Dressing changed every 48 hours with amnion

Allograft Homograft

Donated human cadaver skin harvested within 24 hours after death

Monitored for wound exudate and signs of infection

Rejection can occur within 24 hours

Xenograft Heterograft

Porcine skin harvested after slaughter and preserved for storage

Rejection can occur within 24-72 hours

Xenograft over granulation tissue replaced every 2-5 days until the wound heals naturally or until closure with autograft is complete

BIOSYNTHETIC AND SYNTHETIC

Wound can be inspected visually—dressings are transparent or translucent

Monitored for wound exudate and signs of infection

BOX 40-8

Types of Skin Grafts

SPLIT-THICKNESS GRAFT

Graft of half of the epidermis; applied in sheets or postage stamp–like pieces

FULL-THICKNESS GRAFT

Graft consists of epidermis and dermis; commonly used for reconstructive surgery months or years after the initial injury

PEDICLE FLAP

Commonly used for reconstructive surgery months or years after the initial injury

CULTURED EPITHELIUM

Uses client's unburned skin

Keratinocytes isolated and epithelial cells cultured in a laboratory; these cells are then attached to the burn wound

   e. Monitor for foul-smelling drainage, increased temperature, increased white blood cell count, hematoma, or fluid accumulation
   f. Instruct the client to avoid using fabric softeners and harsh detergents in the laundry
   g. Instruct the client to lubricate healing skin with cocoa butter as prescribed
   h. Instruct the client to protect the affected area from sunlight

   i. Instruct the client to use splints and support garments, as prescribed
5. Care of the donor site
   a. Method of care will vary, depending on physician's preference
   b. A moist gauze dressing is applied at the time of the surgery to maintain pressure and stop any oozing
   c. The physician may prescribe site treatment with single-layer gauze impregnated with petrolatum or with a biosynthetic dressing such as Biobrane
   d. Keep the donor site clean, dry, and free from pressure
   e. Prevent the client from scratching the donor site
   f. Apply lubricating lotions to soften the area and reduce the itching after the donor site is healed
   g. Donor site can be reused once healing has occurred (heals spontaneously within 7 to 14 days with proper care)

F. Physical therapy
1. An individualized program of splinting, positioning, exercises, ambulation, and activities of daily living; implemented early in the acute phase of recovery to maximize functional and cosmetic outcomes
2. Perform range-of-motion exercises as prescribed to reduce edema and maintain strength and joint function
3. Ambulate the client as prescribed to maintain the strength of the lower extremities
4. Apply splints as prescribed to maintain proper joint position and prevent contractures
   a. Static splints immobilize the joint and are applied for periods of immobilization, during sleeping, and for clients who cannot maintain proper positioning
   b. Dynamic splints exercise the affected joint
   c. Do not apply pressure to skin areas with splints, which could lead to further tissue and nerve damage
5. Scarring is controlled by elastic wraps and bandages, which apply continuous pressure to the healing skin during the period when the skin is vulnerable to shearing
6. Antiburn scar support garments are worn 23 hours a day until the **burn** scar tissue has matured, which takes 18 months to 2 years

G. Rehabilitative phase (Box 40-9)
1. Description
   a. Final phase of **burn** care
   b. Overlaps the acute-care phase and goes well beyond hospitalization
   c. Goals of this phase are designed so that the client can gain independence and achieve maximal function

BOX 40-9

Surgical Options for Contractures and Scarring

Split-thickness and full-thickness skin grafts
Skin flaps
Z-plasty
Tissue expansion

2. Goals
   a. Promote wound healing
   b. Minimize deformities
   c. Increase strength and function
   d. Provide emotional support

PRACTICE QUESTIONS

1. Which of the following individuals would be at the greatest risk for development of an integumentary disorder?
   1. An older female
   2. An adolescent
   3. An outdoor construction worker
   4. A physical education teacher

2. A client scheduled for a skin biopsy asks the nurse how painful the procedure is. The nurse makes which response to the client?
   1. "There is no pain associated with this procedure."
   2. "There is some pain, but the physician will prescribe an analgesic following the procedure."
   3. "The local anesthetic may cause a burning or stinging sensation."
   4. "A preoperative medication will be given so you will be sleeping and will not feel any pain."

3. A nurse has reinforced discharge instructions to a client who had a skin biopsy. Which statement by the client indicates a need for further instruction?
   1. "I will call the physician if I see any drainage from the wound."
   2. "I will return in 7 days to have the sutures removed."
   3. "I will use the antibiotic ointment as prescribed."
   4. "I will remove the dressing when I get home and wash the site with tap water."

4. A nurse prepares to help the physician examine the client's skin with a Wood's light. Which of the following would be included in the plan for this procedure?
   1. Obtain an informed consent
   2. Darken the room for the examination
   3. Shave the skin and scrub with povidone-iodine (Betadine) solution
   4. Prepare a local anesthetic

5. A nurse is checking for the presence of cyanosis in a dark-skinned client. Which body area would provide the best information?
   1. Back of the hands
   2. Earlobes

3. Palms of the hands
4. Sacrum

6. A nurse reinforces instructions to a client who is to return to the physician's office in 1 week for a patch test to identify the allergen causing the dermatitis. The nurse provides which instruction to the client?
   1. Remain NPO prior to the test
   2. Shower using an antibacterial soap on the morning of the test
   3. Discontinue the prescribed antihistamine 2 days before the test
   4. Consume fluids only on the day of the test

7. A nurse reinforces discharge instructions to a client following patch testing. Which statement by the client indicates the need for further instruction?
   1. "I will return to the clinic in 2 days for the initial reading."
   2. "If the patch comes off, I need to reapply it."
   3. "I need to avoid activities that will cause me to sweat."
   4. "I need to keep the test sites dry."

8. A nurse reinforces instructions to a client who has complained of chronic dry skin and episodes of pruritus. Which of the following, if stated by the client, indicates a need for further instructions?
   1. "I should drink 8 to 10 glasses of water a day."
   2. "I need to avoid using astringents on my skin."
   3. "I should limit myself to one shower a day and apply emollient to my skin after the shower."
   4. "I should use a dehumidifier, especially during the winter months."

9. The nurse prepares to assist in instructing a client about Lyme disease. Which of the following information would the nurse include in the instructions?
   1. It is contagious by skin contact with an infected individual
   2. It is caused by the inhalation of spores from bird droppings
   3. It is caused by contamination from cat feces
   4. It is caused by a tick carried by deer

10. Following diagnostic evaluation, it has been determined that the client has Lyme disease, stage 2. The nurse understands that which of the following is most indicative of this stage?
   1. Erythematous rash
   2. Neurological deficits
   3. Arthralgias
   4. Joint enlargement

11. The client arrives at the health care clinic and tells the nurse that he was just bitten by a tick and would like to be tested for Lyme disease. Which nursing action is appropriate?
   1. Tell the client that a blood test is needed immediately
   2. Inform the client that there is no test available for Lyme disease

3. Inform the client that he will need to return in 4 to 6 weeks to be tested, because testing before this time is not reliable

4. Tell the client that testing is not necessary unless arthralgia develops

12. A client calls the emergency room and tells the nurse that he has been cleaning a wooded area in the back yard and has discovered that he came directly in contact with poison ivy shrubs. The client tells the nurse that he cannot see anything on the skin and asks the nurse what to do. The nurse makes which statement to the client?

1. "Come to the emergency room."

2. "It is not necessary to do anything if you cannot see anything on your skin."

3. "Take a shower immediately, lathering and rinsing several times."

4. "Apply calamine lotion immediately to the exposed skin areas."

13. A client with acquired immunodeficiency syndrome (AIDS) is diagnosed with cutaneous Kaposi's sarcoma. Based on this diagnosis, the nurse understands that this has been determined by which of the following?

1. Appearance of reddish-blue lesions on the skin

2. Swelling in the lower extremities

3. Punch biopsy of the cutaneous lesions

4. Swelling in the genital area

14. Which of the following individuals is least likely at risk for the development of Kaposi's sarcoma?

1. A male with a history of same-sex partners

2. A renal transplant client

3. A client receiving antineoplastic medications

4. An individual working in an environment where exposure to asbestos exists

15. A nurse prepares to give a bath and change the bed linens for a client with cutaneous Kaposi's sarcoma lesions. The lesions are open and draining a scant amount of serous fluid. Which of the following would the nurse use during the bathing of this client?

1. Gown, gloves, and mask

2. Gown and gloves

3. Gloves

4. Gown and gloves to change the bed linens and gloves only for the bath

16. A client is being admitted to the hospital for treatment of acute cellulitis of the lower left leg. The client asks the nurse to explain what cellulitis means. The nurse bases the response on the understanding that the characteristics of cellulitis include:

1. A skin infection into the deep dermis and subcutaneous fat

2. An acute superficial infection

3. An inflammation of the lymphatics

4. A superficial infection caused by staphylococcus

17. A nurse prepares to care for a client with acute cellulitis of the lower leg. Which of the following would the nurse anticipate to be prescribed for the client?

1. Warm compresses to the affected area

2. Cold compresses to the affected area

3. Intermittent heat lamp treatments four times daily

4. Alternating hot to cold compresses continuously

18. A nurse notes that the physician has documented a diagnosis of herpes zoster in the client's chart. Based on an understanding of the cause of this disorder, the nurse would determine that this diagnosis was made following which diagnostic test?

1. Skin biopsy

2. Wood's light examination

3. Culture of the lesion

4. Patch test

19. A nurse is assigned to care for a client with herpes zoster. Which of the following characteristics would the nurse expect to note when assessing the lesions of this infection?

1. A generalized body rash

2. Small blue-white spots with a red base

3. A fiery red edematous rash on the cheeks

4. Clustered skin vesicles

20. A nurse employed in a long-term care facility is planning the clinical assignments for the day. The nurse avoids assigning which staff member to the client with a diagnosis of herpes zoster?

1. A staff member who has never had mumps

2. An experienced nursing assistant who has never had chickenpox

3. A staff member who has never had roseola

4. A nursing assistant who has never had German measles

21. A client returns to the clinic for follow-up treatment following a skin biopsy of a suspicious lesion performed 1 week ago. The biopsy report indicates that the lesion is a melanoma. The nurse understands that which of the following describes the characteristic of this type of a lesion?

1. Is highly metastatic

2. Metastasis is rare

3. Is characterized by local invasion

4. Is encapsulated

22. A nurse is reviewing the health care record of a client with a lesion diagnosed as malignant melanoma. The nurse would expect to note which characteristic of this type of lesion documented in the client's record?

1. A small papule with a dry, rough scale

2. A firm nodular lesion topped with crust

3. A pearly papule with a central crater and a waxy border

4. An irregularly shaped lesion

23. A nurse reinforces instructions to a group of clients regarding measures that will assist in preventing skin cancer. Which statement by a client indicates a need for further instructions?
    1. "I need to use sunscreen when participating in outdoor activities."
    2. "I need to examine my body monthly for any lesions that may be suspicious."
    3. "I need to wear a hat, opaque clothing, and sunglasses when in the sun."
    4. "I need to avoid sun exposure before 11 AM and after 3 PM."

24. A nurse reviews a client's chart and notes that the physician has documented a diagnosis of paronychia. Based on this diagnosis, which of the following would the nurse expect to note during data collection?
    1. Swelling of the skin near the parotid gland
    2. Red, shiny skin around the nail bed
    3. White, silvery patches on the elbows
    4. White, taut skin in the popliteal area

25. A nurse reinforces instructions to a client diagnosed with impetigo. Which statement by the client indicates a need for further instructions?
    1. "I need to continue with the antibiotics as prescribed."
    2. "I need to separate my dishes and wash them separately from the dishes of other household members."
    3. "I can wash my laundry with other household members' items."
    4. "I need to wash my hands thoroughly and frequently throughout the day."

26. A client arrives at the emergency room and has experienced frostbite to the right hand. Which of the following would the nurse note on data collection of the client's hand?
    1. A fiery red skin with edema in the nail beds
    2. A pink edematous hand
    3. Black fingertips surrounded by an erythematous rash
    4. A white color to the skin, which is insensitive to touch

27. A nurse is assigned to assist in caring for a client with frostbite of the toes. Which of the following would the nurse anticipate to be prescribed for this condition?
    1. Rapid and continuous rewarming of the toes in a warm water bath until flushing of the skin occurs
    2. Rapid and continuous rewarming of the toes in hot water for 15 to 20 minutes
    3. Rapid and continuous rewarming of the toes when flushing occurs
    4. Rapid and continuous rewarming of the toes in cold water for 45 minutes

28. An evening nurse reviews the nursing documentation in the client's chart and notes that the day nurse has documented that the client has a stage 2 pressure ulcer (decubitus) in the sacral area. Which of the following would the nurse expect to note when checking the client's sacral area?
    1. Skin is intact
    2. Partial-thickness skin loss of the epidermis
    3. A deep crater-like appearance
    4. The presence of sinus tracts

29. Which of the following conditions would least likely be a risk factor for the development of skin breakdown?
    1. A client who is unable to move about and is confined to bed
    2. A client incontinent for urine and feces
    3. A client with chronic nutritional deficiencies
    4. A client with a lowered mental awareness status

30. Isotretinoin (Accutane) is prescribed for a client with severe cystic acne. Which of the following, if stated by the client, would indicate a need for further instruction regarding this medication?
    1. "I need to continue to take my vitamin A supplements."
    2. "I need to use emollients and lip balm for my dry skin."
    3. "The medication may cause dryness and burning in my eyes."
    4. "I will need to return for a blood test to check my triglyceride level."

31. A nurse inspects the skin of a client suspected of having scabies. Which of the following findings would the nurse note if this disorder was present?
    1. The appearance of vesicles or pustules with a thick, honey-colored crust
    2. The presence of white patches scattered about the trunk
    3. Multiple straight or wavy threadlike lines beneath the skin
    4. Patchy hair loss and round red macules with scales

32. A nurse is told that an assigned client is suspected of having scabies. Which of the following precautions will the nurse institute during the care of the client?
    1. Wear a mask and gloves
    2. Wear gloves only
    3. Wear a gown and gloves
    4. Avoid touching the client's clothes

33. The client arrives at the emergency room following a burn injury that occurred in the basement at home, and an inhalation injury is suspected. Which of the following would the nurse anticipate to be prescribed for the client?
    1. 100% oxygen via an aerosol mask
    2. Oxygen via nasal cannula at 15 L
    3. 100% oxygen via a tight-fitting, nonrebreather face mask
    4. Oxygen via nasal cannula at 10 L

34. A nurse is caring for a client who has just been admitted to the nursing unit following flame burns to the face and chest. The nurse notes a hoarse cough and that the client is expectorating sputum with black flecks. The client's eyelashes and eyebrows are singed and the eyelids are swollen. The client suddenly becomes restless and his color becomes dusky. The nurse interprets this data as indicating which of the following?
    1. The client is afraid and is having a panic attack due to the unfamiliar surroundings
    2. Pain is present from the burn injury
    3. The client is hypotensive
    4. The burn has probably caused laryngeal edema, which has occluded the airway

35. Which of the following would be the anticipated therapeutic outcome of an escharotomy procedure performed for a circumferential arm burn?
    1. Brisk bleeding from the site
    2. Formation of granulation tissue
    3. Decreasing edema formation
    4. Return of distal pulses

36. A client is undergoing radiation therapy to treat lung cancer. Following the treatment, the nurse notes that the chest and neck are red, and the client is complaining of pain at the radiation site. The nurse interprets this data as:
    1. A superficial injury to tissue from the radiation
    2. An allergic reaction to the radiation
    3. A cutaneous reaction to products formed by lysis of the neoplastic cells
    4. An ischemic injury, much like decubitus formation

37. A nurse is caring for a client with circumferential burns of both legs. Which of the following leg positions is appropriate for this type of a burn?
    1. A dependent position
    2. Flat without elevation
    3. Elevation above the level of the heart
    4. Elevation of the knees

38. A nurse is assisting in caring for a client receiving IV fluids who has sustained second- and third-degree injuries of the back and legs. The nurse understands that which of the following would provide the most reliable indicator for determining the adequacy of the fluid resuscitation?
    1. Vital signs
    2. Urine output
    3. Peripheral pulses
    4. Mental status

39. A nurse is caring for a client following an autograft and grafting to a burn wound on the right knee. Which of the following would the nurse anticipate to be prescribed for the client?
    1. Elevation and immobilization of the affected leg
    2. Placing the affected leg flat
    3. Placing the affected leg in a dependent position
    4. Immobilization in a dependent position

40. A nurse reinforces discharge instructions regarding skin care to a client following grafting to burn injuries sustained to the left chest and left arm. Which statement by the client indicates a need for further instructions?
    1. "I need to bathe using a mild soap and rinsing thoroughly."
    2. "I need to avoid the use of lanolin products to the newly healed skin area."
    3. "I need to avoid direct sunlight on the newly healed skin area."
    4. "I should never wear warm clothing over the newly healed skin area."

ALTERNATE FORMAT QUESTION: FILL IN THE BLANK

The adult client was burned as a result of an explosion. The burn initially affected the client's entire face (anterior half of the head) and the upper half of the anterior torso, and there were circumferential burns to the lower half of both of the arms. The client's clothes caught on fire, and the client ran, causing subsequent burn injuries to the posterior surface of the head, and the upper half of the posterior torso. Using the Rule of Nines, the extent of the burn injury would be which of the following?

Answer:_____

ANSWERS

1. *Answer: 3*

Rationale: Prolonged exposure to the sun, unusual cold, or other conditions can damage the skin. An older client may be at a higher risk than a younger individual because immobility and lack of nutrition would increase the older person's risk. An adolescent may be prone to the development of acne, but this does not occur in all adolescents. The physical education teacher is at low or no risk of developing an integumentary problem.

Test-Taking Strategy: Use the process of elimination. Note the key words, *greatest risk*. Eliminate option 4 first. Eliminate options 1 and 2 next because not all older persons or adolescents are at risk for the development of integumentary disorders. If you had difficulty with this question, review the risk factors associated with integumentary disorders.

Level of Cognitive Ability: Comprehension
Client Needs: Health Promotion and Maintenance
Integrated Process: Nursing Process/Data Collection
Content Area: Adult Health/Integumentary

Reference: Phipps, W., Monahan, F., Sands, J., Marek, J., & Neighbors, M. (2003). *Medical-surgical nursing: Health and illness perspectives* (7th ed.). St. Louis: Mosby, p. 1936.

2. *Answer:* **3**

Rationale: Depending on the size and location of the lesion, a biopsy is usually a quick and almost painless procedure. The most common source of pain is the initial local anesthetic, which can produce a burning or stinging sensation. Options 1, 2, and 4 are incorrect.

Test-Taking Strategy: Use the process of elimination. Eliminate option 1 first because of the absolute word "no." Eliminate option 2 next because this option addresses postprocedure, which is not the issue of the client's question to the nurse. Eliminate option 4 because a preoperative medication that puts the client to sleep is not part of the procedure for a skin biopsy. If you had difficulty with this question, review the procedure related to a skin biopsy.

Level of Cognitive Ability: Application
Client Needs: Psychosocial Integrity
Integrated Process: Nursing Process/Implementation
Content Area: Adult Health/Integumentary
Reference: Linton, A., & Maebius, N. (2003). *Introduction to medical-surgical nursing* (3rd ed.). Philadelphia: W.B. Saunders, p. 1018.

3. *Answer:* **4**

Rationale: Following a skin biopsy, the nurse instructs the client to keep the dressing dry and in place for a minimum of 8 hours. After the dressing is removed, the site is cleaned once a day with tap water or saline to remove any dry blood or crusts. The physician may prescribe an antibiotic ointment to minimize local bacterial colonization. The nurse instructs the client to report any redness or excessive drainage at the site. Sutures are usually removed 7 to 10 days after biopsy.

Test-Taking Strategy: Use the process of elimination and note the key words, *need for further instruction*. These words indicate a false response question and that you need to select the incorrect client statement. Eliminate option 3 first because the client verbalizes a physician's prescription. Eliminate options 1 and 2 next. A client needs to report signs of drainage and needs to return to the physician for follow-up and suture removal. Consider the alteration in skin integrity that occurs with a skin biopsy. This should assist in directing you to the correct option. Review postprocedure instructions following a skin biopsy if you had difficulty with this question.

Level of Cognitive Ability: Comprehension
Client Needs: Health Promotion and Maintenance
Integrated Process: Teaching/Learning
Content Area: Adult Health/Integumentary
References: Black, J., & Hawks, J. (2005). *Medical-surgical nursing: Clinical management for positive outcomes* (7th ed.). Philadelphia: W.B. Saunders, p. 1387.
Pagana, K., & Pagana, T. (2003). *Mosby's diagnostic and laboratory test reference* (6th ed.). St. Louis: Mosby, p. 315.

4. *Answer:* **2**

Rationale: Examination of the skin under a Wood's light is always carried out in a darkened room. This is a noninvasive

examination; therefore an informed consent is not required. A handheld long-wavelength ultraviolet light or Wood's light is used. The skin does not need to be shaved nor is a local anesthetic necessary. Areas of blue-green or red fluorescence are associated with certain skin infections. The procedure is painless.

Test-Taking Strategy: Use the process of elimination. Recalling that this is a noninvasive procedure will assist in eliminating options 1, 3, and 4. Review this procedure if you had difficulty answering this question.

Level of Cognitive Ability: Application
Client Needs: Physiological Integrity
Integrated Process: Nursing Process/Planning
Content Area: Adult Health/Integumentary
Reference: Linton, A., & Maebius, N. (2003). *Introduction to medical-surgical nursing* (3rd ed.). Philadelphia: W.B. Saunders, p. 1018.

5. *Answer:* **3**

Rationale: In a dark-skinned client, the nurse examines the lips, tongue, nail beds, conjunctiva, and palms and soles at regular intervals for subtle color changes. In a client with cyanosis, the lips and tongue are gray, and the palms, soles, conjunctiva, and nail beds have a bluish tinge.

Test-Taking Strategy: Focus on the key word, *dark-skinned*, and use the process of elimination. This will assist in directing you to option 3. Review this important data collection technique if you had difficulty with this question.

Level of Cognitive Ability: Comprehension
Client Needs: Physiological Integrity
Integrated Process: Nursing Process/Data Collection
Content Area: Adult Health/Integumentary
References: Black, J., & Hawks, J. (2005). *Medical-surgical nursing: Clinical management for positive outcomes* (7th ed.). Philadelphia: W.B. Saunders, p. 1383.
Jarvis, C. (2004). *Physical examination and health assessment* (4th ed.). Philadelphia: W.B. Saunders, p. 249.

6. *Answer:* **3**

Rationale: Client preparation for a patch test includes informing the client to discontinue systemic corticosteroids or antihistamines for at least 48 hours before the test. To prevent suppression of the inflammatory response to an allergen, these medications must be discontinued. Options 1, 2, and 4 are unnecessary.

Test-Taking Strategy: Use the process of elimination. Eliminate options 1 and 4 first. These options are similar and there is no need to restrict food or remain NPO prior to the procedure. A "patch" test does not require a body shower with an antibacterial soap. Also, note the relationship between "allergen" in the question and "antihistamine" in the correct option. Review this test if you had difficulty with this question.

Level of Cognitive Ability: Application
Client Needs: Health Promotion and Maintenance
Integrated Process: Nursing Process/Implementation
Content Area: Adult Health/Integumentary
Reference: Linton, A., & Maebius, N. (2003) *Introduction to medical-surgical nursing* (3rd ed.). Philadelphia: W.B. Saunders, p. 1018.

7. *Answer: 2*

Rationale: The nurse instructs the client to keep the test site dry at all times. The nurse also discourages excessive physical activity that will result in sweating. Reapplying the patch can interfere with an accurate interpretation of the allergic reactions. The nurse reinforces the necessity of removing loose or nonadherent test patches for reapplication at a later date. The initial reading is performed 2 days after application, and the final reading is performed 2 to 5 days later.

Test-Taking Strategy: Use the process of elimination and note the key words, *need for further instruction*. These words indicate a false response question and that you need to select the incorrect client statement. Eliminate options 3 and 4 first, because keeping the test site dry and avoiding sweating are similar. From the remaining options, recalling that follow-up is important after any procedure will assist in directing you to option 2. If you had difficulty with this question, review the client teaching points following a patch test.

Level of Cognitive Ability: Comprehension
Client Needs: Health Promotion and Maintenance
Integrated Process: Teaching/Learning
Content Area: Adult Health/Integumentary
Reference: Thompson, J., McFarland, G., Hirsch, J., & Tucker, S. (2002). *Mosby's clinical nursing* (5th ed.). St. Louis: Mosby, p. 1392.

8. *Answer: 4*

Rationale: The client should avoid using a dehumidifier because this will further dry room air. Instead, the client should use a room humidifier during the winter months or whenever the furnace is in use. The client should be taught to maintain a daily fluid intake of 3000 mL unless contraindicated, and should avoid alcohol and caffeine ingestion. The client should avoid applying rubbing alcohol, astringents, or other drying agents to the skin. One bath or one shower per day for 15 to 20 minutes with warm water and a mild soap should be immediately followed by the application of an emollient to prevent evaporation of water from the hydrated epidermis.

Test-Taking Strategy: Use the process of elimination and note the key words, *need for further instructions*. These words indicate a false response question and that you need to select the incorrect client statement. Recalling that a dehumidifier is going to dry the air in the environment will assist in directing you to option 4. If you had difficulty with this question, review client teaching points related to dry skin and pruritus.

Level of Cognitive Ability: Comprehension
Client Needs: Health Promotion and Maintenance
Integrated Process: Teaching/Learning
Content Area: Adult Health/Integumentary
References: Linton, A., & Maebius, N. (2003). *Introduction to medical-surgical nursing* (3rd ed.). Philadelphia: W.B. Saunders, p. 1022.
Thompson, J., McFarland, G., Hirsch, J., & Tucker, S. (2002). *Mosby's clinical nursing* (5th ed.). St. Louis: Mosby, p. 481.

9. *Answer: 4*

Rationale: Lyme disease is a multisystem infection that results from a bite by a tick carried by several species of deer. Persons bitten by the *Ixodes* ticks are infected with the spirochete *Borrelia burgdorferi*. Histoplasmosis is caused by the inhalation of spores from bat or bird droppings. Toxoplasmosis is caused by the ingestion of cysts from contaminated cat feces. Lyme disease cannot be transmitted from one person to another.

Test-Taking Strategy: Use the process of elimination. Recalling that this disease is caused by a bite will assist in eliminating the incorrect options. If you had difficulty with this question, review the cause of Lyme disease.

Level of Cognitive Ability: Application
Client Needs: Health Promotion and Maintenance
Integrated Process: Nursing Process/Implementation
Content Area: Adult Health/Integumentary
Reference: Linton, A., & Maebius, N. (2003). *Introduction to medical-surgical nursing* (3rd ed.). Philadelphia: W.B. Saunders, p. 202.

10. *Answer: 2*

Rationale: Stage 2 of Lyme disease develops within 1 to 6 months in most untreated individuals. The most serious problems include cardiac conduction defects and neurological disorders, such as Bell's palsy and paralysis. These problems are not usually permanent. Arthralgias and joint enlargements are noted in stage 3. A rash appears in stage 1.

Test-Taking Strategy: Use the process of elimination. Eliminate options 3 and 4 first because they are similar. Recalling that a rash appears initially following the tick bite will assist in eliminating option 1. If you had difficulty with this question, review the clinical manifestations associated with each stage of Lyme disease.

Level of Cognitive Ability: Comprehension
Client Needs: Physiological Integrity
Integrated Process: Nursing Process/Data Collection
Content Area: Adult Health/Integumentary
Reference: Thompson, J., McFarland, G., Hirsch, J., & Tucker, S. (2002). *Mosby's clinical nursing* (5th ed.). St. Louis: Mosby, p. 1046.

11. *Answer: 3*

Rationale: There is a blood test available to detect Lyme disease; however, it is not reliable if performed prior to 4 to 6 weeks following the tick bite. Options 1, 2, and 4 are incorrect.

Test-Taking Strategy: Use the process of elimination. Eliminate option 1 first because of the word "immediately." A blood test is available; therefore, eliminate option 2. Eliminate option 4 because treatment should begin before the arthralgia develops. If you had difficulty with this question, review the method of diagnosing Lyme disease.

Level of Cognitive Ability: Application
Client Needs: Physiological Integrity
Integrated Process: Nursing Process/Implementation
Content Area: Adult Health/Integumentary
Reference: Linton, A., & Maebius, N. (2003). *Introduction to medical-surgical nursing* (3rd ed.). Philadelphia: W.B. Saunders, p. 202.

12. *Answer: 3*

Rationale: When an individual comes in contact with a poison ivy plant, the sap from the plant forms an invisible film on the skin. The client should be instructed to shower immediately

and to lather the skin several times and rinse each time in running water. Calamine lotion is a treatment used if dermatitis develops. It is not necessary for the client to be seen in the emergency room at this time.
Test-Taking Strategy: Recall that dermatitis can develop from contact with an allergen. Also, recalling that contact with poison ivy results in an invisible film will assist in directing you to option 3. Review the immediate treatment for contact with poison ivy if you had difficulty with this question.
Level of Cognitive Ability: Application
Client Needs: Health Promotion and Maintenance
Integrated Process: Nursing Process/Implementation
Content Area: Adult Health/Integumentary
Reference: Phipps, W., Monahan, F., Sands, J., Marek, J., & Neighbors, M. (2003). *Medical-surgical nursing: Health and illness perspectives* (7th ed.). St. Louis: Mosby, p. 1957.

13. *Answer: 3*
Rationale: Kaposi's sarcoma lesions begin as red, dark blue, or purple macules on the lower legs that change into plaques. These large plaques ulcerate or open and drain. The lesions spread by metastasis through the upper body, and then to the face and oral mucosa. It can also spread to the lymphatic system, lungs, and gastrointestinal (GI) tract. Late disease results in swelling and pain in the lower extremities, penis, scrotum, or face. Diagnosis is made by punch biopsy of cutaneous lesions and biopsy of pulmonary and GI lesions.
Test-Taking Strategy: Use the process of elimination, eliminating options 2 and 4 first. These symptoms occur late in the development of Kaposi's sarcoma. Note the key words, *this has been determined.* These words should assist in directing you to the option that will confirm the diagnosis, which is biopsy of the lesions. Review this skin disorder if you had difficulty with this question.
Level of Cognitive Ability: Comprehension
Client Needs: Physiological Integrity
Integrated Process: Nursing Process/Data Collection
Content Area: Adult Health/Integumentary
Reference: Linton, A., & Maebius, N. (2003). *Introduction to medical-surgical nursing* (3rd ed.). Philadelphia: W.B. Saunders, p. 1032.

14. *Answer: 4*
Rationale: Kaposi's sarcoma is a vascular malignancy that presents as a skin disorder. It is a common acquired immunodeficiency syndrome (AIDS) indicator. Malignancy is seen most frequently in men with a history of same-sex partners. Although the cause of Kaposi's sarcoma is not known, it is considered to be the result of an alteration or failure in the immune system. The renal transplant client and the client receiving antineoplastic medications are at risk for immunosuppression. Exposure to asbestos is not related to the development of Kaposi's sarcoma.
Test-Taking Strategy: Use the process of elimination. Note the key words, *least likely.* You can easily eliminate option 1 first. Next, note the similarity between options 2 and 3. These clients are at risk for immunosuppression. With this in mind, these options can be eliminated, leaving option 4 as the correct option. If you had difficulty with this question, review the risk factors associated with Kaposi's sarcoma.

Level of Cognitive Ability: Comprehension
Client Needs: Physiological Integrity
Integrated Process: Nursing Process/Data Collection
Content Area: Adult Health/Integumentary
References: Lewis, S., Heitkemper, M., & Dirksen, S. (2004). *Medical-surgical nursing: Assessment and management of clinical problems* (6th ed.). St. Louis: Mosby, p. 284.
Phipps, W., Monahan, F., Sands, J., Marek, J., & Neighbors, M. (2003). *Medical-surgical nursing: Health and illness perspectives* (7th ed.). St. Louis: Mosby, p. 1684.

15. *Answer: 2*
Rationale: Gowns and gloves are required if the nurse anticipates contact with soiled items, such as wound drainage on bed linens. Masks are not required unless droplet or airborne precautions are necessary.
Test-Taking Strategy: Use the process of elimination. Think about the method of transmission when answering a question of this type. Read the question, noting the task presented; in this case, it is bathing and changing linens. Eliminate option 1 because the method of transmission is not respiratory in nature. Eliminate options 3 and 4 because neither provides adequate protection based on the method of transmission. If you had difficulty with this question, review standard precautions.
Level of Cognitive Ability: Application
Client Needs: Safe, Effective Care Environment
Integrated Process: Nursing Process/Implementation
Content Area: Adult Health/Integumentary
Reference: Christensen, B., & Kockrow, E. (2003). *Foundations of nursing* (4th ed.). St. Louis: Mosby, pp. 240-242.

16. *Answer: 1*
Rationale: Cellulitis is a skin infection into deeper dermis and subcutaneous fat; it results in deep red erythema without sharp borders, and spreads widely through tissue spaces. The skin is erythematous, edematous, tender, and sometimes nodular. Erysipelas is an acute superficial rapidly spreading inflammation of the dermis and lymphatics.
Test-Taking Strategy: Knowledge regarding the characteristics of cellulitis is required to answer the question. Remember, cellulitis is a skin infection into deeper dermis and subcutaneous fat. If you had difficulty with this question, review the characteristics of cellulitis and erysipelas.
Level of Cognitive Ability: Comprehension
Client Needs: Physiological Integrity
Integrated Process: Nursing Process/Implementation
Content Area: Adult Health/Integumentary
Reference: Christensen, B., & Kockrow, E. (2003). *Foundations of nursing* (4th ed.). St. Louis: Mosby, pp. 423, 880.

17. *Answer: 1*
Rationale: Warm compresses may be used to decrease the discomfort, erythema, and edema. After tissue and blood cultures are obtained, antibiotics are initiated. Heat lamps can cause more disruption to already inflamed tissue. Continuous cold and hot compresses are not the best measures.
Test-Taking Strategy: Use the process of elimination, noting that option 1 is different from the other options. Option 1 addresses "warm" compresses whereas options 2, 3,

and 4 address either cold or hot measures. If you had difficulty with this question, review the treatment associated with cellulitis.
Level of Cognitive Ability: Application
Client Needs: Physiological Integrity
Integrated Process: Nursing Process/Planning
Content Area: Adult Health/Integumentary
Reference: Lewis, S., Heitkemper, M., & Dirksen, S. (2004). *Medical-surgical nursing: Assessment and management of clinical problems* (6th ed.). St. Louis: Mosby, p. 494.

18. *Answer:* 3
Rationale: Herpes zoster is caused by a reactivation of the varicella-zoster virus, the cause of chickenpox. A viral culture of the lesion provides the definitive diagnosis. In a Wood's light examination, the skin is viewed under ultraviolet light to identify superficial infections of the skin. A patch test is a skin test that involves the administration of an allergen to the skin's surface to identify specific allergies. A biopsy will determine tissue type.
Test-Taking Strategy: Use the process of elimination and focus on the diagnosis. Recall that herpes zoster is caused by a virus. This will assist in eliminating options 2 and 4. From the remaining options, remember that a biopsy will determine tissue type, whereas a culture will identify an organism. Review this skin disorder if you had difficulty with this question.
Level of Cognitive Ability: Comprehension
Client Needs: Physiological Integrity
Integrated Process: Nursing Process/Data Collection
Content Area: Adult Health/Integumentary
Reference: Linton, A., & Maebius, N. (2003). *Introduction to medical-surgical nursing* (3rd ed.). Philadelphia: W.B. Saunders, p. 1029.

19. *Answer:* 4
Rationale: The primary lesion of herpes zoster is a vesicle. The classic presentation is grouped vesicles on a erythematous base along a dermatome. Because they follow nerve pathways, the lesions do not cross the body's midline. Options 1, 2, and 3 are incorrect descriptions.
Test-Taking Strategy: Use the process of elimination. Remembering that these lesions occur as grouped vesicles along a nerve pathway will assist in answering the question. If you had difficulty with this question, review the characteristics of herpes zoster lesions.
Level of Cognitive Ability: Comprehension
Client Needs: Physiological Integrity
Integrated Process: Nursing Process/Data Collection
Content Area: Adult Health/Integumentary
Reference: Linton, A., & Maebius, N. (2003). *Introduction to medical-surgical nursing* (3rd ed.). Philadelphia: W.B. Saunders, p. 1028.

20. *Answer:* 2
Rationale: Herpes zoster is caused by a reactivation of the varicella-zoster virus, the causative virus of chickenpox. Individuals who have not been exposed to the varicella-zoster virus are susceptible to chickenpox. Options 1, 3, and 4 are not associated with the herpes zoster virus.

Test-Taking Strategy: Use the process of elimination and note the key word, *avoids.* Recalling that herpes zoster is caused by a reactivation of the varicella-zoster virus, the causative virus of chickenpox, will assist in answering the question. Review the relationship between herpes zoster and chickenpox if you had difficulty with this question.
Level of Cognitive Ability: Application
Client Needs: Safe, Effective Care Environment
Integrated Process: Nursing Process/Planning
Content Area: Delegating/Prioritizing
Reference: Linton, A., & Maebius, N. (2003). *Introduction to medical-surgical nursing* (3rd ed.). Philadelphia: W.B. Saunders, p. 1028.

21. *Answer:* 1
Rationale: Melanomas are pigmented malignant lesions originating in the melanin-producing cells of the epidermis. This skin cancer is highly metastatic, and a person's survival depends on early diagnosis and treatment. Basal cell carcinomas arise in the basal cell layer of the epidermis. Early malignant basal cell lesions often go unnoticed and, although metastasis is rare, underlying tissue destruction can progress to include vital structures. Squamous cell carcinomas are malignant neoplasms of the epidermis. They are characterized by local invasion and the potential for metastasis.
Test-Taking Strategy: Knowledge regarding the various types of skin cancers, and recalling that melanomas are highly metastatic, will assist in directing you to the correct option. If you had difficulty with this question, review the characteristics of skin cancers.
Level of Cognitive Ability: Comprehension
Client Needs: Physiological Integrity
Integrated Process: Nursing Process/Data Collection
Content Area: Adult Health/Integumentary
Reference: Linton, A., & Maebius, N. (2003). *Introduction to medical-surgical nursing* (3rd ed.). Philadelphia: W.B. Saunders, p. 1032.

22. *Answer:* 4
Rationale: A melanoma is a irregularly shaped pigmented papule or plaque with a red, white, or blue color. Basal cell carcinoma appears as a pearly papule with a central crater and rolled waxy border. Squamous cell carcinoma is a firm nodular lesion topped with a crust or a central area of ulceration. Actinic keratosis, a premalignant lesion, appears as a small macule or papule with a dry, rough, adherent yellow or brown scale.
Test-Taking Strategy: Use the process of elimination. Remembering that irregularly shaped lesions are a cause for concern will assist you in answering the question. If you had difficulty with this question, review the characteristics of malignant skin lesions.
Level of Cognitive Ability: Comprehension
Client Needs: Physiological Integrity
Integrated Process: Nursing Process/Data Collection
Content Area: Adult Health/Integumentary
Reference: Linton, A., & Maebius, N. (2003). *Introduction to medical-surgical nursing* (3rd ed.). Philadelphia: W.B. Saunders, p. 1032.

23. *Answer:* **4**

Rationale: The client should be instructed to avoid sun exposure between the hours of 11 AM and 3 PM. Sunscreen, a hat, opaque clothing, and sunglasses should be worn for outdoor activities. The client should be instructed to examine the body monthly for the appearance of any possible cancerous or any precancerous lesions.

Test-Taking Strategy: Use the process of elimination. Note the key words, *need for further instructions.* These words indicate a false response question and that you need to select the incorrect client statement. Careful reading of the question will direct you to option 4. Review client teaching in the prevention of skin cancer if you had difficulty with this question.

Level of Cognitive Ability: Comprehension
Client Needs: Health Promotion and Maintenance
Integrated Process: Teaching/Learning
Content Area: Adult Health/Integumentary
Reference: Lewis, S., Heitkemper, M., & Dirksen, S. (2004). *Medical-surgical nursing: Assessment and management of clinical problems* (6th ed.). St. Louis: Mosby, p. 490.

24. *Answer:* **2**

Rationale: Paronychia or infection around the nail is characterized by red, shiny skin, often associated with painful swelling. These infections frequently result from trauma, picking at the nail, or disorders such as dermatitis. Often, these become secondarily infected with bacteria or fungus, which later involves the nail. Options 1, 3, and 4 are incorrect descriptions of this disorder.

Test-Taking Strategy: Use the process of elimination. If you knew that this disorder related to an infection of the nail you would easily be directed to the correct option. If you had difficulty with this question, review the definition of this disorder.

Level of Cognitive Ability: Comprehension
Client Needs: Physiological Integrity
Integrated Process: Nursing Process/Data Collection
Content Area: Adult Health/Integumentary
Reference: Christensen, B., & Kockrow, E. (2003). *Foundations of nursing* (4th ed.). St. Louis: Mosby, p. 87.

25. *Answer:* **3**

Rationale: Thorough hand washing, separating laundry, and separate washing of the client's dishes is required because this infection is contagious as long as skin lesions are present. Antibiotics are administered and should be continued, as prescribed.

Test-Taking Strategy: Note the key words, *need for further instructions.* These words indicate a false response question and that you need to select the incorrect client statement. Recalling that this infection is contagious will direct you to option 3. If you had difficulty with this question, review client instructions related to home care and the prevention of transmission of the infection.

Level of Cognitive Ability: Application
Client Needs: Health Promotion and Maintenance
Integrated Process: Teaching/Learning
Content Area: Adult Health/Integumentary
Reference: Phipps, W., Monahan, F., Sands, J., Marek, J., & Neighbors, M. (2003). *Medical-surgical nursing: Health and illness perspectives* (7th ed.). St. Louis: Mosby, p. 1951.

26. *Answer:* **4**

Rationale: Findings in frostbite include a white or blue skin color and skin that is hard, cold, and insensitive to touch. As thawing occurs, flushing of the skin, the development of blisters or blebs, or tissue edema appears. Gangrene can develop in 9 to 15 days.

Test-Taking Strategy: Use the process of elimination and focus on the diagnosis, frostbite. The words "insensitive to touch" should assist in directing you to the correct option. If you had difficulty with this question, review the characteristics associated with frostbite.

Level of Cognitive Ability: Comprehension
Client Needs: Physiological Integrity
Integrated Process: Nursing Process/Data Collection
Content Area: Adult Health/Integumentary
Reference: Christensen, B., & Kockrow, E. (2003). *Foundations of nursing* (4th ed.). St. Louis: Mosby, pp. 630-631.

27. *Answer:* **1**

Rationale: Frost bite is ideally treated with rapid and continuous rewarming of the tissue in a water bath for 15 to 20 minutes, or until flushing of the skin occurs. Hot or cold water is not used in the treatment of frostbite.

Test-Taking Strategy: Use the process of elimination. Eliminate options 2 and 4 first, avoiding options that address "hot" or "cold." Eliminate option 3 because interventions would begin immediately. If you had difficulty with this question, review the interventions associated with frost bite.

Level of Cognitive Ability: Application
Client Needs: Physiological Integrity
Integrated Process: Nursing Process/Planning
Content Area: Adult Health/Integumentary
Reference: Christensen, B., & Kockrow, E. (2003). *Foundations of nursing* (4th ed.). St. Louis: Mosby, pp. 630-631.

28. *Answer:* **2**

Rationale: In a stage 2 pressure ulcer, the skin is not intact. There is partial-thickness skin loss of the epidermis or dermis. The ulcer is superficial and may look like an abrasion, blister, or shallow crater. The skin is intact in stage 1. A deep, crater-like appearance occurs in stage 3, and sinus tracts develop in stage 4.

Test-Taking Strategy: Use the process of elimination and knowledge of the characteristics associated with each stage of pressure ulcers. Remember, in a stage 2 pressure ulcer, the skin is not intact. If you had difficulty with this question, review the characteristics associated with each stage of pressure ulcers.

Level of Cognitive Ability: Comprehension
Client Needs: Physiological Integrity
Integrated Process: Nursing Process/Data Collection
Content Area: Adult Health/Integumentary
Reference: Linton, A., & Maebius, N. (2003). *Introduction to medical-surgical nursing* (3rd ed.). Philadelphia: W.B. Saunders, pp. 272-273.

29. *Answer:* **4**

Rationale: Bed or chair confinement, inability to move, loss of bowel or bladder control, poor nutrition, absent or inconsistent caregiving, and a lowered mental awareness can all

contribute to the development of skin breakdown. The least likely risk as presented in the options is the lowered mental awareness status. Options 1, 2, and 3 identify physiological conditions, which are the risk priorities.
Test-Taking Strategy: Note the key words, *least likely*. Use Maslow's Hierarchy of Needs theory. Remember that physiological needs are the priority. This will assist you in eliminating options 1, 2, and 3. Review the risk factors associated with skin breakdown if you had difficulty with this question.
Level of Cognitive Ability: Comprehension
Client Needs: Physiological Integrity
Integrated Process: Nursing Process/Data Collection
Content Area: Adult Health/Integumentary
Reference: deWit, S. (2005). *Fundamental concepts and skills for nursing* (2nd ed.). Philadelphia: W.B. Saunders, p. 275.

30. *Answer: 1*
Rationale: In severe cystic acne, isotretinoin may be prescribed to inhibit inflammation. Adverse effects include elevated triglycerides, skin dryness, eye discomfort such as dryness and burning, and cheilitis (lip inflammation). Close medical follow-up is required and dry skin and cheilitis can be decreased by the use of emollients and lip balms. Vitamin A supplements are stopped during this treatment.
Test-Taking Strategy: Use the process of elimination and note the key words, *need for further instruction*. These words indicate a false response question and that you need to select the incorrect client statement. Recalling that isotretinoin is a metabolite of vitamin A will direct you to option 1. If you had difficulty with this question review the action, side effects, and adverse effects of this medication.
Level of Cognitive Ability: Comprehension
Client Needs: Health Promotion and Maintenance
Integrated Process: Teaching/Learning
Content Area: Adult Health/Integumentary
Reference: McKenry, L., & Salerno, E. (2003). *Mosby's pharmacology in nursing* (21st ed.). St. Louis: Mosby, p. 1133.

31. *Answer: 3*
Rationale: Scabies can be identified by the multiple straight or wavy threadlike lines noted beneath the skin. The skin lesions are caused by the female, which burrows beneath the skin and lays its eggs. The eggs hatch in a few days and the baby mites find their way to the skin surface where they mate and complete the life cycle. Options 1, 2, and 4 are not characteristics of scabies.
Test-Taking Strategy: Recalling that scabies burrows beneath the skin surface will assist in the process of elimination and provide direction in selecting the correct option. If you had difficulty with this question, review the characteristics associated with scabies.
Level of Cognitive Ability: Comprehension
Client Needs: Physiological Integrity
Integrated Process: Nursing Process/Data Collection
Content Area: Adult Health/Integumentary
Reference: Linton, A., & Maebius, N. (2003). *Introduction to medical-surgical nursing* (3rd ed.). Philadelphia: W.B. Saunders, p. 1031.

32. *Answer: 3*
Rationale: The Centers for Disease Control and Prevention recommend the wearing of gowns and gloves for close contact with a person infested with scabies. Masks are not necessary. Transmission via clothing and other inanimate objects is uncommon. Scabies is usually transmitted from person to person by direct skin contact. All contacts that the client has had should be treated at the same time.
Test-Taking Strategy: Consider the mode of transmission of scabies and use the process of elimination. Because scabies is transmitted by direct skin contact, eliminate options 1, 2, and 4. If you had difficulty with question, review standard precautions and the transmission mode of scabies.
Level of Cognitive Ability: Application
Client Needs: Safe, Effective Care Environment
Integrated Process: Nursing Process/Implementation
Content Area: Adult Health/Integumentary
Reference: deWit, S. (2005). *Fundamental concepts and skills for nursing* (2nd ed.). Philadelphia: W.B. Saunders, p. 837.

33. *Answer: 3*
Rationale: If an inhalation injury is suspected, administration of 100% oxygen via a tight-fitting, nonrebreather face mask is prescribed until the carboxyhemoglobin level falls below 15%. In inhalation injuries, the oropharynx is inspected for evidence of erythema, blisters, or ulcerations. The need for endotracheal intubation is also assessed. Options 1, 2, and 4 are incorrect.
Test-Taking Strategy: Use the process of elimination. Recalling that 100% oxygen is required following an inhalation injury will assist in eliminating options 2 and 4. From the remaining options, recall that a tight-fitting nonrebreather mask is preferred so that the client will not rebreathe exhaled air. If you had difficulty with this question, review care of the client following an inhalation injury.
Level of Cognitive Ability: Analysis
Client Needs: Physiological Integrity
Integrated Process: Nursing Process/Planning
Content Area: Adult Health/Integumentary
Reference: Lewis, S., Heitkemper, M., & Dirksen, S. (2004). *Medical-surgical nursing: Assessment and management of clinical problems* (6th ed.). St. Louis: Mosby, p. 516.

34. *Answer: 4*
Rationale: The client exhibits several warning signs of an inhalation injury—namely, history of a flame burn to the face, hoarseness, cough, carbonaceous sputum, singed facial hair, facial edema, and then color change. Additionally, one of the cardinal signs of hypoxia is restlessness.
Test-Taking Strategy: Use the ABCs to answer the question. The only option that addresses airway is option 4. If you had difficulty with this question, review the clinical manifestations associated with burns to the face.
Level of Cognitive Ability: Analysis
Client Needs: Physiological Integrity
Integrated Process: Nursing Process/Data Collection
Content Area: Adult Health/Integumentary
Reference: Lewis, S., Heitkemper, M., & Dirksen, S. (2004). *Medical-surgical nursing: Assessment and management of clinical problems* (6th ed.). St. Louis: Mosby, p. 396.

35. *Answer:* **4**

Rationale: Escharotomies are performed to alleviate the compartment syndrome that can occur when edema forms under nondistensible eschar in a circumferential burn. Escharotomies are performed through avascular eschar to subcutaneous fat. Although bleeding may occur from the site, it is considered a complication rather than an anticipated therapeutic outcome. Formation of granulation tissue is not the intent of an escharotomy. Escharotomy will not affect the formation of edema.

Test-Taking Strategy: Note the issue of the question, a therapeutic outcome. Use the ABCs to answer the question. The only option that addresses circulation is option 4. If you had difficulty with this question, review the purpose of an escharotomy.

Level of Cognitive Ability: Analysis
Client Needs: Physiological Integrity
Integrated Process: Nursing Process/Evaluation
Content Area: Adult Health/Integumentary
Reference: Lewis, S., Heitkemper, M., & Dirksen, S. (2004). *Medical-surgical nursing: Assessment and management of clinical problems* (6th ed.). St. Louis: Mosby, p. 543.

36. *Answer:* **1**

Rationale: Superficial injury from radiation causes erythema and pain, hyperpigmentation, dry desquamation, or moist desquamation. Options 2, 3, and 4 are not associated with the description presented in the question.

Test-Taking Strategy: Use the process of elimination. Focus on the description in the question and note the word "superficial" in the correct option. If you had difficulty with this question, review the effects of radiation burns.

Level of Cognitive Ability: Comprehension
Client Needs: Physiological Integrity
Integrated Process: Nursing Process/Data Collection
Content Area: Adult Health/Integumentary
Reference: Phipps, W., Monahan, F., Sands, J., Marek, J., & Neighbors, M. (2003). *Medical-surgical nursing: Health and illness perspectives* (7th ed.). St. Louis: Mosby, p. 336.

37. *Answer:* **3**

Rationale: Circumferential burns of the extremities may compromise circulation. Elevating injured extremities above the level of the heart and active exercise help reduce dependent edema formation. Options 1, 2, and 4 are incorrect.

Test-Taking Strategy: Use the process of elimination, remembering that when an injury occurs such as a burn, edema occurs. Option 3 addresses a position that will reduce edema. If you had difficulty with this question, review care of the client experiencing this type of a burn injury.

Level of Cognitive Ability: Application
Client Needs: Physiological Integrity
Integrated Process: Nursing Process/Implementation
Content Area: Adult Health/Integumentary
References: Ignatavicius, D., & Workman, M. (2002). *Medical-surgical: Critical thinking for collaborative care* (4th ed.). Philadelphia: W.B. Saunders, pp. 1573, 1582.
Phipps, W., Monahan, F., Sands, J., Marek, J., & Neighbors, M. (2003). *Medical-surgical nursing: Health and illness perspectives* (7th ed.). St. Louis: Mosby, pp. 2012-2013.

38. *Answer:* **2**

Rationale: Successful or adequate fluid resuscitation in the adult is signaled by stable vital signs, adequate urine output, palpable peripheral pulses, and clear sensorium. The most reliable indicator for determining adequacy of fluid resuscitation is the urine output. For an adult, the hourly urine volume should be 30 to 50 mL.

Test-Taking Strategy: Use the process of elimination. Note the key words, *most reliable*. Note the issue of the question, fluid resuscitation. Urine output is most similar to the issue of administering fluids. Review care of the burn client during fluid resuscitation if you had difficulty with this question.

Level of Cognitive Ability: Analysis
Client Needs: Physiological Integrity
Integrated Process: Nursing Process/Evaluation
Content Area: Adult Health/Integumentary
Reference: Phipps, W., Monahan, F., Sands, J., Marek, J., & Neighbors, M. (2003). *Medical-surgical nursing: Health and illness perspectives* (7th ed.). St. Louis: Mosby, p. 1995.

39. *Answer:* **1**

Rationale: Autografts placed over joints or on the lower extremities are often elevated and immobilized following surgery for 3 to 7 days. This period of immobilization allows the autograft time to adhere and attach to the wound bed.

Test-Taking Strategy: Use the process of elimination. Eliminate options 2 and 3 first, because they are similar. Note that the autograft was placed over a joint. This should direct you to select the option that identifies elevation and immobilization. If you had difficulty with this question, review care of an autograft placed over a joint.

Level of Cognitive Ability: Application
Client Needs: Physiological Integrity
Integrated Process: Nursing Process/Planning
Content Area: Adult Health/Integumentary
Reference: Phipps, W., Monahan, F., Sands, J., Marek, J., & Neighbors, M. (2003). *Medical-surgical nursing: Health and illness perspectives* (7th ed.). St. Louis: Mosby, p. 2001.

40. *Answer:* **4**

Rationale: Newly healed skin is more sensitive to the cold, and the client should be instructed to wear warm clothing. The client should wash using a mild soap, rinsing thoroughly, and patting the skin dry using a clean towel. Newly healed skin sunburns easily and direct sunlight needs to be avoided. Products that contain perfume, alcohol, or lanolin should be avoided because they tend to irritate newly healed skin.

Test-Taking Strategy: Use the process of elimination and note the key words, *need for further instructions*. These words indicate a false response question and that you need to select the incorrect client statement. Read each option carefully, noting that the correct option uses the absolute word "never." If you had difficulty with this question, review home care instructions regarding skin care.

Level of Cognitive Ability: Application
Client Needs: Health Promotion and Maintenance
Integrated Process: Teaching/Learning
Content Area: Adult Health/Integumentary

References: Linton, A., & Maebius, N. (2003). *Introduction to medical-surgical nursing* (3rd ed.). Philadelphia: W.B. Saunders, p. 1037.
Thompson, J., McFarland, G., Hirsch, J., & Tucker, S. (2002). *Mosby's clinical nursing* (5th ed.). St. Louis: Mosby, p. 503.

ALTERNATE FORMAT QUESTION: FILL IN THE BLANK

Answer: 36

Rationale: According to the Rule of Nines, with the initial burn, the anterior half of the head equals 4.5%, the upper half of the anterior torso equals 9%, and the lower halves of both arms equals 9%. The subsequent burn included the posterior half of head, 4.5%, and the upper half of the posterior torso, 9%. This totals 36%.

Test-Taking Strategy: Knowledge regarding the Rule of Nines is required to answer this question. The entire head equals 9%, each arm equals 9% (both arms, 18%), anterior or posterior torso each equals 18% (36% for entire torso), each leg equals 18% (both legs, 36%), and perineum equals 1%. Remember: 9% (head), 18% (arms), 36% (torso), 36% (legs), 1% (perineum), totalling 100%. If you had difficulty with this question, learn the Rule of Nines.
Level of Cognitive Ability: Analysis
Client needs: Physiological Integrity
Integrated Process: Nursing Process/Data Collection
Content Area: Adult Health/Integumentary
Reference: Lewis, S., Heitkemper, M., & Dirksen, S. (2004). *Medical-surgical nursing: Assessment and management of clinical problems* (6th ed.). St. Louis: Mosby, p. 519.

REFERENCES

Black, J., & Hawks, J. (2005). *Medical-surgical nursing: Clinical management for positive outcomes* (7th ed.). Philadelphia: W.B. Saunders.

Christensen, B., & Kockrow, E. (2003). *Foundations of nursing* (4th ed.). St. Louis: Mosby.

deWit, S. (2005). *Fundamental concepts and skills for nursing* (2nd ed.). Philadelphia: W.B. Saunders.

Ignatavicius, D., & Workman, M. (2002). *Medical surgical nursing: Critical thinking for collaborative care* (4th ed.). Philadelphia: W.B. Saunders.

Jarvis, C. (2004). *Physical examination and health assessment* (4th ed.). Philadelphia: W.B. Saunders, pp. 542-543.

Lewis, S., Heitkemper, M., & Dirksen, S. (2004). *Medical-surgical nursing: Assessment and management of clinical problems* (6th ed.). St. Louis: Mosby.

Linton, A., & Maebius, N. (2003). *Introduction to medical-surgical nursing* (3rd ed.). Philadelphia: W.B. Saunders.

McKenry, L., & Salerno, E. (2003). *Mosby's pharmacology in nursing* (21st ed.). St. Louis: Mosby.

Pagana, K., & Pagana, T. (2003). *Mosby's diagnostic and laboratory test reference* (6th ed.). St. Louis: Mosby.

Phipps, W., Monahan, F., Sands, J., Marek, J., & Neighbors, M. (2003). *Medical-surgical nursing: Health and illness perspectives* (7th ed.). St. Louis: Mosby.

Thompson, J., McFarland, G., Hirsch, J., & Tucker, S. (2002). *Mosby's clinical nursing* (5th ed.). St. Louis: Mosby.

Integumentary Medications

I. EMOLLIENTS AND LOTIONS

A. Emollients (Box 41-1)
1. Oily or fatty substances that soften and soothe irritated skin by allowing the skin to retain water
2. Available as creams or ointments
3. Used for dry, scaly, itchy inflammatory conditions

B. Solutions and lotions (Box 41-2)
1. Liquid suspensions or dispersions
2. Require shaking before application
3. Although lotions are predominantly water, they have a drying effect on the skin when the water evaporates
4. Used as a wash for the skin, as soaks, or as wet dressings on ulcers or **burns**
5. Used for subacute inflammatory lesions after the severe exudate phase has ceased
6. Medicated lotions are often used as anti-inflammatory agents because they provide a drying, protective, and cooling effect

II. RUBS AND LINIMENTS (Box 41-3)

A. Used for the temporary relief of muscular aches, rheumatism, arthritis, sprains, and neuralgia
B. Over-the-counter (OTC) products contain combinations of antiseptics, local anesthetics, analgesics, and counterirritants
C. Some products contain salicylates and, if used over a large area of the skin, may cause salicylate side effects such as tinnitus, nausea, or vomiting
D. A heating pad is not used with these products, because irritation or burning of the skin may occur

III. ANTI-INFECTIVE AGENTS

A. Description
1. Includes antiseptics and antibacterial, antifungal, antiviral, and antiparasitic medications
2. Topical antibiotics are safe and effective in certain conditions; extensive use may encourage the emergence of resistant bacteria

B. Antiseptics
1. Sodium hypochlorite (Dakin solution)
a. A chloride solution that loosens, dissolves, and deodorizes necrotic tissue and blood clots
b. It kills most common bacteria, including spores, amebas, fungi, protozoa viruses, and yeast
c. It is used for irrigating and cleaning necrotic or purulent wounds

---

BOX 41-1

Emollients

Cold cream
Glycerin
Lanolin
Lubriderm
Petrolatum
Zinc ointment
Vitamin A and D ointment

BOX 41-2

Solutions and Lotions

Aluminum acetate solution (Burow's solution)
Calamine lotion (Caladryl lotion)

BOX 41-3

Rubs and Liniments

Aspercreme
Ben-Gay
Icy Hot
Myoflex

d. Loses its potency during storage, so fresh solution is prepared frequently

e. It should not be in contact with healing or normal tissue

2. Chlorhexidine gluconate (Hibiclens)

a. Effective for cleaning wounds caused by staphylococci and other gram-positive bacteria

b. Used for irrigating and cleansing wounds, but not for packing wounds because it may cause contact dermatitis

3. Acetic acid

a. Effective for irrigating, cleansing, and packing wounds infected by *Pseudomonas aeruginosa*

b. Healthy skin surrounding the wound must be protected with a petroleum barrier because it excoriates the skin

4. Hydrogen peroxide

a. As a 3% solution, it has effervescent action that releases gas and breaks up necrotic tissue

b. It is used to irrigate and clean necrotic tissue and pus from open wounds

c. It is not used to pack wounds because it decomposes too rapidly

d. When epithelial tissue begins to form, hydrogen peroxide is discontinued because it inhibits tissue formation

5. Hexachlorophene (pHisoHex, Septisol)

a. A combination of hexachlorophene and alcohol

b. Hexachlorophene is a bacteriostatic agent with activity against staphylococci and other gram-positive bacteria

c. Hexachlorophene is heavily absorbed through broken skin and can cause neurotoxicity; it should not be used on wounds

d. The alcohol component dries and irritates tissue, is not a very effective germicide, and forms a film that can actually promote infection

e. All hexachlorophene products are well rinsed from the skin after their use to prevent systemic absorption

C. Antibacterials (Box 41-4)

1. Description: Used for superficial skin infections

2. Mupirocin (Bactroban)

a. Topical antibacterial active against *Staphylococcus aureus*, beta-hemolytic streptococci, or *Streptococcus pyogenes*

b. Applied three times daily; if improvement is not observed within 3 to 5 days, it is discontinued

D. Antifungals

1. May cause erythema, stinging, blistering, peeling, pruritus, urticaria, and general skin irritation

2. Client is re-evaluated if no results are obtained after 4 weeks of treatment

E. Antiviral: Acyclovir (Zovirax)

1. Inhibits DNA replication in the virus

2. Used for herpes simplex virus types 1 and 2, varicella-zoster virus, Epstein-Barr virus, and cytomegalovirus

3. Can cause mild pain and transient burning and stinging.

4. Applied completely over the lesion every 3 hours six times daily for 1 week

5. Rubber gloves are used to apply the ointment to prevent the spread of infection

F. Antiparasitics

1. Used to treat scabies (mites) and pediculosis (lice)

2. May be harmful during pregnancy and in young children

3. May irritate the skin, eyes, and mucous membranes

4. May cause allergic reactions

5. Permethrin 5% (Elimite)

BOX 41-4

Antibacterials, Antifungals, Antiviral, and Antiparasitics

ANTIBACTERIALS
Bacitracin
Chlortetracycline
Chloramphenicol
Erythromycin
Gentamicin
Mupirocin (Bactroban)
Mycitracin Triple Antibiotic (neomycin, bacitracin, polymyxin B)
Neomycin

ANTIFUNGALS
Amphotericin B (Fungizone)
Betamethasone and clotrimazole (Lotrisone)
Ciclopirox olamine (Loprox)
Clioquinol (Vioform)
Clotrimazole (Lotrimin, Mycelex)
Econazole nitrate (Spectazole)
Haloprogin (Halotex)
Ketoconazole (Nizoral)
Miconazole (Micatin)
Nystatin (Mycostatin)
Tolnaftate (Tinactin)
Triacetin (Fungoid)
Undecylenic acid (Desenex)

ANTIVIRAL
Acyclovir (Zovirax)

ANTIPARASITICS
Crotamiton (Eurax)
Lindane (Kwell)
Permethrin 5% (Elimite)
Malathion (Ovide)

a. Wash, rinse, and towel dry the hair; apply sufficient volume to saturate the hair and scalp

b. Allow to remain on the hair 10 minutes and then rinse with water

6. Lindane (Kwell)

a. Applied in a thin layer to the entire body below the head; no more than 30 g (1 oz) should be used

b. The medication is removed by washing 8 to 12 hours later; usually, only one application is required

IV. ANTIPRURITICS (Box 41-5)

A. Used to relieve itching

B. Applied as wet dressings, pastes, lotions, creams, or ointments

C. Persons with dry skin should be instructed to bathe less frequently

V. KERATOLYTICS (Box 41-6)

A. Description

1. Preparations that dissolve keratin

2. Soften scales and loosen the horny layer of the skin, resulting in minimal peeling or extensive desquamation

3. Used to treat superficial fungal infections, dermatitis, psoriasis, and localized dermatitis

B. Salicylic acid

1. Used to treat seborrheic dermatitis, acne, psoriasis, and to thin and remove calluses

2. Can be absorbed systematically and can cause salicylism, characterized by dizziness and tinnitus; is not applied to large surface areas or open wounds

C. Podophyllum resin

1. Used for various types of skin cancer

2. Causes lesions to slough off, leaving a superficial ulcer and moderate dermatitis

3. After the therapy is discontinued, the lesions are treated with a mild antiseptic ointment; healing usually occurs within a few days

D. Cantharidin (Cantharone)

1. Used in treating warts

2. Has an exfoliation effect only on epidermal cells

3. May cause tingling, itching, and burning

4. Site may be very tender for a period of 2 to 6 days

E. Masoprocol (Actinex)

1. Has antiproliferative activity against keratinocytes and is used to treat keratosis

2. Occlusive dressings are not to be used

3. Transient burning may be experienced after administration

BOX 41-5

Antipruritics

Calamine lotion
Cornstarch or oatmeal baths
Solutions of bismuth salts, aluminum acetate, or boric acid

BOX 41-6

Keratolytics

Cantharidin (Cantharone)
Imiquimod (Aldara)
Masoprocol (Actinex)
Podophyllum resin
Podofilox (Condylox)
Resorcinol
Salicylic acid

BOX 41-7

Stimulants and Irritants

Coal tar
Compound benzoin tincture

VI. STIMULANTS AND IRRITANTS (Box 41-7)

A. Description: Produce a mild irritation to the surface of the skin, causing hyperemia and inflammation that promote the healing process

B. Coal tar

1. Used in treating psoriasis, seborrheic dermatitis, and atopic dermatitis

2. Has an unpleasant odor and frequently stains the skin and hair

3. Can cause phototoxicity

C. Compound benzoin tincture

1. Protects the skin when the client has bed sores, ulcers, cracked nipples, and fissures of any orifice

2. Causes a mild irritation that produces increased blood flow and healing

VII. PROTECTIVES (Box 41-8)

A. Description

1. Preparations that provide a film on the skin to protect it from irritations such as light, moisture, air, and dust

2. Promote natural healing without the usual formation of dry crust over the wound

3. Allow exudate to collect beneath the dressing, forming an artificial blister

---

BOX 41-8

Protectives

Benzoin
DuoDerm
Mediskin
Opsite
Polyskin
Tegaderm
Tegasorb
Uniflex
Vigilon
Zinc oxide paste (Unna Boot)

---

4. Designed to be left in place for up to 7 days or until leakage occurs around the dressing
5. Uniflex and PolySkin may be used to cover central and peripheral IV sites
6. Opsite, Tegasorb, Mediskin, and Vigilon may be used for skin **burns**

B. Sunscreens
1. Act by absorbing ultraviolet rays
2. Most effective when applied about 30 to 60 minutes before exposure to the sun; should be reapplied every 2 to 3 hours after swimming or sweating
3. Can cause contact dermatitis and photosensitivity reactions

C. Nonadherent dressings
1. Woven or nonwoven dressings that may be impregnated with saline, petrolatum, or antimicrobials
2. Nonadherent dressings include Adaptic, Exu-Dry, Sofsorb, Telfa, vaseline gauze, and Xeroform

---

VIII. GROWTH FACTORS
A. Description
1. Used to promote wound healing
2. Stimulate cells to divide and migrate, which results in wound healing, formation of granulation tissue, and new epidermis
B. Procuren solution
1. Promotes healing by actively stimulating growth and granulation tissue, capillaries, and epithelium
2. Applied to the wound and covered with petrolatum-impregnated gauze
3. Left in place for 12 hours and then washed off; during the remaining 12 hours of the day, the wound is covered with sulfadiazine (Silvadene)

IX. ENZYMES
A. Description
1. Used to promote healing of wounds and to debride skin ulcers

---

BOX 41-9

Enzymes That Promote Wound Healing

Hyaluronidase (Wydase)
Papain (Panafil, Panafil White)

---

2. Reduce inflammation resulting from trauma and infection
3. Dissolve fibrin clots, which helps reduce the size of surface hematomas
4. To be effective, must be in contact with affected tissue in adequate concentrations for a sufficient length of time
5. Wound may need to be surgically debrided prior to application; if not administered to a clean, debrided wound, healing may be delayed

B. Enzymes that promote wound healing (Box 41-9)
1. Papain (Panafil, Panafil White)
a. Does not injure or affect healthy tissue or cells
b. Enzyme must be in immediate contact with the purulent wound material
c. Wounds are cleansed with prescribed irrigating solution between applications
d. Hydrogen peroxide cannot be used to irrigate the wound, because it inactivates the papain
e. Light dressings and cellophane wrap may be used over the wound to prevent soiling of clothing
f. Dressings are changed frequently to prevent contamination and to remove necrotic debris
2. Hyaluronidase (Wydase)
a. Facilitates the absorption of fluid administered by subcutaneous hypodermoclysis
b. Can be injected subcutaneous into an infiltrated IV site when a potent vasoconstrictor such as norepinephrine (Levophed) or metaraminol (Aramine) has infiltrated
c. It reduces the sloughing of tissue likely to occur secondarily to infiltration
C. Enzymes to debride and remove exudates (Box 41-10)
1. Description
a. Alter the thick, purulent drainage to a thin, liquid material that can be easily wiped or irrigated off the wound
b. Enzyme contact with the wound is necessary to promote wound healing
c. Wound needs to be cleansed; cross-hatching of eschar on **burns** is performed prior to application
2. Sutilains (Travase)
a. Used to remove nonviable or necrotic tissue and purulent enzymes from **burns**, ulcers, traumatic injury, and peripheral vascular disease wounds

BOX 41-10

Enzymes to Debride and Remove Exudates

Collagenase (Santyl)
Dextranomer (Debrisan)
Fibrinolysin and desoxyribonuclease (Elase)
Sutilains (Travase)

b. Inactive on viable tissue
c. The wound is moistened with normal saline or sterile water before application

3. Collagenase (Santyl)
   a. Used as a topical debriding agent
   b. Provides effective debridement of the collagen tissue at the wound edges where necrotic tissue is anchored
   c. Encourages the formation of granulation tissue at the wound edges and quicker epithelization of wounds
   d. Apply with a tongue depressor directly into deep wounds
   e. Prior to application, cleanse wound of debris by gently rubbing with a gauze pad with sterile water or Dakin solution, followed by sterile normal saline
   f. Remove all excess ointment each time dressing is changed
   g. Apply only to injured area; causes erythema in healthy tissues
   h. Protect healthy tissue by applying zinc oxide paste
   i. Discontinued when necrotic tissue is gone

4. Fibrinolysin and desoxyribonuclease (Elase)
   a. Used to debride wounds, including **burns**, **decubitus** ulcers, and inflamed or infected lesions
   b. Clean wound with sterile water, pat dry; flush away necrotic debris with normal saline, then apply a thin layer and cover with petrolatum gauze

D. Dextranomer (Debrisan)
   1. Not a debriding agent but a cleansing agent that actually absorbs peptides and proteins
   2. Effective in wet wounds only
   3. It is not packed tightly into the wound because maceration of surrounding tissue may occur from contact with the agent

X. CORTICOSTEROIDS

A. Have anti-inflammatory, antipruritic, and vasoconstrictive actions
B. Contraindications
   1. Clients demonstrating previous sensitivity to corticosteroids
   2. Those with current systemic fungal, viral, or bacterial infections
   3. Those with current complications related to corticosteroid therapy
C. Local adverse effects
   1. Hypopigmentation
   2. Acneform eruptions
   3. Contact dermatitis
   4. Burning, dryness, irritation, itching
   5. Overgrowth of bacteria, fungi, and viruses
   6. Skin atrophy
D. Systemic adverse effects
   1. Occur rarely
   2. Adrenal suppression
   3. Cushing's syndrome
   4. Striae, skin atrophy
   5. Ocular effects (glaucoma and cataracts)
E. Topical steroids
   1. Monitor plasma cortisol levels if prolonged therapy is necessary
   2. Wash area just prior to application to increase medication penetration
   3. Apply sparingly in a light film, rubbing gently
   4. May apply to skin alone or with a dry occlusive dressing if prescribed by the physician
   5. Instruct the client to report burning, irritation, or signs of infection to the physician

XI. ACNE PRODUCTS (Box 41-11)

A. Description
   1. Mild acne can be treated with bar soaps, soap-free cakes, liquid cleansers, lotions, gels, and creams
   2. For moderate acne, topical anti-inflammatory medication such as benzoyl peroxide, tretinoin (Retin-A), isotretinoin (Accutane), azelaic acid (Azelex), and adapalene (Differin) may be prescribed; antibiotics may also be prescribed
   3. Side effects can include excessive redness, extreme dryness of the skin leading to blistering and crusting, temporary pigmentation changes, and peeling of the skin
   4. All products are kept away from the eyes, inside the nose, mucous membranes, and hair
B. Benzoyl peroxide: A keratolytic agent that is bacteriostatic and may decrease the production of irritant free fatty acids in the follicle
C. Tretinoin (Retin-A) and adapalene (Differin): Acids of vitamin A that are used to treat acne vulgaris; may also be used to treat skin cancer and aging of the skin
D. Tretinoin (Retin-A)
   1. Decreases cohesiveness of the epithelial cells, increasing cell mitosis and turnover; potentially irritating, particularly when used correctly
   2. Within 48 hours of use, the skin generally becomes red and begins to peel
   3. Temporary hyperpigmentation and hypopigmentation can occur

BOX 41-11

Acne Products

CLEANSERS
Acnomel
Brevoxyl
Clearasil
Fostex
pHisoDerm
Stri-Dex

DRYING AGENTS
Acnomel
Ionax
Listerex

MISCELLANEOUS
Adapalene (Differin)
Alpha hydroxy acids
Antibiotics
Azelaic acid (Azelex)
Bensulfoid cream (benzoyl peroxide and sulfur)
Benzamycin gel (benzoyl peroxide and sulfur)
Benzoyl peroxide wash, gel
Isotretinoin (Accutane)
Rosorcinol (as an ingredient in other preparations)
Salicylic acid (as an ingredient in other preparations)
Tazarotene (Tazorac)
Tretinoin (Retin-A)

BOX 41-12

Poison Ivy Treatment Products

Calamine lotion
Calomox
IV-Chex
Ivy-Rid
Rhuli cream, spray, gel

1. Used to treat acne; include clindamycin (Cleocin T), erythromycin, tetracycline (Topicycline), and meclocycline (Meclan)
2. Therapeutic response generally requires 6 to 12 weeks of therapy
3. Side effects include acute contact dermatitis, transient stinging or burning, staining of the skin, erythema, and skin tenderness

XII. POISON IVY TREATMENT (Box 41-12)

XIII. BURN PRODUCTS (Box 41-13)

A. Nitrofurazone (Furacin)
1. Applied topically to the **burn** as a solution, ointment, or cream
2. Has a broad spectrum of antibacterial activity
3. Used in **burns** when bacterial resistance to other agents is a problem
4. Topical: Apply $1/16$-inch film directly to **burn**
5. Side effects: Contact dermatitis, rash
6. Less common side effects: Pruritus, local edema
B. Mafenide (Sulfamylon)
1. A water-soluble cream that is bacteriostatic for both gram-negative and gram-positive organisms
2. Is used to treat **burns** to reduce the bacteria present in avascular tissues
3. Diffuses through the devascularized areas of the skin; may precipitate metabolic acidosis (usually compensated by hyperventilation)
4. Apply $1/16$-inch film directly to the burn
5. Side effects can include local pain, rash
6. Systemic effects include bone marrow depression, hemolytic anemia, metabolic acidosis
7. Keep **burn** covered with mafenide at all times
8. Notify physician if hyperventilation occurs; if acidosis develops, mafenide is washed off the skin
C. Silver sulfadiazine (Silvadene)
1. Has a broad spectrum of activity against gram-negative bacteria, gram-positive bacteria, and yeast
2. Released slowly from the cream, which is selectively toxic to bacteria
3. Used primarily to prevent sepsis in clients with **burns**

4. Client should avoid sun exposure because photosensitivity may occur
5. Applied liberally to the skin; hands are washed thoroughly immediately after applying
6. Therapeutic results should be seen after 2 to 3 weeks but may not be optimal until after 6 weeks
7. Client may use cosmetics, but the skin needs to be cleaned thoroughly before applying the cosmetics
E. Isotretinoin (Accutane)
1. A metabolite of vitamin A
2. Used to treat severe cystic acne; its use is reserved for persons who have not responded to other therapies, including systemic antibiotics
3. Can cause xerosis and facial desquamation, palmoplantar desquamation, pruritus, brittle nails, and hair loss
4. Administered with meals two times daily for a 15- to 20-week course; if another course of therapy is needed, an 8-week interval should occur
5. Photosensitivity may occur, so the client needs to be instructed to decrease sun exposure
6. Alcohol consumption should be eliminated during therapy because alcohol may potentiate serum triglyceride elevation
F. Local antibiotics

BOX 41-13

Burn Products

Mafenide (Sulfamylon)
Nitrofurazone (Furacin)
Silver nitrate
Silver sulfadiazine (Silvadene)

4. Is not a carbonic anhydrase inhibitor and therefore does not cause acidosis
5. Rash and itching occurs from topical application
6. Apply $\frac{1}{16}$-inch film; keep **burn** covered at all times with silver sulfadiazine
7. Systemic effects include leukopenia, interstitial nephritis
8. Monitor complete blood cell (CBC) count, particularly white blood cells (WBCs) frequently; if leukopenia develops, the medication is discontinued

D. Silver nitrate
   1. An antiseptic solution active against gram-negative bacteria
   2. Dressings are applied to the **burn**, which are then kept moist with silver nitrate; this stains anything that it comes into contact with; this discoloration is not usually permanent
   3. Used on extensive **burns** that may precipitate fluid and electrolyte imbalances
   4. Apply to dressing; do not apply to wounds, cuts, or broken skin

PRACTICE QUESTIONS

1. A camp nurse asks the children preparing to swim in the lake if they have applied sunscreen. The nurse tells the children that sunscreen is most effective when applied:
   1. One hour before exposure to the sun
   2. Immediately before exposure to the sun
   3. 15 minutes before exposure to the sun
   4. Immediately after swimming
2. The nurse is assigned to care for a client with a burn injury to the lower legs. Nitrofurazone (Furacin) is prescribed to be applied to the sites of injury. The nurse plans to:
   1. Apply saline-soaked dressings over the medication
   2. Apply 1-inch film directly to the burn sites
   3. Apply $\frac{1}{16}$-inch film directly to the burn sites
   4. Apply $\frac{1}{2}$-inch film directly to the burn sites after cleansing the wounds
3. Mafenide (Sulfamylon) is prescribed for the client with a burn injury. When applying the medication, the client complains of local discomfort and burning. The nurse would:
   1. Discontinue the medication
   2. Notify the registered nurse immediately
   3. Apply a thinner film than prescribed to the burn site
   4. Inform the client that this is normal
4. A burn client is receiving treatments of topical mafenide (Sulfamylon) to the site of injury. The nurse would suspect that a systemic effect has occurred if which of the following is noted in the client?
   1. Local pain at the burn site
   2. Local rash at the burn site
   3. Hyperventilation
   4. Elevated blood pressure
5. Sodium hypochlorite (Dakin solution) is prescribed for a client with a leg wound containing purulent drainage. The nurse is assisting in developing a plan of care for the client and includes which of the following in the plan?
   1. Apply the solution to the wound and on normal skin tissue surrounding the wound
   2. Allow the solution to remain in the wound following irrigation
   3. Soak a sterile dressing with solution and pack into the wound
   4. Ensure that the solution is freshly prepared before use
6. Tretinoin (Retin-A) is prescribed for a client with acne. The client calls the physician's office and tells the nurse that the skin has become very red and is beginning to peel. The nurse responds by telling the client:
   1. To come to the clinic immediately
   2. To discontinue the medication
   3. To notify the physician
   4. That this is a normal occurrence with the use of this medication
7. A nurse provides instructions to a client regarding the use of tretinoin (Retin-A). Which statement by the client indicates the need for further instructions?
   1. "I should wash my hands thoroughly after applying the medication."
   2. "Optimal results will be seen after 6 weeks."
   3. "I should apply a very thin layer to my skin."
   4. "I should cleanse my skin thoroughly before applying the medication."
8. Isotretinoin (Accutane) is prescribed for a client to treat severe cystic acne. The nurse tells the client that the length of the usual prescribed course of treatment is:
   1. 1 month
   2. 8 weeks
   3. 15 to 20 weeks
   4. 1 year
9. Isotretinoin (Accutane) is prescribed for a client with severe acne. Before the administration of this medication, the nurse would expect that which laboratory test will be prescribed?
   1. Complete blood count
   2. White blood cell count
   3. Triglyceride level
   4. Platelet count

10. A client with severe acne is seen at the physician's office. The physician prescribes isotretinoin (Accutane). The nurse reviews the client's health record and would notify the physician if the client is presently taking which of the following medications?
    1. Digoxin (Lanoxin)
    2. Phenytoin (Dilantin)
    3. Vitamin A
    4. Furosemide (Lasix)

11. Fibrinolysin and desoxyribonuclease (Elase) dry powder is prescribed to treat a skin ulcer. The nurse assists in developing a plan of care for the client and includes which intervention in the plan?
    1. Clean the wound with tap water before applying the medication
    2. After applying the medication, cover the wound with a dry, sterile dressing
    3. Apply a thick layer of medication, followed by a second layer
    4. Apply a thin layer of medication and cover with a petrolatum gauze

12. Sutilains (Travase) is prescribed to treat the ulcer. The nurse avoids which action when performing the dressing change?
    1. Cleans the wound with a sterile solution
    2. Dries the wound and covers the Travase application with a dry sterile dressing
    3. Moistens the wound with sterile normal saline and then applies the Travase
    4. Places the Travase in the refrigerator following use

13. A nurse employed in a physician's office is collecting data from a client. The nurse notes that the client is taking azelaic acid (Azelex). Because of the medication prescription, the nurse suspects that the client is being treated for:
    1. Herpes simplex
    2. Acne
    3. Eczema
    4. Hair loss

14. Collagenase (Santyl) is prescribed for a client with a severe burn to the hand. The nurse provides instructions to the client regarding the use of the medication. Which statement by the client indicates an accurate understanding of the use of this medication?
    1. "I will apply the ointment once a day and leave it open to the air."
    2. "I will apply the ointment once a day and cover it with a sterile dressing."
    3. "I will apply the ointment twice a day and leave it open to the air."
    4. "I will apply the ointment at bedtime and in the morning and cover it with a sterile dressing."

15. Dextranomer (Debrisan) is prescribed for a client with a decubiti ulcer. The nursing instructor asks the nursing student preparing to perform the treatment about the medication and the procedure. Which statement, if made by the student, indicates a need for further research?
    1. "It is effective in wet wounds only."
    2. "It should be packed lightly into the wound."
    3. "Maceration of tissue surrounding the wound can occur from the medication."
    4. "The wound bed must be thoroughly dried prior to applying the medication."

16. Coal tar has been prescribed for a client with a diagnosis of psoriasis, and the nurse provides instructions to the client about the medication. Which statement by the client indicates a need for further instructions?
    1. "The medication has an unpleasant odor."
    2. "The medication can stain the skin and hair."
    3. "The medication can cause systemic effects."
    4. "The medication can cause phototoxicity."

17. A client is diagnosed with herpes simplex. The physician tells the nurse that a topical medication for treatment will be prescribed. The nurse expects that which of the following medications will be prescribed?
    1. Triple antibiotic
    2. Acyclovir (Zovirax)
    3. Mupirocin (Bactroban)
    4. Masoprocol (Actinex)

18. Salicylic acid is prescribed for a client with a diagnosis of psoriasis. The nurse suspects the presence of systemic toxicity from this medication if which of the following occurs in the client?
    1. Decreased respirations
    2. Diarrhea
    3. Constipation
    4. Tinnitus

19. A hospitalized client with severe seborrheic dermatitis is receiving treatments of topical glucocorticoid applications followed by the application of an occlusive dressing. The nurse monitors for which systemic effect that can occur from this treatment?
    1. Adrenal suppression
    2. Adrenal hyperactivity
    3. Local infection
    4. Thinning of the skin

20. A nurse is applying a topical glucocorticoid to a client with eczema. The nurse monitors for systemic absorption of the medication if the medication is being applied to which of the following body areas?
    1. Back
    2. Axilla
    3. Palms of the hands
    4. Soles of the feet

21. A topical glucocorticoid is prescribed for a client with dermatitis. The nurse provides instructions to the client regarding the use of the medication.

Which of the following, if stated by the client, would indicate a need for further instruction?
1. "I need to apply the medication in a thin film."
2. "I should gently rub the medication into the skin."
3. "I should place a bandage over the site after applying the medication."
4. "The medication will help to relieve the inflammation and itching."

22. Lindane (Kwell) is prescribed for the treatment of scabies. The nurse would question the order if the medication were prescribed for which of the following clients?
1. A 42-year-old female
2. An older client
3. A 6-year-old child
4. A 52-year-old male with hypertension

23. A client is seen in the clinic for complaints of skin itchiness that has been persistent over the past several weeks. Following data collection, it has been determined that the client has scabies. Lindane (Kwell) is prescribed and the nurse is asked to provide instructions to the client regarding the use of the medication. The nurse tells the client to:
1. Leave the cream on for 8 to 12 hours and then remove by washing
2. Apply a thick layer of cream to the entire body
3. Apply the cream as prescribed for 2 days in a row
4. Apply to the entire body and scalp, excluding the face

24. An outbreak of pediculosis capitus has occurred at the local school. The nurse is helping provide instructions to the mothers of the children attending the school regarding the application of permethrin 5% (Elimite). The nurse tells the mothers to:
1. Apply at bedtime and rinse off in the morning
2. Apply prior to washing the hair
3. Avoid saturating the hair and scalp when applying
4. Allow to remain on the hair 10 minutes and then rinse with water

25. The physician has prescribed Myoflex topical cream for a client with a diagnosis of rheumatism who is complaining of muscular aches. Which of the following information does the nurse provide to the client regarding this medication?
1. Apply a heating pad to the area after applying the medication
2. The medication acts by decreasing muscle spasms
3. The medication is prescribed to cause the skin to peel
4. The medication will act as a local anesthetic

ALTERNATE FORMAT QUESTION: FILL IN THE BLANK

A nurse is caring for a client who has an ulcer on the medial aspect of the left ankle that is being treated with Duoderm. The nurse removes the Duoderm, cleanses the wound as prescribed, and reapplies the Duoderm. The nurse documents that the Duoderm needs to be changed in how many days?

Answer: _____

ANSWERS

1. *Answer*: **1**
Rationale: Sunscreens are most effective when applied about 30 to 60 minutes before exposure to the sun so that they can penetrate the skin. All sunscreens should be reapplied after swimming or sweating.
Test-Taking Strategy: Use the process of elimination. Recalling that sunscreens need to penetrate the skin will assist in eliminating options 2 and 3. From the remaining options, noting the key words, *most effective*, will direct you to option 1. Review protective skin measures if you had difficulty with this question.
Level of Cognitive Ability: Application
Client Needs: Health Promotion and Maintenance
Integrated Process: Nursing Process/Implementation
Content Area: Pharmacology
Reference: McKenry, L., & Salerno, E. (2003). *Mosby's pharmacology in nursing* (21st ed.). St. Louis: Mosby, p. 1125.

2. *Answer*: **3**
Rationale: Furacin is applied topically to the burn and has a broad spectrum of antibiotic activity. It is used in a burn injury when bacterial resistance to other agents is a real or potential problem. A film of $1/16$ inch is applied directly to the burn. Saline-soaked dressings are not used.
Test-Taking Strategy: Use the process of elimination. Option 1 can be eliminated because infection is a major concern with the burn client and a wet dressing can more easily harbor bacteria. Recalling that a very thin film is required will direct you to option 3 from the remaining options. Review the use of this medication for burn therapy if you had difficulty with this question.
Level of Cognitive Ability: Application
Client Needs: Physiological Integrity
Integrated Process: Nursing Process/Planning
Content Area: Pharmacology
Reference: McKenry, L., & Salerno, E. (2003). *Mosby's pharmacology in nursing* (21st ed.). St. Louis: Mosby, p. 1135.

3. *Answer*: **4**
Rationale: Mafenide acetate is bacteriostatic for both gram-negative and gram-positive organisms and is used to treat burn injuries to reduce bacteria present in avascular tissues.

The client should be informed that the medication will cause local discomfort and burning.
Test-Taking Strategy: Use the process of elimination. Eliminate options 1 and 3 because it is not within the scope of nursing practice to alter or discontinue a medication. From the remaining options, recalling that this is a normal expected occurrence will direct you to option 4. If you had difficulty with this question, review this medication.
Level of Cognitive Ability: Application
Client Needs: Physiological Integrity
Integrated Process: Nursing Process/Implementation
Content Area: Pharmacology
Reference: McKenry, L., & Salerno, E. (2003). *Mosby's pharmacology in nursing* (21st ed.). St. Louis: Mosby, p. 1135.

4. *Answer*: 3
Rationale: Mafenide acetate can suppress renal excretion of acid and cause acidosis, evidenced by hyperventilation. Clients receiving this treatment should be monitored for acid-base status and, if the acidosis becomes severe, the medication is discontinued for 1 to 2 days. Options 1 and 2 describe local rather than systemic effects. An elevated blood pressure may be expected in the client with pain.
Test-Taking Strategy: Use the process of elimination. Note the key words, *systemic effect*. Options 1 and 2 can be eliminated because these are local rather than systemic effects. From the remaining options, recall that the client in pain would likely have an elevated blood pressure. This should direct you to option 3. Review the systemic effects of this medication if you had difficulty with this question.
Level of Cognitive Ability: Analysis
Client Needs: Physiological Integrity
Integrated Process: Nursing Process/Data Collection
Content Area: Pharmacology
Reference: McKenry, L., & Salerno, E. (2003). *Mosby's pharmacology in nursing* (21st ed.). St. Louis: Mosby, p. 1135.

5. *Answer*: 4
Rationale: Dakin solution is a chloride solution that is used for irrigating and cleaning necrotic or purulent wounds. It can be used for packing necrotic wounds. It cannot be used to pack purulent wounds, because the solution is inactivated by copious pus. It should not come into contact with healing or normal tissue, and it should be rinsed off immediately if used for irrigation. Solutions are unstable and must be prepared fresh for each use.
Test-Taking Strategy: Use the process of elimination. Note the key words, *purulent drainage*. Eliminate options 2 and 3 first because they are similar. It makes sense to ensure that the solution is freshly prepared; therefore, select option 4. If you are unfamiliar with the use of this solution, review this content.
Level of Cognitive Ability: Application
Client Needs: Physiological Integrity
Integrated Process: Nursing Process/Planning
Content Area: Pharmacology
References: Black, J., & Hawks, J. (2005). *Medical-surgical nursing: Clinical management for positive outcomes* (7th ed.). Philadelphia: W.B. Saunders, p. 409.
McKenry, L., & Salerno, E. (2003). *Mosby's pharmacology in nursing* (21st ed.). St. Louis: Mosby, p. 1202.

6. *Answer*: 4
Rationale: Tretinoin decreases cohesiveness of the epithelial cells, increasing cell mitosis and turnover. It is potentially irritating particularly when used correctly. Within 48 hours of use, the skin generally becomes red and begins to peel.
Test-Taking Strategy: Use the process of elimination. Options 1 and 3 can be eliminated first because they are similar. Eliminate option 2 next because it is not within the scope of nursing practice to advise a client to discontinue a medication. Review the effects of this medication if you had difficulty with this question.
Level of Cognitive Ability: Application
Client Needs: Physiological Integrity
Integrated Process: Nursing Process/Implementation
Content Area: Pharmacology
Reference: Hodgson, B., & Kizior, R. (2005). *Saunders nursing drug handbook 2005*. Philadelphia: W.B. Saunders, p. 1072.

7. *Answer*: 3
Rationale: Tretinoin is applied liberally to the skin. The hands are washed thoroughly immediately after applying. Therapeutic results should be seen after 2 to 3 weeks but may not be optimal until after 6 weeks. The skin needs to be cleansed thoroughly before applying the medication.
Test-Taking Strategy: Use the process of elimination and note the key words, *need for further instructions*. These words indicate a false response question and that you need to select the incorrect client statement. Eliminate options 1 and 4 first using the principles of asepsis. From the remaining options, knowledge regarding the use of the medication will assist in directing you to option 3. Review this medication if you had difficulty with this question.
Level of Cognitive Ability: Comprehension
Client Needs: Health Promotion and Maintenance
Integrated Process: Teaching/Learning
Content Area: Pharmacology
Reference: Hodgson, B., & Kizior, R. (2005). *Saunders nursing drug handbook 2005*. Philadelphia: W.B. Saunders, p. 1071.

8. *Answer*: 3
Rationale: Isotretinoin is administered two times daily for 15 to 20 weeks. If needed, a second course may be given, but not until 2 months have elapsed after completing the first course.
Test-Taking Strategy: Knowledge regarding the use of this medication is required to answer this question. Remember, isotretinoin is administered two times daily for 15 to 20 weeks. Review this medication if you had difficulty with this question.
Level of Cognitive Ability: Application
Client Needs: Health Promotion and Maintenance
Integrated Process: Nursing Process/Implementation
Content Area: Pharmacology
Reference: Hodgson, B., & Kizior, R. (2005). *Saunders nursing drug handbook 2005*. Philadelphia: W.B. Saunders, p. 596.

9. *Answer*: 3
Rationale: Isotretinoin can elevate triglyceride levels. Blood triglyceride levels should be measured prior to treatment and periodically thereafter until the effects of the medication on the triglycerides have been evaluated.

Test-Taking Strategy: Use the process of elimination. Eliminate options 1 and 2 first because a complete blood count will also measure the white blood cell count. From the remaining options, it is necessary to know that the medication can affect triglyceride levels in the client. Review this medication if you had difficulty with this question.
Level of Cognitive Ability: Analysis
Client Needs: Physiological Integrity
Integrated Process: Nursing Process/Planning
Content Area: Pharmacology
Reference: Hodgson, B., & Kizior, R. (2005). *Saunders nursing drug handbook 2005*. Philadelphia: W.B. Saunders, p. 596.

10. *Answer*: 3
Rationale: Vitamin A, a derivative of isotretinoin, can produce generalized intensification of isotretinoin toxicity. Because of the potential for increased toxicity, vitamin A supplements should be discontinued prior to isotretinoin therapy.
Test-Taking Strategy: Use the process of elimination. Recalling that isotretinoin is a derivative of vitamin A will easily direct you to the correct option. If you are unfamiliar with this medication, review the contraindications associated with its use.
Level of Cognitive Ability: Application
Client Needs: Safe, Effective Care Environment
Integrated Process: Nursing Process/Implementation
Content Area: Pharmacology
Reference: Hodgson, B., & Kizior, R. (2005). *Saunders nursing drug handbook 2005*. Philadelphia: W.B. Saunders, p. 597.

11. *Answer*: 4
Rationale: The wound should be cleansed with a sterile solution and gently patted dry. A thin layer of Elase is applied and covered with a petrolatum gauze. If a dry powder is used, the solution should be prepared just prior to use.
Test-Taking Strategy: Use the process of elimination. Noting the word "thin" in option 4 should assist in directing you to this option. Review the method of application of this medication if you had difficulty with this question.
Level of Cognitive Ability: Application
Client Needs: Physiological Integrity
Integrated Process: Nursing Process/Planning
Content Area: Pharmacology
Reference: McKenry, L., & Salerno, E. (2003). *Mosby's pharmacology in nursing* (21st ed.). St. Louis: Mosby, p. 1146.

12. *Answer*: 2
Rationale: The wound should be cleansed with a sterile solution prior to treatment. The nurse then thoroughly moistens the wound with normal saline or sterile water, applies a thin film of Travase extending $1/4$ to $1/2$ inch beyond the area to be debrided, and then applies a loose thin dressing. The ointment should be refrigerated.
Test-Taking Strategy: Note the key word, *avoids*, in the stem of the question. This word indicates a false response question and that you need to select the incorrect action. Recalling that the wound is moistened prior to applying the Travase will direct you to the correct option. Review the method of application of Travase if you had difficulty with this question.
Level of Cognitive Ability: Application
Client Needs: Physiological Integrity

Integrated Process: Nursing Process/Implementation
Content Area: Pharmacology
References: Black, J., & Hawks, J. (2005). *Medical-surgical nursing: Clinical management for positive outcomes* (7th ed.). Philadelphia: W.B. Saunders, pp. 411-412.
McKenry, L., & Salerno, E. (2001). *Mosby's pharmacology in nursing* (21st ed.). St. Louis: Mosby, p. 1146.

13. *Answer*: 2
Rationale: Azelaic acid is a topical medication used to treat mild to moderate acne. It appears to work by suppressing the growth of *Propionibacterium acnes* and by decreasing proliferation of keratinocytes.
Test-Taking Strategy: Knowledge regarding the use of azelaic acid is required to answer this question. Remember, Azelaic acid is a topical medication used to treat mild to moderate acne. Review this medication if you had difficulty with this question.
Level of Cognitive Ability: Analysis
Client Needs: Physiological Integrity
Integrated Process: Nursing Process/Data Collection
Content Area: Pharmacology
Reference: Lehne, R. (2004). *Pharmacology for nursing care* (5th ed.). Philadelphia: W.B. Saunders, p. 1113.

14. *Answer*: 2
Rationale: Collagenase is used to promote debridement of dermal lesions and severe burns. It is applied once daily and covered with a sterile dressing.
Test-Taking Strategy: Note the key words, *indicates an accurate understanding*. Knowledge regarding the use of this medication will direct you to option 2. Review this medication if you had difficulty with this question.
Level of Cognitive Ability: Analysis
Client Needs: Health Promotion and Maintenance
Integrated Process: Teaching/Learning
Content Area: Pharmacology
Reference: McKenry, L., & Salerno, E. (2003). *Mosby's pharmacology in nursing* (21st ed.). St. Louis: Mosby, p. 1145.

15. *Answer*: 4
Rationale: Debrisan is a cleansing rather than a debriding agent. It is effective in wet wounds only. It is not packed tightly into the wound because maceration of surrounding tissue may result.
Test-Taking Strategy: Use the process of elimination. Note the key words, *indicates a need for further research*. These words indicate a false response question and that you need to select the incorrect statement. Noting that option 1 indicates that the wound should be wet and option 4 indicates that the wound should be dry provides the clue that one of these options is correct. If you are unfamiliar with the use of Debrisan, review the procedure associated with its use.
Level of Cognitive Ability: Analysis
Client Needs: Physiological Integrity
Integrated Process: Teaching/Learning
Content Area: Pharmacology
References: Black, J., & Hawks, J. (2005). *Medical-surgical nursing: Clinical management for positive outcomes* (7th ed.). Philadelphia: W.B. Saunders, pp. 411-412.

McKenry, L., & Salerno, E. (2001). *Mosby's pharmacology in nursing* (21st ed.). St. Louis: Mosby, p. 1147.

16. Answer: 3
Rationale: Coal tar is used to treat psoriasis and other chronic disorders of the skin. It suppresses DNA synthesis, mitotic activity, and cell proliferation. It has an unpleasant odor, can frequently stain the skin and hair, and can cause phototoxicity. Systemic toxicity does not occur.
Test-Taking Strategy: Use the process of elimination and note the key words, *need for further instructions*. These words indicate a false response question and that you need to select the incorrect client statement. The name of the medication will assist in eliminating options 1 and 2. From the remaining options, it is necessary to know that the medication does not cause systemic effects. Review this treatment if you had difficulty with this question.
Level of Cognitive Ability: Analysis
Client Needs: Physiological Integrity
Integrated Process: Teaching/Learning
Content Area: Pharmacology
References: Black, J., & Hawks, J. (2005). *Medical-surgical nursing: Clinical management for positive outcomes.* (7th ed.). Philadelphia: W.B. Saunders, p. 1393.
Lehne, R. (2004). *Pharmacology for nursing care* (5th ed.). Philadelphia: W.B. Saunders, p. 1116.

17. Answer: 2
Rationale: Acyclovir is a topical antiviral agent that inhibits DNA replication in the virus. It has activity against herpes simplex virus types 1 and 2, varicella-zoster virus, Epstein-Barr virus, and cytomegalovirus. Triple antibiotic would not be effective in treating herpesvirus. Mupirocin is a topical antibacterial active against impetigo caused by staphylococcus or streptococcus. Masoprocol is a keratolytic.
Test-Taking Strategy: Use the process of elimination. Recalling that herpes simplex is a virus will direct you to the option that identifies an antiviral medication. Review this medication if you had difficulty with this question.
Level of Cognitive Ability: Analysis
Client Needs: Physiological Integrity
Integrated Process: Nursing Process/Planning
Content Area: Pharmacology
Reference: Hodgson, B., & Kizior, R. (2005). *Saunders nursing drug handbook 2005*. Philadelphia: W. B. Saunders, p. 12.

18. Answer: 4
Rationale: Salicylic acid is readily absorbed through the skin and systemic toxicity (salicylism) can result. Symptoms include tinnitus, hyperpnea, dizziness, and psychological disturbances. Constipation and diarrhea are not associated with salicylism.
Test-Taking Strategy: Use the process of elimination. Noting the name of the medication will assist in directing you to the correct option if you can recall the toxic effects that occur with acetyl*salicylic* acid (aspirin). If you are unfamiliar with the toxic effects of salicylic acid, review this content.
Level of Cognitive Ability: Analysis
Client Needs: Physiological Integrity
Integrated Process: Nursing Process/Data Collection

Content Area: Pharmacology
Reference: Lehne, R. (2004). *Pharmacology for nursing care* (5th ed.). Philadelphia: W.B. Saunders, p. 1108.

19. Answer: 1
Rationale: Topical glucocorticoids can be absorbed in sufficient amounts to produce systemic toxicity. Principal concerns are growth retardation (in children), and adrenal suppression in all age groups. Options 3 and 4 identify local rather than systemic reactions.
Test-Taking Strategy: Use the process of elimination. Options 3 and 4 can be eliminated first because they are local reactions. From the remaining options, recalling the concerns related to systemic toxicity is required to answer the question. Review these systemic effects if you had difficulty with this question.
Level of Cognitive Ability: Application
Client Needs: Physiological Integrity
Integrated Process: Nursing Process/Data Collection
Content Area: Pharmacology
References: Lehne, R. (2004). *Pharmacology for nursing care* (5th ed.). Philadelphia: W.B. Saunders, p. 1108.
McKenry, L., & Salerno, E. (2003). *Mosby's pharmacology in nursing* (21st ed.). St. Louis: Mosby, p. 852.

20. Answer: 2
Rationale: Topical glucocorticoids can be absorbed into the systemic circulation. Absorption is higher from regions where the skin is especially permeable (scalp, axilla, face, eyelids, neck, perineum, genitalia), and lower from regions where penetrability is poor (back, palms, soles).
Test-Taking Strategy: Focus on the issue of the question, "systemic absorption." Eliminate options 3 and 4 because these body areas are similar in terms of skin characteristics. From the remaining options, think about permeability of the skin area. This will direct you to option 2. Review this medication if you had difficulty with this question.
Level of Cognitive Ability: Application
Client Needs: Physiological Integrity
Integrated Process: Nursing Process/Data Collection
Content Area: Pharmacology
Reference: Lehne, R. (2004). *Pharmacology for nursing care* (5th ed.). Philadelphia: W.B. Saunders, p. 1108.

21. Answer: 3
Rationale: Clients should be advised not to use occlusive dressings (bandages or plastic wraps) to cover the affected site following the application of the topical glucocorticoid, unless the physician specifically prescribes wound coverage. Options 1, 2, and 4 are accurate statements related to the use of this medication.
Test-Taking Strategy: Use the process of elimination and note the key words, *need for further instruction*. Eliminate option 4 knowing that this is the action for glucocorticoids. The words "thin" in option 1 and "gently" in option 2 should assist you in eliminating these options. If you had difficulty with this question, review this medication.
Level of Cognitive Ability: Analysis
Client Needs: Health Promotion and Maintenance
Integrated Process: Teaching/Learning
Content Area: Pharmacology

Reference: Lehne, R. (2004). *Pharmacology for nursing care* (5th ed.). Philadelphia: W.B. Saunders, p. 1108.

22. Answer: 3
Rationale: Lindane can penetrate the intact skin and can cause convulsions if absorbed in sufficient quantities. Clients at highest risk for convulsions are premature infants, children, and clients with preexisting seizure disorders. Lindane should not be used on pediatric clients unless safer medications have failed to control the infection.
Test-Taking Strategy: Knowledge regarding the contraindications associated with the use of lindane is required to answer this question. Remember, lindane should not be used on pediatric clients unless safer medications have failed to control the infection. If you are unfamiliar with these contraindications, review this content.
Level of Cognitive Ability: Analysis
Client Needs: Safe, Effective Care Environment
Integrated Process: Nursing Process/Implementation
Content Area: Pharmacology
Reference: McKenry, L., & Salerno, E. (2003). *Mosby's pharmacology in nursing* (21st ed.). St. Louis: Mosby, p. 1137.

23. Answer: 1
Rationale: Lindane is applied in a thin layer to the entire body below the head. No more than 30 g (1 oz) should be used. The medication is removed by washing 8 to 12 hours later. Usually, only one application is required.
Test-Taking Strategy: Knowledge regarding the use of lindane is required to answer this question. Remember, the medication is removed by washing 8 to 12 hours after application. If you are unfamiliar with the use of this medication, review this procedure.
Level of Cognitive Ability: Application
Client Needs: Health Promotion and Maintenance
Integrated Process: Nursing Process/Implementation
Content Area: Pharmacology
Reference: McKenry, L., & Salerno, E. (2003). *Mosby's pharmacology in nursing* (21st ed.). St. Louis: Mosby, p. 1136.

24. Answer: 4
Rationale: The instructions for the use of permethrin include wash, rinse, and towel-dry the hair; apply sufficient volume to saturate the hair and scalp; allow to remain on the hair 10 minutes and then rinse with water. Options 1, 2, and 3 are incorrect instructions.
Test-Taking Strategy: Note that both options 1 and 4 address a time frame for allowing the medication to remain on the hair. Recognizing this may provide you with the clue that one of these options is correct. From this point, it is necessary to

know the procedure for this treatment. If you are unfamiliar with this treatment, review this content.
Level of Cognitive Ability: Application
Client Needs: Health Promotion and Maintenance
Integrated Process: Nursing Process/Implementation
Content Area: Pharmacology
Reference: Lehne, R. (2004). *Pharmacology for nursing care* (5th ed.). Philadelphia: W.B. Saunders, p. 1055.

25. Answer: 4
Rationale: Myoflex is one of the many products used for the temporary relief of muscular aches, rheumatism, arthritis, sprains, and neuralgia. These types of products contain combinations of antiseptics, local anesthetics, analgesics, and counterirritants. A heating pad should not be applied because irritation or burning of the skin may occur. These medications do not act in a systemic manner (option 2). They are not prescribed to cause the skin to peel and, if this sort of reaction occurs, the physician should be notified.
Test-Taking Strategy: Use the process of elimination. Noting the key words, *topical cream*, may assist in eliminating option 2. Eliminate option 3, knowing that this is not an expected therapeutic effect. Recalling the principles related to the application of heat will assist in eliminating option 1. Review this medication if you had difficulty with this question.
Level of Cognitive Ability: Application
Client Needs: Physiological Integrity
Integrated Process: Teaching/Learning
Content Area: Pharmacology
Reference: Kee, J., & Hayes, E. (2003). *Pharmacology: A nursing process approach* (4th ed.). Philadelphia: W.B. Saunders, pp. 254-255.

ALTERNATE FORMAT QUESTION: FILL IN THE BLANK
Answer: 7
Rationale: Protective dressings such as Duoderm are designed to be left in place for 7 days unless leakage occurs around the dressing.
Test-Taking Strategy: Note the key word, *Duoderm*. Recalling that these dressings are designed to be left in place for 7 days will assist in answering this question. Review the purpose and procedure for using protective dressings if you had difficulty with this question.
Level of Cognitive Ability: Application
Client Needs: Physiological Integrity
Integrated Process: Nursing Process/Planning
Content Area: Pharmacology
Reference: McKenry, L., & Salerno, E. (2003). *Mosby's pharmacology in nursing* (21st ed.). St. Louis: Mosby, p. 1147.

REFERENCES
Black, J., & Hawks, J., (2005). *Medical-surgical nursing: Clinical management for positive outcomes* (7th ed.). Philadelphia: W.B. Saunders.
Hodgson, B., & Kizior, R. (2005). *Saunders nursing drug handbook 2005*. Philadelphia: W.B. Saunders.
Kee, J., & Hayes, E. (2003). *Pharmacology: A nursing process approach* (4th ed.). Philadelphia: W.B. Saunders.
Lehne, R. (2004). *Pharmacology for nursing care* (5th ed.). Philadelphia: W.B. Saunders.
McKenry, L. & Salerno, E. (2003). *Mosby's pharmacology in nursing* (21st ed.) St. Louis: Mosby.
McKenry, L. & Salerno, E. (2001). *Mosby's pharmacology in nursing* (21st ed.) St. Louis: Mosby.

The Adult Client with an Oncological Disorder

PYRAMID TERMS

benign Usually refers to growths that are encapsulated, remain localized, and are slow-growing.

cancer A neoplastic disorder that can involve all body organs. Cells lose their normal growth-controlling mechanism, and the growth of cells is uncontrolled.

carcinogen A physical, chemical, or biological stressor that causes neoplastic changes in normal cells.

carcinoma A new growth or malignant tumor that originates from epithelial cells, the skin, gastrointestinal (GI) tract, lungs, uterus, breast, and other organs.

carcinoma in situ A lesion with all the histological characteristics of malignancies, except invasion.

hospice A concept of care for terminally ill clients that includes the idea of intensive caring rather than intensive care. The family and the client are the focus of nursing care, and the goal is to relieve pain and facilitate optimal quality of life.

leukemia or myeloma Neoplasms that originate from blood-forming organs.

lymphoma Neoplasms that originate from lymphoid tissue.

malignant Refers to growths that are not encapsulated but metastasize and grow. These growths are cancerous lesions that have the characteristics of disorderly, uncontrolled, and chaotic proliferation of cells.

metastasis The transfer of disease from one organ or part to another not directly connected with it. Secondary malignant lesions, originating from the primary tumor, are located in anatomically distant places.

nadir The period of time during which an antineoplastic medication has its most profound effects on the bone marrow.

neoplasm A new growth, which may be benign or malignant.

sarcoma Neoplasms that originate from muscle, bone, fat, the lymph system, or connective tissues.

staging A method of classifying malignancies based on the presence and extent of the tumor within the body.

tumor marker Specific body substance that seems to indicate tumor progression or regression.

undifferentiated cell A cell that has lost the capacity for specialized functions.

PYRAMID TO SUCCESS

Pyramid points focus on treatment modalities related to an oncological disorder, such as pain management, internal and external radiation, and chemotherapy, and on oncological disorders such as skin cancer, leukemia, breast cancer, and lung cancer. Specific focus relates to the nursing care related to these treatment modalities and disorders, and to client adaptation and the impact of the treatment or the disorder. Specifically, focus on the complications related to chemotherapy and the nursing measures required in monitoring for these complications, and on, preventing life-threatening conditions such as infection and bleeding. Specific laboratory values include the white blood cell count and the platelet count. The Integrated Processes addressed in this unit include Caring, Clinical Problem-Solving Process (Nursing Process), Communication and Documentation, and Teaching/Learning.

CLIENT NEEDS
Safe, Effective Care Environment

Advance directives
Advocacy related to client's decisions
Client rights
Confidentiality regarding diagnosis
Establishing priorities
Ethical practice
Handling hazardous and infectious materials related to radiation and chemotherapy
Informed consent for treatments and procedures
Medical and surgical asepsis
Oncology-related consultations and referrals
Protective precautions
Standard and other precautions

Health Promotion and Maintenance

Client and family instructions regarding home care
Client lifestyle choices
Expected body image changes related to chemotherapy and treatments
Health screening measures for cancer
Health promotion programs regarding risks for cancer

Instructions regarding monthly breast or testicular self-examinations

Prevention of disease related to infection

Psychosocial Integrity

Ability to cope, adapt, and/or problem solve during illness or stressful events

Assisting the client and family to cope with the alteration in body image

End-of-life issues

Grief and loss related to death and the dying process

Mobilizing appropriate support and resource systems

Promoting a positive environment to maintain optimal quality of life

Religious and cultural preferences

Physiological Integrity

Diagnostic tests and laboratory test results, such as white blood cell and platelet counts

Managing pain

Providing basic care and comfort

Monitoring for expected and unexpected responses to radiation and chemotherapy

Promoting nutrition

Protecting the client from the life-threatening side effects of treatments

Radiation therapy

REFERENCES

Black, J., & Hawks, J., (2005). *Medical-surgical nursing: Clinical management for positive outcomes* (7th ed.). Philadelphia: W.B. Saunders.

Chernecky, C., & Berger, B. (2004). *Laboratory tests and diagnostic procedures* (4th ed.). Philadelphia: W.B. Saunders.

Christensen, B., & Kockrow, E. (2003). *Foundations of nursing* (4th ed.). St. Louis: Mosby.

deWit, S. (2005). *Fundamental concepts and skills for nursing* (2nd ed.). Philadelphia: W.B. Saunders.

Ignatavicius, D., & Workman, M. (2002). *Medical surgical nursing: Critical thinking for collaborative care* (4th ed.). Philadelphia: W.B. Saunders.

Jarvis, C. (2004). *Physical examination and health assessment* (4th ed.). Philadelphia; W.B. Saunders, pp. 542-543.

Lewis, S., Heitkemper, M., & Dirksen, S. (2004). *Medical-surgical nursing: Assessment and management of clinical problems* (6th ed.). St. Louis: Mosby.

Linton, A., & Maebius, N. (2003). *Introduction to medical-surgical nursing* (3rd ed.). Philadelphia: W.B. Saunders.

National Council of State Boards of Nursing. (2005). *Detailed test plan for the National Council licensure examination for practical/vocational Nurses.* Chicago: Author.

Pagana, K., & Pagana, T. (2003). *Mosby's diagnostic and laboratory test reference* (6th ed.). St. Louis: Mosby.

Phipps, W., Monahan, F., Sands, J., Marek, J., & Neighbors, M. (2003). *Medical-surgical nursing: Health and illness perspectives* (7th ed.). St. Louis: Mosby.

Thompson, J., McFarland, G., Hirsch, J., & Tucker, S. (2002). *Mosby's clinical nursing* (5th ed.). St. Louis: Mosby.

Oncological Disorders

I. CANCER

A. Description

1. A neoplastic disorder that can involve all body organs
2. Cells lose their normal growth-controlling mechanism, and the growth of cells is uncontrolled
3. **Cancer** produces serious health problems such as impaired immune and hematopoietic (blood-producing) function; altered gastrointestinal (GI) tract structure and function; motor and sensory deficits; and decreased respiratory function

B. **Metastasis** (Box 42-1)

1. **Cancer** cells move from their original location to other sites
2. Routes of **metastasis**

   a. Local seeding: Distribution of shed **cancer** cells in the local area of the primary tumor
   b. Bloodborne **metastasis:** Tumor cells enter the blood; most common cause of **cancer** spread
   c. Lymphatic spread: Primary sites rich in lymphatics are more susceptible to early metastatic spread

C. **Cancer** classification

1. Solid tumors: Associated with the organs from which they develop, such as breast **cancer** or lung **cancer**
2. Hematologic **cancers:** Originate from blood cell-forming tissues, such as the **leukemias** and the **lymphomas**

D. Grading and **staging** (Box 42-2)

1. A method used to describe the tumor

BOX 42-1

Common Sites of Metastasis

BREAST CANCER
Bone
Lung

LUNG CANCER
Brain

COLORECTAL CANCER
Liver

PROSTATE CANCER
Bone
Spine and legs

BRAIN TUMORS
Central nervous system

BOX 42-2

Grading and Staging

GRADING
Grade I: Cells differ slightly from normal cells and are well differentiated (mild dysplasia)
Grade II: Cells are more abnormal and are moderately differentiated (moderate dysplasia)
Grade III: Cells are very abnormal and are poorly differentiated (severe dysplasia)
Grade IV: Cells are immature (anaplasia) and undifferentiated; cell of origin is difficult to determine

STAGING
Stage 0: Cancer in situ
Stage I: Tumor limited to the tissue of origin; localized tumor growth
Stage II: Limited local spread
Stage III: Extensive local and regional spread
Stage IV: Metastasis

2. Includes the extent of the tumor, the extent to which malignancy has increased in size, the involvement of regional nodes, and metastatic development
3. Grading a tumor classifies the cellular aspects of the **cancer**
4. **Staging** classifies the clinical aspects of the **cancer**

E. Factors that influence **cancer** development
   1. Environmental factors
      a. Chemical **carcinogens**: Industrial chemicals, drugs, and tobacco
      b. Physical **carcinogens**: Ionizing radiation (diagnostic and therapeutic x-rays) and ultraviolet radiation (sun, tanning beds, and germicidal lights); chronic irritation and tissue trauma
      c. Viral **carcinogens**: Viruses capable of causing **cancer** are known as oncoviruses (Epstein-Barr virus, hepatitis B virus, human papillomavirus)
   2. Dietary factors: High-fat and low-fiber diets; high animal fat intake; preservatives, contaminants, additives; and nitrates
   3. Genetic predisposition: Inherited predisposition to specific **cancers,** inherited conditions associated with **cancer,** familial clustering, and chromosomal abberations
   4. Age: Advancing age is a significant risk factor for the development of **cancer**
   5. Immune function: Incidences of **cancer** are higher in immunosuppressed individuals, organ transplant recipients who are taking immunosuppressive medication, and individuals with acquired immunodeficiency syndrome (AIDS)

F. Prevention: Avoidance of known or potential **carcinogens** and avoidance or modification of the factors associated with the development of **cancer** cells

G. Early detection (Box 42-3)
   1. Mammography
   2. Papanicolaou ("Pap") test
   3. Stools for occult blood
   4. Sigmoidoscopy
   5. Breast self-examination
   6. Testicular self-examination
   7. Skin inspection

BOX 42-3

Seven Warning Signs of Cancer: "CAUTION"

Change in bowel or bladder habits
Any sore that does not heal
Unusual bleeding or discharge
Thickening or lump in breast or elsewhere
Indigestion
Obvious change in wart or mole
Nagging cough or hoarseness

II. BREAST SELF-EXAMINATION (BSE)

A. Performing BSE
   1. Perform 7 to 10 days after menses
   2. Postmenopausal clients or clients who have had a hysterectomy should select a specific day of the month and perform BSE monthly on that day
B. Procedure (Figure 42-1)

III. TESTICULAR SELF-EXAMINATION (TSE)

A. Performing TSE: Select a day of the month and perform the examination on the same day each month
B. Procedure (Figure 42-2)

IV. DIAGNOSTIC TESTS

A. Diagnostic tests to be performed will depend on the suspected primary or metastatic site(s) of the **cancer** (Box 42-4)
B. Biopsy
   1. Description
      a. Definitive means of diagnosing **cancer** and provides histologic proof of malignancy
      b. Involves the surgical incision of a small piece of tissue for microscopic examination
   2. Types
      a. Needle: Aspiration of cells
      b. Incisional: Wedge of suspected tissue is removed from a larger mass
      c. Excisional: Complete removal of the entire lesion
      d. **Staging:** Multiple needle or incisional biopsies in tissues where **metastasis** is suspected or likely (see Box 42-2)
   3. Tissue examination
      a. Following excision, a frozen section or a permanent paraffin section is obtained to examine the specimen
      b. The advantage of the frozen section is the speed with which the section can be prepared and the diagnosis made, because only minutes are required for this test
      c. Permanent paraffin section takes about 24 hours; however, it provides clearer details than the frozen section
   4. Interventions
      a. The procedure is usually performed in an outpatient surgical setting
      b. Prepare the client for the diagnostic procedure, following the physician's instructions
      c. Obtain an informed consent

V. PAIN CONTROL

A. Causes of pain
   1. Bone destruction
   2. Obstruction of an organ

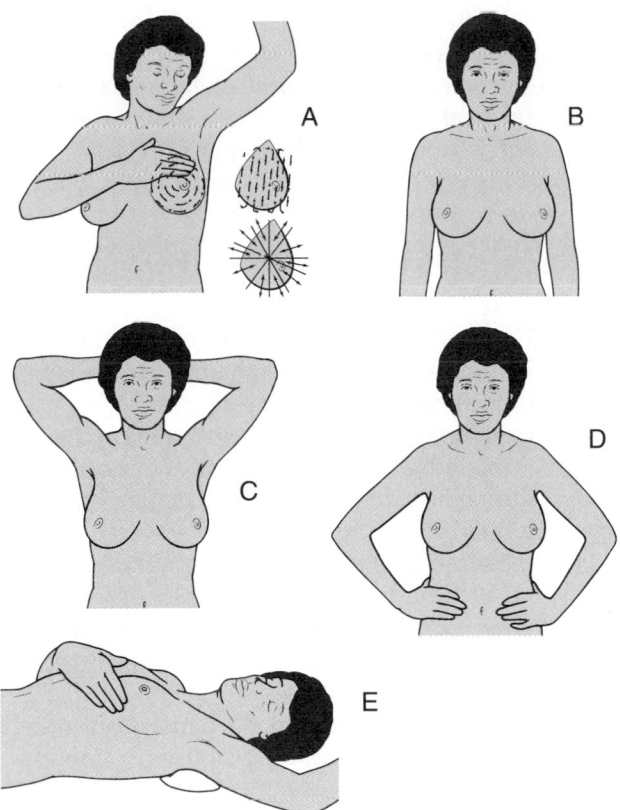

FIG. 42-1 Breast self-examination (BSE). **A,** While in the shower or bath, when the skin is slippery with soap and water, examine your breasts. Use the pads of your second, third, and fourth fingers to firmly press every part of the breast. Use your right hand to examine your left breast and your left hand to examine your right breast. Using the pads of the fingers on your left hand, examine the entire breast using small circular motions in a spiral or in an up-and-down motion so that the entire breast area is examined. Repeat the procedure using your right hand to examine your left breast. Repeat pattern of palpation under the arm. Check for any lump, hard knot, or thickening of the tissue. **B,** Look at your breasts in a mirror. Stand with your arms at your side. **C,** Raise your arms overhead and check for any changes in the shape of your breasts, dimpling of the skin, or any changes in the nipple. **D,** Next, place your hands on your hips and press down firmly, tightening the pectoral muscles. Observe for asymmetry or changes, keeping in mind that your breasts probably do not exactly match. **E,** While lying down, feel your breasts as described in step 1. When examining your right breast, place a folded towel under your right shoulder and put your right hand behind your head. Repeat the procedure while examining your left breast. Mark your calendar that you have completed your BSE; note any changes or unique characteristics that you want to check with your health care provider. From Lewis, S., Heitkemper, M., & Dirksen, S. [2004]. *Medical-surgical nursing: Assessment and management of clinical problems* [6th ed.]. St. Louis: Mosby.)

3. Compression of peripheral nerves
4. Infiltration and distention of tissue
5. Inflammation and necrosis
6. Psychological, such as fear or anxiety

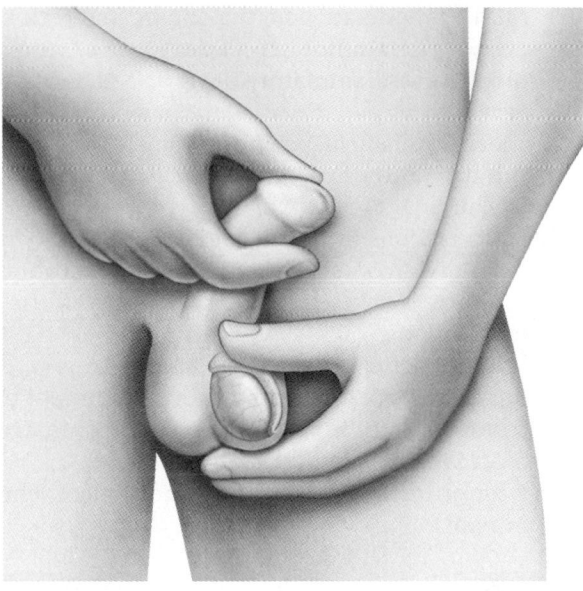

Testicular self-examination
1. The best time to perform this examination is right after a shower when your scrotal skin is moist and relaxed, making the testicles easy to feel.
2. Gently lift each testicle. Each one should feel like an egg, firm but not hard, and smooth with no lumps.
3. Using both hands, place your middle fingers on the underside of each testicle and your thumbs on top.
4. Gently roll the testicle between the thumb and fingers to feel for any lumps, swelling, or mass (see illustration).
5. If you notice any changes from one month to the next, notify your physician or nurse practitioner.

FIG. 42-2 Testicular self-examination. (From Harkreader, H., & Hogan, M.A. [2004]. *Fundamentals of nursing: Caring and clinical judgment* [2nd ed.]. Philadelphia: W.B. Saunders.)

BOX 42-4

Diagnostic Tests

Biopsy
Bone marrow examination (if a hematolymphoid malignancy is suspected)
Chest x-ray
Complete blood count
Computed tomography (CT) scan
Cytology studies (Pap smear)
Liver function studies
Magnetic resonance imaging (MRI)
Presence of oncofetal antigens such as carcinoembryonic antigen (CEA) and alpha fetoprotein (AFP)
Proctoscopic examination (including guaiac for occult blood)
Radiographic studies (mammography)
Radioisotope scans (liver, brain, bone, lung)

B. Interventions
1. Assess the client's pain; pain is what the client describes or says that it is
2. Collaborate with other members of the health care team to develop a pain management program
3. Administer oral preparations if possible and if they provide adequate relief of pain

4. Mild or moderate pain may be treated with salicylates, acetaminophen (Tylenol), and nonsteroidal anti-inflammatory drugs (NSAIDs)
5. Severe pain is treated with narcotics, such as codeine sulfate, meperidine (Demerol), morphine sulfate, and hydromorphone hydrochloride (Dilaudid)
6. Subcutaneous injections and continuous IV infusions of narcotics provide superior pain control
7. Monitor vital signs and for side effects of medications
8. Monitor for effectiveness of medications
9. Provide nonpharmacological techniques of pain control, such as relaxation, guided imagery, biofeedback, and diversion
10. Do not undermedicate the **cancer** client who is in pain

VI. SURGERY

A. Description: Used to diagnose, stage, and treat **cancer**
B. Prophylactic surgery
 1. Performed in clients with an existing premalignant condition or a known family history that strongly predisposes the person to the development of **cancer**
 2. An attempt is made to remove the tissue or organ at risk and thus prevent the development of **cancer**
C. Curative surgery: All gross and microscopic tumor is either removed or destroyed
D. Control (cytoreductive) surgery
 1. A "debulking" procedure that consists of removing part of the tumor
 2. It decreases the number of **cancer** cells and increases the chance that other therapies will be successful
E. Palliative surgery
 1. Performed to improve quality of life during the survival time
 2. Performed to reduce pain, relieve airway obstruction, relieve obstructions in the gastrointestinal or urinary tract, relieve pressure on the brain or spinal cord, prevent hemorrhage, remove infected or ulcerated tumors, or drain abscesses
F. Reconstructive or rehabilitative surgery: Performed to improve quality of life by restoring maximal function and appearance, such as breast reconstruction after mastectomy
G. Side effects of surgery
 1. Loss or loss of function of a specific body part
 2. Reduced function as a result of organ loss
 3. Scarring or disfigurement
 4. Grieving about altered body image or imposed change in lifestyle

VII. CHEMOTHERAPY

A. Description
 1. Kills or inhibits the reproduction of neoplastic cells; also attacks and kills normal cells

2. The effects are systemic; affects both healthy cells and cancerous cells
3. Normal cells most profoundly affected include those of the skin, hair, and lining of the GI tract, spermatocytes, and hematopoietic cells
4. Cell cycle phase–specific medications affect cells only during a certain phase of the reproductive cycle, and cell cycle phase–nonspecific medications affect cells in any phase of the reproductive cycle
5. Usually, several medications are used in combination (combination therapy) to increase the therapeutic response
6. Combination chemotherapy is planned to avoid prescribing medications with **nadirs** (the times during which bone marrow activity and white blood cell counts are at their lowest) at or near the same time to minimize immunosuppression
7. Antineoplastic therapy may be combined with other treatments, such as surgery and radiation
8. The preferred route of administration is by the intravenous (IV) route
9. Side effects include alopecia, nausea and vomiting, mucositis, skin changes, immunosuppression, anemia, and thrombocytopenia
10. Refer to Chapter 43 for information regarding the care of the client receiving chemotherapy

VIII. RADIATION THERAPY

A. Description
 1. Destroys **cancer** cells with minimal exposure of normal cells to the damaging effects of radiation; the cells damaged either die or become unable to divide
 2. Effective on tissues directly within the path of the radiation beam
 3. Side effects include skin changes and irritation, alopecia, fatigue, and altered taste sensation; also, the effects vary according to the site of treatment
 4. Teletherapy and brachytherapy are the types of radiation therapy most commonly used to treat **cancer**
B. Teletherapy (Box 42-5)
 1. Also called beam radiation; the actual radiation source is external to client
 2. The client does not emit radiation and does not pose a hazard to anyone else
C. Brachytherapy
 1. The radiation source comes into direct, continuous contact with tumor tissues for a specific time
 2. The radiation source is within the client; for a period of time, the client emits radiation and can pose a hazard to others
 3. Includes either an unsealed source or a sealed source of radiation
 4. Unsealed radiation source
  a. Administered via the oral or intravenous (IV) route or by instillation into body cavities

BOX 42-5

Teletherapy: Client Education

Wash area with water or mild soap and water, using the hand rather than a washcloth; rinse the soap thoroughly, and pat dry with a soft towel or cloth.

Do not remove the radiation markings from the skin.

Use no powders, ointments, lotions, or creams on the area unless prescribed.

Wear soft clothing over the area, avoiding belts, buckles, straps, or any clothing that binds or rubs the skin.

Avoid sun and heat exposure.

Monitor for moist desquamation (weeping of the skin).

If moist desquamation occurs, cleanse the area with warm water and pat dry, apply antibiotic ointment or steroid cream as prescribed, and expose the site to air.

b. The source is not completely confined to one body area; it enters body fluids and is eventually eliminated via various excreta, which are radioactive and harmful to others; most of the source is eliminated from the body within 48 hours; then, neither the client nor the excreta are radioactive or harmful

5. Sealed radiation source (Boxes 42-6 and 42-7)

a. A sealed, temporary or permanent radiation source (solid implant) implanted within the tumor target tissues

b. The client emits radiation while the implant is in place, but the excreta are not radioactive

6. Removal of sealed radiation sources

a. The client is no longer radioactive

b. Inform the client that sexual partners cannot "catch" **cancer**

c. Inform the female client that she may resume sexual intercourse after 7 to 10 days, if the implant was cervical or vaginal

d. Provide a Betadine douche, if prescribed, if the implant was placed in the cervix

e. Administer a Fleet enema if prescribed

f. Advise the client who had a cervical or vaginal implant to notify the physician if nausea, vomiting, diarrhea, frequent urination, vaginal or rectal bleeding, hematuria, foul-smelling vaginal discharge, abdominal pain or distention, or fever occurs

IX. BONE MARROW TRANSPLANTATION

A. Description

1. Used in the treatment of **leukemia** for clients who have closely matched donors and who are experiencing temporary remission with chemotherapy

2. The goal of treatment is to rid the client of all leukemic or other **malignant** cells through treatment with high doses of chemotherapy and whole-body irradiation

3. Because these treatments are lethal to bone marrow, without the replacement of bone marrow

BOX 42-6

Care of the Client with a Sealed Radiation Source

Place the client in a private room with a private bath.

Place a caution sign on the client's door.

Organize nursing tasks to minimize exposure to the radiation source.

Nursing assignments to a client with a radiation implant should be rotated.

Limit time to 30 minutes per care provider per shift.

Wear a dosimeter film badge to measure radiation exposure.

Wear a lead shield to reduce the transmission of radiation.

A nurse should never care for more than one client with a radiation implant at one time.

Do not allow a pregnant nurse to care for the client.

Do not allow children under the age of 16 years or a pregnant woman to visit the client.

Limit visitors to 30 minutes per day; visitors should be at least 6 feet from the source.

Save bed linens and dressings until the source is removed; then, dispose of in the usual manner.

Other equipment can be removed from the room at any time.

BOX 42-7

Dislodged Radiation Source

Do not touch a dislodged radiation source with bare hands.

If the radiation source dislodges, use long-handled forceps to place the source in the lead container kept in the client's room, and call the physician.

If unable to locate the radiation source, bar visitors and notify the physician.

function through transplantation, the client would die of infection or hemorrhage

B. Transplantation: Bone marrow is administered through the client's central line in a manner similar to a blood transfusion

C. Post-transplantation period

1. The client remains without any natural immunity until the donor marrow begins to proliferate and engraftment occurs

2. Infection and severe thrombocytopenia are major concerns until engraftment occurs

D. Complications: Major complications include failure to engraft and graft-versus-host disease (GVHD)

X. SKIN CANCER (See Chapter 40)

XI. LEUKEMIA (Box 42-8)

A. Description

1. **Malignant** exacerbation in the number of leukocytes, usually at an immature stage, in the bone marrow

BOX 42-8

Classification of Leukemia

ACUTE LYMPHOCYTIC LEUKEMIA (ALL)
Mostly lymphoblasts present in bone marrow
Age of onset is younger than 15 years

ACUTE MYELOGENOUS LEUKEMIA (AML)
Mostly myeloblasts present in bone marrow
Age of onset is between 15 and 39 years

CHRONIC MYELOGENOUS LEUKEMIA (CML)
Mostly granulocytes present in bone marrow
Age of onset is older than 50 years

CHRONIC LYMPHOCYTIC LEUKEMIA (CLL)
Mostly lymphocytes present in bone marrow
Age of onset is older than 50 years

2. May be acute, with a sudden onset and short duration, or chronic, with a slow onset and persistent symptoms over a period of years
3. Affects the bone marrow, causing anemia, leukopenia, the production of immature cells, thrombocytopenia, and a decline in immunity
4. The cause is unknown and appears to involve gene damage of cells, leading to the transformation of cells from a normal state to a **malignant** state
5. Risk factors include genetic, viral, immunological, and environmental factors and exposure to radiation, chemicals, and medications

B. Data collection
 1. Anorexia, fatigue, weakness, weight loss
 2. Bleeding (nosebleeds, gum bleeding, rectal bleeding, hematuria, increased menstrual flow)
 3. Petechiae
 4. Prolonged bleeding after minor abrasions or lacerations
 5. Elevated temperature
 6. Lymphadenopathy and splenomegaly
 7. Normal, elevated, or reduced white blood cell (WBC) count
 8. Decreased hemoglobin and hematocrit levels
 9. Decreased platelet count
 10. Positive bone marrow biopsy identifying leukemic blast phase cells

C. Infection
 1. A major cause of death in the immunosuppressed client
 2. Can occur through autocontamination or cross-contamination
 3. Common sites of infection are the skin, respiratory tract, and GI tract
 4. Initiate protective isolation procedures
 5. Ensure frequent and thorough handwashing
 6. Ensure that anyone entering the client's room is wearing a mask

7. Use strict aseptic technique for all procedures
8. Keep supplies for the client separate from supplies for other clients; keep frequently used equipment in the room for the client's use only
9. Limit the number of caregivers entering the client's room
10. Maintain the client in a private room
11. Place the client in a room with high-efficiency particulate air (HEPA) filtration or laminar airflow system if possible
12. Reduce exposure to environmental organisms by eliminating raw fruits and vegetables (low-bacteria diet) from the diet and fresh flowers from the client's room and by not leaving standing water in the client's room
13. Be sure that the client's room is cleaned daily
14. Assist the client with daily bathing, using an antimicrobial soap
15. Assist the client to perform oral hygiene frequently
16. Initiate a bowel program to prevent constipation and prevent rectal trauma
17. Avoid invasive procedures such as injections, rectal temperatures, and urinary catheterization
18. Change wound dressings daily, and inspect the wounds for redness, swelling, or drainage
19. Monitor the urine for color and cloudiness
20. Monitor skin and oral mucous membranes for signs of infection (Box 42-9)
21. Encourage the client to cough and deep breathe
22. Monitor temperature, pulse, and blood pressure
23. Monitor WBC and neutrophil counts
24. The physician is notified if signs of infection are present; prepare to obtain specimens for culture of open lesions, urine, and sputum
25. Antibiotic, antifungal, and antiviral medication may be prescribed
26. Instruct the client to avoid crowds and those with infections
27. Instruct the client about a low-bacteria diet and to avoid drinking water that has been standing for longer than 15 minutes
28. Instruct the client to avoid activities that expose the client to infection, such as changing a pet's litter box or working with houseplants or in the garden
29. Instruct clients that neither they nor their household contacts should receive immunization with a live virus

D. Bleeding
 1. During the period of greatest bone marrow suppression (the **nadir**), the platelet count may be extremely low, less than 10,000/mm^3
 2. The client is at risk for bleeding when the platelet count falls below 50,000/mm^3; spontaneous bleeding frequently occurs when the platelet count is lower than 20,000/mm^3
 3. Clients with platelet counts below 20,000/mm^3 may need a platelet transfusion

---

BOX 42-9

Mouth Care for the Client with Mucositis

Inspect mouth daily.

Offer complete mouth care before and after every meal and at bedtime.

Brush teeth and tongue with a soft-bristled toothbrush or sponges.

Provide mouth rinses every 12 hours (saline or sodium bicarbonate and water, as prescribed).

Administer topical anesthetic agents to the mouth sores as prescribed.

Avoid the use of alcohol- or glycerin-based mouthwashes or swabs.

Avoid foods that are hard or spicy.

---

4. For clients with anemia and fatigue, packed red blood cells (RBCs) may be prescribed
5. Monitor laboratory values
6. Examine the client for signs and symptoms of bleeding; examine all body fluids and excrement for the presence of blood
7. Handle the client gently; use caution when taking blood pressures to prevent skin injury
8. Measure abdominal girth, which can provide an indication of internal hemorrhage
9. Provide soft foods that are cool to warm
10. Avoid injections if possible, to prevent trauma to the skin and bleeding; apply firm and gentle pressure to a needlestick site for at least 10 minutes
11. Pad side rails and sharp corners of the bed and furniture
12. Avoid rectal suppositories, enemas, and thermometers
13. If the female client is menstruating, count the number of pads or tampons used
14. Blood products may be prescribed
15. Instruct the client to use a soft toothbrush and avoid dental floss
16. Instruct the client to use only an electric razor for shaving
17. Instruct the client to avoid blowing the nose
18. Instruct the client to avoid constrictive or tight clothing or shoes
19. Discourage the client from engaging in activities involving the use of sharp objects
20. Instruct the client to avoid using nonsteroidal antiinflammatory drugs and products that contain aspirin

E. Fatigue and nutrition
1. Assist the client in selecting a well-balanced diet
2. Provide small, frequent meals (high calorie, high protein, high carbohydrate) that require little chewing
3. Assist the client in self-care and mobility activities
4. Allow adequate rest periods during care
5. Do not perform activities unless they are essential
6. Administer blood products for anemia as prescribed

BOX 42-10

Staging in Hodgkin's Disease

STAGE I

Involvement of a single lymph node region or an extra-lymphatic organ or site

STAGE II

Involvement of two or more lymph node regions on the same side of the diaphragm or localized involvement of an extralymphatic organ or site

STAGE III

Involvement of lymph node regions on both sides of the diaphragm

STAGE IV

Diffuse or disseminated involvement of one or more extralymphatic organs with or without associated lymph node involvement

---

F. Additional interventions
1. Chemotherapy
2. Prepare the client for transplantation, as prescribed
3. Administer colony-stimulating factors, as prescribed
4. Provide psychosocial support and support services for home care

XII. HODGKIN'S DISEASE

A. Description
1. A malignancy of the lymph nodes that originates in a single lymph node or a single chain of nodes
2. **Metastasis** occurs to other, adjacent lymph structures and eventually invades nonlymphoid tissue
3. Usually involves lymph nodes, tonsils, spleen, and bone marrow and is characterized by the presence of Reed-Sternberg cells in the nodes
4. Possible causes include viral infections and previous exposure to alkylating chemical agents
5. Prognosis is dependent on the stage of the disease (Box 42-10)

B. Data collection
1. Fever
2. Malaise, fatigue, and weakness
3. Night sweats
4. Loss of appetite and significant weight loss
5. Anemia and thrombocytopenia
6. Enlarged lymph nodes, spleen, and liver
7. Positive biopsy of lymph nodes, with cervical nodes most often affected first
8. Presence of Reed-Sternberg cells in nodes
9. Positive computed tomography (CT) scan of the liver and spleen

C. Interventions
1. For stages I and II without mediastinal node involvement, the treatment of choice is extensive external radiation of the involved lymph node regions

2. With more extensive disease, radiation along with multiagent chemotherapy is utilized
3. Monitor for side effects related to chemotherapy or radiation
4. Monitor for signs of infection and bleeding
5. Maintain infection and bleeding precautions
6. Discuss the possibility of sterility with the male client receiving radiation; inform the client of options related to sperm banks

XIII. MULTIPLE MYELOMA

A. Description
   1. A **malignant** proliferation of plasma cells and tumors within the bone
   2. An excessive number of abnormal plasma cells invade the bone marrow, develop into tumors, and ultimately destroy bone; invasion of the lymph nodes, spleen, and liver occurs
   3. The abnormal plasma cells produce an abnormal antibody (**myeloma** protein, or the Bence Jones protein) that is found in the blood and urine
   4. Causes decreased production of immunoglobulin and antibodies and increased levels of uric acid and calcium, which can lead to renal failure
   5. The cause is unknown
B. Data collection
   1. Bone (skeletal) pain, especially in the pelvis, spine, and ribs
   2. Weakness and fatigue
   3. Recurrent infections
   4. Anemia
   5. Bence Jones proteinuria and elevated total serum protein level
   6. Osteoporosis (bone loss and the development of pathological fractures)
   7. Thrombocytopenia and granulocytopenia
   8. Elevated calcium and uric acid levels
   9. Renal failure
   10. Spinal cord compression and paraplegia
C. Interventions
   1. Administer chemotherapy as prescribed
   2. Provide supportive care to control symptoms and prevent complications, especially bone fractures, renal failure, and infections
   3. Maintain neutropenic and bleeding precautions as necessary
   4. Monitor for signs of bleeding, infection, and skeletal fractures
   5. Encourage fluids up to 3 to 4 L/day to offset potential problems associated with hypercalcemia, hyperuricemia, and proteinuria
   6. Monitor for signs of renal failure
   7. Encourage ambulation to prevent renal problems and to slow down bone resorption
   8. Provide skeletal support during moving, turning, and ambulating to prevent pathological fractures; provide a hazard-free environment

9. IVs and diuretics may be prescribed to increase renal excretion of calcium
10. Blood transfusions may be prescribed for anemia
11. Administer analgesics as prescribed to control pain
12. Administer antibiotics as prescribed for infection
13. Prepare the client for local radiation therapy if prescribed
14. Instruct the client in home care measures and the signs and symptoms of infection

XIV. TESTICULAR CANCER

A. Description
   1. Arises from germinal epithelium from the sperm-producing germ cells or from nongerminal epithelium from other structures in the testicles (Box 42-11)
   2. Most often occurs between the ages of 15 and 40 years
   3. **Metastasis** occurs to the lung, liver, bone, and adrenal glands
B. Prevention: Routine testicular self-examination
C. Data collection
   1. Painless testicular swelling
   2. Dragging sensation in scrotum
   3. Palpable lymphadenopathy, abdominal masses, and gynecomastia may indicate **metastasis**
   4. Late signs include back or bone pain and respiratory symptoms
D. Interventions
   1. Chemotherapy will be prescribed
   2. Prepare the client for radiation therapy, as prescribed
   3. Prepare the client for unilateral orchiectomy, if prescribed, for diagnosis and primary surgical management
   4. Prepare the client for radical retroperitoneal lymph node dissection, if prescribed, to stage the disease and reduce tumor volume so that chemotherapy and radiation therapy are more effective
   5. Discuss reproduction, sexuality, and fertility information and options with the client
   6. Identify reproductive options such as sperm storage, donor insemination, and adoption

---

BOX 42-11

Types of Testicular Cancer

GERMINAL TUMORS
Seminomas
Nonseminomas

NONGERMINAL TUMORS
Interstitial cell tumors
Androblastoma

E. Postoperative interventions
1. Monitor for signs of bleeding and wound infection
2. Monitor intake and output (I&O)
3. The physician is notified if chills, fever, increasing pain or tenderness at the incision site, or drainage of the incision occurs
4. Instruct the client that he may resume normal activities within 1 week, except for lifting objects heavier than 20 pounds or stair climbing
5. Instruct the client to perform monthly TSE on the remaining testicle
6. Inform the client that sutures will be removed 7 to 10 days after surgery

XV. CERVICAL CANCER

A. Description
1. Preinvasive **cancer** is limited to the cervix (Box 42-12)
2. Invasive **cancer** is in the cervix and other pelvic structures
3. **Metastasis** is usually confined to the pelvis, but distant **metastasis** occurs through lymphatic spread
4. Premalignant changes are described on a continuum from dysplasia, which is the earliest premalignancy change, to **carcinoma in situ** (CIS), the most advanced premalignant change

B. Precipitating factors
1. Low socioeconomic group
2. Early first marriage
3. Early and frequent intercourse
4. Multiple sex partners
5. High parity
6. Poor hygiene

C. Data collection
1. Painless vaginal bleeding, postmenstrually and postcoitally
2. Foul-smelling or serosanguineous vaginal discharge
3. Pelvic, lower back, leg, or groin pain
4. Anorexia and weight loss
5. Leakage of urine and feces from the vagina
6. Dysuria
7. Hematuria
8. Cytological changes on Papanicolaou (Pap) test

D. Interventions (Box 42-13)
E. Laser therapy
1. Used when all boundaries of the lesion are visible during colposcopic examination
2. Energy from the beam is absorbed by fluid in the tissues, causing them to vaporize
3. Minimal bleeding is associated with the procedure
4. Slight vaginal discharge is expected following the procedure, and healing occurs in 6 to 12 weeks

F. Cryosurgery
1. Freezing of the tissues by a probe with subsequent necrosis
2. No anesthesia is required, although cramping may occur during the procedure
3. A heavy, watery discharge will occur for several weeks following the procedure
4. Instruct the client to avoid intercourse and the use of tampons while the discharge is present

G. Conization
1. A cone-shaped area of the cervix is removed
2. Performed in women who desire further childbearing
3. Long-term follow-up care is needed as new lesions can develop
4. The risks of the procedure include hemorrhage, uterine perforation, incompetent cervix, cervical stenosis, and preterm labor in future pregnancies

H. Hysterectomy
1. Description
a. For microinvasive **cancer** if childbearing is not desired
b. A vaginal approach is most commonly performed
c. A radical hysterectomy and bilateral lymph node dissection may be performed for **cancer** that has spread beyond the cervix but not to the pelvic wall
2. Postoperative interventions
a. Monitor vital signs
b. Assist with coughing and deep-breathing exercises

BOX 42-12

Preinvasive Cancers: Cervical Intraepithelial Neoplasia (CIN)

CIN I: Mild dysplasia
CIN II: Moderate dysplasia
CIN III: Severe dysplasia to cancer in situ (CIS)

BOX 42-13

Treatment for Cervical Cancer

NONSURGICAL
Chemotherapy
Cryosurgery
External radiation
Internal radiation implants (intracavitary)
Laser therapy

SURGICAL
Conization
Hysterectomy
Pelvic exenteration

c. Assist with range-of-motion (ROM) exercises and provide early ambulation

d. Apply antiembolism stockings as prescribed

e. Monitor I&O, Foley catheter drainage, and hydration status

f. Monitor bowel sounds

g. Monitor vaginal bleeding; more than one saturated pad per hour may indicate excessive bleeding

h. Monitor incision site for signs of infection

i. Administer pain medication as prescribed

j. Instruct the client to avoid stair climbing for 1 month and to avoid tub baths and sitting for long periods

k. Avoid strenuous activity or lifting anything weighing more than 10 to 20 pounds

l. Instruct the client to consume foods that aid in the healing

m. Instruct the client to avoid sexual intercourse for 3 to 6 weeks as prescribed

n. Instruct the client in the signs associated with complications

I. Pelvic exenteration (Box 42-14)

1. Description

a. A radical surgical procedure performed for recurrent **cancer** if there is no evidence of tumor outside the pelvis and no lymph node involvement

b. When the bladder is removed, an ileal conduit will be created and located on the right side of the abdomen to divert urine

c. A colostomy may need to be created and will be located of the left side of the abdomen for the passage of feces

2. Postoperative interventions

a. Nursing care measures are similar to postoperative care after hysterectomy

b. Monitor incision site for infection

c. Administer perineal irrigations with half-normal saline (NS) and hydrogen peroxide, as prescribed

d. Provide sitz baths, as prescribed

BOX 42-14

Types of Pelvic Exenteration

ANTERIOR
Removal of the uterus, ovaries, fallopian tubes, vagina, bladder, urethra, and pelvic lymph nodes

POSTERIOR
Removal of the uterus, ovaries, fallopian tubes, descending colon, rectum, and anal canal

TOTAL
Combination of anterior and posterior

---

e. Instruct the client that the perineal opening, if present, may drain for several months

f. Instruct the client in the care of the ileal conduit and colostomy, if created

g. Provide sexual counseling, as vaginal intercourse is not possible after anterior and total pelvic exenteration

XVI. OVARIAN CANCER

A. Description

1. Grows rapidly, spreads fast, and is often bilateral

2. **Metastasis** occurs by direct spread to the organs in the pelvis, by distal spread through lymphatic drainage, or by peritoneal seeding

3. Prognosis is usually poor because the tumor is usually detected late

4. An exploratory laparotomy is performed to diagnose and stage the tumor

B. Data collection

1. Abdominal discomfort or swelling

2. GI disturbances

3. Dysfunctional vaginal bleeding

4. Abdominal mass

C. Interventions

1. External radiation is used if the tumor has invaded other organs

2. Chemotherapy is used postoperatively for all stages of ovarian **cancer**

3. Intraperitoneal chemotherapy, which involves the instillation of chemotherapy into the abdominal cavity

4. Immunotherapy, which alters the immunological response of the ovary and promotes tumor resistance

5. Total abdominal hysterectomy and bilateral salpingo-oophorectomy

XVII. ENDOMETRIAL CANCER

A. Description

1. A slow-growing tumor associated with the menopausal years

2. **Metastasis** occurs through the lymphatic system to the ovaries and pelvis, via the blood to the lungs, liver, and bone, or intra-abdominally to the peritoneal cavity

B. Precipitating factors

1. History of uterine polyps

2. Nulliparity

3. Polycystic ovary disease

4. Estrogen stimulation

5. Late menopause

6. Family history

C. Data collection

1. Postmenopausal bleeding

2. Watery, serosanguineous discharge

3. Low back, pelvic, or abdominal pain
4. Enlarged uterus in advanced stages
D. Nonsurgical interventions
1. External radiation or internal radiation used alone or in combination with surgery, depending on the stage of cancer
2. Chemotherapy is used to treat advanced or recurrent disease
3. Progestational therapy with medication such as medroxyprogesterone (Depo-Provera) or megestrol acetate (Megace) for estrogen-dependent tumors
4. Tamoxifen (Nolvadex), an antiestrogen, may also be prescribed
E. Surgical interventions: Total abdominal hysterectomy and bilateral salpingo-oophorectomy

XVIII. BREAST CANCER
A. Description
1. Classified as invasive when it penetrates the tissue surrounding the mammary duct and grows in an irregular pattern
2. **Metastasis** occurs via lymph nodes
3. Common sites of **metastasis** are the bone, lungs, brain, and liver
4. Diagnosis is made by breast biopsy through a needle aspiration or by surgical removal of the tumor with microscopic examination for **malignant** cells
B. Precipitating factors
1. Family history
2. Early menarche and late menopause
3. Previous **cancer of** the breast, uterus, or ovaries
4. Nulliparity
5. Obesity
6. High-dose radiation exposure to chest
C. Data collection
1. Mass felt during BSE
2. Mass usually felt in the upper outer quadrant or beneath the nipple
3. A fixed, irregular nonencapsulated mass
4. A painless mass except in the very late stages
5. Nipple retraction or elevation
6. Asymmetry, with the affected breast being higher
7. Bloody or clear nipple discharge
8. Skin dimpling, retraction, or ulceration
9. Skin edema or peau d'orange skin
10. Axillary lymphadenopathy
11. Lymphedema of affected arm
12. Symptoms of bone or lung **metastasis**
13. Presence of the lesion on mammography
D. Prevention: Monthly BSE
E. Nonsurgical interventions
1. Chemotherapy
2. Radiation therapy
3. Hormonal manipulation via the use of medication in postmenopausal women or other medications

such as tamoxifen (Nolvadex) for estrogen receptor-positive tumors
F. Surgical interventions
1. Surgical breast procedures with possible breast reconstruction (Box 42-15)
2. Oophorectomy for estrogen receptor–positive tumors
3. Ablative therapy with adrenalectomy or chemical ablation, which blocks the production of cortisol, androstenedione, and aldosterone
G. Postoperative interventions
1. Monitor vital signs
2. Position in semi-Fowler's; turn from back to unaffected side, with the affected arm elevated above the level of the heart to promote drainage and prevent lymphedema
3. Encourage coughing and deep breathing
4. If a drain (usually Jackson-Pratt) is in place, maintain suction and record the amount of drainage and drainage characteristics
5. Monitor operative site for infection, swelling, or the presence of fluid collection under the skin flaps
6. Monitor incision site for constriction from dressing, impaired sensation, or color changes of the skin
7. If breast reconstruction was performed, the client will return from surgery with a surgical brassiere and the temporary prosthesis in place
8. Place a sign above the bed stating "No IVs, No Injections, No BPs, No Venipunctures in Affected Arm"; the affected arm is protected for life and any intervention that could traumatize the affected arm is avoided
9. Provide the use of a pressure sleeve as prescribed if edema is severe
10. Administer diuretics and provide a low-salt diet as prescribed for severe lymphedema

---

BOX 42-15

Surgical Breast Procedures

LUMPECTOMY
The tumor is excised and removed.
Lymph node dissection may also be performed.

SIMPLE MASTECTOMY
Breast tissue and the nipple are removed.
Lymph nodes are left intact.

MODIFIED RADICAL MASTECTOMY
Breast tissue, nipple, and lymph nodes are removed.
Muscles are left intact.

HALSTED RADICAL MASTECTOMY
Breast tissue, nipple, underlying muscles, and lymph nodes are removed.

11. Consult with the physician and the physical therapist regarding the appropriate exercise program
12. Assist with exercise as prescribed to decrease lymphedema and muscle weakness
13. Instruct the client about home care measures (Box 42-16)

XIX. GASTRIC CANCER

A. Description
1. A **malignant** growth in the stomach
2. Risk factors include a diet high in carbohydrates, grains, and salt, and low in fresh, green leafy vegetables and fresh fruit; smoking; alcohol; the use of nitrates; and a history of gastric ulcers
3. Complications include hemorrhage, obstruction, **metastasis**, and dumping syndrome
4. The goal of treatment is to remove the tumor and provide a nutritional program

B. Data collection
1. Fatigue
2. Anorexia and weight loss
3. Nausea and vomiting
4. Indigestion and epigastric discomfort
5. A sensation of pressure in the stomach
6. Dysphagia
7. Anemia

8. Ascites
9. Palpable mass

C. Interventions
1. Monitor vital signs
2. Monitor hemoglobin and hematocrit; blood transfusions may be prescribed
3. Monitor weight
4. Monitor nutritional status; encourage small, bland, easily digestible meals with vitamin and mineral supplements
5. Administer pain medication as prescribed
6. Prepare the client for chemotherapy or radiation therapy as prescribed
7. Prepare the client for surgical resection of the tumor as prescribed (Box 42-17)

D. Postoperative interventions (see Chapter 46 for information regarding postoperative care)

XX. PANCREATIC CANCER

A. Description
1. The most common neoplasm affecting the pancreas
2. More common in blacks than in whites, in smokers, and in men
3. Occurrence has been linked to diabetes mellitus, alcohol use, history of previous pancreatitis, smoking, ingestion of a high-fat diet, and exposure to environmental chemicals
4. Symptoms usually do not occur until the tumor is large in size; therefore, the prognosis is poor

B. Data collection
1. Nausea and vomiting
2. Jaundice
3. Unexplained weight loss
4. Clay-colored stools
5. Glucose intolerance
6. Abdominal pain

BOX 42-16

Client Instructions Following Mastectomy

Avoid overuse of the arm during the first few months.
To prevent lymphedema, keep the affected arm elevated.
Provide incision care with lanolin to soften and prevent wound contracture.
Encourage use of Reach for Recovery volunteers.
Encourage the client to perform BSE on the remaining breast.
Protect the affected hand and arm.
Avoid exposure of the affected arm to strong sunlight.
Do not let the affected arm hang dependent.
Do not carry a handbag or anything heavy over the affected arm.
Avoid trauma, cuts, bruises, or burns to the affected side.
Avoid wearing constricted clothing or jewelry on the affected side.
Wear gloves when gardening.
Use thick oven mitts when cooking.
Use a thimble when sewing.
Apply lanolin hand cream several times daily.
Use cream cuticle remover.
Call the physician if signs of inflammation occur in the affected arm.
Wear a Medic-Alert bracelet stating lymphedema arm.

BOX 42-17

Surgical Interventions for Gastric Cancer

SUBTOTAL GASTRECTOMY
Billroth I
Also called gastroduodenostomy
Partial gastrectomy; remaining segment is anastomosed to the duodenum
Billroth II
Also called gastrojejunostomy
Partial gastrectomy; remaining segment is anastomosed to the jejunum

TOTAL GASTRECTOMY
Also called esophagojejunostomy
Removal of the stomach, with attachment of the esophagus to the jejunum or duodenum

C. Interventions
1. Radiation
2. Chemotherapy
3. Whipple's procedure, which involves a pancreaticoduodenectomy with removal of the distal third of the stomach, pancreaticojejunostomy, gastrojejunostomy, and choledochojejunostomy
4. Postoperative care measures are similar to care of a client with pancreatitis and the client following gastric surgery

XXI. INTESTINAL TUMORS

A. Description
1. **Malignant** lesions that develop in the cells lining the bowel wall or develop as polyps in the colon or rectum
2. Complications include bowel perforation with peritonitis, abscess and/or fistula formation, hemorrhage, and complete intestinal obstruction
3. **Metastasis** occurs via the circulatory or lymphatic system, or by direct extension to other areas in the colon or other organs

B. Data collection
1. Blood in stools
2. Anorexia, vomiting, and weight loss
3. Malaise
4. Anemia
5. Abnormal stools
   a. Ascending colon tumor: Diarrhea
   b. Descending colon tumor: Constipation or some diarrhea, or flat, ribbon-like stool resulting from a partial obstruction
   c. Rectal tumor: Alternating constipation and diarrhea
6. Guarding or abdominal distention
7. Abdominal mass (a late sign)
8. Cachexia (a late sign)

C. Interventions
1. Monitor for signs of complications, which include bowel perforation with peritonitis, abscess and/or fistula formation, hemorrhage, and complete intestinal obstruction
2. Monitor for signs of intestinal perforation, which include low blood pressure (BP), rapid and weak pulse, distended abdomen, and elevated temperature
3. Monitor for signs of intestinal obstruction, which include vomiting (may be fecal contents), pain, constipation, and abdominal distention
4. Note that an early sign of intestinal obstruction is increased peristaltic activity, which produces an increase in bowel sounds; as the obstruction progresses, hypoactive sounds are heard
5. Prepare for radiation preoperatively to facilitate surgical resection and postoperatively to

decrease the risk of recurrence or to reduce pain, hemorrhage, bowel obstruction, or **metastasis**
6. Chemotherapy is used postoperatively to assist in the control of symptoms and the spread of the disease

D. Surgical interventions: Bowel resection and creation of colostomy or ileostomy

E. Colostomy or ileostomy
1. Preoperative interventions
   a. Consult with the enterostomal therapist to assist in identifying optimal placement of ostomy
   b. Instruct the client to eat a low-residue diet for a day or two prior to surgery as prescribed
   c. Administer intestinal antiseptics and antibiotics as prescribed to decrease the bacterial content of the colon and to reduce the risk of infection from the surgical procedure
   d. Administer laxatives and enemas, as prescribed
2. Postoperative: Colostomy
   a. Place a petroleum jelly gauze over the stoma to keep it moist, covered by a dry sterile dressing if a pouch system is not in place
   b. Place a pouch system on the stoma as soon as possible
   c. Monitor the stoma for size, unusual bleeding, or necrotic tissue
   d. Monitor for color changes in the stoma
   e. Note that the normal stoma color is red or pink, indicating high vascularity
   f. Note that a pale pink stoma indicates low hemoglobin and hematocrit levels, and a purple-black stoma indicates compromised circulation, requiring physician notification
   g. Monitor the pouch system for proper fit and signs of leakage
   h. Assess the functioning of the colostomy
   i. Expect that stool will be liquid postoperatively but will become more solid, depending on the area of the colostomy
   j. Ascending colon colostomy: Expect liquid stool
   k. Transverse colon colostomy: Expect loose to semiformed stool
   l. Descending colon colostomy: Expect close to normal stool
   m. Fecal matter should not be allowed to remain on the skin
   n. Empty pouch when one third full
   o. Administer analgesics and antibiotics as prescribed
   p. Irrigate perineal wound if present and if prescribed, and monitor for signs of infection
   q. Instruct the client to avoid foods that cause excessive gas formation and odor
   r. Instruct the client in stoma care and irrigations as prescribed (Box 42-18)
   s. Instruct the client that normal activities may be resumed when approved by the physician

BOX 42-18

Colostomy Irrigation

PURPOSE

An enema is given through the stoma to stimulate bowel emptying.

DESCRIPTION

500 to 1000 mL of lukewarm tap water is infused through the stoma; the water and stool are allowed to drain into a collection bag.

PROCEDURE

If ambulatory, position the client sitting on toilet.

If on bed rest, position the client on the side.

Hang the irrigation bag so that the bottom of the bag is at the level of the client's shoulder, or slightly higher.

Insert the irrigation tube carefully, without force.

Begin the flow of irrigation.

Clamp tubing if cramping occurs; release tubing as cramping subsides.

Perform irrigation around the same time each day.

Perform irrigation preferably 1 hour after a meal.

3. Postoperative: Ileostomy
   a. Healthy stoma is red; a color change to dark blue or black should be reported to the physician
   b. Postoperative drainage will be dark green and progress to yellow as the client begins to eat
   c. Stool is liquid
   d. Risk for dehydration and electrolyte imbalance exists
   e. Do not give suppositories through ileostomy

XXII. LUNG CANCER

A. Description
   1. **Malignant** tumor of the lung that may be primary or metastatic
   2. The lungs are a common target for **metastasis** from other organs
   3. Bronchiogenic **carcinoma** spreads through direct extension and lymphatic dissemination
   4. The four major types of lung **cancer** include small cell (oat cell), epidermal (squamous cell), adenocarcinoma, and large cell anaplastic **carcinoma**
   5. Diagnosis is made by a chest x-ray, which will show a lesion or mass, and bronchoscopy and sputum studies, which will demonstrate a positive cytology for **cancer** cells

B. Causes
   1. Cigarette smoking
   2. Exposure to environmental pollutants
   3. Exposure to occupational pollutants

C. Data collection
   1. Cough
   2. Dyspnea
   3. Hoarseness
   4. Hemoptysis
   5. Chest pain
   6. Anorexia and weight loss
   7. Weakness

D. Interventions
   1. Monitor vital signs
   2. Monitor breathing patterns and breath sounds and for signs of respiratory impairment
   3. Monitor for tracheal deviation
   4. Administer analgesics as prescribed for pain management
   5. Place in Fowler's position for ease in breathing
   6. Administer oxygen as prescribed and humidification to moisten and loosen secretions
   7. Monitor pulse oximetry
   8. Provide respiratory treatments, as prescribed
   9. Administer bronchodilators and corticosteroids as prescribed to decrease bronchospasm, inflammation, and edema
   10. Provide a high-calorie, high-protein, high-vitamin diet
   11. Provide activity as tolerated, rest periods, and active and passive range-of-motion (ROM) exercises
   12. Monitor for bleeding, infection, and electrolyte imbalances

E. Nonsurgical interventions
   1. Radiation therapy for localized intrathoracic lung **cancers** and for palliation of hemoptysis, obstructions, dysphagia, and pain
   2. Chemotherapy
   3. Immunotherapy directed at enhancing an effective immune response, which favorably affects the course of the disease

F. Surgical interventions
   1. Laser therapy: To relieve endobronchial obstruction
   2. Thoracentesis and pleurodesis: To remove pleural fluid and relieve hypoxia
   3. Thoracotomy with pneumonectomy: Surgical removal of a lung
   4. Thoracotomy with lobectomy: Surgical removal of one lobe of the lung for tumors confined to a single lobe
   5. Thoracotomy with segmental resection: Surgical removal of a lobe segment for clients unable to tolerate lobectomy or pneumonectomy

G. Preoperative interventions
   1. Explain the potential postoperative need for chest tubes
   2. Note that closed chest drainage is not usually used for a pneumonectomy, and the serum fluid that accumulates in the empty thoracic cavity eventually consolidates, preventing shifts of the mediastinum, heart, and remaining lung

H. Postoperative interventions
1. Monitor vital signs
2. Monitor cardiac and respiratory status; monitor for the absence and presence of lung sounds
3. Monitor chest tube drainage system, which will drain air and/or blood that accumulates in the pleural space
4. Monitor chest tube insertion site for crepitus (subcutaneous air) and drainage
5. Administer oxygen as prescribed
6. Check physician's orders regarding client positioning; complete lateral turning is avoided
7. Monitor pulse oximetry
8. Provide activity as tolerated
9. Encourage active ROM exercises of the operative shoulder, as prescribed
10. See Chapter 19 for care of the client with a chest tube

XXIII. LARYNGEAL CANCER

A. Description
1. A **malignant** tumor of the larynx
2. Laryngeal **cancer** presents as **malignant** ulcerations with underlying infiltration
3. **Metastasis** to the lung is common
4. Diagnosis is made by laryngoscopy and biopsy showing a positive cytology for **cancer** cells
B. Causes
1. Cigarette smoking
2. Exposure to environmental pollutants
3. Exposure to radiation
4. Voice strain
C. Data collection
1. Persistent hoarseness and sore throat
2. Painless neck mass
3. A feeling of a lump in the throat
4. Burning sensation in the throat
5. Dysphagia
6. Change in voice quality
7. Dyspnea
8. Weakness and weight loss
9. Hemoptysis
10. Foul breath odor
D. Interventions
1. Place in Fowler's position to promote optimal air exchange
2. Monitor respiratory status
3. Monitor for signs of aspiration of food and fluid
4. Administer oxygen, as prescribed
5. Provide respiratory treatments, as prescribed
6. Provide activity as tolerated
7. Provide a high-calorie, high-protein, high-vitamin diet
8. Prepare to provide nutritional support via total parenteral nutrition (TPN), nasogastric (NG)

tube feedings, or gastrostomy or jejunostomy tube, as prescribed
9. Administer analgesics as prescribed for pain
E. Nonsurgical interventions
1. Radiation therapy if the **cancer** is limited to a small area in one vocal cord
2. Chemotherapy, which may be done in combination with radiation and surgery
F. Surgical interventions
1. Depend on the tumor size and the amount of tissue to be resected
2. Types of resection include cordal stripping, cordectomy, partial laryngectomy, and total laryngectomy
3. A tracheostomy is performed with a total laryngectomy; this airway opening is always permanent and is referred to as a laryngectomy stoma
G. Preoperative interventions
1. Establish methods of communication for the client
2. Encourage the client to express feelings about changes in body image and loss of voice
3. Describe the rehabilitation program and information about the tracheostomy and suctioning
H. Postoperative interventions
1. Monitor vital signs
2. Monitor respiratory status; monitor airway patency and provide frequent suctioning to remove bloody secretions
3. Place the client in high Fowler's position
4. Maintain mechanical ventilator support or a tracheostomy collar with humidification, as prescribed
5. Monitor pulse oximetry
6. Maintain surgical drains in the neck area if present
7. Observe for hemorrhage and edema in the neck
8. Monitor IV fluids or TPN if prescribed until nutrition is administered via NG, gastrostomy, or jejunostomy tube
9. Provide oral hygiene
10. Monitor gag and cough reflexes and ability to swallow
11. Increase activity, as tolerated
12. Monitor the color, amount, and consistency of sputum
13. Provide stoma and laryngectomy care (Box 42-19)
14. Provide consultation with speech and language pathologist, as prescribed
15. Reinforce method of communication established preoperatively
16. Prepare the client for rehabilitation and speech therapy (Box 42-20)

XXIV. CANCER OF THE PROSTATE

A. Description
1. A slow-growing **cancer** of the prostate gland, which is usually an androgen-dependent type of adenocarcinoma

BOX 42-19

Stoma Care Following Laryngectomy

Teach the client clean suctioning technique.

Instruct the client how to clean the incision and provide stoma care.

Protect the neck from injury.

Instruct the client to wear a stoma guard to shield the stoma.

Avoid swimming, showering, and using aerosol sprays.

Demonstrate ways to prevent debris from entering the stoma.

Advise the client to wear loose-fitting, high-collar clothing to hide the stoma.

Advise the client to increase humidity in the home.

Instruct the client in range-of-motion exercises for arms, shoulders, and neck, as prescribed.

Avoid exposure to people with infections.

Alternate rest periods with activity.

Increase fluid intake to 3000 mL/day, as prescribed.

Advise the client to obtain a Medic-Alert bracelet.

BOX 42-20

Speech Rehabilitation Following Laryngectomy

ESOPHAGEAL SPEECH

Client produces esophageal speech by "burping" the air swallowed

Voice produced is monotone, cannot be raised or lowered, carries no pitch

Client must have adequate hearing because the client uses the mouth to shape words as they are heard

MECHANICAL DEVICES

Known as electrolarynges

Placed against the side of the neck; air inside the neck and pharynx is vibrated, and the client articulates

Cooper-Rand device: Consists of a plastic tube that is placed inside the client's mouth and vibrates on articulation

TRACHEOESOPHAGEAL FISTULA (TEF)

Surgical creation of a fistula between the trachea and the esophagus, with eventual placement of a prosthesis used to produce speech

Prosthesis provides the client with a means to divert the air from the lungs through the trachea, into the esophagus, and out of the mouth

Speech is produced by lip and tongue movement

2. The risk increases in men with each decade after age 50

3. Prostate cancer can spread via direct invasion of surrounding tissues or by **metastasis**, through the bloodstream and lymphatics, to the bony pelvis and spine

4. Bone **metastasis** is a concern

B. Data collection
   1. Asymptomatic in early stages
   2. Hard, pea-sized nodule palpated on rectal examination
   3. Hematuria
   4. Late symptoms include weight loss, urinary obstruction, and pain radiating from the lumbosacral area down the leg
   5. Prostate-specific antigen (PSA) test does not necessarily indicate malignancy; used routinely to monitor the client's response to therapy
   6. Elevated serum acid phosphatase level indicates spread and **metastasis**

C. Nonsurgical interventions
   1. Prepare the client for hormone manipulation therapy, as prescribed
   2. Administer luteinizing hormone, such as leuprolide acetate (Lupron), flutamide (Eulexin), or diethylstilbestrol (DES), as prescribed, to slow the rate of growth of the tumor
   3. Goserelin acetate (Zoladex) may be prescribed for palliation in advanced prostatic **cancer** when orchiectomy or estrogen administration is neither acceptable nor indicated for the client
   4. Prepare the client for radiation (internal or external), which may be prescribed alone or in conjunction with surgery; may be prescribed preoperatively or postoperatively to reduce the lesion and limit **metastasis**
   5. Prepare the client for the administration of chemotherapy in cases of hormone-resistant tumors

D. Surgical interventions
   1. Prepare the client for orchiectomy (palliative) if prescribed, which will limit the production of testosterone
   2. Prepare the client for transurethral resection of the prostate (TURP) or prostatectomy if prescribed
   3. Cyrosurgical ablation: A minimally invasive procedure that may be an alternative to radical prostatectomy; liquid nitrogen freezes the gland, and the dead cells are absorbed by the body

E. TURP (transurethral resection of the prostate)
   1. Insertion of a scope into the urethra to excise prostatic tissue
   2. Bleeding is common following TURP, and monitoring for hemorrhage is an important nursing intervention
   3. Continuous bladder irrigation (CBI) will be prescribed postoperatively to maintain the urine at a pink color
   4. Bladder spasms are common following surgery, and antispasmodics may be prescribed
   5. Dribbling or incontinence may occur postoperatively, and it is important for the nurse to instruct the client to monitor for these occurrences

6. Sterility may or may not occur following the surgical procedure
F. Suprapubic prostatectomy
   1. Removal of the prostate by an abdominal incision with a bladder incision
   2. The client will have an abdominal dressing that may drain copious amounts of urine, and the abdominal dressing will need to be changed frequently
   3. Severe hemorrhage is possible, and monitoring for blood loss is an important nursing intervention
   4. Bladder spasms are common, and antispasmodics may be prescribed
   5. Continuous bladder irrigation (CBI) will be prescribed and administered to keep the urine pink
   6. A longer healing process is involved as compared with TURP
   7. Sterility occurs with this procedure
G. Retropubic prostatectomy
   1. Removal of the prostate gland by a low abdominal incision without opening the bladder
   2. Less bleeding occurs with this procedure, as compared with suprapubic prostatectomy, and the client experiences fewer bladder spasms
   3. There is minimal abdominal drainage
   4. CBI may be used
   5. Sterility occurs with this procedure
H. Perineal prostatectomy
   1. The prostate gland is removed through an incision made between the scrotum and anus
   2. Minimal bleeding occurs with this procedure
   3. The client needs to be monitored closely for infection, because the risk of infection is increased with this type of prostatectomy
   4. Urinary incontinence is common
   5. The procedure causes sterility
   6. Teach the client how to perform perineal exercises
   7. Avoid inserting rectal tubes, taking the temperature rectally, or administering enemas
I. Postoperative interventions
   1. Monitor vital signs
   2. Monitor urinary output
   3. Monitor urine for hemorrhage and clots
   4. Increase fluids to 2400 to 3000 mL/day unless contraindicated
   5. Monitor for arterial bleeding as evidenced by bright red urine with numerous clots, and if it occurs, increase CBI; the physician is notified immediately
   6. Monitor for venous bleeding as evidenced by burgundy-colored urine output; if it occurs, the physician is notified, who may apply traction on the catheter
   7. Monitor hemoglobin and hematocrit levels
   8. Expect red to light pink urine for 24 hours, turning to amber in 3 days

9. Ambulate the client as early as possible and as soon as urine begins to clear in color
10. Inform the client that a continuous feeling of an urge to void is normal
11. Instruct the client to avoid attempts to void around the catheter because this will cause bladder spasms
12. Administer antibiotics, analgesics, stool softeners, and antispasmodics as prescribed
13. Monitor three-way Foley catheter, which will have a 30- to 45-mL retention balloon
14. Maintain CBI with sterile bladder irrigation solution as prescribed to keep the catheter free of obstruction and maintain the urine pink in color (Box 42-21)
J. Postoperative: Suprapubic prostatectomy
   1. Monitor suprapubic and Foley catheter drainage
   2. Monitor CBI if prescribed
   3. Note that the Foley catheter will be removed 2 to 4 days postoperatively if the client has a suprapubic catheter
   4. If prescribed, clamp the suprapubic catheter after the Foley catheter is removed, and instruct client to attempt to void; after the client has voided, check the amount of residual urine in the bladder by unclamping the suprapubic catheter and measuring the output
   5. Prepare for removal of suprapubic catheter when client consistently empties bladder and residual urine is 75 mL or less
   6. Monitor suprapubic incision dressing, which may become saturated with urine, until the incision heals
K. Postoperative: Retropubic prostatectomy
   1. Note that because the bladder is not entered, there is no urinary drainage on the abdominal dressing
   2. Check for urinary or purulent drainage on the dressing; if this occurs, notify the physician
   3. Monitor for fever and increased pain, which may indicate an infection
L. Postoperative: Perineal prostatectomy
   1. Note that the client will have an incision, which may or may not have a drain
   2. Avoid rectal thermometers, rectal tubes, and enemas, because they may cause trauma and bleeding

XXV. BLADDER CANCER
A. Description
   1. Papillomatous growths in the bladder urothelium that undergo **malignant** changes and that may infiltrate the bladder wall
   2. Predisposing factors include cigarette smoking, exposure to industrial chemicals, and exposure to radiation
   3. Common sites of **metastasis** include the liver, bones, and lungs

BOX 42-21

Postoperative Care Following Transurethral Resection of the Prostate (TURP)

CONTINUOUS BLADDER IRRIGATION (CBI)

Three-way (lumen) irrigation to decrease bleeding and to keep the bladder free from clots:
- One lumen for inflating the balloon (30 mL)
- One lumen for instillation (inflow)
- One lumen for outflow

INTERVENTIONS

Maintain traction on the catheter, if applied to prevent bleeding, by pulling the catheter taut and taping it to the abdomen or thigh.

Instruct the client to keep the leg straight if traction is applied to the catheter and it is taped to the thigh.

Catheter traction is not released without a physician's order; it is usually released after any bright red drainage has diminished.

Use normal saline or prescribed solution only to prevent water intoxication.

Run the solution at a rate as prescribed to keep the urine pink.

Run the solution rapidly if bright red drainage or clots are present.

Run the solution at about 40 gtt/minute when the bright red drainage clears.

If the urinary catheter becomes obstructed, turn off the CBI and irrigate the catheter with 30 to 50 mL of normal saline if prescribed; notify physician if obstruction does not resolve.

Monitor for transurethral resection syndrome or severe hyponatremia (water intoxication) caused by the excessive absorption of bladder irrigation (altered mental status, bradycardia, increased blood pressure, and confusion).

Discontinue CBI and Foley catheter as prescribed, usually 24 to 48 hours after surgery.

Monitor for continence and urinary retention when the catheter is removed.

Inform the client that some burning, frequency, and dribbling may occur after catheter removal.

Inform the client that he should be voiding 150 to 200 mL of clear yellow urine every 3 to 4 hours by 3 days after surgery.

Inform the client that he may pass small clots and tissue debris for several days.

Teach the client to avoid heavy lifting, stressful exercise, driving, Valsalva's maneuver, and sexual intercourse for 2 to 6 weeks to prevent strain, and to call the physician if bleeding occurs or there is a decrease in urinary stream.

Instruct the client to drink 2400 to 3000 mL of fluid each day, preferably before 8 PM.

Instruct the client to avoid alcohol, caffeinated beverages, and spicy foods to avoid overstimulation of the bladder.

Instruct the client that if the urine becomes bloody, to rest and increase fluid intake, and that if the bleeding does not subside, to notify the physician.

4. As the tumor progresses, it can extend into the rectum, vagina, other pelvic soft tissues, and retroperitoneal structures

B. Data collection
1. Gross, painless hematuria
2. Frequency, urgency, dysuria
3. Clot-induced obstruction
4. Bladder biopsy confirms diagnosis

C. Radiation
1. Most bladder **cancers** are poorly radiosensitive and require high doses of radiation
2. Radiation therapy is more acceptable for advanced disease that cannot be eradicated by surgery
3. Palliative radiation may be used to relieve pain and bowel obstruction and control potential hemorrhage and leg edema secondary to venous or lymphatic obstruction
4. Intracavitary radiation may be prescribed, which protects adjacent tissue
5. External radiation combined with chemotherapy or surgery may be prescribed because the external radiation alone may be ineffective
6. Complications of radiation
   a. Abacterial cystitis
   b. Proctitis
   c. Fistula formation
   d. Ileitis or colitis
   e. Bladder ulceration and hemorrhage

D. Chemotherapy
1. Intravesical instillation
   a. An alkylating chemotherapeutic agent is instilled into the bladder
   b. This method provides a concentrated topical treatment with little systemic absorption
   c. The medication is injected into a urethral catheter and retained for 2 hours
   d. Following instillation, the client's position is rotated every 15 to 30 minutes, starting in the supine position to avoid lying on a full bladder
   e. After 2 hours, the client voids in a sitting position and is instructed to increase fluids to flush the bladder
   f. Treat the urine as a biohazard; send to the radioisotope laboratory for monitoring
   g. For 6 hours following intravesical chemotherapy, disinfect the toilet with household bleach after the client has voided
2. Systemic chemotherapy: Used to treat inoperable or late tumors
3. Complications of chemotherapy
   a. Bladder irritation
   b. Hemorrhagic cystitis

E. Surgical interventions
1. TURP
   a. Local resection and fulguration (destruction of tissue by electrical current through electrodes placed in direct contact with the tissue)

b. Performed for very early tumors for cure or for inoperable tumors for palliation

2. Partial cystectomy
   a. The removal of up to half of the bladder
   b. Done for early tumors and for clients who cannot tolerate a radical cystectomy
   c. During the initial postoperative period, bladder capacity is markedly reduced to about 60 mL; however, as the bladder tissue expands, the capacity increases to 200 to 400 mL
   d. Maintenance of a continuous output of urine following surgery is critical to prevent bladder distention and stress on the suture line
   e. A urethral catheter and a suprapubic catheter may be in place, and the suprapubic catheter may be left in place for 2 weeks until healing occurs

3. Cystectomy and urinary diversion
   a. Removal of the bladder and the urethra in women, and the bladder, the urethra, and usually the prostate and seminal vesicles in men
   b. When the bladder and urethra are removed, permanent urinary diversion is required
   c. The surgery may be performed in two stages if the tumor is extensive, with the creation of the urinary diversion first and the cystectomy several weeks later
   d. If a radical cystectomy is performed, lower extremity lymphedema may occur as a result of lymph node dissection, and impotence may occur in the male client

4. Ileal conduit
   a. Also called ureteroileostomy or Bricker's procedure
   b. Ureters are implanted into a segment of the ileum, with the formation of an abdominal stoma
   c. The urine flows into the conduit and is continually propelled out through the stoma by peristalsis
   d. The client is required to wear an appliance over the stoma to collect the urine
   e. Complications include obstruction, pyelonephritis, leakage at the anastomosis site, stenosis, hydronephrosis, calculi, skin irritation and ulceration, and stomal defects

5. Kock pouch
   a. A continent internal ileal reservoir created from a segment of the ileum and ascending colon
   b. The ureters are implanted into the side of the reservoir, and a special nipple valve is constructed to attach the reservoir to the skin
   c. Postoperatively, the client will have a 24 to 26 Foley catheter in place to drain urine continuously until the pouch has healed
   d. The catheter is irrigated gently with NS to prevent obstruction from mucus or clots
   e. Following removal of the catheter, the client is instructed in how to self-catheterize and to drain the reservoir at 4- to 6-hour intervals

6. Indiana pouch
   a. A continent reservoir is created from the ascending colon and terminal ileum, making a pouch larger than the Kock pouch
   b. Postoperatively, the client will have a 24 to 26 Foley catheter in place to drain urine continuously until the pouch has healed
   c. The Foley catheter is irrigated gently with NS to prevent obstruction from mucus or clots
   d. Following removal of the Foley catheter, the client is instructed in how to self-catheterize and to drain the reservoir at 4- to 6-hour intervals

7. Creation of a neobladder
   a. Similar to the creation of an internal reservoir; different because, instead of emptying through an abdominal stoma, it empties through a pelvic outlet into the urethra
   b. The client empties the neobladder by relaxing the external sphincter and creating abdominal pressure or by intermittent self-catheterization

8. Percutaneous nephrostomy or pyelostomy
   a. Used when the **cancer** is inoperable, to prevent obstruction
   b. Involves a percutaneous or surgical insertion of a nephrostomy tube into the kidney for drainage
   c. Nursing interventions involve stabilizing the tube to prevent dislodgment and monitoring output

9. Ureterostomy
   a. May be performed as a palliative procedure if the ureters are obstructed by the tumor
   b. The ureters are attached to the surface of the abdomen, where the urine flows directly into a drainage appliance without a conduit
   c. Potential problems include infection, skin irritation, and obstruction to urinary flow as a result of strictures at the opening

10. Vesicostomy
    a. The bladder is sutured to the abdomen, and a stoma is created in the bladder wall
    b. The bladder empties through the stoma

F. Preoperative interventions
   1. Administer bowel preparation as prescribed, which may include a clear liquid diet, laxatives and enemas, and antibiotics to lower the bacterial count in the bowel

2. Assist the surgeon and the enterostomal nurse in selecting an appropriate skin site for creation of the abdominal stoma
3. Encourage the client to talk about his or her feelings related to the stoma creation

G. Postoperative interventions
1. Monitor vital signs
2. Monitor incision site
3. Assess stoma (should be red and moist) every hour for the first 24 hours (Box 42-22)

4. Monitor for edema in the stoma, which may be present in the immediate postoperative period
5. If the stoma appears dark and dusky, notify the physician immediately, because this indicates necrosis
6. Monitor for prolapse or retraction of the stoma
7. Monitor for return of bowel function; monitor for peristalsis, which will return in 3 to 4 days
8. Maintain NPO status as prescribed until bowel sounds return
9. Monitor urine flow, which is continuous (30 to 60 mL/hour) following surgery
10. The physician is notified if the urine output is less than 30 mL/hour or if there is no urine output for more than 15 minutes
11. Ureteral stents or catheters may be in place for 2 to 3 weeks or until healing occurs; maintain stability with catheters to prevent dislodgment
12. Monitor urinary output closely and irrigate catheter gently to prevent obstruction, as prescribed, with 60 mL of NS (Box 42-23)
13. Monitor for hematuria
14. Monitor for signs of peritonitis

BOX 42-22

Urinary Stoma Care

Instruct the client to change the appliance in the morning, when urinary production is slowest.

Collect equipment, remove collection bag, use water or commercial solvent to loosen adhesive.

Hold a rolled gauze pad against the stoma to collect and absorb urine during the procedure.

Cleanse the skin around stoma and under the drainage bag with mild nonresidue soap and water.

Inspect the skin for excoriation, and instruct the client to prevent urine from coming into contact with the skin.

After the skin is dry, apply skin adhesive around the appliance.

Instruct the client to cut the stoma opening of the skin barrier just large enough to fit over the stoma (no more that 3 mm larger than the stoma).

Instruct the client that the stoma will begin to shrink, requiring a smaller stoma opening on the skin barrier.

Apply skin barrier before attaching the pouch or faceplate.

Place the appliance over the stoma and secure in place.

Encourage self-care; teach the client to use mirror.

Instruct the client that the pouch may be drained by a bedside bag or leg bag, especially at night.

Instruct the client to empty the urinary collection bag when it is one-third to one-half full to prevent pulling of the appliance and leakage.

Instruct the client to check the appliance seal if perspiring occurs.

Instruct the client to leave the urinary pouch in place as long as it is not leaking and to change every 5 to 7 days.

During appliance changes, leave the skin open to air as long as possible.

Use a nonkaraya gum product, because urine erodes karaya gum.

To control odor, instruct the client to drink adequate fluids, to wash the appliance thoroughly with soap and lukewarm water, and to soak the collection pouch in dilute white vinegar for 20 to 30 minutes or place a special deodorant tablet into the pouch while it is being worn.

Instruct the client who takes baths to keep the level of the water below the stoma and to avoid oily soaps.

If the client plans to shower, instruct the client to direct the flow of water away from the stoma.

BOX 42-23

Self-Irrigation and Catheterization of Stoma

IRRIGATION

Instruct the client to wash hands and use clean technique.

Instruct the client to use a catheter and syringe and to instill 60 mL of NS or water into the reservoir and to gently aspirate or allow to drain.

Instruct the client to irrigate until the drainage remains free of mucus but to be cautious not to overirrigate.

CATHETERIZATION

Instruct the client to wash hands and use clean technique.

Initially, the client is taught to insert a catheter every 2 to 3 hours to drain the reservoir; during each week thereafter, the interval is increased by 1 hour until the catheterization is done every 4 to 6 hours.

Lubricate the catheter well with water-soluble lubricant, and instruct the client never to force the catheter into the reservoir.

If resistance is met, instruct the client to pause, rotate the catheter, and apply gentle pressure to insert.

Instruct the client to notify the physician if he or she is unable to insert the catheter.

When urine has stopped, instruct the client to take several deep breaths and move the catheter in and out 2 to 3 inches to ensure that the pouch is empty.

Instruct the client to withdraw the catheter slowly, and to pinch the catheter when withdrawn so that it does not leak urine.

Instruct the client to carry catheterization supplies with him or her.

15. Monitor for bladder distention following a partial cystectomy
16. Monitor for shock, hemorrhage, thrombophlebitis, and lower extremity lymphedema following a radical cystectomy
17. Monitor the urinary drainage pouch for leaks, and check skin integrity
18. Monitor the pH of the urine (do not place the dipstick into the stoma), because strong alkaline urine can cause skin irritation and facilitate crystal formation
19. Instruct the client regarding the potential for urinary tract infection or the development of calculi
20. Instruct the client to check the skin for irritation and to monitor the urinary drainage pouch for any leakage
21. Encourage the client to express feelings about changes in body image, embarrassment, and sexual dysfunction

XXVI. ONCOLOGICAL EMERGENCIES

A. Sepsis and disseminated intravascular coagulation (DIC)
   1. Description: The client with an oncological disorder is at increased risk for infection; DIC is caused by sepsis
   2. Interventions
      a. Maintain strict aseptic technique with the immunocompromised client and monitor closely for infection
      b. IV antibiotics may be prescribed
      c. Anticoagulants may be prescribed during the early phase of DIC
      d. Cryoprecipitated clotting factors may be prescribed when DIC progresses and hemorrhage is the primary problem
B. Syndrome of inappropriate antidiuretic hormone (SIADH)
   1. Description
      a. Tumors can produce, secrete, or stimulate the brain to synthesize antidiuretic hormone (ADH)
      b. Mild symptoms include weakness, muscle cramps, loss of appetite, and fatigue; serum sodium levels range from 115 to 120 mEq/L
      c. More serious signs and symptoms relate to water intoxication and include weight gain, personality changes, confusion, and extreme muscle weakness
      d. As the serum sodium level approaches 110 mEq/L, seizures, coma, and eventually death will occur, unless the condition is rapidly treated
   2. Interventions
      a. Initiate fluid restriction and increased sodium intake as prescribed

      b. Demeclocycline (Declomycin) may be prescribed, an antagonist to ADH
      c. Monitor serum sodium levels
C. Spinal cord compression
   1. Description
      a. Occurs when a tumor directly enters the spinal cord or when the vertebral column collapses from tumor entry
      b. Causes back pain, usually before neurological deficits occur
      c. Neurological deficits relate to the spinal level of compression and include numbness, tingling, loss of urethral, vaginal, and rectal sensation, and muscle weakness
   2. Interventions
      a. Monitor for back pain and neurological deficits
      b. Prepare the client for radiation and/or chemotherapy to reduce the size of the tumor and relieve compression
      c. Surgery may need to be performed to remove the tumor and relieve the pressure on the spinal cord
      d. Instruct the client in the use of neck or back braces if they are prescribed
D. Hypercalcemia
   1. Description
      a. A late manifestation of extensive malignancy that occurs most often in clients with bone **metastasis**
      b. Decreased physical mobility contributes to or worsens hypercalcemia
      c. Early signs include fatigue, anorexia, nausea, vomiting, constipation, and polyuria
      d. More serious signs and symptoms include severe muscle weakness, diminished deep tendon reflexes, paralytic ileus, dehydration, and electrocardiography (ECG) changes
   2. Interventions
      a. Monitor serum calcium level
      b. Oral or parenteral (normal saline) fluids may be prescribed
      c. Medications to lower the calcium level may be prescribed
      d. Prepare the client for dialysis if the condition becomes life threatening or is accompanied by renal impairment
E. Superior vena cava (SVC) syndrome
   1. Description
      a. Occurs when the SVC is compressed or obstructed by tumor growth
      b. Signs and symptoms result from blockage of blood flow in the venous system of the head, neck, and upper trunk
      c. Early signs and symptoms generally occur in the morning; include edema of the face, especially around the eyes, and tightness of the shirt or blouse collar (Stokes' sign)

d. As the condition worsens, edema in the arms and hands, dyspnea, erythema of the upper body, and epistaxis occur

e. Life-threatening signs and symptoms include hemorrhage, cyanosis, mental status changes, decreased cardiac output, and hypotension

2. Interventions

a. Monitor for signs and symptoms of SVC syndrome

b. Prepare the client for radiation therapy to the mediastinal area

F. Tumor lysis syndrome (TLS)

1. Description

a. Occurs when large quantities of tumor cells are destroyed rapidly and are released into the bloodstream faster than the body's homeostatic mechanisms can handle them

b. TLS is a positive sign that **cancer** treatment is effective; however, if left untreated, it can cause severe tissue damage and death

c. Hyperkalemia and hyperuricemia occur; hyperuricemia can lead to acute renal failure

2. Interventions

a. Encourage oral hydration; IV hydration may be prescribed for the client experiencing nausea

b. Instruct the client regarding the importance of fluid intake during chemotherapy

c. Diuretics may be prescribed to increase the urine flow through the kidneys

d. Medications that increase the excretion of purines, such as allopurinol (Zyloprim), may be prescribed

e. IV infusion of glucose and insulin may be prescribed to treat hyperkalemia

f. Prepare the client for dialysis if hyperkalemia and hyperuricemia persist despite treatment

PRACTICE QUESTIONS

1. A nurse is instructing a client to perform a testicular self-examination (TSE). Which instruction would the nurse provide to the client?
   1. Examine the testicles while lying down
   2. The best time for the examination is after a shower
   3. Gently feel the testicle with one finger to feel for a growth
   4. Testicular examinations should be done at least every 6 months

2. A nurse is assisting in conducting a health promotion program at a local school. The nurse determines that additional teaching is needed if a student identifies which of the following as a risk factor associated with cancer?
   1. Viral factors
   2. Stress
   3. Low-fat and high-fiber diets
   4. Exposure to radiation

3. A client with cancer is receiving chemotherapy and develops thrombocytopenia. Which intervention is the priority in the nursing plan of care?
   1. Ambulate the client three times daily
   2. Monitor the client's temperature
   3. Monitor the client for bleeding
   4. Monitor the client for pathological fractures

4. A nurse inspects the oral cavity of a client with cancer and notes white patches on the mucous membranes. The nurse determines that this occurrence:
   1. Is common
   2. Is characteristic of a thrush infection
   3. Is indicative that oral hygiene needs to be improved
   4. Suggests that the client is anemic

5. A nurse is monitoring the laboratory results of a client preparing to receive chemotherapy. The nurse determines that the white blood cell count (WBC) is normal if which of the following results were present?
   1. $2000/mm^3$
   2. $3000/mm^3$
   3. $5000/mm^3$
   4. $15,000/mm^3$

6. A nurse is instructing a group of female clients about breast self-examination (BSE). The nurse would instruct the clients to perform the examination:
   1. At the onset of menstruation
   2. One week after menstruation begins
   3. Every month during ovulation
   4. Weekly at the same time of day

7. A nurse instructs the client in breast self-examination (BSE). The nurse instructs the client to lie down and to examine the left breast. The nurse instructs the client that while examining the left breast, to place a pillow:
   1. Under the right shoulder
   2. Under the left shoulder
   3. Under the small of the back
   4. Under the right scapula

8. A nurse is teaching breast self-examination (BSE) to a client who has had a hysterectomy. The nurse tells the client to perform the BSE:
   1. 7 to 10 days after menses
   2. Just before the menses begins
   3. At ovulation time
   4. At a specific day of the month and on that same day every month thereafter

9. A client suspected of having an abdominal tumor is scheduled for a computerized tomography (CT) scan with dye injection. The nurse tells the client which of the following about the test?
   1. The test may be painful
   2. The dye injected may cause a warm, flushing sensation
   3. Fluids will be restricted following the test
   4. The test takes approximately 2 to 3 hours

10. A 32-year-old female client has a history of fibro-cystic disorder of the breasts. The nurse gathering data from the client asks whether the breast lumps are more noticeable:
    1. In the spring months
    2. In the autumn
    3. After menses
    4. Before menses

11. A client has undergone mastectomy. The nurse interprets that the client is making the best adjustment to the loss of the breast if which of the following behaviors is observed?
    1. Participating in the care of the surgical drain
    2. Reading postoperative care booklet
    3. Refusing to look at wound
    4. Asking for pain medication when needed

12. A client is preparing for discharge after under-going a radical vulvectomy. The nurse plans to tell the client that which activity is acceptable after discharge because it will not precipitate complications?
    1. Sexual activity
    2. Walking
    3. Sitting for lengthy periods
    4. Driving a car

13. A client has undergone vaginal hysterectomy. The nurse avoids which of the following in the care of this client?
    1. Removal of antiembolism stockings twice daily
    2. Assisting with range-of-motion leg exercises
    3. Elevating the knees while in bed
    4. Checking placement of pneumatic compression boots

14. A client suspected of an ovarian tumor is scheduled for a pelvic ultrasound. The nurse plans to tell the client that preparation for the ultrasound includes which of the following?
    1. NPO before the procedure
    2. A light breakfast only
    3. Drinking six to eight glasses of water without voiding before the test
    4. Wearing comfortable clothing and shoes for the procedure

15. A client is diagnosed as having a bowel tumor and several diagnostic tests are prescribed. The nurse understands that which test will confirm the diagnosis of malignancy?
    1. Magnetic resonance imaging (MRI)
    2. Computerized tomography (CT) scan
    3. Abdominal ultrasound
    4. Biopsy of the tumor

16. A client is diagnosed with multiple myeloma and the client asks the nurse about the diagnosis. The nurse bases the response on which characteristic of the disorder?
    1. Malignant exacerbation in the number of leukocytes
    2. Altered red blood cell production
    3. Altered production of lymph nodes
    4. Malignant proliferation of plasma cells and tumors within the bone

17. A nurse is reviewing the laboratory results of a client diagnosed with multiple myeloma. Which of the following would the nurse expect to specifically note with this diagnosis?
    1. Decreased number of plasma cells in the bone marrow
    2. Increased white blood cells
    3. Increased calcium level
    4. Decreased blood urea nitrogen (BUN) level

18. A nurse is assisting in developing a plan of care for the client with multiple myeloma. A priority nursing intervention for a client with multiple myeloma is which of the following?
    1. Coughing and deep breathing
    2. Encouraging fluids
    3. Monitoring the red blood cell count
    4. Providing frequent oral care

19. A nursing instructor asks a nursing student about the characteristics of Hodgkin's disease. The instructor determines that the student needs to read about the characteristics of this disease if the student states that which of the following is an associated characteristic?
    1. Presence of Reed-Sternberg cells
    2. Involvement of lymph nodes, spleen, and liver
    3. Occurs most often in older adults
    4. Prognosis depends on the stage of the disease

20. A nurse is assisting in conducting a health promo-tion program regarding testicular cancer to commu-nity members. The nurse determines that further teaching is needed if a community member states that which of the following is a sign of testicular cancer?
    1. Painless testicular swelling
    2. Heavy sensation in the scrotum
    3. Alopecia
    4. Back pain

21. A nurse is reviewing the laboratory results of a client with leukemia who has received a regimen of chemotherapy. Which laboratory value would the nurse specifically note as a result of the massive cell destruction that occurs with the chemotherapy?
    1. Anemia
    2. Decreased platelets
    3. Decreased leukocyte count
    4. Increased uric acid level

22. A nurse is preparing a client with a bowel tumor for surgery. The physician has informed the client that the surgery is palliative in the treatment of the tumor. The nurse understands that this type of surgery is performed to:
    1. Restore maximal function and appearance
    2. Eliminate high-risk factors

3. To reduce pain
4. To cure the client

23. A client is receiving external radiation to the neck for cancer of the larynx. The nurse plans care knowing that the most likely side effect to be expected is:
    1. Constipation
    2. Dyspnea
    3. Sore throat
    4. Diarrhea

24. A nurse inspects the skin of a client receiving external radiation therapy and documents a finding noted as moist desquamation. The nurse understands that moist desquamation is best described as which of the following?
    1. Reddened skin
    2. A rash
    3. Weeping of the skin
    4. Dermatitis

25. A nurse is providing instructions to a client receiving external radiation therapy. The nurse determines that the client needs further instructions if the client states an intention to:
    1. Avoid exposure to sunlight
    2. Wash the skin with a mild soap and pat dry
    3. Apply pressure on the radiated area to prevent bleeding
    4. Eat a high-protein diet

26. A nurse is caring for a client with an internal radiation implant. When caring for the client, the nurse should observe which principle?
    1. Limit the time with the client to 1 hour per shift
    2. Do not allow pregnant women into the client's room
    3. Individuals under 16 years may be allowed to go in the room as long as they are 6 feet away from the client
    4. Remove dosimeter badge when entering the client's room

27. A client was hospitalized for a cervical radiation implant for the treatment of cervical cancer. The implant is removed, the client is to be discharged, and the nurse reinforces discharge instructions. Which statement by the client indicates the need for further instructions?
    1. "Cream may be used to relieve dryness or itching."
    2. "Foul-smelling vaginal discharge is expected."
    3. "Sexual intercourse may be resumed after 7 to 10 days."
    4. "I should call my physician if I have vaginal bleeding."

28. A cervical radiation implant is placed in the client for treatment of cervical cancer. What activity order would the nurse most likely expect to note in the physician's orders?
    1. Out of bed in a chair only
    2. Ambulate to the bathroom only

3. Bed rest
4. Out of bed as desired

29. A nurse teaches skin care to the client receiving external radiation therapy. Which of the following statements, if made by the client, would indicate the need for further instruction?
    1. "I will handle the area gently."
    2. "I will avoid the use of deodorants."
    3. "I will limit sun exposure to 1 hour daily."
    4. "I will wear loose-fitting clothing."

30. A client is hospitalized for insertion of an internal cervical radiation implant. While giving care, the nurse finds the radiation implant in the bed. The nurse would immediately:
    1. Call the physician
    2. Pick up the implant with gloved hands and flush it down the toilet
    3. Reinsert the implant into the vagina immediately
    4. Pick up the implant with long-handled forceps and place into a lead container

31. A nurse is assisting in developing a plan of care for a client experiencing hematological toxicity as a result of chemotherapy. The nurse suggests including which of the following in the plan of care?
    1. Restricting all visitors
    2. Restricting fluid intake
    3. Inserting an indwelling urinary catheter to prevent skin breakdown
    4. Restricting fresh fruits and vegetables in the diet

32. A nurse is reviewing the laboratory results of a client receiving chemotherapy and notes that the platelet count is 10,000/mm^3. Based on this laboratory value, the priority action is to monitor which of the following?
    1. Level of consciousness
    2. Temperature
    3. Bowel sounds
    4. Skin turgor

33. A nurse is caring for a postoperative client who had a pelvic exenteration. The physician has changed the client's diet from NPO to clear liquids. The nurse checks which of the following before administering the clear liquids?
    1. Ability to ambulate
    2. Specific gravity of the urine
    3. Incision appearance
    4. Bowel sounds

34. A client is admitted to the hospital with a diagnosis of suspected Hodgkin's disease. Which of the following findings would the nurse most likely expect to note documented in the client's record?
    1. Weakness
    2. Fatigue
    3. Weight gain
    4. Enlarged lymph nodes

35. When reviewing the health care record of a client with ovarian cancer, the nurse recognizes which symptom as typical of the disease?
    1. Hypermenorrhea
    2. Abdominal distention
    3. Diarrhea
    4. Abnormal bleeding

36. A nurse is reviewing the complications of conization with a client who has microinvasive cervical cancer. The nurse determines that the client needs additional information about the complications of the procedure if the client states that which of the following is a complication?
    1. Infection
    2. Infertility
    3. Ovarian perforation
    4. Hemorrhage

37. A nurse is caring for a client dying of ovarian cancer. During care, the client states, "If I can just live long enough to attend my daughter's graduation, I'll be ready to die." Which phase of coping is this client experiencing?
    1. Denial
    2. Bargaining
    3. Depression
    4. Anger

38. A nurse is caring for a client following a modified radical mastectomy. Which of the following findings would indicate that the client is experiencing a complication related to the surgery?
    1. Sanguineous drainage in the drainage tube
    2. Pain at the incisional site
    3. Complaints of decreased sensation near the operative site
    4. Arm edema on the operative side

39. A nurse is reviewing the health record of a client with laryngeal cancer. The nurse would expect to note which most common risk factor for this type of cancer documented in the record?
    1. Use of chewing tobacco
    2. Cigarette smoking
    3. Urban living
    4. Alcohol abuse

40. A female client who has been receiving radiation therapy for bladder cancer tells the nurse that it feels as if she is voiding through the vagina. The nurse interprets that the client may be experiencing:
    1. Extreme stress due to the diagnosis of cancer
    2. Altered perineal sensation as a side effect of radiation therapy
    3. The development of a vesicovaginal fistula
    4. Rupture of the bladder

41. A client with leukemia is receiving busulfan (Myleran). Allopurinol (Zyloprim) is prescribed for the client. The nurse understands that the purpose of the allopurinol (Zyloprim) is to:
    1. Prevent gouty arthritis
    2. Prevent hyperuricemia
    3. Prevent stomatitis
    4. Prevent diarrhea

42. A client receiving chemotherapy is experiencing stomatitis. The nurse advises the client to use which of the following as the best substance to rinse the mouth?
    1. Hydrogen peroxide mixture
    2. Weak salt and bicarbonate mouth rinse
    3. Lemon-flavored mouthwash
    4. Alcohol-based mouthwash

43. A nurse is assisting in conducting a health promotion program and the topic of the discussion relates to the risk factors of gastric cancer. The nurse determines that a client attending the program needs additional teaching if the client states that which of the following is associated with the incidence of this type of cancer?
    1. History of gastric polyps
    2. History of pernicious anemia
    3. A diet of smoked, highly salted, and spiced food
    4. High meat and carbohydrate consumption

44. A nurse is reviewing the preoperative orders of a client with a colon tumor who is scheduled for abdominal perineal resection. The nurse notes that the physician has prescribed neomycin sulfate (Mycifradin) for the client. The nurse determines that this medication has been prescribed:
    1. Because the client has an infection
    2. To prevent an infection
    3. To decrease the bacteria in the bowel
    4. Because the client is allergic to penicillin

45. A nurse caring for a client following a radical neck dissection and creation of a tracheostomy performed for laryngeal cancer is reinforcing discharge instructions to the client. Which statement by the client indicates the need for additional instructions regarding care to the stoma?
    1. "I need to apply a thin layer of petrolatum to the skin around the stoma to prevent cracking."
    2. "I need to protect the stoma from water."
    3. "I need to use an air conditioner to provide cool air to assist in breathing."
    4. "I need to keep powders and sprays away from the stoma site."

46. A nurse is caring for a client with cancer of the prostate following a prostatectomy. The nurse reinforces discharge instructions and plans to include which of the following?
    1. Notify the physician if small blood clots are noticed during urination
    2. Avoid driving the car for 1 week
    3. Restrict fluid intake to prevent incontinence
    4. Avoid lifting objects heavier than 20 pounds for at least 6 weeks

47. A nurse is assisting in providing a teaching session to a community group regarding the risks and

causes of bladder cancer. The nurse determines that additional teaching is needed if a member of the community group states that which of the following is associated with this type of cancer?

1. It most often occurs in women
2. It is generally seen in clients older than age 40
3. Environmental health hazards have been attributed as a cause
4. Using cigarettes, artificial sweeteners, and coffee drinking can increase the risk

48. A nurse is reviewing the history of a client with bladder cancer. The nurse would expect to note which most common symptom of this type of cancer documented in the record?

1. Frequency of urination
2. Urgency on urination
3. Hematuria
4. Dysuria

49. A nurse is inspecting the stoma of a client following a ureterostomy. Which of the following would the nurse expect to note?

1. A pale stoma
2. A red and moist stoma
3. A dry stoma
4. A dark-colored stoma

50. A nurse is caring for a client following a radical mastectomy. Which nursing intervention would assist in preventing lymphedema of the affected arm?

1. Placing cool compresses on the affected arm
2. Elevating the affected arm on a pillow above heart level
3. Maintaining an IV site below the antecubital area on the affected side
4. Avoiding arm exercises in the immediate postoperative period

ALTERNATE FORMAT QUESTION: MULTIPLE RESPONSE

A client with carcinoma of the lung develops syndrome of inappropriate antidiuretic hormone (SIADH) as a complication of the cancer. The nurse anticipates that which of the following may be prescribed?

___ Increased fluid intake
___ Decreased sodium intake
___ Monitoring of serum sodium blood levels
___ Medication that is antagonistic to antidiuretic hormone (ADH)
___ Radiation or chemotherapy

ANSWERS

1. *Answer: 2*
Rationale: The TSE is recommended monthly after a warm bath or shower when the scrotal skin is relaxed. The client should stand to examine the testicles. Using both hands, with fingers under the scrotum and thumbs on top, the client should gently roll the testicles feeling for any lumps.
Test-Taking Strategy: Use the process of elimination. Eliminate option 4 first because of the words "6 months." Next, eliminate option 3 because of the word "one." From the remaining options, eliminate option 1 by trying to visualize the process of the self-examination. If you had difficulty with this question, review this self-examination.
Level of Cognitive Ability: Application
Client Needs: Health Promotion and Maintenance
Integrated Process: Teaching/Learning
Content Area: Adult Health/Oncology
Reference: Potter, P., & Perry, A. (2005). *Fundamentals of nursing* (6th ed.). St. Louis: Mosby, p. 752.

2. *Answer: 3*
Rationale: Viruses may be one of multiple agents acting to initiate carcinogenesis and have been associated with several types of cancer. Increased stress has been associated with causing the growth and proliferation of cancer cells. Two forms of radiation, ultraviolet and ionizing, can lead to cancer. High-fiber diets may reduce the risk of colon cancer. A diet high in fat may increase the risk of developing some cancers.
Test-Taking Strategy: Note the key words, *additional teaching is needed.* These words indicate a false response question and that you need to select the incorrect client statement. Read each option carefully, using the process of elimination. Recalling the risk factors related to cancer will direct you to option 3. Review these risk factors if you had difficulty with this question.
Level of Cognitive Ability: Comprehension
Client Needs: Health Promotion and Maintenance
Integrated Process: Teaching/Learning
Content Area: Adult Health/Oncology
Reference: Lewis, S., Heitkemper, M., & Dirksen, S. (2004). *Medical-surgical nursing: Assessment and management of clinical problems* (6th ed.). St. Louis: Mosby, p. 299.

3. *Answer: 3*
Rationale: Thrombocytopenia indicates a decrease in the number of platelets in the circulating blood. A major concern is monitoring for and preventing bleeding. Option 2 relates to monitoring for infection particularly if leukopenia is present. Options 1 and 4, although important in the plan of care, are not directly related to thrombocytopenia.
Test-Taking Strategy: Use the process of elimination and note the key word, *thrombocytopenia.* Recalling that this condition places the client at risk of bleeding will assist in eliminating options 1, 2, and 4. If you are unfamiliar with the nursing interventions related to this disorder, review this content.
Level of Cognitive Ability: Application
Client Needs: Physiological Integrity
Integrated Process: Nursing Process/Planning
Content Area: Adult Health/Oncology

Reference: Linton, A., & Maebius, N. (2003). *Introduction to medical-surgical nursing* (3rd ed.). Philadelphia: W.B. Saunders, pp. 339, 526.

4. Answer: 2

Rationale: Candidiasis is a fungal infection caused by *Candida albicans*. When it occurs in the mouth, it is called thrush, and appears as white plaques. Although it can occur in an immunocompromised client, it is not considered to be common. Options 3 and 4 are not accurate regarding this infection.

Test-Taking Strategy: Use the process of elimination. Options 1 and 3 can be eliminated first. Recalling that the anemic client is more likely to exhibit pallor will assist in eliminating option 4 and will direct you to option 2. If you are unfamiliar with the manifestations associated with thrush, review this content.

Level of Cognitive Ability: Comprehension
Client Needs: Physiological Integrity
Integrated Process: Nursing Process/Data Collection
Content Area: Adult Health/Oncology
References: Christensen, B., & Kockrow, E. (2003). *Foundations of nursing* (4th ed). St. Louis: Mosby, p. 880.
Lewis, S., Heitkemper, M., & Dirksen, S. (2004). *Medical-surgical nursing: Assessment and management of clinical problems* (6th ed.). St. Louis: Mosby, p. 1008.

5. Answer: 3

Rationale: The normal WBC count ranges from 4500 to 11,000/mm^3. Options 1 and 2 identify values lower than normal. Option 4 identifies a value higher than normal.

Test-Taking Strategy: Recalling the normal WBC count will direct you to the correct option. Review the normal WBC count if you had difficulty with this question.

Level of Cognitive Ability: Comprehension
Client Needs: Physiological Integrity
Integrated Process: Nursing Process/Data Collection
Content Area: Adult Health/Oncology
Reference: Pagana, K., & Pagana, T. (2003). *Mosby's diagnostic and laboratory test reference* (6th ed.). St. Louis: Mosby, p. 940.

6. Answer: 2

Rationale: The BSE should be performed monthly about 7 days after the menstrual period begins. It is not recommended to perform the examination weekly. At the onset of menstruation and during ovulation, hormonal changes occur that may alter breast tissue.

Test-Taking Strategy: Use the process of elimination. Option 4 can be eliminated first because of the word "weekly." Eliminate options 1 and 3 next because of the similarity that exists in regard to the hormonal changes that occur during these times. If you are unfamiliar with the procedure for performing BSE, review this self-examination.

Level of Cognitive Ability: Application
Client Needs: Health Promotion and Maintenance
Integrated Process: Teaching/Learning
Content Area: Adult Health/Oncology
Reference: Potter, P., & Perry, A. (2005). *Fundamentals of nursing* (6th ed.). St. Louis: Mosby, p. 736.

7. Answer: 2

Rationale: The nurse would instruct the client to lie down and place a towel or pillow under the shoulder on the side of the breast to be examined. If the left breast it to be examined, the pillow would be placed under the left shoulder. Options 3 and 4 are incorrect.

Test-Taking Strategy: Visualize this procedure to select the correct option. Remember, to examine the left breast, the pillow is placed under the left shoulder, to examine the right breast, the pillow is placed under the right shoulder. If you are unfamiliar with the procedure for performing BSE, review this self-examination.

Level of Cognitive Ability: Application
Client Needs: Health Promotion and Maintenance
Integrated Process: Teaching/Learning
Content Area: Adult Health/Oncology
Reference: Potter, P., & Perry, A. (2005). *Fundamentals of nursing* (6th ed.). St. Louis: Mosby, p. 736.

8. Answer: 4

Rationale: If the client has had a hysterectomy or is no longer menstruating, the BSE should be performed on the same day every month. Options 1 and 2 are inappropriate because the client who had a hysterectomy would not be menstruating. It is best not to perform the BSE at ovulation time because of the hormonal changes that occur.

Test-Taking Strategy: Use the process of elimination and note the key word, *hysterectomy*. Options 1 and 2 can be easily eliminated. Eliminate option 3 because of the hormonal changes that occur at this time. If you are unfamiliar with the procedure for performing BSE, review this self-examination.

Level of Cognitive Ability: Application
Client Needs: Health Promotion and Maintenance
Integrated Process: Teaching/Learning
Content Area: Adult Health/Oncology
Reference: Potter, P., & Perry, A. (2005). *Fundamentals of nursing* (6th ed.). St. Louis: Mosby, p. 737.

9. Answer: 2

Rationale: The CT scan causes no pain and takes about 15 to 60 minutes to perform. The dye may cause a warm flushing sensation when injected. Fluids are encouraged following the procedure. If an iodine dye is used, the client should be asked about allergies to seafood or iodine.

Test-Taking Strategy: Use the process of elimination and note the key words, *dye injection*. Noting the relationship between these key words and option 2 will assist in answering the question. Review this diagnostic test if you had difficulty with this question.

Level of Cognitive Ability: Comprehension
Client Needs: Physiological Integrity
Integrated Process: Nursing Process/Implementation
Content Area: Adult Health/Oncology
Reference: Pagana, K., & Pagana, T. (2003). *Mosby's diagnostic and laboratory test reference* (6th ed.). St. Louis: Mosby, p. 281.

10. Answer: 4

Rationale: The nurse asks the client with fibrocystic breast disorder about worsening of symptoms (breast lumps, painful breasts, and possible nipple discharge) before the onset of menses. This is associated with cyclical hormone changes. Options 1, 2, and 3 do not provide significant data regarding this disorder.

Test-Taking Strategy: Note the key words, *more noticeable.* This implies that there is a predictable variation in symptoms. Use knowledge of the effects of various hormones in the body to analyze the options and choose correctly. Review fibrocystic disorder, if you had difficulty with this question.

Level of Cognitive Ability: Application
Client Needs: Physiological Integrity
Integrated Process: Nursing Process/Data Collection
Content Area: Adult Health/Oncology
Reference: Christensen, B., & Kockrow, E. (2003). *Adult health nursing* (4th ed.). St. Louis: Mosby, p. 528.

11. *Answer:* **1**

Rationale: The client demonstrates the best adjustment by participating in his or her own care. This would include care of surgical drains that would be in place for a short time after discharge. Asking for pain medication is also an action-oriented option, but it does not relate to acceptance of the loss of the breast. Reading the postoperative care booklet is useful, but is not the best of the options presented. Refusing to look at the wound indicates a lack of adjustment to the loss.

Test-Taking Strategy: Note the key words, *best adjustment.* This tells you that more than one or all of the options may be partially or totally correct. Use prioritizing skills, noting that option 1 is the most action oriented behavior. Review the psychosocial needs of the client following mastectomy if you had difficulty with this question.

Level of Cognitive Ability: Analysis
Client Needs: Psychosocial Integrity
Integrated Process: Nursing Process/Evaluation
Content Area: Adult Health/Oncology
References: Christensen, B., & Kockrow, E. (2003). *Adult health nursing* (4th ed.). St. Louis: Mosby, pp. 534-536.
Phipps, W., Monahan, F., Sands, J., Marek, J., & Neighbors, M. (2003). *Medical-surgical nursing: Health and illness perspectives* (7th ed.). St. Louis: Mosby, p. 1809.

12. *Answer:* **2**

Rationale: The client should resume activity slowly, and walking is a beneficial activity. The client should be instructed to rest when fatigue occurs. Activities to be avoided include driving, heavy housework, wearing tight clothing, crossing the legs, and prolonged standing or sitting. Sexual activity is prohibited for 4 to 6 weeks after surgery.

Test-Taking Strategy: Use the process of elimination and note the key words, *not precipitate complications.* With this in mind, evaluate each of the options in terms of the stress or harm it could cause to the perineal area. This will direct you to option 2. Review home care measures following vulvectomy if you had difficulty with this question.

Level of Cognitive Ability: Application
Client Needs: Physiological Integrity
Integrated Process: Nursing Process/Planning
Content Area: Adult Health/Oncology
Reference: Black, J., & Hawks, J. (2005). *Medical-surgical nursing: Clinical management for positive outcomes* (7th ed.). Philadelphia: W.B. Saunders, p. 1087.

13. *Answer:* **3**

Rationale: The client is at risk of deep vein thrombosis or thrombophlebitis after this surgery, as for any other major surgery. For this reason, the nurse implements measures that will prevent this complication. Range-of-motion exercises, antiembolism stockings, and pneumatic compression boots are all helpful. The nurse should avoid elevating the knees while in the bed, which inhibits venous return, thus placing the client more at risk for deep vein thrombosis or thrombophlebitis.

Test-Taking Strategy: Use the process of elimination and note the key word, *avoids.* This word indicates a false response question and that you need to select the incorrect intervention. Recalling the complications following this type of surgery and the interventions that will prevent these complications will direct you to option 3. Review these postoperative nursing interventions if you had difficulty with this question.

Level of Cognitive Ability: Application
Client Needs: Physiological Integrity
Integrated Process: Nursing Process/Implementation
Content Area: Adult Health/Oncology
Reference: Linton, A., & Maebius, N. (2003). *Introduction to medical-surgical nursing* (3rd ed.). Philadelphia: W.B. Saunders, p. 947.

14. *Answer:* **3**

Rationale: A pelvic ultrasound requires the ingestion of large volumes of water just prior to the procedure. A full bladder is necessary so that this organ will be visualized as such and not mistaken as a possible pelvic growth. An abdominal ultrasound may require that the client abstain from food or fluid for several hours before the procedure. Option 4 is unrelated to this specific procedure.

Test-Taking Strategy: Use the process of elimination. Noting the key word, *pelvic,* will assist in directing you to option 3. Review preparation for a pelvic ultrasound if you had difficulty with this question.

Level of Cognitive Ability: Application
Client Needs: Physiological Integrity
Integrated Process: Nursing Process/Implementation
Content Area: Adult Health/Oncology
Reference: Pagana, K., & Pagana, T. (2003). *Mosby's diagnostic and laboratory test reference* (6th ed.). St. Louis: Mosby, p. 661.

15. *Answer:* **4**

Rationale: A biopsy is done to determine whether a tumor is malignant or benign. An MRI, CT scan, and ultrasound will visualize the presence of a mass but will not confirm a diagnosis of malignancy.

Test-Taking Strategy: Use the process of elimination and note the key word, *confirm.* This key word will direct you to option 4. Review the purpose of these tests if you had difficulty with this question.

Level of Cognitive Ability: Comprehension
Client Needs: Physiological Integrity
Integrated Process: Nursing Process/Data Collection
Content Area: Adult Health/Oncology
Reference: Christensen, B., & Kockrow, E. (2003). *Adult health nursing* (4th ed.). St. Louis: Mosby, p. 720.

16. *Answer: 4*
Rationale: Multiple myeloma is a neoplastic condition characterized by abnormal malignant proliferation of plasma cells and the accumulation of mature plasma cells in the bone marrow. Option 1 describes the leukemic process. Options 2 and 3 are not characteristics of multiple myeloma.
Test-Taking Strategy: Use the process of elimination and knowledge regarding the pathophysiology associated with this disorder to answer the question. Focusing on the name of the diagnosis will assist in directing you to option 4. Review this information if you are unfamiliar with this oncological disorder.
Level of Cognitive Ability: Comprehension
Client Needs: Physiological Integrity
Integrated Process: Nursing Process/Planning
Content Area: Adult Health/Oncology
Reference: Linton, A., & Maebius, N. (2003). *Introduction to medical-surgical nursing* (3rd ed.). Philadelphia: W.B. Saunders, p. 552.

17. *Answer: 3*
Rationale: Findings indicative of multiple myeloma are an increased number of plasma cells in the bone marrow, anemia, hypercalcemia as a result of the release of calcium from the deteriorating bone tissue, and an elevated BUN level. An increased white blood cell count may or may not be present and is not specifically related to multiple myeloma.
Test-Taking Strategy: Knowledge regarding the pathophysiology associated with this disorder and the effects it produces on the body is required to answer the question. Remember, hypercalcemia occurs as a result of the release of calcium from the deteriorating bone tissue. Review this information if you are unfamiliar with this oncological disorder.
Level of Cognitive Ability: Comprehension
Client Needs: Physiological Integrity
Integrated Process: Nursing Process/Data Collection
Content Area: Adult Health/Oncology
Reference: Lewis, S., Heitkemper, M., & Dirksen, S. (2004). *Medical-surgical nursing: Assessment and management of clinical problems* (6th ed.). St. Louis: Mosby, p. 745.

18. *Answer: 2*
Rationale: Hypercalcemia secondary to bone destruction is a priority concern in the client with multiple myeloma. The nurse should encourage fluids in adequate amounts to maintain an output of 1.5 to 2.0 L/day. Clients require about 3 L of fluid per day. The fluid is needed not only to dilute the calcium, but also to prevent protein from precipitating in the renal tubules. Options 1, 3, and 4 may be a component of the plan of care, but are not the priority in this client.
Test-Taking Strategy: Knowledge regarding the clinical manifestations that occur in multiple myeloma is required to answer the question. Recalling that encouraging fluids is specific to the care of a client with this disorder will direct you to option 2. Review the specific manifestations of this disorder if you had difficulty with this question.
Level of Cognitive Ability: Application
Client Needs: Physiological Integrity

Integrated Process: Nursing Process/Planning
Content Area: Adult Health/Oncology
Reference: Lewis, S., Heitkemper, M., & Dirksen, S. (2004). *Medical-surgical nursing: Assessment and management of clinical problems* (6th ed.). St. Louis: Mosby, p. 746.

19. *Answer: 3*
Rationale: Hodgkin's disease is a disorder of young adults and primarily occurs between the ages of 20 to 40. Options 1, 2, and 4 are characteristics of this disease.
Test-Taking Strategy: Use the process of elimination and note the key words, *needs to read about the characteristics of this disease.* Recalling that Hodgkin's disease occurs in the young adult will direct you to option 3. Review the characteristics of this disorder if you had difficulty with this question.
Level of Cognitive Ability: Comprehension
Client Needs: Physiological Integrity
Integrated Process: Nursing Process/Planning
Content Area: Adult Health/Oncology
Reference: Christensen, B., & Kockrow, E. (2003). *Adult health nursing* (4th ed). St. Louis: Mosby, p. 279.

20. *Answer: 3*
Rationale: Alopecia is not a finding in testicular cancer. It may however occur as a result of radiation or chemotherapy. Options 1, 2, and 4 are findings in testicular cancer. Back pain may indicate metastasis to the retroperitoneal lymph nodes.
Test-Taking Strategy: Note the key words, *further teaching is needed.* These words indicate a false response question and that you need to select the incorrect sign. Use the process of elimination, remembering that alopecia occurs as a result of chemotherapy rather than from the disease. Review the manifestations associated with testicular cancer if you had difficulty with this question.
Level of Cognitive Ability: Comprehension
Client Needs: Health Promotion and Maintenance
Integrated Process: Teaching/Learning
Content Area: Adult Health/Oncology
Reference: Christensen, B., & Kockrow, E. (2003). *Adult health nursing* (4th ed). St. Louis: Mosby, p. 541.

21. *Answer: 4*
Rationale: Hyperuricemia is especially common following treatment for leukemias and lymphomas, because the therapy results in massive cell destruction. Although options 1, 2, and 3 may also be noted, an increased uric acid level is specifically related to cell destruction.
Test-Taking Strategy: Note the key words, *specifically note* and *massive cell destruction.* Recalling the cell response to destruction will assist in directing you to option 4. Review this concept if you had difficulty with this question.
Level of Cognitive Ability: Comprehension
Client Needs: Physiological Integrity
Integrated Process: Nursing Process/Data Collection
Content Area: Adult Health/Oncology
Reference: Black, J., & Hawks, J. (2005). *Medical-surgical nursing: Clinical management for positive outcomes* (7th ed.). Philadelphia: W.B. Saunders, pp. 2405-2406.

22. Answer: 3
Rationale: Palliative surgery that can benefit the client with cancer and improve quality of life includes procedures that reduce pain, relieve airway obstructions, relieve obstruction in the gastrointestinal and urinary tracts, relieve pressure on the brain and spinal cord, and prevent hemorrhage. Options 1, 2, and 4 do not describe palliative surgery.
Test-Taking Strategy: Note the key word, *palliative.* Knowledge of the definition of this word will assist in directing you to option 3. Review the various types of surgery if you had difficulty with this question.
Level of Cognitive Ability: Comprehension
Client Needs: Physiological Integrity
Integrated Process: Nursing Process/Planning
Content Area: Adult Health/Oncology
Reference: Christensen, B., & Kockrow, E. (2003). *Adult health nursing* (4th ed.). St. Louis: Mosby, p. 20.

23. Answer: 3
Rationale: In general, only the area in the treatment field is affected by the radiation. Skin reactions, fatigue, nausea, and anorexia may occur with radiation to any site, whereas other side effects occur only when specific areas are involved in treatment. A client receiving radiation to the larynx is most likely to experience a sore throat. Options 1 and 4 may occur with radiation to the gastrointestinal (GI) tract. Dyspnea may occur with lung involvement.
Test-Taking Strategy: Use the process of elimination and note the key words, *most likely.* Eliminate options 1 and 4 first because they are similar and GI related. Consider the anatomical location of the radiation therapy to assist in directing you to option 3. Review the effects of radiation therapy if you had difficulty with this question.
Level of Cognitive Ability: Application
Client Needs: Physiological Integrity
Integrated Process: Nursing Process/Planning
Content Area: Adult Health/Oncology
Reference: Linton, A., & Maebius, N. (2003). *Introduction to medical-surgical nursing* (3rd ed.). Philadelphia: W.B. Saunders, p. 330.

24. Answer: 3
Rationale: Moist desquamation occurs when the basal cells of the skin are destroyed. The dermal level is exposed, which results in the leakage of serum. Reddened skin, a rash, and dermatitis may occur with external radiation but is not described as a moist desquamation.
Test-Taking Strategy: Use the process of elimination. Noting the key word, *moist,* will direct you to option 3. Options 1, 2, and 4 are eliminated because they are similar and describe a dry rather than a moist skin alteration. Review the signs associated with a moist desquamation if you had difficulty with this question.
Level of Cognitive Ability: Comprehension
Client Needs: Physiological Integrity
Integrated Process: Nursing Process/Data Collection
Content Area: Adult Health/Oncology
Reference: Thompson, J., McFarland, G., Hirsch, J., & Tucker, S. (2002). *Mosby's clinical nursing* (5th ed.). St. Louis: Mosby, pp. 1230-1231.

25. Answer: 3
Rationale: The client should avoid pressure on the radiated area and should wear loose-fitting clothing. Options 1, 2, and 4 are accurate instructions regarding radiation therapy.
Test-Taking Strategy: Use the process of elimination and note the key words, *needs further instructions.* These words indicate a false response question and that you need to select the incorrect client statement. The word "pressure" in option 3 should be an indication that this is an inappropriate measure. Review client teaching points related to skin care and radiation therapy if you had difficulty with this question.
Level of Cognitive Ability: Comprehension
Client Needs: Health Promotion and Maintenance
Integrated Process: Teaching/Learning
Content Area: Adult Health/Oncology
Reference: Linton, A., & Maebius, N. (2003). *Introduction to medical-surgical nursing* (3rd ed.). Philadelphia: W.B. Saunders, p. 342.

26. Answer: 2
Rationale: The time that the nurse spends in a room of a client with an internal radiation implant is 30 minutes per 8-hour shift. The dosimeter badge must be worn when in the client's room. Children younger than 16 years of age and pregnant women are not allowed in the client's room.
Test-Taking Strategy: Use the process of elimination. Option 4 can be eliminated first. Knowledge of the time frame related to exposure to the client will assist in eliminating option 1. From the remaining options, select option 2 because of the possible risks associated with exposure to the mother and fetus. Review these principles if you had difficulty with this question.
Level of Cognitive Ability: Application
Client Needs: Safe, Effective Care Environment
Integrated Process: Nursing Process/Implementation
Content Area: Adult Health/Oncology
Reference: Black, J., & Hawks, J. (2005). *Medical-surgical nursing: Clinical management for positive outcomes* (7th ed.). Philadelphia: W.B. Saunders, p. 363.

27. Answer: 2
Rationale: The client is instructed to notify the physician if nausea, vomiting, diarrhea, frequent urination, vaginal or rectal bleeding, hematuria, foul-smelling vaginal discharge, abdominal pain, or fever occurs. Options 1, 3, and 4 are accurate discharge instructions.
Test-Taking Strategy: Note the key words, *need for further instructions.* These words indicate a false response question and that you need to select the incorrect client statement. Recalling that foul-smelling vaginal discharge is a sign of infection will direct you to option 2. Review these points if you had difficulty with this question.
Level of Cognitive Ability: Comprehension
Client Needs: Health Promotion and Maintenance
Integrated Process: Teaching/Learning
Content Area: Adult Health/Oncology
Reference: Linton, A., & Maebius, N. (2003). *Introduction to medical-surgical nursing* (3rd ed.). Philadelphia: W.B. Saunders, pp. 962-963.

28. *Answer: 3*
Rationale: The client with a cervical radiation implant should be maintained on bed rest in the dorsal position to prevent movement of the radiation source. The head of the bed is elevated to a maximum of 10 to 15 degrees for comfort. Turning the client on the side is avoided. If the client needs to be turned, a pillow is placed between the knees and, with the body in straight alignment, the client is logrolled.
Test-Taking Strategy: Consider the anatomical location of the implant and the risk of dislodgment to answer the question. Additionally, note that options 1, 2, and 4 are similar. If you had difficulty with this question, review care of the client with a radiation implant.
Level of Cognitive Ability: Comprehension
Client Needs: Safe, Effective Care Environment
Integrated Process: Nursing Process/Planning
Content Area: Adult Health/Oncology
Reference: Linton, A., & Maebius, N. (2003). *Introduction to medical-surgical nursing* (3rd ed.). Philadelphia: W.B. Saunders, p. 962.

29. *Answer: 3*
Rationale: The client needs to be instructed to avoid exposure to the sun. Options 1, 2, and 4 are accurate measures in the care of a client receiving external radiation therapy.
Test-Taking Strategy: Note the key words, *need for further instruction*. These words indicate a false response question and that you need to select the incorrect client statement. Eliminate option 1 because of the word "gently" and option 4 because of the word "loose." From the remaining options, recalling that sun exposure is to be avoided will assist in answering the question. Review skin care measures for the client receiving external radiation if you had difficulty with this question.
Level of Cognitive Ability: Comprehension
Client Needs: Health Promotion and Maintenance
Integrated Process: Teaching/Learning
Content Area: Adult Health/Oncology
Reference: Linton, A., & Maebius, N. (2003). *Introduction to medical-surgical nursing* (3rd ed.). Philadelphia: W.B. Saunders, p. 342.

30. *Answer: 4*
Rationale: A lead container and long-handled forceps should be kept in the client's room at all times during internal radiation therapy. If the implant becomes dislodged, the nurse should pick up the implant with long-handled forceps and place it into the lead container. Options 1, 2, and 3 are inaccurate interventions.
Test-Taking Strategy: Use the process of elimination. Note the key word, *immediately*. Option 3 is not an appropriate action. Eliminate option 2 next because the implant would not be discarded. Although the physician would be notified, the initial action is option 4. Review the measures related to a dislodged implant if you had difficulty with this question.
Level of Cognitive Ability: Application
Client Needs: Safe, Effective Care Environment
Integrated Process: Nursing Process/Implementation
Content Area: Adult Health/Oncology

Reference: Black, J., & Hawks, J. (2005). *Medical-surgical nursing: Clinical management for positive outcomes* (7th ed.). Philadelphia: W.B. Saunders, p. 362.

31. *Answer: 4*
Rationale: In a client experiencing hematological toxicity, a low-bacteria diet is implemented. This includes avoiding fresh fruits and vegetables and thorough cooking of all foods. Not all visitors are restricted, but the client is protected from people with known infections. Fluids should be encouraged. Invasive measures such as an indwelling urinary catheter should be avoided to prevent infections.
Test-Taking Strategy: Use the process of elimination. Eliminate option 1 because of the word "all." Next, eliminate option 2 because it is not reasonable to restrict fluids in a client receiving chemotherapy who is already at risk for fluid and electrolyte imbalances. Eliminate option 3 because of the risk of infection that exists with this measure. Review interventions for the client with hematological toxicity if you had difficulty with this question.
Level of Cognitive Ability: Application
Client Needs: Safe, Effective Care Environment
Integrated Process: Nursing Process/Planning
Content Area: Adult Health/Oncology
References: Christensen, B., & Kockrow, E. (2003). *Adult health nursing* (4th ed). St. Louis: Mosby, p. 732.
Linton, A., & Maebius, N. (2003). *Introduction to medical-surgical nursing* (3rd ed.). Philadelphia: W.B. Saunders, p. 340.

32. *Answer: 1*
Rationale: A high risk of hemorrhage exists when the platelet count is lower than 20,000/mm^3. Fatal central nervous system (CNS) hemorrhage or massive gastrointestinal (GI) hemorrhage can occur when the platelet count is lower than 10,000/mm^3. The client should be monitored for changes in level of consciousness, which may be an early indication of an intracranial hemorrhage. Option 2 is a priority when the WBC count is low and the client is at risk for an infection. Although options 3 and 4 are important, they are not the priority in this situation.
Test-Taking Strategy: Use the process of elimination and note the key word, *priority*. Recalling the normal platelet count and determining that a low count places the client at risk for bleeding will assist in eliminating options 2, 3, and 4. Review the normal platelet count and the nursing interventions for a client with a low count if you had difficulty with this question.
Level of Cognitive Ability: Analysis
Client Needs: Physiological Integrity
Integrated Process: Nursing Process/Implementation
Content Area: Adult Health/Oncology
References: Lewis, S., Heitkemper, M., & Dirksen, S. (2004). *Medical-surgical nursing: Assessment and management of clinical problems* (6th ed.). St. Louis: Mosby, p. 700.
Pagana, K., & Pagana, T. (2003). *Mosby's diagnostic and laboratory test reference* (6th ed.). St. Louis: Mosby, p. 679.

33. *Answer: 4*
Rationale: The client is kept NPO until peristalsis returns, usually in 4 to 6 days postoperatively. When signs of bowel

function return, clear fluids are given to the client. If no distention occurs, the diet is advanced as tolerated. It is most important to monitor for bowel sounds prior to feeding the client. Options 1, 2, and 3 are unrelated to the issue of the question.

Test-Taking Strategy: Use the process of elimination. Note the key words, *priority* and *NPO to clear liquids*. Option 4 is the only option that relates to gastrointestinal function, which is the issue of the question. Review care of the client following abdominal surgery if you had difficulty with this question.

Level of Cognitive Ability: Application
Client Needs: Physiological Integrity
Integrated Process: Nursing Process/Implementation
Content Area: Adult Health/Oncology
Reference: Lewis, S., Heitkemper, M., & Dirksen, S. (2004). *Medical-surgical nursing: Assessment and management of clinical problems* (6th ed.). St. Louis: Mosby, p. 1062.

34. *Answer: 4*

Rationale: Hodgkin's disease is a chronic progressive neoplastic disorder of lymphoid tissue characterized by the painless enlargement of lymph nodes with progression to extralymphatic sites, such as the spleen and liver. Weight loss is most likely to be noted. Fatigue and weakness may occur, but is not significantly related to the disease.

Test-Taking Strategy: Use the process of elimination and note the key words, *most likely*. Option 3 can be eliminated first because in such a disorder, weight loss is most likely to occur. Options 1 and 2 are similar and rather vague symptoms that can occur in many disorders. Also, recalling that Hodgkin's disease affects the lymph nodes will direct you to option 4. Review the manifestations associated with Hodgkin's disease if you had difficulty with this question.

Level of Cognitive Ability: Comprehension
Client Needs: Physiological Integrity
Integrated Process: Nursing Process/Data Collection
Content Area: Adult Health/Oncology
Reference: Christensen, B., & Kockrow, E. (2003). *Adult health nursing* (4th ed.). St. Louis: Mosby, p. 279.

35. *Answer: 2*

Rationale: Clinical manifestations of ovarian cancer include abdominal distention, urinary frequency and urgency, pain from pressure caused by the growing tumor and the effects of urinary or bowel obstruction, and constipation. Abnormal bleeding, often resulting in hypermenorrhea, is associated with uterine cancer.

Test-Taking Strategy: Use the process of elimination. Eliminate options 1 and 4 first because they are similar. From the remaining options, consider the anatomical location of the diagnosis. This will assist in directing you to option 2. Review the manifestations associated with ovarian cancer if you had difficulty with this question.

Level of Cognitive Ability: Comprehension
Client Needs: Physiological Integrity
Integrated Process: Nursing Process/Data Collection
Content Area: Adult Health/Oncology
Reference: Linton, A., & Maebius, N. (2003). *Introduction to medical-surgical nursing* (3rd ed.). Philadelphia: W.B. Saunders, p. 960.

36. *Answer: 3*

Rationale: Conization is generally not performed on women who desire to bear children because it can lead to incompetence of the cervix or infertility. Other complications of the procedure include hemorrhage, infection and, less frequently, cervical stenosis.

Test-Taking Strategy: Use the process of elimination. Note the key words *needs additional information* and the words "cervical cancer." Select option 3 because this option addresses an "ovarian" condition, not a cervical one. Review the complications associated with this procedure if you had difficulty with this question.

Level of Cognitive Ability: Comprehension
Client Needs: Physiological Integrity
Integrated Process: Nursing Process/Implementation
Content Area: Adult Health/Oncology
Reference: Christensen, B., & Kockrow, E. (2003). *Adult health nursing* (4th ed.). St. Louis: Mosby, p. 524.

37. *Answer: 2*

Rationale: Denial, bargaining, anger, depression, and acceptance are recognized stages that a person facing a life-threatening illness experiences. The client's statement is indicative of bargaining. Denial is expressed as shock and disbelief and may be the first response to hearing bad news. Depression may be manifested by hopelessness, weeping openly, or remaining quiet or withdrawn. Anger may also be a first response to upsetting news and the predominant theme is "Why me?" or the blaming of others.

Test-Taking Strategy: Focus on the client's statement as identified in the question to assist in selecting the correct option. From this point, you should be able to eliminate options 1, 3, and 4. Review these stages if you had difficulty with this question.

Level of Cognitive Ability: Analysis
Client Needs: Psychosocial Integrity
Integrated Process: Nursing Process/Data Collection
Content Area: Adult Health/Oncology
Reference: Christensen, B., & Kockrow, E. (2003). *Adult health nursing* (4th ed.). St. Louis: Mosby, pp. 931-933.

38. *Answer: 4*

Rationale: Arm edema on the operative side (lymphedema) is a complication following mastectomy and can occur immediately, months, or even years after surgery. Options 1, 2, and 3 are expected occurrences following mastectomy and are not indicative of a complication.

Test-Taking Strategy: Use the process of elimination, considering the normal expected occurrences following a mastectomy. This will direct you to the correct option. If you had difficulty with this question, review the complications following mastectomy.

Level of Cognitive Ability: Comprehension
Client Needs: Physiological Integrity
Integrated Process: Nursing Process/Data Collection
Content Area: Adult Health/Oncology
Reference: Linton, A., & Maebius, N. (2003). *Introduction to medical-surgical nursing* (3rd ed.). Philadelphia: W.B. Saunders, pp. 957, 959.

39. *Answer: 2*

Rationale: The most common risk factor associated with laryngeal cancer is cigarette smoking. Approximately 75%

of those diagnosed with this form of cancer smoke, either currently or in the past. Alcohol abuse may have a synergistic effect with cigarette smoking. Air pollution is also a contributing cause, as well as chronic laryngitis and consistent voice strain.

Test-Taking Strategy: Use the process of elimination and note the key words, *most common*. Begin to answer this question by eliminating options 3 and 4. Because cancer of the upper and lower airway is most often related to tobacco, these are the options that are most likely correct. From the remaining options, recalling that cigarettes are the most harmful guides you to choose this option over the option of chewing tobacco. Review these risk factors if you had difficulty with this question.

Level of Cognitive Ability: Comprehension
Client Needs: Health Promotion and Maintenance
Integrated Process: Nursing Process/Data Collection
Content Area: Adult Health/Oncology
Reference: Linton, A., & Maebius, N. (2003). *Introduction to medical-surgical nursing* (3rd ed.). Philadelphia: W.B. Saunders, p. 1111.

40. *Answer:* **3**
Rationale: A vesicovaginal fistula is a genital fistula that occurs between the bladder and the vagina. The fistula is an abnormal opening between these two body parts and, if this occurs, the client may experience drainage of urine through the vagina. The client's complaint is not associated with options 1, 2, and 4.

Test-Taking Strategy: Use the process of elimination. Noting the key words, *voiding through the vagina*, should direct you to option 3. Review the symptoms associated with vesicovaginal fistula if you had difficulty with this question.

Level of Cognitive Ability: Comprehension
Client Needs: Physiological Integrity
Integrated Process: Nursing Process/Data Collection
Content Area: Adult Health/Oncology
Reference: Phipps, W., Monahan, F., Sands, J., Marek, J., & Neighbors, M. (2003). *Medical-surgical nursing: Health and illness perspectives* (7th ed.). St. Louis: Mosby, pp. 1758-1759.

41. *Answer:* **2**
Rationale: Allopurinol decreases uric acid production and reduces uric acid concentrations in both serum and urine. In the client receiving chemotherapy, uric acid levels increase as a result of the massive cell destruction that occurs from the chemotherapy. This medication prevents or treats hyperuricemia secondary to chemotherapy. Although the medication is used to treat gout, it is not the purpose in this client's situation. This medication is not used to prevent stomatitis or diarrhea.

Test-Taking Strategy: Use the process of elimination. Recalling that hyperuricemia occurs as a result of chemotherapy will assist in directing you to option 2. If you had difficulty with this question or are unfamiliar with the action of this medication, review this content.

Level of Cognitive Ability: Analysis
Client Needs: Physiological Integrity
Integrated Process: Nursing Process/Planning
Content Area: Adult Health/Oncology

Reference: McKenry, L., & Salerno, E. (2003). *Mosby's pharmacology in nursing* (21st ed.). St. Louis: Mosby, pp. 686-687.

42. *Answer:* **2**
Rationale: An acidic environment in the mouth is favorable for bacterial growth. Therefore, the client is advised to rinse the mouth at least before every meal and at bedtime with a weak salt and sodium bicarbonate mouth rinse. This lessens the growth of bacteria and limits plaque formation. The other substances are irritating to oral tissue, which is already at risk. If hydrogen peroxide must be used, it should be a very weak solution, because it dries the mucous membranes.

Test-Taking Strategy: Use the process of elimination. Options 3 and 4 can be eliminated first because of the irritating effects of these solutions. From the remaining options, note the word "weak" in the correct option. Review the treatment measures for stomatitis if you had difficulty with this question.

Level of Cognitive Ability: Application
Client Needs: Physiological Integrity
Integrated Process: Nursing Process/Implementation
Content Area: Adult Health/Oncology
Reference: Phipps, W., Monahan, F., Sands, J., Marek, J., & Neighbors, M. (2003). *Medical-surgical nursing: Health and illness perspectives* (7th ed.). St. Louis: Mosby, p. 353.

43. *Answer:* **4**
Rationale: High meat and carbohydrate consumption plays a role in the development of cancer of the pancreas. Options 1, 2, and 3 are risk factors related to gastric cancer.

Test-Taking Strategy: Use the process of elimination. Note that the question asks about the risk factors associated with gastric cancer, and note the key words, *needs additional teaching*. Eliminate options 1 and 2 because they are directly related to gastric disorders. Eliminate option 3 knowing that spicy foods cause gastric irritation. Review the risk factors associated with gastric cancer if you had difficulty with this question.

Level of Cognitive Ability: Comprehension
Client Needs: Health Promotion and Maintenance
Integrated Process: Teaching/Learning
Content Area: Adult Health/Oncology
Reference: Phipps, W., Monahan, F., Sands, J., Marek, J., & Neighbors, M. (2003). *Medical-surgical nursing: Health and illness perspectives* (7th ed.). St. Louis: Mosby, p. 1046.

44. *Answer:* **3**
Rationale: To reduce the risk of contamination at the time of surgery, the bowel is emptied and cleansed. Laxatives and enemas are given to empty the bowel. Intestinal antiinfectives such as neomycin are administered to decrease the bacteria in the bowel.

Test-Taking Strategy: Use the process of elimination. Eliminate options 1 and 4 first because there is no reference made to this information in the question. Recalling the concepts related to the flora of the intestinal tract will assist in directing you to option 3 as the primary purpose of this medication. Review this preoperative intervention if you had difficulty with this question.

Level of Cognitive Ability: Comprehension
Client Needs: Physiological Integrity
Integrated Process: Teaching/Learning

Content Area: Adult Health/Oncology
Reference: Phipps, W., Monahan, F., Sands, J., Marek, J., & Neighbors, M. (2003). *Medical-surgical nursing: Health and illness perspectives* (7th ed.). St. Louis: Mosby, p. 1108.

45. Answer: 3
Rationale: Air conditioners need to be avoided to protect from excessive coldness. A humidifier in the home should be used if excessive dryness is a problem. Options 1, 2, and 4 are appropriate interventions regarding stoma care following radical neck dissection and creation of a tracheotomy.
Test-Taking Strategy: Use the process of elimination. Noting the key words, *need for additional instructions*, will assist in eliminating options 2 and 4. From the remaining options, recalling that a humidifier rather than an air conditioner is recommended will assist in selecting the correct option. If you had difficulty with this question, review discharge instructions following radical neck dissection.
Level of Cognitive Ability: Comprehension
Client Needs: Health Promotion and Maintenance
Integrated Process: Teaching/Learning
Content Area: Adult Health/Oncology
Reference: Phipps, W., Monahan, F., Sands, J., Marek, J., & Neighbors, M. (2003). *Medical-surgical nursing: Health and illness perspectives* (7th ed.). St. Louis: Mosby, p. 509.

46. Answer: 4
Rationale: Small pieces of tissue or blood clots can be passed during urination for up to 2 weeks after surgery. Driving a car and sitting for long periods of time are restricted for at least 3 weeks. A daily fluid intake of 2 to 2.5 L/day should be maintained to limit clot formation and prevent infection. Option 4 is an accurate discharge instruction following prostatectomy.
Test-Taking Strategy: Use the process of elimination. Option 3 can be easily eliminated first. Eliminate option 2 next, because 1 week is a rather short time period. Recalling that blood clots are expected following this type of surgery will assist in directing you to option 4. Review client teaching points following prostatectomy if you had difficulty with this question.
Level of Cognitive Ability: Application
Client Needs: Health Promotion and Maintenance
Integrated Process: Nursing Process/Implementation
Content Area: Adult Health/Oncology
Reference: Phipps, W., Monahan, F., Sands, J., Marek, J. & Neighbors, M. (2003). *Medical-surgical nursing: Health and illness perspectives* (7th ed.). St. Louis: Mosby, p. 1846.

47. Answer: 1
Rationale: The incidence of bladder cancer is three times greater in men than in women and affects the white population twice as often as the black population. Options 2, 3, and 4 are associated with the incidence of bladder cancer.
Test-Taking Strategy: Use the process of elimination and note the key words, *additional teaching is needed*. Basic information regarding the risks associated with cancer will assist in eliminating options 3 and 4. From the remaining options, knowledge regarding the risk factors associated with bladder cancer will direct you to option 1. If you had difficulty with this question, review these risks.

Level of Cognitive Ability: Comprehension
Client Needs: Health Promotion and Maintenance
Integrated Process: Teaching/Learning
Content Area: Adult Health/Oncology
Reference: Lewis, S., Heitkemper, M., & Dirksen, S. (2004). *Medical-surgical nursing: Assessment and management of clinical problems* (6th ed.). St. Louis: Mosby, p. 1194.

48. Answer: 3
Rationale: The most common symptom in clients with cancer of the bladder is hematuria. The client may also experience irritative voiding symptoms such as frequency, urgency, and dysuria, and these symptoms are often associated with cancer in situ.
Test-Taking Strategy: Use the process of elimination and note the key words, *most common*. Options 1, 2, and 4 are symptoms that are associated with bladder infection. Review the clinical manifestations associated with bladder cancer if you had difficulty with this question.
Level of Cognitive Ability: Comprehension
Client Needs: Physiological Integrity
Integrated Process: Nursing Process/Data Collection
Content Area: Adult Health/Oncology
Reference: Phipps, W., Monahan, F., Sands, J., Marek, J., & Neighbors, M. (2003). *Medical-surgical nursing: Health and illness perspectives* (7th ed.). St. Louis: Mosby, p. 1226.

49. Answer: 2
Rationale: After ureterostomy, the stoma should be red and moist. A pale stoma may indicate an inadequate amount of vascular supply. A dry stoma may indicate body fluid deficit. Any sign of darkness or duskiness in the stoma may mean loss of vascular supply and must be corrected immediately or necrosis can occur.
Test-Taking Strategy: Use the process of elimination. You should easily be able to eliminate options 1 and 4. From the remaining options, note the key word, *moist*, in option 2. This should indicate that this is an expected and positive finding. If you had difficulty with this question, review expected and unexpected findings following ureterostomy.
Level of Cognitive Ability: Comprehension
Client Needs: Physiological Integrity
Integrated Process: Nursing Process/Data Collection
Content Area: Adult Health/Oncology
Reference: Linton, A., & Maebius, N. (2003). *Introduction to medical-surgical nursing* (3rd ed.). Philadelphia: W.B. Saunders, p. 363.

50. Answer: 2
Rationale: After mastectomy, the arm should be elevated above the level of the heart. Arm exercises should be encouraged. No blood pressure readings, injections, IV line insertions, or blood draws should be performed on the affected arm. Cool compresses are not a suggested measure to prevent lymphedema from occurring.
Test-Taking Strategy: Note the key words, *assist in preventing*. Use the process of elimination and note the relationship between the words lymph"edema" in the question and "elevating" in the correct option. Review these measures if you had difficulty with this question.

Level of Cognitive Ability: Application
Client Needs: Physiological Integrity
Integrated Process: Nursing Process/Implementation
Content Area: Adult Health/Oncology
Reference: Linton, A., & Maebius, N. (2003). *Introduction to medical-surgical nursing* (3rd ed.). Philadelphia: W.B. Saunders, p. 959.

ALTERNATE FORMAT QUESTION: MULTIPLE RESPONSE

Answers:
Monitoring of serum sodium blood levels
Medication that is antagonistic to antidiuretic hormone (ADH)
Radiation or chemotherapy
Rationale: Cancer is a common cause of SIADH. In SIADH, excessive amounts of water are reabsorbed by the kidney and put into the systemic circulation. The increased water causes hyponatremia (decreased serum sodium levels) and some degree of fluid retention. SIADH is managed by treating the condition and cause and usually includes fluid restriction, increased sodium intake, and medication with a mechanism of action that is antagonistic to ADH. Sodium levels are monitored closely because hypernatremia can suddenly develop as a result of treatment. The immediate institution of appropriate cancer therapy, usually either radiation or chemotherapy, can cause such tumor regression that ADH synthesis and release processes return to normal.
Test-Taking Strategy: Focusing on the client's diagnosis and recalling that, in SIADH, excessive amounts of water are reabsorbed by the kidney and put into the systemic circulation will assist in answering this question. Review the treatment for SIADH if you had difficulty with this question.
Level of Cognitive Ability: Analysis
Client Needs: Physiological Integrity
Integrated Process: Nursing Process/Planning
Content Area: Adult Health/Oncology
Reference: Ignatavicius, D., & Workman, M. (2006). *Medical surgical nursing: Critical thinking for collaborative care* (5th ed.). Philadelphia: W.B. Saunders, pp. 501-502.

REFERENCES

Black, J., & Hawks, J. (2005). *Medical-surgical nursing: Clinical management for positive outcomes* (7th ed.). Philadelphia: W.B. Saunders.

Christensen, B., & Kockrow, E. (2003). *Adult health nursing* (4th ed.). St. Louis: Mosby.

Christensen, B., & Kockrow, E. (2003). *Foundations of nursing* (4th ed.). St. Louis: Mosby.

Ignatavicius, D., & Workman, M. (2006). *Medical surgical nursing: Critical thinking for collaborative care* (5th ed.). Philadelphia: W.B. Saunders.

Lewis, S., Heitkemper, M., & Dirksen, S. (2004). *Medical-surgical nursing: Assessment and management of clinical problems* (6th ed.). St. Louis: Mosby.

Linton, A., & Maebius, N. (2003). *Introduction to medical-surgical nursing* (3rd ed.). Philadelphia: W.B. Saunders.

McKenry, L., & Salerno, E. (2003). *Mosby's pharmacology in nursing* (21st ed.). St. Louis: Mosby.

Pagana, K., & Pagana, T. (2003). *Mosby's diagnostic and laboratory test reference* (6th ed.). St. Louis: Mosby.

Phipps, W., Monahan, F., Sands, J., Marek, J., & Neighbors, M. (2003). *Medical-surgical nursing: Health and illness perspectives* (7th ed.). St. Louis: Mosby.

Potter, P., & Perry, A. (2005). *Fundamentals of nursing* (6th ed.). St. Louis: Mosby.

Thompson, J., McFarland, G., Hirsch, J., & Tucker, S. (2002). *Mosby's clinical nursing* (5th ed.). St. Louis: Mosby.

Antineoplastic Medications

I. ANTINEOPLASTIC MEDICATIONS

A. Description

1. Kill or inhibit the reproduction of neoplastic cells
2. The effect of antineoplastic medications may not be limited to neoplastic cells; normal cells are also affected by the medication
3. Cell cycle phase–specific medications affect cells only during a certain phase of the reproductive cycle
4. Cell cycle phase–nonspecific medications affect cells in any phase of the reproductive cycle
5. Usually, several medications are used in combination to increase the therapeutic response
6. Antineoplastic medications may be combined with other treatments, such as surgery and radiation
7. The routes of antineoplastic medication administration can vary; the intravenous (IV) route is the preferred route
8. Side effects result from the effects of the antineoplastic medication on normal cells

▲ B. Side effects

1. Mucositis
2. Alopecia
3. Anorexia, nausea, and vomiting
4. Diarrhea
5. Anemia
▲ 6. Low white blood cell (WBC) count (neutropenia)
▲ 7. Thrombocytopenia
8. Infertility

▲ C. Interventions

1. Physiological integrity
▲   a. Monitor complete blood count (CBC), WBC count, platelet count, and electrolytes
▲   b. Initiate bleeding precautions if thrombocytopenia occurs

c. When the platelet count is less than 50,000 cells/ μL, any small trauma can lead to episodes of prolonged bleeding; when less than 20,000 cells/ μL, spontaneous and uncontrollable bleeding can occur
▲ d. Monitor for petechiae, ecchymosis, bleeding of the gums, and nosebleeds because the decreased platelet count can precipitate bleeding tendencies
▲ e. Avoid intramuscular injections and venipunctures as much as possible to prevent bleeding
▲ f. Initiate neutropenic precautions if the WBC count decreases
g. Monitor for fever, sore throat, unusual bleeding, or signs and symptoms of infection
h. Inform the client that loss of appetite may also be due to a bitter taste in the mouth from the medications
i. Monitor for nausea and vomiting and provide a high-calorie diet with protein supplements
▲ j. Antiemetics are administered several hours before chemotherapy and for 12 to 48 hours after as prescribed because antineoplastic medications stimulate the vomiting centers
▲ k. Encourage hydration; IV fluids will be administered before and during therapy
▲ l. Promote a fluid intake of at least 2000 mL/day to maintain adequate renal function
▲ m. Administer allopurinol (Zyloprim) as prescribed to lower the serum uric acid level that occurs from the rapid destruction of cells by the antineoplastic medication

2. Safe, effective care environment
▲ a. IV chemotherapy is prepared in an air-vented space (biohazard cabinet area)
b. Gloves, a gown, eye protectors, and a mask are worn when handling IV medications

c. Nurses who are pregnant should not prepare or administer IV chemotherapy

d. IV equipment is discarded in designated (biohazard) containers

e. Antineoplastic medications are usually administered in short, high-dose, intermittent courses as prescribed to maximize antineoplastic effects while allowing normal cells to recover

f. Monitor for phlebitis with IV administration, because these medications irritate the veins

g. Monitor for extravasation (leakage of medication into surrounding skin and subcutaneous tissue), which causes tissue necrosis; notify the physician if this occurs; heat or ice is applied depending on the medication and an antidote may be injected into the site

3. Psychosocial integrity

a. Instruct the client in the potential for hair loss and that varying degrees of hair loss may occur after the first or second treatment

b. Discuss the purchase of a wig before treatment starts

c. Inform the client that new hair growth will occur several months after the final treatment

d. Instruct the client about the need for contraception, because these medications have teratogenic effects

e. Discuss the potential effects of infertility, which may be irreversible

f. Encourage pretreatment counseling

4. Health promotion and maintenance

a. Instruct the client that, if diarrhea is a problem, to avoid hot foods and high-fiber foods, which increase peristalsis

b. Instruct the client to inspect the oral mucosa for erythema and ulcers, to rinse mouth after meals, and to practice good oral hygiene

c. Instruct the client to use saline or sodium bicarbonate mouth rinses for mouth sores

d. Instruct the client in the use of antifungal medications for mouth sores if prescribed for the development of a superinfection

e. Instruct the client to avoid crowds and persons with infections and to report signs of infection such as fever, chills, or sore throat

f. Instruct individuals with colds or infections to wear a mask when visiting or to avoid visiting the client

g. Instruct the client to use a soft toothbrush and an electric razor to minimize the risk of bleeding

h. Instruct the client to avoid aspirin-containing products to minimize the risk of bleeding

i. Instruct the client to avoid alcohol to minimize the risk of toxicity

j. Instruct the client to consult the physician before receiving vaccinations

D. Anaphylactic reactions

1. Precautions

a. Obtain an allergy history

b. A test dose of the medication may be prescribed by the physician

c. Stay with the client during the administration of medication

d. Monitor vital signs

e. Have emergency equipment and medications readily available

f. An IV line is needed for the administration of emergency medications if needed

2. Signs of anaphylactic reaction

a. Dyspnea

b. Chest tightness or pain

c. Pruritus, urticaria

d. Tachycardia

e. Dizziness

f. Anxiety, agitation

g. Flushed appearance

h. Hypotension

i. Decreased sensorium

j. Cyanosis

3. Interventions for anaphylactic reaction

a. Stop medication

b. Maintain airway

c. The physician is notified

d. An IV access is maintained with 0.9% normal saline

e. Place client in supine position with legs elevated if not contraindicated

f. Monitor vital signs

g. Emergency medications may be prescribed

II. ALKYLATING MEDICATIONS (Box 43-1)

A. Description

1. Affect the synthesis of DNA by causing cross-linking of DNA to inhibit cell reproduction

2. Cell cycle phase–nonspecific medications

B. Side effects

1. Anorexia, nausea, and vomiting

2. Stomatitis

3. Skin rash

4. Pain during IV administration

5. Busulfan (Myleran) may cause hyperuricemia

6. Chlorambucil (Leukeran) and mechlorethamine HCl (Mustargen) may cause gonadal suppression and hyperuricemia

7. Cisplatin (Platinol-AQ) may cause ototoxicity, tinnitus, hypokalemia, hypocalcemia, hypomagnesemia, and nephrotoxicity (amifostine [Ethyol] may be administered before cisplatin to reduce the potential for renal toxicity)

8. Cyclophosphamide (Cytoxan) may cause alopecia, gonadal suppression, hemorrhagic cystitis, and hematuria

▲ C. Interventions
1. Monitor vital signs and temperature for signs of infection
2. Monitor CBC, WBC, platelet, uric acid, and electrolyte counts
3. The medication is withheld if the platelet count is less than 75,000 cells/μL or the WBC count is less than 4,000 cells/μL; notify the physician if blood counts are low
4. Pulmonary function test results are monitored
5. Chest radiographs and renal and liver function test results are monitored
6. The client is hydrated with IV and/or oral fluids before administering the antineoplastic medication, as prescribed
7. An antiemetic is administered 30 to 60 minutes before the antineoplastic medication, as prescribed
8. As prescribed, IV site pain is reduced by altering IV rates, diluting the medication, or warming the injection site to distend vein and increase blood flow
9. Monitor IV site for irritation and phlebitis
10. When the client is receiving cisplatin (Platinol-AQ), monitor the client for dizziness, tinnitus, hearing loss, incoordination, and numbness or tingling of extremities
11. Monitor for signs of hemorrhagic cystitis, such as hematuria or dysuria, during cyclophosphamide (Cytoxan) or ifosfamide (Ifex) therapy, and encourage the client to drink increased fluids (2 to 3 L/day)

12. Mesna (Mesnex) may be administered with ifosfamide (Ifex) to reduce the potential of ifosfamide-induced cystitis
13. Instruct the client that cyclophosphamide (Cytoxan), when prescribed orally, is administered without food
14. Instruct the client to follow a diet low in purines to alkalinize urine and lower uric acid blood levels
15. Instruct the client about how to avoid infection
16. Instruct the client to report signs of infection or bleeding
17. Instruct the client about good oral hygiene and use of a soft toothbrush

III. ANTITUMOR-ANTIBIOTIC MEDICATIONS (Box 43-2)

A. Description
1. Interfere with DNA and ribonucleic acid synthesis
2. Cell cycle phase–nonspecific medications

B. Side effects
1. Nausea and vomiting
2. Fever
3. Bone marrow depression
4. Skin rash
5. Alopecia
6. Stomatitis
7. Gonadal suppression
8. Hyperuricemia
9. Vesication (blistering of tissue at IV site) ▲
10. Plicamycin (Mithracin) affects bleeding time
11. Daunorubicin (Cerubidine) may cause congestive heart failure (CHF) and dysrhythmias
12. Doxorubicin (Adriamycin) and idarubicin ▲ (Idamycin) may cause cardiotoxicity, cardiomyopathy, and electrocardiography (ECG) changes; dexrazoxane (Zinecard) may be administered with doxorubicin to reduce cardiomyopathy
13. Pulmonary toxicity can occur with bleomycin ▲ sulfate (Blenoxane)

BOX 43-1

Alkylating Medications

NITROGEN MUSTARFDS
Chlorambucil (Leukeran)
Cyclophosphamide (Cytoxan)
Ifosfamide (Ifex)
Mechlorethamine HCl (Mustargen)
Melphalan (Alkeran)
Uracil mustard

NITROSOUREAS
Carmustine (BiCNU)
Lomustine (CeeNU)
Streptozocin (Zanosar)

OTHER ALKYLATING MEDICATIONS
Altretamine (Hexalen)
Busulfan (Myleran)
Carboplatin (Paraplatin)
Cisplatin (Platinol-AQ)
Dacarbazine (DTIC-Dome)
Thiotepa (Thioplex)

BOX 43-2

Antitumor-Antibiotic Medications

Bleomycin sulfate (Blenoxane)
Dactinomycin (Actinomycin D, Cosmegan)
Daunorubicin (Cerubidine, DaunoXome)
Doxorubicin (Adriamycin)
Idarubicin (Idamycin)
Mitomycin (Mutamycin)
Mitoxantrone (Novantrone)
Pentostatin (Nipent)
Plicamycin (Mithracin)
Valrubicin (Valstar)

C. Interventions
1. Monitor vital signs and temperature for signs of infection
2. Monitor CBC, WBC, platelets, uric acid, bleeding time, and electrolyte counts
3. The medication is withheld if the platelets are less than 75,000 cells/μL or the WBC count is less than 4,000 cells/μL; notify physician
4. Pulmonary function test results are monitored
5. Monitor for ECG changes
6. Monitor lung sounds for wheezes
7. Monitor for signs of congestive heart failure (CHF), including dyspnea, crackles, peripheral edema, and weight gain
8. Chest radiographs and renal and liver function studies are monitored
9. The client is hydrated with IV and/or oral fluids before the antineoplastic medication
10. An antiemetic is administered 30 to 60 minutes before the antineoplastic medication
11. As prescribed, IV site pain is reduced by altering IV rates, diluting the medication, or warming injection site to distend vein and increase blood flow
12. Monitor IV site for irritation, phlebitis, and vesication
13. Monitor for myocardial toxicity, dyspnea, dysrhythmias, hypotension, and weight gain when doxorubicin (Adriamycin) or idarubicin (Idamycin) is administeredd
14. Monitor pulmonary status when administering bleomycin (Blenoxane)
15. Aspirin, anticoagulants, and thrombolytic agents are avoided when plicamycin (Mithracin) is administered

IV. ANTIMETABOLITE MEDICATIONS (Box 43-3)
A. Description
1. Halt the synthesis of cell protein
2. Replace normal proteins required for DNA synthesis
3. Cell cycle phase–specific; affect the S phase

BOX 43-3

Antimetabolite Medications

Capecitabine (Xeloda)
Cladribine (Leustatin)
Cytarabine HCl (ara-C; Cytosar-U)
Floxuridine (FUDR)
Fludarabine (Fludara)
5-Fluorouracil (5-FU; Adrucil)
Hydroxyurea (Hydrea)
6-Mercaptopurine (Purinethol)
Methotrexate (Rheumatrex, Trexall)
Procarbazine HCl (Matulane)
Thioguanine

B. Side effects
1. Anorexia, nausea, and vomiting
2. Diarrhea
3. Alopecia
4. Stomatitis
5. Depression of bone marrow
6. Cytarabine HCl (ara-C, Cytosar-U) may cause alopecia, stomatitis, hyperuricemia, and hepatotoxicity
7. 5-Fluorouracil (5-FU; Adrucil) may cause alopecia, stomatitis, diarrhea, phototoxicity reactions, and cerebellar dysfunction
8. 6-Mercaptopurine (Purinethol) may cause hyperuricemia and hepatotoxicity
9. Methotrexate (Rheumatrex and Trexall) may cause alopecia, stomatitis, hyperuricemia, photosensitivity, hepatotoxicity, hematological, gastrointestinal, and skin toxicity

C. Interventions
1. Monitor vital signs and temperature for signs of infection
2. Monitor the CBC, WBC, uric acid level, and platelet count
3. The medication is withheld if the WBC count is less than 4,000 cells/μL or the platelet count is less than 75,000 cells/μL; notify the physician
4. Monitor renal function studies
5. Monitor for cerebellar dysfunction
6. Monitor for photosensitivity
7. Antiemetics are administered 30 to 60 minutes before the antineoplastic medication as prescribed
8. Monitor IV site for extravasation
9. Encourage fluid intake of 2 to 3 L/day
10. Encourage good oral hygiene
11. Instruct the client how to avoid infections and bleeding
12. When the client is receiving 5-fluorouracil (5-FU; Adrucil), monitor for signs of cerebellar dysfunction, such as dizziness, weakness, and ataxia, and monitor for stomatitis and diarrhea, which may necessitate medication discontinuation
13. When the client is receiving methotrexate (Folex) in large doses, leucovorin (folinic acid, citrovorum factor) may be prescribed to prevent fatal toxicity (known as leucovorin rescue)
14. When the client is receiving 5-fluorouracil (5-FU; Adrucil) or methotrexate (Folex), instruct the client to use sunscreen and wear protective clothing to prevent photosensitivity reactions

V. MIOTIC INHIBITORS (VINCA ALKALOIDS) (Box 43-4)
A. Description
1. Prevent mitosis causing cell death
2. Mitotic inhibitors prevent cell division
3. Cell cycle phase–specific; act on the M phase

B. Side effects
   1. Leukopenia
   2. Neurotoxicity with vincristine sulfate (Oncovin), manifested as numbness and tingling in the fingers and toes
   3. Ptosis
   4. Hoarseness
   5. Motor instability
   6. Anorexia, nausea, and vomiting
   7. Constipation
   8. Peripheral neuropathy
   9. Alopecia
  10. Stomatitis
  11. Hyperuricemia
  12. Phlebitis at IV site

C. Interventions
   1. Monitor vital signs
   2. Monitor WBC, CBC, uric acid level, and platelet counts
   3. Monitor for hoarseness
   4. Check the eyes for ptosis
   5. Monitor motor stability and initiate safety precautions as necessary

---

BOX 43-4

Miotic Inhibitors (Vinca Alkaloids)

Docetaxel (Taxotere)
Etoposide (VePesid)
Teniposide (Vumon)
Vinblastine sulfate (Velban)
Vincristine sulfate (Oncovin)
Vinorelbine (Navelbine)

---

   6. Monitor for neurotoxicity with vincristine sulfate (Oncovin), manifested as numbness and tingling in the fingers and toes

VI. HORMONAL MEDICATIONS AND ENZYMES
(Box 43-5)

A. Description
   1. Suppress the immune system and block normal hormones in hormone-sensitive tumors
   2. Change the hormonal balance and slow the growth rates of certain tumors

B. Side effects
   1. Anorexia, nausea, and vomiting
   2. Leukopenia
   3. Impaired pancreatic function with asparaginase (Elspar)
   4. Gynecomastia
   5. Breast swelling
   6. Hot flashes
   7. Weight gain
   8. Hemorrhagic cystitis, hypouricemia, and hypercholesterolemia, with mitotane (Lysodren)
   9. Hypertension
  10. Thromboembolitic disorders
  11. Edema
  12. Sex characteristic alterations
  13. Electrolyte imbalances
  14. Tamoxifen citrate (Nolvadex) may cause edema, hypercalcemia, and elevated cholesterol and triglyceride levels
  15. Tamoxifen citrate (Nolvadex) decreases the effects of estrogen
  16. Diethylstilbestrol (DES; Stilphostrol) may cause impotence and gynecomastia in men

---

BOX 43-5

Hormonal Medications and Enzymes

ESTROGENS
Diethylstilbestrol (DES; Stilphostrol)
Ethinyl estradiol (Estinyl)
Estramustine (Emcyt)

ANTIESTROGENS
Anastrozole (Arimidex)
Exemestane (Aromasin)
Letrozole (Femara)
Raloxifene (Evista)
Tamoxifen citrate (Nolvadex)
Testolactone (Teslac)
Toremifene (Fareston)

ANDROGENS
Testosterone
Fluoxymesterone (Halotestin)

ANTIANDROGENS
Bicalutamide (Casodex)
Flutamide (Eulexin)
Goserelin acetate (Zoladex)
Nilutamide (Nilandron)
Triptorelin (Trelstar)

PROGESTINS
Medroxyprogesterone (Depo-Provera)
Megestrol acetate (Megace)

OTHER HORMONAL ANTAGONISTS, ENZYMES
Aminoglutethimide (Cytadren)
Asparaginase (Elspar)
Leuprolide acetate (Lupron)
Mitotane (Lysodren)

17. Diethylstilbestrol (DES; Stilphostrol) may alter effects of insulin, oral anticoagulants, and oral hypoglycemic agents

C. Interventions
1. Monitor vital signs
2. Ask the client about the medications currently taking
3. Monitor serum calcium levels with androgens
4. Monitor for signs of alterations in sexual characteristics
5. Monitor pancreatic function with asparaginase (Elspar)
6. Encourage an oral intake of 2 to 3 L of fluids per day
7. Monitor uric acid and cholesterol levels
8. Monitor for signs of hemorrhagic cystitis

VII. IMMUNOMODULATOR AGENTS: BIOLOGICAL RESPONSE MODIFIERS (Box 43-6)

A. Description
1. Stimulate the immune system to recognize cancer cells and take action to eliminate or destroy them
2. Interleukins: Help different immune system cells recognize and destroy abnormal body cells
3. Interferons: Slow down tumor cell division, stimulate proliferation and activation of natural killer cells, and help cancer cells resume a more normal appearance and revert to their previous characteristics

B. Colony-stimulating factors (CSF): Induce more rapid bone marrow recovery after suppression by chemotherapy (Box 43-7)

BOX 43-6

Immunomodulator Agents

Aldesleukin (Proleukin, recombinant interleukin-2)
Interferon alfa-2a (Roferon-A)
Interferon alfa-2b (Intron A)
Interferon alfa-n3 (Alferon N)
Levamisole (Ergamisole)
Rituximab (Rituxan)

BOX 43-7

Colony-Stimulating Factors (CSF)

GRANULOCYTE-MACROPHAGE COLONY-STIMULATING FACTOR (GM-CSF)
Sargramostim (Leukine, Prokine)

GRANULOCYTE COLONY-STIMULATING FACTOR (G-CSF)
Filgrastim (Neupogen)

ERYTHROPOIETIN
Epoetin alfa (Epogen, Procrit)

VIII. OTHER ANTINEOPLASTIC MEDICATIONS

A. Altretamine (Hexalen): Cytotoxic agent used to treat ovarian cancer
B. Denileukin difitox (Ontak): Recombinant DNA–derived medication used to treat cutaneous T-cell lymphoma
C. Gemcitabine (Gemzar): Used to treat non–small cell lung cancer and adenocarcinoma of the pancreas
D. Irinotecan (Camptosar): Used to treat colorectal or rectal cancer
E. Paclitaxel (Taxol): Used to treat ovarian or metastatic breast cancer
F. Pegaspargase (Oncaspar): Used in combination chemotherapies for acute lymphoblastic leukemia in clients unable to take L-asparaginase
G. Topotecan (Hycamtin): Indicated for the treatment of relapsed or refractory metastatic ovarian cancer after other therapies have failed
H. Trastuzumab (Herceptin): Used in combination chemotherapy to treat breast cancer
I. Tretinoin (Vesanoid): Used to treat acute promyelocytic leukemia
J. Bexarotene (Targretin): Use to treat advanced stage cutaneous T-cell lymphoma

PRACTICE QUESTIONS

1. A client with breast cancer is being treated with cyclophosphamide (Cytoxan). The nurse plans care knowing that this medication is:
   1. Cell cycle phase–specific
   2. Cell cycle phase–nonspecific
   3. A hormonal medication
   4. An antimetabolite
2. A client with bladder cancer is receiving cisplatin (Platinol) and vincristine (Oncovin). The nurse plans care knowing that the purpose of administering both of these medications is to:
   1. Prevent gastrointestinal side effects
   2. Prevent alopecia
   3. Decrease the destruction of cells
   4. Decrease medication resistance and reduce medication toxicity
3. A nurse is instructed to initiate bleeding precautions on a client receiving an antineoplastic medication intravenously. The nurse reviews the laboratory results and would expect to note which of the following?
   1. A white blood cell (WBC) of 5000/μL
   2. A platelet count of 70,000 cells/μL
   3. A clotting time of 10 minutes
   4. An ammonia level of 20 mcg/dL
4. A nurse is caring for a client who is receiving an intravenous (IV) infusion of an antineoplastic medication. During the infusion, the client complains of pain at the insertion site. On inspection of the site, the nurse

notes redness and swelling and that the infusion of the medication has slowed in rate. The nurse takes which appropriate action?

1. Elevate the extremity of the IV site and slow the infusion
2. Apply ice and maintain the infusion rate, as prescribed
3. Administer pain medication to reduce the discomfort
4. Notify the registered nurse

5. A client with leukemia is receiving busulfan (Myleran). Allopurinol (Zyloprim) is prescribed for the client. The nurse administers the allopurinol knowing that its purpose is to prevent:
1. Gouty arthritis
2. Hyperuricemia
3. Stomatitis
4. Diarrhea

6. A nurse is reinforcing medication instructions to a client with breast cancer who will be taking cyclophosphamide (Cytoxan). Which of the following would the nurse include in the instructions?
1. Take the medication with food
2. Increase fluid intake to 2000 to 3000 mL/day
3. Decrease sodium intake while taking the medication
4. Increase potassium intake while taking the medication

7. A nurse is assigned to care for a client with non-Hodgkin's lymphoma who is receiving daunorubicin (Cerubidine). Which of the following signs would indicate to the nurse that the client is experiencing a toxic effect related to the medication?
1. Nausea and vomiting
2. Fever
3. Dyspnea
4. Diarrhea

8. A nurse assigned to care for a client with testicular cancer who is receiving plicamycin (Mithracin) is preparing to administer the prescribed daily medications to the client. The nurse would question which of the following medications if noted on the client's medication record?
1. Warfarin (Coumadin)
2. Allopurinol (Zyloprim)
3. Acetaminophen (Tylenol)
4. Ondansetron (Zofran)

9. A client with squamous cell carcinoma of the larynx is receiving bleomycin sulfate (Blenoxane) intravenously. The nurse anticipates that which diagnostic study will be prescribed for this client?
1. Pulmonary function studies
2. Electrocardiography
3. Cervical x-ray studies
4. Echocardiography

10. Cytarabine HCl (Cytosar) is prescribed for the client with acute lymphocytic leukemia. The nurse plans care knowing that this is a:
1. Cell cycle phase–nonspecific medication
2. Hormone medication
3. Cell cycle phase–specific medication
4. A medication that affects cells in any phase of the reproductive cell cycle

11. The nurse is assisting in preparing a teaching plan for the client receiving an antineoplastic medication. The nurse suggests including which of the following in the plan of care?
1. Take aspirin (acetylsalicylic acid, ASA) as needed for headache
2. Drink beverages containing alcohol in moderate amounts
3. Consult with the physician before receiving immunizations
4. Be sure to receive the flu and pneumonia vaccine

12. The client with lung cancer is receiving a high dose of methotrexate (Rheumatrex). Leucovorin (citrovorum factor, folic acid) is also prescribed. The nurse who is assisting in planning care for the client understands that the purpose of administering the leucovorin is to:
1. Preserve normal cells
2. Promote DNA synthesis
3. Promote medication excretion
4. Promote the synthesis of nucleic acids

13. The client with ovarian cancer is being treated with vincristine (Oncovin). The nurse caring for the client monitors for which side effect specific to this medication?
1. Diarrhea
2. Numbness and tingling in the fingers and toes
3. Chest pain
4. Hair loss

14. Asparaginase (Elspar), an antineoplastic agent, is prescribed for a client. The nurse assigned to care for the client collects data from the client. The nurse would report which of the following conditions contraindicated with the administration of asparaginase?
1. Myocardial infarction
2. Chronic obstructive pulmonary disease
3. Diabetes mellitus
4. Pancreatitis

15. Tamoxifen (Nolvadex) is prescribed for the client with metastatic breast carcinoma. The nurse assists in planning care knowing that the primary action of this medication is to:
1. Increase DNA and RNA synthesis
2. Compete with estradiol for binding to estrogen in tissues containing high concentrations of receptors

3. Increase estrogen concentration and estrogen response
4. Promote the biosynthesis of nucleic acids

16. The client with metastatic breast cancer is receiving tamoxifen (Nolvadex). The nurse assigned to care for the client monitors for signs of which of the following during therapy with this medication?
    1. Leukocytosis
    2. Weight loss
    3. Hypercalcemia
    4. Hypotension

17. Megestrol acetate (Megace), an antineoplastic medication, is prescribed for a client with metastatic endometrial carcinoma. The nurse assigned to the client collects data regarding the client's medical history. The nurse would report which of the following conditions that requires caution with the administration of megestrol acetate?
    1. Asthma
    2. Myocardial infarction
    3. Thrombophlebitis
    4. Gout

18. A female client with carcinoma of the breast is admitted to the hospital for treatment with intravenous vincristine (Oncovin). The client tells the nurse that she has been told by her friends that she is going to lose all her hair. The nurse makes which appropriate response to the client?
    1. "You will not lose your hair."
    2. "Your friends are correct."
    3. "Hair loss may occur, but it will grow back just as it is now."
    4. "Hair loss may occur, and it will grow back, but it may have a different color or texture."

19. A nurse is helping prepare instructions for a client who has developed stomatitis following the administration of a course of antineoplastic medications. Which of the following instructions does the nurse suggest to include in the plan of care?
    1. To rinse the mouth with diluted baking soda or saline
    2. To avoid foods and fluids for the next 24 hours
    3. To swab the mouth daily with lemon and glycerin swabs
    4. To brush the teeth and use waxed dental floss three times a day

20. A client with acute myelocytic leukemia is being treated with busulfan (Myleran). The nurse monitors for signs of which of the following that specifically occurs from the administration of this medication?
    1. Hyperglycemia
    2. Renal failure
    3. Hyperkalemia
    4. Congestive heart failure

ALTERNATE FORMAT QUESTION: MULTIPLE RESPONSE

A nurse is assisting in caring for a client with cancer who is receiving cisplatin (Platinol-AQ). Select the toxic effects associated with this medication that the nurse monitors for.

___ Ototoxicity
___ Tinnitus
___ Hyperkalemia
___ Hypercalcemia
___ Hypomagnesemia
___ Nephrotoxicity

ANSWERS

1. *Answer:* **2**
Rationale: Cyclophosphamide is an antineoplastic medication of the alkalating classification. Medications in this classification are cell cycle–phase nonspecific and affect all phases of the reproductive cell cycle. Cell phase–specific medications affect cells only during a certain phase of the reproductive cycle.
Test-Taking Strategy: Knowledge regarding the classification of this medication and the specific action of alkalating agents is needed to answer the question. Remember, alkalating agents are cell cycle phase–nonspecific and affect all phases of the reproductive cell cycle. If you had difficulty with this question, review the action of alkalating medications.
Level of Cognitive Ability: Analysis
Client Needs: Physiological Integrity
Integrated Process: Nursing Process/Planning

Content Area: Pharmacology
Reference: Lilley, L., Harrington, S., & Snyder, J. (2005). *Pharmacology and the nursing process* (4th ed.). St. Louis: Mosby, p. 778.

2. *Answer:* **4**
Rationale: Cisplatin is an alkalating medication and vincristine is a vinca alkaloid. Alkalating medications are cell cycle phase–nonspecific. Vinca alkaloids are cell cycle phase–specific. Combinations of medications are used to enhance tumoricidal effects. Use of combination medications decrease medication resistance, increase destruction of cancer cells, and reduce medication toxicity.
Test-Taking Strategy: Use the process of elimination. Eliminate options 1 and 2 first; it may be possible, with some specific interventions, to reduce gastrointestinal effects and alopecia, but it is unlikely that these occurrences can be prevented.

From the remaining options, recall that the use of combination medications decreases medication resistance, increases destruction of cancer cells, and reduces medication toxicity. Review the purpose of combination therapy if you had difficulty with this question.
Level of Cognitive Ability: Analysis
Client Needs: Physiological Integrity
Integrated Process: Nursing Process/Planning
Content Area: Pharmacology
References: McKenry, L., & Salerno, E. (2001). *Mosby's pharmacology in nursing* (21st ed.) St. Louis: Mosby. p. 931. (2005). *Mosby's 2005 drug consult for nurses.* St. Louis: Mosby, p. 269.

3. *Answer:* **2**
Rationale: Bleeding precautions need to be initiated when the platelet count drops. Bleeding precautions include avoiding all trauma, such as rectal temperatures or injections. The normal platelet count is 150,000 to 450,000 cells/μL. The normal WBC is 5000 to 10,000/μL. When the WBC count drops, neutropenic precautions need to be implemented. The normal clotting time is 8 to 15 minutes. The normal ammonia value is 15 to 45 mcg/dL.
Test-Taking Strategy: Use the process of elimination and knowledge regarding normal laboratory values. Options 1, 3, and 4 identify normal laboratory values. Remember, correlate a low platelet count with the need for bleeding precautions, and a low WBC count with the need for neutropenic precaution. Review these normal laboratory values if you had difficulty with this question.
Level of Cognitive Ability: Analysis
Client Needs: Safe, Effective Care Environment
Integrated Process: Nursing Process/Data Collection
Content Area: Pharmacology
Reference: Lilley, L., Harrington, S., & Snyder, J. (2005). *Pharmacology and the nursing process* (4th ed.). St. Louis: Mosby, p. 801.

4. *Answer:* **4**
Rationale: When antineoplastic medications are administered IV, great care must be taken to prevent the medication from escaping into the tissues surrounding the injection site, because pain, tissue damage, and necrosis can result. The nurse monitors for signs of extravasation, such as redness or swelling at the insertion site and a decreased infusion rate. If extravasation occurs, the registered nurse needs to be notified who will then contact the physician.
Test-Taking Strategy: Use the process of elimination and focus on the data in the question. Eliminate option 1 and 2 first. The nurse would not slow the IV rate, and the nurse would not be able to maintain the prescribed rate in this situation. Administering pain medication to reduce discomfort at an IV site is not an appropriate action. Further investigation of the cause of the discomfort is required. This leaves option 4 as the correct nursing action. Review care of the client receiving IV chemotherapy if you had difficulty with this question.
Level of Cognitive Ability: Application
Client Needs: Physiological Integrity
Integrated Process: Nursing Process/Implementation
Content Area: Pharmacology

Reference: Lilley, L., Harrington, S., & Snyder, J. (2005). *Pharmacology and the nursing process* (4th ed.). St. Louis: Mosby, p. 803.

5. *Answer:* **2**
Rationale: Busulfan is as alkalating medication used in the treatment of acute myelocytic leukemia and in the palliative treatment of chronic myelogenous leukemia. Hyperuricemia can result from the use of this medication because it may produce uric acid nephropathy, renal stones, and acute renal failure. Allopurinol, an antigout medication, is used with chemotherapy to prevent or treat hyperuricemia. It may be prescribed for use in mouthwash following fluorouracil (Adrucil) therapy to prevent stomatitis. Allopurinol is not used to prevent diarrhea.
Test-Taking Strategy: Knowledge regarding the side effects associated with busulfan and the purpose of administering allopurinol during the administration of an antineoplastic medication is needed to answer this question. Recalling that allopurinol is an antigout medication will direct you to the correct option. Review both of these medications if you had difficulty with this question.
Level of Cognitive Ability: Application
Client Needs: Physiological Integrity
Integrated Process: Nursing Process/Implementation
Content Area: Pharmacology
Reference: Hodgson, B., & Kizior, R. (2005). *Saunders nursing drug handbook 2005.* Philadelphia: W.B. Saunders, p. 30.

6. *Answer:* **2**
Rationale: Hemorrhagic cystitis is a toxic effect that can occur with the use of cyclophosphamide. The client needs to be instructed to drink copious amounts of fluid during the administration of this medication. Clients should also monitor urine output for hematuria. The medication should be taken on an empty stomach, unless gastrointestinal upset occurs. Hyperkalemia can result from the use of the medication; therefore, the client would not be encouraged to increase potassium intake. The client would not be instructed to alter his or her sodium intake.
Test-Taking Strategy: Use the process of elimination. If you correlated cyclophosphamide with hemorrhagic cystitis, then, by the process of elimination, option 2 would be selected. If you had difficulty with this question, review the toxic effects associated with this medication.
Level of Cognitive Ability: Analysis
Client Needs: Health Promotion and Maintenance
Integrated Process: Teaching/Learning
Content Area: Pharmacology
Reference: Hodgson, B., & Kizior, R. (2005). *Saunders nursing drug handbook 2005.* Philadelphia: W.B. Saunders, p. 272.

7. *Answer:* **3**
Rationale: Cardiotoxicity and/or cardiomyopathy manifested as congestive heart failure (CHF) is a toxic effect of daunorubicin. Bone marrow depression is also a toxic effect. Nausea and vomiting is a frequent side effect associated with the medication that begins a few hours after administration and lasts 24 to 48 hours. Fever is a frequent side effect and diarrhea can occur occasionally.

Test-Taking Strategy: Use the process of elimination, keeping in mind that the question is asking for a toxic effect. This concept should direct you to the option of addressing a sign of CHF. Additionally, the correct option presents the most serious concern. If you had difficulty with this question, review the toxic effects associated with daunorubicin.
Level of Cognitive Ability: Analysis
Client Needs: Physiological Integrity
Integrated Process: Nursing Process/Data Collection
Content Area: Pharmacology
Reference: Hodgson, B., & Kizior, R. (2005). *Saunders nursing drug handbook 2005.* Philadelphia: W.B. Saunders, p. 291.

8. Answer: 1
Rationale: Plicamycin is an antitumor-antibiotic agent. Because plicamycin affects bleeding time, the use of aspirin, anticoagulants, and thrombolytic agents should be avoided. Warfarin is an anticoagulant and the risk of hemorrhage is increased if it is administered during plicamycin therapy. Allopurinol, an antigout medication, may be used with chemotherapy to prevent or treat hyperuricemia secondary to blood dyscrasias caused by cancer chemotherapy. Acetaminophen may be used to treat mild discomfort. Ondansetron is an antiemetic used to prevent or treat nausea and vomiting during chemotherapy.
Test-Taking Strategy: Knowledge regarding the classifications of the medications identified in the options is needed to answer the question. Remember, plicamycin affects the bleeding time. If you are unfamiliar with plicamycin or the medications identified in the options, review these medications and purposes for use.
Level of Cognitive Ability: Analysis
Client Needs: Physiological Integrity
Integrated Process: Nursing Process/Implementation
Content Area: Pharmacology
Reference: Hodgson, B., & Kizior, R. (2005). *Saunders nursing drug handbook 2005.* Philadelphia: W.B. Saunders, p. 868.

9. Answer: 1
Rationale: Bleomycin sulfate is an antineoplastic medication that can cause interstitial pneumonitis that can progress to pulmonary fibrosis. Pulmonary function studies, along with hematologic, hepatic, and renal function tests, need to be monitored. The nurse needs to monitor for dyspnea, which may indicate pulmonary toxicity. The medication will be discontinued immediately if pulmonary toxicity occurs.
Test-Taking Strategy: Use the process of elimination. Eliminate options 2 and 4 first because they are both cardiac-related and therefore similar. From the remaining options, select option 1 because it relates to airway. If you had difficulty with this question, review the toxic effects of this medication.
Level of Cognitive Ability: Analysis
Client Needs: Physiological Integrity
Integrated Process: Nursing Process/Planning
Content Area: Pharmacology
References: Hodgson, B., & Kizior, R. (2005). *Saunders nursing drug handbook 2005.* Philadelphia: W.B. Saunders, p. 131. Lilley, L., Harrington, S., & Snyder, J. (2005). *Pharmacology and the nursing process* (4th ed.). St. Louis: Mosby, p. 801.

10. Answer: 3
Rationale: Cytarabine is an antimetabolite. Antimetabolites are classified as cell cycle phase–specific. Alkalating medications affect all phases of the cell reproductive cycle. Hormone medications suppress the immune system and block normal hormones in hormone-sensitive tumors.
Test-Taking Strategy: Use the process of elimination. Eliminate options 1 and 4 first because they are similar. From the remaining options, recalling that this medication is an antimetabolite will direct you to the correct option. Review the action of this medication if you had difficulty with this question.
Level of Cognitive Ability: Application
Client Needs: Physiological Integrity
Integrated Process: Nursing Process/Planning
Content Area: Pharmacology
Reference: Hodgson, B., & Kizior, R. (2005). *Saunders nursing drug handbook 2005.* Philadelphia: W.B. Saunders, p. 276.

11. Answer: 3
Rationale: Because antineoplastic medications lower the body's resistance, clients must be informed not to receive immunizations or vaccines without a physician's approval. Aspirin and aspirin-containing products need to be avoided to minimize the risk of bleeding. Alcohol needs to be avoided to minimize the risk of toxicity.
Test-Taking Strategy: Use general guidelines related to medication administration. Also, remembering that antineoplastic medications lower the body's resistance will direct you to option 3. Review client teaching points regarding these medications if you had difficulty with this question.
Level of Cognitive Ability: Application
Client Needs: Health Promotion and Maintenance
Integrated Process: Nursing Process/Planning
Content Area: Pharmacology
Reference: Lilley, L., Harrington, S., & Snyder, J. (2005). *Pharmacology and the nursing process* (4th ed.). St. Louis: Mosby, p. 805.

12. Answer: 1
Rationale: High concentrations of methotrexate damage normal cells. To save normal cells, leucovorin is given, which is known as leucovorin rescue. Options 2, 3, and 4 do not identify the purpose for administering leucovorin.
Test-Taking Strategy: Use the process of elimination. Eliminate options 2 and 4 first because they are similar. Nucleic acids include RNA and DNA. Next, eliminate option 3 because increased fluids and diuretics are usually administered to promote medication excretion. If you had difficulty with this question, review leucovorin rescue.
Level of Cognitive Ability: Comprehension
Client Needs: Physiological Integrity
Integrated Process: Nursing Process/Planning
Content Area: Pharmacology
Reference: Hodgson, B., & Kizior, R. (2005). *Saunders nursing drug handbook 2005.* Philadelphia: W.B. Saunders, p. 623.

13. Answer: 2
Rationale: A side effect specific of vincristine is peripheral neuropathy, which occurs in nearly every client. This can be manifested as numbness and tingling in the fingers and toes.

Constipation rather than diarrhea is most likely to occur with this medication, although diarrhea may occur occasionally. Hair loss occurs with nearly all of the antineoplastic medications. Chest pain is unrelated to this medication.
Test-Taking Strategy: Use the process of elimination. Eliminate options 1 and 4 first because these side effects are associated with many of the antineoplastic agents. Next, note that the question asks for the side effect "specific" to this medication. Correlate peripheral neuropathy with vincristine. Review the side effects of vincristine if you had difficulty with this question.
Level of Cognitive Ability: Application
Client Needs: Physiological Integrity
Integrated Process: Nursing Process/Data Collection
Content Area: Pharmacology
Reference: Hodgson, B., & Kizior, R. (2005). *Saunders nursing drug handbook 2005.* Philadelphia: W.B. Saunders, p. 1111.

14. *Answer:* 4
Rationale: Asparaginase is contraindicated if hypersensitivity exists, in pancreatitis, or if the client has a history of pancreatitis. The medication impairs pancreatic function, and pancreatic function tests should be performed before therapy begins and when a week or more has elapsed between the administration of the doses. The client needs to be monitored for signs of pancreatitis, which include nausea, vomiting, and abdominal pain.
Test-Taking Strategy: Knowledge regarding the contraindications associated with asparaginase is required to answer this question. Remember, asparaginase is contraindicated if hypersensitivity exists, in pancreatitis, or if the client has a history of pancreatitis. Review this medication if you had difficulty answering this question.
Level of Cognitive Ability: Application
Client Needs: Physiological Integrity
Integrated Process: Nursing Process/Implementation
Content Area: Pharmacology
Reference: Hodgson, B. & Kizior, R. (2005). *Saunders nursing drug handbook 2005.* Philadelphia: W.B. Saunders, p. 84.

15. *Answer:* 2
Rationale: Tamoxifen is an antineoplastic medication that competes with estradiol for binding to estrogen in tissues containing high concentrations of receptors. It is used in the treatment of metastatic breast carcinoma in women and men. It is also effective in delaying the recurrence of cancer following mastectomy. It reduces DNA synthesis and estrogen response.
Test-Taking Strategy: Use the process of elimination. Eliminate options 1 and 4 first because they are similar. Nucleic acids include DNA and RNA. From this point, select option 2, because it is unlikely that treatment of metastatic breast carcinoma would focus on increasing estrogen concentration and estrogen response. If you had difficulty with this question, review the action of this medication.
Level of Cognitive Ability: Application
Client Needs: Physiological Integrity
Integrated Process: Nursing Process/Planning
Content Area: Pharmacology
Reference: Hodgson, B., & Kizior, R. (2005). *Saunders nursing drug handbook 2005.* Philadelphia: W.B. Saunders, p. 1005.

16. *Answer:* 3
Rationale: Tamoxifen may increase calcium, cholesterol, and triglyceride levels. The nurse should monitor for hypercalcemia while the client is taking this medication. Signs of hypercalcemia include increased urine volume, excessive thirst, nausea, vomiting, constipation, hypotonicity of muscles, and deep bone or flank pain. Leukopenia, weight gain, and hypertension are most likely to occur.
Test-Taking Strategy: Knowledge regarding the side effects associated with this medication is required to answer this question. Remember, tamoxifen may increase calcium, cholesterol, and triglyceride levels. Review this medication if you had difficulty answering this question.
Level of Cognitive Ability: Analysis
Client Needs: Physiological Integrity
Integrated Process: Nursing Process/Data Collection
Content Area: Pharmacology
Reference: Hodgson, B., & Kizior, R. (2005). *Saunders nursing drug handbook 2005.* Philadelphia: W.B. Saunders, p. 1006.

17. *Answer:* 3
Rationale: Megestrol acetate suppresses the release of luteinizing hormone from the anterior pituitary by inhibiting pituitary function and regressing tumor size. It is used with caution if the client has a history of thrombophlebitis.
Test-Taking Strategy: Knowledge regarding the cautions associated with the administration of this medication is needed to answer this question. Remember, megestrol acetate is used with caution if the client has a history of thrombophlebitis. Review this medication if you had difficulty answering this question.
Level of Cognitive Ability: Application
Client Needs: Physiological Integrity
Integrated Process: Nursing Process/Implementation
Content Area: Pharmacology
Reference: Hodgson, B., & Kizior, R. (2005). *Saunders nursing drug handbook 2005.* Philadelphia: W.B. Saunders, p. 667.

18. *Answer:* 4
Rationale: Alopecia, hair loss, can occur following the administration of many antineoplastic medications. Alopecia is reversible, but new hair growth may have a different color and texture.
Test-Taking Strategy: Use knowledge regarding the side effects of antineoplastic medications and therapeutic communication techniques to answer this question. Option 1 is incorrect and option 2 is a nontherapeutic response. Recalling that new hair growth may have a different color and texture will assist in directing you to option 4. Review content related to hair loss and antineoplastic medications if you had difficulty with this question.
Level of Cognitive Ability: Application
Client Needs: Psychosocial Integrity
Integrated Process: Caring
Content Area: Pharmacology
Reference: Hodgson, B., & Kizior, R. (2005). *Saunders nursing drug handbook 2005.* Philadelphia: W.B. Saunders, p. 1111.

19. *Answer:* 1
Rationale: Stomatitis, ulceration in the mouth, can occur as a result of the administration of antineoplastic medications.

The client should be instructed to examine the mouth daily and to report any signs of ulceration. If stomatitis occurs, the client should be instructed to rinse the mouth with diluted baking soda or saline. Food and fluid is important and should not be restricted. The client should avoid toothbrushing and flossing when stomatitis is severe. Lemon and glycerin swabs may cause pain and further irritation.

Test-Taking Strategy: Use the process of elimination. Recalling that stomatitis involves ulcerations in the mucous membranes of the mouth will assist in eliminating the incorrect options. Eliminate option 2 first, because foods and fluids would not be restricted in a client who received antineoplastic medication. Eliminate option 3, because lemon can be irritating to ulcerated lesions. Eliminate option 4, because a toothbrush and floss will also irritate ulcerations and may cause bleeding. If you had difficulty with this question, review the client teaching points related to stomatitis.
Level of Cognitive Ability: Application
Client Needs: Physiological Integrity
Integrated Process: Nursing Process/Planning
Content Area: Pharmacology
Reference: Christensen, B., & Kockrow, E. (2003). *Adult health nursing* (4th ed.). St. Louis: Mosby, p. 726.

20. *Answer:* 2
Rationale: Busulfan can cause an increase in the uric acid level. Hyperuricemia can produce uric acid nephropathy, renal stones, and acute renal failure. Options 1, 3, and 4 are unrelated to the administration of this medication.
Test-Taking Strategy: Knowledge regarding the adverse effects of this medication is needed to answer this question. Remember, busulfan can cause an increase in the uric acid level. If you had difficulty with this question, review the effects of busulfan.
Level of Cognitive Ability: Application

Client Needs: Physiological Integrity
Integrated Process: Nursing Process/Data Collection
Content Area: Pharmacology
Reference: Hodgson, B., & Kizior, R. (2005). *Saunders nursing drug handbook 2005.* Philadelphia: W.B. Saunders, p. 148.

ALTERNATE FORMAT QUESTION: MULTIPLE RESPONSE

Answers:
Ototoxicity
Tinnitus
Hypomagnesemia
Nephrotoxicity
Rationale: Cisplatin (Platinol-AQ) is an alkalating medication. Alkalating medications are cell cycle phase–nonspecific medications that affect the synthesis of DNA by causing cross-linking of DNA to inhibit cell reproduction. Cisplatin may cause ototoxicity, tinnitus, hypokalemia, hypocalcemia, hypomagnesemia, and nephrotoxicity. Amifostine (Ethyol) may be administered before cisplatin to reduce the potential for renal toxicity.
Teat-Taking Strategy: Note that the medication is an antineoplastic medication. Recall that most antineoplastic medications affect the bone marrow and hematological system. This concept will assist in determining that "hypo" rather than "hyper" conditions would occur. Also, recall that this medication affects the ear (ototoxicity and tinnitus) and the kidneys (nephrotoxicity). Review the toxic effects of this medication if you had difficulty with this question.
Level of Cognitive Ability: Analysis
Client Needs: Physiological Integrity
Integrated Process: Nursing Process/Data Collection
Content Area: Pharmacology
Reference: Mosby's 2005 drug consult for nurses. (2005). St. Louis: Mosby, p. 268.

REFERENCES

Christensen, B., & Kockrow, E. (2003). *Foundations of nursing* (4th ed.). St. Louis: Mosby.

Hodgson, B., & Kizior, R. (2005). *Saunders nursing drug handbook 2005.* Philadelphia:W.B. Saunders.

Lilley, L., Harrington, S., & Snyder, J. (2005). *Pharmacology and the nursing process* (4th ed.). St. Louis: Mosby.

McKenry, L., & Salerno, E. (2001). *Mosby's pharmacology in nursing* (21st ed.). St. Louis: Mosby. p. 931.

Mosby's 2005 drug consult for nurses. (2005). St. Louis: Mosby.

The Adult Client with an Endocrine Disorder

PYRAMID TERMS

addisonian crisis A life-threatening disorder caused by adrenal hormone insufficiency. It is precipitated by infection, trauma, stress, or surgery. Death can occur from shock, vascular collapse, or hyperkalemia.

Addison's disease Hyposecretion of adrenal cortex hormones (glucocorticoids and mineralocorticoids) from the adrenal gland, resulting in deficiency of the steroid hormones. The condition is fatal if left untreated.

adrenalectomy The surgical removal of an adrenal gland. Lifelong replacement of glucocorticoids and mineralocorticoids is necessary with a bilateral adrenalectomy. Temporary replacement may be necessary for up to 2 years for a unilateral adrenalectomy.

Chvostek's sign A spasm of the facial muscles elicited by tapping the facial nerve just anterior to the ear. It is noted in hypocalcemia.

Cushing's syndrome A condition resulting from the hypersecretion of glucocorticoids from the adrenal cortex.

dawn phenomenon Results from a nocturnal release of growth hormone, which may cause blood glucose level elevations before breakfast. Treatment includes administering an evening dose of intermediate-acting insulin at 10 PM.

diabetes insipidus The hyposecretion of antidiuretic hormone (ADH) from the posterior pituitary gland, which results in failure of tubular reabsorption of water in the kidneys.

diabetes mellitus A chronic disorder of glucose intolerance and impaired carbohydrate, protein, and lipid metabolism caused by a deficiency of insulin or resistance to the action of insulin. A deficiency of effective insulin results in hyperglycemia.

diabetic ketoacidosis (DKA) A life-threatening complication of diabetes mellitus that develops when a severe insulin deficiency occurs. Hyperglycemia progresses to ketoacidosis over a period of several hours to several days. It occurs in clients with type 1 diabetes mellitus, undiagnosed diabetics, and persons who stop prescribed treatment for diabetes.

hyperglycemia Elevated blood glucose level.

hyperglycemic hyperosmolar nonketotic syndrome (HHNS) Extreme hyperglycemia without acidosis. It is a complication of type 2 diabetes mellitus, which may result in dehydration or vascular collapse. Onset is usually slow, taking from hours to days.

hyperthyroidism A condition that occurs as a result of excessive thyroid hormone secretion.

hypoglycemia Low blood glucose level (below 60 mg/dL), which results from too much insulin, not enough food, or excess activity.

hypophysectomy Removal of the pituitary gland.

insulin waning A progressive rise in the blood glucose level from bedtime to morning. Treatment includes increasing the evening (predinner or bedtime) dose of intermediate- or long-acting insulin, or instituting a dose of insulin before the evening meal if one has not already been prescribed.

myxedema (hypothyroidism) A hypothyroid state resulting from a hyposecretion of thyroid hormone. The condition occurs in adulthood.

myxedema coma A rare but serious disorder that results from persistently low thyroid production. It can be precipitated by acute illness, rapid withdrawal of thyroid medication, anesthesia and surgery, hypothermia, and the use of sedatives and narcotics.

Somogyi's phenomenon A rebound phenomenon that occurs in clients with type 1 diabetes mellitus. Normal or elevated blood glucose levels are present at bedtime; hypoglycemia occurs at about 2 to 3 AM. Counterregulatory hormones, produced to prevent further hypoglycemia, result in hyperglycemia (evident in the prebreakfast blood glucose level). Treatment includes decreasing the evening (predinner or bedtime) dose of intermediate-acting insulin or increasing the bedtime snack.

thyroid storm An acute, potentially fatal exacerbation of hyperthyroidism. It may result from manipulation of the thyroid gland during surgery, severe infection, or stress.

thyroidectomy Surgical removal of the thyroid gland to treat persistent hyperthyroidism or thyroid tumors.

Trousseau's sign A sign of hypocalcemia. Carpal spasm can be elicited by compressing the brachial artery with a blood pressure cuff for 3 minutes.

PYRAMID TO SUCCESS

The endocrine system is made up of organs or glands that secrete hormones and release them directly into the circulation. The endocrine system can be easily understood if you remember that basically one of two situations can occur: hypersecretion or hyposecretion of hormones from the organ or gland. When an excess of the hormone occurs, treatment is aimed at blocking the hormone release through medication or surgery. When a deficit of the hormone exists, treatment is aimed at replacement therapy. Pyramid points focus on diabetes mellitus, including the prevention and treatment of complications, insulin therapy, hypoglycemic and hyperglycemic reactions, and diabetic ketoacidosis; Addison's disease and addisonian crisis; Cushing's syndrome; thyroid disorders and thyroid storm; and care of the client after thyroidectomy or adrenalectomy. The Integrated Processes addressed in this unit include Caring, Clinical Problem-Solving Process (Nursing Process), Communication and Documentation, and Teaching/Learning.

▲ CLIENT NEEDS
Safe, Effective Care Environment

Accident prevention
Advocacy
Confidentiality
Consultation
Establishing priorities
Handling hazardous and infectious materials
Informed consent
Medical and surgical asepsis

Health Promotion and Maintenance

Disease prevention
Expected body image changes
Health screening
Lifestyle choices
Principles of teaching and learning
Self-care
Techniques of data collection

Psychosocial Integrity

Coping mechanisms
Grief and loss

Sensory and perceptual alterations
Situational role changes
Support systems
Unexpected body image changes

Physiological Integrity

Alterations in body systems
Diagnostic tests
Elimination
Expected outcomes and effects of medication administration
Fluid and electrolyte imbalances
Identifying potential complications
Laboratory values
Nonpharmacological comfort interventions
Nutrition and oral hydration
Potential for complications of diagnostic tests, treatments, and procedures
Unexpected response to therapies

REFERENCES

Black, J., & Hawks, J. (2005). *Medical-surgical nursing: Clinical management for positive outcomes* (7th ed.). Philadelphia: W.B. Saunders.
Chernecky, C., & Berger, B. (2004). *Laboratory tests and diagnostic procedures* (4th ed.). Philadelphia: W.B. Saunders.
Christensen, B., & Kockrow, E. (2003). *Foundations of nursing* (4th ed.). St. Louis: Mosby.
deWit, S. (2005). *Fundamental concepts and skills for nursing* (2nd ed.). Philadelphia: W.B. Saunders.
Jarvis, C. (2004). *Physical examination and health assessment* (4th ed.). Philadelphia: W.B. Saunders, pp. 542-543.
Lewis, S., Heitkemper, M., & Dirksen, S. (2004). *Medical-surgical nursing: Assessment and management of clinical problems* (6th ed.). St. Louis: Mosby.
Linton, A. & Maebius, N. (2003). *Introduction to medical-surgical nursing* (3rd ed.). Philadelphia: W.B. Saunders.
National Council of State Boards of Nursing. (2005). *Detailed test plan for the National Council licensure examination for practical/vocational nurses.* Chicago: Author.
Pagana, K., & Pagana, T. (2003). *Mosby's diagnostic and laboratory test reference* (6th ed.). St. Louis: Mosby.
Phipps, W., Monahan, F., Sands, J., Marek, J., & Neighbors, M. (2003). *Medical-surgical nursing: Health and illness perspectives* (7th ed.). St. Louis: Mosby.
Stuart, G., & Laraia, M. (2005). *Principles and practice of psychiatric nursing* (8th ed.). St. Louis: Mosby.
Thompson, J., McFarland, G., Hirsch, J., & Tucker, S. (2002). *Mosby's clinical nursing* (5th ed.). St. Louis: Mosby.

Endocrine System

I. ANATOMY AND PHYSIOLOGY OF ENDOCRINE GLANDS (Box 44-1)

A. Functions (Box 44-2)
1. Maintenance and regulation of vital functions
2. Response to stress and injury
3. Growth and development
4. Energy metabolism
5. Reproduction
6. Fluid, electrolyte, and acid-base balance

B. Pituitary gland (Box 44-3)
1. The master gland
2. Located at the base of the brain
3. Influenced by the hypothalamus

4. Directly affects the function of the other endocrine glands
5. Promotes growth of body tissue
6. Influences water absorption by the kidney
7. Controls sexual development and function

C. Adrenal gland
1. One on top of each kidney
2. Regulates sodium and electrolyte balance
3. Affects carbohydrate, fat, and protein metabolism
4. Influences the development of sexual characteristics
5. Sustains the "flight-or-fight" response
6. Adrenal cortex
   a. The outer shell of the adrenal gland
   b. Synthesizes glucocorticoids and mineralocorticoids; secretes small amounts of sex hormones (androgens, estrogens) (Box 44-4)
7. Adrenal medulla
   a. The inner core of the adrenal gland

BOX 44-1

Endocrine Glands

Pituitary
Adrenal
Thyroid
Parathyroid
Pancreas
Ovaries
Testes

BOX 44-2

Risk Factors for Endocrine Disorders

Hereditary
Congenital
Trauma
Environmental
Secondary to other disorders

BOX 44-3

Pituitary Gland Hormones

ANTERIOR LOBE PRODUCTION
ACTH (adrenocorticotropic hormone)
TSH (thyroid-stimulating hormone)
STH (somatotropic growth-stimulating hormone)
FSH (follicle-stimulating hormone)
LH (luteinizing hormone)
PRL (prolactin)
GH (growth hormone)
MSH (melanocyte-stimulating hormone)

POSTERIOR LOBE PRODUCTION
ADH (vasopressin, antidiuretic hormone)
Oxytocin

BOX 44-4

Adrenal Cortex

GLUCOCORTICOIDS: CORTISOL, CORTISONE, CORTICOSTERONE
Responsible for glucose metabolism, protein metabolism, fluid and electrolyte balance, suppression of the inflammatory response to injury, protective immune response to invasion by infectious agents, and resistance to stress

MINERALOCORTICOIDS: ALDOSTERONE
Regulates electrolyte balance by promoting sodium retention and potassium excretion

---

    b. Works as part of the sympathetic nervous system
    c. Produces epinephrine and norepinephrine
D. Thyroid gland
  1. Located in the anterior part of the neck
  2. Controls the rate of body metabolism and growth
  3. Produces thyroxine (T_4), triiodothyronine (T_3), and thyrocalcitonin
E. Parathyroid glands
  1. Located on the thyroid gland
  2. Controls calcium and phosphorus metabolism
  3. Produce parathyroid hormone (PTH)
F. Pancreas
  1. Located posterior to the stomach
  2. Influences carbohydrate metabolism
  3. Indirectly influences fat and protein metabolism
  4. Produces insulin and glucagon
G. Ovaries and testes
  1. Ovaries
    a. Located in the pelvic cavity
    b. Produce estrogen and progesterone
  2. Testes
    a. Located in the scrotum
    b. Control the development of the secondary sex characteristics
    c. Produce testosterone

II. DIAGNOSTIC TESTS

A. Stimulation and suppression tests
  1. Stimulation testing
    a. In the client with suspected underactivity of an endocrine gland, a stimulus may be provided to determine whether the gland is capable of normal hormone production
    b. Measured amounts of selected hormones or substances are administered to stimulate the target gland to produce its hormone.
    c. Hormone levels produced by the target gland are measured
    d. Failure of the hormone level to increase with stimulation indicates hypofunction

  2. Suppression tests
    a. Used when hormone levels are high or in the upper range of normal
    b. Failure of hormone production to be suppressed during standardized testing indicates hyperfunction
B. Radioactive iodine (RAI) uptake
  1. A thyroid function test that measures the absorption of the iodine isotope to determine how the thyroid gland is functioning.
  2. A small dose of radioactive iodine is given by mouth or intravenously; the amount of radioactivity is measured in 2 to 4 hours and again at 24 hours
  3. Normal values are 3% to 10% at 2 to 4 hours and 5% to 30% at 24 hours
  4. Elevated values are indicative of **hyperthyroidism**, decreased iodine intake, or increased iodine excretion
  5. Decreased values indicate a low T_4 level, the use of antithyroid medications, thyroiditis, **myxedema**, or **hypothyroidism**
  6. Test is contraindicated in pregnancy
C. T_3 and T_4 resin uptake tests
  1. Blood tests for the diagnosis of thyroid disorders
  2. T_3 and T_4 regulate thyroid-stimulating hormone
  3. Normal values (normal findings vary among laboratories)
    a. T_3: 80 to 230 ng/dL
    b. T_4: 5.0 to 12.0 mcg/dL
    c. Thyroxine, free (FT4): 0.8 to 2.4 ng/dL
  4. T_3 level is elevated in **hyperthyroidism**, decreases with the aging process, and may be decreased in **hypothyroidism**
  5. T_4 level is elevated in **hyperthyroidism** and decreased in **hypothyroidism**
D. Thyroid-stimulating hormone (TSH)
  1. Blood test used to differentiate the diagnosis of primary **hypothyroidism**
  2. Normal value: 0.2 to 5.4 microunits/mL (normal findings vary among laboratories)
  3. Elevated values indicate primary **hypothyroidism**
  4. Decreased values indicate **hyperthyroidism** or secondary **hypothyroidism**
E. Thyroid scan
  1. Performed to identify nodules or growths in the thyroid gland
  2. A radioisotope of iodine or technetium is administered prior to the scanning of the thyroid gland
  3. Reassure the client that the level of radioactive medication is not dangerous to self or others
  4. Determine whether the client has received radiographic contrast agents within the past 3 months, because these may invalidate scan
  5. Check with physician regarding the need to discontinue medications containing iodine for

14 days prior to the test and the need to discontinue thyroid medication 4 to 6 weeks before the test

6. Instruct the client to maintain an NPO status after midnight on the day before the test; if iodine is used, the client will fast for an additional 45 minutes after ingestion of the oral isotope and the scan will be performed in 24 hours

7. If technetium is used, it is administered by the intravenous (IV) route 30 minutes before the scan

F. Needle aspiration of thyroid tissue
1. Aspiration of thyroid tissue for cytological examination
2. No client preparation is necessary
3. Light pressure is applied to the aspiration site after the procedure

G. Glucose tolerance test (GTT)
1. Aids in the diagnosis of **diabetes mellitus**
2. If the glucose levels peak at higher than normal at 1 and 2 hours after injection or ingestion of glucose, and are slower than normal to return to fasting levels, then **diabetes mellitus** is confirmed
3. Client preparation (Box 44-5)

H. Glycosylated hemoglobin
1. Description
   a. Glycosylated hemoglobin is blood glucose bound to hemoglobin
   b. HbA_{1c} (glycosylated hemoglobin A) is a reflection of how well blood glucose levels have been controlled for at least the prior 3 to 4 months
   c. **Hyperglycemia** in a client with **diabetes mellitus** is usually a cause of an increase in HbA_{1c}
2. Values
   a. Values are expressed as a percentage of total hemoglobin
   b. Goal for client with diabetes mellitus is lower than 7%
   c. For clients without diabetes, normal range is 4% to 6%.
3. Nursing consideration: Fasting is not required

III. PITUITARY GLAND DISORDERS (Box 44-6)

A. Hypopituitarism
1. Description: The hyposecretion of one or more of the pituitary hormones caused by tumors, trauma, encephalitis, autoimmunity, or stroke
2. Hormones most often affected are growth hormone (GH) and the gonadotropins (LH and FSH), but thyroid-stimulating hormone (TSH), adrenocorticotropic hormone (ACTH), or antidiuretic hormone (ADH) may be involved
3. Data collection
   a. Mild to moderate obesity (GH, TSH)
   b. Reduced cardiac output (GH, ADH)
   c. Infertility, sexual dysfunction (gonadotropins, ACTH)
   d. Fatigue, low blood pressure

BOX 44-5

Client Preparation: Glucose Tolerance Test

Eat a diet with adequate carbohydrate for 3 days before the test.

Avoid alcohol, coffee, and smoking for 36 hours before testing.

Fast for 10 to 16 hours prior to the test.

Avoid strenuous exercise for 8 hours before and after the test.

Withhold morning insulin or oral hypoglycemic medication (client with diabetes mellitus).

The test will take 3 to 5 hours, requires intravenous or oral administration of glucose, and multiple blood samples.

BOX 44-6

Pituitary Gland Disorders

ANTERIOR PITUITARY
Hypopituitarism
Hyperpituitarism

POSTERIOR PITUITARY
Diabetes insipidus
SIADH (syndrome of inappropriate antidiuretic hormone)

---

   e. Tumors of the pituitary may also cause headaches and visual defects (pituitary is located near the optic nerve)
4. Interventions
   a. Provide emotional support to client and family
   b. Encourage client and family to express feelings related to altered body image or sexual dysfunction
   c. May need hormone replacement for specific deficient hormones

B. Acromegaly
1. Description: The hypersecretion of GH by the anterior pituitary gland in an adult; primarily caused by pituitary tumors
2. Data collection
   a. Large hands and feet
   b. Thickening and protrusion of the jaw
   c. Arthritic changes
   d. Visual disturbances
   e. Diaphoresis
   f. Oily, rough skin
   g. Organomegaly
   h. Hypertension
   i. Dysphagia
   j. Deepening of the voice
3. Interventions
   a. Provide emotional support to client and family; encourage client and family to express feelings related to altered body image

b. Provide frequent skin care

c. Provide pharmacological and nonpharmacological interventions for joint pain

d. Prepare the client for radiation of the pituitary gland if prescribed

e. Prepare the client for **hypophysectomy** if planned

C. **Hypophysectomy** (pituitary adenectomy, transsphenoidal pituitary surgery)

1. Description

a. The removal of the pituitary tumor via craniotomy or via transsphenoidal (endoscopic transnasal) approach (the latter approach is preferred because it is associated with few complications)

b. Complications of craniotomy include increased intracranial pressure (ICP), bleeding, meningitis, and hypopituitarism

c. Complications of transsphenoidal surgery include cerebrospinal fluid (CSF) leak, infection, and hypopituitarism

2. Postoperative interventions

a. Initiate postoperative care similar to craniotomy care

b. Monitor vital signs, neurological status, and level of consciousness (LOC)

c. Elevate the head of the bed

d. Monitor for increased ICP

e. Monitor for bleeding

f. Monitor for any postnasal drip or nasal drainage, which might indicate leakage of CSF in transsphenoidal approach (check the nasal drainage for glucose)

g. Instruct the client to avoid sneezing, coughing, and blowing the nose

h. Monitor electrolyte values for temporary **diabetes insipidus** resulting from antidiuretic hormone (ADH) disturbances

i. Monitor intake and output (I&O) and avoid water intoxication

j. Administer glucocorticoids and other hormone replacements, as prescribed

k. Administer antibiotics, analgesics, and antipyretics, as prescribed

l. Instruct the client in the administration of prescribed medications, which may include vasopressin (synthetic ADH), levothyroxine, gonadotropic hormones, growth hormone (somatotropin), and glucocorticoids if the entire gland has been removed

D. **Diabetes insipidus**

1. Description

a. Hyposecretion of antidiuretic hormone (ADH) caused by stroke or trauma, or idiopathic causes

b. Kidney tubules fail to reabsorb water

2. Data collection

a. Polyuria of 4 to 24 L/day

b. Polydipsia

c. Dehydration

d. Decreased skin turgor, dry mucous membranes

e. Inability to concentrate urine

f. A low urinary specific gravity: 1.006 or less

g. Fatigue

h. Muscle pain and weakness

i. Headache

j. Postural hypotension; may progress to vascular collapse without rehydration

k. Tachycardia

3. Interventions

a. Monitor vital signs and neurological and cardiovascular status

b. Provide a safe environment, particularly in the client with a change in LOC or mental status

c. Monitor electrolyte values and for signs of dehydration

d. Monitor I&O, weight, specific gravity of urine

e. Maintain the intake of adequate fluids, monitor for signs of dehydration

f. Instruct the client to avoid foods or liquids that produce diuresis

g. Administer chlorpropamide (Diabenese) if prescribed for mild diabetes insipidus

h. Administer vasopressin tannate (Pitressin Tannate) or desmopressin acetate (DDAVP, Stimate), as prescribed; used when the ADH deficiency is severe or chronic

i. Instruct the client in the administration of medications as prescribed (DDAVP may be administered by injection, intranasally, or orally)

j. Instruct the client to wear a Medic-Alert bracelet

E. Syndrome of inappropriate antidiuretic hormone (SIADH)

1. Description

a. Excess ADH is released, but not in response to the body's need for it

b. Causes include trauma, stroke, malignancies (often in the lungs or pancreas), medications, stress

c. Results in hyponatremia

2. Data collection

a. Signs of fluid volume overload

b. Changes in LOC and mental status changes

c. Weight gain

d. Hypertension

e. Tachycardia

f. Anorexia, nausea, and vomiting

g. Hyponatremia

3. Interventions

a. Monitor vital signs and cardiac and neurological status

b. Provide a safe environment, particularly for the client with changes in LOC or mental status
c. Monitor I&O and obtain daily weights
d. Monitor fluid and electrolyte balances
e. Restrict fluid intake, as prescribed
f. Diuretics and IV fluids may be prescribed; monitor IV fluids carefully because of the risk for water intoxication
g. Demeclocycline (Declomycin) may be prescribed (inhibits ADH-induced water reabsorption and produces water diuresis)

IV. ADRENAL GLAND DISORDERS (Box 44-7)

A. Addison's disease
1. Description
   a. Hyposecretion of adrenal cortex hormones (glucocorticoids and mineralocorticoids)
   b. The condition is fatal if left untreated
2. Data collection
   a. Lethargy, fatigue, and muscle weakness
   b. Gastrointestinal (GI) disturbances
   c. Weight loss
   d. Menstrual changes in women; impotence in men
   e. **Hypoglycemia**
   f. Hyperkalemia
   g. Postural hypotension
   h. Dehydration
   i. Emotional disturbances
3. Interventions
   a. Monitor vital signs, particularly blood pressure (BP), weight, and I&O
   b. Monitor blood glucose and potassium levels
   c. Administer glucocorticoid or mineralocorticoid medications as prescribed
   d. Observe for **addisonian crisis** secondary to stress, infection, trauma, or surgery
4. Client teaching
   a. Avoid individuals with an infection
   b. Avoid stress
   c. Avoid strenuous exercise
   d. Need for lifelong glucocorticoid therapy
   e. Avoid over-the-counter medications
   f. Wear a Medic-Alert bracelet

B. Addisonian crisis
1. Description (Box 44-8)
2. Data collection
   a. Severe headache
   b. Severe abdominal, leg, and lower back pains
   c. Generalized weakness
   d. Irritability and confusion
   e. Severe hypotension
   f. Shock
3. Interventions
   a. IV glucocorticoids may be prescribed; hydrocortisone sodium succinate (Solu-Cortef) is usually prescribed initially
   b. Following resolution of the crisis, administer oral glucocorticoid and mineralocorticoid, as prescribed
   c. Monitor vital signs, particularly BP
   d. Monitor neurological status, noting irritability and confusion
   e. Monitor I&O
   f. Monitor laboratory values, particularly the sodium, potassium, and blood glucose levels
   g. IV fluids may be prescribed to restore electrolyte balance
   h. Protect the client from infection
   i. Maintain bed rest and provide a quiet environment

C. Cushing's syndrome
1. Description
   a. A condition resulting from the hypersecretion of glucocorticoids from the adrenal cortex
   b. Can be caused by an increased pituitary secretion of adrenocorticotropic hormone (ACTH), a pituitary adenoma, or an adrenal adenoma
2. Data collection
   a. Truncal obesity with thin extremities
   b. Moonface
   c. Buffalo hump
   d. Supraclavicular fat pads
   e. Generalized muscle wasting and weakness
   f. Fragile skin that easily bruises
   g. Reddish-purple striae on the abdomen and upper thighs
   h. Hirsutism (masculine characteristics in female)
   i. Hypertension

BOX 44-7

Adrenal Gland Disorders

ADRENAL CORTEX
Addison's disease
Cushing's syndrome
Primary hyperaldosteronism (Conn's syndrome)

ADRENAL MEDULLA
Pheochromocytoma

BOX 44-8

Addisonian Crisis

Life-threatening disorder caused by acute adrenal insufficiency
Precipitated by stress, infection, trauma, or surgery
Can cause hyponatremia, hyperkalemia, hypoglycemia, and shock

j. Elevated blood glucose and sodium levels and white blood cell (WBC) count

k. Decreased calcium and potassium levels

3. Interventions

a. Monitor vital signs, particularly blood pressure

b. Monitor I&O and weight

c. Monitory laboratory values, particularly the blood glucose, sodium, potassium, and calcium levels and WBC count

d. Provide good skin care

e. Allow the client to discuss feelings related to body appearance

f. Chemotherapeutic agents may be prescribed for inoperable adrenal tumors

g. Prepare the client for radiation as prescribed if the condition results from a pituitary adenoma

h. Prepare the client for removal of pituitary tumor (**hypophysectomy**, transsphenoidal adenectomy) if the condition results from increased pituitary secretion of ACTH

i. Prepare the client for **adrenalectomy** if the condition results from an adrenal adenoma; glucocorticoid replacement may be required following **adrenalectomy**

D. Primary hyperaldosteronism (Conn's syndrome)

1. Description

a. A hypersecretion of aldosterone from the adrenal cortex of the adrenal gland

b. Most commonly caused by an adenoma

2. Data collection

a. Symptoms relate to hypokalemia and hypertension

b. Headache, fatigue, muscle weakness, nocturia

c. Polydipsia and polyuria

d. Paresthesias

e. Visual changes

f. Hypernatremia

g. Low urine specific gravity and increased urinary aldosterone

3. Interventions

a. Monitor vital signs, particularly BP

b. Monitor for signs of hypokalemia

c. Monitor I&O and specific gravity of urine

d. Spironolactone (Aldactone) may be prescribed to promote fluid balance; medication is a potassium-sparing diuretic and aldosterone antagonist

e. Administer potassium supplements, as prescribed

f. Administer antihypertensives, as prescribed

g. Prepare the client for **adrenalectomy**

h. Maintain sodium restriction, if prescribed, preoperatively

i. Administer glucocorticoids preoperatively as prescribed to prevent adrenal hypofunction

j. Instruct the client regarding the need for glucocorticoids following **adrenalectomy**

k. Instruct the client about the need to wear a Medic-Alert bracelet

E. Pheochromocytoma

1. Description

a. A catecholamine-producing tumor usually found in the adrenal medulla, but extra-adrenal locations include the chest, bladder, abdomen, and brain

b. Excessive amounts of epinephrine and norepinephrine are secreted

c. Typically a benign tumor, but can be malignant

d. Surgical excision of adrenal gland is the primary treatment

e. Symptomatic treatment is initiated if surgical excision is not possible

f. Complications associated with pheochromocytoma include hypertensive retinopathy and nephropathy, cardiac enlargement, congestive heart failure (CHF), increased platelet aggregation, and cerebrovascular accident (CVA)

g. Death can occur from shock, CVA, renal failure, dysrhythmias, or dissecting aortic aneurysm

2. Data collection

a. Paroxysmal or sustained hypertension

b. Severe headaches

c. Palpitations

d. Profuse diaphoresis

e. Flushing

f. Pain in the chest or abdomen with nausea and vomiting

g. Heat intolerance

h. Weight loss

i. Tremors

j. **Hyperglycemia** and glycosuria

3. Interventions

a. Monitor vital signs, particularly the BP and heart rate

b. Monitor for hypertensive crisis; monitor for complications that can occur with hypertensive crisis such as stroke, cardiac dysrhythmia, myocardial infarction

c. Be alert to stimuli that can precipitate a hypertensive crisis, such as increased abdominal pressure, urination, and vigorous abdominal palpation (avoid these stimuli)

d. Instruct the client not to smoke, drink caffeine-containing beverages, or change position suddenly

e. Prepare for the administration of an alpha-adrenergic blocking agent, such as phenoxybenzamine (Dibenzyline), as prescribed, to control blood pressure

f. Monitor blood glucose and urine for ketones

g. Promote rest and a nonstressful environment

h. Provide a diet high in calories, vitamins, and minerals

i. Prepare the client for **adrenalectomy**

F. **Adrenalectomy**

1. Description (Box 44-9)
2. Preoperative interventions
   a. Monitor electrolytes and correct electrolyte imbalances
   b. Monitor for cardiac irregularities
   c. Monitor for **hyperglycemia**
   d. Protect the client from infections
   e. Administer glucocorticoids as prescribed
3. Postoperative interventions
   a. Monitor vital signs
   b. Monitor I&O and, if the urinary output is lower than 30 mL/hour, notify the physician, because this may be indicative of renal failure and impending shock
   c. Monitor daily weights
   d. Monitor electrolytes
   e. Monitor for signs of shock and hemorrhage, particularly during first 24 to 48 hours
   f. Check the dressing for drainage
   g. Monitor for paralytic ileus, as manifested by abdominal distention and pain, nausea, vomiting, and diminished or absent bowel sounds (paralytic ileus can develop from internal bleeding)
   h. Monitor IV fluids as prescribed to maintain blood volume
   i. Administer glucocorticoids, as prescribed
   j. Administer pain medication, as prescribed
   k. Instruct the client in the importance of glucocorticoid therapy following surgery
   l. Instruct the client regarding the need to wear a Medic-Alert bracelet

V. THYROID GLAND DISORDERS (Box 44-10)

A. Hypothyroidism (myxedema)

BOX 44-9

Adrenalectomy

This is the surgical removal of an adrenal gland.
Lifelong glucocorticoid replacement is necessary with a bilateral adrenalectomy.
Temporary glucocorticoid replacement, up to 2 years, is necessary for a unilateral adrenalectomy.
Catecholamine levels drop as a result of surgery, which can result in cardiovascular collapse, hypotension, and shock, and the client needs to be monitored closely.
Hemorrhage can also occur because of the high vascularity of the adrenal glands.

BOX 44-10

Disorders of the Thyroid Gland

Hypothyroidism
Hyperthyroidism

---

1. Description
   a. A hypothyroid state resulting from a hyposecretion of the thyroid hormones thyroxine (T_4) and triiodothyronine (T_3)
   b. Characterized by a decreased rate of body metabolism
2. Data collection
   a. Lethargy and fatigue
   b. Weakness, muscle aches, paresthesias
   c. Intolerance to cold
   d. Weight gain
   e. Dry skin and hair
   f. Loss of body hair
   g. Bradycardia
   h. Constipation
   i. Generalized puffiness and edema around the eyes and face
   j. Forgetfulness and loss of memory
   k. Menstrual disturbances
   l. Cardiac enlargement, tendency to develop congestive heart failure
3. Interventions
   a. Monitor vital signs, including heart rate and rhythm
   b. Administer thyroid replacement; levothyroxine sodium (Synthroid) is most commonly prescribed
   c. Instruct the client about thyroid replacement therapy
   d. Instruct the client in low-calorie, low-cholesterol, low-saturated fat diet
   e. Monitor the client for constipation; provide roughage and fluids to prevent constipation
   f. Provide a warm environment for the client
   g. Avoid sedatives and narcotics because of increased sensitivity to these medications
   h. Monitor for overdose of thyroid medications, characterized by tachycardia, restlessness, nervousness, and insomnia
   i. Instruct the client to report episodes of chest pain immediately

B. Myxedema coma

1. Description (Box 44-11)
2. Data collection
   a. Hypotension
   b. Bradycardia

BOX 44-11

Myxedema Coma

A rare but serious disorder that results from persistently low thyroid production
Can be precipitated by acute illness, rapid withdrawal of thyroid medication, anesthesia and surgery, hypothermia, or the use of sedatives and narcotics

c. Hypothermia

d. Hyponatremia

e. **Hypoglycemia**

f. Respiratory failure

g. Coma

3. Interventions

a. Maintain a patent airway

b. Monitor IV fluids, as prescribed

c. Levothyroxine sodium (Synthroid) IV may be prescribed

d. Monitor client's temperature frequently

e. Monitor blood pressure

f. Keep client warm

g. Monitor for changes in mental status

h. Monitor electrolytes and glucose level

▲ **C. Hyperthyroidism**

1. Description

a. A hyperthyroid state resulting from hypersecretion of thyroid hormones (T_3 and T_4)

b. Characterized by an increased rate of body metabolism

c. A common cause is Graves' disease, also known as toxic diffuse goiter

d. Clinical manifestations are referred to as thyrotoxicosis

2. Data collection for **hyperthyroidism** caused by Graves' disease

a. Enlarged thyroid gland (goiter)

b. Palpitations, cardiac dysrhythmias, such as tachycardia or atrial fibrillation

c. Protruding eyeballs (exophthalmos) may be present

d. Hypertension

e. Heat intolerance

f. Diaphoresis

g. Weight loss

h. Diarrhea

i. Smooth, soft skin and hair

j. Nervousness and fine hand tremors

k. Personality changes

l. Irritability and agitation

m. Mood swings

3. Interventions

a. Provide adequate rest

b. Administer sedatives, as prescribed

c. Provide a cool and quiet environment

d. Obtain daily weights

e. Provide a high-calorie diet

f. Avoid the administration of stimulants

g. Administer antithyroid medications (propylthiouracil, PTU) that block thyroid synthesis, as prescribed

h. Administer iodine preparations that inhibit the release of thyroid hormone, as prescribed

i. Administer propranolol (Inderal) for tachycardia, as prescribed

j. Prepare the client for radioactive iodine therapy, as prescribed, to destroy thyroid cells

k. Prepare the client for **thyroidectomy** if prescribed

D. **Thyroid storm**

1. Description (Box 44-12)

2. Data collection

a. Elevated temperature (fever)

b. Tachycardia

c. Systolic hypertension

d. Nausea, vomiting, and diarrhea

e. Agitation, tremors, anxiety

f. Irritability, agitation, restlessness, confusion, and seizures as the condition progresses

g. Delirium and coma

3. Interventions

a. Maintain a patent airway and adequate ventilation

b. Administer antithyroid medications, sodium iodide solution, propranolol (Inderal), and glucocorticoids, as prescribed

c. Monitor vital signs

d. Monitor continually for cardiac dysrhythmias

e. Administer nonsalicylate antipyretics, as prescribed (salicylates increase free thyroid hormone levels)

f. Use a cooling blanket to lower temperature, as prescribed

E. **Thyroidectomy**   ▲

1. Description

a. Removal of the thyroid gland

b. Performed when persistent hyperthryoidism exists

2. Preoperative interventions

a. Obtain vital signs and weight

b. Check electrolyte levels

c. Check for **hyperglycemia** and glycosuria

d. Instruct the client in how to perform coughing and deep-breathing exercises and how to support the neck in the postoperative period when coughing and moving

e. Administer antithyroid medications, sodium iodide solution, propranolol (Inderal), and

---

BOX 44-12

Thyroid Storm

An acute and life-threatening condition that occurs in a client with uncontrollable hyperthyroidism

Can occur from manipulation of the thyroid gland during surgery and the release of thyroid hormone into the bloodstream; can also be caused by severe infection and stress

Antithyroid medications, beta blockers, glucocorticoids, and iodides: administered to the client prior to thyroid surgery to prevent its occurrence

glucocorticoids, as prescribed, to prevent the occurrence of **thyroid storm**

3. Postoperative interventions
   a. Monitor for respiratory distress
   b. Have a tracheotomy set, oxygen, and suction at the bedside
   c. Maintain semi-Fowler's position
   d. Monitor surgical site for edema and for signs of bleeding; check dressing anteriorly and at the back of the neck
   e. Limit client talking, and assess level of hoarseness
   f. Monitor for laryngeal nerve damage, as evidenced by respiratory obstruction, dysphonia, high-pitched voice, stridor, dysphagia, and restlessness
   g. Monitor for signs of hypocalcemia and tetany, which can be due to trauma to the parathyroid gland (Box 44-13)
   h. Prepare to administer calcium gluconate as prescribed for tetany
   i. Monitor for **thyroid storm**

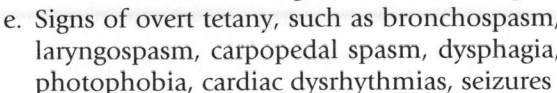 

VI. PARATHYROID GLAND DISORDERS (Box 44-14)

A. Hypoparathyroidism
  1. Description
     a. A condition caused by hyposecretion of parathyroid hormone by the parathyroid gland
     b. Can occur following **thyroidectomy** because of removal of parathyroid tissue
  2. Data collection
     a. Hypocalcemia and hyperphosphatemia
     b. Numbness and tingling in the face

BOX 44-13

Signs of Tetany

Positive Chvostek's sign
Positive Trousseau's sign
Wheezing and dyspnea (bronchospasm, laryngospasm)
Dysphagia
Numbness and tingling of the face and extremities
Carpopedal spasm
Visual disturbances (photophobia)
Muscle and abdominal cramps
Cardiac dysrhythmias
Seizures

BOX 44-14

Parathyroid Gland Disorders

Hypoparathyroidism
Hyperparathyroidism

---

c. Muscle cramps and cramps in the abdomen or in the extremities
   d. Positive **Trousseau's sign** or **Chvostek's sign**
   e. Signs of overt tetany, such as bronchospasm, laryngospasm, carpopedal spasm, dysphagia, photophobia, cardiac dysrhythmias, seizures
   f. Hypotension
   g. Anxiety, irritability, depression
3. Interventions
   a. Monitor vital signs
   b. Monitor for signs of hypocalcemia and tetany
   c. Initiate seizure precautions
   d. Place a tracheotomy set, oxygen, and suctioning at the bedside
   e. Calcium gluconate may be prescribed for hypocalcemia
   f. Provide a high-calcium and low-phosphorus diet
   g. Instruct the client in the administration of calcium supplements, as prescribed
   h. Instruct the client in the administration of vitamin D supplements, as prescribed; vitamin D enhances the absorption of calcium from the GI tract
   i. Instruct the client in the administration of phosphate binders as prescribed to promote the excretion of phosphate through the GI tract
   j. Instruct the client to wear a Medic-Alert bracelet

B. Hyperparathyroidism
  1. Description: A condition caused by hypersecretion of parathyroid hormone by the parathyroid gland
  2. Data collection
     a. Hypercalcemia and hypophosphatemia
     b. Fatigue and muscle weakness
     c. Skeletal pain and tenderness
     d. Bone deformities that result in pathological fractures
     e. Anorexia, nausea, vomiting, epigastric pain
     f. Weight loss
     g. Constipation
     h. Hypertension
     i. Cardiac dysrhythmias
     j. Renal stones
  3. Interventions
     a. Monitor vital signs, particularly the BP
     b. Monitor for cardiac irregularities
     c. Monitor I&O and for signs of renal stones
     d. Monitor for skeletal pain; move client slowly and carefully
     e. Encourage fluids
     f. Administer furosemide (Lasix) as prescribed to lower calcium levels
     g. IV normal saline may be prescribed to maintain hydration
     h. Administer phosphates as prescribed, which interfere with calcium resorption

i. Calcitonin (Calcimar) may be prescribed to decrease skeletal calcium release and increase renal clearance of calcium

j. Monitor calcium and phosphorus levels

k. The physician is notified immediately if a precipitous drop in the calcium level occurs; assess for tingling and numbness in the muscles and signs of hypocalcemia

l. Prepare the client for parathyroidectomy, as prescribed

C. Parathyroidectomy

1. Description: Removal of one or more of the parathyroid glands

2. Preoperative interventions

a. Monitor electrolyte, calcium, phosphate, and magnesium levels

b. Ensure that calcium levels are decreased to near normal

c. Inform the client that talking may be painful for the first day or two after surgery

3. Postoperative interventions

a. Monitor for respiratory distress

b. Place a tracheotomy set, oxygen, and suctioning at the bedside

c. Monitor vital signs

d. Position the client in semi-Fowler's

e. Check the neck dressing for bleeding

f. Monitor for hypocalcemic crisis, as evidenced by tingling and twitching in the extremities and face

g. Monitor for positive **Trousseau's sign** or **Chvostek's sign**, which signals the potential for tetany

h. Monitor for changes in voice pattern and hoarseness

i. Monitor for laryngeal nerve damage

j. Instruct the client in the administration of calcium and vitamin D supplements as prescribed

VII. DISORDERS OF THE PANCREAS

A. **Diabetes mellitus** (Table 44-1)

1. Description

a. A chronic disorder of impaired carbohydrate, protein, and lipid metabolism that is caused by a deficiency of effective insulin

b. A deficiency of effective insulin results in **hyperglycemia**

TABLE 44-1

Major Types of Diabetes Mellitus

Type 1: Insulin-dependent diabetes mellitus
Type 2: Non–insulin-dependent diabetes mellitus

c. Type 1 **diabetes mellitus** is a nearly absolute deficiency of insulin; if insulin is not given, fats are metabolized, resulting in ketonemia (acidosis)

d. Type 2 **diabetes mellitus** is a relative lack of insulin or resistance to the action of insulin; there is usually sufficient insulin to stabilize fat and protein metabolism, but not enough to deal with carbohydrate metabolism

e. Macrovascular complications include coronary disease, cardiomyopathy, hypertension, cerebrovascular disease, peripheral vascular disease, and infection

f. Microvascular complications include retinopathy, nephropathy, and neuropathy

2. Data collection

a. Polyuria, polydipsia, polyphagia (more common in type 1 **diabetes mellitus**)

b. **Hyperglycemia**

c. Weight loss (common in type 1 **diabetes mellitus,** rare in type 2 **diabetes mellitus**)

d. Blurred vision

e. Slow wound healing

f. Vaginal infections

g. Weakness and paresthesias

h. Signs of inadequate circulation to the feet

i. Signs of accelerated atherosclerosis (renal, cerebral, cardiac, peripheral)

3. Diet

a. The total number of calories is individualized on the basis of the client's current or desired weight and the presence of other existing health problems

b. As prescribed by the physician, the client may be advised to follow the food exchange from the American Diabetic Association diet or the dietary guidelines for Americans (My Pyramid see Figure 12-1) issued by the U.S. Departments of Agriculture and Health and Human Services

c. Incorporate diet into individual client needs, lifestyle, and cultural and socioeconomic patterns

4. Exercise

a. Lowers blood glucose level

b. Reduces cardiovascular risks

c. Improves circulation and muscle tone

d. Decreases total cholesterol and triglyceride levels

e. Encourages weight loss

f. Instruct the client in dietary adjustments when exercising; dietary adjustments are individualized

g. Instruct the client to monitor blood glucose before exercising; if the client plans to participate in extended periods of exercise, blood glucose levels should be checked before, during, and after the exercise period

h. Initially, the client who requires insulin should be instructed to eat a 15-g carbohydrate snack (a fruit exchange) or a snack of complex carbohydrate with a protein before engaging in moderate exercise to prevent **hypoglycemia**

i. If the client requires extra food during exercise to prevent **hypoglycemia,** it need not be deducted from the regular meal plan

j. If the blood glucose level is higher than 250 mg/dL and urinary ketones (type 1 **diabetes mellitus**) are present, the client is instructed not to exercise until the blood glucose level is closer to normal and urinary ketones are negative

5. Oral hypoglycemic medications

a. Prescribed for clients with **diabetes mellitus type 2**

b. Determine the client's knowledge of **diabetes mellitus** and the use of oral hypoglycemic agents

c. Monitor vital signs and blood glucose levels

d. Check the medications that the client is currently taking

e. Aspirin, alcohol, sulfonamides, oral contraceptives, and monoamine oxidase inhibitors (MAOIs) increase the hypoglycemic effect, causing a decrease in blood glucose levels

f. Glucocorticoids, thiazide diuretics, and estrogen increase blood glucose levels

g. Teach the client to recognize symptoms of **hypoglycemia** and **hyperglycemia**

h. Teach the client to avoid over-the-counter medications unless prescribed by the physician

i. Teach the client to avoid alcohol if taking sulfonylureas

j. Inform the client with type 2 **diabetes mellitus** that insulin may be needed during stress, surgery, or infection

k. Teach the client about the importance of compliance with the prescribed medication

l. Advise the client to obtain a Medic-Alert bracelet

6. Insulin

a. Used in the treatment of type 1 **diabetes mellitus** and in type 2 **diabetes mellitus** when diet and weight control therapy have failed to maintain satisfactory blood glucose levels

b. Regular insulin is the only insulin that can be administered intravenously in the emergency treatment of **diabetic ketoacidosis**

c. Aspirin, alcohol, oral anticoagulants, oral hypoglycemics, beta blockers, tricyclic antidepressants, tetracycline, and monoamine oxidase inhibitors increase the hypoglycemic effect of insulin, causing further decrease in blood glucose levels

d. Glucocorticoids, thiazide diuretics, thyroid agents, oral contraceptives, and estrogen increase blood glucose levels

e. Illness, infection, and stress increase blood glucose levels and the need for insulin; insulin should not be withheld during illness, infection, or stress, because **hyperglycemia** and ketoacidosis can result

f. Instruct the client to recognize symptoms of **hypoglycemia** and **hyperglycemia**

g. The peak action time of insulin is very important because of the possibility of hypoglycemic reactions occurring during that time

B. Complications of insulin therapy

1. Local allergic reactions

a. Redness, swelling, tenderness, and induration or a wheal at the site of injection 1 to 2 hours after administration

b. Usually occurs during the early stages of insulin therapy

c. Instruct the client to avoid the use of alcohol to cleanse the skin prior to injection

d. The physician may prescribe an antihistamine to be taken 1 hour prior to injection

2. Insulin lipodystrophy

a. Lipoatrophy is loss of subcutaneous fat and appears as slight dimpling or more serious pitting of subcutaneous fat; the use of human insulin helps prevent this complication

b. Lipohypertrophy is the development of fibrous fatty masses at the injection site; caused by repeated use of an injection site

c. Instruct the client to avoid injecting insulin into affected sites

d. Instruct the client about the importance of rotating insulin injection sites

3. Insulin resistance

a. The client receiving insulin develops immune antibodies that bind the insulin, thereby decreasing the insulin available for use in the body

b. Treatment consists of administering a purer insulin preparation

c. Insulin resistance is also the term used for lack of tissue sensitivity to the body's insulin, which results in hyperglycemia

4. **Dawn phenomenon**

a. Results from reduced tissue sensitivity to insulin that develops between 5 and 8 AM (prebreakfast **hyperglycemia** occurs); may be caused by nocturnal release of growth hormone

b. Treatment includes administering an evening dose of intermediate-acting insulin at 10 PM

5. **Somogyi's phenomenon**

a. Normal or elevated blood glucose levels are present at bedtime; **hypoglycemia** occurs at 2 to 3 AM, which causes an increase in the production of counterregulatory hormones

b. By 7 AM, in response to the counterregulatory hormones, the blood glucose rebounds significantly to the hyperglycemic range

c. Treatment includes decreasing the evening (predinner or bedtime) dose of intermediate-acting insulin or increasing the bedtime snack

6. **Insulin waning**

a. A progressive rise in the blood glucose level from bedtime to morning

b. Treatment includes increasing the evening (predinner or bedtime) dose of intermediate- or long-acting insulin, or instituting a dose of insulin before the evening meal if one is not already prescribed

C. Insulin administration

1. Subcutaneous injections and mixing insulin: Refer to Chapter 45

2. Insulin pens

a. A device that uses a small, prefilled insulin cartridge that is loaded into a penlike holder; a disposable needle is attached to the device for injection

b. The client inserts the needle for injection; insulin is delivered by dialing in a dose or pushing a button for every 1- to 2-unit increment administered

3. Jet injectors

a. A device that delivers insulin through the skin under pressure in an extremely fine stream

b. Insulin administered by this device usually absorbs faster

c. Can cause bruising at the site of insulin delivery

4. Insulin pumps

a. Continuous subcutaneous insulin infusion is administered by an externally worn device that contains a syringe attached to a long, thin, narrow-lumen tube with a needle or Teflon catheter attached to the end

b. The client inserts the needle or Teflon catheter into the subcutaneous tissue (usually on the abdomen) and secures it with tape or a transparent dressing; the pump is worn either on a belt or in a pocket; the needle or Teflon catheter is changed at least every 3 days

c. A continuous basal rate of insulin infuses; in addition, based on the blood glucose level, the anticipated food intake, and the activity level, the client delivers a bolus of insulin before each meal

d. The pump uses regular insulin (buffered to prevent the precipitation of insulin crystals within the catheter); some physicians may prescribe the use of insulin lispro

5. Implantable insulin delivery

a. An insulin pump is implanted into the peritoneal cavity, where insulin can be absorbed in a more physiological manner

b. Not widely used because of mechanical problems associated with the pump, catheter, and insulin delivery

6. Pancreas transplants

a. The goal of pancreatic transplantation is to halt or reverse the complications of **diabetes mellitus**

b. Performed on a limited number of clients (most are clients receiving a kidney transplant simultaneously)

c. Immunosuppressive therapy is prescribed to prevent and treat rejection

D. Self-monitoring of blood glucose

1. Provides the client with the current blood glucose level and information to maintain good glycemic control

2. Requires a finger prick to obtain a drop of blood for testing

3. Must be used with caution in clients with diabetic neuropathy

4. Client instructions (Box 44-15)

E. Urine testing

1. Less reliable indicator as compared with blood glucose monitoring

2. Instruct the client in the procedure for testing urine for glucose and ketones

3. Inform the client that the second voided urine specimen is most accurate

4. The presence of ketones may indicate impending **ketoacidosis**

5. Urine ketone testing should be performed during illness and whenever the client with type 1 **diabetes mellitus** has glycosuria or persistently elevated blood glucose levels (higher than 240 mg/dL for two consecutive testing periods)

VIII. ACUTE COMPLICATIONS OF DIABETES MELLITUS

A. **Hypoglycemia**

1. Description

BOX 44-15

Client Instructions: Monitoring of Blood Glucose

Instruct in the proper procedure for obtaining the blood glucose level, and that the procedure must be done precisely to obtain accurate results.

Follow the manufacturer's instructions for the glucometer.

Hand washing must be done before and after performing the procedure to prevent infection.

Calibrate the monitor as instructed by the manufacturer.

Check the expiration date on the test strips.

If the blood glucose results do not seem reasonable, reread the instructions, reassess technique, check the expiration date of the test strips, and perform the procedure again to verify results.

a. Occurs when the blood glucose level falls below 60 mg/dL
b. Caused by too much insulin or oral hypoglycemic agents, too little food, or excessive activity
c. The client needs to be instructed always to carry some form of fast-acting simple carbohydrate with them
d. If the client has a hypoglycemic reaction and does not have any of the recommended emergency foods available, any available food should be eaten; high-fat foods slow the absorption of glucose and the hypoglycemic symptoms may not resolve quickly

2. Data collection (Table 44-2)
   a. Mild **hypoglycemia**: A blood glucose level below 60 mg/dL
   b. Moderate **hypoglycemia**: A blood glucose level below 40 mg/dL
   c. Severe **hypoglycemia**: A blood glucose level below 20 mg/dL; the client is unable to swallow, is unconscious, or experiencing seizures

3. Interventions: Mild **hypoglycemia**
   a. Give 10 to 15 g of a fast-acting simple carbohydrate (Box 44-16)
   b. Retest the blood glucose level in 15 minutes and repeat the treatment if symptoms do not resolve
   c. Once symptoms resolve, a snack containing protein and carbohydrate, such as milk or cheese and crackers, is recommended unless the client plans to eat a regular meal within 60 minutes

4. Interventions: Moderate **hypoglycemia**
   a. Administer 15 to 30 g of a fast-acting simple carbohydrate
   b. Administer additional food such as low fat milk or cheese after 10 to 15 minutes

5. Interventions: Severe **hypoglycemia**
   a. If the client is unconscious and cannot swallow, an injection of glucagon is administered subcutaneously or intramuscularly
   b. Administer a second dose in 10 minutes if the client remains unconscious
   c. A small meal is given to the client when the client awakens as long as the client is not nauseated
   d. The physician is notified if a severe hypoglycemic reaction occurs
   e. In the hospital or emergency department, the client may be treated with an IV injection of 25 to 50 mL of 50% dextrose in water
   f. Family members need to be instructed about the administration of glucagon

B. **Diabetic ketoacidosis (DKA)**
   1. Description
      a. A life-threatening complication of type 1 **diabetes mellitus** that develops when a severe insulin deficiency occurs
      b. The main clinical manifestations include **hyperglycemia**, dehydration and electrolyte loss, and acidosis
      c. The major causes include a decreased or missed dose of insulin, illness or infection, and undiagnosed and untreated type 1 **diabetes mellitus**
      d. Develops over a period over several hours to days
   2. Data collection (Box 44-17)
      a. Blood glucose levels may vary from 300 to 800 mg/dL
      b. Low serum bicarbonate level and a low pH
      c. Sodium and potassium levels may be low, normal, or high, depending on the amount of water loss and dehydration status

TABLE 44-2

Findings in Hypoglycemia

Mild	Moderate	Severe
Sweating	Inability to	Disoriented
Tremor	concentrate	behavior
Tachycardia	Headache	Difficulty
Palpitations	Lightheadedness	arousing
Nervousness	Confusion	from sleep
Hunger	Memory lapses	Loss of
	Numbness of the	consciousness
	lips and tongue	Seizures
	Slurred speech	
	Impaired	
	coordination	
	Emotional changes	
	Irrational or	
	combative behavior	
	Double vision	
	Drowsiness	

BOX 44-16

Simple Carbohydrates to Treat Hypoglycemia

Commercially prepared glucose tablets
6 to 10 Life Savers or hard candy
4 tsp sugar
4 sugar cubes
1 tbsp honey or syrup
½ cup of fruit juice or regular (nondiet) soft drink
8 ounces low-fat milk
6 saltines
3 graham crackers

BOX 44-17

Data Collection Findings in Diabetic Ketoacidosis

Polyuria
Polydipsia
Blurred vision
Weakness
Headache
Hypotension
Weak, rapid pulse
Anorexia, nausea, vomiting, and abdominal pain
Acetone breath (a fruity odor)
Kussmaul respirations
Mental status changes

3. Interventions
    a. Restore circulating volume and protect against cerebral, coronary, or renal hypoperfusion
    b. Dehydration is treated with rapid IV infusions of 0.9% or 0.45% saline as prescribed; dextrose is added to IV fluids (D_5W NS or 5% dextrose in 0.45% saline) when the blood glucose level reaches 250 to 300 mg/dL
    c. **Hyperglycemia** is treated with regular insulin administered intravenously, as prescribed
    d. Correct electrolyte imbalances (potassium level may be elevated as a result of dehydration and acidosis)
    e. Monitor potassium level closely because, when the client receives treatment for the dehydration and acidosis, the serum potassium level will decrease and potassium replacement may be required
4. Insulin IV administration
    a. Regular insulin only is used for IV administration
    b. A dose of 5 to 10 units of regular insulin by IV bolus may be prescribed before a continuous infusion is begun
    c. An IV dose of regular insulin for continuous infusion is mixed in 0.9% or 0.45% saline, as prescribed
    d. The insulin solution is flushed through the entire intravenous infusion set and the first 50 mL of solution is discarded before connecting and administering to the client; insulin molecules adhere to plastic of IV infusion sets
    e. The insulin infusion is always placed on an IV infusion controller
    f. Insulin is infused continuously until subcutaneous administration resumes
    g. Monitor vital signs and for signs of fluid overload
    h. Monitor potassium levels, glucose levels, and urinary output, and for signs of increased intracranial pressure

    i. If the blood glucose level falls too far, too fast before the brain has time to equilibrate, water is pulled from the blood to the cerebrospinal fluid and the brain, causing cerebral edema and increased intracranial pressure
    j. The potassium level will fall rapidly within the first hour of treatment as the dehydration and acidosis are treated
    k. Potassium is administered intravenously in a diluted solution as prescribed when the potassium reaches normal level to prevent hypokalemia; ensure adequate renal function before administering potassium
5. Client education (Box 44-18)
C. **Hyperglycemic hyperosmolar nonketotic syndrome (HHNS)**
    1. Description
        a. Extreme **hyperglycemia** without ketosis and acidosis
        b. Occurs most often in individuals with type 2 **diabetes mellitus**
        c. The major difference between **HHNS** and **DKA** is that ketosis and acidosis do not occur with **HHNS**
        d. Onset is usually slow and takes hours to days to develop
    2. Data collection
        a. Blood glucose level is from 600 to 1200 mg/dL
        b. Hypotension
        c. Dehydration
        d. Tachycardia
        e. Mental status changes
        f. Neurological deficits
        g. Seizures
    3. Interventions
        a. Similar to the treatment for **DKA**
        b. Includes fluid replacement, correction of electrolyte imbalances, and insulin administration
        c. Insulin plays a less critical role in the treatment of **HHNS** than it does for the treatment of **DKA**, because ketosis and acidosis do not occur in **HHNS**

IX. CHRONIC COMPLICATIONS OF DIABETES MELLITUS
A. Diabetic retinopathy
    1. Description
        a. A chronic and progressive impairment of the retinal circulation that eventually causes hemorrhage
        b. Permanent vision changes and blindness can occur
        c. The client has difficulty carrying out the daily tasks of blood glucose testing and insulin injections
    2. Data collection

BOX 44-18

Client Education: Guidelines during Illness

Take insulin or oral antidiabetic medications, as prescribed.

Test blood glucose level and test the urine for ketones every 3 to 4 hours.

If the usual meal plan cannot be followed, substitute soft foods six to eight times a day.

If vomiting, diarrhea, or fever occurs, consume liquids every 30 to 60 minutes to prevent dehydration and to provide calories.

Notify the physician if vomiting, diarrhea, or fever persists, if blood glucose levels are higher than 250 to 300 mg/dL, when ketonuria is present for more than 24 hours, when unable to take food or fluids for a period of 4 hours, or when illness persists for more than 2 days.

---

    a. A change in vision due to the rupture of small microaneurysms in retinal blood vessels
    b. Blurred vision resulting from macular edema
    c. Sudden loss of vision as a result of retinal detachment
    d. Cataracts resulting from lens opacity
  3. Interventions
    a. Maintain safety
    b. Early prevention by the control of hypertension and blood glucose levels
    c. Photocoagulation (laser therapy) to remove hemorrhagic tissue to decrease scarring
    d. Vitrectomy to remove vitreous hemorrhages and thus decrease tension on the retina, preventing detachment
    e. Cataract removal with lens implant
B. Diabetic nephropathy
  1. Description: A progressive decrease in kidney function
  2. Data collection
    a. Microalbuminuria
    b. Thirst
    c. Fatigue
    d. Anemia
    e. Weight loss
    f. Signs of malnutrition
    g. Frequent urinary tract infections
    h. Signs of a neurogenic bladder
  3. Interventions
    a. Early prevention measures include the control of hypertension and blood glucose levels
    b. Monitor vital signs
    c. Monitor I&O
    d. Monitor serum BUN and creatinine levels and urine albumin levels
    e. Restrict dietary protein, sodium, and potassium, as prescribed
    f. Avoid nephrotoxic medications
    g. Prepare the client for dialysis procedures, as prescribed

    h. Prepare the client for kidney transplant, as prescribed
    i. Prepare the client for pancreas transplant, as prescribed
C. Diabetic neuropathy
  1. Description
    a. General deterioration of the nervous system throughout the body.
    b. Complications include the development of nonhealing ulcers of the feet, gastric paresis, erectile dysfunction
  2. Data collection
    a. Paresthesias
    b. Decreased or absent reflexes
    c. Decreased sensation to vibration or light touch
    d. Pain, aching, and burning in the lower extremities
    e. Poor peripheral pulses
    f. Skin breakdown and signs of infection
    g. Weakness or loss of sensation in cranial nerves III, IV, V, or VI
    h. Dizziness and postural hypotension
    i. Nausea and vomiting
    j. Diarrhea or constipation
    k. Incontinence
    l. Dyspareunia
    m. Impotence
    n. Hypoglycemic unawareness
  3. Interventions
    a. Early prevention measures include the control of hypertension and blood glucose levels
    b. Careful foot care to prevent trauma (Box 44-19)
    c. Administer medications as prescribed for pain relief
    d. Initiate bladder-training programs
    e. Instruct in the use of estrogen-containing lubricants for women with dyspareunia
    f. Prepare the male client with impotence for penile injections or an implantable device, as prescribed
    g. Prepare for surgical decompression for compression lesions related to the cranial nerves, as prescribed

X. OPERATIVE CARE FOR THE DIABETIC CLIENT

A. Preoperative care
  1. Check with physician regarding withholding oral hypoglycemic medications or insulin
  2. Some long-acting oral antidiabetic medications are discontinued 24 to 48 hours prior to surgery
  3. Insulin dose may be adjusted or withheld if IV insulin administration during surgery is planned
  4. Monitor blood glucose level
  5. Monitor IV fluids, as prescribed
B. Postoperative care
  1. IV glucose and regular insulin infusions may be prescribed until the client can tolerate oral feedings

BOX 44-19

Preventive Foot Care Instructions

Carry out meticulous skin care and proper foot care.

Inspect feet daily and monitor feet for redness, swelling, or break in skin integrity.

Notify the physician if redness or a break in the skin occurs.

Avoid thermal injuries from hot water, heating pads, and baths.

Wash feet with warm (not hot) water and dry thoroughly (avoid foot soaks).

Do not soak feet.

Do not treat corns, blisters, or ingrown toenails.

Do not cross legs or wear tight garments that may constrict blood flow.

Apply moisturizing lotion to the feet but not between the toes.

Prevent moisture from accumulating between the toes.

Wear loose socks and well-fitting (not tight) shoes, and instruct the client not to go barefoot.

Change into clean cotton socks daily.

Wear socks to keep feet warm.

Do not wear the same pair of shoes 2 days in a row.

Do not wear open-toed shoes or shoes with a strap that goes between the toes.

Check shoes for cracks or tears in the lining and for foreign objects before putting them on.

Break in new shoes gradually.

Cut toenails straight across and smooth nails with an emery board.

Do not smoke.

---

2. Administer supplemental short-acting insulin as prescribed on the basis of blood glucose results
3. Monitor blood glucose levels frequently if the client is receiving total parenteral nutrition
4. When the client is tolerating food, ensure that the client receives an adequate amount of carbohydrates daily to prevent **hypoglycemia** and ketosis

PRACTICE QUESTIONS

1. A nurse is caring for a client following hypophysectomy. The nurse notices clear nasal drainage from the client's nostril. The appropriate nursing action would be to:
   1. Continue to observe drainage
   2. Test the drainage for glucose
   3. Lower the head of the bed
   4. Obtain a culture of the drainage
2. Following several diagnostic tests, a client is diagnosed with diabetes insipidus. The nurse understands that which symptom is indicative of this disorder?
   1. Diarrhea
   2. Polydipsia
   3. Weight gain
   4. Fatigue

3. A nurse caring for a client with Addison's disease would expect to note which of the following?
   1. Obesity
   2. Edema
   3. Hypotension
   4. Hirsutism
4. A client with Cushing's syndrome verbalizes concern to the nurse regarding the appearance of the buffalo hump that has developed. The nurse makes which statement to the client?
   1. "This is permanent, but looks are deceiving and not that important."
   2. "Don't be concerned; this problem can be covered with clothing."
   3. "Try not to worry about it. There are other things to be concerned about."
   4. "Usually, these physical changes slowly improve following treatment."
5. A nurse assists in developing a plan of care for a client with Graves' disease. Which of the following would the nurse include in the plan of care?
   1. Provide three small meals a day
   2. Provide the client with extra blankets
   3. Provide a high-fiber diet
   4. Provide a restful environment
6. A nurse is caring for a client following thyroidectomy and notes that calcium gluconate is prescribed for the client. The nurse determines that this medication has been prescribed to:
   1. Treat thyroid storm
   2. Prevent cardiac irritability
   3. Stimulate the release of parathyroid hormone
   4. Treat hypocalcemic tetany
7. A nurse is collecting data on the client following a thyroidectomy and notes that the client has developed hoarseness and a weak voice. Which of the following nursing actions is appropriate?
   1. Notify the registered nurse immediately
   2. Reassure the client that this is usually a temporary condition
   3. Check for signs of bleeding
   4. Administer calcium gluconate
8. A client is admitted to the emergency room and a diagnosis of myxedema coma is made. Which nursing action would the nurse prepare to carry out initially?
   1. Warm the client
   2. Administer fluids
   3. Maintain a patent airway
   4. Administer thyroid hormone
9. A client is taking NPH insulin daily every morning. The nurse instructs the client that the most likely time for a hypoglycemic reaction to occur is:
   1. 2 to 4 hours after administration
   2. 6 to 14 hours after administration
   3. 16 to 18 hours after administration
   4. 18 to 24 hours after administration

10. A nurse is assisting in preparing a teaching plan for the client with diabetes mellitus regarding proper foot care. Which of the following instructions should be included in the plan?
    1. Soak feet in hot water
    2. Apply a moisturizing lotion to dry feet, but not between the toes
    3. Always have a podiatrist cut your toenails; never cut them yourself
    4. Avoid using soap to wash the feet

11. A nurse provides dietary instructions to a client with diabetes mellitus regarding the prescribed diabetic diet. Which statement, if made by the client, indicates a need for further teaching?
    1. "I need to drink diet soft drinks."
    2. "I'll eat a balanced meal plan."
    3. "I need to buy special dietetic foods."
    4. "I'll snack on fruit instead of cake."

12. An external insulin pump is prescribed for a client with diabetes mellitus and the client asks the nurse about the functioning of the pump. The nurse plans to base the response on the information that the pump:
    1. Gives a small continuous dose of regular insulin subcutaneously, and the client can self-administer an additional dose from the pump before each meal
    2. Is timed to release programmed doses of regular or NPH insulin into the bloodstream at specific intervals
    3. Is surgically attached to the pancreas and infuses regular insulin into the pancreas, which in turn releases the insulin into the bloodstream
    4. Continuously infuses small amounts of NPH insulin into the bloodstream while regularly monitoring blood glucose levels

13. A client newly diagnosed with diabetes mellitus has been stabilized with daily insulin injections. The nurse assists in preparing a discharge teaching plan regarding the insulin and includes which of the following concepts?
    1. Increase the amount of insulin prior to unusual exercise
    2. Acetone in the urine will signify a need for less insulin
    3. Always keep insulin vials refrigerated
    4. Systematically rotate insulin injection sites

14. A nurse reinforces teaching with a client with diabetes mellitus about differentiating between hypoglycemia and ketoacidosis. The client demonstrates an understanding of the teaching by stating that glucose will be taken if which of the following symptoms develop?
    1. Fruity breath odor
    2. Shakiness
    3. Blurred vision
    4. Polyuria

15. A client with diabetes mellitus demonstrates acute anxiety when admitted to the hospital for the treatment of hyperglycemia. The appropriate intervention to decrease the client's anxiety would be to:
    1. Administer a sedative
    2. Make sure the client knows all the correct medical terms so that he or she can understand what is happening
    3. Ignore the signs and symptoms of anxiety so that they will soon disappear
    4. Convey empathy, trust, and respect toward the client

16. A nurse reinforces instructions to a client newly diagnosed with type 1 diabetes mellitus. The nurse determines accurate understanding of measures to prevent diabetic ketoacidosis (DKA) when the client says:
    1. "I will stop taking my insulin if I'm too sick to eat."
    2. "I will decrease my insulin dose during times of illness."
    3. "I will notify my physician if my blood glucose level is higher than 250 mg/dL."
    4. "I will adjust my insulin dose according to the level of glucose in my urine."

17. A physician prescribes levothyroxine (Synthroid), 0.15 mg orally daily, for a client with hypothyroidism. The nurse prepares to administer this medication:
    1. Three times a day in equal doses of 0.5 mg each to ensure consistent serum drug levels
    2. In the morning to prevent sleeplessness
    3. Only when the client complains of fatigue and cold intolerance
    4. At various times of the day to prevent tolerance from occurring

18. A nurse is monitoring a client receiving chlorpropamide (Diabenese). The nurse understands that which of the following is an ineffective therapeutic outcome indicating poor glycemic control?
    1. A decrease in polyuria
    2. A blood glucose level of 110 mg/dL
    3. A decrease in polyphagia
    4. A glycosylated hemoglobin level of 18%

19. A nurse is monitoring a client newly diagnosed with diabetes mellitus for sign of complications. Which of the following, if exhibited in the client, would indicate hyperglycemia and warrant physician notification?
    1. Hypertension
    2. Diaphoresis
    3. Polyuria
    4. Increased pulse rate

20. A nurse is reinforcing instructions with a client with diabetes mellitus recovering from diabetic

ketoacidosis (DKA) in measures to prevent a recurrence. The nurse tells the client to:

1. Eat six small meals daily
2. Receive appropriate follow-up health care
3. Monitor blood glucose levels frequently
4. Test urine for ketone levels

21. A nurse is collecting data from a client with type 2 diabetes mellitus. Which statement by the client indicates an understanding of the medication regimen?

1. "I am taking oral insulin instead of insulin shots."
2. "The medication that I am taking helps release the insulin I already make."
3. "By taking these medications, I am able to eat more."
4. "When I become ill, I need to increase the number of pills I take."

22. A client with type 1 diabetes mellitus is having trouble remembering the type, duration, and onset of the action of insulin and the client's family members have not been supportive. The nurse should make which statement to the client?

1. "You can't always depend on your family to help."
2. "Let me go over the types of insulin with you again."
3. "It's not really necessary for you to remember this."
4. "What is it you don't understand?"

23. A nurse is doing discharge teaching with a client who has Cushing's syndrome. Which of the following statements by the client indicate that the instructions related to dietary management were understood?

1. "I am fortunate that I do not need to follow any special diet."
2. "I will need to limit the amount of protein in my diet."
3. "I am fortunate that I can eat all the salty foods I enjoy."
4. "I can eat foods that have a lot of potassium in them."

24. A client with type 1 diabetes mellitus calls the nurse to report recurrent episodes of hypoglycemia. Which statement by the client indicates an inadequate understanding of NPH insulin and exercise?

1. "The best time for me to exercise is late afternoon."
2. "The best time for me to exercise is after lunch."
3. "The best time for me to exercise is after breakfast."
4. "The best time for me to exercise is in the evening."

25. A nurse is collecting data from an older client who is being admitted to the hospital for a diagnostic workup for primary hyperparathyroidism. The nurse understands that which client complaint would be characteristic of this disorder?

1. Diarrhea
2. Polyuria
3. Polyphagia
4. Weight gain

26. A nurse is caring for a postoperative parathyroidectomy client. Which client complaint would indicate that a serious life-threatening complication may be developing that requires immediate notification of the physician?

1. Difficulty voiding
2. Abdominal cramps
3. Laryngeal stridor
4. Mild to moderate incisional pain

27. A nurse is preparing to discharge a client who has had a parathyroidectomy. The nurse teaches the client about the prescribed oral calcium supplements and tells the client to:

1. Store the calcium in the refrigerator to maintain potency
2. Check the pulse daily, and not to take the calcium if it is below 60 beats per minute
3. Take the calcium 30 to 60 minutes following a meal
4. Avoid sunlight because it can cause skin color change

28. A nurse notes that a client with type 1 diabetes mellitus has lipodystrophy on both upper thighs. The nurse would most appropriately inquire if the client:

1. Cleanses the skin with alcohol before each injection
2. Rotates sites for injection
3. Aspirates for blood prior to injection into the subcutaneous tissue
4. Administers the insulin at a 45-degree angle

29. A nurse is caring for a client with type 1 diabetes mellitus. Which of the following client complaints would alert the nurse of a possible hypoglycemic reaction?

1. Hot, dry skin
2. Muscle cramps
3. Anorexia
4. Tremors

30. A male client with type 1 diabetes mellitus tells the nurse that he might lose his job because he has been having frequent hypoglycemic reactions. When these reactions occur, his boss thinks that he is drunk and has been drinking on the job. Which action by the nurse would best assist this client to meet his needs?

1. Contact the local employment office to help him find another job
2. Ask the client if he indeed has been drinking at work

3. Examine factors that may be causing frequent hypoglycemic episodes

4. Ask the client what he does to treat his hypoglycemia

31. A nurse needs to maintain food and fluid intake to minimize the risk of dehydration in an older client with diabetes mellitus who has gastroenteritis. An appropriate nursing intervention to perform is to:
    1. Offer water only until the client is able to tolerate solid foods
    2. Withhold all fluids until vomiting has ceased for at least 4 hours
    3. Encourage the client to take 8 to 12 ounces of fluid every hour while awake
    4. Maintain a clear liquid diet for at least 5 days before advancing the diet to allow inflammation of the bowel to dissipate

32. A client who is currently taking levothyroxine (Synthroid) complains of cold intolerance, constipation, dry skin, weight gain, and puffy eyes. Based on these findings, the nurse would anticipate which of the following physician prescriptions?
    1. Increased levothyroxine dosage after checking the T_4 level
    2. Decreased levothyroxine dosage after checking the T_4 level
    3. Discontinue the levothyroxine, because the client is having an adverse reaction
    4. No change in medication dosage, because these are common side effects that will diminish with time

33. A nurse is caring for a client with diabetes insipidus receiving vasopressin (Pitressin). The nurse understands that which of the following is a therapeutic effect of this medication?
    1. Decreased gastrointestinal tract smooth muscle tone and contractions
    2. Decreased urine output
    3. Decreased reabsorption of water by the renal tubules
    4. Vasodilation of vascular vessels

34. A client is diagnosed with pheochromocytoma. The nurse helping to prepare a nursing care plan for the client understands that pheochromocytoma is a condition that:
    1. Causes profound hypotension
    2. Causes the release of excessive amounts of catecholamines
    3. Is not a curable condition and is treated symptomatically
    4. Is manifested by severe hypoglycemia

35. A nurse is collecting data on a client admitted to the hospital with a diagnosis of pheochromocytoma. The nurse observes for the major symptom associated with pheochromocytoma when the nurse:
    1. Tests the client's urine for glucose

2. Takes the client's weight
3. Palpates the skin for its temperature
4. Takes the client's blood pressure

36. A nurse is caring for a client with pheochromocytoma. The client is scheduled for an adrenalectomy. In the preoperative period, the priority nursing action would be to monitor:
    1. Vital signs
    2. Urine for glucose and acetone
    3. Intake and output
    4. Blood urea nitrogen (BUN) level

37. A nurse is caring for a client with pheochromocytoma. The client asks for a snack and something warm to drink. The appropriate choice for this client to meet nutritional needs would be which of the following?
    1. Graham crackers and warm milk
    2. Toast with peanut butter and cocoa
    3. Crackers with cheese and tea
    4. Vanilla wafers and coffee with cream and sugar

38. A nurse is caring for a client with pheochromocytoma. Which of the following data would indicate a potential complication associated with this disorder?
    1. A urinary output of 50 mL/hour
    2. Congestion heard on auscultation of the lungs
    3. A blood urea nitrogen (BUN) level of 20 mg/dL
    4. A coagulation time of 5 minutes

39. A client with pheochromocytoma is scheduled for surgery and says to the nurse, "I'm not sure that surgery is the best thing to do." The appropriate response by the nurse is which of the following?
    1. "You have concerns about the surgical treatment for your condition."
    2. "There is no reason to worry. Your doctor is a wonderful surgeon."
    3. "You are very ill. Your physician has made the correct decision."
    4. "I think you are making the right decision to have the surgery."

40. A nurse is caring for a client following thyroidectomy and is monitoring for signs of thyroid storm. The nurse understands that which of the following is a manifestation associated with this disorder?
    1. Low-grade fever
    2. Bradycardia
    3. Hypotension
    4. Constipation

ALTERNATE FORMAT QUESTION: PRIORITIZING (ORDERED RESPONSE)

A hospitalized client with type 1 diabetes mellitus received NPH and regular insulin 2 hours ago (at 7:30 AM). The client calls the nurse and reports that he is feeling hungry, shaky, and weak. The client ate breakfast at 8 AM and is due to eat lunch at 12:00 noon. List in order of priority the actions that the nurse would take. (Number 1 is the first action.)

___ Give the client $1/2$ cup of fruit juice to drink
___ Check the client's blood glucose level
___ Take the client's vital signs
___ Give the client a small snack of carbohydrate and protein
___ Document the client's complaints, actions taken, and outcome

ANSWERS

1. **Answer: 2**
Rationale: Following hypophysectomy, the client should be monitored for rhinorrhea, which could indicate a cerebrospinal fluid (CSF) leak. If this occurs, the drainage should be collected and tested for the presence of CSF. The head of the bed should not be lowered to prevent increased intracranial pressure. Clear nasal drainage would not indicate the need for a culture. Continuing to observe the drainage without taking action could result in a serious complication.
Test-Taking Strategy: Use the process of elimination. Option 3 can be eliminated first. Option 4 can be eliminated because the drainage is clear. Because an action is required, eliminate option 1. Review the complications following hypophysectomy if you had difficulty with this question.
Level of Cognitive Ability: Application
Client Needs: Physiological Integrity
Integrated Process: Nursing Process/Implementation
Content Area: Adult Health/Endocrine
References: Black, J., & Hawks, J. (2005). *Medical-surgical nursing: Clinical management for positive outcomes* (7th ed.). Philadelphia: W.B. Saunders, p. 1234.
Linton, A. & Maebius, N. (2003) *Introduction to medical-surgical nursing* (3rd ed.). Philadelphia: W.B. Saunders, p. 861.

2. **Answer: 2**
Rationale: Polydipsia and polyuria are classic symptoms of diabetes insipidus. The urine is pale in color and its specific gravity is low. Anorexia and weight loss occur.
Test-Taking Strategy: Use the process of elimination. Eliminate option 4 first because this symptom is rather vague and occurs in many conditions. Knowledge of the manifestations of diabetes insipidus will assist in eliminating options 1 and 3. If you had difficulty with this question, review the clinical manifestations associated with diabetes insipidus.
Level of Cognitive Ability: Comprehension
Client Needs: Physiological Integrity
Integrated Process: Nursing Process/Data Collection
Content Area: Adult Health/Endocrine
Reference: Linton, A., & Maebius, N. (2003). *Introduction to medical-surgical nursing* (3rd ed.). Philadelphia: W.B. Saunders, p. 864.

3. **Answer: 3**
Rationale: Common manifestations of Addison's disease include postural hypotension from fluid loss, syncope, muscle weakness, anorexia, nausea and vomiting, abdominal cramps, weight loss, depression, and irritability.
Test-Taking Strategy: Knowledge regarding the clinical manifestations associated with Addison's disease is required to answer this question. Remember that hypotension occurs in Addison's disease. If you had difficulty with this question, review this endocrine disorder.
Level of Cognitive Ability: Comprehension
Client Needs: Physiological Integrity
Integrated Process: Nursing Process/Data Collection
Content Area: Adult Health/Endocrine
Reference: Linton, A., & Maebius, N. (2003). *Introduction to medical-surgical nursing* (3rd ed.). Philadelphia: W.B. Saunders, p. 870.

4. **Answer: 4**
Rationale: The client with Cushing's syndrome should be reassured that most physical changes resolve with treatment. Options 1, 2, and 3 are not therapeutic responses.
Test-Taking Strategy: Use knowledge regarding the physical changes that occur in Cushing's syndrome and therapeutic communication techniques to answer this question. Options 1, 2, and 3 are not therapeutic responses to a client. Review this disorder and therapeutic communication techniques if you had difficulty with this question.
Level of Cognitive Ability: Application
Client Needs: Psychosocial Integrity
Integrated Process: Communication and Documentation
Content Area: Adult Health/Endocrine
Reference: Linton, A., & Maebius, N. (2003). *Introduction to medical-surgical nursing* (3rd ed.). Philadelphia: W.B. Saunders, p. 876.

5. **Answer: 4**
Rationale: Because of the hypermetabolic state, the client with Graves' disease needs to be provided with an environment that is restful both physically and mentally. Six full meals a day that are well balanced and high in calories are required because of the accelerated metabolic rate. Foods that increase peristalsis, such as high-fiber foods, need to be avoided. These clients suffer from heat intolerance and require a cool environment.
Test-Taking Strategy: The key concept to bear in mind when answering this question is that clients with Graves' disease experience an accelerated metabolic rate. This concept should assist in eliminating options 1, 2, and 3. Review care of the client with Graves' disease if you had difficulty with this question.
Level of Cognitive Ability: Application
Client Needs: Physiological Integrity

Integrated Process: Nursing Process/Planning
Content Area: Adult Health/Endocrine
Reference: Linton, A., & Maebius, N. (2003). *Introduction to medical-surgical nursing* (3rd ed.). Philadelphia: W.B. Saunders, pp. 883; 890.

6. *Answer:* 4
Rationale: Hypocalcemia can develop after thyroidectomy if the parathyroid glands are accidentally removed during surgery. Manifestations develop 1 to 7 days after surgery. If the client develops numbness and tingling around the mouth, fingertips or toes, muscle spasms, or twitching, the physician is notified immediately. Calcium gluconate should be kept at the bedside.
Test-Taking Strategy: Noting the name of the medication (calcium gluconate) should easily direct you to option 4. Calcium is given if hypocalcemic tetany occurs. Review this medication if you had difficulty with this question.
Level of Cognitive Ability: Analysis
Client Needs: Physiological Integrity
Integrated Process: Nursing Process/Planning
Content Area: Pharmacology
Reference: Linton, A., & Maebius, N. (2003) *Introduction to medical-surgical nursing* (3rd ed.). Philadelphia: W.B. Saunders, p. 886.

7. *Answer:* 2
Rationale: Weakness and hoarseness of the voice can occur as a result of trauma of the laryngeal nerve. If this develops, the client should be reassured that the problem will subside in a few days. Unnecessary talking should be discouraged. It is not necessary to notify the registered nurse immediately. These signs do not indicate bleeding or the need to administer calcium gluconate.
Test-Taking Strategy: Use the process of elimination. Options 3 and 4 can easily be eliminated, because they are unrelated to the signs presented in the question. From the remaining options recall that these signs indicate a temporary condition. Review the expected findings following thyroidectomy if you had difficulty with this question.
Level of Cognitive Ability: Application
Client Needs: Physiological Integrity
Integrated Process: Nursing Process/Implementation
Content Area: Adult Health/Endocrine
Reference: Black, J., & Hawks, J. (2005). *Medical-surgical nursing: Clinical management for positive outcomes* (7th ed.). Philadelphia: W.B. Saunders, p. 1203.

8. *Answer:* 3
Rationale: The initial nursing action would be to maintain a patent airway. Oxygen would be administered, followed by fluid replacement, keeping the client warm, monitoring vital signs, and administering thyroid hormones.
Test-Taking Strategy: Note the key words, *carry out initially*. All the options are appropriate interventions, but use of the ABCs—airway, breathing, and circulation—will direct you to option 3. Review care of the client with myxedema coma if you had difficulty with this question.
Level of Cognitive Ability: Application
Client Needs: Physiological Integrity

Integrated Process: Nursing Process/Implementation
Content Area: Delegating/Prioritizing
Reference: Black, J., & Hawks, J. (2005). *Medical-surgical nursing: Clinical management for positive outcomes* (7th ed.). Philadelphia: W.B. Saunders, p. 1196.

9. *Answer:* 2
Rationale: NPH is an intermediate-acting insulin. The onset of action is 1 to 2 hours, it peaks in 6 to 14 hours, and its duration of action is 24 hours. Hypoglycemic reactions most likely occur during peak time.
Test-Taking Strategy: Knowledge regarding the onset, peak, and duration of action for NPH insulin is required to answer this question. Remember, hypoglycemic reactions most likely occur during peak time. Review the characteristics of NPH insulin if you had difficulty with this question.
Level of Cognitive Ability: Application
Client Needs: Health Promotion and Maintenance
Integrated Process: Teaching/Learning
Content Area: Pharmacology
References: Linton, A., & Maebius, N. (2003) *Introduction to medical-surgical nursing* (3rd ed.). Philadelphia: W.B. Saunders, p. 908.
McKenry, L. & Salerno, E. (2003). *Mosby's pharmacology in nursing* (21st ed.). St. Louis: Mosby, p. 864.

10. *Answer:* 2
Rationale: The client should use a moisturizing lotion on his or her feet and avoid applying lotion between the toes. The client should also be instructed not to soak the feet and to avoid hot water to prevent burns. The client may cut toenails straight and even with the toe itself, and would consult a podiatrist if the toenails were thick, hard to cut, or if vision is poor. The client should be instructed to wash the feet daily using a mild soap.
Test-Taking Strategy: Use the process of elimination. Eliminate option 3 first because of the word "always" and option 1 because of the word "hot." From the remaining options, recalling the concern related to skin infection will assist in eliminating option 4. Review diabetic foot care instructions if you had difficulty with this question.
Level of Cognitive Ability: Application
Client Needs: Health Promotion and Maintenance
Integrated Process: Nursing Process/Planning
Content Area: Adult Health/Endocrine
References: Linton, A., & Maebius, N. (2003) *Introduction to medical-surgical nursing* (3rd ed.). Philadelphia: W.B. Saunders, p. 904.
Phipps, W., Monahan, F., Sands, J., Marek, J., & Neighbors, M. (2003). *Medical-surgical nursing: Health and illness perspectives* (7th ed.). St. Louis: Mosby, p. 968.

11. *Answer:* 3
Rationale: It is important to emphasize to the client and family that they are not eating a diabetic diet but rather following a balanced meal plan. Adherence to nutrition principles is an important component of diabetic management, and an individualized meal plan should be developed for the client. It is not necessary for the client to purchase special dietetic foods.

Test-Taking Strategy: Note the key words, *indicates a need for further teaching.* These words indicate a false response question and that you need to select the incorrect client statement. Basic principles related to the diabetic diet will direct you to option 3. Review these principles if you had difficulty with this question.
Level of Cognitive Ability: Comprehension
Client Needs: Health Promotion and Maintenance
Integrated Process: Teaching/Learning
Content Area: Adult Health/Endocrine
Reference: Linton, A., & Maebius, N. (2003). *Introduction to medical-surgical nursing* (3rd ed.). Philadelphia: W.B. Saunders, p. 906.

12. *Answer:* 1
Rationale: An insulin pump provides a small continuous dose of regular insulin subcutaneously throughout the day and night, and the client can self-administer an additional dose from the pump before each meal as needed. Regular insulin is used in an insulin pump. An external pump is not surgically attached to the pancreas.
Test-Taking Strategy: Use the process of elimination. Recalling that regular insulin is used in an insulin pump will assist in eliminating options 2 and 4. Careful reading of the question, noting the word "external," will assist in eliminating option 3. Review the use of the insulin pump if you are unfamiliar with it.
Level of Cognitive Ability: Application
Client Needs: Physiological Integrity
Integrated Process: Nursing Process/Planning
Content Area: Adult Health/Endocrine
Reference: Lewis, S., Heitkemper, M., & Dirksen, S. (2004). *Medical-surgical nursing: Assessment and management of clinical problems* (6th ed.). St. Louis: Mosby, pp. 1276-1277.

13. *Answer:* 4
Rationale: Insulin dosages should not be adjusted nor increased prior to unusual exercise. If acetone is found in the urine, it may possibly indicate the need for additional insulin. To minimize the discomfort associated with insulin injections, insulin should be administered at room temperature. Injection sites should be systematically rotated from one area to another. The client should be instructed to give injections in one area, about 1 inch apart, until the whole area has been used, and then change to another site. This prevents dramatic changes in daily insulin absorption.
Test-Taking Strategy: Use the process of elimination. Eliminate option 3 first because of the word "always." Knowledge regarding insulin administration and the significance of acetone in the urine will assist in eliminating options 1 and 2. If you had difficulty with this question, review insulin management.
Level of Cognitive Ability: Application
Client Needs: Health Promotion and Maintenance
Integrated Process: Nursing Process/Planning
Content Area: Pharmacology
Reference: McKenry, L., & Salerno, E. (2003). *Mosby's pharmacology in nursing* (21st ed.). St. Louis: Mosby, p. 863.

14. *Answer:* 2
Rationale: Shakiness is a sign of hypoglycemia and would indicate the need for food or glucose. A fruity breath odor, blurred vision, and polyuria are signs of hyperglycemia.

Test-Taking Strategy: Knowledge regarding the signs and symptoms of hypoglycemia and hyperglycemia is required to answer this question. If you are unfamiliar with these signs, be sure to learn them.
Level of Cognitive Ability: Comprehension
Client Needs: Health Promotion and Maintenance
Integrated Process: Nursing Process/Evaluation
Content Area: Adult Health/Endocrine
Reference: Linton, A., & Maebius, N. (2003). *Introduction to medical-surgical nursing* (3rd ed.). Philadelphia: W.B. Saunders, p. 921.

15. *Answer:* 4
Rationale: The appropriate intervention is to address the client's feelings related to the anxiety. Administering a sedative is not the most appropriate intervention. The nurse should not ignore the client's anxious feelings. A client will not relate to medical terms, particularly when anxiety exists.
Test-Taking Strategy: Use therapeutic communication techniques to answer the question. Remember that client's feelings come first. Keeping this in mind will direct you to option 4. Review these techniques if you had difficulty with this question.
Level of Cognitive Ability: Application
Client Needs: Psychosocial Integrity
Integrated Process: Caring
Content Area: Adult Health/Endocrine
Reference: Potter, P., & Perry, A. (2005). *Fundamentals of nursing* (6th ed.). St. Louis: Mosby, pp. 437-440.

16. *Answer:* 3
Rationale: During illness, the client should monitor the blood glucose level and should notify the physician if the level is higher than 250 mg/dL. Insulin should never be stopped. In fact, insulin may need to be increased during times of illness. Doses should not be adjusted without the physician's advice.
Test-Taking Strategy: Use the process of elimination. Note that options 1, 2, and 4 all relate to adjustment of insulin doses. Therefore, eliminate these options. Review diabetic management during illness if you had difficulty with this question.
Level of Cognitive Ability: Comprehension
Client Needs: Health Promotion and Maintenance
Integrated Process: Teaching/Learning
Content Area: Adult Health/Endocrine
Reference: Linton, A., & Maebius, N. (2003). *Introduction to medical-surgical nursing* (3rd ed.). Philadelphia: W.B. Saunders, p. 905.

17. *Answer:* 2
Rationale: Levothyroxine is a synthetic thyroid hormone that increases cellular metabolism. It should be given in the morning in a single dose to prevent sleeplessness and should be given at the same time each day to maintain a drug level.
Test-Taking Strategy: Use the process of elimination. Options 1 and 3 can be eliminated, because the nurse cannot change or alter a physician's order. From the remaining options, use principles related to medication administration to direct you to option 2. Review this medication if you had difficulty with this question.

Level of Cognitive Ability: Application
Client Needs: Physiological Integrity
Integrated Process: Nursing Process/Implementation
Content Area: Adult Health/Endocrine
References: McKenry, L., & Salerno, E. (2003). *Mosby's pharmacology in nursing* (21st ed.). St. Louis: Mosby, pp. 842-844. Phipps, W., Monahan, F., Sands, J., Marek, J., & Neighbors, M. (2003). *Medical-surgical nursing: Health and illness perspectives* (7th ed.). St. Louis: Mosby, p. 903.

18. *Answer: 4*
Rationale: Chlorpropamide is an oral hypoglycemic agent administered to decrease the serum glucose level and the signs and symptoms of hyperglycemia. Therefore, a decrease in both polyuria and polyphagia would indicate a therapeutic response. Laboratory values are also used to assess a client's response to treatment. A blood glucose level of 110 mg/dL is within normal limits. However, a glycosylated hemoglobin of 18% indicates poor glycemic control.
Test-Taking Strategy: Note the key words, *ineffective therapeutic outcome.* Recalling that chlorpropamide is an oral hypoglycemic agent tells you to look for an option that would indicate hyperglycemia (lack of response to the medication). Options 1 and 3 are similar and are eliminated first. Next, eliminate option 2 because it is a normal blood glucose level. Review this medication if you had difficulty with this question.
Level of Cognitive Ability: Analysis
Client Needs: Physiological Integrity
Integrated Process: Nursing Process/Evaluation
Content Area: Adult Health/Endocrine
Reference: Lehne, R. (2004). *Pharmacology for nursing care* (5th ed.). Philadelphia: W.B. Saunders, p. 612.

19. *Answer: 3*
Rationale: The classic symptoms of hyperglycemia include polydipsia, polyuria, and polyphagia. Options 1, 2, and 4 are not signs of hyperglycemia.
Test-Taking Strategy: Focus on the issue, hyperglycemia. Remember the 3 P's—polyuria, polydipsia, polyphagia. Review the signs of hyperglycemia if you had difficulty with this question.
Level of Cognitive Ability: Comprehension
Client Needs: Physiological Integrity
Integrated Process: Nursing Process/Data Collection
Content Area: Adult Health/Endocrine
Reference: Linton, A., & Maebius, N. (2003) *Introduction to medical-surgical nursing* (3rd ed.). Philadelphia: W.B. Saunders, p. 900.

20. *Answer: 3*
Rationale: Client education following DKA should emphasize the need for home glucose monitoring two to four times per day. It is also important to instruct the client to notify the health care provider when illness occurs. The presence of urinary ketones indicates that DKA has already occurred. The client should eat well-balanced meals with snacks as prescribed.
Test-Taking Strategy: Focus on the issue, preventing DKA. Recall that the treatment of DKA focuses on maintenance of an appropriate blood glucose level. Option 1 is not an accurate component of diabetic care. Option 2 will not prevent DKA, and option 4 does not prevent DKA but actually confirms the diagnosis. Review this complication of diabetes mellitus if you had difficulty with this question.
Level of Cognitive Ability: Application
Client Needs: Health Promotion and Maintenance
Integrated Process: Teaching/Learning
Content Area: Adult Health/Endocrine
Reference: Linton, A., & Maebius, N. (2003). *Introduction to medical-surgical nursing* (3rd ed.). Philadelphia: W.B. Saunders, p. 906.

21. *Answer: 2.*
Rationale: Clients with type 2 diabetes mellitus have decreased or impaired insulin secretion. Oral hypoglycemic agents are given to these clients to facilitate glucose utilization. Insulin injections may be given during times of stress-induced hyperglycemia. Oral insulin is not available or effective because of the breakdown of the insulin by digestion.
Test-Taking Strategy: Focus on the issue, type 2 diabetes mellitus. Eliminate option 1 because there is no "oral insulin." Next, eliminate options 3 and 4 because they are not accepted treatment for diabetes mellitus. Review the treatment for diabetes mellitus if you had difficulty with this question.
Level of Cognitive Ability: Comprehension
Client Needs: Health Promotion and Maintenance
Integrated Process: Nursing Process/Evaluation
Content Area: Adult Health/Endocrine
Reference: Linton, A., & Maebius, N. (2003) *Introduction to medical-surgical nursing* (3rd ed.). Philadelphia: W.B. Saunders, p. 912.

22. *Answer: 2*
Rationale: Reinforcement of knowledge and behaviors is vital to the success of the client's self-care. Option 1 may devalue a client's family. Option 3 places the issue on hold, and option 4 requests an explanation by the client. Option 2 clarifies previous information.
Test-Taking Strategy: Focus on the data in the question. Use therapeutic communication techniques to answer the question. This will direct you to option 2. Review these techniques if you had difficulty with this question.
Level of Cognitive Ability: Application
Client Needs: Psychosocial Integrity
Integrated Process: Communication and Documentation
Content Area: Adult Health/Endocrine
Reference: Potter, P., & Perry, A. (2005). *Fundamentals of nursing* (6th ed.). St. Louis: Mosby, pp. 437-440.

23. *Answer: 4*
Rationale: A diet low in calories, carbohydrates, and sodium, but ample in protein and potassium content, is encouraged for a client with Cushing's syndrome. Such a diet promotes weight loss, reduction of edema and hypertension, control of hypokalemia, and rebuilding of wasted tissue.
Test-Taking Strategy: Note the key words, *instructions related to dietary management were understood.* Eliminate option 1 because it indicates that no dietary change is necessary. Eliminate option 2 next, because protein is usually only

limited with renal disorders. Excess sodium is not healthy in general, so eliminate option 3. Review dietary management of Cushing's syndrome if you had difficulty with this question.
Level of Cognitive Ability: Comprehension
Client Needs: Health Promotion and Maintenance
Integrated Process: Nursing Process/Evaluation
Content Area: Adult Health/Endocrine
Reference: Linton, A., & Maebius, N. (2003). *Introduction to medical-surgical nursing* (3rd ed.). Philadelphia: W.B. Saunders, p. 877.

24. *Answer:* **1**
Rationale: A hypoglycemic reaction may occur in response to increased exercise. Clients should avoid exercise during the peak time of insulin. NPH insulin peaks at 6 to 14 hours; therefore, late afternoon exercise will occur during the peak of the medication.
Test-Taking Strategy: Use the process of elimination and note the key words, *inadequate understanding*. Recalling the peak time of insulin will direct you to option 1. Review the measures to prevent hypoglycemia if you had difficulty with this question.
Level of Cognitive Ability: Comprehension
Client Needs: Health Promotion and Maintenance
Integrated Process: Teaching/Learning
Content Area: Adult Health/Endocrine
References: Lewis, S., Heitkemper, M., & Dirksen, S. (2004). *Medical-surgical nursing: Assessment and management of clinical problems* (6th ed.). St. Louis: Mosby, pp. 1282-1283.
Linton, A., & Maebius, N. (2003). *Introduction to medical-surgical nursing* (3rd ed.). Philadelphia: W.B. Saunders, p. 913.

25. *Answer:* **2**
Rationale: Hypercalcemia is the hallmark of hyperparathyroidism. Elevated serum calcium levels produce osmotic diuresis (polyuria). This diuresis leads to dehydration and the client would lose weight. Both options 1 and 3 are gastrointestinal (GI) symptoms but are not associated with the common GI symptoms typical of hyperparathyroidism (nausea, vomiting, anorexia, constipation).
Test-Taking Strategy: Use the process of elimination. Note that options 1, 3, and 4 are similar and are all GI symptoms. Review the characteristics of hyperparathyroidism if you had difficulty with this question.
Level of Cognitive Ability: Analysis
Client Needs: Physiological Integrity
Integrated Process: Nursing Process/Data Collection
Content Area: Adult Health/Endocrine
Reference: Linton, A., & Maebius, N. (2003). *Introduction to medical-surgical nursing* (3rd ed.). Philadelphia: W.B. Saunders, p. 894.

26. *Answer:* **3**
Rationale: During the postoperative period, the nurse carefully observes the client for signs of hemorrhage, which cause swelling and compression of adjacent tissue. Laryngeal stridor is a harsh, high-pitched sound heard on inspiration and expiration caused by compression of the trachea leading to respiratory distress. It is an acute emergency situation that requires immediate attention to avoid complete obstruction of the airway.
Test-Taking Strategy: Consider the anatomical location of the surgical procedure and use the ABCs—airway, breathing, and circulation—to select the correct option. Options 1, 2, and 4 are usual postoperative problems that are not life-threatening. Option 3 addresses the airway. Review care of the client following parathyroidectomy if you had difficulty with this question.
Level of Cognitive Ability: Analysis
Client Needs: Physiological Integrity
Integrated Process: Nursing Process/Data Collection
Content Area: Adult Health/Endocrine
Reference: Black, J., & Hawks, J. (2005). *Medical-surgical nursing: Clinical management for positive outcomes* (7th ed.). Philadelphia: W.B. Saunders, p. 1213.

27. *Answer:* **3**
Rationale: Oral calcium supplements need to be taken 30 to 60 minutes after meals to enhance their absorption and decrease gastrointestinal irritation. All the other options are unrelated to oral calcium therapy.
Test-Taking Strategy: Knowledge regarding the administration of calcium is required to answer this question. Eliminate those options that seem unusual. Checking the pulse is usually done for cardiac medications. Avoidance of sunlight and refrigeration of tablets are required for some medications, but is not a common intervention. Review this medication if you had difficulty with this question.
Level of Cognitive Ability: Application
Client Needs: Health Promotion and Maintenance
Integrated Process: Teaching/Learning
Content Area: Adult Health/Endocrine
Reference: Hodgson, B., & Kizior, R. (2005). *Saunders nursing drug handbook 2005*. Philadelphia: W.B. Saunders, p. 155.

28. *Answer:* **2**
Rationale: Lipodystrophy (hypertrophy of subcutaneous tissue at the injection site) occurs in some diabetic clients when the same injection sites are used for prolonged periods of time. Thus, clients are instructed to adhere to a rotating injection site plan to avoid tissue changes. Cleansing with alcohol, aspiration, and angle of insulin administration does not produce tissue damage.
Test-Taking Strategy: Recalling the definition of lipodystrophy will direct you to the correct option. If you are unfamiliar with this complication of insulin therapy, review this component of diabetic teaching.
Level of Cognitive Ability: Application
Client Needs: Physiological Integrity
Integrated Process: Nursing Process/Data Collection
Content Area: Adult Health/Endocrine
Reference: Linton, A., & Maebius, N. (2003). *Introduction to medical-surgical nursing* (3rd ed.). Philadelphia: W.B. Saunders, p. 910.

29. *Answer:* **4**
Rationale: Decreased blood glucose levels produce automatic nervous system symptoms, which are classically manifested as nervousness, irritability, and tremors. Option 1 is more likely

to occur with hyperglycemia. Options 2 and 3 are unrelated to the signs of hypoglycemia.

Test-Taking Strategy: Focus on the issue, a hypoglycemic reaction. Recalling the signs associated with this reaction will direct you to option 4. Review this complication if you had difficulty with this question.

Level of Cognitive Ability: Comprehension
Client Needs: Physiological Integrity
Integrated Process: Nursing Process/Data Collection
Content Area: Adult Health/Endocrine
Reference: Linton, A., & Maebius, N. (2003). *Introduction to medical-surgical nursing* (3rd ed.). Philadelphia: W.B. Saunders, p. 921.

30. **Answer: 3**
Rationale: Hypoglycemic reactions present adrenergic symptoms of tremor, shakiness, and nervousness, which are similar to those of alcohol intoxication. The best action to deal with this client's psychosocial need is to identify and then eliminate those factors that precipitate these types of reactions. Option 1 presumes that the problem is unavoidable and thus the client is at fault. Option 2 is nontherapeutic, because it presumes that the client may be drinking, and option 4 avoids the psychosocial aspects of the client's problem.

Test-Taking Strategy: Use the process of elimination. Note the relationship between the issue, "hypoglycemic reactions," and option 3. Review the psychosocial issues related to the complications of diabetes mellitus if you had difficulty with this question.

Level of Cognitive Ability: Application
Client Needs: Psychosocial Integrity
Integrated Process: Nursing Process/Implementation
Content Area: Adult Health/Endocrine
Reference: Linton, A., & Maebius, N. (2003). *Introduction to medical-surgical nursing* (3rd ed.). Philadelphia: W.B. Saunders, pp. 921-922.

31. **Answer: 3**
Rationale: Fluids containing both glucose and electrolytes should be offered to the client every hour. Small amounts of fluid may be tolerated, even when vomiting is present. Water alone is insufficient. Withholding all fluids is inappropriate. A clear liquid diet for 5 days is inappropriate.

Test-Taking Strategy: Use the process of elimination. Eliminate options 1 and 2 because of the words "only" and "all." The time frame in option 4 seems unreasonable; therefore, select option 3. Review care of the diabetic client during illness if you had difficulty with this question.

Level of Cognitive Ability: Application
Client Needs: Physiological Integrity
Integrated Process: Nursing Process/Implementation
Content Area: Adult Health/Endocrine
Reference: Black, J., & Hawks, J. (2005). *Medical-surgical nursing: Clinical management for positive outcomes* (7th ed.). Philadelphia: W.B. Saunders, p. 1286.

32. **Answer: 1**
Rationale: Manifestations of hypothyroidism include cold intolerance, constipation, loss of initiative, thick dry skin,

a notably puffy appearance of the skin around the eyes, slowed intellectual function, including retarded speech and apathy, and a low metabolic rate. Levothyroxine is used to correct hypothyroidism. In this situation, the dosage is subtherapeutic and needs to be increased.

Test-Taking Strategy: Note the key words, *currently taking levothyroxine*. Recalling that the signs presented in the question relate to the manifestations associated with hypothyroidism will direct you to option 1. Review this medication and the signs of hypothyroidism if you had difficulty with this question.

Level of Cognitive Ability: Analysis
Client Needs: Physiological Integrity
Integrated Process: Nursing Process/Planning
Content Area: Adult Health/Endocrine
Reference: McKenry, L., & Salerno, E. (2003). *Mosby's pharmacology in nursing* (21st ed.). St. Louis: Mosby, pp. 840-841.

33. **Answer: 2**
Rationale: Vasopressin, an antidiuretic hormone, causes increased gastrointestinal smooth muscle tone and contractions, increased reabsorption of water by the renal tubules, and vasoconstriction with reduced blood flow in coronary, peripheral, cerebral, and pulmonary vessels.

Test-Taking Strategy: Note the key word, *therapeutic*, in the stem of the question. Recalling the pathophysiology related to diabetes insipidus and the associated clinical manifestations will direct you to the correct option. If you had difficulty with this question, review this disorder.

Level of Cognitive Ability: Analysis
Client Needs: Physiological Integrity
Integrated Process: Nursing Process/Evaluation
Content Area: Adult Health/Endocrine
Reference: McKenry, L., & Salerno, E. (2003). *Mosby's pharmacology in nursing* (21st ed.). St. Louis: Mosby, p. 833.

34. **Answer: 2**
Rationale: Pheochromocytoma is a catecholamine-producing tumor of the adrenal gland and causes secretion of excessive amounts of epinephrine and norepinephrine. Hypertension is the principal manifestation, and the client has episodes of a high blood pressure accompanied by pounding headaches. The excessive release of catecholamine also results in excessive conversion of glycogen into glucose in the liver. Consequently, hyperglycemia and glucosuria occur during attacks. Pheochromocytoma is curable. The primary treatment is surgical removal of one or both of the adrenal glands, depending on whether the tumor is unilateral or bilateral.

Test-Taking Strategy: Knowledge regarding the pathophysiology associated with pheochromocytoma is required to answer this question. Remember, pheochromocytoma is a catecholamine-producing tumor and causes secretion of excessive amounts of epinephrine and norepinephrine. Review this disorder if you had difficulty with this question.

Level of Cognitive Ability: Comprehension
Client Needs: Physiological Integrity
Integrated Process: Nursing Process/Planning
Content Area: Adult Health/Endocrine

Reference: Linton, A.. & Maebius, N. (2003). *Introduction to medical-surgical nursing* (3rd ed.). Philadelphia: W.B. Saunders, p. 877.

35. *Answer:* 4

Rationale: Hypertension is the major symptom associated with pheochromocytoma. The blood pressure status is monitored by taking the client's blood pressure. Glycosuria, weight loss, and diaphoresis are also clinical manifestations of pheochromocytoma, but hypertension is the major symptom.

Test-Taking Strategy: Note the key words, *major symptom*. Use the principles associated with prioritizing and the ABCs—airway, breathing, and circulation. A method of assessing circulation is to take the blood pressure. Review the manifestations of this disorder if you had difficulty with this question.

Level of Cognitive Ability: Application
Client Needs: Physiological Integrity
Integrated Process: Nursing Process/Data Collection
Content Area: Adult Health/Endocrine
Reference: Linton, A., & Maebius, N. (2003). *Introduction to medical-surgical nursing* (3rd ed.). Philadelphia: W.B. Saunders, p. 877.

36. *Answer:* 1

Rationale: Hypertension is the hallmark of pheochromocytoma. Severe hypertension can precipitate a cerebrovascular accident or sudden blindness. Although all the options are accurate nursing interventions for the client with pheochromocytoma, the priority nursing action is to monitor the vital signs, particularly the blood pressure.

Test-Taking Strategy: Note the key words, *priority nursing action*. Use the ABCs—airway, breathing, and circulation. Monitoring vital signs is the nursing action that would assess airway, breathing, and circulation. Also, note that options 2, 3, and 4 all refer to assessment of the renal system. Review care of the client with pheochromocytoma if you had difficulty with this question.

Level of Cognitive Ability: Application
Client Needs: Physiological Integrity
Integrated Process: Nursing Process/Implementation
Content Area: Delegating/Prioritizing
Reference: Linton, A., & Maebius, N. (2003). *Introduction to medical-surgical nursing* (3rd ed.). Philadelphia: W.B. Saunders, p. 877.

37. *Answer:* 1

Rationale: The client with pheochromocytoma needs to be provided with a diet high in vitamins, minerals, and calories. Of particular importance is that food or beverages that contain caffeine, such as chocolate, coffee, tea, or cola, are prohibited. Cocoa, tea, and coffee are caffeine-containing products.

Test-Taking Strategy: Use the process of elimination. Eliminate options 2, 3, and 4 because they are similar and include food items that contain caffeine. Review dietary measures for the client with pheochromocytoma if you had difficulty with this question.

Level of Cognitive Ability: Application
Client Needs: Physiological Integrity
Integrated Process: Nursing Process/Implementation

Content Area: Adult Health/Endocrine
Reference: Christensen, B., & Kockrow, E. (2003). *Adult health nursing* (4th ed.). St. Louis: Mosby, p. 474.

38. *Answer:* 2

Rationale: The complications associated with pheochromocytoma include hypertensive retinopathy and nephropathy, myocarditis, congestive heart failure (CHF), increased platelet aggregation, and cerebrovascular accident (CVA). Death can occur from shock, CVA, renal failure, dysrhythmias, or dissecting aortic aneurysm. Congestion heard on auscultation of the lungs are indicative of CHF. A urinary output of 50 mL/hour is an appropriate output; the nurse would become concerned if the output were below 30 mL/hour. A BUN level of 20 mg/dL is a normal finding. A coagulation time of 5 minutes is normal.

Test-Taking Strategy: Use the ABCs—airway, breathing, and circulation. Congestion heard on auscultation of the lungs is associated with airway. Additionally, if you know the normal hourly urinary output and the normal laboratory values for coagulation time and the BUN level, you can determine that option 2 is correct by the process of elimination. Review the complications associated with pheochromocytoma if you had difficulty with this question.

Level of Cognitive Ability: Analysis
Client Needs: Physiological Integrity
Integrated Process: Nursing Process/Data Collection
Content Area: Adult Health/Endocrine
Reference: Christensen, B., & Kockrow, E. (2003). *Adult health nursing* (4th ed.). St. Louis: Mosby, p. 473.

39. *Answer:* 1

Rationale: Paraphrasing is restating the client's message in the nurse's own words. Option 1 addresses the therapeutic communication technique of paraphrasing. The client is reaching out for understanding. In option 2, the nurse is offering a false reassurance and this type of response will block communication. Option 3 also represents a communication block because it reflects a lack of the client's right to an opinion. In option 4, the nurse is expressing approval, which can be harmful to a nurse-client relationship.

Test-Taking Strategy: Use therapeutic communication techniques and always address the client's concerns and feelings. Option 1 is the only therapeutic option. Review these techniques if you had difficulty with this question.

Level of Cognitive Ability: Application
Client Needs: Psychosocial Integrity
Integrated Process: Communication and Documentation
Content Area: Adult Health/Endocrine
Reference: Potter, P., & Perry, A. (2005). *Fundamentals of nursing* (6th ed.). St. Louis: Mosby, pp. 437-440.

40. *Answer:* 3

Rationale: Clinical manifestations associated with thyroid storm include a fever as high as 106° F (41.1° C), severe tachycardia, profuse diarrhea, extreme vasodilation, hypotension, atrial fibrillation, hyperreflexia, abdominal pain, diarrhea, and dehydration. In this disorder, the client's condition can rapidly progress to coma and cardiovascular collapse.

Test-Taking Strategy: Knowledge regarding the manifestations associated with thyroid storm is required to answer the question. Remember, this condition is a rare but potentially fatal hypermetabolic state. If you are unfamiliar with this disorder, review the content.

Level of Cognitive Ability: Comprehension
Client Needs: Physiological Integrity
Integrated Process: Nursing Process/Data Collection
Content Area: Adult Health/Endocrine
Reference: Lewis, S., Heitkemper, M., & Dirksen, S. (2004). *Medical-surgical nursing: Assessment and management of clinical problems* (6th ed.). St. Louis: Mosby, p. 312.

ALTERNATE FORMAT QUESTION: PRIORITIZING (ORDERED RESPONSE)

Answer: 21345
Rationale: The client is experiencing symptoms of mild hypoglycemia. If symptoms such as hunger, irritability, shakiness, or weakness occur, the nurse would first check the client's blood glucose level to verify that the client is experiencing hypoglycemia. Once this is verified, the nurse would give the client 10 to 15 g of a carbohydrate. The nurse would retest the blood glucose in 15 minutes. In the meantime, the nurse would check the client's vital signs. The nurse would give the client another 10- to 15-g carbohydrate food item if the client's symptoms do not resolve. Otherwise, the nurse would provide a small snack of carbohydrate and protein if the client's next scheduled meal is more than an hour away from the time of occurrence of these symptoms. Following treatment and resolution of the hypoglycemic event, the nurse would document the occurrence, actions taken, and outcome.

Test-Taking Strategy: Focus on the client's symptoms. Noting that the client is hospitalized will assist in determining that the first action would be to check the client's blood glucose level. Once this has been done, it is necessary to treat the hypoglycemia. Recalling that an outcome cannot be determined until treatment has been instituted will assist in selecting the documentation action as the last action. From the remaining two actions, select taking the vital signs as the third action. The nurse would not give the client a carbohydrate and protein food item immediately after giving the client a 10- to 15-g carbohydrate item. Review management of hypoglycemia if you had difficulty with this question.

Level of Cognitive Ability: Application
Client Needs: Physiological Integrity
Integrated Process: Nursing Process/Implementation
Content Area: Delegating/Prioritizing
Reference: Ignatavicius, D., & Workman, M. (2006). *Medical surgical nursing: Critical thinking for collaborative care* (5th ed.). Philadelphia: W.B. Saunders, p. 1541.

REFERENCES

Black, J., & Hawks, J. (2005). *Medical-surgical nursing: Clinical management for positive outcomes* (7th ed.). Philadelphia: W.B. Saunders.

Christensen, B., & Kockrow, E. (2003). *Adult health nursing* (4th ed.). St. Louis: Mosby.

Hodgson, B., & Kizior, R. (2005). *Saunders nursing drug handbook 2005*. Philadelphia: W.B. Saunders.

Lehne, R. (2004). *Pharmacology for nursing care* (5th ed.). Philadelphia: W.B. Saunders.

Lewis, S., Heitkemper, M., & Dirksen, S. (2004). *Medical-surgical nursing: Assessment and management of clinical problems* (6th ed.). St. Louis: Mosby.

Linton, A., & Maebius, N. (2003). *Introduction to medical-surgical nursing* (3rd ed.). Philadelphia: W.B. Saunders.

McKenry, L., & Salerno, E. (2003). *Mosby's pharmacology in nursing* (21st ed.). St. Louis: Mosby.

Phipps, W., Monahan, F., Sands, J., Marek, J., & Neighbors, M. (2003). *Medical-surgical nursing: Health and illness perspectives* (7th ed.). St. Louis: Mosby.

Potter, P., & Perry, A. (2005). *Fundamentals of nursing* (6th ed.). St. Louis: Mosby.

Endocrine Medications

I. PITUITARY MEDICATIONS

A. Description
1. Anterior pituitary gland: Secretes growth hormone (GH), thyroid-stimulating hormone (TSH), adrenocorticotropic hormone (ACTH), and gonadotropins (follicle-stimulating hormone, FSH, and luteinizing hormone, LH)
2. Posterior pituitary gland: Secretes antidiuretic hormones (ADH, vasopressin) and oxytocin

B. Growth hormones and related medications
1. Uses and side effects (Table 45-1)
2. Interventions
   a. Assess child's physical growth and compare growth with standards
   b. Recommend annual bone age determinations for children receiving growth hormones
   c. Monitor blood and urine glucose levels
   d. Teach the client and family about the importance of follow-up regarding blood and urine glucose testing

II. ANTIDIURETIC HORMONES (Box 45-1)

A. Description
1. Enhance reabsorption of water in the kidneys, promoting an antidiuretic effect and regulating fluid balance
2. Used in **diabetes insipidus**

B. Side effects
1. Flushing
2. Headache
3. Nausea and abdominal cramps
4. Water intoxication
5. Hypertension with water intoxication
6. Nasal congestion with nasal administration

C. Interventions
1. Monitor weight
2. Monitor intake and output (I&O) and urine osmolality
3. Monitor electrolytes
4. Restrict fluid intake as prescribed to prevent water intoxication

TABLE 45-1

Growth Hormones and Related Medications

Medication(s)	Use	Side Effects
Somatrem (Protropin)	Growth failure (adults)	Development of antibodies to growth hormone (GH)
Somatropin (Humatrope)	Growth failure (children)	Headache, muscle pain, weakness, mild hyperglycemia, hypertension, allergic reaction (rash, swelling), pain at injection site
Bromocriptine (Parlodel)	Acromegaly	Nausea, headache, dizziness
Octreotide (Sandostatin)	Acromegaly	Diarrhea, nausea, abdominal discomfort, increased or decreased glucose level

5. Monitor for signs of water intoxication, such as drowsiness, listlessness, and headache
6. Monitor blood pressure
7. Instruct the client in how to use the intranasal medication
8. Instruct the client to report signs of water intoxication or symptoms of headache or shortness of breath

III. THYROID HORMONES (Box 45-2)

A. Description
 1. Control the metabolic rate of tissues and accelerate heat production and oxygen consumption
 2. Used to replace thyroid hormone deficit in the treatment of **hypothyroidism, myxedema,** or cretinism
 3. Enhance the action of oral anticoagulants, sympathomimetics, and antidepressants, and decrease the action of insulin, oral hypoglycemics, and digitalis preparations; the action of thyroid hormones is decreased by phenytoin (Dilantin) and carbamazepine (Tegretol)
 4. Should be given at least 4 hours apart from multivitamins, aluminum and magnesium hydroxide, simethicone, calcium carbonate, bile acid sequestrants, iron, and sucralfate, because these medications decrease the absorption of thyroid replacements

B. Side effects
 1. Nausea and decreased appetite
 2. Cramps and diarrhea
 3. Weight loss
 4. Nervousness and tremors
 5. Headache
 6. Hypertension
 7. Tachycardia and dysrhythmias
 8. Sweating and heat intolerance
 9. Insomnia
 10. Toxicity: **Hyperthyroidism**

C. Interventions
 1. Check with the client for a history of medications currently being taken
 2. Monitor vital signs
 3. Monitor weight
 4. Monitor triiodothyronine (T_3), thyroxine (T_4), and thyroid-stimulating hormone (TSH) levels
 5. Instruct the client to take the medication at the same time each day, preferably in the morning without food
 6. Instruct the client in how to monitor pulse rate
 7. Advise the client to report symptoms of **hyperthyroidism,** such as tachycardia, chest pain, palpitations, and excessive sweating
 8. Instruct the client to avoid foods that can inhibit thyroid secretion, such as strawberries, peaches, pears, cabbage, turnips, spinach, kale, brussels sprouts, cauliflower, radishes, and peas
 9. Advise the client to avoid over-the-counter medications
 10. Instruct the client to wear a Medic-Alert bracelet

IV. ANTITHYROID MEDICATIONS (Box 45-3)

A. Description
 1. Inhibit the synthesis of thyroid hormone
 2. Used for **hyperthyroidism,** or Graves' disease

B. Side effects
 1. Nausea and vomiting
 2. Diarrhea
 3. Hypersensitivity with skin rash
 4. Agranulocytosis with leukopenia
 5. Toxicity: **Hypothyroidism**
 6. Iodism: Characterized by vomiting, abdominal pain, metallic taste in the mouth, rash, and sore salivary glands

C. Interventions
 1. Monitor vital signs
 2. Monitor T_3, T_4, and TSH levels
 3. Monitor weight
 4. Instruct the client to take medication with meals to avoid gastrointestinal (GI) upset
 5. Instruct the client about how to monitor the pulse rate
 6. Inform the client of side effects and when to notify the physician
 7. Advise the client to contact the physician if a fever or sore throat develops
 8. Instruct the client in the signs of **hypothyroidism**

BOX 45-1

Antidiuretic Hormones

Desmopressin acetate (DDAVP, Stimate)
Vasopressin (Pitressin Synthetic)

BOX 45-2

Thyroid Hormones

Levothyroxine (Synthroid, Levothroid, Levoxyl)
Liothyronine (Cytomel)
Liotrix (Thyrolar)
Thyroid, desiccated (Thyrar)

BOX 45-3

Antithyroid Medications

Strong iodine solution (Lugol solution)
Methimazole (Tapazole)
Propylthiouracil (PTU)

9. Instruct the client regarding the importance of medication compliance and that abruptly stopping the medication could cause **thyroid storm**

10. Instruct the client to monitor for signs and symptoms of **thyroid storm** (fever, flushed skin, confusion and behavioral changes, tachycardia, dysrhythmias, and signs of heart failure)

11. Instruct the client to monitor for signs of iodism

12. Advise the client to consult physician before eating iodized salt and iodine-rich foods

13. Instruct the client to avoid acetylsalicylic acid (aspirin) and medications containing iodine

V. PARATHYROID MEDICATIONS (Box 45-4)

A. Description

1. Parathyroid hormone regulates serum calcium levels

2. Low serum levels of calcium stimulate parathyroid hormone release

3. Hyperparathyroidism results in a high serum calcium level and bone demineralization, and medication is used to lower the serum calcium level

4. Hypoparathyroidism results in a low serum calcium level, which increases neuromuscular excitability; treatment includes calcium and vitamin D supplements

5. Parathyroid and antihypercalcemic agents may cause hypermagnesemia

6. Calcium salts administered with digoxin (Lanoxin) increase the risk of digoxin toxicity

7. Oral calcium salts reduce the absorption of tetracycline hydrochloride

B. Interventions

1. Monitor electrolyte and calcium levels

2. Monitor for signs and symptoms of hypocalcemia and hypercalcemia

3. Monitor for symptoms of tetany in the client with hypocalcemia

4. Instruct the client in the signs and symptoms of hypercalcemia and hypocalcemia

5. Instruct the client to check over-the-counter medication labels for the possibility of calcium content

6. Instruct the client receiving oral calcium to maintain an adequate intake of vitamin D, because vitamin D enhances absorption of calcium

7. Instruct clients receiving calcium regulators such as alendronate sodium (Fosamax) to swallow tablet whole with water at least 30 minutes before breakfast and not to lie down for at least 30 minutes after taking medication

---

BOX 45-4

Medications to Treat Calcium Disorders

CALCIUM SUPPLEMENTS
Calcium carbonate (Caltrate 600, Rolaids, Tums)
Calcium carbonate, oyster-shell derived (Os-Cal 500, Oysco 500, Oyst-Cal 500)
Calcium citrate (Citracal)
Calcium glubionate (Calcionate, Neo-Calglucon)
Calcium gluconate
Calcium lactate
Dibasic calcium phosphate
Tribasic calcium phosphate (Posture)

VITAMIN D SUPPLEMENTS
Calcifediol (Calderol)
Calcitriol (Calcijex, Rocaltrol)
Dihydrotachysterol (DHT, Hytakerol)
Ergocalciferol (Calciferol, Drisdol)

CALCIUM REGULATORS
Alendronate (Fosamax)
Calcitonin human (Cibacalcin)
Calcitonin salmon (Calcimar, Miacalcin)
Etidronate (Didronel)
Pamidronate (Aredia)
Risedronate (Actonel)
Tiludronate (Skelid)

ANTIHYPERCALCEMICS
Gallium nitrate (Ganite)

VI. ADRENOCORTICOTROPIC HORMONES (ACTH) (Box 45-5)

A. Description

1. Stimulate the adrenal cortex to secrete cortisol

2. Produce an anti-inflammatory effect

3. Used to diagnose adrenocortical disorders (Box 45-6)

4. Used to treat acute multiple sclerosis

B. Side effects

1. Nausea and vomiting

2. Gastric irritation with tendency to develop peptic ulcer disease

---

BOX 45-5

Medications for Adrenal Replacement Therapy

Betamethasone (Celestone)
Cortisone (Cortone)
Fludrocortisone (Florinef)
Hydrocortisone (Cortef)
Triamcinolone (Aristocort, Kenacort)
Dexamethasone (Decadron)
Methylprednisolone (Medrol Dosepak, Depo-Medrol, Solu-Medrol)
Prednisolone (Delta-Cortef, Prelone, Orapred, Pediapred)
Prednisone (Orasone, Deltasone, Meticorten)

3. Mood swings
4. Petechiae
5. Water and sodium retention, hypertension
6. Hypokalemia
7. Hypocalcemia, osteoporosis
8. Increased susceptibility to infection
9. Cataracts
10. Hirsuitism, acne, fragile skin, bruising

C. Interventions
1. Monitor vital signs
2. Monitor I&O, weight, and for edema
3. Monitor for signs of infection
4. Monitor electrolyte and calcium levels
5. Avoid administering to the client with adreno-cortical hyperfunction
6. Instruct the client to decrease salt intake
7. Instruct the client to report side effects such as muscle weakness, edema, petechiae, ecchymosis, decrease in growth, delayed wound healing, and menstrual irregularities
8. Monitor for adverse effects when the medication is discontinued; dose should be tapered and not stopped abruptly, because adrenal hypofunction may result
9. Advise the client to wear Medic-Alert bracelet

VII. CORTICOSTEROIDS (GLUCOCORTICOIDS)
(See Box 45-5)

A. Description
1. Produce metabolic effects
2. Alter the normal immune response and suppress inflammation
3. Promote sodium and water retention and potassium excretion
4. Produce anti-inflammatory, antiallergic, and antistress effects
5. May be used as a replacement for adrenocortical insufficiency

B. Side effects
1. Hyperglycemia
2. Hypokalemia
3. Sodium and water retention
4. Edema
5. Cause muscle wasting, osteoporosis, growth retardation in children, peptic ulcer, increased serum glucose levels, hypertension, convulsions,

mood swings, cataracts, glaucoma, fragile skin, hirsutism, altered fat distribution
6. Mask the signs and symptoms of infection

C. Contraindications and cautions
1. Contraindicated in hypersensitivity, psychosis, and fungal infections
2. Use with caution in **diabetes mellitus**
3. Dexamethasone (Decadron) decreases the effects of oral anticoagulants and oral anti-diabetic agents
4. Increase the potency of medications taken concurrently, such as aspirin and nonsteroidal anti-inflammatory drugs (NSAIDs), thus increasing the risk of GI bleeding and ulceration
5. Use of potassium-wasting diuretics increases potassium loss, resulting in hypokalemia
6. Barbiturates, phenytoin (Dilantin), and rifampin (Rifadin) decrease the effect of prednisone
7. The action of dexamethasone (Decadron) is decreased by the use of phenytoin (Dilantin), theophylline, rifampin (Rifadin), barbiturates, and antacids
8. NSAIDs, aspirin, and estrogen increase the effect of dexamethasone (Decadron)
9. Should be used with extreme caution in clients with infections because they mask the signs and symptoms of an infection
10. Advise the client to wear Medic-Alert bracelet

D. Interventions
1. Monitor vital signs
2. Monitor serum electrolyte and blood glucose levels
3. Monitor for hypokalemia and **hyperglycemia**
4. Monitor I&O, weight, and for edema
5. Monitor for hypertension
6. Check the client's medical history for glaucoma, cataracts, peptic ulcer, mental health disorders, or **diabetes mellitus**
7. Monitor the older client for signs and symptoms of increased osteoporosis
8. Monitor for changes in muscle strength
9. Prepare a schedule for the client on short-term, tapered doses
10. Instruct the client to take at mealtime or with food
11. Advise the client to eat foods high in potassium
12. Instruct the client to avoid individuals with respiratory infections
13. Advise the client to inform all health care providers about taking the medication
14. Instruct the client to report signs and symptoms of a medication overdose or **Cushing's syndrome,** including a moon face, puffy eyelids, edema in the feet, increased bruising, dizziness, bleeding, and menstrual irregularities
15. Note that the client may need additional doses during periods of stress, such as surgery

---

BOX 45-6

Medications Used in Diagnosing Adrenal Gland Dysfunction

Corticotropin repository (H.P. Acthar Gel, ACTH gel)
Cosyntropin (Cortrosyn)

16. Instruct the client not to stop medication abruptly, because abrupt withdrawal can result in severe adrenal insufficiency
17. Advise the client to consult with the physician before receiving vaccinations
18. Advise the client to wear Medic-Alert bracelet

E. Mineralocorticoids
   1. Description
      a. Steroid hormones that enhance the reabsorption of sodium and chloride and promote the excretion of potassium and hydrogen from the renal tubules, thereby helping to maintain fluid and electrolyte balance
      b. Used for replacement therapy in primary and secondary adrenal insufficiency in **Addison's disease**
   2. Medication: Fludrocortisone (Florinef)
   3. Side effects
      a. Sodium and water retention, hypertension
      b. Hypokalemia
      c. Hypocalcemia
      d. Increased susceptibility to infection
      e. Delayed wound healing
      f. GI distress, tendency to develop peptic ulcer
      g. Osteoporosis, compression fractures
      h. Increased appetite and weight gain
      i. Insomnia
      j. Mood swings
      k. Abdominal distention
   4. Interventions
      a. Monitor vital signs
      b. Monitor weight
      c. Monitor electrolyte and calcium levels
      d. Instruct the client to take medication with food or milk
      e. Instruct the client to consume a high-potassium diet
      f. Instruct the client not to stop the medication abruptly
      g. Instruct the client to notify the physician if signs of infection, muscle aches, sudden weight gain, or headaches occur
      h. Instruct the client to avoid exposure to disease or trauma
      i. Instruct the client not to take aspirin or any other medication without consulting the physician
      j. Instruct the client to wear a Medic-Alert bracelet

VIII. ANDROGENS (Box 45-7)

A. Description
   1. Used either to replace deficient hormones or to treat hormone-sensitive disorders
   2. Can cause bleeding if the client is taking oral anticoagulants (increase the effect of anticoagulants)

BOX 45-7

Androgens

Fluoxymesterone (Halotestin)
Methyltestosterone (Android, Testred, Virilon)
Testosterone (Androderm, Testoderm)
Testosterone (Testopel pellets)
Testosterone cypionate (Andronate, Depo-Testosterone)
Testosterone enanthate (Delatestryl)

---

3. Cause decreased serum glucose concentration, thereby reducing insulin requirements in the client with **diabetes mellitus**
4. Hepatotoxic medications are avoided with the use of androgens because of the risk of additive damage to the liver
5. Usually avoided in men with known prostatic or breast carcinoma because androgens often stimulate growth of these tumors

B. Side effects
   1. Masculine secondary sexual characteristics (body hair growth, lowered voice, muscle growth)
   2. Bladder irritation and urinary tract infections
   3. Breast tenderness
   4. Gynecomastia
   5. Priapism
   6. Menstrual irregularities
   7. Virilism
   8. Sodium and water retention with edema
   9. Nausea, vomiting, or diarrhea
   10. Acne
   11. Changes in libido
   12. Hepatotoxicity, jaundice
   13. Hypercalcemia

C. Interventions
   1. Monitor vital signs
   2. Monitor for edema, weight gain, and skin changes
   3. Monitor mental status and neurological function
   4. Monitor for signs of liver dysfunction, including right upper quadrant abdominal pain, malaise, fever, jaundice, pruritus
   5. Monitor for the development of secondary sexual characteristics
   6. Instruct the client to take with meals or a snack
   7. Instruct the client to notify the physician if priapism develops
   8. Instruct the client to notify the physician if fluid retention occurs
   9. Instruct women to use a nonhormonal contraceptive while on therapy
   10. For women, monitor for menstrual irregularities and decreased breast size

---

BOX 45-8

Estrogens

Diethylstilbestrol (DES)
Estradiol (Estrace, Climara, Estraderm, Vivelle)
Estradiol cypionate (Depo-Estradiol)
Estradiol valerate (Delestrogen)
Estrogens, congugated (Premarin)
Estrone (Kestrone 5)
Estropipate (Ogen)

BOX 45-9

Progestins

Medroxyprogesterone, tablets (Provera)
Medroxyprogesterone, injection (Depo-Provera)
Medroxyprogesterone and conjugated estrogens
   (Premphase, Prempro)
Megestrol (Megace)
Norethindrone acetate (Aygestin)
Progesterone, micronized (Prometrium)
Progesterone (Crinone, Progestasert)

IX. ESTROGENS AND PROGESTINS

A. Description
1. Estrogens are steroids that stimulate female reproductive tissues
2. Progestins are steroids that specifically stimulate the uterine lining
3. Estrogen and progestin preparations may be used to stimulate endogenous hormones to restore hormonal balance or to treat hormone-sensitive tumors (suppress tumor growth), or for contraception (Boxes 45-8 and 45-9)
B. Contraindications and cautions
1. Estrogens
   a. Contraindicated in clients with breast cancer, endometrial hyperplasia, endometrial cancer, history of thromboembolism, known or suspected pregnancy , or lactation
   b. Use with caution in hypertension, gall bladder disease, liver, or kidney dysfunction
   c. Increase the risk of toxicity when used with hepatotoxic medications
   d. Barbiturates, phenytoin, (Dilantin), and rifampin (Rifadin) decrease the effectiveness of estrogen
2. Progestins: Contraindicated in clients with thromboembolitic disorders, and avoided in clients with breast tumors or hepatic disease

C. Side effects
1. Breast tenderness, menstrual changes
2. Nausea, vomiting, and diarrhea
3. Malaise, depression, excessive irritability
4. Weight gain
5. Edema and fluid retention
6. Atherosclerosis
7. Hypertension, stroke, myocardial infarction
8. Thromboembolism (estrogen)
9. Migraine headaches and vomiting (estrogen)
D. Interventions
1. Monitor vital signs
2. Monitor for hypertension
3. Monitor for edema and weight gain
4. Advise the client not to smoke
5. Advise the client to undergo routine breast and pelvic examinations

X. ORAL CONTRACEPTIVES

A. Description
1. These medications contain a combination of estrogen and a progestin or a progestin alone
2. Estrogen-progestin combinations suppress ovulation and change the cervical mucus, making it difficult for sperm to enter
3. Medications that contain only progestins are less effective than the combined medications
4. Usually taken for 21 consecutive days and stopped for 7 days; then the administration cycle is repeated
5. Provide reversible prevention of pregnancy
6. Useful in controlling irregular or excessive menstrual cycles
7. Risk factors associated with the development of complications related to the use of oral contraceptives include smoking, obesity, and hypertension
8. Contraindicated in women with hypertension, thromboembolitic disease, cerebrovascular or coronary disease, estrogen-dependent cancers, pregnancy
9. Avoided with the use of hepatotoxic medications
10. Interfere with the activity of bromocriptine (Parlodel) and anticoagulants and increase the toxicity of tricyclic antidepressants
11. May alter blood glucose levels
B. Side effects
1. Breakthrough bleeding
2. Excessive cervical mucus formation
3. Breast tenderness
4. Hypertension
5. Nausea, vomiting
C. Interventions
1. Monitor vital signs and weight
2. Instruct the client in the administration of the medication (it may take up to 1 week for full

contraceptive effect to occur when the medication is begun)

3. Instruct the client with **diabetes mellitus** to monitor blood glucose levels carefully

4. Instruct the client to report signs of thromboembolitic complications

5. Instruct the client to notify the physician if vaginal bleeding or menstrual irregularities occur or if pregnancy is suspected

6. Inform the client that many medications interfere with the effectiveness of birth control pills

7. Instruct the client to perform breast self-examination monthly and about the importance of yearly physical examinations

8. If the client decides to discontinue the oral contraceptive to become pregnant, recommend that the client use an alternative form of birth control for 2 months after discontinuation to ensure more complete excretion of hormonal agents before conception

XI. FERTILITY MEDICATIONS (Box 45-10)

A. Description

1. Act to stimulate follicle development and ovulation in functioning ovaries; combined with human chorionic gonadotropin (hCG) to maintain the follicles once ovulation has occurred

2. Contraindicated in the presence of primary ovarian function, thyroid or adrenal dysfunction, ovarian cysts, pregnancy, or idiopathic uterine bleeding

3. Used with caution in clients with thromboembolitic or respiratory diseases

B. Side effects

1. Risk of multiple births and birth defects

2. Ovarian overstimulation (abdominal pain, distention, ascites, pleural effusion)

3. Headache, irritability

4. Fluid retention and bloating

5. Nausea, vomiting

6. Uterine bleeding

7. Ovarian enlargement

8. Gynecomastia

9. Rash

10. Orthostatic hypotension

11. Febrile reactions

BOX 45-10

Fertility Medications

Bromocriptine (Parlodel)
Chorionic gonadotropin (A.P.L., Profasi)
Clomiphene (Clomid)
Follitropin alfa (Gonal-F)
Follitropin beta (Follistim)
Menotropins (Pergonal)

C. Interventions

1. Instruct the client regarding administration of the medication

2. Provide a calendar of treatment days and instructions on when intercourse should occur to increase therapeutic effectiveness of the medication

3. Provide information about the risks and hazards of multiple births

4. Instruct the client to notify the physician if signs of ovarian stimulation occur

5. Inform the client about the need for regular follow-up for evaluation

XII. MEDICATIONS FOR PENILE ERECTION DYSFUNCTION

A. Description

1. Alprostadil (Caverject, Muse) is a prostaglandin that relaxes smooth muscle and promotes blood flow into the corpus cavernosum

2. Sildenafil (Viagra), tadalafil (Cialis), vardenafil (Levitra) cause smooth muscle relaxation and allow blood flow into the corpus cavernosum

3. Contraindicated in the presence of any anatomical obstruction or condition that might predispose to priapism and in clients with penile implants

4. Caution should be used in clients with bleeding disorders

5. Sildenafil, tadalafil, and vardenafil are used cautiously in clients with coronary artery disease, active peptic ulcer, bleeding disorders, or retinitis pigmentosa

6. Sildenafil, tadalafil, and vardenafil cannot be administered to clients taking nitrates, nitroprusside, or alpha blockers

B. Side effects

1. Alprostadil: Pain at the injection site, infection, priapism, fibrosis, rash, hypertension

2. Sildenafil, tadalafil, and vardenafil: Headache, flushing, dyspepsia, urinary tract infection, diarrhea, dizziness, rash

3. Blurred vision and changes in color vision

C. Interventions

1. Obtain a thorough health and medication history

2. Instruct the client regarding administration of the medication; alprostadil is injected, and sildenafil, tadalafil, and vardenafil are taken orally

3. Inform the client of the side effects necessitating the need to notify the physician

XIII. MEDICATIONS FOR DIABETES MELLITUS

A. Insulin and oral hypoglycemic medications

1. Description

a. Insulin increases glucose transport into cells and promotes conversion of glucose to glycogen, decreasing serum glucose levels

b. Oral hypoglycemic agents stimulate the pancreas to produce more insulin, increase the sensitivity of peripheral receptors to insulin, decrease hepatic glucose output or delay intestinal absorption of glucose, thus decreasing serum glucose levels

2. Contraindications and concerns

a. Insulin is contraindicated in clients with hypersensitivity

b. Oral hypoglycemic agents are contraindicated in type 1 **diabetes mellitus**

c. Sulfonylureas can affect cardiac function and oxygen consumption and lead to cardiac dysrhythmias

d. Use of hypoglycemic medications with beta-adrenergic blocking agents masks signs and symptoms of **hypoglycemia**

e. Anticoagulants, chloramphenicol (Chloromycetin), salicylates, propranolol (Inderal), monoamine oxidase inhibitors (MAOIs), pentamidine (Pentam 300), and sulfonamides may cause **hypoglycemia**

f. Corticosteroids, sympathomimetics, thiazide diuretics, phenytoin (Dilantin), thyroid preparations, oral contraceptives, and estrogen compounds may cause **hyperglycemia**

g. Side effects of the sulfonylureas include gastrointestinal symptoms and dermatological reactions; **hypoglycemia** can occur when an excessive dose is administered or when meals are omitted or delayed, food intake is decreased, or activity is increased

h. Sulfonylureas, such as chlorpropamide (Diabinese), can cause a disulfiram (Antabuse) type of reaction when alcohol is ingested

B. Oral hypoglycemic medications

1. Prescribed for clients with type 2 **diabetes mellitus**

2. Sulfonylureas (Box 45-11)

a. May be classified as first- or second-generation sulfonylureas

b. Stimulate the beta cells to produce more insulin

3. Nonsulfonylureas (see Box 45-11)

a. Affect the hepatic and gastrointestinal production of glucose

b. May be used alone or in combination with a sulfonylurea

4. Interventions

a. Assess the client's knowledge of **diabetes mellitus** and the use of oral antidiabetic agents

b. Obtain a medication history regarding the medications that the client is currently taking

c. Monitor vital signs and blood glucose levels

d. Instruct the client to recognize symptoms of **hypoglycemia** and **hyperglycemia**

e. Instruct the client to avoid over-the-counter medications unless prescribed by the health care provider

f. Instruct the client not to ingest alcohol with sulfonylureas

g. Inform the client that insulin may be needed during stress, surgery, or infection

h. Instruct the client in the necessity of compliance with prescribed medication

i. Advise the client to obtain a Medic-Alert bracelet

C. Insulin (Table 45-2)

1. Primarily acts in the liver, muscle, and adipose tissue by attaching to receptors on cellular membranes and facilitating the passage of glucose, potassium, and magnesium

2. Prescribed for clients with type 1 **diabetes mellitus**

3. Storing insulin (Box 45-12)

4. Insulin injection sites

a. The main areas for injections are the abdomen, arms (posterior surface), thighs (anterior surface), and hips

b. Insulin injected into the abdomen may absorb more evenly and rapidly than at other sites

c. Systematic rotation within one anatomical area is recommended to prevent lipodystrophy; client should be instructed not to use the same site more than once in a 2- to 3-week period

d. Injections should be 1.5 inches apart within the anatomical area

e. Heat, massage, and exercise of the injected area can increase absorption rates and may result in **hypoglycemia**

f. Injection into scar tissue may delay absorption of insulin

---

BOX 45-11

Sulfonylureas and Nonsulfonylureas

SULFONYLUREAS
Acetohexamide (Dymelor)
Chlorpropamide (Diabinese)
Glimepiride (Amaryl)
Glipizide (Glucotrol)
Glyburide (Diabeta, Micronase)
Tolazamide (Tolinase)
Tolbutamide (Orinase)

NONSULFONYLUREAS
Alpha-Glucosidase Inhibitor
Acarbose (Precose)
Miglitol (Glyset)
Biguanide
Metformin (Glucophage)
Meglitinides
Nateglinide (Starlix)
Repaglinide (Prandin)
Thiazolidinediones
Pioglitazone (Actos)
Rosiglitazone (Avandia)

TABLE 45-2

Common Types of Insulin

Type	Onset	Peak (hours)	Duration (hours)
RAPID-ACTING INSULIN			
Insulin lispro (Humalog)	15 minutes	$\frac{1}{2}$ to $1\frac{1}{2}$	4-5
Insulin aspart (NovoLog)	5-10 minutes	1-3	3-5
SHORT-ACTING INSULIN			
Regular (Humulin R, Novolin R)	30-60 minutes	2-4	5-7
INTERMEDIATE-ACTING INSULIN			
NPH (Humulin N, Novolin N)	1-2 hours	6-14	24
Lente (Humulin L, Novolin L)	1-3 hours	6-14	24
LONG-ACTING INSULIN			
Ultralente (Humulin U)	6 hours	18-24	36
Insulin glargine (Lantus)	—	—	24
PREMIXED INSULIN			
70% NPH /30% Regular (Humulin 70/30)	30-60 minutes	2-12	18-24
50% NPH/50% Regular (Humulin 50/50)	30 minutes	3-5	24
75% insulin lispro protamine/ 25% lispro	10-15 minutes	1-6	24

BOX 45-12

Storing Insulin

Exposure to extremes in temperature should be avoided. Insulin should not be frozen or kept in direct sunlight or a hot car.

Before injection, insulin should be at room temperature.

If a vial of insulin will be used up in a month, it may be kept at room temperature; otherwise, the vial should be refrigerated.

5. Administering insulin
   a. To prevent dosage errors, be certain that the insulin concentration noted on the vial matches with the calibration of units on the insulin syringe; the usual concentration of insulin is Units 100 (100 units/mL)
   b. Most insulin syringes have a 27- to 29-gauge needle that is approximately 0.5 inch long
   c. Before use, roll the insulin bottle to ensure that the insulin and ingredients are mixed well; otherwise, an inaccurate dose will be drawn; shaking the bottle will cause bubbles to form
   d. Premixed insulins (NPH and Regular insulin) are available as 70/30 (most commonly used) and 50/50; (premixed insulin lispro protamine and insulin lispro 75/25 are also available)
   e. Mixtures of insulin in prefilled syringes should be kept in the refrigerator, where they will be stable for at least 1 week; prefilled syringes should be kept flat or with the needle in an upright position to avoid clogging the needle
   f. Inject air into the insulin bottle (a vacuum makes it difficult to draw up the insulin)
   g. When mixing insulins, draw up the Regular (shorter acting) insulin first
   h. Regular insulin may be mixed with any other type of insulin
   i. Insulin zinc suspensions may be mixed only with each other and Regular insulin, not with other types of insulin
   j. Administer a mixed dose of insulin within 5 to 15 minutes of preparation; after this time, the Regular insulin binds with the NPH insulin and its action is reduced
   k. Aspiration is generally not recommended with self-injection of insulin
   l. Administer insulin at a 45- to 90-degree angle and at a 45- to 60-degree angle in thin persons
   m. *Remember*: Regular insulin is the only type of insulin that can be administered by IV

D. Glucagon
   1. A hormone secreted by the alpha cells of the islets of Langerhans in the pancreas
   2. Increases blood glucose level by stimulating glycogenolysis in the liver
   3. Can be administered by the subcutaneous, intramuscular, or intravenous route
   4. Used to treat insulin-induced **hypoglycemia** when the client is semiconscious or unconscious and cannot ingest liquids

5. The blood glucose level begins to increase within 5 to 20 minutes after administration
6. Instruct the family in the procedure for administration
7. See Chapter 44 for additional information regarding interventions for severe **hypoglycemia**

E. Diazoxide (Proglycem)
   1. Increases blood glucose level by inhibiting insulin release from the beta cells and stimulating the release of epinephrine from the adrenal medulla
   2. Used to treat chronic **hypoglycemia** caused by hyperinsulinism resulting from islet cell cancer or hyperplasia
   3. It is not used for **hypoglycemic** reactions from insulin

PRACTICE QUESTIONS

1. Somatren (Protropin) is administered to a client with pituitary dwarfism. The expected therapeutic effect of this medication is to:
   1. Promote weight gain
   2. Stimulate linear growth
   3. Increase bone density
   4. Decrease the mobilization of fats

2. A nurse is monitoring a client receiving desmopressin (DDAVP). Which of the following, if noted in the client, would indicate an adverse effect of the medication?
   1. Increased urination
   2. Weight loss
   3. Drowsiness
   4. Insomnia

3. A nurse reinforces instructions to a client taking levothyroxine (Synthroid). The nurse determines that the teaching was effective if the client states that he or she will take the medication:
   1. With food
   2. On an empty stomach
   3. At bed time
   4. At lunch time

4. Thyroid replacement therapy is prescribed for a client diagnosed with hypothyroidism. The client asks the nurse when the medication will no longer be needed. The nurse makes which response to the client?
   1. "You will need to ask your physician."
   2. "Most clients require medication therapy for about 1 year."
   3. "It depends on the results of the laboratory values."
   4. "The medication will need to be continued for life."

5. A nurse reinforces medication instructions to a client taking levothyroxine (Synthroid). The nurse instructs the client to notify the physician if which of the following occurs?
   1. Cold intolerance
   2. Tremors
   3. Excessively dry skin
   4. Fatigue

6. A nurse reviews the health record of a client seen in the physician's office and noted that the client is taking propylthiouracil (PTU) daily. The nurse suspects that the client has a history of:
   1. Cushing's syndrome
   2. Addison's disease
   3. Myxedema
   4. Graves' disease

7. A nurse is reinforcing instructions to a client regarding the administration of lypressin (Diapid). The nurse instructs the client that the medication will be taken by which of the following routes?
   1. Oral
   2. Subcutaneous
   3. Intranasal
   4. Intramuscular

8. A client is seen by the physician for complaints of fatigue, a lack of energy, constipation, and depression. Following diagnostic studies, hypothyroidism is diagnosed. Levothyroxine (Synthroid) is prescribed. The nurse tells the client that the primary expected outcome of the medication is to:
   1. Increase energy levels
   2. Achieve normal thyroid hormone levels
   3. Increase blood glucose levels
   4. Alleviate depression

9. Propylthiouracil (PTU) is prescribed for a client with hyperthyroidism and the nurse reinforces instructions to the client regarding the medication. The nurse informs the client to notify the physician if which of the following signs occur?
   1. Drowsiness
   2. Sore throat
   3. Polyuria
   4. Dry mouth

10. A client is scheduled for subtotal thyroidectomy. Iodine solution (Lugol solution) is prescribed. The nurse understands that the therapeutic effect of this medication is to:
   1. Increase thyroid hormone production
   2. Suppress thyroid hormone production
   3. Replace thyroid hormone
   4. Prevent the oxidation of iodide

11. A nurse reinforces instructions to the client taking fludrocortisone (Florinef). The nurse tells the client to notify the physician if which of the following occurs?
   1. Weight loss
   2. Nausea
   3. Swelling of the feet
   4. Fatigue

12. Calcium carbonate (Os-Cal 500) is prescribed for a client with hypocalcemia. The nurse tells the client to take the medication:
   1. With meals
   2. One hour after meals
   3. One hour before meals
   4. One hour before breakfast

13. Calcitriol (Rocaltrol) is prescribed for the client with hypocalcemia and the nurse provides dietary instructions to the client. Which food item would the nurse instruct the client to avoid while taking this medication?
    1. Oysters
    2. Milk
    3. Whole-grain cereals
    4. Sardines

14. A daily dose of prednisone (Deltasone) is prescribed for a client. A nurse provides instructions to the client regarding administration of the medication and tells the client that the best time to take this medication is:
    1. At bedtime
    2. At noon
    3. Early morning
    4. Any time, at the same time, each day

15. Sildenafil citrate (Viagra) is prescribed to treat a client with erectile dysfunction. A nurse reviews the client's medical record and would question the prescription if which of the following is noted in the client's history?
    1. Neuralgia
    2. Use of nitroglycerin
    3. Use of multivitamins
    4. Insomnia

16. A nurse is teaching the client how to mix Regular insulin and NPH insulin in the same syringe. Which of the following actions, if performed by the client, would indicate the need for further teaching?
    1. Injects air into NPH insulin vial first
    2. Injects the amount of air equal to the desired dose of insulin into the vial
    3. Withdraws the NPH insulin first
    4. Withdraws the Regular insulin first

17. A nurse is reinforcing home care instructions to a client recently diagnosed with diabetes mellitus. The client is taking NPH insulin daily and asks the nurse how to store the unopened vials of insulin. The nurse tells the client to:
    1. Freeze the insulin
    2. Refrigerate the insulin
    3. Keep the insulin at room temperature
    4. Keep in a dark, dry place

18. A client with diabetes mellitus is self-administering NPH insulin from a vial that is kept at room temperature. The client asks the nurse about the length of time an unrefrigerated vial of insulin will maintain its potency. The appropriate response is which of the following?
    1. Two weeks
    2. One month
    3. Two months
    4. Six months

19. Lispro insulin (Humalog), a rapid-acting form of insulin, is prescribed for a client. The nurse instructs the client to administer the insulin:
    1. Immediately before eating
    2. 30 minutes before eating
    3. 45 minutes before eating
    4. 60 minutes before eating

20. Tolbutamide (Orinase) is prescribed for the client with diabetes mellitus. The nurse instructs the client to avoid which of the following while taking this medication?
    1. Carbonated beverages
    2. Organ meats
    3. Alcohol
    4. Whole-grain cereals

ALTERNATE FORMAT QUESTION: FILL IN THE BLANK

A client with diabetes mellitus is preparing for discharge from the hospital and tells the nurse that syringes prefilled with NPH and Regular insulin will be prepared by a home care nurse who will be visiting the client. The client asks the nurse how often the home care nurse will need to visit to prefill syringes. Considering the stability of insulin, the nurse tells the client that how many prefilled syringes can be prepared by the home care nurse?

Answer: _____

ANSWERS

1. *Answer: 2*
Rationale: Protropin is a growth stimulator used in the long-term treatment of growth failure resulting from growth hormone deficiency. It stimulates linear growth, increases the number and size of muscle cells, and red cell mass. It affects carbohydrate metabolism by antagonizing the action of insulin, increasing mobilization of fats, and increasing cellular protein synthesis.
Test-Taking Strategy: Use the client diagnosis in the question to assist in the process of elimination in answering the question. Note the relationship between "dwarfism" in the question and "growth" in the correct option. Review the action of this medication if you had difficulty with this question.
Level of Cognitive Ability: Analysis
Client Needs: Physiological Integrity
Integrated Process: Nursing Process/Evaluation
Content Area: Pharmacology
Reference: Hodgson, B., & Kizior, R. (2005). *Saunders nursing drug handbook 2005.* Philadelphia: W.B. Saunders, p. 981.

2. *Answer: 3*

Rationale: Water intoxication or hyponatremia is an adverse reaction to DDAVP. Early signs include drowsiness, listlessness, and headache. Decreased urination, rapid weight gain, confusion, seizures, and coma may also occur in overhydration.

Test-Taking Strategy: Use the process of elimination. Knowledge that this medication is used in the treatment of diabetes insipidus will assist in eliminating options 1 and 2. Recalling the action of the medication will assist you in determining that water intoxication is an adverse reaction. This thought process will assist in directing you to option 3. Review the adverse effects of reactions related to this medication if you had difficulty with this question.

Level of Cognitive Ability: Analysis
Client Needs: Physiological Integrity
Integrated Process: Nursing Process/Data Collection
Content Area: Pharmacology
Reference: Hodgson, B., & Kizior, R. (2005). *Saunders nursing drug handbook 2005.* Philadelphia: W.B. Saunders, p. 303.

3. *Answer: 2*

Rationale: Oral doses of levothyroxine should be taken on an empty stomach to enhance absorption. The medication should be taken in the morning before breakfast.

Test-Taking Strategy: Use the process of elimination. Eliminate options 1 and 4 first because they are similar. From the remaining options, recalling the purpose of the medication and that it is administered in the morning will direct you to option 2. Review this medication if you had difficulty with this question.

Level of Cognitive Ability: Analysis
Client Needs: Physiological Integrity
Integrated Process: Nursing Process/Evaluation
Content Area: Pharmacology
References: Hodgson, B., & Kizior, R. (2005). *Saunders nursing drug handbook 2005.* Philadelphia: W.B. Saunders, p. 632.
McKenry, L., & Salerno, E. (2003). *Mosby's pharmacology in nursing* (21st ed.). St. Louis: Mosby, p. 842.

4. *Answer: 4*

Rationale: For most hypothyroid clients, replacement therapy must be continued for life. Treatment provides symptomatic relief but does not produce a cure. The client should be told that although therapy will improve symptoms, these improvements do not constitute a reason to interrupt or discontinue the medication.

Test-Taking Strategy: Use the process of elimination. Recalling the physiology associated with hypothyroidism will direct you to option 4. If you are unfamiliar with this disorder and the medication therapy associated with it, review this content.

Level of Cognitive Ability: Application
Client Needs: Physiological Integrity
Integrated Process: Nursing Process/Implementation
Content Area: Pharmacology
Reference: Hodgson, B., & Kizior, R. (2005). *Saunders nursing drug handbook 2005.* Philadelphia: W.B. Saunders, p. 633.

5. *Answer: 2*

Rationale: Excessive doses of levothyroxine can produce signs and symptoms of hyperthyroidism (thyrotoxicosis). These include tachycardia, angina, tremors, nervousness, insomnia, hyperthermia, heat intolerance, and sweating. The client should be instructed to notify the physician if these occur. Options 1, 3, and 4 are signs of hypothyroidism.

Test-Taking Strategy: Use the process of elimination, recalling the symptoms associated with hypothyroidism, the purpose of administering levothyroxine, and the effects of the medication. Options 1, 3, and 4 are symptoms related to hypothyroidism. Review the adverse effects of the medication if you are unfamiliar with it.

Level of Cognitive Ability: Application
Client Needs: Physiological Integrity
Integrated Process: Nursing Process/Implementation
Content Area: Pharmacology
Reference: Hodgson, B., & Kizior, R. (2005). *Saunders nursing drug handbook 2005.* Philadelphia: W.B. Saunders, p. 633.

6. *Answer: 4*

Rationale: PTU inhibits thyroid hormone synthesis and is used to treat hyperthyroidism or Graves' disease. Myxedema indicates hypothyroidism. Cushing's syndrome and Addison's disease are disorders related to adrenal function.

Test-Taking Strategy: Knowledge regarding the action of the medication and the treatment measures for Graves' disease is required to answer the question. Remember, PTU inhibits thyroid hormone synthesis and is used to treat hyperthyroidism or Graves' disease. If you are unfamiliar with either of these, review this content.

Level of Cognitive Ability: Analysis
Client Needs: Physiological Integrity
Integrated Process: Nursing Process/Data Collection
Content Area: Pharmacology
References: Hodgson, B., & Kizior, R. (2005). *Saunders nursing drug handbook 2005.* Philadelphia: W.B. Saunders, p. 904.
McKenry, L., & Salerno, E. (2003). *Mosby's pharmacology in nursing* (21st ed.). St. Louis: Mosby, p. 825.

7. *Answer: 3*

Rationale: Lypressin is administered by the intranasal route. It is used for diabetes insipidus. The usual adult dosage is one or two sprays into each nostril four times daily. Options 1, 2, and 4 are incorrect.

Test-Taking Strategy: Knowledge that lypressin is administered by the nasal route is required to answer the question. Review this medication if you had difficulty with this question.

Level of Cognitive Ability: Application
Client Needs: Physiological Integrity
Integrated Process: Nursing Process/Implementation
Content Area: Pharmacology
Reference: McKenry, L., & Salerno, E. (2003). *Mosby's pharmacology in nursing* (21st ed.). St. Louis: Mosby, p. 833.

8. *Answer: 2*

Rationale: Laboratory determination of the serum thyroid-stimulating hormone level (TSH) is an important means of evaluation of therapy with levothyroxine. Effective therapy will cause the elevated TSH levels to decrease. These levels will begin their decline within hours of the onset of therapy and will continue to drop as plasma levels of thyroid hormone build up. If an adequate dosage is established, TSH levels will remain suppressed for the duration of the therapy. Although energy levels are expected to increase, the primary expected outcome is measured by thyroid hormone levels. Options 3 and 4 are unrelated to this medication.

Test-Taking Strategy: Note the key words, *primary* and *expected outcome*. Relate the diagnosis of hypo"thyroidism" with "thyroid" hormone levels in the correct option. If you had difficulty with this question, review the therapeutic effects of levothyroxine.

Level of Cognitive Ability: Application
Client Needs: Physiological Integrity
Integrated Process: Nursing Process/Implementation
Content Area: Pharmacology
Reference: Hodgson, B., & Kizior, R. (2005). *Saunders nursing drug handbook 2005.* Philadelphia: W.B. Saunders, p. 632.

9. *Answer:* 2
Rationale: An adverse effect of PTU is agranulocytosis. The client needs to be informed of the early signs of this adverse effect, which includes fever or sore throat. Drowsiness is an occasional side effect of the medication. Polyuria and dry mouth are unrelated to this medication.

Test-Taking Strategy: Use the process of elimination. Recalling that agranulocytosis is an adverse effect of PTU will direct you to option 2. Review this medication if you had difficulty with this question.

Level of Cognitive Ability: Application
Client Needs: Health Promotion and Maintenance
Integrated Process: Nursing Process/Implementation
Content Area: Pharmacology
Reference: McKenry, L., & Salerno, E. (2003). *Mosby's pharmacology in nursing* (21st ed.). St. Louis: Mosby, p. 848.

10. *Answer:* 2
Rationale: Lugol solution is administered to hyperthyroid individuals in preparation for thyroidectomy to suppress thyroid function. Initial effects develop within 24 hours; peak effects develop in 10 to 15 days. Options 1, 3, and 4 are incorrect.

Test-Taking Strategy: Use the process of elimination. Eliminate options 1 and 3 first because they are similar. From the remaining options, select option 2 because of its relationship to the issue of the question. If you had difficulty with this question, review the purpose of this medication.

Level of Cognitive Ability: Comprehension
Client Needs: Physiological Integrity
Integrated Process: Nursing Process/Evaluation
Content Area: Pharmacology
Reference: McKenry, L., & Salerno, E. (2003). *Mosby's pharmacology in nursing* (21st ed.). St. Louis: Mosby, p. 845.

11. *Answer:* 3
Rationale: Excessive doses of fludrocortisone cause retention of sodium and water and excessive excretion of potassium, resulting in expansion of blood volume, hypertension, cardiac enlargement, edema, and hypokalemia. The client needs to be informed about the signs of sodium and water retention, such

as unusual weight gain or swelling of the feet or lower legs. If these signs occur, the physician needs to be notified.

Test-Taking Strategy: Use the process of elimination. Recalling that fludrocortisone can cause water retention will direct you to option 3. If you are unfamiliar with the adverse effects associated with this medication, review this content.

Level of Cognitive Ability: Application
Client Needs: Health Promotion and Maintenance
Integrated Process: Nursing Process/Implementation
Content Area: Pharmacology
Reference: Hodgson, B., & Kizior, R. (2005). *Saunders nursing drug handbook 2005.* Philadelphia: W.B. Saunders, p. 445.

12. *Answer:* 2
Rationale: The client should be instructed to take oral calcium 30 to 60 minutes after meals to promote absorption. The client should take the medication with a full glass of water.

Test-Taking Strategy: Use the process of elimination. Eliminate options 3 and 4 first because they are similar. From the remaining options, it is necessary to know that this medication is taken after meals. Review this medication if you had difficulty with this question.

Level of Cognitive Ability: Application
Client Needs: Physiological Integrity
Integrated Process: Teaching/Learning
Content Area: Pharmacology
Reference: *Mosby's 2005 drug consult for nurses.* (2005). St. Louis: Mosby, p. 1279.

13. *Answer:* 3
Rationale: The client taking an antihypocalcemic medication should be instructed to avoid eating foods that can suppress calcium absorption. These foods include Swiss chard, beets, bran, and whole-grain cereals.

Test-Taking Strategy: Use the process of elimination. Note that the client's diagnosis is "hypocalcemia" and note the key word, *avoid*. Eliminate options 1 and 4 first because they are similar. From the remaining options, recalling the food items that can suppress calcium absorption will direct you to option 3. Review these foods if you had difficulty with this question.

Level of Cognitive Ability: Application
Client Needs: Health Promotion and Maintenance
Integrated Process: Nursing Process/Implementation
Content Area: Pharmacology
Reference: Hodgson, B., & Kizior, R. (2004). *Saunders nursing drug handbook 2004.* Philadelphia: W.B. Saunders, p. 1117.

14. *Answer:* 3
Rationale: Glucocorticoids should be administered before 9 AM, and the client should be instructed to do so. Administration at this time helps minimize adrenal insufficiency and mimics the burst of glucocorticoids released naturally by the adrenals each morning.

Test-Taking Strategy: Knowledge regarding the administration of glucocorticoids is required to answer this question. Remember, glucocorticoids should be administered before 9 AM. If you had difficulty with this question, review the guidelines associated with administering glucocorticoids.

Level of Cognitive Ability: Application
Client Needs: Physiological Integrity

Integrated Process: Nursing Process/Implementation
Content Area: Pharmacology
Reference: Hodgson, B., & Kizior, R. (2005). *Saunders nursing drug handbook 2005.* Philadelphia: W.B. Saunders, p. 883.

15. *Answer:* 2
Rationale: Sildenafil citrate (Viagra) enhances the vasodilation effect of nitric oxide in the corpus cavernosus of the penis, thus sustaining an erection. Because of the effect of the medication, it is contraindicated with concurrent use of organic nitrates and nitroglycerin. It is not contraindicated with the use of vitamins. Neuralgia and insomnia are side effects of the medication.
Test-Taking Strategy: Use the process of elimination and note the key words, *would question the prescription.* Recalling the action of the medication will direct you to option 2. If you had difficulty with this question, review the contraindications associated with the use of this medication.
Level of Cognitive Ability: Analysis
Client Needs: Physiological Integrity
Integrated Process: Nursing Process/Implementation
Content Area: Pharmacology
Reference: Mosby's 2005 drug consult for nurses. (2005). St. Louis: Mosby, p. 1358.

16. *Answer:* 3
Rationale: When preparing a mixture of Regular insulin with another insulin preparation, the Regular insulin should be drawn into the syringe first. This sequence will avoid contaminating the vial of Regular insulin with insulin of another type. Options 1, 2, and 4 are correct.
Test-Taking Strategy: Use the process of elimination and note the key words, *need for further teaching.* These words indicate a false response question and that you need to select the incorrect client statement. Recalling the appropriate method of preparing insulin for injection will direct you to option 3. Review this procedure if you had difficulty with this question.
Level of Cognitive Ability: Analysis
Client Needs: Health Promotion and Maintenance
Integrated Process: Teaching/Learning
Content Area: Pharmacology
References: Black, J., & Hawks, J. (2005). *Medical-surgical nursing: Clinical management for positive outcomes* (7th ed.). Philadelphia: W.B. Saunders, p. 1264.
Hodgson, B., & Kizior, R. (2005). *Saunders nursing drug handbook 2005.* Philadelphia: W.B. Saunders, pp. 570-571.
McKenry, L., & Salerno, E. (2003). *Mosby's pharmacology in nursing* (21st ed.). St. Louis: Mosby, p. 870.

17. *Answer:* 2
Rationale: Unopened vials of insulin should be stored under refrigeration until needed. Vials should not be frozen. Open vials in use may be kept at room temperature and should be kept away from heat and direct light.
Test-Taking Strategy: Use the process of elimination and note the key word, *store,* in the question. Remembering that insulin should not be frozen will assist in eliminating option 1. Eliminate options 3 and 4 first because they are similar. Review client teaching points related to insulin if you had difficulty with this question.

Level of Cognitive Ability: Application
Client Needs: Health Promotion and Maintenance
Integrated Process: Teaching/Learning
Content Area: Pharmacology
References: Hodgson, B., & Kizior, R. (2005). *Saunders nursing drug handbook 2005.* Philadelphia: W.B. Saunders, p. 570.
McKenry, L., & Salerno, E. (2003). *Mosby's pharmacology in nursing* (21st ed.). St. Louis: Mosby, p. 868.

18. *Answer:* 2
Rationale: An unrefrigerated insulin vial will maintain its potency for up to 1 month. Direct sunlight and heat must be avoided.
Test-Taking Strategy: Note the key word, *unrefrigerated,* to assist in directing you to the correct option. Review the concepts related to insulin stability if you had difficulty with this question.
Level of Cognitive Ability: Application
Client Needs: Health Promotion and Maintenance
Integrated Process: Nursing Process/Implementation
Content Area: Pharmacology
References: McKenry, L., & Salerno, E. (2003). *Mosby's pharmacology in nursing* (21st ed.). St. Louis: Mosby, p. 868.

19. *Answer:* 1
Rationale: The effect of lispro insulin begins within 5 minutes of subcutaneous injection and persists for 2 to 4 hours. Lispro insulin acts more rapidly than Regular insulin but has a shorter duration of action. Because of its rapid onset, it can be administered immediately before eating. In contrast, Regular insulin is generally administered 30 to 60 minutes before meals.
Test-Taking Strategy: Use the process of elimination. Noting the key words *rapid-acting* will assist in eliminating options 3 and 4. From the remaining options, remember that the question is asking about lispro, not Regular, insulin. Review this type of insulin if you had difficulty with this question.
Level of Cognitive Ability: Application
Client Needs: Health Promotion and Maintenance
Integrated Process: Teaching/Learning
Content Area: Pharmacology
Reference: Black, J., & Hawks, J. (2005). *Medical-surgical nursing: Clinical management for positive outcomes* (7th ed.). Philadelphia: W.B. Saunders, pp. 1254-1255.

20. *Answer:* 3
Rationale: When alcohol is combined with tolbutamide, a disulfiram-like reaction may occur. This syndrome includes flushing, palpitations, and nausea. Also, alcohol can potentiate the hypoglycemic effects of tolbutamide. Clients must be warned about alcohol consumption while taking this medication.
Test-Taking Strategy: Use the process of elimination. Eliminate options 1, 2, and 4 because these food items are allowed in a diabetic diet. From the remaining options, remembering that alcohol can affect the action of many medications will assist in directing you to option 3. Review this medication if you had difficulty with this question.
Level of Cognitive Ability: Application

Client Needs: Physiological Integrity
Integrated Process: Teaching/Learning
Content Area: Pharmacology
Reference: McKenry, L., & Salerno, E. (2003). *Mosby's pharmacology in nursing* (21st ed.). St. Louis: Mosby, p. 1018.

ALTERNATE FORMAT QUESTION: FILL IN THE BLANK

Answer: 7
Rationale: Mixtures of insulin in prefilled syringes should be stored in a refrigerator, where they will be stable for 1 week. The syringe should be stored vertically, with the needle pointing up, to avoid clogging the needle.

Prior to administration, the syringe should be agitated gently to resuspend the insulin.
Test-Taking Strategy: It is necessary to know the concepts related to insulin stability and storage to answer this question. Review these concepts if you are unfamiliar with the principles related to prefilling insulin syringes.
Level of Cognitive Ability: Application
Client Needs: Health Promotion and Maintenance
Integrated Process: Nursing Process/Implementation
Content Area: Pharmacology
Reference: *Mosby's 2005 drug consult for nurses.* (2005). St. Louis: Mosby, p. 1107.

REFERENCES

Black, J., & Hawks, J. (2005). *Medical-surgical nursing: Clinical management for positive outcomes* (7th ed.). Philadelphia: W.B. Saunders.

Hodgson, B., & Kizior, R. (2005). *Saunders nursing drug handbook 2005*. Philadelphia: W.B. Saunders.

McKenry, L., & Salerno, E. (2003). *Mosby's pharmacology in nursing* (21st ed.). St. Louis: Mosby.

Mosby's 2005 drug consult for nurses. (2005). St. Louis: Mosby.

The Adult Client with a Gastrointestinal Disorder

PYRAMID TERMS

ascites The accumulation of fluid within the peritoneal cavity that results in venous congestion of the hepatic capillaries. This leads to plasma leaking directly from the liver surface and portal vein.

asterixis Also termed liver flap. The coarse tremor is characterized by rapid, nonrhythmic extensions and flexions in the wrist and fingers.

Billroth I Also called gastroduodenostomy; partial gastrectomy and remaining segment are anastomosed to the duodenum.

Billroth II Also called gastrojejunostomy; partial gastrectomy and remaining segment are anastomosed to the jejunum.

cholecystectomy Removal of the gallbladder.

cholecystitis An inflammation of the gallbladder that may occur as an acute or chronic process. Acute inflammation is associated with gallstones (cholelithiasis). Chronic cholecystitis results when inefficient bile emptying and gallbladder muscle wall disease result in a fibrotic and contracted gallbladder.

choledochotomy Incision into the common bile duct to remove the stone.

cirrhosis A chronic, progressive disease of the liver characterized by diffuse damage to cells, with fibrosis and nodular regeneration. Repeated destruction of hepatic cells causes the formation of scar tissue.

Crohn's disease An inflammatory disease that can occur anywhere in the gastrointestinal (GI) tract, but most often affects the terminal ileum and leads to thickening and scarring, a narrowed lumen, fistulas, ulcerations, and abscesses. It is characterized by remissions and exacerbations.

Cullen's sign Bluish discoloration of the abdomen and periumbilical area, seen in acute hemorrhagic pancreatitis.

diverticulitis Inflammation of one or more diverticuli. It results when the diverticulum perforates, with local abscess formation. A perforated diverticulum can progress to intra-abdominal perforation, with generalized peritonitis.

diverticulosis Outpouchings or herniations of the intestinal mucosa. This can occur in any part of the intestine but are most common in the sigmoid colon.

dumping syndrome Rapid emptying of the gastric contents into the small intestine. It occurs following gastric resection.

esophageal varices Dilated and tortuous veins in the submucosa of the esophagus. They are caused by portal hypertension, are often associated with liver cirrhosis, and are at high risk for rupture if portal circulation pressure rises.

fetor hepaticus Fruity, musty breath odor associated with chronic liver disease.

gastrectomy Also called esophagojejunostomy. It involves removal of the stomach, with attachment of the esophagus to the jejunum or duodenum.

gastric resection Also called antrectomy. It involves removal of the lower half of the stomach and usually includes a vagotomy.

hiatal hernia Also known as esophageal or diaphragmatic hernia. A portion of the stomach herniates through the diaphragm and into the thorax. It results from weakening of the muscles of the diaphragm and is aggravated by factors that increase abdominal pressure, such as pregnancy, ascites, obesity, tumors, and heavy lifting.

Kock ileostomy (continent ileostomy) An intra-abdominal pouch is constructed from the terminal ileum. The pouch is connected to the stoma with a nipple-like valve constructed from a portion of the ileum. The stoma is flush with the skin.

Murphy's sign A sign of gallbladder disease consisting of pain on taking a deep breath when the examiner's fingers are on the approximate location of the gallbladder.

pancreatitis An acute or chronic inflammation of the pancreas, with associated escape of pancreatic enzymes into surrounding tissue. Acute pancreatitis occurs suddenly as one attack or can be recurrent but resolves. Chronic pancreatitis is a continual inflammation and destruction of the pancreas, with scar tissue replacing pancreatic tissue.

peristalsis Wavelike rhythmic contractions that propel material through the GI tract.

portal hypertension A persistent increase in pressure within the portal vein that develops as a result of obstruction to flow.

pyloroplasty Enlarging the pylorus to prevent or decrease pyloric obstruction, thereby enhancing gastric emptying.

Turner's sign A gray-blue discoloration of the flanks, seen in acute hemorrhagic pancreatitis.

ulcerative colitis Ulcerative and inflammatory disease of the bowel that results in poor absorption of nutrients. Acute ulcerative colitis results in vascular congestion, hemorrhage, edema, and ulceration of the bowel mucosa. Chronic ulcerative colitis causes muscular hypertrophy, fat deposits, and fibrous tissue with bowel thickening, shortening, and narrowing.

vagotomy Surgical division of the vagus nerve to eliminate the vagal impulses that stimulate hydrochloric acid secretion in the stomach.

▲ PYRAMID TO SUCCESS

Pyramid points focus on diagnostic tests, nursing care related to the various gastric or intestinal tubes, gastric surgery, cirrhosis, hepatitis, pancreatitis, and colostomy care. Focus on preprocedure and postprocedure care of the client undergoing a gastrointestinal diagnostic test. Remember that an informed consent is required for any invasive procedure. Focus on diet restrictions before and following the diagnostic test, and remember that the gag reflex or bowel sounds must return before allowing a client to consume food or fluids. Pyramid points include instructions to the client and family regarding the prevention of gastrointestinal disorders and the complications associated with the disorder. Focus on teaching the client and family about diet and nutrition specific to the disorder, tube and wound care, preventing the transmission of infection, and care to a colostomy or ileostomy. Remember that body image disturbances can occur in clients with a GI disorder. Specific focus relates to the client with a diversion, such as an ileostomy or colostomy, and to the social isolation issues that can occur, and coping strategies. The Integrated Processes addressed in this unit include Caring, Clinical Problem-Solving Process (Nursing Process), Communication and Documentation, and Teaching/Learning.

▲ CLIENT NEEDS

Safe, Effective Care Environment

Confidentiality issues related to the GI disorder
Consultation related to nutritional status
Establishing priorities
Handling infectious drainage and secretions
Informed consent for treatments and surgical procedures
Preventing the transmission of disease
Referrals to home care and community services
Standard precautions

Health Promotion and Maintenance

Data collection techniques for the GI system
Health screening related to GI disorders
Health promotion programs related to GI disorders
Teaching related to prescribed dietary and other treatment measures
Teaching related to colostomy or ileostomy care
Teaching related to preventing the transmission of disease

Psychosocial Integrity

Coping mechanisms
End-of-life issues
Grief and loss
Support systems
Unexpected body image changes related to colostomy or ileostomy

Physiological Integrity

Care of GI tubes
Diagnostic tests related to the GI system
Elimination
Fluid and electrolyte imbalances
Infectious diseases of the GI tract
Medication therapy specific to the GI disorder
Monitoring for complications related to tests, procedures, and surgical interventions
Nonpharmacological and pharmacological comfort measures
Nutrition and oral hydration
Personal hygiene
Parenteral fluids
Total parenteral nutrition

REFERENCES

Black, J., & Hawks, J. (2005). *Medical-surgical nursing: Clinical management for positive outcomes* (7th ed.). Philadelphia: W.B. Saunders.

Chernecky, C., & Berger, B. (2004). *Laboratory tests and diagnostic procedures* (4th ed.). Philadelphia: W.B. Saunders.

Christensen, B., & Kockrow, E. (2003). *Foundations of nursing* (4th ed.). St. Louis: Mosby.

deWit, S. (2005). *Fundamental concepts and skills for nursing* (2nd ed.). Philadelphia: W.B. Saunders.

Jarvis, C. (2004). *Physical examination and health assessment* (4th ed.). Philadelphia: W.B. Saunders, pp. 542-543.

Lewis, S., Heitkemper, M., & Dirksen, S. (2004). *Medical-surgical nursing: Assessment and management of clinical problems* (6th ed.). St. Louis: Mosby.

Linton, A., & Maebius, N. (2003). *Introduction to medical-surgical nursing* (3rd ed.). Philadelphia: W.B. Saunders.

National Council of State Boards of Nursing. (2005). *Detailed test plan for the National Council licensure examination for practical/vocational nurses.* Chicago: Author.

Pagana, K., & Pagana, T. (2003). *Mosby's diagnostic and laboratory test reference* (6th ed.). St. Louis: Mosby.

Phipps, W., Monahan, F., Sands, J., Marek, J., & Neighbors, M. (2003). *Medical-surgical nursing: Health and illness perspectives* (7th ed.). St. Louis: Mosby.

Stuart, G., & Laraia, M. (2005). *Principles and practice of psychiatric nursing* (8th ed.). St. Louis: Mosby.

Thompson, J., McFarland, G., Hirsch, J., & Tucker, S. (2002). *Mosby's clinical nursing* (5th ed.). St. Louis: Mosby.

Gastrointestinal System

I. ANATOMY AND PHYSIOLOGY

A. Functions of the gastrointestinal (GI) system
1. Process food substances
2. Absorb the products of digestion into the blood
3. Excrete unabsorbed materials
4. Provide an environment for microorganisms to synthesize nutrients, such as vitamin K
5. For risk factors associated with the GI system, see Box 46-1

B. Mouth
1. Contains the lips, cheeks, palate, tongue, teeth, salivary glands, muscles, and maxillary bones
2. Saliva contains the amylase enzyme (ptyalin) that aids in digestion

C. Esophagus
1. A collapsible muscular tube, about 10 inches long
2. Carries food from the pharynx to the stomach

BOX 46-1

Risk Factors Associated with the GI System

Family history of GI disorders
Chronic laxative use
Tobacco use
Chronic alcohol use
Chronic high stress levels
Allergic reactions to food or medications
Chronic use of aspirin or nonsteroidal anti-inflammatory drugs (NSAIDs)
Long-term GI conditions such as ulcerative colitis; may predispose to colorectal cancer
Previous abdominal surgery or trauma; may lead to adhesions
Neurological disorders; can impair movement, particularly with chewing and swallowing
Cardiac, respiratory, and endocrine disorders; may lead to constipation
Diabetes mellitus; may predispose to oral candidal infections

---

D. Stomach: Contains the cardia, fundus, body, and pylorus
1. Mucous glands
   a. Located in mucosa
   b. Prevent autodigestion by providing an alkaline protective covering
2. Lower esophageal (cardiac) sphincter: Prevents reflux of gastric contents into the esophagus
3. Pyloric sphincter: Regulates the rate of stomach emptying into the small intestine
4. Hydrochloric acid: Kills microorganisms, breaks food into small particles, and provides a chemical environment that is required by the gastric enzymes
5. Pepsin: The chief coenzyme of gastric juice, which converts proteins into proteases and peptones
6. Intrinsic factor: Necessary for the absorption of vitamin B_{12}
7. Gastrin: Controls gastric acidity

E. Small intestine
1. Duodenum: Contains the openings of the bile and pancreatic ducts
2. Jejunum: Approximately 8 feet long
3. Ileum: Approximately 12 feet long
4. The small intestine terminates into the cecum

F. Pancreatic intestinal juice enzymes
1. Amylase digests starch to maltose
2. Maltase reduces maltose to monosaccharide glucose
3. Lactase splits lactose into galactose and glucose
4. Sucrase reduces sucrose to fructose and glucose
5. Nucleoses split nucleic acids to nucleotides
6. Enterokinase converts trypsinogen to trypsin

G. Large intestine
1. Approximately 5 feet long
2. Absorbs water and eliminates wastes
3. Intestinal bacteria play a vital role in the synthesis of some B vitamins and vitamin K

4. Colon
   a. Ascending
   b. Transverse
   c. Descending
   d. Sigmoid
   e. Rectum
5. Ileocecal valve: Prevents contents of large intestine from entering ileum
6. Anal sphincters: Guard the anal canal
H. Peritoneum
   1. Lines the abdominal cavity
   2. Forms the mesentery that supports the intestines and blood supply
I. Liver
   1. The largest gland in the body, weighing 3 to 4 pounds
   2. Contains Kupffer cells, which remove bacteria from the portal venous blood
   3. Removes excess glucose and amino acids from the portal blood
   4. Synthesizes glucose, amino acids, and fats
   5. Aids in the digestion of fats, carbohydrates, and proteins
   6. Stores and filters blood (200 to 400 mL of blood stored)
   7. Stores vitamins A, D, B_{12}, and iron
   8. Secretes bile to emulsify fats (500 to 1000 mL of bile/day)
   9. Hepatic ducts
      a. Deliver bile to the gallbladder via the cystic duct
      b. Deliver bile to the duodenum via the common bile duct
      c. The common bile duct opens into the duodenum, with the pancreatic duct at the ampulla of Vater
      d. The sphincter prevents the reflux of intestinal contents into the common bile duct and pancreatic duct
J. Gallbladder
   1. Stores and concentrates bile
   2. Contracts to force bile into the duodenum during the digestion of fats
   3. The cystic duct joins the hepatic duct to form the common bile duct
   4. The sphincter of Oddi guards the entrance into the duodenum
   5. The presence of fatty materials in the duodenum stimulates the liberation of cholecystokinin, which causes contraction of the gallbladder and relaxation of the sphincter of Oddi
K. Pancreas
   1. Exocrine gland
      a. Secretes sodium bicarbonate to neutralize the acidity of the stomach contents as they enter the duodenum
      b. Pancreatic juices contain enzymes for digesting carbohydrates, fats, and proteins

---

BOX 46-2

GI System Diagnostic Studies

Upper GI tract study (barium swallow)
Lower GI tract study (barium enema)
Gastric analysis
Upper GI fiberoscopy
Anoscopy, proctoscopy, and sigmoidoscopy
Fiberoptic colonoscopy
Laparoscopy (peritoneoscopy)
Cholecystography
Endoscopic retrograde cholangiopancreatography (ERCP)
Percutaneous transhepatic cholangiography
Paracentesis
Liver biopsy
Stool specimens
Liver and pancreas laboratory studies

---

2. Endocrine gland
   a. Insulin secretion is produced by the islets of Langerhans
   b. Insulin is secreted into the bloodstream and is important for carbohydrate metabolism
   c. Secretes glucagon to raise blood glucose levels
   d. Secretes somatostatin to exert a hypoglycemic effect

II. DIAGNOSTIC PROCEDURES (Box 46-2)
A. Upper GI tract study (barium swallow)
   1. Description: An examination of the upper GI tract under fluoroscopy after the client drinks barium sulfate
   2. Preprocedure: Nothing by mouth (NPO) after midnight before the day of the test
   3. Postprocedure
      a. A laxative may be prescribed
      b. Instruct the client to drink increase oral fluids to help pass the barium
      c. Monitor stools for the passage of barium (stools will appear chalky white) because barium can cause a bowel obstruction
B. Lower GI tract study (barium enema)
   1. Description
      a. A fluoroscopic and radiographic examination of the large intestine after rectal instillation of barium sulfate
      b. May be done with or without air
   2. Preprocedure
      a. A low-residue diet for 1 to 2 days before the test
      b. A clear liquid diet and a laxative the evening before the test
      c. NPO after midnight before the day of the test
      d. Cleansing enemas on the morning of the test
   3. Postprocedure
      a. Instruct the client to drink increased oral fluids to help pass the barium

b. Administer a mild laxative as prescribed to facilitate emptying of the barium

c. Monitor stools for the passage of barium

d. Notify the physician if a bowel movement does not occur within 2 days

C. Gastric analysis

1. Description

a. The passage of a nasogastric (NG) tube into the stomach to aspirate gastric contents for the analysis of acidity (pH), appearance, and volume; the entire gastric contents are aspirated and then specimens are collected every 15 minutes for 1 hour

b. Histamine or pentagastrin may be administered subcutaneously to stimulate gastric secretions; may produce a flushed feeling

c. Esophageal reflux of gastric acid may be performed by ambulatory pH monitoring; a probe is placed just above the lower esophageal sphincter, is connected to an external recording device, and provides a computer analysis and graphic display of results

2. Preprocedure

a. Fasting for 8 to 12 hours before the test

b. Avoid tobacco and chewing gum for 6 hours before the test

c. Medications that stimulate gastric secretions are withheld for 24 to 48 hours

3. Postprocedure

a. May resume normal activities

b. Refrigerate gastric samples if not tested within 4 hours

D. Upper GI fiberoscopy

1. Description

a. Also known as esophagogastroduodenoscopy (EGD)

b. Following sedation, an endoscope is passed down the esophagus to view the gastric wall, sphincters, and duodenum; tissue specimens can be obtained

2. Preprocedure

a. NPO for 6 to 12 hours before the test

b. A local anesthetic (spray or gargle) is administered along with midazolam (Versed) IV (provides conscious sedation and relieves anxiety) just before the scope is inserted

c. Atropine sulfate may be administered to reduce secretions, and glucagon may be administered to relax smooth muscle

d. Client is positioned on the left side to facilitate saliva drainage and to provide easy access of the endoscope

e. Airway patency is monitored during the test and pulse oximetry is used to monitor oxygen saturation; emergency equipment should be readily available

3. Postprocedure

a. NPO until the gag reflex returns (1 to 2 hours)

b. Monitor for signs of perforation (pain, bleeding, unusual difficulty swallowing, elevated temperature)

c. Maintain bed rest for the sedated client until alert

d. Lozenges, saline gargles, or oral analgesics can relieve minor sore throat after the gag reflex returns

E. Anoscopy, proctoscopy, and sigmoidoscopy

1. Description

a. Anoscopy: Use of a rigid scope to examine the anal canal; client is placed in the knee-chest position, with his or her back inclined at a 45-degree angle

b. Proctoscopy and sigmoidoscopy: Use of a flexible scope to examine the rectum and sigmoid colon; client is placed on his or her left side with the right leg bent and placed anteriorly

c. Biopsies and polypectomies can be performed

2. Preprocedure: Enemas until the returns are clear

3. Postprocedure: Monitor for rectal bleeding and signs of perforation

F. Fiberoptic colonoscopy

1. Description

a. A fiberoptic endoscopy study in which the lining of the large intestine is visually examined; biopsies and polypectomies can be performed

b. Cardiac and respiratory function are monitored continuously during the test

c. Performed with the client lying on his or her left side with the knees drawn up to the chest; position may be changed during the test to facilitate passing of the scope

2. Preprocedure

a. Adequate cleansing of the colon is necessary, as prescribed by the physician

b. A clear liquid diet is started at noon on the day before the test

c. Consult with the physician regarding medications that must be withheld before the test

d. Client is NPO after midnight on the day before the test

e. Midazolam (Versed) IV is administered to provide sedation

f. Glucagon may be administered to relax smooth muscle

3. Postprocedure

a. Provide bed rest until alert

b. Monitor for signs of perforation

c. Instruct the client to report any bleeding to the physician

G. Laparoscopy (peritoneoscopy): Performed with a fiberoscopic laparoscope that allows direct visualization of organs and structures within the abdomen; biopsies may be obtained

H. Cholecystography
  1. Description: Performed to detect gallstones and to assess the ability of the gallbladder to fill, concentrate its contents, contract, and empty
  2. Preprocedure
     a. Check for allergies to iodine or seafood
     b. Contrast agents such as iopanoic acid (Telepaque), iodipamide meglumine (Cholografin), or sodium ipodate (Oragrafin) may be administered 10 to 12 hours (evening before) before the test
     c. Client is NPO after the contrast agent is administered
     d. Instruct the client that if a rash, itching, hives, or difficulty in breathing occurs after taking the contrast agent, to report to the emergency room
  3. Postprocedure
     a. Inform the client that dysuria is common because the contrast agent is excreted in the urine
     b. A normal diet may be resumed (a fatty meal may enhance excretion of the contrast agent)

I. Endoscopic retrograde cholangiopancreatography (ERCP)
  1. Description
     a. Examination of the hepatobiliary system via a flexible endoscope inserted into the esophagus to the descending duodenum; multiple positions are required during the procedure to pass the endoscope
     b. If medication is administered before the procedure, the client is monitored closely for signs of respiratory and central nervous system depression, hypotension, oversedation, and vomiting
  2. Preprocedure
     a. Client is NPO for several hours before the procedure
     b. Sedation is administered before the procedure
  3. Postprocedure
     a. Monitor vital signs
     b. Monitor for the return of the gag reflex
     c. Monitor for signs of perforation or infection
J. Percutaneous transhepatic cholangiography
  1. Description
     a. Involves the injection of dye directly into the biliary tree
     b. The hepatic ducts within the liver, the entire length of the common bile duct, the cystic duct, and the gallbladder are clearly outlined
  2. Preprocedure
     a. Client is NPO for several hours before the test
     b. Sedating medication is administered
  3. Postprocedure
     a. Monitor vital signs

     b. Monitor for signs of bleeding, peritonitis, and septicemia; report the presence of pain immediately
     c. Administer antibiotics as prescribed to reduce the risk of sepsis
K. Paracentesis
  1. Description: Transabdominal removal of fluid from the peritoneal cavity for analysis
  2. Preprocedure
     a. Void before the start of procedure to empty bladder and to move bladder out of the way of the paracentesis needle
     b. Measure abdominal girth, weight, and baseline vital signs
     c. Note that the client is positioned upright on the edge of the bed with the back supported and the feet resting on a stool (Fowler's position is used for the client confined to bed)
  3. Postprocedure
     a. Monitor vital signs
     b. Measure fluid collected, describe, and record
     c. Label fluid samples and send to the laboratory for analysis
     d. Apply a dry sterile dressing to the insertion site; monitor site for bleeding
     e. Measure abdominal girth and weight
     f. Monitor for hypovolemia, electrolyte loss, mental status changes, or encephalopathy
     g. Monitor for hematuria due to bladder trauma
     h. Instruct the client to notify the physician if the urine becomes bloody, pink, or red
L. Liver biopsy
  1. Description: A needle is inserted through the abdominal wall to the liver to obtain a tissue sample for biopsy and microscopic examination
  2. Preprocedure
     a. Check results of coagulation tests (prothrombin time, partial thromboplastin time, platelet count)
     b. Administer a sedative, as prescribed
     c. Note that the client is placed in the supine or left lateral position during the procedure to expose the right side of the upper abdomen
  3. Postprocedure
     a. Monitor vital signs
     b. Monitor biopsy site for bleeding
     c. Monitor for peritonitis
     d. Maintain bed rest for several hours
     e. Place client on the right side with a pillow under the costal margin to decrease the risk of hemorrhage, and instruct the client to avoid coughing and straining
     f. Instruct the client to avoid heavy lifting and strenuous exercise for 1 week

M. Stool specimens
1. Includes inspecting the specimen for consistency and color and testing for occult blood
2. Tested for fecal urobilinogen, fat, nitrogen, parasites, pathogens, food substances, and other substances; these tests require that the specimen be sent to the laboratory
3. Random specimens are promptly sent to the laboratory
4. Quantitative 24- to 72-hour collections must be kept refrigerated until they are taken to the laboratory
5. Some specimens require that a certain diet be followed or that certain medications be withheld; check agency guidelines regarding specific procedures

N. Liver and pancreas laboratory studies (see Chapter 11)
1. Alkaline phosphatase: Released during liver damage or biliary obstruction
2. Prothrombin time (PT): Prolonged with liver damage
3. Serum ammonia: Assesses the ability of the liver to deaminate protein by-products
4. Liver enzymes (transaminase studies): Elevated with liver damage
5. Cholesterol: Increase indicates **pancreatitis** or biliary obstruction
6. Bilirubin: Increase indicates liver damage or biliary obstruction
7. Amylase and lipase: Elevations indicate **pancreatitis**

III. DATA COLLECTION

A. Abdominal assessment (Box 46-3)
1. Inspect skin for color, abnormalities, contour, and tautness and the abdomen for distention
2. Auscultate for bowel sounds
3. Percuss for air or solids
4. Palpate for tenderness
B. Bowel sounds
1. Auscultate bowel sounds before percussion and palpation
2. Normal bowel sounds occur 5 to 30 times a minute, or every 5 to 15 seconds
3. Auscultate in all abdominal quadrants
4. Listen for at least 5 minutes in each quadrant before assuming sounds are absent

---

BOX 46-3

Order for Performing the Abdominal Assessment

1. Inspect
2. Auscultate
3. Percuss
4. Palpate

IV. GASTROINTESTINAL TUBES (see Chapter 19)

V. GASTROESOPHAGEAL REFLEX DISEASE (GERD)

A. Description
1. The backflow of gastric and duodenal contents into the esophagus
2. Caused by an incompetent lower esophageal sphincter, pyloric stenosis, or motility disorder
3. Symptoms may mimic those of a heart attack
B. Data collection
1. Pyrosis
2. Dyspepsia
3. Regurgitation
4. Pain and difficulty with swallowing
5. Hypersalivation
C. Interventions
1. Instruct the client to avoid factors that decrease lower esophageal sphincter pressure or cause esophageal irritation
2. Instruct the client to eat a low-fat, high-fiber diet; avoid caffeine, tobacco, and carbonated beverages; avoid eating and drinking 2 hours before bedtime; avoid wearing tight clothes; and to elevate the head of the bed on 6- to 8-inch blocks
3. Avoid the use of anticholinergics, which delay stomach emptying
4. Instruct the client regarding prescribed medications, such as antacids, histamine H_2-receptor antagonists, or gastric acid pump inhibitors
5. Instruct the client regarding the administration of prokinetic medications if prescribed, which accelerate gastric emptying
6. If medical management is unsuccessful, surgery may be required and involves a fundoplication (wrapping a portion of the gastric fundus around the sphincter area of the esophagus); may be performed by laparoscopy

VI. HIATAL HERNIA

A. Description
1. Also known as esophageal or diaphragmatic hernia
2. A portion of the stomach herniates through the diaphragm and into the thorax
3. It results from weakening of the muscles of the diaphragm and is aggravated by factors that increase abdominal pressure, such as pregnancy, **ascites**, obesity, tumors, and heavy lifting
4. Complications include ulceration, hemorrhage, regurgitation and aspiration of stomach contents, strangulation, and incarceration of the stomach in the chest with possible necrosis, peritonitis, and mediastinitis

B. Data collection
   1. Heartburn
   2. Regurgitation or vomiting
   3. Dysphagia
   4. Feeling of fullness
C. Interventions
   1. Medical and surgical management is similar to that for GERD
   2. Provide small, frequent meals and limit the amount of liquids consumed with meals
   3. Advise the client not to recline for 1 hour after eating
   4. Avoid anticholinergics, which delay stomach emptying

VII. GASTRITIS
A. Description
   1. Inflammation of the stomach or gastric mucosa
   2. Acute: Caused by the ingestion of food contaminated with disease-causing microorganisms or food that is irritating or too highly seasoned, the overuse of aspirin or other nonsteroidal anti-inflammatory drugs (NSAIDs), excessive alcohol intake, bile reflux, or radiation therapy
   3. Chronic: Caused by benign or malignant ulcers, or by the bacterium *Helicobacter pylori;* may also be caused by autoimmune disease, dietary factors, medications, alcohol, smoking, or reflux
B. Data collection (Box 46-4)
C. Interventions
   1. Acute: Food and fluids may be withheld until symptoms subside; then, ice chips, followed by clear liquids; solid food is then introduced
   2. Monitor for signs of hemorrhagic gastritis such as hematemesis, tachycardia, and hypotension, and notify the physician if these signs occur
   3. Instruct the client to avoid irritating foods, fluids, and other substances such as spicy and highly seasoned foods, caffeine, alcohol, and nicotine

   4. Instruct the client in the use of prescribed medications, such as antibiotics and bismuth salts (Pepto-Bismol)
   5. Provide the client with information about the importance of vitamin B_{12} injections if a deficiency is present

VIII. PEPTIC ULCER DISEASE
A. Description
   1. An ulceration in the mucosal wall of the stomach, pylorus, duodenum, or esophagus, in portions that are accessible to gastric secretions; erosion may extend through the muscle
   2. May be referred to as gastric, duodenal, or esophageal ulcers depending on location
   3. The most common peptic ulcers are gastric ulcers and duodenal ulcers
B. Gastric ulcers
   1. Description
      a. Involves ulceration of the mucosal lining that extends to the submucosal layer of the stomach
      b. Predisposing factors include stress, smoking, the use of corticosteroids, NSAIDs, alcohol, a history of gastritis, a family history of gastric ulcers, or infection with *Helicobacter pylori*
      c. Complications include hemorrhage, perforation, and pyloric obstruction
   2. Data collection (Box 46-5)
   3. Interventions
      a. Monitor vital signs and for signs of bleeding
      b. Administer small, frequent, bland feedings during the active phase
      c. Administer histamine H_2-receptor antagonists as prescribed to decrease the secretion of gastric acid
      d. Administer antacids as prescribed to neutralize gastric secretions
      e. Administer anticholinergics as prescribed to reduce gastric motility
      f. Administer mucosal barrier protectants as prescribed 1 hour before each meal

---

BOX 46-4

Findings in Acute and Chronic Gastritis

ACUTE
Abdominal discomfort
Headache
Anorexia, nausea, and vomiting
Hiccuping

CHRONIC
Anorexia, nausea, and vomiting
Heartburn after eating
Belching
Sour taste in the mouth
Vitamin B_{12} deficiency

BOX 46-5

Data Collection: Gastric and Duodenal Ulcers

GASTRIC
Gnawing, sharp pain in or left of the midepigastric region that is accentuated by the ingestion of food and occurs 30 to 60 minutes after eating
Nausea and vomiting
Hematemesis

DUODENAL
Burning pain in the midepigastric area 2 to 4 hours after eating and during the night
Pain that is often relieved by eating
Melena

g. Administer prostaglandins as prescribed for their protective and antisecretory actions

4. Client education
   a. Avoid consuming alcohol and substances that contain caffeine or chocolate
   b. Avoid smoking
   c. Avoid aspirin or NSAIDs
   d. Obtain adequate rest and reduce stress

5. Interventions during active bleeding
   a. Monitor vital signs closely
   b. Monitor for signs of dehydration, hypovolemic shock, sepsis, and respiratory insufficiency
   c. Maintain NPO status and administer IV fluid replacement as prescribed; monitor input and output (I&O)
   d. Monitor hemoglobin and hematocrit levels
   e. Administer blood transfusions as prescribed
   f. Assist with the insertion of an NG tube for decompression and for lavage access
   g. Assist with normal saline or tap water lavage at room temperature to reduce active bleeding
   h. Prepare to assist with administering vasopressin (Pitressin) by IV as prescribed to induce vasoconstriction and reduce bleeding

6. Surgical interventions
   a. Total **gastrectomy:** Also called esophagojejunostomy; removal of the stomach, with attachment of the esophagus to the jejunum or duodenum
   b. **Vagotomy:** Surgical division of the vagus nerve to eliminate the vagal impulses that stimulate hydrochloric acid secretion in the stomach
   c. **Gastric resection:** Also called antrectomy; involves removal of the lower half of the stomach; usually includes a **vagotomy**
   d. **Billroth I:** Also called gastroduodenostomy; partial **gastrectomy,** with remaining segment anastomosed to duodenum
   e. **Billroth II:** Also called gastrojejunostomy; partial **gastrectomy,** with remaining segment anastomosed to jejunum
   f. **Pyloroplasty:** Enlarges the pylorus to prevent or decrease pyloric obstruction, thereby enhancing gastric emptying

7. Postoperative interventions
   a. Monitor vital signs
   b. Position in Fowler's for comfort and to promote drainage
   c. Administer fluids and electrolyte replacements IV as prescribed; monitor I&O
   d. Monitor bowel sounds
   e. Monitor NG suction as prescribed
   f. Do not irrigate or remove the NG tube
   g. Assist the physician with NG irrigation or removal of the NG tube
   h. Maintain NPO status as prescribed for 1 to 3 days until **peristalsis** returns

i. Progress the diet from NPO to sips of clear water to six small, bland meals a day as prescribed when bowel sounds return
j. Monitor for postoperative complications of hemorrhage, **dumping syndrome,** diarrhea, hypoglycemia, and vitamin B_{12} deficiency

C. Duodenal ulcers
1. Description
   a. A break in the mucosa of the duodenum
   b. Risk factors and causes include alcohol intake, smoking, stress, caffeine, the use of aspirin, corticosteroids, NSAIDs, and infection with *Helicobacter pylori*
   c. Complications include bleeding, perforation, gastric outlet obstruction, and intractable disease
2. Data collection (see Box 46-5)
3. Interventions
   a. Monitor vital signs
   b. Assist with performing abdominal assessment
   c. Instruct the client in a bland diet with small frequent meals
   d. Provide for adequate rest
   e. Encourage the cessation of smoking
   f. Instruct the client to avoid alcohol intake, caffeine, the use of aspirin, corticosteroids, and NSAIDs
   g. Administer antacids as prescribed to neutralize acid secretions
   h. Administer histamine H_2-receptor antagonists as prescribed to block the secretion of acid
4. Surgical interventions: Surgery is performed only if the ulcer is unresponsive to medications or if hemorrhage, obstruction, or perforation occurs

D. Dumping syndrome
1. Description
   a. Rapid emptying of the gastric contents into the small intestine
   b. Occurs following **gastric resection**
2. Data collection
   a. Symptoms occurring 30 minutes after eating
   b. Nausea and vomiting
   c. Feelings of abdominal fullness and abdominal cramping
   d. Diarrhea
   e. Palpitations and tachycardia
   f. Perspiration
   g. Weakness and dizziness
   h. Borborygmi
3. Client education (Box 46-6)

IX. VITAMIN B_{12} DEFICIENCY

A. Description
1. Results from either an inadequate intake of vitamin B_{12} or a lack of absorption of ingested vitamin B_{12} from the intestinal tract

---

BOX 46-6

Client Education: Preventing Dumping Syndrome

Eat a high-protein, high-fat, low-carbohydrate diet.
Eat small meals and avoid consuming fluids with meals.
Avoid sugar and salt.
Lie down after meals.
Take antispasmodic medications as prescribed to delay gastric emptying.

BOX 46-7

Foods Rich in Vitamin B$_{12}$

Brewer's yeast
Citrus fruits
Dried beans
Green leafy vegetables
Liver
Nuts
Organ meats

---

2. Pernicious anemia results from a deficiency of intrinsic factor, which is necessary for intestinal absorption of vitamin B$_{12}$

B. Data collection
   1. Severe pallor
   2. Fatigue
   3. Weight loss
   4. Smooth, beefy red tongue
   5. Slight jaundice
   6. Paresthesias of the hands and feet
   7. Disturbances with gait and balance

C. interventions
   1. Increase dietary intake of foods rich in vitamin B$_{12}$ if the anemia is the result of a dietary deficiency (Box 46-7)
   2. Administer vitamin B$_{12}$ injections as prescribed on a weekly basis initially, and then monthly for maintenance (lifelong) if the anemia is the result of a deficiency of the intrinsic factor

---

X. GASTRIC CANCER (See Chapter 42)

XI. ESOPHAGEAL VARICES

A. Description
   1. Dilated and tortuous veins in the submucosa of the esophagus
   2. Caused by **portal hypertension,** often associated with liver **cirrhosis,** at high risk for rupture if portal circulation pressure rises
   3. Bleeding varices is an emergency
   4. The goal of treatment is to control bleeding, prevent complications, and prevent the reoccurrence of bleeding

B. Data collection
   1. Hematemesis
   2. Melena
   3. Tarry stools
   4. **Ascites**
   5. Jaundice
   6. Hepatomegaly and splenomegaly
   7. Dilated abdominal veins
   8. Hemorrhoids
   9. Signs of shock

C. Interventions
   1. Monitor vital signs
   2. Elevate the head of the bed
   3. Monitor for orthostatic hypotension
   4. Monitor lung sounds and for the presence of respiratory distress
   5. Administer oxygen as prescribed to prevent tissue hypoxia
   6. Monitor level of consciousness (LOC)
   7. Maintain NPO status
   8. Monitor IV fluids administered as prescribed to restore fluid volume and electrolyte imbalances; monitor I&O
   9. Monitor hemoglobin, hematocrit, and coagulation factors
   10. Blood transfusions or clotting factors may be prescribed
   11. Prepare to assist in inserting an NG tube or balloon tamponade, as prescribed
   12. Prepare to assist with the administration of iced saline irrigations to achieve vasoconstriction of the varices
   13. Prepare to assist with administering vasopressin (Pitressin) by IV or intra-arterial infusion as prescribed to induce vasoconstriction and reduce bleeding
   14. Prepare to assist with administering nitroglycerin (Tridil) with the vasopressin (Pitressin) if prescribed to prevent vasoconstriction of the coronary arteries
   15. Instruct the client to avoid activities that will initiate vasovagal responses
   16. Prepare the client for endoscopic procedures or surgical procedures, as prescribed

D. Endoscopic injection (sclerotherapy)
   1. Injection of a sclerosing agent into and around bleeding varices
   2. Complications include chest pain, pleural effusion, aspiration pneumonia, esophageal stricture, and perforation of the esophagus

E. Endoscopic variceal ligation
   1. Ligation of the varices with an elastic rubber band
   2. Sloughing, followed by superficial ulceration, occurs in the area of ligation within 3 to 7 days

F. Surgical shunt procedures
  1. Splenorenal: Involves splenectomy, with anastomosis of the splenic vein to the left renal vein
  2. Portacaval: Shunting of the blood from the portal vein to the inferior vena cava
  3. Mesocaval: Involves a side anastomosis of the superior mesenteric vein to the proximal end of the inferior vena cava
  4. Transjugular intrahepatic portal-systemic
     a. Uses the normal vascular anatomy of the liver to create a shunt with the use of a metallic stent
     b. The shunt is between the portal and systemic venous system within the liver and is aimed at relieving **portal hypertension**

XII. ULCERATIVE COLITIS

A. Description
  1. Ulcerative and inflammatory disease of the bowel that results in poor absorption of nutrients
  2. Commonly begins in the rectum and spreads upward toward the cecum
  3. The colon becomes edematous and may develop bleeding lesions and ulcers; the ulcers may lead to perforation
  4. Scar tissue develops and causes loss of elasticity and loss of ability to absorb nutrients
  5. Characterized by various periods of remissions and exacerbations
  6. Acute **ulcerative colitis** results in vascular congestion, hemorrhage, edema, and ulceration of the bowel mucosa
  7. Chronic **ulcerative colitis** causes muscular hypertrophy, fat deposits, and fibrous tissue with bowel thickening, shortening, and narrowing
  8. Surgical intervention involves creation of an ostomy; the ostomy can be created within the ileum or at various sites within the large bowel
  9. An ileostomy is the surgical creation of an opening into the ileum or small intestine that allows for drainage of fecal matter from the ileum to the outside of the body
  10. A colostomy is the surgical creation of an opening into the colon that allows for drainage of fecal matter from the colon to the outside of the body

B. Data collection
  1. Anorexia
  2. Weight loss
  3. Malaise
  4. Abdominal tenderness and cramping
  5. Severe diarrhea that may contain blood and mucus
  6. Dehydration and electrolyte imbalances
  7. Anemia
  8. Vitamin K deficiency

C. Interventions

  1. Acute phase: Maintain NPO status; IVs, electrolytes, or total parenteral nutrition (TPN) may be prescribed
  2. Restrict the client's activity to reduce intestinal activity
  3. Monitor bowel sounds and for abdominal tenderness and cramping
  4. Monitor stools, noting color, consistency, and the presence or absence of blood
  5. Monitor for perforation, peritonitis, and hemorrhage
  6. Following the acute phase, the diet progresses from clear liquids to low-residue diet as tolerated
  7. Instruct the client to consume a low-residue, high-protein diet; vitamins and iron supplements may be prescribed
  8. Instruct the client to avoid gas-forming foods and milk products, and foods such as whole wheat grains, nuts, raw fruits and vegetables, pepper, alcohol, and caffeine-containing products
  9. Instruct the client to avoid smoking
  10. Administer bulk-forming agents such as bran, psyllium, or methylcellulose as prescribed to decrease diarrhea and relieve symptoms
  11. Administer antimicrobials, corticosteroids, and immunosuppressants as prescribed to prevent infection and reduce inflammation

D. Surgical interventions
  1. Total proctocolectomy with permanent ileostomy
     a. Curative and involves the removal of the entire colon (colon, rectum, and anus with anal closure)
     b. The end of the terminal ileum forms the stoma, which is located in the right lower quadrant
  2. **Kock ileostomy** (continent ileostomy)
     a. An intra-abdominal pouch (that stores the feces) is constructed from the terminal ileum
     b. The pouch is connected to the stoma with a nipple-like valve constructed from a portion of the ileum; the stoma is flush with the skin
     c. A catheter is used to empty the pouch, and a small dressing or adhesive bandage is worn over the stoma between emptyings
  3. Ileoanal reservoir
     a. A two-stage procedure that involves the excision of the rectal mucosa, an abdominal colectomy, construction of a reservoir to the anal canal, and a temporary loop ileostomy
     b. The ileostomy is closed in approximately 3 to 4 months after the capacity of the reservoir is increased
  4. Ileoanal anastomosis (ileorectostomy)
     a. Does not require an ileostomy
     b. A 12- to 15-cm rectal stump is left after the colon is removed; the small intestine is inserted into this rectal sleeve and anastomosed
     c. Requires a large, compliant rectum

5. Preoperative and postoperative care for colostomy and ileostomy (see Chapter 42)

XIII. CROHN'S DISEASE (REGIONAL ENTERITIS)

A. Description
  1. An inflammatory disease that can occur anywhere in the GI tract but most often affects the terminal ileum and leads to thickening and scarring, a narrowed lumen, fistulas, ulcerations, and abscesses
  2. It is characterized by remissions and exacerbations
B. Data collection
  1. Fever
  2. Cramplike and colicky pain after meals
  3. Diarrhea (semisolid); may contain mucus and pus
  4. Abdominal distention
  5. Anorexia, nausea, and vomiting
  6. Weight loss
  7. Anemia
  8. Dehydration
  9. Electrolyte imbalances
C. Interventions: Care is similar to the client with **ulcerative colitis;** however, surgery is avoided as much as possible because recurrence of the disease process in the same region is likely to occur

XIV. PANCREATIC TUMORS, INTESTINAL TUMORS AND BOWEL OBSTRUCTIONS (See Chapter 42)

XV. DIVERTICULOSIS AND DIVERTICULITIS

A. Description
  1. Diverticulosis
    a. Outpouching or herniations of the intestinal mucosa
    b. They can occur in any part of the intestine but are most common in the sigmoid colon
  2. Diverticulitis
    a. Inflammation of one or more diverticuli that results when a diverticulum perforates
    b. A perforated diverticulum can progress to intra-abdominal perforation with generalized peritonitis
B. Data collection
  1. Left lower quadrant abdominal pain that increases with coughing, straining, or lifting
  2. Elevated temperature
  3. Nausea and vomiting
  4. Flatulence
  5. Cramplike pain
  6. Abdominal distention and tenderness
  7. Palpable, tender rectal mass
  8. Blood in the stools
C. Interventions

1. Provide bed rest during the acute phase
2. Maintain NPO status or provide clear liquids during the acute phase as prescribed
3. Introduce a fiber-containing diet gradually, when the inflammation is resolved
4. Prepare to administer antibiotics, analgesics, and anticholinergics to reduce bowel spasms, as prescribed
5. Instruct the client to refrain from lifting, straining, coughing, or bending to avoid increased intra-abdominal pressure
6. Monitor for perforation, hemorrhage, fistulas, abscesses
7. Instruct the client to increase fluid intake to 2500 to 3000 mL/day, unless contraindicated
8. Instruct the client to eat soft high-fiber foods such as whole grains
9. Instruct the client to avoid gas-forming foods or foods containing indigestible roughage, seeds, or nuts because these food substances become trapped in diverticula and cause inflammation
10. Instruct the client to consume a small amount of bran daily and to take bulk-forming laxatives as prescribed to increase stool mass
11. Instruct the client to avoid high-fiber foods when inflammation occurs because these foods will further irritate the mucosa
D. Surgical interventions
  1. Colon resection with primary anastomosis
  2. Temporary or permanent colostomy may be required for increased bowel inflammation

XVI. HEMORRHOIDS

A. Description
  1. Dilated varicose veins of the anal canal
  2. May be either internal, external, or prolapsed
  3. Internal hemorrhoids lie above the anal sphincter and cannot be seen on inspection of the perianal area
  4. External hemorrhoids lie below the anal sphincter and can be seen on inspection
  5. Prolapsed hemorrhoids can become thrombosed or inflamed
  6. Hemorrhoids are caused from **portal hypertension,** straining, irritation, increased venous or abdominal pressure
B. Data collection
  1. Bright red bleeding with defecation
  2. Rectal pain
  3. Rectal itching
C. Interventions
  1. Apply cold packs to the anal-rectal area followed by sitz baths, as prescribed
  2. Apply witch hazel soaks and topical anesthetics, as prescribed

3. Encourage a high-fiber diet and fluids to promote bowel movements without straining
4. Administer stool softeners, as prescribed

D. Endoscopic procedures
1. Sclerotherapy
2. Endoscopic ligation

E. Surgical procedures
1. Cryosurgery
2. Hemorrhoidectomy

F. Postoperative interventions
1. Assist the client to a prone or side-lying position to prevent bleeding
2. Maintain ice packs over the dressing as prescribed until the packing is removed by the physician
3. Monitor for urinary retention
4. Administer stool softeners, as prescribed
5. Instruct the client to increase fluids and high-fiber foods
6. Instruct the client to limit sitting to short periods of time
7. Instruct the client in the use of sitz baths three to four times a day, as prescribed

XVII. APPENDICITIS

A. Description
1. Inflammation of the appendix
2. When the appendix becomes inflamed or infected, rupture may occur within a matter of hours, leading to peritonitis and sepsis

B. Data collection
1. Pain in the periumbilical area that descends to the right lower quadrant
2. Abdominal pain that is most intense at McBurney's point
3. Rebound tenderness and abdominal rigidity
4. Low-grade fever
5. Elevated white blood cell (WBC) count
6. Anorexia, nausea, and vomiting
7. Client in side-lying position, with abdominal guarding and legs flexed
8. Constipation or diarrhea

C. Peritonitis: Inflammation of the peritoneum (Box 46-8); can occur if the appendix ruptures

D. Appendectomy: Surgical removal of the appendix

BOX 46-8

Signs of Peritonitis

Increased fever and chills
Progressive abdominal distention and abdominal pain
Right guarding of the abdomen
Tachycardia and tachypnea
Pallor
Restlessness

---

1. Preoperative interventions
   a. Maintain NPO status
   b. Monitor IV fluids administered to prevent dehydration
   c. Monitor for changes in level of pain
   d. Monitor for signs of ruptured appendix and peritonitis
   e. Position client in right side-lying or low to semi-Fowler's position to promote comfort
   f. Monitor bowel sounds
   g. Apply ice packs to the abdomen for 20 to 30 minutes every hour, as prescribed
   h. Antibiotics may be prescribed
   i. Avoid the application of heat to the abdomen
   j. Avoid laxatives or enemas

2. Postoperative interventions
   a. Monitor temperature for signs of infection
   b. Monitor incision for signs of infection such as redness, swelling, and pain
   c. Maintain NPO status until bowel function has returned
   d. Advance diet gradually as tolerated and as prescribed when bowel sounds return
   e. If rupture of the appendix has occurred, Penrose drain may be inserted or the incision may be left open to heal from the inside out
   f. Expect that drainage from the Penrose drain may be profuse for the first 12 hours
   g. Position the client in right side-lying or low to semi-Fowler's position, with legs flexed, to facilitate drainage
   h. Change the dressing as prescribed and record the type and amount of drainage
   i. Perform wound irrigations if prescribed
   j. Maintain NG suction and patency of NG tube if present
   k. Administer antibiotics and analgesics, as prescribed

XVIII. CIRRHOSIS (Box 46-9)

A. Description
1. A chronic, progressive disease of the liver, characterized by diffuse damage to cells with fibrosis and nodular regeneration
2. Repeated destruction of hepatic cells causes the formation of scar tissue

B. Complications
1. **Portal hypertension:** A persistent increase in pressure within the portal vein that develops as a result of obstruction to flow
2. **Ascites**
   a. The accumulation of fluid within the peritoneal cavity that results in venous congestion of the hepatic capillaries
   b. This leads to plasma leaking directly from the liver surface and portal vein

BOX 46-9

Types of Cirrhosis

LAENNEC'S CIRRHOSIS
Alcohol-induced, nutritional, or portal cirrhosis
Cellular necrosis; causes eventual widespread scar tissue, with fibrotic infiltration of the liver

POSTNECROTIC CIRRHOSIS
Occurs after massive liver necrosis
Results as a complication of acute viral hepatitis or exposure to hepatotoxins
Scar tissue causes destruction of liver lobules and entire lobes

BILIARY CIRRHOSIS
Develops from chronic biliary obstruction, bile stasis, and inflammation, resulting in severe obstructive jaundice

CARDIAC CIRRHOSIS
Associated with severe, right-sided congestive heart failure (CHF); results in an enlarged, edematous, congested liver
Liver becomes anoxic, resulting in liver cell necrosis and fibrosis

3. Bleeding **esophageal varices:** Fragile, thin-walled, distended esophageal veins that become irritated and rupture
4. Coagulation defects
   a. Decreased synthesis of bile fats in the liver prevent the absorption of fat-soluble vitamins
   b. Without vitamin K and clotting factors II, VII, IX, and X, the client is prone to bleeding
5. Jaundice: Occurs because the liver is unable to metabolize bilirubin and because the edema, fibrosis, and scarring of the hepatic bile ducts interfere with normal bile and bilirubin secretion
6. Portal systemic encephalopathy: End-stage hepatic failure and **cirrhosis,** characterized by altered LOC, neurological symptoms, impaired thinking, and neuromuscular disturbances
7. Hepatorenal syndrome
   a. Progressive renal failure associated with hepatic failure
   b. Characterized by a sudden decrease in urinary output, elevated blood urea nitrogen (BUN) and creatinine levels, decreased urine sodium excretion, and increased urine osmolarity
C. Data collection
   1. Anorexia and weight loss
   2. Early morning nausea and vomiting (presence of blood in vomitus)
   3. Dyspepsia
   4. Flatulence and changes in bowel habits
   5. Emaciation
   6. Fatigue

7. Jaundice
8. Abdominal pain or tenderness
9. **Ascites**
10. Peripheral edema
11. Dry skin and rashes
12. Petechiae or ecchymosis
13. Spider angiomas on the nose, cheeks, upper thorax, and shoulders
14. Hepatomegaly
15. Protruding umbilicus
16. Dilated abdominal veins
17. **Fetor hepaticus,** the fruity, musty breath odor of chronic liver disease
18. **Asterixis** (liver flap): A course tremor characterized by rapid, nonrhythmic extension and flexions in the wrist and fingers
19. Delirium
D. interventions
   1. Elevate the head of the bed to minimize shortness of breath
   2. If **ascites** and edema are absent and the client does not exhibit signs of impending coma, a high-protein diet supplemented with vitamins is prescribed
   3. Provide supplemental vitamins (A, B complex, C, K, folic acid, and thiamine), as prescribed
   4. Restrict sodium intake and fluid intake, as prescribed
   5. Initiate enteral feedings or total parenteral nutrition (TPN), as prescribed
   6. Administer diuretics, as prescribed
   7. Monitor I&O and electrolyte balance
   8. Weigh client and measure abdominal girth daily
   9. Monitor LOC; assess for precoma state (tremors, delirium)
   10. Monitor for **asterixis**
   11. Maintain gastric intubation to assess bleeding and/or esophagogastric balloon tamponade to control bleeding varices if prescribed
   12. Blood products may be prescribed
   13. Monitor coagulation laboratory results; administer vitamin K if prescribed
   14. Administer low sodium antacids, as prescribed
   15. Administer lactulose (Chronulac) as prescribed, which decreases the pH of the bowel, decreases production of ammonia by bacteria in the bowel, and facilitates the excretion of ammonia
   16. Administer neomycin (Mycifradin) as prescribed to inhibit protein synthesis in bacteria and decrease the production of ammonia
   17. Avoid medications such as narcotics, sedatives, and barbiturates and any hepatotoxic medications or substances
   18. Instruct the client about the restriction of alcohol intake
   19. Prepare the client for paracentesis to remove abdominal fluid

20. Prepare the client for surgical shunting procedures if prescribed

XIX. CHOLECYSTITIS

A. Description
1. An inflammation of the gallbladder that may occur as an acute or chronic process
2. Acute inflammation is associated with gallstones (cholelithiasis)
3. Chronic **cholecystitis** results when inefficient bile emptying and gallbladder muscle wall disease cause a fibrotic and contracted gallbladder
4. Acalculus **cholecystitis** occurs in the absence of gallstones and is caused by bacterial invasion via the lymphatic or vascular system

B. Data collection
1. Nausea and vomiting
2. Indigestion
3. Belching
4. Flatulence
5. Epigastric pain that radiates to the scapula 2 to 4 hours after eating fatty foods and may persist for 4 to 6 hours
6. Pain localized in right upper quadrant
7. Guarding, rigidity, and rebound tenderness
8. Mass palpated in the right upper quadrant
9. **Murphy's sign** (cannot take a deep breath when the examiner's fingers are passed below the hepatic margin)
10. Elevated temperature
11. Tachycardia
12. Signs of dehydration

C. Biliary obstruction
1. Jaundice
2. Dark orange and foamy urine
3. Steatorrhea and clay-colored feces
4. Pruritus

D. Interventions
1. Maintain NPO status during nausea and vomiting episodes
2. Maintain nasogastric decompression as prescribed for severe vomiting
3. Administer antiemetics as prescribed for nausea and vomiting
4. Administer analgesics as prescribed to relieve pain and reduce spasm (*note*: although morphine sulfate or codeine sulfate may be prescribed, they are generally avoided because they can cause spasm of the sphincter of Oddi and increase pain)
5. Administer antispasmodic (anticholinergics) as prescribed to relax smooth muscle
6. Instruct the client with chronic **cholecystitis** to eat frequent, small low-fat meals more
7. Instruct the client to avoid gas-forming foods

8. Prepare the client for nonsurgical and surgical procedures, as prescribed

E. Nonsurgical interventions
1. Dissolution therapy
   a. To remove cholesterol stones
   b. Medications such as chenodeoxycholic acid (chenodiol) or ursodiol (Actigall) may be administered orally to decrease the size of the stones or to dissolve small stones
   c. Direct contact with repeated injections and aspirations of a dissolution agent via percutaneous catheter may be performed
2. Extracorporeal shock wave lithotripsy
   a. Shock waves are administered that disintegrate stones in the biliary system
   b. Oral dissolution follows

F. Surgical interventions
1. **Cholecystectomy**: Removal of the gallbladder
2. **Choledochotomy**: Incision into the common bile duct to remove the stone
3. Surgical procedures may be performed by laparoscopy

G. Postoperative interventions
1. Monitor for respiratory complications secondary to pain at the incisional site
2. Encourage coughing and deep breathing
3. Encourage early ambulation
4. Instruct the client about splinting the abdomen to prevent discomfort during coughing
5. Administer antiemetics as prescribed for nausea and vomiting
6. Administer analgesics as prescribed for pain relief
7. Maintain NPO status and NG tube suction as prescribed
8. Advance diet from clear liquids to solids when prescribed and as tolerated by the client
9. Maintain and monitor drainage from the T tube, if present (Box 46-10)

XX. PANCREATITIS

A. Description
1. An acute or chronic inflammation of the pancreas, with associated escape of pancreatic enzymes into surrounding tissue
2. Acute **pancreatitis** occurs suddenly as one attack or can be recurrent, but resolves
3. Chronic **pancreatitis** is a continual inflammation and destruction of the pancreas, with scar tissue replacing pancreatic tissue
4. Precipitating factors include trauma, the use of alcohol, biliary tract disease, viral or bacterial disease, hyperlipidemia, hypercalcemia, cholelithiasis, hyperparathyroidism, ischemic vascular disease, and peptic ulcer disease

B. Acute

BOX 46-10

Care of a T Tube

PURPOSE AND DESCRIPTION

A T tube is placed after surgical exploration of the common bile duct. It preserves the patency of the duct and ensures drainage of bile until edema resolves and bile is effectively draining into the duodenum. A gravity drainage bag is attached to the T tube to collect the drainage.

INTERVENTIONS

Position client in semi-Fowler's position to facilitate drainage.

Monitor the amount, color, consistency, and odor of drainage.

Report sudden increases in bile output to the physician.

Monitor for inflammation and protect the skin from irritation.

Keep the drainage system below the level of the gallbladder.

Monitor for foul odor and purulent drainage and report to the physician.

Avoid irrigation, aspiration, or clamping of the T tube without a physician's order.

As prescribed, clamp the tube before eating, and observe for abdominal discomfort and distention, nausea, chills, or fever; unclamp the tube if nausea or vomiting occurs.

1. Data collection
   a. Abdominal pain, including a sudden onset at the midepigastric or left upper quadrant, with radiation to the back
   b. Pain that is aggravated by a fatty meal, alcohol, or lying in a recumbent position
   c. Abdominal tenderness and guarding
   d. Nausea and vomiting
   e. Weight loss
   f. **Cullen's sign** (discoloration of the abdomen and periumbilical area)
   g. **Turner's sign** (bluish discoloration of the flanks)
   h. Absent or decreased bowel sounds
   i. Elevated white blood cell (WBC) count; elevated glucose, bilirubin, alkaline phosphatase, urinary amylase levels
   j. Elevated lipase and amylase levels
2. Interventions
   a. Maintain NPO status and maintain hydration with IV fluids, as prescribed
   b. TPN may be administered for severe nutritional depletion
   c. Administer supplemental preparations and vitamins and minerals to increase caloric intake if prescribed
   d. Maintain NG tube to decrease gastric distention and suppress pancreatic secretion
   e. Administer meperidine hydrochloride (Demerol) as prescribed for pain because it

causes less incidence of smooth muscle spasm of the pancreatic ducts and sphincter of Oddi (*note:* although morphine sulfate or codeine sulfate may be prescribed, they are generally avoided because they can cause spasm of the sphincter of Oddi and increase pain)
   f. Administer antacids as prescribed to neutralize gastric secretions
   g. Administer histamine H_2-receptor antagonists as prescribed to decrease hydrochloric acid production and prevent activation of pancreatic enzymes
   h. Administer anticholinergics as prescribed to decrease vagal stimulation, decrease GI motility, and inhibit pancreatic enzyme secretion
   i. Instruct the client in the importance of avoiding alcohol
   j. Instruct the client in the importance of follow-up visits with the physician
   k. Instruct the client to notify the physician if acute abdominal pain, jaundice, clay-colored stools, or dark urine develops

C. Chronic
1. Data collection
   a. Abdominal pain and tenderness
   b. Left upper quadrant mass
   c. Steatorrhea and foul-smelling stools that may increase in volume as pancreatic insufficiency increases
   d. Weight loss
   e. Muscle wasting
   f. Jaundice
   g. Signs and symptoms of diabetes mellitus
2. Interventions
   a. Instruct the client in the prescribed dietary measures (fat and/or protein intake may be limited)
   b. Instruct the client to avoid heavy meals
   c. Instruct the client about the importance of avoiding alcohol
   d. Provide supplemental preparations and vitamins and minerals to increase caloric intake
   e. Administer pancreatic enzymes as prescribed to aid in the digestion and absorption of fat and protein
   f. Administer insulin or oral hypoglycemic medications as prescribed to control diabetes mellitus, if present
   g. Instruct the client in the use of pancreatic enzyme medications
   h. Instruct the client in the treatment plan for glucose management
   i. Instruct the client to notify the physician if increased steatorrhea, abdominal distention or cramping, or skin breakdown develops
   j. Instruct the client in the importance of follow-up visits

XXI. HEPATITIS

A. Description
   1. An inflammation of the liver caused by a virus, bacteria, or exposure to medications or hepatotoxins
   2. The goals of treatment include resting the inflamed liver to reduce metabolic demands and increase the blood supply, thus promoting cellular regeneration and preventing complications

B. Types of viral hepatitis
   1. Hepatitis A (HAV), infectious hepatitis
   2. Hepatitis B (HBV), serum hepatitis
   3. Hepatitis C (HCV), non-A, non-B hepatitis or post-transfusion hepatitis
   4. Hepatitis D (HDV), delta agent hepatitis
   5. Hepatitis E (HEV), enterically transmitted or epidemic non-A, non-B hepatitis
   6. Hepatitis G (HGV), non-A, non-B, non-C hepatitis

C. Stages of viral hepatitis (Box 46-11)

D. Data collection
   1. Preicteric stage
      a. Flulike symptoms: Malaise, fatigue
      b. Anorexia, nausea, vomiting, diarrhea
      c. Pain: Headache, muscle aches, polyarthritis
      d. Serum bilirubin and enzyme levels are elevated
   2. Icteric stage
      a. Jaundice
      b. Pruritus
      c. Brown-colored urine
      d. Lighter colored stools
      e. Decrease in preicteric phase symptoms
   3. Posticteric stage
      a. Energy levels increase
      b. Pain subsides
      c. GI symptoms are minimal to absent
      d. Serum bilirubin and enzyme levels return to normal

E. Laboratory findings
   1. Alanine aminotransferase (ALT) level: Elevated to more than 1000 milliunits/mL and may rise to as high as 4000 milliunits/mL
   2. Aspartate aminotransferase (AST) level: May rise to 1000 to 2000 milliunits/mL
   3. Alkaline phosphatase levels: May be normal or mildly elevated
   4. Total bilirubin levels: Elevated in both serum and urine

XXII. HEPATITIS A (HAV)

A. Description
   1. Formerly known as infectious hepatitis
   2. Commonly seen during the fall and early winter

B. Increased-risk individuals
   1. Commonly seen in young children
   2. Individuals in institutionalized settings
   3. Health care personnel

BOX 46-11

Stages of Viral Hepatitis

PREICTERIC STAGE
The first stage of hepatitis preceding the appearance of jaundice

ICTERIC STAGE
The second stage of hepatitis; includes the appearance of jaundice and associated symptoms such as elevated bilirubin levels, dark or tea-colored urine, and clay-colored stools

POSTICTERIC STAGE
The convalescent stage, in which the jaundice decreases and the color of the urine and stool return to normal

---

C. Transmission
   1. Fecal-oral route
   2. Person-to-person contact
   3. Parenteral
   4. Contaminated fruits, vegetables, or uncooked shellfish
   5. Contaminated water or milk
   6. Poorly washed utensils

D. Incubation period
   1. Incubation period is 2 to 6 weeks
   2. Infectious period is 2 to 3 weeks before and 1 week after developing jaundice

E. Testing
   1. Infection is established by the presence of hepatitis A virus (HAV) antibodies (anti-HAV) in the blood
   2. Immunoglobulins M and G (IgM and IgG) are normally present in the blood, and increased levels indicate infection and inflammation
   3. Ongoing inflammation of the liver is evidenced by the presence of elevated IgM antibodies, which persist in the blood for 4 to 6 weeks
   4. Previous infection is indicated by the presence of elevated IgG antibodies

F. Complication: Fulminant hepatitis

G. Prevention
   1. Strict hand washing
   2. Stool and needle precautions
   3. Treatment of municipal water supplies
   4. Serologic screening of food handlers
   5. Hepatitis A vaccine (Havrix)
   6. Immune globulin (IG): For individuals exposed to HAV who have never received the hepatitis A vaccine; administer during the period of incubation and within 2 weeks of exposure
   7. IG is recommended for household members and sexual contacts of individuals with Hepatitis A
   8. Pre-exposure prophylaxis with IG is recommended to individuals traveling to countries with poor or uncertain sanitation conditions

XXIII. HEPATITIS B (HBV)
A. Description
1. Is nonseasonal in nature
2. All age-groups are affected
B. Increased-risk individuals
1. Drug addicts
2. Clients undergoing long-term hemodialysis
3. Health care personnel
C. Transmission
1. Blood or body fluid contact
2. Infected blood products
3. Infected saliva or semen
4. Contaminated needles
5. Sexual contact
6. Parenteral
7. Perinatal period
8. Blood or body fluids contact at birth
D. Incubation period: 6 to 24 weeks
E. Testing
1. Infection is established by the presence of hepatitis B antigen-antibody systems in the blood
2. Presence of hepatitis B surface antigen (HBsAg) is the serologic marker to establish the diagnosis of hepatitis B
3. The client is considered infectious if this antigen is present in the blood
4. If the serologic marker (HBsAg) is present after 6 months, it indicates a carrier state or chronic hepatitis
5. Normally, the serologic marker (HBsAg) level declines and disappears after the acute hepatitis B episode
6. The presence of antibodies to HBsAg (anti-HBs) indicates recovery and immunity to hepatitis B
7. Hepatitis B early antigen (HBeAg) is detected in the blood about 1 week after the appearance of HBsAg; its presence determines the infective state of the client
F. Complications
1. Fulminant hepatitis
2. Chronic liver disease
3. **Cirrhosis**
4. Primary hepatocellular carcinoma
G. Prevention
1. Strict hand washing
2. Screening blood donors
3. Testing of all pregnant women
4. Needle precautions
5. Avoiding sexual contact if hepatitis B surface antigen (HBsAg) is positive
6. Hepatitis B vaccine: Engerix-B, Recombivax HB
7. Hepatitis B immune globulin (HBIG): For individuals exposed to HBV either through sexual contact or through the percutaneous or transmucosal routes, who have never had hepatitis B and have never received hepatitis B vaccine

XXIV. HEPATITIS C (HCV)
A. Description
1. Occurs year-round
2. Can occur in any age group
3. Is common among drug abusers and is the major cause of post-transfusion hepatitis
4. Risk factors are similar to those of HBV, because hepatitis C is also parenterally transmitted
B. Increased-risk individuals
1. Parenteral drug users
2. Clients receiving frequent transfusions
3. Health care personnel
C. Transmission: Same as HBV; primarily through blood
D. Incubation period: 5 to 10 weeks
E. Testing: Anti-HCV is the antibody to HCV and is most accurate in detecting chronic states of hepatitis C
F. Complications
1. Chronic liver disease
2. **Cirrhosis**
3. Primary hepatocellular carcinoma
G. Prevention
1. Strict hand washing
2. Needle precautions
3. Screening of blood donors

XXV. HEPATITIS D (HDV)
A. Description
1. Common in the Mediterranean area and Middle East
2. Seen with hepatitis B and may cause infection only in the presence of active HBV infection
3. Coinfection with HDV intensifies the acute symptoms of hepatitis B
4. Transmission and risk of infection are the same as HBV via contact with blood and blood products
5. Prevention of HBV infection with vaccine also prevents HDV infection, because HDV is dependent on HBV for replication
B. High-risk individuals
1. Drug users
2. Clients receiving hemodialysis
3. Clients receiving frequent blood transfusions
C. Transmission: Same as HBV
D. Incubation period: 7 to 8 weeks
E. Testing: Serologic hepatitis delta virus (HDV) determination is made by detection of the hepatitis D antigen (HDAg) early in the course of the infection and by detection of anti-HDV antibody in the later disease stages
F. Complications
1. Chronic liver disease
2. Fulminant hepatitis
G. Prevention: Because hepatitis D must coexist with hepatitis B, the precautions that help prevent hepatitis B are also useful in preventing HDV

XXVI. HEPATITIS E (HEV)

A. Description
1. A waterborne virus
2. Prevalent in areas where sewage disposal is inadequate or where communal bathing in contaminated rivers is practiced
3. Risk of infection is the same as HAV
4. Presents as a mild disease except in infected women in the third trimester of pregnancy, in whom the mortality rate is high

B. Increased-risk individuals
1. Travelers to countries that have a high incidence of hepatitis E such as India, Burma (Myanmar), Afghanistan, Algeria, and Mexico
2. Eating or drinking food or water contaminated with the virus

C. Transmission: Same as HAV

D. Incubation period: 2 to 9 weeks

E. Testing: Specific serologic tests for hepatitis E virus (HEV) include detection of IgM and IgG antibodies to hepatitis E (anti-HEV)

F. Complications
1. High mortality rate in pregnant women
2. Fetal demise

G. Prevention

BOX 46-12

Client and Family Education for Hepatitis

The client needs to perform strict and frequent hand washing.

The client needs to avoid sharing bathrooms unless the client strictly adheres to personal hygiene measures.

Individual washcloths, towels, drinking and eating utensils, as well as toothbrushes and razors, must be labeled and identified.

The client must not prepare food for other family members.

The client should avoid alcohol and over-the-counter medications, particularly acetaminophen (Tylenol) and sedatives, because these medications are hepatotoxic.

The client should increase activity gradually to prevent fatigue.

The client should consume small, frequent, high-carbohydrate, low-fat meals.

The client is not to donate blood.

The client may maintain normal contact with people as long as proper personal hygiene is maintained.

The client is to avoid sexual activity until hepatitis B surface antigen (HBsAg) results are negative.

Close personal contact such as kissing should be discouraged until HBsAg test results are negative.

The client needs to carry a Medic-Alert card noting the date of hepatitis onset.

The client needs to inform other health professionals, such as medical or dental personnel, of the onset of hepatitis.

The client needs to keep follow-up appointments with the health care provider.

---

1. Strict hand washing
2. Treatment of water supplies and sanitation measures

XXVII. HEPATITIS G (HGV)

A. Non-A, non-B, non-C hepatitis

B. Autoantibodies are absent

C. Risk factors are similar to those for hepatitis C

D. Hepatitis G (HGV) has been found in some blood donors, IV drug users, hemodialysis clients, and clients with hemophilia; however, HGV does not appear to cause significant liver disease

XXVIII. INSTRUCTION FOR HOME CARE FOR THE CLIENT AND FAMILY (Box 46-12)

PRACTICE QUESTIONS

1. A client presents to the emergency department with upper gastrointestinal (GI) bleeding and is in moderate distress. Which nursing action would be the priority for this client?
   1. Thorough investigation of the precipitating events
   2. Insertion of a nasogastric tube and hematest the emesis
   3. Complete abdominal physical examination
   4. Determination of vital signs

2. A nurse is caring for a client with possible cholelithiasis who is being prepared for a cholangiogram and provides instructions to the client about the procedure. Which client statement indicates that the client understands the purpose of this test?
   1. "They are going to look at my gallbladder and ducts."
   2. "This procedure will drain my gallbladder."
   3. "My gallbladder will be irrigated."
   4. "They will put medication in my gallbladder."

3. A nurse is caring for a client with acute pancreatitis and a history of alcoholism and is monitoring the client for complications. Which of the following data would be a sign of paralytic ileus?
   1. Firm, nontender mass palpable at the lower right costal margin
   2. Severe, constant pain with rapid onset
   3. Inability to pass flatus
   4. Loss of anal sphincter control

4. A nurse is caring for a client with a resolved intestinal obstruction who has a nasogastric tube in place. The client has tolerated the tube being clamped every 2 hours for 1 hour and the physician has now ordered the nasogastric tube to be discontinued. To determine the client's readiness for discontinuation of the nasogastric tube, the nurse should check for:
   1. Proper nasogastric tube placement
   2. The client's serum electrolyte levels

3. Presence of bowel sounds in all four quadrants
4. The pH of the gastric aspirate

5. A sexually active 20-year-old client has developed viral hepatitis. Which of the following statements if made by the client would indicate a need for teaching?
   1. "A condom should be used for sexual intercourse."
   2. "I can never drink alcohol again."
   3. "I won't go back to work right away."
   4. "My close friends should get the vaccine."

6. A client is admitted to the hospital with severe jaundice and is having diagnostic testing. Because the client has no complaints of fatigue, the client is encouraged to ambulate in the hall to maintain muscle strength. The client paces around the room, but will not enter the hall. Which of the following problems most likely is the reason for the client's reluctance to walk in the hall?
   1. Fear of catching another disease
   2. Not wanting to overexert and get overtired
   3. Feeling self-conscious about appearance
   4. Unfamiliarity with the hospital

7. A client with viral hepatitis has no appetite and food makes the client nauseated. Which nursing intervention would be appropriate?
   1. Explain that high-fat diets are usually better tolerated
   2. Encourage foods low in calories
   3. Explain that the majority of calories need to be consumed in the evening hours
   4. Monitor for fluid and electrolyte imbalances

8. A nurse is participating in a health screening clinic and is preparing teaching materials about colorectal cancer. The nurse would plan to include which risk factor for colorectal cancer in the material?
   1. Age of 20 years
   2. High-fiber, low-fat diet
   3. Distant relative with colorectal cancer
   4. Personal history of ulcerative colitis or gastrointestinal polyps

9. A hospitalized client with gastroesophageal reflux disease (GERD) is complaining of chest discomfort that feels like heartburn following a meal. After administering a prescribed antacid, the nurse would encourage the client to lie in which position?
   1. Supine, with the head of the bed flat
   2. On the stomach, with the head flat
   3. On the left side, with the head of the bed elevated 30 degrees
   4. On the right side, with the head of the bed elevated 30 degrees

10. A nurse is planning to teach a client with gastroesophageal reflux disease (GERD) about substances that will increase the lower esophageal sphincter (LES) pressure. The nurse tells the client to include which item in the diet?
    1. Fatty foods
    2. Nonfat milk
    3. Tea
    4. Coffee

11. A client has undergone esophagogastroduodenoscopy (EGD). The nurse places highest priority on which of the following items as part of the client's care plan?
    1. Checking for return of a gag reflex
    2. Giving warm gargles for a sore throat
    3. Monitoring the temperature
    4. Monitoring for complaints of heartburn

12. A nurse has taught a client about an upcoming endoscopic retrograde cholangiopancreatography (ERCP) procedure. The nurse determines that the client needs additional information if the client makes which statement?
    1. "I know I must sign a consent form."
    2. "I'm glad I don't have to lie still for this procedure."
    3. "I'm glad some medication will be given IV to relax me."
    4. "I hope the throat spray keeps me from gagging."

13. A client being seen in a physician's office has just been scheduled for a barium swallow the next day. The nurse writes down which of the following instructions for the client to follow before the test?
    1. Remove all metal and jewelry before the test
    2. Eat a regular supper and breakfast
    3. Continue to take all oral medications as scheduled
    4. Monitor own bowel movement pattern for constipation

14. A nurse is teaching the client about an upcoming colonoscopy procedure. The nurse would include in the instructions that the client will be placed in which of the following positions for the procedure?
    1. Left Sims' position
    2. Right Sims' position
    3. Knee-chest position
    4. Lithotomy position

15. A nurse has given postprocedure instructions to a client who has undergone a colonoscopy. The nurse determines that the client did not fully understand the directions if the client states that:
    1. Intake should be light at first, then progress to regular intake
    2. It is normal to feel gassy or bloated after the procedure
    3. The abdominal muscles may be tender from stretching during the procedure
    4. It is all right to drive once the client has been home for an hour or so

16. A nurse is preparing to perform an abdominal examination. The initial step would be which of the following?
    1. Auscultation
    2. Inspection
    3. Palpation
    4. Percussion

17. A client is scheduled for an oral cholecystography. The nurse would plan to obtain what type of diet for the evening meal before the test?
    1. Low-protein
    2. High-carbohydrate
    3. Fat-free
    4. Liquid

18. A client with viral hepatitis states to the nurse, "I am so yellow." The nurse would most appropriately:
    1. Assist the client in expressing feelings
    2. Keep the client isolated from other clients and visitors
    3. Provide information to the client about hepatitis
    4. Restrict visitors until the jaundice subsides

19. A nurse provides instructions to a client following a liver biopsy. The nurse tells the client to:
    1. Avoid alcohol for 8 hours
    2. Save all stools to be checked for blood
    3. Remain NPO for 24 hours
    4. Lie on the right side for 2 hours

20. A nurse is caring for a client with a diagnosis of chronic gastritis. The nurse anticipates that this client is at risk for which vitamin deficiency?
    1. Vitamin A
    2. Vitamin B$_{12}$
    3. Vitamin C
    4. Vitamin E

21. A nurse is reviewing the medication record of a client with acute gastritis. Which of the following medications, if noted on the client's record, would the nurse question?
    1. Digoxin (Lanoxin)
    2. Ibuprofen (Motrin)
    3. Furosemide (Lasix)
    4. Propranolol hydrochloride (Inderal)

22. A nurse is monitoring a client with a diagnosis of peptic ulcer. Which finding would most likely indicate perforation of the ulcer?
    1. Bradycardia
    2. Numbness in the legs
    3. Nausea and vomiting
    4. A rigid, boardlike abdomen

23. A client with peptic ulcer disease is scheduled for a pyloroplasty and the client asks the nurse about the procedure. The nurse bases the response on which of the following?
    1. A pyloroplasty involves cutting the vagus nerve
    2. A pyloroplasty involves removing the distal portion of the stomach

3. A pyloroplasty involves removal of the ulcer and a large portion of the cells that produce hydrochloric acid
    4. A pyloroplasty involves an incision and resuturing of the pylorus to relax the muscle and enlarge the opening from the stomach to the duodenum

24. A client with a peptic ulcer is scheduled for a vagotomy and the client asks the nurse about the purpose of this procedure. The nurse tells the client that a vagotomy:
    1. Decreases food absorption in the stomach
    2. Heals the gastric mucosa
    3. Halts stress reactions
    4. Reduces the stimulus to acid secretions

25. A nurse is caring for a client following a Billroth II procedure. On review of the postoperative orders, which of the following, if prescribed, would the nurse question and verify?
    1. Irrigating the nasogastric (NG) tube
    2. Coughing and deep breathing exercises
    3. Leg exercises
    4. Early ambulation

26. The nurse is providing discharge instructions to a client following gastrectomy. Which measure will the nurse instruct the client to follow to help prevent dumping syndrome?
    1. Eat high-carbohydrate foods
    2. Limit the fluids taken with meals
    3. Ambulate following a meal
    4. Sit in a high Fowler's position during meals

27. A nurse is monitoring a client for the early signs and symptoms of dumping syndrome. Which of the following symptoms will indicate this occurrence?
    1. Dry skin and stomach pain
    2. Bradycardia and indigestion
    3. Sweating and pallor
    4. Double vision and chest pain

28. A nurse is instructing the client who had a herniorrhaphy how to reduce postoperative swelling following the procedure. Which of the following would the nurse suggest to the client to prevent swelling?
    1. Apply heat to the abdomen
    2. Elevate the scrotum
    3. Limit fluids
    4. Maintain a low-roughage diet

29. A nurse is reviewing the record of a client with Crohn's disease. Which of the following stool characteristics would the nurse expect to note documented in the record?
    1. Bloody stools
    2. Diarrhea
    3. Constipation
    4. Stool constantly oozing from the rectum

30. A nurse is performing a colostomy irrigation on a client. During the irrigation, the client begins to complain of abdominal cramps. Which of the following is the appropriate nursing action?
    1. Notify the registered nurse immediately
    2. Increase the height of the irrigation
    3. Stop the irrigation temporarily
    4. Medicate for pain and resume irrigation

31. A nurse is teaching a client how to perform a colostomy irrigation. To enhance the effectiveness of the irrigation, what measure should the nurse instruct the client to do?
    1. Increase fluid intake
    2. Reduce the amount of irrigation solution
    3. Massage the abdomen gently
    4. Place heat on the abdomen

32. A nurse is reviewing the record of a client with a diagnosis of cirrhosis and notes that there is documentation of the presence of asterixis. To check for the presence of this sign, the nurse would do which of the following?
    1. Ask the client to extend the arms
    2. Check for the presence of Homans' sign
    3. Instruct the client to lean forward
    4. Measure the abdominal girth

33. A client with ascites is scheduled for a paracentesis. The nurse is assisting the physician in performing the procedure. Which of the following positions will the nurse assist the client to assume for this procedure?
    1. Flat
    2. Left side-lying
    3. Right side-lying
    4. Upright

34. A nurse is reviewing the laboratory results of a client with cirrhosis and notes that the ammonia level is elevated. Which of the following diets would the nurse anticipate would most likely be prescribed for this client?
    1. High-carbohydrate
    2. Moderate-fat
    3. High-protein
    4. Low-protein

35. Lactulose (Chronulac) is prescribed for a client with a diagnosis of hepatic encephalopathy. Which finding indicates that the client is responding to this medication therapy as anticipated?
    1. The fecal pH is acidic
    2. The client experiences diarrhea
    3. The client is able to tolerate a full diet
    4. Vomiting occurs

36. An ultrasound of the gallbladder is scheduled for the client with a suspected diagnosis of cholecystitis. The nurse explains to the client that this test:
    1. Requires the client to lie still for short intervals
    2. Requires that the client be NPO
    3. Is preceded by the administration of oral tablets
    4. Is uncomfortable

37. A nurse is providing preoperative teaching to a client scheduled for a cholecystectomy. Which intervention would be the highest priority in the preoperative teaching plan?
    1. Teaching coughing and deep breathing exercises
    2. Teaching leg exercises
    3. Instructions regarding fluid intake and diet
    4. Checking the client's understanding of the surgical procedure

38. A Penrose drain is in place on the first postoperative day following a cholecystectomy. Serosanguineous drainage is noted on the dressing covering the drain. Which nursing intervention is appropriate?
    1. Notify the registered nurse immediately
    2. Change the dressing
    3. Circle the amount on the dressing with a pen
    4. Continue to monitor the drainage

39. A client is admitted to the hospital for treatment of acute hepatitis B. Which activity order would the nurse expect to be prescribed?
    1. Bed rest
    2. Encourage ambulation
    3. Out of bed in a chair continuously during the day
    4. No activity restrictions

40. It has been determined that a client with hepatitis has contracted the infection from contaminated food. What type of hepatitis is this client most likely experiencing?
    1. Hepatitis A
    2. Hepatitis B
    3. Hepatitis C
    4. Hepatitis D

41. A nurse is reviewing the physician's orders written for a client admitted with acute pancreatitis. Which physician order would the nurse verify if noted on the client's chart?
    1. NPO status
    2. Prepare to insert a nasogastric tube
    3. An anticholinergic medication
    4. Morphine sulfate for pain

42. A client with peptic ulcer disease states that stress frequently causes exacerbation of the disease. The nurse would interpret that which of the following items mentioned by the client is most likely responsible for the exacerbations?
    1. Sleeping 8 to 10 hours a night
    2. Eating five or six small meals per day
    3. Ability to work at home periodically
    4. Frequent need to work overtime on short notice

43. A client with peptic ulcer disease needs dietary modification to reduce episodes of epigastric pain. The nurse would teach the client that which of the

following items does not need to be limited or eliminated with this disease?

1. Wine
2. Baked chicken
3. Coffee
4. Fresh fruit

44. A nurse instructs the ileostomy client to do which of the following as part of essential care of the stoma?
1. Cleanse the peristomal skin meticulously
2. Eat high-fiber foods, such as nuts
3. Massage the area below the stoma every morning and every evening
4. Limit fluid intake to prevent diarrhea

45. A client with hiatal hernia chronically experiences heartburn following meals. The nurse would teach the client to avoid which of the following, which is contraindicated with hiatal hernia?
1. Eating small, frequent, bland meals
2. Lying recumbent following meals
3. Raising the head of the bed on 6-inch blocks
4. Taking histamine receptor antagonist medication, as prescribed

46. A nurse is monitoring for stoma prolapse in a client with a colostomy. The nurse would observe which of the following appearances in the stoma if prolapse occurred?
1. Sunken and hidden
2. Dark and bluish in color
3. Narrowed and flattened
4. Protruding and swollen

47. A client with a new colostomy is concerned about odor from stool in the ostomy drainage bag. The nurse teaches the client to include which of the following foods in the diet to reduce odor?
1. Yogurt
2. Broccoli
3. Cucumbers
4. Eggs

48. A nurse has given instructions to the client with an ileostomy about foods to eat to thicken the stool. The nurse determines that the client did not fully understand the instructions if the client states that he or she eats which of the following foods to make the stool less watery?
1. Pasta
2. Boiled rice
3. Bran
4. Low-fat cheese

49. A nurse is doing preoperative teaching with the client who is about to undergo creation of a Kock pouch. The nurse determines that the client has the best understanding of the nature of the surgery if the client makes which statement?
1. "I will need to drain the pouch regularly with a catheter."
2. "I will need to wear a drainage bag for the rest of my life."

3. "The stool from this type of ostomy will be formed."
4. "I will be able to pass stool by the rectum eventually."

50. The client with chronic pancreatitis needs information on dietary modification to manage health problems. The nurse teaches the client to limit which of the following items in the diet?
1. Carbohydrate
2. Protein
3. Fat
4. Water-soluble vitamins

51. A client with acute pancreatitis is experiencing severe pain from the disorder. The nurse tells the client to avoid which position that could aggravate the pain?
1. Sitting up
2. Lying flat
3. Leaning forward
4. Flexing the left leg

52. A nurse is evaluating the effect of dietary counseling on the client with cholecystitis. The nurse determines that the client understands the instructions given if the client states that which food item is acceptable to include in the diet?
1. Baked scrod
2. Sauces and gravies
3. Fried chicken
4. Fresh whipped cream

53. A client with cirrhosis is beginning to show signs of hepatic encephalopathy. The nurse would plan a dietary consult to limit the amount of which ingredient in the client's diet?
1. Fat
2. Carbohydrate
3. Protein
4. Minerals

54. A client with Crohn's disease has an order to begin taking antispasmodic medication. The nurse should time the medication so that each dose is taken:
1. 30 minutes before meals
2. During meals
3. 60 minutes after meals
4. On arising and at bedtime

55. A client is admitted to the hospital with acute viral hepatitis. Which of the following signs or symptoms would the nurse expect to note based upon this diagnosis?
1. Spider angiomas
2. Fatigue
3. Pale urine
4. Weight gain

56. A client with viral hepatitis who is discussing with the nurse the need to avoid alcohol states, "I'm not sure I can do that." The nurse would respond by saying:
1. "Everything will be all right."
2. "I think you should talk more with the doctor about this."

3. "I don't believe that."

4. "I'm not sure that I understand. Would you please explain?"

57. Of the following infection control methods, which would be the priority to include in the plan of care to prevent hepatitis B in a client considered to be at high risk for exposure?

1. Correct hand washing technique
2. Hepatitis B vaccine
3. Proper personal hygiene
4. Use of immune globulin

58. A nurse provides home care instructions to a client with hepatitis B. Which statement by the client indicates the best understanding of how to prevent transmission of the disease?

1. "I should be vaccinated as soon as possible."
2. "I will never share a towel with anyone else."
3. "It is all right to kiss my wife."
4. "My wife should get the vaccine."

59. A client is admitted to the hospital with viral hepatitis and is complaining of a loss of appetite. In order to provide adequate nutrition, the nurse encourages the client to:

1. Eat a large supper when anorexia is most likely not as severe

2. Eat less often, preferably only three large meals daily
3. Increase intake of fluids including juices
4. Select foods high in fat

60. An African-American client has a diagnosis of acute viral hepatitis. Which of the following specific areas would the nurse inspect for jaundice in this client?

1. Flexor surfaces of the extremities
2. Hard palate of the mouth
3. Nail beds
4. Skin

ALTERNATE FORMAT QUESTION: MULTIPLE RESPONSE

A nurse is reviewing the orders of a client admitted to the hospital with a diagnosis of acute pancreatitis. Select the interventions that the nurse would expect to be prescribed for the client.

___ Small, frequent high calorie feedings
___ Meperidine (Demerol) as prescribed for pain
___ Maintain the client in a supine and flat position
___ Encourage coughing and deep breathing
___ Administer antacids, as prescribed
___ Administer anticholinergics, as prescribed

ANSWERS

1. *Answer:* 4

Rationale: The determination of vital signs indicates whether the client is in shock from blood loss and also provides a baseline blood pressure and pulse by which to monitor the progress of treatment. Signs and symptoms of shock include low blood pressure; rapid, weak pulse; increased thirst; cold, clammy skin; and restlessness. Vital signs should be monitored at least every 15 to 30 minutes, and the physician should be informed of any significant changes. The client may not be able to provide subjective data until the immediate physical needs are met. Although options 2 and 3 may be a component of care, they are not the priority.

Test-Taking Strategy: Note the word "priority" and use the ABCs—airway, breathing, and circulation. A client with an acute upper GI bleed is at risk for shock. Monitoring vital signs is the nursing action that will assess circulation, provide information about the client's circulating volume status, and alert the nurse to early stages of shock. Review care of the client with a GI bleed if you had difficulty with this question.

Level of Cognitive Ability: Application
Client Needs: Physiological Integrity
Integrated Process: Nursing Process/Implementation
Content Area: Adult Health/Gastrointestinal
References: Christensen, B., & Kockrow, E. (2003). *Adult health nursing* (4th ed.). St. Louis: Mosby, p. 192.

Linton, A., & Maebius, N. (2003). *Introduction to medical-surgical nursing* (3rd ed.). Philadelphia: W.B. Saunders, p. 688.

2. *Answer:* 1

Rationale: A cholangiogram is for diagnostic purposes. It outlines both the gallbladder and the ducts, so gallstones that have moved into the ductal system can be detected. X-rays are used to visualize the biliary duct system after an IV injection of radiopaque dye. Options 2, 3, and 4 are incorrect.

Test-Taking Strategy: Use the process of elimination. Eliminate options 2, 3 and 4 because they are similar. Review this procedure if you had difficulty with this question.

Level of Cognitive Ability: Comprehension
Client Needs: Physiological Integrity
Integrated Process: Nursing Process/Evaluation
Content Area: Adult Health/Gastrointestinal
References: Linton, A., & Maebius, N. (2003). *Introduction to medical-surgical nursing* (3rd ed.). Philadelphia: W.B. Saunders, p. 718.

Thompson, J., McFarland, G., Hirsch, J., & Tucker, S. (2002). *Mosby's clinical nursing* (5th ed.). St. Louis: Mosby, pp. 1378-1379.

3. *Answer:* 3

Rationale: An inflammatory reaction such as acute pancreatitis can cause paralytic ileus, the most common form of

nonmechanical obstruction. Inability to pass flatus is a clinical manifestation of paralytic ileus. Option 1 is the description of the physical finding of liver enlargement. The liver is usually enlarged in cases of cirrhosis or hepatitis. Although this client may have an enlarged liver, an enlarged liver is not a sign of paralytic ileus or intestinal obstruction. Pain is associated with paralytic ileus, but the pain usually presents as a more constant generalized discomfort. Pain that is severe, constant, and rapid in onset is more likely caused by strangulation of the bowel. Loss of sphincter control is not a sign of paralytic ileus.
Test-Taking Strategy: Use the process of elimination. Note the relationship between the words "paralytic ileus" and option 3. Review these clinical manifestations if you had difficulty with this question.
Level of Cognitive Ability: Comprehension
Client Needs: Physiological Integrity
Integrated Process: Nursing Process/Data Collection
Content Area: Adult Health/Gastrointestinal
Reference: Linton, A., & Maebius, N. (2003). *Introduction to medical-surgical nursing* (3rd ed.). Philadelphia: W.B. Saunders, p. 223.

4. *Answer:* 3
Rationale: Distention, vomiting, and abdominal pain are a few of the symptoms associated with intestinal obstruction and a nasogastric tube may be used to empty the stomach and relieve distention and vomiting. Bowel sounds return to normal as the obstruction is relieved and normal bowel function is restored. Discontinuing the nasogastric tube before normal bowel function returns may result in a return of the symptoms necessitating reinsertion of the nasogastric tube. Serum electrolyte levels, tube placement, and pH of gastric aspirate are important assessments for the client with a nasogastric tube in place, but would not assist in determining the readiness for removing the nasogastric tube.
Test-Taking Strategy: Use the process of elimination and focus on the issue, removing the nasogastric tube. Recalling the pathophysiology for intestinal obstruction and purpose of a nasogastric tube as a therapy will direct you to option 3. Review care of the client with an intestinal obstruction if you had difficulty with this question.
Level of Cognitive Ability: Comprehension
Client Needs: Physiological Integrity
Integrated Process: Nursing Process/Data Collection
Content Area: Adult Health/Gastrointestinal
References: Linton, A., & Maebius, N. (2003). *Introduction to medical-surgical nursing* (3rd ed.). Philadelphia: W.B. Saunders, pp. 660, 662.
Potter, P., & Perry, A. (2005). *Fundamentals of nursing* (6th ed.). St. Louis: Mosby, pp. 762, 1183.

5. *Answer:* 2
Rationale: To prevent transmission of hepatitis, a condom is advised during sexual intercourse as well as vaccination of the partner or close friends. Alcohol should be avoided for 1 year, because it is detoxified in the liver and may interfere with recovery. Rest is especially important until laboratory studies show that the liver function has returned to normal. The client's activity is increased gradually.

Test-Taking Strategy: Use the process of elimination and note the key words, *need for teaching*. These words indicate a false response question and that you need to select the incorrect client statement. Recalling the pathophysiology related to hepatitis and noting the key word *never* in option 2 will direct you to this option. Review client instructions regarding hepatitis if you had difficulty with this question.
Level of Cognitive Ability: Comprehension
Client Needs: Safe, Effective Care Environment
Integrated Process: Nursing Process/Evaluation
Content Area: Adult Health/Gastrointestinal
Reference: Linton, A., & Maebius, N. (2003). *Introduction to medical-surgical nursing* (3rd ed.). Philadelphia: W.B. Saunders, p. 731.

6. *Answer:* 3
Rationale: Clients with jaundice frequently have a body image disturbance because of a change in appearance. This can be manifested in negative verbal or nonverbal behavior. Options 1, 2, and 4 are unrelated to the data in the question.
Test-Taking Strategy: Use the process of elimination. Noting the key words, *severe jaundice*, will direct you to option 3. Review the psychosocial issues related to jaundice if you had difficulty with this question.
Level of Cognitive Ability: Comprehension
Client Needs: Psychosocial Integrity
Integrated Process: Nursing Process/Data Collection
Content Area: Adult Health/Gastrointestinal
Reference: Linton, A., & Maebius, N. (2003). *Introduction to medical-surgical nursing* (3rd ed.). Philadelphia: W.B. Saunders, p. 723.

7. *Answer:* 4
Rationale: If nausea persists, the client will need to be assessed for fluid and electrolyte imbalances. It is important to explain to the client that the majority of calories should be eaten in the morning hours, because nausea most often occurs in the afternoon and evening. Clients should select a diet high in calories, because energy is required for healing. Changes in bilirubin interfere with fat absorption, so low fat-diets are better tolerated.
Test-Taking Strategy: Use the process of elimination. Recalling the nutritional aspects of care for clients with viral hepatitis will direct you to option 4. Review care of the client with viral hepatitis if you had difficulty answering this question.
Level of Cognitive Ability: Application
Client Needs: Physiological Integrity
Integrated Process: Nursing Process/Implementation
Content Area: Adult Health/Gastrointestinal
Reference: Christensen, B., & Kockrow, E. (2003). *Adult health nursing* (4th ed). St. Louis: Mosby, pp. 233-234.

8. *Answer:* 4
Rationale: Common risk factors for colorectal cancer include age over 40 years, first-degree relative with colorectal cancer, high-fat, low-fiber diet, and history of bowel problems such as ulcerative colitis or familial polyposis.
Test-Taking Strategy: Use the process of elimination. Noting the key words, *personal history*, in option 4 will direct you to this option. Review these risk factors if you had difficulty with this question.

Level of Cognitive Ability: Application
Client Needs: Health Promotion and Maintenance
Integrated Process: Nursing Process/Planning
Content Area: Adult Health/Gastrointestinal
Reference: Linton, A., & Maebius, N. (2003). *Introduction to medical-surgical nursing* (3rd ed.). Philadelphia: W.B. Saunders, p. 682.

9. *Answer: 3*
Rationale: The discomfort of reflux is aggravated by positions that compress the abdomen and the stomach. These include lying flat either on the back or stomach after a meal, or lying on the right side. The left side-lying position with the head of the bed elevated is most likely to give relief to the client.
Test-Taking Strategy: Use the process of elimination. Evaluate each of the positions described in terms of their ability to put pressure on the stomach and cause reflux. Using knowledge of anatomy and these basic nursing positions, you should be able to eliminate each of the incorrect options. Review the measures to relieve reflux if you had difficulty with this question.
Level of Cognitive Ability: Application
Client Needs: Physiological Integrity
Integrated Process: Nursing Process/Implementation
Content Area: Adult Health/Gastrointestinal
Reference: Linton, A., & Maebius, N. (2003). *Introduction to medical-surgical nursing* (3rd ed.). Philadelphia: W.B. Saunders, p. 682.

10. *Answer: 2*
Rationale: Foods that increase the LES pressure will decrease reflux, and lessen the symptoms of GERD. The food item that will increase the LES pressure is nonfat milk. The other items listed decrease the LES pressure, thus increasing reflux symptoms. Aggravating substances include chocolate, coffee, fatty foods and alcohol.
Test-Taking Strategy: Use the process of elimination. Eliminate options 3 and 4 first because they are similar and both contain caffeine. From the remaining options, recalling the effects of fatty foods will direct you to option 2. Review these food items if you had difficulty with this question.
Level of Cognitive Ability: Application
Client Needs: Health Promotion and Maintenance
Integrated Process: Teaching/Learning
Content Area: Adult Health/Gastrointestinal
Reference: Linton, A., & Maebius, N. (2003). *Introduction to medical-surgical nursing* (3rd ed.). Philadelphia: W.B. Saunders, p. 682.

11. *Answer: 1*
Rationale: The nurse places highest priority on managing the client's airway. This includes assessing for return of the gag reflex. The client's vital signs are also monitored and a sudden sharp increase in temperature could indicate perforation of the gastrointestinal tract. This would be accompanied by other signs as well, such as pain. Monitoring for sore throat and heartburn are also important; the client's airway still takes priority however.
Test-Taking Strategy: Use the process of elimination. Note that the question contains the key words, *highest priority*. Use the

ABCs—airway, breathing, and circulation. This will direct you to option 1. Review postprocedure care following EGD if you had difficulty with this question.
Level of Cognitive Ability: Application
Client Needs: Physiological Integrity
Integrated Process: Nursing Process/Data Collection
Content Area: Delegating/Prioritizing
Reference: Chernecky, C., & Berger, B. (2004). *Laboratory tests and diagnostic procedures* (4th ed.). Philadelphia: W.B. Saunders, p. 510.

12. *Answer: 2*
Rationale: The client needs to lie still for ERCP, which takes about an hour to perform. The client also needs to sign a consent form. IV sedation is given to relax the client, and an anesthetic spray is used to help keep the client from gagging as the endoscope is passed.
Test-Taking Strategy: Use the process of elimination. Note the key words, *needs additional information*. These words indicate a false response question and that you need to select the incorrect client statement. Invasive procedures require consent, so option 1 can be eliminated. Noting the name of the procedure and considering the anatomical location will assist in eliminating options 3 and 4. Review this procedure if you had difficulty with this question.
Level of Cognitive Ability: Comprehension
Client Needs: Physiological Integrity
Integrated Process: Nursing Process/Evaluation
Content Area: Adult Health/Gastrointestinal
Reference: Chernecky, C., & Berger, B. (2004). *Laboratory tests and diagnostic procedures* (4th ed.). Philadelphia: W.B. Saunders, p. 501.

13. *Answer: 1*
Rationale: A barium swallow is an x-ray that uses a substance called barium for contrast to highlight abnormalities in the gastrointestinal (GI) tract. The client is told to remove all jewelry before the test, so it won't interfere with x-ray visualization of the field. The client should fast for 8 to 12 hours before the test, depending on the physician's instructions. Most oral medications are also withheld before the test, depending on the physician's instructions. It is important to monitor for constipation following the procedure, which can occur as a result of the presence of barium in the GI tract.
Test-Taking Strategy: Use the process of elimination. Note that the key words in the stem of the question are *barium swallow* and *before*. This tells you that the correct option is an item that the client needs to comply with before the test is done. Eliminate option 4 first, because it is a part of aftercare. Eliminate option 3 next because of the word "all." Recalling that the procedure is a type of x-ray that involves barium for contrast and an NPO status will direct you to option 1. Review preprocedure instructions for this test if you had difficulty with this question.
Level of Cognitive Ability: Application
Client Needs: Physiological Integrity
Integrated Process: Nursing Process/Implementation
Content Area: Adult Health/Gastrointestinal
References: Chernecky, C., & Berger, B. (2004). *Laboratory tests and diagnostic procedures* (4th ed.). Philadelphia: W.B. Saunders, p. 360.

Lewis, S., Heitkemper, M., & Dirksen, S. (2004). *Medical-surgical nursing: Assessment and management of clinical problems* (6th ed.). St. Louis: Mosby, p. 961.

14. Answer: 1
Rationale: The client is placed in the left Sims' position for the procedure. This position takes the best advantage of the client's anatomy for ease in introducing the colonoscope. The other options are incorrect.
Test-Taking Strategy: Use concepts related to gastrointestinal anatomy to answer this question. The position would be the same as would be utilized for giving the client an enema while lying down. When answering factual questions such as these, remember the guiding principles and attempt to visualize the procedure to help you select the correct option. Review this procedure if you had difficulty with this question.
Level of Cognitive Ability: Application
Client Needs: Physiological Integrity
Integrated Process: Nursing Process/Implementation
Content Area: Adult Health/Gastrointestinal
Reference: Chernecky, C., & Berger, B. (2004). *Laboratory tests and diagnostic procedures* (4th ed.). Philadelphia: W.B. Saunders, p. 390.

15. Answer: 4
Rationale: The client should not drive for several hours after this test because the client would have received sedative medications during the procedure. The client should resume intake slowly, and progress as tolerated. The client may experience gas or abdominal tenderness for a short while after the procedure, and this is normal.
Test-Taking Strategy: Use the process of elimination. Note that the question contains the key words, *did not fully understand.* This tells you that the correct option is an incorrect statement on the part of the client. Use knowledge of events during the procedure to choose the correct option. Recalling that sedating medications are administered will direct you to option 4. Review postprocedure instructions if you had difficulty with this question.
Level of Cognitive Ability: Comprehension
Client Needs: Health Promotion and Maintenance
Integrated Process: Teaching/Learning
Content Area: Adult Health/Gastrointestinal
Reference: Chernecky, C., & Berger, B. (2004). *Laboratory tests and diagnostic procedures* (4th ed.). Philadelphia: W.B. Saunders, p. 391.

16. Answer: 2
Rationale: The appropriate technique for abdominal examination is inspection, auscultation, percussion, and palpation. Auscultation is performed after inspection and before percussion and palpation to ensure that the motility of the bowel and bowel sounds are not altered. The sequence of maneuvers is inspect, auscultate, percuss, and palpate.
Test-Taking Strategy: Use the process of elimination and think about the procedure. Remember that the sequence for abdominal examination is different than the usual systematic approach. Review this technique if you had difficulty with this question.
Level of Cognitive Ability: Application

Client Needs: Health Promotion and Maintenance
Integrated Process: Nursing Process/Data Collection
Content Area: Adult Health/Gastrointestinal
Reference: Christensen, B., & Kockrow, E. (2003). *Foundations of nursing* (4th ed.). St. Louis: Mosby, pp. 67-68.

17. Answer: 3
Rationale: Normal dietary intake of fat should be maintained during the days preceding the test in order to empty bile from the gallbladder. A fat-free diet is ordered on the evening before the test. The fat-free supper prevents contraction of the gallbladder and allows accumulation of the contrast substance needed for x-ray visualization. Options 1, 2, and 4 are incorrect.
Test-Taking Strategy: Use the process of elimination. Recalling that an oral cholecystogram is an x-ray of the gallbladder and thinking about the function of the gallbladder will assist in selecting the correct option. Review this test if you had difficulty with this question.
Level of Cognitive Ability: Application
Client Needs: Physiological Integrity
Integrated Process: Nursing Process/Planning
Content Area: Adult Health/Gastrointestinal
Reference: Lewis, S., Heitkemper, M., & Dirksen, S. (2004). *Medical-surgical nursing: Assessment and management of clinical problems* (6th ed.). St. Louis: Mosby, pp. 1144-1145.

18. Answer: 1
Rationale: The client's feelings should be explored to discover how the client feels about the disease process and appearance so appropriate interventions can be planned. Options 2, 3, and 4 are inappropriate.
Test-Taking Strategy: Use the process of elimination and focus on the client's concern. Remembering to address the client's feelings will direct you to option 1. Review the psychosocial issues related to hepatitis if you had difficulty with this question.
Level of Cognitive Ability: Application
Client Needs: Psychosocial Integrity
Integrated Process: Nursing Process/Implementation
Content Area: Adult Health/Gastrointestinal
Reference: Linton, A., & Maebius, N. (2003). *Introduction to medical-surgical nursing* (3rd ed.). Philadelphia: W.B. Saunders, p. 723.

19. Answer: 4
Rationale: In order to splint the puncture site, the client is kept on his or her right side for a minimum of 2 hours. It is not necessary to remain NPO for 24 hours. Permission regarding the consumption of alcohol should be obtained from the physician. It is not necessary to save all stools.
Test-Taking Strategy: Use the process of elimination and focus on the issue, a liver biopsy. Recalling the anatomical location of this procedure will direct you to option 4. Review postprocedure instructions following a liver biopsy if you had difficulty with this question.
Level of Cognitive Ability: Application
Client Needs: Physiological Integrity
Integrated Process: Nursing Process/Implementation
Content Area: Adult Health/Gastrointestinal

Reference: Pagana, K., & Pagana, T. (2003). *Mosby's diagnostic and laboratory test reference* (6th ed.). St. Louis: Mosby, p. 569.

20. Answer: 2
Rationale: Deterioration and atrophy of the lining of the stomach lead to the loss of function of the parietal cells. When the acid secretion decreases, the source of the intrinsic factor is lost, which results in the inability to absorb vitamin B_{12}. This leads to the development of pernicious anemia. Options 1, 3, and 4 are incorrect.
Test-Taking Strategy: Use the process of elimination. Knowledge regarding the pathophysiology related to the lining of the stomach is required to answer this question. If you are unfamiliar with vitamin B_{12} deficiency and its relationship to gastric disorders, review this content.
Level of Cognitive Ability: Comprehension
Client Needs: Physiological Integrity
Integrated Process: Nursing Process/Data Collection
Content Area: Adult Health/Gastrointestinal
Reference: Linton, A., & Maebius, N. (2003). *Introduction to medical-surgical nursing* (3rd ed.). Philadelphia: W.B. Saunders, p. 690.

21. Answer: 2
Rationale: Ibuprofen is a nonsteroidal anti-inflammatory drug (NSAID) and can cause ulceration of the esophagus, stomach, duodenum, or small intestine. It is contraindicated in a client with a gastrointestinal disorder. Furosemide is a loop diuretic. Digoxin is an antidysrhythmic. Propranolol hydrochloride is a beta-adrenergic blocker. Furosemide, digoxin, and propranolol hydrochloride are not contraindicated in clients with gastric disorders.
Test-Taking Strategy: Knowledge regarding the side effects associated with the medications identified in the options is required to answer this question. Remember, a nonsteroidal anti-inflammatory drug (NSAID) can cause ulceration of the esophagus, stomach, duodenum, or small intestine. If you are unfamiliar with these medications, review this content.
Level of Cognitive Ability: Analysis
Client Needs: Safe, Effective Care Environment
Integrated Process: Nursing Process/Implementation
Content Area: Adult Health/Gastrointestinal
Reference: McKenry, L., & Salerno, E. (2003). *Mosby's pharmacology in nursing* (21st ed.). St. Louis: Mosby, p. 290.

22. Answer: 4
Rationale: Perforation is a surgical emergency. It is characterized by sudden, sharp, intolerable severe pain beginning in the midepigastric area and spreading over the abdomen, which becomes rigid and boardlike. Nausea and vomiting may occur. Tachycardia may occur as hypovolemic shock develops. Numbness in the legs is not an associated finding.
Test-Taking Strategy: Use the process of elimination. Note the key words, *most likely*, in the stem of the question. Option 2 can be eliminated first. Eliminate option 1 next because tachycardia rather that bradycardia would develop if the client is bleeding. From the remaining options, focusing on the key words will assist in directing you to option 4. Review the signs of perforation if you had difficulty with this question.
Level of Cognitive Ability: Analysis

Client Needs: Physiological Integrity
Integrated Process: Nursing Process/Data Collection
Content Area: Adult Health/Gastrointestinal
Reference: Linton, A., & Maebius, N. (2003). *Introduction to medical-surgical nursing* (3rd ed.). Philadelphia: W.B. Saunders, pp. 688-689.

23. Answer: 4
Rationale: Option 4 describes the procedure for a pyloroplasty. A vagotomy involves cutting the vagus nerve. A subtotal gastrectomy involves removing the distal portion of the stomach. A Billroth II procedure involves removal of the ulcer and a large portion of the cells that produce hydrochloric acid.
Test-Taking Strategy: Use the process of elimination. Note the relationship between the words "pyloroplasty" in the question and "pylorus" in the correct option. Review this procedure if you had difficulty with this question.
Level of Cognitive Ability: Comprehension
Client Needs: Physiological Integrity
Integrated Process: Nursing Process/Implementation
Content Area: Adult Health/Gastrointestinal
Reference: Linton, A., & Maebius, N. (2003). *Introduction to medical-surgical nursing* (3rd ed.). Philadelphia: W.B. Saunders, p. 687.

24. Answer: 4
Rationale: A vagotomy, or cutting of the vagus nerve, is done to eliminate parasympathetic stimulation of gastric secretion. Options 1, 2, and 3 are incorrect descriptions of a vagotomy.
Test-Taking Strategy: Knowledge regarding the procedure and purpose of a vagotomy is required to answer this question. Remember, a vagotomy is done to eliminate parasympathetic stimulation of gastric secretion. If you are unfamiliar with this procedure, review this content.
Level of Cognitive Ability: Application
Client Needs: Physiological Integrity
Integrated Process: Nursing Process/Implementation
Content Area: Adult Health/Gastrointestinal
Reference: Linton, A., & Maebius, N. (2003). *Introduction to medical-surgical nursing* (3rd ed.). Philadelphia: W.B. Saunders, p. 687.

25. Answer: 1
Rationale: In a Billroth II resection, the proximal remnant of the stomach is anastomosed to the proximal jejunum. Patency of the NG tube is critical for preventing the retention of gastric secretions. The nurse, however, should never irrigate or reposition the gastric tube after gastric surgery unless specifically ordered by the physician. In this situation, the nurse should clarify the order. Options 2, 3, and 4 are appropriate postoperative interventions.
Test-Taking Strategy: Use the process of elimination. Eliminate options 2, 3, and 4 because they are general postoperative measures. Also, consider the anatomical location of the surgical procedure to assist in directing you to option 1. Review these postoperative measures if you had difficulty with this question.
Level of Cognitive Ability: Application
Client Needs: Safe, Effective Care Environment
Integrated Process: Nursing Process/Implementation

Content Area: Adult Health/Gastrointestinal
References: Christensen, B., & Kockrow, E. (2003). *Adult health nursing* (4th ed). St. Louis: Mosby, p. 190.
Linton, A., & Maebius, N. (2003). *Introduction to medical-surgical nursing* (3rd ed.). Philadelphia: W.B. Saunders, p. 689.

26. *Answer:* 2
Rationale: The client should be instructed to decrease the amount of fluid taken at meals. The client should also be instructed to avoid high-carbohydrate foods including fluids, such as fruit nectars; to assume a low Fowler's position during meals; to lie down for 30 minutes after eating to delay gastric emptying; and to take antispasmotics as prescribed.
Test-Taking Strategy: Use the process of elimination. Eliminate options 3 and 4 first because these measures will promote gastric emptying. From the remaining options, select option 2 because this measure will delay gastric emptying. If you are unfamiliar with this syndrome, review these client teaching points.
Level of Cognitive Ability: Application
Client Needs: Health Promotion and Maintenance
Integrated Process: Teaching/Learning
Content Area: Adult Health/Gastrointestinal
Reference: Linton, A., & Maebius, N. (2003). *Introduction to medical-surgical nursing* (3rd ed.). Philadelphia: W.B. Saunders, p. 692.

27. *Answer:* 3
Rationale: Early manifestations occur 5 to 30 minutes after eating. Symptoms include vertigo, tachycardia, syncope, sweating, pallor, palpitations, and the desire to lie down.
Test-Taking Strategy: Knowledge regarding the early manifestations associated with dumping syndrome is required to answer this question. Remember, sweating and pallor occur and are early signs of dumping syndrome. If you are unfamiliar with these manifestations, review this content.
Level of Cognitive Ability: Comprehension
Client Needs: Physiological Integrity
Integrated Process: Nursing Process/Data Collection
Content Area: Adult Health/Gastrointestinal
Reference: Linton, A., & Maebius, N. (2003). *Introduction to medical-surgical nursing* (3rd ed.). Philadelphia: W.B. Saunders, p. 662.

28. *Answer:* 2
Rationale: Following herniorrhaphy, the client should be instructed to elevate the scrotum and apply ice packs while in bed to decrease pain and swelling. The client is also instructed to apply a scrotal support when out of bed. Options 1, 3, and 4 are incorrect.
Test-Taking Strategy: The issue of the question is to prevent swelling. Basic knowledge regarding the effects of heat and cold will assist in eliminating option 1. Options 3 and 4 can be eliminated next by focusing on the issue. Review postoperative care following herniorrhaphy if you had difficulty with this question.
Level of Cognitive Ability: Application
Client Needs: Health Promotion and Maintenance
Integrated Process: Teaching/Learning
Content Area: Adult Health/Gastrointestinal

Reference: Black, J., & Hawks, J. (2005). *Medical-surgical nursing: Clinical management for positive outcomes.* (7th ed.). Philadelphia: W.B. Saunders, p. 841.

29. *Answer:* 2
Rationale: Crohn's disease is characterized by nonbloody diarrhea of usually not more than four or five stools daily. Over time, the diarrhea episodes increase in frequency, duration, and severity. Options 3 and 4 are not characteristics of Crohn's disease.
Test-Taking Strategy: Use the process of elimination. Recalling the pathophysiology related to Crohn's disease will direct you to option 2. If you are unfamiliar with this disorder, review this content.
Level of Cognitive Ability: Comprehension
Client Needs: Physiological Integrity
Integrated Process: Nursing Process/Data Collection
Content Area: Adult Health/Gastrointestinal
Reference: Christensen, B., & Kockrow, E. (2003). *Adult health nursing* (4th ed.). St. Louis: Mosby, p. 202.

30. *Answer:* 3
Rationale: If cramping occurs during colostomy irrigation, the irrigation flow is stopped temporarily and the client is allowed to rest. Cramping may occur from infusion that is too rapid or is causing too much pressure. Increasing the height of the irrigation will cause further discomfort. The registered nurse does not need to be notified immediately. Medicating the client for pain is not the appropriate action.
Test-Taking Strategy: Use the process of elimination and focus on the issue of the question. Using the principles related to administering an enema will direct you to option 3. Review the procedure for colostomy irrigation if you had difficulty with this question.
Level of Cognitive Ability: Application
Client Needs: Physiological Integrity
Integrated Process: Nursing Process/Implementation
Content Area: Adult Health/Gastrointestinal
Reference: Lewis, S., Heitkemper, M., & Dirksen, S. (2004). *Medical-surgical nursing: Assessment and management of clinical problems* (6th ed.). St. Louis: Mosby, p. 1092.

31. *Answer:* 3
Rationale: To enhance effectiveness of the irrigation, the client is instructed to change position, ambulate, massage the abdomen gently, and drink something warm. Options 1, 2, and 4 will not enhance the effectiveness of this procedure.
Test-Taking Strategy: Focus on the issue of the question, which is the measure that will enhance the effectiveness of the irrigation. This focus will assist in eliminating options 1, 2, and 4. Review this procedure if you had difficulty with this question.
Level of Cognitive Ability: Application
Client Needs: Health Promotion and Maintenance
Integrated Process: Teaching/Learning
Content Area: Adult Health/Gastrointestinal
Reference: Phipps, W., Monahan, F., Sands, J., Marek, J., & Neighbors, M. (2003). *Medical-surgical nursing: Health and illness perspectives* (7th ed.). St. Louis: Mosby, p. 1092.

32. *Answer:* 1

Rationale: Asterixis is irregular flapping movements of the fingers and wrists when the hands and arms are outstretched, with the palms down, wrists bent up, and fingers spread. It is the most common sign that hepatic encephalopathy is developing.

Test-Taking Strategy: Use the process of elimination. Recalling the definition of asterixis will direct you to option 1. If you are unfamiliar with this data collection procedure, review this content.

Level of Cognitive Ability: Application
Client Needs: Health Promotion and Maintenance
Integrated Process: Nursing Process/Data Collection
Content Area: Adult Health/Gastrointestinal
Reference: Christensen, B., & Kockrow, E. (2003). *Adult health nursing* (4th ed.). St. Louis: Mosby, p. 229.

33. *Answer:* 4

Rationale: An upright position allows the intestine to float posteriorly and helps prevent intestinal laceration during catheter insertion. Options 1, 2, and 3 are incorrect positions.

Test-Taking Strategy: Use the process of elimination and visualize this procedure in selecting the correct option. Knowing that fluid will be aspirated from the abdominal cavity will assist in directing you to option 4. If you had difficulty with this question, review this procedure.

Level of Cognitive Ability: Application
Client Needs: Physiological Integrity
Integrated Process: Nursing Process/Implementation
Content Area: Adult Health/Gastrointestinal
Reference: Chernecky, C., & Berger, B. (2004). *Laboratory tests and diagnostic procedures* (4th ed.). Philadelphia: W.B. Saunders, p. 843.

34. *Answer:* 4

Rationale: Most of the ammonia in the body is found in the gastrointestinal tract. Protein provided by the diet is transported to the liver by the portal vein. The liver breaks down protein and this results in the formation of ammonia. A low-protein diet would be prescribed. The diets in options 1, 2, and 3 are incorrect.

Test-Taking Strategy: Use the process of elimination. Note that options 3 and 4 are opposite, which should provide you with the clue that one of these options is correct. Recalling the physiology of the liver will direct you to option 4. Review care of the client with cirrhosis if you had difficulty with this question.

Level of Cognitive Ability: Comprehension
Client Needs: Physiological Integrity
Integrated Process: Nursing Process/Planning
Content Area: Adult Health/Gastrointestinal
Reference: Christensen, B., & Kockrow, E. (2003). *Adult health nursing* (4th ed.). St. Louis: Mosby, p. 231.

35. *Answer:* 1

Rationale: Lactulose is an osmotic laxative. The desired effect is two or three soft stools per day, with an acid fecal pH. Lactulose creates an acid environment in the bowel, resulting in a fall of the colon's pH from 7 to 5. This causes ammonia to leave the circulatory system and move into the colon.

Diarrhea may indicate excessive administration of the medication. Options 3 and 4 do not determine that a desired effect has occurred.

Test-Taking Strategy: Knowledge regarding the purpose and action of this medication is required to answer this question. Remember the desired effect is two or three soft stools per day, with an acid fecal pH. Review this medication if you had difficulty with this question.

Level of Cognitive Ability: Analysis
Client Needs: Physiological Integrity
Integrated Process: Nursing Process/Evaluation
Content Area: Adult Health/Gastrointestinal
Reference: Hodgson, B., & Kizior, R. (2005). *Saunders nursing drug handbook 2005*. Philadelphia: W.B. Saunders, pp. 611-612.

36. *Answer:* 1

Rationale: Ultrasound of the gallbladder is a noninvasive procedure and is frequently used for emergency diagnosis of acute cholecystitis. The client does not need to be NPO but may be instructed to avoid carbonated beverages for 48 hours before the test to help decrease intestinal gas. It is a painless test and does not require the administration of oral tablets as preparation.

Test-Taking Strategy: Focus on the issue, an ultrasound. Visualizing this procedure will direct you to option 1. Review this procedure if you had difficulty with this question.

Level of Cognitive Ability: Application
Client Needs: Physiological Integrity
Integrated Process: Nursing Process/Implementation
Content Area: Adult Health/Gastrointestinal
Reference: Chernecky, C., & Berger, B. (2004). *Laboratory tests and diagnostic procedures* (4th ed.). Philadelphia: W.B. Saunders, p. 484.

37. *Answer:* 1

Rationale: After cholecystectomy, breathing tends to be shallow, because deep breathing is painful as a result of the location of the surgical procedure. Teaching the importance of performing coughing and deep breathing exercises is the priority.

Test-Taking Strategy: Note the key words, *highest priority*. Use the process of elimination and recall the anatomical location of this surgical procedure. Use of the ABCs—airway, breathing, and circulation—will direct you to option 1. Review preoperative teaching for a cholecystectomy if you had difficulty with this question.

Level of Cognitive Ability: Application
Client Needs: Physiological Integrity
Integrated Process: Nursing Process/Implementation
Content Area: Delegating/Prioritizing
Reference: Linton, A., & Maebius, N. (2003). *Introduction to medical-surgical nursing* (3rd ed.). Philadelphia: W.B. Saunders, p. 737.

38. *Answer:* 2

Rationale: Serosanguineous drainage with a small amount of bile is expected from the Penrose drain for the first 24 hours. Drainage then decreases and the drain is removed usually in 48 hours. The registered nurse does not need to be notified immediately. A sterile dressing covers the site and should be changed to prevent infection and skin excoriation.

Test-Taking Strategy: Use the process of elimination. Eliminate options 3 and 4 first because they are similar. From the remaining options, recalling the expected findings following this surgical procedure will direct you to option 2. Review care of the client following cholecystectomy if you had difficulty with this question.

Level of Cognitive Ability: Application
Client Needs: Physiological Integrity
Integrated Process: Nursing Process/Implementation
Content Area: Adult Health/Gastrointestinal
Reference: Christensen, B., & Kockrow, E. (2003). *Adult health nursing* (4th ed). St. Louis: Mosby, p. 241.

39. *Answer:* 1
Rationale: Fatigue is a normal response to hepatic cellular damage. During the acute stage, rest is an essential intervention to reduce the liver's metabolic demands and increase its blood supply. Options 2, 3, and 4 are incorrect.

Test-Taking Strategy: Use the process of elimination. Note the key word, *acute*, in the question. Knowing that the liver will need to rest in order to heal will direct you to option 1. If you are unfamiliar with the care of a client with hepatitis, review this content.

Level of Cognitive Ability: Comprehension
Client Needs: Physiological Integrity
Integrated Process: Nursing Process/Implementation
Content Area: Adult Health/Gastrointestinal
Reference: Christensen, B., & Kockrow, E. (2003). *Adult health nursing* (4th ed). St. Louis: Mosby, p. 233.

40. *Answer:* 1
Rationale: Hepatitis A is transmitted by the fecal oral route via contaminated food or infected food handlers. Hepatitis B, C, and D are most commonly transmitted via infected blood or body fluids.

Test-Taking Strategy: Knowledge regarding the modes of transmission of the various types of hepatitis is required to answer this question. Remember, hepatitis A is transmitted by the fecal oral route via contaminated food or infected food handlers. If you are unfamiliar with the modes of transmission of hepatitis, review this content.

Level of Cognitive Ability: Comprehension
Client Needs: Physiological Integrity
Integrated Process: Nursing Process/Data Collection
Content Area: Adult Health/Gastrointestinal
Reference: Christensen, B., & Kockrow, E. (2003). *Adult health nursing* (4th ed.). St. Louis: Mosby, p. 232.

41. *Answer:* 4
Rationale: Meperidine (Demerol) rather than morphine sulfate is the medication of choice, because morphine sulfate can cause spasms in the sphincter of Oddi. Therefore, the nurse would verify this order. Options 1, 2, and 3 are appropriate interventions for the client with acute pancreatitis.

Test-Taking Strategy: Use the process of elimination and note the key word, *acute*, in the question. Recalling the treatment measures for acute pancreatitis and the contraindications in

the care of the client will direct you to option 4. Review these measures if you had difficulty with this question.

Level of Cognitive Ability: Analysis
Client Needs: Safe, Effective Care Environment
Integrated Process: Nursing Process/Implementation
Content Area: Adult Health/Gastrointestinal
Reference: Christensen, B., & Kockrow, E. (2003). *Adult health nursing* (4th ed). St. Louis: Mosby, p. 243.

42. *Answer:* 4
Rationale: Psychological or emotional stressors that exacerbate peptic ulcer disease may be found either at home or in the workplace. The frequent need to work overtime on short notice is the option that is potentially most stressful, because it is the item over which the client has least control. An ability to work at home periodically is not necessarily stressful, because there is increased client control over timing of work and location. Adequate rest and proper dietary pattern (options 1 and 2) should alleviate symptoms, not worsen them.

Test-Taking Strategy: Use the process of elimination. Begin to answer this question by eliminating options 1 and 2, because they are healthy living habits. Recall that psychological stress may be worsened in situations where there is little client control. This will direct you to option 4. Review the causes of exacerbation of this disease if you had difficulty with this question.

Level of Cognitive Ability: Analysis
Client Needs: Physiological Integrity
Integrated Process: Nursing Process/Data Collection
Content Area: Adult Health/Gastrointestinal
Reference: Christensen, B., & Kockrow, E. (2003). *Adult health nursing* (4th ed.). St. Louis: Mosby, pp. 192-193.

43. *Answer:* 2
Rationale: Dietary modification for the client with peptic ulcer disease includes eliminating foods that are irritating to the client. Items that are generally eliminated or avoided are highly spiced foods, alcohol, caffeine, chocolate, and fresh fruits. Other foods may be taken according to the client's tolerance of that specific food.

Test-Taking Strategy: Use the process of elimination and focus on the client's diagnosis. Note the key words, *does not need to be limited or eliminated.* Recalling which types of foods and beverages are irritating to the gastrointestinal mucosa will direct you to option 2. Review the dietary measures for peptic ulcer disease if you had difficulty with this question.

Level of Cognitive Ability: Application
Client Needs: Health Promotion and Maintenance
Integrated Process: Teaching/Learning
Content Area: Adult Health/Gastrointestinal
Reference: Christensen, B., & Kockrow, E. (2003). *Adult health nursing* (4th ed). St. Louis: Mosby, p. 193.

44. *Answer:* 1
Rationale: The peristomal skin must receive meticulous cleansing because ileostomy drainage has more enzymes and is more caustic to the skin than colostomy drainage. Foods such as nuts and those with seeds will pass through the ileostomy. The client should be taught that these foods will

remain undigested. The area below the ileostomy may be massaged as needed if the ileostomy becomes blocked by high-fiber foods. Fluid intake should be maintained by at least six to eight glasses of water per day to prevent dehydration.
Test-Taking Strategy: Use the process of elimination. Note the key words, *essential care* and *stoma*. This tells you that the correct option will be the option that deals with the stoma directly. This focus will direct you to option 1. Review client teaching regarding ileostomy care if you had difficulty with this question.
Level of Cognitive Ability: Application
Client Needs: Health Promotion and Maintenance
Integrated Process: Teaching/Learning
Content Area: Adult Health/Gastrointestinal
Reference: Christensen, B., & Kockrow, E. (2003). *Adult health nursing* (4th ed.). St. Louis: Mosby, pp. 201-202.

45. Answer: 2
Rationale: Hiatal hernia is due to a protrusion of a portion of the stomach above the diaphragm, where the esophagus usually is positioned. The client generally experiences pain caused by reflux resulting from ingestion of irritating foods, lying flat following meals or at night, and consuming large or fatty meals. Relief is obtained by eating small, frequent, and bland meals; by histamine antagonists and antacids; and by elevation of the thorax following meals and during sleep.
Test-Taking Strategy: Use the process of elimination. Note the key word, *contraindicated.* This tells you that the correct answer will be the option that represents an aggravating factor for hiatal hernia discomfort. Visualize each option and think about the anatomical location of a hiatal hernia to direct you to option 2. Review these teaching points if you had difficulty with this question.
Level of Cognitive Ability: Application
Client Needs: Health Promotion and Maintenance
Integrated Process: Teaching/Learning
Content Area: Adult Health/Gastrointestinal
Reference: Linton, A., & Maebius, N. (2003). *Introduction to medical-surgical nursing* (3rd ed.). Philadelphia: W.B. Saunders, p. 682.

46. Answer: 4
Rationale: A prolapsed stoma is one in which bowel protrudes through the stoma, with an elongated and swollen appearance. A stoma retraction is characterized by sinking of the stoma. Ischemia of the stoma would be associated with dusky or bluish color. A stoma with a narrowed opening, either at the level of the skin or fascia, is said to be stenosed.
Test-Taking Strategy: Use the process of elimination. Focusing on the key word, *prolapse,* will direct you to option 4. Review the different complications that can occur with ostomy formation if you had difficulty with this question.
Level of Cognitive Ability: Analysis
Client Needs: Physiological Integrity
Integrated Process: Nursing Process/Data Collection
Content Area: Adult Health/Gastrointestinal
Reference: Linton, A., & Maebius, N. (2003). *Introduction to medical-surgical nursing* (3rd ed.). Philadelphia: W.B. Saunders, p. 355.

47. Answer: 1
Rationale: The client should be taught to include deodorizing foods in the diet, such as beet greens, parsley, buttermilk, and yogurt. Spinach also reduces odor, but is a gas-forming food as well. Broccoli, cucumbers, and eggs are gas-forming foods.
Test-Taking Strategy: Use the process of elimination. Recalling the effect of various foods on the gastrointestinal tract of the client with an ostomy will direct you to option 1. If this question was difficult, review foods that cause odor or gas and those that have a deodorizing effect.
Level of Cognitive Ability: Application
Client Needs: Health Promotion and Maintenance
Integrated Process: Teaching/Learning
Content Area: Adult Health/Gastrointestinal
Reference: Black, J., & Hawks, J. (2005). *Medical-surgical nursing: Clinical management for positive outcomes* (7th ed.). Philadelphia: W.B. Saunders, p. 827.

48. Answer: 3
Rationale: Foods that help to thicken the stool of the client with an ileostomy include pasta, boiled rice, and low-fat cheese. Bran is high in dietary fiber, and thus will increase the output of watery stool by increasing propulsion through the bowel. Ileostomy output is liquid by nature. Addition or elimination of various foods can help thicken or loosen this liquid drainage.
Test-Taking Strategy: Use the process of elimination and note the key words, *did not fully understand.* These words indicate a false response question and that you need to select the incorrect food item. Recalling that high-fiber foods such as bran can aggravate watery stools will direct you to option 3. Review dietary measures for the client with an ileostomy if you had difficulty with this question.
Level of Cognitive Ability: Comprehension
Client Needs: Health Promotion and Maintenance
Integrated Process: Teaching/Learning
Content Area: Adult Health/Gastrointestinal
Reference: Black, J., & Hawks, J. (2005). *Medical-surgical nursing: Clinical management for positive outcomes* (7th ed.). Philadelphia: W.B. Saunders, p. 827.

49. Answer: 1
Rationale: A Kock pouch is a continent ileostomy. As the ileostomy begins to function, the client drains it with a catheter every 3 to 4 hours, which is then decreased to about three times a day or as needed when full. The client does not need to wear a drainage bag, but should wear an absorbent dressing to absorb mucous drainage from the stoma. Ileostomy drainage is liquid in nature. The client would only be able to pass stool from the rectum if an ileal-anal pouch or anastomosis were created.
Test-Taking Strategy: To answer this question accurately, it is necessary to understand the different surgical procedures that are performed with ileostomy and their consequences on the bowel habits of the client. Remember, a Kock pouch is a continent ileostomy. If this question was difficult, review this content.
Level of Cognitive Ability: Comprehension
Client Needs: Physiological Integrity
Integrated Process: Nursing Process/Evaluation

Content Area: Adult Health/Gastrointestinal
References: Christensen, B., & Kockrow, E. (2003). *Adult health nursing* (4th ed.). St. Louis: Mosby, p. 447.
Linton, A., & Maebius, N. (2003). *Introduction to medical-surgical nursing* (3rd ed.). Philadelphia: W.B. Saunders, pp. 362-363.

50. Answer: 3
Rationale: The client should limit fat in the diet. The client should also eat small meals. This will also reduce the amount of carbohydrate and protein that the client must digest at any one time. The client does not need to limit water-soluble vitamins in the diet.
Test-Taking Strategy: Use the process of elimination. Recalling the pathophysiology related to pancreatic function will direct you to option 3. Review these dietary measures if you had difficulty with this question.
Level of Cognitive Ability: Application
Client Needs: Health Promotion and Maintenance
Integrated Process: Teaching/Learning
Content Area: Adult Health/Gastrointestinal
Reference: Linton, A., & Maebius, N. (2003). *Introduction to medical-surgical nursing* (3rd ed.). Philadelphia: W.B. Saunders, p. 745.

51. Answer: 2
Rationale: Positions such as sitting up, leaning forward, and flexing the legs (especially the left leg) may alleviate some of the pain associated with pancreatitis. The pain is aggravated by lying supine or walking. This is because the pancreas is located retroperitoneally, and the edema and inflammation intensify the irritation of the posterior peritoneal wall with these positions.
Test-Taking Strategy: Use the process of elimination. Eliminate options 1 and 3 first because they are similar. From the remaining options, visualize the pancreas and the potential effects of stretching associated with the various positions listed. This will direct you to option 2. Review care of the client with pancreatitis if you had difficulty with this question.
Level of Cognitive Ability: Application
Client Needs: Physiological Integrity
Integrated Process: Nursing Process/Implementation
Content Area: Adult Health/Gastrointestinal
Reference: Christensen, B., & Kockrow, E. (2003). *Adult health nursing* (4th ed.). St. Louis: Mosby, p. 243.

52. Answer: 1
Rationale: The client with cholecystitis should decrease overall intake of dietary fat. Foods that should be generally avoided to achieve this end include sauces and gravies, fatty meats, fried foods, products made with cream, and heavy desserts. The correct food item is baked scrod, which is low in fat.
Test-Taking Strategy: Use the process of elimination and recall that clients with cholecystitis should decrease fat intake. Also note that options 2, 3, and 4 are similar and are high in fat. Review dietary instructions for the client with cholecystitis if you had difficulty with this question.
Level of Cognitive Ability: Comprehension
Client Needs: Health Promotion and Maintenance

Integrated Process: Nursing Process/Evaluation
Content Area: Adult Health/Gastrointestinal
Reference: Nix, S. (2005). *Williams basic nutrition and diet therapy* (11th ed.). St. Louis: Mosby, p. 343.

53. Answer: 3
Rationale: Ammonia is formed as a product of protein metabolism. Clients with hepatic encephalopathy have high serum ammonia levels, which is responsible for the encephalopathy symptoms. Limiting protein intake will curb the elevation in the serum ammonia level and prevent further deterioration of the client's mental status.
Test-Taking Strategy: Use the process of elimination. Recalling the relationships between cirrhosis, encephalopathy, and protein intake will direct you to option 3. Review dietary measures for the client with cirrhosis if you had difficulty with this question.
Level of Cognitive Ability: Application
Client Needs: Health Promotion and Maintenance
Integrated Process: Nursing Process/Planning
Content Area: Adult Health/Gastrointestinal
Reference: Nix, S. (2005). *Williams basic nutrition and diet therapy* (11th ed.). St. Louis: Mosby, pp. 342-343.

54. Answer: 1
Rationale: In order to be effective in decreasing bowel motility, antispasmodic medications should be administered 30 minutes before mealtime. The other options are incorrect.
Test-Taking Strategy: Use the process of elimination. Recalling that antispasmodics slow down gut motility, it can be reasoned that they should be taken before meals, which normally stimulates increased gastrointestinal motility. Review the purpose of antispasmodic medications if you had difficulty with this question.
Level of Cognitive Ability: Application
Client Needs: Physiological Integrity
Integrated Process: Nursing Process/Implementation
Content Area: Adult Health/Gastrointestinal
Reference: Black, J., & Hawks, J. (2005). *Medical-surgical nursing: Clinical management for positive outcomes* (7th ed.). Philadelphia: W.B. Saunders, p. 848.

55. Answer: 2
Rationale: Common signs of acute viral hepatitis include weight loss, dark urine, and fatigue. The client is anorexic and finds food distasteful. The urine darkens because of excess bilirubin being excreted by the kidneys. Fatigue occurs during all phases of hepatitis. Spider angiomas, small, dilated blood vessels, are commonly seen in cirrhosis of the liver.
Test-Taking Strategy: Use the process of elimination. Recalling the function of the liver will direct you to option 2. Remember, lethargy is a classic symptom associated with hepatitis. If you had difficulty with this question, review the manifestations associated with hepatitis.
Level of Cognitive Ability: Analysis
Client Needs: Physiological Integrity
Integrated Process: Nursing Process/Data Collection
Content Area: Adult Health/Gastrointestinal

Reference: Christensen, B., & Kockrow, E. (2003). *Adult health nursing* (4th ed.). St. Louis: Mosby, p. 232.

56. *Answer:* 4
Rationale: Clarifying the meaning of what has been said increases understanding for both the client and the nurse. Providing false reassurance is inappropriate. Telling the client what to do implies that the nurse knows what is best and discourages independent thinking. Refusing to consider the client's ideas may cause the client to discontinue interaction with the nurse for fear of further rejection. Placing the client's feelings on hold by referring the client to the physician for further information is a block to communication.
Test-Taking Strategy: Use therapeutic communication techniques. Remember always to focus on the client's feelings first. This will direct you to option 4. Review therapeutic communication techniques if you had difficulty with this question.
Level of Cognitive Ability: Application
Client Needs: Psychosocial Integrity
Integrated Process: Communication and Documentation
Content Area: Adult Health/Gastrointestinal
Reference: Potter, P., & Perry, A. (2005). *Fundamentals of nursing* (6th ed.). St. Louis: Mosby, p. 437.

57. *Answer:* 2
Rationale: Immunization is the most effective method of preventing hepatitis B infection. Other general measures include hand washing. Immune globulin is used to prevent hepatitis A and is used for prophylaxis if traveling to endemic areas. Personal hygiene, such as hand washing after a bowel movement and before eating, also helps prevent the transmission of hepatitis A.
Test-Taking Strategy: Use the process of elimination and note the key word, *priority.* Although more than one of the options are correct for preventing transmission of hepatitis B, the priority is immunization with hepatitis B vaccine. If you had difficulty with this question, review content associated with hepatitis.
Level of Cognitive Ability: Application
Client Needs: Safe, Effective Care Environment
Integrated Process: Nursing Process/Planning
Content Area: Adult Health/Gastrointestinal
Reference: Linton, A., & Maebius, N. (2003). *Introduction to medical-surgical nursing* (3rd ed.). Philadelphia: W.B. Saunders, p. 723.

58. *Answer:* 4
Rationale: Hepatitis B is transmitted through body fluids. The vaccine is recommended for both sexual and household contacts of clients with hepatitis B. Hepatitis B can be transmitted through intimate contact, such as kissing or sexual intercourse. The vaccine is used for prevention.
Test-Taking Strategy: Use the process of elimination. Eliminate option 2 because of the absolute word "never." Recalling the mode of transmission and the measures to prevent hepatitis will direct you to option 4. Review this content if you had difficulty with this question.
Level of Cognitive Ability: Comprehension
Client Needs: Health Promotion and Maintenance
Integrated Process: Nursing Process/Evaluation

Content Area: Adult Health/Gastrointestinal
Reference: Linton, A., & Maebius, N. (2003). *Introduction to medical-surgical nursing* (3rd ed.). Philadelphia: W.B. Saunders, p. 723.

59. *Answer:* 3
Rationale: Although no special diet is required in the treatment of viral hepatitis, it is generally recommended that clients have a diet with low fat content, because fat may be poorly tolerated because of decreased bile production. Small, frequent meals are preferable and may even prevent nausea. Frequently, the appetite is better in the morning, so it is easier to eat a healthy breakfast. An adequate fluid intake of 2500 to 3000 mL/day that includes nutritional fluids is also important.
Test-Taking Strategy: Use the process of elimination and focus on the issue, a lack of appetite. Eliminate option 4 because of the words "high in fat." Eliminate options 1 and 2 next because of the word "large." Review dietary measures for the client with hepatitis if you had difficulty with this question.
Level of Cognitive Ability: Application
Client Needs: Physiological Integrity
Integrated Process: Nursing Process/Implementation
Content Area: Adult Health/Gastrointestinal
References: Christensen, B., & Kockrow, E. (2003). *Adult health nursing* (4th ed.). St. Louis: Mosby, p. 231.
Lewis, S., Heitkemper, M., & Dirksen, S. (2004). *Medical-surgical nursing: Assessment and management of clinical problems* (6th ed.). St. Louis: Mosby, p. 1113.

60. *Answer:* 2
Rationale: Jaundice occurs in the skin and mucous membranes. In light-skinned persons, it is first seen in the sclera of the eyes and later in the skin. In dark-skinned persons, jaundice is observed in the inner canthus of the eyes and hard palate of the mouth. Pallor is detected in the nail beds, and flushing is detected in the flexor surfaces of the extremities.
Test-Taking Strategy: Use the process of elimination and focus on the client. Recalling that jaundice occurs in the skin and mucous membranes will direct you to option 2. Review data collection techniques for jaundice if you had difficulty with this question.
Level of Cognitive Ability: Application
Client Needs: Health Promotion and Maintenance
Integrated Process: Nursing Process/Data Collection
Content Area: Adult Health/Gastrointestinal
Reference: Linton, A., & Maebius, N. (2003). *Introduction to medical-surgical nursing* (3rd ed.). Philadelphia: W.B. Saunders, p. 715.

ALTERNATE FORMAT QUESTION: MULTIPLE RESPONSE

Answers:
Meperidine (Demerol) as prescribed for pain
Encourage coughing and deep breathing
Administer antacids, as prescribed
Administer anticholinergics, as prescribed
Rationale: The client with acute pancreatitis is normally placed on an NPO status to rest the pancreas and suppress

GI secretions. Because abdominal pain is a prominent symptom of pancreatitis, pain medication such as meperidine will be prescribed. Some clients experience lessened pain by assuming positions that flex the trunk and draw the knees up to the chest. A side-lying position with the head elevated 45 degrees decreases tension on the abdomen and may also help ease the pain. The client is susceptible to respiratory infections because the retroperitoneal fluid raises the diaphragm, which causes the client to take shallow, guarded abdominal breaths. Therefore, measures such as turning, coughing, and deep breathing are instituted. Antacids and anticholinergics may be prescribed to suppress GI secretions.

Test-Taking Strategy: Focus on the pathophysiology associated with pancreatitis and note the word "acute" in the question. This will assist in selecting the correct interventions. Review treatment measures for acute pancreatitis if you had difficulty with this question.
Level of Cognitive Ability: Analysis
Client Needs: Physiological Integrity
Integrated Process: Nursing Process/Planning
Content Area: Adult Health/Gastrointestinal
Reference: Lewis, S., Heitkemper, M., & Dirksen, S. (2004). *Medical-surgical nursing: Assessment and management of clinical problems* (6th ed.). St. Louis: Mosby, p. 1138.

REFERENCES

Black, J., & Hawks, J. (2005). *Medical-surgical nursing: Clinical management for positive outcomes* (7th ed.). Philadelphia: W.B. Saunders.

Chernecky, C., & Berger, B. (2004). *Laboratory tests and diagnostic procedures* (4th ed.). Philadelphia: W.B. Saunders.

Christensen, B., & Kockrow, E. (2003). *Foundations of nursing* (4th ed.). St. Louis: Mosby.

Hodgson, B., & Kizior, R. (2005). *Saunders nursing drug handbook 2005*. Philadelphia: W.B. Saunders.

Lewis, S., Heitkemper, M., & Dirksen, S. (2004). *Medical-surgical nursing: Assessment and management of clinical problems* (6th ed.). St. Louis: Mosby,

Linton, A., & Maebius, N. (2003). *Introduction to medical-surgical nursing* (3rd ed.). Philadelphia: W.B. Saunders.

McKenry, L., & Salerno, E. (2003). *Mosby's pharmacology in nursing* (21st ed.) St. Louis: Mosby.

Nix, S. (2005). *Williams basic nutrition and diet therapy* (12th ed.). St Louis: Mosby.

Pagana, K., & Pagana, T. (2003). *Mosby's diagnostic and laboratory test reference* (6th ed.). St. Louis: Mosby.

Phipps, W., Monahan, F., Sands, J., Marek, J., & Neighbors, M. (2003). *Medical-surgical nursing: Health and illness perspectives* (7th ed.). St. Louis: Mosby,

Potter, P., & Perry, A. (2005). *Fundamentals of nursing* (6th ed.). St. Louis: Mosby.

Thompson, J., McFarland, G., Hirsch, J., & Tucker, S. (2002). *Mosby's clinical nursing* (5th ed.). St. Louis: Mosby.

Gastrointestinal Medications

I. ANTACIDS AND MUCOSAL PROTECTIVE MEDICATIONS (Box 47-1)

A. Description
1. React with gastric acid to produce neutral salts or salts of low acidity
2. Inactivate pepsin and enhance mucosal protection but do not coat the ulcer crater to protect it from the acid and pepsin
3. Used for peptic ulcer disease and gastroesophageal reflux disease (GERD)
4. Should be taken on a regular schedule
5. Some antacids are prescribed to be taken seven times a day, 1 and 3 hours after each meal and at bedtime
6. To provide maximum benefit, treatment should elevate the gastric pH above 5
7. Antacid tablets should be chewed thoroughly and followed with a glass of water or milk
8. Liquid preparations should be shaken before dispensing
9. Interactions with other medications can be minimized by allowing 1 hour between antacid administration and the administration of other medications

---

BOX 47-1

Antacids and Mucosal Protective Medications

Aluminum carbonate gel (Basaljel)
Aluminum hydroxide gel (Amphojel, Alu-Cap, Dialume)
Bismuth subsalicylate (Pepto-Bismol)
Calcium carbonate (Tums)
Magnesium hydroxide (Milk of magnesia, MOM)
Misoprostol (Cytotec)
Sulcralfate (Carafate)

---

10. Can interfere with the action of sucralfate (Carafate); to minimize this interaction, the medications should be administered 1 hour apart from each other

B. Sucralfate (Carafate)
1. Creates a protective barrier against acid and pepsin
2. Administered orally; should be taken on an empty stomach
3. Administer at least 60 minutes apart from an antacid
4. May cause constipation
5. May impede absorption of warfarin sodium (Coumadin), phenytoin (Dilantin), theophylline, digoxin (Lanoxin), and some antibiotics; should be administered at least 2 hours apart from these medications

C. Misoprostol (Cytotec)
1. Used to prevent gastric ulcers caused by long-term therapy with nonsteroidal anti-inflammatory drugs (NSAIDs)
2. Suppresses secretion of gastric acid
3. Promotes secretion of bicarbonate and cytoprotective mucus
4. Maintains submucosal blood flow by promoting vasodilation
5. Administered with meals
6. Causes diarrhea and abdominal pain
7. Contraindicated for use in pregnancy

D. Magnesium hydroxide
1. Rapid-acting
2. Also referred to as milk of magnesia
3. Most prominent side effect is diarrhea
4. Usually administered in combination with aluminum hydroxide, an antacid that assists in preventing diarrhea
5. Contraindicated in clients with intestinal obstruction, appendicitis, or undiagnosed abdominal pain
6. In clients with renal impairment, magnesium can accumulate to high levels, causing signs of toxicity

E. Aluminum hydroxide (Amphojel, Alu-Cap, Dialume)
1. Slow-acting
2. Contains significant amounts of sodium
3. Used with caution in clients with hypertension and heart failure
4. Most common side effect is constipation
5. Can reduce the effects of tetracyclines, warfarin sodium (Coumadin), and digoxin (Lanoxin)
6. Can reduce phosphate absorption and thereby cause hypophosphatemia
F. Calcium carbonate (Tums)
1. Rapid-acting
2. Common side effect is constipation
3. Should not be administered with milk, milk products, or foods or supplements high in vitamin D because milk-alkali syndrome (headache, urinary frequency, anorexia, nausea, vomiting, fatigue) can occur
G. Sodium bicarbonate
1. Rapid onset
2. Liberates carbon dioxide, increases intradominal pressure, and promotes flatulence
3. Used with caution in clients with hypertension and heart failure
4. Can cause systemic alkalosis in clients with renal impairment
5. Is useful for treating acidosis and elevating urinary pH to promote excretions of acidic medications following overdose

II. HISTAMINE H$_2$-RECEPTOR ANTAGONISTS (Box 47-2)

A. Description
1. Suppress secretions of gastric acid
2. Alleviate symptoms of heartburn and assist in preventing complications of peptic ulcer disease
3. Prevent stress ulcers and reduce the recurrence of all ulcers
4. Promotes healing in GERD
5. Contraindicated in hypersensitivity
6. Used with caution in clients with impaired renal or hepatic function
B. Cimetidine (Tagamet)
1. Can be administered orally, intramuscularly, and intravenously
2. Food reduces the rate of absorption; if taken with meals, absorption will be slowed
3. Antacids can decrease the absorption of cimetidine
4. Cimetidine and antacids should be administered at least 1 hour apart from each other
5. Passes the blood-brain barrier, and central nervous system (CNS) side effects can occur
6. May cause mental confusion, agitation, psychosis, depression, anxiety, and disorientation
7. Dosage should be reduced in clients with renal impairment
8. Intravenous administration can cause hypotension and dysrhythmias
9. If administered with warfarin sodium (Coumadin), phenytoin (Dilantin), theophylline, or lidocaine, the dosages of these medications should be reduced
C. Ranitidine (Zantac)
1. Can be administered orally or by the intramuscular or intravenous route
2. Side effects are uncommon
3. Unlike cimetidine, it does not penetrate the blood-brain barrier
4. Zantac is not affected by food
D. Famotidine (Pepcid) and nizatidine (Axid)
1. Similar to Zantac and Tagamet
2. Do not need to be administered with food
E. Ranitidine bismuth citrate
1. Used to treat active duodenal ulcers associated with *Helicobacter pylori*
2. Administered with the antibiotic clarithromycin (Biaxin) (Box 47-3)

III. PROTON PUMP INHIBITORS (Box 47-4)

A. Suppress gastric acid secretion
B. Used with active ulcer disease, erosive esophagitis, and pathological hypersecretory conditions
C. Contraindicated in hypersensitivity

BOX 47-3

Antimicrobials Effective Against *Helicobacter pylori*

Amoxicillin (Amoxil)
Clarithromycin (Biaxin)
Metronidazole (Flagyl)
Tetracycline (Achromycin)

BOX 47-2

Histamine H$_2$-Receptor Antagonists

Cimetidine (Tagamet)
Famotidine (Pepcid)
Nizatidine (Axid)
Ranitidine (Zantac)
Ranitidine bismuth citrate

BOX 47-4

Proton Pump Inhibitors

Esomeprazole (Nexium)
Lansoprazole (Prevacid)
Omeprazole (Prilosec)
Pantoprazole (Protonix)
Rabeprazole (Aciphex)

D. Common side effects include headache, diarrhea, abdominal pain, and nausea

IV. GASTROINTESTINAL STIMULANTS (Box 47-5)

A. Stimulate motility of the upper gastrointestinal (GI) tract and increase rate of gastric emptying without stimulating gastric, biliary, or pancreatic secretions

B. Used for gastroesophageal reflux

C. May cause restlessness, drowsiness, extrapyramidal reactions, dizziness, insomnia, headache

D. Usually administered 30 minutes before meals and at bedtime

E. Contraindicated in clients with sensitivity

F. Contraindicated in clients with mechanical obstruction, perforation, or GI hemorrhage

G. Can precipitate hypertensive crisis in clients with pheochromocytoma

H. Safety in pregnancy is not established

I. Reglan can cause parkinsonian reactions, and if this occurs the medication is discontinued

J. Anticholinergics and narcotic analgesics antagonize the effects of metoclopramide (Reglan)

K. Alcohol, sedatives, cyclosporine (Sandimmune), and tranquilizers produce an additive effect

V. BILE ACID SEQUESTRANTS (Box 47-6)

A. Description
1. Used to treat pruritus associated with biliary disease
2. Acts by absorbing and combining with intestinal bile salts, which are then secreted in the feces, preventing intestinal reabsorption
3. May be used in the treatment of hypercholesterolemia in adults
4. Used cautiously in clients with bowel obstruction or severe constipation because of the adverse GI effects
5. Taste and palatability are often reasons for noncompliance and can be improved by the use of flavored products or mixing the medication with various juices
6. Stool softeners and other sources of fiber can be used to abate the GI side effects

B. Side effects
1. Constipation
2. Bloating
3. Flatulence
4. Nausea
5. Fecal impaction and intestinal obstruction
6. Exacerbation of hemorrhoids
7. Hypoprothrombinemia
8. Decreased vitamin absorption

VI. MEDICATIONS FOR CHOLELITHIASIS (Box 47-7)

A. Chenodiol (Chenix)
1. Decreases cholesterol production, lowering content of bile, thus facilitating dissolution of gallstones
2. Can cause diarrhea and possible hepatotoxicity
3. Baseline liver function studies should be performed
4. Client should be instructed to contact the physician if abdominal pain, sudden right upper quadrant pain, nausea, or vomiting occurs
5. Administer with food or milk
6. Avoid aluminum-containing antacids

B. Ursodiol (Actigall)
1. A naturally occurring bile salt
2. Suppresses hepatic synthesis and secretion of cholesterol and inhibits intestinal absorption of cholesterol
3. Requires months of therapy for dissolution of gallstone to occur
4. Ultrasound images are obtained within 6 months to determine effectiveness of therapy
5. Clients should be instructed to report nausea, vomiting, diarrhea, or rash to the physician
6. Administer with food or milk
7. Avoid aluminum-containing antacids

C. Monoctanoin (Moctanin)
1. Used when stones made of calcium are resistant to dissolution by oral chenodiol
2. Administered through a T tube, nasal biliary catheter, or percutaneous transhepatic catheter
3. Effective only when in contact with the stone
4. Major side effects include diarrhea, nausea, and abdominal pain

---

BOX 47-5

Gastrointestinal Stimulants

Bethanechol chloride (Urecholine, Duvoid)
Dexpanthenol (Ilopan)
Metoclopramide (Reglan)
Neostigmine methylsulfate (Prostigmin)

BOX 47-6

Bile Acid Sequestrants

Cholestyramine (Questran, Prevalite)
Colestipol (Colestid)

BOX 47-7

Medications for Cholelithiasis

Chenodiol (Chenix)
Monoctanoin (Moctanin)
Ursodiol (Actigall)

BOX 47-8

Medications To Treat Hepatic Encephalopathy

Lactulose (Cholac)
Neomycin (Mycifradin)

BOX 47-9

Pancreatic Enzyme Replacements

Pancreatin
Pancrelipase (Pancrease, Viokase)

BOX 47-10

Commonly Administered Antiemetics

Diphenidol hydrochloride (Vontrol)
Dolesetron (Anzemet)
Dronabinol (Marinol)
Granisetron (Kytril)
Hydroxyzine hydrochloride (Atarax)
Hydroxyzine pamoate (Vistaril)
Meclizine hydrochloride (Antivert)
Metoclopramide (Reglan)
Ondansetron (Zofran)
Prochlorperazine (Compazine)
Promethazine hydrochloride (Phenergan)
Scopolamine hydrobromide, transdermal (Transderm Scōp)
Thiethylperazine malate (Torecon)
Trimethobenzamide hydrochloride (Tigan)

BOX 47-11

Laxatives

BULK-FORMING LAXATIVES
Methylcellulose (Citrucel)
Calcium polycarbophil (Fibercon)
Psyllium hydrophilic mucilloid (Metamucil, Fiberall, Konsyl, Serutan)

STIMULANT CATHARTICS
Bisacodyl (Dulcolax)
Cascara sagrada
Castor oil, emulsified (Neoloid)
Sennosides (Ex-Lax, Senexon, Senna-Gen)

OSMOTIC CATHARTICS
Glycerin suppositories
Lactulose (Cholac)
Magnesium citrate
Magnesium hydroxide (milk of magnesia, MOM)
Magnesium sulfate (Epsom Salts)
Polyethylene glycol (PEG)–electrolytes (GoLYTELY)
Potassium bitartrate and sodium bicarbonate
Sodium phosphates (Fleet Phospho-Soda)

STOOL SOFTENERS
Docusate calcium (Surfak)
Docusate sodium (Colace)
Docusate with casanthranol (Peri-Colace)

LUBRICANT
Mineral oil

VII. MEDICATIONS TO TREAT HEPATIC ENCEPHALOPATHY (Box 47-8)

A. Lactulose (Cholac)
   1. Reduces ammonia levels
   2. Improves protein tolerance in clients with advanced hepatic **cirrhosis**
   3. Lowers the colonic pH from 7 to 5; this acidification pulls ammonia into the bowel to be excreted in the feces, thus lowering the ammonia level
   4. Administered orally in the form of a syrup
B. Neomycin (Mycifradin)
   1. Reduces the number of colonic bacteria that normally convert urea and amino acids into ammonia
   2. Administered orally or via nasogastric (NG) tube
   3. Used with caution in clients with kidney impairment

VIII. PANCREATIC ENZYME REPLACEMENTS (Box 47-9)

A. Used to supplement or replace pancreatic enzymes
B. Taken with meals or a snack (food helps buffer the stomach acid)

C. A high-fiber diet may increase the efficacy of the medication
D. Side effects include abdominal cramps or pain, nausea, and diarrhea
E. Products that contain calcium carbonate or magnesium hydroxide interfere with the action of the medication

IX. ANTIEMETICS (Box 47-10)

A. Medications used to control vomiting
B. The choice of the antiemetic is determined by the cause of the nausea and vomiting
C. Monitor for drowsiness and protect the client from injury
D. Monitor vital signs and input and output (I&O)
E. Limit odors in the client's room when the client is nauseated and/or vomiting
F. Limit oral intake to clear liquids when the client is nauseated and/or vomiting

X. LAXATIVES (Box 47-11)

A. Bulk-forming laxatives
   1. Description

a. Absorb water into the feces and increase bulk to produce large and soft stools
b. For short-term use
c. Contraindicated in bowel obstruction
2. Side effects
a. GI disturbances
b. Dehydration
c. Electrolyte imbalance
d. Dependency with chronic use
B. Stimulant cathartics
1. Description: Stimulate motility of large intestine
2. Biscodyl (Dulcolax): Do not administer within 60 minutes of an antacid or milk
3. Cascara (castor oil): Administer with juice; produces results in 2 to 6 hours
C. Saline cathartics
1. Attract water into the large intestine to produce bulk
2. Stimulate **peristalsis**
3. Achieve results in 2 to 6 hours
D. Stool softeners
1. Inhibit absorption of water so fecal mass remains large and soft
2. Used to avoid straining
E. Lubricants
1. Act to soften the feces
2. Ease the strain of passing stool
3. Lessen irritation to hemorrhoids
4. Mineral oil
a. Can cause lipid pneumonia if accidentally aspirated
b. Interferes with absorption of fat-soluble vitamins A, D, E, and K

XI. MEDICATIONS TO CONTROL DIARRHEA
(Box 47-12)
A. Opioids
1. Decrease intestinal motility and **peristalsis**
2. When poisons, infections, or bacterial toxins are the cause of the diarrhea, opioids worsen the condition by delaying the elimination of toxins
3. Tincture of opium has an unpleasant taste and can be diluted with 15 to 30 mL of water for administration
B. Other antidiarrheals: See Box 47-12

XII. ANTISPASMODIC (Box 47-13)
A. Description: Relaxes smooth muscle of the GI tract
B. Side effects
1. Constipation or diarrhea
2. Rash
3. Euphoria
4. Dizziness
5. Drowsiness
6. Headache

BOX 47-12

Medications to Control Diarrhea

OPIOIDS AND RELATED MEDICATIONS
Codeine phosphate; codeine sulfate
Difenoxin with atropine (Motofen)
Diphenoxylate hydrochloride with atropine (Lomotil)
Loperamide hydrochloride (Imodium)
Tincture of opium

ABSORBENT ANTIDIARRHEALS
Bismuth subsalicylate (Pepto-Bismol)
Kaolin and pectin (Kao-Spen, Kapectolin)
Octreotide (Sandostatin)

BOX 47-13

Antispasmodic

Dicyclomine hydrochloride (Antispas, Bentyl)

---

7. Nausea
8. Weakness

PRACTICE QUESTIONS

1. A client has been started on psyllium (Metamucil). The nurse would teach the client to take this medication with:
   1. Gelatin, applesauce, or pudding
   2. A full glass of liquid, followed by a second glass
   3. A multivitamin and mineral supplement
   4. A dose of antacid
2. A nurse teaches a client taking metoclopramide (Reglan) to discontinue the medication immediately and call the physician if which side effect occurs with long-term use?
   1. Anxiety or irritability
   2. Dry mouth not helped by the use of sugar-free hard candy
   3. Excessive excitability
   4. Uncontrolled rhythmic movements of the face or limbs
3. A client has just taken a dose of trimethobenzamide (Tigan). The nurse plans to monitor this client for relief of:
   1. Nausea and vomiting
   2. Abdominal pain
   3. Heartburn
   4. Constipation
4. A client has a PRN order for ondansetron (Zofran). The nurse would administer this medication to the postoperative client for relief of:
   1. Urinary retention
   2. Incisional pain

  3. Nausea and vomiting
  4. Paralytic ileus
5. A client has an order to take magnesium citrate to prevent constipation following a barium study of the upper gastrointestinal (GI) tract. The nurse plans to administer this medication:
  1. With a full glass of water
  2. With fruit juice only
  3. Chilled
  4. At room temperature
6. A nurse is administering a dose of prochlorperazine (Compazine) to a client for nausea and vomiting. The nurse would monitor the client for which frequent side effect of this medication?
  1. Diarrhea
  2. Drooling
  3. Excessive lacrimation
  4. Blurred vision
7. A client has begun medication therapy with pancrelipase (Pancrease). The nurse determines that the medication is having the optimal intended benefit if which effect is observed?
  1. Reduction of steatorrhea
  2. Absence of abdominal pain
  3. Relief of heartburn
  4. Weight loss
8. A nurse is giving a client directions for proper use of aluminum hydroxide tablets (Alu-Caps). The nurse tells the client to:
  1. Chew the tablets thoroughly and follow with 4 ounces of water
  2. Swallow the tablets whole with a full glass of water
  3. Take the tablets at the same time as other medications
  4. Take each dose with a laxative to prevent constipation
9. A client with a history of duodenal ulcer is taking calcium carbonate chewable tablets. The nurse determines that the client is experiencing optimal effects of the medication if:
  1. Muscle twitching stops
  2. Heartburn is relieved
  3. Serum calcium levels rise
  4. Serum phosphorus levels decrease
10. A hospitalized client asks the nurse for sodium bicarbonate to relieve heartburn following a meal. The nurse reviews the client's medical record, knowing that the medication is contraindicated in which of the following conditions?
  1. Urinary calculi
  2. Chronic bronchitis
  3. Metabolic alkalosis
  4. Respiratory acidosis
11. An older client has recently been started on cimetidine (Tagamet). The nurse monitors the client for which frequent central nervous system (CNS) side effect of this medication?
  1. Confusion
  2. Dizziness
  3. Tremors
  4. Hallucinations
12. A client with a gastric ulcer has an order for sucralfate (Carafate), 1 g orally four times a day. The nurse schedules the medication for which of the following times?
  1. With meals and at bedtime
  2. One hour before meals and at bedtime
  3. Every 6 hours around the clock
  4. One hour after meals and at bedtime
13. A physician has written an order for ranitidine (Zantac), 300 mg once daily. The nurse schedules the medication for which of the following times?
  1. Before breakfast
  2. After lunch
  3. With supper
  4. At bedtime
14. A client has been taking omeprazole (Prilosec) for 4 weeks. The nurse determines that the client is receiving the optimal intended effect of the medication if the client reports absence of which of the following symptoms?
  1. Constipation
  2. Heartburn
  3. Diarrhea
  4. Flatulence
15. A client is taking cascara sagrada and develops abdominal cramps. The nurse determines that the client is most likely experiencing:
  1. A common side effect of this medication
  2. Partial bowel obstruction
  3. A case of influenza
  4. Peptic ulcer disease
16. A physician prescribes bisacodyl (Dulcolax) for a client in preparation for a diagnostic test and wants the client to achieve a rapid effect from the medication. The nurse then tells the client to take the medication:
  1. With a large meal
  2. On an empty stomach
  3. At bedtime with a snack
  4. With two glasses of juice
17. A client has a PRN order for loperamide (Imodium). The nurse should plan to administer this medication if the client has:
  1. Hematest-positive nasogastric tube drainage
  2. Abdominal pain
  3. Constipation
  4. An episode of diarrhea
18. A nurse has given instructions to the client who just received a prescription for diphenoxylate

with atropine (Lomotil). The nurse determines that the client understands the use of the medication and its properties if the client states that he or she will:

1. Stay within the prescribed dose because it can be habit-forming
2. Take the medication with a bulk-forming laxative
3. Expect increased salivation while taking the medication
4. Anticipate side effects related to central nervous system excitability

19. A client has received a dose of dimenhydrinate (Dramamine). The nurse determines that the medication has been effective if the client states relief of:

1. Headache
2. Chills
3. Nausea and vomiting
4. Buzzing sound in the ears

20. A client is taking docusate sodium (Colace). The nurse monitors which of the following to determine whether the client is having a therapeutic effect from this medication?

1. Abdominal pain
2. Hematest-negative stools
3. Reduction in steatorrhea
4. Regular bowel movements

ALTERNATE FORMAT QUESTION: FILL IN THE BLANK

The client with gastroesophageal reflux has been given a prescription for metoclopramide (Reglan). The nurse tells the client to take the medication how many minutes before meals?

Answer: _____

ANSWERS

1. *Answer: 2*
Rationale: Metamucil is a bulk-forming laxative. It should be taken with a full glass of water or juice, followed by another glass of liquid. This will help prevent impaction of the medication in the stomach or small intestine. The other options are incorrect.
Test-Taking Strategy: Use the process of elimination. Option 4 can be eliminated first because most medications are not taken with antacids. Eliminate options 1 and 3 next because they have no physiological benefit for medication effect. Review the administration of this medication if you had difficulty with this question.
Level of Cognitive Ability: Application
Client Needs: Physiological Integrity
Integrated Process: Teaching/Learning
Content Area: Pharmacology
Reference: Hodgson, B., & Kizior, R. (2005). *Saunders nursing drug handbook 2005.* Philadelphia: W.B. Saunders, p. 908.

2. *Answer: 4*
Rationale: If the client experiences tardive dyskinesia (rhythmic movements of the face or limbs), the client should stop the medication and call the physician. These side effects may be irreversible. Excitability is not a side effect of this medication. Anxiety, irritability, and dry mouth are side effects that are not as harmful to the client.
Test-Taking Strategy: Use the process of elimination and focus on the issue, to call the physician. Recalling that the medication can cause tardive dyskinesia will direct you to option 4. Review the side effects of this medication if you had difficulty with this question.
Level of Cognitive Ability: Application
Client Needs: Physiological Integrity
Integrated Process: Teaching/Learning

Content Area: Pharmacology
Reference: Hodgson, B., & Kizior, R. (2005). *Saunders nursing drug handbook 2005.* Philadelphia: W.B. Saunders, p. 701.

3. *Answer: 1*
Rationale: Trimethobenzamide is an antiemetic agent that is used in the treatment of nausea and vomiting. The other options are incorrect.
Test-Taking Strategy: Use the process of elimination. Recalling that trimethobenzamide is an antiemetic will direct you to option 1. Review the action and use of this medication if you had difficulty with this question.
Level of Cognitive Ability: Application
Client Needs: Physiological Integrity
Integrated Process: Nursing Process/Planning
Content Area: Pharmacology
Reference: Hodgson, B., & Kizior, R. (2005). *Saunders nursing drug handbook 2005.* Philadelphia: W.B. Saunders, p. 1081.

4. *Answer: 3*
Rationale: Ondansetron is an antiemetic that is used in the treatment of postoperative nausea and vomiting, as well as nausea and vomiting associated with chemotherapy. The other options are incorrect.
Test-Taking Strategy: Use the process of elimination. Recalling that ondansetron is an antiemetic will direct you to option 3. Review the action and use of this medication if you had difficulty with this question.
Level of Cognitive Ability: Application
Client Needs: Physiological Integrity
Integrated Process: Nursing Process/Implementation
Content Area: Pharmacology
Reference: Hodgson, B., & Kizior, R. (2005). *Saunders nursing drug handbook 2005.* Philadelphia: W.B. Saunders, p. 802.

5. Answer: 3
Rationale: Magnesium citrate is available as an oral solution. It is used commonly as a laxative following certain studies of the GI tract. It should be served chilled, and should not be allowed to stand for prolonged periods. This would reduce the carbonation and make the solution even less palatable. Options 1, 2, and 4 are incorrect.
Test-Taking Strategy: Use the process of elimination. Eliminate options 1 and 2 first, knowing that magnesium citrate is itself a liquid. From the remaining options, it is necessary to know it should be given cold to enhance palatability. Review this medication if you had difficulty with this question.
Level of Cognitive Ability: Application
Client Needs: Physiological Integrity
Integrated Process: Nursing Process/Planning
Content Area: Pharmacology
References: Hodgson, B., & Kizior, R. (2005). *Saunders nursing drug handbook 2005.* Philadelphia: W.B. Saunders, p. 660.
McKenry, L., & Salerno, E. (2003). *Mosby's pharmacology in nursing* (21st ed.). St. Louis: Mosby, p. 218.

6. Answer: 4
Rationale: The nurse would monitor the client for blurred vision as a frequent side effect of prochlorperazine. Other frequent side effects of this phenothiazine-type antiemetic and antipsychotic are dry eyes, dry mouth, and constipation.
Test-Taking Strategy: Focus on the name of the medication. Recalling that this medication is a phenothiazine-type antiemetic and antipsychotic will assist with answering this question. Remember, frequent side effects of this phenothiazine-type antiemetic and antipsychotic are blurred vision, dry eyes, dry mouth, and constipation. Review this medication if you had difficulty with this question.
Level of Cognitive Ability: Application
Client Needs: Physiological Integrity
Integrated Process: Nursing Process/Data Collection
Content Area: Pharmacology
References: Hodgson, B., & Kizior, R. (2005). *Saunders nursing drug handbook 2005.* Philadelphia: W.B. Saunders, p. 892.
McKenry, L., & Salerno, E. (2003). *Mosby's pharmacology in nursing* (21st ed.). St. Louis: Mosby, p. 400.

7. Answer: 1
Rationale: Pancrelipase is a pancreatic enzyme used in clients with pancreatitis as a digestive aid. The medication should reduce the amount of fatty stools (steatorrhea). Another intended effect could be improved nutritional status. It is not used to treat abdominal pain or heartburn. It could result in weight gain, but should not result in weight loss if it is aiding in digestion.
Test-Taking Strategy: Use the process of elimination. The name of the medication gives an indication of the possible uses of this medication. Use knowledge of the physiology of the pancreas to assist in directing you to the correct option. Review this medication if you had difficulty with this question.
Level of Cognitive Ability: Analysis
Client Needs: Physiological Integrity
Integrated Process: Nursing Process/Evaluation

Content Area: Pharmacology
Reference: Hodgson, B., & Kizior, R. (2005). *Saunders nursing drug handbook 2005.* Philadelphia: W.B. Saunders, p. 824.

8. Answer: 1
Rationale: Aluminum hydroxide tablets should be chewed thoroughly before swallowing. This prevents them from entering the small intestine undissolved. They should not be swallowed whole. Antacids should be taken at least 1 hour apart from other medications to prevent interactive effects. Constipation is a side effect of use of aluminum products, but it is not correct for the client to take a laxative with each dose of aluminum hydroxide tablets. This promotes laxative abuse; the client should first try other means to prevent constipation.
Test-Taking Strategy: Use the process of elimination. Eliminate option 4 first, because this action does not promote healthy bowel function. Next, eliminate option 3 using general knowledge of antacid interactive effects. Using principles of digestion and medication use, select from the remaining options. Review the administration of this medication if you had difficulty with this question.
Level of Cognitive Ability: Application
Client Needs: Physiological Integrity
Integrated Process: Teaching/Learning
Content Area: Pharmacology
Reference: Hodgson, B., & Kizior, R. (2005). *Saunders nursing drug handbook 2005.* Philadelphia: W.B. Saunders, p. 41.

9. Answer: 2
Rationale: Calcium carbonate is used as an antacid for the relief of heartburn and indigestion in a client with a duodenal ulcer. It can also be used as a calcium supplement (option 3) or to bind phosphorus in the gastrointestinal tract with renal failure (option 4). Option 1 is incorrect, although proper calcium levels are needed for proper neurological function.
Test-Taking Strategy: Focus on the client's diagnosis. The key words in the question are *duodenal ulcer* and *optimal effects.* Knowledge of the concepts related to duodenal ulcer will direct you to option 2. Review the actions and use of this medication if you had difficulty with this question.
Level of Cognitive Ability: Analysis
Client Needs: Physiological Integrity
Integrated Process: Nursing Process/Evaluation
Content Area: Pharmacology
Reference: Hodgson, B., & Kizior, R. (2005). *Saunders nursing drug handbook 2005.* Philadelphia: W.B. Saunders, p. 155.

10. Answer: 3
Rationale: Sodium bicarbonate is an electrolyte modifier and antacid. It would further aggravate metabolic alkalosis. The conditions identified in the other options are not contraindications for the use of sodium bicarbonate.
Test-Taking Strategy: Note the key word, *contraindicated,* and use knowledge of acid-base concepts to answer this question. Focus on the name of the medication to assist in eliminating options 1, 2, and 4. Review the contraindications associated with the use of this medication if you had difficulty with this question.
Level of Cognitive Ability: Analysis
Client Needs: Physiological Integrity

Integrated Process: Nursing Process/Data Collection
Content Area: Pharmacology
Reference: Hodgson, B., & Kizior, R. (2005). *Saunders nursing drug handbook 2005.* Philadelphia: W.B. Saunders, p. 974.

11. *Answer:* 1
Rationale: Older clients are especially susceptible to the central nervous system (CNS) side effects of cimetidine. The most frequent of these is confusion. Less common CNS side effects include headache, dizziness, drowsiness, and hallucinations.
Test-Taking Strategy: Use the process of elimination. Note the key words, *most frequent.* Use knowledge of the concepts related to the older client and medication administration, and knowledge of this medication to answer the question. Review this medication if you had difficulty with this question.
Level of Cognitive Ability: Application
Client Needs: Physiological Integrity
Integrated Process: Nursing Process/Implementation
Content Area: Pharmacology
Reference: Hodgson, B., & Kizior, R. (2005). *Saunders nursing drug handbook 2005.* Philadelphia: W.B. Saunders, p. 227.

12. *Answer:* 2
Rationale: The medication should be scheduled for administration 1 hour before meals and at bedtime. The medication is timed to allow it to form a protective coating over the ulcer before food intake stimulates gastric acid production and mechanical irritation. The other options are incorrect.
Test-Taking Strategy: Use the process of elimination. Focusing on the client's diagnosis and recalling the action of the medication will direct you to option 2. Review this medication if you had difficulty with this question.
Level of Cognitive Ability: Application
Client Needs: Physiological Integrity
Integrated Process: Nursing Process/Implementation
Content Area: Pharmacology
Reference: Hodgson, B., & Kizior, R. (2005). *Saunders nursing drug handbook 2005.* Philadelphia: W.B. Saunders, p. 994.

13. *Answer:* 4
Rationale: A single daily dose of ranitidine is scheduled to be given at bedtime. This allows for a prolonged effect, and the greatest protection of the gastric mucosa. The other options are incorrect.
Test-Taking Strategy: Specific knowledge of the timing of this medication is needed to answer this question. Also, recalling that ranitidine suppresses secretions of gastric acids will direct you to option 4. If you had difficulty with this question, review this medication.
Level of Cognitive Ability: Application
Client Needs: Physiological Integrity
Integrated Process: Nursing Process/Implementation
Content Area: Pharmacology
Reference: Hodgson, B., & Kizior, R. (2005). *Saunders nursing drug handbook 2005.* Philadelphia: W.B. Saunders, p. 926.

14. *Answer:* 2
Rationale: Omeprazole is a gastric pump inhibitor and is classified as an antiulcer agent. The intended effect of the medication is relief of pain from gastric irritation, often referred to as heartburn by clients. Options 1, 3, and 4 are incorrect.
Test-Taking Strategy: Use the process of elimination. Recalling the action and use of omeprazole will direct you to option 2. Review this medication if you had difficulty with this question.
Level of Cognitive Ability: Analysis
Client Needs: Physiological Integrity
Integrated Process: Nursing Process/Evaluation
Content Area: Pharmacology
References: Hodgson, B., & Kizior, R. (2005). *Saunders nursing drug handbook 2005.* Philadelphia: W.B. Saunders, p. 801. McKenry, L., & Salerno, E. (2003). *Mosby's pharmacology in nursing* (21st ed.). St. Louis: Mosby, p. 771.

15. *Answer:* 1
Rationale: Cascara sagrada is a laxative that causes nausea and abdominal cramps as the most frequent side effects. Other health problems are not determined based on a single symptom.
Test-Taking Strategy: Use the process of elimination. Remember that options that are similar are not likely to be correct. This will allow you to eliminate the two gastrointestinal disorders (options 2 and 4). From the remaining options, recalling that laxatives can cause abdominal cramping will direct you to option 1. Review the effects of this medication if you had difficulty with this question.
Level of Cognitive Ability: Analysis
Client Needs: Physiological Integrity
Integrated Process: Nursing Process/Data Collection
Content Area: Pharmacology
Reference: Hodgson, B., & Kizior, R. (2005). *Saunders nursing drug handbook 2005.* Philadelphia: W.B. Saunders, p. 174.

16. *Answer:* 2
Rationale: Most rapid results from bisacodyl occur when it is taken on an empty stomach. It will not have a rapid effect if taken with a large meal. If it is taken at bedtime, the client will have a bowel movement in the morning. Taking the medication with two glasses of juice will not add to its effect.
Test-Taking Strategy: Use the process of elimination. Focus on the key words, *rapid effect.* Recalling that food generally slows the absorption of medication will assist in directing you to option 2. Review the administration of laxatives if you had difficulty with this question.
Level of Cognitive Ability: Application
Client Needs: Physiological Integrity
Integrated Process: Nursing Process/Implementation
Content Area: Pharmacology
Reference: Hodgson, B., & Kizior, R. (2005). *Saunders nursing drug handbook 2005.* Philadelphia: W.B. Saunders, p. 124.

17. *Answer:* 4
Rationale: Loperamide is an antidiarrheal agent. It is commonly administered after loose stools. It is used in the management of acute diarrhea and also in chronic diarrhea, such as with inflammatory bowel disease. It can also be used to reduce the volume of drainage from an ileostomy. The other options are incorrect.

Test-Taking Strategy: Use the process of elimination. Knowledge that this medication is an antidiarrheal will direct you to the correct option. Review the action of this medication if you had difficulty with this question.
Level of Cognitive Ability: Application
Client Needs: Physiological Integrity
Integrated Process: Nursing Process/Planning
Content Area: Pharmacology
Reference: Hodgson, B., & Kizior, R. (2005). *Saunders nursing drug handbook 2005.* Philadelphia: W.B. Saunders, p. 647.

18. *Answer:* 1
Rationale: The client should not exceed the recommended dose because it may be habit-forming. The medication is an antidiarrheal, and therefore should not be taken with a laxative. Side effects of the medication include dry mouth and drowsiness.
Test-Taking Strategy: To answer this question accurately, it is necessary to be familiar with this medication and its habit-forming properties. Noting that atropine is an ingredient will help to eliminate options 3 and 4. From the remaining options, recalling that the medication is an antidiarrheal will assist in eliminating option 2. Review this medication if you had difficulty with this question.
Level of Cognitive Ability: Analysis
Client Needs: Physiological Integrity
Integrated Process: Nursing Process/Evaluation
Content Area: Pharmacology
References: Hodgson, B., & Kizior, R. (2005). *Saunders nursing drug handbook 2005.* Philadelphia: W.B. Saunders, p. 336.
McKenry, L., & Salerno, E. (2003). *Mosby's pharmacology in nursing* (21st ed.). St. Louis: Mosby, p. 784.

19. *Answer:* 3
Rationale: Dimenhydrinate is used to treat and prevent the symptoms of dizziness, vertigo, nausea, and vomiting that accompany motion sickness. The other options are incorrect.
Test-Taking Strategy: Use the process of elimination. Recalling that dimenhydrinate is used to treat motion sickness will direct you to option 3. Review this medication if you had difficulty with this question.
Level of Cognitive Ability: Analysis

Client Needs: Physiological Integrity
Integrated Process: Nursing Process/Evaluation
Content Area: Pharmacology
Reference: McKenry, L., & Salerno, E. (2003). *Mosby's pharmacology in nursing* (21st ed.). St. Louis: Mosby, p. 741.

20. *Answer:* 4
Rationale: Docusate sodium is a stool softener that promotes the absorption of water into the stool, producing a softer consistency of stool. The intended effect is relief or prevention of constipation. The medication does not relieve abdominal pain, stop gastrointestinal bleeding, or decrease the amount of fat in the stools.
Test-Taking Strategy: Use the process of elimination. Recalling that docusate is a stool softener will direct you to option 4. Review the action of this medication if you had difficulty with this question.
Level of Cognitive Ability: Application
Client Needs: Physiological Integrity
Integrated Process: Nursing Process/Implementation
Content Area: Pharmacology
Reference: Hodgson, B., & Kizior, R. (2005). *Saunders nursing drug handbook 2005.* Philadelphia: W.B. Saunders, p. 346.

ALTERNATE FORMAT QUESTION: FILL IN THE BLANK

Answer: 30
Rationale: The client should be taught to take this medication 30 minutes before meals. This allows the medication time to begin working before the client takes in food, which requires digestion and movement. A dose is also usually prescribed to be taken at bedtime.
Test-Taking Strategy: Focusing on the client's diagnosis will assist in answering this question. Review administration of this medication if you had difficulty with this question.
Level of Cognitive Ability: Application
Client Needs: Physiological Integrity
Integrated Process: Teaching/Learning
Content Area: Pharmacology
Reference: *Mosby's 2005 drug consult for nurses.* (2005). St. Louis: Mosby, p. 713.

REFERENCES

Hodgson, B., & Kizior, R. (2005). *Saunders nursing drug handbook 2005.* Philadelphia: W.B. Saunders.
McKenry, L., & Salerno, E. (2003). *Mosby's pharmacology in nursing* (21st ed.). St. Louis: Mosby.

Mosby's 2005 drug consult for nurses. (2005). St. Louis: Mosby.

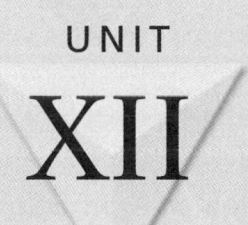
The Adult Client with a Respiratory Disorder

PYRAMID TERMS

bacille Calmette-Guérin (BCG) vaccine A vaccine containing attenuated tubercle bacilli that may be given to people in foreign countries or to those traveling to foreign countries to produce increased resistance to tuberculosis (TB).

chronic airflow limitation (CAL), chronic obstructive lung disease (COLD), chronic obstructive pulmonary disease (COPD) A group of diseases that includes emphysema, asthma, bronchiectasis, and bronchitis; characterized by progressive airflow limitations into and out of the lungs, elevated airway resistance, irreversible lung distention, and arterial blood gas imbalance; can lead to pulmonary insufficiency, pulmonary hypertension, and cor pulmonale. In emphysema, the stimulus to breathe is a low Po_2 instead of an increased Pco_2.

emphysema A chronic pulmonary disease marked by a narrowing of the small airways and the trapping of air, with destructive changes in their walls; also known as chronic obstructive pulmonary disease (COPD).

Mantoux test The most reliable determinant of infection with tuberculosis (TB). A small amount (0.1 mL) of intermediate-strength purified protein derivative (PPD) containing 5 tuberculin units is given intradermally in the forearm. An area of induration measuring 15 mm or more in diameter in an individual at low risk, 48 to 72 hours after injection, indicates that the individual has been exposed to TB.

mechanical ventilation The use of a ventilator if a client is unable to ventilate enough on his or her own to maintain proper levels of oxygen and carbon dioxide in the blood. Types of ventilators include negative-pressure and positive-pressure ventilators. Various ventilator modes are adjusted to the client's individual needs.

multidrug-resistant TB strain (MDR-TB) A multidrug-resistant strain of TB can occur as a result of improper or noncompliant use of treatment programs and the development of mutations in the tubercle bacilli.

Mycobacterium tuberculosis The causative organism (bacillus) of tuberculosis; an aerobic bacterium that is a nonmotile, nonsporulating, acid-fast rod that secretes niacin.

pneumothorax The accumulation of atmospheric air in the pleural space, which results in a rise in intrathoracic pressure and reduced vital capacity. The loss of negative intrapleural pressure results in collapse of the lung. Diagnosis of pneumothorax is made by chest x-ray.

suctioning A sterile procedure that involves the removal of respiratory secretions that accumulate in the tracheobronchial airway when the client cannot expectorate secretions; performed to maintain a patent airway.

tuberculosis (TB) A highly communicable disease caused by *Mycobacterium tuberculosis*. It is transmitted by the airborne route via droplet infection.

PYRAMID TO SUCCESS

The Pyramid to Success focuses on maintaining a patent airway. Pyramid points focus on infectious diseases, particularly tuberculosis, and on the client with pneumonia, respiratory failure, chronic obstructive pulmonary disease, or pneumothorax. The Pyramid to Success includes the care of the client with tuberculosis, especially with regard to the importance of the medication regimen, providing adequate nutrition and adequate rest to promote the healing process, and preventing disease progression. Focus on assisting the client to cope with the social isolation issues that exist during the period of illness and on teaching the client and family the critical measures of screening and of preventing respiratory disease and the transmission of disease. The Integrated Processes addressed in this unit include Caring, the Clinical Problem-Solving Process (Nursing Process), Communication and Documentation, and Teaching/Learning.

CLIENT NEEDS
Safe, Effective Care Environment

Asepsis when caring for wounds or tracheostomy sites and during mechanical ventilation or suctioning

Client rights

Confidentiality related to the respiratory disorder

Consultations and referrals related to the respiratory disorder

Establishing priorities

Handling infectious materials such as sputum or body fluids

Informed consent related to diagnostic and surgical procedures
Respiratory precautions
Standard precautions

Health Promotion and Maintenance

Teaching related to the prevention of transmission of infection
Teaching related to medication administration
Teaching related to breathing exercises and respiratory therapy and care
Teaching related to adequate fluid and nutritional intake
Teaching related to the need for follow-up care
Health promotion programs
Health screening related to risks for respiratory disorders
Respiratory data collection techniques
Prevention of respiratory disorders and infectious diseases

Psychosocial Integrity

Body image changes related to tracheostomy if performed
Coping mechanisms
Community resources
Grief and loss
End-of-life issues
Religious, cultural, and spiritual influences
Situational role changes
Support systems

Physiological Integrity

Alterations in body systems
Comfort interventions

Infectious diseases
Mechanical ventilation
Medical emergencies
Nutrition and oral hygiene
Oxygen delivery systems
Personal hygiene and rest and sleep
Pharmacological therapy
Respiratory care

REFERENCES

Black, J., & Hawks, J. (2005). *Medical-surgical nursing: Clinical management for positive outcomes* (7th ed.). Philadelphia: W.B. Saunders.

Chernecky, C., & Berger, B. (2004). *Laboratory tests and diagnostic procedures* (4th ed.). Philadelphia: W.B. Saunders.

Christensen, B., & Kockrow, E. (2003). *Adult health nursing* (4th ed.). St. Louis: Mosby.

Christensen, B., & Kockrow, E. (2003). *Foundations of nursing* (4th ed.). St. Louis: Mosby.

Harkreader, H., & Hogan, M.A. (2004). *Fundamentals of nursing: Caring and clinical judgment* (2nd ed.). Philadelphia: W.B. Saunders.

Hodgson, B., & Kizior, R. (2005). *Saunders nursing drug handbook 2005.* Philadelphia: W.B. Saunders.

Lewis, S., Heitkemper, M., & Dirksen, S. (2004). *Medical-surgical nursing: Assessment and management of clinical problems* (6th ed.). St. Louis: Mosby.

Linton, A., & Maebius, N. (2003). *Introduction to medical-surgical nursing* (3rd ed.). Philadelphia: W.B. Saunders.

McKenry, L., & Salerno, E. (2003). *Mosby's pharmacology in nursing* (21st ed.). St. Louis: Mosby.

National Council of State Boards of Nursing. (2005). *Detailed test plan for the National Council licensure examination for practical/vocational nurses.* Chicago: Author.

Pagana, K., & Pagana, T. (2003). *Mosby's diagnostic and laboratory test reference* (6th ed.). St. Louis: Mosby.

Perry, A., & Potter, P. (2002). *Clinical nursing skills and techniques* (5th ed.). St. Louis: Mosby.

Potter, P., & Perry, A. (2003). *Essentials for practice* (5th ed.). St. Louis: Mosby.

Phipps, W., Monahan, F., Sands, J., Marek, J., & Neighbors, M. (2003). *Medical-surgical nursing: Health and illness perspectives* (7th ed.). St. Louis: Mosby.

Respiratory System

I. ANATOMY AND PHYSIOLOGY

A. Primary functions
1. Provides oxygen for metabolism in the tissues
2. Removes carbon dioxide, the waste product of metabolism

B. Secondary functions
1. Facilitates sense of smell
2. Produces speech
3. Maintains acid-base balance
4. Maintains body water levels
5. Maintains heat balance

C. Upper respiratory tract
1. Nose: Humidifies, warms, and filters inspired air
2. Sinuses
   a. Air-filled cavities within the hollow bones that surround the nasal passages
   b. Provide resonance during speech
3. Pharynx
   a. Located behind the oral and nasal cavities
   b. Divided into the nasopharynx, oropharynx, and laryngopharynx
   c. Passageway for both the respiratory and digestive tracts
4. Larynx
   a. Located above the trachea and just below the pharynx at the root of the tongue
   b. Commonly called the voice box
   c. Contains two pairs of vocal cords, the false and true cords
   d. The opening between the true vocal cords is the glottis
   e. The glottis plays an important role in coughing, which is the most fundamental defense mechanism of the lungs
5. Epiglottis
   a. Leaf-shaped elastic structure that is attached along one end to the top of the larynx
   b. It prevents food from entering the tracheobronchial tree by closing over the glottis during swallowing

D. Lower respiratory tract
1. Trachea
   a. Located in front of the esophagus
   b. Branches into the right and left main stem bronchi at the carina
2. Main stem bronchi
   a. Begin at the carina
   b. The right bronchus is slightly wider, shorter, and more vertical than the left bronchus
   c. The main stem bronchi divide into five secondary or lobar bronchi that enter each of the five lobes of the lung
   d. The bronchi are lined with cilia, which propel mucus up and away from the lower airway to the trachea, where it can be expectorated or swallowed
3. Bronchioles
   a. Branch from the secondary bronchi and subdivide into the small terminal and respiratory bronchioles
   b. They contain no cartilage and depend on the elastic recoil of the lung for patency
   c. The terminal bronchioles contain no cilia and do not participate in gas exchange
4. Alveolar ducts and alveoli
   a. *Acinus* (pl., *acini*) is a term used to indicate all structures distal to the terminal bronchiole
   b. Alveolar ducts branch from the respiratory bronchioles
   c. Alveolar sacs, which arise from the ducts, contain clusters of alveoli, which are the basic units of gas exchange
   d. Cells in the walls of the alveoli secrete surfactant, a phospholipid protein that reduces the

surface tension in the alveoli; without surfactant, the alveoli would collapse

5. Lungs
   a. Located in the pleural cavity in the thorax
   b. Extend from just above the clavicles to the diaphragm, the major muscle of inspiration
   c. The right lung, which is larger than the left, is divided into three lobes, the upper, middle, and lower lobes
   d. The left lung, which is somewhat narrower than the right lung to accommodate the heart, is divided into two lobes
   e. Innervation of the respiratory structures is accomplished by the phrenic nerve, the vagus nerve, and the thoracic nerves
   f. The parietal pleura lines the inside of the thoracic cavity, including the upper surface of the diaphragm
   g. The visceral pleura covers the pulmonary surfaces
   h. A thin fluid layer, which is produced by the cells lining the pleura, lubricates the visceral pleura and the parietal pleura, allowing them to glide smoothly and painlessly during respiration
   i. Blood flow through the lungs occurs via the pulmonary system and the bronchial system

6. Accessory muscles of respiration: Include the scalene muscles, which elevate the first two ribs; the sternocleidomastoid muscles, which raise the sternum; and the trapezius and pectoralis muscles, which fix the shoulders

7. The respiratory process
   a. The diaphragm descends into the abdominal cavity during inspiration, causing negative pressure in the lungs
   b. The negative pressure draws air from the area of greater pressure, the atmosphere, into the area of lesser pressure, the lungs
   c. In the lungs, air passes through the terminal bronchioles into the alveoli to oxygenate the body tissues
   d. At the end of inspiration, the diaphragm and intercostal muscles relax and the lungs recoil
   e. As the lungs recoil, pressure within the lungs becomes greater than atmospheric pressure, causing the air, which now contains the cellular waste products of carbon dioxide and water, to move from the alveoli in the lungs to the atmosphere
   f. Expiration is a passive process

II. DIAGNOSTIC TESTS

A. Risk factors for respiratory disorders (Box 48-1)
B. Chest x-ray (CXR; radiography)
   1. Description: Provides information regarding the anatomic location and appearance of the lungs

---

BOX 48-1

Risk Factors for Respiratory Disease

Smoking
Use of chewing tobacco
Allergies
Frequent respiratory illnesses
Chest injury
Surgery
Exposure to chemicals and environmental pollutants
Crowded living conditions
Family history of infectious disease
Geographic residence and travel to foreign countries

BOX 48-2

Suctioning Procedure

Use aseptic technique.
Hyperoxygenate by a resuscitation bag, increasing the oxygen flow rate, or asking the client to take deep breaths.
Lubricate the catheter with sterile water.
For tracheal suctioning, insert the catheter 4 inches.
For nasotracheal suctioning, insert the catheter to induce cough reflex.
Do not apply suction while inserting the catheter.
Apply suction intermittently for 10 seconds; rotate the catheter and withdraw.
Hyperoxygenate the client and encourage deep breaths.

---

2. Preprocedure
   a. Remove all jewelry and other metal objects from the chest area
   b. Determine the client's ability to inhale and hold breath
   c. Question females regarding pregnancy or the possibility of pregnancy
3. Postprocedure: Assist the client to dress

C. Sputum specimen
   1. Description: A specimen obtained by expectoration or tracheal **suctioning** to assist in the identification of organisms or abnormal cells (Box 48-2)
   2. Preprocedure
      a. Determine specific purpose of collection and check with institutional policy for appropriate collection of specimen
      b. Obtain an early morning sterile specimen from **suctioning** or expectoration after a respiratory treatment, if a treatment is prescribed
      c. Obtain 15 mL of sputum
      d. Instruct the client to rinse the mouth with water before collection
      e. Instruct the client to take several deep breaths and then cough deeply to obtain sputum
      f. Always collect the specimen before starting antibiotics

3. Postprocedure
   a. If a culture of sputum is prescribed, transport specimen to laboratory immediately
   b. Assist the client with mouth care
D. Bronchoscopy
   1. Description: Direct visual examination of the larynx, trachea, and bronchi with a fiberoptic bronchoscope
   2. Preprocedure
      a. Obtain informed consent
      b. Nothing by mouth (NPO) from midnight before the procedure
      c. Obtain vital signs
      d. Check the results of coagulation studies
      e. Remove dentures or eyeglasses
      f. Prepare suction equipment
      g. Administer medication for sedation as prescribed
      h. Have emergency resuscitation equipment readily available
   3. Postprocedure
      a. Monitor vital signs
      b. Maintain semi-Fowler's position
      c. Check for the return of the gag reflex
      d. Maintain NPO status until gag reflex returns
      e. Have an emesis basin readily available for client to expectorate sputum
      f. Monitor for bloody sputum
      g. Monitor respiratory status, particularly if sedation was administered
      h. Monitor for complications, such as bronchospasm, bronchial perforation indicated by facial or neck crepitus, dysrhythmias, fever, bacteremia, hemorrhage, hypoxemia, and **pneumothorax**
      i. The physician is notified if fever, difficulty in breathing, or other signs of complications occur following the procedure
E. Pulmonary angiography
   1. Description
      a. An invasive fluoroscopic procedure in which a catheter is inserted through the antecubital or femoral vein into the pulmonary artery or one of its branches
      b. Involves an injection of iodine or radiopaque or contrast material
   2. Preprocedure
      a. Obtain informed consent
      b. Check for allergies to iodine, seafood, or other radiopaque dyes
      c. Maintain NPO status for 8 hours before the procedure
      d. Monitor vital signs
      e. Assess results of coagulation studies
      f. An IV access will be established
      g. Administer sedation as prescribed
      h. Instruct the client that he or she must lie still during the procedure

i. Instruct the client that he or she may feel an urge to cough, flushing, nausea, or a salty taste following injection of the dye
j. Have emergency resuscitation equipment available
   3. Postprocedure
      a. Monitor vital signs
      b. Avoid taking blood pressures for 24 hours in the extremity used for the injection
      c. Monitor peripheral neurovascular status of the affected extremity
      d. Monitor insertion site for bleeding
      e. Monitor for delayed reaction to the dye
F. Thoracentesis
   1. Description: Removal of fluid or air from the pleural space via a transthoracic aspiration
   2. Preprocedure
      a. Obtain informed consent
      b. Obtain vital signs
      c. Prepare the client for ultrasound or chest radiography, if prescribed, before procedure
      d. Check results of coagulation studies
      e. Note that the client is positioned sitting upright, with the arms and head supported by a table at the bedside during the procedure
      f. If the client cannot sit up, the client is placed lying in bed on the unaffected side, with the head of the bed elevated 45 degrees
      g. Instruct the client not to cough, breath deeply, or move during the procedure
   3. Postprocedure
      a. Monitor vital signs
      b. Monitor respiratory status
      c. Apply a pressure dressing, and assess the puncture site for bleeding and crepitus
      d. Monitor for signs of **pneumothorax**, air embolism, and pulmonary edema
G. Pulmonary function test (PFTs)
   1. Description: Include a number of different tests used to evaluate lung mechanics, gas exchange, and acid-base disturbance through spirometric, lung volume, and arterial blood gas measurement
   2. Preprocedure
      a. Determine if an analgesic that may depress the respiratory function is being administered
      b. The physician is consulted regarding holding bronchodilators before testing
      c. Instruct the client to void before procedure and to wear loose clothing
      d. Remove dentures
      e. Instruct the client to refrain from smoking or eating a heavy meal for 4 to 6 hours before the test
   3. Postprocedure: Resume normal diet and any bronchodilators and respiratory treatments that were held before the procedure

H. Lung biopsy
  1. Description
     a. A percutaneous lung biopsy is performed to obtain tissue for analysis by culture or cytological examination
     b. A needle biopsy is done to identify pulmonary lesions, changes in lung tissue, and the cause of pleural effusion
  2. Preprocedure
     a. Obtain informed consent
     b. Maintain NPO status before the procedure
     c. Inform the client that a local anesthetic will be used, but that a sensation of pressure during needle insertion and aspiration may be felt
     d. Administer analgesics and sedatives, as prescribed
  3. Postprocedure
     a. Monitor vital signs
     b. Apply a dressing to the biopsy site and monitor for drainage or bleeding
     c. Monitor for signs of respiratory distress; the physician is notified if they occur
     d. Monitor for signs of **pneumothorax** and air emboli; the physician is notified if they occur
     e. Prepare the client for chest x-ray if prescribed
I. Ventilation perfusion lung scan
  1. Description
     a. In the perfusion scan, blood flow to the lungs is evaluated
     b. The ventilation scan determines the patency of the pulmonary airways and detects abnormalities in ventilation
     c. A radionuclide may be injected for the procedure
  2. Preprocedure
     a. Obtain informed consent
     b. Check for allergies to dye, iodine, or seafood
     c. Remove jewelry around the chest area
     d. Review breathing methods that may be required during testing
     e. An intravenous (IV) access is established
     f. Administer sedation if prescribed
     g. Have emergency resuscitation equipment available
  3. Postprocedure
     a. Monitor client for reaction to the radionuclide
     b. Instruct client to wash hands carefully with soap and water for 24 hours following the procedure
J. Skin tests
  1. Description: An intradermal injection used to assist in diagnosing various infectious diseases
  2. Preprocedure: Determine hypersensitivity or previous reactions to skin tests
  3. Procedure
     a. Use a test site that is free of excessive body hair, dermatitis, and blemishes
     b. Apply at the upper third of inner surface of left arm

     c. Circle and mark the injection test site
     d. Document the date, time, and test site
  4. Postprocedure
     a. Advise the client not to scratch the test site to prevent infection and abscess formation
     b. Instruct the client to avoid washing the test site
     c. Interpret the reaction at the injection site 24 to 72 hours after administration of the test antigen
     d. Check the test site for the amount of induration (hard swelling) in millimeters and the presence of erythema and vesiculation (small blister-like elevations)
K. Arterial blood gases (ABGs)
  1. Description: Measurement of the dissolved oxygen and carbon dioxide in the arterial blood; reveals the acid-base status and how well the oxygen is being carried to the body (Box 48-3)
  2. Preprocedure and postprocedure care: See Chapter 10
L. Pulse oximetry
  1. Description
     a. A noninvasive test that registers the oxygen saturation of the client's hemoglobin
     b. This arterial oxygen saturation (SaO_2) is recorded as a percentage
     c. The normal value is 95% to 100%
     d. After a hypoxic client uses up the readily available oxygen (measured as the arterial oxygen pressure, PaO_2, on arterial blood gas testing), the reserve oxygen, the oxygen attached to the hemoglobin (SaO_2), is drawn on to provide oxygen to the tissues
     e. A pulse oximeter reading can alert the nurse to hypoxemia before clinical signs occur
  2. Procedure
     a. A sensor is placed on the client's finger, toe, nose, earlobe, or forehead to measure oxygen saturation, which is then displayed on a monitor
     b. Maintain the transducer at heart level
     c. Do not select an extremity with an impediment to blood flow
     d. Results lower than 91% necessitate immediate treatment
     e. If the SaO_2 is below 85%, the body's tissues have a difficult time becoming oxygenated; an SaO_2 of less than 70% is life-threatening

---

BOX 48-3

Normal Arterial Blood Gas (ABG) Values

pH: 7.35 to 7.45
PCO_2: 35 to 45 mm Hg
HCO_3^-: 22 to 27 mEq/L
PO_2: 80 to 100 mm Hg
O_2 saturation: 96% to 100%
Oxyhemoglobin dissociation curve: No shift

III. RESPIRATORY TREATMENTS

A. Chest physiotherapy (CPT)
1. Description: Percussion and vibration over the thorax to loosen secretions in the affected area of the lungs
2. Interventions
   a. A layer of material (gown or pajamas) is placed between the hands and the client's skin
   b. Best time to perform is in the morning on arising, 1 hour before meals, or 2 to 3 hours after meals
   c. If client is receiving a tube feeding, stop the feeding and aspirate the residual before beginning CPT
   d. Stop CPT if pain occurs
   e. Dispose of sputum properly
   f. Provide mouth care after procedure
3. Contraindications
   a. When bronchospasm is increased by its use
   b. History of pathological fractures
   c. Rib fractures
   d. Chest incisions
B. Postural drainage
1. Description
   a. Use of gravity to drain secretions from segments of the lungs
   b. May be combined with CPT
2. Interventions
   a. Position the client properly (lung segment to be drained is uppermost)
   b. Best time for the procedure is in the morning on arising, 1 hour before meals, or 2 to 3 hours after meals
   c. If client is receiving a tube feeding, stop the feeding and aspirate the residual before beginning postural drainage
   d. Stop postural drainage if cyanosis or exhaustion occurs
   e. Maintain position 5 to 20 minutes after procedure
   f. Dispose of sputum properly
   g. Provide mouth care after the procedure
3. Contraindications
   a. Unstable vital signs
   b. Increased intracranial pressure
C. Incentive spirometry (Box 48-4)

IV. OXYGEN

A. Interventions
1. Check color and vital signs before and during treatment
2. Place an "Oxygen in Use" sign at the client's bedside
3. Check for the presence of chronic lung problems
4. Humidify the oxygen

B. Nasal cannula (nasal prongs) (Box 48-5)
1. Description
   a. Used at flow rates of 1 to 6 L/minute, providing approximate oxygen concentrations of 24% (at 1 L/minute) to 44% (at 6 L/minute)
   b. Flow rates higher than 6 L/minute do not significantly increase oxygenation, because the anatomic reserve or dead space (oral and nasal cavities) is full
   c. Used for the client with chronic airflow limitation (**CAL**) and for long-term oxygen use; however, the **CAL** client who is hypoxemic and also has chronic hypercarbia requires lower levels of oxygen, usually 1 to 2 L/minute.
   d. Effective oxygen concentration can be delivered to both nose breathers and mouth breathers with the use of a nasal cannula
2. Interventions
   a. Place the nasal prongs in the nostrils, with the openings facing the client
   b. Add humidification as prescribed when a flow rate higher than 2 L/minute is prescribed
   c. Check the water level and change the humidifier as needed
   d. Monitor the client for changes in respiratory rate or depth
   e. Check the mucosa because high flow rates have a drying effect and increase mucosal irritation
   f. Monitor skin integrity, because the oxygen tubing can irritate the skin
   g. Provide water-soluble jelly to the nares PRN

BOX 48-4

Client Instructions for Incentive Spirometry

Instruct the client to assume a sitting or upright position.
Instruct the client to place his or her mouth tightly around the mouthpiece.
Instruct the client to inhale slowly to raise and maintain the flow rate indicator between the 600 and 900 marks.
Instruct the client to hold his or her breath for 5 seconds and then to exhale through pursed lips.
Instruct the client to repeat this process ten times every hour.

BOX 48-5

Fio$_2$ Delivered via Nasal Cannula

24% at 1 L/minute
28% at 2 L/minute
32% at 3 L/minute
36% at 4 L/minute
40% at 5 L/minute
44% at 6 L/minute

BOX 48-6

Fio₂ Delivered via Simple Face Mask

40% at 5 L/minute
45% to 50% at 6 L/minute
55% to 60% at 8 L/minute
Pyramid point: Flow rate must be set to at least 5 L/minute to flush the mask of carbon dioxide.

BOX 48-7

Fio₂ Delivered via Partial Rebreather Mask

70% to 90% Fio₂: Delivered at 6 to 15 L/minute
Pyramid point: A flow rate high enough to maintain the bag two-thirds full during inspiration is needed.

C. Simple face mask (Box 48-6)
  1. Description
    a. A face mask used to deliver oxygen concentrations of 40% to 60% for short-term oxygen therapy or to deliver oxygen in an emergency
    b. A minimal flow rate of 5 L/minute is needed to prevent the rebreathing of exhaled air
  2. Interventions
    a. Be sure the mask fits securely over the nose and mouth because a poorly fitting mask reduces the Fio₂ (fraction of inspired oxygen) delivered
    b. Monitor skin and provide skin care to the area covered by the mask, because pressure and moisture under the mask may cause skin breakdown
    c. Monitor the client closely for risk of aspiration, because the mask limits the client's ability to clear the mouth, especially if vomiting occurs
    d. Provide emotional support to decrease anxiety in the client who feels claustrophobic
    e. Consult with the physician regarding switching the client from a mask to a nasal cannula during eating
D. Partial rebreather mask (Box 48-7)
  1. Description
    a. A partial rebreather mask consists of a mask with a reservoir bag that provides an oxygen concentration of 70% to 90%, with flow rates of 6 to 15 L/minute
    b. The client rebreathes one third of the exhaled tidal volume, which is high in oxygen, thus providing a high Fio₂
  2. Interventions
    a. Make sure that the reservoir does not twist or kink, which results in a deflated bag
    b. Adjust the flow rate to keep the reservoir bag inflated two-thirds full during inspiration, because deflation results in decreased oxygen delivered and rebreathing of exhaled air
E. Nonrebreather mask
  1. Description
    a. A nonrebreather mask provides the highest concentration of the low-flow systems and can deliver an Fio₂ greater than 90%, depending on the client's ventilatory pattern

    b. It is most frequently used in the client with deteriorating respiratory status who might require intubation
    c. The nonrebreather mask has a one-way valve between the mask and the reservoir and two flaps over the exhalation ports
    d. The valve allows the client to draw the entire quantity of oxygen from the reservoir bag
    e. The flaps prevent room air from entering through the exhalation ports
    f. During exhalation, air leaves through these exhalation ports while the one-way valve prevents exhaled air from re-entering the reservoir bag
  2. Fio₂ delivered: 60% to 100% Fio₂ at a liter flow that maintains the bag two-thirds full
  3. Interventions
    a. Remove mucus or saliva from the mask
    b. Monitor the client closely
    c. Ensure that the valve and flaps are intact and functional during each breath
    d. Valves should open during expiration and close during inhalation
    e. Suffocation can occur if the reservoir bag kinks or if the oxygen source disconnects ▲
F. Face tent
  1. Fits over the client's chin, with the top extending halfway across the face
  2. The oxygen concentration varies, but the face tent is useful instead of a tight-fitting mask for the client who has facial trauma or burns
G. Aerosol mask: Used for the client who requires high humidity after extubation or upper airway surgery, or for the client who has thick secretions
H. Tracheostomy collar and T piece
  1. The tracheostomy collar can be used to deliver high humidity and the desired oxygen to the client with a tracheostomy
  2. A special adapter, called the T piece, can be used to deliver any desired Fio₂ to the client with a tracheostomy, laryngectomy, or endotracheal tube
  3. See Chapter 19 for information on endotracheal and tracheostomy tubes
I. Interventions for face tent, aerosol mask, tracheostomy collar, and T piece
  1. Change delivery system to a nasal cannula during mealtimes
  2. Ensure that the aerosol mist escapes from the vents of the delivery system during inspiration and expiration

3. Empty condensation from the tubing to prevent the client from being lavaged with water and to promote an adequate flow rate
   a. Ensure that there is sufficient water in the canister, and change the aerosol water container as needed
   b. Keep the exhalation port on the T piece open and uncovered (if the port is occluded, the client can suffocate)
   c. Position the T piece so that it does not pull on the tracheostomy or endotracheal tube and cause erosion of skin at the tracheostomy insertion site
   d. Make sure the humidifier creates enough mist; a mist should be seen during inspiration and expiration
J. Venturi mask
   1. Description
      a. A high-flow oxygen delivery system
      b. Its operation is based on a mechanism that pulls in a specific proportional amount of room air for each liter flow of oxygen
      c. An adapter is located between the bottom of the mask and the oxygen source; the adapter contains holes of different sizes that allow only specific amounts of air to mix with the oxygen
      d. The adapter allows selection of the amount of oxygen desired
   2. FiO_2 delivered: 24% to 55% FiO_2 with flow rates of 4 to 10 L/minute
   3. Interventions
      a. Monitor closely to ensure an accurate flow rate for specific FiO_2
      b. Keep the orifice for the Venturi adapter open and uncovered to ensure adequate oxygen delivery
      c. Ensure that the mask fits snugly and that tubing is free of kinks, because the FiO_2 is altered if kinking occurs or if the mask fits poorly
      d. Monitor the client for dry mucous membranes; humidity or aerosol can be added to the system

V. MECHANICAL VENTILATION

A. Description: Used to overcome the client's inability to ventilate or oxygenate adequately
B. Interventions
   1. Assess the client first and the ventilator second
   2. Monitor vital signs, lung sounds, respiratory status, and breathing patterns (the client will never breathe at a rate less than the rate set on the ventilator)
   3. Monitor skin color, particularly in the lips and nail beds
   4. Monitor chest for bilateral expansion
   5. Obtain pulse oximetry readings

BOX 48-8

Causes of Ventilator Alarms

HIGH-PRESSURE ALARM
Increased secretions in the airway
Wheezing or bronchospasm, causing decreased airway size
Displacement of the endotracheal tube
Obstructed endotracheal tube as a result of water or a kink in the tubing
Client coughs, gags, or bites on the oral endotracheal tube
Client is anxious or fights the ventilator

LOW-PRESSURE ALARM
Disconnection or leak in the ventilator system or in the client's airway cuff
Client stops spontaneous breathing

---

   6. Monitor ABG results
   7. Monitor the need for **suctioning** and observe the type, color, and amount of secretions
   8. Check ventilator settings
   9. Monitor the level of water in humidifier and temperature of the humidification system because extremes in temperature can cause damage to the mucosal airway
   10. Ensure that the alarms are set
   11. If a cause for an alarm cannot be determined, ventilate the client manually with a resuscitation bag until the problem is corrected
   12. Empty the ventilator tubing when moisture collects
   13. Turn the client at least every 2 hours or get the client out of bed as prescribed to prevent complications of immobility
   14. Have resuscitation equipment available at the bedside
C. Causes of alarms (Box 48-8)
D. Complications
   1. Hypotension caused by the application of positive pressure, which increases intrathoracic pressure and inhibits blood return to the heart
   2. Respiratory complications such as **pneumothorax** or subcutaneous **emphysema** as a result of positive pressure
   3. Gastrointestinal alterations such as stress ulcers
   4. Malnutrition if nutrition is not maintained
   5. Infections
   6. Muscular deconditioning
   7. Ventilator dependence or inability to wean
E. Weaning: The process of going from ventilator dependence to spontaneous breathing

VI. CHEST INJURIES

A. Rib fracture
   1. Description

a. Results from direct blunt chest trauma and causes a potential for intrathoracic injury, such as **pneumothorax** or pulmonary contusion

b. Pain with movement and chest splinting result in impaired ventilation and inadequate clearance of secretions

2. Data collection
   a. Pain at injury site that increases with inspiration
   b. Tenderness at site
   c. Shallow respirations
   d. Client splints chest
   e. Fractures noted on chest x-ray film

3. Interventions
   a. Note that ribs usually unite spontaneously
   b. Position the client in high Fowler's position
   c. Administer pain medication as prescribed to maintain adequate ventilatory status
   d. Monitor for increased respiratory distress
   e. Instruct the client to self-splint with hands and arms
   f. Prepare the client for an intercostal nerve block as prescribed if the pain is severe

B. Flail chest
1. Description
   a. A blunt chest trauma associated with accidents, which may result in hemothorax and rib fractures
   b. The loose segment of the chest wall becomes paradoxical to the expansion and contraction of the rest of the chest wall

2. Data collection
   a. Paradoxical respirations (inward movement of a segment of the thorax during inspiration with outward movement during expiration)
   b. Severe pain in chest
   c. Dyspnea
   d. Cyanosis
   e. Tachycardia
   f. Hypotension
   g. Tachypnea, shallow respirations
   h. Diminished breath sounds

3. Interventions
   a. Position the client in high Fowler's
   b. Administer humidified oxygen, as prescribed
   c. Monitor for increased respiratory distress
   d. Encourage coughing and deep breathing
   e. Administer pain medication as prescribed
   f. Maintain bed rest and limit activity to reduce oxygen demands
   g. Prepare for intubation with **mechanical ventilation**

C. Pulmonary contusion
1. Description
   a. Characterized by interstitial hemorrhage associated with intraalveolar hemorrhage, resulting in decreased pulmonary compliance
   b. The major complication is acute respiratory distress syndrome (ARDS)

2. Data collection
   a. Dyspnea
   b. Hypoxemia
   c. Increased bronchial secretions
   d. Hemoptysis
   e. Restlessness
   f. Decreased breath sounds
   g. Crackles and wheezes

3. Interventions
   a. Maintain airway and ventilation
   b. Position the client in high Fowler's
   c. Administer oxygen as prescribed
   d. Monitor for increased respiratory distress
   e. Maintain bed rest and limit activity to reduce oxygen demands
   f. Prepare for **mechanical ventilation**

D. Pneumothorax
1. Description
   a. The accumulation of atmospheric air in the pleural space, which results in a rise in intrathoracic pressure and reduced vital capacity
   b. The loss of negative intrapleural pressure results in collapse of the lung
   c. A spontaneous **pneumothorax** occurs with the rupture of a bleb
   d. An open **pneumothorax** occurs when an opening through the chest wall allows the entrance of positive atmospheric pressure into the pleural space
   e. A tension **pneumothorax** occurs from a blunt chest injury or from **mechanical ventilation** with positive end-expiratory pressure when there is a buildup of positive pressure in the pleural space
   f. Diagnosis of **pneumothorax** is made by chest x-ray

2. Data collection (Box 48-9)
3. Interventions
   a. Apply a dressing over an open chest wound
   b. Administer oxygen as prescribed

BOX 48-9

Data Collection Findings: Pneumothorax

Dyspnea
Tachycardia
Tachypnea
Sharp chest pain
Absent breath sounds on affected side
Decreased chest expansion unilaterally
Cyanosis
Hypotension
Subcutaneous emphysema, as evidenced by crepitus on palpation
Sucking sound with open chest wound
Tracheal deviation to the unaffected side with tension pneumothorax

c. Position the client in high Fowler's

d. Prepare for chest tube placement until the lung has fully expanded

e. Monitor chest tube drainage system

f. Monitor for subcutaneous **emphysema**

g. See Chapter 19 for information on chest tubes

VII. RESPIRATORY FAILURE

A. Description

1. Occurs when the client cannot eliminate carbon dioxide from the alveoli

2. The carbon dioxide retention results in hypoxemia

3. Oxygen reaches the alveoli but cannot be absorbed or used properly

4. The lungs can move air sufficiently but cannot oxygenate the pulmonary blood properly

5. Respiratory failure occurs as a result of a mechanical abnormality of the lungs or chest wall, a defect in the respiratory control center in the brain, or an impairment in the function of the respiratory muscles

6. The $Paco_2$ level is higher than 45 mm Hg

B. Data collection

1. Dyspnea

2. Headache

3. Restlessness

4. Confusion

5. Tachycardia

6. Cyanosis

7. Dysrhythmias

8. Decreased level of consciousness

9. Alterations in respirations and breath sounds

C. Interventions

1. Identify and treat the cause of respiratory failure

2. Administer oxygen as prescribed to maintain the Pao_2 level above 60 to 70 mm Hg

3. Position the client in high Fowler's

4. Encourage deep breathing

5. Administer bronchodilators as prescribed

6. Prepare the client for **mechanical ventilation** if supplemental oxygen cannot maintain acceptable Pao_2 levels

VIII. ACUTE RESPIRATORY DISTRESS SYNDROME (ARDS)

A. Description

1. A form of acute respiratory failure that occurs as a complication of some other condition, is caused by a diffuse lung injury, and leads to extravascular lung fluid

2. The major site of injury is the alveolar capillary membrane

3. The interstitial edema causes compression and obliteration of the terminal airways and leads to reduced lung volume and compliance

4. The ABGs identify respiratory acidosis and hypoxemia that does not respond to an increased percentage of oxygen

5. The chest x-ray shows interstitial edema

6. Some of the causes include sepsis, fluid overload, shock, trauma, neurological injuries, burns, disseminated intravascular coagulation (DIC), drug ingestion, and the inhalation of toxic substances

B. Data collection

1. Tachypnea

2. Dyspnea

3. Decreased breath sounds

4. Deteriorating blood gas levels

5. Hypoxemia despite high concentrations of delivered oxygen

6. Decreased pulmonary compliance

7. Pulmonary infiltrates

C. Interventions

1. Identify and treat cause of the ARDS

2. Administer oxygen as prescribed

3. Position client in high Fowler's

4. Restrict fluid intake as prescribed

5. Provide respiratory treatments as prescribed

6. Administer diuretics, anticoagulants, or corticosteroids as prescribed

7. Prepare the client for intubation and **mechanical ventilation**

IX. CHRONIC OBSTRUCTIVE PULMONARY DISEASE (COPD)

A. Description

1. Also known as **chronic obstructive lung disease (COLD)** and **chronic airflow limitation (CAL)**

2. A group of diseases that includes **emphysema**, asthma, bronchiectasis, and bronchitis

3. Characterized by progressive airflow limitations into and out of the lungs, elevated airway resistance, irreversible lung distention, and arterial blood gas imbalance

4. **COPD** leads to pulmonary insufficiency, pulmonary hypertension, and cor pulmonale

5. In **emphysema**, the stimulus to breathe is a low Po_2 instead of an increased Pco_2

B. Data collection

1. Cough

2. Exertional dyspnea

3. Wheezing and crackles

4. Sputum production

5. Weight loss

6. Barrel chest (**emphysema**)

7. Use of accessory muscles for breathing

8. Cyanosis

9. Clubbing of fingers

10. Orthopnea

11. Cardiac dysrhythmias

12. Congestion and hyperinflation on chest x-ray film
13. ABGs indicate respiratory acidosis and hypoxemia
14. PFTs demonstrate decreased vital capacity

C. Interventions
1. Monitor vital signs
2. Administer a low concentration of oxygen (1 to 2 L/minute) as prescribed; the stimulus to breathe is a low Po_2 instead of an increased Pco_2
3. Monitor pulse oximetry
4. Provide respiratory treatments and chest physiotherapy
5. Instruct the client in diaphragmatic or abdominal and pursed lip breathing techniques
6. Record the color, amount, and consistency of sputum
7. Suction the client, if necessary, to clear airway and prevent infection
8. Monitor weight
9. Encourage small, frequent meals to prevent dyspnea
10. Provide a high-calorie, high-protein diet with supplements
11. Encourage fluids up to 3000 mL/day to keep secretions thin, unless contraindicated
12. Position in high Fowler's and leaning forward to aid in breathing
13. Allow activity as tolerated
14. Administer bronchodilators as prescribed, and instruct the client in the use of both oral and inhalant medications
15. Administer corticosteroids as prescribed to reduce inflammation
16. Administer mucolytics as prescribed to thin secretions
17. Administer antibiotics for infection if prescribed

D. Client education (Box 48-10)

X. SEVERE ACUTE RESPIRATORY SYNDROME (SARS)

A. A respiratory illness caused by the coronavirus, called SARS-associated coronavirus (SARS-CoV)
B. Begins with a fever, an overall feeling of discomfort, body aches, and mild respiratory symptoms
C. After 2 to 7 days, the client may develop a dry cough and dyspnea
D. It is spread by close person-to-person contact by direct contact with infectious material (respiratory secretions or by contact with people or objects infected with infectious droplets)
E. Prevention includes avoiding contact with those suspected of having SARS, avoiding travel to countries where an outbreak of SARS exists, avoiding close contact with crowds in areas where SARS exists, and frequent hand washing if in an area where SARS exists

---

BOX 48-10

Client Education: Chronic Obstructive Pulmonary Disease (COPD)

Stop smoking.
Recognize the signs and symptoms of respiratory infection and hypoxia.
Adhere to activity limitations, alternating rest periods with activity.
Avoid exposure to individuals with infections and avoid crowds.
Use pursed lip and diaphragmatic or abdominal breathing.
Understand proper use of medications and inhalers.
Use oxygen therapy, as recommended.
Ensure diet containing nutritional requirements.
Avoid eating gas-producing foods, spicy foods, and extremely hot or cold foods.
Stress importance of receiving immunizations as recommended.
When dusting, use a wet cloth.
Avoid powerful odors.
Avoid extremes in temperature.
Avoid fireplaces, pets, feather pillows, and other environmental allergens.

F. Interventions are supportive; antibiotics and antiviral agents are not able to kill the virus or prevent its replication

---

XI. PNEUMONIA

A. Description
1. An infection of the pulmonary tissue, including the interstitial spaces, the alveoli, and the bronchioles
2. The edema associated with inflammation stiffens the lung, decreases lung compliance and vital capacity, and causes hypoxemia
3. Can be community acquired or hospital acquired
4. The chest x-ray indicates diffuse patches throughout the lungs or consolidation in a lobe
5. A sputum culture identifies the organism
6. The white blood cells (WBCs) and the erythrocyte sedimentation rate (ESR) are elevated

B. Data collection
1. Chills
2. Elevated temperature
3. Pleuritic pain
4. Congestion, rhonchi, and wheezes
5. Use of accessory muscles for breathing
6. Cyanosis
7. Mental status changes
8. Sputum production

C. Interventions
1. Administer oxygen, as prescribed
2. Monitor respiratory status
3. Monitor for labored respirations, cyanosis, cold and clammy skin

4. Encourage coughing and deep breathing and use of incentive spirometer
5. Position in semi-Fowler's to facilitate breathing and lung expansion
6. Change position frequently and ambulate as tolerated to mobilize secretions
7. Provide chest physiotherapy
8. Perform nasotracheal **suctioning** if the client is unable to clear secretions
9. Monitor pulse oximetry
10. Monitor and record color, consistency, and amount of sputum
11. Provide a high-calorie, high-protein diet with small frequent meals
12. Encourage fluids up to 3 L/day to thin secretions unless contraindicated
13. Provide a balance of rest and activity, increasing activity gradually
14. Administer antibiotics as prescribed
15. Administer antipyretics, bronchodilators, cough suppressants, mucolytic agents, and expectorants, as prescribed
16. Prevent the spread of infection by handwashing and the proper disposal of secretions

D. Client education
1. The importance of rest, proper nutrition, and adequate fluid intake
2. Avoid chilling and exposure to individuals with respiratory infections or viruses
3. Instruct the client regarding medications and the use of inhalants as prescribed
4. Instruct the client to notify physician if chills, fever, dyspnea, hemoptysis, or increased fatigue occurs
5. Instruct the client about the importance of receiving immunizations as recommended

XII. PLEURAL EFFUSION

A. Description
1. The collection of fluid in the pleural space
2. Any condition that interferes with either secretion or drainage of this fluid will lead to pleural effusion

B. Data collection
1. Pleuritic pain that is sharp and increases with inspiration
2. Dyspnea on exertion
3. Dry nonproductive cough caused by bronchial irritation or mediastinal shift
4. Tachycardia
5. Elevated temperature
6. Decreased breath sounds
7. Chest x-ray shows pleural effusion and a mediastinal shift away from the fluid

C. Interventions
1. Identify and treat underlying cause
2. Monitor breath sounds

3. Position the client in high Fowler's
4. Encourage coughing and deep breathing
5. Prepare the client for thoracentesis
6. If pleural effusion is recurrent, prepare the client for pleurectomy or pleurodesis

D. Pleurectomy
1. Consists of surgically stripping the parietal pleura away from the visceral pleura
2. This produces an intense inflammatory reaction that promotes adhesion formation between the two layers during healing

E. Pleurodesis
1. Involves the instillation of a sclerosing substance into the pleural space via a thoracotomy tube
2. This creates an inflammatory response that scleroses tissues together

XIII. EMPYEMA

A. Description
1. The collection of pus within the pleural cavity
2. The fluid is thick, opaque, and foul smelling
3. The most common cause is pulmonary infection and lung abscess caused by thoracic surgery or chest trauma, in which bacteria are introduced directly into the pleural space
4. Treatment focuses on emptying the empyema cavity, re-expanding the lung, and controlling the infection

B. Data collection
1. Recent febrile illnesses or trauma
2. Chest pain
3. Cough
4. Dyspnea
5. Anorexia and weight loss
6. Malaise
7. Elevated temperature and chills
8. Night sweats
9. Diminished chest wall movement on the affected side
10. Pleural exudate on chest x-ray

C. Interventions
1. Monitor breath sounds
2. Position client in semi-Fowler's or high Fowler's
3. Encourage coughing and deep breathing
4. Administer antibiotics as prescribed
5. Instruct the client to splint chest as necessary
6. Assist with chest tube insertion to promote drainage and lung expansion
7. If marked pleural thickening occurs, prepare the client for decortication, if prescribed; this is a surgical procedure that involves removal of the restrictive mass of fibrin and inflammatory cells

XIV. PLEURISY

A. Description

1. Inflammation of the visceral and parietal membranes
2. These membranes rub together during respiration and cause pain
3. May be caused by pulmonary infarction or pneumonia
4. It usually occurs on one side of the chest, usually in the lower lateral portions in the chest wall

B. Data collection
1. Knifelike pain that is aggravated on deep breathing and coughing
2. Dyspnea
3. Pleural friction rub heard on auscultation
4. Apprehension

C. Interventions
1. Identify and treat cause
2. Monitor lung sounds
3. Administer analgesics, as prescribed
4. Apply hot or cold applications, as prescribed
5. Encourage coughing and deep breathing
6. Instruct the client to lie on affected side to splint chest

XV. PULMONARY EMBOLISM

A. Description
1. Occurs when a thrombus that forms in a deep vein detaches and travels to the right side of the heart then lodges in a branch of the pulmonary artery
2. Clients prone to pulmonary embolism are those at risk for deep vein thrombosis, including those with prolonged immobilization, surgery, obesity, pregnancy, congestive heart failure (CHF), advanced age, or prior history of thromboembolism
3. Fat emboli can occur as a complication following a fracture of a flat long bone
4. Treatment is aimed at preventing venous status; includes range-of-motion exercises and early ambulation following surgery, the use of antiembolism or pneumatic compression stockings, and preventing pressure under the popliteal space

B. Data collection (Box 48-11)

C. Interventions
1. Administer oxygen as prescribed
2. Position client in high Fowler's
3. Monitor lung sounds
4. Maintain bed rest and active and passive range-of-motion exercises, as prescribed
5. Encourage use of incentive spirometry, as prescribed
6. Monitor pulse oximetry
7. Prepare for intubation and **mechanical ventilation** for severe hypoxemia
8. Anticoagulation with IV heparin (bolus), followed by continuous infusion, may be prescribed during the acute phase

---

BOX 48-11

Data Collection Findings: Pulmonary Embolism

Chest pain
Dyspnea accompanied by anginal and pleuritic pain, exacerbated by inspiration
Tachypnea and tachycardia
Hypotension
Shallow respirations
Wheezes on auscultation
Cough
Blood-tinged sputum
Distended neck veins
Cyanosis

---

9. Administer warfarin (Coumadin) orally as prescribed when heparin infusion is discontinued
10. Monitor prothrombin time (PT) and partial thromboplastin time (PTT) closely
11. Prepare the client for embolectomy, vein ligation, or insertion of an umbrella filter, as prescribed

XVI. LUNG CANCER AND LARYNGEAL CANCER
(See Chapter 42)

XVII. CARBON MONOXIDE POISONING

A. Description
1. Carbon monoxide is a colorless, odorless, and tasteless gas that has an affinity for hemoglobin 200 times greater than that of oxygen
2. Oxygen molecules are displaced and carbon monoxide reversibly binds to hemoglobin to form carboxyhemoglobin; tissue hypoxia occurs

B. Data collection (Table 48-1)

C. Interventions
1. Remove victim from exposure
2. Administer oxygen
3. Assess need for basic life support
4. Monitor vital signs
5. Monitor carbon monoxide levels

XVIII. HISTOPLASMOSIS

A. Description
1. A pulmonary fungal infection caused by spores of *Histoplasma capsulatum*
2. Transmission occurs by the inhalation of spores, which are commonly located in contaminated soil
3. Spores are also usually found in bird droppings

B. Data collection
1. Dyspnea
2. Chills
3. Elevated temperature
4. Chest pain

TABLE 48-1

Data Collection: Levels of Carbon Monoxide

Level (%)	Assessment Finding
5 to 10	Impaired visual acuity
11 to 20	Flushing
21 to 30	Nausea and impaired dexterity
31 to 40	Vomiting, dizziness, and syncope
41 to 50	Tachypnea and tachycardia
Higher than 50	Coma and death

5. Pulmonary infiltrates on chest x-ray
6. Elevated white blood cell (WBC) count
7. Positive skin test for histoplasmosis
8. Positive agglutination test
9. Splenomegaly, hepatomegaly

C. Interventions
1. Administer oxygen, as prescribed
2. Monitor breath sounds
3. Administer antiemetics, antihistamines, antipyretics, and corticosteroids, as prescribed
4. Administer fungicidal medications, as prescribed
5. Encourage coughing and deep breathing
6. Position client in semi-Fowler's
7. Monitor vital signs
8. Monitor for nephrotoxicity from fungicidal medications
9. Instruct the client to spray area with water before sweeping barn and chicken coops

XIX. SARCOIDOSIS

A. Description
1. Epitheloid cell tubercles in lung
2. Cause is unknown
3. High titer of Epstein-Barr virus may be identified
4. Virus incidence is highest in blacks and young adults

B. Data collection
1. Night sweats
2. Fever
3. Weight loss
4. Cough
5. Skin nodules
6. Polyarthritis
7. Kveim test: Sarcoid node antigen is injected intradermally and causes local nodular lesion in approximately 1 month

C. Interventions
1. Administer corticosteroids to control symptoms
2. Monitor temperature
3. Increase fluid intake
4. Provide frequent periods of rest
5. Encourage small, frequent nutritious meals

XX. OCCUPATIONAL LUNG DISEASE: SILICOSIS

A. Description
1. Known as asbestosis and coal worker's pneumoconiosis
2. Fibrotic disease of the lungs caused by the inhalation of inorganic dusts over long periods of time
3. Common in miners and sandblasters

B. Data collection
1. Uncomplicated or simple: Asymptomatic with evidence of fibrosis on chest x-ray
2. Chronic complicated: Malaise, anorexia, weight loss, severe dyspnea on exertion, evidence of massive fibrosis on chest x-ray

C. Interventions
1. Administer antitussive for cough
2. Administer medication for **tuberculosis** (a complication) as prescribed
3. Eliminate the toxic substances
4. Administer oxygen as prescribed
5. Encourage coughing and deep breathing

XXI. TUBERCULOSIS

A. Description
1. A highly communicable disease caused by *Mycobacterium tuberculosis*
2. *Mycobacterium tuberculosis* is a nonmotile, nonsporulating, acid-fast rod that secretes niacin; when the bacillus reaches a susceptible site, it multiplies freely
3. Because *Mycobacterium tuberculosis* is an aerobic bacterium, it primarily affects the pulmonary system, especially the upper lobes, where the oxygen content is highest, but can also affect other areas of the body, such as the brain, intestines, peritoneum, kidney, joints, and liver
4. An exudative-type response causes a nonspecific pneumonitis and the development of granulomas in the lung tissue
5. **Tuberculosis (TB)** has an insidious onset, and many clients are not aware of symptoms until the disease is well advanced
6. A **multidrug-resistant strain (MDR-TB)** of **TB** can exist as a result of improper use of or noncompliance with medication therapy causing the development of mutations in the tubercle bacilli
7. The goal of treatment is to prevent transmission, control symptoms, and prevent progression of the disease

B. Risk factors (Box 48-12)

C. Transmission
1. Via airborne route by droplet infection
2. When an infected individual coughs, laughs, sneezes, or sings, droplet nuclei containing **TB** bacteria enter the air and may be inhaled by others

Risk Factors for Tuberculosis

Alcoholism
Intravenous drug use
Malnutrition
Infection
The elderly
The homeless
Refugees
Minority groups
Individuals from a lower socioeconomic group
Children younger than 5 years of age
Individuals living in crowded areas, such as long-term care facilities, prisons, and mental health facilities
Individuals in constant, frequent contact with an untreated or undiagnosed individual
Individuals with immune dysfunction or human immunodeficiency virus (HIV) infection or individuals who are immunosuppressed as a result of medication therapy
Drinking unpasteurized milk if the cow is infected with bovine tuberculosis

3. Identification of those individuals in close contact with the infected individual is important so that they can be tested and treated as necessary
4. When contacts have been identified, these people are assessed with a tuberculin test and chest x-ray to determine infection with **TB**
5. After the infected individual has received **TB** medication for 2 to 3 weeks, the risk of transmission is greatly reduced

D. Disease progression
1. Droplets enter the lungs, and the bacteria form a tubercle lesion
2. The body's defense systems encapsulate the tubercle, leaving a scar
3. If encapsulation does not occur, bacteria may enter the lymph system, travel to the lymph nodes, and cause an inflammatory response called granulomatous inflammation
4. Primary lesions form; the primary lesions may become dormant, but can be reactivated and become a secondary infection when reexposed to the bacterium
5. In an active phase, **TB** can cause necrosis and cavitation in the lesions, leading to rupture and the spread of necrotic tissue, and damage to various parts of the body

E. Client history
1. Past exposure to **TB**
2. Client's country of origin and travel to foreign countries in which there is a high incidence of **TB**
3. Recent history of influenza, pneumonia, febrile illness, cough, or foul-smelling sputum production
4. Previous tests for **TB** and what the results were

5. Recent **bacille Calmette-Guérin (BCG) vaccine** (a vaccine containing attenuated tubercle bacilli that may be given to people in foreign countries or to persons traveling to foreign countries, to produce increased resistance to **TB**)
6. An individual who has received **BCG** will have a positive skin test and should be evaluated for **TB** with a chest x-ray

F. Clinical manifestations
1. May be asymptomatic in primary infection
2. Fatigue
3. Lethargy
4. Anorexia
5. Weight loss
6. Low-grade fever
7. Chills
8. Night sweats
9. Persistent cough and the production of mucoid and mucopurulent sputum, which is occasionally streaked with blood
10. Chest tightness and a dull, aching chest pain may accompany the cough

G. Chest assessment
1. A physical examination of the chest does not provide conclusive evidence of **TB**
2. Chest x-ray is not definitive, but the presence of multinodular infiltrates with calcification in the upper lobes suggests **TB**
3. If the disease is active, caseation and inflammation may be seen on the chest x-ray
4. Advanced disease
   a. Dullness with percussion over involved parenchymal areas, bronchial breath sounds, rhonchi and/or crackles
   b. Partial obstruction of a bronchus, caused by endobronchial disease or compression by lymph nodes, may produce localized wheezing and dyspnea

H. Sputum cultures
1. Sputum specimens are obtained for an acid-fast smear
2. A sputum culture identifying *Mycobacterium tuberculosis* confirms the diagnosis
3. After medications are started, sputum samples are obtained again to determine the effectiveness of therapy
4. Most clients have negative cultures after 3 months of treatment

I. Mantoux test
1. The most reliable determinant of infection with **TB**
2. A positive reaction does not mean that active disease is present but indicates exposure to **TB** or the presence of inactive (dormant) disease
3. Once the test result is positive, it will be positive in any future tests
4. A small amount (0.1 mL) of intermediate-strength purified protein derivative (PPD)

BOX 48-13

Client Education: Tuberculosis

Provide the client and family with information about TB and allay concerns about the contagious aspect of the infection.

Instruct the client to follow the medication regimen exactly as prescribed and always to have a supply of the medication on hand.

Advise the client of the side effects of the medication and ways of minimizing them to ensure compliance.

Reassure the client that, after 2 to 3 weeks of medication therapy, it is unlikely that the client will infect anyone.

Inform the client that activities should be resumed gradually.

Instruct the client about the need for adequate nutrition and a well-balanced diet to promote healing and to prevent recurrence of infection.

Instruct the client to increase foods rich in iron, protein, and vitamin C.

Inform the client and family that respiratory isolation is not necessary because family members have already been exposed.

Instruct the client to cover the mouth and nose when coughing or sneezing and to keep used tissues in plastic bags.

Instruct the client and family about thorough hand washing.

Inform the client that a sputum culture is needed every 2 to 4 weeks once medication therapy is initiated.

Inform the client that when the results of three sputum cultures are negative, the client is no longer considered infectious and can usually return to his or her former employment.

Advise the client to avoid excessive exposure to silicone or dust because these substances can cause further lung damage.

Instruct the client regarding the importance of compliance with treatment, follow-up care, and sputum cultures, as prescribed.

---

containing 5 tuberculin units is administered intradermally in the forearm

5. An area of induration measuring 15 mm or more in diameter in low-risk groups, 48 to 72 hours after injection, indicates that the individual has been exposed to **TB**

6. For individuals with HIV infection or who are immunocompromised, a reaction of 5 mm or greater is considered positive

7. Once an individual's skin test is positive, a chest x-ray is necessary to rule out active **TB** or to detect old, healed lesions

J. The hospitalized client

1. The client with active **TB** is placed in respiratory isolation precautions in a negative pressure room; to maintain negative pressure, the door of the room must be tightly closed

2. The room should have at least six exchanges of fresh air per hour and should be ventilated to the outside environment if possible

3. The nurse wears a particulate respirator (a special individually fitted mask) when caring for the client and a gown when there is a possibility of contamination of clothing

4. Hands are always thoroughly washed before and after caring for the client

5. If the client needs to leave the room for a test or procedure, the client is required to wear a mask

6. Isolation is discontinued when the client is no longer considered infectious

7. After the infected individual has received **TB** medication for 2 to 3 weeks, the risk of transmission is greatly reduced

K. Client education (Box 48-13)

L. Medications (see Chapter 49)

PRACTICE QUESTIONS

1. A nurse is assisting in planning care for a client scheduled for insertion of a tracheostomy. What equipment would the nurse plan to have at the bedside when the client returns from surgery?
   1. Oral airway
   2. Epinephrine
   3. Obturator
   4. Tracheostomy tube with the next larger size

2. A nursing instructor is observing a nursing student suctioning a client through a tracheostomy tube. The nursing instructor intervenes if the student performed which incorrect action?
   1. Hyperventilating the client with 100% oxygen before suctioning
   2. Using sterile technique to perform the procedure
   3. Applying suction during insertion of the catheter
   4. Applying suction during withdrawal of the catheter

3. A nurse is caring for a client with an endotracheal tube attached to a ventilator. The high-pressure alarm sounds on the ventilator. The nurse prepares to perform which nursing intervention?
   1. Check for a disconnection
   2. Evaluate the tube cuff for a leak
   3. Notify the respiratory therapist
   4. Suction the client

4. A nurse is preparing to obtain a sputum specimen from the client. Which nursing action will facilitate obtaining the specimen?
   1. Limiting fluids
   2. Having the client take three deep breaths
   3. Asking the client to spit into the collection container
   4. Asking the client to obtain the specimen after eating

5. A nurse is caring for a client following a bronccoscopy and biopsy. Which sign if noted in the client should be reported immediately?
   1. Blood-streaked sputum
   2. Dry cough
   3. Hematuria
   4. Stridor

6. An emergency room nurse is caring for a client who sustained a blunt injury to the chest wall. Which sign if noted in the client would indicate the presence of a pneumothorax?
   1. Bradypnea
   2. Shortness of breath
   3. A low respiratory rate
   4. The presence of a barrel chest

7. A nurse is checking the respiratory status of a client who has suffered a fractured rib. The nurse would expect to note which of the following?
   1. Pain, especially with inspiration
   2. Slow, deep respirations
   3. Rapid, deep respirations
   4. Paradoxical respirations

8. An oxygen delivery system is prescribed for a client with chronic airflow limitation (CAL) to deliver a precise oxygen concentration. Which type of oxygen delivery system would the nurse anticipate to be prescribed?
   1. Venturi mask
   2. Aerosol mask
   3. Face tent
   4. Tracheostomy collar

9. A nurse is caring for a client hospitalized with acute exacerbation of chronic obstructive pulmonary disease (COPD). Which of the following would the nurse expect to note in evaluating this client?
   1. Increased oxygen saturation with exercise
   2. Hypocapnia
   3. A hyperinflated chest on x-ray
   4. A widened diaphragm noted on chest x-ray

10. A nurse is reinforcing instructions with a hospitalized client with a diagnosis of emphysema about positions that will enhance the effectiveness of breathing during dyspneic periods. Which position will the nurse instruct the client to assume?
    1. Side-lying in bed
    2. Sitting in a recliner chair
    3. Sitting up in bed
    4. Sitting on the side of the bed, leaning on an overbed table

11. A nurse is gathering data on a client with a diagnosis of tuberculosis (TB). The nurse reviews the results of which diagnostic test that will confirm this diagnosis?
    1. Bronchoscopy
    2. Chest x-ray
    3. Sputum culture
    4. Tuberculin skin test

12. A nursing instructor asks a nursing student to describe the route of transmission of tuberculosis (TB). The nursing instructor determines that the student understands this route of transmission if the student states that TB is transmitted by:
    1. The airborne route
    2. Blood and body fluids
    3. The enteric route
    4. Hand to mouth

13. A nurse is caring for a client with emphysema who is receiving oxygen. The nurse checks the oxygen flow rate to ensure that it does not exceed:
    1. 1 L/minute
    2. 2 L/minute
    3. 6 L/minute
    4. 10 L/minute

14. A nurse is instructing a client about pursed lip breathing and the client asks the nurse about its purpose. The nurse tells the client that the primary purpose of pursed lip breathing is to:
    1. Promote oxygen intake
    2. Strengthen the diaphragm
    3. Strengthen the intercostal muscles
    4. Promote carbon dioxide elimination

15. The low-pressure alarm sounds on the ventilator. The nurse checks the client and then attempts to determine the cause of the alarm but is unsuccessful. Which initial action will the nurse take?
    1. Check the client's vital signs
    2. Ventilate the client manually
    3. Administer oxygen
    4. Start cardiopulmonary resuscitation (CPR)

16. A nurse is caring for a client who is on strict bed rest. The nurse assists in developing a plan of care and suggests goals related to the prevention of deep vein thrombosis (DVT) and pulmonary emboli. Which nursing action would be most helpful to prevent these disorders from developing?
    1. Applying a heating pad to the lower extremities
    2. Active range-of-motion (ROM) exercises
    3. Placing a pillow under the knees
    4. Restricting fluids

17. A nurse has taught a client about the use of a respiratory inhaler. Which statement by the client indicates a need for further teaching?
    1. "I need to remove the cap and shake the inhaler well before use."
    2. "I need to press the canister down with my finger as I breathe in."
    3. "I need to inhale the mist and quickly exhale."
    4. "I need to wait 1 minute between puffs if more than one puff has been prescribed."

18. A nurse is assigned to care for a client following a left pneumonectomy. The nurse would avoid positioning the client:
    1. On the side
    2. In a semi-Fowler's

3. In a low Fowler's

4. With the head of the bed elevated 40 degrees

19. A female client is scheduled to have a chest x-ray. Which question is most important to ask the client during data collection?
    1. "Is there any possibility that you could be pregnant?"
    2. "Are you wearing any metal chains or jewelry?"
    3. "Can you hold your breath easily?"
    4. "Are you able to hold your arms above your head?"

20. A nurse is caring for a client following pulmonary angiography via catheter insertion into the left groin. The nurse monitors for an allergic reaction to the contrast medium by noting the presence of:
    1. Hematoma in the left groin
    2. Discomfort in the left groin
    3. Respiratory distress
    4. Hypothermia

21. A nurse is teaching the client with chronic respiratory failure how to use a metered-dose inhaler correctly. The nurse instructs the client to:
    1. Inhale through the nose
    2. Inhale quickly
    3. Take two inhalations during one breath
    4. Hold the breath after inhalation

22. A nurse is caring for a client who is suspected of having lung cancer. The nurse monitors the client for which most frequent early sign of lung cancer?
    1. Blood-streaked sputum
    2. Cough
    3. Wheezing
    4. Pleuritic pain

23. A client who has had a radical neck dissection begins to hemorrhage at the incision site. Which action by the nurse would be contraindicated?
    1. Lowering the head of the bed to a flat position
    2. Applying manual pressure over the site
    3. Monitoring the client's airway
    4. Calling the physician immediately

24. A nurse is reinforcing discharge instructions to the client with pulmonary sarcoidosis. The nurse determines that the client understands the information if the client verbalizes to report which early sign of exacerbation?
    1. Fever
    2. Weight loss
    3. Fatigue
    4. Shortness of breath

25. A nurse working on a respiratory nursing unit is caring for several clients with respiratory disorders. The nurse would identify which of the following clients as being at the least risk for developing infection with tuberculosis?
    1. A woman newly immigrated from Korea
    2. An uninsured man who is homeless

3. An older woman admitted from a long-term care facility

4. A man who is an inspector for the United States Postal Service

26. A nurse is reading the results of a Mantoux skin test on a client with no documented health problems. The site has no induration and a 1 mm area of ecchymosis. The nurse interprets that the result is:
    1. Positive
    2. Negative
    3. Uncertain
    4. Borderline

27. A nurse reads a client's Mantoux skin test as positive. The nurse notes that previous tests were negative. The client becomes upset and asks the nurse what this means. The nurse's response is based on the understanding that the client has:
    1. No evidence of tuberculosis
    2. Systemic tuberculosis
    3. Pulmonary tuberculosis
    4. Exposure to tuberculosis

28. A nurse is caring for a client who had a Mantoux skin test implantation 48 hours ago on admission to the nursing unit and reads the result of the skin test as positive. Which action by the nurse is the priority?
    1. Report the findings
    2. Call the radiology department for a chest x-ray
    3. Document the finding in the client's record
    4. Call the employee health service department

29. A nurse is caring for a client with tuberculosis who is fearful of the disease and anxious about the prognosis. In planning nursing care, the nurse would incorporate which of the following as the best strategy to assist the client in coping with the disease?
    1. Encourage the client to visit with the pastoral care department chaplain
    2. Ask family members if they wish a psychiatric consult
    3. Provide reassurance that continued compliance with medication therapy is the most proactive way to cope with the disease
    4. Allow the client to deal with the disease in an individual fashion

30. A nurse has instructed a client diagnosed with tuberculosis (TB) about how to prevent the spread of infection after discharge. The nurse determines that the client needs further reinforcement of information if the client makes which of the following statements?
    1. "It's very important to wash my hands after I touch my mask, tissues, or body fluids."
    2. "I should cough into tissues and throw them away carefully."
    3. "It's important to cover my mouth if I laugh, sneeze, or cough."
    4. "I should use disposable plates, forks, and knives."

31. A nurse is caring for the client diagnosed with tuberculosis (TB). Which of the following findings, if made by the nurse, would be inconsistent with the usual clinical presentation of tuberculosis?
    1. Nonproductive or productive cough
    2. Anorexia and weight loss
    3. Chills and night sweats
    4. High-grade fever

32. A client being discharged from the hospital to home with a diagnosis of tuberculosis (TB) is worried about the possibility of infecting the family and others. The nurse determines that the client would get the most reassurance from the knowledge that:
    1. The family does not need therapy, and the client will not be contagious after 1 month of medication therapy
    2. The family does not need therapy, and the client will not be contagious after 6 consecutive weeks of medication therapy
    3. The family will receive prophylactic therapy, and the client will not be contagious after 1 continuous week of medication therapy
    4. The family will be treated prophylactically, and the client will not be contagious after 2 to 3 consecutive weeks of medication therapy

33. A client diagnosed with tuberculosis (TB) is distressed over the loss of physical stamina and fatigue. The nurse plans to tell the client that this is:
    1. A short-lived problem, which should be gone within 1 week of medication therapy
    2. An unexpected finding with TB, but it should resolve within about 1 month
    3. Expected, and the client should very gradually increase activity as tolerated
    4. Expected, and will last for at least a year

34. A nurse is teaching a client with tuberculosis (TB) about dietary elements that should be increased in the diet. The nurse suggests that the client increase the intake of:
    1. Meats and citrus fruits
    2. Grains and broccoli
    3. Eggs and spinach
    4. Potatoes and fish

35. A nurse has reinforced discharge teaching with a client who was diagnosed with tuberculosis (TB) and has been on medication for $1^1/_2$ weeks. The nurse determines that the client has understood the information if the client makes which statement?
    1. "I need to continue medication therapy for 2 months."
    2. "I should not be contagious after 2 to 3 weeks of medication therapy."
    3. "I can't shop at the mall for the next 6 months."
    4. "I can return to work if a sputum culture comes back negative."

36. A client with tuberculosis asks a nurse about precautions to take after discharge from the hospital to prevent infection of others. The nurse develops a response to the client's question based on the understanding that:
    1. The client should maintain enteric precautions only
    2. The disease is transmitted by droplet nuclei
    3. Clothing and sheets should be bleached after each use
    4. Deep pile carpet should be removed from the home

37. A nurse is preparing to give a bed bath to the immobilized client with tuberculosis (TB). The nurse should plan to wear which of the following items when performing this care?
    1. Particulate respirator, gown, and gloves
    2. Particulate respirator and protective eyewear
    3. Surgical mask and gloves
    4. Surgical mask, gown, and protective eyewear

38. A client with tuberculosis (TB), whose status is being monitored in an ambulatory care clinic, asks the nurse when it is permissible to return to work. The nurse replies that the client may resume employment when:
    1. Three sputum cultures are negative
    2. Five sputum cultures are negative
    3. A sputum culture and a chest x-ray are negative
    4. A sputum culture and a Mantoux test are negative

39. A client with acquired immunodeficiency syndrome (AIDS) has histoplasmosis. A nurse checks the client for which sign/symptom?
    1. Weight gain
    2. Dyspnea
    3. Hypothermia
    4. Headache

40. A nurse is taking the nursing history of a client with silicosis. The nurse checks whether the client wears which of the following items during periods of exposure to silica particles?
    1. Mask
    2. Gown
    3. Gloves
    4. Eye protection

ALTERNATE FORMAT QUESTION: MULTIPLE RESPONSE

The nurse is preparing a list of home care instructions for the client who has been hospitalized and treated for tuberculosis. Select the instructions that the nurse will include on the list.

___ Avoid contact with other individuals, except family members, for at least 6 months

___ Activities should be resumed gradually

___ Consume a well-balanced diet and foods rich in iron, protein, and vitamin C

___ Respiratory isolation is not necessary because family members have already been exposed

___ Cover the mouth and nose when coughing or sneezing and confine used tissues to plastic bags

___ A sputum culture is needed every 2 to 4 weeks once medication therapy is initiated

___ When one sputum cultures is negative, the client is no longer considered infectious and can usually return to his or her former employment

ANSWERS

1. *Answer: 3*

Rationale: A replacement tracheostomy tube of the same size and an obturator is kept at the bedside at all times in case the tracheostomy tube is dislodged. Additionally, a curved hemostat that could be used to hold the trachea open if dislodgment occurs should also be kept at the bedside. An oral airway and epinephrine would not be needed.

Test-Taking Strategy: Use the process of elimination. Eliminate option 4 first because a tracheostomy tube of the next larger size would not be appropriate for the client. Next, eliminate option 2 because it is unrelated to the issue of the question. From the remaining options, recall that the airway has been altered because of the tracheostomy, so an oral airway would not be necessary. Remember that a replacement tracheostomy tube, an obturator, and a curved hemostat should be kept at the bedside of a client with a tracheostomy. Review care of the client with a tracheostomy if you had difficulty with this question.

Level of Cognitive Ability: Application
Client Needs: Physiological Integrity
Integrated Process: Nursing Process/Planning
Content Area: Adult Health/Respiratory
Reference: Christensen, B., & Kockrow, E. (2003). *Foundations of nursing* (4th ed.). St. Louis: Mosby, p. 457.

2. *Answer: 3*

Rationale: The client should be hyperoxygenated with 100% oxygen prior to suctioning. Sterile technique is always used. Suction is not applied during insertion of the catheter, and intermittent suction and a twirling motion of the catheter are used during withdrawal.

Test-Taking Strategy: Use the process of elimination and note the key words, *incorrect action.* These words indicate a false response question and that you need to select the incorrect action. Visualize the procedure and think about the mechanical trauma that suctioning can cause to the tissues. This will direct you to option 3. Review this procedure if you had difficulty with this question.

Level of Cognitive Ability: Comprehension
Client Needs: Physiological Integrity
Integrated Process: Teaching/Learning
Content Area: Adult Health/Respiratory
Reference: Christensen, B., & Kockrow, E. (2003). *Foundations of nursing* (4th ed.). St. Louis: Mosby, p. 457.

3. *Answer: 4*

Rationale: When the high-pressure alarm sounds on a ventilator, it is most likely caused by an obstruction. The obstruction can be caused by the client biting on the tube, kinking of the tubing, or mucus plugging requiring suctioning. It is also important to check the tubing for the presence of any water and determine if the client is out of rhythm with breathing with the ventilator. A disconnection or a cuff leak can result in sounding of the low-pressure alarm. The respiratory therapist would be notified if the nurse could not determine the cause of the alarm.

Test-Taking Strategy: Use the process of elimination. Note the key words, *high-pressure alarm,* in the question. Recalling that the high-pressure alarm indicates a possible obstruction will assist in directing you to the correct option. Review nursing interventions related to care of a client on a ventilator if you had difficulty with this question.

Level of Cognitive Ability: Application
Client Needs: Physiological Integrity
Integrated Process: Nursing Process/Implementation
Content Area: Adult Health/Respiratory
Reference: Black, J., & Hawks, J. (2005). *Medical-surgical nursing: Clinical management for positive outcomes* (7th ed.). Philadelphia: W.B. Saunders, p. 1887.

4. *Answer: 2*

Rationale: To obtain a sputum specimen, the client should brush his or her teeth to reduce mouth contamination. The client should then take three deep breaths and cough into a sputum specimen container. The client should be encouraged to cough and not spit so sputum can be obtained. Sputum can be thinned by fluids or by a respiratory treatment, such as inhalation of nebulized saline or water. The optimal time to obtain a specimen is on arising in the morning.

Test-Taking Strategy: Use the process of elimination. Option 1 can be eliminated first recalling that fluids assist in loosening or thinning secretions. Eliminate option 3 because of the word "spit." Spit is very different from saliva. Next, eliminate option 4 because of the words "after eating." Review this procedure if you had difficulty with this question.

Level of Cognitive Ability: Application
Client Needs: Physiological Integrity
Integrated Process: Nursing Process/Implementation
Content Area: Adult Health/Respiratory
Reference: Chernecky, C., & Berger, B. (2004). *Laboratory tests and diagnostic procedures* (4th ed.). Philadelphia: W.B. Saunders, p. 1020.

5. *Answer: 4*

Rationale: If a biopsy was performed during a broncoscopy, blood-streaked sputum is expected for several hours. Frank blood is indicative of hemorrhage. A dry cough may be expected. The client should be assessed for signs of complications, which can include cyanosis, dyspnea, stridor, hemoptysis, hypotension, tachycardia, and dysrhythmias. Hematuria is unrelated to this procedure.

Test-Taking Strategy: Use the process of elimination. Eliminate option 3 first, because it is unrelated to the procedure. Next, eliminate option 2 because a dry cough may be expected. Noting that a biopsy has been performed will assist in eliminating option 1 because blood streaked sputum would be expected. Note that option 4, the correct option, relates to airway. If you had difficulty with this question, review postprocedure care following broncoscopy with biopsy.

Level of Cognitive Ability: Analysis
Client Needs: Physiological Integrity
Integrated Process: Nursing Process/Data Collection
Content Area: Adult Health/Respiratory
References: Chernecky, C., & Berger, B. (2004). *Laboratory tests and diagnostic procedures* (4th ed.). Philadelphia: W.B. Saunders, p. 297.
Pagana, K., & Pagana, T. (2003). *Mosby's diagnostic and laboratory test reference* (6th ed.). St. Louis: Mosby, p. 196.

6. *Answer:* **2**
Rationale: This client has sustained a blunt or a closed chest injury. Basic symptoms of a closed pneumothorax are shortness of breath and chest pain. A larger pneumothorax may present with tachypnea, cyanosis, diminished breath sounds, and subcutaneous emphysema. There may also be hyperresonance on the affected side.

Test-Taking Strategy: Use the process of elimination. Option 4 can be eliminated because a barrel chest is a characteristic finding in a client with chronic obstructive pulmonary disease. Next, eliminate options 1 and 3 because they are similar. Review the signs of pneumothorax if you had difficulty with this question.

Level of Cognitive Ability: Analysis
Client Needs: Physiological Integrity
Integrated Process: Nursing Process/Data Collection
Content Area: Adult Health/Respiratory
Reference: Linton, A., & Maebius, N. (2003). *Introduction to medical-surgical nursing* (3rd ed.). Philadelphia: W.B. Saunders, p. 486.

7. *Answer:* **1**
Rationale: Rib fractures are a common injury, especially in the older client, and result from a blunt injury or a fall. Typical signs and symptoms include pain and tenderness that is localized at the fracture site and is exacerbated by inspiration and palpation; shallow respirations; splinting or guarding the chest protectively to minimize chest movement; and possible bruising at the fracture site. Paradoxical respirations are seen with flail chest.

Test-Taking Strategy: Use the process of elimination. Focusing on the anatomical location of the injury will direct you to option 1. Review the findings in rib fractures, if you had difficulty with this question.

Level of Cognitive Ability: Analysis
Client Needs: Physiological Integrity
Integrated Process: Nursing Process/Data Collection
Content Area: Adult Health/Respiratory

Reference: Black, J., & Hawks, J. (2005). *Medical-surgical nursing: Clinical management for positive outcomes* (7th ed.). Philadelphia: W.B. Saunders, pp. 1900-1901.

8. *Answer:* **1**
Rationale: The Venturi mask delivers the most accurate oxygen concentration. It is the best oxygen delivery system for the client with CAL because it delivers a precise oxygen concentration. The face tent, aerosol mask, and tracheostomy collar are also high-flow oxygen delivery systems but are most often used to administer high humidity.

Test-Taking Strategy: Use the process of elimination and note the key words, *precise oxygen concentration.* Eliminate options 2, 3, and 4 because they are similar in that they are used to provide high humidity. Review these types of oxygen delivery systems if you had difficulty with this question.

Level of Cognitive Ability: Comprehension
Client Needs: Physiological Integrity
Integrated Process: Nursing Process/Planning
Content Area: Adult Health/Respiratory
Reference: Linton, A., & Maebius, N. (2003). *Introduction to medical-surgical nursing* (3rd ed.). Philadelphia: W.B. Saunders, pp. 470-471.

9. *Answer:* **3**
Rationale: Clinical manifestations of COPD include hypoxemia, hypercapnia, dyspnea on exertion and at rest, oxygen desaturation with exercise, and the use of accessory muscles of respiration. Chest x-ray will reveal a hyperinflated chest and a flattened diaphragm if the disease is advanced.

Test-Taking Strategy: Use the process of elimination. Eliminate option 1 because oxygen desaturation rather than saturation would occur. Next, eliminate option 2 because in the client with COPD, hypercapnia would be noted. From the remaining options, reading carefully will assist in directing you to option 3. If you are unfamiliar with the manifestations associated with COPD, review this content.

Level of Cognitive Ability: Analysis
Client Needs: Physiological Integrity
Integrated Process: Nursing Process/Data Collection
Content Area: Adult Health/Respiratory
Reference: Lewis, S., Heitkemper, M., & Dirksen, S. (2004). *Medical-surgical nursing: Assessment and management of clinical problems* (6th ed.). St. Louis: Mosby, p. 662.

10. *Answer:* **4**
Rationale: Positions that will assist the client with breathing include sitting up and leaning on an overbed table, sitting up and resting with the elbows on the knees, or standing or leaning against the wall. The positions in options 1, 2, and 3 will not enhance the effectiveness of breathing.

Test-Taking Strategy: Use the process of elimination. Eliminate option 1 because side-lying will not promote appropriate lung expansion. Next, eliminate options 2 and 3 because they are similar. If you had difficulty with this question, review the positions that will decrease the work of breathing in a client with emphysema.

Level of Cognitive Ability: Application
Client Needs: Physiological Integrity
Integrated Process: Teaching/Learning

Content Area: Adult Health/Respiratory
Reference: Linton, A., & Maebius, N. (2003). *Introduction to medical-surgical nursing* (3rd ed.). Philadelphia: W.B. Saunders, p. 502.

11. *Answer: 3*
Rationale: A definitive diagnosis of TB is confirmed through culture and isolation of *Mycobacterium tuberculosis.* A presumptive diagnosis is made on the basis of a tuberculin skin test, a sputum smear that is positive for acid-fast bacteria, a chest x-ray, and histologic evidence of graunulomatous disease on biopsy.
Test-Taking Strategy: Use the process of elimination and note the key word, *confirm,* in the stem of the question. Confirmation is made by identifying *Mycobacterium tuberculosis.* If you had difficulty with this question, review the diagnostic procedures related to TB.
Level of Cognitive Ability: Application
Client Needs: Physiological Integrity
Integrated Process: Nursing Process/Data Collection
Content Area: Adult Health/Respiratory
Reference: Linton, A., & Maebius, N. (2003). *Introduction to medical-surgical nursing* (3rd ed.). Philadelphia: W.B. Saunders, p. 505.

12. *Answer: 1*
Rationale: Tuberculosis is an infectious disease caused by the bacillus *Mycobacterium tuberculosis* and spread primarily by the airborne route. Options 2, 3, and 4 are incorrect.
Test-Taking Strategy: Use the process of elimination. Recalling that TB is a respiratory disease will direct you to option 1. If you had difficulty with this question, review the transmission of this disease.
Level of Cognitive Ability: Comprehension
Client Needs: Physiological Integrity
Integrated Process: Teaching/Learning
Content Area: Adult Health/Respiratory
Reference: Linton, A., & Maebius, N. (2003). *Introduction to medical-surgical nursing* (3rd ed.). Philadelphia: W.B. Saunders, p. 506.

13. *Answer: 2*
Rationale: One to 3 L/minute of oxygen by nasal cannula may be required to raise the PaO_2 level to 60 to 80 mm Hg. However, oxygen is used cautiously in the client with emphysema and should not exceed 2 L/minute. Because of the long-standing hypercapnia that occurs in this disorder, the respiratory drive is triggered by low oxygen levels rather than by increased carbon dioxide levels, which is the case in a normal respiratory system.
Test-Taking Strategy: Recalling the physiology associated with emphysema is required to answer this question. If you are unfamiliar with this disorder, review this content.
Level of Cognitive Ability: Analysis
Client Needs: Physiological Integrity
Integrated Process: Nursing Process/Data Collection
Content Area: Adult Health/Respiratory
Reference: Linton, A., & Maebius, N. (2003). *Introduction to medical-surgical nursing* (3rd ed.). Philadelphia: W.B. Saunders, p. 500.

14. *Answer: 4*
Rationale: Pursed lip breathing facilitates maximal expiration for clients with obstructive lung disease and promotes carbon dioxide elimination. This type of breathing allows better expiration by increasing airway pressure, which keeps air passages open during exhalation. Options 1, 2, and 3 are not the purposes of this type of breathing.
Test-Taking Strategy: Use the process of elimination. Visualize the use of this breathing technique to assist in answering correctly. Recalling the respiratory conditions in which this type of breathing is helpful will also assist in directing you to option 4. Review the purpose of this breathing technique if you had difficulty with this question.
Level of Cognitive Ability: Application
Client Needs: Health Promotion and Maintenance
Integrated Process: Teaching/Learning
Content Area: Adult Health/Respiratory
References: Black, J., & Hawks, J. (2005). *Medical-surgical nursing: Clinical management for positive outcomes* (7th ed.). Philadelphia: W.B. Saunders, p. 1812.
Linton, A., & Maebius, N. (2003). *Introduction to medical-surgical nursing* (3rd ed.). Philadelphia: W.B. Saunders, p. 467.

15. *Answer: 2*
Rationale: If an alarm is sounding at any time and the nurse cannot quickly ascertain the problem, the client is disconnected from the ventilator and a manual resuscitation device is used to support respirations until the problem can be corrected. There is no reason to begin CPR. Checking vital signs is not the initial action. Although oxygen is helpful, it will not provide ventilation to the client.
Test-Taking Strategy: Use the process of elimination. Read the question carefully and note that the issue relates to adequate ventilation of the client. Focusing on this issue will direct you to option 2. If you are unfamiliar with the management of a client on a ventilator, review this content.
Level of Cognitive Ability: Application
Client Needs: Physiological Integrity
Integrated Process: Nursing Process/Implementation
Content Area: Adult Health/Respiratory
References: Black, J., & Hawks, J. (2005). *Medical-surgical nursing: Clinical management for positive outcomes* (7th ed.). Philadelphia: W.B. Saunders, p. 1885.
Linton, A., & Maebius, N. (2003). *Introduction to medical-surgical nursing* (3rd ed.). Philadelphia: W.B. Saunders, pp. 472-473.

16. *Answer: 2*
Rationale: Persons at greatest risk for pulmonary emboli are immobilized clients. Basic preventive measures include early ambulation, leg elevation, active leg exercises, elastic stockings, and intermittent pneumatic calf compression. Keeping the client well hydrated is essential because dehydration predisposes to clotting. A pillow under the knees may cause venous stasis. Heat should not be applied without a physician's prescription.
Test-Taking Strategy: Use the process of elimination and knowledge regarding preventive measures related to preventing DVT and pulmonary emboli to answer this question. Basic principles related to care of the immobile client will assist

in directing you to option 2. If you are unfamiliar with these basic measures, review this content.
Level of Cognitive Ability: Application
Client Needs: Physiological Integrity
Integrated Process: Nursing Process/Planning
Content Area: Adult Health/Respiratory
Reference: Linton, A., & Maebius, N. (2003). *Introduction to medical-surgical nursing* (3rd ed.). Philadelphia: W.B. Saunders, p. 489.

17. *Answer:* **3**
Rationale: The client should be instructed to hold his or her breath for at least 5 to 10 seconds before exhaling the mist. Options 1, 2, and 4 are accurate instructions regarding the use of the inhaler.
Test-Taking Strategy: Use the process of elimination and note the key words, *need for further teaching.* These words indicate a false response question and that you need to select the incorrect client statement. Visualizing this procedure will direct you to option 3. If you are unfamiliar with the client teaching points related to the use of an inhaler, review this content.
Level of Cognitive Ability: Comprehension
Client Needs: Health Promotion and Maintenance
Integrated Process: Teaching/Learning
Content Area: Adult Health/Respiratory
Reference: McKenry, L., & Salerno, E. (2003). *Mosby's pharmacology in nursing* (21st ed.). St. Louis: Mosby, p. 715.

18. *Answer:* **1**
Rationale: Complete lateral positioning should be avoided following pneumonectomy. Because the mediastinum is no longer held in place on both sides by lung tissue, lateral positioning may cause mediastinal shift and compression of the remaining lung.
Test-Taking Strategy: Use the process of elimination and note the key word, *avoid.* This word indicates a false response question and that you need to select the incorrect position. Eliminate options 2, 3, and 4 because they are similar. If you had difficulty with this question, review care of the client following pneumonectomy.
Level of Cognitive Ability: Application
Client Needs: Physiological Integrity
Integrated Process: Nursing Process/Implementation
Content Area: Adult Health/Respiratory
Reference: Christensen, B., & Kockrow, E. (2003). *Adult health nursing* (4th ed.). St. Louis: Mosby, p. 389.

19. *Answer:* **1**
Rationale: The most important question to ask is about the client's pregnancy status, because pregnant women should not be exposed to radiation. Clients are also asked to remove any chains or metal objects that could interfere with obtaining an adequate film. A chest x-ray is most often done at full inspiration, which gives optimal lung expansion. If a lateral view of the chest is ordered, the client is asked to raise the arms above the head. Most films are taken in the posterior-anterior (PA) view.
Test-Taking Strategy: Note the key words, *most important.* Recalling the teratogenic effects of radiation on the fetus will

direct you to option 1. Review this procedure if you had difficulty with this question.
Level of Cognitive Ability: Application
Client Needs: Physiological Integrity
Integrated Process: Nursing Process/Data Collection
Content Area: Adult Health/Respiratory
Reference: Chernecky, C., & Berger, B. (2004). *Laboratory tests and diagnostic procedures* (4th ed.). Philadelphia: W.B. Saunders, p. 360.

20. *Answer:* **3**
Rationale: Signs of allergic reaction to the contrast medium include localized itching and edema, respiratory distress, stridor, and decreased blood pressure. Hypothermia is an unrelated event. Discomfort is expected. Hematoma formation is a complication of the procedure, but does not indicate an allergic reaction.
Test Taking Strategy: Use the ABCs—airway, breathing, and circulation—and focus on the issue, an allergic reaction. This will direct you to option 3. Review the signs of an allergic reaction to the contrast medium if you had difficulty with this question.
Level of Cognitive Ability: Application
Client Needs: Physiological Integrity
Integrated Process: Nursing Process/Data Collection
Content Area: Adult Health/Respiratory
Reference: Chernecky, C., & Berger, B. (2004). *Laboratory tests and diagnostic procedures* (4th ed.). Philadelphia: W.B. Saunders, p. 929.

21. *Answer:* **4**
Rationale: Instructions for using a metered-dose inhaler include shake the canister, hold it right-side up, inhale slowly and evenly through the mouth, deliver one spray per breath, and hold the breath after inhalation.
Test Taking Strategy: Specific knowledge regarding the use of an inhaler is required to answer this question. Visualizing this procedure will direct you to option 4. Review this procedure if you had difficulty with this question.
Level of Cognitive Ability: Application
Client Needs: Health Promotion and Maintenance
Integrated Process: Teaching/Learning
Content Area: Adult Health/Respiratory
Reference: McKenry, L., & Salerno, E. (2003). *Mosby's pharmacology in nursing* (21st ed.). St. Louis: Mosby, p. 715.

22. *Answer:* **2**
Rationale: Cough is the most frequent early sign of lung cancer, which begins as nonproductive and hacking and progresses to productive. In the smoker who already has a cough, a change in the character and frequency of the cough usually occurs. Wheezing and blood-streaked sputum are later signs. Pain is a very late sign and is usually pleuritic in nature.
Test Taking Strategy: Use the process of elimination and note the key word, *early.* Focusing on the client's diagnosis, lung cancer, will direct you to option 2. Review the early signs of lung cancer if you had difficulty with this question.
Level of Cognitive Ability: Application
Client Needs: Physiological Integrity
Integrated Process: Nursing Process/Data Collection

Content Area: Adult Health/Respiratory
References: Christensen, B., & Kockrow, E. (2003). *Adult health nursing* (4th ed.). St. Louis: Mosby, p. 388.
Linton, A., & Maebius, N. (2003). *Introduction to medical-surgical nursing* (3rd ed.). Philadelphia: W.B. Saunders, p. 508.

23. Answer: 1
Rationale: If the client begins to hemorrhage from the surgical site following radical neck dissection, the nurse elevates the head of the bed to maintain airway patency and prevent aspiration. The nurse applies pressure over the bleeding site, and calls the physician immediately.
Test Taking Strategy: Use the process of elimination and note the key word, *contraindicated*. This word indicates a false response question and that you need to select the incorrect action. Option 1 would not maintain airway patency. Review care of the client following radical neck dissection if you had difficulty with this question.
Level of Cognitive Ability: Application
Client Needs: Physiological Integrity
Integrated Process: Nursing Process/Implementation
Content Area: Adult Health/Respiratory
Reference: Christensen, B., & Kockrow, E. (2003). *Adult health nursing* (4th ed.). St. Louis: Mosby, p. 366.

24. Answer: 4
Rationale: Shortness of breath is an early sign of exacerbation of pulmonary sarcoidosis. Others include chest pain, hemoptysis, and pneumothorax. Systemic signs and symptoms that occur later include weakness and fatigue, malaise, fever, and weight loss.
Test Taking Strategy: Note the key word, *early*, in the stem of the question. Because sarcoidosis is a pulmonary problem, eliminate options 1 and 2 first. Choose option 4 over option 3, because the shortness of breath (and impaired ventilation) appears first, and would cause the fatigue as a secondary symptom. Review this disorder if you had difficulty with this question.
Level of Cognitive Ability: Analysis
Client Needs: Health Promotion and Maintenance
Integrated Process: Teaching/Learning
Content Area: Adult Health/Respiratory
References: Black, J., & Hawks, J. (2005). *Medical-surgical nursing: Clinical management for positive outcomes* (7th ed.). Philadelphia: W.B. Saunders, p. 1871.
Linton, A., & Maebius, N. (2003). *Introduction to medical-surgical nursing* (3rd ed.). Philadelphia: W.B. Saunders, p. 507.

25. Answer: 4
Rationale: People at high risk for acquiring tuberculosis include immigrants from Asia, Africa, Latin America, and Central and South Pacific regions; medically underserved populations (ethnic minorities, homeless); those with human immunodeficiency virus or other immunosuppressive disorders; residents in group settings (long-term care, correctional facilities); and health care workers.
Test-Taking Strategy: Use the process of elimination and note the key words, *least risk*. Begin to answer this question by eliminating options 1 and 2, because immigrants and the medically underserved are more frequently affected by this infection. From the remaining options, note that the postal

inspector may or may not come in contact with many people, depending on job description. The client from the long-term care facility, however, lives in a group setting, where a large number of people share a common environment 24 hours a day. Review the risks associated with TB if you had difficulty with this question.
Level of Cognitive Ability: Analysis
Client Needs: Health Promotion and Maintenance
Integrated Process: Nursing Process/Data Collection
Content Area: Adult Health/Respiratory
References: Black, J., & Hawks, J. (2005). *Medical-surgical nursing: Clinical management for positive outcomes* (7th ed.). Philadelphia: W.B. Saunders, pp. 1844-1845.
Christensen, B., & Kockrow, E. (2003). *Adult health nursing* (4th ed.). St. Louis: Mosby, p. 373.
Linton, A., & Maebius, N. (2003). *Introduction to medical-surgical nursing* (3rd ed.). Philadelphia: W.B. Saunders, p. 504.

26. Answer: 2
Rationale: A positive Mantoux reading has an induration measuring 15 mm or more in diameter in low-risk individuals. A small area of ecchymosis is insignificant and is probably related to injection technique.
Test-Taking Strategy: To answer this question accurately, it is necessary to know that induration is necessary for a positive response. Because the client in this question has no induration, the result is negative. Review Mantoux skin test results if you had difficulty with this question.
Level of Cognitive Ability: Comprehension
Client Needs: Physiological Integrity
Integrated Process: Nursing Process/Data Collection
Content Area: Adult Health/Respiratory
References: Black, J., & Hawks, J. (2005). *Medical-surgical nursing: Clinical management for positive outcomes* (7th ed.). Philadelphia: W.B. Saunders, p. 1846.
Chernecky, C., & Berger, B. (2004). *Laboratory tests and diagnostic procedures* (4th ed.). Philadelphia: W.B. Saunders, p. 766.

27. Answer: 4
Rationale: A client who tests positive on a Mantoux skin test has either been exposed to tuberculosis or has inactive (dormant) tuberculosis. The client must then be tested by chest x-ray and sputum culture to confirm the diagnosis.
Test-Taking Strategy: Use the process of elimination, eliminating options 2 and 3 first, because they are similar, indicating the presence of TB. In selecting between options 1 and 4, review the question, noting that the Mantoux skin test is positive. From this information, it is best to eliminate option 1. Review this test if you had difficulty with this question.
Level of Cognitive Ability: Application
Client Needs: Psychosocial Integrity
Integrated Process: Nursing Process/Implementation
Content Area: Adult Health/Respiratory
Reference: Chernecky, C., & Berger, B. (2004). *Laboratory tests and diagnostic procedures* (4th ed.). Philadelphia: W.B. Saunders, p. 766.

28. Answer: 1
Rationale: The nurse who interprets a Mantoux test as positive notifies the physician immediately. The physician would

order a chest x-ray to determine whether the client has clinically active tuberculosis (TB) or old, healed lesions. A sputum culture would be done to confirm the diagnosis of active TB. The client is placed on TB precautions prophylactically until a final diagnosis is made. The findings are documented in the client's record but this action is not the highest priority. Calling the employee health service would be of no benefit to the client.

Test-Taking Strategy: Use the process of elimination and note the key word, *priority.* Because the nurse may not order diagnostic tests, eliminate option 2 first. Similarly, option 4 can be eliminated, because calling the employee health service is of no benefit to the client. From the remaining options, notifying the physician should have a higher priority than the documentation, even though they may both be done in the same narrow time period. Review nursing interventions related to Mantoux testing if you had difficulty with this question.

Level of Cognitive Ability: Application
Client Needs: Safe, Effective Care Environment
Integrated Process: Nursing Process/Implementation
Content Area: Adult Health/Respiratory
Reference: Pagana, K., & Pagana, T. (2003). *Mosby's diagnostic and laboratory test reference* (6th ed.). St. Louis: Mosby, p. 895.

29. *Answer: 3*

Rationale: A primary role of the nurse in working with the client with tuberculosis is to teach the client about medication therapy. The anxious client may not absorb information optimally. The nurse continues to reinforce teaching using a variety of methods (repetition, teaching aids) and teaches the family about the medications as well. The most effective way of coping with the disease is to learn about the therapy, which will eradicate it. This gives the client a measure of power over the situation and outcome.

Test-Taking Strategy: Use the process of elimination. The question asks for the best strategy for coping with anxiety about the disease and its prognosis. Options 2 and 4 are the least useful options and may be eliminated first. Option 2 does not involve the client, and option 4 gives no active assistance to the client. To choose from the remaining options, recall that TB is a controllable disease and not necessarily a fatal one. Review the psychosocial issues related to TB if you had difficulty with this question.

Level of Cognitive Ability: Application
Client Needs: Psychosocial Integrity
Integrated Process: Nursing Process/Planning
Content Area: Adult Health/Respiratory
Reference: Linton, A., & Maebius, N. (2003). *Introduction to medical-surgical nursing* (3rd ed.). Philadelphia: W.B. Saunders, p. 506.

30. *Answer: 4*

Rationale: Because tuberculosis is transmitted by droplets, it cannot be carried on clothing, eating utensils, or other possessions. It is important to perform proper hand washing after contact with body substances, tissues, or face masks. The client should cover the mouth with a tissue when laughing, coughing, or sneezing, and dispose of tissues the carefully.

Test-Taking Strategy: Note the key words, *needs further reinforcement of information.* These words indicate a false

response question and that you need to select the incorrect client statement. Recall that TB is an airborne disease and that organisms cannot be carried on inanimate objects. This will direct you to option 4. Review client teaching points related to the prevention of the spread of TB if you had difficulty with this question.

Level of Cognitive Ability: Comprehension
Client Needs: Safe, Effective Care Environment
Integrated Process: Teaching/Learning
Content Area: Adult Health/Respiratory
Reference: Linton, A., & Maebius, N. (2003). *Introduction to medical-surgical nursing* (3rd ed.). Philadelphia: W.B. Saunders, p. 506.

31. *Answer: 4*

Rationale: The client with tuberculosis usually experiences cough (either productive or nonproductive), fatigue, anorexia, weight loss, dyspnea, hemoptysis, chest discomfort or pain, chills and sweating (which may occur at night), and a low-grade fever.

Test-Taking Strategy: Note the key word, *inconsistent.* Options 1 and 2 can be eliminated first because they are symptoms that are common in the client with TB. From the remaining options, you need to know either that the client may get night sweats or that the fever is low grade. Review the clinical manifestations associated with TB if you had difficulty with this question.

Level of Cognitive Ability: Analysis
Client Needs: Physiological Integrity
Integrated Process: Nursing Process/Data Collection
Content Area: Adult Health/Respiratory
Reference: Linton, A., & Maebius, N. (2003). *Introduction to medical-surgical nursing* (3rd ed.). Philadelphia: W.B. Saunders, p. 505.

32. *Answer: 4*

Rationale: Family members or others who have been in close contact with a client diagnosed with TB are placed on prophylactic therapy with isoniazid (INH) for 6 to 12 months. The client is usually not contagious after taking medication for 2 to 3 consecutive weeks. However, the client must take the full course of therapy (for 6 months or longer) to prevent reinfection or drug resistant TB.

Test-Taking Strategy: Use the process of elimination. Recalling that the family requires prophylactic therapy allows you to eliminate options 1 and 2. From the remaining options, it is necessary to know that the client is not contagious after 2 to 3 weeks of therapy. Review the concepts related to the prevention of the spread of TB if you had difficulty with this question.

Level of Cognitive Ability: Comprehension
Client Needs: Psychosocial Integrity
Integrated Process: Nursing Process/Planning
Content Area: Adult Health/Respiratory
Reference: Linton, A., & Maebius, N. (2003). *Introduction to medical-surgical nursing* (3rd ed.). Philadelphia: W.B. Saunders, p. 505.

33. *Answer: 3*

Rationale: The client with TB has significant fatigue and loss of physical stamina. This can be very frightening for the client.

The nurse teaches the client that this will resolve as the therapy progresses, and that the client should gradually increase activity as energy levels permit.
Test-Taking Strategy: Use the process of elimination. A helpful concept to remember in answering this question is that fatigue caused by respiratory problems may not resolve easily, and is an expected occurrence, because of tissue hypoxia. Knowing this, you can eliminate options 1 and 2 first. Choose between options 3 and 4 in this way: because the client will be on medication therapy for 6 to 9 months, or even up to 12 months, it is not reasonable that the fatigue would last for "at least a year." This will direct you to option 3. Review the manifestations associated with TB if you had difficulty with this question.
Level of Cognitive Ability: Application
Client Needs: Physiological Integrity
Integrated Process: Nursing Process/Planning
Content Area: Adult Health/Respiratory
Reference: Linton, A., & Maebius, N. (2003). *Introduction to medical-surgical nursing* (3rd ed.). Philadelphia: W.B. Saunders, p. 506.

34. **Answer: 1**
Rationale: The nurse teaches the client with TB to increase intake of protein, iron, and vitamin C. Foods rich in vitamin C include citrus fruits, berries, melons, pineapple, broccoli, cabbage, green peppers, tomatoes, potatoes, chard, kale, asparagus, and turnip greens. Food sources that are rich in iron include liver and other meats, from which 10% to 30% of available iron is absorbed. Less than 10% of iron is absorbed from eggs and less than 5% is absorbed from grains and vegetables.
Test-Taking Strategy: To answer correctly, you must recall that the diet in TB should be high in protein, vitamin C, and calories. Recalling which types of foods contain these various nutrients will direct you to option 1. If you had difficulty with this question, review these nutritional concepts.
Level of Cognitive Ability: Application
Client Needs: Health Promotion and Maintenance
Integrated Process: Nursing Process/Implementation
Content Area: Adult Health/Respiratory
Reference: Linton, A., & Maebius, N. (2003). *Introduction to medical-surgical nursing* (3rd ed.). Philadelphia: W.B. Saunders, p. 506.

35. **Answer: 2**
Rationale: The client is continued on medication therapy for 6 to 12 months, depending on the situation. The client is generally considered to be not contagious after 2 to 3 weeks of medication therapy. The client is instructed to wear a mask if there will be exposure to crowds, until the medication is effective in preventing transmission. The client is allowed to return to employment when the results of three sputum cultures are negative.
Test-Taking Strategy: Use the process of elimination. Knowing that the medication therapy lasts for at least 6 months helps you eliminate option 1 first. Knowing that three sputum cultures must be negative helps you eliminate option 4 next. From the remaining options, recalling that the client is not contagious after 2 to 3 weeks of therapy helps you choose

option 2. If you had difficulty with this question, review the infectious period of TB.
Level of Cognitive Ability: Comprehension
Client Needs: Physiological Integrity
Integrated Process: Nursing Process/Evaluation
Content Area: Adult Health/Respiratory
References: Christensen, B., & Kockrow, E. (2003). *Adult health nursing* (4th ed.). St. Louis: Mosby, p. 375.
Linton, A., & Maebius, N. (2003). *Introduction to medical-surgical nursing* (3rd ed.). Philadelphia: W.B. Saunders, p. 505.

36. **Answer: 2**
Rationale: Tuberculosis is spread by droplet nuclei or the airborne route. The disease is not carried on objects such as clothing, eating utensils, linens, or furniture. Bleaching of clothing and linens is unnecessary, although the client and family members should use good hand washing technique. It is unnecessary to remove carpeting from the home.
Test-Taking Strategy: Use the process of elimination. Knowing that TB is not carried on inanimate objects helps you eliminate options 3 and 4 first. From the remaining options, recalling that the disease is transmitted by the airborne route will direct you to option 2. If you had difficulty with this question, review the transmission mode of TB.
Level of Cognitive Ability: Comprehension
Client Needs: Safe, Effective Care Environment
Integrated Process: Nursing Process/Planning
Content Area: Adult Health/Respiratory
Reference: Linton, A., & Maebius, N. (2003). *Introduction to medical-surgical nursing* (3rd ed.). Philadelphia: W.B. Saunders, p. 506.

37. **Answer: 1**
Rationale: The nurse who is in contact with a client with TB should wear an individually fitted particulate respirator. The nurse would also wear gloves as per standard precautions. The nurse wears a gown whenever there is a possibility that the clothing could become contaminated, such as when giving a bed bath.
Test-Taking Strategy: Use the process of elimination. Knowing that the nurse should wear a particulate respirator mask helps you eliminate options 3 and 4 first. Recalling standard precautions helps you choose option 1 over option 2. Review care of the client with TB if you had difficulty with this question.
Level of Cognitive Ability: Application
Client Needs: Safe, Effective Care Environment
Integrated Process: Nursing Process/Planning
Content Area: Adult Health/Respiratory
References: Christensen, B., & Kockrow, E. (2003). *Adult health nursing* (4th ed.). St. Louis: Mosby, pp. 240-241, 375.
Linton, A., & Maebius, N. (2003). *Introduction to medical-surgical nursing* (3rd ed.). Philadelphia: W.B. Saunders, p. 506.

38. **Answer: 1**
Rationale: The client must have sputum cultures tested every 2 to 4 weeks after initiation of antituberculosis medication therapy. The client may return to work when the results of three sputum cultures are negative, because the client is considered noninfectious at that point. The Mantoux test will not revert

to negative once it is positive. The chest x-ray may or may not be negative.
Test-Taking Strategy: Use the process of elimination. Knowing that a positive Mantoux test result never reverts to negative helps you eliminate option 4. To discriminate among the remaining options, it is necessary to know that three negative sputum cultures are required. If this question was difficult, review these concepts.
Level of Cognitive Ability: Application
Client Needs: Safe, Effective Care Environment
Integrated Process: Nursing Process/Implementation
Content Area: Adult Health/Respiratory
Reference: Black, J., & Hawks, J. (2005). *Medical-surgical nursing: Clinical management for positive outcomes* (7th ed.). Philadelphia: W.B. Saunders, p. 1846.

39. *Answer: 2*
Rationale: Histoplasmosis is an opportunistic fungal infection that can occur in the client with AIDS. The infection begins as a respiratory infection and can progress to disseminated infection. Typical signs and symptoms include fever, dyspnea, cough, and weight loss. There may be enlargement of the client's lymph nodes, liver, and spleen as well.
Test-Taking Strategy: Use the process of elimination. Recalling that histoplasmosis is an infectious process helps you eliminate option 3. Because the client has AIDS as well as another infection, weight gain is an unlikely symptom and can be eliminated next. Knowing that histoplasmosis begins as a respiratory infection helps you choose dyspnea over headache as the correct option. Review the signs of histoplasmosis if you had difficulty with this question.
Level of Cognitive Ability: Application
Client Needs: Physiological Integrity
Integrated Process: Nursing Process/Data Collection
Content Area: Adult Health/Respiratory
Reference: Ignatavicius, D., & Workman, M. (2006). *Medical surgical nursing: Critical thinking for collaborative care* (5th ed.). Philadelphia: W.B. Saunders, pp.1851, 2391.

40. *Answer: 1*
Rationale: Silicosis results from chronic, excessive inhalation of particles of free crystalline silica dust. The client should wear a mask to limit inhalation of this substance, which can cause restrictive lung disease after years of exposure. Options 2, 3, and 4 are not necessary.
Test-Taking Strategy: Use the process of elimination. Recalling that exposure to silica dust causes the illness and that the dust is inhaled into the respiratory tract will direct you to option 1. If you had difficulty with this question, review the protective measures associated with silicosis.
Level of Cognitive Ability: Comprehension
Client Needs: Safe, Effective Care Environment

Integrated Process: Nursing Process/Data Collection
Content Area: Adult Health/Respiratory
Reference: Phipps, W., Monahan, F., Sands, J., Marek, J. & Neighbors, M. (2003). *Medical-surgical nursing: Health and illness perspectives* (7th ed.). St. Louis: Mosby, p. 547.

ALTERNATE FORMAT QUESTION: MULTIPLE RESPONSE
Answers:
Activities should be resumed gradually
Consume a well-balanced diet and foods rich in iron, protein, and vitamin C
Respiratory isolation is not necessary because family members have already been exposed
Cover the mouth and nose when coughing or sneezing and confine used tissues to plastic bags
A sputum culture is needed every 2 to 4 weeks once medication therapy is initiated
Rationale: The nurse should provide the client and family with information about tuberculosis and allay concerns about the contagious aspect of the infection. The client is to follow the medication regimen exactly as prescribed and always to have a supply of the medication on hand. The client is advised of the side effects of the medication and ways of minimizing them to ensure compliance. The client is reassured that, after 2 to 3 weeks of medication therapy, it is unlikely that the client will infect anyone. The client is informed that activities should be resumed gradually and about the need for adequate nutrition and a well-balanced diet that is rich in iron, protein, and vitamin C to promote healing and prevent recurrence of infection. The client and family are informed that respiratory isolation is not necessary, because family members have already been exposed. The client is instructed about thorough hand washing and to cover the mouth and nose when coughing or sneezing and confine used tissues to plastic bags. The client is informed that a sputum culture is needed every 2 to 4 weeks once medication therapy is initiated and, when the results of three sputum cultures are negative, the client is no longer considered infectious and can usually return to his or her former employment.
Test-Taking Strategy: Knowledge regarding the pathophysiology, transmission, and treatment of tuberculosis is needed to answer this question. Review home care instructions for the client with tuberculosis if you had difficulty with this question.
Level of Cognitive Ability: Application
Client Needs: Health Promotion and Maintenance
Integrated Process: Teaching/Learning
Content Area: Adult Health/Respiratory
Reference: Ignatavicius, D., & Workman, M. (2006). *Medical surgical nursing: Critical thinking for collaborative care* (5th ed.). Philadelphia: W.B. Saunders, pp. 644-645.

REFERENCES

Black, J., & Hawks, J. (2005). *Medical-surgical nursing: Clinical management for positive outcomes* (7th ed.). Philadelphia: W.B. Saunders.

Chernecky, C., & Berger, B. (2004). *Laboratory tests and diagnostic procedures* (4th ed.). Philadelphia: W.B. Saunders.

Christensen, B., & Kockrow, E. (2003). *Adult health nursing* (4th ed.). St. Louis: Mosby.

Christensen, B., & Kockrow, E. (2003). *Foundations of nursing* (4th ed.). St. Louis: Mosby.

Hodgson, B. & Kizior, R. (2005). *Saunders nursing drug handbook 2005.* Philadelphia: W.B. Saunders.

Ignatavicius, D., & Workman, M. (2002). *Medical surgical nursing: Critical thinking for collaborative care* (4th ed.). Philadelphia: W.B. Saunders.

Lewis, S., Heitkemper, M., & Dirksen, S. (2004). *Medical-surgical nursing: Assessment and management of clinical problems* (6th ed.). St. Louis: Mosby.

Linton, A., & Maebius, N. (2003). *Introduction to medical-surgical nursing* (3rd ed.). Philadelphia: W.B. Saunders.

McKenry, L., & Salerno, E. (2003). *Mosby's pharmacology in nursing* (21st ed.). St. Louis: Mosby.

Pagana, K., & Pagana, T. (2003). *Mosby's diagnostic and laboratory test reference* (6th ed.). St. Louis: Mosby.

Phipps, W., Monahan, F., Sands, J., Marek, J. & Neighbors, M. (2003). *Medical-surgical nursing: Health and illness perspectives* (7th ed.). St. Louis: Mosby.

Respiratory Medications

I. BRONCHODILATORS

A. Description

1. Sympathomimetic bronchodilators dilate the airways of the respiratory tree, making air exchange and respiration easier for the client, and relax the smooth muscle of the bronchi (Box 49-1)

2. Xanthine bronchodilators stimulate the central nervous system and respiration, dilate coronary and pulmonary vessels, cause diuresis, and relax smooth muscle (Box 49-2)

3. Used to treat allergic rhinitis and sinusitis, acute bronchospasm, acute and chronic asthma, bronchitis, **chronic obstructive pulmonary disease, and emphysema**

BOX 49-1

Bronchodilators: Sympathomimetics

BETA-RECEPTOR AGONISTS
Albuterol (Proventil, Ventolin)
Bitolterol mesylate
Epinephrine (AsthmaHaler Mist)
Epinephrine (Adrenalin, Primatene)
Formoterol fumarate (Foradil)
Isoproterenol (Isuprel)
Levalbuterol (Xopenex)
Metaproterenol sulfate (Alupent)
Pirbuterol acetate (Maxair)
Salmeterol (Serevent)
Terbutaline sulfate (Brethine, Brethaire)

ANTICHOLINERGIC
Ipratropium bromide (Atrovent, Combivent)

---

4. Contraindicated in individuals with hypersensitivity, peptic ulcer disease, severe cardiac disease and cardiac dysrhythmias, hyperthyroidism, or uncontrolled seizure disorders

5. Used with caution in clients with hypertension, diabetes mellitus, or narrow-angle glaucoma

6. Theophylline increases the risk of digitalis toxicity and decreases the effects of lithium and phenytoin (Dilantin)

7. If theophylline and a beta-adrenergic agonist are administered together, cardiac dysrhythmias may result

8. Beta blockers, cimetidine (Tagamet), and erythromycin increase the effects of theophylline

9. Barbiturate and carbamazepine (Tegretol) decrease the effects of theophylline

10. Xanthine bronchodilators are not used as frequently as previously; may be introduced later in therapy

B. Side effects

1. Palpitations and tachycardia

2. Dysrhythmias

3. Restlessness, nervousness, tremors

4. Anorexia, nausea, and vomiting

5. Headaches and dizziness

BOX 49-2

Bronchodilators: Xanthines

Aminophylline
Theophylline (Bronkodyl, Elixophyllin)
Theophylline (Aerolate, Slo-Phyllin, Theolair)
Theophylline (Theo-Dur, Slo-Bid, Theo-24, Uni-Dur, Uniphyl)

---

6. Hyperglycemia
7. Decreased clotting time
8. Mouth dryness and throat irritation with inhalers
9. Tolerance and paradoxical bronchoconstriction with inhalers

C. Interventions
1. Monitor vital signs
2. Monitor for cardiac dysrhythmias
3. Monitor for cough, wheezing, decreased breath sounds, and sputum production
4. Monitor for restlessness and confusion
5. Provide adequate hydration
6. Administer the medication at regular intervals around the clock to maintain a sustained therapeutic level
7. Administer oral medications with or after meals to decrease gastrointestinal (GI) irritation
8. Instruct the client not to crush enteric-coated or sustained-release tablets or capsules
9. Instruct the client to avoid caffeine products, such as coffee, tea, cola, and chocolate
10. Instruct the client in the side effects of bronchodilators
11. Instruct the client in how to monitor the pulse and to report any abnormalities to the physician
12. Instruct the client in how to use an inhaler or nebulizer and how to monitor the amount of medication remaining in an inhaler canister
13. Instruct the client to avoid over-the-counter medications
14. Instruct the client to stop smoking and provide information regarding support resources
15. Instruct the client with diabetes mellitus to monitor blood glucose level
16. Instruct the client with asthma to wear a Medic-Alert bracelet
17. Monitor for a therapeutic serum theophylline level of 10 to 20 mcg/mL
18. Note that toxicity is likely to occur when the serum level is higher than 20 mcg/mL
19. IV aminophylline or theophylline preparations should be administered slowly and always via an infusion pump

II. GLUCOCORTICOIDS (CORTICOSTEROIDS) (Box 49-3)

A. Act as anti-inflammatory agents and reduce edema of the airways
B. See Chapter 45 for information on glucocorticoids

III. INHALED NONSTEROIDAL ANTIALLERGY AGENTS (Box 49-4)

A. Description

1. Antiasthmatic, antiallergic, and mast cell stabilizers that inhibit mast cell release after exposure to antigens
2. Used for the treatment of allergic rhinitis, bronchial asthma, and exercise-induced bronchospasm
3. Contraindicated in clients with known hypersensitivity
4. Oral cromolyn sodium is used with caution in clients with impaired hepatic or renal function

B. Side effects
1. Cough or bronchospasm following inhalation
2. Nasal sting or sneezing following inhalation
3. Unpleasant taste in the mouth

C. Interventions
1. Monitor vital signs
2. Monitor respirations and assess lung sounds for rhonchi and wheezing
3. Instruct the client to drink a few sips of water before and after inhalation to prevent cough and unpleasant taste in the mouth
4. Administer oral capsules (cromolyn sodium) at least 30 minutes before meals
5. Instruct the client not to discontinue the medication abruptly because a rebound asthmatic attack can occur

IV. LEUKOTRIENE MODIFIERS (Box 49-5)

A. Description

BOX 49-3

Glucocorticoids (Corticosteroids)

Beclomethasone dipropionate (Beconase AQ)
Budesonide (Pulmicort)
Flunisolide (AeroBid)
Fluticasone (Flonase, Flovent)
Fluticasone and salmeterol (Advair Diskus)
Mometasone intranasal (Nasonex)
Triamcinolone (Azmacort)

BOX 49-4

Inhaled Nonsteroidal Antiallergy Agents: Mast Cell Stabilizers

Cromolyn sodium (Intal)
Nedocromil (Tilade)

BOX 49-5

Leukotriene Modifiers

Montelukast (Singulair)
Zafirlukast (Accolate)
Zileuton (Zyflo)

1. Used in the prophylaxis and treatment of chronic bronchial asthma
2. Not used for acute asthma episodes
3. Inhibit bronchoconstriction caused by specific antigens
4. Reduce airway edema and smooth muscle constriction
5. Contraindicated with hypersensitivity and in breast-feeding mothers
6. Used with caution in clients with impaired hepatic function
7. Co-administration of inhaled glucocorticoids increases the risk of upper respiratory infection

B. Side effects
1. Headache
2. Nausea and vomiting
3. Dyspepsia
4. Diarrhea
5. Generalized pain, myalgia
6. Fever
7. Dizziness

C. Interventions
1. Monitor vital signs
2. Monitor lung sounds for rhonchi, wheezing, and crackles
3. Check liver function laboratory values
4. Monitor for cyanosis
5. Instruct the client to take medication 1 hour before or 2 hours after meals
6. Instruct the client to increase fluid intake
7. Instruct the client not to discontinue medication and to take as prescribed, even during symptom-free periods

V. ANTIHISTAMINES (Box 49-6)
A. Description
1. Called histamine antagonists or H_1 blockers; these medications compete with histamine for receptor sites, thus preventing a histamine response

---

BOX 49-6

Antihistamines

Azelastine hydrochloride (Astelin)
Brompheniramine maleate (Brovex)
Cetirizine hydrochloride (Zyrtec)
Chlorpheniramine maleate (Aller-Chlor, Chlor-Trimeton)
Clemastine fumarate (Tavist)
Dexchlorpheniramine maleate (Polaramine)
Dimenhydrinate (Dramamine)
Diphenhydramine (Benadryl)
Doxylamine succinate (Unisom Nighttime Sleep-Aid)
Fexofenadine (Allegra)
Loratadine (Claritin)
Phenindamine tartrate (Nolahist)
Tripelennamine (Pyribenzamine)

---

2. When the H_1 receptor is stimulated, the extravascular smooth muscles, including those lining the nasal cavity, are constricted
3. Decrease nasopharyngeal secretions by blocking the H_1 receptor and decrease nasal itching that causes sneezing
4. Used for the common cold, rhinitis, nausea and vomiting, motion sickness, urticaria, and as a sleep aid
5. Can cause central nervous system (CNS) depression if taken with alcohol, narcotics, hypnotics, or barbiturates
6. Used with caution in clients with **chronic obstructive pulmonary disease (COPD)** because of their drying effect
7. Diphenhydramine (Benadryl) has an anticholinergic effect and should be avoided in clients with narrow-angle glaucoma

B. Side effects
1. Drowsiness and fatigue
2. Dizziness
3. Urinary retention
4. Blurred vision
5. Wheezing
6. Constipation
7. Dry mouth
8. Gastrointestinal (GI) irritation
9. Hypotension
10. Hearing disturbances
11. Photosensitivity
12. Nervousness and irritability
13. Confusion
14. Nightmares

C. Interventions
1. Monitor vital signs
2. Monitor for signs of urinary dysfunction
3. Administer with food or milk
4. Avoid subcutaneous injection and administer intramuscular injection in a large muscle if the intramuscular route is prescribed
5. Instruct the client to avoid hazardous activities, alcohol, and other CNS depressants
6. Instruct the client taking medication for motion sickness to take the medication 30 minutes before the event, and then before meals and at bedtime during the event
7. Instruct the client to suck on hard candy or ice chips for dry mouth

VI. NASAL DECONGESTANTS (Box 49-7)
A. Description
1. Stimulate the alpha-adrenergic receptors, thus producing vasoconstriction of the capillaries within the nasal mucosa
2. Shrink nasal mucosal membranes and reduce fluid secretion

3. Used for allergic rhinitis, hay fever, and acute coryza (profuse nasal discharge)

4. Contraindicated or used with extreme caution in clients with hypertension, cardiac disease, hyperthyroidism, or diabetes mellitus

5. Nasal decongestants can cause tolerance and rebound nasal congestion (vasodilation), caused by irritation of the nasal mucosa, and should not be used for more than 48 hours

B. Side effects

1. Frequent use of decongestants, especially nasal sprays or drops, can result in tolerance and rebound nasal congestion (vasodilation), caused by irritation of the nasal mucosa

2. Nervousness

3. Restlessness

4. Hypertension

5. Hyperglycemia

C. Interventions

1. Ask the client about existing medical disorders

2. Monitor for cardiac dysrhythmias

3. Monitor blood glucose levels

4. Instruct the client to avoid caffeine in large amounts because it can increase restlessness and palpitations

5. Instruct the client in the importance of limiting the use of nasal sprays and drops

VII. EXPECTORANTS AND MUCOLYTIC AGENTS (Box 49-8)

A. Description

1. Loosen bronchial secretions so that they can be eliminated with coughing

2. Used for dry, unproductive cough and to stimulate bronchial secretions

---

BOX 49-7

Nasal Decongestants

Oxymetazoline hydrochloride (Afrin)
Phenylephrine hydrochloride (Neo-Synephrine)
Pseudoephedrine (Dimetapp, Sudafed)

BOX 49-8

Expectorants and Mucolytic Agents

EXPECTORANTS
Dornase alfa (Pulmozyme)
Guaifenesin (glyceryl guaiacolate) (Humibid, Robitussin)

MUCOLYTIC AGENT
Acetylcysteine (Mucomyst)

---

3. Mucolytic agents with dextromethorphan should not be used by clients with **COPD** because they suppress the cough

4. Acetylcysteine (Mucomyst) can increase airway resistance and should not be used in clients with asthma

B. Side effects

1. GI irritation

2. Skin rash

3. Oropharyngeal irritation

C. Interventions

1. Instruct the client to take medication with a full glass of water to loosen mucus

2. Instruct the client to maintain an adequate fluid intake

3. Encourage the client to cough and deep breathe

4. Acetylcysteine (Mucomyst), administered by nebulization, should not be mixed with another medication

5. If acetylcysteine (Mucomyst) is administered with a bronchodilator, the bronchodilator should be administered 5 minutes before the acetylcysteine

6. Monitor for side effects of acetylcysteine (Mucomyst), such as nausea and vomiting, stomatitis, and runny nose

VIII. ANTITUSSIVES (Box 49-9)

A. Description

1. Act on the cough control center in the medulla to suppress the cough reflex

2. Used for a cough that is nonproductive and irritating

B. Side effects

1. Dizziness, drowsiness, sedation

2. GI irritation, nausea

3. Dry mouth

4. Constipation

5. Respiratory depression

C. Interventions

1. Instruct the client that if the cough lasts longer than 1 week and a fever or rash occurs, the physician should be notified

2. Encourage the client to take adequate fluids with the medication

---

BOX 49-9

Antitussives

NARCOTICS
Codeine, codeine phosphate, codeine sulfate
Hydrocodone bitartrate (Hycodan)

NON-NARCOTICS
Diphenhydramine hydrochloride (Benadryl)

BOX 49-10

Narcotic Antagonist

Naloxone hydrochloride (Narcan)

3. Encourage the client to sleep with the head of the bed elevated
4. Instruct the client to avoid hazardous activities
5. Note that drug dependency can occur
6. Avoid administration to the client with a head injury or postoperative cranial surgery
7. Avoid administration to the client using narcotics, sedative hypnotics, barbiturates, or antidepressants, because CNS depression can occur
8. Instruct the client to avoid the use of alcohol

IX. NARCOTIC ANTAGONIST (Box 49-10)

A. Description
  1. Reverses respiratory depression in narcotic overdose
  2. Avoid use in non-narcotic respiratory depression
B. Side effects
  1. CNS depression
  2. Nausea, vomiting
  3. Tremors
  4. Sweating
  5. Increased blood pressure
  6. Tachycardia
C. Interventions
  1. Monitor vital signs, especially respirations
  2. Have oxygen and resuscitative equipment available during administration

X. USE OF AN INHALER

A. Client instructions (Figure 49-1)
B. If two different inhaled medications are prescribed, and one of the medications contains a glucocorticoid (corticosteroid), administer the bronchodilator first and the corticosteroid second
C. Wait 5 minutes following the bronchodilator before inhaling the corticosteroid

XI. TUBERCULOSIS (TB) MEDICATIONS

A. Description
  1. The most effective method for treating the disease and preventing transmission
  2. Treatment of identified lesions depends on whether the individual has active disease or has been exposed to the disease
  3. Treatment is difficult because the bacterium has a waxy substance on the capsule, which makes penetration and destruction difficult

4. The use of a multiple-medication regimen destroys organisms as quickly as possible and minimizes the emergence of medication-resistant organisms
5. Active **TB** is treated with a combination of medications to which the organism is susceptible
6. Individuals with active **TB** are treated for 6 to 9 months; however, clients with human immunodeficiency virus (HIV) infection will be treated for a longer period
7. After the infected individual has received medication for 2 to 3 weeks, the risk of transmission is greatly reduced
8. Most clients have negative sputum cultures after 3 months of compliance with medication therapy
9. Individuals who have been exposed to active **TB** are treated with preventive isoniazid (INH) for 9 to 12 months
B. First-line or second-line medications
  1. First-line medications provide the most effective antituberculosis activity
  2. Second-line medications are used in combination with first-line medications, but are more toxic
  3. Current infecting organisms are proving resistant to standard first-line medications, and the resistant organisms develop because individuals with the disease fail to complete the course of treatment; surviving bacteria adapt to the medication and become resistant
  4. Multidrug therapies are instituted because of the resistant organisms
C. **Multidrug-resistant tuberculosis (MDR-TB)**
  1. Occurs when a client receiving two medications (first-line and second-line medications) discontinues one of the medications without the physician's knowledge
  2. The client briefly experiences some response from the single medication, but then large numbers of resistant organisms begin to grow
  3. The client, infectious again, transmits the drug-resistant organism to other individuals
  4. As this event is repeated, an organism develops that is resistant to many of the first-line **tuberculosis** medications

XII. FIRST-LINE MEDICATIONS FOR TB (Box 49-11)

A. Isoniazid (INH) (Nydrazid)
  1. Description
    a. Bactericidal
    b. Inhibits synthesis of mycolic acids and acts to kill actively growing organisms in the extracellular environment
    c. Inhibits growth of dormant organisms in the macrophages and caseating granulomas
    d. Active only during cell division

1. Insert the medicine canister into the inhaler unit and remove the cover from the mouthpiece. Shake the unit gently according to the manufacturer's recommendations.

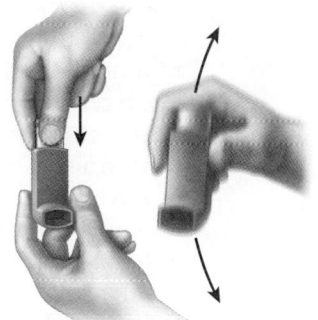

4. Press the top of the canister as you breathe in slowly through your mouth. (Failing to coordinate respiration with inhalation will decrease the amount of medication that reaches your lungs.)

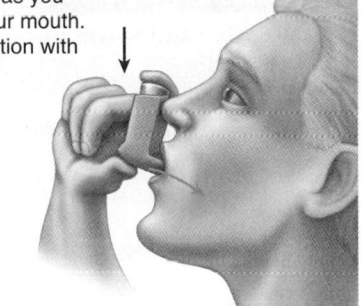

2. Hold the inhaler ready for inspiration. Exhale slowly. (Do not breathe into the inhaler; that could clog the inhaler valve.)

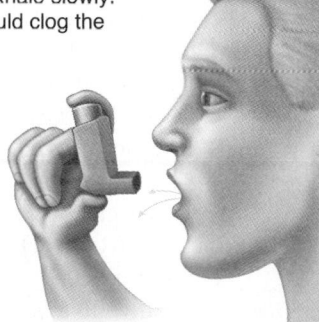

5. Remove the inhaler. Hold your breath for 10 seconds, then breathe out slowly through pursed lips.

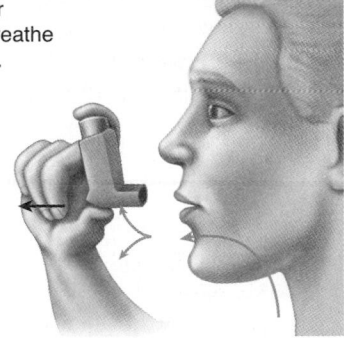

3. Place the mouthpiece into your mouth and seal it with your lips. Tilt your head slightly back and keep your tongue away from the mouth of the inhaler. (Alternatively, hold the inhaler 1 to 2 inches in front of your mouth and keep your mouth open. With steroids, do not put the inhaler in your mouth. Ineffective use results from medication bouncing off teeth, tongue, or palate.)

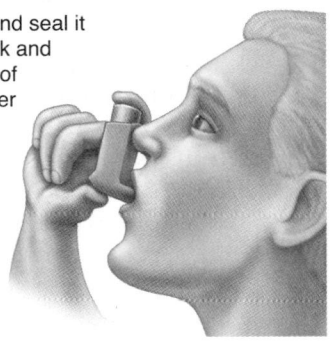

6. Keep the cap in place between uses to prevent dirt from getting into the inhaler. To clean the inhaler, remove the metal canister and rinse the holder in warm water. Dry the holder thoroughly before using it again.

FIG. 49-1 Teaching for self-care using a metered-dose inhaler. (From Harkreader, H., & Hogan, M.A. [2004]. *Fundamentals of nursing: Caring and clinical judgment.* [2nd ed.]. Philadelphia: W.B. Saunders.)

e. Used in combination with other antitubercular medications
2. Contraindications and cautions
   a. Contraindicated in clients with hypersensitivity or with acute liver disease
   b. Use with caution in clients with chronic liver disease, alcoholism, or renal impairment
   c. Use with caution in clients taking niacin, nicotinic acid (Nicobid)
   d. Use with caution in clients taking hepatotoxic medications because the risk for hepatotoxicity increases
   e. Alcohol increases the risk of hepatotoxicity

f. Isoniazid (INH) may increase the risk of toxicity of carbamazepine (Tegretol) and phenytoin (Dilantin)
   g. Isoniazid (INH) may decrease ketoconazole (Nizoral) concentration
3. Side effects
   a. Hypersensitivity reactions
   b. Peripheral neuritis
   c. Neurotoxicity
   d. Hepatotoxicity
   e. Pyridoxine (vitamin B_6) deficiency
   f. Irritation at injection site with IM administration
   g. Nausea and vomiting

BOX 49-11

First-Line and Second-Line Medications for Tuberculosis

FIRST-LINE AGENTS
Isoniazid (INH, Nydrazid)
Rifampin (Rifadin)
Ethambutol (Myambutol)
Streptomycin
Pyrazinamide (PZA)

SECOND-LINE AGENTS
Capreomycin (Capastat)
Ethionamide (Trecator-SC)
Kanamycin (Kantrex)
Para-aminosalicylate (PAS)
Cycloserine (Seromycin)

OTHER MEDICATIONS
Rifabutin (Mycobutin): Antimycobacterial used for the prophylaxis for disseminated *Mycobacterium avium* complex (MAC) in persons with acquired immunodeficiency syndrome
Rifampin and isoniazid (Rifamate): For treatment of tuberculosis after dosage of separate medications has been established

h. Dry mouth
i. Dizziness
j. Hyperglycemia
k. Increased liver function test results
l. Hepatitis
4. Interventions
   a. Monitor for hypersensitivity
   b. Monitor for hepatic dysfunction
   c. Check for sensitivity to niacin, nicotinic acid (Nicobid)
   d. Monitor liver function tests
   e. Monitor for signs of hepatitis, such as anorexia, nausea, vomiting, weakness, fatigue, dark urine, or jaundice; if these symptoms occur, withhold the medication and notify the physician
   f. Monitor for tingling, numbness, or burning of the extremities
   g. Monitor mental status
   h. Monitor for visual changes, and notify the physician if they occur
   i. Monitor for dizziness and initiate safety precautions
   j. Monitor complete blood cell (CBC) count and blood glucose level
   k. Administer 1 hour before or 2 hours after a meal, because food may delay absorption
   l. Administer at least 1 hour before antacids, especially those antacids that contain aluminum
5. Client education
   a. Instruct the client not to skip doses and to take medication for the full length of the prescribed therapy

b. Instruct the client not to take any other medication without consulting the physician
c. Advise the client of the importance of follow-up physician visits, vision testing, and laboratory tests
d. Instruct the client to avoid alcohol
e. Advise the client to take medication on an empty stomach with 8 ounces of water, 1 hour before or 2 hours after meals, and to avoid taking antacids with the medication
f. Instruct the client to avoid tyramine-containing foods because they may cause a reaction such as red and itching skin, pounding heartbeat, lightheadedness, hot or clammy feeling, or headache and, if this does occur, to notify the physician
g. Instruct the client in the signs of neurotoxicity, hepatitis, and hepatotoxicity
h. Instruct the client to notify the physician if signs of neurotoxicity, hepatitis and hepatotoxicity, or visual changes occur

B. Rifampin (Rifadin)
1. Description
   a. Inhibits bacterial RNA synthesis
   b. Binds to DNA-dependent RNA polymerase and blocks RNA transcription
   c. Used in conjunction with at least one other antitubercular medication
2. Contraindications and cautions
   a. Contraindicated in clients with hypersensitivity
   b. Use with caution in clients with hepatic dysfunction or alcoholism
   c. Use of alcohol or hepatotoxic medications may increase the risk of hepatotoxicity
   d. Decreases the effects of several medications, including oral anticoagulants, oral hypoglycemics, chloramphenicol (Chloromycetin), digoxin (Lanoxin), disopyramide phosphate (Norpace), mexiletine (Mexitil), quinidine, fluconazole (Difulcan), methadone hydrochloride (Dolophine), phenytoin (Dilantin), and verapamil hydrochloride (Calan)
3. Side effects
   a. Hypersensitivity reaction including fever, chills, shivering, headache, muscle and bone pain, and dyspnea
   b. Heartburn
   c. Nausea, vomiting, diarrhea
   d. Increased liver function tests
   e. Hepatotoxicity and hepatitis
   f. Increased uric acid level
   g. Blood dyscrasias
   h. Colitis
4. Interventions
   a. Monitor for hypersensitivity
   b. Evaluate CBC, uric acid level, and liver function tests
   c. Monitor for signs of hepatitis and, if they occur, withhold the medication and notify the physician

d. Monitor stools for signs of colitis

e. Monitor mental status

f. Monitor for visual changes

5. Client education

a. Instruct the client not to skip doses and to take medication for the full length of the prescribed therapy

b. Instruct the client not to take any other medication without consulting the physician

c. Advise the client of the importance of follow-up physician visits and laboratory tests

d. Instruct the client to avoid alcohol

e. Advise the client to take medication on an empty stomach with 8 ounces of water, 1 hour before or 2 hours after meals, and to avoid taking antacids with the medication

f. Instruct the client that urine, feces, sweat, and tears will be red-orange in color and that soft contact lenses can become permanently discolored

g. Instruct the client to notify the physician if jaundice (yellow eyes or skin) develops or if weakness, fatigue, nausea, vomiting, sore throat, fever, or unusual bleeding occurs

C. Ethambutol (Myambutol)

1. Description

a. Bacteriostatic

b. Interferes with cell metabolism and multiplication by inhibiting one or more metabolites in susceptible organism

c. Inhibits bacterial RNA synthesis

d. Active only during cell division

e. Is slow-acting and must be used in combination with other bactericidal agents

2. Contraindications and cautions

a. Contraindicated in clients with hypersensitivity or optic neuritis and in children younger than 13 years of age

b. Use with caution in clients with renal dysfunction, gout, ocular defects, diabetic retinopathy, cataracts, or ocular inflammatory conditions

c. Use with caution in clients taking neurotoxic medications, because the risk for neurotoxicity increases

3. Side effects

a. Hypersensitivity reactions

b. Anorexia, nausea, vomiting

c. Dizziness

d. Malaise

e. Mental confusion

f. Joint pain

g. Dermatitis

h. Optic neuritis

i. Peripheral neuritis

j. Thrombocytopenia

k. Increased uric acid levels

l. Anaphylactoid reaction

4. Interventions

a. Monitor for hypersensitivity

b. Evaluate results of CBC, uric acid, and renal and liver function tests

c. Obtain baseline visual acuity and color discrimination, especially to the color green

d. Monitor for visual changes such as altered color perception and decreased visual acuity; if changes occur, withhold the medication and notify the physician

e. Administer once every 24 hours and administer with food to decrease GI upset

f. Monitor uric acid concentrations and assess for painful or swollen joints or signs of gout

g. Monitor input and output (I&O) and for adequate renal function

h. Monitor mental status

i. Monitor for dizziness and initiate safety precautions

j. Assess for peripheral neuritis (numbness, tingling or burning of the extremities); if it occurs, notify the physician

5. Client education

a. Inform the client that he or she can prevent nausea related to the medication by taking the daily dose at bedtime or by taking prescribed antinausea medications

b. Instruct the client not to skip doses and to take the medication for the full length of the prescribed therapy

c. Instruct the client not to take any other medication without consulting the physician

d. Advise the client of the importance of follow-up physician visits, vision testing, and laboratory tests

e. Instruct the client to notify the physician immediately if a visual problem, rash, swelling and pain in the joints, or numbness, tingling, or burning in the hands or feet occurs

D. Streptomycin

1. Description

a. An aminoglycoside antibiotic that is used in conjunction with at least one other antitubercular medication

b. Bactericidal, because of receptor-binding action, interfering with protein synthesis in susceptible organisms

2. Contraindications and cautions

a. Contraindicated in clients with hypersensitivity, myasthenia gravis, parkinsonism, or eighth cranial nerve damage

b. Use with caution in the older client, in neonates because of renal insufficiency and immaturity, and in young infants because the medication may cause CNS depression

c. The risk of toxicity increases when taken with other aminoglycosides or nephrotoxicity- or ototoxicity-producing medications

3. Side effects (Box 49-12)

a. Hypersensitivity

BOX 49-12

Side Effects of Streptomycin

NEPHROTOXICITY
Changes in urine output
Increased thirst
Decreased appetite
Nausea, vomiting

NEUROTOXICITY
Muscle numbness
Tingling
Twitching
Seizures

VESTIBULAR OTOTOXICITY
Dizziness
Clumsiness
Loss of hearing

AUDITORY OTOTOXICITY
Ringing in the ears
Unsteadiness
A full feeling in the ears

   b. Visual changes
   c. Increased liver and renal function tests
   d. Peripheral neuritis
4. Interventions
   a. Monitor for hypersensitivity
   b. Monitor liver and renal function tests
   c. Monitor for ototoxic, neurotoxic, and nephrotoxic reactions
   d. Perform baseline audiometric testing and repeat every 1 to 2 months, because the medication impairs the eighth cranial nerve
   e. Monitor hearing acuity
   f. Monitor for visual changes
   g. Monitor hydration status and maintain adequate hydration during therapy
   h. Monitor I&O
   i. Check urinalysis results
   j. Monitor for signs of peripheral neuritis
5. Client education
   a. Instruct the client not to skip doses and to take medication for the full length of the prescribed therapy
   b. Instruct the client not to take any other medication without consulting the physician
   c. Advise the client of the importance of follow-up physician visits and laboratory tests
   d. Instruct the client to notify the physician if hearing loss, changes in vision, or urinary problems occur
E. Pyrazinamide (PZA)
   1. Description
      a. Exact mechanism of action is unknown

   b. May be bacteriostatic or bactericidal, depending on its concentration at the infection site and susceptibility of infecting organism
   c. Used in conjunction with at least one other antitubercular medication after failure or ineffectiveness of the primary medications occurs
2. Contraindications and cautions
   a. Contraindicated in clients with hypersensitivity
   b. Use with caution in clients with diabetes mellitus, renal impairment, or gout, and in children
   c. May decrease the effects of allopurinol (Zyloprim), colchicine, probenecid (Benemid), sulfinpyrazone (Anturane)
   d. Cross-sensitivity is possible with isoniazid (INH), ethionamide (Trecator-SC), niacin, nicotinic acid (Nicobid)
3. Side effects
   a. Increases liver function and uric acid level
   b. Arthralgia, myalgia
   c. Photosensitivity
   d. Hepatotoxicity
   e. Thrombocytopenia
4. Interventions
   a. Monitor for hypersensitivity
   b. Evaluate CBC, liver function tests, and uric acid level
   c. Observe for hepatotoxic effects; if they occur, withhold the medication and notify the physician
   d. Monitor for painful or swollen joints
   e. Evaluate blood glucose level because diabetes mellitus may be difficult to control while on medication
5. Client education
   a. Instruct the client to take the medication with food to reduce GI distress
   b. Instruct the client to avoid sunlight or ultraviolet light until photosensitivity is determined
   c. Instruct the client to notify the physician if any side effects occur
   d. Instruct the client not to skip doses and to take the medication for the full length of the prescribed therapy
   e. Instruct the client not to take any other medication without consulting the physician
   f. Advise the client of the importance of follow-up physician visits and laboratory tests

XIII. SECOND-LINE MEDICATIONS FOR TB
A. Capreomycin sulfate (Capastat Sulfate)
   1. Description
      a. Mechanism of action is unknown
      b. Used to treat **MDR-TB** when significant resistance to other medications is expected
      c. Must be given intramuscularly

2. Contraindications and cautions
   a. The risk of nephrotoxicity, ototoxicity, and neuromuscular blockade is increased with the use of aminoglycosides or loop diuretics
   b. Use with caution in clients with renal insufficiency, acoustic nerve impairment, hepatic disorder, myasthenia gravis, or parkinsonism
   c. Do not administer to clients receiving streptomycin
3. Side effects
   a. Nephrotoxicity
   b. Ototoxicity
   c. Neuromuscular blockade
4. Interventions
   a. Perform baseline audiometric testing
   b. Check renal, hepatic, and electrolyte levels before administration
   c. Monitor I&O
   d. Reconstituted medication may be stored for 48 hours at room temperature
   e. Administer deep intramuscular in a large muscle mass
   f. Rotate injection sites
   g. Observe injection site for redness, excessive bleeding, and inflammation
5. Client education
   a. Instruct the client not to perform tasks that require mental alertness
   b. Instruct the client to report any hearing loss, balance disturbances, respiratory difficulty, weakness, or signs of hypersensitivity reactions

B. Kanamycin (Kantrex)
1. Description
   a. An aminoglycoside antibiotic that is used in conjunction with at least one other antitubercular medication
   b. Bactericidal, because of receptor-binding action, interfering with protein synthesis in susceptible microorganisms
2. Contraindications and cautions
   a. Contraindicated in clients with hypersensitivity, neuromuscular disorders, or eighth cranial nerve damage
   b. Use with caution in the older client, in neonates because of renal insufficiency and immaturity, and in young infants because it may cause CNS depression
   c. The risk of toxicity increases when taken with other aminoglycosides or nephrotoxicity- or ototoxicity-producing medications
3. Side effects
   a. Hypersensitivity
   b. Pain and irritation at the injection site
   c. Nephrotoxicity, as evidenced by increased blood urea nitrogen (BUN) and serum creatinine levels
   d. Ototoxicity, as evidenced by tinnitus, dizziness, ringing or roaring in the ears, and reduced hearing

e. Neurotoxicity, as evidenced by headache, dizziness, lethargy, tremors, and visual disturbances
   f. Superinfections
4. Interventions
   a. Monitor for hypersensitivity
   b. Monitor for ototoxic, neurotoxic, and nephrotoxic reactions
   c. Monitor liver and renal function tests
   d. Perform baseline audiometric testing and repeat every 1 to 2 months, because the medication impairs the eighth cranial nerve
   e. Monitor hearing acuity
   f. Monitor for visual changes
   g. Monitor hydration status and maintain adequate hydration during therapy
   h. Monitor I&O
   i. Check urinalysis results
   j. Monitor for superinfection
5. Client education
   a. Instruct the client not to skip doses and to take medication for the full length of the prescribed therapy
   b. Instruct the client not to take any other medication without consulting the physician
   c. Advise the client of the importance of follow-up physician visits and laboratory tests
   d. Instruct the client to notify the physician if hearing loss, changes in vision, or urinary problems occur

C. Ethionamide (Trecator-SC)
1. Description
   a. Mechanism of action is unknown
   b. Used to treat **MDR-TB** when significant resistance to other medications is expected
2. Contraindications and cautions
   a. Contraindicated in clients with hypersensitivity
   b. Use with caution in clients with diabetes mellitus or renal dysfunction
3. Side effects
   a. Anorexia, nausea, vomiting
   b. Metallic taste in the mouth
   c. Orthostatic hypotension
   d. Jaundice
   e. Mental changes
   f. Peripheral neuritis
   g. Rash
4. Interventions
   a. Monitor liver and renal function tests
   b. Monitor glucose level in the client with diabetes mellitus
   c. Administer pyridoxine as prescribed to reduce the risk of neurotoxicity
5. Client education
   a. Instruct the client to take medication with food or meals to minimize GI irritation
   b. Instruct the client to change positions slowly

c. Instruct the client to report signs of a rash, which can progress to exfoliative dermatitis if the medication is not discontinued

d. Instruct the client to avoid alcohol

e. Instruct the client to report signs of jaundice and other side effects of the medication if they occur

D. Aminosalicylate sodium

1. Description
   a. Inhibits folic acid metabolism in mycobacteria
   b. Used to treat **MDR-TB** when significant resistance to other medications is expected

2. Contraindications and cautions
   a. Contraindicated with hypersensitivity to aminosalicylates, salicylates, or compounds containing para-aminophenyl group
   b. Aminobenzoates block the absorption of aminosalicylate sodium

3. Side effects
   a. Hypersensitivity
   b. Bitter taste in the mouth
   c. GI tract irritation
   d. Exfoliative dermatitis
   e. Blood dyscrasias
   f. Crystalluria
   g. Changes in thyroid function

4. Interventions
   a. Monitor for hypersensitivity
   b. Offer clear water to rinse the mouth and chewing gum or hard candy to alleviate the bitter taste
   c. Encourage fluid intake to prevent crystalluria
   d. Monitor I&O

5. Client education
   a. Instruct the client to discard the medication if a purplish-brown discoloration occurs
   b. Instruct the client to take the medication with food or antacid
   c. Inform the client that urine may turn red on contact with hypochlorite bleach if bleach was used to clean a toilet
   d. Instruct the client not to take aspirin or over-the-counter medications without the physician's approval
   e. Inform the client with diabetes mellitus that a false-positive result can occur in glucose monitoring
   f. Instruct the client to report signs of a blood dyscrasia, such as a sore throat or mouth, malaise, fatigue, bruising, or bleeding

E. Cycloserine (Seromycin)

1. Description
   a. Interferes with cell wall biosynthesis
   b. Used to treat **MDR-TB** when significant resistance to other medications is expected

2. Contraindications and cautions
   a. Use of alcohol or ethionamide (Trecator-SC) increases the risk of seizures

b. Use with caution in clients with epilepsy, depression, severe anxiety, psychosis, or renal insufficiency, or the client who uses alcohol

3. Side effects
   a. Hypersensitivity
   b. CNS reactions
   c. Neurotoxicity
   d. Seizures
   e. Congestive heart failure (CHF)
   f. Headache
   g. Vertigo
   h. Altered level of consciousness (LOC)
   i. Irritability, nervousness, anxiety
   j. Confusion
   k. Mood changes, depression, thoughts of suicide

4. Interventions
   a. Monitor level of consciousness
   b. Monitor for changes in mental status and thought processes
   c. Monitor renal and hepatic function tests
   d. Monitor serum drug level to avoid the risk of neurotoxicity; peak concentrations, measured 2 hours after dosing, should be 25 to 35 mcg/mL

5. Client education
   a. Instruct the client to take the medication after meals to prevent GI upset
   b. Instruct the client to avoid alcohol
   c. Instruct the client to report signs of a rash or signs of CNS toxicity
   d. Instruct the client to avoid driving or performing tasks that require alertness until the reaction to the medication has been determined
   e. Advise the client of the need for serum drug levels weekly, as prescribed

PRACTICE QUESTIONS

1. A nurse is preparing to administer albuterol (Proventil) to a client. The nurse checks for which of the following before and during therapy?
   1. Increased urine output
   2. Nausea and vomiting
   3. Respiratory distress
   4. Complaints of headache

2. A nurse is administering a dose of isoproterenol (Isuprel) to a client. The nurse plans to monitor for which side effect of this medication?
   1. Increased pulse and blood pressure
   2. Drowsiness
   3. Hyperglycemia
   4. Hypokalemia

3. A nurse has an order to give a client metaproterenol sulfate (Alupent), two puffs, and beclomethasone (Beconase AQ), two puffs, by metered-dose

inhaler. The nurse administers the medication by giving the:

1. Beclomethasone first and then the metaproterenol
2. Metaproterenol first and then the beclomethasone
3. Alternating a single puff of each, beginning with the beclomethasone
4. Alternating a single puff of each, beginning with the metaproterenol

4. A client has begun therapy with theophylline (Theo-Dur). The nurse tells the client to limit the intake of which of the following while taking this medication?
1. Oysters, lobster, and shrimp
2. Coffee, cola, and chocolate
3. Cottage cheese, cream cheese, and dairy creamers
4. Oranges and pineapple

5. A client with an order to take theophylline (Slo-bid) daily has been given medication instructions by the nurse. The nurse determines that the client needs further information about the medication if the client states that he or she will:
1. Avoid changing brands of the medication without physician approval
2. Avoid over-the-counter (OTC) cough and cold medications unless approved by the physician
3. Drink at least 2 L fluid per day
4. Take the daily dose at bedtime

6. A client is taking brompheniramine maleate (Dimetane). The nurse checks for which of the following side effects of this medication?
1. Excitability
2. Drowsiness
3. Excess salivation
4. Diarrhea

7. A client taking brompheniramine maleate (Dimetane) is scheduled for allergy skin testing and tells the nurse in the physician's office that a dose was taken this morning. The nurse determines that:
1. A lower dose of allergen will need to be injected
2. A higher dose of allergen will need to be injected
3. The client should have the skin test read a day later than usual
4. The client should reschedule the appointment

8. A client is receiving acetylcysteine (Mucomyst), 20% solution diluted in 0.9% normal saline by nebulizer. The nurse should have which item available for possible use after giving this medication?
1. Suction equipment
2. Nasogastric tube
3. Intubation tray
4. Ambu bag

9. A nurse is assisting to administer acetylcysteine (Mucomyst) to a client admitted with acetaminophen (Tylenol) overdose. Before giving this medication, the nurse would ensure that the:
1. Client knows how to use a nebulizer
2. Antidote to acetaminophen is readily available

3. Stomach is empty from emesis or lavage
4. Solution is given full strength

10. A client has an order to take guaifenesin (Humibid) every 4 hours, as needed. The nurse determines that the client understands the most effective use of this medication if the client states that he or she will:
1. Take the tablet with a full glass of water
2. Take an extra dose if the cough is accompanied by fever
3. Watch for irritability as a side effect
4. Crush the sustained-release tablet if immediate relief is needed

11. A postoperative client has received a dose of naloxone (Narcan) for respiratory depression shortly after transfer to the nursing unit from the postanesthesia care unit. Following administration of the medication, the nurse checks the client for:
1. Pupillary changes
2. Sudden episodes of diarrhea
3. Sudden increase in pain
4. Scattered lung wheezes

12. A client with suspected narcotic overdose has received a dose of naloxone (Narcan). The client subsequently becomes restless, starts to vomit, and complains of abdominal cramping. The blood pressure increases from 110/72 to 160/86 mm Hg. The nurse provides emotional support and reassurance while administering care to the client, knowing that:
1. These effects will only last a few moments
2. These are signs of opioid withdrawal
3. The client may otherwise sign out against medical advice
4. The client may become suicidal

13. A nurse is assisting in caring for a client who is receiving a dose of naloxone (Narcan) intravenously to treat narcotic overdose. The nurse plans to have which of the following available as supportive equipment in case it is needed?
1. Nasogastric tube
2. Paracentesis tray
3. Central line insertion tray
4. Resuscitation equipment

14. A nurse is reinforcing instructions to a client about the effects of diphenhydramine (Benadryl), which has been ordered as a cough suppressant. Which statement by the client indicates the need for further instructions?
1. "I need to avoid driving or other activities requiring mental alertness while taking this medication."
2. "I need to use sugarless gum, candy, or oral rinses to decrease dry mouth."
3. "I need to avoid alcohol while taking this medication."
4. "I need to take the medication on an empty stomach."

15. A client has been taking isoniazid (INH) for 1½ months. The client complains to a nurse about numbness, paresthesias, and tingling in the extremities. The nurse interprets that the client is experiencing:
    1. Small blood vessel spasm
    2. Impaired peripheral circulation
    3. Hypercalcemia
    4. Peripheral neuritis

16. A client is to begin a 6-month course of therapy with isoniazid (INH). A nurse plans to teach the client to:
    1. Drink alcohol in small amounts only
    2. Report yellow eyes or skin immediately
    3. Increase intake of Swiss or aged cheeses
    4. Avoid vitamin supplements during therapy

17. A client has been started on long-term therapy with rifampin (Rifadin). A nurse teaches the client that the medication:
    1. Should be double-dosed if one dose is forgotten
    2. May be discontinued independently if symptoms are gone in 3 months
    3. Causes orange discoloration of sweat, tears, urine, and feces
    4. Should always be taken with food or antacids

18. A nurse has given a client taking ethambutol (Myambutol) information about the medication. The nurse determines that the client understands the instructions if the client states that he or she will immediately report:
    1. Gastrointestinal (GI) side effects
    2. Impaired sense of hearing
    3. Orange-red discoloration of body secretions
    4. Problems with visual acuity

19. Cycloserine (Seromycin) is added to the medication regimen for a client with tuberculosis. Which of the following would the nurse include in the client teaching plan regarding this medication?
    1. To take the medication before meals
    2. To return to the clinic weekly for serum drug level testing
    3. It is not necessary to call the physician if a skin rash occurs
    4. It is not necessary to restrict alcohol intake with this medication

20. A client with tuberculosis is being started on antituberculosis therapy with isoniazid (INH). Before giving the client the first dose, a nurse ensures that which of the following baseline studies has been completed?
    1. Coagulation times
    2. Electrolyte levels
    3. Serum creatinine level
    4. Liver enzyme levels

ALTERNATE FORMAT QUESTION: MULTIPLE RESPONSE

A client with chronic obstructive pulmonary disease is receiving theophylline (Theo-Dur) and the nurse is monitoring the client for side effects of the medication. Select the side effects of this medication.

____ Bradycardia

____ Restlessness

____ Headaches

____ Tremors

ANSWERS

1. *Answer:* 3

Rationale: Albuterol is a bronchodilator of the adrenergic type. The nurse checks the respiratory pattern, pulse, and blood pressure before and during therapy. The color, character and amount of sputum are also noted. Options 1, 2, and 4 are not directly related to this medication.

Test-Taking Strategy: Use the ABCs—airway, breathing, and circulation—to answer the question. Option 3 is the only option that addresses airway. Review this medication if you had difficulty with this question.

Level of Cognitive Ability: Application
Client Needs: Physiological Integrity
Integrated Process: Nursing Process/Data Collection
Content Area: Pharmacology
Reference: Hodgson, B., & Kizior, R. (2005). *Saunders nursing drug handbook 2005.* Philadelphia: W.B. Saunders, p. 22.

2. *Answer:* 1

Rationale: Isoproterenol is an adrenergic bronchodilator. Side effects can include tachycardia, hypertension, chest pain, dysrhythmias, nervousness, restlessness, and headache, among others. The nurse monitors for these effects during therapy. Options 2, 3, and 4 are not side effects.

Test-Taking Strategy: Use the process of elimination, recalling that this medication is a bronchodilator. Remembering that tachycardia is a side effect should assist in selecting the option that identifies an increased pulse, option 1. Review the side effects of this medication if you had difficulty with this question.

Level of Cognitive Ability: Application
Client Needs: Physiological Integrity
Integrated Process: Nursing Process/Data Collection
Content Area: Pharmacology
References: Hodgson, B., & Kizior, R. (2005). *Saunders nursing drug handbook 2005.* Philadelphia: W.B. Saunders, p. 133C.

McKenry, L., & Salerno, E. (2003). *Mosby's pharmacology in nursing* (21st ed.). St. Louis: Mosby, p. 467.

3. Answer: 2
Rationale: Metaproterenol is a bronchodilator. Beclomethasone is a glucocorticoid. Bronchodilators are always administered before glucocorticoids, when both are to be given on the same time schedule. This allows for widening of the air passages by the bronchodilator, which then makes the glucocorticoid more effective.
Test-Taking Strategy: To answer this question correctly, it is necessary to know two different things. First, you must know that a bronchodilator is always given before a glucocorticoid. This would allow you to eliminate options 3 and 4, because you would not alternate the medications. To select between options 1 and 2, it is necessary to know that metaproterenol is a bronchodilator, whereas beclomethasone is a glucocorticoid. Review these medications if you had difficulty with this question.
Level of Cognitive Ability: Application
Client Needs: Physiological Integrity
Integrated Process: Nursing Process/Implementation
Content Area: Pharmacology
Reference: McKenry, L., & Salerno, E. (2003). *Mosby's pharmacology in nursing* (21st ed.). St. Louis: Mosby, pp. 705-706.

4. Answer: 2
Rationale: Theophylline is a xanthine bronchodilator. The nurse teaches the client to limit the intake of xanthine-containing foods while taking this medication. These include coffee, cola, and chocolate.
Test-Taking Strategy: Focus on the name of the medication to determine that theophylline is a xanthine bronchodilator. Recalling which food items are naturally high in xanthines will direct you to option 2. Review the foods naturally high in xanthines if you had difficulty with this question.
Level of Cognitive Ability: Application
Client Needs: Health Promotion and Maintenance
Integrated Process: Nursing Process/Implementation
Content Area: Pharmacology
Reference: McKenry, L., & Salerno, E. (2003). *Mosby's pharmacology in nursing* (21st ed.). St. Louis: Mosby, p. 724.

5. Answer: 4
Rationale: The client taking a single daily dose of theophylline, a xanthine bronchodilator, should take the medication early in the morning. This enables the client to have maximal benefit from the medication during daytime activities. Additionally, this medication causes insomnia. The client should take in at least 2 L of fluid per day to decrease viscosity of secretions. The client should check with the physician before changing brands of the medication. The client also checks with the physician before taking OTC cough, cold, or other respiratory preparations because they could cause interactive effects, increasing the side effects of theophylline and causing dysrhythmias.
Test-Taking Strategy: Use the process of elimination. Note the key words, *needs further information*. These words indicate a false response question and that you need to select the

incorrect client statement. General principles related to medication therapy will assist in eliminating options 1 and 2. Additionally, recalling that option 3 is an important measure to thin secretions will direct you to option 4. Review this medication if you had difficulty with this question.
Level of Cognitive Ability: Analysis
Client Needs: Health Promotion and Maintenance
Integrated Process: Teaching/Learning
Content Area: Pharmacology
Reference: McKenry, L., & Salerno, E. (2003). *Mosby's pharmacology in nursing* (21st ed.). St. Louis: Mosby, pp. 723-724.

6. Answer: 2
Rationale: A frequent side effect of brompheniramine, an antihistamine, is drowsiness or sedation. Others include blurred vision, hypertension (and sometimes hypotension), dry mouth, constipation, urinary retention, and sweating.
Test-Taking Strategy: Focus on the name of the medication to determine that this medication is an antihistamine. Recalling that antihistamines typically cause drowsiness will direct you to option 2. Review the side effects of antihistamines if you had difficulty with this question.
Level of Cognitive Ability: Application
Client Needs: Physiological Integrity
Integrated Process: Nursing Process/Data Collection
Content Area: Pharmacology
Reference: McKenry, L., & Salerno, E. (2003). *Mosby's pharmacology in nursing* (21st ed.). St. Louis: Mosby, p. 225.

7. Answer: 4
Rationale: Brompheniramine is an antihistamine, which provides relief of symptoms caused by allergy. Antihistamines should be discontinued for at least 3 days (72 hours) before allergy skin testing to avoid false negative readings. This client should have the appointment rescheduled for 3 days after discontinuing the medication.
Test-Taking Strategy: Focus on the name of the medication to determine that this medication is an antihistamine. It is also necessary to know that antihistamines reduce the allergic response. With this in mind, option 1 is eliminated first, because it makes no sense. Options 2 and 3 are also eliminated, because the medication would still interfere with the test results. Review this medication if you had difficulty with this question.
Level of Cognitive Ability: Analysis
Client Needs: Physiological Integrity
Integrated Process: Nursing Process/Planning
Content Area: Pharmacology
Reference: McKenry, L., & Salerno, E. (2003). *Mosby's pharmacology in nursing* (21st ed.). St. Louis: Mosby, p. 227.

8. Answer: 1
Rationale: Acetylcysteine can be given orally or by nasogastric tube to treat acetaminophen overdose, or it may be given by inhalation for use as a mucolytic. The nurse administering this medication as a mucolytic should have suction equipment available in case the client cannot manage to clear the increased volume of liquefied secretions.
Test-Taking Strategy: To answer this question, it is necessary to know that acetylcysteine may be given for either acetaminophen

overdose or as a mucolytic agent. It is also necessary to know that the inhalation route is only used for mucolytic effects. With this in mind, options 3 and 4 are eliminated because the client does not need resuscitation. Option 2 is eliminated also, because a nasogastric tube may be used in the client with acetaminophen overdose. If you had difficulty with this question, review the purpose of this medication and the related nursing interventions.
Level of Cognitive Ability: Application
Client Needs: Physiological Integrity
Integrated Process: Nursing Process/Implementation
Content Area: Pharmacology
Reference: Skidmore-Roth, L. (2005). *Mosby's drug guide for nurses* (6th ed.). St. Louis: Mosby, p. 10.

9. *Answer:* **3**
Rationale: Acetylcysteine can be given orally or by nasogastric tube to treat acetaminophen overdose, or it may be given by inhalation for use as a mucolytic. Prior to giving the medication as an antidote to acetaminophen, the nurse ensures that the client's stomach is empty through emesis or gastric lavage. The solution is diluted in cola, water, or juice to make the solution more palatable. It is then administered orally or by nasogastric tube.
Test-Taking Strategy: Use the process of elimination. Begin to answer this question by eliminating options 1 and 2. This medication is not given by the inhalation route to treat acetaminophen overdose, and acetylcysteine is the antidote (to acetaminophen). To select between the remaining options, remember that the solution must be diluted and that the stomach must be emptied for maximal effect of the antidote. Review this medication if you had difficulty with this question.
Level of Cognitive Ability: Application
Client Needs: Physiological Integrity
Integrated Process: Nursing Process/Implementation
Content Area: Pharmacology
Reference: Skidmore-Roth, L. (2005). *Mosby's drug guide for nurses* (6th ed.). St. Louis: Mosby, p. 10.

10. *Answer:* **1**
Rationale: Guaifenesin is an expectorant. It should be taken with a full glass of water to decrease viscosity of secretions. Sustained-release preparations should not be broken open, crushed, or chewed. The medication may occasionally cause dizziness, headache, or drowsiness as side effects. The client should contact the physician if the cough lasts longer than 1 week or is accompanied by fever, rash, sore throat, or persistent headache.
Test-Taking Strategy: Use the process of elimination. Begin to answer this question by eliminating option 4 first. Sustained-released preparations are not crushed or broken. Option 2 is eliminated next, because fever indicates infection, and an "extra dose" of an expectorant is not helpful in treating infection. From the remaining options, recalling that increased fluids helps liquefy secretions for more effective coughing will direct you to option 1. Review this medication if you had difficulty with this question.
Level of Cognitive Ability: Analysis
Client Needs: Health Promotion and Maintenance
Integrated Process: Nursing Process/Evaluation

Content Area: Pharmacology
Reference: Skidmore-Roth, L. (2005). *Mosby's drug guide for nurses* (6th ed.). St. Louis: Mosby, p. 410.

11. *Answer:* **3**
Rationale: Naloxone is an antidote to opioids, and may also be given to the postoperative client to treat respiratory depression. When given to the postoperative client for respiratory depression, it may also reverse the effects of analgesics. Therefore, the nurse must check the client for a sudden increase in the level of pain experienced. Options 1, 2, and 4 are not associated with this medication.
Test-Taking Strategy: Use the process of elimination. Recalling that this medication is an antidote to narcotic analgesics will assist in directing you to option 3. Remember that this medication will cause sudden pain in the postoperative client or return of pain in the client who received narcotic analgesics. If you had difficulty with this question, review this medication.
Level of Cognitive Ability: Application
Client Needs: Physiological Integrity
Integrated Process: Nursing Process/Data Collection
Content Area: Pharmacology
Reference: Hodgson, B., & Kizior, R. (2005). *Saunders nursing drug handbook 2005.* Philadelphia: W.B. Saunders, p. 749.

12. *Answer:* **2**
Rationale: Signs of opioid withdrawal include increased temperature and blood pressure, abdominal cramping, vomiting, and restlessness. They can occur at any time, from a few minutes to a few hours after administration of naloxone, depending on the opioid involved, the degree of dependence, and the dose of naloxone. Options 1, 3, and 4 are incorrect interpretations.
Test-Taking Strategy: Use the process of elimination. Eliminate option 1 first, because the symptoms identified in the question are not likely to disappear in a few moments. Option 4 is eliminated next, because there is no supporting information in the question. From the remaining options, knowing that the client with narcotic overdose may have a history of prior chronic use will direct you to option 2. Review the signs of opioid withdrawal if you had difficulty with this question.
Level of Cognitive Ability: Analysis
Client Needs: Psychosocial Integrity
Integrated Process: Nursing Process/Implementation
Content Area: Pharmacology
Reference: Hodgson, B., & Kizior, R. (2005). *Saunders nursing drug handbook 2005.* Philadelphia: W.B. Saunders, p. 749.

13. *Answer:* **4**
Rationale: The nurse should have resuscitation equipment readily available to support naloxone therapy, if it is needed. Other adjuncts that may be needed include oxygen, a mechanical ventilator, and emergency medications.
Test-Taking Strategy: Use the process of elimination and note the key words, *narcotic overdose.* Recalling the effects of narcotics will direct you to option 4. Also, note that option 4 is the umbrella (global) option. Review care of the client receiving naloxone if you had difficulty with this question.

Level of Cognitive Ability: Application
Client Needs: Physiological Integrity
Integrated Process: Nursing Process/Planning
Content Area: Pharmacology
Reference: Skidmore-Roth, L. (2005). *Mosby's drug guide for nurses* (6th ed.). St. Louis: Mosby, p. 600.

14. Answer: 4
Rationale: Diphenhydramine has several uses, including as an antihistamine, antitussive, antidyskinetic, and sedative/hypnotic. Instructions for use include taking the medication with food or milk to decrease gastrointestinal upset and to use oral rinses, sugarless gum, or hard candy to minimize dry mouth. Because the medication causes drowsiness, the client should avoid the use of alcohol or central nervous system depressants, operating a car, or engaging in other activities requiring mental acuity during use.
Test-Taking Strategy: Use the process of elimination and note the key words, *need for further instructions*. These words indicate a false response question and that you need to select the incorrect client statement. Knowing that the medication has a sedative effect helps you eliminate options 1 and 3 first. Next, recalling that the medication causes dry mouth helps you eliminate option 2. If you had difficulty with this question, review the client teaching points related to this medication.
Level of Cognitive Ability: Analysis
Client Needs: Health Promotion and Maintenance
Integrated Process: Teaching/Learning
Content Area: Pharmacology
Reference: McKenry, L., & Salerno, E. (2003). *Mosby's pharmacology in nursing* (21st ed.). St. Louis: Mosby, p. 743.

15. Answer: 4
Rationale: A common side effect of INH is peripheral neuritis. This is manifested by numbness, tingling, and paresthesias in the extremities. This side effect can be minimized by pyridoxine (vitamin B_6) intake. Options 1, 2, and 3 are incorrect.
Test-Taking Strategy: Use the process of elimination. Options 1 and 2 would not cause the symptoms presented in the question, but instead would cause pallor and coolness. From the remaining options, you should know either that peripheral neuritis is a side effect of the medication or that these signs and symptoms do not correlate with hypercalcemia. Review the side effects associated with INH if you had difficulty with this question.
Level of Cognitive Ability: Analysis
Client Needs: Physiological Integrity
Integrated Process: Nursing Process/Data Collection
Content Area: Pharmacology
Reference: Kee, J., & Hayes, E. (2003). *Pharmacology: A nursing process approach* (4th ed.). Philadelphia: W.B. Saunders, pp. 435-436.

16. Answer: 2
Rationale: INH is hepatotoxic, and therefore the client is taught to report signs and symptoms of hepatitis immediately (which include yellow skin and sclera). For the same reason, alcohol should be avoided during therapy. The client should avoid intake of Swiss cheese, fish such as tuna, and foods containing tyramine because they may cause a reaction characterized by redness and itching of the skin, flushing, sweating, tachycardia, headache, or lightheadedness. The client can avoid developing peripheral neuritis by increasing the intake of pyridoxine (vitamin B_6) during the course of INH therapy.
Test-Taking Strategy: Use the process of elimination. Alcohol intake is prohibited with the use of many medications, so option 1 should be eliminated first. Because the client receiving this medication typically is supplemented with vitamin B_6, option 4 is incorrect and is eliminated next. From the remaining options, recalling that the medication is hepatotoxic will direct you to option 2. If you had difficulty with this question, review this medication.
Level of Cognitive Ability: Application
Client Needs: Physiological Integrity
Integrated Process: Teaching/Learning
Content Area: Pharmacology
Reference: Hodgson, B., & Kizior, R. (2004). *Saunders nursing drug handbook 2004*. Philadelphia: W.B. Saunders, p. 560.

17. Answer: 3
Rationale: Rifampin should be taken exactly as directed. Doses should not be doubled or skipped. The client should not stop therapy until directed to do so by a physician. The medication should be administered on an empty stomach unless it causes gastrointestinal upset, and then it may be taken with food. Antacids, if prescribed, should be taken at least 1 hour before the medication. Rifampin causes orange-red discoloration of body secretions and will permanently stain soft contact lenses.
Test-Taking Strategy: Use the process of elimination. Use of general medication administration principles will assist in eliminating options 1 and 2. Eliminate option 4 next because of the absolute word "always." If you had difficulty with this question, review the side effects associated with this medication.
Level of Cognitive Ability: Application
Client Needs: Physiological Integrity
Integrated Process: Teaching/Learning
Content Area: Pharmacology
Reference: Kee, J., & Hayes, E. (2003). *Pharmacology: A nursing process approach* (4th ed.). Philadelphia: W.B. Saunders, p. 436.

18. Answer: 4
Rationale: Ethambutol causes optic neuritis, which decreases visual acuity and the ability to discriminate between the colors red and green. This poses a potential safety hazard when a client is driving a motor vehicle. The client is taught to report this symptom immediately. The client is also taught to take the medication with food if GI upset occurs. Impaired hearing results from antitubercular therapy with streptomycin. Orange-red discoloration of secretions occurs with rifampin (Rifadin).
Test-Taking Strategy: Use the process of elimination. Option 1 is the least likely symptom to report; rather, it should be managed by taking the medication with food. To select from the other options, it is necessary to know that this

medication causes optic neuritis, resulting in difficulty with red-green discrimination. If this question was difficult, review antitubercular medications, because incorrect options for this question are typical side effects of other antitubercular medications.
Level of Cognitive Ability: Analysis
Client Needs: Physiological Integrity
Integrated Process: Nursing Process/Evaluation
Content Area: Pharmacology
Reference: Hodgson, B., & Kizior, R. (2004). *Saunders nursing drug handbook 2004.* Philadelphia: W.B. Saunders, pp. 388, 389.

19. *Answer: 2*
Rationale: Cycloserine (Seromycin) is an antitubercular medication that requires weekly serum drug level determinations to monitor for the potential of neurotoxicity. Serum drug levels lower than 30 mg/mL reduce the incidence of neurotoxicity. The medication needs to be taken after meals to prevent gastrointestinal irritation. The client needs to be instructed to notify the physician if a skin rash or signs of central nervous system toxicity are noted. Alcohol needs to be avoided because it increases the risk of seizure activity.
Test-Taking Strategy: Use the process of elimination. Eliminate options 3 and 4 first, using guidelines related to general medication administration principles. From this point, knowing that the medication level needs to be monitored will assist in selecting the correct option. If you had difficulty with this question, review this medication.
Level of Cognitive Ability: Application
Client Needs: Physiological Integrity
Integrated Process: Teaching/Learning
Content Area: Pharmacology
Reference: Kee, J., & Hayes, E. (2003). *Pharmacology: A nursing process approach* (4th ed.). Philadelphia: W.B. Saunders, p. 435.

20. *Answer: 4*
Rationale: INH therapy can cause an elevation of hepatic enzyme levels and hepatitis. Therefore, liver enzyme levels are monitored when therapy is initiated and during the first 3 months of therapy. They may be monitored longer in the client who is over age 50 or abuses alcohol.

Test-Taking Strategy: Use the process of elimination. In order to answer this question correctly, it is necessary to know that this medication can be toxic to the liver. Review the adverse effects of the various antitiberculosis medications if this is an area that is unfamiliar to you.
Level of Cognitive Ability: Analysis
Client Needs: Physiological Integrity
Integrated Process: Nursing Process/Data Collection
Content Area: Pharmacology
Reference: Kee, J., & Hayes, E. (2003). *Pharmacology: A nursing process approach* (4th ed.). Philadelphia: W.B. Saunders, p. 433.

ALTERNATE FORMAT QUESTION: MULTIPLE RESPONSE
Answers:
Restlessness
Headaches
Tremors
Rationale: Theophylline (Theo-Dur) is a xanthine bronchodilator that dilates the airways of the respiratory tree and relaxes the smooth muscles of the bronchi. Xanthine bronchodilators stimulate the central nervous system and respiratory sytem, dilate coronary and pulmonary vessels, causing diuresis, and relax smooth muscle. Side effects include palpitations and tachycardia, dysrhythmias, restlessness, nervousness, tremors, and gastrointestinal effects such as anorexia, nausea, and vomiting. Other side effects include headaches and dizziness.
Test-Taking Strategy: Note the type of medication that the client is receiving. Recalling the action of a xanthine bronchodilator will assist in determining the side effects. Review the side effects of a xanthine bronchodilator if you had difficulty with this question.
Level of Cognitive Ability: Analysis
Client Needs: Physiological Integrity
Integrated Process: Nursing Process/Data Collection
Content Area: Pharmacology
Reference: *Mosby's 2005 drug consult for nurses.* (2005). St. Louis: Mosby, p. 1389.

REFERENCES

Hodgson, B., & Kizior, R. (2004). *Saunders nursing drug handbook 2004.* Philadelphia: W.B. Saunders.
Hodgson, B., & Kizior, R. (2005). *Saunders nursing drug handbook 2005.* Philadelphia: W.B. Saunders.
Kee, J., & Hayes, E. (2003). *Pharmacology: A nursing process approach* (4th ed.). Philadelphia: W.B. Saunders.

McKenry, L., & Salerno, E. (2003). *Mosby's pharmacology in nursing* (21st ed.). St. Louis: Mosby.
Mosby's 2005 drug consult for nurses. (2005). St. Louis: Mosby.
Skidmore-Roth, L. (2005). *Mosby's drug guide for nurses* (6th ed.). St. Louis: Mosby.

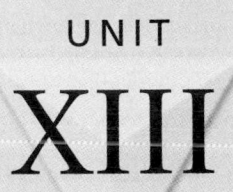

The Adult Client with a Cardiovascular Disorder

PYRAMID TERMS

arterial anastomosis Ensures that when one of the blood-supplying arteries is damaged, flow is maintained from the other arteries. Blood flow to the hands, feet, brain, and other organs is protected by arterial anastomosis.

blood pressure (BP) Measures the force exerted by the blood against the walls of the blood vessels. If the BP falls too low, blood flow to the tissues, heart, brain, and other organs become inadequate. If the BP becomes too high, the risk of vessel rupture and damage increases.

cardiac output The total volume of blood pumped through the heart in 1 minute. The normal cardiac output is 4 to 8 L/minute; cardiac output = stroke volume × heart rate.

contractility Refers to the inherent ability of the myocardium to alter contractile force and velocity. Sympathetic stimulation increases myocardial contractility, thus increasing stroke volume. Conditions that decrease myocardial contractility reduce stroke volume.

diastole The phase of the cardiac cycle in which the heart relaxes between contractions. It represents the period of time when the two ventricles are dilated by the blood flowing into them.

diastolic pressure The force of the blood exerted against the artery walls when the heart relaxes or fills.

postural (orthostatic) hypotension A blood pressure decrease of more than 10 to 15 mm Hg of the systolic pressure or a decrease of more than 10 mm Hg of the diastolic pressure and a 10% to 20% increase in heart rate; occurs when the client's blood pressure is not adequately maintained when moving from a lying to a sitting or standing position.

pulse pressure The difference between the systolic and diastolic pressures; normal pulse pressure is 30 to 40 mm Hg.

systole The phase of contraction of the heart, especially of the ventricles, during which blood is forced into the aorta and pulmonary artery.

systolic pressure The maximum pressure of blood exerted against the artery walls when the heart contracts.

venous pressure The force exerted by the blood against the vein walls. Normal venous pressures are highest in the extremities (5 to 14 cm H_2O in the arm), and lowest closest to the heart (6 to 8 cm H_2O in the inferior vena cava).

PYRAMID TO SUCCESS

Pyramid points focus on data collection related to cardiovascular risks, health screening and promotion, complications of the various cardiovascular disorders, emergency implementation measures, and client education. Focus on the findings in angina, myocardial infarction (MI), heart failure and pulmonary edema, hypertension, and arterial and vascular disorders. Focus also on the care of the client following diagnostic treatments and surgical procedures. Note appropriate and therapeutic client positions, particularly with arterial and venous disorders of the extremities. Focus on treatments and medications prescribed for the various cardiovascular disorders and client teaching related to prescribed treatment plans. Be familiar with the components related to cardiac rehabilitation. The Integrated Processes addressed in this unit include Caring, Clinical Problem-Solving Process (Nursing Process), Communication and Documentation, and Teaching/ Learning.

CLIENT NEEDS
Safe, Effective Care Environment

Cardiovascular consultations and referrals
Client rights
Consultation with members of the health care team
Establishing priorities
Informed consent related to treatments and procedures
Medical and surgical asepsis
Standard precautions

Health Promotion and Maintenance

Alterations in lifestyle
Cardiac rehabilitation
Cardiovascular data collection techniques
Health screening and health promotion programs

Mobilization of appropriate community resources

Prevention of cardiovascular disease

Teaching related to diet therapy, exercise, and medications

Psychosocial Integrity

Accepting lifestyle changes

Coping mechanisms

End-of-life issues

Fear, anxiety, and denial

Grief and loss

Religious, spiritual, and cultural influences on health

Situational role changes

Support systems

Unexpected body image changes

Physiological Integrity

Assisting with basic care measures

Activity limitations and rest and sleep

Interventions required in emergencies

Medical emergencies

Monitoring cardiac enzymes, troponin levels, and laboratory values related to the cardiovascular system

Monitoring for complications related to cardiovascular disorders

Monitoring for therapeutic effects of medications

Nonpharmacological and pharmacological comfort interventions

REFERENCES

Black, J., & Hawks, J. (2005). *Medical-surgical nursing: Clinical management for positive outcomes* (7th ed.). Philadelphia: W.B. Saunders.

Chernecky, C., & Berger, B. (2004). *Laboratory tests and diagnostic procedures* (4th ed.). Philadelphia: W.B. Saunders.

Christensen, B., & Kockrow, E. (2003). *Adult health nursing* (4th ed.). St. Louis: Mosby.

Christensen, B., & Kockrow, E. (2003). *Foundations of nursing* (4th ed.). St. Louis: Mosby.

Fortinash, K., & Holoday-Worret, P. (2004). *Psychiatric mental health nursing* (3rd ed.). St. Louis: Mosby.

Harkreader, H., & Hogan, M.A. (2004). *Fundamentals of nursing: Caring and clinical judgment.* (2nd ed.). Philadelphia: W.B. Saunders.

Hodgson, B., & Kizior, R. (2005). *Saunders nursing drug handbook 2005.* Philadelphia: W.B. Saunders.

Lewis, S., Heitkemper, M., & Dirksen, S. (2004). *Medical-surgical nursing: Assessment and management of clinical problems* (6th ed.). St. Louis: Mosby.

Linton, A., & Maebius, N. (2003). *Introduction to medical-surgical nursing* (3rd ed.). Philadelphia: W.B. Saunders.

McKenry, L., & Salerno, E. (2003). *Mosby's pharmacology in nursing* (21st ed.). St. Louis: Mosby.

National Council of State Boards of Nursing. (2005). *Detailed test plan for the National council licensure examination for practical/vocational nurses.* Chicago: Author.

Pagana, K., & Pagana, T. (2003). *Mosby's diagnostic and laboratory test reference* (6th ed.). St. Louis: Mosby.

Perry, A., & Potter, P. (2002). *Clinical nursing skills and techniques* (5th ed.). St. Louis: Mosby.

Phipps, W., Monahan, F., Sands, J., Marek, J., & Neighbors, M. (2003). *Medical-surgical nursing: Health and illness perspectives* (7th ed.). St. Louis: Mosby.

Potter, P., & Perry, A. (2003). *Essentials for practice* (5th ed.). St. Louis: Mosby.

Cardiovascular System

I. ANATOMY AND PHYSIOLOGY

A. Heart and heart layers
1. The heart is located in the left side of the mediastinum
2. The epicardium covers the outer surface of the heart
3. The myocardium is the middle layer and is the actual contracting muscle of the heart
4. The endocardium is the innermost layer and lines the inner chambers and heart valves

B. Pericardium
1. The pericardium encases and protects the heart from trauma and infection
2. The parietal pericardium is the tough, fibrous outer membrane that attaches anteriorly to the lower half of the sternum, posteriorly to the thoracic vertebrae, and inferiorly to the diaphragm
3. The visceral pericardium is the thin inner layer that closely adheres to the heart
4. The pericardial space is between the parietal and visceral layers; it holds 5 to 20 mL of pericardial fluid, which lubricates the pericardial surfaces and cushions the heart

C. Heart chambers
1. The right atrium receives deoxygenated blood from the body via the superior and inferior vena cava
2. The right ventricle receives blood from the right atrium and pumps it to the lungs via the pulmonary artery
3. The left atrium receives oxygenated blood from the lungs via four pulmonary veins
4. The left ventricle is the largest and most muscular chamber; it receives oxygenated blood from the lungs via the left atrium and pumps blood into the systemic circulation via the aorta

D. Heart valves
1. The atrioventricular (AV) valves lie between the atria and the ventricles
2. The AV valves close at the beginning of ventricular contraction and prevent blood from flowing back into the atria from the ventricles; these valves open when the ventricle relaxes
3. The bicuspid or mitral valve is located on the left side of the heart
4. The tricuspid valve is located on the right side of the heart
5. The pulmonic semilunar valve lies between the right ventricle and the pulmonary artery
6. The aortic semilunar valve lies between the left ventricle and the aorta
7. The semilunar valves prevent blood from flowing back into the ventricles during relaxation; they open during ventricular contraction and close when the ventricles begin to relax.

E. Atrioventricular (AV) node
1. The AV node is located in the lower aspect of the atrial septum
2. The AV node receives electrical impulses from the sinoatrial (SA) node

F. The bundle of His (AV bundle)
1. The bundle of His fuses with the AV node to form another pacemaker site
2. It branches into the right bundle branch (RBB), which extends down the right side of the interventricular septum, and the left bundle branch (LBB), which extends into the left ventricle
3. The right and left bundle branches terminate in Purkinje fibers
4. If the SA node fails, the bundle of His can initiate and sustain the heart rate at 40 to 60 beats per minute

G. Purkinje fibers
 1. Purkinje fibers are a diffuse network of conducting strands located beneath the ventricular endocardium
 2. These fibers spread the wave of depolarization through the ventricles
H. Coronary arteries: supply the capillaries of the myocardium with blood (Box 50-1)
I. Sinoatrial (SA) node
 1. The SA node or pacemaker initiates each heart beat
 2. It is located at the junction of the superior vena cava and the right atrium
 3. It generates electrical impulses approximately 60 to 100 times per minute; controlled by the sympathetic and parasympathetic systems
J. Heart sounds
 1. The first heart sound (S_1) is heard as the AV valves close
 2. The second heart sound (S_2) is heard when the semilunar valves close
K. Heart rate (Box 50-2)
 1. The faster the heart rate, the less time the heart has for filling, and the **cardiac output** decreases
 2. An increase in heart rate increases oxygen consumption
L. Autonomic nervous system
 1. Stimulation of sympathetic nerve fibers releases the neurotransmitter norepinephrine, producing an increased heart rate, increased conduction speed through the AV node, increased atrial and ventricular **contractility**, and peripheral

vasoconstriction; stimulation occurs when a decrease in pressure is detected
 2. Stimulation of the parasympathetic nerve fibers releases the neurotransmitter acetylcholine, which decreases the heart rate and lessens atrial and ventricular **contractility** and conductivity; stimulation occurs when an increase in pressure is detected
M. Blood pressure control
 1. Baroreceptors, also called pressoreceptors, are located in the walls of the aortic arch and carotid sinuses
 2. Baroreceptors are specialized nerve endings that are affected by changes in the arterial blood pressure
 3. Increases in arterial pressure stimulate baroreceptors, and the heart rate and arterial pressure decrease
 4. Decreases in arterial pressure reduce stimulation of the baroreceptors, and vasoconstriction occurs, as does an increase in heart rate
 5. Stretch receptors, located in the vena cava and the right atrium, respond to pressure changes that affect circulatory blood volume
 6. When the **blood pressure** decreases as a result of hypovolemia, a sympathetic response occurs, causing an increased heart rate and blood vessel constriction; when the **blood pressure** increases as a result of hypervolemia, an opposite effect occurs
 7. Antidiuretic hormone (ADH) influences **blood pressure** indirectly by regulating vascular volume
 8. Increases in blood volume result in decreased ADH release, increasing diuresis and decreasing blood volume, and thus a decrease in **blood pressure**
 9. Decreases in blood volume result in increased ADH release; this promotes an increase in blood volume and thus an increase in **blood pressure**
 10. Renin, a potent vasoconstrictor, causes the **blood pressure** to increase
 11. Renin converts angiotensinogen to angiotensin I; angiotensin I is then converted to angiotensin II in the lungs
 12. Angiotensin II stimulates the release of aldosterone, which promotes water and sodium retention by the kidneys; this action increases blood volume and **blood pressure**
N. The vascular system
 1. Arteries are vessels through which the blood passes away from the heart to various parts of the body; they convey highly oxygenated blood from the left side of the heart to the tissues
 2. Arterioles control the blood flow into the capillaries
 3. Capillaries allow the exchange of fluid and nutrients between the blood and the interstitial spaces
 4. Venules receive blood from the capillary bed and move blood into the veins
 5. Veins transport deoxygenated blood from the tissues back to the heart and lungs for oxygenation

---

BOX 50-1

Coronary Arteries

Right coronary artery (RCA): Supplies the right atrium and ventricle, the inferior portion of the left ventricle, the posterior septal wall, and the SA and AV nodes

Left coronary artery (LCA): Consists of two major branches, the left anterior descending (LAD) and the circumflex arteries

LAD artery: Supplies blood to the anterior wall of the left ventricle, the anterior ventricular septum, and the apex of the left ventricle

Circumflex artery: Supplies blood to the left atrium and the lateral and posterior surfaces of the left ventricle

---

BOX 50-2

Heart Rate

The normal heart rate is 60 to 100 beats per minute.
Sinus tachycardia is a heart rate higher than 100 beats per minute.
Sinus bradycardia is a heart rate lower than 60 beats per minute.

6. Valves help return blood to the heart against the force of gravity

7. The lymphatics drain the tissues and return the tissue fluid to the blood

II. DIAGNOSTIC TESTS AND PROCEDURES
(Box 50-3)

A. Cardiac enzymes

1. CK-MB (creatine kinase, myocardial muscle)
   a. An elevation in value indicates myocardial damage
   b. An elevation occurs within 4 to 6 hours and peaks 18 to 24 hours following an acute ischemic attack
   c. Normal value is 0% to 5% of total; total CK is 26 to 174 units/L

2. Lactic dehydrogenase (LDH)
   a. Elevations in LDH level occur 24 hours following myocardial infarction and peak in 48 to 72 hours
   b. When the serum concentration of LDH_1 is higher than that for LDH_2, the pattern is indicated as "flipped," signifying myocardial necrosis
   c. Normal value in conventional units is 140 to 280 international units/L

3. Troponin
   a. Composed of three proteins: cardiac troponin, troponin I, and troponin T
   b. Troponin I, especially, has a high affinity for myocardial injury; its level increases within 3 hours and persists for up to 7 days

c. Normal values are quite low, with troponin T levels normally ranging from 0.0 to 0.2 ng/mL and troponin I lower than 0.6 ng/mL; thus, any increase can indicate myocardial cell damage

4. Myoglobin
   a. An oxygen-binding protein found in cardiac and skeletal muscle
   b. Level rises within 1 hour after cell death, peaks in 4 to 6 hours, and returns to normal within 24 to 36 hours (and in some clients even faster)

B. Complete blood cell (CBC) count

1. The red blood cell (RBC) count decreases in rheumatic heart disease and infective endocarditis; increases in conditions characterized by inadequate tissue oxygenation

2. The white blood cell (WBC) count increases in infectious and inflammatory diseases of the heart and after myocardial infarction (MI), because large numbers of WBCs are needed to dispose of the necrotic tissue resulting from the infarction

3. An elevated hematocrit value can result from vascular volume depletion

4. Decreases in hematocrit and hemoglobin values can indicate anemia

C. Blood coagulation factors: An increase in coagulation factors can occur during and after MI, which places the client at greater risk of thrombophlebitis and development of clots into the coronary artery

D. Serum lipids

1. The lipid profile measures serum cholesterol, triglyceride, and lipoprotein levels

2. The lipid profile is used to assess the risk of developing coronary artery disease

3. The desirable range for the serum cholesterol level is lower than 200 mg/dL, with the low-density lipoprotein (LDH) cholesterol level lower than 130 mg/dL and the high-density lipoprotein (HDL) cholesterol level ranging from 30 to 70 mg/dL

E. Electrolytes

1. Potassium
   a. Hypokalemia causes increased cardiac electrical instability, ventricular dysrhythmias, and increased risk of digitalis toxicity
   b. In hypokalemia, the electrocardiogram would show flattening and inversion of the T wave, the appearance of a U wave, and sagging of the ST segment
   c. Hyperkalemia causes asystole and ventricular dysrhythmias

2. Sodium
   a. The serum sodium level decreases with the use of diuretics
   b. The serum sodium level decreases in heart failure, indicating water excess

---

BOX 50-3

Diagnostic Tests and Procedures

LABORATORY TESTS
Blood coagulation factors
Blood urea nitrogen level
Calcium, phosphorus, and magnesium levels
Cardiac enzyme levels
Chest x-ray
Complete blood cell count
Electrolyte levels
Lipid levels
Myoglobin level
Troponin levels

PROCEDURES
Cardiac catheterization
Digital subtraction angiography
Echocardiography
Exercise testing
Electrocardiography
Holter monitoring

F. Calcium
 1. Hypocalcemia can cause ventricular dysrhythmias, prolonged QT interval, and cardiac arrest
 2. Hypercalcemia can cause a shortened QT interval, AV block, tachycardia or bradycardia, digitalis hypersensitivity, and cardiac arrest
G. Phosphorus level: Phosphorus levels should be interpreted with calcium levels because the kidneys retain or excrete one electrolyte in an inverse relationship to the other
H. Magnesium
 1. A low magnesium level can cause ventricular tachycardia and fibrillation
 2. A high magnesium level can cause muscle weakness, hypotension, bradycardia, and a prolonged PR interval and wide QRS complex
I. Blood urea nitrogen (BUN): The BUN level is elevated in heart disorders that adversely affect renal circulation, such as heart failure and cardiogenic shock
J. Blood glucose: An acute cardiac episode can elevate the blood glucose level
K. Chest x-ray (radiography)
 1. Description
  a. Done to determine the size, silhouette, and position of the heart
  b. Specific pathological changes are difficult to determine via x-ray, but anatomical changes can be seen
 2. Interventions
  a. Prepare the client for x-ray, explaining the purpose and procedure
  b. Remove jewelry
L. Electrocardiography (ECG)
 1. Description: A common noninvasive diagnostic test that evaluates the heart's function by recording electrical activity
 2. Interventions
  a. Determine the client's ability to lie still; advise the client to lie still, breathe normally, and refrain from talking during the test
  b. Reassure the client that an electrical shock will not occur
  c. Document any cardiac medications the client is taking
M. Holter monitoring
 1. Description
  a. A noninvasive test in which the client wears a Holter monitor and an ECG tracing is recorded continuously over a period of 24 hours or more
  b. It identifies dysrhythmias if they occur; evaluates the effectiveness of antidysrhythmics or pacemaker therapy
 2. Interventions: Instruct the client to resume normal daily activities and to maintain a diary documenting activities and any symptoms that may develop

N. Echocardiography
 1. Description
  a. A noninvasive procedure based on the principles of ultrasound
  b. It evaluates structural and functional changes in the heart
 2. Interventions: Determine the client's ability to lie still, and advise the client to lie still, breathe normally, and refrain from talking during the test
O. Exercise testing (stress test)
 1. Description
  a. A noninvasive test that studies the heart during activity and detects and evaluates coronary artery disease
  b. Treadmill testing is the most commonly used method of stress testing
  c. Stress testing may be used in conjunction with myocardial radionuclide testing (perfusion imaging), at which point the procedure becomes invasive because a radionuclide must be injected
  d. If the client is unable to tolerate exercise, an IV infusion of dipyridamole (Persantine) is given to dilate the coronary arteries and stimulate the effect of exercise; caffeine and theophylline products are held for 12 hours before the test and calcium channel blockers and beta blockers may be held for 24 hours per physician's order
  e. Informed consent is required if a radionuclide is injected
 2. Preprocedure interventions
  a. Obtain an informed consent if required
  b. Provide adequate rest the night before the procedure
  c. Instruct the client to eat a light meal 1 to 2 hours before the procedure
  d. Instruct the client to avoid smoking, alcohol, and caffeine before the procedure
  e. Ask the physician about taking prescribed medication on the day of the procedure
  f. Instruct the client to wear nonconstrictive, comfortable clothing and supportive shoes
 3. Postprocedure interventions
  a. Instruct the client to notify the physician if any chest pain, dizziness, or shortness of breath occurs
  b. Instruct the client to avoid taking a hot bath or shower for at least 1 to 2 hours
P. Digital subtraction angiography
 1. Description
  a. Combines x-ray techniques and a computerized subtraction technique with fluoroscopy for visualization of the cardiovascular system
  b. A contrast medium (dye) is injected
 2. Preprocedure interventions
  a. Assess the client for allergy to contrast medium (dye), iodine, or seafood

b. Obtain informed consent
3. Postprocedure interventions
a. Monitor vital signs (VS)
b. Monitor injection site for bleeding or discomfort

Q. Nuclear cardiology
1. Description
a. The use of radionuclide techniques and scanning in cardiovascular assessment
b. The most common tests include technetium pyrophosphate scanning, thallium imaging, and multigated cardiac blood pool imaging (MUGA)
2. Preprocedure interventions
a. Obtain informed consent
b. Inform the client that a small amount of radioisotope will be injected, and that the radiation exposure and risks are minimal
3. Postprocedure interventions
a. Monitor vital signs (VS)
b. Monitor injection site for bleeding or discomfort
c. Inform the client that fatigue may be experienced

R. Cardiac catheterization
1. Description
a. Involves insertion of a catheter into the heart and surrounding vessels
b. Obtains information about the structure and performance of the heart valves and circulatory system
2. Preprocedure interventions
a. Obtain informed consent
b. Assess for allergies to seafood, iodine, or radiopaque dyes
c. Withhold solid food for 6 to 8 hours and liquids for 4 hours to prevent vomiting and aspiration during the procedure
d. Document the client's height and weight, because these data will be needed to determine the amount of dye to be administered
e. Document baseline vital signs, and note the quality and presence of peripheral pulses for postprocedure comparison
f. Inform the client that a local anesthetic will be administered before catheter insertion
g. Inform the client that he or she may feel fatigued because of the need to lie still and quiet on a relatively hard table for up to 2 hours
h. Inform the client that he or she may feel a fluttery feeling as the catheter passes through the heart, a flushed, warm feeling when the dye is injected, a desire to cough, and palpitations caused by heart irritability
i. Prepare insertion site by shaving and cleaning with an antiseptic solution if prescribed
j. Administer preprocedure medications if prescribed
k. Prepare the client for insertion of an intravenous (IV) line if prescribed

3. Postprocedure interventions
a. Monitor VS and cardiac rhythm for dysrhythmias at least every 30 minutes for 2 hours initially
b. Monitor for chest pain and, if dysrhythmias or chest pain occurs, the physician is notified
c. Monitor peripheral pulses and the color, warmth, and sensation of the extremity distal to the insertion site at least every 30 minutes for 2 hours initially
d. The physician is notified if the client complains of numbness and tingling, if the extremity becomes cool, pale, or cyanotic, or if loss of the peripheral pulses occurs
e. Monitor the pressure dressing for bleeding or hematoma formation
f. Apply a sandbag or compression device to the insertion site to provide additional pressure if required
g. Monitor for bleeding and, if bleeding occurs, apply pressure immediately and notify the physician
h. Monitor for hematoma and, if a hematoma develops, notify the physician
i. Keep extremity extended for 4 to 6 hours, keeping the leg straight to prevent arterial occlusion
j. Maintain strict bed rest for 6 to 12 hours; however, the client may turn from side to side; do not elevate the head of the bed more than 15 degrees
k. If the antecubital vessel was used, immobilize the arm with an arm board
l. Encourage fluids, if not contraindicated, to promote renal excretion of the dye
m. Monitor for nausea, vomiting, rash, or other signs of hypersensitivity to the dye

III. THERAPEUTIC MANAGEMENT

A. Percutaneous transluminal coronary angioplasty (PTCA)
1. Description
a. One or more arteries are dilated with a balloon catheter to open the vessel lumen and improve arterial blood flow
b. The client can experience reocclusion after the procedure; thus, the procedure may need to be repeated
c. Complications can include arterial dissection or rupture, immobilization of plaque fragments, spasm, and acute MI
d. Firm commitment is needed on the client's part to stop smoking, lose weight, alter exercise pattern, and stop any behaviors that lead to progression of artery occlusion
2. Preprocedure interventions
a. Maintain NPO status after midnight

b. Prepare the groin area with antiseptic soap and shave per institutional procedure and as prescribed

c. Check baseline VS and peripheral pulses

3. Postprocedure interventions

a. Monitor VS closely

b. Monitor distal pulses in both extremities

c. Maintain bed rest as prescribed, keeping the limb straight for 6 to 8 hours

d. Anticoagulants and antiplatelet agents may be prescribed to prevent thrombus formation

e. Intravenous nitroglycerin may be prescribed to prevent coronary artery spasm

f. Instruct the client in the administration of nitrates, calcium channel blockers, antiplatelet agents, and anticoagulants, as prescribed

g. Instruct the client to take daily aspirin permanently if prescribed

h. Assist the client with planning lifestyle modifications

B. Laser-assisted angioplasty

1. Description

a. A laser probe is advanced through a cannula similar to that used for PTCA

b. Used also for clients with small occlusions in the distal superficial femoral, proximal popliteal, and common iliac arteries

c. Heat from the laser vaporizes the plaque to open the occluded artery

2. Preprocedure and postprocedure care

a. Similar to that for PTCA

b. Monitor for complications of coronary dissection, acute occlusion, perforation, embolism, and MI

C. Coronary artery stents

1. Description

a. Used instead of PTCA to eliminate the risk of acute coronary vessel closure and to improve long-term patency of the vessel

b. A balloon catheter bearing the stent is inserted into the coronary artery and positioned at the site of occlusion

c. When placed in the coronary artery, the stent reopens the blocked artery

2. Postprocedure interventions

a. Acute thrombosis is a major concern following the procedure; the client is placed on antiplatelet and anticoagulation therapy for several months following the procedure

b. Monitor for complications of the procedure, such as stent migration or occlusion, coronary artery dissection, and bleeding resulting from anticoagulation

D. Atherectomy

1. Description

a. Removes plaque from an artery by the use of a cutting chamber on the inserted catheter or a rotating blade that pulverizes the plaque

b. Used to improve blood flow to ischemic limbs in individuals with peripheral arterial disease

2. Postprocedure interventions: Monitor for complications of perforation, embolus, and reocclusion

E. Transmyocardial revascularization

1. Used for clients with widespread atherosclerosis involving vessels that are too small and numerous for replacement or balloon catheterization

2. Uses a high-powered laser that creates 15 to 30 holes (channels) in the heart

3. Blood enters these small channels, providing the affected region of the heart with oxygenated blood

4. Performed through a small chest incision

5. The opening on the heart's surface heals over; however, the main channels remain and perfuse the myocardium

F. Arterial revascularization

1. Description

a. Performed to increase arterial blood flow to the affected limb

b. Inflow procedures involve bypassing the arterial occlusion above the superficial femoral arteries

c. Outflow procedures involve bypassing the arterial occlusions at or below the superficial femoral arteries

d. Graft material is sutured above and below the occlusion to facilitate blood flow around the occlusion

2. Preoperative interventions

a. Check baseline VS and peripheral pulses

b. Prepare the client for insertion of an IV and urinary catheter, as prescribed

c. Maintain central venous catheter and/or arterial line if inserted

3. Postoperative interventions

a. Monitor vital signs

b. Monitor the **blood pressure** and notify the physician if changes occur

c. Monitor for hypotension, which may indicate hypovolemia

d. Monitor for hypertension, which may place stress on the graft and facilitate clot formation

e. Maintain bed rest for 24 hours, as prescribed

f. Instruct the client to keep affected extremity straight, limit movement, and avoid bending the knee and hip

g. Monitor for warmth, redness, and edema, which are often expected outcomes because of increased blood flow

h. Monitor for graft occlusion, which often occurs within the first 24 hours

i. Monitor peripheral pulses and for adverse changes in color and temperature of the extremity

j. Monitor for a sharp increase in pain, because pain is frequently the first indicator of postoperative graft occlusion

k. If signs of graft occlusion occur, the physician is notified immediately

l. Encourage coughing and deep breathing and the use of incentive spirometry

m. Maintain NPO status, with progression to clear liquids, as prescribed

n. Use strict aseptic technique when in contact with the incision

o. Monitor the incision for drainage, warmth, or swelling

p. Monitor for excessive bleeding (a small amount of bloody drainage is expected)

q. Monitor the area over the graft for hardness, tenderness, and warmth, which may indicate infection; if this occurs, the physician is notified immediately

r. Instruct the client about proper foot care and measures to prevent ulcer formation

s. Instruct the client to take medications as prescribed

t. Instruct the client in how to care for incision

u. Assist the client in modifying lifestyle to prevent further plaque formation

G. Coronary artery bypass graft (CABG)

1. Description

a. The occluded coronary arteries are bypassed with the client's own venous or arterial blood vessels

b. The saphenous vein, radial artery, or internal mammary artery is used to bypass lesions in the coronary arteries

c. Performed when the client does not respond to medical management of coronary artery disease (CAD) or when disease progression is evident

2. Preoperative interventions

a. Familiarize the client and family with the cardiac surgical critical care unit

b. Instruct the client in how to splint the chest incision, cough and deep breathe, and perform arm and leg exercises

c. Instruct the client to inform the nurse of any postoperative pain, because pain medication will be available

d. Inform the client that a sternal incision, possible breast incision, arm or leg incision(s), one or two chest tubes, a Foley catheter, and several IV fluid catheters may be present

e. Inform the client that an endotracheal (ET) tube will be in place and connected to a ventilator for 6 to 24 hours

f. Advise the client to breathe with the ventilator and not fight it

g. Inform the family that the client will not be able to talk while the ET tube is in place

h. Encourage the client and family to discuss anxieties and fears related to surgery

i. Note that prescribed medications are to be discontinued preoperatively (usually diuretics 2 to 3 days before surgery, digoxin [Lanoxin] 12 hours before surgery, and aspirin and anticoagulants 1 week before surgery)

j. Administer medications as prescribed, which may include potassium chloride, antihypertensives, antidysrhythmics, and antibiotics

3. Transfer from the cardiac surgical unit

a. Monitor VS, level of consciousness (LOC), and peripheral perfusion

b. Monitor for dysrhythmias

c. Auscultate lungs and monitor respiratory status

d. Encourage the client to splint the incision, cough, deep breathe, and use incentive spirometer to raise secretions and prevent atelectasis

e. Monitor temperature and WBC count, which, if elevated after 3 to 4 days, indicates infection

f. Provide adequate fluids and hydration as prescribed to liquefy secretions

g. Monitor suture line and chest tube insertion sites for redness, purulent discharge, and signs of infection

h. Monitor sternal suture line (if present) for instability, which may indicate an infection

i. Guide the client to gradually resume activity

j. Monitor the client for tachycardia, **orthostatic hypotension**, and fatigue before, during, and after activity

k. Discontinue activities if the **BP** drops more than 10 to 20 mm Hg or if the pulse increases more than 10 beats per minute

l. Monitor episodes of pain closely

m. See Box 50-4 for home care instructions

BOX 50-4

Home Care Instructions Following Cardiac Surgery

Progress with activities at home.

Limit pushing or pulling activities for 6 weeks following discharge.

Perform incisional care and record signs of redness, swelling, or drainage.

Sternotomy incision heals in about 6 to 8 weeks.

Avoid crossing legs, wear elastic hose as prescribed until edema subsides, and elevate surgical limb when sitting in a chair.

Use prescribed medications.

Follow dietary measures, including the avoidance of saturated fats and cholesterol and the use of salt.

Sexual intercourse can be resumed on the advice of the physician after exercise tolerance is assessed; if the client can walk one block or climb two flights of stairs without symptoms, he or she can safely resume sexual activity.

H. Heart transplant
   1. A donor heart from an individual with a comparable body weight and ABO compatibility is transplanted into a recipient within less than 6 hours of procurement
   2. The surgeon removes the diseased heart, leaving the posterior portion of the atria to serve as an anchor for the new heart
   3. Because a remnant of the client's atria remains, two unrelated P waves are noted on the ECG
   4. The transplanted heart is denervated and unresponsive to vagal stimulation; because the heart is denervated, clients do not experience angina
   5. Symptoms of heart rejection include hypotension, dysrhythmias, weakness, fatigue, and dizziness
   6. Endomyocardial biopsies are performed at regular scheduled intervals and whenever rejection is suspected
   7. Clients require lifetime immunosuppressive therapy
   8. The heart rate approximates 100 beats per minute and responds slowly to exercise or stress with regard to increases in heart rate, **contractility**, and **cardiac output**

IV. MANAGEMENT OF DYSRHYTHMIAS

A. Vagal maneuvers
   1. Description: Induce vagal stimulation of the cardiac conduction system; used to terminate supraventricular tachydysrhythmias
   2. Carotid sinus massage
      a. The physician instructs the client to turn the head away from the side to be massaged
      b. The physician massages over the carotid artery for 6 to 8 seconds until there is a change in cardiac rhythm
      c. Observe the cardiac monitor for a change in rhythm
      d. Record an ECG rhythm strip before, during, and after the procedure
      e. Have a defibrillator and resuscitative equipment available
      f. Monitor VS, cardiac rhythm, and level of consciousness (LOC) following the procedure
   3. Valsalva maneuvers
      a. The physician instructs the client to bear down or induces a gag reflex in the client, both of which stimulate a vagal reflex
      b. Monitor the heart rate, rhythm, and **BP**
      c. Observe the cardiac monitor for a change in rhythm
      d. Record an ECG rhythm strip before, during, and after the procedure
      e. Provide an emesis basin if the gag reflex is stimulated, and initiate precautions to prevent aspiration

f. Have a defibrillator and resuscitative equipment available
B. Cardioversion
   1. Description
      a. Synchronized countershock to convert an undesirable rhythm to a stable rhythm
      b. An elective procedure performed by the physician
      c. A lower amount of energy is used than with defibrillation
      d. Defibrillator is synchronized to the client's R wave to avoid discharging the shock during the vulnerable period (T wave)
      e. If the defibrillator were not synchronized, it would discharge on the T wave and cause ventricular fibrillation (VF)
   2. Preprocedure interventions
      a. Obtain an informed consent
      b. Administer sedation, as prescribed
      c. Hold digoxin (Lanoxin) 48 hours preprocedure as prescribed to prevent postcardioversion ventricular irritability
   3. During the procedure
      a. Ensure that the skin is clean and dry in the area where the electrode paddles will be placed
      b. Stop the oxygen during the procedure to avoid the hazard of fire
      c. Be sure that no one is touching the bed or the client when delivering the countershock
   4. Postprocedure interventions
      a. Maintain airway patency
      b. Administer oxygen as prescribed
      c. Monitor vital signs
      d. Monitor LOC
      e. Monitor cardiac rhythm
      f. Monitor for indications of successful response, such as conversion to sinus rhythm, strong peripheral pulses, and an adequate **BP**
C. Defibrillation
   1. Description
      a. An asynchronous countershock used to terminate pulseless ventricular tachycardia (VT) or VF
      b. Three rapid consecutive shocks are delivered, with the first at an energy of 200 J (joules)
      c. If unsuccessful, the shock is repeated at 200 to 300 J
      d. The third and subsequent shock will be at 360 J
   2. During the procedure
      a. Stop the oxygen during the procedure to avoid the hazard of fire
      b. Be sure that no one is touching the bed or the client when delivering the countershock
D. Use of paddle electrodes
   1. Apply conductive pads
   2. One paddle is placed at the third intercostal space to the right of the sternum; the other is placed at the fifth intercostal space on the left midaxillary line

3. Apply firm pressure with the paddles
4. Be sure that no one is touching the bed or the client when delivering the countershock
▲ E. Automatic external defibrillator (AED)
   1. Used by laypersons and emergency medical technicians for prehospital cardiac arrest
   2. Place the client on a firm dry surface
   3. Stop cardiopulmonary resuscitation (CPR)
   4. Ensure that no one is touching the client to avoid motion artifact during rhythm analysis
   5. Place the electrode paddles in the correct position on the client's chest
   6. Press the analyzer button to identify the rhythm, which may take 30 seconds; the machine will advise whether a shock is necessary
   7. Shocks are recommended for pulseless VF only
   8. If shock is recommended, the shock is initially delivered at an energy of 200 joules
   9. If unsuccessful, the shock is repeated at 200 to 300 joules
   10. The third and subsequent shock will be at 360 joules
   11. If unsuccessful, CPR is continued for 1 minute, and then another series of three shocks is delivered, each at 360 J F.
F. Implantable cardioverter defibrillator (ICD)
   1. Description
      a. Monitors cardiac rhythm and detects and terminates episodes of VT and VF
      b. It senses VT or VF and delivers 25 to 30 J, up to four times if necessary
      c. Used in clients with episodes of spontaneous sustained VT or VF unrelated to an MI or in clients whose medication therapy has been unsuccessful in controlling life-threatening dysrhythmias
      d. Electrodes are placed in the right atrium and ventricle and apical pericardium
      e. The generator is implanted in the abdomen
   ▲ 2. Client education (Box 50-5)

V. PACEMAKERS

A. Description: A temporary or permanent device that provides electrical stimulation and maintains the heart rate when the client's intrinsic pacemaker fails to provide a perfusing rhythm
B. Settings
   1. Synchronous or demand pacemaker: Senses the client's rhythm and paces only if the client's intrinsic rate falls below the set pacemaker rate
   2. Asynchronous or fixed rate: Paces at a preset rate regardless of the client's intrinsic rhythm
   3. Overdrive pacing: Suppresses the underlying rhythm in tachydysrhythmias, so that the sinus node will regain control of the heart

---

BOX 50-5

Implantable Cardioverter Defibrillator (ICD): Client Education

Know basic functioning of the ICD.
Know how to perform cough CPR.
Know how to take the pulse; the pulse is taken daily and a diary of pulse rates is maintained.
Wear loose-fitting clothing.
Avoid contact sports and strenuous activities.
Report any fever, redness, swelling, or drainage from the insertion site.
Report symptoms of fainting, nausea, weakness, blackouts, and rapid pulse rates to the physician.
During shock discharge, expect to feel faint or short of breath.
Sit or lie down if a shock is felt, and notify the physician.
Know how to access the emergency medical system.
Have the family learn CPR.
Maintain a diary of any shocks that are delivered, including the date, preceding activity, the number of shocks, and if the shocks were successful.
Avoid electromagnetic fields directly over the ICD, because they can inactivate the device.
Move away from the magnetic field immediately if beeping tones are heard, and notify the physician.
Keep a pacemaker ID in the wallet, and obtain and wear a Medic-Alert bracelet.
Inform all health care providers that an ICD has been inserted.

C. Spikes ▲
   1. When a pacing stimulus is delivered to the heart, a spike (straight vertical line) is seen on the monitor or ECG strip
   2. The spike should be followed by a P wave indicating atrial depolarization or by a QRS complex indicating ventricular depolarization; this pattern is referred to as "capture," indicating that the pacemaker has successfully depolarized, or captured, the chamber
   3. If the electrode is in the ventricle, the spike is in front of the QRS complex; if the electrode is in the atrium, the spike is before the P wave
   4. If the electrode is in both the atrium and the ventricle, the spike is before both the P wave and the QRS complex
D. Temporary pacemakers
   1. Noninvasive temporary pacing (NTP)
      a. Used as an emergency measure or when a client is being transported and the risk of bradydysrhythmia exists
      b. A large electrode patch is placed on the chest and back
      c. Wash the skin with soap and water before applying electrodes
      d. Do not shave the hair or apply alcohol or tinctures to the skin

e. Place the posterior electrode between the spine and left scapula, behind the heart, avoiding placement over bone

f. Place the anterior electrode between the V_2 and V_5 positions over the heart

g. Do not place the anterior electrode over female breast tissue; rather, displace breast tissue and place under the breast

h. Do not take the pulse or **BP** on the left side; the results will not be accurate because of the muscle twitching and electrical current

i. Ensure that electrodes are in good contact with the skin

j. If loss of capture occurs, assess the skin contact of the electrodes and increase the current until "capture" is regained

2. Transvenous invasive temporary pacing

a. Pacing lead wire is placed through antecubital, femoral, jugular, or subclavian vein into the right atrium for atrial pacing, or through the right ventricle, and positioned in contact with the endocardium

b. Monitor cardiac rhythm continuously

c. Monitor vital signs

d. Monitor pacemaker insertion site

e. Restrict client movement to prevent lead wire displacement

3. Epicardial invasive temporary pacing: Applied by using a transthoracic approach; the lead wires are loosely threaded on the epicardial surface of the heart after cardiac surgery

4. Reducing the risk of microshock

a. Use only inspected and approved equipment

b. Insulate the exposed portion of wires with plastic or rubber material (fingers of rubber gloves) when wires are not attached to the pulse generator, and cover with nonconductive tape

c. Ground all electrical equipment, using a three-pronged plug

d. Wear gloves when handling exposed wires

e. Keep dressings dry

E. Permanent pacemakers

1. Pulse generator is internal and surgically implanted in a subcutaneous pocket under the clavicle or abdominal wall

2. The leads are passed transvenously via the cephalic or subclavian vein to the endocardium on the right side of the heart

3. May be single chambered, in which the lead wire is placed in the chamber to be paced, or may be dual chambered, with lead wires placed in the atrium and right ventricle

4. It is programmed when inserted and can be reprogrammed if necessary by noninvasive transmission from an external programmer to the implanted generator

5. Pacemakers are powered by a lithium battery that has an average life span of 10 years, are nuclear-powered with a life span of 20 years or longer, or are designed to be recharged externally

6. Pacemaker function can be checked in the physician's office or clinic by a pacemaker interrogater/programmer or from home using a telephone transmitter device

7. The client may be provided with a device that is placed over the pacemaker battery generator with an attachment to the telephone; the heart rate can then be transmitted to the clinic

8. Provide client teaching: See Box 50-6

VI. CORONARY ARTERY DISEASE (CAD)

A. Description

1. A narrowing or obstruction of one or more coronary arteries as a result of atherosclerosis, an accumulation of lipid-containing plaque in the arteries

2. Causes decreased perfusion of myocardial tissue and inadequate myocardial oxygen supply

3. Leads to hypertension, angina, dysrhythmias, myocardial infarction, heart failure, and death

---

BOX 50-6

Pacemakers: Client Education

Know about the pacemaker, including the programmed rate.

Know about the signs of battery failure and when to notify the physician.

Report any fever, redness, swelling, or drainage from the insertion site.

Report signs of dizziness, weakness or fatigue, swelling of the ankles or legs, chest pain, or shortness of breath.

Keep a pacemaker identification card in the wallet, and obtain and wear a Medic-Alert bracelet.

Know about how to take the pulse, to take the pulse daily, and to maintain a diary of pulse rates.

Wear loose-fitting clothing.

Avoid contact sports.

Inform all health care providers that a pacemaker has been inserted.

Inform airport security that he or she has a pacemaker, because the pacemaker may set off the security detector.

Know that most electrical appliances can be used without any interference with the functioning of the pacemaker; however, advise the client not to operate electrical appliances directly over the pacemaker site.

Avoid transmitter towers and antitheft devices in stores.

Know that, if any unusual feelings occur when near any electrical devices, to move 5 to 10 feet away and check the pulse.

Know the methods of monitoring the function of the device.

Follow-up with the physician.

4. Collateral circulation, more than one artery supplying a muscle with blood, is normally present in the coronary arteries, especially in older persons

5. The development of collateral circulation takes time and develops when chronic ischemia occurs, to meet the metabolic demands; therefore, an occlusion of a coronary artery in a younger individual is more likely to be lethal than in an older individual

6. Symptoms occur when the coronary artery is occluded to the point that inadequate blood supply to the muscle occurs, causing ischemia

7. Coronary artery narrowing is significant if the lumen diameter of the left main artery is reduced at least 50% or if any major branch is reduced at least 75%

8. The goal of treatment is to alter the atherosclerotic progression

B. Data collection
   1. Findings may be normal during asymptomatic periods
   2. Chest pain
   3. Palpitations
   4. Dyspnea
   5. Syncope
   6. Cough or hemoptysis
   7. Excessive fatigue

C. Diagnostic studies
   1. ECG
      a. When blood flow is reduced and ischemia occurs, ST-segment depression or T-wave inversion is noted; the ST segment returns to normal when the blood flow returns
      b. With infarction, cell injury results in ST segment elevation, followed by T-wave inversion
   2. Cardiac catheterization
      a. Provides the most definitive source for diagnosis
      b. Shows the presence of atherosclerotic lesions
   3. Blood lipid levels
      a. May be elevated
      b. Cholesterol-lowering medications may be prescribed to reduce the development of atherosclerotic plaques

D. Interventions
   1. Instruct the client regarding the purpose of diagnostic medical and surgical procedures and preprocedure and postprocedure expectations
   2. Assist the client to identify risk factors that can be modified
   3. Assist the client to set goals to promote lifestyle changes that will reduce the impact of risk factors
   4. Assist the client in identifying barriers to compliance with the therapeutic plan and methods to overcome barriers
   5. Instruct the client regarding a low-calorie, low-sodium, low-cholesterol, and low-fat diet, with an increase in dietary fiber

6. Stress to the client that dietary changes are not temporary and must be maintained for life; instruct the client regarding prescribed medications

7. Provide community resources to the client regarding exercise, smoking reduction, and stress reduction

E. Surgical procedures
   1. PTCA to compress the plaque against the walls of the artery and dilate the vessel
   2. Laser angioplasty to vaporize the plaque
   3. Atherectomy to remove the plaque from the artery
   4. Vascular stent to prevent the artery from closing and to prevent restenosis
   5. Coronary artery bypass graft to improve blood flow to the myocardial tissue at risk for ischemia or infarction because of the occluded artery

F. Medications
   1. Nitrates to dilate the coronary arteries
   2. Calcium channel blockers to dilate coronary arteries and reduce vasospasm
   3. Cholesterol-lowering medications to reduce the development of atherosclerotic plaques
   4. Beta blockers to reduce **blood pressure** in individuals who are hypertensive

VII. ANGINA

A. Description
   1. Chest pain resulting from myocardial ischemia caused by inadequate myocardial blood and oxygen supply
   2. Caused by an imbalance between oxygen supply and demand
   3. Causes include obstruction of coronary blood flow because of atherosclerosis, coronary artery spasm, and conditions increasing myocardial oxygen consumption
   4. The goal of treatment is to provide relief of an acute attack, correct the imbalance between myocardial oxygen supply and demand, and prevent the progression of the disease and further attacks to reduce the risk of MI

B. Patterns of angina
   1. Stable angina
      a. Also called exertional angina
      b. Occurs with activities that involve exertion or emotional stress; relieved with rest or nitroglycerin
      c. It usually has a stable pattern of onset, duration, severity, and relieving factors
   2. Unstable angina
      a. Also called preinfarction angina
      b. Occurs with an unpredictable degree of exertion or emotion and increases in occurrence, duration, and severity over time
      c. Pain may not be relieved with nitroglycerin

3. Variant angina
   a. Also called Prinzmetal's or vasospastic angina
   b. Results from coronary artery spasm; similar to classic angina, but lasts longer
   c. May occur at rest
   d. Attacks may be associated with ST-segment elevation noted by ECG
4. Intractable angina: A chronic, incapacitating angina that is unresponsive to interventions
5. Preinfarction angina
   a. Associated with acute coronary insufficiency
   b. Lasts longer than 15 minutes
   c. A symptom of worsening cardiac ischemia
6. Postinfarction angina: Occurs after an MI, when residual ischemia may cause episodes of angina

C. Data collection
   1. Pain (Table 50-1)
      a. Can develop slowly or quickly
      b. Usually described as mild or moderate pain
      c. Substernal, crushing, squeezing pain
      d. May radiate to the shoulders, arms, jaw, neck, back
      e. Usually lasts less than 5 minutes; however, can last up to 15 to 20 minutes
      f. Relieved by nitroglycerin or rest
   2. Dyspnea
   3. Pallor
   4. Sweating
   5. Palpitations and tachycardia
   6. Dizziness and faintness
   7. Hypertension
   8. Digestive disturbances

D. Diagnostic studies
   1. ECG: Normal during rest, with ST depression or elevation and/or T-wave inversion during an episode of pain

---

TABLE 50-1

Characteristics of Pain: Angina and Myocardial Infarction

ANGINA
Can develop slowly or quickly
Usually described as mild or moderate pain
Substernal, crushing, squeezing pain
May radiate to the shoulders, arms, jaw, neck, back
Usually lasts less than 5 minutes; however, can last up to 15 to 20 minutes
Relieved by nitroglycerin or rest

MYOCARDIAL INFARCTION
Crushing substernal pain
May radiate to the jaw, back, and left arm
Occurs without cause, primarily early in the morning
Is unrelieved by rest or nitroglycerin, and relieved only by opioids
Lasts 30 minutes or longer

---

2. Stress test: Chest pain or changes noted by ECG or vital signs during testing may indicate ischemia
3. Cardiac enzymes and troponins: Normal findings in angina
4. Cardiac catheterization: Provides a definitive diagnosis by providing information about the patency of the coronary arteries

E. Interventions
   1. Immediate management
      a. Assess pain
      b. Provide bed rest
      c. Administer oxygen at 2 to 4 L by nasal cannula, as prescribed
      d. Administer nitroglycerin as prescribed to dilate the coronary arteries, reduce the oxygen requirements of the myocardium, and relieve the chest pain
      e. Obtain a 12-lead electrocardiogram
      f. Provide continuous cardiac monitoring
   2. Following acute episode
      a. Instruct the client regarding the purpose of diagnostic medical and surgical procedures and the preprocedure and postprocedure expectations
      b. Assist the client to identify angina-precipitating events
      c. Instruct the client to stop activity and rest if chest pain occurs and to take nitroglycerin as prescribed
      d. Instruct the client to seek medical attention if pain persists
      e. Instruct the client regarding prescribed medications
      f. Provide diet instructions to the client, stressing that dietary changes are not temporary and must be maintained for life
      g. Assist the client to identify risk factors that can be modified
      h. Assist the client to set goals that will promote changes in lifestyle to reduce the impact of risk factors
      i. Assist the client to identify barriers to compliance with the therapeutic plan and to identify methods to overcome barriers
      j. Provide community resources to the client regarding exercise, smoking reduction, and stress reduction

F. Surgical procedures: Refer to the section coronary artery disease

G. Medications
   1. Refer to the section coronary artery disease
   2. Antiplatelet therapy to inhibit platelet aggregation and reduce the risk of developing an acute MI

VIII. MYOCARDIAL INFARCTION (MI)

A. Description
   1. Occurs when myocardial tissue is abruptly and severely deprived of oxygen

2. Ischemia can lead to necrosis of myocardial tissue if blood flow is not restored

3. Infarction does not occur instantly, but evolves over several hours

4. Obvious physical changes do not occur in the heart until 6 hours after the infarction, when the infarcted area appears blue and swollen

5. After 48 hours, the infarct turns gray with yellow streaks as neutrophils invade the tissue

6. By 8 to 10 days after infarction, granulation tissue forms

7. Over 2 to 3 months, the necrotic area develops into a scar; scar tissue permanently changes the size and shape of the entire left ventricle

8. Not all clients experience the classic symptoms of an MI

9. Women may experience atypical discomfort, shortness of breath, or fatigue

10. An older client may experience shortness of breath, pulmonary edema, dizziness, altered mental status, or a dysrhythmia

B. Location of MI
1. Obstruction of the left anterior descending (LAD) artery results in anterior or septal MI or both
2. Obstruction of the circumflex artery results in posterior wall MI or lateral wall MI
3. Obstruction of the right coronary artery results in inferior wall MI

C. Risk factors
1. Atherosclerosis
2. CAD
3. Elevated cholesterol levels
4. Smoking
5. Hypertension
6. Obesity
7. Physical inactivity
8. Impaired glucose tolerance
9. Stress

D. Diagnostic studies
1. Total creatine kinase levels
   a. Rise within 3 hours after the onset of chest pain
   b. Peak within 24 hours after damage and death of cardiac tissue
2. CK-MB isoenzyme
   a. Peak elevation occurs 18 to 24 hours after the onset of chest pain
   b. Levels return to normal 48 to 72 hours later
3. Troponin levels
   a. Rise within 3 hours
   b. Remain elevated for up to 7 days
4. Myoglobin: Rises within 1 hour after cell death, peaks in 4 to 6 hours, and returns to normal within 24 to 36 hours or less
5. LDH levels
   a. Rise within 24 hours after MI
   b. Peak between 48 and 72 hours and fall to normal in 7 days

c. Serum levels of LDH_1 isoenzyme rise higher than serum levels of LDH_2

6. WBC count: An elevated white blood cell count of 10,000 to 20,000 cells/mm^3 appears on the second day following the MI and lasts up to 1 week

7. ECG
   a. ST-segment elevation, T-wave inversion, abnormal Q wave
   b. Hours to days after the MI, ST- and T-wave changes will return to normal but the Q wave usually remains permanently

8. Diagnostic tests following the acute stage
   a. Exercise tolerance test or stress test may be prescribed to assess for electrocardiographic changes and ischemia and to evaluate for medical therapy or identify clients who may need invasive therapy
   b. Thallium scans may be prescribed to assess for ischemia or necrotic muscle tissue
   c. MUGA scans: May be used to evaluate left ventricular function
   d. Cardiac catheterization: Performed to determine the extent and location of obstructions of the coronary arteries

E. Data collection
1. Pain (see Table 50-1)
   a. Crushing substernal pain
   b. May radiate to the jaw, back, and left arm
   c. Occurs without cause, primarily early in the morning
   d. Is unrelieved by rest or nitroglycerin, and relieved only by opioids
   e. Lasts 30 minutes or longer
2. Nausea and vomiting
3. Diaphoresis
4. Dyspnea
5. Dysrhythmias
6. Feelings of fear and anxiety
7. Pallor, cyanosis, coolness of extremities

F. Complications of MI
1. Dysrhythmias
2. Heart failure
3. Pulmonary edema
4. Cardiogenic shock
5. Thrombophlebitis
6. Pericarditis
7. Mitral valve insufficiency
8. Postinfarction angina
9. Ventricular rupture
10. Dressler's syndrome (a combination of pericarditis, pericardial effusion, and pleural effusion, which can occur several weeks to months following an MI)

G. Interventions, acute stage
1. Obtain a description of the chest discomfort
2. Monitor vital signs

3. Monitor cardiovascular status and maintain cardiac monitoring
4. Obtain a 12-lead electrocardiogram
5. Administer nitroglycerin, as prescribed
6. Administer morphine sulfate as prescribed to relieve chest discomfort that is unresponsive to nitroglycerin
7. Administer oxygen at 2 to 4 L by nasal cannula, as prescribed
8. Place the client in semi-Fowler's position to enhance comfort and tissue oxygenation
9. Prepare to establish an IV access route
10. Intravenous nitroglycerin and antidysrhythmics may be prescribed
11. Monitor thrombolytic therapy, which may be prescribed within the first 6 hours of the coronary event
12. Monitor for signs of bleeding if the client is receiving thrombolytics
13. Monitor laboratory values, as prescribed
14. Assist with administering beta blockers to slow the heart rate and increase myocardial perfusion, while reducing the force of myocardial contraction, as prescribed
15. Monitor for complications related to the MI
16. Monitor for cardiac dysrhythmias, because tachycardia and premature ventricular contractions (PVC) frequently occur in the first few hours after MI
17. Monitor distal peripheral pulses and skin temperature, because poor **cardiac output** may be identified by cool diaphoretic skin and diminished or absent pulses
18. Monitor I&O
19. Monitor respiratory rate and breath sounds for signs of heart failure, as indicated by the presence of crackles or wheezes or dependent edema
20. Monitor the **BP** closely after the administration of medications; if the **BP** is lower than 100 systolic or 25 mm Hg lower than the previous reading, lower the head of the bed (the physician is notified)
21. Provide reassurance to the client and family

H. Interventions following acute episode
1. Maintain bed rest for the first 24 to 36 hours
2. Allow the client to stand to void or use a bedside commode if prescribed
3. Provide range-of-motion exercises to prevent thrombus formation and maintain muscle strength
4. Progress to dangling at the side of the bed or out of bed to the chair for 30 minutes three times, a day as prescribed
5. Progress to ambulation in the client's room and to the bathroom, and then in the hallway, three times a day
6. Monitor for complications
7. Encourage the client to verbalize feelings regarding the MI

I. Cardiac rehabilitation: Process of actively assisting the client with cardiac disease to achieve and maintain a vital and productive life within the limitations of the heart disease

IX. HEART FAILURE

A. Description
1. The inability of the heart to maintain adequate circulation to meet the metabolic needs of the body because of an impaired pumping capability
2. **Cardiac output** is diminished, and peripheral tissue is not adequately perfused
3. Congestion of the lungs and periphery may occur

B. Classification
1. Acute: Occurs suddenly
2. Chronic: Develops over time; however, a client with chronic heart failure can develop an acute episode

C. Types of heart failure
1. Right-sided and left-sided heart failure
   a. Because the two ventricles of the heart represent two separate pumping systems, it is possible for one to fail alone for a short period
   b. Most heart failure begins with left ventricular failure and progresses to failure of both ventricles
   c. Acute pulmonary edema, a medical emergency, results from left ventricular failure
   d. If pulmonary edema is not treated, death will occur from suffocation as the client literally drowns in own fluids
2. Forward and backward failure
   a. In forward failure, an inadequate output of the affected ventricle causes decreased perfusion to vital organs
   b. In backward failure, blood backs up behind the affected ventricle, causing increased pressure in the atrium behind the affected ventricle
3. Low- and high-output failure
   a. In low-output failure, not enough **cardiac output** is available to meet the demands of the body
   b. High-output failure occurs when a condition causes the heart to work harder to meet the demands of the body
4. Systolic and diastolic failure
   a. Systolic failure leads to problems with contraction and the ejection of blood
   b. Diastolic failure leads to problems with the heart relaxing and filling with blood

D. Compensatory mechanisms
1. Act to restore **cardiac output** to near-normal levels
2. Initially these mechanisms increase **cardiac output**; however, they eventually have a damaging effect on pump action

TABLE 50-2

Data Collection: Right-Sided and Left-Sided Heart Failure

RIGHT-SIDED HEART FAILURE
Signs evident in the systemic circulation
Pitting, dependent edema in the feet, legs, sacrum, back, buttocks
Distended neck veins
Ascites from portal hypertension
Tenderness of right upper quadrant, organomegaly
Abdominal pain, bloating
Anorexia, nausea

LEFT-SIDED HEART FAILURE
Signs evident in the pulmonary system
Cough, which may become productive with frothy sputum
Dyspnea on exertion
Orthopnea
Paroxysmal nocturnal dyspnea
Crackles on auscultation
Confusion and disorientation
Signs of cerebral anoxia

3. Contribute to an increase in myocardial oxygen consumption; when this occurs, myocardial reserve is exhausted and clinical manifestations of heart failure develop
4. Include increased heart rate, improved stroke volume, arterial vasoconstriction, sodium and water retention, and myocardial hypertrophy

▲ E. Data collection (Table 50-2)
    1. Right-sided heart failure: Signs of right-sided failure will be evident in the systemic circulation
    2. Left-sided heart failure: Signs of left-sided failure will be evident in the pulmonary system
    3. Additional signs of right- and left-sided heart failure include pulsus alternans (regular alteration of weak and strong beats noted in the pulse), fatigue, weight gain, nocturnal diuresis, tachycardia, pallor, and cyanosis
    4. Acute pulmonary edema
       a. Severe dyspnea and orthopnea
       b. Pallor
       c. Tachycardia
       d. Expectoration of large amounts of blood-tinged, frothy sputum
       e. Wheezing and crackles
       f. Bubbling respirations
       g. Acute anxiety, apprehension, restlessness
       h. Profuse sweating
       i. Cold, clammy skin
       j. Cyanosis
       k. Nasal flaring
       l. Use of accessory breathing muscles
       m. Tachypnea
       n. Hypocapnia, evidenced by muscle cramps, weakness, dizziness, and paresthesias

F. Immediate management
    1. Place the client in high Fowler's position, with the legs in a dependent position, to reduce pulmonary congestion and relieve edema
    2. Administer oxygen in high concentrations by mask or cannula as prescribed to improve gas exchange and pulmonary function
    3. Prepare for intubation and ventilator support if required; monitor lung sounds for crackles and decreased breath sounds
    4. Suction as needed to maintain a patent airway
    5. Monitor level of consciousness
    6. Provide reassurance to the client
    7. Monitor vital signs closely, noting tachycardia or pulsus alternans
    8. Monitor for hypotension resulting from decreased tissue perfusion or hypertension resulting from anxiety or history of hypertension
    9. Monitor heart rate and dysrhythmias by using a cardiac monitor
    10. Check for edema in dependent areas and in the sacral, lumbar, and posterior thigh region in the client on bed rest
    11. Insert a Foley catheter as prescribed and monitor urine output closely following administration of a diuretic
    12. Monitor I&O
    13. Avoid the administration of unnecessary IV fluids
    14. Morphine sulfate may be prescribed to provide sedation and vasodilation; monitor for respiratory depression or hypotension after administration
    15. Prepare for the administration of diuretics as prescribed to reduce preload, enhance renal excretion of sodium and water, reduce circulating blood volume, and reduce pulmonary congestion
    16. Prepare for the administration of digitalis as prescribed to increase ventricular **contractility** and improve **cardiac output**
    17. Prepare for the administration of bronchodilators as prescribed for severe bronchospasm or bronchoconstriction
    18. Prepare for the administration of additional inotropic medications, such as dopamine (Intropin) or dobutamine (Dobutrex) as prescribed to facilitate myocardial **contractility** and enhance stroke volume
    19. Prepare for the administration of vasodilators as prescribed to reduce afterload, increase the capacity of the systemic venous bed, and decrease venous return to the heart
    20. Monitor weight to determine response to treatment
    21. Monitor for hepatomegaly and ascites, and measure and record abdominal girth
    22. Monitor peripheral pulses

23. Check arterial blood gas results, and check electrolyte levels for imbalances
24. Monitor potassium level closely, which may decrease as a result of diuretic therapy, and administer potassium supplements as prescribed to prevent digitalis toxicity

G. Following the acute episode
1. Encourage the client to verbalize feelings about the lifestyle changes required as a result of the heart failure
2. Assist the client to identify precipitating risk factors of heart failure and methods of eliminating these risk factors
3. Instruct the client in the prescribed medication regimen, which may include digoxin (Lanoxin), a diuretic, and vasodilators
4. Advise the client to notify the physician if side effects occur from the medications
5. Advise the client to avoid over-the-counter medications
6. Instruct the client to contact the physician if he or she cannot take medications because of illness
7. Instruct the client to avoid large amounts of caffeine, found in coffee, tea, cocoa, chocolate, and some carbonated beverages
8. Instruct the client about the prescribed low-sodium, low-fat, and low-cholesterol diet
9. Provide the client with a list of potassium-rich foods, because diuretics will cause hypokalemia (except for potassium-sparing diuretics)
10. Instruct the client regarding fluid restriction, if prescribed, advising the client to spread the fluid out during the day and to suck on hard candy to reduce thirst
11. Instruct the client to space periods of activity and rest
12. Advise the client to avoid isometric activities, which increase pressure in the heart
13. Instruct the client to monitor daily weight
14. Instruct the client to report signs of fluid retention, such as edema or weight gain

X. CARDIOGENIC SHOCK (Box 50-7)

BOX 50-7

Cardiogenic Shock

Failure of the heart to pump adequately, thereby reducing cardiac output and compromising tissue perfusion
Necrosis of more than 40% of the left ventricle, usually as a result of occlusion of major coronary vessels occurs
Goal of treatment: maintain tissue oxygenation and perfusion and improve the pumping ability of the heart

---

XI. INFLAMMATORY DISEASES OF THE HEART

A. Pericarditis
1. Description
   a. An acute or chronic inflammation of the pericardium
   b. Chronic pericarditis, a chronic inflammatory thickening of the pericardium, constricts the heart, causing compression
   c. The pericardial sac becomes inflamed
   d. Can result in loss of pericardial elasticity or an accumulation of fluid within the sac
   e. Heart failure or cardiac tamponade may result
2. Data collection
   a. Precordial pain in the anterior chest that radiates to the left side of the neck, shoulder, or back
   b. Pain that is aggravated by breathing (particularly inspiration), coughing, and swallowing
   c. Pain is worse when in the supine position and may be relieved by leaning forward
   d. Pericardial friction rub (scratchy, high-pitched sound) heard on auscultation; produced by rubbing of the inflamed pericardial layers
   e. Fever and chills
   f. Fatigue and malaise
   g. Elevated WBC count
   h. Electrocardiographic changes
   i. Signs of right-sided heart failure in clients with chronic constrictive pericarditis
3. Interventions
   a. Assess the nature of the pain
   b. Position the client side-lying, high Fowler's, or upright and leaning forward
   c. Administer analgesics, nonsteroidal anti-inflammatory drugs (NSAIDs), or corticosteroids for pain, as prescribed
   d. The administration of aspirin and anticoagulants is avoided because they increase the risk of cardiac tamponade (see Box 50-8)
   e. Auscultate for a pericardial friction rub
   f. Evaluate the blood culture report
   g. Prepare for the administration of antibiotics for bacterial infection, as prescribed
   h. Prepare for the administration of diuretics and digoxin (Lanoxin) as prescribed to the client with chronic constrictive pericarditis
   i. Monitor for signs of cardiac tamponade, including pulsus paradoxus, jugular vein distention with clear lung sounds, muffled heart sounds, narrowed **pulse pressure**, tachycardia, and decreased **cardiac output**
   j. The physician is notified if signs of cardiac tamponade occur

B. Myocarditis

1. Description: An acute or chronic inflammation of the myocardium as a result of pericarditis, systemic infection, or allergic response
2. Data collection
   a. Fever
   b. Pericardial friction rub
   c. A gallop rhythm
   d. A murmur that sounds like fluid passing an obstruction
   e. Pulsus alternans
   f. Signs of heart failure
   g. Fatigue
   h. Dyspnea
   i. Tachycardia
   j. Chest pain
3. Interventions
   a. Assist the client to a position of comfort, such as sitting up and leaning forward
   b. Administer analgesics, salicylates, or NSAIDs as prescribed to reduce fever and pain
   c. Administer oxygen, as prescribed
   d. Provide adequate rest periods
   e. Limit activities to avoid overexertion and to decrease the workload of the heart
   f. Administer digoxin (Lanoxin) as prescribed and monitor for signs of digoxin toxicity
   g. Prepare for the administration of antidysrhythmics, as prescribed
   h. Prepare for the administration of antibiotics as prescribed to treat the causative organism
   i. Monitor for complications, which can include thrombus, heart failure, or cardiomyopathy

C. Endocarditis
1. Description
   a. An inflammation of the inner lining of the heart and valves
   b. Occurs primarily in clients who are IV drug abusers, have had valve replacements, or have mitral valve prolapse or other structural defects
   c. Ports of entry for the infecting organism include the oral cavity (especially if the client has had a dental procedure in the previous 3 to 6 months), cutaneous invasion, infections, or invasive procedures or surgery
2. Data collection
   a. Fever
   b. Anorexia
   c. Weight loss
   d. Fatigue
   e. Cardiac murmurs
   f. Heart failure
   g. Embolic complications from vegetation fragments traveling through the circulation
   h. Petechiae
   i. Splinter hemorrhages in the nailbeds
   j. Osler's nodes (reddish, tender lesions) on the pads of the fingers, hands, and toes
   k. Janeway lesions (nontender hemorrhagic lesions) on the fingers, toes, nose, or earlobes
   l. Splenomegaly
   m. Clubbing of the fingers
3. Interventions
   a. Provide adequate rest balanced with activity to prevent thrombus formation
   b. Maintain antiembolism stockings
   c. Monitor cardiovascular status
   d. Monitor for signs of heart failure
   e. Monitor for signs of emboli
   f. Monitor for splenic emboli, as evidenced by sudden abdominal pain radiating to the left shoulder, and the presence of rebound abdominal tenderness on palpation
   g. Monitor for renal emboli, as evidenced by flank pain radiating to the groin, hematuria, and pyuria
   h. Monitor for confusion, aphasia, or dysphagia, which may be indicative of central nervous system (CNS) emboli
   i. Monitor for pulmonary emboli, as evidenced by pleuritic chest pain, dyspnea, and cough
   j. Check skin, mucous membranes, and conjunctiva for petechiae
   k. Check nail beds for splinter hemorrhages
   l. Check for Osler's nodes on the pads of the fingers, hands, and toes
   m. Check for Janeway lesions on the fingers, toes, nose, or earlobes
   n. Check for clubbing of the fingers
   o. Evaluate blood culture results
   p. Prepare for the administration of IV antibiotics, as prescribed
   q. Assist to plan and arrange for discharge, providing resources required for the continued administration of IV antibiotics
4. Client education
   a. Instruct the client about the signs and symptoms of complications and to notify the physician if they occur
   b. Inform the client about the importance of good oral hygiene
   c. Instruct the client to brush teeth twice daily with a soft toothbrush, followed by oral rinses
   d. Instruct the client to avoid irrigation devices, electric toothbrushes, and flossing, because these activities can cause the gums to bleed, allowing bacteria to enter the mucous membranes and bloodstream
   e. Advise the client of the importance of prophylactic antibiotics before any invasive procedure and the importance of informing all health care professionals of his or her disease history

BOX 50-8

Cardiac Tamponade

A pericardial effusion occurs when the space between the parietal and visceral layers of the pericardium fill with fluid.

Pericardial effusion places the client at risk for cardiac tamponade, an accumulation of fluid in the pericardial cavity.

Tamponade restricts ventricular filling, and cardiac output drops.

Acute tamponade occurs when a small volume (20 to 50 mL) of fluid accumulates in the pericardium.

XII. CARDIAC TAMPONADE (Box 50-8)

XIII. VALVULAR HEART DISEASE

A. Description
   1. Occurs when the heart valves cannot fully open (stenosis) or close completely (insufficiency or regurgitation)
   2. Prevents efficient blood flow through the heart
B. Types
   1. Mitral stenosis: Valvular tissue thickens and narrows the valve opening
   2. Mitral insufficiency or regurgitation: Valve is incompetent, preventing complete valve closure
   3. Mitral valve prolapse: Valve leaflets protrude into the left atrium during **systole**
   4. Aortic stenosis: Valvular tissue thickens and narrows the valve opening
   5. Aortic insufficiency: Valve is incompetent, preventing complete valve closure
C. Repair procedures
   1. Balloon valvuloplasty
      a. An invasive, nonsurgical procedure
      b. The passage of a balloon catheter from the femoral vein through the atrial septum to the mitral valve, or through the femoral artery to the aortic valve
      c. The balloon is inflated to enlarge the orifice
      d. Institute precautions for arterial puncture if appropriate
      e. Monitor for bleeding from the catheter insertion site
      f. Monitor for signs of systemic emboli
      g. Monitor for signs of a regurgitant valve by monitoring cardiac rhythm, heart sounds, and **cardiac output**
   2. Mitral annuloplasty: Tightening and suturing the malfunctioning valve annulus to eliminate or markedly reduce regurgitation
   3. Commissurotomy-valvotomy

a. Accomplished with cardiopulmonary bypass during open heart surgery
      b. The valve is visualized, thrombi are removed from the atria, fused leaflets are incised, and calcium is debrided from the leaflets, thus widening the orifice
D. Valve replacement procedures
   1. Mechanical prosthetic valves
      a. Prosthetic valves are very durable but can fail
      b. Thromboembolism is a problem following the valve replacement, and lifetime anticoagulant therapy is required
   2. Bioprosthetic valves
      a. Biological grafts are xenografts (valves from other species): porcine valves (pig), bovine valves (cow), or homografts (human cadavers)
      b. There is little risk of clot formation; therefore, long-term anticoagulation is not indicated
   3. Preoperative interventions: Consult with the physician regarding discontinuing anticoagulants 72 hours before surgery
   4. Postoperative interventions
      a. Monitor closely for signs of bleeding
      b. Monitor **cardiac output** and for signs of heart failure
      c. Administer digoxin (Lanoxin) as prescribed to maintain **cardiac output** and prevent atrial fibrillation
      d. Provide client teaching (Box 50-9)

XIV. CARDIOMYOPATHY

A. Description
   1. A subacute or chronic disorder of the heart muscle
   2. Treatment is palliative, not curative, and the client needs to deal with numerous lifestyle changes and a shortened life span
B. Dilated cardiomyopathy (DCM)
   1. Description
      a. Most common type
      b. Heart ejects less than 40% of the blood in the left ventricle (normal, 70%), and reduced **cardiac output** leads to heart failure
   2. Data collection
      a. Symptoms of left ventricular heart failure
      b. Weakness and fatigue
      c. Activity intolerance
      d. Chest pain
      e. Dysrhythmias
      f. Eventual signs of right-sided heart failure
   3. Interventions
      a. Symptomatic treatment of heart failure
      b. Diuretics, cardiac glycosides, and vasodilators to increase **cardiac output**
      c. Antidysrhythmics to control dysrhythmias
      d. Instruct the client to report any signs of dizziness or fainting, which may indicate a dysrhythmia

BOX 50-9

Valve Replacement: Client Education

Adequate rest is important and fatigue is usual.

There may be a need for anticoagulant therapy if a mechanical prosthetic valve was inserted.

Hazards may be related to anticoagulant therapy; notify the physician if bleeding or excessive bruising occurs.

Know the importance of good oral hygiene to reduce the risk of infective endocarditis.

Brush teeth twice daily with a soft toothbrush, followed by oral rinses.

Avoid irrigation devices, electric toothbrushes, and flossing, because these can cause the gums to bleed, allowing bacteria to enter the mucous membranes and bloodstream.

Monitor incision and report any drainage or redness.

Avoid any dental procedures for 6 months.

Heavy lifting (greater than 10 pounds) is to be avoided, and exercise caution when in an automobile to prevent injury to the sternal incision.

If a prosthetic valve was inserted, a soft audible clicking sound may be heard.

Know the importance of prophylactic antibiotics prior to any invasive procedure and the importance of informing all health care professionals of the valvular disease history.

Obtain and wear a Medic-Alert bracelet.

---

e. Instruct the client to avoid ingestion of alcohol because of its cardiac depressant effect
f. Heart transplant
C. Hypertropic cardiomyopathy (HCM)
1. Description
   a. Characterized by massive ventricular hypertrophy, leading to hypercontraction of the left ventricle and rigid ventricle walls
   b. Causes obstruction of the left ventricular outflow
2. Data collection
   a. Exertional dyspnea
   b. Syncope
   c. Chest pain that occurs at rest, is prolonged, is unrelated to exertion, and is not relieved by nitrates
   d. Dysrhythmias
3. Interventions
   a. Symptomatic treatment, similar to the care of a client with MI
   b. Conversion of atrial fibrillation if it occurs
   c. Instruct the client to report any signs of dizziness or fainting, which may indicate a dysrhythmia
   d. Instruct the client to avoid ingestion of alcohol because of its cardiac depressant effect
   e. Beta blockers and calcium antagonists may be prescribed to decrease the outflow obstruction and decrease the heart rate

f. Vasodilators and cardiac glycosides are contraindicated because vasodilator and positive inotropic effects augment the obstruction
g. Ventriculomyotomy or muscle resection with mitral valve replacement may be necessary
D. Restrictive cardiomyopathy
1. Description: Characterized by restriction of filling of the ventricles
2. Data collection
   a. Exertional dyspnea
   b. Weakness
3. Interventions
   a. Symptomatic treatment of heart failure
   b. Exercise restriction
   c. Diuretics, cardiac glycosides, and vasodilators may be prescribed to increase **cardiac output**
   d. Antidysrhythmics to control dysrhythmias
   e. Instruct the client to report any signs of dizziness or fainting, which may indicate a dysrhythmia
   f. Instruct the client to avoid ingestion of alcohol because of its cardiac depressant effect

XV. VASCULAR DISORDERS
A. Venous thrombosis
1. Description
   a. Thrombus can be associated with an inflammatory process
   b. When a thrombus develops, inflammation occurs, thickening the vein wall and leading to embolization
2. Types
   a. Thrombophlebitis: A thrombus associated with inflammation
   b. Phlebothrombus: A thrombus without inflammation
   c. Phlebitis: Vein inflammation associated with invasive procedures such as IVs
   d. Deep vein thrombophlebitis (DVT): More serious than a superficial thrombophlebitis because of the risk for pulmonary embolism
3. Risk factors for thrombus formation
   a. Venous stasis from varicose veins, heart failure, immobility
   b. Hypercoagulability disorders
   c. Injury to the venous wall from IV injections, fractures, trauma
   d. Following surgery, particularly hip surgery and open prostate surgery
   e. Pregnancy
   f. Ulcerative colitis
   g. Use of oral contraceptives
B. Phlebitis
1. Data collection
   a. Red, warm area radiating up an extremity
   b. Pain and soreness
   c. Swelling

2. Interventions
   a. Apply warm moist soaks as prescribed to dilate the vein and promote circulation
   b. Check temperature of soak before applying
   c. Monitor for signs of complications, such as tissue necrosis, infection, or pulmonary embolus

C. Deep vein thrombophlebitis
   1. Data collection
      a. Calf or groin tenderness or pain with or without swelling
      b. Positive Homans' sign
      c. Warm skin that is tender to touch
   2. Interventions
      a. Provide bed rest
      b. Elevate the affected extremity above the level of the heart as prescribed
      c. Avoid elevation of the knees and placing a pillow under the knees
      d. Do not massage the extremity
      e. Provide thigh-high compression or antiembolism stockings as prescribed to reduce venous stasis and to assist in the venous return of blood to the heart
      f. Administer intermittent or continuous warm, moist compresses, as prescribed
      g. Palpate the site gently, monitoring for warmth and edema
      h. Measure and record the circumferences of the thighs and calves
      i. Monitor for shortness of breath and chest pain, which can indicate pulmonary emboli
      j. Prepare for the administration of thrombolytic therapy (t-PA, tissue plasminogen activator) if prescribed, which must be initiated within 5 days after the onset of symptoms
      k. Prepare for the administration of heparin therapy as prescribed to prevent enlargement of the existing clot and prevent the formation of new clots
      l. Monitor activated partial thromboplastin time (aPTT) during heparin therapy
      m. Prepare for the administration of warfarin (Coumadin) as prescribed when the symptoms of DVT have resolved
      n. Monitor prothrombin time (PT) and international normalized ratio (INR) during warfarin (Coumadin) therapy
      o. Monitor for the hazards and side effects associated with anticoagulant therapy
      p. Administer analgesics as prescribed to reduce pain
      q. Administer diuretics as prescribed to reduce lower extremity edema
      r. Provide client teaching (Box 50-10)
D. Venous insufficiency
   1. Description
      a. Results from prolonged venous hypertension, which stretches the veins and damages the valves

---

BOX 50-10

Deep Vein Thrombosis: Client Education

Know the hazards of anticoagulation therapy.
Recognize the signs and symptoms of bleeding.
Avoid prolonged sitting or standing, constrictive clothing, or crossing legs when seated.
Elevate the legs for 10 to 20 minutes every few hours each day.
Plan a progressive walking program.
Inspect the legs for edema, and measure the circumference of the legs.
Wear antiembolism stockings, as prescribed.
Avoid smoking.
Avoid any medications unless prescribed by the physician.
Physician visits and laboratory studies are important follow-up measures.
Obtain and wear a Medic-Alert bracelet.

---

   b. The resultant edema and venous stasis cause venous stasis ulcers, swelling, and cellulitis
   c. Treatment focuses on decreasing edema and promoting venous return from the affected extremity
   d. Treatment for venous stasis ulcers focuses on healing the ulcer and preventing stasis and ulcer recurrence
   2. Data collection
      a. Stasis dermatitis or discoloration along the ankles and extending up to the calf
      b. Edema
      c. The presence of ulcer formation
   3. Interventions
      a. Instruct the client to wear elastic or compression stockings during the day and evening, as prescribed
      b. Instruct the client to put elastic stockings on when awakening, before getting out of bed
      c. Advise the client to put a clean pair of elastic stockings on each day and that it will probably be necessary to wear the stockings for the rest of his or her life
      d. Instruct the client to avoid prolonged sitting or standing, constrictive clothing, or crossing legs when seated
      e. Instruct the client to elevate the legs for 10 to 20 minutes every few hours each day
      f. Instruct the client to elevate legs above the level of the heart when in bed
      g. Instruct the client in the use of an intermittent sequential pneumatic compression system, if prescribed; instruct the client to apply the compression system twice daily for 1 hour in the morning and 1 hour in the evening
      h. Advise the client with an open ulcer that the compression system is applied over a dressing

4. Wound care
    a. Provide care to the wound as prescribed by the physician
    b. Determine the client's ability to care for the wound, and initiate home care resources as necessary
    c. If an Unna boot (a dressing constructed of gauze moistened with zinc oxide) is prescribed, it will be changed by the physician weekly
    d. The wound is cleansed with normal saline before application of the Unna boot; providone-iodine (Betadine) or hydrogen peroxide is not used because it destroys granulation tissue
    e. The Unna boot is covered with an elastic wrap that hardens to promote venous return and prevent stasis
    f. Monitor for signs of arterial occlusion from an Unna boot, which may be too tight
    g. Keep tape off the client's skin
5. Medications
    a. Apply topical agents to wound as prescribed to debride the ulcer, eliminate necrotic tissue, and promote healing
    b. When applying topical agents, apply an oil-based agent such as petroleum jelly (Vaseline) on surrounding skin, because debriding agents can injure healthy tissue
    c. Administer antibiotics as prescribed if infection or cellulitis occurs

E. Varicose veins
    1. Description
        a. Distended protruding veins that appear darkened and tortuous
        b. Vein walls weaken and dilate, and valves become incompetent
    2. Data collection
        a. Pain in the legs with dull aching after standing
        b. A feeling of fullness in the legs
        c. Ankle edema
    3. Trendelenburg test
        a. Place the client in a supine position with the legs elevated
        b. When the client sits up, if varicosities are present, veins fill from the proximal end; veins normally fill from the distal end
    4. Interventions
        a. Assist with the Trendelenburg test
        b. Emphasize the importance of antiembolism stockings as prescribed
        c. Instruct the client to elevate the legs as much as possible
        d. Instruct the client to avoid constrictive clothing and pressure on the legs
        e. Prepare the client for sclerotherapy or vein stripping, as prescribed

5. Sclerotherapy
    a. A solution is injected into the vein, followed by the application of a pressure dressing
    b. Incision and drainage of the trapped blood in the sclerosed vein is performed 14 to 21 days after the injection, followed by the application of a pressure dressing for 12 to 18 hours
6. Vein stripping
    a. Varicose veins are removed if they are larger than 4 mm in diameter or if they are in clusters
    b. Preoperatively assist the physician with vein marking
    c. Evaluate pulses as a baseline for comparison postoperatively
    d. Maintain elastic (Ace) bandages on the client's legs postoperatively
    e. Monitor the groin and leg for bleeding through the elastic bandages
    f. Monitor the extremity for edema, warmth, color, and pulses
    g. Elevate the legs above the level of the heart postoperatively
    h. Encourage range-of-motion exercises of the legs
    i. Instruct the client to avoid leg dangling or chair sitting
    j. Instruct the client to elevate the legs when sitting
    k. Emphasize the importance of wearing elastic stockings after bandage removal

XVI. ARTERIAL DISORDERS
A. Peripheral arterial disease (PAD)
    1. Description
        a. A chronic disorder in which partial or total arterial occlusion deprives the lower extremities of oxygen and nutrients
        b. Tissue damage occurs below the level of the arterial occlusion
        c. Atherosclerosis is the most common cause of PAD
    2. Data collection
        a. Intermittent claudication (pain in the muscles resulting from an inadequate blood supply)
        b. Rest pain, characterized by numbness, burning, or aching in the distal portion of the lower extremities, which awakens the client at night and is relieved by placing the extremity in a dependent position
        c. Lower back or buttock discomfort
        d. Loss of hair and dry scaly skin on the lower extremities
        e. Thickened toenails
        f. Cold and gray-blue color of skin in the lower extremities
        g. Elevational pallor and dependent rubor in the lower extremities

h. Decreased or absent peripheral pulses
i. Signs of arterial ulcer formation occurring on or between the toes, or on the upper aspect of the foot, that are characterized as painful
j. **Blood pressure** measurements at the thigh, calf, and ankle are lower than the brachial pressure (normally, **BP** readings in the thigh and calf are higher than those in the upper extremities)

3. Interventions
   a. Monitor pain level
   b. Monitor the extremities for color, motion, sensation, and pulses
   c. Obtain **BP** measurements
   d. Monitor for signs of ulcer formation or signs of gangrene
   e. Assist in developing an individualized exercise program, which is initiated gradually and slowly increased
   f. Encourage prescribed exercise, which will improve arterial flow through the development of collateral circulation
   g. Instruct the client to walk to the point of claudication, stop and rest, and then walk a little further
   h. Swelling in the extremities prevents arterial blood flow; therefore, instruct the client to elevate the feet at rest, but to refrain from elevating them above the level of the heart, because extreme elevation slows arterial blood flow to the feet
   i. In severe cases of PAD, clients with edema may sleep with the affected limb hanging from the bed or they may sit upright in a chair for comfort
   j. Instruct the client with PAD to avoid crossing the legs, which interferes with blood flow
   k. Instruct the client to avoid exposure of the extremities to cold (causes vasoconstriction) and to wear socks or insulated shoes for warmth at all times
   l. Instruct the client never to apply direct heat to the limb, such as with a heating pad or hot water, because the decreased sensitivity in the limb will cause burning
   m. Instruct the client to inspect the skin on the extremities daily and to report any signs of skin breakdown
   n. Instruct the client to avoid tobacco and caffeine because of their vasoconstrictive effects
   o. Instruct the client in the use of hemorrheologic and antiplatelet medications, as prescribed
   p. Inform the client of the importance of taking all medications prescribed by the physician

4. Procedures to improve arterial blood flow
   a. Percutaneous transluminal angioplasty
   b. Laser-assisted angioplasty
   c. Atherectomy
   d. Bypass surgery (aortofemoral or femoral-popliteal)

B. Raynaud's disease
   1. Description
      a. Vasospasms of the arterioles and arteries of the upper and lower extremities
      b. Vasospasm causes constriction of the cutaneous vessels
      c. Attacks are intermittent and occur with exposure to cold or stress
      d. Affects primarily fingers, toes, ears, and cheeks
   2. Data collection
      a. Blanching of the extremity, followed by cyanosis during vasoconstriction
      b. Reddened tissue when the vasospasm is relieved
      c. Numbness, tingling, swelling, and a cold temperature at the affected body part
   3. Interventions
      a. Monitor pulses
      b. Administer vasodilators, as prescribed
      c. Instruct the client regarding medication therapy
      d. Assist the client to identify and avoid precipitating factors such as cold and stress
      e. Instruct the client to avoid smoking
      f. Instruct the client to wear warm clothing, socks, and gloves in cold weather
      g. Advise the client to avoid injuries to fingers and hands

C. Buerger's disease (thromboangiitis obliterans)
   1. Description
      a. An occlusive disease of the median and small arteries and veins
      b. The distal upper and lower limbs are most commonly affected
   2. Data collection
      a. Intermittent claudication
      b. Ischemic pain occurring in the digits while at rest
      c. Aching pain that is more severe at night
      d. Cool, numb, or tingling sensation
      e. Diminished pulses in the distal extremities
      f. Extremities are cool and red in the dependent position
      g. Development of ulcerations in the extremities
   3. Interventions
      a. Instruct the client to stop smoking
      b. Monitor pulses
      c. Instruct the client to avoid injury to the upper and lower extremities
      d. Administer vasodilators, as prescribed
      e. Instruct the client regarding medication therapy

XVII. AORTIC ANEURYSMS
A. Description
   1. Abnormal dilation of the arterial wall, caused by localized weakness and stretching in the medial layer or wall of an artery

2. The aneurysm can be located anywhere along the abdominal aorta
3. The goal of treatment is to limit the progression of the disease by modifying risk factors, controlling the **BP** to prevent strain on the aneurysm, recognizing symptoms early, and preventing rupture

B. Types
  1. Fusiform: Diffuse dilation that involves the entire circumference of the arterial segment
  2. Saccular: Distinct localized outpouching of the artery wall
  3. Dissecting: Created when blood separates the layers of the artery wall, forming a cavity between them
  4. False (pseudoaneurysm)
    a. Occurs when the clot and connective tissue are outside the arterial wall
    b. Formed after complete rupture and subsequent formation of a scar sac

C. Data collection
  1. Thoracic
    a. Pain extending to neck, shoulders, lower back, or abdomen
    b. Syncope
    c. Dyspnea
    d. Increased pulse
    e. Cyanosis
    f. Weakness
  2. Abdominal
    a. Prominent, pulsating mass in abdomen, at or above the umbilicus
    b. Systolic bruit over the aorta
    c. Tenderness on deep palpation
    d. Abdominal or lower back pain
  3. Rupturing aneurysm
    a. Severe abdominal or back pain
    b. Lumbar pain radiating to the flank and groin
    c. Hypotension
    d. Increased pulse rate
    e. Signs of shock
  4. Diagnostic tests
    a. Done to confirm the presence, size, and location of the aneurysm
    b. Includes abdominal ultrasound, CT scanning, and arteriography
  5. Interventions
    a. Monitor vital signs
    b. Determine risk factors for the arterial disease process
    c. Obtain information regarding back or abdominal pain
    d. Question the client regarding the sensation of palpation in the abdomen
    e. Inspect the skin for the presence of vascular disease or breakdown
    f. Check peripheral circulation, including pulses, temperature, and color

    g. Observe for signs of rupture
    h. Note any tenderness over the abdomen
    i. Monitor for abdominal distention
  6. Nonsurgical interventions
    a. Modify risk factors
    b. Instruct the client regarding the procedure for monitoring **BP**
    c. Instruct the client on the importance of regular physician visits to monitor the size of the aneurysm
    d. Instruct the client that, if severe back or abdominal pain or fullness, soreness over the umbilicus, sudden development of discoloration in the extremities, or a persistent elevation of **BP** occurs, to notify the physician immediately
    e. Instruct the client with a thoracic aneurysm to immediately report the occurrence of chest or back pain, shortness of breath, difficulty swallowing, or hoarseness

D. Pharmacological interventions
  1. Administer antihypertensives to maintain the **BP** within normal limits and to prevent strain on the aneurysm
  2. Instruct the client in the purpose of the medications
  3. Instruct the client about the side effects and schedule of the medication

E. Abdominal aneurysm resection
  1. Description: Surgical resection or excision of the aneurysm; the excised section is replaced with a graft that is sewn end to end
  2. Preoperative interventions
    a. Assess all peripheral pulses as a baseline for postoperative comparison
    b. Instruct the client on coughing and deep breathing exercises
    c. Administer bowel preparation, as prescribed
  3. Postoperative interventions
    a. Monitor vital signs
    b. Monitor peripheral pulses distal to the graft site
    c. Monitor for signs of graft occlusion, including changes in pulses, cool to cold extremities below the graft, white or blue extremities or flanks, severe pain, or abdominal distention
    d. Limit elevation of the head of the bed to 45 degrees to prevent flexion of the graft
    e. Monitor for hypovolemia and renal failure resulting from significant blood loss during surgery
    f. Monitor urine output hourly, and notify the physician if it is less than 30 to 50 mL/hour
    g. Monitor serum creatinine and BUN levels daily
    h. Monitor respiratory status and auscultate breath sounds to identify respiratory complications
    i. Encourage turning, coughing and deep breathing, and splinting the incision

j. Ambulate, as prescribed

k. Maintain nasogastric tube to low suction until bowel sounds return

l. Check for bowel sounds and report their return to the physician

m. Monitor for pain and administer medication, as prescribed

n. Check incision site for bleeding or signs of infection

o. Prepare the client for discharge by providing instructions regarding pain management, wound care, and activity restrictions

p. Instruct the client not to lift objects heavier than 15 to 20 pounds for 6 to 12 weeks

q. Advise the client to avoid activities requiring pushing, pulling, or straining

r. Instruct the client not to drive a vehicle until the activity is approved by the physician

▲ F. Thoracic aneurysm repair

1. Description

a. A thoracotomy or median sternotomy approach is used to enter the thoracic cavity

b. The aneurysm is exposed and excised, and a graft or prosthesis is sewn onto the aorta

c. Total cardiopulmonary bypass is necessary for excision of aneurysms in the ascending aorta

d. Partial cardiopulmonary bypass is used for clients with an aneurysm in the descending aorta

2. Postoperative interventions

a. Monitor vital signs

b. Monitor for signs of hemorrhage, such as a drop in **BP** and increased pulse rate and respirations, and report to the physician immediately

c. Monitor chest tubes for an increase in chest drainage, which may indicate bleeding or separation at the graft site

d. Monitor sensation and motion of all extremities; the physician is notified if deficits occur, which can be due to a lack of blood supply during surgery

e. Monitor respiratory status and auscultate breath sounds to identify respiratory complications

f. Encourage turning, coughing and deep breathing, and splinting the incision

g. Monitor cardiac status for dysrhythmias

h. Monitor for pain and administer medication, as prescribed

i. Check the incision site for bleeding or signs of infection

j. Prepare the client for discharge by providing instructions regarding pain management, wound care, and activity restrictions

k. Instruct the client not to lift objects heavier than 15 to 20 pounds for 6 to 12 weeks

l. Advise the client to avoid activities requiring pushing, pulling, or straining

m. Instruct the client not to drive a vehicle until the activity is approved by the physician

XVIII. HYPERTENSION

A. Description

1. The classification of prehypertension describes an individual with a systolic blood pressure between 120 and 139 mm Hg or a diastolic pressure between 80 and 89 mm Hg

2. In an individual over the age of 50, the systolic pressure is a more important value to note than the diastolic pressure in regard to the need for treatment

3. Major risk factor for coronary, cerebral, renal, and peripheral vascular disease

4. The disease is initially asymptomatic

5. The goals of treatment include reducing the **blood pressure** and preventing or lessening the extent of organ damage (Table 50-3)

6. Nonpharmacological approaches, such as lifestyle changes, may be initially prescribed; if the **BP** cannot be decreased after a reasonable period (1 to 3 months), then the client may require pharmacological treatment

B. Primary or essential hypertension

1. No known etiology

2. Risk factors

a. Aging

b. Family history

c. Black race, with higher prevalence in males

d. Obesity

e. Smoking

f. Stress

C. Secondary hypertension

1. Treatment depends on the cause and the organs involved

2. Occurs as a result of other disorders or conditions

3. Precipitating disorders or conditions

a. Cardiovascular disorders

b. Renal disorders

c. Endocrine system disorders

d. Pregnancy

e. Medications

TABLE 50-3

Hypertension

Organ Involvement	Complications
Eyes	Visual changes
Brain	Cerebrovascular accident (CVA)
Cardiovascular system	Heart failure, hypertensive crisis
Kidneys	Renal failure

D. Data collection
1. May be asymptomatic
2. Headache
3. Visual disturbances
4. Dizziness
5. Chest pain
6. Tinnitus
7. Flushed face
8. Epistaxis
E. Interventions
1. Goals
   a. To reduce the **blood pressure**
   b. To prevent or lessen the extent of organ damage
2. Question the client regarding the signs and symptoms indicative of hypertension
3. Obtain the **blood pressure (BP)** two or more times on both arms, with the client supine and standing
4. Compare the **blood pressure** with prior documentation
5. Determine family history of hypertension
6. Identify current medication therapy
7. Obtain weight
8. Evaluate dietary patterns and sodium intake
9. Check for visual changes or retinal damage
10. Check for cardiovascular changes, such as distended neck veins, increased heart rate, dysrhythmias
11. Evaluate chest x-ray for heart enlargement
12. Check neurological system
13. Evaluate renal function
14. Evaluate results of diagnostic and laboratory studies
F. Nonpharmacological interventions
1. Weight reduction, if necessary, or maintenance of ideal weight
2. Dietary sodium restriction to 2 g daily, as prescribed
3. Moderate intake of alcohol and caffeine-containing products
4. Initiation of a regular exercise program
5. Avoidance of smoking
6. Relaxation techniques and biofeedback therapy
7. Elimination of unnecessary medications that may contribute to the hypertension
G. Stepped care approach
1. Description
   a. If a pharmacological approach to treating hypertension is required, a single medication is prescribed and monitored for its effectiveness
   b. Medications are added to the treatment regimen until the **BP** is controlled
   c. See Chapter 51 for medications to treat hypertension
2. Step 1: A single medication is prescribed, which may be a diuretic, beta blocker, calcium channel blocker, or angiotensin-converting enzyme (ACE) inhibitor
3. Step 2
   a. Step 1 therapy is evaluated after 1 to 3 months
   b. If the response is not adequate, compliance is evaluated
   c. The medication may be increased or a new medication is prescribed, or a second medication is added the treatment plan
4. Step 3
   a. Compliance is evaluated
   b. Further evaluation of Step 2
   c. If a therapeutic response is not adequate, a second medication is substituted or a third medication is added to the treatment plan
5. Step 4
   a. Compliance is evaluated
   b. Factors limiting the antihypertensive response are carefully assessed
   c. A third or fourth medication may be added to the treatment plan
H. Client education: See Box 50-11

XIX. HYPERTENSIVE CRISIS
A. Description
1. Any clinical condition requiring immediate reduction in **blood pressure (BP)**
2. An acute and life-threatening condition
3. The accelerated hypertension requires emergency treatment, because target organ damage (brain, heart, kidneys, retina of the eye) can occur quickly
4. Death can be caused by stroke, renal failure, or cardiac disease
B. Data collection
1. An extremely high **BP**; usually the **diastolic pressure** is above 120 mm Hg
2. Headache
3. Drowsiness and confusion
4. Blurred vision
5. Changes in neurological status
6. Tachycardia and tachypnea
7. Dyspnea
8. Cyanosis
9. Seizures can occur
C. Interventions
1. Maintain a patent airway
2. Intravenous antihypertensive medications may be prescribed
3. Monitor vital signs, checking the **BP** every 5 minutes
4. Monitor for hypotension during the administration of antihypertensives
5. Place the client in a supine position if hypotension occurs
6. Have emergency medications and resuscitation equipment readily available
7. Maintain bed rest, with the head of the bed elevated at 45 degrees

BOX 50-11

Hypertension: Client Education

Describe the importance of compliance with the treatment plan.

Describe the disease process, explaining that symptoms usually do not develop until organs have suffered damage.

Initiate and assist the client in planning a regular exercise program, avoiding heavy weight lifting and isometric exercises.

Emphasize the importance of beginning the exercise program gradually.

Encourage the client to express feelings about daily stress.

Assist the client to identify ways to reduce stress.

Teach relaxation techniques.

Instruct the client in how to incorporate relaxation techniques into the daily living pattern.

Instruct the client and family in the technique for monitoring blood pressure.

Instruct the client to maintain a diary of blood pressure readings.

Emphasize the importance of lifelong medication and the need for follow-up treatment.

Instruct the client and family about dietary restrictions, which may include sodium, fat, calories, and cholesterol.

Instruct the client in how to shop for and prepare low-sodium meals.

Provide a list of products that contain sodium.

Instruct the client to read labels of products to determine sodium content, focusing on substances listed as sodium, sodium chloride (NaCl), or monosodium glutamate (MSG).

Instruct the client to bake, roast, or boil foods, avoid salt in preparation of foods, and avoid using salt at the table.

Instruct the client that fresh foods are best to consume and to avoid canned foods.

Instruct the client about the actions, side effects, and scheduling of medications.

Advise the client that, if uncomfortable side effects occur, to contact the physician and not to stop the medication.

Instruct the client to avoid over-the-counter medications.

Stress the importance of follow-up care.

8. Monitor IV therapy, assessing for fluid overload
9. Monitor I&O
10. Insert Foley catheter, as prescribed
11. Monitor urinary output; if oliguria or anuria occurs, notify the physician

PRACTICE QUESTIONS

1. A client is scheduled for a cardiac catheterization using a radiopaque dye. The nurse checks which most critical item before the procedure?
   1. Intake and output
   2. Peripheral pulse rates
   3. Height and weight
   4. Allergy to iodine or shellfish

2. A client is scheduled for a dipyridamole (Persantine) thallium scan. The nurse would check to make sure that the client has not had which of the following before the procedure?
   1. Milk products
   2. Caffeine
   3. Excess sugar
   4. Fatty meal

3. A client with no history of cardiovascular disease presents to the ambulatory clinic with flu-like symptoms. While at the clinic, the client suddenly develops chest pain. Which question would best help the nurse to discriminate pain caused by a noncardiac problem?
   1. "Have you ever had this pain before?"
   2. "Can you describe the pain to me?"
   3. "Does the pain get worse when you breathe in?"
   4. "Can you rate the pain on a scale of 1 to 10, with 10 being the worst?"

4. A client with myocardial infarction (MI) has been transferred from the coronary care unit (CCU) to the general medical unit with cardiac monitoring via telemetry. The nurse assisting in caring for the client expects to note which type of activity prescribed?
   1. Strict bed rest for 24 hours
   2. Bathroom privileges and self-care activities
   3. Unsupervised hallway ambulation with distances less than 200 feet
   4. Ad lib activities, because the client is monitored

5. A nurse notes bilateral 2+ edema in the lower extremities of a client with myocardial infarction admitted 2 days ago. The nurse would plan to do which of the following next?
   1. Review the intake and output records for the last 2 days
   2. Change the time of diuretic administration from morning to evening
   3. Request a sodium restriction of 1 g/day from the physician
   4. Order daily weights starting on the following morning

6. A nurse is collecting data from a client with a primary diagnosis of heart failure. Which disorder reported by the client is unassociated with exacerbating the heart failure?
   1. Recent upper respiratory infection
   2. Nutritional anemia
   3. Peptic ulcer disease
   4. Atrial fibrillation

7. A nurse is collecting data from a client with heart failure who is being sent directly to the hospital from the physician's office. The nurse reviews the physician's orders and expects to note an order for which medication?
   1. Diltiazem (Cardizem)
   2. Digoxin (Lanoxin)
   3. Propranolol (Inderal)
   4. Metoprolol (Lopressor)

8. A nurse checks the sternotomy incision of a client on the second postoperative day after cardiac surgery. The incision shows some slight "puffiness" along the edges, is nonreddened, with no apparent drainage. The client's temperature is 99° F (37.2° C) orally. The white blood cell (WBC) count is 7500/mm³. The nurse interprets that the incision line:
   1. Is slightly edematous but shows no active signs of infection
   2. Shows no sign of infection although the WBC count is elevated
   3. Shows early signs of infection although the temperature is near normal
   4. Shows early signs of infection supported by an elevated WBC count

9. A postcardiac surgery client has a urine output averaging 20 mL/hour for 2 hours. The client received a single bolus of 500 mL of IV fluid. Urine output for the subsequent hour was 25 mL. Daily laboratory results indicate that the blood urea nitrogen (BUN) level is 45 mg/dL and the serum creatinine level is 2.2 mg/dL. The nurse interprets that the client is at risk for:
   1. Hypovolemia
   2. Urinary tract infection
   3. Glomerulonephritis
   4. Acute renal failure

10. A nurse is preparing to ambulate a postoperative client following cardiac surgery. The nurse plans to do which of the following to enable the client to best tolerate the ambulation?
   1. Encourage the client to cough and deep breathe
   2. Premedicate the client with an analgesic
   3. Provide the client with a walker
   4. Remove the telemetry equipment

11. A client is wearing a continuous cardiac monitor, which begins to alarms. The nurse sees no electrocardiographic complexes on the screen. The nurse would first:
   1. Check the client status and lead placement
   2. Press the recorder button on the ECG console
   3. Call the physician
   4. Call a code blue

12. A client with a diagnosis of rapid rate atrial fibrillation asks the nurse why the physician is going to perform carotid massage. The nurse responds that this procedure may stimulate the:
   1. Vagus nerve to slow the heart rate
   2. Vagus nerve to increase the heart rate
   3. Diaphragmatic nerve to slow the heart rate
   4. Diaphragmatic nerve to increase the heart rate

13. A nurse is caring for a client on a cardiac monitor who is alone in a room at the end of the hall. The client has a short burst of ventricular tachycardia followed by ventricular fibrillation (VF). The client immediately loses consciousness. The nurse would immediately:
   1. Call for help and initiate cardiopulmonary resuscitation (CPR)
   2. Start oxygen by cannula at 10 L/minute and lower the head of the bed
   3. Go to the nurse's station quickly and call a code
   4. Run to get a defibrillator from an adjacent nursing unit

14. A nurse is monitoring a client following cardioversion. Which of the following observations would be of highest priority to the nurse?
   1. Oxygen flow rate
   2. Status of airway
   3. Blood pressure
   4. Level of consciousness

15. An automatic external defibrillator is available to treat the client who goes into cardiac arrest and is receiving cardiopulmonary resuscitation (CPR). With this device, the nurse checks the cardiac rhythm by:
   1. Applying standard electrocardiographic monitoring leads to the client and observing the rhythm
   2. Holding the defibrillator paddles firmly against the chest
   3. Applying the adhesive patch electrodes to the skin and moving away from the client
   4. Connecting standard electrocardiographic electrodes to a transtelephonic monitoring device

16. The nurse is caring for the client immediately after insertion of a permanent demand pacemaker via the right subclavian vein. The nurse takes care not to dislodge the pacing catheter by:
   1. Limiting movement and abduction of the right arm
   2. Limiting movement and abduction of the left arm
   3. Assisting the client to get out of bed and ambulate with a walker
   4. Having the physical therapist do active range of motion to the right arm

17. A client diagnosed with thrombophlebitis 1 day ago suddenly complains of chest pain and shortness of breath, and is visibly anxious. The nurse immediately checks the client for other signs and symptoms of:
   1. Myocardial infarction
   2. Pneumonia
   3. Pulmonary embolism
   4. Pulmonary edema

18. A client seeks treatment in the physician's office for unsightly varicose veins, and sclerotherapy is recommended. Before leaving the examining room, the client says to the nurse, "Can you tell me again how this sclerotherapy is done?" In formulating a response, the nurse informs the client that sclerotherapy consists of:
   1. Injecting an agent into the vein to damage the vein wall and close off the vein

2. Tying off the vein at the upper end to prevent stasis from occurring
3. Tying off the vein at the lower end to prevent stasis from occurring
4. Surgical removal of the varicosity

19. A client is having a follow-up physician office visit after vein ligation and stripping. The client describes a sensation of "pins and needles" in the affected leg. Based on evaluation of this comment, the nurse:
    1. Reassures the client that this is only temporary
    2. Advises the client to take acetaminophen (Tylenol) until it is gone
    3. States that warm packs should help
    4. Reports the complaint to the physician

20. A 24-year-old man seeks medical attention for complaints of claudication in the arch of the foot. The nurse also notes superficial thrombophlebitis of the lower leg. The nurse would next check the client for:
    1. Familial tendency toward peripheral vascular disease
    2. Smoking history
    3. Recent exposure to allergens
    4. History of recent insect bites

21. A nurse has given instructions to the client with Raynaud's disease about self-management of the disease process. The nurse determines that the client needs further reinforcement if the client states that:
    1. Smoking cessation is very important
    2. Sources of caffeine should be eliminated from the diet
    3. Taking nifedipine (Procardia) as prescribed will decrease vessel spasm
    4. Moving to a warmer climate should help

22. A nurse is checking the blood pressure of a client diagnosed with primary hypertension. The nurse ensures accurate measurement by avoiding which of the following?
    1. Seating the client with arm bared, supported, and at heart level
    2. Measuring the blood pressure after the client is seated quietly for 5 minutes
    3. Using a cuff with a rubber bladder that encircles at least 80% of the limb
    4. Taking the blood pressure within 10 minutes following nicotine or caffeine ingestion

23. A client with myocardial infarction suddenly becomes tachycardic, shows signs of air hunger, and begins coughing frothy, pink-tinged sputum. A nurse listens to breath sounds, expecting to hear bilateral:
    1. Rhonchi
    2. Diminished breath sounds
    3. Crackles
    4. Wheezes

24. A nurse caring for a client in one room is told by another nurse that a second client has developed severe pulmonary edema. On entering the second client's room, the nurse would expect the client to be:
    1. Slightly anxious
    2. Mildly anxious
    3. Moderately anxious
    4. Extremely anxious

25. A nurse is collecting data on a client with a diagnosis of right-sided heart failure. The nurse would expect to note which specific characteristic of this condition?
    1. Dyspnea
    2. Crackles on lung auscultation
    3. Hacking cough
    4. Dependent edema

26. A client is admitted to the hospital with an arterial ischemic leg ulcer. The nurse assesses the ulcer, expecting to note that it:
    1. Has a pink-colored base
    2. Is superficial, with uneven edges
    3. Has little granulation tissue
    4. Has brown pigmentation surrounding it

27. A nurse is checking the neurovascular status of a client who returned to the surgical nursing unit 4 hours ago after undergoing aortoiliac bypass graft. The affected leg is warm, and the nurse notes redness and edema. The pedal pulse is palpable and unchanged from admission. The nurse interprets that the neurovascular status is:
    1. Normal, caused by increased blood flow through the leg
    2. Slightly deteriorating, and should be monitored for another hour
    3. Moderately impaired, and the surgeon should be called
    4. Adequate from an arterial approach, but venous complications are arising

28. A client with an abdominal aortic aneurysm (AAA) is not a candidate for surgery because the aneurysm is not yet large enough. The client is fearful that the aneurysm will rupture, causing death. The nurse plans to assist the client in coping with this fear by emphasizing what the client can do for self-monitoring. Which of the following items would be unnecessary for the nurse to include in discussions with the client?
    1. Antibiotic prophylaxis before invasive procedures
    2. Importance of follow-up computerized tomography (CT) scans
    3. Management of hypertension
    4. Reporting abdominal or back pain

29. A client has an Unna boot applied for treatment of a venous stasis leg ulcer. The nurse notes that the client's toes are mottled and cool, and the client

verbalizes some numbness and tingling of the foot. The nurse interprets that the boot:
1. Is controlling leg edema
2. Has been applied too tightly
3. Is impairing venous return
4. Has not yet dried

30. A nurse is planning care for an ambulatory client with a venous stasis leg ulcer. The nurse anticipates that which type of dressing will be used in the care of this client?
1. Damp to dry isotonic saline dressings
2. Half-strength betadine dressings
3. Dry sterile dressings
4. Zinc oxide dressings (Unna boot)

31. A nurse is caring for a client receiving digoxin (Lanoxin) for the treatment of heart failure. The nurse would monitor the client for which signs that indicate toxicity?
1. Thrombocytopenia and weight gain
2. Anorexia, nausea, and visual disturbances
3. Diarrhea and hypotension
4. Fatigue and muscle twitching

32. A client with angina complains that the anginal pain is prolonged and severe and occurs at the same time each day, most often in the morning. On further data collection, the nurse notes that the pain occurs in the absence of precipitating factors. This type of anginal pain is best described as:
1. Stable angina
2. Unstable angina
3. Variant angina
4. Nonanginal pain

33. A nurse is assisting in monitoring the condition of a client after pericardiocentesis for cardiac tamponade. Which observation would indicate that the procedure was unsuccessful?
1. Clear breath sounds
2. A fall in blood pressure (BP)

3. Client expressions of relief
4. Clearly audible heart sounds

34. A nurse is monitoring a client with an abdominal aortic aneurysm (AAA). Which finding is probably unrelated to the AAA?
1. Pulsatile abdominal mass
2. Hyperactive bowel sounds in the area
3. Systolic bruit over the area of the mass
4. Subjective sensation of "heart beating" in the abdomen

35. A client arrives in the emergency department after complaining of unrelieved chest pain for 2 days. The pain has subsided slightly, but has not disappeared completely. When the nurse approaches the client with a nitroglycerin sublingual tablet, the client states, "I don't need that. My dad takes that for his heart. There's nothing wrong with my heart." Which of the following best describes the client's response?
1. Obsessive-compulsive
2. Denial
3. Phobic
4. Angry

ALTERNATE FORMAT QUESTION: MULTIPLE RESPONSE

A nurse in a medical unit is caring for a client with heart failure. The client suddenly develops extreme dyspnea, tachycardia, and lung crackles, and the nurse suspects pulmonary edema. The nurse immediately asks another nurse to contact the physician and prepares the client for which priority interventions?

_____ Administration of furosemide (Lasix)
_____ Transport to the coronary care unit
_____ Administration of oxygen
_____ Placing the client in a low Fowler's side-lying position
_____ Administration of intravenous morphine sulfate

ANSWERS

1. *Answer: 4*
Rationale: This procedure requires a signed consent, because it involves injection of a radiopaque dye into the blood vessel. The risk of allergic reaction and possible anaphylaxis is serious, and must be assessed before the procedure. Although options 1, 2, and 3 may be a component of data collection, they are not the most critical items.
Test-Taking Strategy: Use prioritization skills and note the key words, *most critical.* Recalling the risk of anaphylaxis if an allergy exists will direct you to option 4. Review preprocedure interventions for a cardiac catheterization if you had difficulty with this question.
Level of Cognitive Ability: Application
Client Needs: Physiological Integrity

Integrated Process: Nursing Process/Data Collection
Content Area: Delegating/Prioritizing
Reference: Chernecky, C., & Berger, B. (2004). *Laboratory tests and diagnostic procedures* (4th ed.). Philadelphia: W.B. Saunders, p. 327.

2. *Answer: 2*
Rationale: This test is an alternative to the exercise stress test. Dipyridamole (Persantine) dilates the coronary arteries as exercise would. Before the procedure, any form of caffeine should be withheld, as well as aminophylline or theophylline. Aminophylline is the antagonist to dipyridamole.
Test-Taking Strategy: Use the process of elimination and note the key words, *has not had.* Remember, factors that put a strain on the heart, such as nicotine and caffeine, can interfere with

cardiac diagnostic test results. Review preprocedure interventions for this test if you had difficulty with this question.
Level of Cognitive Ability: Application
Client Needs: Physiological Integrity
Integrated Process: Nursing Process/Data Collection
Content Area: Adult Health/Cardiovascular
Reference: Chernecky, C., & Berger, B. (2004). *Laboratory tests and diagnostic procedures* (4th ed.). Philadelphia: W.B. Saunders, p. 1026.

3. *Answer: 3*
Rationale: Chest pain is assessed using the standard pain assessment parameters, (characteristics, location, intensity, duration, precipitating and alleviating factors, and associated symptoms). Options 1, 2, and 4 may or may not help determine the origin of pain. Pain of pleuropulmonary origin usually worsens on inspiration.
Test-Taking Strategy: Focus on the issue, a method of discriminating among the causes of pain. The three incorrect options, although appropriate to use in clinical practice, are general assessment questions only. Option 3 will discriminate between a cardiac and noncardiac cause of pain. Review pain data collection techniques if you had difficulty with this question.
Level of Cognitive Ability: Analysis
Client Needs: Physiological Integrity
Integrated Process: Nursing Process/Data Collection
Content Area: Adult Health/Cardiovascular
Reference: Linton, A., & Maebius, N. (2003). *Introduction to medical-surgical nursing* (3rd ed.). Philadelphia: W.B. Saunders, p. 457.

4. *Answer: 2*
Rationale: Upon transfer from the CCU, the client is allowed self-care activities and bathroom privileges. Supervised ambulation in the hall for brief distances is encouraged, with distances gradually increased (50, 100, 200 feet).
Test-Taking Strategy: Use the process of elimination. Eliminate options 3 and 4 first because they are excessive, given that the client has just transferred from the CCU. Option 1 is not correct, because the client would be doing less activity than in the CCU prior to transfer. Review activity prescriptions for the client with an MI if you had difficulty with this question.
Level of Cognitive Ability: Comprehension
Client Needs: Physiological Integrity
Integrated Process: Nursing Process/Planning
Content Area: Adult Health/Cardiovascular
Reference: Christensen, B., & Kockrow, E. (2003). *Adult health nursing* (4th ed.). St. Louis: Mosby, p. 313.

5. *Answer: 1*
Rationale: Edema, the accumulation of excess fluid in the interstitial spaces, can be measured by intake greater than output and by a sudden increase in weight. Diuretics should be given in the morning whenever possible to avoid nocturia. Strict sodium restrictions are reserved for clients with severe symptoms.
Test-Taking Strategy: Use the process of elimination. The question asks what the nurse would do next. Focusing on the issue will direct you to option 1. Option 1 can give the nurse

immediate information about fluid balance. Review data collection methods for the client with edema if you had difficulty with this question.
Level of Cognitive Ability: Application
Client Needs: Physiological Integrity
Integrated Process: Nursing Process/Implementation
Content Area: Adult Health/Cardiovascular
Reference: Christensen, B., & Kockrow, E. (2003). *Adult health nursing* (4th ed.). St. Louis: Mosby, p. 320.

6. *Answer: 3*
Rationale: Heart failure is precipitated or exacerbated by physical or emotional stress, dysrhythmias, infections, anemia, thyroid disorders, pregnancy, Paget's disease, nutritional deficiencies (thiamine, alcoholism), pulmonary disease, and hypervolemia.
Test-Taking Strategy: Use the process of elimination and note the key word, *unassociated*. This word indicates a false response question and that you need to select the item that is not related to the heart failure. Because heart failure is exacerbated by factors that increase the workload of the heart, options 1, 2, and 4 can be eliminated. Review the precipitating factors associated with heart failure if you had difficulty with this question.
Level of Cognitive Ability: Analysis
Client Needs: Physiological Integrity
Integrated Process: Nursing Process/Data Collection
Content Area: Adult Health/Cardiovascular
References: Christensen, B., & Kockrow, E. (2003). *Adult health nursing* (4th ed.). St. Louis: Mosby, pp. 320-321.
Linton, A., & Maebius, N. (2003). *Introduction to medical-surgical nursing* (3rd ed.). Philadelphia: W.B. Saunders, pp. 580-581.

7. *Answer: 2*
Rationale: Digoxin exerts a positive inotropic effect on the heart while slowing the overall rate through a variety of mechanisms. It is the medication of choice used to treat heart failure. Diltiazem (calcium channel blocker), propranolol, and metoprolol (beta-adrenergic blockers) have a negative inotropic effect, and would worsen the failing heart.
Test-Taking Strategy: Use the process of elimination. Eliminate options 3 and 4 first because they are similar and are both beta blockers. From the remaining options, it is necessary to know that digoxin is used to treat heart failure. Review the treatment for this disorder if you had difficulty with this question.
Level of Cognitive Ability: Analysis
Client Needs: Physiological Integrity
Integrated Process: Nursing Process/Planning
Content Area: Adult Health/Cardiovascular
Reference: Hodgson, B., & Kizior, R. (2005). *Saunders nursing drug handbook 2005*. Philadelphia: W.B. Saunders, p. 324.

8. *Answer: 1*
Rationale: Sternotomy incision sites are assessed for signs and symptoms of infection, such as redness, swelling, and induration. An elevated temperature and elevated WBC count after

3 to 4 days usually indicate infection. A WBC count of 7500/mm³ is within the normal range.

Test-Taking Strategy: Use the process of elimination. Eliminate options 2 and 4 because the WBC count is normal. The lack of drainage and redness helps you choose option 1 over 3. Review the signs of an incisional infection if you had difficulty with this question.

Level of Cognitive Ability: Analysis
Client Needs: Physiological Integrity
Integrated Process: Nursing Process/Data Collection
Content Area: Adult Health/Cardiovascular
References: Black, J., & Hawks, J. (2005). *Medical-surgical nursing: Clinical management for positive outcomes* (7th ed.). Philadelphia: W.B. Saunders, p. 406.
Linton, A., & Maebius, N. (2003). *Introduction to medical-surgical nursing* (3rd ed.). Philadelphia: W.B. Saunders, p. 579.

9. *Answer:* **4**
Rationale: The client who undergoes cardiac surgery is at risk for renal injury from poor perfusion, hemolysis, low cardiac output, or vasopressor medication therapy. Renal insult is signaled by a decreased urine output and increased BUN and creatinine levels. The client may need medications to increase renal perfusion, and could possibly need peritoneal dialysis or hemodialysis.

Test-Taking Strategy: Use the process of elimination. The question provides no evidence of any infection, so eliminate options 2 and 3 first. Hypovolemia is eliminated next because of the high BUN and creatinine values and the poor response to the bolus of fluid. Review laboratory values and postcardiac surgery complications if you had difficulty with this question.

Level of Cognitive Ability: Analysis
Client Needs: Physiological Integrity
Integrated Process: Nursing Process/Data Collection
Content Area: Adult Health/Cardiovascular
Reference: Linton, A., & Maebius, N. (2003). *Introduction to medical-surgical nursing* (3rd ed.). Philadelphia: W.B. Saunders, p. 585.

10. *Answer:* **2**
Rationale: The nurse should encourage regular use of pain medication for the first 48 to 72 hours after cardiac surgery, because analgesia will promote rest, decrease myocardial oxygen consumption due to pain, and allow better participation in activities such as coughing, deep breathing, and ambulation.

Test-Taking Strategy: Use the process of elimination. The question asks for the best action of the nurse to help a client tolerate ambulation. Coughing and deep breathing will not actively help endurance, so eliminate option 1. Eliminate option 4 because removal of telemetry equipment is contraindicated unless ordered. From the remaining options, noting that the client is postoperative will direct you to option 2. Review postoperative instructions if you had difficulty with this question.

Level of Cognitive Ability: Application
Client Needs: Physiological Integrity
Integrated Process: Nursing Process/Planning
Content Area: Adult Health/Cardiovascular

Reference: Linton, A., & Maebius, N. (2003). *Introduction to medical-surgical nursing* (3rd ed.). Philadelphia: W.B. Saunders, p. 578.

11. *Answer:* **1**
Rationale: Sudden loss of electrocardiographic complexes indicates ventricular asystole or possibly electrode displacement. Assessment of the client and equipment is the first action by the nurse.

Test-Taking Strategy: Use the steps of the nursing process and remember that data collection is the first step. Options 3 and 4 are incorrect because they indicate calling for assistance prior to collecting data. Option 2 may sound reasonable, but the electrocardiographic monitor automatically starts recording when an alarm sounds. Option 1 is the best option, because you should always check the client directly before taking any action. Review care of a client on a cardiac monitor if you had difficulty with this question.

Level of Cognitive Ability: Application
Client Needs: Physiological Integrity
Integrated Process: Nursing Process/Implementation
Content Area: Adult Health/Cardiovascular
Reference: Christensen, B., & Kockrow, E. (2003). *Adult health nursing* (4th ed.). St. Louis: Mosby, pp. 293-294.

12. *Answer:* **1**
Rationale: Carotid sinus massage is one maneuver used for vagal stimulation to decrease a rapid heart rate and possibly terminate a tachydysrhythmia. The other maneuvers are the Valsalva maneuver of inducing the gag reflex and asking the client to strain or bear down. Medication therapy is often needed as an adjunct to keep the rate down or maintain the normal rhythm.

Test-Taking Strategy: Use the process of elimination. Eliminate options 2 and 4 first because these options indicate increasing an already rapid rate. From the remaining options, use knowledge of anatomy and physiology. A rapid-rate dysrhythmia would need to be slowed, which is the function of the vagus nerve. The diaphragmatic nerve affects respiration. If you are unfamiliar with the functions of these nerves, review this content.

Level of Cognitive Ability: Application
Client Needs: Physiological Integrity
Integrated Process: Nursing Process/Implementation
Content Area: Adult Health/Cardiovascular
Reference: Mosby's medical, nursing, and allied health dictionary (6th ed.). (2002). St. Louis: Mosby, p. 301.

13. *Answer:* **1**
Rationale: When VF occurs, the nurse remains with the client and initiates CPR until a defibrillator is available and attached to the client. Options 2, 3, and 4 are incorrect.

Test-Taking Strategy: Use the process of elimination. Eliminate options 3 and 4 first because you would never leave the client alone. From the remaining options, lowering the head of bed is appropriate (for resuscitation), but the oxygen by cannula at 10 L/minute is incorrect. Option 1 is the correct option. Review care of the client with VF if you had difficulty with this question.

Level of Cognitive Ability: Application

Client Needs: Physiological Integrity
Integrated Process: Nursing Process/Implementation
Content Area: Adult Health/Cardiovascular
Reference: Christensen, B., & Kockrow, E. (2003). *Adult health nursing* (4th ed.). St. Louis: Mosby, p. 299.

14. *Answer: 2*

Rationale: Nursing responsibilities after cardioversion include maintenance of a patent airway, oxygen administration, assessment of vital signs and level of consciousness, and dysrhythmia detection.

Test-Taking Strategy: Use the ABCs—airway, breathing, and circulation—to answer the question. This will direct you to option 2. Remember, airway comes first. Review care of the client following cardioversion if you had difficulty with this question.

Level of Cognitive Ability: Analysis
Client Needs: Physiological Integrity
Integrated Process: Nursing Process/Data Collection
Content Area: Delegating/Prioritizing
Reference: Linton, A., & Maebius, N. (2003). *Introduction to medical-surgical nursing* (3rd ed.). Philadelphia: W.B. Saunders, pp. 577, 586.

15. *Answer: 3*

Rationale: The nurse or rescuer puts two large adhesive patch electrodes on the client's chest in the usual defibrillator position. The nurse stops cardiopulmonary resuscitation and orders anyone near the client to move away and not touch the client. The defibrillator then analyzes the rhythm, which may take up to 30 seconds. The machine then indicates if it is necessary to defibrillate. Although automatic external defibrillation can be done transtelephonically, it is done through the use of patch electrodes (not standard electrocardiographic electrodes) that interact via telephone lines to a base station that controls any actual defibrillation. It is not necessary to hold defibrillator paddles against the client's chest with this device.

Test-Taking Strategy: If you are not familiar with this piece of equipment, look first at the word "automatic" in the name. This implies that someone is not as involved in the process as with a conventional defibrillator, and may help you eliminate option 2. Because standard electrocardiographic monitoring leads are not used (options 1 and 4), you can eliminate these similar, and incorrect, options. Although automatic external defibrillation can be done transtelephonically, it is done through the use of patch electrodes. Review the use of this device if you had difficulty with this question.

Level of Cognitive Ability: Application
Client Needs: Physiological Integrity
Integrated Process: Nursing Process/Implementation
Content Area: Adult Health/Cardiovascular
Reference: Phipps, W., Monahan, F., Sands, J., Marek, J., & Neighbors, M. (2003). *Medical-surgical nursing: Health and illness perspectives* (7th ed.). St. Louis: Mosby, p. 701.

16. *Answer: 1*

Rationale: In the first several hours after insertion of either a permanent or temporary pacemaker, the most common complication is pacing electrode dislodgment. The nurse helps prevent this complication by limiting the client's activities.

Test-Taking Strategy: Use the process of elimination. The question tells you that the pacemaker was inserted on the right side. Therefore, to prevent pacing electrode dislodgment, motion must be limited on that side. Options 3 and 4 involve movement of the right arm. Limiting the movement of the left arm (option 2) is of no benefit to the client. Thus, option 1 is correct. Review care of the client following pacemaker insertion if you had difficulty with this question.

Level of Cognitive Ability: Application
Client Needs: Physiological Integrity
Integrated Process: Nursing Process/Implementation
Content Area: Adult Health/Cardiovascular
Reference: Christensen, B., & Kockrow, E. (2003). *Adult health nursing* (4th ed.). St. Louis: Mosby, p. 302.

17. *Answer: 3*

Rationale: Pulmonary embolism is a life-threatening complication of deep vein thrombosis and thrombophlebitis. Chest pain is the most common symptom, which is sudden in onset and may be aggravated by breathing. Other signs and symptoms include dyspnea, cough, diaphoresis, and apprehension.

Test-Taking Strategy: Use the process of elimination. This question tests your ability to analyze signs and symptoms of pulmonary embolism in a client at risk. Each of the incorrect options should be eliminated because myocardial infarction and pulmonary edema are cardiac related problems and are therefore similar, and pneumonia is an infectious process. Review the complications of thrombophlebitis if you had difficulty with this question.

Level of Cognitive Ability: Analysis
Client Needs: Physiological Integrity
Integrated Process: Nursing Process/Data Collection
Content Area: Adult Health/Cardiovascular
Reference: Christensen, B., & Kockrow, E. (2003). *Adult health nursing* (4th ed.). St. Louis: Mosby, p. 391.

18. *Answer: 1*

Rationale: Sclerotherapy is the injection of a sclerosing agent into a varicosity. The agent damages the vessel and causes aseptic thrombosis, which results in vein closure. With no blood flow through the vessel, there is no distention. The surgical procedure for varicose veins is vein ligation and stripping. This procedure involves tying off the varicose vein and large tributaries, and then removal of the vein with the use of hook and wires via multiple small incisions in the leg.

Test-Taking Strategy: If you are uncertain of the response to this question, look at the word "sclerotherapy." A vessel that is sclerosed is blocked. This may help you select the correct option. At the very least, you should be able to eliminate options 2 and 3 readily, because neither of these makes sense using principles of blood flow and gravity. Also, they are similar, and so are likely to be incorrect. Review this procedure if you had difficulty with this question.

Level of Cognitive Ability: Comprehension
Client Needs: Physiological Integrity
Integrated Process: Nursing Process/Implementation
Content Area: Adult Health/Cardiovascular

References: Christensen, B., & Kockrow, E. (2003). *Adult health nursing* (4th ed.). St. Louis: Mosby, p. 344.
Linton, A., & Maebius, N. (2003). *Introduction to medical-surgical nursing* (3rd ed.). Philadelphia: W.B. Saunders, p. 621.

19. *Answer:* 4
Rationale: Hypersensitivity or a sensation of "pins and needles" in the surgical limb may indicate temporary or permanent nerve injury following surgery. The saphenous vein and the saphenous nerve run close together in the distal third of the leg. Because complications from this surgery are relatively rare, this symptom should be reported. Options 1, 2, and 3 are incorrect actions.
Test-Taking Strategy: Use the process of elimination. Pins and needles sensations usually indicate nerve irritation or damage. Knowing this, options 2 and 3 can be eliminated as the least likely correct options. Reassuring the client about something being "only temporary" is not often a good choice, unless this is known to be absolutely true. By the process of elimination, therefore, the physician should be notified. Review the complications following vein ligation and stripping if you had difficulty with this question.
Level of Cognitive Ability: Application
Client Needs: Physiological Integrity
Integrated Process: Nursing Process/Implementation
Content Area: Adult Health/Cardiovascular
Reference: Linton, A., & Maebius, N. (2003). *Introduction to medical-surgical nursing* (3rd ed.). Philadelphia: W.B. Saunders, pp. 620-621.

20. *Answer:* 2
Rationale: The mixture of arterial and venous manifestations (claudication and phlebitis, respectively) in the young male client suggests thromboangiitis obliterans (Buerger's disease). This is a relatively uncommon disorder, characterized by inflammation and thrombosis of smaller arteries and veins. This disorder is typically found in young men who smoke. The cause is unknown, but is suspected to have an autoimmune component.
Test-Taking Strategy: Use the process of elimination. You can first eliminate options 3 and 4 because they would most likely cause local skin reactions. The question asks which item you should check "next." It is often better to assess a modifiable factor before a nonmodifiable one. This will direct you to option 2. Review the causes of Buerger's disease if you had difficulty with this question.
Level of Cognitive Ability: Analysis
Client Needs: Health Promotion and Maintenance
Integrated Process: Nursing Process/Data Collection
Content Area: Adult Health/Cardiovascular
Reference: Linton, A., & Maebius, N. (2003). *Introduction to medical-surgical nursing* (3rd ed.). Philadelphia: W.B. Saunders, p. 629.

21. *Answer:* 4
Rationale: Raynaud's disease responds favorably to the elimination of nicotine and caffeine. Medications such as calcium channel blockers may inhibit vessel spasm and prevent symptoms. Avoiding exposure to cold through a variety of means is very important. However, moving to a warmer climate may not necessarily be beneficial, because the symptoms could still occur with the use of air conditioning and during periods of cooler weather.
Test-Taking Strategy: Note the key words, *needs further reinforcement.* These words indicate a false response question and that you need to select the incorrect client statement. All of the options seem reasonable. However, when you analyze each of them, note that relocation is the least favorable of all the options, from the viewpoints of practicality and encountering new environmental concerns. Review treatment measures for this disorder if you had difficulty with this question.
Level of Cognitive Ability: Comprehension
Client Needs: Health Promotion and Maintenance
Integrated Process: Nursing Process/Evaluation
Content Area: Adult Health/Cardiovascular
Reference: Linton, A., & Maebius, N. (2003). *Introduction to medical-surgical nursing* (3rd ed.). Philadelphia: W.B. Saunders, pp. 628-629.

22. *Answer:* 4
Rationale: The blood pressure should be taken with the client seated with the arm bared, positioned with support and at heart level. The client should sit with the legs on floor, feet uncrossed, and should not speak during the recording. The client should not have smoked tobacco or taken in caffeine during the 30 minutes preceding the measurement. The client should rest quietly for 5 minutes before the reading is taken. The cuff bladder should encircle at least 80% of the limb being measured. Gauges other than a mercury sphygmomanometer should be calibrated every 6 months to ensure accuracy. Finally, two or more readings should be averaged.
Test-Taking Strategy: Note the key word, *avoiding.* This word indicates a false response question and that you need to select the incorrect action. Because blood pressure measurement is a basic skill, this should be fairly easy to answer. However, remember that in questions worded such as these, variables that interfere with accuracy (such as caffeine and nicotine in this instance) are likely to be the correct option. Review this procedure if you had difficulty with this question.
Level of Cognitive Ability: Application
Client Needs: Physiological Integrity
Integrated Process: Nursing Process/Data Collection
Content Area: Adult Health/Cardiovascular
Reference: Christensen, B., & Kockrow, E. (2003). *Foundations of nursing* (4th ed.). St. Louis: Mosby, p. 223.

23. *Answer:* 3
Rationale: Pulmonary edema is characterized by extreme breathlessness, dyspnea, air hunger, and production of frothy, pink-tinged sputum. Auscultation of the lungs reveals crackles. Wheezes, rhonchi, and diminished breath sounds are not associated with pulmonary edema.
Test-Taking Strategy: Use the process of elimination. Recall that fluid produces sounds that are called crackles. This will assist in eliminating options 1, 2, and 4. If you had difficulty with this question, review the manifestations found in pulmonary edema.
Level of Cognitive Ability: Analysis
Client Needs: Physiological Integrity
Integrated Process: Nursing Process/Data Collection

Content Area: Adult Health/Cardiovascular
Reference: Lewis, S., Heitkemper, M., & Dirksen, S. (2004). *Medical-surgical nursing: Assessment and management of clinical problems* (6th ed.). St. Louis: Mosby, p. 842.

24. Answer: 4
Rationale: Pulmonary edema causes the client to be extremely agitated and anxious. The client may complain of a sense of drowning, suffocation, or smothering.
Test-Taking Strategy: Use the process of elimination. Noting the key word, *severe,* will direct you to option 4. Review the clinical manifestations associated with severe pulmonary edema if you had difficulty with this question.
Level of Cognitive Ability: Analysis
Client Needs: Psychosocial Integrity
Integrated Process: Nursing Process/Data Collection
Content Area: Adult Health/Cardiovascular
Reference: Phipps, W., Monahan, F., Sands, J., Marek, J., & Neighbors, M. (2003). *Medical-surgical nursing: Health and illness perspectives* (7th ed.). St. Louis: Mosby, p. 730.

25. Answer: 4
Rationale: Right-sided heart failure is characterized by signs of systemic congestion that occur as a result of right ventricular failure, fluid retention, and pressure buildup in the venous system. Edema develops in the lower legs and ascends to the thighs and abdominal wall. Other characteristics include jugular (neck vein) congestion, enlarged liver and spleen, anorexia and nausea, distended abdomen, swollen hands and fingers, polyuria at night, and weight gain. Left-sided heart failure produces pulmonary signs. These include dyspnea, crackles on lung auscultation, and a hacking cough.
Test-Taking Strategy: Focus on the issue, right-sided heart failure. Eliminate options 1, 2, and 3 because they are similar and are pulmonary signs. Review the signs of right- and left-sided heart failure if you had difficulty with this question.
Level of Cognitive Ability: Analysis
Client Needs: Physiological Integrity
Integrated Process: Nursing Process/Data Collection
Content Area: Adult Health/Cardiovascular
Reference: Ignatavicius, D., & Workman, M. (2006). *Medical surgical nursing: Critical thinking for collaborative care* (5th ed.). Philadelphia: W.B. Saunders, p. 753.

26. Answer: 3
Rationale: Arterial leg ulcers tend to be deep and pale, with uneven edges and little granulation tissue. The client usually has rest pain, and the ulcer site is painful. Options 1, 2, and 4 are incorrect.
Test-Taking Strategy: Use the process of elimination. This question is asking you to differentiate between signs and symptoms of arterial and venous leg ulcers. Because arterial ulcers are caused by marked reduction in blood flow and tissue malnutrition, you can eliminate options 1 and 2. Brown discoloration (option 4) indicates clogging of peripheral tissue with waste products of metabolism, and indicates a venous problem. The answer is option 3, which is also consistent with tissue malnutrition. Review the characteristics of an arterial ischemic ulcer if you had difficulty with this question.
Level of Cognitive Ability: Analysis

Client Needs: Physiological Integrity
Integrated Process: Nursing Process/Data Collection
Content Area: Adult Health/Cardiovascular
Reference: Christensen, B., & Kockrow, E. (2003). *Adult health nursing* (4th ed.). St. Louis: Mosby, p. 345.

27. Answer: 1
Rationale: An expected outcome of surgery is warmth, redness, and edema in the surgical extremity cause by increased blood flow. Options 2, 3, and 4 are incorrect.
Test-Taking Strategy: Use the process of elimination. Option 3 can be eliminated because the pedal pulse is unchanged. Venous complications from immobilization due to surgery would not be apparent within 4 hours, so eliminate option 4 next. To choose between options 1 and 2, think about the effects of sudden reperfusion in an ischemic limb. There would be redness from new blood flow and edema from the sudden change in pressure in the blood vessels. Thus option 1 is correct. Review the expected findings following aortoiliac bypass graft if you had difficulty with this question.
Level of Cognitive Ability: Analysis
Client Needs: Physiological Integrity
Integrated Process: Nursing Process/Data Collection
Content Area: Adult Health/Cardiovascular
Reference: Christensen, B., & Kockrow, E. (2003). *Adult health nursing* (4th ed.). St. Louis: Mosby, p. 336.

28. Answer: 1
Rationale: Psychosocial care of the client with medical management of an AAA includes listening to the client's concerns and reinforcing the rationales for ongoing medical surveillance. This includes periodic CT scanning to monitor the size of the aneurysm and careful adherence to medication and diet therapy for hypertension. The client is instructed to report any sensation of abdominal fullness or abdominal or back pain to the physician without delay.
Test-Taking Strategy: Use the process of elimination and note the key word, *unnecessary.* Options 2 and 4 can be eliminated because they are obviously good actions. From the remaining options, remember that increased blood pressure (option 3) could cause strain and rupture. This will direct you to option 1. Review care of the client with an AAA if you had difficulty with this question.
Level of Cognitive Ability: Application
Client Needs: Physiological Integrity
Integrated Process: Nursing Process/Implementation
Content Area: Adult Health/Cardiovascular
Reference: Christensen, B., & Kockrow, E. (2003). *Adult health nursing* (4th ed.). St. Louis: Mosby, p. 340.

29. Answer: 2
Rationale: An Unna boot that is applied too tightly can cause signs of arterial occlusion. The nurse assesses the circulation to the foot and teaches the client to do the same. Options 1, 3, and 4 are incorrect interpretations.
Test-Taking Strategy: Note that the symptoms described in the question are signs of arterial compromise. Option 2 is the only option that is consistent with this circumstance. Review the signs of arterial compromise if you had difficulty with this question.

Level of Cognitive Ability: Analysis
Client Needs: Physiological Integrity
Integrated Process: Nursing Process/Data Collection
Content Area: Adult Health/Cardiovascular
Reference: Christensen, B., & Kockrow, E. (2003). *Adult health nursing* (4th ed.). St. Louis: Mosby, pp. 345-346.

30. *Answer:* 4
Rationale: For the ambulatory client, the physician may apply a gauze dressing moistened with zinc oxide to the leg, which hardens like a cast (Unna boot). This dressing then prevents venous stasis and provides a sterile environment for the wound. The dressing is changed on a weekly basis. Betadine is not used; it is a strong agent that could cause further damage to friable tissues. Dry sterile dressings do not keep the wound moist. Damp to dry dressings may be used when mechanical debridement is needed.
Test-Taking Strategy: Focus on the issue, a venous stasis ulcer. Recalling the treatment associated with this type of ulcer will direct you to option 4. Review this form of treatment if you had difficulty with this question.
Level of Cognitive Ability: Analysis
Client Needs: Physiological Integrity
Integrated Process: Nursing Process/Planning
Content Area: Adult Health/Cardiovascular
Reference: Christensen, B., & Kockrow, E. (2003). *Adult health nursing* (4th ed.). St. Louis: Mosby, p. 346.

31. *Answer:* 2
Rationale: The first signs and symptoms of digoxin toxicity in adults include abdominal pain, nausea, vomiting, visual disturbances (blurred, yellow or green vision, halos around lights), bradycardia, and other dysrhythmias. Options 1, 3, and 4 are not associated with this medication.
Test-Taking Strategy: Focus on the issue, toxicity. Remember gastrointestinal disturbances and visual disturbances are signs of toxicity. Digoxin is a commonly used medication, so review the signs of toxicity if you had difficulty with this question.
Level of Cognitive Ability: Application
Client Needs: Physiological Integrity
Integrated Process: Nursing Process/Data Collection
Content Area: Adult Health/Cardiovascular
Reference: Hodgson, B., & Kizior, R. (2005). *Saunders nursing drug handbook 2005.* Philadelphia: W.B. Saunders, pp. 325-326.

32. *Answer:* 3
Rationale: Stable angina is induced by exercise and relieved by rest or nitroglycerin tablets. Unstable angina occurs at lower and lower levels of activity, or at rest, is less predictable, and is often a precursor of myocardial infarction. Variant angina, or Prinzmetal's angina, is prolonged and severe, and occurs at the same time each day, most often in the morning.
Test-Taking Strategy: Focus on the data in the question and use knowledge regarding the various types of angina to answer the question. This will assist in eliminating options 1, 2, and 4. Review the characteristics of the various types of angina if you had difficulty with this question.
Level of Cognitive Ability: Comprehension
Client Needs: Physiological Integrity
Integrated Process: Nursing Process/Data Collection

Content Area: Adult Health/Cardiovascular
Reference: Black, J., & Hawks, J. (2005). *Medical-surgical nursing: Clinical management for positive outcomes* (7th ed.). Philadelphia: W.B. Saunders, p. 1704.

33. *Answer:* 2
Rationale: Following pericardiocentesis, a rise in blood pressure is expected. The client usually expresses immediate relief. Heart sounds are no longer muffled or distant. Clear breath sounds are a positive sign. A drop in the central venous pressure is also expected.
Test-Taking Strategy: Note the key word, *unsuccessful.* Successful therapy is measured by the disappearance of the original signs and symptoms of cardiac tamponade. Therefore, look for the option that identifies a sign consistent with continued tamponade. Review signs of cardiac tamponade and the expected effects of pericardiocentesis if you had difficulty with this question.
Level of Cognitive Ability: Analysis
Client Needs: Physiological Integrity
Integrated Process: Nursing Process/Evaluation
Content Area: Adult Health/Cardiovascular
Reference: Chernecky, C., & Berger, B. (2004). *Laboratory tests and diagnostic procedures* (4th ed.). Philadelphia: W.B. Saunders, pp. 860-861.

34. *Answer:* 2
Rationale: Not all clients with AAA exhibit symptoms. Those who do may describe a feeling of the "heart beating" in the abdomen when supine, or being able to feel the mass throbbing. A pulsatile mass may be palpated in the middle and upper abdomen. A systolic bruit may be auscultated over the mass. Hyperactive bowel sounds is not specifically related to an AAA.
Test-Taking Strategy: Use the process of elimination. Note the key word, *unrelated.* Note that options 1, 3, and 4 are similar in that they identify a circulatory component. Review the signs of AAA if you had difficulty with this question.
Level of Cognitive Ability: Analysis
Client Needs: Physiological Integrity
Integrated Process: Nursing Process/Data Collection
Content Area: Adult Health/Cardiovascular
Reference: Linton, A., & Maebius, N. (2003). *Introduction to medical-surgical nursing* (3rd ed.). Philadelphia: W.B. Saunders, p. 629.

35. *Answer:* 2
Rationale: Denial is the most common reaction when a client has a myocardial infarction or anginal pain. No angry behavior was identified in the question. Phobias and obsessive-compulsive disorders are mental health diagnoses.
Test-Taking Strategy: Use the process of elimination. Eliminate options 1 and 3 first because these are medical diagnoses. Recalling that denial is the most common reaction when a person has chest pain will direct you to option 2. Review psychosocial responses in the client experiencing chest pain if you had difficulty with this question.
Level of Cognitive Ability: Analysis
Client Needs: Psychosocial Integrity
Integrated Process: Nursing Process/Data Collection

Content Area: Pharmacology
References: Black, J., & Hawks, J. (2005). *Medical-surgical nursing: Clinical management for positive outcomes* (7th ed.). Philadelphia: W.B. Saunders, p. 526.
Christensen, B., & Kockrow, E. (2003). *Foundations of nursing* (4th ed.). St. Louis: Mosby, p. 931.

ALTERNATE FORMAT QUESTION: MULTIPLE RESPONSE

Answers:
Administration of furosemide (Lasix)
Administration of oxygen
Administration of intravenous morphine sulfate
Rationale: Pulmonary edema is a life-threatening event that can result from severe heart failure. In pulmonary edema, the left ventricle fails to eject sufficient blood, and pressure increases in the lungs because of the accumulated blood. Oxygen is always prescribed and the client is placed in a high Fowler's position to ease the work of breathing. Furosemide, a rapid-acting diuretic, will eliminate accumulated fluid.

Intravenous morphine sulfate reduces venous return (preload), decreases anxiety, and reduces the work of breathing. Transporting the client to the coronary care unit is not a priority intervention. In fact, this may not be necessary at all if the client's response to treatment is successful.
Test-Taking Strategy: Note the key words, *priority interventions*, and focus on the client's diagnosis. Recalling the pathophysiology associated with pulmonary edema and using the ABCs—airway, breathing, and circulation—will assist in determining the priority interventions. Review priority interventions for the client with pulmonary edema if you had difficulty with this question.
Level of Cognitive Ability: Application
Client Needs: Physiological Integrity
Integrated Process: Nursing Process/Implementation
Content Area: Adult Health/Cardiovascular
Reference: Ignatavicius, D., & Workman, M. (2006). *Medical surgical nursing: Critical thinking for collaborative care* (5th ed.). Philadelphia: W.B. Saunders, p. 760.

REFERENCES

Black, J., & Hawks, J. (2005). *Medical-surgical nursing: Clinical management for positive outcomes* (7th ed.). Philadelphia: W.B. Saunders.

Chernecky, C., & Berger, B. (2004). *Laboratory tests and diagnostic procedures* (4th ed.). Philadelphia: W.B. Saunders.

Christensen, B., & Kockrow, E. (2003). *Adult health nursing* (4th ed.). St. Louis: Mosby.

Christensen, B., & Kockrow, E. (2003). *Foundations of nursing* (4th ed.). St. Louis: Mosby.

Hodgson, B., & Kizior, R. (2005). *Saunders nursing drug handbook 2005.* Philadelphia: W.B. Saunders.

Ignatavicius, D. & Workman, M. (2006). *Medical surgical nursing: Critical thinking for collaborative care* (5th ed.). Philadelphia: W.B. Saunders.

Lewis, S., Heitkemper, M., & Dirksen, S. (2004). *Medical-surgical nursing: Assessment and management of clinical problems* (6th ed.). St. Louis: Mosby.

Linton, A., & Maebius, N. (2003). *Introduction to medical-surgical nursing* (3rd ed.). Philadelphia: W.B. Saunders.

Mosby's medical, nursing, and allied health dictionary (6th ed.). (2002). St. Louis: Mosby.

Phipps, W., Monahan, F., Sands, J., Marek, J., & Neighbors, M. (2003). *Medical-surgical nursing: Health and illness perspectives* (7th ed.). St. Louis: Mosby.

Cardiovascular Medications

I. ANTICOAGULANTS (Box 51-1)

A. Description
1. Prevent the extension and formation of clots by inhibiting factors in the clotting cascade and decreasing blood coagulability
2. Used for thrombosis, pulmonary embolism, and myocardial infarction (MI)
3. Contraindicated with active bleeding, except for disseminated intravascular coagulation (DIC), bleeding disorders or blood dyscrasias, ulcers, liver and kidney disease, and spinal cord or brain injuries

B. Side effects (Box 51-2)
1. Hemorrhage
2. Hematuria
3. Epistaxis
4. Ecchymosis
5. Bleeding gums
6. Thrombocytopenia
7. Hypotension

C. Heparin sodium (Liquaemin)
1. Description
   a. Prevents thrombin from converting fibrinogen to fibrin
   b. Prevents thromboembolism
   c. The therapeutic dose does not dissolve clots, but prevents new thrombus formation
2. Blood levels
   a. Normal activated partial thromboplastin time (aPTT) is 20 to 36 seconds
   b. Maintain aPTT at 1.5 to 2.5 times normal
   c. At therapeutic levels, heparin will increase the aPTT by a factor of 1.5 to 2
   d. aPTT therapy should be measured every 4 to 6 hours during initial therapy, and then on a daily basis
   e. If the aPTT is too long, more than 80 seconds, the dosage should be lowered
   f. If aPTT is too short, less than 60 seconds, the dosage should be increased
   g. Normal clotting time is 8 to 15 minutes; maintain the clotting time at 15 to 20 minutes

---

BOX 51-1

Anticoagulants

ORAL
Anisindione (Miradon)
Warfarin sodium (Coumadin)

PARENTERAL
Ardeparin (Normiflo)
Dalteparin (Fragmin)
Danaparoid (Orgaran)
Enoxaparin (Lovenox)
Heparin sodium (Liquaemin)
Tinzaparin (Innohep)

BOX 51-2

Substances to Avoid with Anticoagulants

Green, leafy vegetables and foods high in vitamin K
Allopurinol (Zyloprim)
Cimetidine (Tagamet)
Corticosteroids
Nonsteroidal anti-inflammatory drugs (NSAIDs)
Oral hypoglycemic agents
Phenytoin (Dilantin)
Salicylates
Sulfonamides

3. Interventions
   a. Monitor clotting time and aPTT
   b. Monitor platelet count
   c. Observe for bleeding gums, bruises, nose-bleeds, hematuria, hematemesis, occult blood in the stool, and petechiae
   d. When administering heparin subcutaneously, inject into the abdomen with a small needle (25- to 28 gauge) at a 90-degree angle and do not aspirate or rub the injection site
   e. Instruct the client regarding measures to prevent bleeding
   f. Antidote: protamine sulfate
D. Warfarin sodium (Coumadin)
   1. Description
      a. Decreases prothrombin activity and prevents the use of vitamin K by the liver
      b. Used for long-term anticoagulation
      c. Prolongs clotting time and is monitored by the prothrombin time (PT)
      d. Used mainly to prevent thromboembolitic conditions such as thrombophlebitis, pulmonary embolism, and embolism formation caused by atrial fibrillation, thrombosis, myocardial infarction (MI), or heart valve damage
      e. Usually given for 2 to 3 months after an MI to decrease the incidence of deep vein thrombosis and thromboembolism
   2. Blood levels
      a. Average PT is 9.6 to 11.8 seconds
      b. Warfarin sodium prolongs the PT
   3. International normalized ratio (INR)
      a. The normal INR is 1.3 to 2
      b. The INR is determined by multiplying the observed PT ratio (the ratio of the client's PT to a control PT) by a correction factor specific to a particular thromboplastin preparation used in the testing
      c. The treatment goal is to raise the INR to an appropriate value
      d. An INR of 2 to 3 is appropriate for most clients, although, for some clients, the target INR is 3 to 4.5
      e. If the INR is below the recommended range, warfarin sodium should be increased
      f. If the INR is above the recommended range, warfarin sodium should be reduced
   4. Interventions
      a. Monitor PT and INR
      b. Observe for bleeding gums, bruises, nose-bleeds, hematuria, hematemesis, occult blood in the stool, and petechiae
      c. Instruct the client regarding measures to prevent bleeding
      d. Antidote: Vitamin K phytonadione (Aqua-MEPHYTON)

II. THROMBOLYTIC MEDICATIONS (Box 51-3)

A. Description
   1. Activate plasminogen; plasminogen generates plasmin (the enzyme that dissolves clots)
   2. Used early in the course of myocardial infarction (within 4 to 6 hours of the onset of the infarct) to restore blood flow, limit myocardial damage, preserve left ventricular function, and prevent death
B. Contraindications
   1. Active internal bleeding
   2. History of cerebrovascular accident (CVA)
   3. Intracranial problems
   4. Intracranial surgery or trauma within the previous 2 months
   5. History of thoracic, pelvic, or abdominal surgery in the previous 10 days
   6. History of hepatic or renal disease
   7. Uncontrolled hypertension
   8. Recent required, prolonged cardiopulmonary resuscitation (CPR)
C. Side effects
   1. Bleeding
   2. Dysrhythmias
   3. Fever
   4. Allergic reactions
D. Interventions
   1. Obtain aPTT, PT, fibrinogen level, hematocrit, and platelet count
   2. Monitor vital signs
   3. Monitor pulses
   4. Monitor for bleeding
   5. Monitor all excretions for occult blood
   6. Monitor for neurological changes such as slurred speech, lethargy, confusion, and hemiparesis
   7. Monitor for hypotension and tachycardia
   8. Avoid injections if possible
   9. Apply direct pressure over a puncture site for 20 to 30 minutes
   10. Handle the client as little as possible when moving
   11. Instruct the client to use an electric razor for shaving and to brush teeth gently
   12. Discontinue the medication if bleeding develops, and notify the physician

---

BOX 51-3

Thrombolytic Medications

Alteplase (Activase, tissue plasminogen activator [t-PA])
Anistreplase (APSAC, Eminase)
Reteplase (Retavase)
Streptokinase (Kabikinase, Streptase)
Urokinase (Abbokinase)

13. Antidote
    a. Aminocaproic acid (Amicar)
    b. Used only in acute, life-threatening conditions

III. ANTIPLATELET MEDICATIONS (Box 51-4)

A. Description
    1. Inhibit the aggregation of platelets in the clotting process, thereby prolonging the bleeding time
    2. May be used in conjunction with anticoagulants
    3. Used in the prophylaxis of long-term complications following MI, coronary revascularization, and CVAs
    4. Contraindicated in bleeding disorders and known sensitivity
B. Side effects
    1. Gastrointestinal (GI) bleeding
    2. Bruising
    3. Hematuria
    4. Tarry stools
C. Interventions
    1. Determine sensitivity prior to administration
    2. Monitor vital signs
    3. Instruct the client to take medication with food if GI upset occurs
    4. Monitor bleeding time
    5. Monitor for side effects related to bleeding
    6. Instruct the client in the use of the medication
    7. Instruct the client to monitor for side effects related to bleeding and in the measures to prevent bleeding

IV. CARDIAC GLYCOSIDES (Box 51-5)

A. Description
    1. Inhibit sodium-potassium pump, thus increasing intracellular calcium level, which causes the heart muscle fibers to contract more efficiently
    2. Produce a positive inotropic action, which increases the force of myocardial contractions
    3. Produce a negative chronotropic action, which depresses the sinoatrial (SA) node, reduces conduction of the impulse through the atrioventricular (AV) node, and slows the heart rate
    4. Produce a negative dromotropic action that decreases the conduction of the heart cells

---

BOX 51-4

Antiplatelet Medications

Abciximab (ReoPro)
Aspirin (acetylsalicylic acid [ASA])
Clopidogrel bisulfate (Plavix)
Dipyridamole (Persantine)
Eptifibatide (Integrilin)
Ticlopidine hydrochloride (Ticlid)
Tirofiban (Aggrastat)

---

5. The increase in myocardial **contractility** increases cardiac, peripheral, and kidney function by increasing **cardiac output**, decreasing preload, improving blood flow to the periphery and kidneys, decreasing edema, and increasing fluid excretion; as a result, fluid retention in the lungs and extremities is decreased
6. Used for congestive heart failure (CHF), atrial tachycardia, atrial fibrillation, and atrial flutter
7. Contraindicated in ventricular dysrhythmias and second- or third-degree heart block
8. Used with caution in clients with renal disease, hypothyroidism, and hypokalemia
B. Side effects
    1. Anorexia, nausea, vomiting
    2. Headache
    3. Visual disturbances: diplopia, blurred vision, yellow-green halos
    4. Photophobia
    5. Drowsiness
    6. Bradycardia
    7. Fatigue, weakness
C. Interventions
    1. Monitor for toxicity, as evidenced by anorexia, nausea, vomiting, visual disturbances, confusion, bradycardia, heart block, premature ventricular contractions (PVCs), and tachydysrhythmias
    2. Monitor serum digoxin level, electrolyte levels, and renal function tests
    3. Therapeutic digoxin range is 0.5 to 2 ng/mL; levels above 2 ng/mL are toxic
    4. An increased risk of toxicity exists in clients with hypercalcemia, hypokalemia, hypomagnesemia, or hypothyroidism
    5. Monitor potassium level; if hypokalemia occurs (potassium below 3.5 mEq/L), notify the physician
    6. Instruct the client to avoid over-the-counter medications
    7. Monitor the client taking a potassium-wasting diuretic or corticosteroids closely for hypokalemia, because the hypokalemia can cause digoxin toxicity
    8. Note that older clients are more sensitive to toxicity
    9. Advise the client to eat foods high in potassium, such as fresh and dried fruits, fruit juices, vegetables, and potatoes
    10. Monitor the apical pulse

BOX 51-5

Cardiac Glycosides

Digoxin (Lanoxicaps, Lanoxin)

11. If the apical pulse rate is below 60 beats per minute, the medication should be held and the physician notified
12. Teach the client how to measure pulse
13. Teach the client to notify physician if the pulse rate is below 60 or above 100 beats per minute,
14. Teach the client the signs and symptoms of toxicity
15. Antidote: Digoxin immune Fab (Digibind) is used in extreme toxicity

V. ANTIHYPERTENSIVE MEDICATIONS (Box 51-6)
A. Thiazide diuretics (Box 51-7)
1. Description
   a. Increase sodium and water excretion by inhibiting sodium reabsorption in the distal tubule of the kidney
   b. Used for hypertension and peripheral edema
   c. Used in clients with normal renal function
   d. Not effective for immediate diuresis
   e. Contraindicated in renal failure
   f. Used with caution in the client taking lithium, because lithium toxicity can occur
   g. Used with caution in the client taking digoxin, corticosteroids, or antidiabetic medications
2. Side effects
   a. Hypercalcemia, hyperglycemia, hyperuricemia
   b. Hypokalemia, hyponatremia
   c. Hypovolemia
   d. Hypotension
   e. Headaches
   f. Nausea, vomiting
   g. Constipation
   h. Rashes
   i. Photosensitivity
   j. Blood dyscrasias

BOX 51-6

Classifications of Diuretics

Thiazide diuretics
Loop diuretics
Osmotic diuretics
Potassium-sparing diuretics
Carbonic anhydrase inhibitors

BOX 51-7

Thiazide and Thiazide-like Diuretics

Chlorothiazide (Diuril)
Chlorthalidone (Hygroton, Thalitone)
Hydrochlorothiazide (Esidrix, Oretic, HydroDIURIL)
Indapamide (Lozol)
Metolazone (Zaroxolyn)

---

3. Interventions
   a. Monitor vital signs
   b. Monitor weight
   c. Monitor urine output
   d. Monitor electrolyte, glucose, calcium, and uric acid levels
   e. Check peripheral extremities for edema
   f. Instruct the client to take the medication in the morning to avoid nocturia and sleep interruption
   g. Instruct the client in how to record the BP
   h. Instruct the client to eat foods rich in potassium
   i. Instruct the client in how to take potassium supplements if prescribed
   j. Instruct the client to take medication with food to avoid GI upset
   k. Instruct the client to change positions slowly to prevent orthostatic hypotension
   l. Instruct the client to use sunscreen when in direct sunlight
   m. Instruct the client with diabetes mellitus to have the blood glucose level checked periodically

B. Loop diuretics (Box 51-8)
1. Description
   a. Inhibit sodium and chloride reabsorption from the loop of Henle and the distal tubule
   b. They have little effect on the blood glucose level; however, they cause marked depletion of water and electrolytes, increased uric acid levels, and the excretion of calcium
   c. Are more potent than the thiazide diuretics, causing rapid diuresis, thus decreasing vascular fluid volume, cardiac output, and blood pressure
   d. Used for hypertension, edema associated with CHF, hypercalcemia, and renal disease
   e. Use with caution in the client taking digoxin or lithium
   f. Use with caution in the client on aminoglycosides, anticoagulants, corticosteroids, or amphotericin B
2. Side effects
   a. Hypokalemia, hyponatremia, hypocalcemia, hypomagnesemia
   b. Hypochloremia
   c. Thrombocytopenia
   d. Hyperuricemia
   e. Orthostatic hypotension
   f. Skin disturbances

BOX 51-8

Loop Diuretics

Furosemide (Lasix)
Bumetanide (Bumex)
Ethacrynic acid (Edecrin)
Torsemide (Demadex)

g. Ototoxicity and deafness

h. Thiamine deficiency

i. Dehydration

3. Interventions

a. Monitor vital signs

b. Monitor weight

c. Monitor urine output

d. Monitor electrolyte, calcium, magnesium, and uric acid levels

e. Check the peripheral extremities for edema

f. Monitor for signs of digoxin or lithium toxicity if the client is on these medications

g. Instruct the client to take the medication in the morning to avoid nocturia and sleep interruption

h. Instruct the client in how to record the BP

i. Instruct the client to eat foods rich in potassium

j. Instruct the client in how to take potassium supplements if prescribed

k. Instruct the client to take medication with food to avoid GI upset

l. Instruct the client to change positions slowly to prevent orthostatic hypotension

C. Osmotic diuretics

1. See Chapter 57 for information regarding osmotic diuretics

2. See Box 51-9 for a list of these medications

D. Carbonic anhydrase inhibitors (Box 51-10)

1. Description

a. Block the action of the enzyme carbonic anhydrase, needed to maintain acid-base balance

b. Inhibition of this enzyme, carbonic anhydrase, causes increased sodium, potassium, and bicarbonate excretion

c. Metabolic acidosis can occur with prolonged use

d. Used to decrease intraocular pressure in open-angle (chronic) glaucoma, and to produce diuresis, manage epilepsy, and treat high-altitude sickness

e. Used to treat metabolic alkalosis

f. Contraindicated in narrow-angle or acute glaucoma

2. Side effects

a. Hyperglycemia, hyperuricemia, hypercalcemia

b. Hypokalemia

c. Anorexia, nausea, vomiting

d. Orthostatic hypotension

e. Renal calculi

f. Hemolytic anemia

3. Interventions

a. Monitor vital signs

b. Monitor weight

c. Monitor urine output

d. Monitor electrolyte, glucose, calcium, and uric acid levels

e. Monitor mental status

f. Instruct the client to monitor for signs of renal calculi

E. Potassium-sparing diuretics (Box 51-11)

1. Description

a. Act on the distal tubule to promote sodium and water excretion and potassium retention

b. Used for edema and hypertension to increase urine output, to treat fluid retention and overload associated with CHF, hepatic cirrhosis, or nephrotic syndrome, and for diuretic-induced hypokalemia

c. Contraindicated in severe kidney or hepatic disease or in severe hyperkalemia

d. Used with caution in the client with diabetes mellitus

e. Used with caution in the client taking antihypertensives or lithium

f. Used with caution in the client taking angiotensin-converting enzyme (ACE) inhibitors, because hyperkalemia can result

g. Used with caution in the client taking potassium supplements

2. Side effects

a. Hyperkalemia

b. Nausea, vomiting, diarrhea

c. Rash

d. Dizziness, weakness

e. Headache

f. Dry mouth

g. Photosensitivity

BOX 51-9

Osmotic Diuretics

Glycerin (Osmoglyn)
Mannitol (Osmitrol)
Urea (Ureaphil)

BOX 51-10

Carbonic Anhydrase Inhibitors

Acetazolamide (Diamox)
Dichlorphenamide (Daranide)
Methazolamide (Neptazane)

BOX 51-11

Potassium-Sparing Diuretics

Spironolactone (Aldactone)
Amiloride (Midamor)
Triamterene (Dyrenium)
Amiloride hydrochloride and hydrochlorothiazide (Moduretic)
Spironolactone and hydrochlorothiazide (Aldactazide)

BOX 51-12

Peripherally Acting Alpha-Adrenergic Blockers

Doxazosin mesylate (Cardura)
Prazosin (Minipress)
Terazosin (Hytrin)
Guanadrel (Hylorel)
Guanethidine (Ismelin)
Reserpine (Serpasil)
Phenoxybenzamine (Dibenzyline)
Phentolamine (Regitine)

BOX 51-13

Centrally Acting Sympatholytics

Clonidine (Catapres)
Methyldopa (Aldomet)
Guanabenz (Wytensin)

h. Anemia
    i. Thrombocytopenia
3. Interventions
    a. Monitor vital signs
    b. Monitor urine output
    c. Monitor for signs and symptoms of hyper-kalemia, such as nausea, diarrhea, abdominal cramps, tachycardia followed by bradycardia, peaked narrow T wave on the electrocardiogram, or oliguria
    d. Monitor for a potassium level higher than 5.3 mEq/L, which indicates hyperkalemia
    e. Instruct the client to avoid foods high in potassium
    f. Instruct the client to avoid exposure to direct sunlight
    g. Instruct the client to monitor for signs of hyperkalemia
    h. Instruct the client to avoid salt substitutes because they contain potassium
    i. Instruct the client to take with or after meals to decrease GI irritation

VI. PERIPHERALLY ACTING ALPHA-ADRENERGIC BLOCKERS (Box 51-12)

A. Description
    1. Decrease sympathetic vasoconstriction by reducing the effects of norepinephrine at peripheral nerve endings, resulting in vasodilation and decreased **BP**
    2. Used to maintain renal blood flow
    3. Used to treat hypertension
B. Side effects
    1. Orthostatic hypotension
    2. Reflex tachycardia
    3. Sodium and water retention
    4. GI disturbances
    5. Nausea
    6. Drowsiness
    7. Nasal congestion
    8. Edema
    9. Weight gain
    10. Reserpine (Serpasil) can cause depression, GI irritation, and impotence

C. Interventions
    1. Monitor vital signs
    2. Monitor for fluid retention and edema
    3. Instruct the client to change positions slowly to prevent **orthostatic hypotension**
    4. Instruct the client in how to monitor the **BP**
    5. Instruct the client to monitor for edema
    6. Instruct the client to decrease salt intake
    7. Instruct the client to avoid over-the-counter medications

VII. CENTRALLY ACTING SYMPATHOLYTICS (ADRENERGIC BLOCKERS) (Box 51-13)

A. Description
    1. Stimulate alpha receptors in the central nervous system (CNS) to inhibit vasoconstriction, thus reducing peripheral resistance
    2. Used to treat hypertension
    3. Contraindicated in impaired liver function
B. Side effects
    1. Sodium and water retention
    2. Drowsiness, dizziness
    3. Dry mouth
    4. Bradycardia
    5. Edema
    6. Impotence
    7. Hypotension
    8. Depression
C. Interventions
    1. Monitor vital signs
    2. Instruct the client not to discontinue medication, because abrupt withdrawal can cause severe rebound hypertension
    3. Monitor liver function tests

VIII. ANGIOTENSIN-CONVERTING ENZYME (ACE) INHIBITORS (Box 51-14)

A. Description
    1. Prevent peripheral vasoconstriction by blocking conversion of angiotensin I to angiotensin II
    2. Used to treat hypertension
    3. Avoid use with potassium supplements and potassium-sparing diuretics
B. Side effects
    1. Nausea, vomiting, diarrhea
    2. Persistent cough

BOX 51-14

Angiotensin-Converting Enzyme (ACE) Inhibitors

Benazepril (Lotensin)
Captopril (Capoten)
Enalapril (Vasotec)
Fosinopril (Monopril)
Lisinopril (Prinivil, Zestril)
Moexipril (Univasc)
Perindopril (Aceon)
Quinapril (Accupril)
Ramipril (Altace)
Trandolapril (Mavik)

BOX 51-15

Antiangina Medications

Isosorbide mononitrate (Imdur, Monoket)
Isosorbide dinitrate (Isordil)
Nitroglycerin (Nitrostat, Nitrolingual, Nitrogard)
Nitroglycerin ointment, 2% (Nitro-Bid, Nitrol, Nitrong)
Nitroglycerin, transdermal patch (Nitrodisc, Nitro-Dur, Transderm-Nitro)

---

3. Hypotension
4. Hyperkalemia
5. Tachycardia
6. Headache
7. Dizziness, fatigue
8. Insomnia
9. Hypoglycemic reaction in the client with diabetes mellitus
10. Bruising, petechiae, bleeding
11. Diminished taste

C. Interventions
1. Monitor vital signs
2. Monitor protein, albumin, blood urea nitrogen (BUN), creatinine, white blood cell (WBC), and potassium levels
3. Monitor for hypoglycemic reactions in the client with diabetes mellitus
4. Instruct the client to take captopril (Capoten) 20 to 60 minutes before a meal
5. Monitor for bruising, petechiae, or bleeding with captopril
6. Instruct the client not to discontinue medications because rebound hypertension can occur
7. Instruct the client not to take over-the-counter medications
8. Instruct the client in how to take the BP
9. Instruct the client that if dizziness occurs and persists, to notify the physician
10. Inform the client that the taste of food may be diminished during the first month of therapy

---

IX. **ANTIANGINAL MEDICATIONS** (Box 51-15)
A. Nitrates
1. Description
   a. Produce vasodilation
   b. Decrease preload and afterload and reduce myocardial oxygen consumption
   c. Contraindicated in the client with marked hypotension, increased intracranial pressure (ICP), or severe anemia
   d. Used with caution with severe renal or hepatic disease

e. Avoid abrupt withdrawal of long-acting preparations to prevent the rebound effect of severe pain from myocardial ischemia
2. Side effects
   a. Headache
   b. **Orthostatic hypotension**
   c. Dizziness, weakness
   d. Faintness
   e. Nausea, vomiting
   f. Flushing or pallor
   g. Confusion
   h. Rash
   i. Dry mouth
   j. Reflex tachycardia
   k. Paradoxical bradycardia
3. Sublingual medications
   a. Monitor vital signs
   b. Offer sips of water before giving, because dryness may inhibit medication absorption
   c. Instruct the client to place under the tongue and leave until fully dissolved
   d. Instruct the client not to swallow the medication
   e. Instruct the client to take one tablet for pain, and repeat every 5 minutes for a total of three doses
   f. Instruct the client to seek medical help immediately if pain is not relieved in 15 minutes following the three doses
   g. Inform the client that a stinging or biting sensation may indicate that the tablet is fresh
   h. Instruct the client to store medication in a dark, tightly closed bottle
   i. Instruct the client to check the expiration date on the medication bottle, because medication could reach this date within 6 months of obtaining medication
   j. Instruct the client to take acetaminophen (Tylenol) for a headache
4. Translingual medications
   a. Instruct the client to direct spray against the oral mucosa
   b. Instruct the client to avoid inhaling the spray

5. Sustained-released medications: Instruct the client to swallow and not to chew or crush the medication
6. Transmucosal-buccal medications
   a. Instruct the client to place between the upper lip and gum or in the buccal area between the cheek and gum
   b. Inform the client that the medication will adhere to the oral mucosa and slowly dissolve
7. Transdermal patch
   a. Instruct the client to apply the patch to a hairless area, using a new patch and a different site each day
   b. As prescribed, instruct the client to remove the patch after 12 to 14 hours, allowing 10 to 12 "patch-free" hours each day to prevent tolerance
   c. Do not apply the patch on the chest in the area of defibrillator-cardioverter paddle placement, because skin burns can result if the paddles need to be used
8. Topical ointments
   a. Instruct the client to remove the ointment on the skin from the previous dose
   b. Instruct the client to squeeze a ribbon of ointment of the prescribed length onto the applicator paper
   c. Instruct the client to spread the ointment over a 6- × 6-inch area, using the chest, back, abdomen, upper arm, or anterior thigh (avoiding hairy areas), and cover with a plastic wrap
   d. Instruct the client to rotate sites and to avoid touching the ointment when applying
   e. Do not apply the ointment on the chest in the area of defibrillator-cardioverter paddle placement, because skin burns can result if the paddles need to be used

X. BETA-ADRENERGIC BLOCKERS (Box 51-16)

A. Description
1. Inhibit response to beta-adrenergic stimulation, thus decreasing **cardiac output**
2. Block the release of the catecholamines, epinephrine, and norepinephrine, thus decreasing the heart rate and **blood pressure**
3. Decrease the workload of the heart and decrease oxygen demands
4. Used for angina, dysrhythmias, hypertension, migraine headaches, prevention of MI, and glaucoma
5. Contraindicated in the client with asthma, bradycardia, CHF, severe renal or hepatic disease, hyperthyroidism, or CVA
6. Used with caution in the client with diabetes mellitus, because it may mask symptoms of hypoglycemia
7. Used with caution in the client on antihypertensives

BOX 51-16

Beta-Adrenergic Blockers

Acebutolol (Sectral)
Atenolol (Tenormin)
Betaxolol (Kerlone)
Bisoprolol fumarate (Zebeta)
Carteolol (Cartrol)
Carvedilol (Coreg)
Labetalol (Normodyne, Trandate, Vescal)
Metoprolol (Lopressor, Toprol-XL)
Nadolol (Corgard)
Penbutolol
Pindolol (Visken)
Propranolol (Inderal)
Sotalol (Betapace)
Timolol (Blocadren)

B. Side effects
1. Bradycardia
2. Bronchospasm
3. Hypotension
4. Weakness, fatigue
5. Nausea, vomiting
6. Dizziness
7. Hyperglycemia
8. Agranulocytosis
9. Behavioral or psychotic response
10. Depression
11. Nightmares
C. Interventions
1. Monitor vital signs
2. Hold the medication if the pulse or **BP** is not within the prescribed parameters
3. Monitor for signs of CHF
4. Monitor for respiratory distress and for signs of wheezing and dyspnea
5. Instruct the client to report dizziness, lightheadedness, or nasal congestion
6. Instruct the client not to stop the medication, because rebound hypertension, rebound tachycardia, or an anginal attack can occur
7. Advise the client on insulin that early signs of hypoglycemia, such as tachycardia and nervousness, can be masked by the beta blocker
8. Instruct the client on insulin to monitor the blood glucose level
9. Instruct the client in how to take pulse and **BP**
10. Instruct the client to change positions slowly to prevent **orthostatic hypotension**
11. Instruct the client to avoid over-the-counter cold medications and nasal decongestants

XI. CALCIUM CHANNEL BLOCKERS (Box 51-17)

A. Description

BOX 51-17

Calcium Channel Blockers

Amlodipine (Norvasc)
Diltiazem (Cardizem, Cardizem SR)
Felodipine (Plendil)
Isradipine (DynaCirc)
Nicardipine (Cardene)
Nifedipine (Procardia, Procardia XL, Adalat CC)
Nimodipine (Nimotop)
Nisoldipine (Sular)
Verapamil (Calan, Isoptin)

BOX 51-18

Peripheral Vasodilators

ALPHA-ADRENERGIC BLOCKER
Tolazoline (Priscoline)

BETA-ADRENERGIC AGONISTS
Isoxsuprine (Vasodilan)

DIRECT-ACTING PERIPHERAL VASODILATOR
Ergoloid mesylate (Hydergine)

ALPHA BLOCKERS
Doxazosin mesylate (Cardura)
Prazosin hydrochloride (Minipress)
Terazosin hydrochloride (Hytrin)

CALCIUM CHANNEL BLOCKERS
Nifedipine (Procardia)
Nimodipine (Nimotop)

HEMORRHEOLOGIC AGENT
Pentoxifylline (Trental): Increases microcirculation and tissue perfusion

1. Decrease cardiac **contractility** (negative inotropic effect by relaxing smooth muscle) and the workload of the heart, thus decreasing the need for oxygen
2. Promote vasodilatation of the coronary and peripheral vessels
3. Used for angina, dysrhythmias, or hypertension
4. Used with caution in the client with CHF, bradycardia, or AV block

B. Side effects
1. Bradycardia
2. Hypotension
3. Reflex tachycardia as a result of hypotension
4. Headache
5. Dizziness, lightheadedness
6. Fatigue
7. Peripheral edema
8. Constipation
9. Flushing of the skin
10. Changes in liver and kidney function

C. Interventions
1. Monitor vital signs
2. Monitor for signs of CHF
3. Monitor liver enzyme levels
4. Monitor kidney function tests
5. Instruct the client not to discontinue the medication
6. Instruct the client in how to take a pulse
7. Instruct the client to notify the physician if dizziness or fainting occurs
8. Instruct the client not to crush or chew sustained-released tablets

XII. PERIPHERAL VASODILATORS (Box 51-18)

A. Description
1. Decrease peripheral resistance by exerting a direct action on the arteries or on both the arteries and the veins
2. Increase blood flow to the extremities
3. Used in peripheral vascular disorders of venous and arterial vessels
4. Most effective for disorders resulting from vasospasm (Raynaud's disease)
5. These medications may decrease some of the symptoms of cerebral vascular insufficiency

B. Side effects
1. Lightheadedness, dizziness
2. **Postural hypotension**
3. Tachycardia
4. Palpitations
5. Flushing
6. GI distress

C. Interventions
1. Monitor vital signs, especially the **BP** and the heart rate
2. Monitor for **orthostatic hypotension** and tachycardia
3. Monitor for signs of inadequate blood flow to the extremities, such as pallor, coldness of the extremities, and pain
4. Instruct the client that it may take up to 3 months for a desired therapeutic response
5. Advise the client not to smoke because smoking increases vasospasm
6. Instruct the client to avoid aspirin or aspirin-like compounds unless approved by the physician
7. Instruct the client to take the medication with meals if GI disturbances occur
8. Instruct the client to avoid alcohol because it may cause a hypotensive reaction
9. Encourage the client to change positions slowly to avoid **orthostatic hypotension**

BOX 51-19

Bile Acid Sequestrants

Cholestyramine (Questran)
Colesevelam (WelChol)
Colestipol (Colestid)

BOX 51-20

HMG-CoA Reductase Inhibitors

Atorvastatin (Lipitor)
Fluvastatin (Lescol)
Lovastatin (Mevacor)
Pravastatin (Pravachol)
Simvastatin (Zocor)

BOX 51-21

Other Antilipemic Medications

Dextrothyroxine (Choloxin)
Exetimibe (Zetia)
Fenofibrate (Tricor)
Gemfibrozil (Lopid)
Niacin (Niacor)

XIII. ANTILIPEMIC MEDICATIONS

A. Description
   1. Reduce serum levels of cholesterol, triglycerides, or low-density lipoprotein (LDL)
   2. When cholesterol, triglyceride, and LDL levels are elevated, the client is at increased risk for coronary artery disease
   3. In many cases diet alone will not lower blood lipid levels; therefore, antilipemic medications will be prescribed

B. Bile sequestrants (Box 51-19)
   1. Description
      a. Bind with acids in the intestines
      b. Bile acid sequestrants should not be used as the only therapy in clients with elevated triglyceride levels, because they typically raise triglyceride levels
   2. Side effects
      a. Constipation
      b. Peptic ulcer
   3. Interventions
      a. Cholestyramine (Questran) comes in a gritty powder that must be mixed thoroughly in juice or water before administration
      b. Monitor the client for early signs of peptic ulcer, such as nausea and abdominal discomfort followed by abdominal pain and distention
      c. Instruct the client that the medication must be taken with and followed by sufficient fluids

C. HMG-CoA reductase inhibitors (Box 51-20)
   1. Description
      a. Lovastatin (Mevacor) is highly protein-bound and should not be administered with anticoagulants
      b. Lovastatin should not be administered with gemfibrozil (Lopid)
      c. Administer lovastatin with caution to the client on immunosuppressive medications
   2. Side effects
      a. Nausea
      b. Diarrhea or constipation
      c. Abdominal pain or cramps
      d. Flatulence
      e. Dizziness
      f. Headache
      g. Blurred vision
      h. Rash
      i. Pruritus
      j. Elevated liver enzymes
      k. Causes GI disturbances, headaches, muscle cramps, and fatigue
   3. Interventions
      a. Monitor serum liver enzyme levels
      b. Instruct the client to receive an annual eye examination because the medication causes cataract formation
      c. If lovastatin is not effective in lowering the lipid level after 3 months, it should be discontinued

D. Other antilipemic medications (Box 51-21)
   1. Description
      a. Gemfibrozil should not be taken with anticoagulants because they compete for protein sites; if the client is on an anticoagulant, the anticoagulant dose should be reduced during antilipemic therapy and the INR monitored closely
      b. Do not administer gemfibrozil with lovastatin
   2. Interventions
      a. Monitor vital signs
      b. Monitor liver enzyme levels
      c. Monitor serum cholesterol and triglyceride levels
      d. Instruct the client to restrict intake of fats, cholesterol, carbohydrates, and alcohol
      e. Instruct the client to follow an exercise program

f. Instruct the client that it will take several weeks before the lipid level declines

g. Instruct the client to have an annual eye examination and to report any changes in vision

h. Instruct the client with diabetes mellitus who is taking gemfibrozil to monitor blood glucose levels regularly

i. Instruct the client to increase fluid intake

j. Note that nicotinic acid has numerous side effects, which include GI disturbances, flushing of the skin, elevated liver enzyme levels, hyperglycemia, and hyperuricemia

k. Instruct the client that aspirin may assist in reducing the side effects of nicotinic acid

l. Instruct the client to take nicotinic acid with meals to reduce GI discomfort

PRACTICE QUESTIONS

1. A nurse reinforces discharge instructions to a postoperative client taking warfarin sodium (Coumadin). Which statement by the client indicates the need for further teaching?
   1. "I will take Ecotrin for my headaches because it is coated."
   2. "I will be certain to limit my alcohol consumption."
   3. "I will take my pills every day at the same time."
   4. "I have already called my family to pick up a Medic-Alert bracelet."

2. A client taking digoxin (Lanoxin) has a serum potassium level of 3.0 mEq/L and is complaining of anorexia. The physician orders a digoxin level to be obtained to rule out digoxin toxicity. The nurse checks the results of the test, knowing that the therapeutic serum level for digoxin is which of the following?
   1. 0.1 to 0.5 ng/mL
   2. 0.3 to 0.8 ng/mL
   3. 0.5 to 2 ng/mL
   4. 1 to 3 ng/mL

3. Heparin sodium (Liquaemin) by subcutaneous injection is prescribed for a client. When administering the medication, the nurse would:
   1. Use a 23- to 25-gauge, 1-inch needle
   2. Aspirate before injection
   3. Apply heat after the injection
   4. Administer with a 25- to 27-gauge, $^5/_8$-inch needle

4. A client is taking hydrochlorothiazide (hydroDIURIL, HCTZ) without taking any form of electrolyte supplement. The nurse would encourage intake of which of the following foods?
   1. Canned pears
   2. Oranges
   3. Cranberry juice
   4. Applesauce

5. A 51-year-old client is admitted to the hospital with a diagnosis of myocardial infarction and is started on streptokinase (Streptase) therapy. The nurse determines that the client's wife understands the purpose of the medication if she states that it is used to:
   1. Thin the blood
   2. Slow the clotting of the blood
   3. Dissolve any clots in the coronary arteries
   4. Prevent further clots from forming in the coronary arteries

6. A client is being treated for moderate hypertension and has been taking diltiazem (Cardizem) for several months. The client is seen by the physician, and Prinzmetal's angina is diagnosed. The nurse planning care for the client understands that which action of the medication will provide a therapeutic effect for this new diagnosis?
   1. Increases oxygen demands within the myocardium
   2. Prevents influx of calcium ions in vascular smooth muscle
   3. Leads to an increase in calcium absorption in the vascular smooth muscle
   4. Increases the force of contraction of ventricular tissues

7. A nurse is caring for a client who is taking propranolol (Inderal). Which data would indicate an adverse reaction associated with this medication?
   1. A baseline blood pressure of 150/80 mm Hg followed by a blood pressure of 138/72 mm Hg after two doses of the medication
   2. A baseline resting heart rate of 88 beats per minute followed by a resting heart rate of 72 beats per minute after two doses of the medication
   3. The development of audible expiratory wheezes
   4. The development of complaints of insomnia

8. A client is admitted to the emergency department with an acute anterior wall myocardial infarction. Streptokinase (Streptase) therapy is prescribed for the client and the client's spouse is concerned about the dangers of this treatment. The nurse should make which statement to the client's spouse?
   1. "Your loved one is very ill. The physician has made the best decision for you."
   2. "There is no reason to worry. We use this medication all of the time."
   3. "I'm certain you made the correct decision to use this medication."
   4. "You have concerns about whether this treatment is the best option."

9. A physician prescribed digoxin (Lanoxin), 0.25 mg, for a client with atrial fibrillation. The medication is available as 0.125-mg tablets. The nurse calculates that the client will receive two tablets of digoxin.

When the nurse administers the medication, the client looks at the medication and states, "Every time I get chest pain, I will take one of these heart pills." After double-checking the dosage calculation, the nurse decides to:

1. Not administer the medication as prescribed and calculated
2. Administer one half-tablet of the medication instead of the dosage calculated
3. Administer the medication as prescribed and calculated, and monitor for untoward effects such as seizures
4. Administer the medication as prescribed and calculated and proceed with further client teaching

10. A nurse is caring for an older client who will be discharged home. Furosemide (Lasix) is prescribed for the client and the nurse reinforces instructions to the client about the medication. Which statement by the client indicates the need for further instructions?
    1. "I will take my medication every morning with breakfast."
    2. "I will call my doctor if my ankles swell or my rings get tight."
    3. "I need to drink lots of coffee and tea to keep myself healthy."
    4. "I will sit up slowly before standing each morning."

11. Isosorbide mononitrate (Imdur) is prescribed for a client with angina pectoris. The client tells the nurse that the medication is causing a chronic headache. The nurse appropriately suggests that the client:
    1. Contact the physician
    2. Discontinue the medication
    3. Cut the dose in half
    4. Take the medication with food

12. A client is being discharged with a prescription for propanolol (Inderal). When reinforcing instruction to the client about the medication, the nurse would include which of the following?
    1. Gentle exercising will prevent orthostatic hypotension
    2. Hot baths and showers are advised to increase vasodilation
    3. Medication should be taken on an empty stomach to enhance absorption
    4. Medication should be withheld if the pulse rate drops below 60 beats per minute

13. Heparin sodium (Liquaemin) is prescribed for the client. The nurse expects that the physician will order which of the following to monitor for a therapeutic effect of the medication?
    1. Prothrombin time (PT)
    2. Activated partial thromboplastin time (aPTT)
    3. Hematocrit level
    4. Hemoglobin level

14. A client has suffered an acute myocardial infarction and is receiving tissue plasminogen activator (t-PA). Which of the following is a priority nursing intervention while caring for the client?
    1. Have heparin sodium (Liquaemin) available
    2. Monitor for renal failure
    3. Monitor for signs of bleeding
    4. Monitor psychosocial status

15. A nurse is reinforcing instructions to the client about the use of a nitrate patch for the treatment of angina pectoris. Which of the following will the nurse include in the instructions to prevent client tolerance to nitrates?
    1. Do not remove the patches
    2. Have a 12-hour "no-nitrate" time
    3. Have a 24-hour "no-nitrate" time
    4. Keep nitrates on 24 hours, then off 24 hours

16. A hypertensive client who has been taking metoprolol (Lopressor) has been ordered to decrease the dose of the medication. The client asks the nurse why this must be done over a period of 1 to 2 weeks. In formulating a response, the nurse incorporates the understanding that abrupt withdrawal could:
    1. Give the client insomnia
    2. Cause enhanced side effects of other prescribed medications
    3. Result in hypoglycemia
    4. Precipitate rebound hypertension

17. A client with a diagnosis of congestive heart failure is seen in the clinic. The client is being treated with a variety of medications, including digoxin (Lanoxin) and furosemide (Lasix). Which findings on data collection would lead the nurse to suspect that the client is hypokalemic?
    1. Constipation
    2. Intermittent intestinal colic
    3. Muscle weakness and leg cramps
    4. Tingling of fingers and toes

18. A nurse is reinforcing dietary instructions to a client who is taking triamterene (Dyrenium). The nurse instructs the client that it is acceptable to consume which of the following food items daily?
    1. Avocado
    2. Banana
    3. Baked potato
    4. Apple

19. Hydrochlorothiazide (HydroDIURIL) is prescribed for the client. The nurse checks the client's record for documentation of which of the following before administering the medication?
    1. Penicillin allergy
    2. Hyperkalemia
    3. Sulfa allergy
    4. History of osteoporosis

20. Cholestyramine resin (Questran) is prescribed for a client with an elevated triglyceride level and

a serum cholesterol level of 398 mg/dL. The nurse reinforces instructions to the client about the medication. Which statement by the client indicates the need for further instructions?

1. "Constipation and bloating might be a problem."
2. "I'll continue to watch my diet and reduce my fats."
3. "I'll continue my nicotinic acid from the health food store."
4. "Walking a mile each day will help the whole process."

21. A client is experiencing impotence after taking guanfacine (Tenex). The client states, "I would sooner have a stroke than keep living with the side effects of this medication." The nurse makes which appropriate response to the client?
    1. "I can understand completely."
    2. "That doctor should change your prescription."
    3. "You wouldn't really want to have a stroke."
    4. "You are concerned about the side effects of your medication."

22. A physician tells the nurse that a potassium-sparing diuretic is being prescribed for the client with congestive heart failure. The nurse reviews the physician's orders, expecting that which of the following medications will be prescribed?
    1. Spironolactone (Aldactone)
    2. Furosemide (Lasix)
    3. Ethacrynic acid (Edecrin)
    4. Hydrochlorothiazide (HydroDIURIL)

23. A client with coronary artery disease complains of substernal chest pain. After checking the client's heart rate and blood pressure, the nurse administers nitroglycerin, 0.4 mg sublingually. After 5 minutes, the client states, "My chest still hurts." If the vital signs have remained stable, the nurse should:
    1. Wait another 10 minutes and then administer a second nitroglycerin tablet
    2. Apply 10 L of oxygen via nasal cannula
    3. Administer another nitroglycerin tablet
    4. Call the resuscitation team immediately

24. A nurse is caring for the client with history of mild heart failure who is receiving diltiazem (Cardizem) for hypertension. The nurse would check the client for:
    1. Tachycardia and rebound hypertension
    2. Wheezing and shortness of breath
    3. Bradycardia, weight gain, and peripheral edema
    4. Chest pain and tachycardia

25. A client receiving nifedipine (Procardia) for angina complains of feeling listless, with generalized weakness and no energy. To support the client most effectively, the nurse must understand that these symptoms:
    1. Are unrelated to taking the medication
    2. Are an expected effect of the medication

3. Indicate a toxic reaction to the medication
4. Indicate underdosing of the medication

26. A nurse has an order to administer a dose of nitroglycerin ointment (Nitro-Bid) to a client. The nurse would avoid doing which of the following in preparing the medication for administration?
    1. Using the manufacturer's applicator papers
    2. Using the fingers to spread the ointment
    3. Applying the dose in an even layer
    4. Washing off the previous application

27. A 66-year-old client is seen in the clinic complaining of not feeling well. The client is taking several medications for the control of heart disease and hypertension. These medications include atenolol (Tenormin), digoxin (Lanoxin), and chlorothiazide (Diuril). A tentative diagnosis of digoxin toxicity is made. The nurse collects data from the client, knowing that which of the following would support this diagnosis?
    1. Chest pain, hypotension, and paresthesia
    2. Constipation, dry mouth, and sleep disorder
    3. Double vision, loss of appetite, and nausea
    4. Dyspnea, edema, and palpitations

28. A 79-year-old client is being treated for congestive heart failure with bumetanide (Bumex). The client's vital signs are blood pressure, 100/60 mm Hg, pulse, 96 beats per minute, and respirations, 24 breaths per minute. The nurse checks which priority item before administering the medication?
    1. Blood pressure
    2. Weight
    3. Urine output
    4. Temperature

29. Atorvastatin (Lipitor) has been prescribed for a client with an elevated cholesterol level. The nurse collects a health history from the client, knowing that the medication is contraindicated in which of the following conditions?
    1. Cirrhosis
    2. Coronary artery disease
    3. Diabetes mellitus
    4. Hypothyroidism

30. Warfarin sodium (Coumadin) is prescribed for the client. The nurse expects that the physician will order which of the following to monitor for a therapeutic effect of the medication?
    1. Prothrombin time (PT)
    2. Activated partial thromboplastin time (aPTT)
    3. Red blood cell (RBC) count
    4. Platelet count

ALTERNATE FORMAT QUESTION: MULTIPLE RESPONSE

A client with coronary artery disease complains of substernal chest pain. After assessing the client's heart rate and blood pressure, a nurse administers nitroglycerin, 0.4 mg, sublingually. After 5 minutes, the client states that the pain is unrelieved. Select the appropriate actions that the nurse should take.

___ Assess the client's pain level

___ Check the client's blood pressure

___ Contact the physician

___ Call a code blue

___ Administer a second nitroglycerin, 0.4 mg, sublingually

ANSWERS

1. Answer: 1

Rationale: Ecotrin is an aspirin-containing product and should be avoided. Excessive alcohol consumption should be avoided when taking warfarin sodium. Taking prescribed medication at the same time increases client compliance. The Medic-Alert bracelet provides health care personnel emergency information.

Test-Taking Strategy: Use the process of elimination. Note the key words, *need for further teaching*. These words indicate a false response question and that you need to select the incorrect client statement. Recalling that warfarin sodium is an anticoagulant and that Ecotrin is an aspirin-containing product will direct you to option 1. Review client teaching points related to warfarin sodium if you had difficulty with this question.

Level of Cognitive Ability: Analysis

Client Needs: Health Promotion and Maintenance

Integrated Process: Nursing Process/Evaluation

Content Area: Pharmacology

Reference: Hodgson, B., & Kizior, R. (2005). *Saunders nursing drug handbook 2005.* Philadelphia: W.B. Saunders, p. 1122.

2. Answer: 3

Rationale: The therapeutic serum digoxin level ranges from 0.5 to 2 ng/mL.

Test-Taking Strategy: Knowledge of the therapeutic serum digoxin level is necessary to answer the question. Review this level if you had difficulty with this question.

Level of Cognitive Ability: Comprehension

Client Needs: Physiological Integrity

Integrated Process: Nursing Process/Data Collection

Content Area: Pharmacology

References: Chernecky, C., & Berger, B. (2004). *Laboratory tests and diagnostic procedures* (4th ed.). Philadelphia: W.B. Saunders, p. 477.

Hodgson, B., & Kizior, R. (2005). *Saunders nursing drug handbook 2005.* Philadelphia: W.B. Saunders, p. 326.

3. Answer: 4

Rationale: For subcutaneous heparin sodium injection, a 25- to 27-gauge, $^5/_8$-inch needle is used to prevent tissue trauma and inadvertent intramuscular injection. A 1-inch needle would inject the heparin sodium into the muscle. The application of heat may affect the absorption of the heparin. Aspiration before injection is avoided with heparin sodium.

Test-Taking Strategy: Use the process of elimination. Recalling the anatomy of muscle and subcutaneous layers of tissue will

assist in directing you to option 4. If you had difficulty with this question, review the principles related to heparin administration.

Level of Cognitive Ability: Application

Client Needs: Physiological Integrity

Integrated Process: Nursing Process/Implementation

Content Area: Pharmacology

Reference: McKenry, L., & Salerno, E. (2003). *Mosby's pharmacology in nursing* (21st ed.). St. Louis: Mosby, p. 625.

4. Answer: 2

Rationale: Hydrochlorothiazide is a potassium-losing diuretic, and clients are at risk for hypokalemia. Potassium is found in many foods, especially unprocessed foods, many vegetables, fruits, and fresh meats. Because potassium is very water-soluble, foods that are prepared in water are often lower in potassium than the same foods cooked another way (e.g., boiled versus baked potato). Clients who need potassium added to the diet are encouraged to take in these foods. Many salt substitutes are also high in potassium.

Test-Taking Strategy: Focus on the name of the medication to assist in determining that it is a diuretic. Evaluating food choices in terms of their water content and according to how highly processed they are may be a helpful approach for some questions related to potassium. In this question, note that each of the incorrect options is processed to some degree and has a high water content. Review foods high in potassium if you had difficulty with this question.

Level of Cognitive Ability: Application

Client Needs: Physiological Integrity

Integrated Process: Nursing Process/Implementation

Content Area: Adult Health/Cardiovascular

References: Lehne, R. (2004). *Pharmacology for nursing care* (5th ed.). Philadelphia: W.B. Saunders, p. 409.

Nix, S. (2005). *Williams basic nutrition and diet therapy* (11th ed.). St. Louis: Mosby, p. 137.

5. Answer: 3

Rationale: Streptokinase converts plasminogen in the blood to plasmin. Plasmin is an enzyme that digests or dissolves fibrin clots wherever they exist. Option 1, 2, and 4 describe mechanisms of action of heparin sodium (Liquaemin) and warfarin sodium (Coumadin).

Test-Taking Strategy: Focus on the name of the medication, recalling that it is a thrombolytic. Remember that streptokinase dissolves clots. This will direct you to option 3. Review this medication if you had difficulty with this question.

Level of Cognitive Ability: Analysis

Client Needs: Physiological Integrity

Integrated Process: Nursing Process/Evaluation
Content Area: Pharmacology
Reference: Hodgson, B., & Kizior, R. (2005). *Saunders nursing drug handbook 2005.* Philadelphia: W.B. Saunders, p. 989.

6. Answer: 2
Rationale: Diltiazem is a calcium channel blockers that inhibits calcium influx through the slow channels of the membrane of smooth muscle cells. Calcium channel blockers decrease myocardial oxygen demands and blocks calcium channels, thereby decreasing the force of contraction of the ventricular tissue.
Test-Taking Strategy: Focus on the name of the medication and recall that it is a calcium channel blocker. Note the relation of the medication classification and option 2. Review the action of calcium channel blockers if you had difficulty with this question.
Level of Cognitive Ability: Analysis
Client Needs: Physiological Integrity
Integrated Process: Nursing Process/Planning
Content Area: Pharmacology
Reference: Hodgson, B., & Kizior, R. (2005). *Saunders nursing drug handbook 2005.* Philadelphia: W.B. Saunders, p. 328.

7. Answer: 3
Rationale: Audible expiratory wheezes may indicate a serious adverse reaction, bronchospasm. Beta blockers may induce this reaction particularly in clients with chronic obstructive pulmonary disease (COPD) or asthma. A normal decrease in blood pressure and heart rate is expected. Insomnia is a frequent mild side effect and should be monitored.
Test-Taking Strategy: Use the process of elimination. Eliminate options 1 and 2 first because these are expected responses from the medication. From the remaining options, noting the key words, *adverse reaction*, will assist in directing you to option 3. Review the adverse effects of this medication if you had difficulty with this question.
Level of Cognitive Ability: Analysis
Client Needs: Physiological Integrity
Integrated Process: Nursing Process/Data Collection
Content Area: Pharmacology
References: Hodgson, B., & Kizior, R. (2005). *Saunders nursing drug handbook 2005.* Philadelphia: W.B. Saunders, p. 903.
McKenry, L., & Salerno, E. (2003). *Mosby's pharmacology in nursing* (21st ed.). St. Louis: Mosby, p. 561.

8. Answer: 4
Rationale: Paraphrasing is restating the client's or family member's own words. Option 1 represents a communication block that denies the person's right to an opinion. Option 2 is offering a false reassurance. In option 3, the nurse is expressing approval, which can be harmful to the client-nurse or family-nurse relationship.
Test-Taking Strategy: Use therapeutic communication techniques. Remembering to address client feelings first will direct you to option 4. Review these therapeutic techniques if you had difficulty with this question.
Level of Cognitive Ability: Application
Client Needs: Psychosocial Integrity
Integrated Process: Communication and Documentation

Content Area: Pharmacology
References: Hodgson, B., & Kizior, R. (2005). *Saunders nursing drug handbook 2005.* Philadelphia: W. B. Saunders, p. 989.
Potter, P., & Perry, A. (2005). *Fundamentals of nursing* (6th ed.). St. Louis: Mosby, p. 437.

9. Answer: 4
Rationale: It is appropriate to treat atrial fibrillation with the prescribed and calculated dose of digoxin, as indicated in the question. The issue of the question is that the client verbalizes inaccurate and unsafe knowledge regarding this medication and the treatment for chest pain. This client needs further teaching regarding the safe administration of medications for episodes of chest pain. Options 1, 2, and 3 are incorrect actions.
Test-Taking Strategy: Perform the calculation first and determine that the dose that the nurse is to give is a correct dose. From this point, eliminate options 1 and 2. From the remaining options, note the issue of the question, the need for client teaching. This should direct you to option 4. Review the client teaching points related to digoxin if you had difficulty with this question.
Level of Cognitive Ability: Application
Client Needs: Health Promotion and Maintenance
Integrated Process: Nursing Process/Planning
Content Area: Pharmacology
Reference: Hodgson, B., & Kizior, R. (2005). *Saunders nursing drug handbook 2005.* Philadelphia: W.B. Saunders, p. 325.

10. Answer: 3
Rationale: Tea and coffee are stimulants as well as mild diuretics. These are a poor choice for hydration. Taking the medication at the same time each day improves compliance. Because furosemide is a diuretic, the morning is the best time to take the medication so as not to interrupt sleep. Notification of the health care provider is appropriate if edema is noted in the hands, feet, or face, or if the client is short of breath. Sitting up slowly prevents postural hypotension.
Test-Taking Strategy: Note the key words, *need for further instructions*. These words indicate a false response question and that you need to select the incorrect client statement. Tea and coffee are stimulants and diuretics and can potentially worsen dehydration. Additionally, coffee and tea are not healthy foods. This should alert you that this is the correct option for this question, as stated. Review client teaching points related to this medication if you had difficulty with this question.
Level of Cognitive Ability: Comprehension
Client Needs: Health Promotion and Maintenance
Integrated Process: Teaching/Learning
Content Area: Pharmacology
Reference: Hodgson, B., & Kizior, R. (2005). *Saunders nursing drug handbook 2005.* Philadelphia: W.B. Saunders, pp. 479-480.

11. Answer: 4
Rationale: Isosorbide mononitrate is an antianginal medication. Headache is a frequent side effect of isosorbide mononitrate and usually disappears during continued therapy. If a headache occurs during therapy, the client should be

instructed to take the medication with food or meals. It is not necessary to contact the physician unless the headaches persist with therapy. It is not appropriate to instruct the client to discontinue therapy or adjust the dosages.

Test-Taking Strategy: Use the process of elimination. Eliminate options 2 and 3 first because it is not within the scope of nursing practice to instruct a client to discontinue or adjust dosages. From the remaining options, recalling that the headache can be relieved with the administration of food with the medication will assist in directing you to option 4. Review this medication if you had difficulty with this question.

Level of Cognitive Ability: Application
Client Needs: Health Promotion and Maintenance
Integrated Process: Teaching/Learning
Content Area: Pharmacology
References: Hodgson, B., & Kizior, R. (2005). *Saunders nursing drug handbook 2005.* Philadelphia: W.B. Saunders, pp. 594-595. McKenry, L., & Salerno, E. (2003). *Mosby's pharmacology in nursing* (21st ed.). St. Louis: Mosby, p. 679.

12. *Answer:* 4

Rationale: Most beta blockers may be administered with food or on an empty stomach but propranolol is best absorbed if taken with meals or directly after eating. Exercise will not prevent orthostatic hypotension. Hot showers and baths are not advised because of their vasodilating effect. The client needs to be instructed how to take his or her pulse rate and to notify the physician if the heart rate falls below 60 beats per minute.

Test-Taking Strategy: Focus on the name of the medication and recall that medication names that end with the letters "lol" are beta blockers. Recalling that bradycardia can occur with the use of beta blockers will direct you to option 4. If you had difficulty with question, review this medication.

Level of Cognitive Ability: Application
Client Needs: Health Promotion and Maintenance
Integrated Process: Teaching/Learning
Content Area: Pharmacology
Reference: Hodgson, B., & Kizior, R. (2005). *Saunders nursing drug handbook 2005.* Philadelphia: W.B. Saunders, p. 903.

13. *Answer:* 2

Rationale: The PT will assess for the therapeutic effect of warfarin sodium (Coumadin) and the aPTT will assess the therapeutic effect of heparin sodium. Heparin sodium doses are determined based on these laboratory results. The hemoglobin and hematocrit values assess red blood cell concentrations.

Test-Taking Strategy: Use the process of elimination. Eliminate options 3 and 4 because these laboratory values are unrelated to heparin sodium therapy. From the remaining options, knowledge of the appropriate test for monitoring therapeutic values of both heparin sodium and warfarin sodium is required to answer this question. Review this content if you had difficulty with this question.

Level of Cognitive Ability: Comprehension
Client Needs: Physiological Integrity
Integrated Process: Nursing Process/Data Collection
Content Area: Pharmacology
Reference: Hodgson, B., & Kizior, R. (2005). *Saunders nursing drug handbook 2005.* Philadelphia: W.B. Saunders, p. 523.

14. *Answer:* 3

Rationale: t-PA is a thrombolytic. Hemorrhage is a complication of any type of thrombolytic medication. The client should be monitored for bleeding. Monitoring for renal failure and the client's psychosocial status is important; however, they are not the priority. Heparin sodium is given following thrombolytic therapy, but the question is not asking for the associated medications following t-PA therapy.

Test-Taking Strategy: Use the process of elimination and note the key word, *priority.* Use the principles of prioritizing and knowledge regarding this medication to direct you to option 3. Additionally, remember that bleeding is a priority. Review this medication if you had difficulty with this question.

Level of Cognitive Ability: Application
Client Needs: Physiological Integrity
Integrated Process: Nursing Process/Implementation
Content Area: Pharmacology
Reference: Lehne, R. (2004). *Pharmacology for nursing care* (5th ed.). Philadelphia: W.B. Saunders, p. 560.

15. *Answer:* 2

Rationale: To help prevent tolerance, clients need a 12-hour "no-nitrate" time. In addition to having a 12-hour no-nitrate time, the client must rotate the nitrate patch and wash his or her hands to prevent topical absorption through the fingers. Options 1, 3, and 4 are incorrect.

Test-Taking Strategy: Use the process of elimination. Option 1 can be easily eliminated based on the issue of the question. Eliminate options 3 and 4 next because they are similar. Review the administration of nitrate patches if you had difficulty with this question.

Level of Cognitive Ability: Application
Client Needs: Health Promotion and Maintenance
Integrated Process: Teaching/Learning
Content Area: Pharmacology
Reference: Hodgson, B., & Kizior, R. (2005). *Saunders nursing drug handbook 2005.* Philadelphia: W.B. Saunders, p. 779.

16. *Answer:* 4

Rationale: Beta-adrenergic blocking agents should be tapered slowly. This will avoid abrupt withdrawal syndrome, characterized by headache, malaise, palpitations, tremors, sweating, rebound hypertension, dysrhythmias, and possibly myocardial infarction (in clients with cardiac disorders, including angina pectoris). Options 1, 2, and 3 are incorrect.

Test-Taking Strategy: Focus on the name of the medication and recall that medication names that end with the letters "lol" are beta blockers. Next, recall that all beta-adrenergic blocking agents should be tapered slowly to prevent withdrawal symptoms, as well as to prevent return of the symptoms for which the medication was prescribed. Also, note that the question guides you to the correct option by telling you that the client was taking this medication for hypertension. Review this medication if you had difficulty with this question.

Level of Cognitive Ability: Comprehension
Client Needs: Physiological Integrity
Integrated Process: Nursing Process/Implementation
Content Area: Adult Health/Cardiovascular

Reference: Hodgson, B., & Kizior, R. (2005). *Saunders nursing drug handbook 2005.* Philadelphia: W.B. Saunders, p. 705.

17. *Answer: 3*
Rationale: Clients on potassium-wasting diuretics are at high risk of hypokalemia. Clinical manifestations of hypokalemia include fatigue, anorexia, nausea, vomiting, muscle weakness, leg cramps, decreased bowel motility, paresthesias, and dysrhythmias. Diarrhea and intestinal colic are signs of hyperkalemia. Tingling of the fingers and toes are signs of hypocalcemia.
Test-Taking Strategy: Knowledge regarding the signs of hypokalemia is required to answer the question. Remember, muscle weakness and leg cramps are associated with hypokalemia. If you had difficulty with this question, review the signs of this electrolyte imbalance.
Level of Cognitive Ability: Comprehension
Client Needs: Physiological Integrity
Integrated Process: Nursing Process/Data Collection
Content Area: Pharmacology
Reference: Hodgson, B., & Kizior, R. (2005). *Saunders nursing drug handbook 2005.* Philadelphia: W.B. Saunders, p. 480.

18. *Answer: 4*
Rationale: Triamterene is a potassium-sparing diuretic, which means that the client must avoid the intake of foods high in potassium. Options 1, 2, and 3 are high-potassium food items.
Test-Taking Strategy: Focus on the name of the medication and recall that triamterene is a potassium-sparing diuretic. Next, recalling the food items high in potassium will direct you to option 4. If you are unfamiliar with this medication and those foods high in potassium, review this content.
Level of Cognitive Ability: Application
Client Needs: Physiological Integrity
Integrated Process: Teaching/Learning
Content Area: Pharmacology
Reference: Hodgson, B., & Kizior, R. (2005). *Saunders nursing drug handbook 2005.* Philadelphia: W.B. Saunders, p. 1075.

19. *Answer: 3*
Rationale: Thiazide diuretics such as hydrochlorothiazide are sulfa-based medications, and a client with a sulfa allergy is at risk for an allergic reaction. Options 1, 2, and 4 are not associated with the use of this medication.
Test-Taking Strategy: Knowledge of the chemical make-up of thiazide diuretics is necessary to answer this question. Recalling that these medications contain a sulfa ring in their structure will direct you to option 3. Review the contraindications associated with the thiazide diuretics if you had difficulty with this question.
Level of Cognitive Ability: Application
Client Needs: Safe, Effective Care Environment
Integrated Process: Nursing Process/Data Collection
Content Area: Pharmacology
References: Hodgson, B., & Kizior, R. (2005). *Saunders nursing drug handbook 2005.* Philadelphia: W.B. Saunders, p. 530.
Skidmore-Roth, L. (2005). *Mosby's drug guide for nurses* (6th ed.). St. Louis: Mosby, p. 419.

20. *Answer: 3*
Rationale: Nicotinic acid should be avoided because it may lead to liver abnormalities. All lipid-lowering medications can also cause liver abnormalities, so a combination of nicotinic acid and cholestyramine is to be avoided. Constipation and bloating are the two most common side effects. Both walking and the reduction of fats in the diet are therapeutic measures to reduce cholesterol and triglyceride levels.
Test-Taking Strategy: Note the key words, *need for further instructions.* These words indicate a false response question and that you need to select the incorrect client statement. Recalling that over-the-counter medications should be avoided when a client is taking a prescription medication will direct you to option 3. Review client teaching points related to this medication if you had difficulty with this question.
Level of Cognitive Ability: Analysis
Client Needs: Health Promotion and Maintenance
Integrated Process: Nursing Process/Evaluation
Content Area: Pharmacology
Reference: Skidmore-Roth, L. (2005). *Mosby's drug guide for nurses* (6th ed.). St. Louis: Mosby, pp. 186-187.

21. *Answer: 4*
Rationale: Reflection of the client's own comment lets the client know that you are hearing his or her concerns without judging. The nurse cannot understand what the client is experiencing (option 1). Option 2 devalues the physician's judgement. Option 3 is confrontative and unsupportive.
Test-Taking Strategy: Use therapeutic communication techniques. Select nonjudgmental responses that reflect the fact that you are listening to the client's concerns. Review these techniques if you had difficulty with this question.
Level of Cognitive Ability: Application
Client Needs: Psychosocial Integrity
Integrated Process: Communication and Documentation
Content Area: Pharmacology
Reference: Potter, P., & Perry, A. (2005). *Fundamentals of nursing* (6th ed.). St. Louis: Mosby, p. 437.

22. *Answer: 1*
Rationale: Spironolactone is a potassium-sparing diuretic that promotes sodium excretion while conserving potassium. Options 2, 3, and 4 identify diuretics that do not conserve potassium.
Test-Taking Strategy: Knowledge that spironolactone is a potassium-sparing diuretic is required to answer this question. Review the potassium-sparing diuretics if you are unfamiliar with them and had difficulty with this question.
Level of Cognitive Ability: Analysis
Client Needs: Physiological Integrity
Integrated Process: Nursing Process/Planning
Content Area: Pharmacology
Reference: Hodgson, B., & Kizior, R. (2005). *Saunders nursing drug handbook 2005.* Philadelphia: W.B. Saunders, p. 985.

23. *Answer: 3*
Rationale: Nitroglycerin tablets are usually ordered one every 5 minutes PRN for chest pain, for a total dose of three tablets. Waiting 10 minutes is inappropriate if the client is having

chest pain. Oxygen at 10 L is an unsafe dose. There is no need to call the resuscitation team at this time.

Test-Taking Strategy: Focus on the information provided in the question and use knowledge regarding the administration of nitroglycerin for chest pain. Recalling that a nitroglycerin tablet can be administered for three doses 5 minutes apart if the vital signs remain stable will direct you to option 3. Review the administration of nitroglycerin if you had difficulty with this question.

Level of Cognitive Ability: Application
Client Needs: Physiological Integrity
Integrated Process: Nursing Process/Implementation
Content Area: Pharmacology
Reference: Hodgson, B., & Kizior, R. (2005). *Saunders nursing drug handbook 2005.* Philadelphia: W.B. Saunders, p. 780.

24. *Answer: 3*
Rationale: Calcium channel blocking agents, such as diltiazem, are used cautiously in clients with conditions that could be worsened by the medication, such as aortic stenosis, bradycardia, heart failure, acute myocardial infarction, and hypotension. The nurse would assess for signs and symptoms that indicate worsening of these underlying disorders. In this question, the nurse assesses for signs and symptoms indicating heart failure.

Test-Taking Strategy: Focus on the medication name to determine that diltiazem is a calcium channel blocker, and recall that these medications decrease the rate and force of cardiac contraction. This helps you to eliminate options 1 and 4, because bradycardia is expected. Option 2 is eliminated next, because these signs could indicate bronchoconstriction, which does not occur with calcium channel blockers but does occur with some beta-adrenergic blockers. Review this medication if you had difficulty with this question.

Level of Cognitive Ability: Analysis
Client Needs: Physiological Integrity
Integrated Process: Nursing Process/Data Collection
Content Area: Adult Health/Cardiovascular
Reference: Hodgson, B., & Kizior, R. (2005). *Saunders nursing drug handbook 2005.* Philadelphia: W.B. Saunders, p. 330.

25. *Answer: 2*
Rationale: The client receiving a calcium channel blocking agent such as nifedipine may develop weakness and lethargy as expected effects of the medication. Options 1, 3, and 4 are incorrect.

Test-Taking Strategy: Focus on the name of the medication. Recall that nifedipine is a calcium channel blocking agent, and that this medication decreases the rate and force of cardiac contraction, lowering the oxygen demand and also the cardiac output. By thinking through this process, you can reach the conclusion that decreased energy would then be an expected effect of the medication. Review this medication if you had difficulty with this question.

Level of Cognitive Ability: Analysis
Client Needs: Physiological Integrity
Integrated Process: Nursing Process/Planning
Content Area: Adult Health/Cardiovascular
Reference: Hodgson, B., & Kizior, R. (2005). *Saunders nursing drug handbook 2005.* Philadelphia: W.B. Saunders, p. 772.

26. *Answer: 2*
Rationale: The ointment is readily absorbed through the skin, so using the fingers will result in the nurse becoming hypotensive. Proper administration of nitroglycerin ointment involves the use of the dose-measuring applicator paper supplied by the manufacturer and application in a thin, uniform even layer to a nonhairy area of the chest, abdomen, anterior thigh, or forearm. The previous dose is removed before applying, and sites are rotated to avoid inflammation.

Test-Taking Strategy: Use the process of elimination and note the key word, *avoid.* This word indicates a false response question and that you need to select the incorrect action. This question tests fundamental principles of medication administration for nitroglycerin ointment. Visualizing each action will direct you to the correct option. Review this medication if you had difficulty with this question.

Level of Cognitive Ability: Application
Client Needs: Physiological Integrity
Integrated Process: Nursing Process/Implementation
Content Area: Adult Health/Cardiovascular
Reference: Lehne, R. (2004). *Pharmacology for nursing care* (5th ed.). Philadelphia: W.B. Saunders, p. 534.

27. *Answer: 3*
Rationale: Double vision, loss of appetite, and nausea are signs of digoxin toxicity. Additional signs of digoxin toxicity include bradycardia, visual alterations such as green and yellow vision, seeing spots or halos, confusion, vomiting, diarrhea, decreased libido, and impotence.

Test-Taking Strategy: Knowledge regarding the signs of digoxin toxicity is required to answer the question. Remembering that gastrointestinal and visual disturbances are signs of toxicity will direct you to option 3. If you had difficulty with this question, review the signs of digoxin toxicity.

Level of Cognitive Ability: Analysis
Client Needs: Physiological Integrity
Integrated Process: Nursing Process/Data Collection
Content Area: Pharmacology
Reference: Hodgson, B., & Kizior, R. (2005). *Saunders nursing drug handbook 2005.* Philadelphia: W.B. Saunders, pp. 218, 326, 373.

28. *Answer: 1*
Rationale: Hypotension is a common side effect with this medication, and an increased risk exists in an older client. Options 2 and 3 will also require monitoring but are not the priority. The temperature is unrelated to administering this medication.

Test-Taking Strategy: Use the process of elimination and focus on the key word, *priority.* Use the ABCs—airway, breathing, and circulation. Blood pressure reflects circulation. Review the side effects of this medication if you had difficulty with this question.

Level of Cognitive Ability: Application
Client Needs: Physiological Integrity
Integrated Process: Nursing Process/Data Collection
Content Area: Pharmacology
Reference: Hodgson, B., & Kizior, R. (2005). *Saunders nursing drug handbook 2005.* Philadelphia: W.B. Saunders, p. 143.

29. *Answer:* **1**

Rationale: Atorvastin is an antihyperlipidemic medication. It is contraindicated in pregnancy, lactation, liver disease, biliary cirrhosis or obstruction, and severe renal dysfunction, and in clients who are hypersensitive to the medication. Options 2, 3, and 4 are not contraindications to the use of this medication.

Test-Taking Strategy: Knowledge regarding the contraindications associated with use of this medication is required to answer this question. Remember, atorvastin is contraindicated in the client with liver disease. Review these contraindications if you had difficulty with this question.

Level of Cognitive Ability: Analysis
Client Needs: Physiological Integrity
Integrated Process: Nursing Process/Data Collection
Content Area: Pharmacology
Reference: Hodgson, B., & Kizior, R. (2005). *Saunders nursing drug handbook 2005.* Philadelphia: W.B. Saunders, p. 93.

30. *Answer:* **1**

Rationale: The PT will assess for the therapeutic effect of warfarin sodium (Coumadin) and the aPTT will assess the therapeutic effect of heparin sodium. The RBC and platelet counts will assess red blood cell concentration and the client's potential for bleeding, respectively. Warfarin sodium doses are determined based the results of the PT.

Test-Taking Strategy: Use the process of elimination. Eliminate options 3 and 4 first, because these laboratory values are unrelated to warfarin sodium therapy. From the remaining options, knowledge of the appropriate test for monitoring the therapeutic values of both heparin sodium and warfarin sodium is required to answer this question. Review this medication if you had difficulty with this question.

Level of Cognitive Ability: Analysis
Client Needs: Physiological Integrity
Integrated Process: Nursing Process/Data Collection
Content Area: Pharmacology

Reference: Hodgson, B., & Kizior, R. (2005). *Saunders nursing drug handbook 2005.* Philadelphia: W.B. Saunders, p. 1122.

ALTERNATE FORMAT QUESTION: MULTIPLE RESPONSE

Answers:
Assess the client's pain level
Check the client's blood pressure
Administer a second nitroglycerin, 0.4 mg, sublingually

Rationale: The usual guidelines for administering nitroglycerin tablets for chest pain is to administer one tablet every 5 minutes PRN for chest pain, for a total dose of three tablets. If the client does not obtain relief after taking a third dose of nitroglycerin, the physician is notified. Because the client is still complaining of chest pain, the nurse would administer a second nitroglycerin tablet. The nurse would assess the client's pain level and check the client's blood pressure before administering each nitroglycerin dose. There is no data in the question that indicates the need to call a code blue.

Test-Taking Strategy: Focus on the data in the question. Use the steps of the clinical problem-solving process (nursing process) to determine that assessing the client's pain level and checking the client's blood pressure are appropriate actions. Next, recalling the usual guidelines for administering nitroglycerin tablets will assist in determining that an appropriate action is to administer a second nitroglycerin, 0.4 mg, sublingually. Review care of the client with chest pain and the guidelines for the administration of nitroglycerin if you had difficulty with this question.

Level of Cognitive Ability: Application
Client Needs: Physiological Integrity
Integrated Process: Nursing Process/Implementation
Content Area: Pharmacology
Reference: Kee, J., & Hayes, E. (2003). *Pharmacology: A nursing process approach* (4th ed.). Philadelphia: W.B. Saunders, p. 576.

REFERENCES

Chernecky, C., & Berger, B. (2004). *Laboratory tests and diagnostic procedures* (4th ed.). Philadelphia: W.B. Saunders.

Hodgson, B., & Kizior, R. (2005). *Saunders nursing drug handbook 2005.* Philadelphia: W.B. Saunders.

Kee, J., & Hayes, E. (2003). *Pharmacology: A nursing process approach* (4th ed.). Philadelphia: W.B. Saunders.

Lehne, R. (2004). *Pharmacology for nursing care* (5th ed.). Philadelphia: W.B. Saunders.

McKenry, L., & Salerno, E. (2003). *Mosby's pharmacology in nursing* (21st ed.). St. Louis: Mosby.

Nix, S. (2005). *Williams basic nutrition and diet therapy* (11th ed.). St. Louis: Mosby.

Potter, P., & Perry, A. (2005). *Fundamentals of nursing* (6th ed.). St. Louis: Mosby.

Skidmore-Roth, L. (2005). *Mosby's drug guide for nurses* (6th ed.). St. Louis: Mosby.

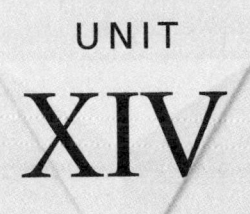

The Adult Client with a Renal Disorder

PYRAMID TERMS

acute renal failure (ARF) The sudden loss of kidney function caused by renal cell damage from ischemia or toxic substances. ARF occurs abruptly and can be reversible. It leads to hypoperfusion, cell death, and decompensation in renal function. The prognosis depends on the cause and the condition of the client. Near-normal or normal kidney function may resume gradually.

anuria Urine output of less than 100 mL/day.

arterial steal syndrome Can develop following the insertion of an arteriovenous (AV) fistula when too much blood is diverted to the vein and arterial perfusion to the hand is compromised.

azotemia The retention of nitrogenous waste products in the blood.

chronic renal failure (CRF) The progressive loss and ongoing deterioration in kidney function that occurs slowly over a period of time. It is irreversible and results in uremia or end-stage renal disease. Chronic renal failure requires dialysis or kidney transplantatation to maintain life.

disequilibrium syndrome A rapid change in the composition of the extracellular fluid (ECF) occurs during hemodialysis. Solutes are removed from the blood faster than from the cerebrospinal fluid (CSF) and brain. Fluid is pulled into the brain, causing cerebral edema.

hemodialysis The process of cleansing the client's blood; the diffusion of dissolved particles from one fluid compartment into another across a semipermeable membrane. The client's blood flows through one fluid compartment and the dialysate is in another fluid compartment.

internal arteriovenous fistula (AV fistula) Created surgically in which an artery in the arm is anastomosed to a vein. This creates an opening, or fistula, between a large artery and a large vein. The flow of arterial blood into the venous system causes the vein to become engorged (maturity). Maturity is necessary so that the engorged vein can be punctured for the dialysis procedure, using a large-bore needle.

nephrolithiasis Refers to the formation of kidney stones, which are formed in the renal parenchyma.

oliguria Urine output of less than 400 mL/day.

peritoneal dialysis The peritoneum is the dialyzing membrane (semipermeable membrane) and substitutes for kidney function during kidney failure; works on the principles of diffusion and osmosis. The dialysis occurs via the transfer of fluid and solute from the bloodstream through the peritoneum.

renal failure The loss of kidney function. The types of renal failure include acute and chronic renal failure; the signs and symptoms are caused by the retention of wastes, the retention of fluids, and the inability of the kidneys to regulate electrolytes.

urolithiasis Refers to the formation of urinary stones or calculi. Urinary calculi are formed in the ureter.

PYRAMID TO SUCCESS

Pyramid points focus on the preprocedure and postprocedure care of the client undergoing diagnostic tests and procedures related to the renal system. Be familiar with renal failure, dialysis procedures such as hemodialysis and continuous ambulatory peritoneal dialysis (CAPD), dialysis access devices, and postoperative care following urinary or renal surgery. Be familiar with urinary diversions, care of the client following prostatectomy, and treatment measures for the client with urinary or renal calculi. Additionally, pyramid points address measures that promote urinary elimination, prevent infection, and maintain skin integrity. The Integrated Processes addressed in this unit include Caring, Clinical Problem-Solving Process (Nursing Process), Communication and Documentation, and Teaching/Learning.

CLIENT NEEDS
Safe, Effective Care Environment

Accident prevention related to complications associated with disorder

Asepsis related to wound care and dialysis access devices

Client rights

Confidentiality related to the renal disorder

Consultations with members of the health care team

Establishing priorities

Informed consent related to diagnostic and surgical

procedures
Renal organ donation
Standard precautions related to care of the client

Health Promotion and Maintenance

Expected body image changes
Instructions regarding care of a urinary diversion, dialysis access device, and dialysis procedures
Instructions regarding prescribed treatments related to a urinary or renal disorder
Instructions regarding the prevention of recurrence of a urinary and renal disorder
Instructions regarding postoperative management
Urinary and renal data collection techniques

Psychosocial Integrity

Body image disturbances
Community resources
Coping mechanisms
End of life
Grief and loss
Loss of function of a body part that occurs in clients with a renal disorder
Religious and spiritual influences
Support systems

Physiological Integrity

Adequate rest and sleep
Findings indicating rejection of renal transplant
Care related to dialysis access devices
Care related to hemodialysis and peritoneal dialysis
Care of the client following prostatectomy
Comfort interventions
Diagnostic tests and laboratory results
Elimination measures
Fluid and electrolyte disorders

Medication administration
Personal hygiene
Prescribed nutrition and fluid measures
Skin integrity
Treatment measures for the client with urinary or renal calculi
Urinary diversions

REFERENCES

Black, J., & Hawks, J. (2005). *Medical-surgical nursing: Clinical management for positive outcomes* (7th ed.). Philadelphia: W.B. Saunders.

Chernecky, C., & Berger, B. (2004). *Laboratory tests and diagnostic procedures* (4th ed.). Philadelphia: W.B. Saunders.

Christensen, B., & Kockrow, E. (2003). *Adult health nursing* (4th ed.). St. Louis: Mosby.

Christensen, B., & Kockrow, E. (2003). *Foundations of nursing* (4th ed.). St. Louis: Mosby.

Fortinash, K., & Holoday-Worret, P. (2004). *Psychiatric mental health nursing* (3rd ed.). St. Louis: Mosby.

Harkreader, H., & Hogan, M.A. (2004). *Fundamentals of nursing: Caring and clinical judgment* (2nd ed.). Philadelphia: W.B. Saunders.

Hodgson, B., & Kizior, R. (2005). *Saunders nursing drug handbook 2005*. Philadelphia: W.B. Saunders.

Lewis, S., Heitkemper, M., & Dirksen, S. (2004). *Medical-surgical nursing: Assessment and management of clinical problems* (6th ed.). St. Louis: Mosby.

Linton, A., & Maebius, N. (2003). *Introduction to medical-surgical nursing* (3rd ed.). Philadelphia: W.B. Saunders.

McKenry, L., & Salerno, E. (2003). *Mosby's pharmacology in nursing* (21st ed.). St. Louis: Mosby.

National Council of State Boards of Nursing. (2005). *Detailed test plan for the National Council licensure examination for practical/vocational nurses*. Chicago: Author.

Pagana, K., & Pagana, T. (2003). *Mosby's diagnostic and laboratory test reference* (6th ed.). St. Louis: Mosby.

Perry, A., & Potter, P. (2002). *Clinical nursing skills and techniques* (5th ed.). St. Louis: Mosby.

Phipps, W., Monahan, F., Sands, J., Marek, J., & Neighbors, M. (2003). *Medical-surgical nursing: Health and illness perspectives* (7th ed.). St. Louis: Mosby.

Potter, P., & Perry, A. (2003). *Essentials for practice* (5th ed.). St. Louis: Mosby.

Renal System

I. ANATOMY AND PHYSIOLOGY

A. Kidneys
1. There are two; each is attached to the abdominal wall at the level of the last thoracic and first three lumbar vertebrae
2. Enclosed in the renal capsule
3. The cortex is the outer layer of the renal capsule
4. The medulla is surrounded by the cortex
5. The nephron makes up the functional unit of the kidneys
6. Functions of kidneys
   a. Maintain homeostasis of the blood and acid-base balance
   b. Excrete end products of body metabolism
   c. Control fluid and electrolyte balance
   d. Excrete bacterial toxins, water-soluble drugs, and drug metabolites
   e. Secrete renin and erythropoietin, which play a role in the function of the parathyroid hormones and vitamin D
7. Nephron
   a. Functional renal unit
   b. Composed of glomerulus and tubules
8. Glomerulus
   a. Is encased in Bowman's capsule
   b. Filters the fluid out of blood
9. Tubules
   a. Include proximal, distal, and Henle's loops
   b. Fluid is converted to urine in the tubules; then the urine moves to the pelvis of the kidney
   c. The urine flows from the pelvis of the kidney through the ureter, and empties into the bladder

B. Bladder
1. The ureterovesical sphincter prevents reflux of urine from the bladder to the ureter
2. The total capacity of the bladder is 1 L

C. Prostate gland
1. Surrounds the male urethra
2. Contains a duct that opens into the prostatic portion of the urethra and secretes the alkaline portion of seminal fluid

D. Urine production
1. As fluid flows through the proximal tubules, water and solutes are reabsorbed
2. Water and solutes that are not reabsorbed become urine
3. The process of selective reabsorption determines the amount of water and solutes to be secreted

E. Homeostasis of water
1. The antidiuretic hormone (ADH) is primarily responsible for the reabsorption of water by the kidneys
2. ADH is produced by the hypothalamus and secreted from the posterior lobe of the pituitary gland
3. Secretion of ADH is stimulated by dehydration or high sodium intake and by a decrease in blood volume
4. ADH increases the permeability of the distal convoluted tubules and collecting duct to water
5. Water is drawn out of the tubules by osmosis into a high-salt concentration of fluid in the medulla and its capillaries; water returns to the blood, and concentrated urine remains in the tubule to be excreted
6. When the client lacks ADH, he or she develops diabetes insipidus
7. Clients with diabetes insipidus produce very large amounts of dilute urine; without treatment, have difficulty drinking sufficient water to survive

F. Homeostasis of sodium
1. When the amount of sodium increases, extra water is retained to preserve osmotic pressure

2. An increase in sodium and water produces an increase in the blood volume and blood pressure (BP)

3. When the BP increases, glomerular filtration increases, and extra water and sodium are lost; blood volume is reduced and the BP returns to normal

4. Reabsorption of sodium in the distal convoluted tubules is controlled by the hormones of the renin-angiotensin system

5. Renin is secreted when the BP or concentration of fluid in the distal convoluted tubule is low

6. Renin is an enzyme that splits angiotensin I from angiotensinogen, which converts to angiotensin II as blood flows through the lung

7. Angiotensin II, a potent vasoconstrictor, stimulates the secretion of aldosterone

8. Aldosterone stimulates the distal convoluted tubules to reabsorb sodium and secrete potassium

9. The additional sodium increases water reabsorption and increases blood volume and BP, returning the BP to normal; the stimulus for the secretion of renin is then removed

G. Homeostasis of potassium

1. Increases in potassium stimulate the secretion of aldosterone

2. Aldosterone stimulates the distal convoluted tubules to secrete potassium; this acts to return the potassium concentration to normal

H. Homeostasis of acidity (pH)

1. Blood pH is controlled by maintaining the concentration of buffer systems

2. Carbonic acid and sodium bicarbonate form the most important buffer for neutralizing acids in the plasma

3. The concentration of carbonic acid is controlled by the respiratory system

4. The concentration of sodium bicarbonate is controlled by the kidneys

5. Normal pH is 7.35 to 7.45, maintained by keeping the ratio of concentration of sodium bicarbonate to carbon dioxide constant at 20:1

6. Strong acids are neutralized by sodium bicarbonate to produce carbonic acid and the sodium salts of the strong acid; this process quickly restores the ratio and thus blood pH

7. The carbonic acid produced dissociates into carbon dioxide and water; because the concentration of carbon dioxide is maintained at a constant level by the respiratory system, the excess carbonic acid is rapidly excreted

8. Sodium combined with the strong acid is actively reabsorbed in the distal convoluted tubules in exchange for hydrogen or potassium ions; the strong acid is neutralized by the secretion of ammonia and is excreted as ammonia or potassium salts

I. Risk factors (Box 52-1)

BOX 52-1

Risk Factors Associated with Renal Disorders

Associated medical conditions
Contact sports
Family history of renal disease
Frequent urinary tract infections
High-sodium diet
History of hypertension
Medication use
Trauma and injury

BOX 52-2

Normal Values for Renal Function Tests

BUN (blood urea nitrogen), 8 to 25 mg/dL
Serum creatinine, 0.6 to 1.3 mg/dL
Creatinine clearance, 100 to 120 mL/min
Serum uric acid, 2.5 to 8.0 ng/dL
Uric acid, urine, 250 to 750 mg/24 hr

II. DIAGNOSTIC TESTS (Box 52-2)

A. See Chapter 11 for information regarding normal values for renal function studies

B. Urinalysis

1. Description: A urine test for evaluation of the renal system and for determining renal disease

2. Interventions

a. Wash perineal area and use a clean container

b. Obtain 10 to 15 mL of the first morning sample

c. Note that refrigerated samples may alter the specific gravity

d. If the client is menstruating, indicate this on the laboratory requisition form

C. Specific gravity determination

1. Description: A urine test that measures the kidney's ability to concentrate urine

2. Interventions

a. Can be measured by multiple-test dipstick (most common method), refractometer (an instrument used in the laboratory setting), or urinometer (least accurate method)

b. Factors that interfere with an accurate reading include radiopaque contrast agents, glucose, and proteins

c. Cold specimens may produce a false high reading

d. Normal value is 1.016 to 1.022 (may vary depending on the laboratory)

e. An increase in specific gravity (more concentrated urine) occurs with insufficient fluid intake, decreased renal perfusion, or presence of ADH

f. A decrease in specific gravity (less concentrated urine) occurs with increased fluid intake, diuretic administration, and diabetes insipidus

D. Urine culture and sensitivity
1. Description: A urine test that identifies the presence of microorganisms and determines the specific antibiotics that will appropriately treat the existing microorganism
2. Interventions
   a. Clean perineal area and urinary meatus with bacteriostatic solution
   b. Collect midstream sample in a sterile container
   c. Send the collected specimen to the laboratory immediately
   d. Note that urine from the client who forced fluids may be too dilute to provide a positive culture
   e. Identify any sources of potential contaminants during the collection of the specimen, such as the hands, skin, clothing, hair, or vaginal or rectal secretions
E. Creatinine clearance test
1. Description
   a. Test of a blood and timed urine specimen that evaluates kidney function
   b. Blood is drawn at the start of the test and the morning of the day that the 24-hour urine specimen collection is complete
2. Interventions
   a. Encourage adequate fluids before and during the test
   b. Instruct the client to avoid tea, coffee, and medications during testing, as prescribed
   c. If the client is taking corticosteroids or thyroid medication, check with the physician regarding the administration of these medications during testing
   d. Maintain the urine specimen on ice or refrigerate, and check with the laboratory regarding the addition of a preservative to the specimen during collection
F. Vanillylmandelic acid (VMA) test
1. Description
   a. A 24-hour urine collection to diagnose pheochromocytoma, a tumor of the adrenal gland
   b. The test identifies level of catecholamines in the urine
2. Interventions
   a. Instruct the client to avoid foods such as caffeine, cocoa, vanilla, cheese, gelatin, licorice, and fruits for at least 2 days prior to beginning the urine collection and during the collection, and to avoid taking medications for 2 to 3 days prior to beginning the test, as prescribed
   b. Instruct the client to avoid stress and to maintain intake of adequate food and fluids during the test
   c. Save all urine, label the container, add preservative, and place the specimen on ice or refrigerate

d. Check with the laboratory regarding medication restrictions
G. Uric acid test
1. Description: A 24-hour urine collection to diagnose gout and kidney disease
2. Interventions
   a. Encourage fluids and a regular diet during testing
   b. Place the specimen on ice or refrigerate, and check with the laboratory regarding the addition of a preservative
H. KUB (kidneys, ureters, and bladder) radiography
1. Description: An x-ray that views the urinary system and adjacent structures; used to detect urinary calculi
2. Interventions: There is no specific preparation
I. Bladder ultrasonography
1. A noninvasive method of measuring the volume of urine in the bladder
2. May be performed for evaluating urinary frequency or inability to urinate
J. Computed tomography (CT) and magnetic resonance imaging (MRI)
1. Description: Provide cross-sectional views of the kidney and urinary tract
2. Interventions: See Chapter 56
K. Intravenous pyelography (IVP)
1. Description
   a. The injection of a radiopaque dye that outlines the renal system
   b. Performed to identify abnormalities in the system
2. Preprocedure interventions
   a. Obtain an informed consent
   b. Assess the client for allergies to iodine, seafood, and radiopaque dyes
   c. Withhold food and fluids after midnight on the night before the test
   d. Administer laxatives, as prescribed
   e. Inform the client about possible throat irritation, flushing of the face, warmth, or a salty taste that may be experienced during the test
3. Postprocedure interventions
   a. Monitor vital signs
   b. Instruct the client to drink at least 1 L of fluid unless contraindicated
   c. Monitor the venipuncture site for bleeding
   d. Monitor urinary output
   e. Monitor for signs of a possible reaction to the dye used during the test
L. Renal angiography
1. Description: The injection of a radiopaque dye through a catheter for examination of the renal arterial supply
2. Preprocedure interventions
   a. Obtain an informed consent

b. Assess the client for allergies to iodine, seafood, and radiopaque dyes

c. Inform the client about the possible burning feeling or the feeling of heat along the vessel when the dye is injected

d. Withhold food and fluids after midnight on the night before the test

e. Instruct the client to void immediately before the procedure

f. Administer enemas as prescribed

g. Shave injection sites as prescribed

h. Check and mark the peripheral pulses

3. Postprocedure interventions

a. Monitor vital signs and peripheral pulses

b. Provide bed rest and use of a sandbag at the insertion site for 4 to 8 hours

c. Monitor the color and temperature of the involved extremity

d. Inspect the catheter insertion site for bleeding or swelling

e. Encourage increased fluids unless contraindicated

f. Monitor urinary output

M. Renal scan

1. Description: An intravenous (IV) injection of a radioisotope for visual imaging of renal blood flow

2. Preprocedure interventions

a. Obtain an informed consent

b. Assess for allergies

c. Assist with administering radioisotope as necessary

d. Instruct the client that he or she will be required to remain motionless

e. Instruct the client that imaging may be repeated at various intervals before the test is complete

3. Postprocedure interventions

a. Encourage fluids unless contraindicated

b. Monitor the client for signs of delayed allergic reaction, such as itching and hives

c. Note that the radioactivity is eliminated in 24 hours

d. Follow standard precautions when caring for incontinent clients and double-bag client linens per agency policy

N. Cystometrography (CMG)

1. Description: A graphic recording of the pressures exerted at various degrees of filling of the bladder

2. Preprocedure interventions: Inform the client of the voiding requirements during the procedure

3. Postprocedure interventions: Monitor the client's voiding after the procedure

O. Cystoscopy and biopsy

1. Description: The bladder mucosa is examined for inflammation, calculi, or tumors by means of a cystoscope; a biopsy may be obtained

2. Preprocedure interventions

a. Obtain an informed consent

b. If a biopsy is planned, withhold food and fluids after midnight on the night before the test

c. If a cystoscopy alone is planned, no special preparation is necessary and the procedure may be performed in the physician's office; postprocedure includes increasing fluid intake

3. Postprocedure interventions following biopsy

a. Monitor vital signs

b. Increase fluids, as prescribed

c. Monitor intake and output

d. Encourage deep breathing exercises to relieve bladder spasms

e. Administer analgesics, as prescribed

f. Administer sitz baths for back and abdominal pain

g. Note that leg cramps are common because the lithotomy position is maintained during the procedure

h. Monitor the urine for color and consistency

i. Note that pink-tinged or tea-colored urine is common

j. Monitor for bright red urine or clots, and notify the physician if this occurs

P. Renal biopsy

1. Description: Insertion of a needle into the kidney to obtain a sample of tissue for examination

2. Preprocedure interventions

a. Check vital signs

b. Check baseline clotting studies

c. Obtain an informed consent

d. Withhold food and fluids after midnight on the night before the test

3. Interventions during the procedure: Position the client prone with a pillow under the abdomen and shoulders

4. Postprocedure interventions

a. Monitor vital signs

b. Monitor hemoglobin and hematocrit

c. Place the client in the supine position and on bed rest for 8 hours, as prescribed

d. Provide pressure to the biopsy site for 30 minutes

e. Check the biopsy site for bleeding

f. Encourage fluids to 1500 to 2000 mL, as prescribed

g. Instruct the client to avoid heavy lifting and strenuous activity for 2 weeks

III. RENAL FAILURE

A. Description

1. The loss of kidney function

2. The types of **renal failure** include **acute renal failure** and **chronic renal failure**

3. The signs and symptoms of **renal failure** are caused by the retention of wastes, the retention

---

BOX 52-3

Phases of Acute Renal Failure

Oliguric
Diuretic
Recovery (convalescent)

---

of fluids, and the inability of the kidneys to regulate electrolytes

B. Acute renal failure (ARF) (Box 52-3)
  1. Description
    a. The sudden loss of kidney function; caused by renal cell damage from ischemia or toxic substances
    b. **ARF** occurs abruptly and can be reversible
    c. It leads to hypoperfusion, cell death, and decompensation in renal function
    d. The prognosis is dependent on the cause and the condition of the client
    e. Near-normal or normal kidney function may resume gradually
  2. Causes
    a. Infection
    b. Renal artery occlusion
    c. Obstruction
    d. Acute kidney disease
    e. Dehydration
    f. Diuretic therapy
    g. Ischemia from hypovolemia, heart failure, septic shock, or blood loss
    h. Toxic substances such as medications, particularly antibiotics
  3. Oliguric phase (Table 52-1)
    a. Duration is 8 to 15 days, and the longer the duration, the less chance of recovery
    b. Sudden drop in urine output; urine output less than 400 mL/day
    c. Urine specific gravity of 1.010 to 1.016
    d. Anorexia, nausea, and vomiting
    e. Hypertension
    f. Decreased skin turgor
    g. Pruritus
    h. Tingling of the extremities
    i. Drowsiness progressing to disorientation to coma
    j. Edema
    k. Dysrhythmias
    l. Signs of congestive heart failure (CHF) and pulmonary edema
    m. Signs of pericarditis
    n. Signs of acidosis
  4. Diuretic phase (see Table 52-1)
    a. Urine output rises slowly and then diuresis occurs (4 to 5 L/day)
    b. Excessive urine output indicates recovery of damaged nephrons

---

TABLE 52-1

Acute Renal Failure

OLIGURIC PHASE
Glomerular filtration rate decreases
Hyperkalemia
Sodium level normal or decreased
Fluid overload
Elevated blood urea nitrogen (BUN) and creatinine levels

DIURETIC PHASE
Glomerular filtration rate begins to increase
Hypokalemia
Hyponatremia
Hypovolemia
Gradual decline in BUN and creatinine levels

RECOVERY PHASE (CONVALESCENT)
BUN level is stable and normal
Complete recovery may take 1 to 2 years

---

    c. Hypotension
    d. Tachycardia
    e. Improvement in level of consciousness (LOC)
  5. Recovery phase (convalescence) (see Table 52-1)
    a. A slow process; complete recovery may take 1 to 2 years
    b. Urine volume is normal
    c. Increase in strength
    d. Increase in LOC
    e. Blood urea nitrogen (BUN) level is stable and normal
    f. Client can develop **chronic renal failure**
C. **Chronic renal failure (CRF)**
  1. Description
    a. The progressive loss and ongoing deterioration in kidney function that occurs slowly over a period of time
    b. It occurs in stages, is irreversible, and results in uremia or end-stage renal disease (Table 52-2)
    c. **CRF** affects all the major body systems and requires dialysis or kidney transplantation to maintain life
    d. Hypervolemia can occur because of the inability of the kidneys to excrete sodium and water, or hypovolemia can occur because of the inability of the kidneys to conserve sodium and water
  2. Causes
    a. May follow **ARF**
    b. Renal artery occlusion
    c. Chronic urinary obstruction
    d. Recurrent infections
    e. Hypertension
    f. Metabolic disorders
    g. Diabetes mellitus
    h. Autoimmune disorders

TABLE 52-2

Stages of Chronic Renal Failure

STAGE I: DIMINISHED RENAL RESERVE
Renal function is reduced
No accumulation of metabolic wastes
The healthier kidney compensates
Nocturia and polyuria occur as a result of decreased ability
 to concentrate urine

STAGE II: RENAL INSUFFICIENCY
Metabolic wastes begin to accumulate
Oliguria and edema occur as a result of decreased
 responsiveness to diuretics

STAGE III: END STAGE
Excessive accumulation of metabolic wastes
Kidneys are unable to maintain homeostasis
Dialysis or other renal replacement therapy is required

BOX 52-4

Special Problems in Renal Failure

Hypertension
Hypervolemia
Hypovolemia
Potassium retention
Phosphorus retention
Low calcium level
Metabolic acidosis
Anemia
GI bleeding
Infection and injury
Pruritis
Muscle cramps
Ocular irritation
Insomnia and fatigue
Neurological changes
Psychosocial problems

3. Data collection
 a. Anorexia and nausea
 b. Headache
 c. Weakness and fatigue
 d. Hypertension
 e. Confusion and lethargy, followed by convulsions and coma
 f. Kussmaul respirations
 g. Diarrhea or constipation
 h. Muscle twitching and numbness of the extremities
 i. Decreased urine output
 j. Decreased urine specific gravity
 k. Proteinuria
 l. Anemia
 m. **Azotemia**
 n. Fluid overload and signs of heart failure
 o. Uremic frost: A layer of urea crystals from evaporated perspiration that appears on the face, eyebrows, axilla, and groin in clients with advanced uremic syndrome

D. Interventions
 1. Monitor vital signs
 2. Monitor urine and intake and output (I&O); monitor hourly in **ARF**
 3. Monitor weight, noting that an increase of 0.5 to 1 pound daily indicates fluid retention
 4. Monitor BUN, creatinine, and electrolyte levels
 5. Monitor for acidosis and treat with sodium bicarbonate, as prescribed
 6. Check urinalysis for protein, hematuria, casts, and specific gravity
 7. Monitor LOC
 8. Monitor for signs of infection, because the client may not demonstrate a temperature or an increased white blood cell (WBC) count

 9. Monitor for dysrhythmias, because a potassium level above 6 mEq/L will cause peaked T waves and a widened QRS complex
 10. Monitor for fluid overload; check lungs for wheezes and rhonchi
 11. Monitor for edema
 12. Administer prescribed diet; usually a moderate protein intake (to decrease the workload on the kidneys) and a high-carbohydrate, low-potassium, low-phosphorus diet is prescribed
 13. Restrict sodium intake as prescribed, based on the electrolyte level
 14. Daily fluid allowances may be 400 to 1000 mL plus measured urinary putput
 15. Administer sodium polystyrene sulfonate (Kayexalate) to lower the potassium level as prescribed
 16. Be alert to the mechanism for metabolism and excretion of all prescribed medication
 17. Be alert to nephrotoxic medications, such as antibiotics, which may be prescribed
 18. Prepare the client for dialysis if prescribed
E. Special problems in **renal failure** (Box 52-4)
 1. Hypertension
 a. Failure of the kidneys to maintain homeostasis of the blood pressure
 b. Monitor vital signs
 c. Maintain fluid and sodium restrictions as prescribed
 d. Administer diuretics and antihypertensives as prescribed
 e. Administer propranolol (Inderal), a beta-adrenergic antagonist, as prescribed, which decreases renin release (renin causes vasoconstriction)
 2. Hypervolemia
 a. Monitor vital signs

b. Monitor I&O and weight

c. Monitor for edema

d. Monitor electrolytes

e. Monitor for hypertension

f. Monitor for CHF and pulmonary edema

g. Enforce fluid restriction

h. Avoid the administration of IV fluids

i. Administer diuretics as prescribed

j. Instruct the client to avoid foods with sodium

k. Instruct the client to avoid antacids or cold remedies containing sodium bicarbonate

3. Hypovolemia

a. Monitor vital signs

b. Monitor I&O and weight

c. Monitor electrolytes

d. Monitor for hypotension

e. Monitor for dehydration

f. Provide replacement therapy based on the electrolyte results

g. Provide sodium supplements as prescribed, depending on the electrolyte value

4. Potassium retention

a. Monitor vital signs and apical rate

b. Monitor potassium level

c. Monitor for dysrhythmias (peaked T waves and widened QRS complex) indicating hyperkalemia

d. Provide a low-potassium diet

e. Administer medications as prescribed to lower the potassium level

f. Prepare the client for dialysis

5. Phosphorus retention

a. Phosphorus level increases and calcium level decreases, which leads to stimulation of parathyroid hormone, causing bone demineralization

b. Treatment is aimed at lowering serum phosphorus level

c. Administer aluminum hydroxide preparations or other phosphate binders as prescribed that bind phosphorus in the intestine and allow the phosphorus to be eliminated

d. Administer aluminum hydroxide preparations at meals and not with other medications, because they bind medications in the intestinal tract

e. Administer stool softeners and laxatives as prescribed to prevent constipation, because aluminum hydroxide preparations are constipating

f. Enforce phosphorus restriction in the diet

6. Low calcium level

a. Occurs because of the high phosphorus level and because of the inability of the diseased kidney to activate vitamin D

b. The absence of vitamin D causes a poor absorption of calcium from the intestinal tract

c. Monitor calcium level

d. Administer calcium supplements, as prescribed

e. Administer activated vitamin D, as prescribed

7. Metabolic acidosis

a. The kidneys are unable to excrete hydrogen ions or manufacture bicarbonate, resulting in acidosis

b. Administer alkalizers such as sodium bicarbonate, as prescribed

c. Note that clients with **CRF** adjust to low bicarbonate levels and do not become acutely ill

8. Anemia

a. A decreased rate of production of red blood cells (RBCs) occurs as a result of the diseased kidney and the decreased secretion of erythropoietin

b. Monitor hemoglobin and hematocrit

c. Administer epoetin alfa (Epogen) as prescribed to stimulate the production of red blood cells (RBCs)

d. Administer folic acid (vitamin B_9) as prescribed, instead of oral iron, because oral iron is not well absorbed by the gastrointestinal tract (GI) tract in **CRF** and causes nausea and vomiting

e. Administer blood transfusions if prescribed, but blood transfusions are prescribed only when necessary because they decrease the stimulus to produce RBCs

f. Monitor bleeding

g. Instruct the client to use a soft toothbrush

h. Administer stool softeners as prescribed

i. Avoid the administration of acetylsalicylic acid (aspirin) because the medication is excreted by the kidneys; if administered, high toxic levels will occur and prolong bleeding time

9. GI bleeding

a. Urea is broken down to ammonia by the intestinal bacteria; ammonia is a mucosal irritant that causes ulceration and bleeding

b. Monitor hemoglobin and hematocrit levels

c. Monitor stools for occult blood

10. Infection and injury

a. Infection and injury need to be monitored and avoided because tissue breakdown causes increased potassium levels

b. Monitor for signs of infection

c. Avoid urinary catheters and provide strict asepsis during insertion and catheter care

d. Instruct the client to avoid fatigue, which decreases body resistance

e. Instruct the client to avoid persons with infections

f. Administer antibiotics as prescribed, monitoring for nephrotoxic effects

11. Pruritus
    a. Urate crystals are excreted through the skin to rid of excess wastes
    b. This deposit of crystals is called uremic frost; is seen in advanced stages of **renal failure**
    c. Monitor for skin breakdown, rash, and uremic frost
    d. Provide good skin care and oral hygiene
    e. Avoid the use of soaps
    f. Administer antipruritics as prescribed
12. Muscle cramps
    a. Occur in the extremities and hands and can be caused by electrolyte imbalances
    b. Monitor electrolytes
    c. Administer electrolyte replacements, as prescribed
    d. Administer heat and massage, as prescribed
13. Ocular irritation
    a. Calcium deposits in the conjunctiva cause burning and watering of the eyes
    b. Administer medications to control the calcium and phosphate levels, as prescribed
    c. Administer lubricating eyedrops
14. Insomnia and fatigue
    a. The diseased kidneys cause a buildup of wastes, causing fatigue in the client
    b. Provide adequate rest periods
    c. Administer mild central nervous system (CNS) depressants, as prescribed
15. Neurological changes
    a. The buildup of active particles and fluids causes changes in the brain cells and leads to confusion and impairment in decision-making ability
    b. Monitor for confusion and monitor LOC
    c. Protect the client from injury
    d. Provide a safe and hazard-free environment
    e. Use side rails as needed
    f. Provide a calm and restful environment
    g. Provide comfort measures and back rubs
16. Psychosocial problems: Monitor the client for psychological problems such as depression, anxiety, suicidal behavior, denial, dependence/independence conflict, and changes in body image

IV. HEMODIALYSIS
A. Description
    1. The diffusion of dissolved particles from one fluid compartment into another across a semipermeable membrane
    2. The client's blood flows through one fluid compartment, and the dialysate is in another fluid compartment
B. Functions of **hemodialysis**
    1. Cleanses the blood of accumulated waste products

    2. Removes the by-products of protein metabolism, such as urea, creatinine, and uric acid
    3. Removes excessive fluids
    4. Maintains or restores the body's buffer system
    5. Maintains or restores electrolyte levels
C. Principles of **hemodialysis**
    1. The semipermeable membrane is made of a thin, porous cellophane
    2. The pore size of the membrane allows small particles to pass through, such as urea, creatinine, uric acid, and water molecules
    3. Proteins, bacteria, and some blood cells are too large to pass through the membrane
    4. The client's blood flows into the dialyzer; the movement of substances occurs from the blood to the dialysate
    5. Diffusion: The movement of particles from an area of higher concentration to one of lower concentration
    6. Osmosis: The movement of fluids across a semipermeable membrane from an area of lower concentration of particles to an area of higher concentration of particles
    7. Ultrafiltration: The movement of fluid across a semipermeable membrane as a result of an artificially created pressure gradient
D. Dialysate bath
    1. Composed of water and major electrolytes
    2. The dialysate need not be sterile because bacteria are too large to pass through; however, the dialysate must meet specific standards, and water treatment systems are used to ensure a safe water supply
E. Interventions
    1. Monitor vital signs
    2. Monitor laboratory values before, during, and after dialysis
    3. Monitor the client for fluid overload before the procedure
    4. Monitor patency of the blood access device
    5. Weigh the client before and after the procedure to determine fluid loss
    6. Hold antihypertensives and other medications that can affect the BP before the procedure, as prescribed
    7. Hold medications that could be dialyzed off, such as water-soluble vitamins and certain antibiotics
    8. Monitor for shock and hypovolemia during the procedure
    9. Provide adequate nutrition (client may eat before the procedure)

V. COMPLICATIONS OF HEMODIALYSIS (Box 52-5)
A. Disequilibrium syndrome
    1. Description
        a. A rapid change in the composition of the extracellular fluid (ECF) occurs during **hemodialysis**

b. Solutes are removed from the blood faster than from the cerebrospinal fluid (CSF) and brain; fluid is pulled into the brain, causing cerebral edema
2. Data collection
   a. Nausea
   b. Vomiting
   c. Headache
   d. Hypertension
   e. Restlessness and agitation
   f. Confusion
   g. Seizures
3. Interventions
   a. Monitor for signs of disequilibrium syndrome
   b. The physician is notified if signs of disequilibrium syndrome occur
   c. Reduce environmental stimuli
   d. Prepare to dialyze the client for a shorter period at reduced blood flow rates to prevent occurrence
B. Dialysis encephalopathy
   1. Description: An aluminum toxicity that occurs as a result of aluminum in the H_2O sources used in the dialysate and the ingestion of aluminum-containing antacids (phosphate binders)
   2. Data collection
      a. Progressive neurological impairment
      b. Mental cloudiness
      c. Speech disturbances
      d. Dementia
      e. Muscle incoordination
      f. Bone pain
      g. Seizures
   3. Interventions
      a. Monitor for signs of dialysis encephalopathy
      b. The physician is notified if signs of dialysis encephalopathy occur
      c. Administer aluminum-chelating agents as prescribed so that the aluminum is freed up and dialyzed from the body

VI. ACCESS FOR HEMODIALYSIS
A. Subclavian and femoral catheter
   1. Description

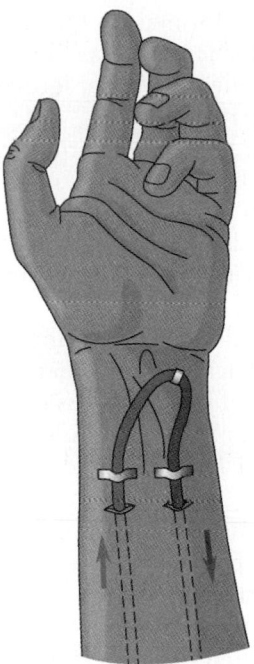

FIG. 52-1   An arteriovenous shunt (AV shunt) in the forearm. (From Ignatavicius, D., & Workman, M. [2006]. *Medical surgical nursing: Critical thinking for collaborative care* [5th ed.]. Philadelphia: W.B. Saunders.)

   a. A subclavian (subclavian vein) or femoral (femoral vein) catheter may be inserted for short-term or temporary use in **ARF**
   b. May be used until a fistula or graft matures or develops, or when the client has fistula or graft access failure because of infection or clotting
2. Interventions
   a. Monitor insertion site for hematoma, bleeding, dislodging, and infection
   b. Do not use these catheters for any reason other than dialysis
   c. Maintain an occlusive dressing over site
3. Subclavian vein catheter
   a. Is usually filled with heparin and capped to maintain patency between dialysis treatments
   b. The catheter should not be uncapped
   c. The catheter may be left in place for up to 6 weeks if complications do not occur
4. Femoral vein catheter
   a. The client should not sit up more than 45 degrees or lean forward, or the catheter may kink and occlude
   b. Monitor extremity for circulation, temperature, and pulses
   c. Prevent pulling or disconnecting of the catheter when giving care
B. External arteriovenous shunt (AV shunt) (Figure 52-1)
   1. Description

a. Access is formed by the surgical insertion of two Silastic cannulas into an artery and a vein in the forearm or leg to form an external blood path

b. The cannulas are connected to form a U shape; blood flows from the client's artery through the shunt into the vein

c. A tube leading to the membrane compartment of the dialyzer is connected to the arterial cannula

d. Blood fills the membrane compartment and flows back to the client through a tube connected to the venous cannula

e. When dialysis is complete, the cannulas are clamped and reattached to form their U shape

2. Advantages

a. Can be used immediately following creation

b. No venipuncture is necessary for dialysis

3. Disadvantages

a. External danger of disconnecting or dislodging

b. Risk of hemorrhage, infection, or clotting

c. Skin erosion around the catheter site can occur

4. Interventions

a. Avoid wetting the shunt

b. A dressing is completely wrapped around the shunt and kept dry and intact

c. Cannula clamps need to be available at the client's bedside

d. Do not take a blood pressure, draw blood, place an IV, or administer injections in the shunt extremity

e. Monitor for hemorrhage, infection, and clotting

f. Monitor skin integrity around the insertion site

g. Note that the shunt is patent if it is warm to touch

h. Auscultate and palpate for a bruit, although a bruit may not be heard and is not always felt with the shunt

i. The physician is notified immediately if signs of clotting, hemorrhage, or infection occur

5. Signs of clotting

a. Fold back the dressing to expose the shunt tubing and check for signs of clotting

b. Fibrin-white flecks noted in the tubing

c. The separation of serum and cells

d. The absence of a previously heard bruit

e. Coolness of the tubing or extremity

f. Client complaints of a tingling sensation

C. **Internal arteriovenous (AV) fistula** (Figure 52-2)

1. Description

a. Access of choice for chronic dialysis clients

b. Created surgically by anastomosis of an artery in the arm to a vein; this creates an opening or fistula between a large artery and a large vein

c. The flow of arterial blood into the venous system causes the veins to become engorged (matured or developed)

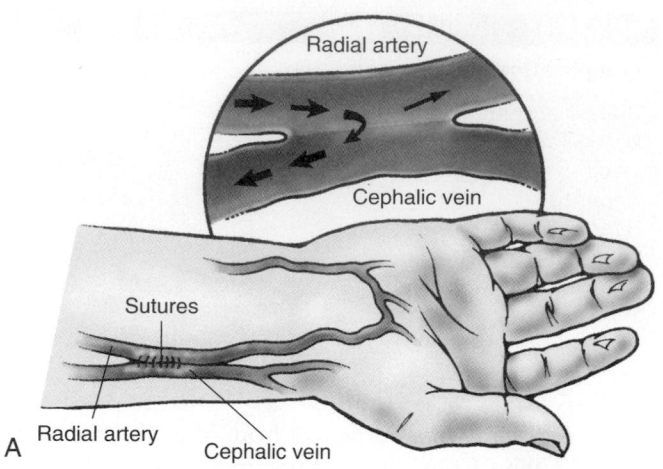

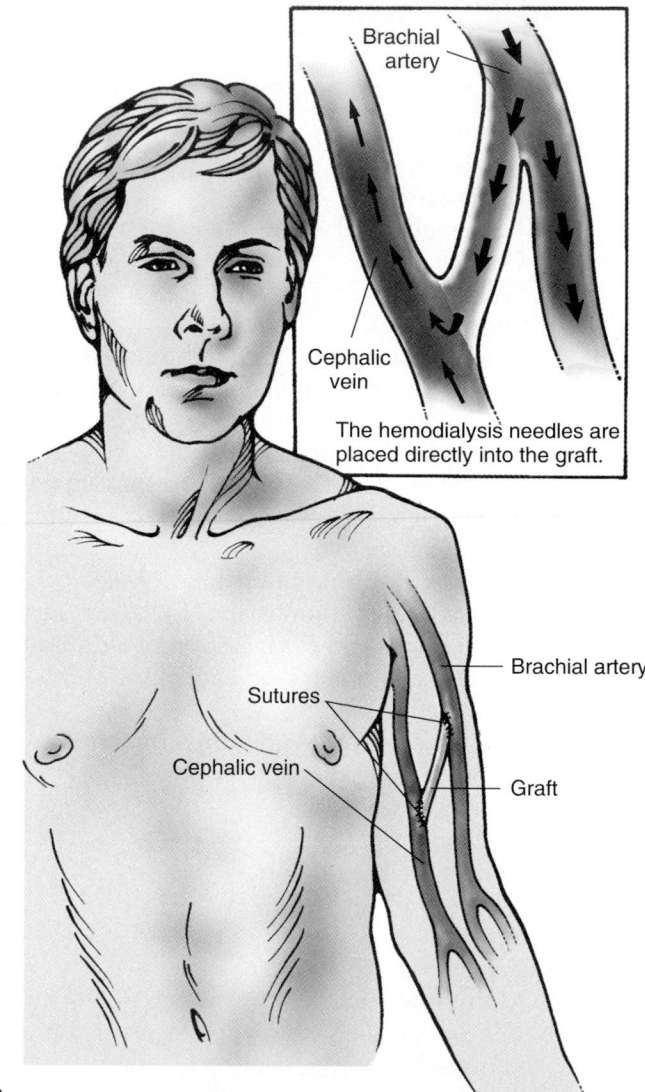

FIG. 52-2 Options for long-term vascular access for hemodialysis. **A,** Surgically created venous fistula. **B,** Surgically placed straight vascular graft in the upper arm. **Inset,** Shunt between arterial and venous blood. (From Ignatavicius, D., & Workman, M. [2006]. *Medical surgical nursing: Critical thinking for collaborative care* [5th ed.]. Philadelphia: W.B. Saunders.)

d. Maturity takes about 1 to 2 weeks and is required before the fistula can be used, so that the engorged vein can be punctured with a large-bore needle for the dialysis procedure

e. Subclavian or femoral catheters, **peritoneal dialysis,** or an external AV shunt can be used for dialysis while the fistula is maturing or developing

2. Advantages
   a. Because the fistula is internal, there is less danger of clotting and bleeding
   b. The fistula can be used indefinitely
   c. Decreased incidence of infection
   d. No external dressing is required
   e. Allows freedom of movement

3. Disadvantages
   a. Cannot be used immediately after insertion
   b. Needle insertions are required for dialysis
   c. Infiltration of the needles during dialysis can occur and cause hematomas
   d. An aneurysm can form in the fistula
   e. **Arterial steal syndrome** can develop (too much blood is diverted to the vein, and arterial perfusion to the hand is compromised)
   f. CHF can occur from the increased blood flow in the venous system

D. Internal arteriovenous graft (AV graft) (see Figure 52-2)
   1. Description
      a. The internal graft is used primarily for chronic dialysis clients who do not have adequate blood vessels for the creation of a fistula
      b. An artificial graft made of Gore-Tex or a bovine (cow) carotid artery is used to create an artificial vein for blood flow
      c. The procedure involves the anastomosis of the graft to the artery, a tunneling under the skin, and anastomosis to a vein
      d. The graft can be used 2 weeks after insertion
      e. Complications of the graft include clotting, aneurysms, and infection
   2. Advantages
      a. Because the graft is internal, there is less danger of clotting and bleeding
      b. The graft can be used indefinitely
      c. Decreased incidence of infection
      d. No external dressing is required
      e. Allows freedom of movement
   3. Disadvantages
      a. Cannot be used immediately after insertion
      b. Needle insertions are required for dialysis
      c. Infiltration of the needles during dialysis can occur and cause hematomas
      d. An aneurysm can form in the graft
      e. **Arterial steal syndrome** can develop (too much blood is diverted to the vein, and arterial perfusion to the hand is compromised)
      f. CHF can occur from the increased blood flow in the venous system

E. Interventions for **AV fistula** and AV graft
   1. Do not measure a blood pressure, draw blood, place an IV, or administer injections in the fistula or graft extremity
   2. Monitor for clotting
      a. Complaints of tingling or discomfort in the extremity
      b. Inability to palpate a thrill or auscultate a bruit over the fistula or graft
   3. Monitor for **arterial steal syndrome**
   4. Palpate or auscultate for bruit or thrill over the fistula or graft
   5. Palpate pulses below the fistula or graft, and monitor for hand swelling as an indication of ischemia
   6. Note temperature and capillary refill of the extremity
   7. Monitor for infection
   8. Monitor lung and heart sounds for signs of CHF
   9. The physician is notified immediately if signs of clotting, infection, or **arterial steal syndrome** occur

VII. PERITONEAL DIALYSIS

A. Description
   1. The peritoneum is the dialyzing membrane (semipermeable membrane) and substitutes for kidney function during kidney failure
   2. Works on the principles of diffusion and osmosis; dialysis occurs via the transfer of fluid and solute from the bloodstream through the peritoneum
   3. The peritoneal membrane is large and porous, allowing solutes and fluid to move via an osmotic gradient from an area of higher concentration in the body to an area of lower concentration in the dialyzing fluid
   4. The peritoneal cavity is rich in capillaries; therefore, it provides a ready access to blood supply

B. Contraindications to **peritoneal dialysis**
   1. Peritonitis
   2. Recent abdominal surgery
   3. Abdominal adhesions
   4. Impending renal transplant

C. Dialysate solution
   1. Solution is sterile
   2. The higher the glucose concentration, the greater the amount of fluid removed during an exchange
   3. Increasing the glucose concentration increases the concentration of active particles that cause osmosis and increases the rate of ultrafiltration and the amount of fluid removed
   4. Potassium: If hyperkalemia is not a problem, potassium may be added to each bag of solution
   5. Heparin: Added to the dialysate solution to prevent clotting of the catheter
   6. Antibiotics: Prophylactic antibiotics may be added to dialysate to prevent peritonitis

7. Insulin: May be added to the dialysate for the client with diabetes mellitus

VIII. ACCESS FOR PERITONEAL DIALYSIS
(Figure 52-3)

A. Description
1. A surgical insertion of a siliconized rubber catheter into the abdominal cavity is required to allow infusion of dialysis fluid
2. The preferred insertion site is 3 to 5 cm below the umbilicus because this area is relatively avascular and has less fascial resistance
3. The catheters are tunneled under the skin to stabilize the catheter and reduce the risk of infection
4. Over a period of 1 to 2 weeks following insertion, there is an ingrowth of fibroblasts and blood vessels into the cuffs of the catheter, which fix the catheter in place and provide an extra barrier against dialysate leakage and bacterial invasion

B. Types of **peritoneal dialysis**
1. Continuous ambulatory **peritoneal dialysis** (CAPD)
   a. Closely resembles renal function because it is a continuous process
   b. Does not require a machine for the procedure
   c. Promotes client independence
   d. The client performs self-dialysis 24 hours a day, 7 days a week
   e. Usually, four dialysis cycles are administered in 24 hours, including an 8-hour dwell time overnight
   f. Four times daily, 1½ to 2 L of dialysate is instilled into the abdomen and allowed to dwell, as prescribed
   g. The dialysis bag, attached to the catheter, is folded and carried in the client's clothing until time for outflow
   h. After dwell, the bag is placed lower than the insertion site so that fluid drains by gravity flow
   i. When full, the bag is changed, new dialysate is instilled into the abdomen, and the process continues
2. Automated **peritoneal dialysis** (APD) (Box 52-6)
   a. Similar to CAPD in that it is a continuous dialysis process
   b. Requires a peritoneal cycling machine
   c. Can be done as intermittent **peritoneal dialysis** (IPD), continuous cycling **peritoneal dialysis** (CCPD), or nightly **peritoneal dialysis** (NPD)

C. **Peritoneal dialysis** infusion
1. Description
   a. One infusion—inflow, dwell, and outflow—is considered one exchange
   b. Uses an open system that presents a risk of infection
   c. Inflow: The infusion of 1 to 2 L of dialysate as prescribed is infused by gravity into the peritoneal space, which usually takes approximately 10 to 20 minutes

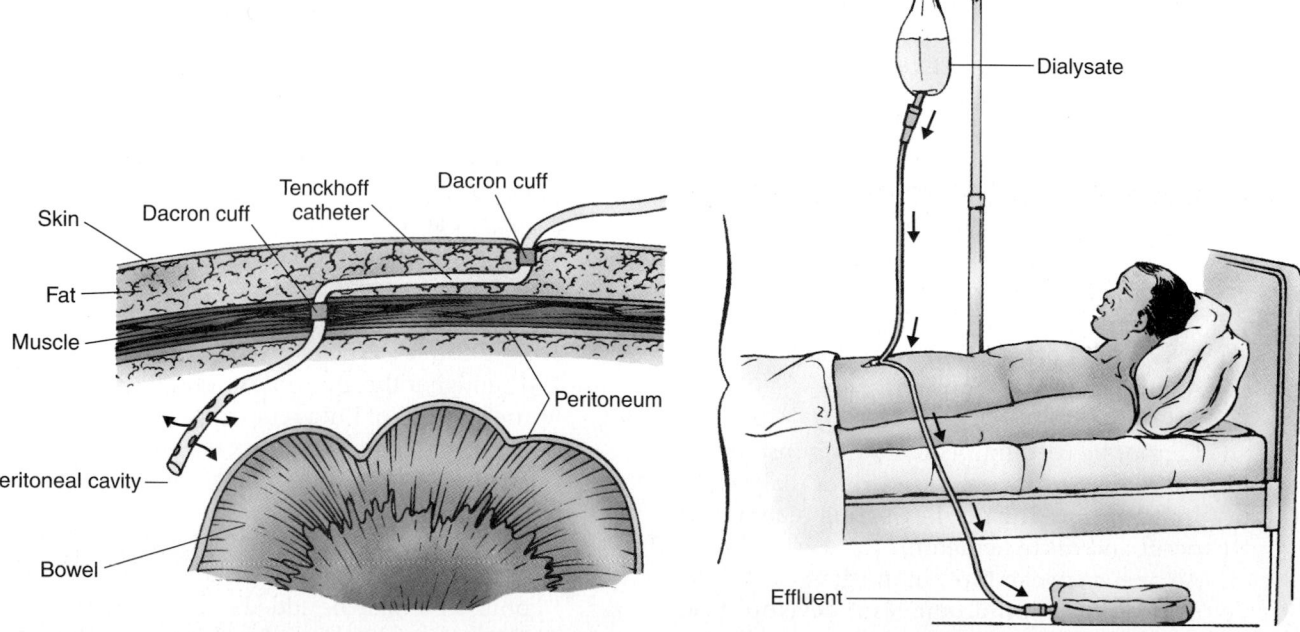

FIG. 52-3 Access for peritoneal dialysis. **A,** Implanted abdominal catheter (Tenckhoff catheter). **B,** Infusion of dialypate into the abdominal cavity; peritoneal effluent (outflow) following dwell time. (From Ignatavicius, D., & Workman, M. [2006]. *Medical surgical nursing: Critical thinking for collaborative care* [5th ed.]. Philadelphia: W.B. Saunders.)

d. Dwell time: The amount of time that the dialysate solution remains in the peritoneal cavity; prescribed by the physician; can last 20 to 30 minutes to 8 or more hours, depending on the type of dialysis used

e. Outflow: Fluid drains out of the body by gravity into the drainage bag

2. Interventions before treatment
   a. Monitor vital signs
   b. Obtain weight
   c. Have the client void, if possible
   d. Check electrolyte and glucose levels

3. Interventions during treatment
   a. Monitor vital signs
   b. Monitor for signs of infection
   c. Monitor for respiratory distress, pain, or discomfort
   d. Monitor for signs of pulmonary edema
   e. Monitor for hypotension and hypertension
   f. Monitor for malaise, nausea, vomiting
   g. Check the catheter site dressing for wetness or bleeding
   h. Monitor dwell time as prescribed by the physician and initiate outflow
   i. Do not allow dwell time to extend beyond the physician's order because this increases the risk for hyperglycemia
   j. Turn the client from side to side or have the client sit upright if the flow is slow to start
   k. Monitor outflow, which should be a continuous stream after the clamp is opened
   l. Monitor outflow for color and clarity
   m. Monitor I&O accurately
   n. If outflow is less than inflow, the difference is equal to the amount absorbed or retained by the client during dialysis and should be counted as intake

---

BOX 52-6

Types of Automated Peritoneal Dialysis

CONTINUOUS CYCLING PERITONEAL DIALYSIS (CCPD)
Requires a peritoneal cycling machine
Usually consists of three cycles done at night, and one cycle with an 8-hour dwell done in the morning
Peritoneal cavity is opened only for the on-and-off procedures, which reduces the risk of infection
Client does not need to do exchanges during the day

INTERMITTENT PERITONEAL DIALYSIS (IPD)
Requires a peritoneal cycling machine
Not a continuous dialysis procedure
Performed for 10 to 14 hours, three to four times a week

NIGHTLY PERITONEAL DIALYSIS (NPD)
Performed 8 to 12 hours each night with no daytime exchanges or dwells

---

IX. COMPLICATIONS OF PERITONEAL DIALYSIS (Box 52-7)

A. Peritonitis
   1. Maintain meticulous sterile technique when hooking up or clamping off bags, and when caring for the catheter insertion site
   2. Follow institutional procedure for hooking up or clamping off bags, which may include scrubbing the connection sites with an antiseptic solution
   3. Monitor temperature closely
   4. Monitor for fever, cloudy outflow, and rebound abdominal tenderness
   5. If peritonitis is suspected, obtain a culture of the outflow to determine the infective organism
   6. Administer antibiotics, as prescribed

B. Abdominal pain
   1. Pain during inflow is common during the first few exchanges, is caused by peritoneal irritation, and usually disappears after a week or two of dialysis treatments
   2. The cold temperature of the dialysate aggravates the discomfort, and the dialysate should be warmed before use only with a special dialysate warmer pad
   3. Place a heating pad on the abdomen during the inflow to relieve discomfort; if a heating pad is used, it is placed on low setting and the client is monitored closely

C. Insufficient outflow
   1. May be caused by catheter migration out of the peritoneal area; if this occurs, the catheter must be repositioned by the physician
   2. Insufficient outflow can also be caused by a full colon
   3. Maintain the drainage bag below the client's abdomen
   4. Change the client's outflow position by turning or ambulating
   5. Check for kinks in the tubing
   6. Encourage a high-fiber diet
   7. Administer stool softeners, as prescribed

D. Leakage around the catheter site
   1. Over a period of 1 to 2 weeks following insertion of the catheter, an ingrowth of fibroblasts and blood vessels into the cuffs of the catheter occurs, which fix the catheter in place and provide an extra barrier against dialysate leakage and bacterial invasion

---

BOX 52-7

Complications of Peritoneal Dialysis

Peritonitis
Abdominal pain
Insufficient outflow
Leakage around the catheter site
Bladder or bowel perforation

2. It may take up to 2 weeks for the client to tolerate a full 2-L exchange without leaking around the catheter site

E. Characteristics of outflow
1. During the first or initial exchanges, the outflow may be bloody; outflow should be clear and colorless thereafter
2. A brown outflow indicates bowel perforation
3. If the outflow is same color as urine, this indicates bladder perforation
4. Cloudy outflow indicates peritonitis

X. UREMIC SYNDROME

A. Description
1. The accumulation of nitrogenous waste products in the blood because of the inability of the kidneys to filter out these waste products
2. It may occur as a result of **acute** or **chronic renal failure**

B. Data collection
1. Oliguria
2. The presence of protein, red blood cells, and casts in the urine
3. A urine specific gravity of 1.010
4. Elevated levels of urea, uric acid, potassium, and magnesium in the urine
5. Hypotension or hypertension
6. Alterations in LOC
7. Electrolyte imbalances
8. Stomatitis
9. Nausea or vomiting
10. Diarrhea or constipation

C. Interventions
1. Monitor vital signs
2. Monitor electrolyte levels
3. Monitor I&O
4. Provide a diet limited in protein, as prescribed (protein provided should be high quality)
5. Limit sodium, nitrogen, potassium, and phosphate intake, as prescribed

XI. CYSTITIS–URINARY TRACT INFECTIONS (UTI) (Box 52-8)

A. Description
1. Inflammation of the bladder from infection or obstruction of the urethra
2. The most common causative organisms are *Escherichia coli*, *Enterobacter*, *Pseudomonas*, and *Serratia*
3. More common in women because women have a shorter urethra than men; location of the urethra in the woman is close to the rectum
4. Sexually active and pregnant women are most vulnerable to cystitis

B. Data collection

BOX 52-8

Causes of Cystitis

Allergens or irritants, such as soaps, sprays, bubble bath, perfumed sanitary napkins
Bladder distention
Calculus
Hormonal changes influencing alterations in vaginal flora
Indwelling urethral catheters
Invasive urinary tract procedures
Loss of bactericidal properties of prostatic secretions in the male
Poor-fitting diaphragms
Sexual intercourse
Synthetic underwear and panty hose
Urinary stasis
Use of spermicides
Wet bathing suits

---

1. Frequency and urgency
2. Burning on urination
3. Voiding in small amounts
4. Inability to void
5. Incomplete emptying of the bladder
6. Lower abdominal discomfort or back discomfort
7. Cloudy, dark, foul-smelling urine
8. Hematuria
9. Bladder spasms
10. Malaise, chills, fever
11. Nausea and vomiting

C. Interventions
1. Obtain a urine specimen for culture and sensitivity, if prescribed, to identify bacterial growth before administering prescribed antibiotics
2. Instruct the client to increase fluids up to 3000 mL/day, especially if the client is taking a sulfonamide, because these medications can form crystals in concentrated urine
3. Administer medications as prescribed, which may include analgesics, antiseptics, antispasmodics, antibiotics, and antimicrobials
4. Maintain an acid urine pH (5.5) by an acid ash diet; instruct the client in foods to consume on an acid ash diet
5. Note that if the client is prescribed an aminoglycoside, a sulfonamide, or nitrofurantoin (Macrodantin), the actions of these medications are diminished by acidic urine
6. Use strict aseptic technique when inserting a urinary catheter into a client
7. Maintain closed urinary drainage systems for the client with an indwelling catheter
8. Provide meticulous perineal care for the client with an indwelling catheter
9. Discourage caffeine products such as coffee, tea, and cola
10. Instruct the client to avoid alcohol

BOX 52-9

Prevention of Cystitis

Teach the female client good perineal care and to wipe from front to back.

Instruct the female client to avoid bubble baths and tub baths and avoid vaginal deodorants or sprays.

Instruct the client to void every 2 to 3 hours.

Instruct the female client to void and drink a glass of water after intercourse.

Instruct the female client to wear cotton pants and to avoid wearing tight-fitting clothes or panty hose with slacks and to avoid sitting in a wet bathing suit for prolonged periods.

Teach pregnant women to void every 2 hours.

Encourage menopausal women to use estrogen vaginal creams to restore pH.

Instruct the female client to use water-soluble lubricants for coitus, especially after menopause.

---

11. Provide heat to the abdomen or sitz baths for complaints of discomfort
12. Instruct the client to take medications, as prescribed
13. Instruct the client to take antibiotics on schedule and to take entire course of medications as prescribed, which may be a course of 10 to 14 days
14. Instruct the client in the importance of a follow-up urine culture following treatment
15. Preventive measures are listed in Box 52-9

XII. UROSEPSIS

A. Description
   1. A gram-negative bacteremia originating in the urinary tract
   2. The most common responsible organism is *Escherichia coli*
   3. The most common cause is the presence of an indwelling urinary catheter or an untreated UTI in a client who is medically compromised
   4. The major problem is the ability of this bacterium to develop resistant strains
   5. Urosepsis can lead to septic shock if not treated aggressively
B. Data collection: Fever is the most common and earliest manifestation
C. Interventions
   1. Obtain a urine specimen for urine culture and sensitivity
   2. Intravenous antibiotics are prescribed, usually until the client has been afebrile for 3 to 5 days
   3. Administer oral antibiotics as prescribed after the 3- to 5-day afebrile period

XIII. URETHRITIS

A. Description
   1. An inflammation of the urethra commonly associated with sexually transmitted diseases (STDs); may be seen with cystitis
   2. In men, it is most often caused by gonorrhea or chlamydial infection
   3. In women, it is most often caused by feminine hygiene sprays, perfumed toilet paper or sanitary napkins, spermicidal jellies, UTIs, or changes in the vaginal mucosal lining
B. Data collection
   1. Males
      a. Burning on urination
      b. Frequency
      c. Urgency
      d. Nocturia
      e. Difficulty voiding
      f. Discharge from the penis
   2. Females
      a. Frequency
      b. Urgency
      c. Nocturia
      d. Painful urination
      e. Difficulty voiding
      f. Lower abdominal discomfort
C. Interventions
   1. Encourage fluids
   2. Prepare the client for testing to determine if an STD is present
   3. Administer antibiotics, as prescribed
   4. Instruct the client in the administration of sitz baths
   5. If stricture occurs, prepare the client for dilation of the urethra and instillation of an antiseptic solution
   6. Instruct the client to avoid intercourse until the symptoms subside or treatment of the STD is complete
   7. Instruct the female client to avoid the use of perfumed toilet paper or sanitary napkins and feminine hygiene sprays

XIV. URETERITIS AND PYELONEPHRITIS

A. Ureteritis
   1. An inflammation of the ureter that is commonly associated with pyelonephritis
   2. Chronic pyelonephritis causes the ureter to become fibrotic and narrowed by strictures
B. Pyelonephritis
   1. An inflammation of the renal pelvis and the parenchyma, commonly caused by bacterial invasion
   2. Acute pyelonephritis often occurs after bacterial contamination of the urethra or following an invasive procedure of the urinary tract

3. Chronic pyelonephritis most commonly occurs following chronic urinary flow obstruction with reflux
4. *Escherichia coli* is the most common bacterial causative organism

C. Acute pyelonephritis
1. Usually, a short course that recurs as a relapse of a previous infection or as a new infection
2. Can progress to bacteremia or chronic pyelonephritis
3. Data collection
   a. Fever and chills
   b. Nausea
   c. Flank pain on the affected side
   d. Costovertebral angle (CVA) tenderness
   e. Headache
   f. Muscular pain
   g. Dysuria
   h. Frequency and urgency
   i. Cloudy, bloody, or foul-smelling urine
   j. Increased white blood cells in the urine

D. Chronic pyelonephritis
1. A slow, progressive disease that is usually associated with recurrent acute attacks
2. Causes contraction of the kidney and dysfunctioning of the nephrons, which are replaced by scar tissue
3. Can lead to **renal failure**
4. Data collection
   a. Frequently diagnosed incidentally when a client is being evaluated for hypertension
   b. Poor urine-concentrating ability
   c. Pyuria
   d. Azotemia
   e. Proteinuria
   f. Anemia
   g. Acidosis

E. Interventions
1. Monitor vital signs
2. Monitor I&O
3. Monitor weight
4. Encourage fluids up to 3000 mL/day
5. Encourage adequate rest
6. Instruct the client in a high-calorie, low-protein diet
7. Provide warm moist compresses to the flank area
8. Encourage the client to take warm baths
9. Administer analgesics, antipyretics, antibiotics, urinary antiseptics, and antiemetics, as prescribed
10. Monitor for signs of **renal failure**

XV. GLOMERULONEPHRITIS
A. Description
1. A term that includes a variety of disorders, most of which are caused by an immunological reaction

2. It results in proliferative and inflammatory changes within the glomerular structure
3. Destruction, inflammation, and sclerosis of the glomeruli of both kidneys occur
4. The inflammation of the glomeruli results from an antigen-antibody reaction produced from an infection elsewhere in the body
5. Loss of kidney function develops

B. Causes
1. Immunological or autoimmune diseases
2. Group A beta-hemolytic streptococcal infection
3. History of pharyngitis or tonsillitis 2 to 3 weeks prior to symptoms

C. Types
1. Acute: Occurs 2 to 3 weeks after a streptococcal infection
2. Chronic: Can occur after the acute phase or slowly over time

D. Complications
1. Heart failure
2. Hypertensive encephalopathy
3. Pulmonary edema
4. **Renal failure**

E. Data collection
1. Gross hematuria
2. Dark, smoky, cola-colored or red-brown urine
3. Proteinuria that produces a persistent and excessive foam in the urine
4. Urinary debris
5. Moderately elevated to high specific gravity
6. Low urinary pH
7. **Oliguria** or **anuria**
8. Headache
9. Chills and fever
10. Fatigue and weakness
11. Anorexia, nausea, and vomiting
12. Pallor
13. Edema in the face, periorbital area, feet, or generalized
14. Shortness of breath, ascites, pleural effusion, and CHF
15. Abdominal or flank pain
16. Hypertension
17. Reduced visual acuity
18. Increased BUN and creatinine levels
19. Increased antistreptolysin O titer (used to diagnose disorders caused by streptococcal infections)

F. Interventions
1. Monitor vital signs
2. Monitor I&O and urine closely
3. Monitor daily weight
4. Monitor for edema
5. Monitor for fluid overload, ascites, pulmonary edema, and CHF
6. Restrict fluid intake as prescribed
7. Provide a high-calorie and low-protein diet

8. Restrict sodium intake as prescribed if edema is present
9. Provide bed rest and limited activity
10. Instruct the client to obtain treatment for infections, specifically sore throats and upper respiratory infections
11. Administer diuretics, antihypertensives, and antibiotics as prescribed
12. Monitor for signs of **renal failure,** cardiac failure, hypertensive encephalopathy
13. Instruct the client to report signs of bloody urine, headache, or edema

XVI. NEPHROTIC SYNDROME

A. Description: A set of clinical manifestations arising from protein wasting secondary to diffuse glomerular damage
B. Data collection
1. Proteinuria
2. Hypoalbuminemia
3. Edema
4. Hyperlipidemia
5. Waxy pallor to the skin
6. Anemia
7. Anorexia
8. Malaise
9. Irritability
10. Amenorrhea or abnormal menses
11. Hematuria may be present
C. Interventions
1. Monitor vital signs
2. Monitor I&O
3. Bed rest if severe edema is present
4. Normal to low-protein diet as prescribed, with adequate carbohydrate and calorie intake
5. Monitor daily weights
6. Provide a mild sodium restriction, as prescribed
7. Monitor potassium level; potassium may be restricted from the diet if the potassium level increases
8. Administer diuretics, as prescribed
9. Administer corticosteroids and cytotoxic medications, as prescribed
10. Plasma volume expanders, such as albumin, plasma, and dextran may be prescribed to raise the osmotic pressure
11. Administer anticoagulants as prescribed for those clients who develop renal vein thrombosis

XVII. HYDRONEPHROSIS

A. Description
1. Distention of the renal pelvis and calices, caused by an obstruction of normal urine flow
2. The urine becomes trapped proximal to the obstruction

3. The causes include calculus, tumors, scar tissue, and ureter obstructions, and hypertrophy of the prostate
B. Data collection
1. Hypertension
2. Headache
3. Flank pain
4. Electrolyte imbalances
C. Interventions
1. Monitor vital signs frequently
2. Monitor for fluid and electrolyte imbalances, including dehydration after the obstruction is relieved
3. Monitor for diuresis, which can lead to fluid depletion
4. Monitor daily weights
5. Monitor urine for specific gravity, albumin, and glucose
6. Administer fluid replacement as prescribed

XVIII. POLYCYSTIC KIDNEY DISEASE

A. Description
1. A cystic formation and hypertrophy of the kidneys, which lead to cystic rupture, infection, the formation of scar tissue, and damaged nephrons
2. There is no known way to arrest the progress of the destructive cysts
3. The ultimate result of this disease is **renal failure**
B. Types
1. Infantile polycystic disease: An inherited autosomal recessive trait that results in the death of the infant within a few months after birth
2. Adult polycystic disease: An autosomal dominant trait that results in end-stage renal disease
C. Data collection
1. Flank, lumbar, or abdominal pain
2. Fever and chills
3. UTIs
4. Hematuria, proteinuria, pyuria
5. Calculi
6. Hypertension
7. Palpable abdominal masses and enlarged kidneys
D. Interventions
1. Monitor for gross hematuria, which indicates cyst rupture
2. Increase sodium and water intake because sodium loss rather than retention occurs
3. Provide bed rest if ruptured cysts and bleeding occur
4. Prepare the client for percutaneous cyst puncture for relief of obstruction or for draining an abscess
5. Administer antihypertensives, as prescribed
6. Prepare the client for dialysis or renal transplantation
7. Encourage the client to seek genetic counseling

XIX. UROLITHIASIS AND NEPHROLITHIASIS

A. Description
1. Calculi or stones can form anywhere in the urinary tract; however, the most frequent site is the kidneys
2. The problems that can occur as a result of calculi are pain, obstruction, and tissue trauma, with secondary hemorrhage and infection
3. Kidneys, ureters, and bladder (KUB) x-ray, intravenous pyelography (IVP), computed tomography (CT) scan, and renal ultrasonography will determine the stone location
4. A stone analysis will be done after passage to determine the type of stone and assist in determining treatment
5. **Urolithiasis** refers to the formation of urinary stones; urinary calculi are formed in the ureters
6. **Nephrolithiasis** refers to the formation of kidney stones; kidney stones are formed in the renal parenchyma
7. When a calculus occludes the ureter and blocks the flow of urine, the ureter dilates, producing a condition known as hydroureter
8. If the obstruction is not removed, urinary stasis results in infection, impairment of renal function on the side of the blockage, and resultant hydronephrosis and irreversible kidney damage

B. Causes
1. Family history of stone formation
2. Diet high in calcium, vitamin D, milk, protein, oxalate, purines, or alkali
3. A high intake of purine-rich food
4. Obstruction and urinary stasis
5. Dehydration
6. Use of diuretics, which can cause volume depletion
7. UTIs and prolonged urinary catheterization
8. Immobilization
9. Hypercalcemia and hyperparathyroidism
10. Elevated uric acid, such as in gout

C. Data collection
1. Renal colic originates in the lumbar region and radiates around the side and down toward the testicle in men and toward the bladder in women
2. Ureteral colic radiates toward the genitalia and thigh
3. Sharp, severe pain of sudden onset
4. Dull, aching kidney
5. Nausea and vomiting, pallor, and diaphoresis during acute pain
6. Urinary frequency with alternating retention
7. Signs of a UTI
8. Low-grade fever
9. RBCs, WBCs, and bacteria in the urine
10. Hematuria

D. Interventions
1. Monitor vital signs
2. Monitor I&O
3. Monitor for fever, chills, and infection
4. Monitor for nausea, vomiting, and diarrhea
5. Encourage fluids up to 3000 mL/day, unless contraindicated, to facilitate the passage of the stone and prevent infection
6. Strain all urine for the presence of stones
7. Send stones to the laboratory for analysis
8. Provide warm baths and heat to the flank area
9. Administer analgesics at regularly scheduled intervals as prescribed to relieve pain
10. Monitor the client's response to pain medication
11. Intravenous fluids may be prescribed to increase the flow of urine and facilitate the passage of the stone
12. Assist the client in performing relaxation techniques to assist in relieving pain
13. Instruct the client in the diet specific to the stone composition
14. Maintain urinary pH, depending on the type of stone
15. Turn and reposition immobilized clients
16. Prepare the client for surgical procedures if prescribed

E. Stone composition (Boxes 52-10 and 52-11)
1. A special diet, such as an alkaline ash or acid ash diet may be prescribed, depending on the physician's preference
2. Calcium phosphate stones
   a. Caused by supersaturation of urine with calcium and phosphate

---

BOX 52-10

Alkaline Ash Diet

OUTCOME
Increases the pH
Reduces the acidity of the urine

FOODS TO INCLUDE:
Milk
Fruits, except cranberries, plums, and prunes
Rhubarb
Most vegetables
Small amounts of beef, halibut, veal, trout, and salmon allowed

---

BOX 52-11

Acid Ash Diet

OUTCOME
Decreases the pH
Makes the urine more acidic

FOODS TO INCLUDE:
Cheese, eggs
Meat, fish, oysters, poultry
Bread, cereal, whole grains
Pastries
Cranberries, prunes, plums, tomatoes
Corn and legumes

b. Diet includes acid ash foods, because calcium stones are alkaline

c. Dietary prescription may include decreasing intake of foods high in calcium and phosphate to reduce urinary calcium content, and avoiding excess vitamin D intake to prevent stones from forming

3. Calcium oxalate stones

a. Caused by supersaturation of urine with calcium and oxalate

b. Diet includes acid ash foods because calcium stones are alkaline

c. Dietary prescription may include decreasing intake of foods high in calcium

d. Dietary prescription may include avoiding oxalate food sources to reduce urinary oxalate content and the formation of stones

e. Oxalate-rich foods to be avoided include tea, almonds, cashews, chocolate, cocoa, beans, spinach, and rhubarb

4. Struvite stones

a. Also called triple-phosphate stones; composed of magnesium and ammonium phosphate

b. Caused by urea splitting by bacteria

c. Struvite stones tend to form in alkaline urine

d. Diet includes acid ash foods

e. Dietary prescription includes limiting high-phosphate foods, such as dairy products, red and organ meats, and whole grains, to reduce urinary phosphate content

5. Uric acid stones

a. Caused by excess dietary purine or gout

b. Uric acid stones tend to form in acidic urine

c. Dietary prescription may include alkaline ash foods and decreased intake of purine sources, such as organ meats, gravies, red wines, and sardines, to reduce urinary purine content

d. Allopurinol (Zyloprim) may be prescribed to lower uric acid levels

6. Cystine stones

a. Caused by cystine crystal formation

b. Cystine stones tend to form in acidic urine

c. Diet includes alkaline ash foods

d. Dietary prescription may also include a low intake of methionine, an essential amino acid that forms cystine; client would be instructed to avoid meat, milk, cheese, and eggs

e. Dietary measures also focus on encouraging fluid intake up to 3 L/day, unless contraindicated, to help dilute the urine and prevent cystine crystals from forming

XX. SURGICAL MANAGEMENT OF KIDNEY STONES

A. Cystoscopy

1. May be done for stones located in the bladder or lower ureter

2. There is no incision

3. One or two ureteral catheters are inserted past the stone

4. The stone may be manipulated and dislodged by the procedure

5. The catheters may mechanically guide the stones downward as they are removed

6. Catheters are left in place for 24 hours to drain the urine trapped proximal to the stone and to dilate the ureter

7. A continuous chemical irrigation may be prescribed to dissolve the stone

B. Extracorporeal shock wave lithotripsy (ESWL)

1. Noninvasive mechanical procedure for breaking up stones that are located in the kidney or upper ureter so that they can pass spontaneously or be removed by other methods

2. Fluoroscopy is used to visualize the stone

3. There is no incision or drains

4. Ultrasonic waves are delivered through a warm water bath to the area of the stone to disintegrate it

5. Stones are passed in the urine within a few days

6. Preprocedure: NPO for 8 hours prior to procedure

7. Postprocedure

a. Monitor vital signs

b. Monitor I&O

c. Monitor for bleeding

d. Monitor for pain and signs of urinary obstruction

e. Instruct the client to increase fluid intake to wash out the stone fragments

f. Inform the client that ambulation is important

C. Percutaneous lithotripsy

1. Performed for stones in the bladder, ureter, or kidney

2. An invasive procedure in which a guide is inserted under fluoroscopy near the area of the stone

3. An ultrasonic wave is aimed at the stone to break it into fragments

4. May be performed via cystoscopy or nephroscopy

5. No incision is required for cystoscopy; however, a small flank incision is needed for nephroscopy

6. The client may possibly have an indwelling catheter

7. A nephrostomy tube may be placed to administer chemical irrigations to break up the stone; nephrostomy tube may remain in place for 1 to 5 days

8. Encourage the client to drink 3000 to 4000 mL of fluid/day following the procedure

9. Monitor for and instruct the client to monitor for complications of infection, hemorrhage, and extravasation of fluid into the retroperitoneal cavity

D. Ureterolithotomy

1. An open surgical procedure, performed if lithotripsy is not effective

2. Performed if the stone is in the ureter

3. Incision into the ureter is made through a lower abdominal or flank incision to remove the stone

4. The client may have a Penrose drain, a ureteral stent catheter, and an indwelling bladder catheter

E. Pyelolithotomy
   1. A flank incision into the kidney is made to remove stones from the renal pelvis
   2. A large flank incision is required
   3. The client will have a Penrose drain and an indwelling catheter

F. Nephrolithotomy
   1. Incision into the kidney is made to remove the stone
   2. A large flank incision is required
   3. The client may have a nephrostomy tube and an indwelling catheter

G. Partial or total nephrectomy
   1. Performed if there is extensive kidney damage, renal infection, or severe obstruction, and to prevent stone recurrence
   2. Postoperative interventions
      a. Care will be planned based on the incision location and the type of drainage tubes used
      b. Monitor incision, particularly if a Penrose drain is in place, because it will drain large amounts of urine
      c. Protect the skin from urinary drainage
      d. Place an ostomy pouch over the Penrose drain to protect the skin if urinary drainage is excessive
      e. Monitor the nephrostomy tube, which may be attached to a drainage bag for a free flow of urine
      f. Drainage cathers are not irrigated unless specifically prescribed
      g. Monitor indwelling Foley catheter for drainage
      h. Encourage fluid intake to ensure a urine output of 2500 to 3000 mL/day or more
      i. Monitor I&O closely
      j. Determine the composition of stone from laboratory analysis
      k. Instruct the client in dietary restrictions if required
      l. Instruct the client about medications that may be needed over the long term to reduce the development of calculi
      m. Medications prescribed for calcium stones may include phosphates, thiazide diuretics, and allopurinol (Zyloprim)
      n. Pyridoxine or magnesium oxide may be prescribed for clients with oxalate stones
      o. Allopurinol (Zyloprim) may be prescribed for oxalate and uric acid stones
      p. Long-term antibiotics may be prescribed for struvite or cystine stones

XXI. KIDNEY TUMORS
A. Description
   1. May be benign or malignant, bilateral or unilateral

2. Common sites of metastasis include bone, lungs, liver, spleen, or other kidney
3. The exact cause of renal carcinoma is unknown

B. Data collection
   1. Dull flank pain
   2. Palpable renal mass
   3. Painless gross hematuria

C. Radical nephrectomy
   1. Description
      a. Removal of the entire kidney, adjacent adrenal gland, and renal artery and vein
      b. Radiation therapy and possibly chemotherapy may follow radical nephrectomy
   2. Postoperative interventions
      a. Monitor vital signs
      b. Monitor abdomen for distention caused by bleeding
      c. Observe bed linens under the client for bleeding
      d. Monitor for hypotension, decreases in urinary output, and alterations in LOC, as indicating signs of hemorrhage
      e. Monitor for signs of adrenal insufficiency
      f. In clients with adrenal insufficiency, a large urinary output followed by hypotension and subsequent **oliguria** occurs
      g. Intravenous fluids and packed red blood cells may be prescribed
      h. Monitor I&O and daily weight
      i. Monitor for a urinary output of 30 to 50 mL/hour to ensure adequate renal function
      j. Monitor specific gravity of urine
      k. Maintain client in semi-Fowler's position
      l. Monitor for signs of respiratory complications related to surgery
      m. Encourage coughing and deep breathing exercises
      n. Monitor bowel sounds for paralytic ileus
      o. Apply antiembolism stockings, as prescribed
      p. Do not irrigate (unless specifically prescribed) or manipulate the nephrostomy tube if in place
      q. Administer pain medications as prescribed

XXII. BLADDER TRAUMA
A. Description
   1. Occurs following a blunt or penetrating injury to the lower abdomen
   2. Penetrating wounds occur as a result of stabbing, gunshot wound, or other objects piercing the abdominal wall
   3. A fractured pelvis that causes bone fragments to puncture the bladder is the most common cause of bladder trauma
   4. A blunt trauma causes compression of the abdominal wall and the bladder

B. Data collection
1. Anuria
2. Hematuria
3. Pain over the costovertebral area (CVA)
4. Nausea and vomiting
C. Interventions
1. Monitor vital signs
2. Monitor for hematuria, hemorrhage, and signs of shock
3. Promote bed rest
4. Monitor pain level
5. Prepare the client for insertion of a suprapubic catheter to aid in urinary drainage if prescribed
6. Prepare the client for surgical repair of the laceration if prescribed

XXIII. EPIDIDYMITIS

A. Description
1. An acute or chronic inflammation of the epididymis that occurs as a result of a UTI, sexually transmitted diseases, prostatitis, or long-term use of a Foley catheter
2. The infective organism passes upward through the urethra and ejaculatory duct, along the vas deferens to the epididymis
B. Data collection
1. Scrotal pain
2. Groin pain
3. Swelling in scrotum and groin
4. Pus and bacteria in the urine
5. Fever and chills
6. Abscess development
C. Interventions
1. Encourage fluid intake
2. Encourage bed rest with the scrotum elevated to prevent traction on the spermatic cord, to facilitate drainage, and to relieve pain
3. Instruct the client in the intermittent application of cold compresses to scrotum
4. Instruct the client in the use of sitz baths
5. Instruct the client in the administration of antibiotics for self and sexual partner if chlamydial or gonorrheal infection is the cause
6. Instruct the client to avoid lifting, straining, and sexual contact until the infection subsides

XXIV. PROSTATITIS

A. Description
1. An inflammation of the prostate gland, which can be caused by an infectious agent (bacterial) or by tissue hyperplasia (abacterial)
2. Bacterial type occurs as a result of the organism reaching the prostate via the urethra or the bloodstream
3. Abacterial type usually occurs following a viral illness or a decrease in sexual activity
B. Data collection
1. Bacterial
a. Fever and chills
b. Dysuria
c. Urethral discharge
d. Boggy, tender prostate
e. Urethral discharge on palpation of prostate
f. WBCs found in prostatic secretions
2. Abacterial
a. Backache
b. Dysuria
c. Perineal pain
d. Frequency
e. Hematuria
f. Irregularly enlarged, firm, and tender prostate
C. Interventions
1. Encourage adequate fluid intake
2. Instruct the client in the use of sitz baths to promote comfort
3. Administer antibiotics, analgesics, antispasmodics, and stool softeners as prescribed
4. Inform the client of activities to drain the prostate, such as intercourse, masturbation, and prostatic massage
5. Instruct the client to avoid spicy foods, coffee, alcohol, prolonged automobile rides, and sexual intercourse during an acute inflammation

XXV. BENIGN PROSTATIC HYPERTROPHY OR HYPERPLASIA (BPH)

A. Description
1. A slow enlargement of the prostate gland, with hypertrophy and hyperplasia of normal tissue
2. The enlargement causes narrowing of the urethra and results in partial or complete obstruction
3. The cause is unknown, and the disorder usually occurs in men older than 50 years
B. Data collection
1. Urgency, frequency, and hesitancy
2. Changes in size and force of urinary stream
3. Retention
4. Dribbling
5. Nocturia
6. Hematuria
7. Urinary stasis
8. UTIs
C. Interventions
1. Encourage fluids of up to 2000 to 3000 mL/day unless contraindicated
2. Prepare for bladder drainage via urinary catheterization for distention
3. Avoid administering medications that cause urinary retention, such as anticholinergics, antihistamines, and decongestants

BOX 52-12

Surgical Interventions for BPH

Transurethral resection of prostate (TURP)
Retropubic prostatectomy
Suprapubic prostatectomy
Perineal prostatectomy

4. Administer finasteride (Proscar) as prescribed to shrink the prostate gland and improve urine flow
5. Prepare the client for surgery as prescribed (Box 52-12)

D. Surgical interventions and postoperative care (see Chapter 42)

XXVI. KIDNEY TRANSPLANTATION

A. Description
  1. Implantation of a human kidney from a compatible donor into a recipient
  2. Performed for irreversible kidney failure
  3. Immunosuppressive medications must be taken by the recipient for life

B. Living related donors
  1. Most desirable source of kidney for transplant is a living related donor who matches the client closely
  2. Screened for ABO blood group, tissue-specific antigen, human leukocyte antigen (HLA) compatibility, and mixed lymphocyte culture index (histocompatibility)
  3. Donor must be in excellent health, with two properly functioning kidneys
  4. The emotional well-being of the donor is determined
  5. Complete understanding of the donation process and outcome is necessary

C. Cadaver donors
  1. Must meet criteria of brain death
  2. Must be younger than 60 years of age
  3. Must have normal renal function
  4. No malignant disease outside the central nervous system (CNS) can be present
  5. No generalized infection can be present
  6. No abdominal or renal trauma can be present
  7. Potential donor must have a negative hepatitis B antigen and negative HIV antibody
  8. Continuous ventilation and heartbeat are maintained until the kidneys are surgically removed
  9. Normal BP must be present
  10. Once the potential donor has demonstrated cerebral death, it is crucial to restore intravascular volume, wean from vasopressors, and establish diuresis

D. Warm ischemic time
  1. The time elapsed between the cessation of perfusion and cooling of the kidney and the time required for anastomosis of the kidney
  2. Maximal allowable warm ischemic time is 30 to 60 minutes
  3. Kidney can be cooled; then the maximum time for transplantation is increased by 24 to 48 hours

E. Preoperative interventions
  1. Verify histocompatibility tests of identical twin or family member
  2. Administer immunosuppressive medications to recipient as prescribed, for 2 days before the transplantation, if this is possible
  3. Maintain protective isolation
  4. Verify that **hemodialysis** of the recipient was completed 24 hours before the transplantation
  5. Ensure that the client is free of any infections
  6. Check renal function studies
  7. Encourage discussion of feelings of both the donor and the recipient

F. Postoperative interventions
  1. Kidney begins to function immediately, or may be delayed a few days
  2. **Hemodialysis** is performed until adequate kidney function is established
  3. Monitor vital signs
  4. Monitor I&O
  5. Monitor urine output every hour
  6. Monitor daily laboratory studies, urine for blood and specific gravity, daily weight, pulse oximetry, and BUN and creatinine levels
  7. Maintain the client in semi-Fowler's position
  8. Monitor for patency of the Foley catheter
  9. Note that urine is pink and bloody initially but gradually returns to normal within several days to weeks
  10. Monitor for gross hematuria and clots, which are not expected; physician is notified if they occur
  11. Monitor the three-way bladder irrigation, if prescribed, to prevent blood clot formation
  12. Note that the Foley catheter should be removed as soon as possible to prevent infection
  13. Maintain protective isolation precautions and monitor for infection
  14. Monitor IV fluids closely and for fluid overload
  15. Begin oral fluids, as prescribed
  16. Monitor for bowel sounds and initiate diet as prescribed when bowel sounds return
  17. Maintain good oral hygiene, monitoring for stomatitis and bacterial and fungal infections
  18. Encourage coughing and deep breathing exercises
  19. Maintain strict aseptic technique with wound care
  20. Administer medications as prescribed, which may include antifungal medications, antibiotics, immunosuppressive agents, and corticosteroids
  21. Monitor for organ rejection
  22. Promote live donor and recipient relationship
  23. Monitor client and recipient for depression

G. Graft rejection: Except for identical twin donor and recipient, the major postoperative complication is graft rejection

BOX 52-13

Client Instructions Following Kidney Transplantation

Avoid prolonged periods of sitting.

Recognize the signs and symptoms of infection and rejection.

Avoid contact sports.

Avoid exposure to people with infections.

Use medications as prescribed, and maintain immunosuppressive therapy for life.

Recognize signs and symptoms that require the need to contact the physician.

Perform follow-up care.

1. Data collection
   a. Fever
   b. Malaise
   c. Elevated WBC count
   d. Graft tenderness
   e. Signs of deteriorating renal function
   f. Acute hypertension
   g. Anemia
2. Hyperacute rejection
   a. Occurs immediately after surgery to 48 hours postoperatively
   b. Interventions: Removal of rejected kidney
3. Acute rejection
   a. Typically occurs within 6 weeks but can occur as late as 2 years
   b. Potentially reversible with increased immunosuppression
   c. Interventions: High doses of corticosteroids; if corticosteroids are ineffective, monoclonal antibodies may be administered
4. Chronic rejection
   a. Occurs slowly months to years after transplantation
   b. Can be irreversible
   c. Mimics **CRF**
   d. Interventions: Immunosuppressive medications
5. Client instructions following kidney transplantation (Box 52-13)

PRACTICE QUESTIONS

1. A nurse has an order to obtain a sample for urinalysis from a client with an indwelling urinary catheter. The nurse would avoid which of the following, which could contaminate the specimen?
   1. Obtaining the specimen from the urinary drainage bag
   2. Clamping the tubing of the drainage bag
   3. Aspirating a sample from the port on the tubing attached to the drainage bag
   4. Wiping the port on the tubing with an alcohol swab before inserting the syringe

2. A nurse is caring for the client who has had a renal biopsy. Which intervention would the nurse avoid in the care of the client after this procedure?
   1. Encouraging fluids to at least 3 L in the first 24 hours
   2. Administering pain medication as prescribed
   3. Testing serial urine samples with dipsticks for occult blood
   4. Ambulating the client in the room and hall for short distances

3. A client with a diagnosis of cystitis has an indwelling urinary catheter and is being cared for by a nursing assistant. The nurse observes the nursing assistant care for the client and intervenes if the nursing assistant:
   1. Uses soap and water to cleanse the perineal area
   2. Keeps the urinary drainage bag below the level of the bladder
   3. Uses the drainage tubing port to obtain urine samples
   4. Lets the drainage tubing rest under the leg

4. A nurse is assisting the client with cystitis with diet selection for an acid ash diet. The nurse encourages the client to eat which of the following foods?
   1. Low-fat milk
   2. Baked haddock
   3. Garden peas
   4. Apples

5. A client who has a history of gout is also diagnosed with urolithiasis. The stones are determined to be of the uric acid type. The nurse tells the client to limit the intake of which food item?
   1. Liver
   2. Apples
   3. Carrots
   4. Milk

6. A nurse is caring for a client who has been diagnosed as having a kidney mass. The client asks the nurse the reason for a renal biopsy, when other tests such as computerized tomography (CT) and ultrasound are available. In formulating a response, the nurse incorporates the knowledge that a renal biopsy:
   1. Helps differentiate between a solid mass and a fluid-filled cyst
   2. Provides an outline of the renal vascular system
   3. Gives specific cytological information about the lesion
   4. Determines if the mass is growing rapidly or slowly

7. A female client is admitted to the emergency room following a fall from a horse. The physician orders insertion of a Foley catheter. The nurse notes blood at the urinary meatus while preparing for the procedure. The nurse should:
   1. Use extra povidone-iodine solution in cleansing the meatus
   2. Use a smaller catheter
   3. Administer pain medication before inserting the catheter
   4. Notify the physician

8. A male client has a tentative diagnosis of urethritis. The nurse collects data from the client, knowing that which of the following are manifestations of the disorder?
   1. Hematuria and penile discharge
   2. Hematuria and pyuria
   3. Dysuria and proteinuria
   4. Dysuria and penile discharge

9. A nurse is assisting in planning a teaching session with the female client diagnosed with urethritis caused by infection with chlamydia. The nurse would plan to include which of the following points in the teaching session?
   1. The most serious complication of this infection is sterility
   2. The infection can be prevented by using spermicide to alter the pH in the perineal area
   3. Medication therapy should be continued for 2 weeks without interruption
   4. Sexual partners during the last 12 months should be notified and treated

10. A male client who is hospitalized is diagnosed with urethritis caused by chlamydial infection. The nursing assistant assigned to the client asks the nurse what measures are necessary to prevent contraction of the infection during care. The nurse tells the assistant that:
    1. Enteric precautions should be instituted for the client
    2. Contact isolation should be initiated, because the disease is highly contagious
    3. Standard precautions are sufficient, because the disease is transmitted sexually
    4. Gloves and mask should be used when in the client's room

11. A client with chlamydial infection has received instructions on self-care and prevention of further infection. The nurse determines that the client needs further reinforcement if the client states that he or she will:
    1. Reduce the chance of reinfection by limiting the number of sexual partners
    2. Use latex condoms to prevent disease transmission
    3. Return to the clinic as requested for follow-up culture in 1 week
    4. Use doxycycline prophylactically to prevent symptoms of chlamydia

12. A nurse is caring for a client with epididymitis. The nurse anticipates noting which of the following findings on data collection?
    1. Fever, diarrhea, groin pain, and ecchymosis
    2. Fever, nausea and vomiting, and painful scrotal edema
    3. Diarrhea, groin pain, and scrotal edema
    4. Nausea, vomiting, and scrotal edema with ecchymosis

13. A nurse is caring for the client with epididymitis. The nurse would avoid using which of the following treatment modalities in the care of the client?
    1. Bed rest
    2. Scrotal elevation
    3. Sitz bath
    4. Use of heating pad

14. A client has epididymitis as a complication of urinary tract infection. The nurse is giving the client instructions to prevent a recurrence. The nurse determines that the client needs further instruction if the client states to:
    1. Drink increased amounts of fluids
    2. Continue to take antibiotics until all symptoms are gone
    3. Limit the force of the stream during voiding
    4. Use condoms to eliminate risk from chlamydia and gonorrhea

15. A nurse is collecting data from a client who has had benign prostatic hyperplasia (BPH) in the past. To determine if the client is currently experiencing exacerbation of BPH, the nurse asks the client about the presence of which early symptom?
    1. Urge incontinence
    2. Nocturia
    3. Decreased force of the stream of urine
    4. Urinary retention

16. A client who has a cold is seen in the emergency room with inability to void. Because the client has a history of benign prostatic hyperplasia (BPH), the nurse questions the client about use of which medication?
    1. Diuretics
    2. Antibiotics
    3. Antitussives
    4. Decongestants

17. A client who had a prostatectomy has learned perineal exercises to gain control of the urinary sphincter. The nurse determines that the client needs further instruction if the client states that he or she will perform which of the following as part of these exercises?
    1. Tightening the muscles as if trying to prevent urination
    2. Contracting the abdominal, gluteal, and perineal muscles
    3. Tightening the rectal sphincter while relaxing abdominal muscles
    4. Performing the Valsalva maneuver

18. A nurse is working with the client newly diagnosed with chronic renal failure to set up a schedule for hemodialysis. The client states, "This is impossible! How can I even think about leading a normal life again if this is what I'm going to have to do?" The nurse determines that the client is exhibiting:
    1. Withdrawal
    2. Depression
    3. Anger
    4. Projection

19. A client newly diagnosed with chronic renal failure has recently begun hemodialysis. Knowing that the client is at risk for disequilibrium syndrome, the nurse monitors the client during dialysis for:
    1. Hypertension, tachycardia, and fever
    2. Hypotension, bradycardia, and hypothermia
    3. Restlessness, irritability, and generalized weakness
    4. Headache, deteriorating level of consciousness, and twitching

20. A client with chronic renal failure has been on dialysis for 3 years. The client is receiving the usual combination of medications for the disease, including aluminum hydroxide as a phosphate-binding agent. The client now presents with mental cloudiness, dementia, and complaints of bone pain. The nurse interprets that this data is compatible with:
    1. Phosphate overdose
    2. Aluminum intoxication
    3. Advancing uremia
    4. Folic acid deficiency

21. A hemodialysis client with a left arm fistula is at risk for arterial steal syndrome. The nurse monitors this client for which manifestation of this disorder?
    1. Warmth, redness, and pain in the left hand
    2. Pallor, diminished pulse, and pain in the left hand
    3. Edema and purplish discoloration of the left arm
    4. Aching pain, pallor, and edema of the left arm

22. A nurse is reviewing the medical record of a client with a diagnosis of pyelonephritis. Which disorder, if noted on the client's record, would the nurse identify as a risk factor for this disorder?
    1. Hypoglycemia
    2. Coronary artery disease
    3. Diabetes mellitus
    4. Orthostatic hypotension

23. A nurse is reviewing the client's record and notes that the physician has documented that the client has a renal disorder. On review of the laboratory results, the nurse would most likely expect to note which of the following?
    1. Elevated blood urea nitrogen (BUN) level
    2. Decreased hemoglobin level
    3. Decreased red blood cell (RBC) count
    4. Decreased white blood cell (WBC) count

24. Which of the following would the nurse include in the plan of care for a client following a renal scan?
    1. Place the client on radiation precautions for 18 hours
    2. Save all urine in a radiation-safe container for 18 hours
    3. Limit contact with the client for 20 minutes per hour
    4. No special precautions, except to wear gloves if coming in contact with the client's urine

25. A client is scheduled for intravenous pyelography (IVP). Before the test, the priority nursing action would be to:
    1. Administer an oral preparation of radiopaque dye
    2. Restrict fluids
    3. Determine a history of allergies
    4. Administer a sedative

26. Following a renal biopsy, the client complains of pain at the biopsy site, which radiates to the front of the abdomen. The nurse interprets this complaint and further monitors the client for:
    1. Bleeding
    2. Infection
    3. Renal colic
    4. Normal, expected pain

27. A nurse is monitoring an 88-year-old woman suspected of having a urinary tract infection (UTI) for signs of the infection. Which of the following would alert the nurse to the possibility of the presence of a UTI?
    1. Fever
    2. Frequency
    3. Confusion
    4. Urgency

28. A nurse is performing an admission assessment on a client with a diagnosis of bladder cancer. Which of the following would the nurse most likely expect to note on data collection of this client?
    1. Hematuria
    2. Burning on urination
    3. Urgency
    4. Frequency

29. A client with benign prostatic hypertrophy (BPH) undergoes a transurethral resection of the prostate (TURP) and is receiving continuous bladder irrigations postoperatively. The nurse monitors the client for signs of transurethral resection (TUR) syndrome. Which of the following data would indicate the onset of this syndrome?
    1. Bradycardia and confusion
    2. Tachycardia and diarrhea
    3. Decreased urinary output and bladder spasms
    4. Increased urinary output and anemia

30. A client with prostatitis secondary to kidney infection has received instructions on management of the condition at home and prevention of recurrence. The nurse determines that the client understood the instructions if the client has verbalized that he will:
    1. Keep fluid intake to a minimum to decrease the need to void
    2. Exercise as much as possible to stimulate circulation
    3. Stop antibiotic therapy when pain subsides
    4. Use warm sitz baths and analgesics to increase comfort

31. A nurse is assessing the patency of an arteriovenous fistula in the left arm of a client who is receiving hemodialysis for the treatment of chronic renal failure. Which finding indicates that the fistula is patent?
    1. Absence of a bruit on auscultation of the fistula
    2. Palpation of a thrill over the fistula
    3. Presence of a radial pulse in the left wrist
    4. Capillary refill less than 3 seconds in the nail beds of the fingers on the left hand

32. A client newly diagnosed with renal failure will be receiving peritoneal dialysis. During the infusion of the dialysate, the client complains of abdominal pain. Which action by the nurse is appropriate?
    1. Slow the infusion
    2. Decrease the amount to be infused
    3. Explain that the pain will subside after the first few exchanges
    4. Stop the dialysis

33. The nurse is instructing a client with diabetes mellitus about peritoneal dialysis. The nurse tells the client that it is important to maintain the dwell time for the dialysis at the prescribed time because of the risk of:
    1. Infection
    2. Hyperglycemia
    3. Fluid overload
    4. Disequilibrium syndrome

34. A client is diagnosed with polycystic kidney disease and the nurse provides information to the client about the treatment plan. The nurse determines that the client needs additional information if the client states that which of the following is a component of the treatment plan?
    1. Sodium restriction
    2. Antihypertensive medications
    3. Increased water intake
    4. Genetic counseling

35. The client with chronic renal failure who is scheduled for hemodialysis this morning is due to receive a daily dose of enalapril (Vasotec). The nurse should plan to administer this medication:
    1. Just prior to dialysis
    2. During dialysis
    3. On return from dialysis
    4. The day after dialysis

ALTERNATE FORMAT QUESTION: MULTIPLE RESPONSE

The nurse is monitoring a client receiving peritoneal dialysis and notes that a client's outflow is less than the inflow. Select the actions that the nurse should take.

___ Place the client in a high-Fowler's position
___ Check the level of the drainage bag
___ Contact the physician
___ Check the peritoneal dialysis system for kinks
___ Reposition the client to his or her side

ANSWERS

1. Answer: 1
Rationale: A urine specimen is not taken from the urinary drainage bag. Urine undergoes chemical changes while sitting in the bag, and does not necessarily reflect current client status. In addition, it may become contaminated with bacteria from opening the system. Options 2, 3, and 4 are correct actions.
Test-Taking Strategy: Note the key word, *avoid*. This word indicates a false response question and that you need to select the incorrect action. Recalling the basic principles of asepsis will direct you to option 1. Review this procedure if you had difficulty with this question.
Level of Cognitive Ability: Application
Client Needs: Safe, Effective Care Environment
Integrated Process: Nursing Process/Implementation
Content Area: Adult Health/Renal
Reference: deWit, S. (2005). *Fundamental concepts and skills for nursing.* Philadelphia: W.B. Saunders, p. 533.

2. Answer: 4
Rationale: After renal biopsy, the nurse ensures that the client remain in bed for at least 24 hours. Vital signs and puncture site assessments are done frequently during this time. Encouraging fluids is done to reduce possible clot formation at the biopsy site. A Hematest is done on serial urine samples with urine dipsticks to evaluate bleeding. Analgesics are often needed to manage the renal colic pain that some clients feel after this procedure.
Test-Taking Strategy: Begin to answer this question by recalling that pain and bleeding are potential concerns after this procedure. This will help eliminate options 2 and 3. From the remaining options, you need to recall that encouraging fluids will reduce clotting at the site, wheras ambulation could initiate or enhance bleeding at the biopsy site. Review care of the client following a renal biopsy if you had difficulty with this question.
Level of Cognitive Ability: Application
Client Needs: Physiological Integrity
Integrated Process: Nursing Process/Implementation
Content Area: Adult Health/Renal
Reference: Christensen, B., & Kockrow, E. (2003). *Adult health nursing* (4th ed.). St. Louis: Mosby, p. 416.

3. Answer: 4
Rationale: Proper care of an indwelling catheter is especially important to prevent prolonged infection or reinfection in the client with cystitis. The nurse and all caregivers must use strict aseptic technique when emptying the drainage bag or obtaining urine specimens. The perineal area is cleansed thoroughly using mild soap and water at least twice a day and following a bowel movement. The drainage bag is kept below the level

of the bladder to prevent urine from being trapped in the bladder and, for the same reason, the drainage tubing is not placed under the client's leg. The tubing must drain freely at all times.

Test-Taking Strategy: Note the key word, *intervenes*. This word indicates a false response question and that you need to select the incorrect action. Eliminate option 1 first, because this is a basic standard of care for the client with an indwelling catheter. Option 3 is also consistent with principles of asepsis, and is eliminated next. From the remaining options, note that option 2 promotes drainage and option 4 could impede drainage. Review care of the client with an indwelling catheter if you had difficulty with this question.

Level of Cognitive Ability: Comprehension
Client Needs: Safe, Effective Care Environment
Integrated Process: Nursing Process/Implementation
Content Area: Leadership/Management
Reference: deWit, S. (2005). *Fundamental concepts and skills for nursing.* Philadelphia: W.B. Saunders, p. 550.

4. *Answer:* 2
Rationale: Foods that are allowed on an acid ash diet include meat, fish, shellfish, cheese, eggs, poultry, grains, cranberries, prunes, plums, corn, lentils, and foods with high amounts of chlorine, phosphorus, and sulfur. Foods that are not included are all milk and milk products (option 1); all other vegetables except corn and lentils (option 3); all fruits except cranberries, plums and prunes (option 4); and foods containing high amounts of sodium, potassium, calcium, and magnesium.

Test-Taking Strategy: This question is difficult to answer without specific knowledge of the types of foods that may be included in the acid ash diet. Recalling that most fruits and vegetables are not included on the list may help you eliminate options 3 and 4. From the remaining options, it is necessary to know that foods such as meat, fish, cheese, and eggs are included, but milk and milk products are not. Review this diet if you had difficulty with this question.

Level of Cognitive Ability: Application
Client Needs: Health Promotion and Maintenance
Integrated Process: Nursing Process/Implementation
Content Area: Adult Health/Renal
References: Nix, S. (2005). *Williams basic nutrition and diet therapy* (11th ed.). St. Louis: Mosby, pp. 406-407.
Peckenpaugh, N. (2003). *Nutrition essentials and diet therapy* (9th ed.). Philadelphia: W.B. Saunders, p. 301.

5. *Answer:* 1
Rationale: Foods containing high amounts of purines should be avoided in the client with uric acid stones. This includes limiting or avoiding organ meats, such as liver, brain, heart, kidney, and sweetbreads. Other foods to avoid include herring, sardines, anchovies, meat extracts, consommés, and gravies. Foods that are low in purines include all fruits, many vegetables, milk, cheese, eggs, refined cereals, sugars and sweets, coffee, tea, chocolate, and carbonated beverages.

Test-Taking Strategy: To answer this question, begin by examining the options and classifying the types of food sources they represent. Options 2 and 3 represent foods that are grown, whereas options 1 and 4 represent foods that derive from animal sources. Because purines are end products of

protein metabolism, you would eliminate options 2 and 3 first. To select between options 1 and 4, you would need to know that organ meats such as liver provide more protein than milk. This will direct you to option 1. Review the foods that are high in purines if you had difficulty with this question.

Level of Cognitive Ability: Application
Client Needs: Health Promotion and Maintenance
Integrated Process: Nursing Process/Implementation
Content Area: Adult Health/Renal
Reference: Black, J., & Hawks, J. (2005). *Medical-surgical nursing: Clinical management for positive outcomes* (7th ed.). Philadelphia: W.B. Saunders, p. 885.

6. *Answer:* 3
Rationale: Renal biopsy is a definitive test that gives specific information about whether the lesion is benign or malignant. An ultrasound discriminates between a fluid-filled cyst and a solid mass. Renal arteriography outlines the renal vascular system.

Test-Taking Strategy: Use the process of elimination. Remember that with a biopsy the cells are examined under a microscope. This examination then yields specific information about the type of neoplastic cell. Review the purpose of this test if you had difficulty with this question.

Level of Cognitive Ability: Application
Client Needs: Physiological Integrity
Integrated Process: Nursing Process/Implementation
Content Area: Adult Health/Renal
Reference: Pagana, K., & Pagana, T. (2003). *Mosby's diagnostic and laboratory test reference* (6th ed.). St. Louis: Mosby, pp. 754-757.

7. *Answer:* 4
Rationale: The presence of blood at the urinary meatus may indicate urethral trauma or disruption. The nurse notifies the physician, knowing that the client should not be catheterized until the cause of the bleeding is determined by diagnostic testing.

Test-Taking Strategy: Focus on the data in the question, that the client experienced a traumatic injury. This will direct you to option 4. Review this procedure and the indications of urethral trauma if you had difficulty with this question.

Level of Cognitive Ability: Application
Client Needs: Physiological Integrity
Integrated Process: Nursing Process/Implementation
Content Area: Adult Health/Renal
Reference: Christensen, B., & Kockrow, E. (2003). *Foundations of nursing* (4th ed.). St. Louis: Mosby, pp. 464-465.

8. *Answer:* 4
Rationale: Urethritis in the male client often results from chlamydial infection and is characterized by dysuria, which is accompanied by a clear to mucopurulent discharge. Because this disorder often coexists with gonorrhea, diagnostic tests are done for both and include culture and rapid assays.

Test-Taking Strategy: Use the process of elimination. Begin to answer this question by eliminating options 1 and 2. Urethritis is generally accompanied by dysuria in the male client. Knowing that the problem originates in the urethra, not the kidney, you would then eliminate the option with

proteinuria, which indicates a problem with kidney function. This leaves option 4 as the correct option. The male client with urethritis has dysuria and discharge from the penis. Review the signs of urethritis if you had difficulty with this question.
Level of Cognitive Ability: Comprehension
Client Needs: Physiological Integrity
Integrated Process: Nursing Process/Data Collection
Content Area: Adult Health/Renal
Reference: Linton, A., & Maebius, N. (2003). *Introduction to medical-surgical nursing* (3rd ed.). Philadelphia: W.B. Saunders, p. 769.

9. *Answer:* **1**
Rationale: The most serious complication of chlamydial infection is sterility. The infection can be prevented by the use of latex condoms. It is treated with doxycycline for 7 days or with azithromycin (Zithromax) as a single dose. All sexual partners during the 30 days before diagnosis should be notified, examined, and treated as necessary.
Test-Taking Strategy: Use the process of elimination. Eliminate option 2 first, using principles of infection control. Knowing that most courses of antibiotic therapy generally extend from 7 to 10 days may help you eliminate option 3 next. From the remaining options, it is necessary to know either that sterility is a serious and permanent complication or that sexual partners within the last month should be notified and treated as needed. Review the complications of this infection if you had difficulty with this question.
Level of Cognitive Ability: Application
Client Needs: Health Promotion and Maintenance
Integrated Process: Teaching/Learning
Content Area: Adult Health/Renal
References: Black, J., & Hawks, J. (2005). *Medical-surgical nursing: Clinical management for positive outcomes* (7th ed.). Philadelphia: W.B. Saunders, p. 1131.
Linton, A., & Maebius, N. (2003). *Introduction to medical-surgical nursing* (3rd ed.). Philadelphia: W.B. Saunders, p. 996.

10. *Answer:* **3**
Rationale: Chlamydia is a sexually transmitted disease, and is frequently called non-gonococcal urethritis in the male client. It requires no special precautions. Caregivers cannot acquire the disease during administration of care, and following standard precautions is the only measure that needs to be used.
Test-Taking Strategy: A basic knowledge of infection control and disease transmission guides you to select option 3 as correct. Also, note that option 3 is the umbrella (global) option. If this question was difficult, review transmission of this disorder and standard precautions.
Level of Cognitive Ability: Application
Client Needs: Safe, Effective Care Environment
Integrated Process: Nursing Process/Implementation
Content Area: Adult Health/Renal
Reference: Linton, A., & Maebius, N. (2003). *Introduction to medical-surgical nursing* (3rd ed.). Philadelphia: W.B. Saunders, p. 139.

11. *Answer:* **4**
Rationale: Antibiotics are not taken prophylactically to prevent acquisition of urethritis from chlamydia. The risk of

reinfection can be reduced by limiting the number of sexual partners, and by the use of condoms. In some instances, follow-up culture is requested in 4 to 7 days to confirm a cure.
Test-Taking Strategy: Note the key words, *needs further reinforcement*. These words indicate a false response question and that you need to select the incorrect client statement. Options 1 and 2 are the most obviously correct and are therefore eliminated as possible answers to the question. From the remaining options, recalling the basic principles of antibiotic therapy allows you to eliminate option 4, because antibiotics are not used intermittently at random for prophylaxis of this infection. Review the client teaching points related to this infection if you had difficulty with this question.
Level of Cognitive Ability: Comprehension
Client Needs: Health Promotion and Maintenance
Integrated Process: Teaching/Learning
Content Area: Adult Health/Renal
Reference: Linton, A., & Maebius, N. (2003). *Introduction to medical-surgical nursing* (3rd ed.). Philadelphia: W.B. Saunders, p. 998.

12. *Answer:* **2**
Rationale: Typical signs and symptoms of epididymitis include scrotal pain and edema, which are often accompanied by fever, nausea and vomiting, and chills. It is most often caused by infection, although sometimes it can be caused by trauma. It needs to be correctly distinguished from testicular torsion.
Test-Taking Strategy: Use the process of elimination. Any disorder that ends in "itis" results from inflammation or infection. Therefore, an expected finding would be elevated temperature. With this in mind, you can eliminate options 3 and 4 because they do not contain fever as part of the option. From the remaining options, recalling that ecchymosis results from bleeding, which is not part of this clinical picture, directs you to option 2. Review the signs of this infection if you had difficulty with this question.
Level of Cognitive Ability: Comprehension
Client Needs: Physiological Integrity
Integrated Process: Nursing Process/Data Collection
Content Area: Adult Health/Renal
Reference: Linton, A., & Maebius, N. (2003). *Introduction to medical-surgical nursing* (3rd ed.). Philadelphia: W.B. Saunders, p. 978.

13. *Answer:* **4**
Rationale: Common interventions used in the treatment of epididymitis include bed rest, elevation of the scrotum, ice packs, sitz baths, analgesics, and antibiotics. A heating pad would not be used because direct application of heat could increase blood flow to the area and increase the swelling.
Test-Taking Strategy: Note the key word, *avoid*. Eliminate options 1 and 2, because they are obviously the most helpful in the care of the client. Note that both remaining options address the application of heat to the client. A sitz bath provides heat that is moist and soothing. Knowing that direct heat may increase inflammation with tissue that is already at risk will guide you to option 4 as the item to avoid. Review care of the client with epididymitis if you had difficulty with this question.

Level of Cognitive Ability: Application
Client Needs: Physiological Integrity
Integrated Process: Nursing Process/Implementation
Content Area: Adult Health/Renal
Reference: Christensen, B., & Kockrow, E. (2003). *Adult health nursing* (4th ed.). St. Louis: Mosby, p. 539.

14. *Answer: 2*
Rationale: The client who experiences epididymitis from urinary tract infection (UTI) should increase intake of fluids to flush the urinary system. Because organisms can be forced into the vas deferens and epididymis from strain or pressure during voiding, the client should limit the force of the stream. Condom use can help prevent urethritis and epididymitis from sexually transmitted diseases. Antibiotics are always taken until the full course of therapy is completed.
Test-Taking Strategy: Note the key words, *needs further instruction.* These words indicate a false response question and that you need to select the incorrect client statement. Because option 1 is consistent with good practices in the prevention of UTI, this option can be eliminated first. From the remaining options, it is necessary to know that the force of stream should be limited to prevent backflow into the epididymis, and that condoms are helpful in preventing this disorder from occurring as a complication of a sexually transmitted disease. Remember that antibiotics are not stopped when symptoms subside, but must be taken until the full course of therapy is completed. Review care of the client with epididymitis if you had difficulty with this question.
Level of Cognitive Ability: Comprehension
Client Needs: Health Promotion and Maintenance
Integrated Process: Teaching/Learning
Content Area: Adult Health/Renal
Reference: Christensen, B., & Kockrow, E. (2003). *Adult health nursing* (4th ed.). St. Louis: Mosby, p. 539.

15. *Answer: 3*
Rationale: Decreased force in the stream of urine is an early sign of BPH. The stream later becomes weak and dribbling. The client may then develop hematuria, frequency, urgency, urge incontinence, and nocturia. If untreated, complete obstruction and urinary retention can occur.
Test-Taking Strategy: Note the key words, *early symptom.* Option 4 identifies the most severe symptom and therefore is eliminated first. From the remaining options, focusing on the key words and recalling the pathophysiology related to BPH will direct you to option 3. Review the signs of benign prostatic hypertrophy if you had difficulty with this question.
Level of Cognitive Ability: Application
Client Needs: Physiological Integrity
Integrated Process: Teaching/Learning
Content Area: Adult Health/Renal
Reference: Linton, A., & Maebius, N. (2003). *Introduction to medical-surgical nursing* (3rd ed.). Philadelphia: W.B. Saunders, p. 978.

16. *Answer: 4*
Rationale: In the client with BPH, episodes of urinary retention can be triggered by certain medications, such as decongestants, anticholinergics, and antidepressants. The client

should be questioned about use of these medications if presenting with urinary retention. Retention can also be precipitated by other factors, such as alcoholic beverages, infection, bed rest, becoming chilled, and taking alcoholic beverages.
Test-Taking Strategy: Use the process of elimination and focus on the issue, medications that could exacerbate or contribute to urinary retention in the client with BPH. Diuretics should help voiding; therefore, eliminate option 1. Next, eliminate option 2, because antibiotics should have no effect at all on voiding. From the remaining options, recall that medications that contain anticholinergics may cause urinary retention. This will guide you to option 4. Also, antitussives have no effect on urinary retention. Review the causes of urinary retention in the client with BPH if you had difficulty with this question.
Level of Cognitive Ability: Analysis
Client Needs: Physiological Integrity
Integrated Process: Nursing Process/Data Collection
Content Area: Adult Health/Renal
Reference: Linton, A., & Maebius, N. (2003). *Introduction to medical-surgical nursing* (3rd ed.). Philadelphia: W.B. Saunders, p. 978.

17. *Answer: 4*
Rationale: The Valsalva maneuver is avoided following prostatectomy, because it increases the risk of bleeding in the postoperative period. An acceptable exercise is tightening the abdominal, gluteal, and perineal muscles, as if trying to prevent urination. Another acceptable exercise is tightening the rectal sphincter while relaxing the abdominal muscles; this prevents the Valsalva maneuver from occurring.
Test-Taking Strategy: Note the key words, *needs further instruction.* These words indicate a false response question and that you need to select the incorrect client statement. Note that the type of movement in the exercises described in options 1, 2, and 3 are all muscle tightening types of movements. On the other hand, the Valsalva maneuver in option 4 involves bearing down or pushing types of movements. Review the purpose of perineal exercises if you had difficulty with this question.
Level of Cognitive Ability: Comprehension
Client Needs: Health Promotion and Maintenance
Integrated Process: Teaching/Learning
Content Area: Adult Health/Renal
References: Black, J., & Hawks, J. (2005). *Medical-surgical nursing: Clinical management for positive outcomes* (7th ed.). Philadelphia: W.B. Saunders, pp. 1025-1026.
Linton, A., & Maebius, N. (2003). *Introduction to medical-surgical nursing* (3rd ed.). Philadelphia: W.B. Saunders, p. 982.

18. *Answer: 3*
Rationale: Psychosocial reactions to chronic renal failure and hemodialysis are varied, and may include anger. Other reactions include personality changes, emotional lability, withdrawal, and depression. The individual client's response may vary depending on the client's personality and support systems. The client in this question is exhibiting anger. The client has not projected blame on the nurse nor does the client statement reflect withdrawal or depression.
Test-Taking Strategy: Use the process of elimination. Focusing on the client's statement will direct you to option 3. Review the

psychosocial aspects of care for the client with CRF if you had difficulty with this question.
Level of Cognitive Ability: Analysis
Client Needs: Psychosocial Integrity
Integrated Process: Nursing Process/Data Collection
Content Area: Adult Health/Renal
Reference: Linton, A., & Maebius, N. (2003). *Introduction to medical-surgical nursing* (3rd ed.). Philadelphia: W.B. Saunders, pp. 788-789.

19. *Answer:* **4**
Rationale: Disequilibrium syndrome is characterized by headache, mental confusion, decreasing level of consciousness, nausea, vomiting, twitching and possible seizure activity. It is caused by rapid removal of solutes from the body during hemodialysis. At the same time, the blood-brain barrier interferes with the efficient removal of wastes from brain tissue. As a result, water goes into cerebral cells because of the osmotic gradient, causing brain swelling and onset of symptoms. It most often occurs in clients who are new to dialysis, and is prevented by dialyzing for shorter times or at reduced blood flow rates.
Test-Taking Strategy: Use the process of elimination. Noting the relation between the words "disequilibrium syndrome" and the signs in option 4 will direct you to this option. Review this syndrome if you had difficulty with this question.
Level of Cognitive Ability: Application
Client Needs: Physiological Integrity
Integrated Process: Nursing Process/Data Collection
Content Area: Adult Health/Renal
Reference: Linton, A., & Maebius, N. (2003). *Introduction to medical-surgical nursing* (3rd ed.). Philadelphia: W.B. Saunders, p. 784.

20. *Answer:* **2**
Rationale: Aluminum intoxication may occur when there is accumulation of aluminum, an ingredient in many phosphate-binding antacids. It results in mental cloudiness, dementia, and bone pain from infiltration of the bone with aluminum. This condition was formerly known as dialysis dementia. It may be treated with aluminum-chelating agents, which make aluminum available to be dialyzed from the body. It can be prevented by avoiding or limiting the use of phosphate-binding agents that contain aluminum.
Test-Taking Strategy: Use the process of elimination. Note the relation between the medication name in the question and option 2. Review the signs of aluminum intoxication if you had difficulty with this question.
Level of Cognitive Ability: Analysis
Client Needs: Physiological Integrity
Integrated Process: Nursing Process/Data Collection
Content Area: Adult Health/Renal
References: Black, J., & Hawks, J. (2005). *Medical-surgical nursing: Clinical management for positive outcomes* (7th ed.). Philadelphia: W.B. Saunders, p. 958.
McKenry, L., & Salerno, E. (2003). *Mosby's pharmacology in nursing* (21st ed.). St. Louis: Mosby, p. 213.

21. *Answer:* **2**
Rationale: Arterial steal syndrome results from vascular insufficiency after creation of a fistula. The client exhibits pallor

and diminished pulse distal to the fistula and complains of pain distal to the fistula, which is caused by tissue ischemia. Warmth, redness, and pain would more likely characterize a problem with infection. Options 3 and 4 are not characteristics of steal syndrome.
Test-Taking Strategy: Use the process of elimination. Recalling that arterial steal syndrome results from vascular insufficiency will direct you to option 2. Review these signs if you had difficulty with this question.
Level of Cognitive Ability: Analysis
Client Needs: Physiological Integrity
Integrated Process: Nursing Process/Data Collection
Content Area: Adult Health/Renal
Reference: Black, J., & Hawks, J. (2005). *Medical-surgical nursing: Clinical management for positive outcomes* (7th ed.). Philadelphia: W.B. Saunders, pp. 2097-2098.

22. *Answer:* **3**
Rationale: Risk factors associated with pyelonephritis include diabetes mellitus, hypertension, chronic renal calculi, chronic cystitis, structural abnormalities of the urinary tract, presence of urinary stones, and indwelling or frequent urinary catheterization.
Test-Taking Strategy: Use the process of elimination. Eliminate options 1 and 4 first as least likely being associated as risk factors. From the remaining options, remember that diabetes mellitus can cause renal complications. This will direct you to the correct option. Review these risk factors if you had difficulty with this question.
Level of Cognitive Ability: Analysis
Client Needs: Health Promotion and Maintenance
Integrated Process: Nursing Process/Data Collection
Content Area: Adult Health/Renal
Reference: Christensen, B., & Kockrow, E. (2003). *Adult health nursing* (4th ed.). St. Louis: Mosby, p. 426.

23. *Answer:* **1**
Rationale: BUN testing is a frequently used laboratory test to determine renal function. The BUN level starts to rise when the glomerular filtration rate falls below 40% to 60%. A decreased hemoglobin and RBC count may be noted if bleeding from the urinary tract occurs or if erythropoietic function by the kidney is impaired. An increased WBC is most likely to be noted in renal disease.
Test-Taking Strategy: Use the process of elimination. Focus on the client's diagnosis and note the key words, *most likely expect to note*. Eliminate option 4 first because it is unassociated with the renal system. Although options 2 and 3 may be noted in some renal disorders, option 1 is the most likely laboratory finding. Remember, the BUN level is a frequently used laboratory test to determine renal function. Review the laboratory tests to determine renal function if you had difficulty with this question.
Level of Cognitive Ability: Analysis
Client Needs: Physiological Integrity
Integrated Process: Nursing Process/Data Collection
Content Area: Adult Health/Renal
Reference: Linton, A., & Maebius, N. (2003). *Introduction to medical-surgical nursing* (3rd ed.). Philadelphia: W.B. Saunders, p. 783.

24. Answer: 4

Rationale: There are no specific precautions following a renal scan. The nurse wears gloves to maintain standard precautions. Options 1, 2, and 3 are unnecessary measures.

Test-Taking Strategy: Use the process of elimination. Recalling that there is generally no danger from the small amount of radioactive material used in this procedure will direct you to option 4. Review this procedure if you had difficulty with this question.

Level of Cognitive Ability: Application
Client Needs: Safe, Effective Care Environment
Integrated Process: Nursing Process/Implementation
Content Area: Adult Health/Renal
Reference: Chernecky, C., & Berger, B. (2004). *Laboratory tests and diagnostic procedures* (4th ed.). Philadelphia: W.B. Saunders, pp. 964-965.

25. Answer: 3

Rationale: The iodine-based dye may be used during the IVP and can cause allergic reactions such as itching, hives, rash, tight feeling in the throat, shortness of breath, and bronchospasm. Assessing for allergies is the priority. Options 1, 2, and 4 are unnecessary.

Test-Taking Strategy: Note the key word, *priority*, and use the nursing process as a guide. Options 1, 2, and 4 address implementation. Option 3 is the only option that addresses data collection. Review this test if you had difficulty with this question.

Level of Cognitive Ability: Application
Client Needs: Physiological Integrity
Integrated Process: Nursing Process/Implementation
Content Area: Adult Health/Renal
Reference: Chernecky, C., & Berger, B. (2004). *Laboratory tests and diagnostic procedures* (4th ed.). Philadelphia: W.B. Saunders, p. 696.

26. Answer: 1

Rationale: If pain originates at the biopsy site and begins to radiate to the flank area and around the front of the abdomen, bleeding should be suspected. Hypotension, a decreasing hematocrit, and gross or microscopic hematuria would also indicate bleeding. Signs of infection would not appear immediately following a biopsy. Pain of this nature is not normal. There are no data to support the presence of renal colic.

Test-Taking Strategy: Use the process of elimination. Focusing on the data in the question will assist in eliminating options 3 and 4. Recalling that signs of infection may not appear immediately following biopsy will assist in directing you to option 1 from the remaining options. Review the complications following renal biopsy if you had difficulty with this question.

Level of Cognitive Ability: Analysis
Client Needs: Physiological Integrity
Integrated Process: Nursing Process/Data Collection
Content Area: Adult Health/Renal
Reference: Pagana, K., & Pagana, T. (2003). *Mosby's diagnostic and laboratory test reference* (6th ed.). St. Louis: Mosby, p. 757.

27. Answer: 3

Rationale: In an older client, the only symptom of a UTI may be something as vague as increasing mental confusion or frequent unexplained falls. Frequency and urgency may commonly occur in an older client and fever can be associated with a variety of conditions.

Test-Taking Strategy: Use the process of elimination. Note the client's age in the question. Eliminate options 2 and 4 because they may commonly occur in an older client. Eliminate option 1 next, because fever can be associated with a variety of conditions. Review the clinical manifestations of UTI that occur in the older client if you had difficulty with this question.

Level of Cognitive Ability: Comprehension
Client Needs: Physiological Integrity
Integrated Process: Nursing Process/Data Collection
Content Area: Adult Health/Renal
Reference: Potter, P., & Perry, A. (2005). *Fundamentals of nursing* (6th ed.). St. Louis: Mosby, p. 783.

28. Answer: 1

Rationale: Gross, painless hematuria is most frequently the first manifestation of bladder cancer. As the disease progresses the client may experience burning, frequency, and urgency.

Test-Taking Strategy: Use the process of elimination and focus on the issue, a manifestation of bladder cancer. Eliminate options 2, 3, and 4 because they are common signs of a urinary tract infection. Review the specific manifestations associated with bladder cancer if you had difficulty with this question.

Level of Cognitive Ability: Comprehension
Client Needs: Physiological Integrity
Integrated Process: Nursing Process/Data Collection
Content Area: Adult Health/Renal
Reference: Linton, A., & Maebius, N. (2003). *Introduction to medical-surgical nursing* (3rd ed.). Philadelphia: W.B. Saunders, p. 778.

29. Answer: 1

Rationale: TUR syndrome is caused by increased absorption of nonelectrolyte irrigating fluid used during surgery. The client may show signs of cerebral edema and increased intracranial pressure such as increased blood pressure, bradycardia, confusion, disorientation, muscle twitching, visual disturbances, and nausea and vomiting.

Test-Taking Strategy: Knowledge regarding TUR syndrome is required to answer this question. Recalling that increased intracranial pressure is the concern will direct you to option 1. Review this disorder if you had difficulty with this question.

Level of Cognitive Ability: Analysis
Client Needs: Physiological Integrity
Integrated Process: Nursing Process/Data Collection
Content Area: Adult Health/Renal
Reference: Phipps, W., Monahan, F., Sands, J., Marek, J., & Neighbors, M. (2003). *Medical-surgical nursing: Health and illness perspectives* (7th ed.). St. Louis: Mosby, p. 1836.

30. Answer: 4

Rationale: Treatment of prostatitis includes medication with antibiotics, analgesics, and stool softeners. The client is also taught to rest, increase fluid intake, and use sitz baths for comfort. Antimicrobial therapy is always continued until the prescription is completely finished.

Test-Taking Strategy: Use the process of elimination. Eliminate option 3 first, because stopping medication therapy before the end of the course is contraindicated. Option 1 is also eliminated, because fluid intake should be increased. From the remaining options, it is necessary to understand that sitz baths provide comfort and that rest is helpful in the healing process. Knowledge of either of these concepts will direct you to option 4. Review the measures to prevent prostatitis if you had difficulty with this question.
Level of Cognitive Ability: Analysis
Client Needs: Health Promotion and Maintenance
Integrated Process: Nursing Process/Evaluation
Content Area: Adult Health/Renal
Reference: Lewis, S., Heitkemper, M., & Dirksen, S. (2004). *Medical-surgical nursing: Assessment and management of clinical problems* (6th ed.). St. Louis: Mosby, p. 1443.

31. *Answer:* 2
Rationale: The nurse assesses the patency of the fistula by palpating for the presence of a thrill or auscultating for a bruit. The presence of a thrill and bruit indicate patency of the fistula. Although the presence of a radial pulse in the left wrist and capillary refill less than 3 seconds in the nail beds of the fingers on the left hand are normal findings, they do not assess fistula patency.
Test-Taking Strategy: Use the process of elimination. Eliminate options 3 and 4 first because they are similar and assess for adequate circulation in the distal portion of the extremity (not the fistula). From the remaining options, focusing on the issue (patency) and noting the word "absence" in option 1 will assist in eliminating this option. Review the expected findings when assessing an arteriovenous fistula if you had difficulty with this question.
Level of Cognitive Ability: Analysis
Client Needs: Physiological Integrity
Integrated Process: Nursing Process/Data Collection
Content Area: Adult Health/Renal
Reference: Ignatavicius, D., & Workman, M. (2006). *Medical-surgical nursing: Critical thinking for collaborative care* (5th ed.). Philadelphia: W.B. Saunders, p. 1754.

32. *Answer:* 3
Rationale: Pain during the inflow of dialysate is common during the first few exchanges because of peritoneal irritation; however, it disappears after a week or two. The infusion amount should not be decreased, and the infusion should not be slowed or stopped.
Test-Taking Strategy: Use the process of elimination. Eliminate options 1, 2, and 4 because they are similar actions. Review the complications associated with peritoneal dialysis and the appropriate nursing actions, if you had difficulty with this question.
Level of Cognitive Ability: Application
Client Needs: Physiological Integrity
Integrated Process: Nursing Process/Implementation
Content Area: Adult Health/Renal
Reference: Ignatavicius, D., & Workman, M. (2006). *Medical-surgical nursing: Critical thinking for collaborative care* (5th ed.). Philadelphia: W.B. Saunders, p. 1758.

33. *Answer:* 2
Rationale: An extended dwell time increases the risk of hyperglycemia in the client with diabetes mellitus as a result of absorption of glucose from the dialysate and electrolyte changes. Diabetic clients may require extra insulin when receiving peritoneal dialysis. Options 1, 3, and 4 are not associated with dwell time.
Test-Taking Strategy: Use the process of elimination. Noting the client's diagnosis and recalling that the dialysate solution contains glucose will direct you to option 2. Review the complications associated with peritoneal dialysis if you had difficulty with this question.
Level of Cognitive Ability: Application
Client Needs: Physiological Integrity
Integrated Process: Teaching/Learning
Content Area: Adult Health/Renal
Reference: Lewis, S., Heitkemper, M., & Dirksen, S. (2004). *Medical-surgical nursing: Assessment and management of clinical problems* (6th ed.). St. Louis: Mosby, p. 1232.

34. *Answer:* 1
Rationale: Individuals with polycystic kidney disease seem to waste rather than retain sodium. Thus, they need an increased sodium and water intake. Aggressive control of hypertension is essential. Genetic counseling is advisable because of the hereditary nature of the disease.
Test-Taking Strategy: Note the key words, *needs additional information.* These words indicate a false response question and that you need to select the incorrect client statement. Recalling that sodium is wasted in polycystic kidney disease will direct you to option 1. Review the manifestations associated with this disease if you had difficulty with this question.
Level of Cognitive Ability: Analysis
Client Needs: Physiological Integrity
Integrated Process: Teaching/Learning
Content Area: Adult Health/Renal
Reference: Phipps, W., Monahan, F., Sands, J., Marek, J., & Neighbors, M. (2003). *Medical-surgical nursing: Health and illness perspectives* (7th ed.). St. Louis: Mosby, p. 1204.

35. *Answer:* 3
Rationale: Antihypertensive medications such as enalapril are given to the client following hemodialysis. This prevents the client from becoming hypotensive during dialysis and from having the medication removed from the bloodstream by dialysis. There is no rationale for waiting a full day to resume the medication. This would lead to ineffective control of the blood pressure.
Test-Taking Strategy: Use the process of elimination. Begin to answer this question by thinking about the effects of an antihypertensive medication on the blood pressure when fluid is being removed from the body. Because hypotension is much more likely to occur in this circumstance, eliminate options 1 and 2. Eliminate option 4 because this action would lead to ineffective blood pressure control. Review preprocedure hemodialysis measures if you had difficulty with this question.
Level of Cognitive Ability: Application
Client Needs: Physiological Integrity
Integrated Process: Nursing Process/Planning

Content Area: Adult Health/Renal

References: Lewis, S., Heitkemper, M., & Dirksen, S. (2004). *Medical-surgical nursing: Assessment and management of clinical problems* (6th ed.). St. Louis: Mosby, p. 1222.

Phipps, W., Monahan, F., Sands, J., Marek, J., & Neighbors, M. (2003). *Medical-surgical nursing: Health and illness perspectives* (7th ed.). St. Louis: Mosby, p. 766.

ALTERNATE FORMAT QUESTION: MULTIPLE RESPONSE

Answers:

Check the level of the drainage bag

Check the peritoneal dialysis system for kinks

Reposition the client to his or her side

Rationale: If outflow drainage is inadequate, the nurse attempts to stimulate outflow by changing the client's position. Turning the client to the other side or making sure that the client is in good body alignment may assist with outflow drainage. A low Fowler's position reduces intra-abdominal pressure; increased intra-abdominal pressure can affect outflow and also contributes to leakage at the peritoneal dialysis catheter site. The drainage bag needs to be lower than the client's abdomen to enhance gravity drainage. The connecting tubing and the peritoneal dialysis system is also checked for kinks or twisting and the clamps on the system are checked to ensure that they are open. There is no reason to contact the physician.

Test-Taking Strategy: Use the principles related to gravity flow and preventing obstruction to flow to answer this question. This will assist in determining the correct interventions. Review the nursing interventions related to insufficient flow of dialysate if you had difficulty with this question.

Level of Cognitive Ability: Application

Client Needs: Physiological Integrity

Integrated Process: Nursing Process/Implementation

Content Area: Adult Health/Renal

Reference: Ignatavicius, D., & Workman, M. (2006). *Medical-surgical nursing: Critical thinking for collaborative care* (5th ed.). Philadelphia: W.B. Saunders, p. 1759.

REFERENCES

Black, J., & Hawks, J. (2005). *Medical-surgical nursing: Clinical management for positive outcomes* (7th ed.). Philadelphia: W.B. Saunders.

Chernecky, C., & Berger, B. (2004). *Laboratory tests and diagnostic procedures* (4th ed.). Philadelphia: W.B. Saunders.

Christensen, B., & Kockrow, E. (2003). *Adult health nursing* (4th ed). St. Louis: Mosby.

Christensen, B., & Kockrow, E. (2003). *Foundations of nursing* (4th ed.). St. Louis: Mosby.

deWit, S. (2005). *Fundamental concepts and skills for nursing.* Philadelphia: W.B. Saunders.

Hodgson, B., & Kizior, R. (2005). *Saunders nursing drug handbook 2005.* Philadelphia: W.B. Saunders.

Ignatavicius, D., & Workman, M. (2006). *Medical surgical nursing: Critical thinking for collaborative care* (5th ed.). Philadelphia: W.B. Saunders.

Lewis, S., Heitkemper, M., & Dirksen, S. (2004). *Medical-surgical nursing: Assessment and management of clinical problems* (6th ed.). St. Louis: Mosby.

Linton, A., & Maebius, N. (2003). *Introduction to medical-surgical nursing* (3rd ed.). Philadelphia: W.B. Saunders.

McKenry, L., & Salerno, E. (2003). *Mosby's pharmacology in nursing* (21st ed.). St. Louis: Mosby.

Nix, S. (2005). *Williams basic nutrition and diet therapy* (11th ed.). St. Louis: Mosby.

Pagana, K., & Pagana, T. (2003). *Mosby's diagnostic and laboratory test reference* (6th ed.). St. Louis: Mosby.

Peckenpaugh, N. (2003). *Nutrition essentials and diet therapy* (9th ed.). Philadelphia: W.B. Saunders.

Renal Medications

I. URINARY TRACT ANTISEPTICS (Box 53-1)

A. Description
1. Inhibit the growth of bacteria in the urine
2. Act as disinfectants within the urinary tract
3. Used to treat urinary tract infections
4. These medications do not achieve effective antibacterial concentrations in blood or tissues and therefore cannot be used for infections at sites outside the urinary tract

B. Side effects and nursing considerations
1. Nitrofurantoin (Furadantin, Macrodantin, Macrobid)
   a. Gastrointestinal effects such as anorexia, nausea, vomiting, and diarrhea; administration with milk or meals will minimize gastrointestinal (GI) distress
   b. Pulmonary reactions such as dyspnea, chest pain, chills, fever, cough, and alveolar infiltrates; these resolve in 2 to 4 days following cessation of treatment
   c. Hematological effects such as agranulocytosis, leukopenia, thrombocytopenia, and megaloblastic anemia
   d. Peripheral neuropathy such as muscle weakness, tingling sensations, and numbness
   e. Neurological effects such as headache, vertigo, drowsiness, nystagmus

f. Imparts a harmless brown color to the urine
g. Contraindicated in clients with renal impairment
h. Instruct the client in the expected side effects and those warranting notifying the physician
2. Methenamine mandelate (Mandelamine) and methenamine hippurate (Hiprex)
   a. Relatively safe and well tolerated
   b. May cause gastric distress
   c. Chronic high-dose therapy can cause bladder irritation
   d. Can cause crystalluria and should not be used in clients with renal impairment
   e. Decomposition of medication generates ammonia; thus, should not be used for clients with liver dysfunction
   f. Requires acidic urine with pH of 5.5 or less
   g. Ingestion of large amounts of fluid will reduce antibacterial effects by diluting the medication and raising the urinary pH
   h. Should not be combined with sulfonamides because of the risk of crystalluria and urinary tract injury
   i. Clients taking this medication should not be given alkalinizing agents
3. Nalidixic acid (NegGram)
   a. Gastrointestinal disturbances: Nausea, vomiting, and abdominal discomfort
   b. Rash
   c. Visual disturbances
   d. Photosensitivity reactions
   e. May produce intracranial hypertension in pediatric clients and should not be administered to children under age 3 months
   f. When used for more than 2 weeks, complete blood cell (CBC) counts and liver function tests should be performed
   g. Can intensify the effects of oral anticoagulants

BOX 53-1

Urinary Tract Antiseptics

Cinoxacin (Cinobac)
Methenamine (Mandelamine)
Methenamine hippurate (Hiprex)
Nalidixic acid (NegGram)
Nitrofurantoin (Furadantin, Macrodantin, Macrobid)

h. Contraindicated in clients with a history of convulsive disorders

4. Cinoxacin (Cinobac)
   a. Side effects are similar to those of nalidixic acid
   b. Dosage should be reduced in clients with renal impairment; failure to do so could result in accumulation of the medication to toxic levels

II. FLUOROQUINOLONES (Box 53-2)

A. Significant side effects include dizziness, drowsiness, gastric distress, diarrhea, vaginitis (trovafloxacin), nausea, and vomiting

B. Adverse effects include psychoses, hallucinations, confusion, tremors, hypersensitivity, and interstitial nephritis

C. Used with caution in clients with hepatic, renal, or central nervous system disorders

D. Monitor client for side effects or signs of adverse reactions

E. Administer with a full glass of water and ensure that client maintains a urine output of at least 1200 to 1500 mL/day to minimize the occurrence of crystalluria

F. Enoxacin (Penetrex) and norfloxacin (Noroxin) are to be taken on an empty stomach

G. Ciprofloxacin (Cipro), lomefloxacin (Maxaquin), ofloxacin (Floxin), and sparfloxacin (Zagam) may be taken with or without food

H. Advise client to report dizziness, lightheadedness, visual disturbances, increased light sensitivity, and feelings of depression, because these signs could indicate central nervous system toxicity

I. Inform client of signs of hepatic and renal toxicity and the importance of reporting these signs to the physician

III. SULFONAMIDES (Box 53-3)

A. Description
   1. Suppress bacterial growth by inhibiting the synthesis of folic acid
   2. Active against a broad spectrum of microbes

B. Side effects and nursing considerations
   1. Hypersensitivity reactions: Rash, fever, and photosensitivity
   2. Stevens-Johnson syndrome, the most severe hypersensitivity response, produces symptoms that include widespread lesions of the skin and mucous membranes, with fever, malaise, and toxemia
   3. Should be discontinued if a rash is observed
   4. Can cause hemolytic anemia, agranulocytosis, leukopenia, and thrombocytopenia
   5. Instruct the client to take medication on an empty stomach with a full glass of water
   6. Instruct the client to avoid prolonged exposure to sunlight, wear protective clothing, and apply a sunscreen to exposed skin
   7. Adults should maintain a daily urine output of 1200 mL by consuming 8 to 10 glasses of water each day to minimize the risk of renal damage from the medication
   8. Can intensify the effects of warfarin sodium (Coumadin), phenytoin (Dilantin), and oral hypoglycemics
   9. Administer with caution in clients with renal impairment
   10. Contraindicated if a hypersensitivity exists to sulfonamides, sulfonylureas, or thiazide or loop diuretics
   11. Contraindicated in infants younger than 2 months and in pregnant women or mothers who are breast-feeding

IV. CHOLINERGIC AGENT (Box 53-4)

A. Description
   1. Used to treat nonobstructive urinary retention and neurogenic bladder
   2. Used to increase bladder tone and function

B. Side effects
   1. Headache
   2. Hypotension
   3. Flushing and sweating

BOX 53-2

Fluoroquinolones

Alatrofloxacin, infusion (Trovan)
Ciprofloxacin (Cipro)
Enoxacin (Penetrex)
Gatifloxacin (Tequin)
Levofloxacin (Levaquin)
Lomefloxacin (Maxaquin)
Moxifloxacin (Avelox)
Norfloxacin (Noroxin)
Ofloxacin (Floxin)
Sparfloxacin (Zagam)
Trovafloxacin, tablets (Trovan)

BOX 53-3

Sulfonamides

Sulfadiazine
Sulfamethizole (Thiosulfil Forte)
Sulfamethoxazole
Sulfisoxazole
Trimethoprim-sulfamethoxazole (Bactrim)

BOX 53-4

Cholinergic Agent

Bethanechol chloride (Urecholine)

4. Increased salivation
5. Abdominal cramps
6. Nausea and vomiting
7. Diarrhea
8. Urinary urgency
9. Bronchoconstriction

C. Nursing considerations
1. Do not administer if the client has a urinary obstruction
2. Is never administer by the intramuscular or intravenous route
3. Monitor intake and output (I&O)
4. Monitor for increased bladder tone and function
5. Monitor for cholinergic overdose
6. Have atropine sulfate (antidote) readily available

V. ANTISPASMODICS

A. Description
1. Oxybutynin chloride (Ditropan) relaxes smooth muscles of the urinary tract
2. Propantheline bromide (Pro-Banthine) decreases bladder muscle spasms

B. Oxybutynin chloride (Ditropan)
1. Side effects
a. Leukopenia
b. Anxiety
c. Anorexia, nausea, vomiting
d. Palpitations
e. Sinus bradycardia
2. Nursing considerations
a. Do not administer to clients with known hypersensitivity, GI or genitourinary (GU) obstruction, glaucoma, severe colitis, or myasthenia gravis
b. Instruct the client to avoid hazardous activities

C. Propantheline bromide (Pro-Banthine)
1. Side effects
a. Palpitations
b. Blurred vision
c. Confusion in elderly clients
d. Tachycardia
e. Constipation
f. Dry mouth
g. Urinary hesitancy and urgency
h. Decreased sweating
2. Nursing considerations
a. Monitor I&O
b. Provide gum or hard candy for dry mouth
c. Do not administer to clients with narrow-angle glaucoma, obstructive uropathy, GI disease, or ulcerative colitis

VI. URINARY TRACT ANALGESIC (Box 53-5)

A. Description
1. Used for pain from urinary tract irritation or infection

BOX 53-5

Urinary Tract Analgesic

Phenazopyridine hydrochloride (Pyridium)

BOX 53-6

Hematopoietic Growth Factor

Epoetin alfa (Epogen, Procrit)

---

2. Administered with an antibiotic because it does not treat infection, but only treats pain

B. Side effects
1. Nausea
2. Headache
3. Vertigo

C. Nursing considerations
1. Instruct the client that the urine will turn red or orange
2. Contraindicated in renal or hepatic disease

VII. HEMATOPOIETIC GROWTH FACTOR
(Box 53-6)

A. Description
1. Used to stimulate red blood cell (RBC) production
2. Reverses anemia associated with **chronic renal failure**
3. Initial effects can be seen within 1 to 2 weeks; hematocrit reaches normal levels (30% to 33%) in 2 to 3 months

B. Side effect: Major side effect is hypertension

C. Nursing considerations
1. Monitor the complete blood count
2. Monitor vital signs, especially the blood pressure, for hypertension
3. The extent of hypertension is directly related to the rate of rise in the hematocrit
4. Contraindicated in clients with uncontrolled hypertension or hypersensitivity to mammalian cell–derived products or human albumin
5. Use with caution in clients with cancers of myeloid origin

VIII. PREVENTING ORGAN REJECTION (Box 53-7)

A. Description
1. Cyclosporine acts on T lymphocytes to suppress production of interleukin-2 (IL-2), interferon gamma, and other cytokines
2. Tracrolimus inhibits calcineurin and thereby prevents T cells from producing IL-2, interferon gamma, and other cytokines
3. Azathioprine (Imuran) suppresses cell-mediated and humoral immune responses by inhibiting the proliferation of B and T lymphocytes

BOX 53-7

Preventing Organ Rejection

IMMUNOSUPPRESSANTS
Cyclosporine (Sandimmune, Neoral)
Tacrolimus (Prograf)

CYTOTOXIC MEDICATIONS
Azathioprine (Imuran)
Mycophenolate mofetil (CellCept)

GLUCOCORTICOID
Prednisone (Deltasone)

ANTIBODIES
Basiliximab (Simulect)
Daclizumab (Zenapax)
Muromonab-CD3 (Orthoclone OKT3)

4. Mycophenolate mofetil causes selective inhibition of B and T lymphocyte proliferation
5. Muromonab-CD3 blocks all T-cell functions
6. Daclizumab and basiliximab bind to IL-2 receptors on lymphocytes, resulting in diminished cell-mediated immune reactions

B. Cyclosporine (Sandimmune, Neoral)
1. Used to prevent rejection of allogeneic kidney transplant
2. Prednisone is usually administered concurrently
3. Oral administration is preferred; intravenous administration is reserved for clients who cannot take the medication orally
4. Blood levels should be measured periodically
5. The most common adverse effects are nephrotoxicity, infection, hypertension, tremor, and hirsutism
6. The client should be informed about the possibility of renal damage and liver damage and the need for periodic blood urea nitrogen (BUN), creatinine, and liver function tests
7. The client should be instructed to monitor for early signs of infection and to report these signs immediately
8. Instruct the client to dispense the oral liquid into a glass container by using a specially calibrated pipette, mix well, and drink immediately; rinse the glass container with diluent and drink it to ensure ingestion of the complete dose; dry the outside of the pipette and return to its cover for storage
9. Instruct the client to mix the concentrated medication solution with milk, chocolate milk, or orange juice just before administration
10. Assure the client that hirsutism is reversible
11. Grapefruit juice can raise cyclosporine levels, thereby increasing the risk of toxicity

12. Phenytoin (Dilantin), phenobarbital, rifampin (Rifadin), and trimethoprim-sulfamethoxazole (TMP-SMZ) can decrease cyclosporine levels
13. Ketoconazole (Nizoral), erythromycin, and amphotericin B (Fungizone) can elevate cyclosporine levels
14. Renal damage can be intensified by the concurrent use of other nephrotoxic medications
15. Contraindicated in the presence of hypersensitivity, pregnancy and breast-feeding, recent inoculation with live virus vaccines, and recent contact with an active infection such as chickenpox or herpes zoster
16. Is embryotoxic; women of childbearing age should use a mechanical form of contraception and avoid oral contraceptives

C. Tacrolimus (Prograf)
1. Nephrotoxicity is the major concern
2. Other common reactions include neurotoxicity, gastrointestinal (GI) effects, hypertension, hyperkalemia, and hyperglycemia
3. Increases the risk of infection and lymphomas
4. Concurrent use of glucocorticoids is recommended

D. Azathioprine (Imuran)
1. Used as an adjunct to cyclosporine and glucocorticoids to help suppress transplant rejection
2. Can cause neutropenia and thrombocytopenia from bone marrow suppression
3. Contraindicated in pregnancy; associated with an increased incidence of neoplasms

E. Mycophenolate mofetil (CellCept)
1. Used in combination with cyclosporine and glucocorticoids
2. Major adverse effects include diarrhea, severe neutropenia, vomiting, and sepsis
3. Associated with an increased risk of infection and malignancies
4. Absorption is decreased by the use of magnesium and aluminum antacids and by cholestyramine (Questran, Prevalite)
5. Contraindicated in pregnancy

F. Muromonab-CD3 (Orthoclone OKT3)
1. Used to prevent acute allograft rejection of kidney transplants
2. Adverse reactions include fever, chills, dyspnea, chest pain, and nausea and vomiting

G. Daclizumab (Zenapax) and basiliximab (Simulect)
1. Used to prevent acute rejection of transplanted kidneys
2. Used in combination with other immunosuppressants such as cyclosporine and glucocorticoids
3. Administered by the intravenous route
4. Contraindicated in the client with an allergy to protein
5. Daclizumab (Zenapax)
   a. Initial dose administered within 24 hours prior to transplantation

b. Side effects include chest pain, GI distress, edema, shortness of breath, pain in the joints, and slow wound healing

6. Basiliximab (Simulect)
   a. Initial dose administered within 2 hours prior to transplant
   b. Side effects are similar to those for daclizumab; in addition, headache, insomnia, dizziness, and tremor can occur

PRACTICE QUESTIONS

1. Cinoxacin (Cinobac) is prescribed for the client with a urinary tract infection. The nurse tells the client to take the medication:
   1. 1 hour before meals
   2. With meals
   3. At bedtime
   4. In the morning before breakfast

2. Laboratory analysis of a urine for culture and sensitivity reveals a gram-negative bacterial infection. Nalidixic acid (NegGram) is prescribed for the client. The nurse questions the prescription if the client has which of the following disorders?
   1. Diabetes mellitus
   2. Seizure disorder
   3. Coronary artery disease
   4. Peptic ulcer disease

3. Methenamine mandelate (Mandelamine) is prescribed for the client with a gram-positive urinary tract infection. The nurse questions the prescription if which of the following pre-existing disorders is noted in the client's record?
   1. Cirrhosis
   2. Diabetes mellitus
   3. Peripheral vascular disease
   4. Hypothyroidism

4. A client receiving nitrofurantoin (Macrodantin) calls the physician's office complaining of side effects related to the medication. Which side effect indicates the need to stop treatment with this medication?
   1. Anorexia
   2. Nausea
   3. Cough and chest pain
   4. Diarrhea

5. Nalidixic acid (NegGram) is prescribed for the client with a urinary tract infection. Reviewing the client's record, the nurse notes that the client is taking warfarin (Coumadin) on a daily basis. Which of the following prescriptions would the nurse anticipate because the client is on this oral anticoagulant?
   1. An increase in the anticoagulation dosage
   2. A reduction in the anticoagulation dosage
   3. The need to discontinue the warfarin (Coumadin) during therapy

   4. The need to administer an alternative medication to treat the urinary tract infection

6. A nurse is reinforcing discharge instructions to a client receiving sulfisoxazole. Which of the following would be included in the plan of care for instructions?
   1. Discontinue the medication when feeling better
   2. Maintain a high fluid intake
   3. Decrease the dosage when symptoms are improving to prevent an allergic response
   4. If the urine turns dark brown, call the physician immediately

7. Trimethoprim-sulfamethoxazole (Bactrim) is prescribed for the client. The nurse tells the client to report which of the following symptoms if it develops during the course of this medication therapy?
   1. Headache
   2. Nausea
   3. Diarrhea
   4. Sore throat

8. Phenazopyridine (Pyridium) is prescribed for the client for symptomatic relief of pain resulting from a lower urinary tract infection. The nurse tells the client:
   1. To take the medication on an empty stomach
   2. That a reddish-orange discoloration of the urine may occur
   3. To discontinue the medication if a headache occurs
   4. To take the medication at bedtime on an empty stomach

9. Bethanechol (Urecholine) is prescribed for the client with urinary retention. The nurse reviews the client's record, knowing that which of the following preexisting disorders would be a contraindication to the administration of this medication?
   1. Neurogenic atony
   2. Urinary strictures
   3. Gastroesophageal reflux
   4. Gastric atony

10. Bethanechol (Urecholine) is prescribed for the client. The nurse tells the client to take the medication:
    1. With meals
    2. Two hours after meals
    3. With a snack in the afternoon
    4. At bedtime with crackers and cheese

11. Oxybutynin (Ditropan) is prescribed for the client with neurogenic bladder. The nurse monitors the client, knowing that which of the following would indicate a possible toxic effect related to this medication?
    1. Bradycardia
    2. Pallor
    3. Restlessness
    4. Drowsiness

12. Propantheline bromide (Pro-Banthine) is prescribed for the client with bladder spasms. Which of the following disorders, if noted in the

client's record, alerts the nurse to question the prescription for this medication?
1. Glaucoma
2. Hypothyroidism
3. Myxedema
4. Coronary artery disease

13. Following kidney transplant, cyclosporine (Sandimmune) is prescribed for the client. Which of the following laboratory results indicates an adverse effect from the use of this medication?
1. Decreased white blood cell (WBC) count
2. Decreased hemoglobin level
3. Elevated blood urea nitrogen (BUN) level
4. Decreased creatinine level

14. A nurse is providing dietary instructions to a client who has been prescribed cyclosporine (Sandimmune). Which of the following food items would the nurse instruct the client to avoid?
1. Orange juice
2. Grapefruit juice
3. Red meats
4. Green leafy vegetables

15. A nurse reinforces instructions to the client prescribed to take cyclosporine (Sandimmune) oral solution. Which of the following instructions would the nurse reinforce?
1. Dilute the medication in a Styrofoam cup before administration
2. Avoid diluting the concentrate for administration
3. Mix the concentration with chocolate milk
4. Mix the concentration with grapefruit juice

16. A nurse is monitoring a client receiving cyclosporine (Sandimmune). Which of the following indicates to the nurse that the client is experiencing an adverse effect from this medication?
1. Nausea
2. Alopecia
3. Tremor
4. Hypotension

17. Tacrolimus (Prograf) is prescribed for the client. Which of the following disorders, if noted on the client's record, indicates that the medication needs to be administered with caution?
1. Diabetes insipidus
2. Coronary artery disease
3. Renal insufficiency
4. Ulcerative colitis

18. A nurse is reviewing the laboratory results documented in the record of a client receiving tacrolimus (Prograf). Which of the following indicates to the nurse that the client is experiencing an adverse effect of the medication?
1. White blood cell (WBC) count, 6000/μL
2. Blood glucose level, 200 mg/dL
3. Potassium level, 3.8 mEq/L
4. Platelet count, 300,000 cells/μL

19. Mycophenolate mofetil (CellCept) is prescribed for a client as prophylaxis for organ rejection following allogeneic renal transplant. Which of the following instructions does the nurse reinforce regarding administration of this medication?
1. Administer following meals
2. Open the capsule and mix with food for administration
3. Contact the physician if a sore throat occurs
4. Take the medication with a magnesium type antacid

20. A client with chronic renal failure (CRF) is receiving epoetin alfa (Epogen). The nurse is reviewing the laboratory results and notes that which of the following results indicates a therapeutic effect of the medication?
1. White blood cell (WBC) count, 6000/μL
2. Hematocrit level, 32%
3. Platelet count, 400,000 cells/μL
4. Blood urea nitrogen (BUN) level, 15 mg/dL

21. A nurse is monitoring the client receiving epoetin alfa (Epogen) for adverse effects of the medication. The nurse notes that which of the following indicates an adverse effect?
1. Hypotension
2. Hypertension
3. Depression
4. Bradycardia

22. A nurse is reviewing the laboratory studies of a client receiving epoetin alfa (Epogen). The nurse expects to note a therapeutic effect of this medication:
1. After 1 week of therapy
2. Immediately
3. 3 days after therapy
4. 2 months after therapy

23. A nurse is reinforcing instructions to a client regarding how to administer epoetin alfa (Epogen) subcutaneously. The nurse tells the client to:
1. Shake the medicine bottle before use
2. Freeze the medication before use
3. Refrigerate the medication
4. Obtain syringes with $\frac{1}{2}$- and 1-inch needles from the pharmacy

24. Aluminum hydroxide (Amphojel) is prescribed for the client with chronic renal failure (CRF). The nurse instructs the client to take this medication:
1. On an empty stomach
2. At bedtime
3. With meals
4. In the morning on arising

25. A nurse is administering 5 mg of bethanechol (Urecholine) subcutaneously to a client with urinary retention. Which of the following would the nurse prepare to have readily available when administering this medication?
1. Protamine sulfate
2. Vitamin K

3. Atropine sulfate
4. Mucomyst

ALTERNATE FORMAT QUESTION: CHART-EXHIBIT

CLIENT'S CHART

Laboratory Test Result
Blood glucose, 102 mg/dL

Client's History
Renal insufficiency

Medication History
Folic acid (vitamin B$_6$) orally daily

Diagnostic Test Result
Chest x-ray: Normal

Cinoxacin (Cinobac), a urinary antiseptic, is prescribed for the client. The nurse reviews the client's medical record and would contact the physician regarding which documented finding to verify the prescription?

1. Laboratory test results
2. Client's history
3. Medication history
4. Diagnostic test result

ANSWERS

1. *Answer:* 2
Rationale: Cinobac is a urinary antiseptic and is administered with meals to decrease GI side effects. Options 1, 3, and 4 are incorrect.
Test-Taking Strategy: Use the process of elimination. Eliminate options 1, 3, and 4 because they are similar in that all these options indicate taking the medication on an empty stomach. Review this medication if you had difficulty with this question.
Level of Cognitive Ability: Application
Client Needs: Health Promotion and Maintenance
Integrated Process: Nursing Process/Implementation
Content Area: Pharmacology
Reference: McKenry, L., & Salerno, E. (2003). *Mosby's pharmacology in nursing* (21st ed.). St. Louis: Mosby, p. 1008.

2. *Answer:* 2
Rationale: NegGram is used for acute and chronic urinary tract infections, especially gram-negative bacterial infections. The medication is contraindicated in clients with a history of seizures. It is used with caution in clients with liver or renal disorders.
Test-Taking Strategy: Knowledge regarding the contraindications associated with this medication is required to answer the question. Remember, NegGram is contraindicated in clients with a history of seizures. Review this medication if you had difficulty with this question.
Level of Cognitive Ability: Application
Client Needs: Safe, Effective Care Environment
Integrated Process: Nursing Process/Implementation
Content Area: Pharmacology
Reference: Lehne, R. (2004). *Pharmacology for nursing care* (5th ed.). Philadelphia: W.B. Saunders, p. 937.

3. *Answer:* 1
Rationale: Mandelamine is contraindicated in clients with renal or hepatic disease or clients with severe dehydration. The nurse would question the physician's prescription for this medication in the client with cirrhosis.

Test-Taking Strategy: Use the process of elimination. Remember that this medication is contraindicated in hepatic disease. Review this medication if you had difficulty with this question.
Level of Cognitive Ability: Application
Client Needs: Safe, Effective Care Environment
Integrated Process: Nursing Process/Implementation
Content Area: Pharmacology
Reference: Lehne, R. (2004). *Pharmacology for nursing care* (5th ed.). Philadelphia: W.B. Saunders, p. 937.

4. *Answer:* 3
Rationale: Gastrointestinal effects are the most frequent adverse reactions to this medication and can be minimized by administering the medication with milk or meals. Pulmonary reactions, manifested as dyspnea, chest pain, chills, fever, cough, and the presence of alveolar infiltrates on the x-ray, would indicate the need to stop the treatment. These symptoms resolve in 2 to 4 days following discontinuation of this medication.
Test-Taking Strategy: Use the process of elimination. Eliminate options 1, 2, and 4 because they are gastrointestinal related side effects. Also, use the ABCs—airway, breathing, and circulation—to direct you to option 3. Review this medication if you had difficulty with this question.
Level of Cognitive Ability: Analysis
Client Needs: Physiological Integrity
Integrated Process: Nursing Process/Data Collection
Content Area: Pharmacology
Reference: Hodgson, B., & Kizior, R. (2005). *Saunders nursing drug handbook 2005*. Philadelphia: W.B. Saunders, p. 777.

5. *Answer:* 2
Rationale: Nalidixic acid can intensify the effects of oral anticoagulants. When an oral anticoagulant is combined with nalidixic acid, a reduction in the anticoagulant dosage may be needed.
Test-Taking Strategy: Use the process of elimination. Recalling that nalidixic acid can intensify the effects of oral anticoagulants will direct you to option 2. Review this medication if you had difficulty with this question.

Level of Cognitive Ability: Analysis
Client Needs: Physiological Integrity
Integrated Process: Nursing Process/Implementation
Content Area: Pharmacology
Reference: Lehne, R. (2004). *Pharmacology for nursing care* (5th ed.). Philadelphia: W.B. Saunders, p. 937.

6. *Answer:* **2**
Rationale: Each dose of sulfisoxazole should be administered with a full glass of water, and the client should maintain a high fluid intake. The medication is more soluble in alkaline urine. The client should not be instructed to taper or discontinue the dose. Some forms of sulfisoxazole, cause the urine to turn dark brown or red. This does not indicate the need to notify the physician.
Test-Taking Strategy: Use the process of elimination. General principles related to medication administration will assist in eliminating options 1 and 3. From the remaining options, recalling that this medication is a sulfonamide will direct you to option 2. Review this medication if you had difficulty with this question.
Level of Cognitive Ability: Application
Client Needs: Health Promotion and Maintenance
Integrated Process: Teaching/Learning
Content Area: Pharmacology
Reference: Lehne, R. (2004). *Pharmacology for nursing care* (5th ed.). Philadelphia: W.B. Saunders, p. 931.

7. *Answer:* **4**
Rationale: Clients taking trimethoprim-sulfamethoxazole should be informed about early signs of blood disorders that can occur from this medication. These signs include sore throat, fever, or pallor, and the client should be instructed to notify the physician if these symptoms occur. The other options do not require physician notification.
Test-Taking Strategy: Focus on the issue, the symptoms to report. Recalling that this medication can cause blood dyscrasias will direct you to option 4. Review this medication if you had difficulty with this question.
Level of Cognitive Ability: Application
Client Needs: Physiological Integrity
Integrated Process: Nursing Process/Implementation
Content Area: Pharmacology
References: Hodgson, B., & Kizior, R. (2005). *Saunders nursing drug handbook 2005.* Philadelphia: W.B. Saunders, p. 265.
Lehne, R. (2004). *Pharmacology for nursing care* (5th ed.). Philadelphia: W.B. Saunders, p. 932.

8. *Answer:* **2**
Rationale: The client should be instructed that a reddish-orange discoloration of urine may occur. The client should also be instructed that this discoloration can stain fabric. The medication should be taken after meals to reduce the possibility of GI upset. A headache is an occasional side effect of the medication and does not warrant discontinuation of the medication.
Test-Taking Strategy: Use the process of elimination. Eliminate options 1 and 4 first because they are similar. From the remaining options, eliminate option 3 because the nurse would not advise the client to discontinue this medication.

Review this medication if you had difficulty with this question.
Level of Cognitive Ability: Application
Client Needs: Health Promotion and Maintenance
Integrated Process: Nursing Process/Implementation
Content Area: Pharmacology
Reference: Hodgson, B., & Kizior, R. (2005). *Saunders nursing drug handbook 2005.* Philadelphia: W.B. Saunders, p. 848.

9. *Answer:* **2**
Rationale: Urecholine can be hazardous to clients with urinary tract obstruction or weakness of the bladder wall. The medication has the ability to contract the bladder and thereby increase pressure within the urinary tract. Elevation of pressure within the urinary tract could rupture the bladder in clients with these conditions
Test-Taking Strategy: Focus on the data in the question. Noting that the medication is used for urinary retention will assist in directing you to option 2. Review this medication if you had difficulty with this question.
Level of Cognitive Ability: Analysis
Client Needs: Physiological Integrity
Integrated Process: Nursing Process/Data Collection
Content Area: Pharmacology
Reference: Hodgson, B., & Kizior, R. (2005). *Saunders nursing drug handbook 2005.* Philadelphia: W.B. Saunders, p. 120.

10. *Answer:* **2**
Rationale: Administration of bethanechol with meals can cause nausea and vomiting in the client. To avoid this problem, oral doses should be administered 1 hour before meals or 2 hours after meals.
Test-Taking Strategy: Use the process of elimination. Note that options 1, 3, and 4 are similar in that they all suggest administering the medication with a food item. Review this medication if you had difficulty with this question.
Level of Cognitive Ability: Application
Client Needs: Physiological Integrity
Integrated Process: Nursing Process/Implementation
Content Area: Pharmacology
Reference: Lehne, R. (2004). *Pharmacology for nursing care* (5th ed.). Philadelphia: W.B. Saunders, p. 114.

11. *Answer:* **3**
Rationale: Toxicity produces central nervous system excitation, such as nervousness, restlessness, hallucinations, and irritability. Other signs of toxicity include either hypotension or hypertension, confusion, tachycardia, flushed or red face, and signs of respiratory depression. Drowsiness is a frequent side effect of the medication, but does not indicate toxicity.
Test-Taking Strategy: Knowledge regarding the manifestations related to toxicity is required to answer this question. Remember, central nervous system excitation is a sign of toxicity. Review this medication if you had difficulty with this question.
Level of Cognitive Ability: Analysis
Client Needs: Physiological Integrity
Integrated Process: Nursing Process/Data Collection
Content Area: Pharmacology

Reference: Hodgson, B., & Kizior, R. (2005). *Saunders nursing drug handbook 2005.* Philadelphia: W.B. Saunders, p. 814.

12. Answer: 1
Rationale: Pro-Banthine is contraindicated in clients with narrow angle glaucoma, obstructive uropathy, gastrointestinal disease or ulcerative colitis. Options 2, 3, and 4 are not contraindications to the use of this medication.
Test-Taking Strategy: Use the process of elimination. Eliminate options 2 and 3 because they are similar. From the remaining options, it is necessary to know the contraindications associated with the medication. Remember, Pro-Banthine is contraindicated in clients with glaucoma. Review these contraindications if you had difficulty with this question.
Level of Cognitive Ability: Analysis
Client Needs: Physiological Integrity
Integrated Process: Nursing Process/Data Collection
Content Area: Pharmacology
Reference: Lehne, R. (2004). *Pharmacology for nursing care* (5th ed.). Philadelphia: W.B. Saunders, p. 120.

13. Answer: 3
Rationale: Nephrotoxicity can occur from the use of Sandimmune. Nephrotoxicity is evaluated by monitoring for elevated BUN and serum creatinine levels. Sandimmune does not depress the bone marrow.
Test-Taking Strategy: Use the process of elimination. Eliminate options 1 and 2 first because they are unrelated to renal function. Next, eliminate option 4 because the creatinine level would be elevated, not decreased. Option 3 is the only option that indicates an increased level of a renal function test. Review these contraindications if you had difficulty with this question.
Level of Cognitive Ability: Analysis
Client Needs: Physiological Integrity
Integrated Process: Nursing Process/Data Collection
Content Area: Pharmacology
Reference: Lehne, R. (2004). *Pharmacology for nursing care* (5th ed.). Philadelphia: W.B. Saunders, pp. 728, 732.

14. Answer: 2
Rationale: A compound present in grapefruit juice inhibits metabolism of cyclosporine. As a result, consuming grapefruit juice can raise cyclosporine levels by 50% to 100%, thereby greatly increasing the risk of toxicity.
Test-Taking Strategy: Note the key word, *avoid.* Knowledge regarding substances that inhibit the metabolism of cyclosporine is required to answer this question. Remember, grapefruit juice inhibits the metabolism of cyclosporine. Review this medication if you had difficulty with this question.
Level of Cognitive Ability: Application
Client Needs: Physiological Integrity
Integrated Process: Teaching/Learning
Content Area: Pharmacology
Reference: Lehne, R. (2004). *Pharmacology for nursing care* (5th ed.). Philadelphia: W.B. Saunders, p. 733.

15. Answer: 3
Rationale: To improve palatability, the client should be taught to mix the concentrated medication solution with chocolate milk or orange juice just before administration. Grapefruit juice can raise cyclosporine levels. Instruct the client to dispense the oral liquid into a glass container using a specially calibrated pipette; mix well and drink immediately; rinse the container with diluent and drink it to ensure ingestion of the complete dose; dry the outside of the pipette and return to its cover for storage.
Test-Taking Strategy: Use the process of elimination. Recalling that the medication is diluted will assist in eliminating option 2. General guidelines related to medication administration will assist in eliminating option 4. From the remaining options, remember that a glass, not a Styrofoam cup, is used. Review this procedure if you had difficulty with this question.
Level of Cognitive Ability: Application
Client Needs: Physiological Integrity
Integrated Process: Teaching/Learning
Content Area: Pharmacology
Reference: Lehne, R. (2004). *Pharmacology for nursing care* (5th ed.). Philadelphia: W.B. Saunders, p. 732.

16. Answer: 3
Rationale: The most common adverse effects of cyclosporine are nephrotoxicity, infection, hypertension, tremor, and hirsutism. Of these, nephrotoxicity and infection are the most serious.
Test-Taking Strategy: Knowledge regarding the adverse effects associated with cyclosporine is required to answer this question. Review these effects if you had difficulty with this question.
Level of Cognitive Ability: Analysis
Client Needs: Physiological Integrity
Integrated Process: Nursing Process/Data Collection
Content Area: Pharmacology
Reference: Lehne, R. (2004). *Pharmacology for nursing care* (5th ed.). Philadelphia: W.B. Saunders, p. 728.

17. Answer: 3
Rationale: Tacrolimus is used with caution in immunosuppressed clients and in clients with renal or hepatic function impairment. It is contraindicated in clients with hypersensitivity to this medication or hypersensitivity to cyclosporine.
Test-Taking Strategy: Many medications affect renal and hepatic function. If you had to select an option and were unsure of the correct answer, select the option that addresses renal or hepatic function. Review the cautions and contraindications associated with the administration of this medication if you had difficulty with this question.
Level of Cognitive Ability: Analysis
Client Needs: Physiological Integrity
Integrated Process: Nursing Process/Data Collection
Content Area: Pharmacology
Reference: Lehne, R. (2004). *Pharmacology for nursing care* (5th ed.). Philadelphia: W.B. Saunders, p. 729.

18. Answer: 2
Rationale: Nephrotoxicity is a major concern with this medication. Other common reactions include neurotoxicity evidenced by headache, tremor, and insomnia, gastrointestinal effects (such as diarrhea, nausea, and vomiting), hypertension, hyperkalemia, and hyperglycemia.

Test-Taking Strategy: Use the process of elimination, noting that options 1, 3, and 4 represent normal values. Option 2 is the only abnormal value reflecting an elevation. Review these normal laboratory values if you had difficulty with this question.
Level of Cognitive Ability: Analysis
Client Needs: Physiological Integrity
Integrated Process: Nursing Process/Data Collection
Content Area: Pharmacology
Reference: Lehne, R. (2004). *Pharmacology for nursing care* (5th ed.). Philadelphia: W.B. Saunders, p. 729.

19. *Answer:* **3**
Rationale: Mycophenolate mofetil should be administered on an empty stomach. The capsules should not be opened or crushed. The client should contact the physician if unusual bleeding or bruising, sore throat, mouth sores, abdominal pain, or fever occurs. Antacids containing magnesium and aluminum may decrease the absorption of the medication and therefore should not be taken with the medication. The medication is given in combination with corticosteroids and cyclosporine.
Test-Taking Strategy: Knowledge regarding the teaching points associated with the administration of this medication is required to answer this question. Recalling that neutropenia can occur with this medication will direct you to option 3. Review this medication if you had difficulty with this question.
Level of Cognitive Ability: Application
Client Needs: Health Promotion and Maintenance
Integrated Process: Teaching/Learning
Content Area: Pharmacology
Reference: Hodgson, B., & Kizior, R. (2005). *Saunders nursing drug handbook 2005.* Philadelphia: W.B. Saunders, pp. 740-741.

20. *Answer:* **2**
Rationale: Epoetin alfa is used to reverse anemia associated with CRF. A therapeutic effect is seen when the hematocrit is between 30% and 33%.
Test-Taking Strategy: Use the process of elimination. Relate the name of the medication, "Epogen," to the potential action or effect. The only laboratory test that would reflect the effect of this medication is identified in option 2. Review the therapeutic effect of this medication if you had difficulty with this question.
Level of Cognitive Ability: Analysis
Client Needs: Physiological Integrity
Integrated Process: Nursing Process/Evaluation
Content Area: Pharmacology
Reference: Lehne, R. (2004). *Pharmacology for nursing care* (5th ed.). Philadelphia: W.B. Saunders, p. 588.

21. *Answer:* **2**
Rationale: Epoetin alfa is generally well tolerated. The most significant adverse effect is hypertension. Occasionally, a tachycardia may occur as a side effect. It may also cause an improved sense of well-being.
Test-Taking Strategy: Knowledge regarding the significant adverse effect associated with epoetin alfa is required to

answer this question. Noting that options 1 and 2 identify opposite conditions will assist in answering the question. Remember, hypertension is an adverse effect. Review this medication if you had difficulty with this question.
Level of Cognitive Ability: Analysis
Client Needs: Physiological Integrity
Integrated Process: Nursing Process/Data Collection
Content Area: Pharmacology
Reference: Lehne, R. (2004). *Pharmacology for nursing care* (5th ed.). Philadelphia: W.B. Saunders, pp. 588, 592.

22. *Answer:* **4**
Rationale: Epoetin alfa stimulates erythropoiesis. Initial effects are noted within 1 to 2 weeks and hematocrit levels reach normal levels in 2 to 3 months. Therefore, this medication is not intended for clients who require immediate correction of severe anemia, and it is not a substitute for emergency transfusions.
Test-Taking Strategy: Recalling that the medication stimulates erythropoiesis will assist in directing you to option 4. Review this medication and its therapeutic effects if you had difficulty with this question.
Level of Cognitive Ability: Analysis
Client Needs: Physiological Integrity
Integrated Process: Nursing Process/Evaluation
Content Area: Pharmacology
Reference: Lehne, R. (2004). *Pharmacology for nursing care* (5th ed.). Philadelphia: W.B. Saunders, p. 589.

23. *Answer:* **3**
Rationale: The client should be instructed not to shake the medicine bottle. The medication should be refrigerated but not frozen. Syringes with a 5/8 inch needle are used to administer subcutaneous injections.
Test-Taking Strategy: Use the process of elimination. Recalling that this medication needs to be refrigerated will direct you to option 3. Review the teaching points related to this medication if you had difficulty with this question.
Level of Cognitive Ability: Application
Client Needs: Health Promotion and Maintenance
Integrated Process: Teaching/Learning
Content Area: Pharmacology
Reference: Lehne, R. (2004). *Pharmacology for nursing care* (5th ed.). Philadelphia: W.B. Saunders, p. 588.

24. *Answer:* **3**
Rationale: The client who is receiving Amphojel should take the medication with meals. The phosphate-binding effect is best when it is taken with food. If tablets are used, they should be chewed well before swallowing.
Test-Taking Strategy: Use the process of elimination. Note that options 1, 2, and 4 are similar in that they all suggest administering the medication without a food item. Review this medication if you had difficulty with this question.
Level of Cognitive Ability: Application
Client Needs: Physiological Integrity
Integrated Process: Nursing Process/Implementation
Content Area: Pharmacology
Reference: Lehne, R. (2004). *Pharmacology for nursing care* (5th ed.). Philadelphia: W.B. Saunders, p. 831.

25. *Answer:* **3**

Rationale: Cholinergic overdose can occur with bethanechol. The antidote is atropine sulfate administered subcutaneous or by the intravenous route, which should be readily available for use should overdose occur. Protamine sulfate is the antidote for heparin. Vitamin K is the antidote for Coumadin. Mucomyst is the antidote for acetaminophen (Tylenol) overdose.

Test-Taking Strategy: Knowledge regarding the antidotes for certain medication overdoses is required to answer this question. Review these antidotes if you had difficulty with this question.

Level of Cognitive Ability: Application
Client Needs: Physiological Integrity
Integrated Process: Nursing Process/Implementation
Content Area: Pharmacology
Reference: Hodgson, B., & Kizior, R. (2005). *Saunders nursing drug handbook 2005*. Philadelphia: W.B. Saunders, p. 121.

ALTERNATE FORMAT QUESTION: CHART-EXHIBIT

Answer: **2**

Rationale: Cinoxacin should be administered with caution in clients with renal impairment. The dosage should be reduced, and failure to do so could result in accumulation of cinoxacin to toxic levels. Therefore, the nurse would verify the prescription with the physician if the client had a documented history of renal insufficiency. The laboratory test result and diagnostic test result are normal findings. Folic acid (vitamin B_6) may be prescribed for a client with renal insufficiency to prevent anemia.

Test-Taking Strategy: Focus on the issue, the need to contact the physician. Eliminate options 1 and 4 because the laboratory test result and diagnostic test result are normal findings. From the remaining options, note the disorder in the client's history. This will direct you to option 2. Review the contraindications associated with this medication if you had difficulty with this question.

Level of Cognitive Ability: Analysis
Client Needs: Physiological Integrity
Integrated Process: Nursing Process/Implementation
Content Area: Pharmacology
Reference: Lehne, R. (2004). *Pharmacology for nursing care* (5th ed.). Philadelphia: W.B. Saunders, p. 937.

REFERENCES

Hodgson, B., & Kizior, R. (2005). *Saunders nursing drug handbook 2005*. Philadelphia: W.B. Saunders.

Lehne, R. (2004). *Pharmacology for nursing care* (5th ed.). Philadelphia: W.B. Saunders.

McKenry, L., & Salerno, E. (2003). *Mosby's pharmacology in nursing* (21st ed.). St. Louis: Mosby.

The Adult Client with an Eye or Ear Disorder

PYRAMID TERMS

accommodation Process by which a clear visual image is maintained as the gaze is shifted from a distant to a near point.

astigmatism Corneal curvature; eye may be hyperopic or myopic.

cataracts An opacity of the lens that distorts the image projected onto the retina; can progress to blindness.

conductive hearing loss When sound waves are blocked to the inner ear fibers because of external ear or middle ear disorders. Disorders can often be corrected with no damage to hearing, or minimal permanent hearing loss.

cycloplegia Refers to the paralysis of the ciliary muscles by medications that block muscarinic receptors. Cycloplegia causes blurred vision because the shape of the lens can no longer be adjusted to near-vision.

emmetropia A state of normal vision characterized by ideal refraction of the eye.

fenestration Removal of the stapes with a small hole drilled in the footplate, and a prosthesis is connected between the incus and foot plate. Sounds cause the prosthesis to vibrate in the same manner as did the stapes.

glaucoma Increased intraocular pressure as a result of inadequate drainage of aqueous humor from the canal of Schlemm or overproduction of aqueous humor. The condition damages the optic nerve and can result in blindness.

hyperopia Farsightedness; objects converge to a point behind the retina. Vision beyond 20 feet is normal, but near-vision is poor. Correction is done by a convex lens.

legally blind If the best visual acuity with corrective lenses in the better eye is 20/200 or less, or if visual acuity is less than 20 degrees of the visual field in the better eye.

Meniere's syndrome A syndrome, also called endolymphatic hydrops, which refers to dilation of the endolymphatic system by overproduction or decreased reabsorption of endolymphatic fluid. It is characterized by tinnitus, unilateral sensorineural hearing loss, and vertigo.

miosis Refers to a constricted pupil; achieved primarily by stimulating the muscarinic receptors of the sphincter muscles.

miotics Medications that cause contraction of the pupil.

mydriasis Refers to a dilated pupil; achieved by blocking the muscarinic receptors of the sphincter muscles or by stimulating the alpha receptors of the dilator muscles.

mydriatics Medications that dilate the pupil.

myopia Nearsightedness; rays coming from an object are focused in front of the retina. Near-vision is normal but distant vision is defective. A biconcave lens is used for correction.

otosclerosis Disease of the labyrinthine capsule of the middle ear that results in a bony overgrowth of tissue surrounding the ossicles; causes the development of irregular areas of new bone formation and fixation of the bones. Stapes fixation leads to a conductive hearing loss.

presbycusis Common cause of sensorineural hearing loss associated with aging.

refraction Process of bending light rays so as to focus an image on the retina.

retinal detachment Occurs when the layers of the retina separate because of the accumulation of fluid between them, or when both retinal layers elevate away from the choroid as a result of a tumor. Partial separation becomes complete if untreated. When detachment becomes complete, blindness occurs.

sensorineural hearing loss A pathological process of the inner ear or of the sensory fibers that lead to the cerebral cortex; is often permanent. Measures must be taken to reduce further damage or to attempt to amplify sound as a means of improving hearing to some degree.

PYRAMID TO SUCCESS

Pyramid points focus on nursing interventions for clients with impairment in sight or hearing and on the nursing care related to disorders such as cataracts, glaucoma, and retinal detachment. Pyramid points also focus on emergency interventions for eye and ear disorders and injuries. Review nursing care related to organ donation for the donor and recipient. Pyramid points also focus on client instructions related to medication administration, sensory perceptual alterations and safety issues, and available support systems. The Integrated Processes addressed in this unit include Caring, Clinical Problem Solving Process (Nursing Process), Communication and Documentation, and Teaching/Learning.

▲ CLIENT NEEDS

Safe, Effective Care Environment

Accident prevention related to sensory impairments
Asepsis with procedures and treatments
Client rights
Communication techniques for impaired vision and hearing
Consultation with members of the health care team
Establishing priorities
Informed consent for invasive procedures
Organ donation
Standard precautions

Health Promotion and Maintenance

Aging process
Data collection related to eye and ear disorders
Expected body image changes
Home care instructions following procedures related to the eye and ear
Instructions regarding the administration of eye and ear medications
Reinforcement regarding the importance of compliance to the prescribed therapy
The prevention and early detection of health problems and diseases related to the eye and the ear

Psychosocial Integrity

Ability to cope with feelings of isolation and loss of independence
Available community resources
Family support systems
Role changes
Sensory perceptual alterations
Threat to vision or hearing loss

Physiological Integrity

Care of assistive devices such as glasses, contact lenses, and hearing aids

Complications related to procedures
Expected responses to therapy
Medical emergencies
Pharmacological therapy
Self-care limitations

REFERENCES

Black, J., & Hawks, J. (2005). *Medical-surgical nursing: Clinical management for positive outcomes* (7th ed.). Philadelphia: W.B. Saunders.

Chernecky, C., & Berger, B. (2004). *Laboratory tests and diagnostic procedures* (4th ed.). Philadelphia: W.B. Saunders.

Christensen, B., & Kockrow, E. (2003). *Adult health nursing* (4th ed.). St. Louis: Mosby.

Christensen, B., & Kockrow, E. (2003). *Foundations of nursing* (4th ed.). St. Louis: Mosby.

Fortinash, K., & Holoday-Worret, P. (2004). *Psychiatric mental health nursing* (3rd ed.). St. Louis: Mosby.

Harkreader, H., & Hogan, M.A. (2004). *Fundamentals of nursing: Caring and clinical judgment* (2nd ed.). Philadelphia: W.B. Saunders.

Hodgson, B., & Kizior, R. (2005). *Saunders nursing drug handbook 2005.* Philadelphia: W.B. Saunders.

Lewis, S., Heitkemper, M., & Dirksen, S. (2004). *Medical-surgical nursing: Assessment and management of clinical problems* (6th ed.). St. Louis: Mosby.

Linton, A., & Maebius, N. (2003). *Introduction to medical-surgical nursing* (3rd ed.). Philadelphia: W.B. Saunders.

McKenry, L., & Salerno, E. (2003). *Mosby's pharmacology in nursing* (21st ed.). St. Louis: Mosby.

National Council of State Boards of Nursing. (2005). *Detailed test plan for the National Council licensure examination for practical/vocational nurses.* Chicago: Author.

Pagana, K., & Pagana, T. (2003). *Mosby's diagnostic and laboratory test reference* (6th ed.). St. Louis: Mosby.

Perry, A., & Potter, P. (2002). *Clinical nursing skills and techniques* (5th ed.). St. Louis: Mosby.

Phipps, W., Monahan, F., Sands, J., Marek, J., & Neighbors, M. (2003). *Medical-surgical nursing: Health and illness perspectives* (7th ed.). St. Louis: Mosby.

Potter, P., & Perry, A. (2003). *Essentials for practice* (5th ed.). St. Louis: Mosby.

The Eye and the Ear

▲

I. ANATOMY AND PHYSIOLOGY OF THE EYE

A. The eye
   1. The eye is 1 inch in diameter
   2. It is located in the anterior portion of the orbit
   3. The orbit is the bony structure of the skull that surrounds the eye and offers protection to the eye

B. Layers of the eye
   1. External layer
      a. The fibrous coat that supports the eye
      b. Contains the sclera, which is an opaque white tissue
      c. Contains the cornea, which is a dense transparent layer
   2. Middle layer
      a. The second layer of the eyeball
      b. Is vascular and heavily pigmented
      c. Consists of the choroid, the ciliary body, and the iris
      d. The choroid is the dark brown membrane located between the sclera and the retina
      e. The choroid lines most of the sclera and is attached to the retina, but can easily detach from the sclera
      f. The choroid contains many blood vessels and supplies nutrients to the retina
      g. The ciliary body connects the choroid with the iris and secretes aqueous humor that helps give the eye its shape
      h. The iris is the colored portion of the eye, is located in front of the lens, and has a central circular opening called the pupil
   3. Internal layer
      a. Consists of the retina
      b. The retina is a thin, delicate structure in which the fibers of the optic nerve are distributed
      c. The retina is bordered externally by the choroid and sclera and internally by the vitreous
      d. The retina contains blood vessels and photoreceptors called rods and cones

C. Vitreous body
   1. Contains a gelatinous substance that occupies the vitreous chamber, which is the space between the lens and the retina
   2. It transmits light and gives shape to the posterior eye

D. Vitreous
   1. A gel-like substance that maintains the shape of the eye
   2. Provides additional physical support to the retina

E. Rods and cones
   1. Rods are responsible for peripheral vision and function at reduced levels of illumination
   2. Cones function at bright levels of illumination and are responsible for color vision and central vision

F. Optic disk
   1. A creamy pink to white depressed area in the retina
   2. The optic nerve enters and exits the eyeball at this area
   3. This area is called the blind spot because it contains only nerve fibers, lacks photoreceptor cells, and is insensitive to light

G. Macula lutea
   1. A small, oval, yellowish-pink area located laterally and temporally to the optic disk
   2. The central depressed part of the macula is the fovea centralis, where most acute vision occurs

H. Aqueous humor
   1. A clear watery fluid that fills the anterior and posterior chambers of the eye
   2. Produced by the ciliary processes; the fluid drains into the canal of Schlemm

3. The anterior chamber lies between the cornea and the iris
4. The posterior chamber lies between the iris and the lens

I. Canal of Schlemm
   1. A passageway that extends completely around the eye
   2. Permits fluid to drain out of the eye into the systemic circulation so a constant intraocular pressure is maintained

J. Lens
   1. A transparent circular structure behind the iris and in front of the vitreous body
   2. Bends rays of light so that the light falls on the retina

K. Pupils
   1. Control the amount of light that enters the eye and reaches the retina
   2. Darkness produces dilation
   3. Light produces constriction

L. Conjunctivae
   1. The thin, transparent mucous membranes
   2. Line the posterior surface of each eyelid and is located over the sclera

M. Lacrimal gland
   1. Produces tears
   2. Tears are drained through the punctum into the lacrimal duct and sac

N. Eye muscles
   1. Muscles do not work independently but work in conjunction with the muscle that produces the opposite movement
   2. Rectus muscles: Exert their pull when the eye turns temporally
   3. Oblique muscles: Exert their pull when the eye turns nasally

O. Nerves
   1. Cranial nerve II: Optic nerve (nerve of sight)
   2. Cranial nerve III: Oculomotor
   3. Cranial nerve IV: Trochlear
   4. Cranial nerve VI: Abducens

P. Blood vessels
   1. Ophthalmic artery: Major artery supplying the structures in the eye
   2. Ophthalmic veins: Venous drainage occurs through the veins

II. ASSESSMENT OF VISION (Box 54-1)

A. Acuity
   1. Visual acuity tests measure the client's distance and near vision
   2. Snellen chart
      a. A simple tool to record visual acuity
      b. The client stands 20 feet from the chart, covers one eye, and uses the other eye to read the line that appears most clearly

---

BOX 54-1

Assessment of Vision

Snellen chart
Confrontational test
Extraocular muscle function
Color vision
Ophthalmoscopy

---

      c. If the client can do this accurately, the client reads the next lower line
      d. This sequence is repeated until the client is unable to identify more than half of the characters on the line correctly
      e. The procedure is repeated for the other eye
      f. The findings are recorded as a comparison between what the client can read at 20 feet and the number of feet normally required by an individual to read the same line
      g. A result of 20/50 means that the client is able to read at 20 feet from the chart what a healthy eye can read at 50 feet
      h. Clients who wear corrective lenses other than for reading should have their vision tested with the lens in place

B. Confrontational test
   1. Performed to examine visual fields or peripheral vision
   2. The examiner and the client sit facing each other
   3. The client is asked to look directly into the eyes of the examiner throughout the test
   4. The examiner covers their right eye while the client covers his or her left eye
   5. The examiner moves a finger from a nonvisible area into the client's line of vision
   6. Both examiner and client should see the object at approximately the same time
   7. When the client sees the object coming into the line of vision, the client informs the examiner
   8. The procedure is repeated on the opposite eye
   9. The test assumes that the examiner has normal peripheral vision

C. Extraocular muscle function
   1. Six cardinal positions of gaze
      a. Client's right (lateral position)
      b. Upward and right (temporal position)
      c. Down and right
      d. Client's left (lateral position)
      e. Upward and left (temporal position)
      f. Down and left
   2. Client holds head still and is asked to move eyes and to follow a small object
   3. The examiner notes for any parallel movements of the eye or for nystagmus, an involuntary, rhythmic, rapid twitching of the eyeballs

D. Color vision
   1. Tests for color vision involve picking numbers or letters out of a complex and colorful picture
   2. Ishihara chart
      a. Consists of numbers that are composed of colored dots located within a circle of colored dots
      b. Client is asked to read the numbers on the chart
      c. Each eye is tested separately
      d. The test is sensitive for the diagnosis of red-green blindness but not effective for the detection of blue discrimination
E. Pupils
   1. Round and of equal size
   2. Increasing light causes pupillary constriction
   3. Decreasing light causes pupillary dilation
   4. Constriction of both pupils is a normal response to direct light
   5. The client is asked to look straight ahead while the examiner quickly brings a beam of light (flashlight) in from the side and directs it onto the eye
   6. The constriction of the eye is a direct response to the shining of a light into that eye; constriction of the opposite eye is known as a consensual response
F. Sclera and cornea
   1. Normal sclera color is white
   2. A yellow color to the sclera may indicate jaundice or systemic problems
   3. In a dark-skinned person, the sclera may normally appear yellow; pigmented dots may be present
   4. The cornea is transparent, smooth, shiny, and bright
   5. Cloudy areas or specks on the cornea may be the result an accident or eye injury
G. Ophthalmoscopy
   1. An instrument is used to examine the external structures and the interior of the eye
   2. The room is darkened so that the pupil will dilate

▲

III. DIAGNOSTIC TESTS FOR THE EYE (Box 54-2)

A. Fluorescein angiography
   1. Description: Detailed imaging and recording of ocular circulation by a series of photographs after the administration of a dye
   2. Interventions preprocedure
      a. Assess the client for allergies and previous reactions to dyes
      b. Obtain informed consent
      c. A mydriatic medication, which causes pupil dilation, is instilled in the eye 1 hour before the test
      d. The dye is injected into a vein of the client's arm
      e. Inform the client that the dye may cause the skin to appear yellow for several hours after the

---

BOX 54-2

Diagnostic Tests for the Eye

Fluorescein angiography
Computed tomography
Slit lamp
Corneal staining
Tonometry

---

test and is gradually eliminated through the urine
      f. The client may experience nausea, vomiting, sneezing, paresthesia of the tongue, or pain at the injection site
      g. If hives appear, oral or intramuscular (IM) antihistamines such as diphenhydramine (Benadryl) is administered, as prescribed
   3. Postprocedure interventions
      a. Encourage rest
      b. Encourage fluids to assist in eliminating the dye from the client's system
      c. Remind the client that the yellow skin appearance will disappear
      d. Instruct the client that the urine will appear bright green until the dye is excreted
      e. Instruct the client to avoid direct sunlight for a few hours after the test
      f. Instruct the client that the photophobia will continue until pupil size returns to normal
B. Computed tomography
   1. Description
      a. An x-ray beam scans the skull and orbits of the eye
      b. A cross-sectional image is formed by the use of a computer
      c. Contrast material is not usually administered
   2. Interventions
      a. No special client preparation or follow-up care is required
      b. Instruct the client that he or she will be positioned in a confined space and needs to keep the head still during the procedure
C. Slit lamp
   1. Description
      a. Allows examination of the anterior ocular structures under microscopic magnification
      b. The client leans on a chin rest to stabilize the head while a narrowed beam of light is aimed so it illuminates only a narrow segment of the eye
   2. Interventions
      a. Explain the procedure to the client
      b. Advise the client about the brightness of the light and the need to look forward at a point over the examiner's ear

▲ D. Corneal staining
  1. Description
     a. Instillation of a topical dye into the conjuctival sac to outline irregularities of the corneal surface that are not easily visible
     b. The eye is viewed through a blue filter; a bright green color indicates areas of a nonintact corneal epithelium
  2. Interventions
     a. If the client wears contact lens, they must be removed
     b. The client is instructed to blink after the dye has been applied to distribute the dye evenly across the cornea
▲ E. Tonometry
  1. Description
     a. The test is primarily used to assess for an increase of intraocular pressure and potential **glaucoma**
     b. Normal ocular pressure is 10 to 21 mm Hg
  2. Interventions
     a. Each eye is anesthetized
     b. The client is asked to stare forward at a point above the examiner's ear
     c. A flattened cone is brought into contact with the cornea
     d. The amount of pressure needed to flatten the cornea is measured
     e. The client must be instructed to avoid rubbing the eye following the examination if the eye has been anesthetized because the potential for scratching the cornea exists

▲

▲ **IV. DISORDERS OF THE EYE**
  A. Risk factors related to eye disorders (Box 54-3)
  B. **Legally blind**
  1. Description: If the best visual acuity with corrective lenses in the better eye is 20/200 or less, or if visual acuity is less than 20 degrees of the visual field in the better eye
▲ 2. Interventions
     a. When speaking to the client who has limited sight or is blind, the nurse uses a normal tone of voice
     b. Alert the client when approaching

BOX 54-3

Risk Factors of Eye Disorders

Aging process
Congenital
Diabetes mellitus
Hereditary
Medications
Trauma
---

     c. Orient the client to the environment
     d. Use a focal point and provide further orientation to the environment from that focal point
     e. Allow the client to touch objects in the room
     f. Use the clock placement of foods on the meal tray to orient the client
     g. Promote independence as much as is possible
     h. Provide radios, televisions, and clocks that give the time orally, or provide a Braille watch
     i. When ambulating, allow the client to grasp the nurse's arm at the elbow; the nurse keeps his or her arm close to the body so that the client can detect the direction of movement
     j. Instruct the client to remain one step behind the nurse when ambulating
     k. Instruct the client in the use of the cane used for the blind client, which is differentiated from other canes by its straight shape, white color, and red tip
     l. Instruct the client that the cane is held in the dominant hand several inches off the floor
     m. Instruct the client that the cane sweeps the ground where the client's foot will be placed next to determine the presence of obstacles
C. **Cataracts**   ▲
  1. Description
     a. An opacity of the lens that distorts the image projected onto the retina, which can progress to blindness
     b. Causes include the aging process (senile **cataracts**), inherited (congenital **cataracts**), and injury (traumatic **cataracts**); can also occur as a result of another eye disease (secondary **cataracts**)
     c. Intervention is indicated when visual acuity has been reduced to a level that the client finds unacceptable or is adversely affecting lifestyle
  2. Data collection
     a. Opaque or cloudy white pupil
     b. Gradual loss of vision
     c. Blurred vision
     d. Decreased color perception
     e. Vision that is better in dim light with pupil dilation
     f. Photophobia
     g. Absence of the red reflex
  3. Interventions
     a. Surgical removal of the lens, one eye at a time
     b. Extracapsular extraction: The lens is lifted out without removing the lens capsule; may be performed by phacoemulsification, in which the lens is broken up by ultrasonic vibrations and extracted
     c. Intracapsular extraction: The lens is removed within its capsule through a small incision

d. A partial iridectomy may be performed with the lens extraction to prevent acute secondary **glaucoma**

e. A lens implantation may be performed at the time of the surgical procedure

4. Preoperative interventions

a. Instruct the client regarding the postoperative measures to prevent or decrease intraocular pressure

b. Administer preoperative eye medications including **mydriatics** and **cycloplegics**, as prescribed

5. Postoperative interventions

a. Elevate the head of the bed 30 to 45 degrees

b. Turn the client to the back or unoperative side

c. Maintain an eye patch; orient the client to the environment

d. Position the client's personal belongings to the unoperative side

e. Use side rails for safety

f. Assist with ambulation

6. Client education (Box 54-4)

 D. Glaucoma

1. Description

a. Increased intraocular pressure as a result of inadequate drainage of aqueous humor from the canal of Schlemm or overproduction of aqueous humor

b. The condition damages the optic nerve and can result in blindness

2. Types (Box 54-5)

3. Data collection

a. Progressive loss of peripheral vision followed by loss of central vision

b. Elevated intraocular pressure (normal pressure is 10 to 21 mm Hg)

c. Vision worsening in the evening with difficulty adjusting to dark rooms

d. Blurred vision

e. Halos around white lights

f. Frontal headaches

g. Eye pain

h. Photophobia

i. Lacrimation

j. Progressive loss of central vision

4. Interventions for acute **glaucoma**

a. Treat as a medical emergency

b. Administer medications as prescribed to lower intraocular pressure

c. Prepare the client for peripheral iridectomy, which allows aqueous humor to flow from the posterior to anterior chamber

5. Interventions for chronic **glaucoma**

a. Instruct the client on the importance of medications (**miotics**) to constrict the pupils, (carbonic anhydrase inhibitors) to decrease the production of aqueous humor, and (beta blockers) to decrease the production of aqueous humor and intraocular pressure

b. Instruct the client on the need for lifelong medication use

c. Instruct the client to wear a Medic-Alert bracelet

d. Instruct the client to avoid anticholinergic medications

e. Instruct the client to report eye pain, halos around the eyes, and changes in vision to the physician

f. Instruct the client that when maximal medical therapy has failed to halt the progression of visual field loss and optic nerve damage, surgery will be recommended

---

BOX 54-4

Client Education Following Cataract Surgery

Avoid eye straining.

Avoid rubbing or placing pressure on the eyes.

Avoid rapid movements, straining, sneezing, coughing, bending, vomiting, or lifting objects over 5 pounds.

Use measures to prevent constipation.

Change dressing and use eyedrops and medications, as prescribed.

Wipe excess drainage or tearing with a sterile wet cotton ball from the inner to the outward canthus.

Use an eye shield at bedtime.

If a lens implantation procedure is not performed, the eye cannot accommodate and glasses must be worn at all times.

Cataract glasses replace central vision only and cause objects to appear closer; therefore, the client needs to accommodate, judge distance, and climb stairs carefully.

Contact lenses provide sharp visual acuity, but dexterity is needed to insert them.

Contact the physician for any decrease in vision, severe eye pain, or increase in eye discharge.

BOX 54-5

Types of Glaucoma

Acute closed-angle or narrow-angle glaucoma: Results from obstruction to outflow to aqueous humor

Chronic closed-angle glaucoma: Follows an untreated attack of acute closed-angle glaucoma

Chronic open-angle glaucoma: Results from overproduction or obstruction to the outflow of aqueous humor

Acute glaucoma: A rapid onset of intraocular pressure higher than 50 to 70 mm Hg

Chronic glaucoma: A slow, progressive, gradual onset of intraocular pressure higher than 30 to 50 mm Hg

g. Prepare the client for trabeculoplasty as prescribed to facilitate aqueous humor drainage

h. Prepare the client for trabeculectomy as prescribed, which allows drainage of aqueous humor into the conjunctival spaces by the creation of an opening

▲ E. Retinal detachment

1. Description

   a. Occurs when the layers of the retina separate because of the accumulation of fluid between them, or when both retinal layers elevate away from the choroid as a result of a tumor

   b. Partial separation becomes complete if untreated

   c. When detachment becomes complete, blindness occurs

2. Data collection

   a. Flashes of light

   b. Floaters

   c. Increase in blurred vision

   d. Sense of a curtain being drawn

   e. Loss of a portion of the visual field

3. Immediate interventions

   ▲ a. Provide bed rest

   ▲ b. Cover both eyes with patches to prevent further detachment

   c. Speak to the client before approaching

   d. Position the client's head as prescribed

   e. Protect the client from injury

   f. Avoid jerky head movements

   g. Minimize eye stress

   h. Prepare the client for the surgical procedure as prescribed

4. Surgical procedures

   a. Draining of fluid from the subretinal space so that the retina can return to the normal position

   b. Sealing retinal breaks by cryosurgery, a cold probe applied to the sclera, to stimulate an inflammatory response leading to adhesions

   c. Diathermy, the use of an electrode needle and heat through the sclera, to stimulate an inflammatory response

   d. Laser therapy, to stimulate an inflammatory response by sealing small retinal tears before the detachment occurs

   e. Scleral buckling, to hold the choroid and retina together with a splint until scar tissue forms, closing the tear

   f. Insertion of gas or silicone oil to encourage attachment, because these agents have a specific gravity lower than that of the vitreous humor or air, and can float against the retina

   ▲ 5. Postoperative interventions

   a. Maintain eye patches bilaterally as prescribed

   b. Monitor for hemorrhage

c. Prevent nausea and vomiting and monitor for restlessness, which can cause hemorrhage

d. Monitor for sudden, sharp eye pain (notify the physician)

e. Encourage deep breathing but avoid coughing

f. Provide bed rest for 1 to 2 days, as prescribed

g. Position the client, as prescribed

h. If gas has been inserted, position as prescribed on the abdomen and turn the head so unaffected eye is down

i. Administer eye medications, as prescribed

j. Assist the client with activities of daily living

k. Avoid sudden head movements or anything that increases intraocular pressure

l. Instruct the client to limit reading for 3 to 5 weeks

m. Instruct the client to avoid squinting, straining and constipation, lifting heavy objects, and bending from the waist

n. Instruct the client to wear dark glasses during the day and an eye patch at night

o. Encourage follow-up care because of the danger of recurrence or occurrence in the other eye

F. Hyphema (Box 54-6)

1. Description

   a. The presence of blood in the anterior chamber

   b. Occurs as a result of an injury

   c. The condition usually resolves in 5 to 7 days

2. Interventions

   a. Encourage rest with the client in semi-Fowler's position

   b. Avoid sudden eye movements for 3 to 5 days to decrease the likelihood of bleeding

   c. Administer cycloplegic eyedrops as prescribed to place the eye at rest

   d. Instruct the client in the use of eye shields or eye patches, as prescribed

   e. Instruct the client to restrict reading and watching television

G. Contusions

1. Description

   a. Bleeding into the soft tissue as a result of an injury

   b. Causes a black eye; the discoloration disappears in approximately 10 days

   c. Pain, photophobia, edema, and diplopia may occur

BOX 54-6

Types of Eye Injuries

Hyphema
Contusion
Foreign body
Penetrating object
Chemical burn

2. Interventions
   a. Place ice on the eye immediately
   b. Instruct the client to receive an eye examination
H. Foreign bodies
   1. Description: An object such as dust that enters the eye
   2. Interventions
      a. Have the client look upward, expose the lower lid, wet a cotton-tipped applicator with sterile normal saline, and gently twist the swab over the particle and remove it
      b. If the particle cannot be seen, have the client look downward, place a cotton applicator horizontally on the outer surface of the upper eye lid, grasp the lashes, and pull the upper lid outward and over the cotton applicator; if the particle is seen, gently twist swab over it to remove
I. Penetrating objects
   1. Description: An injury that occurs to the eye in which an object penetrates the eye
   2. Interventions
      a. Never remove the object because it may be holding ocular structures in place; the object must be removed by the physician
      b. Cover the object with a cup
      c. Do not allow the client to bend
      d. Do not place pressure on eye
      e. Client is to be seen by a physician immediately
J. Chemical burns
   1. Description: An eye injury in which a caustic substance enters the eye
   2. Interventions
      a. Treatment should begin immediately
      b. Flush the eyes at the site of injury with water for at least 15 to 20 minutes
      c. At the scene of the injury, obtain a sample of the chemical involved
      d. At the emergency room, the eye is irrigated with normal saline solution or an ophthalmic irrigation solution
      e. The solution is directed across the cornea and toward the lateral canthus
      f. Prepare for visual acuity assessment
      g. Apply an antibiotic ointment, as prescribed
      h. Cover the eye with a patch, as prescribed
K. Enucleation and exenteration
   1. Description
      a. Enucleation: Removal of the entire eyeball
      b. Exenteration: Removal of the eyeball and surrounding tissues and bone
      c. Performed for the removal of ocular tumors
      d. After the eye is removed, a ball implant is inserted to provide a firm base for socket prosthesis and to facilitate the best cosmetic result
      e. A prosthesis is fitted approximately 1 month after surgery

2. Preoperative interventions
   a. Provide emotional support to the client
   b. Encourage the client to verbalize feelings related to loss
3. Postoperative interventions
   a. Monitor vital signs
   b. Check the pressure patch or dressing for drainage or bleeding
   c. Report changes in vital signs or the presence of bright red drainage on the pressure patch or dressing
L. Organ donation
   1. Donor eyes
      a. Obtained from cadavers
      b. Must be enucleated soon after death because of rapid endothelial cell death
      c. Must be stored in a preserving solution
      d. Storage, handling, and coordination of donor tissue with surgeons is provided by a network of state eye bank associations across the country
   2. Care of the deceased client as a potential eye donor
      a. Discuss the option of eye donation with the physician and family
      b. Raise the head of the bed 30 degrees
      c. Instill antibiotic eyedrops, as prescribed
      d. Close the eyes and apply a small ice pack to the closed eyes
   3. Preoperative care to the recipient
      a. Recipient may be told of tissue availability only several hours to 1 day before the surgery
      b. Assist in alleviating client anxiety
      c. Monitor eye for signs of infection
      d. Report the presence of any redness, watery or purulent drainage, or edema around the eye to the physician
      e. Instill antibiotic drops into the eye as prescribed to reduce the number of microorganisms present
      f. Monitor intravenour (IV) fluids and medications, as prescribed
   4. Postoperative care of the recipient
      a. Eye is covered with a pressure patch and protective shield that are left in place until the next day
      b. Do not remove or change the dressing without a physician's order
      c. Monitor vital signs
      d. Monitor level of consciousness
      e. Check dressing
      f. Position the client on the nonoperative side to reduce intraocular pressure
      g. Orient the client frequently
      h. Monitor for complications of bleeding, wound leakage, infection, and graft rejection
      i. Instruct the client how to apply a patch and eye shield

j. Instruct the client to wear the eye shield at night for 1 month and whenever around small children or pets

k. Advise the client not to rub the eye

5. Graft rejection (Box 54-7)

a. Can occur at any time

b. Inform the client of the signs of rejection

c. Signs include *r*edness, *s*welling, decreased *v*ision, and *p*ain (**RSVP**)

d. Treated with topical corticosteroids

V. ANATOMY AND PHYSIOLOGY OF THE EAR

A. Functions

1. Hearing

2. Maintenance of balance

B. External ear

1. Embedded in the temporal bone bilaterally at the level of the eyes

2. Extends from the auricle through the external canal to the tympanic membrane or eardrum

3. Includes the mastoid process, which is the body ridge located over the temporal bone

C. Middle ear

1. Consists of the medial side of the tympanic membrane

2. Contains three bony ossicles

a. Malleus

b. Incus

c. Stapes

3. The tympanic membrane is a thick transparent sheet of tissue that provides a barrier between the external and middle ear

4. The middle ear is protected from the inner ear by the round and the oval window membranes

5. The eustachian tube opens into the middle ear and allows for equalization of pressure on both sides of the tympanic membrane

D. Inner ear

1. Contains the semicircular canals, the cochlea, and the distal end of the eighth cranial nerve

2. The semicircular canals contain fluid and hair cells connected to sensory nerve fibers of the vestibular portion of the eighth cranial nerve

3. Maintains sense of balance or equilibrium

4. Cochlea: Spiral-shaped organ of hearing

5. Organ of Corti: Receptor and organ of hearing

6. Eighth cranial nerve

a. Cochlear branch: Transmits neuroimpulses from the cochlea to the brain, where they are interpreted as sound

b. Vestibular branch: Maintains balance and equilibrium

E. Hearing and equilibrium

1. The external ear conducts sound waves to the middle ear

2. The middle ear, also called the tympanic cavity, conducts sound waves to the inner ear

3. The middle ear is filled with air, which is kept at atmospheric pressure by the opening of the eustachian tube

4. The inner ear contains sensory receptors for sound and for equilibrium

5. The receptors in the inner ear transmit sound waves and changes in body position to the nerve impulses

VI. ASSESSMENT OF THE EAR (Box 54-8)

A. Otoscopic examination

1. The speculum is introduced into the external canal to visualize the tympanic membrane

2. The normal external canal is pink and intact without lesions; contains various amounts of cerumen and fine little hairs

3. The tympanic membrane is transparent, opaque, pearly gray, and slightly concave

B. Auditory assessment

1. Sound is transmitted by air conduction and bone conduction

2. Air conduction takes two to three times longer than bone conduction

3. Hearing loss is categorized as **conductive**, **sensorineural**, and mixed **conductive** and **sensorineural**

4. **Conductive hearing loss** is caused by any physical obstruction to the transmission of sound waves

---

BOX 54-7

Signs of Graft Rejection of a Corneal Transplant: "RSVP"

Redness
Swelling
Visual acuity decreased
Pain

BOX 54-8

Assessment of Hearing

Otoscopic examination
Voice test
Watch test
Tuning fork tests:
    Weber tuning fork test
    Rinne tuning fork test
Vestibular assessment:
    Test for falling
    Test for past pointing
    Gaze nystagmus evaluation
    Hallpike maneuver

5. **Sensorineural hearing loss** is caused by a defect in the organ of hearing, in the eightth cranial nerve, or in the brain itself
6. A mixed **conductive-sensorineural hearing loss** results in profound hearing loss
7. Tuning fork tests: Weber and the Rinne tuning fork tests assist in distinguishing **conductive hearing loss** from **sensorineural hearing loss**
8. The voice test and the watch test assesses for hearing acuity

C. Vestibular assessment
   1. Test for falling: A significant sway is a positive Romberg sign
   2. Test for past pointing
      a. The normal test response is that the client can easily return to the point of reference
      b. The client with a vestibular function problem lacks a normal sense of position and is unable to return the extended fingers to the point of reference; instead, the fingers deviate either to the right or left of the reference point
   3. Gaze nystagmus evaluation: Any spontaneous nystagmus, a constant and involuntary cyclic movement of the eyeball in any direction, represent a problem with the vestibular system
   4. Hallpike maneuver
      a. Assesses for positional vertigo or induced dizziness
      b. The client assumes a supine position and the head is rotated to one side for 1 minute
      c. A positive test results in nystagmus after 5 to 10 seconds

▲

VII. DIAGNOSTIC TESTS FOR THE EAR (Box 54-9)

A. Tomography
   1. Description
      a. May be performed with or without contrast medium
      b. Assesses the mastoid, middle ear, and inner ear structures
      c. Multiple x-rays of the head are obtained
      d. Especially helpful in the diagnosis of acoustic tumors
   2. Interventions
      a. All jewelry is removed
      b. Lead eye shields are used to cover the cornea to diminish the radiation dose to the eyes
      c. The client must remain still, in a supine position
      d. No follow-up care is required

B. Audiometry
   1. Description
      a. Measures hearing acuity
      b. Uses two types, pure tone audiometry and speech audiometry

   c. Pure tone audiometry is used to identify problems with hearing, speech, music, and other sounds in the environment
   d. In speech audiometry, the client's ability to hear spoken words is measured
   e. After testing, audiographic patterns are depicted on a graph to determine the type and level of the hearing loss
   2. Interventions
      a. Inform the client regarding the procedure
      b. Instruct the client to identify the sounds as they are heard

C. Electronystagmography
   1. Description
      a. A vestibular test that evaluates spontaneous and induced eye movements known as nystagmus
      b. Used to distinguish between normal nystagmus and either medication-induced nystagmus or nystagmus caused by a lesion in the central or peripheral vestibular pathway
      c. Records changing electrical fields with the movement of the eye, as monitored by electrodes placed on the skin around the eye
   2. Interventions
      a. The client is instructed to remain NPO for 3 hours before testing
      b. Unnecessary medications are omitted for 24 hours before testing
      c. Instruct the client that this is a long and tiring procedure
      d. The client should bring prescription eyeglasses to the examination
      e. Client sits and is instructed to gaze at lights, focus on a moving pattern, focus on a moving point, and then sit with his or her eyes closed
      f. While sitting in a chair, the client may be rotated to provide information about vestibular function
      g. In addition, the client's ears are irrigated with both cool and warm water, which may cause nausea and vomiting
      h. Following the procedure, the client begins taking clear fluids slowly and cautiously, because nausea and vomiting may occur
      i. Assistance with ambulation may also be necessary following the procedure

---

BOX 54-9

Diagnostic Tests for The Ear

Tomography
Audiometry
Electronystagmography

BOX 54-10

Risk Factors of Ear Disorders

Aging process
Infection
Medications
Ototoxicity
Trauma
Tumors

BOX 54-11

Signs of Hearing Loss

Frequently asking people to repeat statements
Straining to hear
Turning head or leaning forward to favor one ear
Shouting in conversation
Ringing in the ears
Failing to respond when not looking in the direction of the sound
Answering questions incorrectly
Raising the volume of the television or radio
Avoiding large groups
Better understanding of speech when in a small group
Withdrawing from social interactions

VIII. DISORDERS OF THE EAR

A. Risk factors related to ear disorders (Box 54-10)

B. **Conductive hearing loss**
   1. Description
      a. When sound waves are blocked to the inner ear fibers because of external ear or middle ear disorders
      b. Disorders can often be corrected with no damage to hearing, or minimal permanent hearing loss
   2. Causes
      a. Any inflammatory process or obstruction of the external or middle ear
      b. Tumors
      c. **Otosclerosis**
      d. A buildup of scar tissue on the ossicles from previous middle ear surgery

C. **Sensorineural hearing loss**
   1. Description
      a. A pathological process of the inner ear or of the sensory fibers that lead to the cerebral cortex
      b. Is often permanent; measures must be taken to reduce further damage or to attempt to amplify sound to improve hearing to some degree
   2. Causes
      a. Damage to the inner ear structures
      b. Damage to cranial nerve VIII
      c. Prolonged exposure to loud noise
      d. Medications
      e. Trauma
      f. Inherited disorders
      g. Metabolic and circulatory disorders
      h. Infections
      i. Surgery
      j. **Meniere's syndrome**
      k. Diabetes mellitus
      l. Myxedema

D. Mixed hearing loss
   1. Also known as **conductive-sensorineural hearing loss**
   2. Client has both **sensorineural** and **conductive hearing loss**

E. Signs of hearing loss and facilitating communication (Boxes 54-11 and 54-12)

BOX 54-12

Facilitating Communication

Use of written words if the client can see, read, and write
Providing plenty of light in the room
Getting the attention of the client before you begin to speak
Facing the client when speaking
Talking in a room without distracting noises
Moving close to the client and speaking slowly and clearly
Keeping hands and other objects away from the mouth when talking to the client
Talking in lower tones, because shouting is not helpful
Rephrasing sentences and repeating information
Validating with the client the understanding of statements made by asking the client to repeat what was said
Reading lips
Encouraging the client to wear glasses when talking to someone to improve vision for lip reading
Using sign language, which combines speech with hand movements that signify letters, words, or phrases
Using telephone amplifiers
Flashing lights that are activated by ringing of the telephone or doorbell
Specially trained dogs that help the client to be aware of sound and to alert the client of potential dangers

---

F. Cochlear implantation
   1. Used for **sensorineural hearing loss**
   2. A small computer converts sound waves into electrical impulses
   3. Electrodes are placed near the internal ear, with a computer device attached to the external ear
   4. Electronic impulses directly stimulate nerve fibers

G. Hearing aids
   1. Used for the client with **conductive hearing loss**
   2. Can help the client with **sensorineural loss**, although it is not as effective
   3. A difficulty that exists with its use is amplification of background noise as well as voices
   4. Client education (Box 54-13)

BOX 54-13

Client Education Regarding a Hearing Aid

Encourage client to begin using the hearing aid slowly to develop an adjustment to the device.

Adjust the volume to the minimal hearing level to prevent feedback squeaking.

Teach the client to concentrate on the sounds that are to be heard and to filter out background noise.

Instruct the client to clean ear mold with mild soap and water.

Avoid excessive wetting of the hearing aid and try to keep the hearing aid dry.

Clean the ear cannula of the hearing aid with a toothpick or pipe cleaner.

Turn off the hearing aid and remove the battery when not in use.

Keep extra batteries on hand.

Keep the hearing aid in a safe place.

Prevent hair sprays, oils, or other hair and face products from coming into contact with the receiver of the hearing aid.

BOX 54-14

Client Education Following Myringotomy

Avoid strenuous activities.

Avoid rapid head movements, bouncing, and bending over.

Avoid straining on bowel movement.

Avoid drinking through a straw.

Avoid traveling by air.

Avoid forceful coughing.

Avoid contact with persons with colds.

Avoid washing hair, showering, or getting the head wet for 1 week, as prescribed.

Instruct the client that if he or she needs to blow the nose, blow one side at a time with the mouth open.

Instruct the client to keep the ears dry by keeping a ball of cotton coated with petroleum jelly in the ear and to change the cotton ball daily.

Instruct the client to report excessive ear drainage to the physician.

H. **Presbycusis**
1. Description
    a. Associated with aging
    b. Leads to degeneration or atrophy of the ganglion cells in the cochlea and a loss of elasticity of the basilar membranes
    c. Leads to compromise of the vascular supply to the inner ear with changes in several areas of the ear structure
2. Data collection
    a. Hearing loss is gradual and bilateral
    b. Client states that he or she has no problem with hearing, but cannot understand what the words are
    c. Client thinks that the speaker is mumbling
I. External otitis
1. Description
    a. Infective inflammatory or allergic responses involving the structure of the external auditory canal or the auricles
    b. An irritating or infective agent comes into contact with the epithelial layer of the external ear
    c. This leads to either an allergic response or signs and symptoms of an infection
    d. The skin becomes red, swollen, and tender to touch on movement
    e. The extensive swelling of the canal can lead to **conductive hearing loss** because of obstruction
    f. It is more common in children, is termed *swimmer's ear*; occurs more often in hot, humid environments
    g. Prevention includes the elimination of irritating or infecting agents

2. Data collection
    a. Pain
    b. Itching
    c. Plugged feeling in the ear
    d. Redness and edema
    e. Exudate
    f. Hearing loss
3. Interventions
    a. Apply heat locally for 20 minutes three times a day
    b. Encourage rest to assist in reducing pain
    c. Administer antibiotics or steroids as prescribed
    d. Administer analgesics such as aspirin or acetaminophen (Tylenol) for the pain, as prescribed
    e. Instruct the client that the ears should be kept clean and dry
    f. Instruct the client to use earplugs for swimming
    g. Instruct the client that cotton-tipped applicators should not be used to dry ears because their use can lead to trauma to the canal
    h. Instruct the client that use of irritating agents such as hair products or headphones should be discontinued
J. Otitis media: See Chapter 31
    1. Myringotomy
        a. See Chapter 31
        b. Client education (Box 54-14)
K. Chronic otitis media
    1. Description
        a. A chronic infective, inflammatory, or allergic response involving the structure of the middle ear
        b. Surgical treatment is necessary to restore hearing

c. The type of surgery can vary and include either a simple reconstruction of the tympanic membrane, a myringoplasty, or replacement of the ossicles within the middle ear

d. A tympanoplasty, a reconstruction of the middle ear, may be attempted to improve **conductive hearing loss**

2. Preoperative interventions

a. Administer antibiotic drops, as prescribed

b. Clean the ear of debris as prescribed; irrigate the ear with a solution of equal parts of vinegar and sterile water as prescribed to restore the normal ear pH

c. Instruct the client to avoid persons with upper respiratory infections

d. Instruct the client to obtain adequate rest, eat a balanced diet, and drink adequate fluids

e. Instruct the client in deep breathing and coughing; forceful coughing, which increases pressure in middle ear, is avoided postoperatively

3. Postoperative interventions

a. Inform the client that initial hearing after surgery is diminished because of the packing in the ear canal and that hearing improvement will occur after the ear canal packing is removed

b. Keep dressing clean and dry

c. Keep the client flat, with operative ear up, for at least 12 hours

d. Administer antibiotics, as prescribed

e. Instruct the client that they may return to work in approximately 3 weeks postoperatively, as prescribed

L. **Mastoiditis**

1. Description

a. May be acute or chronic and results from untreated or inadequately treated chronic or acute otitis media

b. The pain is not relieved by myringotomy

2. Data collection

a. Swelling behind the ear and pain with minimal movement of the head

b. Cellulitus on the skin or external scalp over the mastoid process

c. A reddened, dull, thick, immobile tympanic membrane with or without perforation

d. Tender and enlarged postauricular lymph nodes

e. Low-grade fever

f. Malaise

g. Anorexia

3. Interventions

a. Prepare the client for surgical removal of infected material

b. Monitor for complications

c. Simple or modified radical mastoidectomy with tympanoplasty is the most common treatment

d. Once infected tissue has been removed, tympanoplasty is performed to reconstruct the ossicles and the tympanic membranes in an attempt to restore normal hearing

4. Complications

a. Damage to the abducens and facial cranial nerves

b. Damage exhibited by inability to look laterally (cranial nerve VI) and a drooping of the mouth on the affected side (cranial nerve VII)

c. Meningitis

d. Brain abscess

e. Chronic purulent otitis media

f. Wound infections

g. Vertigo, if the infection spreads into the labyrinth

5. Postoperative interventions

a. Monitor for dizziness

b. Monitor for signs of meningitis, as evidenced by a stiff neck and vomiting

c. Prepare for a wound dressing change 24 hours postoperatively

d. Monitor the surgical incision for edema, drainage, and redness

e. Position the client flat, with the operative side up

f. Restrict the client to bed with bedside commode privileges for 24 hours, as prescribed

g. Assist the client with getting out of bed to prevent falling or injuries from dizziness

h. With reconstruction of the ossicles via a graft, precautions are taken to prevent dislodging of the graft

M. **Otosclerosis**

1. Description

a. Disease of the labyrinthine capsule of the middle ear that results in a bony overgrowth of the tissue surrounding the ossicles

b. Causes the development of irregular areas of new bone formation and causes the fixation of the bones

c. Stapes fixation leads to a **conductive hearing loss**

d. If the disease involves the inner ear, **sensorineural hearing loss** is present

e. It is not uncommon to have bilateral involvement, although hearing loss may be worse in one ear

f. The cause is unknown, although it is believed to have a familial tendency

g. Nonsurgical intervention promotes the improvement of hearing through amplification

h. Surgical intervention involves removal of the bony growth that is causing the hearing loss

i. A partial stapedectomy or complete stapedectomy with a prosthesis (**fenestration**) may be surgically performed

2. Data collection
   a. Slowly progressing **conductive hearing loss**
   b. Bilateral hearing loss
   c. A ringing or roaring type of constant tinnitus
   d. Loud sounds heard in the ear when chewing
   e. Pinkish discoloration (Schwartze's sign) of the tympanic membrane, which indicates vascular changes within the ear

N. **Fenestration**
   1. Description
      a. Removal of the stapes with a small hole drilled in the footplate; a prosthesis is connected between the incus and footplate
      b. Sounds cause the prosthesis to vibrate in the same manner as did the stapes
      c. Complications include complete hearing loss, prolonged vertigo, infection, or facial nerve damage
   2. Preoperative interventions
      a. Instruct the client in measures to prevent middle ear or external ear infections
      b. Instruct the client to avoid excessive nose blowing
      c. Instruct the client not to clean the ear canal with cotton-tipped applicators
      d. Instruct the client to remove the hearing aid 2 weeks before surgery to ensure the integration of local tissue
   3. Postoperative interventions
      a. Inform the client that hearing is initially worse after the surgical procedure because of swelling and that no noticeable improvement in hearing may occur for as long as 6 weeks
      b. Inform the client that the Gelfoam ear packing interferes with hearing but is used to decrease bleeding
      c. Assist with ambulation during the first 1 to 2 days after surgery
      d. Provide side rails when the client is in bed
      e. Administer antibiotics, antivertiginous, and pain medications, as prescribed
      f. Monitor for facial nerve damage, weakness, changes in tactile sensation, changes in taste sensation, vertigo, nausea, and vomiting
      g. Instruct the client to move the head slowly when changing positions to prevent vertigo
      h. Instruct the client to avoid persons with upper respiratory tract infections
      i. Instruct the client to avoid showering and getting the head and wound wet
      j. Instruct the client to refrain from using small objects to clean the external ear canal
      k. Instruct the client to avoid rapid, extreme changes in pressure caused by quick head movements, sneezing, nose blowing, straining, and changes in altitude
      l. Instruct the client to avoid changes in middle ear pressure, because they could dislodge the graft or prosthesis

O. Labyrinthitis
   1. Description: Infection of the labyrinth that occurs as a complication of acute or chronic otitis media
   2. Data collection
      a. Hearing loss that may be permanent on the affected side
      b. Tinnitus
      c. Spontaneous nystagmus to the affected side
      d. Vertigo
      e. Nausea and vomiting
   3. Interventions
      a. Monitor for signs of meningitis, the most common complication, as evidenced by headache, stiff neck, lethargy
      b. Administer systemic antibiotics, as prescribed
      c. Advise the client to rest in bed in a darkened room
      d. Administer antiemetics and antivertiginous medications, as prescribed
      e. Instruct the client that the vertigo subsides as the inflammation resolves
      f. Instruct the client that balance problems that persist may require gait training through physical therapy

P. **Meniere's syndrome**
   1. Description
      a. Also called endolymphatic hydrops, which refers to dilation of the endolymphatic system by overproduction or decreased reabsorption of endolymphatic fluid
      b. It is characterized by tinnitus, unilateral **sensorineural hearing loss,** and vertigo
      c. Symptoms occur in attacks and last for several days; the client becomes totally incapacitated during the attacks
      d. Initial hearing loss is reversible but, as the frequency of attacks continues, hearing loss becomes permanent
      e. Repeated damage to the cochlea caused by increased fluid pressure leads to permanent hearing loss
   2. Causes
      a. Any factor that increases endolymphatic secretion in the labyrinth
      b. Viral and bacterial infections
      c. Allergic reactions
      d. Biochemical disturbances
      e. Vascular disturbance producing changes in the microcirculation in the labyrinth
   3. Data collection
      a. Feelings of fullness in the ear
      b. Tinnitus, as a continuous low-pitched roar or humming sound, is present much of the time, but worsens just before and during severe attacks

c. Hearing loss is worse during an attack

d. Vertigo, as periods of whirling, which might cause the client to fall to the ground

e. Vertigo, which is so intense that, even while lying down, the client holds the bed or ground in an attempt to prevent the whirling

f. Nausea and vomiting

g. Nystagmus

h. Severe headaches

4. Nonsurgical interventions

a. Preventing injury during vertigo attacks

b. Providing bed rest in a quiet environment

c. Providing assistance with walking

d. Instruct the client to move the head slowly to prevent worsening of the vertigo

e. Initiate sodium and fluid restrictions, as prescribed

f. Instruct the client to stop smoking

g. Administer nicotinic acid (niacin) as prescribed for its vasodilatory effect

h. Administer antihistamines as prescribed, which will reduce the production of histamine and the inflammation

i. Administer antiemetics, as prescribed

j. Administer tranquilizers and sedatives as prescribed to calm the client, allow the client to rest, and control vertigo, nausea, and vomiting

5. Surgical interventions

a. Performed when medical therapy is ineffective and the functional level of the client has decreased significantly

b. Endolymphatic drainage and insertion of a shunt may be performed early in the course of the disease to assist with the drainage of excess fluids

c. Resection of the vestibular nerve or total removal of the labyrinth (labyrinthectomy) may be performed

6. Postoperative interventions

a. Check ear packing and dressing on the ear

b. Speak to the client on the side of the unaffected ear

c. Perform neurological assessment

d. Maintain side rails

e. Assist with ambulating

f. Encourage the use of a bedside commode

g. Administer antivertiginous and antiemetic medications, as prescribed

Q. Acoustic neuroma

1. Description

a. A benign tumor of the vestibular or acoustic nerve

b. The tumor may cause damage to hearing and to facial movements and sensations

c. Treatment includes surgical removal of the tumor via craniotomy

d. Care is taken to preserve the function of the facial nerve

e. The tumor rarely recurs after surgical removal

f. Postoperative nursing care is similar to postoperative craniotomy care

2. Data collection

a. Symptoms usually begin with tinnitus and progress to gradual **sensorineural hearing loss**

b. As the tumor enlarges, damage to adjacent cranial nerves occurs

R. Trauma

1. Description

a. The tympanic membrane has a limited stretching ability and gives way under high pressure

b. Foreign objects placed in the external canal may exert pressure on the tympanic membrane and cause perforation

c. If the object continues through the canal, the bony structure of the stapes, incus, and malleus may be damaged

d. A blunt injury to the basal skull and ear can damage the middle ear structures via fractures extending to the middle ear

e. Excessive nose blowing and rapid changes of pressure that occur with nonpressurized air flights can increase pressure in the middle ear

f. Depending on the damage to the ossicles, hearing loss may or may not return

2. Interventions

a. Tympanic membrane perforations usually heal within 24 hours

b. Surgical reconstruction of the ossicles and tympanic membrane through tympanoplasty or myringoplasty may be performed to improve hearing

S. Cerumen and foreign bodies

1. Description

a. Cerumen or wax is the most common cause of impacted canals

b. Foreign bodies can include vegetables, beads, pencil erasers, or insects

2. Data collection

a. Sensation of fullness in the ear with or without hearing loss

b. Pain, itching, or bleeding

3. Cerumen

a. Removal of wax by irrigation is a slow process

b. Irrigation is contraindicated in clients with a history of tympanic membrane perforation

c. To soften cerumen, add three drops of glycerin to the ear at bedtime, and three drops of hydrogen peroxide twice a day

d. After several days, the ear is irrigated

e. 50 to 70 mL of solution is the maximal amount a client can tolerate during an irrigation procedure

4. Foreign bodies
   a. With a foreign object of vegetable matter, irrigation is used with care, because this material expands with hydration
   b. Insects are killed before removal, unless they can be coaxed out by a flashlight or a humming noise
   c. Mineral oil or alcohol is instilled to suffocate the insect, which is then removed using ear forceps
   d. Use a small ear forceps to remove the object and avoid pushing the object further into the canal and damaging the tympanic membrane

PRACTICE QUESTIONS

1. A nurse is asked to test the visual acuity of a client using a Snellen chart. The nurse prepares to perform the test knowing that which of the following identifies the accurate procedure for this visual acuity test?
   1. Both eyes are tested together, followed by the testing of the right and then the left eye
   2. The right eye is tested, followed by the left eye, and then both eyes are tested
   3. The client is asked to stand at a distance of 40 feet from the chart and to read the largest line on the chart
   4. The client is asked to stand at a distance of 40 feet from the chart and to read the line that can be read 200 feet away by an individual with unimpaired vision

2. A client's vision is tested with a Snellen chart. The results of the test is documented as 20/60. The nurse interprets this as:
   1. The client can read at a distance of 60 feet what a client with normal vision can read at 20 feet
   2. The client is legally blind
   3. The client's vision is normal
   4. The client can read at a distance of 20 feet what a client with normal vision can read at 60 feet

3. A clinic notes that following several eye examinations the physician has documented a diagnosis of legal blindness in the client's chart. Which of the following would the nurse expect to note documented as the result of the Snellen chart test?
   1. 20/20 vision
   2. 20/40 vision
   3. 20/60 vision
   4. 20/200 vision

4. A nurse is preparing the client for eye testing and the examiner is planning to test the eyes using the confrontational method. The nurse tells the client that this test is performed to:
   1. Examine visual fields or peripheral vision
   2. Check for glaucoma
   3. Check for color blindness
   4. Examine pupil constriction

5. Tonometry is performed on the client with a suspected diagnosis of glaucoma. The nurse reviews the test results as documented in the client's chart and understands that normal intraocular pressure is:
   1. 2 to 7 mm Hg
   2. 10 to 21 mm Hg
   3. 22 to 30 mm Hg
   4. 31 to 35 mm Hg

6. A nurse is assisting in developing a plan of care for the client scheduled for cataract surgery. The nurse makes suggestions regarding the plan, knowing that which problem is most specifically associated with this type of surgery?
   1. Self-care deficit
   2. Imbalanced nutrition
   3. Sensory perceptual alteration
   4. Anxiety

7. A nurse is reviewing the health record of a client diagnosed with a cataract. The chief clinical manifestation that the nurse would expect to note in the early stages of cataract formation is:
   1. Eye pain
   2. Floating spots
   3. Blurred vision
   4. Diplopia

8. A nurse is assigned to administer the prescribed eyedrops for a client preparing for cataract surgery. Which type of eyedrops will the nurse expect to be prescribed?
   1. An osmotic diuretic
   2. A miotic agent
   3. A mydriatic medication
   4. A thiazide diuretic

9. A nurse is assigned to care for a client following a cataract extraction. The nurse plans to position the client:
   1. On the operative side
   2. On the nonoperative side
   3. Prone
   4. Supine

10. During the early postoperative stage, the cataract extraction client complains of nausea and severe eye pain over the operative site. The nurse takes which action?
    1. Reports the client's complaints
    2. Administers the ordered pain medication and antiemetic
    3. Reassures the client that this is normal
    4. Turns the client on his or her operative side

11. A client is being discharged from the ambulatory care unit following cataract removal and the nurse reinforces instructions regarding home care. Which of the following, if stated by the client, indicates an understanding of the instructions?
    1. "I will take aspirin if I have any discomfort."
    2. "I will sleep on the side that I was operated on."

3. "I will wear my eye shield at night and my glasses during the day."

4. "I will not lift anything if it weighs more than 10 pounds."

12. A client is diagnosed with glaucoma. Which data gathered by the nurse indicates a risk factor associated with glaucoma?
   1. A history of migraine headaches
   2. Frequent urinary tract infections
   3. Cardiovascular disease
   4. Frequent upper respiratory infections

13. A client with glaucoma asks the nurse if complete vision will return. The nurse makes which response to the client?
   1. "Although some vision has been lost and cannot be restored, further loss may be prevented by adhering to the treatment plan."
   2. "Your vision will return as soon as the medication begins to work."
   3. "Your vision will never return to normal."
   4. "Your vision loss is temporary and will return in about 3 to 4 weeks."

14. A nurse is assisting in developing a teaching plan for the client with glaucoma. Which instruction would the nurse suggest to include in the plan of care?
   1. Decrease fluid intake to control the intraocular pressure
   2. Avoid reading the newspaper and watching the television
   3. Decrease the amount of salt in the diet
   4. Eye medications will need to be administered for the rest of your life

15. A nurse is assigned to care for a client with a detached retina. Which finding would the nurse expect to be documented in the client's record?
   1. Pain in the effected eye
   2. Blurred vision
   3. A sense of a curtain falling across the field of vision
   4. A yellow discoloration of the sclera

16. A nurse is assigned to care for a client with a diagnosis of detached retina. Which finding would indicate that bleeding has occurred as a result of retinal detachment?
   1. Complaints of a burst of black spots or floaters
   2. A sudden sharp pain in the eye
   3. Total loss of vision
   4. A reddened conjunctiva

17. A client with retinal detachment is admitted to the nursing unit in preparation for a scleral buckling procedure. Which of the following would the nurse anticipate to be prescribed?
   1. Bathroom privileges only
   2. Elevating the head of the bed to 45 degrees
   3. Placing an eye patch over the client's affected eye
   4. Wearing dark glasses to read or watch television

18. A client arrives in the emergency room following an automobile crash. The client's forehead hit the steering wheel and a hyphema has been diagnosed. The nurse would prepare to position the client:
   1. Flat on bed rest
   2. On bed rest in a semi-Fowler's position
   3. In the lateral position on the affected side
   4. In lateral position on the unaffected side

19. A client sustains a contusion of the eyeball following a traumatic injury with a blunt object. The nurse takes which action immediately?
   1. Notifies the physician
   2. Irrigates the eye with cool water
   3. Applies ice to the affected eye
   4. Accompanies the client to the emergency room

20. A client arrives in the emergency room with a penetrating eye injury caused by wood chips while the client was cutting wood. The nurse checks the eye and notes the piece of wood protruding from the eye. The nurse immediately prepares the client for which of the following?
   1. Removal of the piece of wood using a sterile eye clamp
   2. Application of an eye patch
   3. Visual acuity tests
   4. Irrigation of the eye with sterile saline

21. A client sustains a chemical eye injury from a splash of battery acid. The nurse prepares the client for which immediate measure?
   1. Assessment of visual acuity
   2. Irrigation of the eye with sterile normal saline
   3. Swabbing the eye with antibiotic ointment
   4. Covering the eye with a pressure patch

22. A nurse is caring for a client following enucleation and notes the presence of bright red drainage on the dressing. The nurse takes which appropriate action?
   1. Reports the findings
   2. Continues to monitor vital signs
   3. Documents the finding
   4. Marks the drainage on the dressing and monitors for any increase in bleeding

23. A nurse is preparing to administer ear drops to an adult client. The nurse administers the ear drops by:
   1. Pulling the pinna up and back
   2. Pulling the earlobe down and back
   3. Instructing the client to stand and lean to one side
   4. Tilting the client's head forward and down

24. A nurse is assisting the physician with performing a Weber test on a client. The nurse understands that this test checks for:
   1. Visual loss
   2. Cataract development
   3. Hearing loss
   4. Nystagmus

25. A nurse is caring for a client who is hearing-impaired and takes which approach to facilitate communication?
    1. Speaks frequently
    2. Speaks loudly
    3. Speaks directly into the impaired ear
    4. Speaks in a normal tone

26. A client arrives at the emergency room with a foreign body in the left ear that has been determined to be an insect. Which intervention would the nurse anticipate to be prescribed initially?
    1. Irrigation of the ear
    2. Instillation of diluted alcohol
    3. Instillation of antibiotic ear drops
    4. Instillation of corticosteroid ointment

27. A nurse notes that the physician has documented a diagnosis of presbycusis on the client's chart. The nurse understands that this condition is most accurately described as:
    1. A sensorineural loss that occurs with aging
    2. A conductive hearing loss that occurs with aging
    3. Tinnitus that occurs with aging
    4. Nystagmus that occurs with aging

28. A nurse is reinforcing discharge instructions for a client who has had a fenestration procedure for the treatment of otosclerosis. Which of the following, if stated by the client, would indicate an understanding of the instructions?
    1. "I should drink liquids through a straw for the next 2 to 3 weeks."
    2. "It is all right to take a shower and wash my hair."
    3. "I will take stool softeners as prescribed by my doctor."
    4. "I can resume my tennis lessons starting next week."

29. A client with Meniere's disease is experiencing severe vertigo. The nurse instructs the client to do which of the following to assist in controlling the vertigo?
    1. Increase fluid intake to 3000 mL/day
    2. Avoid sudden head movements
    3. Lie still and watch television
    4. Increase sodium in the diet

30. A nurse is assigned to care for a client hospitalized with Meniere's disease. The nurse expects that which of the following would most likely be prescribed for the client?
    1. Low-cholesterol diet
    2. Low-sodium diet
    3. Low-carbohydrate diet
    4. Low-fat diet

31. A nurse is caring for a client following craniotomy for removal of an acoustic neuroma. The nurse understands that assessment of which of the following cranial nerves would identify a complication specifically associated with this surgery?
    1. Cranial nerve I, olfactory
    2. Cranial nerve III, oculomotor
    3. Cranial nerve IV, trochlear
    4. Cranial nerve VII, facial nerve

32. A nurse is monitoring a client with a blunt head injury sustained from a motor vehicle crash. Which of the following would indicate a basal skull fracture as a result of the injury?
    1. Purulent drainage from the auditory canal
    2. Bloody or clear drainage from the auditory canal
    3. Epistaxis
    4. Periorbital edema

33. A nurse is reviewing the record of a client with mastoiditis. The nurse would expect to note which of the following documented regarding the results of the otoscopic examination?
    1. A pink tympanic membrane
    2. A pearl-colored tympanic membrane
    3. A red, dull, thick and immobile tympanic membrane
    4. A transparent and clear tympanic membrane

34. A client is diagnosed with a disorder involving the inner ear. The nurse caring for the client understands that which of the following is the most common client complaint associated with a disorder involving the inner ear?
    1. Hearing loss
    2. Pruritus
    3. Tinnitus
    4. Burning in the ear

35. A nurse is assigned to care for a client with a diagnosis of Meniere's disease. The nurse plans care knowing that this condition is a disorder of the:
    1. External ear canal
    2. Tympanic membrane
    3. Middle ear
    4. Inner ear

36. A nurse is caring for a client who will be undergoing surgical treatment for Meniere's disease. The nurse plans care understanding that surgical treatment for this disorder is performed to:
    1. Provide relief from accumulation of inner ear fluid in the endolymphatic sac
    2. Repair the tympanic membrane
    3. Replace the stapes footplate
    4. Provide relief from accumulation of fluid in the middle ear

37. A nurse is reviewing the health care record of a client with a diagnosis of otosclerosis. The nurse would expect to note documentation of which early symptom of this disorder?
    1. Ringing in the ears
    2. Blurred vision
    3. Headache
    4. Vertigo

38. Surgery has been recommended for the client with otosclerosis. The client tells the nurse that surgery is not desired and asks the nurse about alternative

methods to improve hearing. The nurse makes which appropriate response to the client?
1. "There are no other methods to improve hearing."
2. "You need to have surgery, because it has been recommended."
3. "A hearing aid may improve your hearing."
4. "Your physician is the best. You need to do what the physician suggests."

39. A nurse is caring for a client hospitalized with an acute attack from Meniere's disease. The client verbalizes concern because the client has experienced a hearing loss as a result of the attack. Which response would the nurse make to the client regarding the hearing loss?
1. "It will take several weeks before the hearing returns."
2. "The hearing loss will fluctuate for a period of 1 week."
3. "The attack leaves a hearing loss in the involved ear."
4. "The hearing will return to normal."

40. A nurse is reviewing the physician's orders for a client admitted to the hospital with a diagnosis of an acute attack of Meniere's disease. Which order, if noted on the client's chart, would the nurse question?
1. The administration of a sedative
2. The administration of an antihistamine
3. The administration of a vasoconstrictor
4. Bed rest

41. A nurse is reinforcing discharge instructions to the client who was hospitalized for an acute attack of Meniere's disease. Which statement, if made by the client, indicates a need for further education?
1. "I need to take the diuretics to decrease the fluid in the ear."
2. "I need to take the antihistamine as prescribed."
3. "I need to take a vasodilator."
4. "It is not necessary to restrict salt in my diet."

42. A client with a diagnosis of otosclerosis is admitted to the ambulatory care unit for stapedectomy and the nurse reinforces instructions with the client regarding home care following the procedure. Which statement by the client indicates a need for further education?
1. "I need to keep water out of my ear canal for at least 3 weeks."
2. "I need to avoid air travel for at least 6 months."
3. "I need to notify the physician if I experience any persistent dizziness."
4. "I need to avoid bending and lifting heavy objects for at least 3 weeks."

43. A nurse is reinforcing discharge instructions with a client who is being discharged following a fenestration procedure for the treatment of otosclerosis. Which of the following will be included in the list of instructions prepared for the client?
1. "It is all right to begin your golf lessons."
2. "It is all right to take a shower daily."
3. "You need to avoid air travel."
4. "You need to avoid bending activities for 1 week."

44. A myringotomy is performed on a client in the ambulatory care center. The ambulatory care nurse calls the client 24 hours after the procedure to evaluate the status of the client. The client reports to the nurse that a small amount of brownish drainage has been coming from the ear. Which instruction would the nurse provide to the client?
1. Contact the physician
2. Lie on the unaffected side to prevent the drainage from occurring
3. Continue to monitor the drainage, because this is normal and may occur for 24 to 48 hours following the surgery
4. Place a cotton plug in the ear to absorb the drainage

45. A nurse is reinforcing instructions to a client regarding the use of a hearing aid. Which statement by the client indicates a need for further education?
1. "I should keep an extra battery available at all times."
2. "I should wash the ear mold frequently with mild soap and water."
3. "I should turn the hearing aid off after removing it from my ear."
4. "I should not wear the hearing aid during an ear infection."

ALTERNATE FORMAT QUESTION: MULTIPLE RESPONSE

The nurse is assisting in preparing a teaching plan for a client who is undergoing cataract extraction with intraocular implant. Which home care measures will the nurse include in the plan?
___ To contact the surgeon if eye scratchiness occurs
___ That episodes of sudden severe pain in the eye are expected
___ To place an eye shield on the surgical eye at bedtime
___ To avoid activities that require bending over
___ To contact the surgeon if a decrease in visual acuity occurs

ANSWERS

1. *Answer:* 2

Rationale: Visual acuity is tested in one eye at a time, and then in both eyes together, with the client comfortably seated. Begin with the right eye while the left eye is covered and then test the left eye with the right eye covered, followed by testing both eyes together. Visual acuity is measured with or without corrective lenses, with the client standing at a distance of 20 feet from the chart.

Test-Taking Strategy: Use the process of elimination. Remember that normal visual acuity as measured by a Snellen chart is 20/20 vision. This should assist you to eliminate options 3 and 4. It is best to test each eye separately first, and then test both eyes together. This most accurately assesses visual acuity. Review this data collection technique if you had difficulty with this question.

Level of Cognitive Ability: Application
Client Needs: Health Promotion and Maintenance
Integrated Process: Nursing Process/Data Collection
Content Area: Adult Health/Eye
Reference: deWit, S. (2005). *Fundamental concepts and skills for nursing.* Philadelphia: W.B. Saunders, p. 363.

2. *Answer:* 4

Rationale: Vision that is 20/20 is normal—that is, the client can read from 20 feet what a person with normal vision can read from 20 feet. A client with a visual acuity of 20/60 can only read at a distance of 20 feet what a person with normal vision can read at 60 feet.

Test-Taking Strategy: Understanding how to interpret the results of this visual acuity test is necessary to answer this question. Remember that 20/20 vision is normal—that is, the client is able to read from 20 feet what a person with normal vision can read from 20 feet. Review this visual acuity test if you had difficulty with this question.

Level of Cognitive Ability: Comprehension
Client Needs: Physiological Integrity
Integrated Process: Nursing Process/Evaluation
Content Area: Adult Health/Eye
Reference: Christensen, B., & Kockrow, E. (2003). *Adult health nursing* (4th ed.). St. Louis: Mosby, p. 561.

3. *Answer:* 4

Rationale: Legal blindness is defined as the best visual acuity with corrective lenses in the better eye as 20/200 or less, or if visual acuity is less than 20 degrees of the visual field in the better eye. Options 1, 2, and 3 are incorrect descriptions.

Test-Taking Strategy: Focus on the issue, legal blindness. Select the option that identifies the worst visual impairment. This will direct you to option 4. Review this definition if you had difficulty with this question.

Level of Cognitive Ability: Comprehension
Client Needs: Physiological Integrity
Integrated Process: Nursing Process/Data Collection
Content Area: Adult Health/Eye
Reference: Christensen, B., & Kockrow, E. (2003). *Adult health nursing* (4th ed.). St. Louis: Mosby, p. 563.

4. *Answer:* 1

Rationale: The confrontational method of eye testing is used to examine visual fields or peripheral vision. Tonometry is used to check for glaucoma. An Ishihara chart is used to check color vision. A flashlight is used to test pupillary response to light.

Test-Taking Strategy: Knowledge regarding the procedure for checking peripheral vision by the confrontational method is required to answer this question. Remember, the confrontational method of eye testing is used to examine visual fields or peripheral vision. Review the purpose of this test if you had difficulty with this question.

Level of Cognitive Ability: Application
Client Needs: Health Promotion and Maintenance
Integrated Process: Nursing Process/Implementation
Content Area: Adult Health/Eye
Reference: Jarvis, C. (2004). *Physical examination and health assessment* (4th ed.). Philadelphia: W.B. Saunders, p. 308.

5. *Answer:* 2

Rationale: Tonometry is the method of measuring intraocular fluid pressure using a calibrated instrument that indents or flattens the corneal apex. Pressures between 10 and 21 mm Hg are considered within the normal range.

Test-Taking Strategy: Knowledge regarding the normal intraocular pressure is required to answer this question. Remember, pressures between 10 and 21 mm Hg are considered within the normal range. Review this normal value if you had difficulty with this question.

Level of Cognitive Ability: Comprehension
Client Needs: Physiological Integrity
Integrated Process: Nursing Process/Data Collection
Content Area: Adult Health/Eye
Reference: Linton, A., & Maebius, N. (2003). *Introduction to medical-surgical nursing* (3rd ed.). Philadelphia: W.B. Saunders, p. 1051.

6. *Answer:* 3

Rationale: The most specific associated problem for the client scheduled for cataract surgery is sensory perceptual alteration (visual) related to lens extraction and replacement. Options 1 and 2 may also be concerns but would occur as a result of a sensory perceptual alteration. Option 4 can occur with any type of surgical procedure.

Test-Taking Strategy: Use the process of elimination, focusing on the type of surgery. Remember, disorders of the eye or ear relate to sensory perceptual alterations. Review the problems associated with these disorders if you had difficulty with this question.

Level of Cognitive Ability: Comprehension
Client Needs: Psychosocial Integrity
Integrated Process: Nursing Process/Planning
Content Area: Adult Health/Eye
Reference: Linton, A., & Maebius, N. (2003). *Introduction to medical-surgical nursing* (3rd ed.). Philadelphia: W.B. Saunders, p. 1064.

7. *Answer:* 3

Rationale: A gradual, painless blurring of central vision is the chief clinical manifestation of a cataract. Early symptoms include slightly blurred vision and a decrease in color perception. Options 1, 2, and 4 are not specifically associated with a cataract.

Test-Taking Strategy: Note the key word, *chief.* Recall the pathophysiology related to cataract development. As a cataract develops, the lens of the eye becomes opaque. This description will assist in directing you to the correct option. If you had difficulty with this question, review the signs associated with cataract development.
Level of Cognitive Ability: Comprehension
Client Needs: Physiological Integrity
Integrated Process: Nursing Process/Data Collection
Content Area: Adult Health/Eye
Reference: Christensen, B., & Kockrow, E. (2003). *Adult health nursing* (4th ed.). St. Louis: Mosby, p. 570.

8. *Answer: 3*
Rationale: A mydriatic medication produces mydriasis or dilation of the pupil. Mydriatic medications are used preoperatively in the cataract client. These medications act by dilating the pupils. They also constrict blood vessels. A miotic agent would constrict the pupil. An osmotic agent would act to decrease intraocular pressure. A thiazide diuretic would promote the excretion of body fluid. A thiazide diuretic is not likely to be prescribed for a client with a cataract.
Test-Taking Strategy: Use the process of elimination. Read the question carefully, noting that the client is being prepared for eye surgery. Remember, dilation of the eye is necessary prior to cataract extraction. Review the preparation of a client for cataract surgery if you had difficulty with this question.
Level of Cognitive Ability: Analysis
Client Needs: Physiological Integrity
Integrated Process: Nursing Process/Planning
Content Area: Adult Health/Eye
References: Christensen, B., & Kockrow, E. (2003). *Adult health nursing* (4th ed.). St. Louis: Mosby, p. 571.
Linton, A., & Maebius, N. (2003). *Introduction to medical-surgical nursing* (3rd ed.). Philadelphia: W.B. Saunders, p. 1065.

9. *Answer: 2*
Rationale: Postoperatively, cataract extraction clients should be positioned on their backs in semi-Fowler's position or on the nonoperative side to prevent edema in the surgical site. Options 1, 3, and 4 are incorrect positions and will cause swelling at the surgical site.
Test-Taking Strategy: Use the process of elimination. Remember, edema at the surgical site can occur following the trauma of surgery. Think about the principles of gravity and the prevention of the accumulation of fluid around the surgical site. This will assist in directing you to the correct option. If you had difficulty with this question, review postoperative care of a client following cataract surgery.
Level of Cognitive Ability: Application
Client Needs: Physiological Integrity
Integrated Process: Nursing Process/Planning
Content Area: Adult Health/Eye
References: Christensen, B., & Kockrow, E. (2003). *Adult health nursing* (4th ed.). St. Louis: Mosby, p. 571.
Linton, A., & Maebius, N. (2003). *Introduction to medical-surgical nursing* (3rd ed.). Philadelphia: W.B. Saunders, p. 1065.

10. *Answer: 1*
Rationale: Severe pain or pain accompanied by nausea is an indicator of increased intraocular pressure and should be reported to the physician immediately. Options 2, 3, and 4 are incorrect.
Test-Taking Strategy: Note the key word, *severe.* Eliminate option 3 because this is not a normal condition. The client should not be turned to the operative side; therefore, eliminate option 4. From the remaining options, noting the key word will direct you to the correct option. If you had difficulty with this question, review the postoperative complications of cataract surgery requiring physician notification.
Level of Cognitive Ability: Application
Client Needs: Physiological Integrity
Integrated Process: Nursing Process/Implementation
Content Area: Adult Health/Eye
Reference: Black, J., & Hawks, J. (2005). *Medical-surgical nursing: Clinical management for positive outcomes* (7th ed.). Philadelphia: W.B. Saunders, p. 1951.

11. *Answer: 3*
Rationale: The client is instructed to wear a metal or plastic shield to protect the eye from accidental injury and is instructed not to rub the eye. Glasses may be worn during the day. Aspirin or medications containing aspirin are not to be administered or taken by the client and the client is instructed to take acetaminophen (Tylenol), as needed, for pain. The client is instructed not to sleep on the side of the body that was operated on. The client is not to lift more than 5 pounds.
Test-Taking Strategy: Note the key words, *indicates an understanding.* Use the process of elimination and knowledge regarding the postoperative care following this procedure. If you had difficulty with this question, review these client instructions.
Level of Cognitive Ability: Comprehension
Client Needs: Health Promotion and Maintenance
Integrated Process: Teaching/Learning
Content Area: Adult Health/Eye
Reference: Christensen, B., & Kockrow, E. (2003). *Adult health nursing* (4th ed.). St. Louis: Mosby, p. 573.

12. *Answer: 3*
Rationale: Hypertension, cardiovascular disease, diabetes mellitus, and obesity are associated with the development of glaucoma. Smoking, ingestion of caffeine or large amounts alcohol, illicit drugs, corticosteroids, altered hormone levels, posture, and eye movements may cause varying transient increases in intraocular pressure.
Test-Taking Strategy: Use knowledge regarding the risk factors associated with glaucoma to answer this question. Remember, cardiovascular disease is associated with the development of glaucoma. If you had difficulty with this question, review the risk factors associated with this disorder.
Level of Cognitive Ability: Comprehension
Client Needs: Health Promotion and Maintenance
Integrated Process: Nursing Process/Data Collection
Content Area: Adult Health/Eye
Reference: Black, J., & Hawks, J. (2005). *Medical-surgical nursing: Clinical management for positive outcomes* (7th ed.). Philadelphia: W.B. Saunders, p. 1945.

13. *Answer:* **1**
Rationale: Vision loss to glaucoma is irreparable. The client needs to be reassured that, although some vision has been lost and cannot be restored, further loss may be prevented by adhering to the treatment plan. Options 2, 3, and 4 are incorrect.
Test-Taking Strategy: Use the process of elimination and read the options carefully. Eliminate option 3, because this option does not provide a reassuring response and will produce anxiety in the client as it is stated. From the remaining options, note that option 1 is the umbrella (global) option addressing the importance of compliance with the treatment plan. Review this disorder if you had difficulty with this question.
Level of Cognitive Ability: Application
Client Needs: Psychosocial Integrity
Integrated Process: Nursing Process/Implementation
Content Area: Adult Health/Eye
Reference: Linton, A., & Maebius, N. (2003). *Introduction to medical-surgical nursing* (3rd ed.). Philadelphia: W.B. Saunders, pp. 1067; 1070.

14. *Answer:* **4**
Rationale: The administration of eyedrops is a critical component of the treatment plan for the client with glaucoma. The client needs to be instructed that medications will need to be taken for the rest of their life. Limiting fluids and reducing salt will not decrease intraocular pressure. Option 2 is not necessary.
Test-Taking Strategy: Use the process of elimination. Knowing that medications are an integral component of the treatment plan will assist in directing you to the correct option. Review the treatment associated with the care of the client with glaucoma if you had difficulty with this question.
Level of Cognitive Ability: Application
Client Needs: Health Promotion and Maintenance
Integrated Process: Nursing Process/Planning
Content Area: Adult Health/Eye
Reference: Christensen, B., & Kockrow, E. (2003). *Adult health nursing* (4th ed.). St. Louis: Mosby, p. 580.

15. *Answer:* **3**
Rationale: A characteristic clinical manifestation of retinal detachment described by clients is the feeling that a shadow or curtain is falling across the field of vision. There is no pain associated with detachment of the retina. A retinal detachment is an ophthalmic emergency and even more so if visual acuity is still normal. Options 2 and 4 are not specifically associated with a detached retina.
Test-Taking Strategy: Use the process of elimination. Remember that a characteristic clinical manifestation is the feeling that a shadow or curtain is falling across the field of vision. Retinal detachment can occur suddenly and is an ophthalmic emergency. Review the clinical manifestations associated with this condition if you had difficulty with this question.
Level of Cognitive Ability: Comprehension
Client Needs: Physiological Integrity
Integrated Process: Nursing Process/Data Collection
Content Area: Adult Health/Eye

Reference: Linton, A., & Maebius, N. (2003). *Introduction to medical-surgical nursing* (3rd ed.). Philadelphia: W.B. Saunders, p. 1070.

16. *Answer:* **1**
Rationale: Complaints of a sudden burst of black spots or floaters indicate that bleeding has occurred as a result of the detachment. Options 2, 3, and 4 are not specifically associated with bleeding as a result of detached retina.
Test-Taking Strategy: Use the process of elimination. Hemorrhage is a serious complication associated with retinal detachment. Remember, complaints of a sudden burst of black spots or floaters indicate that bleeding has occurred as a result of the detachment. Review the clinical manifestations associated with the complications of a detached retina if you had difficulty with this question.
Level of Cognitive Ability: Analysis
Client Needs: Physiological Integrity
Integrated Process: Nursing Process/Data Collection
Content Area: Adult Health/Eye
Reference: Christensen, B., & Kockrow, E. (2003). *Adult health nursing* (4th ed.). St. Louis: Mosby, p. 574.

17. *Answer:* **3**
Rationale: The nurse places an eye patch over the client's affected eye to reduce eye movement. Some clients may need bilateral patching. Depending on the location and size of the retinal break, activity restrictions including watching television, may be needed immediately. These restrictions are necessary to prevent further tearing or detachment and to promote drainage of any subretinal fluid. The nurse positions the client as prescribed by the physician.
Test-Taking Strategy: Use the process of elimination. Eliminate options that suggest activity such as in options 1 and 4. Remember that the eye needs to be protected and rested. This should direct you to option 3 from the remaining options. If you had difficulty with this question review care to the client with retinal detachment.
Level of Cognitive Ability: Comprehension
Client Needs: Physiological Integrity
Integrated Process: Nursing Process/Planning
Content Area: Adult Health/Eye
Reference: Christensen, B., & Kockrow, E. (2003). *Adult health nursing* (4th ed.). St. Louis: Mosby, p. 575.

18. *Answer:* **2**
Rationale: A hyphema is the presence of blood in the anterior chamber. It is produced when a force is sufficient to break the integrity of the blood vessels in the eye. It can be caused by direct injury, such as penetrating injury from a BB pellet, or indirectly, such as from striking the forehead on a steering wheel during an accident. The client is treated by bed rest in a semi-Fowler's position to assist gravity in keeping the hyphema away from the optical center of the cornea.
Test-Taking Strategy: Use the process of elimination. Eliminate options 1, 3, and 4 because they are similar. Placing the client flat will produce an increase in pressure at the injured site. Review care of the client with hyphema, if you had difficulty with this question.
Level of Cognitive Ability: Application

Client Needs: Physiological Integrity
Integrated Process: Nursing Process/Implementation
Content Area: Adult Health/Eye
References: Jarvis, C. (2004). *Physical examination and health assessment* (4th ed.). Philadelphia: W.B. Saunders, p. 336. Lewis, S., Heitkemper, M., & Dirksen, S. (2004). *Medical-surgical nursing: Assessment and management of clinical problems* (6th ed.). St. Louis: Mosby, p. 422.

19. Answer: 3
Rationale: Treatment for a contusion begins at the time of injury. Ice is applied immediately. The client should receive a thorough eye examination to rule out the presence of other eye injuries. Eye irrigation is not indicated in a contusion. Options 1 and 4 will delay immediate treatment. Following the application of ice, the physician would be notified.
Test-Taking Strategy: Use the process of elimination, noting the key word, *immediately*. Noting that the client sustained a contusion to the eye will direct you to option 3. Review immediate treatment of an eye contusion if you had difficulty with this question.
Level of Cognitive Ability: Application
Client Needs: Physiological Integrity
Integrated Process: Nursing Process/Implementation
Content Area: Adult Health/Eye
Reference: Christensen, B., & Kockrow, E. (2003). *Adult health nursing* (4th ed.). St. Louis: Mosby, p. 155.

20. Answer: 3
Rationale: If the laceration is the result of a penetrating injury, an object may be noted protruding from the eye. This object must never be removed except by the ophthalmologist, because it may be holding ocular structures in place. Application of an eye patch or irrigation of the eye may disrupt the foreign body and cause further tearing of the cornea.
Test-Taking Strategy: Note the key word, *penetrating*. This should indicate that a laceration has occurred and that interventions are directed at preventing further disruption of the integrity of the eye. The only option that will prevent further disruption of the integrity of the eye is to prepare for testing visual acuity. Review care of the client with a penetrating eye injury if you had difficulty with this question.
Level of Cognitive Ability: Application
Client Needs: Physiological Integrity
Integrated Process: Nursing Process/Implementation
Content Area: Adult Health/Eye
Reference: Christensen, B., & Kockrow, E. (2003). *Adult health nursing* (4th ed.). St. Louis: Mosby, p. 581.

21. Answer: 2
Rationale: Emergency care following a chemical burn to the eye includes irrigating the eye immediately with sterile normal saline or ocular irrigating solution. The irrigation should be maintained for at least 10 minutes. Following this emergency treatment, visual acuity is assessed. Options 3 and 4 are not immediate measures.
Test-Taking Strategy: Use the process of elimination. Read the question carefully, noting the type of injury to the eye. The question asks about emergency care; therefore, in this type

of injury, it is necessary to irrigate the eye first. Review this content if you had difficulty with this question.
Level of Cognitive Ability: Application
Client Needs: Physiological Integrity
Integrated Process: Nursing Process/Implementation
Content Area: Adult Health/Eye
Reference: Black, J., & Hawks, J. (2005). *Medical-surgical nursing: Clinical management for positive outcomes* (7th ed.). Philadelphia: W.B. Saunders, p. 1446.

22. Answer: 1
Rationale: If the nurse notes the presence of bright red drainage on the dressing, it must be reported to the physician, because this can indicate hemorrhage. Options 2, 3, and 4 will delay necessary treatment.
Test-Taking Strategy: Note the key words, *bright red*. Bright red drainage indicates active bleeding. The physician needs to be notified if this type of drainage occurs. Review postoperative complications associated with an enucleation if you had difficulty with this question.
Level of Cognitive Ability: Application
Client Needs: Physiological Integrity
Integrated Process: Nursing Process/Implementation
Content Area: Adult Health/Eye
Reference: Linton, A., & Maebius, N. (2003). *Introduction to medical-surgical nursing* (3rd ed.). Philadelphia: W.B. Saunders, p. 1072.

23. Answer: 1
Rationale: The nurse tilts the client's head slightly away and pulls the pinna up and back. Asking the client to stand and lean to one side is inappropriate and unsafe.
Test-Taking Strategy: Use the process of elimination, noting that the question addresses an adult client. Use basic knowledge regarding the administration of ear medications in selecting the correct option. In the adult, the pinna is pulled up and back. Review this procedure if you had difficulty with this question.
Level of Cognitive Ability: Application
Client Needs: Physiological Integrity
Integrated Process: Nursing Process/Implementation
Content Area: Adult Health/Ear
Reference: Linton, A., & Maebius, N. (2003). *Introduction to medical-surgical nursing* (3rd ed.). Philadelphia: W.B. Saunders, p. 1080.

24. Answer: 3
Rationale: The Weber tuning fork test assesses for conductive or sensorineural hearing loss. Options 1, 2, and 4 are incorrect.
Test-Taking Strategy: Use the process of elimination. Recalling that this is a test to determine the type of hearing loss will direct you to option 3. Review the purpose of this test if you had difficulty with this question.
Level of Cognitive Ability: Comprehension
Client Needs: Health Promotion and Maintenance
Integrated Process: Nursing Process/Data Collection
Content Area: Adult Health/Ear
Reference: Christensen, B., & Kockrow, E. (2003). *Adult health nursing* (4th ed.). St. Louis: Mosby, p. 584.

25. *Answer:* **4**

Rationale: It is important to speak in a normal tone to the client with impaired hearing and to avoid shouting. The nurse should talk directly to the client while facing the client and speak clearly. If the client does not seem to understand what is said, the nurse should express it differently. Moving closer to the client and toward the better ear may facilitate communication, but it is important to avoid talking directly into the impaired ear.

Test-Taking Strategy: Knowledge regarding effective communication techniques for the hearing impaired is required to answer this question. Thinking about the effect of each action identified in the options will direct you to option 4. If you had difficulty with this question, review these techniques

Level of Cognitive Ability: Application
Client Needs: Psychosocial Integrity
Integrated Process: Communication and Documentation
Content Area: Adult Health/Ear
Reference: Christensen, B., & Kockrow, E. (2003). *Adult health nursing* (4th ed.). St. Louis: Mosby, p. 587.

26. *Answer:* **2**

Rationale: Insects are killed before removal unless they can be coaxed out by a flashlight or a humming noise. Mineral oil or diluted alcohol is instilled into the ear to suffocate the insect, which is then removed by using ear forceps. When the foreign object is vegetable matter, irrigation is not used, because this material expands with hydration and the impaction becomes worse. Options 1, 3, and 4 may be prescribed after the initial treatment if necessary and if inflammation or infection is a concern.

Test Taking Strategy: Use the process of elimination and knowledge regarding care of the client with a foreign body in the ear to answer this question. Remember, insects are killed before removal with mineral oil or diluted alcohol. If you had difficulty with this question, review the treatment for this occurrence.

Level of Cognitive Ability: Comprehension
Client Needs: Physiological Integrity
Integrated Process: Nursing Process/Planning
Content Area: Adult Health/Ear
Reference: Christensen, B., & Kockrow, E. (2003). *Adult health nursing* (4th ed.). St. Louis: Mosby, p. 592.

27. *Answer:* **1**

Rationale: Presbycusis is a type of hearing loss that occurs with aging. It is a gradual sensorineural loss caused by nerve degeneration in the inner ear or auditory nerve. Options 2, 3, and 4 are not accurate descriptions.

Test-Taking Strategy: Knowledge regarding the description of presbycusis is required to answer this question. Remember presbycusis is a sensorineural hearing loss that occurs with aging. If you are unfamiliar with this condition, review this age related disorder.

Level of Cognitive Ability: Comprehension
Client Needs: Physiological Integrity
Integrated Process: Nursing Process/Data Collection
Content Area: Adult Health/Ear
Reference: Linton, A., & Maebius, N. (2003). *Introduction to medical-surgical nursing* (3rd ed.). Philadelphia: W.B. Saunders, pp. 1092-1093.

28. *Answer:* **3**

Rationale: Following ear surgery, clients need to avoid straining when having a bowel movement. Clients need to be instructed to avoid drinking with a straw for 2 to 3 weeks, avoid air travel, and avoid coughing excessively. Clients need to avoid getting their head wet, washing their hair, and showering for 1 week. Clients need to avoid rapidly moving the head, bouncing, and bending over for 3 weeks.

Test-Taking Strategy: Use the process of elimination. Note the key words, *an understanding of the instructions.* Consider the anatomical area of the client's condition and the surgical procedure to eliminate the incorrect options. If you had difficulty with this question, review client instructions following ear surgery.

Level of Cognitive Ability: Comprehension
Client Needs: Health Promotion and Maintenance
Integrated Process: Nursing Process/Evaluation
Content Area: Adult Health/Ear
References: Christensen, B., & Kockrow, E. (2003). *Adult health nursing* (4th ed.). St. Louis: Mosby, p. 595.
Linton, A., & Maebius, N. (2003). *Introduction to medical-surgical nursing* (3rd ed.). Philadelphia: W.B. Saunders, p. 233.

29. *Answer:* **2**

Rationale: The nurse instructs the client to make slow head movements to prevent worsening of the vertigo. Dietary changes such as salt and fluid restrictions that reduce the amount of endolymphatic fluid are sometimes prescribed. Watching television can increase the vertigo.

Test-Taking Strategy: Identify the issue of the question. The issue is severe vertigo. Note the relation between severe vertigo and the correct option, avoiding sudden head movements. If you had difficulty with this question, review measures that will reduce vertigo in the client with Meniere's disease.

Level of Cognitive Ability: Application
Client Needs: Physiological Integrity
Integrated Process: Nursing Process/Implementation
Content Area: Adult Health/Ear
Reference: Linton, A., & Maebius, N. (2003). *Introduction to medical-surgical nursing* (3rd ed.). Philadelphia: W.B. Saunders, p. 1091.

30. *Answer:* **2**

Rationale: Dietary changes such as salt and fluid restrictions that reduce the amount of endolymphatic fluid are sometimes prescribed. Options 1, 3, and 4 are not specific dietary prescriptions for this condition.

Test-Taking Strategy: Use the process of elimination. Recalling the pathophysiology related to Meniere's disease will direct you to option 2. Review the pathophysiology related to this condition and the treatment if you had difficulty with this question.

Level of Cognitive Ability: Comprehension
Client Needs: Physiological Integrity
Integrated Process: Nursing Process/Planning
Content Area: Adult Health/Ear
Reference: Christensen, B., & Kockrow, E. (2003). *Adult health nursing* (4th ed.). St. Louis: Mosby, p. 593.

31. *Answer:* **4**
Rationale: Treatment for acoustic neuroma is surgical removal via a craniotomy. Extreme care is taken to preserve remaining hearing and preserve the function of the facial nerve. Acoustic neuromas rarely occur following surgical removal.
Test-Taking Strategy: Use the process of elimination. Recalling the anatomical location of acoustic neuromas will direct you to option 4. If you had difficulty with this question, review the complications associated with this surgical procedure.
Level of Cognitive Ability: Analysis
Client Needs: Physiological Integrity
Integrated Process: Nursing Process/Data Collection
Content Area: Adult Health/Ear
References: Black, J., & Hawks, J. (2005). *Medical-surgical nursing: Clinical management for positive outcomes* (7th ed.). Philadelphia: W.B. Saunders, p. 2085.
Christensen, B., & Kockrow, E. (2003). *Adult health nursing* (4th ed.). St. Louis: Mosby, p. 603.

32. *Answer:* **2**
Rationale: Bloody or clear watery drainage from the auditory canal indicates a cerebrospinal fluid leak following trauma and suggests a basal skull fracture. This warrants immediate attention. Option 1 is indicative of an infectious process. Options 3 and 4 are not specifically associated with a basal skull fracture.
Test-Taking Strategy: Knowledge regarding the signs associated with a basal skull fracture is required to answer this question. Remember, bloody or clear watery drainage from the auditory canal indicates a cerebrospinal fluid leak following trauma and suggests a basal skull fracture. If you had difficulty with this question, review these signs.
Level of Cognitive Ability: Analysis
Client Needs: Physiological Integrity
Integrated Process: Nursing Process/Data Collection
Content Area: Adult Health/Ear
Reference: Linton, A., & Maebius, N. (2003). *Introduction to medical-surgical nursing* (3rd ed.). Philadelphia: W.B. Saunders, p. 194.

33. *Answer:* **3**
Rationale: Otoscopic examination in a client with mastoiditis reveals a red, dull, thick and immobile tympanic membrane with or without perforation. Postauricular lymph nodes are tender and enlarged. Clients also have a low-grade fever, malaise, anorexia, swelling behind the ear, and pain with minimal movement of the head. Options 1, 2, and 4 are not findings that would be noted in this examination in the client with mastoiditis.
Test-Taking Strategy: Focus on the name of the disorder, mastoiditis. Recalling that "-itis" indicates inflammation or infection will direct you to option 3. If you had difficulty with this question, review these findings.
Level of Cognitive Ability: Comprehension
Client Needs: Physiological Integrity
Integrated Process: Nursing Process/Data Collection
Content Area: Adult Health/Ear
Reference: Linton, A., & Maebius, N. (2003). *Introduction to medical-surgical nursing* (3rd ed.). Philadelphia: W.B. Saunders, pp. 1087-1088.

34. *Answer:* **3**
Rationale: Tinnitus is the most common complaint of clients with otologic disorders, especially disorders involving the inner ear. Symptoms of tinnitus range from mild ringing in the ear that can go unnoticed during the day to a loud roaring in the ear that can interfere with the client's thinking process and attention span. Hearing loss may or may not occur. Options 2 and 4 are not specifically associated with inner ear problems.
Test-Taking Strategy: Use the process of elimination. Recalling the functions of the inner ear will direct you to the correct option. Review inner ear problems and the associated findings if you had difficulty with this question.
Level of Cognitive Ability: Comprehension
Client Needs: Physiological Integrity
Integrated Process: Nursing Process/Data Collection
Content Area: Adult Health/Ear
Reference: Black, J., & Hawks, J. (2005). *Medical-surgical nursing: Clinical management for positive outcomes* (7th ed.). Philadelphia: W.B. Saunders, p. 1974.

35. *Answer:* **4**
Rationale: Meniere's disease is a disorder of the labyrinth of the inner ear. This disorder does not affect the external ear, tympanic membrane, or the middle ear.
Test-Taking Strategy: Use the process of elimination. Recalling that a symptom of Meniere's disease is tinnitus will assist in directing you to option 4. Review this disorder if you had difficulty with this question.
Level of Cognitive Ability: Comprehension
Client Needs: Physiological Integrity
Integrated Process: Nursing Process/Planning
Content Area: Adult Health/Ear
Reference: Linton, A., & Maebius, N. (2003). *Introduction to medical-surgical nursing* (3rd ed.). Philadelphia: W.B. Saunders, p. 1089.

36. *Answer:* **1**
Rationale: Surgical treatment for Meniere's disease involves relief from accumulation of inner ear fluid in the endolymphatic sac. Procedures may be directed toward relief of pressure by the bony structures surrounding the sac or toward opening the sac and diverting the flow of endolymph by a shunt to the mastoid bone or to the subarachnoid space. Options 2, 3, and 4 are procedures that are unrelated to Meniere's disease.
Test-Taking Strategy: Use the process of elimination. Recalling that Meniere's disease affects the inner ear will assist in directing you to option 1. If you are unfamiliar with this disorder and the surgical procedures, review this content.
Level of Cognitive Ability: Comprehension
Client Needs: Physiological Integrity
Integrated Process: Nursing Process/Planning
Content Area: Adult Health/Ear
Reference: Linton, A., & Maebius, N. (2003). *Introduction to medical-surgical nursing* (3rd ed.). Philadelphia: W.B. Saunders, p. 1090.

37. *Answer:* **1**
Rationale: Otosclerosis involves the formation of spongy bone in the capsule of the labyrinth of the ear, often causing

the auditory ossicles to become fixed and less able to pass on vibrations when sound enters the ear. An early symptom is ringing in the ears, but the most noticeable symptom is progressive hearing loss. Options 2, 3, and 4 are not associated with this condition.
Test-Taking Strategy: Use the process of elimination and note the key word, *early*. Recalling that this disorder involves the ear will assist in eliminating options 2 and 3. Focusing on the key word will assist in directing you to option 1 from the remaining options. If you had difficulty with this question review this disorder.
Level of Cognitive Ability: Comprehension
Client Needs: Physiological Integrity
Integrated Process: Nursing Process/Data Collection
Content Area: Adult Health/Ear
Reference: Black, J., & Hawks, J. (2005). *Medical-surgical nursing: Clinical management for positive outcomes* (7th ed.). Philadelphia: W.B. Saunders, pp. 1973-1974.

38. *Answer:* **3**
Rationale: Clients with otosclerosis who do not desire surgery may have their hearing loss relieved by the use of a hearing aid. Options 1, 2, and 4 are inappropriate responses.
Test-Taking Strategy: Use therapeutic communication techniques. Eliminate options 2 and 4 first because they are similar and provide advice to the client. Next, eliminate option 1 because it is incorrect and nontherapeutic. Review the surgical treatment for otosclerosis if you had difficulty with this question.
Level of Cognitive Ability: Application
Client Needs: Psychosocial Integrity
Integrated Process: Nursing Process/Implementation
Content Area: Adult Health/Ear
Reference: Christensen, B., & Kockrow, E. (2003). *Adult health nursing* (4th ed.). St. Louis: Mosby, p. 593.

39. *Answer:* **3**
Rationale: After the acute phase, remission occurs but symptoms will recur, with two or three acute attacks per year. As this pattern of attacks and remissions develops, fewer symptoms occur during the acute phase. A complete remission eventually occurs with some degree of hearing loss, varying from slight to complete. It takes several weeks before all symptoms subside after an attack, leaving a loss of hearing in the involved ear. Options 1, 2, and 4 are incorrect.
Test-Taking Strategy: Use the process of elimination. Remember that a hearing loss occurs to some degree for an acute attack of Meniere's disease. If you are unfamiliar with the effects of Meniere's disease on hearing, review this content.
Level of Cognitive Ability: Application
Client Needs: Physiological Integrity
Integrated Process: Nursing Process/Implementation
Content Area: Adult Health/Ear
Reference: Christensen, B., & Kockrow, E. (2003). *Adult health nursing* (4th ed.). St. Louis: Mosby, p. 593.

40. *Answer:* **3**
Rationale: Medical interventions during the acute phase of Meniere's disease include using atropine or diazepam (Valium) to decrease the autonomic nervous system function. Diphenhydramine (Benadryl) may be prescribed for its antihistamine effects, and a vasodilator will also be prescribed. The client will remain on bed rest during the acute attack and, when allowed to be out of bed, the client will need assistance with walking, sitting, or standing.
Test-Taking Strategy: Note the key words, *would the nurse question*. These words indicate a false response question and that you need to select the incorrect intervention. Recalling the pathophysiology associated with Meniere's disease will direct you to option 3. If you are unfamiliar with the treatment measures for this disorder, review this content.
Level of Cognitive Ability: Analysis
Client Needs: Physiological Integrity
Integrated Process: Nursing Process/Implementation
Content Area: Adult Health/Ear
Reference: Christensen, B., & Kockrow, E. (2003). *Adult health nursing* (4th ed.). St. Louis: Mosby, p. 593.

41. *Answer:* **4**
Rationale: Management during remission includes diuretics to decrease the fluid and thereby decrease pressure in the endolymphatic system. Antihistamines, vasodilators, and diuretics may be prescribed for the client. A low-salt diet is prescribed for the client to reduce fluids. The major goal of treatment is to preserve the client's hearing; careful medical management helps achieve this in most clients with Meniere's disease.
Test-Taking Strategy: Note the key words, *need for further education*. These words indicate a false response question and that you need to select the incorrect client statement. Recalling that Meniere's disease occurs as a result of a disturbance in the fluid of the endolymphatic system will direct you to option 4. If you are unfamiliar with the management of this disorder during remission, review this content.
Level of Cognitive Ability: Comprehension
Client Needs: Health Promotions and Maintenance
Integrated Process: Teaching/Learning
Content Area: Adult Health/Ear
Reference: Linton, A., & Maebius, N. (2003). *Introduction to medical-surgical nursing* (3rd ed.). Philadelphia: W.B. Saunders, p. 1091.

42. *Answer:* **2**
Rationale: Following stapedectomy, the client is instructed to keep water out of the ear canal for at least 3 weeks and to avoid swimming for 6 weeks. The client is also instructed to avoid coughing and sneezing and to avoid bending and lifting heavy objects or other strenuous activities for at least 3 weeks. Air travel is avoided for 4 weeks. If the client develops sudden hearing loss, fever or severe persistent vertigo or dizziness the physician should be notified.
Test-Taking Strategy: Note the key words, *indicates a need for further education*. Read each option carefully, noting the time frame and the activities described in the options. Eliminate options 1 and 4 first because of the similar time frames. Eliminate option 3 next, because of the word "persistent." Review the client teaching points following this procedure if you had difficulty with this question.
Level of Cognitive Ability: Comprehension
Client Needs: Health Promotion and Maintenance

Integrated Process: Teaching/Learning
Content Area: Adult Health/Ear
Reference: Christensen, B., & Kockrow, E. (2003). *Adult health nursing* (4th ed.). St. Louis: Mosby, pp. 594-595.

43. *Answer: 3*
Rationale: Following ear surgery, clients need to avoid straining when having a bowel movement. Clients need to be instructed to avoid drinking with a straw for 2 to 3 weeks, avoid air travel, and avoid coughing excessively. Clients need to avoid getting their head wet, washing their hair and showering for 1 week. Clients need to avoid rapidly moving the head, bouncing, and bending over for 3 weeks.
Test-Taking Strategy: Use the process of elimination. Note that the question asks for the instruction that will be included in the plan of care. Consider the anatomical area of the client's condition and the surgical procedure in eliminating the incorrect options. If you had difficulty with this question, review client instructions following ear surgery.
Level of Cognitive Ability: Application
Client Needs: Health Promotion and Maintenance
Integrated Process: Teaching/Learning
Content Area: Adult Health/Ear
Reference: Christensen, B., & Kockrow, E. (2003). *Adult health nursing* (4th ed.). St. Louis: Mosby, p. 595.

44. *Answer: 3*
Rationale: A small amount of brownish or reddish drainage is normal for 24 to 48 hours following the surgery. Excessive drainage, especially clear fluid should be reported immediately. Options 1, 2, and 4 are inaccurate instructions.
Test-Taking Strategy: Read each option carefully and use the process of elimination. Remember, a small amount of brownish or reddish drainage is normal for 24 to 48 hours following the surgery. If you are unfamiliar with the normal findings following myringotomy, review this content.
Level of Cognitive Ability: Application
Client Needs: Physiological Integrity
Integrated Process: Nursing Process/Implementation
Content Area: Adult Health/Ear
Reference: Christensen, B., & Kockrow, E. (2003). *Adult health nursing* (4th ed.). St. Louis: Mosby, p. 597.

45. *Answer: 3*
Rationale: Nurses should have a basic knowledge of the care of a hearing aid to assist the client in its use. The client should be instructed to turn the hearing aid off before removing it from the ear to prevent squealing feedback. The hearing aid

should be turned off when not in use and the client should keep an extra battery available at all times. The client should wash the ear mold frequently with mild soap and water, using a pipe cleaner to cleanse the cannula. The client should not wear the hearing aid during an ear infection.
Test-Taking Strategy: Use the process of elimination and note the key words, *need for further education.* These words indicate a false response question and that you need to select the incorrect client statement. Recalling the causes of squealing feedback will direct you to the correct option. If you had difficulty with this question, review the use of the hearing aid.
Level of Cognitive Ability: Comprehension
Client Needs: Health Promotion and Maintenance
Integrated Process: Teaching/Learning
Content Area: Adult Health/Ear
Reference: Christensen, B., & Kockrow, E. (2003). *Adult health nursing* (4th ed.). St. Louis: Mosby, p. 586.

ALTERNATE FORMAT QUESTION: MULTIPLE RESPONSE

Answers:
To place an eye shield on the surgical eye at bedtime
To avoid activities that require bending over
To contact the surgeon if a decrease in visual acuity occurs
Rationale: Following eye surgery, some scratchiness may occur in the operative eye, which is usually relieved by mild analgesics. If the eye pain becomes severe, the client should notify the surgeon, because this may indicate hemorrhage, infection, or increased intraocular pressure. The nurse would also instruct the client to notify the surgeon if there is increased purulent drainage, increased redness, or any decrease in visual acuity. The client is instructed to place an eye shield over the operative eye at bedtime to protect the eye from injury during sleep and to avoid activities that increase intraocular pressure, such as bending over.
Test-Taking Strategy: Note that the client has had eye surgery. Recalling that the eye needs to be protected and that a concern is increased intraocular pressure will assist in determining the home care measures to be included in the plan. Review these measures if you had difficulty with this question.
Level of Cognitive Ability: Application
Client Needs: Physiological Integrity
Integrated Process: Teaching/Learning
Content Area: Adult Health/Ear
Reference: Lewis, S., Heitkemper, M., & Dirksen, S. (2004). *Medical-surgical nursing: Assessment and management of clinical problems* (6th ed.). St. Louis: Mosby, p. 452.

REFERENCES

Black, J., & Hawks, J. (2005). *Medical-surgical nursing: Clinical management for positive outcomes* (7th ed.). Philadelphia: W.B. Saunders.

Christensen, B., & Kockrow, E. (2003). *Adult health nursing* (4th ed.). St. Louis: Mosby.

deWit, S. (2005). *Fundamental concepts and skills for nursing* (2nd ed.). Philadelphia: W.B. Saunders.

Jarvis, C. (2004). *Physical examination and health assessment* (4th ed.). Philadelphia: W.B. Saunders.

Lewis, S., Heitkemper, M., & Dirksen, S. (2004). *Medical-surgical nursing: Assessment and management of clinical problems* (6th ed.). St. Louis: Mosby.

Linton, A., & Maebius, N. (2003). *Introduction to medical-surgical nursing* (3rd ed.). Philadelphia: W.B. Saunders.

Ophthalmic and Otic Medications

I. OPHTHALMIC MEDICATION ADMINISTRATION

A. Guidelines for the use of eye medications

1. Eye medications are usually in the form of drops or ointments
2. To prevent overflow of medication into the nasal and pharyngeal passages, thus reducing systemic absorption, instruct the client to apply pressure over the inner canthus next to the nose for 30 to 60 seconds following administration of the medication
3. If both an eyedrop and an eye ointment are scheduled to be administered at the same time, administer the eyedrop first
4. Wash hands and don gloves before administering eye medications to avoid contaminating the eye, medication dropper, or applicator
5. Use a separate bottle or tube of medication for each client to avoid accidental cross contamination
6. Place prescribed dose of eye medication in the lower conjunctival sac, never directly onto the cornea
7. Avoid touching any part of the eye with the dropper or applicator
8. Administer glucocorticoid preparations before other medications
9. Monitor the pulse of the client receiving an ophthalmic beta blocker and instruct the client to do the same; if the pulse is below 50 to 60 beats per minute (adult), withhold the next dose of eye medication and notify the physician
10. Instruct the client how to instill medication correctly and supervise instillation until the client can do it safely
11. Instruct the client to read the medication labels carefully to ensure administration of the correct medication and correct strength
12. Remind the client to keep these medications out of the reach of children
13. Instruct the client to avoid driving or operating hazardous equipment if vision is blurred
14. Inform the client that he or she may be unable to drive home after eye examinations when medications to dilate the pupil (**mydriatics**) or medications to paralyze the ciliary muscle (**cycloplegics**) are used
15. If photophobia occurs, instruct the client to wear sunglasses and avoid bright lights
16. Instruct the client to administer a missed dose of the eye medication as soon as remembered, unless the next dose is scheduled to be administered in 1 to 2 hours
17. Inform the client with **glaucoma** that the disorder cannot be cured, only controlled
18. Reinforce the importance of using medications to treat **glaucoma** as prescribed and not to discontinue these medications without consulting the physician
19. Inform the client that medications used to treat **glaucoma** may cause pain and blurred vision, especially when therapy is begun
20. Instruct the client to report the development of any eye irritation
21. Inform the client using eye gel to store the gel at room temperature or in the refrigerator but not to freeze it
22. Instruct the client to discard unused eye gel kept at room temperature after 8 weeks
23. Inform the client that soft contact lenses may absorb certain eye medications and that preservatives in eye medications may discolor the contact lenses
24. Advise the client wearing contact lenses to question the physician carefully about special precautions to observe

25. In infants, inform the parents that atropine sulfate eyedrops may contribute to abdominal distention
26. Instruct the parents to keep a record of the bowel movements of the infant being administered atropine sulfate eyedrops
27. Auscultate bowel sounds of the infant or child receiving atropine sulfate eyedrops

B. Instillation of eye medications
   1. Drops
      a. Wash hands
      b. Put gloves on
      c. Check the name, strength, and expiration date of the medication
      d. Instruct the client to tilt the head backward, open the eyes, and look up
      e. Pull the lower lid down against the cheekbone
      f. Hold the bottle like a pencil, with the tip downward
      g. Holding the bottle, gently rest the wrist of the hand on the client's cheek
      h. Squeeze the bottle gently to allow the drop to fall into the conjunctival sac
      i. Instruct the client to close the eyes gently and not to squeeze the eyes shut
      j. Wait 3 to 5 minutes before instilling another drop, if more than one drop is prescribed, to promote maximal absorption of the medication
      k. Do not allow the medication bottle, dropper, or applicator to come into contact with the eyeball
   2. Ointments
      a. Hold the ointment tube near, but not touching, the eye or eyelashes
      b. Squeeze a thin ribbon of ointment along the lining of the lower conjunctival sac from the inner to the outer canthus
      c. Instruct the client to close the eyes gently
      d. Instruct the client that vision may be blurred by the ointment

II. MYDRIATIC-CYCLOPLEGIC AND ANTICHOLINERGIC MEDICATIONS (Box 55-1)
A. Description
   1. **Mydriatics** and **cycloplegics** dilate the pupils (**mydriasis**) and relax the ciliary muscles (**cycloplegia**)
   2. Anticholinergics block responses of the sphincter muscle in the ciliary body, producing **mydriasis** and **cycloplegia**
   3. Used preoperatively or for eye examinations to produce **mydriasis**
   4. Contraindicated in clients with **glaucoma** because of the risk of increased intraocular pressure
   5. **Mydriatics** are contraindicated in cardiac dysrhythmias and cerebral atherosclerosis and

---

BOX 55-1

Mydriatic-Cycloplegic Eye Medications

Atropine sulfate (Isopto Atropine, Atropisol)
Cyclopentolate hydrochloride (Cyclogyl, AK-Pentolate, Pentolair)
Homatropine hydrobromide (Isopto Homatrine)
Scopolamine hydrobromide (Isopto Hyoscine)
Tropicamide (Mydriacyl, Tropicacyl)

---

should be used with caution in the older client and in clients with prostatic hypertrophy, diabetes mellitus, or parkinsonism
B. Side effects
   1. Tachycardia
   2. Photophobia
   3. Conjunctivitis
   4. Dermatitis
C. Atropine toxicity
   1. Dry mouth
   2. Blurred vision
   3. Photophobia
   4. Tachycardia
   5. Fever
   6. Urinary retention
   7. Constipation
   8. Headache, brow pain
   9. Confusion
   10. Hallucinations, delirium
   11. Coma
   12. Worsening of narrow-angle **glaucoma**
D. Systemic reactions of anticholinergics
   1. Dry mouth and skin
   2. Fever
   3. Thirst
   4. Confusion
   5. Hyperactivity
E. Interventions
   1. Monitor for allergic response
   2. Assess for risk of injury
   3. Monitor for constipation and urinary retention
   4. Instruct the client that a burning sensation may occur on instillation
   5. Instruct the client not to drive or operate machinery for 24 hours after instillation of the medication unless otherwise directed by the physician
   6. Instruct the client to wear sunglasses until the effects of the medication wear off
   7. Instruct the client to notify the physician if blurring of vision, loss of sight, difficulty breathing, sweating, or flushing occurs
   8. Instruct the client to report eye pain to the physician

BOX 55-2

Anti-infective Eye Medications

ANTIBACTERIALS
Chloramphenicol (Chloromycetin, Chloroptic)
Erythromycin (Ilotycin)

AMINOGLYCOSIDES
Gentamicin sulfate (Garamycin, Genoptic)
Tobramycin (Nebcin, Tobrex)

ANTIFUNGAL
Natamycin (Natacyn)

ANTIVIRAL
Idoxuridine (Herplex)
Trifluridine (Viroptic)
Vidarabine (Vira-A)

SULFONAMIDES
Sulfacetamide (Bleph-10, Sulamyd Sodium)
Sulfisoxazole (Gantrisin)

BOX 55-3

Anti-inflammatory Eye Medications

CORTICOSTEROIDS
Dexamethasone (Maxidex)
Fluorometholone (FML S.O.P., FML)
Medrysone (HMS)
Prednisolone (Pred Forte)

NONSTEROIDAL ANTI-INFLAMMATORY DRUGS (NSAIDs)
Diclofenac (Voltaren)
Flurbiprofen sodium (Ocufen)
Ketorolac tromethamine (Acular)

ANTIALLERGIC AGENTS
Cromolyn sodium (Opticrom)
Ketotifen fumarate (Zaditor)
Levocabastine (Livostin)
Lodoxamide (Alomide)

BOX 55-4

Topical Anesthetics for the Eye

Proparacaine hydrochloride (Ophthaine, Ophthetic)
Tetracaine hydrochloride (Pontocaine)

F. Alpha-adrenergic blocker
   1. Medication: Dapiprazole hydrochloride (Rev-Eyes)
   2. Used to counteract **mydriasis**

III. ANTI-INFECTIVE EYE MEDICATIONS (Box 55-2)
A. Description: Kill or inhibit the growth of bacteria, fungi, and viruses
B. Side effects
   1. Superinfection
   2. Global irritation
C. Interventions
   1. Assess for risk of injury
   2. Instruct the client how to apply the eye medication
   3. Instruct the client to continue treatment, as prescribed
   4. Instruct the client to wash hands thoroughly and frequently
   5. Advise the client to notify the physician if improvement does not occur

IV. ANTI-INFLAMMATORY EYE MEDICATIONS (Box 55-3)
A. Description
   1. Control inflammation, thereby reducing vision loss and scarring
   2. Used for uveitis, allergic conditions, and inflammation of the conjunctiva, cornea, and lids
B. Side effects
   1. Cataracts
   2. Increased intraocular pressure
   3. Impaired healing
   4. Masking signs and symptoms of infection

C. Interventions
   1. See earlier, "Anti-Infective Eye Medications, Interventions"
   2. Note that dexamethasone (Maxidex) should not be used for eye abrasions and wounds

V. TOPICAL ANESTHETICS FOR THE EYE (Box 55-4)
A. Description
   1. Produce corneal anesthesia
   2. Used for anesthesia for eye examinations, surgery, or removal of foreign bodies from the eye
B. Side effects
   1. Temporary stinging or burning of the eye
   2. Temporary loss of corneal reflex
C. Interventions
   1. Assess for risk of injury
   2. Note that the medications should not be given to the client for home use and are not to be self-administered by the client
   3. Note that the blink reflex is temporarily lost and that the corneal epithelium needs to be protected
   4. Provide an eye patch to protect the eye from injury until the corneal reflex returns

VI. EYE LUBRICANTS (Box 55-5)
A. Description
   1. Replace tears or add moisture to the eyes

BOX 55-5

Eye Lubricants

Hydroxypropyl methylcellulose (Lacril, Isopto Plain)
Petroleum-based ointment (Artificial Tears)
Polyvinyl alcohol (Liquifilm Tears)

---

    2. Moisten contact lenses or an artificial eye
    3. Protect the eyes during surgery or diagnostic procedures
    4. Used for keratitis, during anesthesia, or in a disorder that results in unconsciousness or decreased blinking
  B. Side effects
    1. Burning on instillation
    2. Discomfort or pain on instillation
  C. Interventions
    1. Inform the client that burning may occur on instillation
    2. Be alert to allergic responses to the preservatives in the lubricants

VII. MIOTICS (Box 55-6)
  A. Description
    1. Reduce intraocular pressure by constricting the pupil and contracting the ciliary muscle, thereby increasing the blood flow to the retina and decreasing retinal damage and loss of vision
    2. Open the anterior chamber angle and increase the outflow of aqueous humor
    3. **Miotic** cholinergic medications reduce intraocular pressure by mimicking the action of acetylcholine
    4. **Miotic** acetylcholine inhibitors reduce intraocular pressure by inhibiting the action of cholinesterase
    5. Used for chronic open-angle **glaucoma** or acute and chronic closed-angle **glaucoma**
    6. Used to achieve **miosis** during eye surgery
    7. Contraindicated in clients with **retinal detachment**, adhesions between the iris and lens, or inflammatory disease
    8. Use with caution in clients with asthma, hypertension, corneal abrasion, hyperthyroidism, coronary vascular disease, urinary tract obstruction, gastrointestinal (GI) obstruction, ulcer disease, parkinsonism, and bradycardia
  B. Side effects
    1. **Myopia**
    2. Headache
    3. Eye pain
    4. Decreased vision in poor light
    5. Local irritation
    6. Systemic effects
      a. Flushing
      b. Diaphoresis
      c. GI upset and diarrhea

BOX 55-6

Miotics

Carbachol (Carboptic)
Pilocarpine hydrochloride (Isopto Carpine)
Demecarium bromide (Humorsol)
Echothiophate (Phospholine Iodide)
Isoflurophate (Floropryl)

---

      d. Frequent urination
      e. Increased salivation
      f. Muscle weakness
      g. Respiratory difficulty
    7. Toxicity
      a. Vertigo and syncope
      b. Bradycardia
      c. Hypotension
      d. Cardiac dysrhythmias
      e. Tremors
      f. Seizures
  C. Interventions
    1. Monitor vital signs
    2. Assess for risk of injury
    3. Assess the client for the degree of diminished vision
    4. Monitor for side effects and toxic effects
    5. Monitor for postural hypotension and instruct the client to change positions slowly
    6. Check breath sounds for crackles and rhonchi, because cholinergic medications can cause bronchospasms and increased bronchial secretions
    7. Maintain oral hygiene because of the increase in salivation
    8. Have atropine sulfate available as an antidote for pilocarpine
    9. Instruct the client or family regarding the correct administration of eye medications
    10. Instruct the client not to stop the medication suddenly
    11. Instruct the client to avoid activities such as driving while vision is impaired
    12. Instruct clients with glaucoma to read labels on over-the-counter medications and to avoid atropine-like medications, because atropine will increase intraocular pressure

VIII. OCUSERT SYSTEM
  A. Description
    1. Ocusert is a thin eye wafer (disk) impregnated with time-release pilocarpine
    2. It is devised to overcome the frequent application of pilocarpine
    3. It is placed in the upper or lower cul-de-sac of the eye
    4. The pilocarpine is released over 1 week

5. The disk is replaced every 7 days
6. Drawbacks of its use include sudden leakage of pilocarpine, migration of the system over the cornea, and unnoticed loss of the system

B. Interventions
1. Determine the client's ability to insert the medication disk
2. Store the medication in the refrigerator
3. Instruct the client to discard damaged or contaminated disks
4. Inform the client that temporary stinging is expected but to notify the physician if blurred vision or brow pain occurs
5. Instruct the client to check for the presence of the disk in the conjunctival sac daily, at bedtime and on arising
6. Because vision may change in the first few hours after the eye system is inserted, instruct the client to replace the disk at bedtime

IX. BETA-ADRENERGIC BLOCKER EYE MEDICATIONS (Box 55-7)

A. Description
1. Reduce intraocular pressure by decreasing sympathetic impulses and decreasing aqueous humor production without affecting **accommodation** or pupil size
2. Used to treat chronic open-angle **glaucoma**
3. Contraindicated in the client with asthma because systemic absorption can cause increased airway resistance
4. Use with caution in the client receiving oral beta blockers

B. Side effects
1. Ocular irritation
2. Visual disturbances
3. Bradycardia
4. Hypotension
5. Bronchospasm

C. Interventions
1. Monitor vital signs, especially blood pressure and pulse before administering medication
2. If the pulse is 60 beats per minute or less or if the systolic blood pressure is below 90 mm Hg, withhold the medication and contact the physician
3. Monitor for shortness of breath
4. Assess for risk of injury
5. Monitor input and output (I&O)
6. Instruct the client to notify the physician if shortness of breath occurs
7. Instruct the client not to discontinue the medication abruptly
8. Instruct the client to change positions slowly to avoid orthostatic hypotension
9. Instruct the client to avoid hazardous activities

BOX 55-7

Beta-Adrenergic Blocker Eye Medications

Betaxolol hydrochloride (Betoptic)
Carteolol hydrochloride (Ocupress)
Levobunolol hydrochloride (Betagan Liquifilm)
Metipranolol (OptiPranolol)
Timolol maleate (Timoptic)

BOX 55-8

Adrenergic Medications

Epinephrine (Epifrin, Glaucon)
Hydroxyamphetamine (Paredrine)
Naphazoline (Allerest, VasoClear)
Oxymetazoline (OcuClear)
Phenylephrine (Ak-Nefrin, Prefrin Liquifilm)
Tetrahydrozoline (Murine Plus, Visine)

BOX 55-9

Carbonic Anhydrase Inhibitor Medications for the Eye

Acetazolamide (Diamox)
Dichlorphenamide (Daranide)
Methazolamide (Neptazane)
Dorzolamide hydrochloride (Trusopt)

---

10. Instruct the client to avoid over-the-counter medications; these should not be taken without the physician's approval

D. Adrenergic medications (Box 55-8)
1. Decrease the production of aqueous humor and lead to a decrease in intraocular pressure
2. Used to treat **glaucoma**

X. CARBONIC ANHYDRASE INHIBITORS (Box 55-9)

A. Description
1. Interfere with the production of carbonic acid, which leads to decreased aqueous humor formation and decreased intraocular pressure
2. Used for long-term treatment of open-angle **glaucoma**
3. Contraindicated in the client allergic to sulfonamides

B. Side effects
1. Appetite loss
2. GI upset
3. Paresthesias in the fingers, toes, and face
4. Polyuria
5. Hypokalemia
6. Renal calculi
7. Photosensitivity
8. Lethargy and drowsiness
9. Depression

C. Interventions
1. Monitor vital signs
2. Assess visual acuity
3. Assess for risk of injury
4. Monitor I&O
5. Monitor weight
6. Maintain oral hygiene
7. Monitor for side effects such as lethargy, anorexia, drowsiness, polyuria, nausea, and vomiting
8. Monitor electrolytes for hypokalemia
9. Increase fluid intake unless contraindicated
10. Advise the client to avoid prolonged exposure to sunlight
11. Encourage the use of artificial tears for dry eyes
12. Instruct the client not to discontinue the medication abruptly
13. Instruct the client to avoid hazardous activities while vision is impaired

XI. OSMOTIC MEDICATIONS (Box 55-10)
A. Description
1. Lower intraocular pressure
2. Used in emergency treatment of acute closed-angle **glaucoma**
3. Used preoperatively and postoperatively to decrease vitreous humor volume
B. Side effects
1. Headache
2. Nausea, vomiting, diarrhea
3. Disorientation
4. Electrolyte imbalances
C. Interventions
1. Monitor vital signs
2. Assess visual acuity
3. Assess for risk of injury
4. Monitor I&O
5. Monitor weight
6. Monitor electrolyte imbalances
7. Increase fluid intake unless contraindicated
8. Monitor for changes in level of orientation

XII. OTIC MEDICATION ADMINISTRATION (Box 55-11)
A. Administering drops
1. In an adult, pull the pinna up and back to straighten the external canal to instill ear drops
2. Pull the pinna down and back for infants and children younger than 3 years of age, up and back for older children
B. Irrigation of the ear
1. Needs to be prescribed by the physician
2. Ensure that there is direct visualization of the tympanic membrane
3. Use warm irrigating solution to 98° F (36.6° C), because solutions that are not close to the client's

---

BOX 55-10

Osmotic Medications for the Eye

Glycerin (Osmoglyn)
Mannitol (Osmitrol)

BOX 55-11

Medications that Affect Hearing

ANTIBIOTICS
Amikacin (Amikin)
Chloramphenicol (Chloromycetin, Chloroptic)
Erythromycin (E-Mycin, ERYC, Ery-Tab, PCE Dispertabs, Ilotycin)
Gentamicin (Garamycin)
Streptomycin sulfate (Streptomycin)
Tobramycin sulfate (Nebcin)
Vancomycin (Vancocin)

DIURETICS
Acetazolamide (Diamox)
Furosemide (Lasix)
Ethacrynic acid (Edecrin)

OTHERS
Cisplatin (Platinol, Platinol-AQ)
Nitrogen mustard
Quinine
Quinidine

---

body temperature will cause ear injury, nausea, and vertigo
4. Irrigation must be done gently to avoid damage to the eardrum
5. When irrigating, do not direct irrigation solution directly toward the eardrum
6. If a perforation of the eardrum is suspected, irrigation is not done

XIII. ANTI-INFECTIVE EAR MEDICATIONS (Box 55-12)
A. Description
1. Kill or inhibit the growth of bacteria
2. Used for otitis media or otitis externa
3. Contraindicated if a prior hypersensitivity exists
B. Side effects: Overgrowth of nonsusceptible organisms
C. Interventions
1. Monitor vital signs
2. Check for allergies
3. Monitor pain level
4. Monitor for nephrotoxicity
5. Instruct the client to report dizziness, fatigue, fever, or sore throat, which may be indicative of a superimposed infection

BOX 55-12

Anti-infective Ear Medications

Acetic acid and aluminum acetate (Otic Domeboro)
Amoxicillin (Amoxil)
Ampicillin trihydrate
Cefaclor (Ceclor)
Clarithromycin (Biaxin)
Chloramphenicol (Chloromycetin Otic)
Clindamycin hydrochloride (Cleocin)
Erythromycin (Ilotycin, E-Mycin)
Gentamicic sulfate otic solution (Garamycin)
Loracarbef (Lorabid)
Penicillin V potassium (Veetids)
Trimethoprim (TMP) and sulfamethoxazole (SMZ) (Bactrim, Cotrim, Septra)

BOX 55-13

Antihistamines and Decongestants

Triprolidine and pseudoephedrine (Actifed Cold & Allergy)
Naphazoline hydrochloride (Allerest, Albalon)
Chlorpheniramine (Chlor-Trimeton, Teldrin)
Brompheniramine (Bromphen)
Clemastine (Tavist Allergy)
Cetirizine (Zyrtec)
Astemizole (Hismanal)

6. Instruct the client to complete the entire course of the medication
7. Instruct the client to keep ear canals dry

XIV. ANTIHISTAMINES AND DECONGESTANTS
(Box 55-13)
A. Description
  1. Produce vasoconstriction
  2. Stimulate the receptors of the respiratory mucosa
  3. Reduce respiratory tissue hyperemia and edema in open, obstructed eustachian tubes
  4. Used for acute otitis media
B. Side effects
  1. Drowsiness
  2. Blurred vision
  3. Dry mucous membranes
C. Interventions
  1. Inform the client that drowsiness, blurred vision, and a dry mouth may occur
  2. Instruct the client to increase fluid intake unless contraindicated and to suck on hard candy to alleviate the dry mouth
  3. Instruct the client to avoid hazardous activities if drowsiness occurs

BOX 55-14

Ceruminolytic Medications

Carbamide peroxide (Debrox)
Boric acid (Ear-Dry)
Trolamine polypeptide oleate-condensate (Cerumenex)

XV. LOCAL ANESTHETICS
A. Description
  1. Block nerve conduction at or near the application site to control pain
  2. Used for pain associated with ear infections
B. Medication: Benzocaine (Americaine Otic; Tympagesic)
C. Side effects
  1. Allergic reaction
  2. Irritation
D. Interventions
  1. Monitor for effectiveness if used for pain relief
  2. Assess for irritation or allergic reaction

XVI. CERUMINOLYTIC MEDICATIONS (Box 55-14)
A. Description
  1. Emulsify and loosen cerumen deposits
  2. Used to loosen and remove impacted wax from the ear canal
B. Side effects
  1. Irritation
  2. Redness or swelling of the ear canal
C. Interventions
  1. Instruct the client not to use drops more often than prescribed
  2. Moisten a cotton plug with medication before insertion
  3. Keep the container tightly closed and away from moisture
  4. Avoid touching the ear with the dropper
  5. Thirty minutes after instillation, gently irrigate the ear as prescribed with warm water using a soft, rubber bulb ear syringe
  6. Irrigation may be done with hydrogen peroxide solution as prescribed to flush cerumen deposits out of the ear canal
  7. For a chronic cerumen impaction, one or two drops of mineral oil will soften the wax
  8. Instruct the client to notify physician if redness, pain, or swelling persists

PRACTICE QUESTIONS

1. In preparation for cataract surgery, the nurse is to administer cyclopentolate hydrochloride (Cyclogyl) eye drops. The nurse administers the medication knowing that the purpose of the medication is to:
  1. Provide lubrication to the operative eye
  2. Produce miosis of the operative eye

   3. Dilate the pupil of the operative eye
   4. Constrict the pupil of the operative eye
2. A nurse is reinforcing instructions to the client regarding the administration of the prescribed eyedrops. Which of the following statements by the client indicates a need for further instructions?
   1. "I can tilt my head back, pull down on the lower lid, and place the drop in the lower lid."
   2. "I can lie down, pull down on the lower lid, and place the drop in the lower lid."
   3. "I can lie down, pull up on the upper lid, and place the drop in the lower lid."
   4. "I can lie on my side opposite to the eye in which I am going to place the drop, put the drop in the corner of the lid nearest my nose, and then slowly turn to my other side while blinking."
3. A nurse is preparing to administer ear drops to an infant. The nurse plans to:
   1. Pull up and back on the ear and direct the solution onto the eardrum
   2. Pull down and back on the ear and direct the solution onto the eardrum
   3. Pull down and back on the ear and direct the solution toward the wall of the canal
   4. Pull up and back on the ear lobe and direct the solution toward the wall of the canal
4. To minimize the systemic effects that eyedrops can produce, the nurse plans to instruct the client to:
   1. Eat before instilling the drops
   2. Swallow several times after instilling the drops
   3. Blink vigorously to encourage tearing after instilling the drops
   4. Occlude the nasolacrimal duct with a finger for several minutes after instilling the drops
5. A client is receiving both epinephrine hydrochloride (Epifrin, Glaucon) and timolol maleate (Timoptic) eyedrops. When instructing the client on the administration of the eyedrops, the nurse plans to tell the client to:
   1. Administer the epinephrine hydrochloride first, followed by the timolol maleate
   2. Administer the timolol maleate first, followed by the epinephrine HCl
   3. Administer epinephrine hydrochloride in the morning and the timolol maleate in the evening
   4. Wait 3 minutes between the instillation of each medication
6. A licensed practical nurse (LPN) is assigned to care for a client with glaucoma. The LPN reviews the client's medication record and would notify the registered nurse (RN) if which medication was noted on the client's record?
   1. Carbachol (Carboptic)
   2. Pilocarpine hydrochloride (Isopto Carpine)

   3. Pilocarpine nitrate (Ocusert Pilo-20, Ocusert Pilo-40)
   4. Atropine sulfate (Isopto Atropine)
7. A miotic medication has been prescribed for the client with glaucoma and the client asks the nurse about the purpose of the medication. The nurse tells the client that:
   1. "The medication will lower the pressure in your eye and increase the blood flow to the retina."
   2. "The medication will help dilate the eye to prevent pressure from occurring."
   3. "The medication will relax the muscles of the eye and prevent blurred vision."
   4. "The medication will help block the responses that are sent to the muscles in the eye."
8. Pilocarpine hydrochloride (Isopto Carpine) is prescribed for the client with glaucoma. Which medication does the nurse plan to have available in the event of systemic toxicity?
   1. Naloxone hydrochloride (Narcan)
   2. Pindolol (Visken)
   3. Atropine sulfate
   4. Mesoridazine besylate (Serentil)
9. Betaxolol hydrochloride (Betoptic) eyedrops have been prescribed for the client with glaucoma. Which nursing action is appropriate related to monitoring for the side effects of this medication?
   1. Monitor temperature
   2. Monitor blood pressure
   3. Monitor urine for sugar and acetone
   4. Monitor peripheral pulses
10. A nurse is assisting the physician with performing an ear irrigation on an assigned client. The nurse would plan to:
   1. Position the client to turn his or her head so that the ear to be irrigated is facing upward
   2. Warm the irrigating solution to 98° F (36.6° C)
   3. Cool the irrigating solution to 85° F (29.4° C)
   4. Position the client with the affected side up following the irrigation

ALTERNATE FORMAT QUESTION: MULTIPLE RESPONSE

The nurse is preparing to administer eyedrops. Select the interventions that the nurse takes to administer the drops.

___ Wash hands
___ Put gloves on
___ Instruct the client to tilt the head forward, open the eyes, and look down
___ Place the drop into the conjunctival sac
___ Instruct the client to squeeze the eyes shut after instilling the eyedrop

ANSWERS

1. *Answer:* 3

Rationale: Cyclopentolate is a rapidly acting mydriatic and cycloplegic medication. It is effective in 25 to 75 minutes, and accommodation returns in 6 to 24 hours. Cyclopentolate is used for preoperative mydriasis. Options 1, 2, and 4 are not actions of this medication.

Test-Taking Strategy: Use the process of elimination. Options 2 and 4 are similar because miosis refers to constricted pupil. Note that the question identifies a client being prepared for eye surgery. The pupil would need to be dilated for the surgical procedure. Review the action and purpose of this medication if you had difficulty with this question.

Level of Cognitive Ability: Analysis
Client Needs: Physiological Integrity
Integrated Process: Nursing Process/Implementation
Content Area: Adult Health/Eye
Reference: Lehne, R. (2004). *Pharmacology for nursing care* (5th ed.). Philadelphia: W.B. Saunders, p. 1104.

2. *Answer:* 3

Rationale: The client can either lie down or sit with the head tilted back. The lower lid should be pulled downward with the thumb or fingers. The client holds the bottle like a pencil, with the tip downward, and squeezes the bottle gently, allowing one drop to fall into the sac. The client gently closes the eye. An alternative method for clients who blink very easily is to place the client in the supine position with the head turned to one side. The eye to receive the eyedrops should be uppermost. With the eye closed, drop the prescribed dose on the inner canthus of the eye. Have the client turn from side to midline and to the other side while blinking. The eyedrops will move via gravity and surface tension into the conjunctival sac.

Test-Taking Strategy: Note the key words, *a need for further instructions*. These words indicate a false response question and that you need to select the incorrect client statement. Knowing that the client places drops into the eye by pulling down on the lower lid will direct you to the correct option. Review the procedure for the administration of eye medications if you had difficulty with this question.

Level of Cognitive Ability: Comprehension
Client Needs: Health Promotion and Maintenance
Integrated Process: Teaching/Learning
Content Area: Adult Health/Eye
References: deWit, S. (2005). *Fundamental concepts and skills for nursing* (2nd ed.). Philadelphia: W.B. Saunders, pp. 650-651.
McKenry, L., & Salerno, E. (2003). *Mosby's pharmacology in nursing* (21st ed.). St. Louis: Mosby, p. 793.

3. *Answer:* 3

Rationale: When administering ear drops to an infant, the ear is pulled down and straight back. In the adult or a child older than 3 years, the ear is pulled up and back to straighten the auditory canal. The medication is administered by aiming it at the wall of the canal rather than directly onto the eardrum.

Test-Taking Strategy: Use the process of elimination. Eliminate options 1 and 2 because you would not direct ear solution directly onto the eardrum. Remember that, in a child younger than 3 years, pulling the ear down and straight back is the correct procedure for administering ear medications. Review the procedure for the administration of ear medications if you had difficulty with this question.

Level of Cognitive Ability: Application
Client Needs: Physiological Integrity
Integrated Process: Nursing Process/Implementation
Content Area: Child Health
Reference: deWit, S. (2005). *Fundamental concepts and skills for nursing* (2nd ed.). Philadelphia: W.B. Saunders, p. 652.

4. *Answer:* 4

Rationale: Applying pressure on the nasolacrimal duct prevents systemic absorption of the medication. Options 1, 2, and 3 will not prevent this.

Test-Taking Strategy: Use the process of elimination. Eliminate options 1 and 2 because eating and swallowing are similar and are unrelated to the systemic absorption of an eye medication. Blinking vigorously to produce tearing may result in the loss of the administered medication. Review this procedure if you had difficulty with this question.

Level of Cognitive Ability: Application
Client Needs: Health Promotion and Maintenance
Integrated Process: Teaching/Learning
Content Area: Adult Health/Eye
References: Christensen, B., & Kockrow, E. (2003). *Adult health nursing* (4th ed.). St. Louis: Mosby, p. 680.
Christensen, B., & Kockrow, E. (2003). *Foundations of nursing* (4th ed.). St. Louis: Mosby, p. 587.

5. *Answer:* 4

Rationale: When two or more medications are to be administered, the client should wait 3 to 5 minutes between instillations. Options 1, 2, and 3 are incorrect.

Test-Taking Strategy: Use the process of elimination and focus on the issue, the administration of two different prescribed eyedrops. Note that option 4 is different from the other options and provides specific information related to the question. Also, remember that when two or more medications are to be administered, the client should wait 3 to 5 minutes between instillations. Review the administration of eye medications if you had difficulty with this question.

Level of Cognitive Ability: Application
Client Needs: Health Promotion and Maintenance
Integrated Process: Teaching/Learning
Content Area: Adult Health/Eye
Reference: Potter, P., & Perry, A. (2005). *Fundamentals of nursing* (6th ed.). St. Louis: Mosby, p. 862.

6. *Answer:* 4

Rationale: Atropine sulfate is a mydriatic and cycloplegic medication and its use is contraindicated in clients with glaucoma. Mydriatic medications dilate the pupil and can cause an increase in intraocular pressure in the eye. Options 1, 2, and 3 are miotic agents used in the treatment of glaucoma.

Test-Taking Strategy: Focus on the classifications of the medications identified in the options to assist you in answering the question. Remember that my"d"riatics "d"ilate, and these medications are contraindicated in glaucoma. Review these medications if you had difficulty with this question.

Level of Cognitive Ability: Analysis
Client Needs: Safe, Effective Care Environment
Integrated Process: Nursing Process/Implementation
Content Area: Adult Health/Eye
References: Lehne, R. (2004). *Pharmacology for nursing care* (5th ed.). Philadelphia: W.B. Saunders, p. 1106.
McKenry, L., & Salerno, E. (2003). *Mosby's pharmacology in nursing* (21st ed.). St. Louis: Mosby, p. 445.

7. *Answer:* 1
Rationale: Miotics are used to lower the intraocular pressure, thereby increasing blood flow to the retina and decreasing retinal damage and loss of vision. Options 2, 3, and 4 all describe actions related to mydriatic medications, which primarily dilate the pupils and relax the ciliary muscles.
Test-Taking Strategy: Use the process of elimination. Note that the client has glaucoma. This should provide you with the clue to direct you to the correct option. Remember, prevention of increased intraocular pressure is the goal in clients with glaucoma. Review this type of medication if you had difficulty with this question.
Level of Cognitive Ability: Application
Client Needs: Health Promotion and Maintenance
Integrated Process: Nursing Process/Implementation
Content Area: Adult Health/Eye
Reference: McKenry, L., & Salerno, E. (2003). *Mosby's pharmacology in nursing* (21st ed.). St. Louis: Mosby, p. 796.

8. *Answer:* 3
Rationale: Systemic absorption of pilocarpine HCl can produce toxicity and includes manifestations of vertigo, bradycardia, tremors, hypotension, and seizures. Atropine sulfate must be available in the event of systemic toxicity. Mesoridazine besylate is an antipsychotic medication. Pindolol is a beta-adrenergic blocker. Naloxone hydrochloride is an opioid antagonist used to reverse narcotic-induced respiratory depression.
Test-Taking Strategy: Knowledge regarding antidotes related to various medications is required to answer this question. Remember, atropine sulfate is the antidote for systemic reactions that occur with pilocarpine. Review antidotes if you had difficulty with this question.
Level of Cognitive Ability: Analysis
Client Needs: Physiological Integrity
Integrated Process: Nursing Process/Planning
Content Area: Adult Health/Eye
Reference: Lilley, L., Harrington, S., & Snyder, J. (2005). *Pharmacology and the nursing process* (4th ed.). St. Louis: Mosby, p. 974.

9. *Answer:* 2
Rationale: This medication is an antiglaucoma medication and a beta-adrenergic blocker. Hypotension manifested as dizziness, nausea, diaphoresis, headache, and fatigue are systemic effects of the medication. The nurse would monitor the client's blood pressure. Options 1, 3, and 4 are not related to side effects associated with this medication.
Test-Taking Strategy: Focus on the name of the medication and recall that medication names that end with "lol" are beta

blockers. Also, use the ABCs—airway, breathing, and circulation. Although option 4 is also related to circulation monitoring, the blood pressure is the umbrella (global) option. Review the side effects of this medication if you had difficulty with this question.
Level of Cognitive Ability: Application
Client Needs: Physiological Integrity
Integrated Process: Nursing Process/Implementation
Content Area: Adult Health/Eye
Reference: Hodgson, B., & Kizior, R. (2005). *Saunders nursing drug handbook 2005*. Philadelphia: W.B. Saunders, p. 120.

10. *Answer:* 2
Rationale: Irrigation solutions that are not close to the client's body temperature can be uncomfortable and may cause injury, nausea, and vertigo. The client is positioned so that the ear to be irrigated is facing downward; this allows gravity to assist in the removal of the ear wax and solution. Following the irrigation, the client is to lie on the affected side for a period of time to finish the drainage of the irrigating solution.
Test-Taking Strategy: Use the process of elimination. Visualizing the procedure will assist in eliminating options 1 and 4. Recalling that the irrigating solution should be close to body temperature will assist in eliminating option 3. Review this procedure if you had difficulty with this question.
Level of Cognitive Ability: Application
Client Needs: Physiological Integrity
Integrated Process: Nursing Process/Planning
Content Area: Adult Health/Ear
Reference: deWit, S. (2005). *Fundamental concepts and skills for nursing* (2nd ed.). Philadelphia: W.B. Saunders, p. 775.

ALTERNATE FORMAT QUESTION: MULTIPLE RESPONSE

Answers:
Wash hands
Put gloves on
Place the drop in the conjunctival sac
Rationale: To administer eye medications, the nurse would wash hands and put gloves on. The client is instructed to tilt the head backward, open the eyes, and look up. The nurse pulls the lower lid down against the cheekbone and holds the bottle like a pencil, with the tip downward. Holding the bottle, the nurse gently rests the wrist of the hand on the client's cheek and squeezes the bottle gently to allow the drop to fall into the conjunctival sac. The client is instructed to close the eyes gently and not to squeeze the eyes shut to prevent the loss of medication.
Test-Taking Strategy: Use guidelines related to standard precautions and visualize this procedure. This will assist in determining the correct interventions. If you are unfamiliar with the procedure for administering eye medications, review these guidelines.
Level of Cognitive Ability: Application
Client Needs: Physiological Integrity
Integrated Process: Nursing Process/Implementation
Content Area: Adult Health/Eye
Reference: deWit, S. (2005). *Fundamental concepts and skills for nursing* (2nd ed.). Philadelphia: W.B. Saunders, p. 666.

REFERENCES

Christensen, B., & Kockrow, E. (2003). *Adult health nursing* (4th ed.). St. Louis. Mosby.

Christensen, B., & Kockrow, E. (2003). *Foundations of nursing* (4th ed.). St. Louis: Mosby.

deWit, S. (2005). *Fundamental concepts and skills for nursing* (2nd ed.). Philadelphia: W.B. Saunders.

Hodgson, B., & Kizior, R. (2005). *Saunders nursing drug handbook 2005*. Philadelphia: W.B. Saunders.

Lehne, R. (2004). *Pharmacology for nursing care* (5th ed.). Philadelphia: W.B. Saunders.

McKenry, L., & Salerno, E. (2003). *Mosby's pharmacology in nursing* (21st ed.). St. Louis: Mosby.

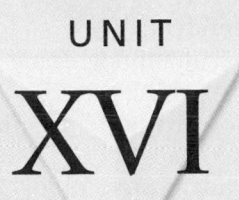

The Adult Client with a Neurological Disorder

PYRAMID TERMS

agnosia The inability to use an object correctly.

apraxia The inability to carry out a purposeful activity.

autonomic dysreflexia Also known as hyperreflexia; caused by visceral distention from a distended bladder or impacted rectum. This is a neurological emergency and must be treated immediately to prevent a hypertensive stroke. It occurs after the period of spinal shock is complete, and occurs with lesions above T6.

Babinski's reflex Indicates a disruption of the pyramidal tract; dorsiflexion of the ankle and great toe with fanning of the other toes.

Brudzinski's sign Flexion of the head causes flexion of both thighs at the hips and knee flexion; indicates meningeal irritation.

decerebrate posturing Client stiffly extends one or both arms and possibly the legs; indicates a brainstem lesion.

decorticate posturing Client flexes one or both arms on the chest and may extend the legs stiffly; indicates a nonfunctioning cortex.

flaccid posturing Client displays no motor response in any extremity.

Glasgow Coma Scale A method of assessing a client's neurological condition; a scoring system based on a scale of 1 to 15 points. A score below 8 indicates that coma is present. The client's ability to open his or her eyes is the most important indicator.

halo traction Pins or screws are inserted into the client's skull, and a circular fixation device and halo jacket or cast is applied.

hemianopsia Blindness in half the visual field.

homonymous hemianopsia Blindness in the same visual field of both eyes.

increased intracranial pressure An increase in intracranial pressure caused by trauma, hemorrhage, growths or tumors, hydrocephalus, edema, or inflammation. It can impede circulation to the brain and absorption of cerebrospinal fluid (CSF), and affect the functioning of nerve cells and lead to brainstem compression and death.

Kernig's sign Flexion of the thigh and knee to right angles; when they are extended extended, spasm of hamstring and pain occur; indicates meningeal iritation.

skull tongs Tongs that are are inserted into the outer aspect of the client's skull, just above the ears, and traction is applied.

spinal shock Also know as neurogenic shock; sudden depression of reflex activity in the spinal cord below the level of injury (areflexia) that occurs within the first hour of injury and lasts for days to months. The muscles become completely paralyzed and flaccid, and reflexes are absent.

unconscious client A state of depressed cerebral functioning with unresponsiveness to sensory and motor function. Some causes include head trauma, cerebral toxins, shock, hemorrhage, tumor, and infection.

unilateral neglect Also known as neglect syndrome; occurs most commonly in clients who have had a right cerebral stroke. The client experiences an inability to recognize his or her physical impairment.

PYRAMID TO SUCCESS

Pyramid points related to neurological disorders focus on safety issues, care of the unconscious client, monitoring for increased intracranial pressure, monitoring level of consciousness, positioning clients, implementation during a seizure, cerebrovascular accident (CVA), Parkinson's disease, and care of the client with myasthenia gravis. Altered body image and psychosocial issues that occur as a result of the neurological disorder are also a focus of the Pyramid to Success. The Integrated Processes addressed in this unit include Caring, Clinical Problem-Solving Process (Nursing Process), Communication and Documentation, and Teaching/Learning.

CLIENT NEEDS
Safe, Effective Care Environment

Accident prevention related to neurological deficits
Advance directives
Advocacy
Asepsis with procedures and treatments
Client rights

Confidentiality
Consultation with members of the health care team
Establishing priorities
Informed consent for invasive procedures
Referrals
Standard precautions

Health Promotion and Maintenance

Expected body image changes resulting from neurological deficits
Home care instructions regarding care related to neurological disorder
Neurological data collection
Prevention and early detection of health problems associated with neurological deficits
Reinforcement regarding the importance of prescribed therapy

Psychosocial Integrity

Ability to cope with feelings of isolation and loss of independence
Cultural, religious, and spiritual influences
End-of-life issues
Grief and loss
Mobilizing coping mechanisms
Sensory and perceptual alterations
Support systems and utilization of community resources
Unexpected body image changes

Physiological Integrity

Alterations in body systems
Complications related to procedures
Emergency care

Fluid and electrolyte imbalances
Measures to promote comfort
Pharmacological therapy
Promoting normal elimination patterns
Promoting self-care measures
Use of assistive devices for mobility

REFERENCES

Black, J., & Hawks, J. (2005). *Medical-surgical nursing: Clinical management for positive outcomes* (7th ed.). Philadelphia: W.B. Saunders.

Chernecky, C., & Berger, B. (2004). *Laboratory tests and diagnostic procedures* (4th ed.). Philadelphia: W.B. Saunders.

Christensen, B., & Kockrow, E. (2003). *Adult health nursing* (4th ed.). St. Louis: Mosby.

Christensen, B., & Kockrow, E. (2003). *Foundations of nursing* (4th ed.). St. Louis: Mosby.

Fortinash, K., & Holoday-Worret, P. (2004). *Psychiatric mental health nursing* (3rd ed.). St. Louis: Mosby.

Harkreader, H., & Hogan, M.A. (2004). *Fundamentals of nursing: Caring and clinical judgment* (2nd ed.). Philadelphia: W.B. Saunders.

Hodgson, B., & Kizior, R. (2005). *Saunders nursing drug handbook 2005*. Philadelphia: W.B. Saunders.

Lewis, S., Heitkemper, M., & Dirksen, S. (2004). *Medical-surgical nursing: Assessment and management of clinical problems* (6th ed.). St. Louis: Mosby.

Linton, A., & Maebius, N. (2003). *Introduction to medical-surgical nursing* (3rd ed.). Philadelphia: W.B. Saunders.

McKenry, L., & Salerno, E. (2003). *Mosby's pharmacology in nursing* (21st ed.). St. Louis: Mosby.

National Council of State Boards of Nursing. (2005). *Detailed test plan for the National Council licensure examination for practical/vocational nurses*. Chicago: Author.

Pagana, K., & Pagana, T. (2003). *Mosby's diagnostic and laboratory test reference* (6th ed.). St. Louis: Mosby.

Perry, A., & Potter, P. (2002). *Clinical nursing skills and techniques* (5th ed.). St. Louis: Mosby.

Phipps, W., Monahan, F., Sands, J., Marek, J., & Neighbors, M. (2003). *Medical-surgical nursing: Health and illness perspectives* (7th ed.). St. Louis: Mosby.

Potter, P., & Perry, A. (2003). *Essentials for practice* (5th ed.). St. Louis: Mosby.

Neurological System

I. ANATOMY AND PHYSIOLOGY OF THE BRAIN AND SPINAL CORD

A. Cerebrum
1. Consists of the right and left hemispheres
2. Each hemisphere receives sensory information from the opposite side of the body and controls the skeletal muscles of the opposite side
3. Governs sensory and motor activity
4. Governs thought and learning

B. Cerebral cortex (Box 56-1)
1. Outer gray layer
2. Divided into four lobes
3. Responsible for the conscious activities of the cerebrum

C. Basal ganglia
1. Cell bodies in white matter
2. Assist cerebral cortex in producing smooth voluntary movements

D. Diencephalon
1. Thalamus
   a. Relays sensory impulses to the cortex
   b. Provides a thalamic pain gate
   c. Part of the reticular activating system
2. Hypothalamus
   a. Regulates autonomic responses of the sympathetic and parasympathetic nervous systems
   b. Regulates stress response, sleep, appetite, body temperature, fluid balance, and emotions
   c. Responsible for the production of hormones secreted by the pituitary gland and hypothalamus

E. Brainstem
1. Midbrain
   a. Responsible for motor coordination
   b. Visual reflex and auditory relay centers
2. Pons
   a. Contains respiratory centers
   b. Regulates breathing
3. Medulla oblongata
   a. Contains all afferent and efferent tracts
   b. Contains cardiac, respiratory, vomiting, and vasomotor centers
   c. Controls heart rate, respiration, blood vessel diameter, sneezing, swallowing, vomiting, and coughing

F. Cerebellum
1. Coordinates smooth muscle movement
2. Coordinates posture, equilibrium, and muscle tone

G. Spinal cord
1. Provides neuron and synapse networks to produce involuntary responses to sensory stimulation
2. Allows for control of the number of pain impulses that pass through the spinal cord on their way to the brain
3. Carries sensory information to, and motor information from, the brain

---

BOX 56-1

Cerebral Cortex

FRONTAL LOBE
Broca's area for speech
Prefontal lobe: Controls morals, emotions, and judgments

PARIETAL LOBE
Interprets pain, touch, temperature, and pressure

TEMPORAL LOBE
Auditory center
Wenicke's area for sensory and speech

OCCIPITAL LOBE
Visual area

---

4. Extends from the first cervical to the second lumbar vertebrae
5. Protected by the meninges, cerebrospinal fluid, and adipose tissue
6. Horns
   a. Inner column of gray matter contains two anterior and two posterior horns
   b. Posterior horns connect with afferent (sensory) nerve fibers
   c. Anterior horns contain efferent (motor) nerve fibers
7. Nerve tracts
   a. White matter contains the nerve tract
   b. Ascending tract (sensory pathway)
   c. Descending tract (motor pathway)
H. Meninges
   1. Dura mater is the tough and fibrous membrane
   2. Arachnoid membrane is the delicate membrane and contains subarachnoid fluid
   3. Pia mater is the vascular membrane
   4. Subarachnoid space is formed by the arachnoid membrane and the pia mater
I. Cerebrospinal fluid
   1. Secreted in the ventricles and circulates through the ventricles to the subarachnoid layer of the meninges, where it is reabsorbed
   2. Circulates in the subarachnoid space
   3. Normal pressure is 50 to 175 mm H_2O
   4. Normal volume is 125 to 150 mL
   5. Acts as a protective cushion
   6. Aids in the exchange of nutrients and wastes
J. Ventricles
   1. Four ventricles
   2. Communicate between the subarachnoid spaces
   3. Produce and circulate cerebrospinal fluid
K. Blood supply
   1. Right and left internal carotids
   2. Right and left vertebral arteries
   3. These arteries supply the brain via an anastomosis at the base of the brain called the circle of Willis
L. Neurotransmitters
   1. Acetylcholine
   2. Norepinephrine
   3. Dopamine
   4. Serotonin
   5. Amino acids
   6. Polypeptides
M. Neurons
   1. The cell body
   2. Contains the axons and dendrites
   3. Neurons carrying impulses to the central nervous system (CNS) are called sensory neurons
   4. Neurons carrying impulses away from the central nervous system (CNS) are called motor neurons
   5. Synapse is the chemical transmission of impulses from one neuron to another

N. Axons and dendrites
   1. The axon conducts impulses from the cell body
   2. The dendrites receive stimuli from the body and transmit them to the axon
   3. Protected and insulated by Schwann cells
   4. The Schwann cell sheath is called the neurolemma
   5. Neurons do not reproduce after the neonatal period
   6. If an axon or dendrite is damaged, it will die and be slowly replaced only if the neurolemma is intact and the cell body has not died
O. Spinal nerves
   1. Thirty-one pairs of spinal nerves
   2. Mixed nerve fibers are formed by the joining of the anterior motor and posterior sensory roots
   3. Posterior roots contain afferent (sensory) nerve fibers
   4. Anterior roots contain efferent (motor) nerve fibers
P. Autonomic nervous system
   1. Sympathetic (adrenergic) fibers dilate pupils, increase heart rate and rhythm, contract blood vessels, and relax smooth muscles of the bronchi
   2. Parasympathetic (cholinergic) fibers produce the opposite effect

II. DIAGNOSTIC TESTS

A. Skull and spinal x-rays
   1. Description
      a. X-rays of the skull reveal the size and shape of the skull bones, suture separation in infants, fractures or bony defects, erosion, or calcification
      b. Spinal x-rays identify fractures, dislocation, compression, curvature, erosion, narrowed spinal cord, and degenerative processes
   2. Preprocedure interventions
      a. Provide nursing support for the confused, combative, or ventilator-dependent client
      b. Maintain immobilization of the neck if a spinal fracture is suspected
      c. Remove metal items from body parts
      d. If the client has thick and heavy hair, this should be documented, because it may affect interpretation of the x-ray film
   3. Postprocedure interventions: Maintain immobilization until results are known
B. Computed tomography (CT)
   1. Description
      a. A type of brain scanning that may or may not require injection of a dye
      b. Used to detect intracranial bleeding, space-occupying lesions, cerebral edema, infarctions, hydrocephalus, cerebral atrophy, and shifts of brain structures

2. Preprocedure interventions
   a. Obtain an informed consent if a dye is used
   b. Check for allergies to iodine, contrast dyes, or shellfish if a dye is used
   c. Instruct the client in the need to lie still and flat during the test
   d. Inform the client that he or she may be requested to hold his or her breath
   e. Prepare the client for insertion of an IV if prescribed
   f. Remove objects from the head, such as wigs, barrettes, earrings, and hairpins
   g. Ask the client about a history of claustrophobia
   h. Inform the client of possible mechanical noises during the scanning
   i. Inform the client that he or she may feel hot and flushed and a metallic taste in the mouth when the dye is injected
   j. Note that some clients may be given the dye, even if they report an allergy, and are treated with an antihistamine and corticosteroids prior to the injection to reduce the severity of a reaction
3. Postprocedure interventions
   a. Provide replacement fluids, because diuresis from the dye is expected
   b. Monitor for an allergic reaction to the dye
   c. Monitor dye injection site for bleeding or hematoma, and monitor extremity for color, warmth, and the presence of distal pulses

C. Magnetic resonance imaging (MRI)
   1. Description
      a. A noninvasive procedure that identifies types of tissues, tumors, and vascular abnormalities
      b. Similar to CT scanning but provides more detailed pictures and does not expose the client to ionizing radiation
   2. Preprocedure interventions
      a. Remove all metal objects from the client
      b. Determine if the client has a pacemaker, implanted defibrillator, or metal implant, such as a hip prosthesis or vascular clips, because these clients cannot have this test performed
      c. Remove intravenous (IV) fluid pumps during the test
      d. Provide precautions for the client who is attached to pulse oximetry because it can cause a burn during testing if coiled around the body or a body part
      e. Ask the client about a history of claustrophobia
      f. Administer medication as prescribed for the client with claustrophobia
      g. Determine if a contrast agent is to be used, and follow the prescription related to the administration of food, fluids, and medications
      h. Instruct the client that he or she will need to remain still during the procedure

3. Postprocedure interventions
   a. Client may resume normal activities
   b. Expect diuresis if a contrast agent is used

D. Lumbar puncture
   1. Description
      a. Insertion of a spinal needle through L3-L4 interspace into the lumbar subarachnoid space to obtain cerebrospinal fluid (CSF), measure CSF fluid or pressure, or instill air, dye, or medications
      b. Contraindicated in clients with **increased intracranial pressure**, because the procedure will cause a rapid decrease in pressure within the CSF around the spinal cord, leading to brain herniation
   2. Preprocedure interventions
      a. Obtain an informed consent
      b. Have the client empty the bladder
   3. Interventions during the procedure
      a. Position the client in a lateral recumbent position and draw the knees up to the abdomen and chin onto the chest
      b. Assist with the collection of specimens (label the specimens in sequence)
      c. Maintain strict asepsis
   4. Postprocedure interventions
      a. Monitor vital signs and neurological signs
      b. Position the client flat, as prescribed
      c. Encourage fluid intake
      d. Monitor input and output (I&O)

E. Myelography
   1. Description: Injection of dye or air into the subarachnoid space to detect abnormalities of the spinal cord and vertebrae
   2. Preprocedure interventions
      a. Obtain an informed consent
      b. Provide hydration for at least 12 hours before the test
      c. Assess for allergies to iodine or other contrast media
      d. If the client is taking a phenothiazine, the medication is held as prescribed because this medication lowers the seizure threshold
      e. Premedicate for sedation, as prescribed
   3. Postprocedure interventions
      a. Vital signs are monitored and neurological assessment is done frequently, as prescribed
      b. If a water-based dye is used (type used most often), elevate the head 15 to 30 degrees for 6 to 8 hours, as prescribed
      c. If an oil-based dye is used, keep the client flat 6 to 8 hours, as prescribed
      d. If air is used, keep the head lower than the trunk for up to 48 hours, as prescribed
      e. Administer analgesics for headache or backache, as prescribed
      f. Encourage fluid intake

g. Monitor I&O

h. Check for bladder distention and voiding

F. Cerebral angiography

1. Description: Injection of contrast through the femoral artery into the carotid arteries to visualize the cerebral arteries and assess for lesions

2. Preprocedure interventions

a. Obtain an informed consent

b. Assess the client for allergies to iodine and shellfish

c. Encourage hydration for 2 days before the test

d. NPO 4 to 6 hours before the test, as prescribed

e. Obtain a baseline neurological assessment

f. Mark the peripheral pulses

g. Remove metal items from the hair

h. Administer premedication, as prescribed

3. Postprocedure interventions

a. Monitor neurological status and vital signs frequently until stable

b. Monitor for swelling in the neck and for difficulty swallowing and notify the physician if these symptoms occur

c. Maintain bed rest for 12 hours, as prescribed

d. Elevate the head of the bed 15 to 30 degrees only if prescribed

e. Keep the bed flat if the femoral artery is used, as prescribed

f. Monitor peripheral pulses

g. Immobilize the puncture site for 12 hours, as prescribed

h. Apply sandbags and a pressure dressing to the injection site, as prescribed

i. Place ice on the puncture site, as prescribed

j. Encourage fluid intake

G. Electroencephalography (EEG)

1. Description: A graphic recording of the electrical activity of the superficial layers of the cerebral cortex

2. Preprocedure interventions

a. Wash the client's hair

b. Inform the client that electrodes are attached to the head and that electricity does not enter the head

c. Withhold stimulants, antidepressants, tranquilizers, and anticonvulsants for 24 to 48 hours before the test, as prescribed

d. Allow the client to have breakfast if prescribed

e. Premedicate for sedation, as prescribed

3. Postprocedure interventions

a. Wash the client's hair

b. Maintain side rails and safety precautions if the client has been sedated

H. Caloric testing (oculovestibular reflex)

1. Description: Provides information about the function of the vestibular portion of the eighth cranial nerve and aids in the diagnosis of cerebellum and brainstem lesions

2. Procedure

a. Patency of the external auditory canal is confirmed

b. The client is positioned supine with the head of the bed elevated 30 degrees

c. Cold water is instilled into the auditory canal to stimulate the semicircular canals

d. A normal response that indicates intact function of cranial nerves III, VI, and VIII is conjugate eye movements toward the side being irrigated, followed by rapid nystagmus to the opposite side

e. Absent or dysconjugate eye movements indicate brainstem damage

III. NEUROLOGICAL DATA COLLECTION

A. Risk factors

1. Trauma
2. Hemorrhage
3. Tumors
4. Infection
5. Toxicity
6. Metabolic disorders
7. Hypoxic conditions
8. Deficiency conditions
9. Hypertension
10. Cigarette smoking
11. Stress

B. Cranial nerves

1. Cranial nerve I (olfactory): Sensory, smell

a. Have the client close his or her eyes and occlude one nostril with finger

b. Ask the client to identify nonirritating odors such as coffee, tea, cloves, soap, chewing gum, and peppermint

c. Repeat the test on the other nostril

2. Cranial nerve II (optic): Sensory, vision

a. Check visual acuity with a Snellen chart or newspaper, or ask the client to count how many fingers the examiner is holding up

b. Check visual fields by confrontation

c. Have the client sit directly in front of examiner and stare at examiner's nose

d. Examiner slowly moves his or her finger from the periphery toward the center until the client says it can be seen

e. Check color vision by asking the client to name the colors of several nearby objects

3. Cranial nerve III (oculomotor); cranial nerve IV (trochlear); cranial nerve VI (abducens)

a. The motor functions of these nerves overlap; therefore, they need to be tested together

b. First, inspect the eyelids for ptosis (drooping); then check ocular movements and note any eye deviation

c. Test accommodation and direct and consensual light reflexes

d. Cranial nerve III (oculomotor): Motor; checks pupillary constriction, upper eyelid elevation, and most eye movement

e. Cranial nerve IV (trochlear): Motor; checks downward and inward eye movement

f. Cranial nerve VI (abducens): Checks lateral eye movement

4. Cranial nerve V (trigeminal): Sensory and motor

a. Checks sensation to the cornea, nasal and oral mucosa, facial skin, and mastication

b. To test motor function, ask the client to close jaws tightly and then try to separate the clenched jaw

c. Test the corneal reflex by lightly touching the client's cornea with a cotton wisp

d. Check sensory function by asking the client to close the eyes; then lightly touch the forehead, cheeks, and chin, noting if the touch can be felt equally on both sides

5. Cranial nerve VII (facial): Sensory and motor

a. Test taste perception on the anterior two thirds of the tongue

b. Have the client show the teeth

c. Attempt to close the client's eyes against resistance, and ask the client to puff out the cheeks

d. Place sugar, salt, or vinegar on the front of the tongue, and have the client identify these substances by their taste

6. Cranial nerve VIII (acoustic): Sensory

a. The ability to hear tests the cochlear portion

b. The sense of equilibrium tests the vestibular portion

c. Check the client's ability to hear a watch ticking or a whisper

d. Observe the client's balance, and observe for swaying when walking or standing

7. Cranial nerve IX (glossopharyngeal): Sensory and motor

a. Checks swallowing ability

b. Checks sensation to the pharyngeal soft palate and tonsillar mucosa, taste perception on the posterior third of the tongue, and salivation

8. Cranial nerve X (vagus): Sensory and motor

a. Checks swallowing and phonation, sensation to the exterior ear's posterior wall, and sensation behind the ear

b. Checks sensation to the thoracic and abdominal viscera

9. Cranial nerve IX (glossopharyngeal); cranial nerve X (vagus)

a. Have the client identify a taste at the back of the tongue

b. Inspect the soft palate and observe for symmetrical elevation when the client says "aah"

c. Touch the posterior pharyngeal wall with a tongue depressor to elicit a gag reflex

10. Cranial nerve XI (spinal accessory): Motor

a. Checks uvula and soft palate movement, sternocleidomastoid and trapezius muscles

b. Checks upper portion of the trapezius muscle, which governs shoulder movement and neck rotation

c. Palpate and inspect the sternocleidomastoid muscle as the client pushes the chin against the examiner's hand

d. Palpate and inspect the trapezius muscle as the client shrugs his or her shoulders against the examiner's resistance

11. Cranial nerve XII (hypoglossal): Motor

a. Checks tongue movements involved in swallowing and speech

b. Observe the tongue for asymmetry, atrophy, deviation to one side, and fasciculations

c. Ask the client to push the tongue against a tongue depressor, and then have the client move the tongue rapidly in and out and from side to side

C. Data collection

1. Level of consciousness

a. Determines cerebral function

b. Client behavior is checked to determine level of consciousness, such as confusion, delirium, unconsciousness, stupor, and coma

2. Vital signs: Monitor for blood pressure or pulse changes, which may indicate **increased intracranial pressure (ICP)**

3. Respirations (Box 56-2)

BOX 56-2

Data Collection: Respirations

CHEYNE-STOKES RESPIRATIONS
Rhythmic, with periods of apnea
Can indicate a metabolic dysfunction or dysfunction in the cerebral hemisphere or basal ganglia

NEUROGENIC HYPERVENTILATION
Regular rapid and deep sustained respirations
Indicates a dysfunction in the low midbrain and middle pons

APNEUSTIC RESPIRATIONS
Irregular respirations, with pauses at the end of inspiration and expiration
Indicates a dysfunction in the middle or caudal pons

ATAXIC RESPIRATIONS
Totally irregular in rhythm and depth
Indicates a dysfunction in the medulla

CLUSTER RESPIRATIONS
Clusters of breaths with irregularly spaced pauses
Indicates a dysfunction in the medulla and pons

4. Temperature
   a. An elevated temperature increases the brain's metabolic rate
   b. An elevation in temperature may indicate a dysfunction of the hypothalamus or brainstem
   c. A slow rise in temperature may indicate infection
5. Pupils (Figure 56-1)
   a. Size
   b. Equality
   c. Reactions to light: described as brisk, slow, or fixed
   d. Unusual eye movements
   e. Unilateral pupil dilation indicates compression of the third cranial nerve
   f. Midposition fixed pupil indicates midbrain injury
   g. Pinpoint fixed pupil indicates pontine damage
6. Motor function
   a. Muscle tone, including strength and equality
   b. Voluntary and involuntary movements
   c. Purposeful and nonpurposeful movements
7. Posturing (Figure 56-2)
   a. Posturing indicates a deterioration of the condition
   b. Flexor (**decorticate posturing**)
      1) Client flexes one or both arms on the chest and may stiffly extend the legs
      2) Indicates a nonfunctioning cortex
   c. Extensor (**decerebrate posturing**)
      1) Client stiffly extends one or both arms and possibly the legs
      2) Indicates a brainstem lesion
   d. **Flaccid posturing**: Client displays no motor response in any extremity
8. Reflexes (Box 56-3)
9. Meningeal irritation (Box 56-4)
   a. Nuchal rigidity
   b. Irritability
   c. Fever
10. Autonomic system
   a. Sympathetic functions/adrenergic responses
      1) Increased pulse and blood pressure
      2) Dilated pupils
      3) Decreased peristalsis
      4) Increased perspiration

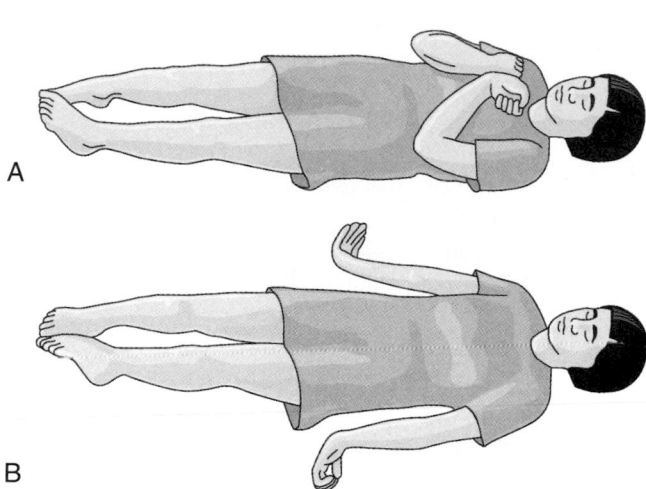

FIG. 56-2   Posturing. **A,** Decorticate posturing. **B,** Decerebrate posturing. (From Ignatavicius, D., & Workman, M. [2006]. *Medical surgical nursing: Critical thinking for collaborative care* [5th ed.]. Philadelphia: W.B. Saunders.)

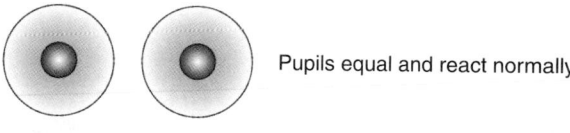
Pupils equal and react normally

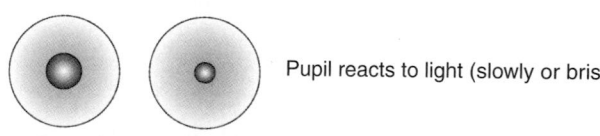
Pupil reacts to light (slowly or briskly)

Dilated pupil (compressed cranial nerve III)

Bilateral dilated, fixed pupils (ominous sign)

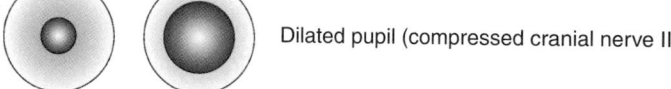
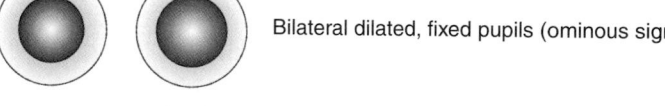
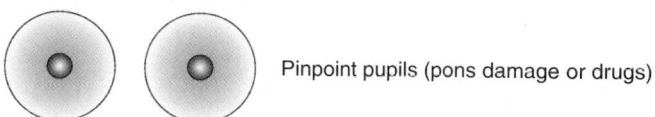
Pinpoint pupils (pons damage or drugs)

FIG. 56-1   Pupillary check for size and response. (From Lewis, S., Heitkemper, M., & Dirksen, S. [2004]. *Medical-surgical nursing: Assessment and management of clinical problems* [6th ed.]. St. Louis: Mosby.)

BOX 56-3

Data Collection: Reflexes

BABINSKI REFLEX
Dorsiflexion of the ankle and great toe, with fanning of the other toes
Indicates a disruption of the pyramidal tract

CORNEAL REFLEX
Loss of the blink reflex
Indicates a dysfunction of cranial nerve V

GAG REFLEX
Loss of the gag reflex
Indicates a dysfunction of cranial nerves IX and X

b. Parasympathetic function/cholinergic responses
  1) Decreased pulse and blood pressure
  2) Constricted pupils
  3) Increased salivation
  4) Increased peristalsis
  5) Dilated blood vessels
  6) Bladder contraction
11. Sensory function
  a. Touch
  b. Pressure
  c. Pain
  d. Bladder control
  e. Bowel control
D. **Glasgow Coma Scale** (Box 56-5)
  1. A method of assessing a client's neurological condition
  2. A scoring system based on a scale of 1 to 15 points
  3. A score below 8 indicates that coma is present
  4. Eye opening is the most important indicator

BOX 56-4

Data Collection: Meningeal Irritation

BRUDZINSKI'S SIGN
Flexion of the head causes flexion of both thighs at the hips, and knee flexion

KERNIG'S SIGN
Flexion of the thigh and knee to right angles; when extended, causes spasm of hamstring and pain

---

BOX 56-5

Glasgow Coma Scale

MOTOR RESPONSE POINTS
Obeys a simple response = 6
Localizes painful stimuli = 5
Normal flexion (withdrawal) = 4
Abnormal flexion (decorticate posturing) = 3
Extensor response (decerebrate posturing) = 2
No motor response to pain = 1

VERBAL RESPONSE POINTS
Oriented = 5
Confused conversation = 4
Inappropriate words = 3
Responds with incomprehensible sounds = 2
No verbal response = 1

EYE-OPENING POINTS
Spontaneous = 4
In response to sound = 3
In response to pain = 2
No response even to painful stimuli = 1

IV. THE UNCONSCIOUS CLIENT
A. Description
  1. A state of depressed cerebral functioning with unresponsiveness to sensory and motor function
  2. Some causes include head trauma, cerebral toxins, shock, hemorrhage, tumor, and infection
B. Data collection
  1. Unarousable
  2. Primitive or no response to painful stimuli
  3. Altered respirations
  4. Decreased cranial nerve and reflex activity
C. Interventions (Box 56-6)

V. INCREASED INTRACRANIAL PRESSURE (ICP)
A. Description
  1. An increase in **ICP** caused by trauma, hemorrhage, growths or tumors, hydrocephalus, edema, or inflammation
  2. Can impede circulation to the brain, impede the absorption of CSF, affect the functioning of nerve cells, and lead to brainstem compression and death
B. Data collection
  1. Check level of consciousness (LOC), which is the most sensitive and earliest indication of **increased intracranial pressure**
  2. Declining LOC from restlessness to confusion and coma
  3. Headache
  4. Abnormal respirations
  5. Increase in blood pressure, with widening pulse pressure
  6. Slowing of pulse
  7. Elevated temperature
  8. Vomiting
  9. Pupil changes
  10. Changes in motor function from weakness to hemiplegia, a positive **Babinski reflex, decorticate** or **decerebrate posturing,** and seizures
  11. Late signs of **increased ICP** include increased systolic blood pressure, widened pulse pressure, and slowed heart rate
C. Interventions
  1. Elevate the head of the bed 30 to 40 degrees, as prescribed
  2. Avoid Trendelenburg position
  3. Prevent flexion of the neck and hips
  4. Monitor respiratory status and prevent hypoxia
  5. Avoid the administration of morphine sulfate to prevent the occurrence of hypoxia
  6. Maintain mechanical ventilation as prescribed, maintaining the $PaCO_2$ at 30 to 35 mm Hg, which will result in vasoconstriction of the cerebral blood vessels, decreased blood flow, and therefore decreased ICP
  7. Maintain body temperature

BOX 56-6

Care of the Unconscious Client

Assess patency of airway and keep an airway and emergency equipment at the bedside.

Monitor blood pressure, pulse, and heart sounds.

Monitor respiratory and circulatory status.

Maintain a patent airway and ventilation, because a high CO_2 level increases intracranial pressure.

Check lung sounds for the accumulation of secretions.

Suction PRN.

Monitor neurological status, including LOC, pupillary reactions, motor and sensory function.

Place the client in semi-Fowler's position.

Change position of the client every 2 hours, avoiding injury when turning.

Avoid Trendelenburg position.

Use side rails at all times.

Monitor for edema.

Monitor for dehydration.

Monitor I&O and daily weight.

Maintain NPO status until consciousness returns.

Maintain nutrition as prescribed, and monitor fluid and electrolyte balance.

Check the gag and swallowing reflex before resuming diet, and begin with ice chips and fluids.

Provide intravenous or enteral feedings, as prescribed.

Monitor bowel sounds.

Monitor elimination patterns.

Monitor for constipation, impaction, and paralytic ileus.

Maintain urinary output to prevent stasis, infection, and calculus formation.

Monitor the status of skin integrity.

Initiate measures to prevent skin breakdown.

Provide frequent mouth care.

Remove dentures and contact lenses.

Check the eyes for corneal reflex and irritation, and instill artificial tears or cover the eyes with eye patches.

Monitor drainage from the ears or nose for the presence of cerebrospinal fluid.

Assume that the unconscious client can hear.

Avoid restraints.

Do not leave the client unattended if unstable.

Initiate seizure precautions if necessary.

Provide range-of-motion exercises to prevent contractures.

Use a footboard or high-top sneakers to prevent foot drop.

Use splints to prevent wrist deformities.

Initiate physical therapy as appropriate.

BOX 56-7

Medications for Increased Intracranial Pressure (ICP)

MANNITOL (OSMITROL)

This hyperosmotic agent increases intravascular pressure by drawing fluid from the interstitial spaces and from the brain cells.

Monitor renal function.

Diuresis is expected.

CORTICOSTEROIDS

These agents stabilize the cell membrane, reduce the leakiness in the blood-brain barrier, and decrease cerebral edema.

A histamine blocker may be administered to counteract the excess gastric secretion that occurs with the corticosteroid.

Clients must be withdrawn slowly from corticosteroid therapy to reduce the risk of adrenal crisis.

BLOOD PRESSURE MEDICATION

This may be required to maintain cerebral perfusion at a normal level.

Notify the physician if the blood pressure range is below 100 or above 150 mm Hg systolic.

ANTIPYRETICS AND MUSCLE RELAXANTS

Temperature reduction decreases metabolism, cerebral blood flow, and thus ICP.

Muscle relaxants prevent shivering.

ANTICONVULSANTS

These may be given prophylactically to prevent seizures.

Seizures increase metabolic requirements and cerebral blood flow and volume, thus increasing ICP.

IV FLUIDS

These are administered via infusion pump to control the amount of IV fluid administered.

Hypertonic IV solutions are avoided because of the risk of promoting additional cerebral edema.

8. Prevent shivering, which can raise **ICP**
9. Decrease environmental stimuli
10. Monitor electrolyte levels and acid-base balance
11. Monitor I&O
12. Limit fluid intake to 1200 mL/day
13. Instruct the client to avoid straining activities such as coughing and sneezing
14. Instruct the client to avoid Valsalva maneuver

D. Medications (Box 56-7)

E. Surgical intervention (Box 56-8)

VI. HYPERTHERMIA

A. Description
   1. A temperature of 106° F (41.1° C), which increases the cerebral metabolism and increases the risk of hypoxia
   2. The causes include infection, heat stroke, exposure to high environmental temperatures, and dysfunction of the thermoregulatory center

B. Data collection
   1. Temperature of 106° F (41.1° C)
   2. Shivering
   3. Nausea and vomiting

C. Interventions
   1. Maintain a patent airway
   2. Initiate seizure precautions

BOX 56-8

Surgical Intervention for ICP

VENTRICULOPERITONEAL SHUNT
Description
This shunts CSF from the ventricles into the peritoneum.
Postprocedure Interventions
Position the client supine and turn from back to non-operative side.
Monitor for signs of increasing ICP resulting from shunt failure.
Monitor for signs of infection.

---

3. Monitor I&O and assess skin and mucous membranes for signs of dehydration
4. Monitor lung sounds
5. Monitor for dysrhythmias
6. Check peripheral pulses for systemic blood flow
7. Induce normothermia with fluids, cool baths, fans, or hypothermia blanket

D. Inducing normothermia
   1. Prevent shivering, which will increase CSF pressure and oxygen consumption
   2. Administer medications as prescribed to prevent shivering
   3. Monitor neurological status
   4. Monitor for infection and respiratory complications, because hypothermia may mask signs of infection
   5. Monitor for cardiac irregularities
   6. Monitor I&O
   7. Prevent trauma to the skin and tissues
   8. Apply lotion to the skin frequently
   9. Inspect for frostbite
E. Medications to prevent shivering (Box 56-9)

VII. HEAD INJURY
A. Description
   1. Trauma to the skull resulting in mild to extensive damage to the brain
   2. Immediate complications include cerebral bleeding, hematomas, uncontrolled **increased ICP**, infections, and seizures
   3. Changes in personality or behavior, cranial nerve deficits, and any other residual deficits depend on the area of the brain damage and the extent of the damage
B. Types of head injuries (Box 56-10)
   1. Open
      a. Scalp lacerations
      b. Fractures in the skull
      c. Interruption of the dura mater
   2. Closed
      a. Concussions
      b. Contusions
      c. Fractures

BOX 56-9

Medications to Prevent Shivering

CHLORPROMAZINE HYDROCHLORIDE (THORAZINE)
This depresses thermoregulation in the hypothalamus and reduces peripheral vasoconstriction, muscle tone, and shivering.

MEPERIDINE HYDROCHLORIDE (DEMEROL)
This relaxes the smooth muscle and reduces shivering.

BOX 56-10

Types of Head Injuries

CONCUSSION
A jarring of the brain within the skull with temporary loss of consciousness

CONTUSION
A bruising type of injury to the brain
May occur with subdural or extradural collections of blood

SKULL FRACTURES
Linear
Depressed
Compound
Comminuted

EPIDURAL HEMATOMA
The most serious type of hematoma; forms rapidly and results from an arterial bleed
Forms between the dura and the skull from a tear in the meningeal artery
A surgical emergency

SUBDURAL HEMATOMA
Forms slowly and results from a venous bleed
Occurs under the dura as a result of tears in the veins crossing the subdural space

SUBARACHNOID HEMORRHAGE
Bleeding directly into the brain, the ventricles, or the subarachnoid space

INTRACEREBRAL HEMORRHAGE
Multiple hemorrhages around a contused area

C. Hematoma
   1. Description: Can occur as a result of a subarachnoid hemorrhage or an intracerebral hemorrhage
   2. Data collection
      a. Findings will be dependent on the injury
      b. Clinical manifestations usually result from **increased ICP**
      c. Changing neurological signs in the client
      d. Changes in level of consciousness
      e. Airway and breathing pattern

f. Vital signs for signs of **increased ICP**
g. Headache, nausea, and vomiting
h. Visual disturbances, pupillary changes, papilledema, and extraocular eye movements
i. Nuchal rigidity
j. CSF drainage from the ears or nose
k. Weakness and paralysis
l. Posturing
m. Decreased sensation or absence of feeling
n. Reflex activity
o. Seizure activity

3. Interventions
a. Monitor respiratory status and maintain a patent airway because increased CO_2 levels increase cerebral edema
b. Monitor neurological status and vital signs, including temperature
c. Monitor for **increased ICP**
d. Maintain head elevation to reduce venous pressure
e. Prevent neck flexion
f. Initiate normothermia measures for increased temperature
g. Check cranial nerve function, reflexes, and motor and sensory function
h. Initiate seizure precautions
i. Monitor for pain and restlessness
j. Avoid the administration of morphine sulfate because it is a respiratory depressant and may lead to **increased ICP**
k. Monitor for drainage from the nose or ears because this fluid may be CSF
l. Do not attempt to clean the nose, suction, or allow the client to blow the nose if drainage occurs
m. Do not clean the ear if drainage is noted, but apply a loose, dry sterile dressing
n. Check drainage for the presence of CSF
o. The physician is notified if drainage from the ears or nose is noted
p. Instruct the client to avoid coughing because this increases **ICP**
q. Monitor for signs of infection
r. Prevent complications of immobility

D. Craniotomy
1. Description
a. A surgical procedure that involves an incision through the cranium to remove accumulated blood or a tumor
b. Complications of the procedure include **increased ICP** from cerebral edema, hemorrhage, or obstruction of the normal flow of CSF
c. Additional complications include hematomas, hypovolemic shock, hydrocephalus, respiratory and neurogenic complications, pulmonary edema, and wound infections
d. Complications related to fluid and electrolyte imbalances include diabetes insipidus and

---

BOX 56-11

Nursing Care Following Craniotomy

Monitor vital signs and neurological status every 30 to 60 minutes.

Monitor for increased ICP.

Monitor for decreased LOC, motor weakness or paralysis, aphasia, visual changes, and personality changes.

Maintain mechanical ventilation and slight hyperventilation for the first 24 to 48 hours as prescribed to prevent increased ICP.

Check the physician's orders regarding client positioning.

Avoid extreme hip or neck flexion, and maintain the head in a midline neutral position.

Provide a quiet environment.

Monitor the head dressing frequently for signs of drainage.

Mark the area of drainage once each nursing shift for baseline comparison.

Monitor the Hemovac or Jackson-Pratt drain, which may be in place for 24 hours.

Maintain suction on the Hemovac or Jackson-Pratt drain.

Measure drainage from the Hemovac or Jackson-Pratt drain every 8 hours, and record the amount and color.

The physician is notified if drainage is greater than the normal amount of 30 to 50 mL per shift.

The physician is notified immediately of excessive amounts of drainage or a saturated head dressing.

Record strict measurement of hourly I&O.

Maintain fluid restriction at 1500 mL/day, as prescribed.

Monitor electrolyte values.

Monitor for dysrhythmias, which may occur as a result of fluid and electrolyte imbalances.

Apply ice packs or cool compresses as prescribed for periorbital edema and ecchymosis of one or both eyes, which is not an unusual occurrence.

Provide range-of-motion exercises every 8 hours.

Place antiembolism stockings on the client, as prescribed.

Administer anticonvulsants, antacids, corticosteroids, and antibiotics, as prescribed.

Administer analgesics such as codeine sulfate and acetaminophen (Tylenol) as prescribed for pain.

---

inappropriate secretion of antidiuretic hormone

2. Preoperative interventions
a. Explain the procedure to the client and family
b. Ensure that an informed consent has been obtained
c. Prepare to shave the client's head as prescribed and cover the head appropriately
d. Stabilize the client before surgery

3. Postoperative interventions (Box 56-11)

4. Postoperative positioning (Box 56-12)

VIII. SPINAL CORD INJURY

A. Description
1. Trauma to the spinal cord causing partial or complete disruption of the nerve tracts and neurons

Client Positioning Following Craniotomy

Positions prescribed following craniotomy vary with the type of surgery and the specific postoperative physician's orders.

Always check the physician's orders regarding client positioning.

Incorrect positioning may cause serious and possibly fatal complications.

REMOVAL OF A BONE FLAP FOR DECOMPRESSION

To facilitate brain expansion, the client should be turned from the back to the nonoperative side, but not to the side operated on.

POSTERIOR FOSSA SURGERY

To protect the operative site from pressure and minimize tension on the suture line, position the client on the side, with a pillow under the head for support, and not on the back.

INFRATENTORIAL SURGERY

This involves surgery below the brain's tentorium.

The physician may order a flat position without head elevation or may order the head of the bed to be elevated at 30 to 45 degrees.

Do not elevate the head of the bed in the acute phase of care following surgery without a physician's order.

SUPRATENTORIAL SURGERY

This involves surgery above the brain's tentorium.

The physician may order the head of the bed to be elevated to 30 degrees to promote venous outflow through the jugular veins.

Do not lower the head of the bed in the acute phase of care following surgery without a physician's order.

2. The injury can involve contusion, laceration, or compression of the cord
3. Spinal cord edema develops; necrosis of the spinal cord can develop as a result of compromised capillary circulation and venous return
4. Loss of motor function, sensation, reflex activity, and bowel and bladder control may result
5. The most common causes include motor vehicle accidents, falls, sporting and industrial accidents, and gunshot or stab wounds
6. Complications related to the injury include respiratory failure, **autonomic dysreflexia**, **spinal shock**, further cord damage, and death

B. Most frequently involved vertebrae
  1. Cervical: C5, C6, and C7
  2. Thoracic: T12
  3. Lumbar: L1

C. Transection of the cord
  1. Complete transection of the cord
    a. The spinal cord is completely severed, with total loss of sensation, movement, and reflex activity below the level of injury

    b. If the cord has not suffered irreparable damage, early treatment is needed to prevent partial damage from developing into total and permanent damage
  2. Partial transection of the cord
    a. The spinal cord is partially damaged or severed
    b. The symptoms depend on the extent and location of the damage

D. Types of injuries
  1. Anterior cord syndrome
    a. Damage to the anterior portion of the gray and white matter of the spinal cord
    b. Motor function, pain, and temperature sensation are lost below the level of injury; however, the sensations of touch, position, and vibration remain intact
  2. Posterior cord injury
    a. Damage to the posterior portion of the gray and white matter of the spinal cord
    b. Motor function remains intact, but the client experiences a loss of vibratory sense, crude touch, and position sensation
  3. Central cord syndrome
    a. Occurs from a lesion in the central portion of the spinal cord
    b. Loss of motor function is more pronounced in the upper extremities, and varying degrees and patterns of sensation remain intact
  4. Brown-Séquard syndrome
    a. Results from penetrating injuries that cause hemisection of the spinal cord or injuries that affect half the cord
    b. Motor function, proprioception, vibration, and deep touch sensations are lost on the same side of the body (ipsilateral) as the lesion
    c. On the opposite side of the body (contralateral) from the injury, the sensations of pain, temperature, and light touch are affected
  5. Conus medullaris syndrome
    a. Follows damage to the lumbar nerve roots and conus medullaris in the spinal cord
    b. Client experiences bowel and bladder areflexia and flaccid lower extremities
    c. If damage is limited to the upper sacral segments of the spinal cord, bulbospongiosis penile (erection) and micturition reflexes will remain
  6. Cauda equina syndrome
    a. Occurs from injury to the lumbosacral nerve roots below the conus medullaris
    b. The client experiences areflexia of the bowel, bladder, and lower reflexes

E. Data collection: See Box 56-13
  1. Depends on the level of the cord injury
  2. The level of the spinal cord injury is the lowest spinal cord segment with intact motor and sensory function
  3. Respiratory status changes

BOX 56-13

Effects of the Spinal Cord Injury

QUADRIPLEGIA

Injury occurring from C1 through C8
Paralysis involving all four extremities

PARAPLEGIA

Injury occurring from T1 through L4
Paralysis involving only the lower extremities

    4. Motor and sensory changes below the level of injury
    5. Total sensory loss and motor paralysis below the level of injury
    6. Loss of reflexes below the level of injury
    7. Loss of bladder and bowel control
    8. Urinary retention and bladder distention
    9. Presence of sweat, which does not occur on paralyzed areas

F. Cervical injuries
    1. C2 to C3 injury is usually fatal
    2. C4 is the major innervation to the diaphragm by the phrenic nerve
    3. Involvement above C4 causes respiratory difficulty and paralysis of all four extremities
    4. Client may have movement in the shoulder if the injury is at C5 or below

G. Thoracic level injuries
    1. Loss of movement of the chest, trunk, bowel, bladder, and legs, depending on the level of injury
    2. Leg paralysis (paraplegia)
    3. **Autonomic dysreflexia** with lesions or injuries above T6 and in cervical lesions
    4. Visceral distention from a distended bladder or impacted rectum may cause reactions such as sweating, bradycardia, hypertension, nasal stuffiness, and gooseflesh

H. Lumbar and sacral level injuries
    1. Loss of movement and sensation of the lower extremities
    2. S2 and S3 center on micturation; therefore, below this level, the bladder will contract but not empty (neurogenic bladder)
    3. Injury above S2 in males allows them to have an erection, but they are unable to ejaculate because of sympathetic nerve damage
    4. Injury between S2 and S4 damages the sympathetic and parasympathetic response, preventing erection or ejaculation

I. Emergency interventions
    1. Emergency management is critical, because improper handling can cause further damage and loss of neurological function
    2. Maintain a patent airway
    3. Always suspect spinal cord injury until this injury is ruled out

    4. Immobilize the client on a spinal backboard with the head in a neutral position to prevent an incomplete injury from becoming complete
    5. Prevent head flexion, rotation, or extension
    6. During immobilization, maintain traction and alignment on the head by placing hands on either side of the head, by the ears
    7. Maintain an extended position
    8. Logroll the client
    9. No part of the body should be twisted or turned, and the client is not allowed to assume a sitting position
   10. In the emergency room, a client who has sustained a severe cervical injury should be placed immediately in skeletal traction via **skull tongs** or **halo traction** to immobilize the cervical spine and reduce the fracture and dislocation

J. Interventions during hospitalization
    1. Respiratory system
      a. Monitor respiratory status because paralysis of the intercostal and abdominal muscles occurs with C4 injuries
      b. Monitor arterial blood gases and maintain mechanical ventilation if prescribed to prevent respiratory arrest, especially with cervical injuries
      c. Encourage deep breathing and the use of an incentive spirometer
      d. Monitor for signs of infection, particularly pneumonia
    2. Cardiovascular system
      a. Monitor for cardiac dysrhythmias
      b. Monitor for signs of hemorrhage or bleeding around the fracture site
      c. Monitor for signs of shock, such as hypotension, tachycardia, and a weak and thready pulse
      d. Monitor the lower extremities for deep vein thrombosis
      e. Measure circumferences of calf and thigh
      f. Apply thigh-high antiembolism stockings, as prescribed
      g. Remove antiembolism stockings daily to assess the skin
      h. Monitor for orthostatic hypotension when repositioning the client
    3. Neuromuscular system
      a. Monitor neurological status
      b. Monitor motor and sensory status to determine the level of injury
      c. Monitor motor ability by testing the client's ability to squeeze hands, spread the fingers, move the toes, and turn the feet
      d. Monitor sensation by pinching skin or pricking with a pin, starting at the shoulders and working down the extremities
      e. Monitor for signs of **autonomic dysreflexia** and **spinal shock**

f. Immobilize the client to promote healing and prevent further injury

g. Check for pain

h. Initiate measures to reduce pain

i. Administer analgesics, as prescribed

j. Monitor for complications of immobility

k. Prepare the client for decompression laminectomy, spinal fusion, or insertion of steel rods if prescribed

l. Collaborate with the physical therapist and occupational therapist to determine appropriate exercise techniques, assess the need for hand and wrist splints, and develop an appropriate plan to prevent footdrop

4. Gastrointestinal system

a. Monitor abdomen for distention and hemorrhage

b. Monitor bowel sounds and assess for paralytic ileus

c. Prevent bowel retention

d. Initiate a bowel control program as appropriate

e. Maintain adequate nutrition and a high-fiber diet

5. Renal system

a. Prevent bladder retention

b. Initiate a bladder control program as appropriate

c. Maintain fluid and electrolyte balance

d. Maintain adequate fluid intake of 2000 mL/day

e. Monitor for urinary tract infection and calculi

6. Integumentary system

a. Monitor skin integrity

b. Turn the client every 2 hours

7. Psychosocial integrity

a. Monitor psychosocial status

b. Encourage the client to express feelings of anger and depression

c. Discuss the sexual concerns of the client

d. Promote self-care, setting realistic goals based on the client's potential functional level

e. Encourage contact with appropriate community resources

K. **Spinal shock**

1. Description

a. Also known as neurogenic shock

b. A sudden depression of reflex activity in the spinal cord below the level of injury (areflexia)

c. Occurs within the first hour of injury and can last days to months

d. The muscles become completely paralyzed and flaccid, and reflexes are absent

e. **Spinal shock** ends when the reflexes are regained

2. Data collection

a. Flaccid paralysis

b. Hypotension

c. Bradycardia

d. Loss of reflex activity below the level of injury

e. Paralytic ileus

3. Interventions

a. Monitor for signs of **spinal shock** following a spinal cord injury

b. Monitor for hypotension and bradycardia

c. Monitor for reflex activity

d. Check for bowel sounds

e. Monitor for bowel and bladder retention

f. Provide supportive measures as prescribed based on the presence of symptoms

g. Monitor for the return of reflexes

L. **Autonomic dysreflexia**

1. Description

a. Also known as hyperreflexia

b. Commonly caused by visceral distention from a distended bladder or impacted rectum

c. Neurological emergency; must be treated immediately to prevent a hypertensive stroke

d. It generally occurs after the period of **spinal shock** is resolved

e. Occurs with lesions or injuries above T6 and in cervical lesions

2. Data collection

a. Hypertension

b. Bradycardia

c. Flushing of the face and neck

d. Severe, throbbing headache

e. Nasal stuffiness

f. Piloerection (gooseflesh)

g. Sweating

h. Nausea

i. Restlessness

j. Dilated pupils and blurred vision

3. Interventions

a. The physician is notified if signs of **autonomic dysreflexia** occur

b. Raise the head of the bed to high Fowler's position

c. Check for the potential cause and remove the stimulus

d. Loosen tight clothing

e. Check for bladder distention, and prepare for urinary catheterization

f. If a urinary catheter is present, check for kinks in the tubing and for drainage

g. Check for a fecal impaction and disimpact immediately

h. Monitor vital signs, particularly blood pressure, every 15 minutes

i. Administer antihypertensives, as prescribed

M. Cervical traction for cervical injuries (Figure 56-3)

1. Description

a. Skeletal traction is used to stabilize fractures or dislocations of the cervical or upper thoracic spine

b. Two types of equipment used for cervical traction—**skull (cervical) tongs** and **halo traction** (halo fixation device)

Gardner-Wells tongs

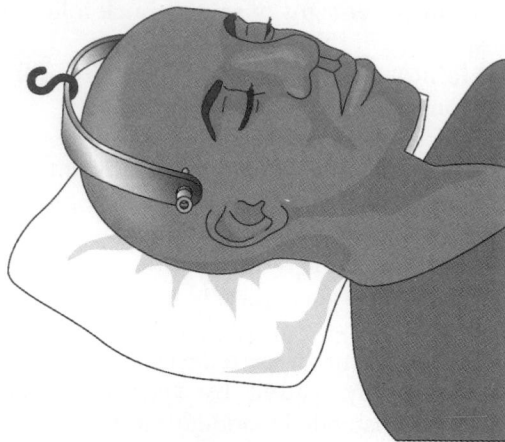

Halo fixation device with jacket

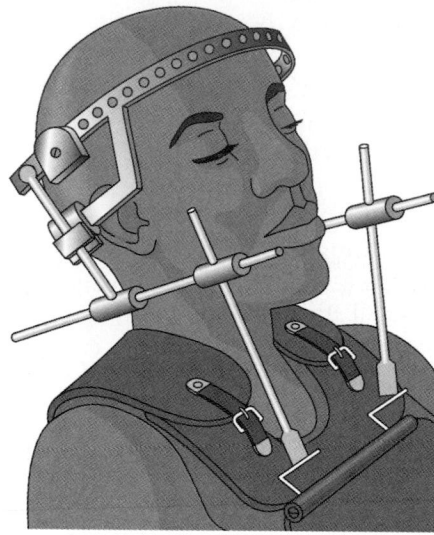

FIG. 56-3   Types of cervical spine traction. (From Ignatavicius, D., & Workman, M. [2006]. *Medical surgical nursing: Critical thinking for collaborative care* [5th ed.]. Philadelphia: W.B. Saunders.)

2. **Skull tongs**
   a. **Skull tongs** are inserted into the outer aspect of the client's skull, and traction is applied
   b. Weights are attached to the tongs and the client is used as countertraction
   c. Monitor neurological status of the client
   d. Determine the amount of weight prescribed to be added to the traction
   e. Ensure that weights hang securely and freely at all times
   f. Ensure that the ropes for the traction remain within the pulley
   g. Maintain body alignment and maintain care of the client on a special bed (RotoRest bed, Stryker, or Foster frame), as prescribed
   h. Turn the client every 2 hours

   i. Monitor insertion site of the tongs for infection
   j. Provide sterile pin site care as prescribed
3. **Halo traction**
   a. A static traction device that consists of a head-piece with four pins, two anterior and two posterior, inserted into the client's skull
   b. The metal halo ring may be attached to a vest (jacket) or cast when the spine is stable, allowing increased client mobility
   c. Monitor the client's neurological status for changes in movement or decreased strength
   d. Never move or turn the client by holding or pulling on the halo device
   e. Check for tightness of the jacket by ensuring that one finger can be placed under the jacket
   f. Monitor skin integrity to ensure that the jacket or cast is not causing pressure
   g. Provide sterile pin site care as prescribed
4. Client education for **halo traction** device (Box 56-14)
N. Interventions for thoracic and lumbar-sacral injuries
   1. Bed rest
   2. Immobilization with a body cast
   3. Use of a brace or corset when the client is out of bed

O. Surgical interventions for thoracic and lumbar-sacral injuries
1. Decompressive laminectomy
    a. Removal of one or more laminae
    b. Allows for cord expansion from edema
    c. Performed if conventional methods fail to prevent neurological deterioration
2. Spinal fusion
    a. Used for thoracic spinal injuries
    b. Bone is grafted between the vertebrae for support and to strengthen the back
3. Postoperative interventions
    a. Monitor for respiratory impairment
    b. Monitor vital signs, motor function, sensation, and circulatory status in the lower extremities
    c. Encourage breathing exercises
    d. Monitor for signs of fluid and electrolyte imbalance
    e. Observe for complications of immobility
    f. Keep the client flat
    g. Provide cast care if the client is in a full body cast
    h. Turn and reposition frequently by logrolling side to back to side, using turning sheets and pillows between the legs to maintain alignment
    i. Administer pain medication as prescribed
    j. Maintain NPO status until the client is actively passing flatus
    k. Monitor bowel sounds
    l. Provide the use of a fracture bedpan
    m. Monitor I&O
    n. Maintain nutritional status
P. Medications
1. Dexamethasone (Decadron)
    a. Used for its anti-inflammatory and edema-reducing effects
    b. May interfere with healing
2. Dextran
    a. A plasma expander
    b. Used to increase capillary blood flow within the spinal cord and to prevent or treat hypotension
3. Dantrolene (Dantrium)-baclofen (Lioresal)
    a. Used for clients with upper motor neuron injuries
    b. Controls muscle spasticity

IX. CEREBRAL ANEURYSM
A. Description
1. Dilation of the walls of a weakened cerebral artery
2. Can lead to rupture
B. Data collection
1. Headache
2. Pain
3. Diplopia
4. Blurred vision
5. Tinnitus
6. Nausea

7. Hemiparesis
8. Nuchal rigidity
9. Irritability
10. Seizures
C. Interventions
1. Maintain a patent airway (suction only with a physician's order)
2. Administer oxygen, as prescribed
3. Monitor vital signs and for hypertension or dysrhythmias
4. Avoid rectal temperatures
5. Maintain bed rest in semi-Fowler's position or side-lying position
6. Maintain a darkened room without stimulation
7. Limit visitors
8. Maintain fluid restrictions
9. Monitor I&O
10. Avoid stimulants in the diet

X. SEIZURES
A. Description
1. An abnormal sudden excessive discharge of electrical activity within the brain
2. Epilepsy is a disorder characterized by chronic seizure activity and indicates brain or central nervous system (CNS) irritation
3. Causes include genetic factors, trauma, tumors, circulatory or metabolic disorders, toxicity, and infections
4. Status epilepticus involves a rapid succession of epileptic spasms without intervals of consciousness; it is a potential complication that can occur with any type of seizure, and brain damage may result
B. Types of seizures (Table 56-1)
1. Generalized seizures
    a. Tonic-clonic (grand mal)
    b. Absence (petit mal)
    c. Myoclonic
    d. Atonic or akinetic (drop attacks)
2. Partial seizures
    a. Simple partial
    b. Complex partial
C. Data collection
1. Seizure history
2. Type of seizure
3. Occurrences before, during, and after the seizure
4. Prodromal signs, such as mood changes, irritability, and insomnia
5. Aura, a sensation that warns the client of the impending seizure
6. Loss of motor activity or bowel and bladder function, or loss of consciousness during the seizure
7. Occurrences during the postictal state, such as headache, loss of consciousness, sleepiness, and impaired speech or thinking

TABLE 56-1

Types of Seizures

Generalized Seizures	Partial Seizures
TONIC-CLONIC May begin with an aura The tonic phase involves the stiffening or rigidity of the muscles of the arms and legs and usually lasts 10 to 20 seconds, followed by loss of consciousness The clonic phase consists of hyperventilation and jerking of the extremities; usually lasts about 30 seconds Full recovery from the seizure may take several hours The client loses consciousness for a few seconds	**SIMPLE PARTIAL** Produces sensory symptoms accompanied by motor symptoms that are localized or confined to a specific area The client remains conscious and may report an aura **COMPLEX PARTIAL** A psychomotor seizure The area of the brain most involved is the temporal lobe Characterized by periods of altered behavior of which the client is not aware
ABSENCE Brief seizure lasting seconds; individual may or may not lose consciousness No loss or change in muscle tone occurs Seizures may occur several times during a day The victim appears to be daydreaming This type of seizure is more common in children	
MYOCLONIC A seizure that presents as a brief generalized jerking or stiffening of extremities The victim may fall to ground as a result of the seizure	
ATONIC OR AKINETIC (DROP ATTACKS) A sudden momentary loss of muscle tone The victim may fall to ground as a result of the seizure	

▲ D. Interventions

1. Note the time and duration of the seizure
2. Assess behavior at the onset of the seizure—whether the client experienced an aura, whether a change in facial expression occurred, or whether a sound or cry occurred from the client
3. If the client is standing, place the client on the floor and protect the head and body
4. Maintain a patent airway (do not force the jaws open)
5. Administer oxygen
6. Prepare to suction
7. Turn the client's head to the side
8. Prevent injury during the seizure
9. Remain with the client
10. Do not restrain the client
11. Loosen restrictive clothing
12. Note the type, character, and progression of the movements during the seizure
13. Monitor for incontinence
14. Medications such as IV diazepam (Valium), phenytoin (Dilantin), and phenobarbital sodium (Luminal) may be prescribed to stop the seizure
15. Document the characteristics of the seizure
16. Monitor behavior following the seizure, such as the state of consciousness, motor ability, and speech ability
17. Instruct the client about the importance of life-long medication and the need for follow-up medication blood levels
18. Instruct the client to avoid alcohol, excessive stress, and fatigue
19. Encourage the client to contact available community resources, such as the Epilepsy Foundation of America

XI. CEREBROVASCULAR ACCIDENT (CVA)

A. Description

1. A sudden focal neurological deficit caused by cerebrovascular disease
2. A syndrome in which the cerebral circulation is interrupted, causing neurological deficits
3. Cerebral anoxia lasting longer than 10 minutes causes cerebral infarction, with irreversible changes

4. Cerebral edema and congestion cause further dysfunction
5. Diagnosis is determined by CT scan, EEG, and cerebral arteriography
6. The permanent disability cannot be determined until the cerebral edema subsides
7. The order in which function may return is facial, swallowing, lower limb, speech, and arms
8. Carotid endarterectomy is a surgical intervention used in stroke management; targeted at stroke prevention, especially in clients with symptomatic carotid stenosis

B. Causes
1. Thrombosis
2. Embolism
3. Hemorrhage from rupture of a vessel
4. Transient ischemic attack (TIA)

C. Risk factors
1. Atherosclerosis
2. Hypertension
3. Anticoagulation therapy
4. Diabetes mellitus
5. Stress
6. Obesity
7. Oral contraceptives

D. Data collection (Figure 56-4; Boxes 56-15 and 56-16)
1. Findings depend on the area of the brain affected
2. Lesions in the cerebral hemisphere result in manifestations on the contralateral side, which is the side of the body opposite the cerebrovascular accident
3. Airway patency is always a priority
4. Pulse (may be slow and bounding)
5. Respirations (Cheyne-Stokes)
6. Blood pressure (hypertension)
7. Headache, nausea, and vomiting
8. Facial drooping
9. Nuchal rigidity
10. Visual changes
11. Ataxia
12. Dysarthria
13. Dysphagia
14. Speech changes
15. Decreased sensation to pressure, heat, and cold
16. Bowel and bladder dysfunctions
17. Paralysis

E. Aphasia
1. Expressive
   a. Damage in Broca's area of the frontal brain
   b. Client understands what is said but is unable to communicate verbally
2. Receptive
   a. Injury involving Wernicke's area in the temporoparietal area
   b. Client is unable to understand the spoken and often the written word

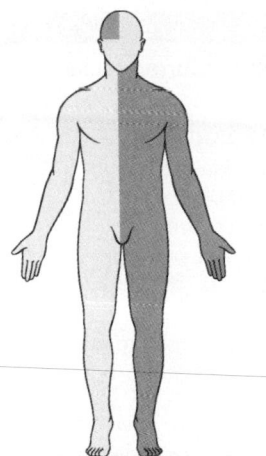
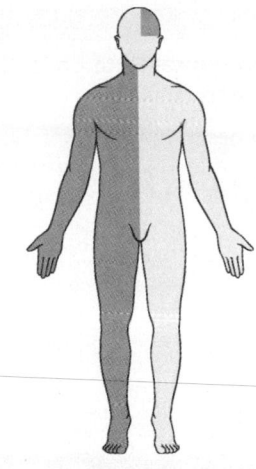

Right-brain damage (stroke on right side of the brain)	**Left-brain damage** (stroke on left side of the brain)
• Paralyzed left side: hemiplegia	• Paralyzed right side: hemiplegia
• Left-sided neglect	• Impaired speech/language aphasias
• Spatial-perceptual deficits	• Impaired right/left discrimination
• Tends to deny or minimize problems	• Slow performance, cautious
• Rapid performance, short attention span	• Aware of deficits: depression, anxiety
• Impulsive, safety problems	• Impaired comprehension related to language, math
• Impaired judgment	
• Impaired time concepts	

FIG. 56-4 Manifestations of right brain and left brain stroke. (From Lewis, S., Heitkemper, M., & Dirksen, S. [2004]. *Medical-surgical nursing: Assessment and management of clinical problems* [6th ed.]. St. Louis: Mosby.)

3. Global or mixed: Language dysfunction in both areas of expression and reception
4. Interventions for aphasia
   a. Provide repetitive directions
   b. Break tasks down to one step at a time
   c. Repeat names of objects frequently used
   d. Use a picture board or communication board

F. Interventions during the acute phase of CVA
1. Maintain a patent airway and administer oxygen, as prescribed
2. Monitor vital signs
3. Maintain a blood pressure of 150/100 mm Hg to maintain cerebral perfusion
4. Suction as prescribed, but never suction nasally and for no longer than 10 seconds, to prevent **increased ICP**
5. Monitor for **increased ICP**, because the client is at most risk during the first 72 hours following the CVA
6. Position the client on the side, with head of bed elevated 15 to 30 degrees, as prescribed

Neurological Data Collection in Cerebrovascular Accident (CVA)

Changes in level of consciousness (LOC)
Signs of increasing intracranial pressure (ICP)
Assessment of cranial nerves V, VII, IX, X, XII
    Cranial nerve V: Difficulty with chewing
    Cranial nerve VII: Facial paralysis or paresis
    Cranial nerves IX and X: Dysphagia
    Cranial nerve IX: Absent gag reflex
    Cranial nerve XII: Impaired tongue movement

Findings in a CVA

AGNOSIA
Inability to use an object correctly

APRAXIA
Inability to carry out a purposeful activity

HEMIANOPSIA
Blindness in half of the visual field

HOMONYMOUS HEMIANOPSIA
Blindness in the same side of both eyes

NEGLECT SYNDROME
Client unaware of the existence of his or her paralyzed side

PROPRIOCEPTION ALTERATIONS
Altered position sense places the client at increased risk of injury
Pyramid point: With visual problems, the client must turn his or her head to scan the complete range of vision.

7. Monitor LOC, pupillary response, motor and sensory response, cranial nerve function, and reflexes
8. Maintain a quiet environment and provide minimal handling of the client to prevent further bleeding
9. Insert a Foley catheter as prescribed
10. IV fluids may be prescribed and need to be monitored closely
11. Maintain fluid and electrolyte balance
12. Prepare to administer anticoagulants, antiplatelets, diuretics, antihypertensives, and anticonvulsants as prescribed
13. Establish a form of communication
G. Interventions in the postacute phase of a CVA
  1. Continue with interventions from the acute phase
  2. Position the client for 2 hours on the unaffected side, 20 minutes on the affected side

3. Position the client in the prone position if prescribed, for 30 minutes three times daily
4. Provide skin, mouth, and eye care
5. Perform passive range-of-motion exercises to prevent contractures
6. Place antiembolism stockings on client
7. Measure thighs and calves for an increase in size, and assess for positive Homans' sign
8. Monitor gag reflex and ability to swallow
9. Provide sips of fluids and slowly advance diet to foods that are easy to chew and swallow
10. Provide soft and semisoft foods and fluids rather than liquids, because the CVA client is better able to tolerate these types of food
11. When the client is eating, position the client sitting in a chair or sitting up in bed, with the head and neck positioned slightly forward and flexed
12. Place food in the back of the mouth on the unaffected side to prevent trapping of food in the affected cheek
H. Interventions in the chronic phase of CVA
  1. Neglect syndrome
    a. Client is unaware of the existence of his or her paralyzed side (places the client at risk for injury)
    b. Teach the client to touch and use both sides of the body
  2. Hemianopsia
    a. Blindness in half of the visual field
    b. Homonymous hemianopsia: blindness in the same side of both eyes
    c. Client is encouraged to turn the head to scan the complete range of vision; otherwise he or she does not see half the visual field
  3. Approach the client from the unaffected side
  4. Place the client's personal objects within the visual field
  5. Provide eye care for visual deficits
  6. Place a patch over the affected eye if the client has diplopia
  7. Increase mobility as tolerated
  8. Encourage fluids and a high-fiber diet
  9. Administer stool softeners, as prescribed
  10. Encourage the client to express feelings
  11. Encourage independence in activities of daily living
  12. Determine the need for assistive devices such as a cane, walker, splints, or braces
  13. Teach transfer technique from bed to chair and chair to bed
  14. Provide gait training
  15. Initiate physical and occupational therapy
  16. Refer to speech and language pathologist

XII. MULTIPLE SCLEROSIS (MS)

A. Description
1. A chronic, progressive, noncontagious, degenerative disease of the CNS, characterized by demyelinization of the neurons
2. It usually occurs between the ages of 20 and 40 years and consists of periods of remissions and exacerbations
3. The causes are unknown, but the disease is thought to be a result of an autoimmune response or viral infection
4. Precipitating factors include pregnancy, fatigue, stress, infection, and trauma
5. Electroencephalograhic findings are abnormal
6. A lumbar puncture indicates increased gamma globulin level, but the serum globulin level is normal

B. Data collection
1. Fatigue and weakness
2. Ataxia and vertigo
3. Tremors and spasticity of the lower extremities
4. Parasthesias
5. Blurred vision and diplopia
6. Nystagmus
7. Dysphasia
8. Decreased perception to pain, touch, and temperature
9. Bladder and bowel disturbances, including urgency, frequency, retention, and incontinence
10. Abnormal reflexes, including hyperreflexia, absent reflexes, and a positive **Babinski reflex**
11. Emotional changes such as apathy, euphoria, irritability, and depression
12. Memory changes and confusion

C. Interventions
1. Provide bed rest during exacerbation
2. Protect the client from injury by providing safety measures
3. Place an eye patch on the eye for diplopia
4. Monitor for potential complications such as urinary tract infections, calculi, decubitus ulcers, respiratory tract infections, and contractures
5. Promote regular elimination by bladder and bowel training
6. Encourage independence
7. Assist the client to establish a regular exercise and rest program
8. Instruct the client to balance moderate activity with rest periods
9. Determine the need for and provide assistive devices
10. Initiate physical and speech therapy
11. Instruct the client to avoid fatigue, stress, infection, overheating, and chilling
12. Instruct the client to increase fluids and eat a balanced diet, including low-fat, high-fiber foods and foods high in potassium
13. Instruct the client in safety measures related to sensory loss, such as regulating the temperature of bath water and avoiding heating pads
14. Instruct the client in safety measures related to motor loss, such as avoiding the use of scatter rugs and using assistive devices
15. Instruct the client in the self-administration of prescribed medications (Box 56-17)
16. Provide information about the National Multiple Sclerosis Society

---

BOX 56-17

Medications Used with Multiple Sclerosis

CORTICOSTEROIDS
Examples
Corticotropin (ACTH) (Acthar)
Methylprednisolone sodium succinate (Solu-Medrol)
Uses
Reduce edema and the inflammatory response
Decrease the length of time the client's symptoms are exacerbated and improve the degree of recovery

IMMUNOSUPPRESSIVES
Used for the treatment of chronic progressive MS to stabilize the disease process

OTHER AGENTS
Baclofen (Lioresal), dantrolene (Dantrium), or diazepam (Valium): Used to lessen muscle spasticity
Carbamazepine (Tegretol): Used to treat paresthesia
Propranolol (Inderal) and clonazepam (Klonopin): Used to treat cerebellar ataxia
Bethanechol (Urecholine): Used to prevent urinary retention
Oxybutynin chloride (Ditropan): Used to increase bladder capacity

---

XIII. MYASTHENIA GRAVIS

A. Description
1. A neuromuscular disease characterized by marked weakness and abnormal fatigue of the voluntary muscles
2. A defect in the transmission of nerve impulses at the myoneural junction
3. Causes include insufficient secretion of acetylcholine, excessive secretion of cholinesterase, and unresponsiveness of the muscle fibers to acetylcholine

B. Data collection
1. Weakness and fatigue
2. Difficulty chewing
3. Dysphagia
4. Ptosis

5. Diplopia
6. Weak, hoarse voice
7. Difficulty breathing
8. Diminished breath sounds
9. Respiratory paralysis and failure
C. Interventions
1. Monitor respiratory status and ability to cough and deep breathe adequately
2. Monitor for respiratory failure
3. Maintain suctioning and emergency equipment at the bedside
4. Monitor vital signs
5. Monitor speech and swallowing abilities to prevent aspiration
6. Encourage the client to sit up when eating
7. Check muscle status
8. Instruct the client to conserve strength
9. Plan short activities that coincide with times of maximal muscle strength
10. Monitor for myasthenic and cholinergic crises
11. Administer anticholinesterase medications, as prescribed
12. Instruct the client to avoid stress, infection, fatigue, and over-the-counter medications
13. Instruct the client to wear a Medic-Alert bracelet
14. Inform the client about services from the Myasthenia Gravis Foundation
D. Anticholinesterase medications
1. Action: Increase levels of acetycholine at the myoneural junction
2. Medications
a. Neostigmine bromide (Prostigmin)
b. Pyridostigmine bromide (Mestinon, Regonol)
c. Edrophonium chloride (Tensilon)
3. Side effects
a. Sweating
b. Salivation
c. Nausea
d. Diarrhea and abdominal cramps
e. Bradycardia
f. Hypotension
4. Interventions
a. Administer medications on time
b. Administer medication 30 minutes before meals with milk and crackers to reduce gastrointestinal upset
c. Monitor and record muscle strength
d. Note that excessive doses lead to cholinergic crisis
e. Have antidote (atropine sulfate) available
E. Myasthenic crisis
1. Description
a. Acute exacerbation of disease
b. Caused by a rapid, unrecognized progression of the disease, an inadequate amount of medication, infection, fatigue, or stress

2. Data collection
a. Restlessness
b. Weakness
c. Dyspnea
d. Dysphagia
e. Difficulty speaking
3. Interventions
a. Monitor for signs of myasthenic crisis
b. Increase anticholinesterase medication
F. Cholinergic crisis
1. Description
a. Depolarization of the motor end plates
b. Caused by overmedication with anticholinesterase
2. Data collection
a. Restlessness
b. Weakness
c. Dysphagia
d. Dyspnea
e. Nausea, vomiting, and diarrhea
f. Fasciculations
g. Sweating
h. Salivation
i. Increased bronchial secretions
3. Interventions
a. Hold anticholinesterase medication
b. Prepare to administer the antidote, atropine sulfate, if prescribed
G. Tensilon test
1. Description: Performed to diagnose myasthenia gravis and to differentiate between myasthenic crisis and cholinergic crisis
2. To diagnose myasthenia gravis
a. Tensilon injection is administered to the client
b. Positive for myasthenia gravis: Client shows improvement in muscle strength after the administration of Tensilon
c. Negative for myasthenia gravis: Client shows no improvement in muscle strength, and strength may even deteriorate after injection of Tensilon
3. To differentiate crisis
a. Myasthenic crisis: Tensilon is administered and, if strength improves, the client needs more medication
b. Cholinergic crisis: Tensilon is administered and, if weakness is more severe, the client is overmedicated; administer atropine sulfate, the antidote, as prescribed

XIV. PARKINSON'S DISEASE

A. Description
1. A degenerative disease caused by the depletion of dopamine, which interferes with the inhibition of excitatory impulses
2. It results in a dysfunction of the extrapyramidal system

3. It is a slow, progressive disease that results in a crippling disability
4. The debilitation can result in falls, self-care deficits, failure of body systems, and depression
5. Mental deterioration occurs late in the disease

B. Data collection
1. Bradykinesia, abnormal slowness of movement, and sluggishness of physical and mental responses
2. Aching shoulders and arms
3. Monotonous speech
4. Handwriting that becomes progressively smaller
5. Tremors in hands and fingers at rest (pill rolling)
6. Tremors increasing when fatigued and decreasing with purposeful activity or sleep
7. Rigidity with jerky, interrupted movements
8. Restlessness and pacing
9. Blank facial expression
10. Drooling
11. Difficulty swallowing and speaking
12. Loss of coordination and balance
13. Shuffling steps, stooped position, and propulsive gait

C. Interventions
1. Check neurological status
2. Check ability to swallow and chew
3. Provide high-calorie, high-protein, high-fiber soft diet with small, frequent feedings
4. Increase fluids to 2000 mL/day
5. Monitor for constipation
6. Promote independence along with safety measures
7. Avoid rushing the client with activities
8. Assist with ambulation
9. Provide assistive devices
10. Instruct the client to wear low-heeled shoes
11. Encourage the client to lift feet when walking and to avoid prolonged sitting
12. Provide a firm mattress and position the client prone, without a pillow, to facilitate proper posture
13. Instruct in proper posture by teaching the client to hold the hands behind the back to keep the spine and neck erect
14. Promote physical therapy and rehabilitation
15. Administer anticholinergic medications as prescribed to treat tremors and rigidity and to inhibit the action of acetylcholine
16. Administer antiparkinsonian medications to increase the level of dopamine in the CNS
17. Instruct the client to avoid foods high in vitamin B_6 because they block the effects of antiparkinsonian medications
18. Instruct the client to avoid monoamine oxidase (MAO) inhibitors because they will precipitate hypertensive crisis
19. See Chapter 57 regarding medication to treat Parkinson's disease

XV. TRIGEMINAL NEURALGIA

A. Description
1. A sensory disorder of the fifth cranial nerve
2. Results in severe, recurrent, sharp, facial pain along the trigeminal nerve

B. Data collection
1. Pain on the lips, gums, or nose, or across the cheeks
2. Situations that stimulate symptoms include cold, washing the face, chewing, or ingesting food or fluids of extreme temperatures

C. Interventions
1. Instruct the client to avoid hot or cold foods and fluids
2. Provide small feedings of liquid and soft foods
3. Instruct the client to chew food on the unaffected side
4. Administer medications, as prescribed (Box 56-18)

D. Surgical interventions
1. An alcohol injection along the affected portion of the nerve to produce anesthesia of the nerve may provide relief of pain for up to 16 months
2. Retrogasserian rhizotomy or total severance of the sensory root of the trigeminal nerve
3. Jannetta procedure, which surgically relocates the artery that is compressing the trigeminal nerve
4. Electrocoagulation or percutaneous radiofrequency rhizotomy to create a heat lesion

XVI. BELL'S PALSY (FACIAL PARALYSIS)

A. Description
1. A lower motor neuron lesion of the seventh cranial nerve that may occur as a result of trauma, hemorrhage, meningitis, or tumor
2. It results in paralysis of one side of the face
3. Recovery usually occurs in a few weeks without residual effects

B. Data collection
1. Flaccid facial muscles
2. Inability to raise the eyebrows, frown, smile, close the eyelids, or puff out the cheeks
3. Upward movement of the eye occurs when attempting to close the eyelid
4. Loss of taste

BOX 56-18

Medications to Treat Trigeminal Neuralgia

Carbamazepine (Tegretol)
Phenytoin (Dilantin)
Baclofen (Lioresal)
Amitriptyline (Elavil)
Diazepam (Valium)

C. Interventions

1. Encourage facial exercises to prevent the loss of muscle tone (a face sling may be prescribed to prevent stretching of weak muscles)
2. Protect the eyes from dryness and prevent injury
3. Promote frequent oral care
4. Instruct the client to chew on the unaffected side

XVII. GUILLAIN-BARRÉ SYNDROME

A. Description

1. An acute infectious neuronitis of the cranial and peripheral nerves
2. The immune system overreacts to the infection and destroys the myelin sheath
3. It is usually preceded by a mild upper respiratory infection or gastroenteritis
4. The recovery is a slow process and can take years
5. The major concern is difficulty breathing

B. Data collection

1. Paresthesias
2. Weakness of lower extremities
3. Gradual progressive weakness of upper extremities and facial muscles
4. Can progress to respiratory failure
5. Cardiac dysrhythmias
6. Cerebrospinal fluid reveals an elevated protein level
7. Electroencephalogram is abnormal

C. Interventions

1. Care is directed toward the treatment of symptoms
2. Monitor respiratory status
3. Provide respiratory treatments
4. Prepare to initiate respiratory support
5. Monitor cardiac status
6. Monitor for complications of immobility
7. Provide the client and family with support

XVIII. AMYOTROPHIC LATERAL SCLEROSIS

A. Description

1. Also known as Lou Gehrig's disease
2. A progressive degenerative disease involving the motor system
3. The sensory and autonomic systems are not involved, and mental status changes do not result from the disease
4. The cause of the disease may be related to an excess of glutamate, a chemical responsible for relaying messages between the motor neurons
5. As the disease progresses, muscle weakness and atrophy develop until a flaccid quadriplegia develops
6. Eventually the respiratory muscles become affected, leading to respiratory compromise, pneumonia, and death
7. There is no known cure; treatment is symptomatic

B. Data collection

1. Fatigue
2. Fatigue while talking
3. Muscle weakness and atrophy
4. Tongue atrophy
5. Dysphagia
6. Weakness of the hands and arms
7. Fasciculations of the face
8. Nasal quality of speech
9. Dysarthria

C. Interventions

1. Care is directed toward the treatment of symptoms
2. Monitor respiratory status
3. Provide respiratory treatments
4. Prepare to initiate respiratory support
5. Monitor for complications of immobility
6. Provide the client and family with support

XIX. ENCEPHALITIS

A. Description

1. An inflammation of the brain parenchyma and often the meninges
2. Affects the cerebrum, the brainstem, and/or the cerebellum
3. Most often caused by a viral agent, although bacteria, fungi, or parasites may also be involved
4. Viral encephalitis is almost always preceded by a viral infection

B. Transmission

1. Arboviruses can be transmitted to humans through the bite of an infected mosquito or tick
2. Echovirus, coxsackievirus, poliovirus, herpes zoster, and viruses that cause mumps and chickenpox are common enteroviruses associated with encephalitis
3. Herpes simplex type 1 virus can cause viral encephalitis
4. Amebic meningoencephalitis can enter the nasal mucosa of people swimming in warm fresh water, ponds, and lakes

C. Data collection

1. Presence of cold sores, lesions, or ulcerations of the oral cavity
2. History of insect bites and swimming in fresh water
3. Exposure to infectious diseases
4. Travel to areas where the disease in prevalent
5. Fever
6. Nausea and vomiting
7. Stiff neck
8. Changes in LOC and mental status
9. Signs of **increased ICP**
10. Motor dysfunction and focal neurological deficits

D. Interventions
1. Monitor vital and neurological signs
2. Check LOC using the **Glasgow Coma Scale**
3. Monitor for mental status changes and personality and behavior changes
4. Monitor for signs of **increased ICP**
5. Monitor for the presence of nuchal rigidity and a positive **Kernig** or **Brudzinski sign**, indicating meningeal irritation
6. Assist the client to turn, cough, and deep breathe frequently
7. Elevate the head of the bed 30 to 45 degrees
8. Monitor for muscle and neurological deficits
9. Administer acyclovir (Zovirax), as prescribed
10. Initiate rehabilitation as needed for motor dysfunction or neurological deficits

XX. WEST NILE VIRUS

A. Description
1. A potentially serious illness that affects the central nervous system
2. It is primarily contracted by the bite of an infected mosquito (mosquitoes become carriers when they feed on infected birds)
3. Symptoms typically develop between 3 and 14 days after being bitten by the infected mosquito
4. Neurological effects can be permanent
B. Data collection
1. Many individuals will not experience any symptoms
2. Mild symptoms include fever, headache and body aches, nausea, vomiting, swollen glands, or a rash on the chest, stomach, or back
3. Severe symptoms include a high fever, headache, neck stiffness, stupor, disorientation, tremors, muscle weakness, vision loss, numbness, paralysis, seizures, or coma
C. Interventions: Supportive; there is no specific treatment for the virus
D. Prevention
1. Use insect repellents containing DEET (N,N-diethylmetatoluamide) when outdoors and wear long sleeves, pants, and light-colored clothing
2. Stay indoors at dusk and dawn when mosquitoes are most active
3. Ensure that mosquito breeding sites are eliminated such as standing water and water in bird baths, and keep wading pools empty and on their sides when not in use

XXI. MENINGITIS

A. Description
1. Inflammation of the arachnoid and pia mater of the brain and spinal cord
2. Caused by bacterial and viral organisms, although fungal and protozoal meningitis also occurs

3. Predisposing factors include skull fractures, brain or spinal surgery, sinus or upper respiratory infections, the use of nasal sprays, and individuals with a compromised immune system
4. CSF fluid is analyzed to determine the diagnosis and the type of meningitis
B. Transmission
1. Direct contact, including droplet spread
2. Occurs in areas of high population density, crowded living areas, and prisons
C. Data collection
1. Mild lethargy
2. Memory changes
3. Short attention span
4. Personality and behavior changes
5. Severe headache
6. Generalized muscle aches and pains
7. Nausea and vomiting
8. Fever and chills
9. Tachycardia
10. Deterioration in the LOC
11. Photophobia
12. Signs of meningeal irritation such as nuchal rigidity and positive **Kernig's sign** and **Brudzinski's sign**
13. Red, macular rash with meningococcal meningitis
14. Abdominal and chest pain with viral meningitis
D. Interventions
1. Monitor vital signs and neurological signs
2. Monitor for signs of **increased ICP**
3. Initiate seizure precautions
4. Monitor for seizure activity
5. Monitor for signs of meningeal irritation
6. Check the cranial nerves
7. Check vascular status
8. Maintain isolation precautions as necessary with bacterial meningitis
9. Maintain urine and stool precautions with viral meningitis
10. Maintain respiratory isolation for the client with pneumococcal meningitis
11. Elevate the head of the bed 30 degrees, and avoid neck flexion and extreme hip flexion
12. Prevent stimulation and restrict visitors
13. Administer analgesics, as prescribed
14. Administer antibiotics, as prescribed

PRACTICE QUESTIONS

1. A client has an impairment of cranial nerve II. Specific to this impairment, the nurse would plan to do which of the following to ensure client safety?
   1. Provide a clear path for ambulation without obstacles
   2. Test the temperature of the shower water
   3. Speak loudly to the client
   4. Check the temperature of the food on the dietary tray

2. The client has a cerebellar lesion. The nurse determines that the client was adapting successfully to this problem if the client demonstrated proper use of which of the following items?
   1. Adaptive eating utensils
   2. Walker
   3. Raised toilet seat
   4. Slider board

3. A nurse is planning care for a client who displays confusion secondary to a neurological problem. Which approach by the nurse would be least helpful in assisting this client?
   1. Giving simple, clear directions
   2. Providing a stable environment
   3. Providing sensory cues
   4. Encouraging multiple visitors at one time

4. A client with a neurological impairment experiences urinary incontinence. Which nursing action would help the client adapt to this alteration?
   1. Establishing a toileting schedule
   2. Inserting a Foley catheter
   3. Using adult diapers
   4. Padding the bed with an absorbent cotton pad

5. The nurse has obtained a personal and family history from the client with a neurological disorder. Which finding in the client's history does not give the client added risk for neurological problems?
   1. Previous back injury
   2. Allergy to pollen
   3. History of hypertension
   4. History of headaches

6. A client with right leg hemiplegia has a nursing diagnosis of Impaired Physical Mobility. The nurse determines that the family needs reinforcement of teaching if the nurse observes which of the following being done by the family?
   1. Encouraging the client to stand unassisted on the leg
   2. Active range of motion (ROM) to the affected leg
   3. Passive ROM to the affected leg
   4. Applying premolded splint

7. A nurse is preparing a client who is scheduled to have cerebral angiography performed. The nurse would check the client for:
   1. Allergy to salmon
   2. Allergy to iodine or shellfish
   3. Claustrophobia
   4. Excessive weight

8. A client admitted to the hospital with a neurological problem indicates to the nurse that magnetic resonance imaging (MRI) may be done. The nurse interprets that the client may be ineligible for this diagnostic procedure based on the client's history of:
   1. Hypertension
   2. Chronic obstructive pulmonary disorder
   3. Heart failure
   4. Prosthetic valve replacement

9. A client is having a lumbar puncture (LP) performed. The nurse would place the client in which position for the procedure?
   1. Side-lying, with legs pulled up and head bent down onto the chest
   2. Supine, in semi-Fowler's
   3. Prone, in slight Trendelenburg's
   4. Prone, with a pillow under the abdomen

10. The client is somewhat nervous about having magnetic resonance imaging (MRI). Which statement by the nurse would provide reassurance to the client about the procedure?
    1. "It is necessary to remove any metal or metal-containing objects before having the MRI done to avoid the metal being drawn into the magnetic field."
    2. "The MRI machine is a long, hollow narrow tube, and may make you feel somewhat claustrophobic."
    3. "Even though you are alone in the scanner, you will be in voice communication with the technologist during the procedure."
    4. "You will be able to eat before the procedure unless you get nauseous easily. If so, you should eat lightly."

11. A client has just undergone computerized tomography (CT) scanning with a contrast medium. The nurse determines that the client understands postprocedure care if the client verbalizes that he or she will:
    1. Eat lightly for the remainder of the day
    2. Rest quietly for the remainder of the day
    3. Hold medications for at least 4 hours
    4. Drink extra fluids for the day

12. A nurse is admitting the client to the ambulatory care unit following a myelogram. A water based contrast agent was used for the procedure. The nurse would plan which activity restriction for the client?
    1. Bed rest for 6 to 8 hours, with the head of the bed elevated 15 to 30 degrees
    2. Bed rest for 2 to 4 hours, with the head of the bed elevated 15 to 30 degrees
    3. Bed rest for 6 to 8 hours, with the head of the bed flat
    4. Bed rest for 2 to 4 hours, with the head of the bed flat

13. A nurse is administering mouth care to an unconscious client. The nurse should avoid doing which of the following?
    1. Positioning the client on the side
    2. Using products with lemon or alcohol
    3. Cleansing the mucous membranes with Toothettes
    4. Brushing the teeth with a small toothbrush

14. A nurse is trying to help the family of an unconscious client cope with the situation. Which intervention

would the nurse plan to incorporate into the care routine for the client?

1. Discouraging the family from touching the client
2. Explaining equipment and procedures on an ongoing basis
3. Ensuring adherence to visiting hours to ensure client's rest
4. Encouraging the family not to "give in" to their feelings of grief

15. The nurse is suctioning an unconscious client who has a tracheostomy. The nurse should avoid which action during this procedure?
    1. Keeping a supply of suction catheters at the bedside
    2. Auscultating breath sounds to determine need for suctioning
    3. Hyperoxygenating the client before, during, and after suctioning
    4. Making sure not to suction for longer than 30 seconds

16. A nurse has applied a hypothermia blanket to a client with a fever. The nurse would inspect the skin frequently to detect which complication of hypothermia blanket use?
    1. Skin breakdown
    2. Frostbite
    3. Arterial insufficiency
    4. Venous insufficiency

17. A nurse is caring for an unconscious client who is experiencing persistent hyperthermia with no signs and symptoms of infection. The nurse understands that there may be damage to the client's thermoregulatory center in the:
    1. Cerebrum
    2. Cerebellum
    3. Hippocampus
    4. Hypothalamus

18. A client seeking treatment for an episode of hyperthermia is being discharged to home. The nurse determines that the client needs clarification of discharge instructions if the client stated that he or she will:
    1. Stay in a cool environment when possible
    2. Increase fluid intake for the next 24 hours
    3. Monitor voiding for adequacy of urine output
    4. Resume full activity level immediately

19. A nurse is caring for a client with increased intracranial pressure (ICP). The nurse would monitor for which of the following trends in vital signs that would occur if the intracranial pressure is rising?
    1. Increasing temperature, increasing pulse, increasing respirations, decreasing blood pressure (BP)
    2. Increasing temperature, decreasing pulse, decreasing respirations, increasing BP

3. Decreasing temperature, decreasing pulse, increasing respirations, decreasing BP
4. Decreasing temperature, increasing pulse, decreasing respirations, increasing BP

20. A nurse is positioning the client with increased intracranial pressure (ICP). Which position would the nurse avoid?
    1. Head turned to the side
    2. Head midline
    3. Neck in neutral position
    4. Head of bed elevated 30 to 45 degrees

21. A client recovering from a head injury is arousable and participating in care. The nurse determines that the client understands measures to prevent elevations in intracranial pressure if the nurse observes the client doing which of the following activities?
    1. Exhaling during repositioning
    2. Isometric exercises
    3. Blowing the nose
    4. Coughing vigorously

22. A family of an unconscious client with increased intracranial pressure is talking at the client's bedside. They are discussing the gravity of the client's condition, and wondering if the client will ever recover. The nurse intervenes, based on the understanding that:
    1. The family needs immediate crisis intervention
    2. The family could benefit from a conference with the physician
    3. It is possible the client can hear the family
    4. The client might have wanted a visit from the hospital chaplain

23. A nurse is providing care to a client with increased intracranial pressure (ICP). Which approach may not be beneficial in controlling the client's ICP from an environmental viewpoint?
    1. Maintaining a calm atmosphere
    2. Reducing environmental noise
    3. Clustering nursing activities to be done all at once
    4. Allowing the client uninterrupted time for sleep

24. A client has clear fluid leaking from the nose following a basilar skull fracture. The nurse determines that this is cerebrospinal fluid (CSF) if the fluid:
    1. Clumps together on the dressing and has a pH of 7
    2. Separates into concentric rings and tests positive for glucose
    3. Is grossly bloody in appearance and has a pH of 6
    4. Is clear in appearance and tests negative for glucose

25. A client is admitted to the hospital for observation with a probable minor head injury after an automobile crash. The nurse would plan on leaving the cervical collar in place until:
    1. The physician makes rounds
    2. The family comes to visit

3. The result of spinal x-rays are known
4. The nurse needs to do physical care

26. A client was seen and treated in the emergency room for treatment of a concussion. The nurse determines that the family needs reinforcement of the discharge instructions if they verbalize to call the physician for which of the client's signs and symptoms?
    1. Difficulty speaking
    2. Difficulty awakening
    3. Vomiting
    4. Minor headache

27. A nurse is caring for a client who has undergone craniotomy with a supratentorial incision. The nurse would plan to place the client in which position postoperatively?
    1. Head of bed flat, head and neck midline
    2. Head of bed flat, head turned to the nonoperative side
    3. Head of bed elevated 30 to 45 degrees, head and neck midline
    4. Head of bed elevated 30 to 45 degrees, head turned to the operative side

28. A nurse is preparing to give the postcraniotomy client medication for incisional pain. The family asks the nurse why the client is receiving codeine sulfate and not "something stronger." In formulating a response, the nurse incorporates the understanding that codeine:
    1. Is one of the strongest narcotic analgesics available
    2. Cannot lead to physical or psychological dependence
    3. Does not cause gastrointestinal upset or constipation as do other narcotics
    4. Does not alter respirations or mask neurological signs as do other narcotics

29. A nurse reinforces home care instructions to the postcraniotomy client. Which statement by the client indicates the need for further instructions?
    1. "A tub bath or shower is permitted, but I need to keep my scalp dry until the sutures are removed."
    2. "I need to use a check-off system for my anticonvulsant medications to avoid missing doses."
    3. "I will not hear sounds clearly unless they are loud."
    4. "If I tend to have seizures or gets dizzy spells, someone should be with me while walking."

30. A nurse notes documentation of a nursing diagnosis of Disturbed Body Image for a client after craniotomy. The nurse determines that the client has not met the outcome criteria by discharge if the client:
    1. Wears a turban to cover the incision
    2. States an intention to purchase a hairpiece until the hair has grown back

3. Verbalizes that periorbital bruising will disappear over time
4. Indicates that facial puffiness will be a permanent problem

31. A client with a cervical spine injury has Crutchfield tongs applied in the emergency room. The nurse would avoid which of the following when planning care for this client?
    1. Use of a Stryker frame bed
    2. Assessment of the integrity of the weights and pulleys
    3. Comparing the amount of ordered traction with the amount in use
    4. Removing the weights to reposition the client

32. A client with spinal cord injury becomes angry and belligerent whenever the nurse tries to administer care. The nurse should:
    1. Advise the client that rehabilitation progresses more quickly with cooperation
    2. Acknowledge the client's anger and continue to encourage participation in care
    3. Leave the client alone until ready to participate
    4. Ask the family to deliver the care

33. A nurse has completed reinforcing discharge instructions with a client with an application of a halo device. The nurse determines that the client needs further clarification of the instructions if the client states that he or she will:
    1. Use caution, because the device alters balance
    2. Wash the skin daily under the lamb's wool liner of the vest
    3. Use a straw for drinking
    4. Drive only during the daytime

34. A client with a spinal cord injury expresses little interest in food, and is very particular about the choice of meals that are actually eaten. The nurse interprets that:
    1. Meal choices represent an area of client control, and should be encouraged as much as is nutritionally reasonable
    2. Anorexia is a sign of clinical depression, and a referral to a psychologist is needed
    3. The client has compulsive habits, which should be ignored as long as they are not harmful
    4. The client probably has a naturally slow metabolism, and the decreased nutritional intake won't matter

35. A nursing student is planning care for a client with paraplegia who has a Risk for Injury related to spasticity of his leg muscles. The registered nurse intervenes if the student plans to include which intervention to minimize the risk of injury to the client?
    1. Removing potentially harmful objects near the spastic limbs
    2. Performing range of motion to the affected limbs

3. Use of padded restraints to immobilize the limb

4. Use of PRN orders for muscle relaxants such as baclofen (Lioresal)

36. A nurse is teaching the paraplegic client measures to promote skin integrity. Which instruction will be least helpful to the client?

1. Shifting weight every 2 hours while in a wheelchair

2. Using a mirror to inspect for redness and breakdown twice a week

3. Checking the bottom sheet for wetness and wrinkles

4. Using a pressure relief pad while in a wheelchair

37. A client who is paraplegic after spinal cord injury has been taught muscle strengthening exercises for the upper body. The nurse determines that the client will derive the least muscle-strengthening benefit from which activity?

1. Doing push-ups in a prone position

2. Extending the arms while holding weights

3. Doing active range of motion to finger joints

4. Squeezing rubber balls

38. A nurse is caring for the client who has suffered spinal cord injury. The nurse further monitors the client for signs of autonomic dysreflexia and suspects this complication if which of the following is noted?

1. Severe, throbbing headache

2. Pallor of the face and neck

3. Sudden tachycardia

4. Severe and sudden hypotension

39. A client with diplopia has been taught to use an eye patch to promote better vision and prevent injury. The nurse determines that the client understands how to use the patch if the client states that he or she will:

1. Use the patch only when vision is especially troublesome

2. Wear the patch for 1 hour at a time

3. Wear the patch continuously, alternating eyes each day

4. Wear the patch continuously, alternating eyes each week

40. A client with spinal cord injury is prone to experiencing autonomic dysreflexia. The nurse would avoid which measure to minimize the risk of recurrence?

1. Strict adherence to a bowel retraining program

2. Limiting bladder catheterization to once every 12 hours

3. Keeping the linen wrinkle-free under the client

4. Avoiding unnecessary pressure on the lower limbs

41. A client with spinal cord injury suddenly experiences an episode of autonomic dysreflexia. After checking vital signs, the nurse immediately:

1. Lowers the head of the bed and administers an antihypertensive agent

2. Removes the noxious stimulus and administers an antihypertensive agent

3. Lowers the head of the bed and removes the noxious stimulus

4. Raises the head of the bed and removes the noxious stimulus

42. A nurse is planning care for the client in spinal shock. Which of the following actions would be least helpful in minimizing the effects of vasodilation below the level of the injury?

1. Monitoring vital signs before and during position changes

2. Using vasopressor medications, as prescribed

3. Moving the client quickly as one unit

4. Applying Teds or compression stockings

43. A nurse is caring for a client with an intracranial aneurysm who was previously alert. Which finding would be an early indication that the level of consciousness (LOC) is deteriorating?

1. Clear speech

2. Ptosis of the left eyelid

3. Drowsiness

4. Frequent spontaneous speech

44. A nurse is planning to put aneurysm precautions in place for the client with a cerebral aneurysm. Which item would be included as part of the precautions?

1. Allowing out of bed activities as tolerated

2. Maintaining the head of bed at 15 degrees

3. Limiting cigarettes to three per day

4. Allowing one cup of caffeinated coffee per day

45. A nursing instructor asks a nursing student about the points to document if the client has had a seizure. The instructor determines that the student needs to read about seizures and documentation points if the student stated that it is important to document:

1. Duration of the seizure

2. What the client ate in the 2 hours preceding seizure activity

3. Seizure progression and type of movements

4. Changes in pupil size or eye deviation

46. A nurse is planning to institute seizure precautions for a client who is being admitted from the Emergency Department. Which of the following measures would the nurse avoid in planning for the client's safety?

1. Placing an airway, oxygen, and suction equipment at the bedside

2. Padding the side rails of the bed

3. Putting a padded tongue blade at the head of the bed

4. Having intravenous (IV) equipment ready for insertion of IV access

47. A nurse is caring for a client who begins to experience seizure activity while in bed. Which action by the nurse would be contraindicated?

1. Loosening restrictive clothing

2. Removing the pillow and raising the padded side rails

3. Restraining the client's limbs
4. Positioning the client to the side, if possible, with head flexed forward

48. A nurse has given medication instructions to the client receiving phenytoin (Dilantin). The nurse determines that the client understands the instructions if the client states:
    1. The medication dose may be self-adjusted, depending on side effects
    2. Alcohol is not contraindicated while taking this medication
    3. Good oral hygiene is needed, including brushing and flossing
    4. The morning dose of the medication should be taken before a sample for a serum drug level is drawn

49. A nurse is planning care for the client with hemiparesis of the right arm and leg. The nurse incorporates in the care plan placement of objects:
    1. Within the client's reach, on the right side
    2. Within the client's reach, on the left side
    3. Just out of the client's reach, on the right side
    4. Just out of the client's reach, on the left side

50. A client with a cerebrovascular accident (CVA) has residual dysphagia. When a diet order is initiated, the nurse avoids doing which of the following?
    1. Giving the client thin liquids
    2. Thickening liquids to the consistency of oatmeal
    3. Placing food on the unaffected side of the mouth
    4. Allowing plenty of time for chewing and swallowing

51. A nurse has instructed the family of a cerebrovascular accident (CVA) client who has homonymous hemianopsia about measures to help the client overcome the deficit. The nurse determines that the family understands the measures to use if they state that they will:
    1. Place objects in the client's impaired field of vision
    2. Approach the client from the impaired field of vision
    3. Remind the client to turn the head to scan the lost visual field
    4. Discourage the client from wearing own eyeglasses

52. A nurse is trying to communicate with a cerebrovascular accident (CVA) client with aphasia. Which action by the nurse would be least helpful to the client?
    1. Speaking to the client at a slower rate
    2. Completing the sentences that the client cannot finish
    3. Looking directly at the client during attempts at speech
    4. Allowing plenty of time for the client to respond

53. A family of a spinal cord–injured client rushes to the nursing station, saying that the client needs immediate help. On entering the room, the nurse notes that the client is diaphoretic, with a flushed face and neck, and complains of a severe headache. The pulse is 40 beats per minute and the blood pressure (BP) is 230/100 mm Hg. The nurse acts quickly, knowing that the client is experiencing:
    1. Spinal shock
    2. Malignant hypertension
    3. Pulmonary embolism
    4. Autonomic dysreflexia

54. A client receives a dose of edrophonium (Tensilon) intravenously. The client shows improvement in muscle strength for a period of time following the injection. The nurse interprets that this finding is compatible with:
    1. Multiple sclerosis
    2. Amyotrophic lateral sclerosis
    3. Myasthenia gravis
    4. Muscular dystrophy

55. A client with myasthenia gravis is having difficulty speaking. The client's speech is dysarthritic and has a nasal tone. The nurse would avoid using which communication strategy when working with this client?
    1. Repeating what the client said to verify the message
    2. Encouraging the client to speak quickly
    3. Using a communication board when necessary
    4. Asking yes and no questions when able

56. A client has experienced an episode of myasthenic crisis. The nurse collects data to determine whether the client has precipitating factors such as:
    1. Too little exercise
    2. Increased intake of fatty foods
    3. Omitted doses of medication
    4. Increased doses of medication

57. A nurse is teaching the client with myasthenia gravis about prevention of myasthenic and cholinergic crises. The nurse tells the client that this is most effectively done by:
    1. Doing all chores early in the day while less fatigued
    2. Taking medications on time to maintain therapeutic blood levels
    3. Doing muscle-strengthening exercises
    4. Eating large, well-balanced meals

58. A nurse has instructed the client with myasthenia gravis about ways to manage his or her own health at home. The nurse determines that the client needs more information if the client makes which of the following statements?
    1. "I should take my medications an hour before mealtime."
    2. "I've made arrangements to get a portable resuscitation bag and home suction equipment."

3. "Going to the beach will be a nice, relaxing form of activity."
4. "Here's the Medic-Alert bracelet I obtained."

59. A client with Parkinson's disease is embarrassed about the symptoms of the disorder, and is bored and lonely. The nurse would plan which approach as most therapeutic in assisting the client to cope with the disease?
    1. Plan only a few activities for the client during the day
    2. Assist the client with activities of daily living (ADLs) as much as possible
    3. Encourage and praise perseverance in exercising and performing ADLs
    4. Cluster activities at the end of the day when the client is most bored

60. A client with Parkinson's disease is experiencing a parkinsonian crisis. The nurse would immediately place the client:
    1. In a quiet, dim room with respiratory and cardiac support available
    2. In a high Fowler's position, with a nasogastric tube at the bedside
    3. In a room near the nursing station, which is near the code cart
    4. In a bed with padded side rails, with limb restraints nearby

61. A nurse has given instructions to the client with Parkinson's disease about maintaining mobility. The nurse determines that the client understands the directions if the client states that he or she will:
    1. Exercise in the evening to combat fatigue
    2. Rock back and forth to start movement with bradykinesia

3. Sit in soft, deep chairs
4. Buy clothes with many buttons to maintain finger dexterity

62. A nurse has given suggestions to the client with trigeminal neuralgia about strategies to minimize episodes of pain. The nurse determines that the client needs reinforcement of information if the client made which of the following statements?
    1. "I will wash my face with cotton pads."
    2. "I'll have to start chewing on the unaffected side."
    3. "I should rinse my mouth if toothbrushing is painful."
    4. "I'll try to eat my food either very warm or very cold."

ALTERNATE FORMAT QUESTION: PRIORITIZING (ORDERED RESPONSE)

The client with a spinal cord injury suddenly experiences an episode of autonomic dysreflexia. After checking the client's vital signs, list the nurse's actions in order of priority. (Number 1 is the first priority action and number 5 is the last priority action.)
___ Check for bladder distention and catheterize if present
___ Raise the head of the bed
___ Contact the physician
___ Loosen tight clothing on the client
___ Administer an antihypertensive medication, as prescribed

ANSWERS

1. *Answer: 1*
Rationale: Cranial nerve II is the optic nerve, which governs vision. The nurse can provide safety for the visually impaired client by clearing the path of obstacles when ambulating. Testing the shower water temperature would be useful if there were impairment of peripheral nerves. Speaking loudly may help overcome a deficit of cranial nerve VIII (vestibulocochlear). Cranial nerves VII (facial) and IX (glossopharyngeal) control taste from the anterior two thirds and posterior one third of the tongue, respectively.
Test-Taking Strategy: Focus on the issue, impairment of cranial nerves. Recalling that this is the optic nerve will direct you to option 1. Review these cranial nerves if you had difficulty with this question.
Level of Cognitive Ability: Application
Client Needs: Safe, Effective Care Environment
Integrated Process: Nursing Process/Planning

Content Area: Adult Health/Neurological
Reference: Potter, P., & Perry, A. (2005). *Fundamentals of nursing* (6th ed.). St. Louis: Mosby, pp. 974-975.

2. *Answer: 2*
Rationale: The cerebellum is responsible for balance and coordination. A walker would provide stability for the client during ambulation. Adaptive eating utensils may be beneficial when the client has partial paralysis of the hand. A raised toilet seat is useful when the client does not have the mobility or ability to flex the hips. A slider board is used in transferring a client from a bed to stretcher or wheelchair.
Test-Taking Strategy: Use the process of elimination. Recall that the cerebellum controls balance and coordination. This will help you eliminate options 3 and 4. To choose between options 1 and 2, remember that adaptive eating utensils are used when there is loss of fine motor coordination, such as with a cerebrovascular accident. The walker would help the

client maintain balance. Review care of the client with a cerebellar lesion if you had difficulty with this question.
Level of Cognitive Ability: Comprehension
Client Needs: Health Promotion and Maintenance
Integrated Process: Nursing Process/Evaluation
Content Area: Adult Health/Neurological
Reference: Linton, A., & Maebius, N. (2003). *Introduction to medical-surgical nursing* (3rd ed.). Philadelphia: W.B. Saunders, pp. 408, 426.

3. *Answer:* 4
Rationale: Clients with cognitive impairment from neurological dysfunction respond best to a stable environment, which is limited in the amounts and type of sensory input. The nurse can provide sensory cues and give clear, simple directions in a positive manner. Confusion and agitation can be minimized by reducing environmental stimuli (such as television, multiple visitors) and keeping familiar personal articles (such as family pictures) at the bedside.
Test-Taking Strategy: Use the process of elimination, noting the key words, *least helpful*. These words indicate a false response question and that you need to select the incorrect action. The client who is confused can handle limited amounts of information at one time, which makes option 4 the correct answer to this question. Review care of the neurological client if you had difficulty with this question.
Level of Cognitive Ability: Application
Client Needs: Psychosocial Integrity
Integrated Process: Nursing Process/Implementation
Content Area: Adult Health/Neurological
Reference: Christensen, B., & Kockrow, E. (2003). *Adult health nursing* (4th ed.). St. Louis: Mosby, pp. 615-616.

4. *Answer:* 1
Rationale: A bladder retraining program, such as use of a toileting schedule, may be helpful to clients experiencing urinary incontinence. A Foley catheter should be used only when necessary because of risk of infection. Use of diapers or pads is the least acceptable alternative, because the risk of skin breakdown exists.
Test-Taking Strategy: This question can be answered most easily by looking at it from a client safety viewpoint. Because Foley catheters carry a risk of infection, and the use of diapers or pads carries the risk of skin breakdown, the only acceptable answer is the toileting schedule. Review care of the client with a neurological impairment if you had difficulty with this question.
Level of Cognitive Ability: Application
Client Needs: Physiological Integrity
Integrated Process: Nursing Process/Implementation
Content Area: Adult Health/Neurological
Reference: Christensen, B., & Kockrow, E. (2003). *Adult health nursing* (4th ed.). St. Louis: Mosby, p. 421.

5. *Answer:* 2
Rationale: Previous neurological problems such as headaches or back injuries place the client more at risk for development of a neurological disorder. Chronic diseases such as hypertension and diabetes mellitus also place the client at greater risk. Assessment of allergies is a routine part of the health history,

regardless of the nature of the client's problem. Additionally, an allergy to pollen would not place the client at risk for a neurological problem.
Test-Taking Strategy: Note the key words, *does not give.* These words indicate a false response question and that you need to select the finding that is not associated with a neurological problem. Each of the incorrect options has an actual or potential neurological association. Allergies indicate a disturbance of the immune system. Review the risks associated with neurological problems if you had difficulty with this question.
Level of Cognitive Ability: Comprehension
Client Needs: Physiological Integrity
Integrated Process: Nursing Process/Data Collection
Content Area: Adult Health/Neurological
Reference: Christensen, B., & Kockrow, E. (2003). *Adult health nursing* (4th ed.). St. Louis: Mosby, p. 607.

6. *Answer:* 1
Rationale: The question is worded to elicit an unsafe action on the part of the family. Depending on the client's functional ability, either passive or active ROM is indicated to keep the joint moving freely. Application of a premolded splint would also keep the limb aligned and in good position. The client should not attempt to stand unsupported on a weak or paralyzed limb. The inability to bear weight will cause the client to fall.
Test-Taking Strategy: Note the key words, *needs reinforcement of teaching.* These words indicate a false response question and that you need to select the incorrect action by the family. Noting that the client has hemiplegia of the leg will direct you to option 1. Review care of the client with hemiplegia if you had difficulty with this question.
Level of Cognitive Ability: Analysis
Client Needs: Health Promotion and Maintenance
Integrated Process: Nursing Process/Evaluation
Content Area: Adult Health/Neurological
References: Christensen, B., & Kockrow, E. (2003). *Adult health nursing* (4th ed.). St. Louis: Mosby, pp. 620-621.
Linton, A., & Maebius, N. (2003). *Introduction to medical-surgical nursing* (3rd ed.). Philadelphia: W.B. Saunders, p. 421.

7. *Answer:* 2
Rationale: The client undergoing cerebral angiography is assessed for possible allergy to the contrast dye, which can be determined by questioning the client about allergies to iodine or shellfish. Allergy to salmon is not associated with this procedure. Claustrophobia and excessive weight are areas of concern with magnetic resonance imaging.
Test-Taking Strategy: Use the process of elimination. Recalling that a contrast dye is used in this procedure will direct you to option 2. Review this diagnostic test if you had difficulty with this question.
Level of Cognitive Ability: Application
Client Needs: Physiological Integrity
Integrated Process: Nursing Process/Data Collection
Content Area: Adult Health/Neurological
Reference: Pagana, K., & Pagana, T. (2003). *Mosby's diagnostic and laboratory test reference* (6th ed.). St. Louis: Mosby, p. 124.

8. *Answer: 4*

Rationale: The client having an MRI has all metallic objects removed, because of the magnetic field generated by the device. A careful history is done to determine if any metal objects are inside the client, such as orthopedic hardware, pacemakers, artificial heart valves, aneurysm clips, or intrauterine devices. These may heat up, become dislodged, or malfunction during this procedure. The client may be ineligible if there is significant risk.

Test-Taking Strategy: Note the key word, *ineligible*. An important concept with regard to MRI is the avoidance of any metal objects in the vicinity of the machine. You will note that each of the incorrect options is a medical disorder. The correct answer is the name of a surgical procedure where an artificial valve (sometimes metal) is implanted. Review the contraindications related to this procedure if you had difficulty with this question.

Level of Cognitive Ability: Comprehension

Client Needs: Physiological Integrity

Integrated Process: Nursing Process/Data Collection

Content Area: Adult Health/Neurological

Reference: Pagana, K., & Pagana, T. (2003). *Mosby's diagnostic and laboratory test reference* (6th ed.). St. Louis: Mosby, p. 606.

9. *Answer: 1*

Rationale: The client undergoing LP is positioned lying on the side, with the legs pulled up to the abdomen and the head bent down onto the chest. This position helps open the spaces between the vertebrae.

Test-Taking Strategy: Use the process of elimination. Recalling that an LP is the introduction of a needle into the subarachnoid space, it is reasonable that the position of the client must facilitate this. The correct answer is the only position that flexes the vertebrae for easier needle insertion. Review positioning procedures for an LP if you had difficulty with this question.

Level of Cognitive Ability: Application

Client Needs: Physiological Integrity

Integrated Process: Nursing Process/Implementation

Content Area: Adult Health/Neurological

Reference: Pagana, K., & Pagana, T. (2003). *Mosby's diagnostic and laboratory test reference* (6th ed.). St. Louis: Mosby, pp. 580-581.

10. *Answer: 3*

Rationale: The MRI scanner is a hollow tube, which gives some clients a feeling of claustrophobia. Metal objects must be removed before the procedure, so they are not drawn into the magnetic field. The client may eat and take all prescribed medications before the procedure. If a contrast medium is used, the client may wish to eat lightly if the client has a tendency to get nauseated easily. The client lies supine on a padded table, which moves into the imager. The client must lie still during the procedure. The imager makes tapping noises while scanning. The client is alone in the imager, but the nurse can reassure the client that the technician is in voice communication with the client at all times during the procedure.

Test-Taking Strategy: Use the process of elimination. The statements in each of the options are correct. However, the question asks which of them will provide reassurance to the client. Although all statements are factually true, the correct option is the only one that provides a measure of reassurance to the client. Review MRI if you had difficulty with this question.

Level of Cognitive Ability: Application

Client Needs: Psychosocial Integrity

Integrated Process: Nursing Process/Implementation

Content Area: Adult Health/Neurological

Reference: Pagana, K., & Pagana, T. (2003). *Mosby's diagnostic and laboratory test reference* (6th ed.). St. Louis: Mosby, pp. 606-607.

11. *Answer: 4*

Rationale: After CT scanning, the client may resume all usual activities. The client should be encouraged to take in extra fluids to replace those lost with diuresis from the contrast dye. Options 1, 2, and 3 are unnecessary.

Test-Taking Strategy: Use the process of elimination. Recalling that there is no special aftercare following this procedure and noting the words "contrast medium" in the question will direct you to option 4. Review the procedure related to CT scanning if you had difficulty with this question.

Level of Cognitive Ability: Comprehension

Client Needs: Health Promotion and Maintenance

Integrated Process: Nursing Process/Evaluation

Content Area: Adult Health/Neurological

Reference: deWit, S. (2005). *Fundamental concepts and skills for nursing*. Philadelphia: W.B. Saunders, pp. 390-391, 404.

12. *Answer: 1*

Rationale: Following myelography, the client is placed on bed rest for 6 to 8 hours after the procedure. When a water-based contrast medium is used, the client is positioned with the head of the bed elevated 15 to 30 degrees. With use of an oil-based medium, the head of the bed is positioned flat (even though the contrast is aspirated out after the procedure).

Test-Taking Strategy: Note that a water-based contrast medium was used for the procedure. Also, note that this question is asking for knowledge of two separate items, length of bed rest and head position. With a myelographic procedure, remember that the longer the bed rest, the less likelihood of complications; this will assist in eliminating options 2 and 4. If you can remember that "oil rises, so keep the head low," you will be able to choose correctly from the remaining options. Review postprocedure care following myelography if you had difficulty with this question.

Level of Cognitive Ability: Application

Client Needs: Physiological Integrity

Integrated Process: Nursing Process/Planning

Content Area: Adult Health/Neurological

References: Linton, A., & Maebius, N. (2003). *Introduction to medical-surgical nursing* (3rd ed.). Philadelphia: W.B. Saunders, p. 436.

Pagana, K., & Pagana, T. (2003). *Mosby's diagnostic and laboratory test reference* (6th ed.). St. Louis: Mosby, p. 623.

13. *Answer: 2*

Rationale: The unconscious client is positioned on the side during mouth care to prevent aspiration. The teeth are

brushed at least twice daily using a small toothbrush. The gums, tongue, roof of mouth, and oral mucous membranes are cleansed with Toothettes to avoid encrustation and infection. The lips are coated with water-soluble lubricant to prevent drying, cracking, and encrustation. The use of products with lemon or alcohol should be avoided, because they have a drying effect.
Test-Taking Strategy: Note the key word, *avoid*. This word indicates a false response question and that you need to select the incorrect nursing action. Standard mouth care procedures include use of toothbrush and Toothettes, so options 3 and 4 are eliminated first. Recalling that the unconscious client is at risk of aspiration tells you that option 1 is a correct action also. This leaves option 2 as incorrect, because repeated use of these products could dry and crack the oral mucous membranes. Review care of the unconscious client if you had difficulty with this question.
Level of Cognitive Ability: Application
Client Needs: Physiological Integrity
Integrated Process: Nursing Process/Implementation
Content Area: Adult Health/Neurological
References: Black, J., & Hawks, J. (2005). *Medical-surgical nursing: Clinical management for positive outcomes* (7th ed.). Philadelphia: W.B. Saunders, pp. 2061-2062.
deWit, S. (2005). *Fundamental concepts and skills for nursing.* Philadelphia: W.B. Saunders, pp. 290-291.

14. *Answer: 2*
Rationale: Families often need assistance to cope with the sudden, severe illness of a loved one. The nurse can help the family of an unconscious client by assisting them to work through their feelings of grief. The nurse should explain all equipment, treatments, and procedures, and supplement or reinforce information given by the physician. The family should be encouraged to touch and speak to the client, and to become involved in the client's care to the extent that they are comfortable. The nurse should allow the family to stay with the client as much as possible, and should encourage them to eat and sleep adequately to maintain their strength.
Test-Taking Strategy: Use the process of elimination and focus on the issue, assisting the family to cope. Each incorrect option either inhibits the family's coping or distances the family from the client or the client's care. Review the psychosocial needs of the family of an unconscious client if you had difficulty with this question.
Level of Cognitive Ability: Application
Client Needs: Psychosocial Integrity
Integrated Process: Nursing Process/Implementation
Content Area: Adult Health/Neurological
Reference: Black, J., & Hawks, J. (2005). *Medical-surgical nursing: Clinical management for positive outcomes* (7th ed.). Philadelphia: W.B. Saunders, pp. 2065-2065.

15. *Answer: 4*
Rationale: Suction equipment should be kept at the bedside of an unconscious client, regardless of whether or not an artificial airway is present. The nurse auscultates breath sounds every 2 to 4 hours, or more frequently if there is a need. The client should be hyperoxygenated before, during, and after suctioning to minimize cerebral hypoxia. The client

should not be suctioned for longer than 10 seconds at one time to prevent cerebral hypoxia and an increase in intracranial pressure.
Test-Taking Strategy: Use the process of elimination and note the key word, *avoid*. This word indicates a false response question and that you need to select the incorrect nursing action. Options 1, 2, and 3 are part of standard suctioning procedure. The only option that is different, and unsafe, is option 4. If you had difficulty with this question, review suctioning procedure.
Level of Cognitive Ability: Application
Client Needs: Physiological Integrity
Integrated Process: Nursing Process/Implementation
Content Area: Adult Health/Neurological
Reference: Linton, A., & Maebius, N. (2003). *Introduction to medical-surgical nursing* (3rd ed.). Philadelphia: W.B. Saunders, p. 1100.

16. *Answer: 1*
Rationale: When a hypothermia blanket is used, the skin is inspected frequently for pressure points, which over time could lead to skin breakdown. Options 2, 3, and 4 are not complications of hypothermia blanket use.
Test-Taking Strategy: Use the process of elimination. Options 3 and 4 may be eliminated first, because they are other health problems. The temperature of the blanket is not cold enough to produce frostbite. This leaves skin breakdown as the correct option. Review the complications associated with the use of a hypothermia blanket if you had difficulty with this question.
Level of Cognitive Ability: Application
Client Needs: Physiological Integrity
Integrated Process: Nursing Process/Implementation
Content Area: Adult Health/Neurological
Reference: deWit, S. (2005). *Fundamental concepts and skills for nursing.* Philadelphia: W.B. Saunders, pp. 779-780.

17. *Answer: 4*
Rationale: Hypothalamic damage causes hyperthermia, which may also be called "central fever." It is characterized by a persistent high fever with no diurnal variation. There is also an absence of sweating. Options 1, 2, and 3 are not associated with temperature regulation.
Test-Taking Strategy: Knowledge of the location of the brain's thermoregulatory center is needed to answer this question. Eliminate options 1 and 2 first, because they are responsible for higher mental functions and balance, respectively. From the remaining options, remember that body temperature is regulated by the hypothalamus. Review the anatomy and physiology of the brain if you had difficulty with this question.
Level of Cognitive Ability: Comprehension
Client Needs: Physiological Integrity
Integrated Process: Nursing Process/Data Collection
Content Area: Adult Health/Neurological
Reference: deWit, S. (2005). *Fundamental concepts and skills for nursing.* Philadelphia: W.B. Saunders, pp. 324-325.

18. *Answer: 4*
Rationale: Discharge instructions for the client hospitalized for hyperthermia include prevention of heat-related disorders, increased fluid intake for 24 hours, self-monitoring of voiding,

and the importance of staying in a cool environment and resting.

Test-Taking Strategy: Note the key words, *needs clarification of discharge instructions.* These words indicate a false response question and that you need to select the incorrect client statement. Options 2 and 3 relate to maintaining and monitoring fluid balance, and are therefore eliminated. A cool environment is appropriate, so option 1 is eliminated also. Resumption of full activity is not helpful; rather, rest periods are indicated. Review home care instructions for the client with hyperthermia if you had difficulty with this question.

Level of Cognitive Ability: Comprehension
Client Needs: Health Promotion and Maintenance
Integrated Process: Teaching/Learning
Content Area: Adult Health/Neurological
References: deWit, S. (2005). *Fundamental concepts and skills for nursing.* Philadelphia: W.B. Saunders, p. 329.
Potter, P., & Perry, A. (2003). *Essentials for practice* (5th ed.). St. Louis: Mosby, p. 187.

19. *Answer: 2*
Rationale: A change in vital signs may be a late sign of increased ICP. Trends include increasing temperature and blood pressure and decreasing pulse and respirations. Respiratory irregularities may also arise.

Test-Taking Strategy: Use the process of elimination. This question looks complex, but can be logically answered. If you remember that temperature rises, then you are able to eliminate options 3 and 4. If you know that the client becomes bradycardic, or know that the BP rises, you are able to select the correct option. Review the signs of increased intracranial pressure if you had difficulty with this question.

Level of Cognitive Ability: Analysis
Client Needs: Physiological Integrity
Integrated Process: Nursing Process/Data Collection
Content Area: Adult Health/Neurological
Reference: Linton, A., & Maebius, N. (2003). *Introduction to medical-surgical nursing* (3rd ed.). Philadelphia: W.B. Saunders, pp. 382-383.

20. *Answer: 1*
Rationale: The head of the client with increased ICP should be positioned so that the head is in a neutral, midline position. The nurse should avoid flexing or extending the neck or turning the head side to side. The head of the bed should be raised to 30 to 45 degrees. Use of proper positions promotes venous drainage from the cranium to keep intracranial pressure down.

Test-Taking Strategy: Note the key word, *avoid.* This word indicates a false response question and that you need to select the incorrect position. This would be one that interferes with arterial circulation to the brain or with venous drainage from the brain. The only position that meets one of those criteria is option 1. Review client positioning with ICP if you had difficulty with this question.

Level of Cognitive Ability: Application
Client Needs: Physiological Integrity
Integrated Process: Nursing Process/Implementation
Content Area: Adult Health/Neurological

Reference: Linton, A., & Maebius, N. (2003). *Introduction to medical-surgical nursing* (3rd ed.). Philadelphia: W.B. Saunders, p. 383.

21. *Answer: 1*
Rationale: Activities that increase intrathoracic and intraabdominal pressures cause indirect elevation of the ICP. Some of these activities include isometric exercises, Valsalva maneuver, coughing, sneezing, and blowing the nose. Exhaling during activities such as repositioning or pulling up in bed opens the glottis, which prevents intrathoracic pressure from rising.

Test-Taking Strategy: Use the process of elimination. Evaluate each option in terms of the tension it puts on the body. Doing so will help you eliminate each of the incorrect options. Review the measures that will reduce or prevent increased intracranial pressure if you had difficulty with this question.

Level of Cognitive Ability: Comprehension
Client Needs: Health Promotion and Maintenance
Integrated Process: Nursing Process/Evaluation
Content Area: Adult Health/Neurological
References: Black, J., & Hawks, J. (2005). *Medical-surgical nursing: Clinical management for positive outcomes* (7th ed.). Philadelphia: W.B. Saunders, p. 2195.
Linton, A., & Maebius, N. (2003). *Introduction to medical-surgical nursing* (3rd ed.). Philadelphia: W.B. Saunders, p. 390.

22. *Answer: 3*
Rationale: Some clients who have awakened from an unconscious state report that they remember hearing specific voices and conversations. Family and staff should assume that the client's sense of hearing is still intact, and act accordingly. Research has also demonstrated that positive outcomes are associated with coma stimulation—that is, speaking to and touching the client.

Test-Taking Strategy: Use the process of elimination. The nurse would not infer that the client wants a visit from the chaplain based on the family speaking over the client at the bedside, so option 4 can be eliminated first. The family demonstrates no evidence of crisis, and they seem to be well informed. This eliminates options 1 and 2. Review care of the unconscious client if you had difficulty with this question.

Level of Cognitive Ability: Application
Client Needs: Psychosocial Integrity
Integrated Process: Nursing Process/Implementation
Content Area: Adult Health/Neurological
Reference: Black, J., & Hawks, J. (2005). *Medical-surgical nursing: Clinical management for positive outcomes* (7th ed.). Philadelphia: W.B. Saunders, pp. 2064-2065.

23. *Answer: 3*
Rationale: Nursing interventions should be spaced out over the shift to minimize the risk of a rise in ICP. If possible, activities known to raise ICP should be avoided when possible. Other interventions to control the ICP include maintaining a calm, quiet environment and avoiding emotional stress and interruption of sleep.

Test-Taking Strategy: Focus on the issue, controlling ICP. Recalling that stimulation raises the ICP will direct you to option 3. Review nursing care of the client with increased intracranial pressure if you had difficulty with this question.

Level of Cognitive Ability: Application
Client Needs: Physiological Integrity
Integrated Process: Nursing Process/Implementation
Content Area: Adult Health/Neurological
Reference: Christensen, B., & Kockrow, E. (2003). *Adult health nursing* (4th ed.). St. Louis: Mosby, p. 619.

24. *Answer: 2*
Rationale: Leakage of CSF from the ears or nose may accompany basilar skull fracture. It can be distinguished from other body fluids because the drainage will separate into bloody and yellow concentric rings on dressing material, which is known as the halo sign. It also tests positive for glucose. Options 1, 3, and 4 are not characteristics of CSF.
Test-Taking Strategy: Use the process of elimination. Recalling that CSF contains glucose, whereas other secretions such as mucus do not, will direct you to option 2. Also, remember that CSF separates into rings. Review testing for CSF fluid if you had difficulty with this question.
Level of Cognitive Ability: Analysis
Client Needs: Physiological Integrity
Integrated Process: Nursing Process/Evaluation
Content Area: Adult Health/Neurological
References: Christensen, B., & Kockrow, E. (2003). *Adult health nursing* (4th ed.). St. Louis: Mosby, pp. 609, 649.
Lewis, S., Heitkemper, M., & Dirksen, S. (2004). *Medical-surgical nursing: Assessment and management of clinical problems* (6th ed.). St. Louis: Mosby, pp. 1506-1507.
Linton, A., & Maebius, N. (2003). *Introduction to medical-surgical nursing* (3rd ed.). Philadelphia: W.B. Saunders, p. 194.

25. *Answer: 3*
Rationale: There is a significant association between cervical spine injury and head injury. For this reason, the nurse leaves any form of spinal immobilization in place until lateral cervical spine x-rays rule out fracture or other damage.
Test-Taking Strategy: Focus on the data in the question and note the client's injury. Remember that the reason for spinal immobilization is to protect the spine from movement, which could cause further damage if the cervical spine were injured. If x-ray results are negative, there is no reason to leave the collar in place. Review emergency care of the client with a suspected cervical injury if this question was difficult.
Level of Cognitive Ability: Application
Client Needs: Physiological Integrity
Integrated Process: Nursing Process/Implementation
Content Area: Adult Health/Neurological
References: Black, J., & Hawks, J. (2005). *Medical-surgical nursing: Clinical management for positive outcomes* (7th ed.). Philadelphia: W.B. Saunders, pp. 2148-2149.
Linton, A., & Maebius, N. (2003). *Introduction to medical-surgical nursing* (3rd ed.). Philadelphia: W.B. Saunders, pp. 194-195.

26. *Answer: 4*
Rationale: A concussion after head injury is a temporary loss of consciousness (from a few seconds to a few minutes) without evidence of structural damage. After concussion, the family is taught to monitor the client and call the physician or return the client to the emergency room if certain signs and symptoms are noted. These include confusion, difficulty awakening or speaking, one-sided weakness, vomiting, or severe headache. Minor headache is expected.
Test-Taking Strategy: Note the key words, *needs reinforcement of the discharge instructions*. These words indicate a false response question and that you need to select the incorrect family statement. Noting the word "minor" in option 4 will direct you to this option. Review care of the client with a concussion if you had difficulty with this question.
Level of Cognitive Ability: Analysis
Client Needs: Health Promotion and Maintenance
Integrated Process: Teaching/Learning
Content Area: Adult Health/Neurological
Reference: Christensen, B., & Kockrow, E. (2003). *Adult health nursing* (4th ed.). St. Louis: Mosby, pp. 648-649.

27. *Answer: 3*
Rationale: Following supratentorial surgery, the head is kept at a 30- to 45-degree angle. The head and neck should not be angled either anteriorly or laterally, but rather should be kept in a neutral (midline) position. This will promote venous return through the jugular veins, which will help prevent a rise in intracranial pressure.
Test-Taking Strategy: This question tests knowledge of differences in positioning the craniotomy client with an infratentorial versus supratentorial incision. If you remember that with *supra-* one should "keep the head up," and with *infra-* one should "keep the head down," options 1 and 2 can be eliminated. Knowing how to position the head for optimal venous drainage helps you select option 3 over option 4. Review client positioning following craniotomy if you had difficulty with this question.
Level of Cognitive Ability: Application
Client Needs: Physiological Integrity
Integrated Process: Nursing Process/Planning
Content Area: Adult Health/Neurological
Reference: Linton, A., & Maebius, N. (2003). *Introduction to medical-surgical nursing* (3rd ed.). Philadelphia: W.B. Saunders, p. 382.

28. *Answer: 4*
Rationale: Codeine sulfate is the narcotic analgesic often used for clients after craniotomy. It is frequently combined with a non-narcotic analgesic such as acetaminophen for added effect. It does not alter the respiratory rate or mask neurological signs as do other narcotics. Side effects of codeine include gastrointestinal upset and constipation. The medication can lead to physical and psychological dependence with chronic use. It is not the strongest narcotic analgesic available.
Test-Taking Strategy: Use the process of elimination. General knowledge about narcotic analgesics helps you eliminate options 2 and 3. Because codeine is not the strongest narcotic available, eliminate option 1 next. This leaves the correct option, which is codeine's advantage of not masking neurological signs. Review this medication if you had difficulty with this question.
Level of Cognitive Ability: Application
Client Needs: Physiological Integrity
Integrated Process: Nursing Process/Implementation
Content Area: Pharmacology

References: Hodgson, B., & Kizior, R. (2005). *Saunders nursing drug handbook 2005.* Philadelphia: W.B. Saunders, p. 254. McKenry, L., & Salerno, E. (2003). *Mosby's pharmacology in nursing* (21st ed.). St. Louis: Mosby, p. 279.

29. *Answer:* 3

Rationale: Seizures are a potential complication that can occur for up to 1 year after surgery. For this reason, the client must diligently take anticonvulsant medications. The client and family are encouraged to keep track of doses administered. The family should learn seizure precautions, and accompany the client while ambulating if dizziness or seizures tend to occur. The suture line is kept dry until sutures are removed to prevent infection. The postcraniotomy client is typically sensitive to loud noises and can find them irritating (e.g., loud television). Awareness control of environmental noise by others is helpful to this client.

Test-Taking Strategy: Note the key words, *need for further instructions.* These words indicate a false response question and that you need to select the incorrect client statement. Begin to answer this question by eliminating option 1 first, because it is a general measure after many types of surgery. If you know that seizures are a potential postoperative risk up to 1 year after surgery, this eliminates options 2 and 4 as well. This leaves option 3 as the correct answer. Many clients after craniotomy have sensitivity to or are irritated by loud noises. Review home care instructions following craniotomy if you had difficulty with this question.

Level of Cognitive Ability: Comprehension
Client Needs: Health Promotion and Maintenance
Integrated Process: Teaching/Learning
Content Area: Adult Health/Neurological
Reference: Black, J., & Hawks, J. (2005). *Medical-surgical nursing: Clinical management for positive outcomes* (7th ed.). Philadelphia: W.B. Saunders, p. 2091.

30. *Answer:* 4

Rationale: After craniotomy, the client may experience difficulty with his or her altered personal appearance. The nurse can help by listening to client concerns and by clarifying any misconceptions about facial edema, periorbital bruising, and hair loss (which are temporary). The nurse can encourage the client to participate in self-grooming and use personal articles of clothing. Finally, the nurse can suggest the use of a turban, followed by a hairpiece, to help the client adapt to the temporary change in appearance.

Test-Taking Strategy: Note the key words, *has not met.* These words indicate a false response question and that you need to select the maladaptive response. Options 1 and 2 both indicate adaptive responses and are therefore eliminated. From the remaining options, recalling that facial edema and bruising are temporary will direct you to option 4. Review care of the client following craniotomy if you had difficulty with this question.

Level of Cognitive Ability: Analysis
Client Needs: Psychosocial Integrity
Integrated Process: Nursing Process/Evaluation
Content Area: Adult Health/Neurological
References: Lewis, S., Heitkemper, M., & Dirksen, S. (2004). *Medical-surgical nursing: Assessment and management of clinical problems* (6th ed.). St. Louis: Mosby, p. 1517.

Linton, A., & Maebius, N. (2003). *Introduction to medical-surgical nursing* (3rd ed.). Philadelphia: W.B. Saunders, 390.

31. *Answer:* 4

Rationale: Crutchfield tongs are applied after drilling holes in the client's skull under local anesthesia. Weights are attached to the tongs, which exert pulling pressure on the longitudinal axis of the cervical spine. Serial x-rays of the cervical spine are taken, with weights being gradually added until radiography reveals that the vertebral column is realigned. Weights may then be gradually reduced to a point that maintains alignment. The client with Crutchfield tongs is placed on a Stryker frame or RotoRest bed. The nurse ensures that weights hang freely and the amount of weight matches the current order. The nurse also inspects the integrity and position of the ropes and pulleys. The nurse does not remove the weights to administer care.

Test-Taking Strategy: Note the key word, *avoid.* This word indicates a false response question and that you need to select the item that would be contraindicated. Recalling the basics of traction and recalling that weights are not removed will direct you to option 4. Review nursing care related to the client with cervical tongs if you had difficulty with this question.

Level of Cognitive Ability: Application
Client Needs: Physiological Integrity
Integrated Process: Nursing Process/Planning
Content Area: Adult Health/Neurological
Reference: Linton, A., & Maebius, N. (2003). *Introduction to medical-surgical nursing* (3rd ed.). Philadelphia: W.B. Saunders, pp. 441-442.

32. *Answer:* 2

Rationale: Adjusting to paralysis is difficult both physically and psychosocially for the client and family. The nurse recognizes that the client goes through the grieving process in adjusting to the loss, and may move back and forth among the stages of grief. The nurse acknowledges the client's feelings while continuing to meet the client's physical needs and encouraging independence.

Test-Taking Strategy: Use the process of elimination. This question can be answered easily by examining the impact or outcome of each of the options. The nurse cannot neglect the client until the client is ready (option 3), so this can be eliminated first. The family is also in crisis and needs the nurse's support (option 4), and should not be relied on for care. Option 1 represents a factual but noncaring approach to the client, which is not therapeutic. This leaves option 2 as the answer. Also, option 2 acknowledges the client's feelings. Review the psychosocial needs of a client with a spinal cord injury if you had difficulty with this question.

Level of Cognitive Ability: Application
Client Needs: Psychosocial Integrity
Integrated Process: Nursing Process/Implementation
Content Area: Adult Health/Neurological
Reference: Linton, A., & Maebius, N. (2003). *Introduction to medical-surgical nursing* (3rd ed.). Philadelphia: W.B. Saunders, p. 448.

33. *Answer:* 4

Rationale: The halo device alters balance and can cause fatigue due to its weight. The client should cleanse the skin daily under the vest or the device to protect the skin from ulceration, and should use powder or lotions sparingly or not at all. The wool liner should be changed if odor becomes a problem. The client should have food cut into small pieces to facilitate chewing and use a straw for drinking. Pin care is done as instructed. The client should not drive, because the device impairs the range of vision.

Test-Taking Strategy: Note the key words, *needs further clarification.* These words indicate a false response question and that you need to select the incorrect client statement. Recall that a halo device is used to allow mobility for the client who needs continuous cervical traction; it maintains the head and spine in a neutral position. With this in mind, it will be easy to select option 4 as the correct answer to the question as stated. The inability to turn the head without turning the torso would make driving contraindicated. Review client teaching points related to a halo device if you had difficulty with this question.

Level of Cognitive Ability: Comprehension
Client Needs: Health Promotion and Maintenance
Integrated Process: Teaching/Learning
Content Area: Adult Health/Neurological
Reference: Phipps, W., Monahan, F., Sands, J., Marek, J., & Neighbors, M. (2003). *Medical-surgical nursing: Health and illness perspectives* (7th ed.). St. Louis: Mosby, pp. 1414-1413, 1477.

34. *Answer: 1*
Rationale: Depression is frequently seen in the client with spinal cord injury, and may be exhibited as a loss of appetite. The client should be allowed to choose the types of food eaten and to eat as much as is feasible, because it is one of the few areas of control that the client has left.

Test-Taking Strategy: Use the process of elimination. The nurse does not make the diagnosis of clinical depression, which makes option 2 incorrect. For the same reason, option 3 should be eliminated. There is no information in the question to demonstrate that the client has a slow metabolic rate, so option 4 is eliminated next. Option 1 provides the client as much control as possible. Review the psychosocial needs of the client with a spinal cord injury if you had difficulty with this question.

Level of Cognitive Ability: Analysis
Client Needs: Psychosocial Integrity
Integrated Process: Nursing Process/Data Collection
Content Area: Adult Health/Neurological
References: Black, J., & Hawks, J. (2005). *Medical-surgical nursing: Clinical management for positive outcomes* (7th ed.). Philadelphia: W.B. Saunders, p. 2218.
Linton, A., & Maebius, N. (2003). *Introduction to medical-surgical nursing* (3rd ed.). Philadelphia: W.B. Saunders, pp. 448-449.

35. *Answer: 3*
Rationale: Range-of-motion exercises are beneficial in stretching muscles, which may diminish spasticity. Removing potentially harmful objects is an important safety measure. Use of muscle relaxants is also indicated if the spasms cause discomfort to the client or pose a risk to the client's safety. Use of limb restraints will not alleviate spasticity and could harm the client.

Test-Taking Strategy: Note the key word, *intervenes.* This word indicates a false response question and that you need to select the action that is potentially harmful to the client. This will direct you to option 3. Remember, restraints should be avoided. Review the safety needs for the client with paraplegia if you had difficulty with this question.

Level of Cognitive Ability: Application
Client Needs: Safe, Effective Care Environment
Integrated Process: Nursing Process/Implementation
Content Area: Leadership/Management
Reference: Linton, A., & Maebius, N. (2003). *Introduction to medical-surgical nursing* (3rd ed.). Philadelphia: W.B. Saunders, pp. 444, 449.

36. *Answer: 2*
Rationale: To prevent pressure ulcers from developing, the paraplegic client should shift weight in the wheelchair every 2 hours and use a pressure relief pad. While in bed, the bottom sheet should be free of wrinkles and wetness. The client should use a mirror to inspect the skin twice a day (morning and evening) to assess for redness, edema, and breakdown. General measures include a nutritious diet and meticulous skin care.

Test-Taking Strategy: Note the key words, *least helpful.* Each option appears reasonable on first inspection. With a closer look, however, you will notice that the time frame for inspecting the skin is much too infrequent, making this the correct option. Review care of the paraplegic client if you had difficulty with this question.

Level of Cognitive Ability: Application
Client Needs: Health Promotion and Maintenance
Integrated Process: Teaching/Learning
Content Area: Adult Health/Neurological
Reference: Linton, A., & Maebius, N. (2003). *Introduction to medical-surgical nursing* (3rd ed.). Philadelphia: W.B. Saunders, p. 449.

37. *Answer: 3*
Rationale: Range-of-motion exercises of the finger joints prevent contractures, but do not actively strengthen muscle groups needed for self-mobilization with paraplegia. Other activities that are more effective include push-ups from a prone position, sit-ups from a sitting position, extending the arms while holding weights, and squeezing rubber balls or crumpling newspaper.

Test-Taking Strategy: Use the process of elimination and note the key words, *least muscle-strengthening benefit.* This question can be answered by thinking about the energy expenditure of the muscle groups involved in the activities listed in each option. The one that will involve the least energy expenditure (and therefore the least amount of muscle development) is the range-of-motion exercises, which makes it the correct answer to this question. Review care of the paraplegic client if you had difficulty with this question.

Level of Cognitive Ability: Analysis
Client Needs: Health Promotion and Maintenance
Integrated Process: Nursing Process/Evaluation
Content Area: Adult Health/Neurological
Reference: Linton, A., & Maebius, N. (2003). *Introduction to medical-surgical nursing* (3rd ed.). Philadelphia: W.B. Saunders, p. 449.

38. *Answer:* 1

Rationale: The client with spinal cord injury above the level of T7 is at risk for autonomic dysreflexia. It is characterized by severe, throbbing headache, flushing of the face and neck, bradycardia, and sudden severe hypertension. Other signs include nasal stuffiness, blurred vision, nausea, and sweating. It is a life-threatening syndrome triggered by a noxious stimulus below the level of the injury.

Test-Taking Strategy: Use the process of elimination. To answer this question correctly, it is necessary to know what causes autonomic dysreflexia. Remember, it results from the sudden exaggerated response of the sympathetic nervous system to a noxious stimulus. A massive sympathetic nervous system response causes severe hypertension. This would account for the throbbing headache (the correct answer), and cause flushing of the face and neck. Baroreceptors sense the sudden hypertension, causing a reflex bradycardia. Also, remember that the pulse and blood pressure changes with autonomic dysreflexia are actually the opposite of what would occur with hypovolemic shock. Review the signs of autonomic dysreflexia if you had difficulty with this question.

Level of Cognitive Ability: Analysis
Client Needs: Physiological Integrity
Integrated Process: Nursing Process/Data Collection
Content Area: Adult Health/Neurological
Reference: Linton, A., & Maebius, N. (2003). *Introduction to medical-surgical nursing* (3rd ed.). Philadelphia: W.B. Saunders, pp. 446-447.

39. *Answer:* 3

Rationale: Placing an eye patch over one eye in the client with diplopia removes the second image and restores more normal vision. The patch is worn continuously and is alternated on a daily basis to maintain the strength of the extraocular muscles of the eyes.

Test-Taking Strategy: Use the process of elimination. Knowing that an eye patch will help diplopia only while it is worn will assist in eliminating options 1 and 2. From the remaining options, recall that the extraocular muscles weaken with eye patch use. This will direct you to option 3, alternating the eye patch each day. Review care of the client with diplopia if you had difficulty with this question.

Level of Cognitive Ability: Comprehension
Client Needs: Physiological Integrity
Integrated Process: Nursing Process/Evaluation
Content Area: Adult Health/Neurological
References: Linton, A., & Maebius, N. (2003). *Introduction to medical-surgical nursing* (3rd ed.). Philadelphia: W.B. Saunders, p. 422.
Swearingen, P. (2003). *Manual of medical-surgical nursing care* (5th ed.). St. Louis: Mosby, p. 404.

40. *Answer:* 2

Rationale: The most frequent cause of autonomic dysreflexia is a distended bladder. Straight catheterization should be done every 4 to 6 hours, and Foley catheters should be checked frequently for kinks in the tubing. Constipation and fecal impaction are other causes, so maintaining bowel regularity is important. Other causes include stimulation of the skin from tactile, thermal, or painful stimuli. The nurse administers care to minimize risk in these areas.

Test-Taking Strategy: Note the key word, *avoid*. Remember that autonomic dysreflexia is caused by noxious stimuli to the bowel, bladder, or skin. With this in mind, you can eliminate each of the incorrect options. Review the measures to minimize the risk of autonomic dysreflexia if you had difficulty with this question.

Level of Cognitive Ability: Application
Client Needs: Physiological Integrity
Integrated Process: Nursing Process/Implementation
Content Area: Adult Health/Neurological
Reference: Linton, A., & Maebius, N. (2003). *Introduction to medical-surgical nursing* (3rd ed.). Philadelphia: W.B. Saunders, p. 447.

41. *Answer:* 4

Rationale: Key nursing actions are to sit the client up in bed, remove the noxious stimulus, and bring the blood pressure under control with antihypertensive medication per protocol. The nurse can also clearly label the client's chart identifying the risk for autonomic dysreflexia. Client and family should be taught to recognize, and later manage, the signs and symptoms of this syndrome.

Test-Taking Strategy: Note the key word, *immediately*, in the question. This is a clue that the first item in each option must be the first action. If you know to raise the head of the client's bed first (to try to minimize cerebral hypertension), then this eliminates each of the incorrect options. Review immediate nursing interventions for the client experiencing autonomic dysreflexia if you had difficulty with this question.

Level of Cognitive Ability: Application
Client Needs: Physiological Integrity
Integrated Process: Nursing Process/Implementation
Content Area: Adult Health/Neurological
Reference: Linton, A., & Maebius, N. (2003). *Introduction to medical-surgical nursing* (3rd ed.). Philadelphia: W.B. Saunders, p. 446.

42. *Answer:* 3

Rationale: Reflex vasodilation below the level of spinal cord injury places the client at risk of orthostatic hypotension, which may be profound. Measures to minimize this include measuring vital signs before and during position changes, use of a tilt table in early mobilization, and changing the client's position slowly. Venous pooling can be reduced by using Teds or compression stockings. Vasopressor medications are used as per protocol and as prescribed.

Test-Taking Strategy: Note the key words, *least helpful*, and recall that reflex vasodilation below the level of the injury causes hypotension. Venous compression (option 4) is helpful and is eliminated. Options 1 and 2 are helpful and are eliminated next. Knowing that quick position changes and movement would aggravate hypotension helps you be sure that you have selected the correct option. Review care of the client with spinal shock if you had difficulty with this question.

Level of Cognitive Ability: Application
Client Needs: Physiological Integrity
Integrated Process: Nursing Process/Implementation
Content Area: Adult Health/Neurological

References: Black, J., & Hawks, J. (2005). *Medical-surgical nursing: Clinical management for positive outcomes* (7th ed.). Philadelphia: W.B. Saunders, p. 2218.

Christensen, B., & Kockrow, E. (2003). *Adult health nursing* (4th ed.). St. Louis: Mosby, p. 650.

43. *Answer:* 3

Rationale: Ptosis of the eyelid is due to pressure on and dysfunction of cranial nerve III and does not relate to LOC. Early changes in LOC relate to alertness and verbal responsiveness. Less frequent speech, slight slurring of speech, and mild drowsiness are early signs of decreasing LOC.

Test-Taking Strategy: Use the process of elimination. Recalling that LOC includes orientation, awareness, and verbal responsiveness will direct you to option 3. Review the early signs of decreasing LOC if you had difficulty with this question.

Level of Cognitive Ability: Analysis
Client Needs: Physiological Integrity
Integrated Process: Nursing Process/Data Collection
Content Area: Adult Health/Neurological
Reference: Linton, A., & Maebius, N. (2003). *Introduction to medical-surgical nursing* (3rd ed.). Philadelphia: W.B. Saunders, p. 371.

44. *Answer:* 2

Rationale: Aneurysm precautions include placing the client on bed rest with the head of the bed elevated in a quiet setting. Lights are kept dim to minimize environmental stimulation. Any activity that increases blood pressure (BP) or impedes venous return from the brain is prohibited, such as pushing, pulling, sneezing, coughing, or straining. The nurse provides all physical care to minimize increases in BP. For the same reason, visitors, radio, television, and reading materials are prohibited or limited. Stimulants such as caffeine and nicotine are prohibited; decaffeinated coffee or tea may be given.

Test-Taking Strategy: Use the process of elimination. Recall that a global principle in aneurysm precautions is to limit the amount of stimulation (in any form) that the client receives, and to prevent increased intracranial pressure (ICP). This will direct you to option 2. Review aneurysm precautions if you had difficulty with this question.

Level of Cognitive Ability: Application
Client Needs: Physiological Integrity
Integrated Process: Nursing Process/Implementation
Content Area: Adult Health/Neurological
Reference: Phipps, W., Monahan, F., Sands, J., Marek, J., & Neighbors, M. (2003). *Medical-surgical nursing: Health and illness perspectives* (7th ed.). St. Louis: Mosby, p. 1385.

45. *Answer:* 2

Rationale: Typically, seizure assessment includes the time the seizure began, part(s) of the body affected, the type of movements and progression of the seizure, changes in pupil size, eye deviation or nystagmus, client condition during the seizure, and postictal status.

Test-Taking Strategy: Note the key words, *needs to read*. These words indicate a false response question and that you need to select the incorrect student statement. Note that options 1, 3, and 4 relate to seizures and neurological assessment whereas option 2 does not. Review nursing assessment during a seizure if you had difficulty answering this question.

Level of Cognitive Ability: Comprehension
Client Needs: Physiological Integrity
Integrated Process: Teaching/Learning
Content Area: Adult Health/Neurological
Reference: Linton, A., & Maebius, N. (2003). *Introduction to medical-surgical nursing* (3rd ed.). Philadelphia: W.B. Saunders, pp. 386-387.

46. *Answer:* 3

Rationale: Seizure precautions may vary somewhat from agency to agency, but they generally have some commonalities. Usually an airway, oxygen, and suctioning equipment are kept available at the bedside. The side rails of the bed are padded, and the bed is kept in the lowest position. The client has a IV access in place to have a readily accessible route if IV anticonvulsant medications must be administered. The use of padded tongue blades is highly controversial, and they should not be kept at the bedside. Forcing a tongue blade into the mouth during a seizure will more likely harm the client who bites down during seizure activity. Other risks include blocking the airway from improper placement, chipping the client's teeth, and subsequent risk of aspirating tooth fragments. If the client has an aura before the seizure, it may give the nurse enough time to place an oral airway before seizure activity begins.

Test-Taking Strategy: Note the key word, *avoid*. This word indicates a false response question and that you need to select the action that is contraindicated. No harm can come to the client from any of the options except for the tongue blade. Review seizure precautions if you had difficulty with this question.

Level of Cognitive Ability: Application
Client Needs: Safe, Effective Care Environment
Integrated Process: Nursing Process/Implementation
Content Area: Adult Health/Neurological
Reference: Linton, A., & Maebius, N. (2003). *Introduction to medical-surgical nursing* (3rd ed.). Philadelphia: W.B. Saunders, p. 387.

47. *Answer:* 3

Rationale: Nursing actions during a seizure include providing for privacy, loosening restrictive clothing, removing the pillow and raising the padded side rails in bed, and placing the client on one side with the head flexed forward, if possible, to allow the tongue to fall forward and facilitate drainage. The limbs are never restrained, because the strong muscle contractions could cause the client harm. If the client is not in bed when seizure activity begins, the nurse lowers the client to the floor, if possible, protects the head against injury, and moves furniture that may injure the client.

Test-Taking Strategy: Note the key word, *contraindicated*. This word indicates a false response question and that you need to select the harmful action. No harm can come to the client from any of the options except for restraining the limbs. Remember to avoid restraints. Review care of a client during a seizure if you had difficulty with this question.

Level of Cognitive Ability: Application
Client Needs: Physiological Integrity
Integrated Process: Nursing Process/Implementation

Content Area: Adult Health/Neurological
Reference: Linton, A., & Maebius, N. (2003). *Introduction to medical-surgical nursing* (3rd ed.). Philadelphia: W.B. Saunders, p. 397.

48. *Answer: 3*
Rationale: Typical anticonvulsant medication instructions include taking the prescribed dose daily to keep the blood level of the drug constant; having a serum drug level drawn before taking the morning dose; avoiding abruptly stopping the medication; avoiding alcohol; checking with the physician before taking over-the-counter medications; avoiding activities where alertness and coordination are required until medication effects are known; providing good oral hygiene and getting regular dental care; and wearing a Medic-Alert bracelet or tag.
Test-Taking Strategy: Use the process of elimination. Options 1 and 2 can be eliminated using general medication administration guidelines. From the remaining options, remember that medications are not generally taken just before drawing samples for checking therapeutic serum levels, because the results would be artificially high. This leaves oral hygiene as the correct answer, because of the risk of gingival hyperplasia associated with this medication. Review client teaching related to phenytoin (Dilantin) if you had difficulty with this question.
Level of Cognitive Ability: Analysis
Client Needs: Health Promotion and Maintenance
Integrated Process: Nursing Process/Evaluation
Content Area: Adult Health/Neurological
Reference: Hodgson, B., & Kizior, R. (2005). *Saunders nursing drug handbook 2005*. Philadelphia: W.B. Saunders, p. 858.

49. *Answer: 2*
Rationale: Hemiparesis is a weakness of the face, arm, and leg on one side. The client with one-sided hemiparesis benefits from having objects placed on the unaffected side and within reach. Other helpful activities with hemiparesis include range-of-motion exercises to the affected side and muscle strengthening exercises to the unaffected side.
Test-Taking Strategy: Focus on the client's diagnosis. Begin to answer this question by eliminating options 3 and 4, because they are hazardous to the client. This question also tests your ability to distinguish between hemiparesis and unilateral neglect. The client with hemiparesis has weakness on one side, and therefore objects should be place on the stronger side. With unilateral neglect, objects are placed on the affected side to train the client to attend to that part of the environment. Knowing this, you would select option 2 as the correct answer. Review care of the client with hemiparesis if you had difficulty with this question.
Level of Cognitive Ability: Application
Client Needs: Safe, Effective Care Environment
Integrated Process: Nursing Process/Planning
Content Area: Adult Health/Neurological
Reference: Linton, A., & Maebius, N. (2003). *Introduction to medical-surgical nursing* (3rd ed.). Philadelphia: W.B. Saunders, p. 382.

50. *Answer: 1*
Rationale: Before the client with dysphagia is started on a diet, the gag and swallow reflexes must have returned. The client is assisted with meals as needed, and is given ample time to chew and swallow. Food is placed on the unaffected side of the mouth. Liquids are thickened to avoid aspiration.
Test-Taking Strategy: Note the key word, *avoids*. This indicates a false response question and that you need to select the incorrect action. Option 4 is generally a good action for all clients. Option 3 is appropriate because the client has better sensation and motion on the unaffected side of the mouth. This narrows your options to two opposing concepts, thin versus thick liquids. Thickened liquids are easier for the client with impaired facial motion and swallowing ability to manage. Knowing this enables you to select option 1 as the action to avoid. Review care of the client with residual dysphagia if you had difficulty with this question.
Level of Cognitive Ability: Application
Client Needs: Physiological Integrity
Integrated Process: Nursing Process/Implementation
Content Area: Adult Health/Neurological
Reference: Linton, A., & Maebius, N. (2003). *Introduction to medical-surgical nursing* (3rd ed.). Philadelphia: W.B. Saunders, p. 415.

51. *Answer: 3*
Rationale: Homonymous hemianopsia is loss of half of the visual field. The client with homonymous hemianopsia should have objects placed in the intact field of vision, and the nurse should approach the client from the intact side. The nurse instructs the client to scan the environment to overcome the visual deficit and does client teaching from within the intact field of vision. The nurse encourages the use of personal eyeglasses, if they are available.
Test-Taking Strategy: To answer this question accurately, you need to be able to distinguish between homonymous hemianopsia and unilateral neglect. Clients are approached differently with these two deficits. Remember that the similarity is that the client must be taught to scan the environment, which is the answer to this question. Review care of the client with homonymous hemianopsia if you had difficulty with this question.
Level of Cognitive Ability: Analysis
Client Needs: Health Promotion and Maintenance
Integrated Process: Nursing Process/Evaluation
Content Area: Adult Health/Neurological
Reference: Linton, A., & Maebius, N. (2003). *Introduction to medical-surgical nursing* (3rd ed.). Philadelphia: W.B. Saunders, p. 416.

52. *Answer: 2*
Rationale: Clients with aphasia after CVA often fatigue easily and have a short attention span. General guidelines when trying to communicate with the aphasic client include speaking more slowly and allowing adequate response time, listening to and watching attempts to communicate, and trying to put the client at ease with a caring and understanding manner. The nurse should avoid shouting (because the client is not deaf), appearing rushed for a response, and letting family members give all the responses for the client.
Test-Taking Strategy: Note the key words, *least helpful*. These words indicate a false response question and that you need to select the inappropriate nursing action. Visualizing each

action will direct you to option 2. If this question was difficult, review these communication strategies.
Level of Cognitive Ability: Application
Client Needs: Psychosocial Integrity
Integrated Process: Nursing Process/Implementation
Content Area: Adult Health/Neurological
Reference: Linton, A., & Maebius, N. (2003). *Introduction to medical-surgical nursing* (3rd ed.). Philadelphia: W.B. Saunders, pp. 414-415.

53. *Answer:* 4

Rationale: The client with spinal cord injury above the level of T7 is at risk for autonomic dysreflexia. It is characterized by severe, throbbing headache, flushing of the face and neck, bradycardia, and sudden severe hypertension. Other signs include nasal stuffiness, blurred vision, nausea, and sweating. It is a life-threatening syndrome triggered by a noxious stimulus below the level of the injury.
Test-Taking Strategy: Use the process of elimination. Begin to answer this question by eliminating options 1 and 3. The client in spinal shock would be hypotensive (not hypertensive), and the client's clinical picture does not match pulmonary embolism. (It may be useful to know also that autonomic dysreflexia does not occur until spinal shock resolves.) The word "hypertension" may have caught your eye in option 2, but knowing that malignant hypertension occurs with anesthesia will help you eliminate this option as well. Review the signs of autonomic dysreflexia if you had difficulty with this question.
Level of Cognitive Ability: Analysis
Client Needs: Physiological Integrity
Integrated Process: Nursing Process/Data Collection
Content Area: Adult Health/Neurological
Reference: Linton, A., & Maebius, N. (2003). *Introduction to medical-surgical nursing* (3rd ed.). Philadelphia: W.B. Saunders, p. 446.

54. *Answer:* 3

Rationale: Myasthenia gravis can often be diagnosed based on clinical signs and symptoms. The diagnosis can be confirmed by injecting the client with a dose of Tensilon. This medication inhibits the breakdown of an enzyme in the neuromuscular junction, so more acetylcholine binds to receptors. If the muscle is strengthened for 3 to 5 minutes after this injection, it confirms a diagnosis of myasthenia gravis. Another medication, neostigmine (Prostigmin), may also be used because its effect lasts for 1 to 2 hours, providing a better analysis. For either medication, atropine sulfate should be available as the antidote.
Test-Taking Strategy: Knowledge of the purpose and expected findings of the Tensilon test is needed to answer this question. Remember, the Tensilon test is used in diagnosing myasthenia gravis. Review this test if you had difficulty with this question.
Level of Cognitive Ability: Analysis
Client Needs: Physiological Integrity
Integrated Process: Nursing Process/Data Collection
Content Area: Pharmacology
Reference: Chernecky, C., & Berger, B. (2004). *Laboratory tests and diagnostic procedures* (4th ed.). Philadelphia: W.B. Saunders, pp. 1035-1036.

55. *Answer:* 2

Rationale: The client has speech that is nasal in tone and dysarthritic because of cranial nerve involvement of the muscles governing speech. The nurse listens attentively and verbally, verifies what the client has said, asks questions requiring a yes or no response, and develops alternative communication methods (e.g., letter board, picture board, pen and paper, flash cards). Encouraging the client to speak quickly is an ineffective communication strategy and is counterproductive.
Test-Taking Strategy: Note the key word, *avoid*. This word indicates a false response question and that you need to select the incorrect communication strategy. There are some techniques that are useful in communicating with clients with speech impairment, regardless of the specific cause of the difficulty. Options 3 and 4 are examples of alternative communication methods that are useful, so eliminate these options as strategies to avoid. From the remaining options, remember that speaking quickly is difficult for a client with a speech impairment. Review these communication strategies if you had difficulty with this question.
Level of Cognitive Ability: Application
Client Needs: Psychosocial Integrity
Integrated Process: Communication and Documentation
Content Area: Adult Health/Neurological
Reference: Christensen, B., & Kockrow, E. (2003). *Adult health nursing* (4th ed.). St. Louis: Mosby, p. 640.

56. *Answer:* 3

Rationale: Myasthenic crisis is often caused by undermedication and responds to administration of cholinergic medications such as neostigmine (Prostigmin) and pyridostigmine (Mestinon). Cholinergic crisis (the opposite problem) is caused by excess medication and responds to withholding of medications. Too little exercise and fatty food intake are incorrect options. Overexertion and overeating could possibly trigger myasthenic crisis.
Test-Taking Strategy: Focus on the client's diagnosis and recall that myasthenic crisis is treated with medication. Remember, undermedication is a cause of myasthenic crisis. Review the causes of this type of crisis if you are unfamiliar with them.
Level of Cognitive Ability: Analysis
Client Needs: Physiological Integrity
Integrated Process: Nursing Process/Data Collection
Content Area: Adult Health/Neurological
Reference: Linton, A., & Maebius, N. (2003). *Introduction to medical-surgical nursing* (3rd ed.). Philadelphia: W.B. Saunders, pp. 403-404.

57. *Answer:* 2

Rationale: Clients with myasthenia gravis are taught to space out activities over the day to conserve energy and restore muscle strength. It is very important to take medications correctly to maintain blood levels that are not too low or too high. Muscle-strengthening exercises are not helpful and can fatigue the client. Overeating is a cause of exacerbation of symptoms, as well as exposure to heat, crowds, erratic sleep habits, and emotional stress.
Test-Taking Strategy: Use the process of elimination and note the key words, *most effectively*. If you know that common

causes of myasthenic and cholinergic crises are undermedication and overmedication, respectively, you should be able to eliminate each of the incorrect options easily. Remember, it is extremely important that these clients take medications on time to maintain therapeutic blood levels. Review measures to prevent myasthenic and cholinergic crises if you are unfamiliar with them.
Level of Cognitive Ability: Application
Client Needs: Physiological Integrity
Integrated Process: Nursing Process/Implementation
Content Area: Adult Health/Neurological
Reference: Linton, A., & Maebius, N. (2003). *Introduction to medical-surgical nursing* (3rd ed.). Philadelphia: W.B. Saunders, p. 404.

58. *Answer:* **3**
Rationale: Most ongoing treatment for myasthenia gravis is done in outpatient settings, and the client needs to be aware of the lifestyle changes needed to maintain independence. Taking medications 1 hour before mealtime gives greater muscle strength for chewing, and is indicated. The client should have portable suction equipment and a portable resuscitation bag available in case of respiratory distress. The client should carry medical identification about the condition. The client should avoid activities that could worsen the symptoms, including stress, infection, heat, surgery, or alcohol.
Test-Taking Strategy: Note the key words, *needs more information.* These words indicate a false response question and that you need to select the incorrect client statement. Options 2 and 4 are reasonable courses of action and are eliminated first. To select from the remaining options, you would need to know that premedication 1 hour before meals gives strength to the muscles (for chewing and swallowing), and that heat and infection (crowds at the beach) trigger myasthenic crisis. Review client education points with myasthenia gravis if you had difficulty with this question.
Level of Cognitive Ability: Comprehension
Client Needs: Health Promotion and Maintenance
Integrated Process: Teaching/Learning
Content Area: Adult Health/Neurological
Reference: Linton, A., & Maebius, N. (2003). *Introduction to medical-surgical nursing* (3rd ed.). Philadelphia: W.B. Saunders, p. 404.

59. *Answer:* **3**
Rationale: The client with Parkinson's disease tends to become withdrawn and depressed, and should become an active participant in his or her own care to prevent this. There should be planned activities throughout the day to inhibit daytime sleeping and boredom. The nurse gives the client encouragement and praises the client for perseverance. Exercise helps prevent progression of the disease and self-care improves self-esteem.
Test-Taking Strategy: Use the process of elimination. Eliminate option 1 because of the absolute word "only." Option 2 is well-intentioned but is not therapeutic in helping the client cope with the disease and promotes dependence. From the remaining options, eliminate option 4 because it will promote fatigue. Review care of the client with Parkinson's disease if you had difficulty with this question.

Level of Cognitive Ability: Application
Client Needs: Psychosocial Integrity
Integrated Process: Nursing Process/Planning
Content Area: Adult Health/Neurological
Reference: Linton, A., & Maebius, N. (2003). *Introduction to medical-surgical nursing* (3rd ed.). Philadelphia: W.B. Saunders, p. 398.

60. *Answer:* **1**
Rationale: Parkinsonian crisis can occur with emotional trauma or sudden withdrawal of medications. The client exhibits severe tremors, rigidity, and bradykinesia. The client also displays anxiety, is diaphoretic, and has tachycardia and hyperpnea. The client should be placed in a quiet, dim room and respiratory and cardiac support should be available.
Test-Taking Strategy: Use the process of elimination. Option 4 is not indicated and is eliminated first. Option 3 is not an immediate concern and is also eliminated. From the remaining options, note that there is nothing about parkinsonian crisis that warrants placement of a nasogastric tube. This leaves the correct option, which is to put the client in a dim, quiet room and provide for support of cardiac and respiratory symptoms. Also, use of the ABCs—airway, breathing, and circulation—will direct you to the correct option. Review nursing care for parkinsonian crisis if you had difficulty with this question.
Level of Cognitive Ability: Application
Client Needs: Safe, Effective Care Environment
Integrated Process: Nursing Process/Implementation
Content Area: Adult Health/Neurological
Reference: Swearingen, P. (2003). *Manual of medical-surgical nursing care* (5th ed.). St. Louis: Mosby, p. 305.

61. *Answer:* **2**
Rationale: The client with Parkinson's disease should exercise in the morning, when energy levels are highest. The client should avoid sitting in soft, deep chairs, because they are difficult to get up from. The client can rock back and forth to initiate movement. The client should buy clothes with Velcro fasteners and slide-locking buckles to support the ability to dress herself or himself.
Test-Taking Strategy: Use the process of elimination. Option 1 is not useful to clients with fatigue from any disorder, so this option can be eliminated first. Knowing that the client with Parkinson's has difficulty with movement and dexterity helps you eliminate options 3 and 4 next. Review client teaching points with Parkinson's disease if you had difficulty with this question.
Level of Cognitive Ability: Comprehension
Client Needs: Health Promotion and Maintenance
Integrated Process: Nursing Process/Evaluation
Content Area: Adult Health/Neurological
Reference: Linton, A., & Maebius, N. (2003). *Introduction to medical-surgical nursing* (3rd ed.). Philadelphia: W.B. Saunders, p. 378.

62. *Answer:* **4**
Rationale: Facial pain can be minimized by using cotton pads to wash the face, using room temperature water. The client should chew on the unaffected side of the mouth, eat a soft

diet, and take in foods and beverages at room temperature. If toothbrushing triggers pain, sometimes an oral rinse after meals is helpful instead.

Test-Taking Strategy: Note the key words, *needs reinforcement of information.* These words indicate a false response question and that you need to select the incorrect client statement. Recalling that the pain of trigeminal neuralgia is triggered by mechanical or thermal stimuli will direct you to the correct option. Remember, very hot or cold foods are likely to trigger the pain, not relieve it. Review these client teaching points if you had difficulty with this question.

Level of Cognitive Ability: Comprehension
Client Needs: Health Promotion and Maintenance
Integrated Process: Teaching/Learning
Content Area: Adult Health/Neurological
References: Christensen, B., & Kockrow, E. (2003). *Adult health nursing* (4th ed.). St. Louis: Mosby, p. 643.
Linton, A., & Maebius, N. (2003). *Introduction to medical-surgical nursing* (3rd ed.). Philadelphia: W.B. Saunders, p. 405.

ALTERNATE FORMAT QUESTION: PRIORITIZING (ORDERED RESPONSE)

Answers: 31425

Rationale: Autonomic dysreflexia is characterized by severe hypertension, bradycardia, severe headache, nasal stuffiness, and flushing. The cause is a noxious stimulus, most often a distended bladder or constipation. It is a neurological emergency and must be treated promptly to prevent a hypertensive stroke. Immediate nursing actions are to sit the client up in bed in a high-Fowler's position and remove the noxious stimulus. The nurse would loosen any tight clothing, and check for bladder distention, and catheterize the client if distention is present. If the client has a Foley catheter, the nurse would check for kinks in the tubing. The nurse would also check for a fecal impaction and disimpact the client, if necessary. The physician is contacted if these actions do not relieve the signs and symptoms. Antihypertensive medication may be prescribed by the physician to minimize cerebral hypertension.

Test-Taking Strategy: Recalling that this syndrome causes severe hypertension will assist in determining that elevating the head of the bed is the first action. Next, recalling that the syndrome is caused by a noxious stimulus will assist in determining that loosening tight clothing, checking for bladder distention, and catheterizing if necessary would be the next actions. Because loosening any tight clothing would take less time than checking for bladder distention and catheterizing, this action would be taken next. Antihypertensives require a physician's order; therefore, calling the physician would be the next action. Review immediate nursing interventions for the client experiencing autonomic dysreflexia if you had difficulty with this question.

Level of Cognitive Ability: Application
Client Needs: Physiological Integrity
Integrated Process: Nursing Process/Implementation
Content Area: Delegating/Prioritizing
References: Ignatavicius, D., & Workman, M. (2006). *Medical-surgical nursing: Critical thinking for collaborative care* (5th ed.). Philadelphia: W.B. Saunders, p. 988.
Lewis, S., Heitkemper, M., & Dirksen, S. (2004). *Medical-surgical nursing: Assessment and management of clinical problems* (6th ed.). St. Louis: Mosby, p. 1625.

REFERENCES

Black, J., & Hawks, J. (2005). *Medical-surgical nursing: Clinical management for positive outcomes* (7th ed.). Philadelphia: W.B. Saunders.

Chernecky, C., & Berger, B. (2004). *Laboratory tests and diagnostic procedures* (4th ed.). Philadelphia: W.B. Saunders.

Christensen, B., & Kockrow, E. (2003). *Adult health nursing* (4th ed.). St. Louis: Mosby.

deWit, S. (2005). *Fundamental concepts and skills for nursing.* Philadelphia: W.B. Saunders.

Hodgson, B., & Kizior, R. (2005). *Saunders nursing drug handbook 2005.* Philadelphia: W.B. Saunders.

Ignatavicius, D., & Workman, M. (2006). *Medical surgical nursing: Critical thinking for collaborative care* (5th ed.). Philadelphia: W.B. Saunders.

Lewis, S., Heitkemper, M., & Dirksen, S. (2004). *Medical-surgical nursing: Assessment and management of clinical problems* (6th ed.). St. Louis: Mosby.

Linton, A., & Maebius, N. (2003). *Introduction to medical-surgical nursing* (3rd ed.). Philadelphia: W.B. Saunders.

McKenry, L., & Salerno, E. (2003). *Mosby's pharmacology in nursing* (21st ed.). St. Louis: Mosby.

Pagana, K., & Pagana, T. (2003). *Mosby's diagnostic and laboratory test reference* (6th ed.). St. Louis: Mosby.

Phipps, W., Monahan, F., Sands, J., Marek, J., & Neighbors, M. (2003). *Medical-surgical nursing: Health and illness perspectives* (7th ed.). St. Louis: Mosby.

Potter, P., & Perry, A. (2003). *Essentials for practice* (5th ed.). St. Louis: Mosby.

Potter, P., & Perry, A. (2005). *Fundamentals of nursing* (6th ed.). St. Louis: Mosby.

Swearingen, P. (2003). *Manual of medical-surgical nursing care* (5th ed.). St. Louis: Mosby.

Neurological Medications

I. ANTIMYASTHENIC MEDICATIONS

A. Description

1. Relieve muscle weakness associated with myasthenia gravis by blocking acetycholine breakdown at the neuromuscular junction
2. Used to treat or diagnose myasthenia gravis or to distinguish cholinergic crisis from myasthenic crisis
3. Neostigmine bromide (Prostigmin), pyridostigmine bromide (Mestinon), ambenonium (Mytelase) are used to control myasthenic symptoms
4. Edrophonium chloride (Tensilon) is used to diagnose myasthenia gravis and to distinguish cholinergic crisis from myasthenic crisis

B. Medications (Box 57-1)

C. Side effects: Cholinergic crisis (Box 57-2)

D. Interventions

1. Monitor neuromuscular status, including reflexes, muscle strength, and gait
2. Monitor the client for signs and symptoms of medication overdose (cholinergic crisis) and underdose (myasthenic crisis)
3. Instruct the client to take medications on time to prevent weakness, because weakness can impair the client's ability to breathe and swallow
4. Instruct the client to take the medication before meals for best absorption
5. Instruct the client to wear a Medic-Alert bracelet
6. Note that antimyasthenic therapy is lifelong therapy
7. Evaluate for medication effectiveness, which is based on the improvement of neuromuscular symptoms or strength without cholinergic signs and symptoms
8. When administering edrophonium (Tensilon), have emergency resuscitation equipment on hand and atropine sulfate available for cholinergic crisis

E. Tensilon test

1. Tensilon is injected by the intravenous route
2. The Tensilon test can cause ventricular fibrillation and cardiac arrest
3. Atropine sulfate is the antidote for overdose
4. Diagnosis of myasthenia gravis: Most myasthenic clients will show a marked improvement in muscle tone within 30 to 60 seconds after injection, and the muscle improvement lasts 4 to 5 minutes

---

BOX 57-1

Antimyasthenic Medications

Edrophonium chloride (Tensilon, Enlon)
Neostigmine bromide (Prostigmin)
Pyridostigmine bromide (Mestinon)
Ambenonium chloride (Mytelase)

BOX 57-2

Signs of Cholinergic Crisis

Gastrointestinal (GI) disturbances
Abdominal cramps
Nausea, vomiting, diarrhea
Increased salivation and tearing
Increased bronchial secretions
Sweating
Miosis
Hypertension

5. Diagnosis of cholinergic crisis (overdose with anticholinesterase) or myasthenic crisis (under-medication)
   a. In cholinergic crisis, muscle tone does not improve after the administration of Tensilon, and muscle twitching may be noted around the eyes and face
   b. A Tensilon injection makes the client in cholinergic crisis temporarily worse (negative Tensilon test)
   c. A Tensilon injection temporarily improves the condition when the client is in myasthenic crisis (positive Tensilon test)

II. ANTIPARKINSONIAN MEDICATIONS

A. Description
   1. Restore the balance of the neurotransmitters acetylcholine and dopamine in the central nervous system (CNS), decreasing the signs and symptoms of Parkinson's disease
   2. These medications include the dopaminergics, which stimulate the dopamine receptors, and the anticholinergics, which block the cholinergic receptors
   3. Used for drug-induced parkinsonism, in which neuroleptic agents block dopamine receptors in the CNS, leading to functional loss of dopamine activity
   4. Used for Parkinson's disease, in which dopamine-containing neurons in the basal ganglia are destroyed or deficient, which causes loss of fine motor control

B. Dopaminergic medications
   1. Description
      a. Stimulate the dopamine receptors
      b. Increase the amount of dopamine available in the CNS or enhance neurotransmission of dopamine
      c. Contraindicated in cardiac, renal or psychiatric disorders
      d. Levodopa taken with a monoamine oxidase inhibitor (MAOI) antidepressant can cause a hypertensive crisis
   2. Medications (Box 57-3)
   3. Side effects
      a. Dyskinesia
      b. Involuntary body movements
      c. Tachycardia
      d. Nausea and vomiting
      e. Urinary retention
      f. Constipation
      g. Dizziness
      h. Orthostatic hypotension
      i. Confusion
      j. Mood changes
      k. Hallucinations

BOX 57-3

Medications to Treat Parkinson's Disease

MEDICATIONS AFFECTING THE AMOUNT OF DOPAMINE
Amantadine (Symmetrel)
Bromocriptine (Parlodel)
Carbidopa-levodopa (Sinemet)
Levodopa (Larodopa, Dopar)
Pergolide mesylate (Permax)
Pramipexole (Mirapex)
Ropinirole (Requip)
Selegiline hydrochloride (Carbex, Eldepryl)
Tolcapone (Tasmar)

ANTICHOLINERGICS
Benztropine mesylate (Cogentin)
Biperiden hydrochloride (Akineton)
Procyclidine hydrochloride (Kemadrin)
Trihexyphenidyl hydrochloride (Artane)

CATHECHOL O-METHYLTRANSFERASE (COMT) INHIBITORS
Diphenhydramine hydrochloride (Benadryl)
Entacapone (Comtan)
Tolcapone (Tasmar)

4. Interventions
   a. Monitor vital signs
   b. Assess for risk of injury
   c. Instruct the client to take the medication with food if nausea and vomiting occur
   d. Monitor for signs and symptoms of parkinsonism, such as rigidity, tremors, akinesia, and bradykinesia; a stooped forward posture; shuffling gait; and masked facies
   e. Monitor for signs of dyskinesia
   f. Instruct the client taking carbidopa-levodopa (Sinemet) to eat low-protein foods, because high-protein diets interfere with medication transport to the CNS
   g. Instruct the client to change positions slowly to minimize orthostatic hypotension
   h. Instruct the client not to discontinue the medication abruptly
   i. Instruct the client to report side effects and symptoms of dyskinesia
   j. Instruct the client to avoid alcohol
   k. Monitor the client for improvement in signs and symptoms of parkinsonism without the development of severe side effects from the medications
   l. Inform the client that urine or perspiration may be discolored and that this is harmless, but it may stain the clothing
   m. Advise the client with diabetes mellitus that glucose testing should not be done through urine testing because the results will not be reliable
   n. When administering levodopa, instruct the client to avoid excessive vitamin B_6 intake to prevent medication reactions

C. Anticholinergic medications
  1. Description
      a. Block the cholinergic receptors in the CNS, thereby suppressing acetylcholine activity
      b. Reduce the rigidity and some of the tremors but have a minimal effect on the bradykinesia
      c. Contraindicated in clients with glaucoma
      d. The client with chronic obstructive lung disease can develop dry, thick mucous secretions
  2. Medications (see Box 57-3)
  3. Side effects
      a. Blurred vision
      b. Dry mouth and dry secretions
      c. Increased pulse rate
      d. Constipation
      e. Urinary retention
      f. Restlessness and confusion
      g. Photophobia
  4. Interventions
      a. Monitor vital signs
      b. Assess for risk of injury
      c. Monitor for signs and symptoms of parkinsonism such as rigidity, tremors, akinesia, and bradykinesia; a stooped forward posture; shuffling gait; and masked facies
      d. Monitor the client for improvement in signs and symptoms
      e. Monitor the client's bowel and urinary function and monitor for urinary retention and constipation
      f. Monitor for involuntary movements
      g. Encourage the client to avoid alcohol, smoking, caffeine, and aspirin to decrease gastric acidity
      h. Instruct the client to consult with the physician before taking any nonprescription medications
      i. Instruct the client to minimize dry mouth by increasing fluid intake and by using ice chips, hard candy, or gum
      j. Instruct the client to prevent constipation by increasing fluid and fiber in the diet
      k. Instruct the client to use sunglasses in direct sun because of possible photophobia
      l. Instruct the client to have routine eye examinations to assess for intraocular pressure

III. ANTICONVULSANT MEDICATIONS (Table 57-1)

A. Description
  1. Used to depress abnormal neuronal discharges and prevent the spread of seizures
  2. Used with caution in clients on anticoagulants, aspirin, sulfonamides, cimetidine (Tagamet), and antipsychotics
  3. Absorption is decreased with the use of antacids, calcium preparations, and antineoplastic medications

TABLE 57-1

Anticonvulsant Medications

Medication	Therapeutic Serum Range
Phenytoin (Dilantin)	10-20 mcg/mL
Carbamazepine (Tegretol)	3-14 mcg/mL
Phenobarbital (Luminal)	15-40 mcg/mL
Amobarbital (Amytal)	1-5 mcg/mL
Clonazepam (Klonopin)	20-80 ng/mL
Lorazepam (Ativan)	50-240 ng/mL

BOX 57-4

Client Education: Anticonvulsants

Take anticonvulsant with food to decrease GI irritation but avoid milk and antacids, which impair absorption.
If taking liquid medication, shake well before ingesting.
Do not discontinue medication.
Avoid alcohol.
Avoid over-the-counter medications.
Wear a Medic-Alert bracelet.
Use caution when driving or performing activities that require alertness.
Maintain good oral hygiene and use a soft toothbrush.
It is important to have preventative dental checkups.
It is important to follow-up with periodic blood studies related to determining toxicity.
Monitor serum glucose levels (diabetes mellitus).
Urine may be a harmless pink-red or red-brown color.
Report symptoms of sore throat, bruising, and nosebleeds, which may indicate a blood dyscrasia.
Inform the physician if adverse reactions occur, such as gingivitis, nystagmus, slurred speech, rash, or dizziness.

B. Interventions for clients on anticonvulsants
  1. Initiate seizure precautions
  2. Monitor urinary output
  3. Monitor liver and renal function test results
  4. Monitor for signs of medication toxicity, which would include CNS depression, ataxia, nausea, vomiting, drowsiness, dizziness, restlessness, and visual disturbances
  5. If a seizure occurs, assess seizure activity, including location and duration
  6. Protect client from hazards in the environment during a seizure
C. Client education (Box 57-4)
D. Hydantoins (Box 57-5)
  1. Used to treat seizures
  2. Phenytoin (Dilantin) is also used to treat dysrhythmias
  3. Side effects
      a. Gingival hyperplasia
      b. Reddened gums that bleed easily
      c. Slurred speech
      d. Confusion

BOX 57-5

Hydantoins

Phenytoin (Dilantin)
Ethotoin (Peganone)
Fosphenytoin (Cerebyx)

BOX 57-7

Benzodiazepines

Clonazepam (Klonopin)
Clorazepate (Tranxene)
Diazepam (Valium)
Lorazepam (Ativan)

BOX 57-6

Barbiturates

Phenobarbital
Primidone (Mysoline)
Amobarbital (Amytal)
Mephobarbital (Mebaral)

BOX 57-8

Succinimides

Ethosuximide (Zarontin)
Methsuximide (Celontin)
Phensuximide (Milontin)

BOX 57-9

Oxazolidinediones

Paramethadione
Trimethadione (Tridione)

BOX 57-10

Valproates

Valproic acid (Depakene)
Divalproex sodium (Depakote)

     e. Depression
     f. Nausea and vomiting
     g. Constipation
     h. Headaches
     i. Blood dyscrasias: decreased platelet count and decreased white blood cell (WBC) count
     j. Elevated blood glucose level
     k. Alopecia
     l. Hirsutism
  4. Interventions
     a. Oral tube feedings may interfere with the absorption of oral phenytoin and diminish the medication's effectiveness; therefore, feedings should be scheduled as far as possible from the phenytoin administration
     b. Monitor therapeutic serum levels to assess for toxicity
     c. Monitor for signs of toxicity
     d. Instruct the client about the importance of good oral hygiene and regular dental examinations
     e. Instruct the client to consult with the physician before taking other medications to ensure compatibility with anticonvulsants
E. Barbiturates (Box 57-6)
  1. Used for tonic-clonic seizures and acute episodes of seizures due to status epilepticus
  2. May also be used as adjuncts to anesthesia
  3. Side effects
     a. Drowsiness
     b. Dizziness
     c. Hypotension
     d. Respiratory depression
     e. Tolerance to the medication
F. Benzodiazepines (Box 57-7)
  1. Used to treat absence seizures
  2. Diazepam (Valium) is used to treat status epilepticus, anxiety, and skeletal muscle spasms
  3. Clorazepate (Tranxene) is used as adjunctive therapy for partial seizures

  4. Side effects
     a. Ataxia
     b. Respiratory and cardiac depression
     c. Medication tolerance and drug dependency
G. Succinimides (Box 57-8)
  1. Used to treat absence seizures
  2. Side effects
     a. Anorexia, nausea, vomiting
     b. Blood dyscrasias
H. Oxazolidinediones (Box 57-9)
  1. Used for absence seizures
  2. Side effects
     a. Sedation
     b. Photophobia
I. Valproates (Box 57-10)
  1. Used to treat tonic-clonic, partial, myoclonic, and psychomotor seizures
  2. Side effects
     a. Nausea
     b. Vomiting
     c. Abdominal cramps
     d. Diarrhea
     e. Constipation
     f. Hepatotoxicity

BOX 57-11

Other Anticonvulsants

Carbamazepine (Tegretol)
Gabapentin (Neurontin)
Lamotrigine (Lamictal)
Tiagabine (Gabitril)
Topiramate (Topamax)

BOX 57-12

Amphetamines

Amphetamine sulfate
Dextroamphetamine sulfate (Dexedrine)
Methamphetamine hydrochloride (Desoxyn)
Methylphenidate hydrochloride (Ritalin)
Pemoline (Cylert)

J. Iminostilbenes (Box 57-11)
   1. Used to treat seizure disorders that have not responded to other anticonvulsants
   2. Used to treat trigeminal neuralgia
   3. Side effects
      a. Drowsiness
      b. Dizziness
      c. Nausea
      d. Vomiting
      e. Constipation or diarrhea
      f. Visual abnormalities
      g. Dry mouth
      h. Headache

BOX 57-13

Anorexiants

Diethylpropion hydrochloride (Tenuate)
Phendimetrazine (Bontril, Melfiat-105)
Phentermine hydrochloride (Fastin, Adipex-P, Zantril)
Benzphetamine hydrochloride (Didrex)
Sibutramine (Meridia)

BOX 57-14

Treating Respiratory Depression

Aminophylline
Caffeine
Doxapram (Dopram)
Theophylline

IV. CENTRAL NERVOUS SYSTEM STIMULANTS

A. Description
   1. Amphetamines and caffeine stimulate the cerebral cortex of the brain (Box 57-12)
   2. Analeptics and caffeine act on the brainstem and medulla to stimulate respiration
   3. Anorexiants act on the cerebral cortex and hypothalamus to suppress appetite (Box 57-13)
   4. Used to treat narcolepsy and attention deficit hyperactivity disorders
   5. Used to treat respiratory depression (Box 57-14)
   6. Used as adjunctive therapy for exogenous obesity

B. Side effects
   1. Irritability
   2. Restlessness
   3. Tremors
   4. Insomnia
   5. Heart palpitations
   6. Tachycardia
   7. Hypertension
   8. Dry mouth
   9. Anorexia
   10. Weight loss
   11. Diarrhea or constipation
   12. Impotence
   13. Dependence and tolerance

C. Interventions
   1. Monitor vital signs
   2. Monitor mental status
   3. Monitor height, weight, and growth of the child
   4. Monitor complete blood count (CBC) and white blood cell (WBC) and platelet counts before and during therapy
   5. Monitor for side effects
   6. Monitor sleep patterns
   7. Monitor for withdrawal symptoms such as nausea, vomiting, weakness, and headache
   8. Instruct the client to take the medication before meals
   9. Instruct the client to avoid foods and beverages containing caffeine to prevent additional stimulation
   10. Instruct the client to read labels on over-the-counter products because many contain caffeine
   11. Instruct the client to avoid alcohol
   12. Instruct the client not to discontinue the medication abruptly
   13. Instruct the client to take the last daily dose of the CNS stimulant at least 6 hours before bedtime to prevent insomnia
   14. Monitor for drug dependence and abuse with amphetamines
   15. If a child is taking a CNS stimulant, instruct the parents to notify the school nurse
   16. Monitor for calming effects of CNS stimulants within 3 to 4 weeks in children with attention-deficit/hyperactivity disorder (ADHD)

17. Monitor growth in the child on long-term therapy with methylphenidate hydrochloride (Ritalin)

V. NON-NARCOTIC ANALGESICS

A. Nonsteroidal anti-inflammatory drugs (NSAIDs) (Box 57-15)
1. Description
   a. NSAIDs are aspirin and aspirin-like medications that inhibit the synthesis of prostaglandins
   b. They act as an analgesic to relieve pain, as an antipyretic to reduce body temperature, and as an anticoagulant to inhibit platelet aggregation
   c. Used to relieve inflammation and pain and to treat of rheumatoid arthritis, bursitis, tendinitis, osteoarthritis, and acute gout
   d. Contraindicated in hypersensitivity or liver or renal disease
   e. Aspirin should not be taken by children with flu symptoms because of the risk of Reye's syndrome
   f. Aspirin should not be taken if the client is on an anticoagulant
   g. Aspirin and an NSAID should not be taken together, because aspirin decreases the blood level and the effectiveness of the NSAID
   h. NSAIDs can increase the effects of warfarin (Coumadin), sulfonamides, cephalosporins, and phenytoin (Dilantin)
   i. Hypoglycemia can result if ibuprofen (Motrin) is taken with insulin or an oral hypoglycemic medication
   j. A high risk of toxicity exists if ibuprofen is taken concurrently with calcium blockers
2. Side effects (Table 57-2)
3. Interventions
   a. Assess client for allergies
   b. Obtain a medication history and medical history on the client
   c. Monitor for history of gastric upset or bleeding or liver disease
   d. Monitor the client for GI upset during medication administration
   e. Monitor for edema
   f. Monitor serum salicylate (aspirin) level when the client is taking high doses
   g. Monitor for signs of bleeding such as tarry stools, bleeding gums, petechiae, ecchymosis, and purpura
   h. Instruct the client to take the medication with water, milk, or food
   i. Enteric-coated form or buffered form of aspirin can be taken to decrease gastric distress
   j. Instruct the client that enteric-coated tablets cannot be crushed or broken

---

BOX 57-15

Nonsteroidal Anti-inflammatory Drugs (NSAIDs)

ACETAMINOPHEN
Acetaminophen (Tylenol)

ASPIRIN
Aspirin (acetylsalicylic acid [ASA], Aspergum, Bayer Aspirin, Ecotrin)
Aspirin (acetylsalicylic acid), buffered (Alka-Seltzer, Bufferin)

PROPIONIC ACID DERIVATIVES
Fenoprofen (Nalfon)
Flurbipofen (Ansaid)
Ibuprofen (Motrin, Advil, Nuprin)
Ketoprofen (Orudis)
Naproxen (Anaprox, Naprosyn)
Oxaprozin (Daypro)

CYCLOOXYGENASE-2 INHIBITORS
Celecoxib (Celebrex)

OTHER NSAIDs
Diclofenac (Voltaren)
Diflunisal (Dolobid)
Etodolac (Lodine)
Indomethacin (Indocin)
Ketorolac tromethamine (Toradol)
Moloxicam (Mobic)
Nabumetone (Relafen)
Piroxicam (Feldene)
Sulindac (Clinoril)
Tolmetin (Tolectin)
Valdecoxib (Bextra)

TABLE 57-2

Side Effects of Aspirin and NSAIDs

Aspirin	NSAIDs
Drowsiness	Hypotension
Tinnitus	Sodium and water retention
Headaches	Gastric irritation
Flushing	Blood dyscrasias
Dizziness	Dizziness
GI symptoms	Tinnitus
Visual changes	Pruritus

k. Advise the client to inform other health care professionals if they are taking high doses of aspirin
l. Note that aspirin should be discontinued 3 to 7 days prior to surgery to reduce the risk of bleeding
m. Instruct the client to avoid alcoholic beverages

B. Acetaminophen (Tylenol)
1. Description
   a. Inhibits prostaglandin synthesis
   b. Used to decrease pain and fever
   c. Contraindicated in hepatic or renal disease, alcoholism, and hypersensitivity

2. Side effects
   a. Anorexia, nausea, vomiting
   b. Rash
   c. Hypoglycemia
   d. Oliguria
   e. Hepatotoxicity
3. Interventions
   a. Monitor vital signs
   b. Ask client about a history of liver dysfunction
   c. Monitor for hepatic damage, which includes nausea, vomiting, diarrhea, and abdominal pain
   d. Monitor liver enzyme tests
   e. Instruct the client that self-medication should not be used longer than 10 days for an adult and 5 days for a child
   f. Note that the antidote for Tylenol is acetylcysteine (Mucomyst)
   g. Evaluate for the effectiveness of the medication

VI. NARCOTIC ANALGESICS

A. Description
   1. Suppress pain impulses but can suppress respiration and coughing by acting on the respiratory and cough center in the medulla of the brainstem
   2. Can produce euphoria and sedation
   3. Can cause physical dependence
   4. Used for relief of mild, moderate, or severe pain
B. Medications (Box 57-16)
   1. Codeine sulfate
      a. Effective cough suppressant at low doses
      b. Can cause constipation
   2. Hydromorphone hydrochloride (Dilaudid)
      a. Can decrease respiration
      b. Can cause constipation
   3. Meperidine hydrochloride (Demerol)
      a. Can cause hypotension and dizziness
      b. Used for acute pain and as a preoperative medication
      c. Can cause **increased intracranial pressure** in head injuries
      d. Contraindicated in head injuries and **increased intracranial pressure**, respiratory disorders, hypotension, shock, severe hepatic and renal disease, and in clients taking monoamine oxidase inhibitors
      e. Should not be taken with alcohol or sedative hypnotics because it may increase the CNS depression
   4. Morphine sulfate
      a. Can cause respiratory depression, orthostatic hypotension, and constipation
      b. May cause nausea and vomiting because of increased vestibular sensitivity
      c. Used for acute pain due to myocardial infarction (MI) or cancer, for dyspnea due to pulmonary edema, and as a preoperative or postoperative medication
      d. Contraindicated in severe respiratory disorders, head injuries, **increased intracranial pressure**, severe renal disease, or seizure activity
      e. Used with caution in clients with shock or blood loss
   5. Oxycodone with aspirin (Percodan)
      a. Should not be taken by a client allergic to aspirin
      b. Can cause gastric irritation and should be taken with food or plenty of liquids
   6. Propoxyphene hydrochloride (Darvon) and propoxyphene napsylate (Darvon-N)
      a. Darvon compound contains aspirin and should not be taken by a client allergic to aspirin
      b. Darvocet-N contains acetaminophen
   7. Nalbuphine hydrochloride (Nubain): Preferable for treating the pain of an MI because it reduces the oxygen needs of the heart without reducing blood pressure
   8. Methadone hydrochloride (Dolophine)
      a. Dilute doses of oral concentrate with at least 90 mL of water
      b. Dilute dispersible tablets in at least 120 mL of water, orange juice, or acidic fruit beverage
      c. Used as a replacement medication for opiate dependence or to facilitate withdrawal
   9. Hydrocodone (Hycodan): Frequently used for cough suppression

---

BOX 57-16

Narcotic Analgesics

Codeine sulfate; codeine phosphate
Hydromorphone hydrochloride (Dilaudid)
Meperidine hydrochloride (Demerol)
Morphine Sulfate
Oxycodone hydrochloride with Acetaminophen (Percocet)
Oxycodone with aspirin (Percodan)
Propoxyphene napsylate (Darvon-N)
Buprenorphine hydrochloride (Buprenex)
Butorphanol tartrate (Stadol, Stadol NS)
Nalbuphine hydrochloride (Nubain)
Methadone hydrochloride (Dolophine, Methadose)
Pentazocine hydrochloride (Talwin)
Hydrocodone (Hycodan)
Levorphanol tartrate (Levo-Dromoran)
Fentanyl (Duragesic, Sulimaze)
Sufentanil Citrate (Sufenta)
Oxycodone (Roxicodone)
Oxymorphone hydrochloride (Numorphan)
Tramadol hydrochloride (Ultram)

C. Interventions for narcotic analgesics
1. Monitor vital signs
2. Assess the client thoroughly before administering pain medication
3. Initiate nursing measures such as massage, distraction, deep breathing and relaxation exercises, the application of heat or cold as prescribed, and providing care and comfort prior to administering the narcotic analgesic
4. Administer medications 30 to 60 minutes before painful activities
5. Monitor respiratory rate; if the rate is less than 12 breaths per minute in an adult, withhold the medication unless ventilatory support is being provided
6. Monitor pulse; if bradycardia develops, hold the dose and notify the physician
7. Monitor blood pressure for hypotension
8. Auscultate breath sounds because narcotic analgesics suppress the cough reflex
9. Encourage activities such as turning, deep breathing, and incentive spirometry to prevent atelectasis and pneumonia
10. Monitor level of consciousness (LOC)
11. Initiate safety precautions such as side rails, a night light, and supervised ambulation
12. Monitor input and output (I&O)
13. Assess for urinary retention
14. Instruct the client to take oral doses with milk or a snack to reduce gastric irritation
15. Instruct the client to avoid alcohol
16. Instruct the client to avoid activities that require alertness
17. Note effectiveness of medication
18. Have the narcotic antagonist, oxygen, and resuscitation equipment available

D. Morphine sulfate
1. Side effects
   a. Respiratory depression
   b. Orthostatic hypotension
   c. Urinary retention
   d. Nausea
   e. Vomiting
   f. Constipation
   g. Cough suppression
   h. Reduction in pupillary size
   i. Miosis
2. Interventions
   a. Have naxolone (Narcan) available for overdose
   b. Monitor vital signs
   c. Note rate and depth of respirations
   d. Withhold the medication if the respiratory rate is less than 12 breaths per minute; respirations less than 10 breaths per minute can indicate respiratory distress
   e. Monitor urinary output, which should be at least 600 mL/day

---

BOX 57-17

Narcotic Antagonists

Nalmefene (Revex)
Naloxone hydrochloride (Narcan)
Naltrexone (ReVia)

---

   f. Monitor bowel sounds for decreased peristalsis because constipation can occur
   g. Monitor for pupil changes, because pinpoint pupils can indicate morphine overdose
   h. Avoid alcohol or CNS depressants because they can cause respiratory depression
   i. Instruct the client to report dizziness or difficulty breathing

E. Meperidine hydrochloride (Demerol)
1. Side effects
   a. Respiratory depression
   b. Hypotension
   c. Drowsiness
   d. Constipation
   e. Urinary retention
   f. Nausea
   g. Vomiting
   h. Tremors
2. Interventions
   a. Monitor vital signs
   b. Monitor for respiratory dysfunction and hypotension
   c. Have naloxone (Narcan) available for overdose
   d. Monitor for urinary retention
   e. Monitor bowel sounds and for constipation

VII. NARCOTIC ANTAGONISTS (Box 57-17)

A. Used to treat respiratory depression from narcotic overdose
B. Interventions
1. Monitor blood pressure, pulse, and respiratory rate every 5 minutes initially, tapering to every 15 minutes, then every 30 minutes until stable
2. Place the client on a cardiac monitor and monitor cardiac rhythm
3. Auscultate breath sounds
4. Have resuscitation equipment available
5. Do not leave the client unattended
6. Monitor the client closely for several hours because when the effects of the antagonist wear off, the client may again display signs of narcotic overdose

VIII. OSMOTIC DIURETICS (Box 57-18)

A. Description
1. Increase osmotic pressure of the glomerular filtrate, inhibiting reabsorption of water and electrolytes

BOX 57-18

Osmotic Diuretics

Mannitol (Osmitrol)
Urea (Ureaphil)

2. Used for oliguria and to prevent renal failure
3. Used to decrease intracranial pressure
4. Used to decrease intraocular pressure in narrow-angle glaucoma
5. Mannitol is used with chemotherapy to induce diuresis

B. Side effects
1. Fluid and electrolyte imbalances
2. Pulmonary edema from the rapid shifts of fluid
3. Nausea and vomiting
4. Tachycardia from the rapid fluid loss
5. Hyponatremia and dehydration

C. Interventions
1. Monitor vital signs
2. Monitor weight
3. Monitor urine output
4. Monitor electrolyte levels
5. Monitor lungs and heart sounds for signs of pulmonary edema
6. Monitor for signs of dehydration
7. Monitor neurological status
8. Monitor for signs of decreasing intracranial pressure if appropriate
9. Change the client's position slowly to prevent orthostatic hypotension

PRACTICE QUESTIONS

1. A nurse is caring for a client diagnosed with Bell's palsy. The client has been taking acetaminophen (Tylenol) for discomfort and an acetaminophen overdose is suspected. The nurse anticipates that the antidote to be prepared for administration is:
   1. Auranofin (Ridaura)
   2. Fludarabine (Fludara)
   3. Acetylcysteine (Mucomyst)
   4. Pentostatin (Nipent)

2. A client with trigeminal neuralgia tells the nurse that acetaminophen (Tylenol) is taken on a frequent daily basis for relief of generalized discomfort. The nurse reviews the client's laboratory results and determines that which of the following indicates toxicity associated with the medication?
   1. Platelet count of 400,000 cells/μl
   2. A direct bilirubin level of 2 mg/dL
   3. Prothrombin time of 12 seconds
   4. Sodium of 140 mEq/L

3. A nurse is assisting in preparing to administer acetyl-cysteine (Mucomyst) to the client with an overdose of acetaminophen (Tylenol). The nurse prepares to administer the medication by:
   1. Mixing the medication in a flavored ice drink and allowing the client to drink the medication through a straw
   2. Administering the medication by the intramuscular route, mixed in 10 mL of normal saline
   3. Administering the medication by the intramuscular route in the gluteal muscle
   4. Administering the medication subcutaneously in the deltoid muscle

4. A client is receiving baclofen (Lioresal) for muscle spasms due to a spinal cord injury. The nurse monitors the client, knowing that which of the following is a side effect of this medication?
   1. Photosensitivity
   2. Slurred speech
   3. Hypertension
   4. Muscle pain

5. A client is suspected of having myasthenia gravis and the physician administers edrophonium (Tensilon) intravenously to determine the diagnosis. Following administration of this medication, which of the following would indicate the presence of myasthenia gravis?
   1. An increase in muscle strength
   2. A decrease in muscle strength
   3. Joint pain
   4. Feelings of faintness, dizziness, hypotension, and signs of flushing in the client

6. A client with myasthenia gravis is suspected of having cholinergic crisis. Which of the following would indicate that this crisis exists?
   1. Hypotension
   2. Hypertension
   3. Mouth sores
   4. Ataxia

7. A client with myasthenia gravis is receiving pyridostig-mine (Mestinon). The nurse monitors for signs and symptoms of cholinergic crisis caused by overdose of the medication. The nurse checks the medication supply to ensure that which medication is available for administration if a cholinergic crisis occurs?
   1. Vitamin K
   2. Protamine sulfate
   3. Acetylcysteine (Mucomyst)
   4. Atropine sulfate

8. A client with myasthenia gravis becomes increasingly weaker. The physician prepares to identify whether the client is reacting to an overdose of the medication (cholinergic crisis) or to increasing severity of the disease (myasthenic crisis). An injection of edrophonium (Tensilon) is administered. Which of the following would indicate that the client is in cholinergic crisis?
   1. An improvement of the weakness
   2. A temporary worsening of the condition

3. No change is the condition

4. Complaints of muscle spasms

9. A client with myasthenia gravis verbalizes complaints of feeling much weaker than normal. The physician plans to implement a diagnostic test to determine if the client is experiencing a myasthenic crisis and administers edrophonium (Tensilon). Which of the following would indicate that the client is experiencing a myasthenic crisis?

1. Increasing weakness

2. No change in the condition

3. A temporary improvement in the condition

4. An increase in muscle spasms

10. Levodopa (Carbidopa) is prescribed for a client with Parkinson's disease, and the nurse monitors the client for adverse reactions to the medication. Which of the following would indicate that the client is experiencing an adverse reaction?

1. Pruritus

2. Hypertension

3. Tachycardia

4. Impaired voluntary movements

11. Phenytoin (Dilantin), 100 mg PO three times daily, has been prescribed for a client for seizure control. The nurse reinforces instructions regarding the medication to the client. Which statement by the client would indicate an understanding of the instructions?

1. "It's all right to break the capsules to make it easier for me to swallow them."

2. "I will use a soft toothbrush to brush my teeth."

3. "If I forget to take my medication, I can wait until the next dose and eliminate that dose."

4. "If my throat becomes sore, it's a normal effect of the medication and it's nothing to be concerned about."

12. A client is taking phenytoin (Dilantin) for seizure control and a sample for a serum drug level is drawn. Which of the following would indicate a therapeutic serum drug range?

1. 5 to 10 mcg/mL

2. 10 to 20 mcg/mL

3. 20 to 30 mcg/mL

4. 30 to 40 mcg/mL

13. Ibuprofen (Motrin) is prescribed for a client. The nurse tells the client to take the medication:

1. 60 minutes before breakfast

2. At bedtime on an empty stomach

3. With 8 oz of milk

4. In the morning after arising

14. A nurse is caring for a client who is taking phenytoin (Dilantin) for control of seizures. During data collection, the nurse notes that the client is taking birth control pills. Which of the following information should the nurse provide to the client?

1. The increased risk of thrombophlebitis exists while taking phenytoin (Dilantin) and birth control pills together

2. The potential for decreased effectiveness of the birth control pills exists while taking phenytoin (Dilantin)

3. The client may stop taking the phenytoin (Dilantin) if it is causing severe gastrointestinal effects

4. Pregnancy should be avoided while taking phenytoin (Dilantin)

15. A client with trigeminal neuralgia is being treated with carbamazepine (Tegretol). Which laboratory result would indicate that the client is experiencing an adverse reaction to the medication?

1. White blood cell count, 3000/µl

2. Blood urea nitrogen (BUN) level, 15 mg/dL

3. Sodium level, 140 mEq/L

4. Uric acid level, 5.0 ng/dL

16. A client with multiple sclerosis is receiving diazepam (Valium), a centrally acting skeletal muscle relaxant. Which of the following would indicate that the client is experiencing a side effect related to this medication?

1. Headache

2. Increased salivation

3. Urinary retention

4. Drowsiness

17. A nurse is caring for a client receiving morphine sulfate subcutaneously for pain. Because morphine sulfate has been prescribed for this client, which nursing action would be included in the plan of care?

1. Monitor the client's temperature

2. Encourage fluid intake

3. Maintain the client in a supine position

4. Encourage the client to cough and deep breath

18. Meperidine (Demerol) is prescribed for the client with pain. Which of the following would the nurse monitor for as a side effect of this medication?

1. Hypertension

2. Bradycardia

3. Diarrhea

4. Urinary retention

19. A nurse is caring for a client with severe back pain and codeine sulfate has been prescribed for the client. Which of the following would the nurse include in the plan of care while the client is taking this medication?

1. Monitor for hypertension

2. Restrict fluid intake

3. Monitor bowel activity

4. Monitor peripheral pulses

20. Dantrolene (Dantrium) is prescribed for a client with a spinal cord injury for discomfort resulting from spasticity. The nurse tells the client about the importance of follow-up and the need for which blood study?

1. Sedimentation rate

2. White blood cell count

3. Liver function studies
4. Creatinine level

21. A client with epilepsy is taking the prescribed dose of phenytoin (Dilantin) to control seizures. A phenytoin (Dilantin) blood level is drawn, and the results reveal a level of 35 mcg/mL. Which of the following symptoms would be expected as a result of this laboratory result?
    1. No symptoms, because this is a normal therapeutic level
    2. Slurred speech
    3. Tachycardia
    4. Nystagmus

22. A physician initiates levodopa (Larodopa) therapy for the client with Parkinson's disease. A few days after the client starts the medication, the client complains of nausea and vomiting. The nurse tells the client that:
    1. This is an expected side effect of the medication
    2. Taking the medication with food will help to prevent the nausea
    3. Taking an antiemetic is the best measure to prevent the nausea
    4. The nausea and vomiting will decrease when the dose of levodopa is stabilized

23. Mannitol (Osmitrol) is being administered to a client with increased intracranial pressure following a head injury. The nurse assisting in caring for the client knows that which of the following indicates the therapeutic action of this medication?
    1. Induces diuresis by raising the osmotic pressure of glomerular filtrate, thereby inhibiting tubular reabsorption of water and solutes
    2. Decreases water loss by promoting the reabsorption of sodium and water in the loop of Henle
    3. Prevents the filtration of sodium and water through the kidneys
    4. Prevents the filtration of sodium and potassium through the kidneys

24. Carbamazepine (Tegretol) is prescribed for a client with a diagnosis of psychomotor seizures. The nurse reviews the client's health history, knowing that this medication is contraindicated if which of the following disorders is present?
    1. Liver disease
    2. Headaches
    3. Hypothyroidism
    4. Diabetes mellitus

25. A client is admitted to the hospital with complaints of back spasms. The client states, "I have been taking two to three aspirin every 4 hours for the last week and it hasn't helped my back." Aspirin intoxication is suspected. Which of the following complaints would indicate aspirin intoxication?
    1. Abdominal cramps
    2. Constipation
    3. Tinnitus
    4. Photosensitivity

ALTERNATE FORMAT QUESTION: MULTIPLE RESPONSE

A client is receiving meperidine hydrochloride (Demerol) for pain. Select the side effects of this medication.
___ Increased respiratory rate
___ Drowsiness
___ Hypotension
___ Urinary frequency
___ Diarrhea

ANSWERS

1. *Answer: 3*
Rationale: The antidote for acetaminophen (Tylenol) is acetylcysteine (Mucomyst). Auranofin (Ridaura) is a gold preparation used in rheumatoid arthritis. Fludarabine (Fludara) and pentostatin (Nipent) are antineoplastic agents.
Test-Taking Strategy: Knowledge regarding the antidote for acetaminophen (Tylenol) and the medication classifications noted in the options will assist you in answering this question. Remember, the antidote for acetaminophen (Tylenol) is acetylcysteine (Mucomyst). If you had difficulty with this question, review antidotes.
Level of Cognitive Ability: Analysis
Client Needs: Physiological Integrity
Integrated Process: Nursing Process/Planning
Content Area: Pharmacology
Reference: Hodgson, B., & Kizior, R. (2005). *Saunders nursing drug handbook 2005.* Philadelphia: W.B. Saunders, p. 9.

2. *Answer: 2*
Rationale: In adults, overdose of acetaminophen (Tylenol) causes liver damage. Option 2 is an indicator of liver function, and is the only option that indicates an abnormal laboratory value. The normal direct bilirubin is 0 to 0.4 mg/dL. The normal platelet count is 150,000 to 400,000 cells/μl. The normal prothrombin time is 10 to 13 seconds. The normal sodium level is 135 to 145 mEq/L.
Test-Taking Strategy: Knowledge that acetaminophen (Tylenol) causes liver damage and knowledge of the normal laboratory results will be helpful in answering this question. Reviewing the laboratory values in the options will direct you to option 2, the only abnormal value. Also, of all the options, the bilirubin is the laboratory value most directly related to liver function. Review the indicators of toxicity if you had difficulty with this question.
Level of Cognitive Ability: Analysis
Client Needs: Physiological Integrity

Integrated Process: Nursing Process/Data Collection
Content Area: Pharmacology
Reference: Hodgson, B., & Kizior, R. (2005). *Saunders nursing drug handbook 2005.* Philadelphia: W.B. Saunders, p. 8.

3. Answer: 1
Rationale: Because acetylcysteine (Mucomyst) has a pervasive odor of rotten eggs, it must be disguised in a flavored ice drink, and is preferably drunk through a straw to minimize contact with the mouth. It is not administered by the intramuscular or subcutaneous route.
Test-Taking Strategy: Use the process of elimination. Knowing that the medication is a solution that is also used for nebulization treatments will assist you to select the option that indicates an oral route. Note that options 2, 3, and 4 indicate parenteral administration and option 1, the correct option, indicates oral administration. Review this medication if you had difficulty with this question.
Level of Cognitive Ability: Application
Client Needs: Physiological Integrity
Integrated Process: Nursing Process/Implementation
Content Area: Pharmacology
Reference: Hodgson, B., & Kizior, R. (2005). *Saunders nursing drug handbook 2005.* Philadelphia: W.B. Saunders, p. 1142.

4. Answer: 2
Rationale: Side effects of baclofen (Lioresal) include drowsiness, dizziness, weakness, and nausea. Occasional side effects include headache, paresthesia of the hands and feet, constipation or diarrhea, anorexia, hypotension, confusion, and nasal congestion. Paradoxical central nervous system excitement and restlessness can occur, along with slurred speech, tremor, dry mouth, nocturia, and impotence. Options 1, 3, and 4 are not side effects of this medication.
Test-Taking Strategy: Note the client's diagnosis. Option 2 is the option that is most closely associated with a neurological disorder. If you had difficulty with this question, review the side effects related to baclofen (Lioresal).
Level of Cognitive Ability: Application
Client Needs: Physiological Integrity
Integrated Process: Nursing Process/Data Collection
Content Area: Pharmacology
Reference: Hodgson, B., & Kizior, R. (2005). *Saunders nursing drug handbook 2005.* Philadelphia: W.B. Saunders, p. 108.

5. Answer: 1
Rationale: Edrophonium (Tensilon) is a short-acting acetylcholinesterase inhibitor used as a diagnostic agent. When a client with suspected myasthenia gravis is given the medication intravenously, an increase in muscle strength would be seen in 1 to 3 minutes. If no response occurs, another dose of edrophonium (Tensilon) is given over the next 2 minutes and muscle strength is again tested. If no increase in muscle strength occurs with this higher dose, the muscle weakness is not caused by myasthenia gravis. Clients receiving injections of this medication commonly demonstrate a drop of blood pressure, feel faint and dizzy, and are flushed.
Test-Taking Strategy: Recalling the pathophysiology associated with myasthenia gravis and the action of edrophonium (Tensilon) will direct you to option 1. Review this medication

as a diagnostic tool for suspected myasthenia gravis you had difficulty with this question.
Level of Cognitive Ability: Analysis
Client Needs: Physiological Integrity
Integrated Process: Nursing Process/Evaluation
Content Area: Pharmacology
Reference: Skidmore-Roth, L. (2005). *Mosby's drug guide for nurses* (6th ed.). St. Louis: Mosby, p. 303.

6. Answer: 2
Rationale: Cholinergic crisis occurs as a result of an overdose of medication. Indications of cholinergic crisis includes gastrointestinal disturbances, nausea, vomiting, diarrhea, abdominal cramps, increased salivation and tearing, miosis, hypertension, sweating, and increased bronchial secretions.
Test-Taking Strategy: Use the process of elimination. Note that options 1 and 2 identify opposite effects. This indicates that one of them may be the correct option. Remember, hypertension occurs with cholinergic crisis. Review both cholinergic and myasthenic crisis if you had difficulty with this question.
Level of Cognitive Ability: Analysis
Client Needs: Physiological Integrity
Integrated Process: Nursing Process/Data Collection
Content Area: Pharmacology
References: Lilley, L., Harrington, S., & Snyder, J. (2005). *Pharmacology and the nursing process* (4th ed.). St. Louis: Mosby, p. 326.
Linton, A. & Maebius, N. (2003). *Introduction to medical-surgical nursing* (3rd ed.). Philadelphia: W.B. Saunders, p. 403.

7. Answer: 4
Rationale: The antidote for cholinergic crisis is atropine sulfate. Vitamin K is the antidote for warfarin (Coumadin). Protamine sulfate is the antidote for heparin, and acetylcysteine (Mucomyst) is the antidote for acetaminophen (Tylenol).
Test-Taking Strategy: Knowledge regarding antidotes for various medications is needed to answer this question. Remember that atropine sulfate is the antidote for cholinergic crisis. Review antidotes if you had difficulty with this question.
Level of Cognitive Ability: Application
Client Needs: Physiological Integrity
Integrated Process: Nursing Process/Implementation
Content Area: Pharmacology
Reference: Lilley, L., Harrington, S., & Snyder, J. (2005). *Pharmacology and the nursing process* (4th ed.). St. Louis: Mosby, p. 327.

8. Answer: 2
Rationale: An edrophonium (Tensilon) injection makes the client in cholinergic crisis temporarily worse. This is known as a negative Tensilon test. An improvement of weakness would occur if the client were experiencing myasthenia gravis. Options 3 and 4 would not occur in either crisis.
Test-Taking Strategy: Focus on the data in the question. Noting the words "overdose of the medication (cholinergic crisis)" will direct you to option 2. It makes sense that administering additional medication will worsen the condition. Review this diagnostic test and the differences between

cholinergic and myasthenic crisis if you had difficulty with this question.
Level of Cognitive Ability: Analysis
Client Needs: Physiological Integrity
Integrated Process: Nursing Process/Evaluation
Content Area: Pharmacology
Reference: Chernecky, C., & Berger, B. (2004). *Laboratory tests and diagnostic procedures* (4th ed.). Philadelphia: W.B. Saunders, p. 1035.

9. *Answer:* **3**
Rationale: Edrophonium (Tensilon) is administered to determine whether the client is reacting to an overdose of a medication (cholinergic crisis) or to an increasing severity of the disease (myasthenic crisis). When the edrophonium (Tensilon) injection is given and the condition improves temporarily, the client is in myasthenic crisis. This is known as a positive Tensilon test. Increasing weakness would occur in cholinergic crisis. Options 3 and 4 would not occur in either crisis.
Test-Taking Strategy: Use the process of elimination. Recalling that myasthenia crisis is an increasing severity of the disease that will improve with medication will direct you to option 3. Review this diagnostic test and the differences between cholinergic and myasthenic crisis if you had difficulty with this question.
Level of Cognitive Ability: Analysis
Client Needs: Physiological Integrity
Integrated Process: Nursing Process/Evaluation
Content Area: Pharmacology
Reference: McKenry, L., & Salerno, E. (2003). *Mosby's pharmacology in nursing* (21st ed.). St. Louis: Mosby, pp. 506-507.

10. *Answer:* **4**
Rationale: Dyskinesia and impaired voluntary movement may occur with high levodopa dosages. Nausea, anorexia, dizziness, orthostatic hypotension, bradycardia, and akinesia (the temporary muscle weakness that lasts 1 minute to 1 hour, also known as the "on-off phenomenon") are frequent side effects of the medication.
Test-Taking Strategy: Use the process of elimination. Options 2 and 3 are cardiac-related options, so these options can be eliminated first. Note that the question asks for an adverse reaction; therefore, select option 4 over option 1 as the correct answer. Review the adverse effects of carbidopa and levodopa if you had difficulty with this question.
Level of Cognitive Ability: Analysis
Client Needs: Physiological Integrity
Integrated Process: Nursing Process/Data Collection
Content Area: Pharmacology
Reference: Hodgson, B., & Kizior, R. (2005). *Saunders nursing drug handbook 2005.* Philadelphia: W.B. Saunders, p.168.

11. *Answer:* **2**
Rationale: Phenytoin (Dilantin) it an anticonvulsant. Gingival hyperplasia, bleeding, swelling, and tenderness of the gums can occur with the use of this medication. The client needs to be taught good oral hygiene, gum massage, and the need for regular dentist visits. The client should not skip medication doses, because this could precipitate a seizure.

Capsules should not be chewed or broken and they must be swallowed. The client needs to be instructed to report a sore throat, fever, glandular swelling, or any skin reaction, because this indicates hematological toxicity.
Test-Taking Strategy: Use the process of elimination. Note the key words, *an understanding of the instructions.* Eliminate option 3 because the client needs to be encouraged to take medications on time. Also, eliminate option 4 because the client needs to report these symptoms to the physician. From the remaining options, recalling that capsules should not be broken will direct you to option 2. Review the side effects related to phenytoin (Dilantin) if you had difficulty with this question.
Level of Cognitive Ability: Analysis
Client Needs: Health Promotion and Maintenance
Integrated Process: Nursing Process/Evaluation
Content Area: Pharmacology
Reference: Hodgson, B., & Kizior, R. (2005). *Saunders nursing drug handbook 2005.* Philadelphia: W.B. Saunders, p. 858.

12. *Answer:* **2**
Rationale: The therapeutic serum drug level range for phenytoin (Dilantin) is 10 to 20 mcg/mL.
Test-Taking Strategy: Knowledge regarding the therapeutic serum range of this medication is required to answer the question. A helpful hint may be to remember that the theophylline therapeutic range and the acetaminophen (Tylenol) therapeutic range are the same as the phenytoin (Dilantin) therapeutic range. Remembering this may assist you when answering questions related to any of these three medications. Review this therapeutic level if you had difficulty with this question.
Level of Cognitive Ability: Comprehension
Client Needs: Physiological Integrity
Integrated Process: Nursing Process/Data Collection
Content Area: Pharmacology
Reference: Hodgson, B., & Kizior, R. (2005). *Saunders nursing drug handbook 2005.* Philadelphia: W.B. Saunders, p. 858.

13. *Answer:* **3**
Rationale: Ibuprofen (Motrin) is a nonsteroidal anti-inflammatory drug (NSAID). NSAIDs should be given with milk or food to prevent gastrointestinal irritation. Options 1, 2, and 4 are incorrect.
Test-Taking Strategy: Use the process of elimination. Note the similarity in options 1, 2, and 4. Each of these options indicates administering the medication without food. Remember, NSAIDs can cause gastric irritation. Review this medication if you had difficulty with this question.
Level of Cognitive Ability: Application
Client Needs: Health Promotion and Maintenance
Integrated Process: Teaching/Learning
Content Area: Pharmacology
References: Hodgson, B., & Kizior, R. (2005). *Saunders nursing drug handbook 2005.* Philadelphia: W.B. Saunders, p. 87.
Lilley, L., Harrington, S., & Snyder, J. (2005). *Pharmacology and the nursing process* (4th ed.). St. Louis: Mosby, p. 742.

14. *Answer:* **2**
Rationale: Phenytoin (Dilantin) enhances the rate of estrogen metabolism, which can decrease the effectiveness of some birth control pills. Options 1, 3, are 4 are not accurate.

Test-Taking Strategy: Use the process of elimination. Option 1 would cause anxiety in the client. A client should not be instructed to stop anticonvulsant medication. Pregnancy does not need to be "avoided." Review medication interactions related to phenytoin (Dilantin) if you had difficulty with this question.
Level of Cognitive Ability: Application
Client Needs: Health Promotion and Maintenance
Integrated Process: Nursing Process/Implementation
Content Area: Pharmacology
Reference: Lehne, R. (2004). *Pharmacology for nursing care* (5th ed.). Philadelphia: W.B. Saunders, p. 208.

15. *Answer:* 1
Rationale: Adverse effects of carbamazepine (Tegretol) appear as blood dyscrasias, including aplastic anemia, agranulocytosis, thrombocytopenia, leukopenia, cardiovascular disturbances, thrombophlebitis, dysrhythmias, and dermatological effects. Options 2, 3, and 4 identify normal laboratory values.
Test-Taking Strategy: Use the process of elimination. If you are familiar with normal laboratory values, you will note that the only option that indicates an abnormal value is option 1. Review the signs of adverse reactions related to this medication if you had difficulty with this question.
Level of Cognitive Ability: Analysis
Client Needs: Physiological Integrity
Integrated Process: Nursing Process/Data Collection
Content Area: Pharmacology
Reference: Lehne, R. (2004). *Pharmacology for nursing care* (5th ed.). Philadelphia: W.B. Saunders, p. 198.

16. *Answer:* 4
Rationale: Incoordination and drowsiness are common side effects resulting from this medication. Options 1, 2, and 3 are incorrect.
Test-Taking Strategy: Note that the question addresses a centrally acting skeletal muscle relaxant. This may assist you in the process of elimination and direct you to the correct option, drowsiness. If you had difficulty with this question, review the side effects associated with diazepam (Valium).
Level of Cognitive Ability: Analysis
Client Needs: Physiological Integrity
Integrated Process: Nursing Process/Data Collection
Content Area: Pharmacology
Reference: Hodgson, B., & Kizior, R. (2005). *Saunders nursing drug handbook 2005.* Philadelphia: W.B. Saunders, p. 316.

17. *Answer:* 4
Rationale: Morphine sulfate suppresses the cough reflex. Clients need to be encouraged to cough and deep breathe to prevent pneumonia. Options 1, 2, and 3 are not specifically associated with this medication.
Test-Taking Strategy: Use the process of elimination. Recalling that morphine sulfate suppresses the cough reflex and the respiratory reflex will direct you to the correct option. Additionally, use the ABCs—airway, breathing, and circulation—to direct you to option 4. Review this medication if you had difficulty with this question.
Level of Cognitive Ability: Application

Client Needs: Physiological Integrity
Integrated Process: Nursing Process/Planning
Content Area: Pharmacology
Reference: Hodgson, B., & Kizior, R. (2005). *Saunders nursing drug handbook 2005.* Philadelphia: W.B. Saunders, p. 734.

18. *Answer:* 4
Rationale: Side effects of this medication include respiratory depression, orthostatic hypotension, tachycardia, drowsiness and mental clouding, constipation, and urinary retention.
Test-Taking Strategy: Knowledge regarding side effects associated with narcotic analgesics will assist you in answering the question. Remember, a side effect of meperidine is urinary retention. If you had difficulty with this question, review this medication.
Level of Cognitive Ability: Analysis
Client Needs: Physiological Integrity
Integrated Process: Nursing Process/Data Collection
Content Area: Pharmacology
Reference: Hodgson, B., & Kizior, R. (2005). *Saunders nursing drug handbook 2005.* Philadelphia: W.B. Saunders, p. 675.

19. *Answer:* 3
Rationale: While the client is taking codeine sulfate, the nurse would monitor vital signs and monitor for hypotension. The nurse should also increase fluid intake, palpate the bladder for urinary retention, auscultate bowel sounds, and monitor the pattern of daily bowel activity and stool consistency. The nurse should monitor respiratory status and initiate breathing and coughing exercises. Additionally, the nurse monitors the effectiveness of the pain medication.
Test-Taking Strategy: Use the process of elimination. Recalling that codeine sulfate can cause constipation will direct you to option 3. If you had difficulty with this question, review nursing measures related to the administration of codeine sulfate.
Level of Cognitive Ability: Application
Client Needs: Physiological Integrity
Integrated Process: Nursing Process/Planning
Content Area: Pharmacology
Reference: Hodgson, B., & Kizior, R. (2005). *Saunders nursing drug handbook 2005.* Philadelphia: W.B. Saunders, p. 254.

20. *Answer:* 3
Rationale: Dantrolene can cause liver damage, and the nurse should monitor liver function studies. Baseline liver function studies are done before therapy starts, and regular liver function studies are performed throughout therapy. Dantrolene is discontinued if no relief of spasticity is achieved in 6 weeks.
Test-Taking Strategy: Use the process of elimination. Recalling that this medication is hepatotoxic will direct you to the correct option. If you had difficulty with this question, review this medication.
Level of Cognitive Ability: Application
Client Needs: Physiological Integrity
Integrated Process: Nursing Process/Implementation
Content Area: Pharmacology
Reference: Hodgson, B., & Kizior, R. (2005). *Saunders nursing drug handbook 2005.* Philadelphia: W.B. Saunders, p. 286.

21. *Answer:* **2**

Rationale: The therapeutic phenytoin (Dilantin) level is 10 to 20 mcg/mL. At a level higher than 20 mcg/mL, involuntary movements of the eyeballs (nystagmus) appears. At a level higher than 30 mcg/mL, ataxia and slurred speech occur.

Test-Taking Strategy: Knowledge regarding the therapeutic phenytoin (Dilantin) level and the manifestations that occur when the level is elevated is required to answer this question. Review the therapeutic levels and associated signs if you had difficulty with this question.

Level of Cognitive Ability: Analysis
Client Needs: Physiological Integrity
Integrated Process: Nursing Process/Data Collection
Content Area: Pharmacology
Reference: Hodgson, B., & Kizior, R. (2005). *Saunders nursing drug handbook 2005.* Philadelphia: W.B. Saunders, p. 857.

22. *Answer:* **2**

Rationale: If levodopa is causing nausea and vomiting, the nurse would tell the client that taking the medication with food will prevent the nausea. Antiemetics from the phenothiazine class should not be used because they block the therapeutic action of dopamine. The other options are incorrect.

Test-Taking Strategy: Use the process of elimination. Eliminate option 3 first, because it is best to use nonpharmacological approaches initially to alleviate the nausea. Next, eliminate options 1 and 4 because they are similar. Review this medication if you had difficulty with this question.

Level of Cognitive Ability: Application
Client Needs: Physiological Integrity
Integrated Process: Nursing Process/Implementation
Content Area: Pharmacology
Reference: Lehne, R. (2004). *Pharmacology for nursing care* (5th ed.). Philadelphia: W.B. Saunders, p. 183.

23. *Answer:* **1**

Rationale: Mannitol (Osmitrol) is an osmotic diuretic that induces diuresis by raising the osmotic pressure of glomerular filtrate, thereby inhibiting tubular reabsorption of water and solutes. It is used to reduce intracranial pressure in the client with head trauma.

Test-Taking Strategy: Use the process of elimination. Read the question carefully, noting that it presents a client with increased intracranial pressure. The only option that suggests an action that will produce diuresis, and thus reduce intracranial pressure, is option 1. If you had difficulty with this question, review the action of mannitol (Osmitrol).

Level of Cognitive Ability: Analysis
Client Needs: Physiological Integrity
Integrated Process: Nursing Process/Evaluation
Content Area: Pharmacology
Reference: Hodgson, B., & Kizior, R. (2005). *Saunders nursing drug handbook 2005.* Philadelphia: W.B. Saunders, p. 662.

24. *Answer:* **1**

Rationale: Carbamazepine (Tegretol) is contraindicated in liver disease, and liver function tests are routinely prescribed for baseline purposes and are monitored during therapy. It is also contraindicated if the client has a history of blood dyscrasias. It is not contraindicated in the conditions noted in options 2, 3, and 4.

Test-Taking Strategy: Knowledge regarding the contraindications associated with carbamazepine (Tegretol) is required to answer this question. Remember, carbamazepine (Tegretol) is contraindicated in liver disease. Review this medication if you are unfamiliar with it.

Level of Cognitive Ability: Analysis
Client Needs: Physiological Integrity
Integrated Process: Nursing Process/Data Collection
Content Area: Pharmacology
Reference: Skidmore-Roth, L. (2005). *Mosby's drug guide for nurses* (6th ed.). St. Louis: Mosby, p. 136.

25. *Answer:* **3**

Rationale: Mild intoxication with acetylsalicylic acid (Aspirin) is called salicylism and is commonly experienced when the daily dosage is higher than 4 g. Tinnitus (ringing in the ears) is the most frequently occurring effect noted with intoxication. Hyperventilation may occur because salicylate stimulates the respiratory center. Fever may result because salicylate interferes with the metabolic pathways involved with oxygen consumption and heat production. Options 1, 2, and 4 are incorrect.

Test-Taking Strategy: Use the process of elimination. Focus on the issue of the question, aspirin intoxication. Eliminate options 1 and 2, because they both relate to gastrointestinal symptoms. Option 3, the correct answer, is the indicator of toxicity. If you had difficulty with this question, review aspirin intoxication.

Level of Cognitive Ability: Analysis
Client Needs: Physiological Integrity
Integrated Process: Nursing Process/Data Collection
Content Area: Pharmacology
Reference: Skidmore-Roth, L. (2005). *Mosby's drug guide for nurses* (6th ed.). St. Louis: Mosby, p. 76.

ALTERNATE FORMAT QUESTION: MULTIPLE RESPONSE

Answers:
Drowsiness
Hypotension

Rationale: Meperidine hydrochloride is a narcotic analgesic. Side effects include respiratory depression, hypotension, drowsiness, constipation, urinary retention, nausea, vomiting, and tremors.

Test-Taking Strategy: Focus on the name of the medication. Recalling that this medication is a narcotic analgesic and recalling the effects of a narcotic analgesic will assist in identifying the side effects. Review the side effects of this medication if you had difficulty with this question.

Level of Cognitive Ability: Analysis
Client Needs: Physiological Integrity
Integrated Process: Nursing Process/Data Collection
Content Area: Pharmacology
Reference: *Mosby's 2005 drug consult for nurses.* (2005). St. Louis: Mosby, p. 812.

REFERENCES

Chernecky, C., & Berger, B. (2004). *Laboratory tests and diagnostic procedures* (4th ed.). Philadelphia: W.B. Saunders.

Hodgson, B., & Kizior, R. (2005). *Saunders nursing drug handbook 2005.* Philadelphia: W.B. Saunders.

Lehne, R. (2004). *Pharmacology for nursing care* (5th ed.). Philadelphia: W.B. Saunders.

Lilley, L., Harrington, S., & Snyder, J. (2005). *Pharmacology and the nursing process* (4th ed.). St. Louis: Mosby.

Linton, A., & Maebius, N. (2003). *Introduction to medical-surgical nursing* (3rd ed.). Philadelphia: W.B. Saunders.

McKenry, L., & Salerno, E. (2003). *Mosby's pharmacology in nursing* (21st ed.). St. Louis: Mosby.

Mosby's 2005 drug consult for nurses. (2005). St. Louis: Mosby.

Skidmore-Roth, L. (2005). *Mosby's drug guide for nurses* (6th ed.). St. Louis: Mosby.

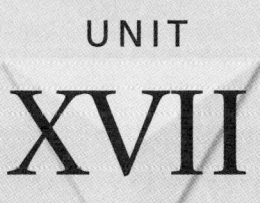

The Adult Client with a Musculoskeletal Disorder

PYRAMID TERMS

cast   Made of plaster or fiberglass to provide immobilization of bone and joints after a fracture or injury.

compartment syndrome   Increased pressure within one or more compartments causing massive compromise of circulation to an area and irreversible neuromuscular damage within 4 to 6 hours of onset if not treated.

external fixation   Stabilization of a fracture by the use of an external frame, with multiple pins applied through the bone.

fat embolism   An embolism that can occur 24 to 48 hours or within the first 72 hours following a fracture.

internal fixation   Stabilization of a fracture that involves the application of screws, plates, pins, or nails to hold the fragments in alignment.

Reduction   The procedure that restores the bone to proper alignment.

Traction   Force applied in two directions to reduce and immobilize a fracture.

▲ PYRAMID TO SUCCESS

The Pyramid to Success focuses on the emergency care for a client who sustains a fracture or other musculoskeletal injury, monitoring for complications related to fractures, and interventions if complications occur. Nursing care related to casts and traction is emphasized. Skill related to instructing the client in the use of an assistive device such as a cane, walker, or crutches is a pyramid point. Pyramid points also include postoperative care following hip surgery or amputation, and care of the client with rheumatoid arthritis or osteoporosis. Focus on the points related to the psychosocial effects as a result of the musculoskeletal disorder, such as unexpected body image changes, and the appropriate and available support services needed for the client. The Integrated Processes addressed in this unit include Caring, Clinical Problem-Solving Process (Nursing Process), Communication and Documentation, and Teaching/Learning.

CLIENT NEEDS   ▲

Safe, Effective Care Environment

Asepsis related to wounds
Client rights
Confidentiality regarding disorder and plan of care
Dietary consultation
Handling hazardous and infectious materials
Informed consent for diagnostic treatments and surgical procedures
Physical therapy and occupational therapy referrals
Preventing injury from accidents
Standard precautions

Health Promotion and Maintenance

Aging process and disease prevention
Data collection related to the musculoskeletal system
Expected body image changes
Health promotion related to diet and activity
Home care instructions regarding care related to musculoskeletal disorder
Reinforcement regarding the importance of prescribed therapy

Psychosocial Integrity

Ability to cope with feelings of isolation and loss of independence
Available support systems and utilization of community resources
Cultural, religious, and spiritual influences
Grief and loss related to mobility limitations and restrictions
Mobilizing coping mechanisms
Sensory and perceptual alterations
Situational role changes as a result of musculoskeletal disorder

Unexpected body image changes as a result of injury or disease

Physiological Integrity

Care related to casts and traction
Complications of a fracture
Complications related to procedures or injuries
Emergency care for a fracture or other injury
Measures to promote comfort
Pharmacological therapy
Postoperative interventions
Promoting normal elimination patterns
Promoting self-care measures
Use of assistive devices for mobility such as canes, walkers, and crutches

REFERENCES

Black, J., & Hawks, J. (2005). *Medical-surgical nursing: Clinical management for positive outcomes* (7th ed.). Philadelphia: W.B. Saunders.

Chernecky, C., & Berger, B. (2004). *Laboratory tests and diagnostic procedures* (4th ed.). Philadelphia: W.B. Saunders.

Christensen, B., & Kockrow, E. (2003). *Adult health nursing* (4th ed.). St. Louis: Mosby.

Christensen, B., & Kockrow, E. (2003). *Foundations of nursing* (4th ed.). St. Louis: Mosby.

Fortinash, K., & Holoday-Worret, P. (2004). *Psychiatric mental health nursing* (3rd ed.). St. Louis: Mosby.

Harkreader, H., & Hogan, M.A. (2004). *Fundamentals of nursing: Caring and clinical judgment* (2nd ed.). Philadelphia: W.B. Saunders.

Hodgson, B., & Kizior, R. (2005). *Saunders nursing drug handbook 2005.* Philadelphia: W.B. Saunders.

Lewis, S., Heitkemper, M., & Dirksen, S. (2004). *Medical-surgical nursing: Assessment and management of clinical problems* (6th ed.). St. Louis: Mosby.

Linton, A., & Maebius, N. (2003). *Introduction to medical-surgical nursing* (3rd ed.). Philadelphia: W.B. Saunders.

McKenry, L., & Salerno, E. (2003). *Mosby's pharmacology in nursing* (21st ed.). St. Louis: Mosby.

National Council of State Boards of Nursing. (2005). *Detailed test plan for the National Council licensure examination for practical/vocational nurses.* Chicago: Author.

Pagana, K., & Pagana, T. (2003). *Mosby's diagnostic and laboratory test reference* (6th ed.). St. Louis: Mosby.

Perry, A., & Potter, P. (2002). *Clinical nursing skills and techniques* (5th ed.). St. Louis: Mosby.

Phipps, W., Monahan, F., Sands, J., Marek, J., & Neighbors, M. (2003). *Medical-surgical nursing: Health and illness perspectives* (7th ed.). St. Louis: Mosby.

Potter, P., & Perry, A. (2003). *Essentials for practice* (5th ed.). St. Louis: Mosby.

Musculoskeletal System

I. ANATOMY AND PHYSIOLOGY

A. Skeleton
1. Axial portion
   a. Cranium
   b. Vertebrae
   c. Ribs
2. Appendicular portion
   a. Limbs
   b. Shoulders
   c. Hips

B. Types of bones (Box 58-1)
1. Spongy bone
   a. Located in the ends of long bones and the center of flat and irregular bones
   b. Can withstand forces applied in many directions
2. Dense (compact) bone
   a. Covers spongy bone
   b. Cylinder around a central marrow cavity
   c. Can withstand force predominantly in one direction
3. Characteristics of the bones
   a. Support and protect structures of the body
   b. Provide attachments for muscles, tendons, and ligaments
   c. Contain tissue in the central cavities, which aids in the formation of blood cells
   d. Assists in regulating calcium and phosphate concentrations

4. Bone growth
   a. The length of bone growth is a result of the ossification of the epiphyseal cartilage at the ends of bones; bone growth stops between the ages of 18 and 25 years
   b. The width of bone growth is a result of the activity of osteoblasts and occurs throughout life, but slows down with the aging process
   c. Bone absorption around the bone marrow continues throughout life; therefore, bones become weaker with aging

C. Types of joints (Table 58-1)
1. Characteristics of the joints
   a. Allow the movement between bones
   b. Formed where two bones join
   c. Surfaces are covered with cartilage
   d. Enclosed in a capsule
   e. Contain a cavity filled with synovial fluid
   f. Ligaments hold the bone and joint in the correct position
   g. Articulation is the meeting point of two or more joints

---

BOX 58-1

Types of Bones

Long
Short
Flat
Irregular

TABLE 58-1

Types of Joints

Type	Description
Synarthrosis	Fibrous or fixed joints
	No movement associated with these joints
Amphiarthrosis	Cartilaginous joints
	Slightly movable joints
Diarthrosis	Synovial joints
	Ball-and-socket joints
Condyloid	Freely movable joints
	Allow frictionless, painless movement

2. Synovial fluid
   a. Found in the joint capsule
   b. Formed by synovial membrane, which lines the joint capsule
   c. Lubricates the cartilage
   d. Cushion for shocks
D. Muscles
   1. Characteristics of muscles
      a. Made up of bundles of muscle fibers
      b. Provide the force to move bones
      c. Assist in maintaining posture
      d. Assist with heat production
   2. The process of contraction and relaxation
      a. Muscle contraction and relaxation require large amounts of adenosine triphosphate (ATP)
      b. Contraction also requires calcium, which functions as a catalyst
      c. Acetylcholine released by the motor end plate of the motor neuron initiates an action potential
      d. Acetylcholine is then destroyed by acetyl-cholinesterase
      e. Calcium is required to contract muscle fibers; acts as a catalyst for the enzyme needed for the sliding together action of actin and myosin
      f. Following contraction, ATP transports calcium out to allow actin and myosin to slide apart and allow the muscle to relax
   3. Skeletal muscles
      a. Attached to two bones and cross at least one joint
      b. The point of origin is the point of attachment on the bone closest to the trunk
      c. The point of insertion is the point of attachment on the bone farthest from the trunk
      d. Skeletal muscles act in groups
      e. Prime movers contract to produce movement
      f. Antagonists relax
      g. Synergists contract to stabilize
      h. Nerves activate and control the muscles

II. RISK FACTORS ASSOCIATED WITH MUSCULOSKELETAL DISORDERS (Box 58-2)

III. DIAGNOSTIC TESTS
A. X-rays
   1. Description: A commonly used procedure to diagnose disorders of the musculoskeletal system
   2. Interventions
      a. Handle injured area carefully
      b. Administer analgesics as prescribed prior to the procedure, particularly if the client is in pain
      c. Remove any radiopaque objects, such as jewelry
      d. Ask the client about pregnancy; shield the clients ovaries or testes

---

BOX 58-2

Risk Factors Associated with Musculoskeletal Disorders

Autoimmune disorders
Calcium deficiency
Degenerative conditions
Falls
Hyperuricemia
Infection
Medications
Metabolic disorders
Neoplastic disorders
Obesity
Postmenopausal states
Trauma and injury

---

      e. The client must lie still during an x-ray
      f. Inform the client that exposure to radiation is minimal and not dangerous
      g. Health care provider is to wear a lead apron if staying in the room with the client
B. Arthrocentesis
   1. Description
      a. Involves aspirating synovial fluid, blood, or pus via a needle inserted into a joint cavity
      b. Medication may be instilled into the joint if necessary to alleviate inflammation
   2. Interventions
      a. Obtain an informed consent
      b. Apply a compress bandage post procedure, as prescribed
      c. Instruct the client to rest the joint for 8 to 24 hours post procedure
      d. Instruct the client to notify the physician if fever or swelling of the joint occurs
C. Arthrography
   1. Description
      a. A radiographic examination of the soft tissues of the joint structures; used to diagnose trauma to the joint capsule or ligaments
      b. A local anesthetic is used for the procedure
      c. A contrast medium or air is injected into the joint cavity; the joint is moved through range of motion as a series of x-rays is taken
   2. Interventions
      a. Instruct the client to fast from food and fluids for 8 hours prior to the procedure
      b. Assess the client for allergies to iodine or seafood prior to the procedure
      c. Obtain an informed consent
      d. Inform the client of the need to remain as still as possible, except when asked to reposition
      e. Minimize the use of the joint for 12 hours after the procedure
      f. Instruct the client that the joint may be edematous and tender for 1 to 2 days after

the procedure; may be treated with ice packs and analgesics, as prescribed

    g. Instruct the client that, if edema and tenderness last longer than 2 days, to notify the physician

    h. If knee arthrography has been performed, an Ace wrap over the knee may be prescribed for 3 to 4 days

    i. If air was used for injection, crepitus may be felt in the joint for up to 2 days

▲ D. Arthroscopy

  1. Description

    a. Provides an endoscopic examination of various joints

    b. Articular cartilage abnormalities can be assessed, loose bodies can be removed, and cartilage can be trimmed

    c. A biopsy may be performed during the procedure

  2. Interventions

    a. Instruct the client to fast for 8 to 12 hours prior to the procedure

    b. Obtain an informed consent

    c. Administer pain medication as prescribed post procedure

    d. An elastic wrap should be worn for 2 to 4 days as prescribed post-procedure

    e. Instruct the client that walking without weight-bearing is usually permitted after sensation returns but to limit activity for 1 to 4 days as prescribed following the procedure

    f. Instruct the client to elevate the extremity as often as possible for 2 days following the procedure, and to place ice on the site to minimize swelling

    g. Reinforce instructions regarding the use of crutches, which may be used for 5 to 7 days post-procedure when walking

    h. Advise the client to notify the physician if fever or increased knee pain occurs or if edema continues for more than 3 days post-procedure

E. Bone mineral density (BMD) measurements

  1. Dual energy x-ray absorptiometry (DEXA)

    a. Measures bone mass of spine, other bones, and the total body

    b. Minimal radiation exposure

    c. Used to diagnosis metabolic bone disease and to monitor changes in bone density with treatment

    d. Inform client that procedure is painless

  2. Quantitative ultrasound (QUS)

    a. Evaluates strength, density, and elasticity of various bones using ultrasound rather than radiation

    b. Inform client that procedure is painless

F. Bone scanning

  1. Description

    a. Radioisotope is injected IV and will collect in areas that indicate abnormal bone metabolism and some fractures, if they exist

    b. The isotope is excreted in the urine and feces within 48 hours and is not harmful to others

  2. Interventions

    a. Hold fluids for 4 hours prior to the procedure

    b. Obtain an informed consent

    c. Remove all jewelry and metal objects

    d. Following the injection of the radioisotope, the client must drink 32 ounces of water (if not contraindicated) to promote renal filtering of the excess isotope

    e. From 1 to 3 hours after the injection, have the client void; the scanning procedure is then performed

    f. Inform the client of the need to lie supine during the procedure and that the procedure is not painful

    g. No special precautions are required after the procedure because a minimal amount of radioactivity exists in the radioisotope

    h. Monitor the injection site for redness and swelling

    i. Encourage oral fluid intake following the procedure

G. Bone or muscle biopsy

  1. Description: May be done during surgery, or through aspiration or punch or needle biopsy

  2. Interventions

    a. Obtain an informed consent

    b. Monitor for bleeding, swelling, hematoma, and severe pain

    c. Elevate the site for 24 hours following the procedure to reduce edema

    d. Apply ice packs as prescribed following the procedure to prevent the development of a hematoma

    e. Monitor for signs of infection following the procedure

    f. Inform the client that mild to moderate discomfort is normal following the procedure

H. Electromyography (EMG)

  1. Description

    a. Measures electrical potential associated with skeletal muscle contractions

    b. Needles are inserted into the muscle, and recordings of muscular electrical activity are traced on recording paper through an oscilloscope

  2. Interventions

    a. Obtain an informed consent

    b. Instruct the client that the needle insertion is uncomfortable

    c. Instruct the client not to take any stimulants or sedatives for 24 hours prior to the procedure

    d. Inform the client that slight bruising may occur at the needle insertion sites

I. Myelography

  1. Description: Injection of dye or air into the subarachnoid space to detect abnormalities of the spinal cord and vertebrae

2. Preprocedure interventions
   a. Obtain an informed consent
   b. Provide hydration for at least 12 hours before the test
   c. Assess for allergies to iodine or seafood (shellfish)
   d. Premedicate for sedation as prescribed
3. Postprocedure interventions
   a. Perform vital signs and neurological assessment frequently, as prescribed
   b. If a water-based dye is used, elevate the head 15 to 30 degrees for 8 hours, as prescribed
   c. If an oil-based dye is used, keep the client flat 6 to 8 hours, as prescribed
   d. If air is used, keep the head lower than the trunk
   e. Force fluids and monitor input and output (I&O)

IV. INJURIES

A. Strains
   1. An excessive stretching of a muscle or tendon
   2. Management involves cold and heat applications, activity limitations, anti-inflammatory medications, and muscle relaxants
   3. Surgical repair may be required for a severe strain (ruptured muscle or tendon)
B. Sprains
   1. An excessive stretching of a ligament; usually caused by a twisting motion
   2. Characterized by pain and swelling
   3. Management involves rest, ice, and a compression bandage to reduce swelling and provide joint support
   4. Casting may be required for moderate sprains to allow the tear to heal
   5. Surgery may be necessary for severe ligament damage
C. Rotator cuff injuries
   1. Musculotendinous or rotator cuff of the shoulder sustains a tear, usually as a result of trauma
   2. Characterized by shoulder pain and the inability to maintain abduction of the arm at the shoulder (drop arm test)
   3. Management involves nonsteroidal anti-inflammatory drugs (NSAIDs), physical therapy, sling support, and ice-heat applications
   4. Surgery may be required if medical management is unsuccessful or for those who have a complete tear

V. FRACTURES

A. Description: A break in the continuity of the bone caused by trauma, twisting as a result of muscle spasm or indirect loss of leverage, or bone decalcification and disease that result in osteopenia
B. Types of fractures (Box 58-3)

C. Data collection of a fracture of an extremity
   1. Pain or tenderness over the involved area
   2. Loss of function
   3. Obvious deformity
   4. Crepitation
   5. Erythema, edema, ecchymosis
   6. Muscle spasm and impaired sensation
D. Initial care of a fracture of an extremity
   1. Immobilize affected extremity
   2. If a compound fracture exists, splint the extremity and cover the wound with a sterile dressing
E. Interventions for a fracture (Box 58-4)
F. **Reduction:** Restoring the bone to proper alignment
   1. Closed **reduction**
      a. Performed by manual manipulation
      b. May be performed under local or general anesthesia
      c. A **cast** may be applied following **reduction**
   2. Open **reduction**
      a. Involves a surgical intervention
      b. May be treated with **internal fixation** devices
      c. The client may be placed in **traction** or a **cast** following the procedure

---

BOX 58-3

Types of Fractures

Closed or simple: Skin over the fractured area remains intact
Greenstick: One side of the bone is broken and the other is bent; most commonly seen in children
Transverse: Bone is fractured straight across
Oblique: Break extends in an oblique direction
Spiral: Break partially encircles bone
Comminuted: Bone is splintered or crushed, with three or more fragments
Complete: Bone is completely separated by a break into two parts
Incomplete: A partial break in the bone
Open or compound: Bone is exposed to air through a break in the skin; soft tissue injury and infection are common
Impacted: Part of the fractured bone is driven into another bone
Depressed: Bone fragments are driven inward
Compression: A fractured bone compressed by other bone
Pathological: A fracture that results from weakening of the bone structure by pathological processes, such as neoplasia or osteomalacia; also called spontaneous fracture

---

BOX 58-4

Interventions for a Fracture

Reduction
Fixation
Traction
Casts

G. Fixation
  1. Internal fixation (Figure 58-1)
     a. Follows open **reduction**
     b. Involves the application of screws, plates, pins, or nails to hold the fragments in alignment
     c. May involve the removal of damaged bone and replacement with a prosthesis
     d. Provides immediate bone strength
     e. Risk of infection is associated with the procedure
  2. External fixation (Figure 58-2)
     a. An external frame is utilized with multiple pins applied through the bone
     b. Provides more freedom of movement than with **traction**
H. **Traction** (Figure 58-3)
  1. Description
     a. The exertion of a pulling force applied in two directions to reduce and immobilize a fracture
     b. Provides proper bone alignment and reduces muscle spasms
  2. Interventions
     a. Maintain proper body alignment
     b. Ensure that the weights hang freely and do not touch the floor
     c. Do not remove or lift the weights without a physician's order

  d. Ensure that pulleys are not obstructed and that ropes in the pulleys move freely
  e. Place knots in the ropes to prevent slipping
  f. Check the ropes for fraying
I. Skeletal **traction** (Figure 58-4)
  1. Description: Mechanically applied to the bone with pins, wires, or tongs
  2. Interventions
     a. Monitor color, motion, and sensation (CMS) of the affected extremity
     b. Monitor the insertion sites for redness, swelling, or drainage
     c. Provide insertion site care as prescribed
  3. Cervical tongs and a halo fixation device (see Chapter 56 regarding care of the client with these types of devices)
J. Skin **traction** (Box 58-5)
  1. Description: **Traction** applied by the use of elastic bandages or adhesive
  2. Cervical (head halter) skin **traction** (see Figure 58-3)
     a. Relieves muscle spasms and compression in the upper extremities and neck
     b. Uses a head halter and a chin pad to attach the **traction**
     c. Use powder to protect the ears from friction rub
     d. Position the client with the head of the bed elevated 30 to 40 degrees, and attach the weights to a pulley system over the head of the bed
  3. Buck's skin **traction** (see Figure 58-3)
     a. Used to alleviate muscle spasms; immobilizes a lower limb by maintaining a straight pull on the limb with the use of weights

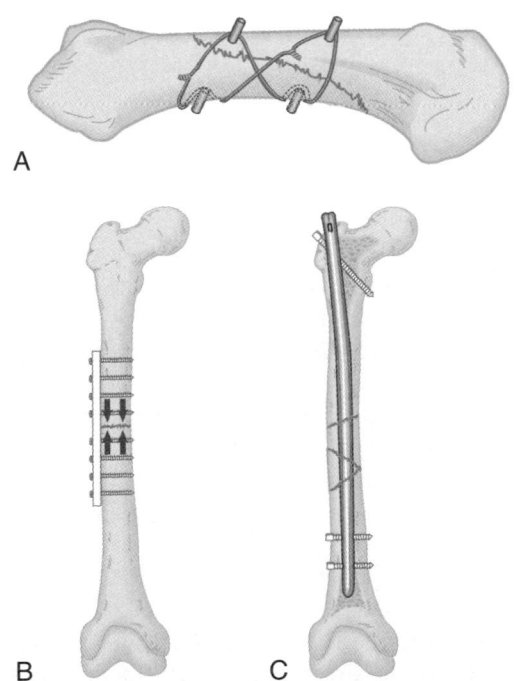

FIG. 58-1 Different internal fixation devices. **A,** Tension band wiring technique using Kirschner wires for fracture of the phalanx. **B,** Compression plate applied to the lateral aspect of the femur. **C,** Intramedullary nail fixed to both proximal and distal fragments of the femur. (From Linton, A., & Maebius, N. [2003]. *Introduction to medical-surgical nursing* [3rd ed.]. Philadelphia: W.B. Saunders.)

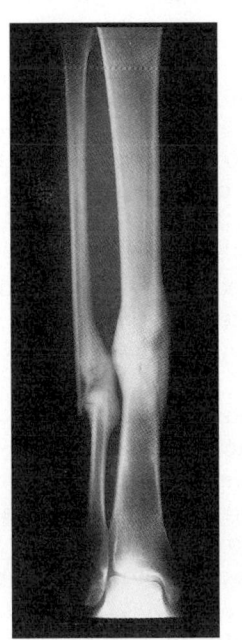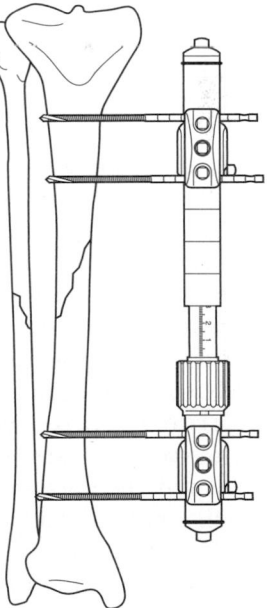

FIG. 58-2 External fixation to provide immobilization of a fracture. (From Black, J., & Hawks, J. [2005]. *Medical-surgical nursing: Clinical management for positive outcomes* [7th ed.]. Philadelphia: W.B. Saunders.)

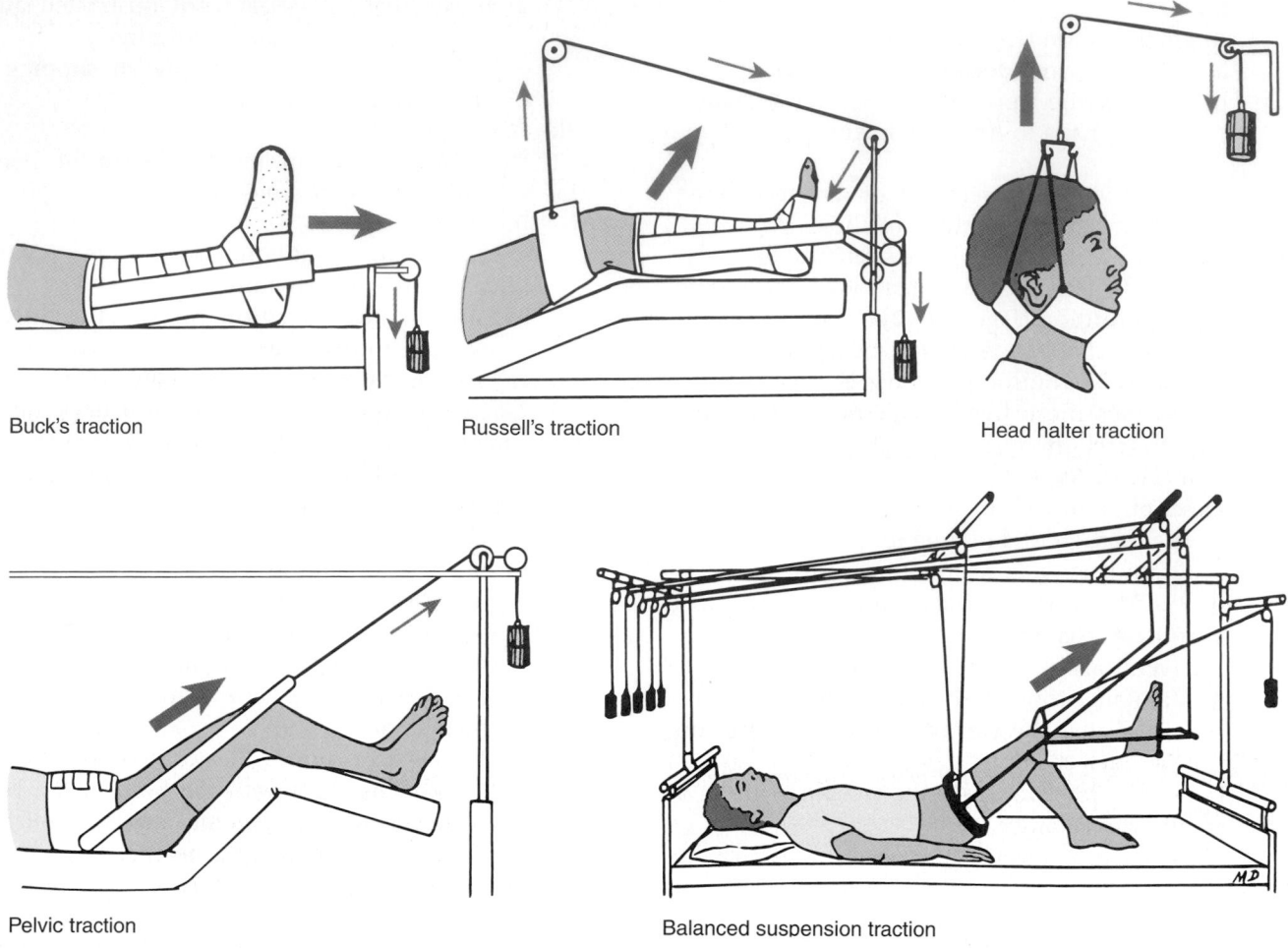

Buck's traction

Russell's traction

Head halter traction

Pelvic traction

Balanced suspension traction

FIG. 58-3 Types of skin traction. (From Linton, A., & Maebius, N. [2003]. *Introduction to medical-surgical nursing* [3rd ed.]. Philadelphia: W.B. Saunders.)

b. A boot appliance is applied to attach to the **traction**

c. Weight is attached to a pulley; allow the weights to hang freely over the edge of bed

d. Not more than 8 to 10 pounds of weight should be applied

e. Elevate the foot of the bed to provide the **traction**

4. Russell's skin **traction** (see Figure 58-3; also see Chapter 36 regarding information related to these types of **traction**)

5. Pelvic skin **traction** (see Figure 58-3)

a. Used to relieve low back, hip, or leg pain and to reduce muscle spasm

b. Apply the **traction** snugly over the pelvis and iliac crest and attach to the weights

c. Use measures as prescribed to prevent the client from slipping down in bed

K. Balanced suspension (see Figure 58-3)

1. Description

a. Used with skin or skeletal **traction**

b. Used to approximate fractures of the femur, tibia, or fibula

c. Produced by a counterforce other than client

2. Interventions

a. Position the client in low Fowler's, on either the side or the back

b. Maintain a 20-degree angle from the thigh to the bed

c. Protect the skin from breakdown

d. Provide pin care if pins are used with the skeletal **traction**

e. Clean the pin sites with sterile normal saline and hydrogen peroxide or Betadine as prescribed or per agency procedure

L. Dunlop's **traction**

1. Description: Horizontal **traction** to align fractures of the humerus; vertical **traction** maintains the forearm in proper alignment

2. Interventions: Nursing care is similar to that for Buck's **traction**

M. Casts

1. Description: Made of plaster or fiberglass to provide immobilization of bone and joints after a fracture or injury

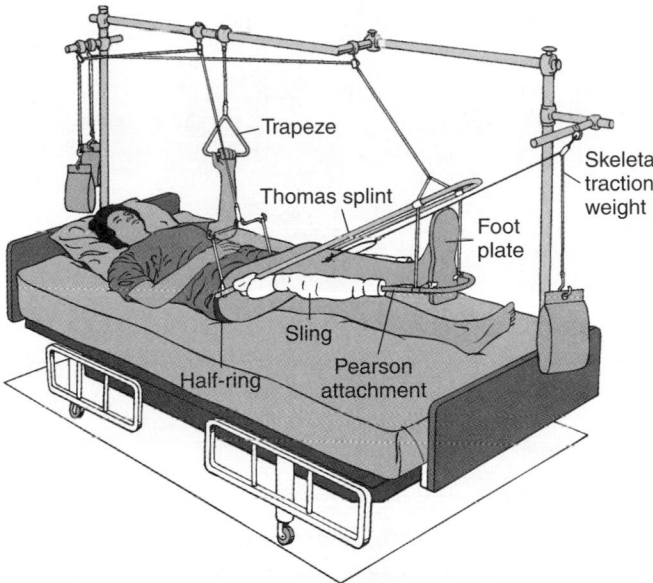

FIG. 58-4 Balanced suspension skeletal traction. (From Elkin, M., Perry, A., & Potter, P. [2004]. *Nursing interventions and clinical skills* [3rd ed.]. St. Louis: Mosby.)

Labels on figure: Trapeze; Thomas splint; Skeletal traction weight; Foot plate; Sling; Pearson attachment; Half-ring

---

BOX 58-5

Types of Skin Traction

Cervical traction
Buck's traction
Bryant's traction
Pelvic traction
Russell's traction

---

2. Interventions
   a. Keep the **cast** and extremity elevated
   b. Allow a wet **cast** 24 to 48 hours to dry (synthetic **casts** dry in 20 minutes)
   c. Handle a wet **cast** with the palms of the hand until dry
   d. Turn the extremity unless contraindicated, so that all sides of the wet **cast** will dry
   e. Cool setting on hair dryer can be used to dry plaster **cast** (heat cannot be used on plaster **cast** because the **cast** heats up and burns the skin)
   f. The **cast** will change from a dull to a shiny substance when dry
   g. Examine the skin and **cast** for pressure areas
   h. Monitor the extremity for circulatory impairment such as pain, swelling, discoloration, tingling, numbness, coolness, or diminished pulse
   i. Notify the physician immediately if circulatory compromise occurs
   j. Prepare for bivalving or cutting the **cast** if circulatory impairment occurs

---

BOX 58-6

Complications of Fractures

Compartment syndrome
Fat emboli
Infection and osteomyelitis
Avascular necrosis
Pulmonary emboli

---

   k. Petal the **cast**; maintain smooth edges around the **cast** to prevent crumbling of the **cast** material
   l. Monitor the client's temperature
   m. Monitor for the presence of a foul odor, which may indicate infection
   n. Monitor drainage and circle the area of drainage on the **cast**
   o. Monitor for warmth on the **cast**
   p. Monitor for wet spots, which may indicate a need for drying, or the presence of drainage under the **cast**
   q. If an open draining area exists on the affected extremity, a cut-out portion of the **cast** or a window will be made by the physician
   r. Instruct the client not to stick objects inside the **cast**
   s. Teach the client to keep the **cast** clean and dry
   t. Instruct the client in isometric exercises to prevent muscle atrophy

VI. COMPLICATIONS OF FRACTURES (Box 58-6)
A. **Fat** embolism
   1. Description
      a. An embolism originating in the bone marrow that occurs after a fracture
      b. Clients with long bone fractures are at the greatest risk for the development of **fat** embolism
      c. Usually occurs within 48 hours following the injury
   2. Data collection
      a. Restlessness
      b. Mental status changes
      c. Tachycardia, tachypnea, and hypotension
      d. Dyspnea
      e. Petechial rash over the upper chest and neck
   3. Interventions
      a. The physician is notified immediately
      b. Treat symptoms as prescribed to prevent respiratory failure and death
B. **Compartment syndrome**
   1. Description
      a. Increased pressure within one or more compartments causing massive compromise of circulation to an area
      b. Leads to decreased perfusion and tissue anoxia

c. Within 4 to 6 hours after the onset of **compartment syndrome**, neuromuscular damage is irreversible

2. Data collection
   a. Unrelieved or increased pain
   b. Swelling
   c. Pain with passive motion
   d. Inability to move joints
   e. Loss of sensation (paresthesia)
   f. Pulselessness

3. Interventions: The physician is notified immediately

C. Infection and osteomyelitis
   1. Description: Can be caused by the interruption of the integrity of the skin; the infection invades bone tissue
   2. Data collection
      a. Fever
      b. Pain
      c. Erythema in the area surrounding the fracture
      d. Tachycardia
      e. Elevated white blood cell (WBC) count
   3. Interventions
      a. The physician is notified immediately
      b. Prepare the client for aggressive IV antibiotic therapy

D. Avascular necrosis
   1. Description: An interruption in the blood supply to the bony tissue, which results in the death of the bone
   2. Data collection
      a. Pain
      b. Decreased sensation
   3. Interventions
      a. The physician is notified if pain or decreased sensation occurs
      b. Prepare the client for removal of necrotic tissue, because it serves as a locus of infection

E. Pulmonary embolism
   1. Description: Caused by immobility precipitated by a fracture
   2. Data collection
      a. Restlessness and apprehension
      b. Dyspnea
      c. Diaphoresis
      d. Arterial blood gas changes
   3. Interventions
      a. The physician is notified if signs of emboli are present
      b. Prepare to administer anticoagulant therapy

VII. CRUTCH WALKING

A. Description
   1. An accurate measurement of the client for crutches is important, because an incorrect measurement could damage the brachial plexus

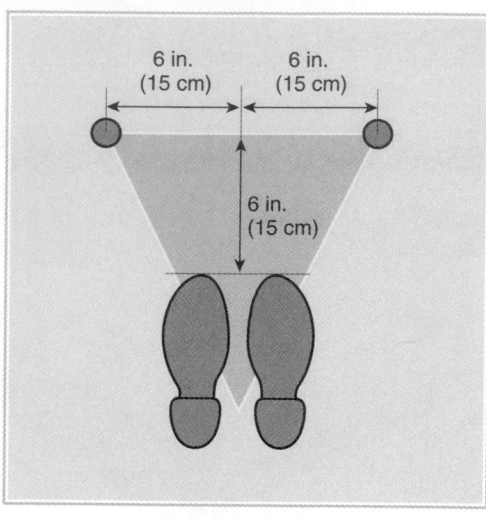

FIG. 58-5   Basic crutch stance, tripod position. (From Harkreader, H., & Hogan, M.A. [2004]. *Fundamentals of nursing: Caring and clinical judgment* [2nd ed.]. Philadelphia: W.B. Saunders.)

6 in.
(15 cm)

6 in.
(15 cm)

6 in.
(15 cm)

2. The distance between the axillae and the arm pieces on the crutches should be two finger-widths in the axilla space
3. The elbows should be slightly flexed, 20 to 30 degrees, when the client is walking
4. When ambulating with the client, stand on the affected side
5. Instruct the client never to rest the axilla on the axillary bars
6. Instruct the client to look up and outward when ambulating
7. Instruct the client to stop ambulation if numbness or tingling in the hands or arms occurs

B. Crutch gaits
   1. Basic crutch stance, tripod position (Figure 58-5)
   2. Two-point gait (Figure 58-6)
   3. Three-point gait (Figure 58-7)
   4. Four-point gait (Figure 58-8)

C. Assisting the client with crutches to sit and stand
   1. Place the unaffected leg against the front of the chair
   2. Move the crutches to the affected side, and grasp the chair's arm with the hand on the unaffected side
   3. Flex the knee of the unaffected leg to lower himself or herself into the chair while placing the affected leg straight out in front
   4. Reverse the steps to move from a sitting to a standing position

D. Going up and down stairs
   1. Up the stairs
      a. The client moves the unaffected leg up first
      b. The client moves the affected leg and the crutches up

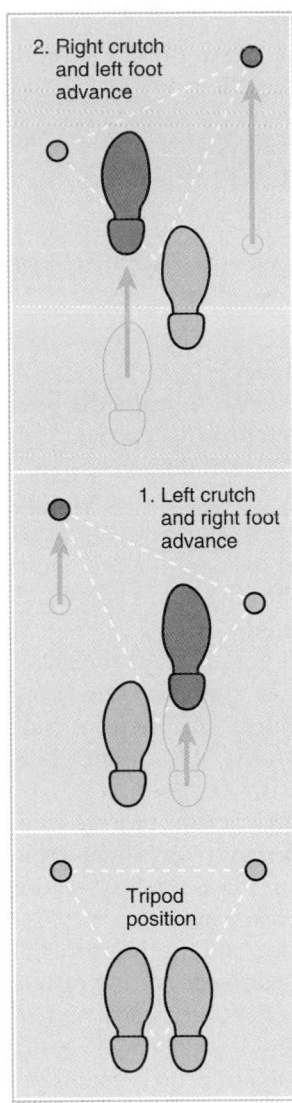

FIG. 58-6   Two-point gait. (From Harkreader, H., & Hogan, M.A. [2004]. *Fundamentals of nursing: Caring and clinical judgment* [2nd ed.]. Philadelphia: W.B. Saunders.)

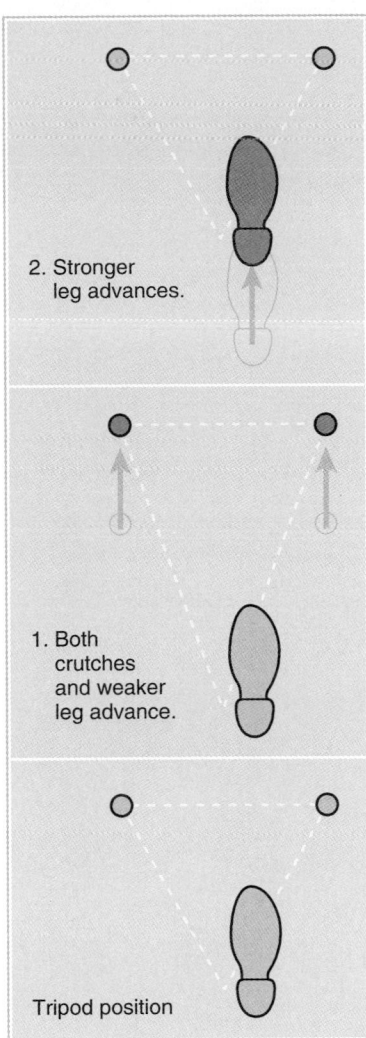

FIG. 58-7   Three-point gait. (From Harkreader, H., & Hogan, M.A. [2004]. *Fundamentals of nursing: Caring and clinical judgment* [2nd ed.]. Philadelphia: W.B. Saunders.)

2. Down the stairs
   a. The client moves the crutches and the affected leg down
   b. The client moves the unaffected leg down

VIII. CANES AND WALKERS

A. Description: Made of a lightweight material, with a rubber tip at the bottom

B. Interventions
   1. Stand at the affected side of the client when ambulating
   2. The handle should be at the level of the client's greater trochanter
   3. The client's elbow should be flexed at a 25- to 30-degree angle
   4. Instruct the client to hold the cane close to the body

5. Instruct the client to hold the cane in the hand on the unaffected side so that the cane and weaker leg can work together with each step
6. Instruct the client to move the cane at the same time as the affected leg
7. Instruct the client to inspect the rubber tips regularly for worn places

C. Hemicanes or quadripod canes
   1. Used for clients who have the use of only one upper extremity
   2. Hemicanes provide more security than a quadripod cane; however, both types provide more security than a single-tipped cane
   3. Position the cane at the client's unaffected side, with the straight, nonangled side adjacent to the body
   4. Position the cane 6 inches from client's side, with the hand grips level with the greater trochanter

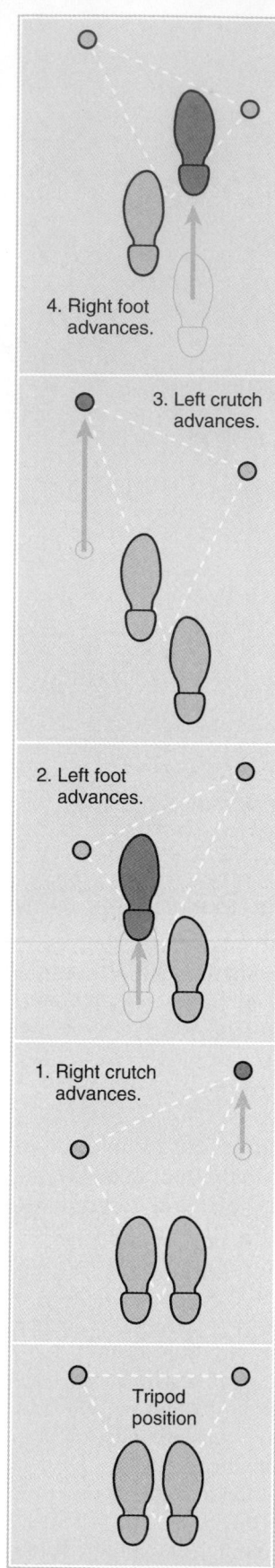

4. Right foot advances.

3. Left crutch advances.

2. Left foot advances.

1. Right crutch advances.

Tripod position

FIG. 58-8 Four-point gait. (From Harkreader, H., & Hogan, M.A. [2004]. *Fundamentals of nursing: Caring and clinical judgment* [2nd ed.]. Philadelphia: W.B. Saunders.)

D. Walker
  1. Stand adjacent to the client on the affected side
  2. Instruct the client to put all four points of the walker flat on the floor before putting weight on the hand pieces
  3. Instruct the client to move the walker forward and to walk into it

IX. FRACTURED HIP

A. Types
  1. Intracapsular
     a. Bone is broken inside the joint
     b. Skin **traction** is applied preoperatively to immobilize and prevent pain
     c. Treatment includes a total hip replacement or **internal fixation**, with replacement of the femoral head with a prosthesis
     d. Avoid hip flexion to prevent displacement
  2. Extracapsular
     a. Fracture can occur at the greater trochanter or can be an intertrochanteric fracture
     b. Trochanteric fracture is outside the joint
     c. Preoperative treatment includes balanced suspension **traction**
     d. Avoid hip flexion to prevent displacement
     e. Surgical treatment includes **internal fixation** with nail plate, screws, or wires

B. Postoperative interventions
  1. Maintain leg and hip in proper alignment
  2. Prevent flexion or external or internal rotation
  3. Turn the client from his or her back to unaffected side
  4. Do not position to the affected side unless prescribed by the physician
  5. Maintain leg abduction to prevent internal or external rotation
  6. Use a trochanter roll to prevent external rotation
  7. Ensure that the hip flexion angle does not exceed 60 to 80 degrees
  8. Elevate the head of the bed 30 to 45 degrees for meals only
  9. Ambulate as prescribed by the physician
  10. Avoid weight-bearing on the affected leg as prescribed; instruct the client in the use of a walker to avoid weight-bearing
  11. Keep the operative leg extended, supported, and elevated when getting client out of bed
  12. Avoid hip flexion greater than 90 degrees and avoid low chairs when out of bed
  13. Monitor the wound for infection or hemorrhage
  14. Monitor circulation and sensation of the affected side
  15. Maintain the Hemovac or Jackson-Pratt drain, if in place; maintain compression to facilitate drainage and monitor and record output of drainage

16. Drainage should continuously decrease in amount; by 48 hours postoperatively, drainage should be approximately 30 mL in an 8-hour period
17. Maintain the use of antiembolism stockings, and encourage the client to flex and extend the feet and ankles
18. Instruct the client to avoid crossing the legs and bending over activities
19. Physical therapy will begin postoperatively as prescribed by the physician

▲

X. TOTAL KNEE REPLACEMENT

A. Description: Implantation of a device to substitute for the femoral condyles and the tibial joint surfaces
B. Postoperative interventions
   1. Monitor the incision for drainage and infection
   2. Maintain the Hemovac or Jackson-Pratt drain if in place
   3. Begin continuous passive motion (CPM) 24 to 48 hours postoperatively as prescribed to exercise the knee and provide moderate flexion and extension
   4. Administer analgesics before CPM to decrease pain
   5. The leg should not be dangled, to prevent dislocation
   6. Prepare the client for out-of-bed activities, as prescribed
   7. Avoid weight-bearing and instruct the client in crutch walking

▲

XI. HERNIATION: INTERVERTEBRAL DISK

A. Description: Nucleus of the disk protrudes into the annulus, causing nerve compression
B. Cervical disk
   1. Occurs at C5 to C6 and C6 to C7 interspaces
   2. Causes pain and stiffness in the neck, top of the shoulders, scapula, upper extremities, and head
   3. Produces paresthesia and numbness of the upper extremities
   4. Interventions
      a. Provide bed rest to relieve pressure and reduce inflammation and edema
      b. Provide immobilization as prescribed via cervical collar, **traction**, or brace
      c. Apply hot, moist compresses as prescribed to increase the blood flow and relax spasms
      d. Instruct the client to avoid flexing, extending, or rotating the neck
      e. Instruct the client that, while sleeping, to avoid the prone position and keep the head, spine, and hip in alignment
      f. Instruct the client to avoid long periods of sitting

g. Instruct the client in the use of analgesics, sedatives, anti-inflammatory agents, and corticosteroids, as prescribed
      h. Prepare the client for a corticosteroid injection into the epidural space if prescribed
      i. Assist the client with the application of a cervical collar or cervical **traction**, as prescribed
   5. Cervical collar
      a. Used for cervical disk herniation
      b. Holds the head in a neutral or slightly flexed position
      c. The client may have to wear a cervical collar 24 hours a day
      d. Inspect the skin under the collar for irritation
      e. When the pain subsides, the client is taught cervical isometric exercises to strengthen the muscles
C. Lumbar disk
   1. Most often occurs at L4 to L5 or L5 to S1 interspaces
   2. Postural deformity occurs
   3. Produces muscle weakness, sensory loss, and alteration of the tendon reflexes
   4. The client experiences low back pain and muscle spasms, with radiation of the pain into one hip and down the leg (sciatica)
   5. Pain is aggravated by bending, lifting, straining, sneezing, and coughing; relieved by bed rest
   6. Interventions
      a. Provide bed rest, as prescribed
      b. Apply moist heat and massage, as prescribed
      c. Instruct the client to sleep on the side, with the knees and hips in a position of flexion and with a pillow between the legs
      d. Apply pelvic **traction** as prescribed to relieve muscle spasms
      e. Begin ambulation gradually as the inflammation and edema subside
      f. Instruct the client in the use of muscle relaxants, anti-inflammatory medications, and corticosteroids, as prescribed
      g. Instruct the client in the use of a corset or brace, as prescribed
      h. Instruct the client regarding correct posture while sitting, standing, walking, and working
      i. Instruct the client to lift objects by bending the knees and keeping the back straight, avoiding lifting anything above the elbows
      j. Instruct the client regarding a weight-control program, as prescribed
      k. Instruct the client in an exercise program as prescribed to strengthen abdominal and back muscles
D. Disk surgery (Box 58-7)
   1. Preoperative interventions
      a. Reassure the client that surgery will not weaken the back

Types of Disk Surgery

Chemolysis: Injections to dissolve affected disk
Diskectomy: Removal of herniated disk tissue and related matter
Diskectomy with fusion: Fusion of vertebrae with bone graft
Laminotomy: Division of the lamina of a vertebra
Laminectomy: Removal of the lamina

b. Instruct the client regarding coughing and deep breathing exercises
c. Instruct the client about logrolling and range-of-motion exercises
2. Postoperative interventions: Cervical disk
   a. Monitor for respiratory difficulty
   b. Encourage coughing and deep breathing
   c. Monitor for hoarseness and inability to cough effectively because this may indicate laryngeal nerve damage
   d. Use throat sprays or lozenges for sore throat; do not use those that could numb the throat to avoid choking
   e. Monitor the wound for drainage
   f. Provide a soft diet if the client complains of dysphagia
   g. Monitor for sudden return of radicular pain, which may indicate that the cervical spine has become unstable
3. Postoperative interventions: Lumbar disk
   a. Monitor for wound hemorrhage
   b. Monitor sensation and motor ability of the lower extremities as well as color, temperature, and sensation of toes
   c. Monitor for urinary retention, paralytic ileus, and constipation
   d. Initiate measures to prevent constipation, such as a high-fiber diet, increased fluids, and stool softeners, as prescribed
   e. When turning and repositioning the client, place the bed in a flat position and a pillow between the legs; turn the client as a unit (logroll) without twisting the client's back
   f. When positioning the client, a pillow is placed under the head with the knees slightly flexed
   g. Avoid extreme knee flexion when the client is lying on the side
   h. To assist the client out of bed, raise the head of the bed while the client lies on the side; the client's head and shoulders are supported by the first nurse, the client pushes himself or herself to a sitting position, and the second nurse eases the client's legs over the side of the bed
   i. Instruct the client to avoid sitting because it places a strain on the surgical site

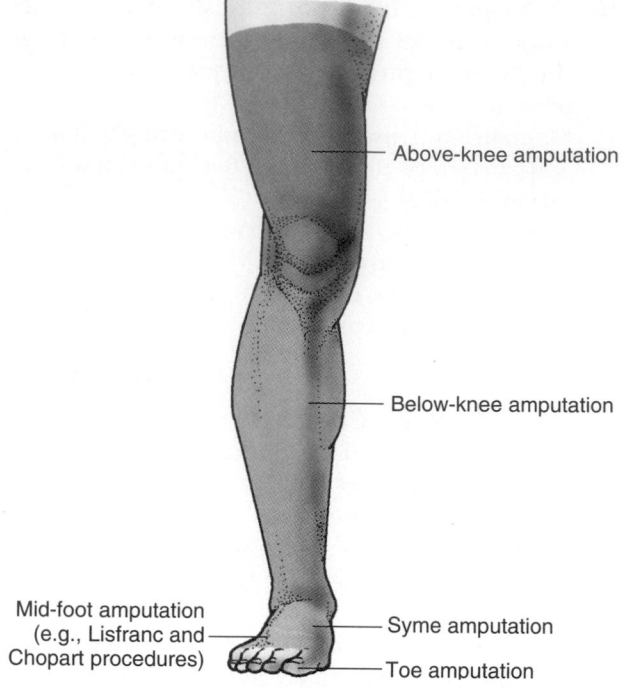

FIG. 58-9 Common levels of lower extremity amputations. (From Ignatavicius, D., & Workman, M. [2006]. *Medical surgical nursing: Critical thinking for collaborative care* [5th ed.]. Philadelphia: W.B. Saunders.)

j. Administer narcotics and sedatives as prescribed to relieve pain and anxiety
k. Encourage early ambulation
l. Assist the client with the use of a back brace or corset if prescribed

XII. AMPUTATION OF A LOWER EXTREMITY
   (Figure 58-9)
A. Description: The surgical removal of a lower limb or part of the limb
B. Postoperative interventions
   1. Monitor vital signs
   2. Monitor for infection and hemorrhage
   3. Mark bleeding and drainage on the dressing if it occurs
   4. Keep a tourniquet at the bedside
   5. Monitor for pulmonary emboli
   6. Observe for and prevent contractures
   7. Monitor for signs of necrosis and neuroma
   8. Evaluate for phantom limb sensation and pain; explain sensation and pain to the client, and medicate the client, as prescribed
   9. Check the physician's orders regarding positioning
   10. If prescribed, during the first 24 hours, elevate the foot of the bed to reduce edema; then keep the bed flat to prevent hip flexion contractures

11. Do not elevate the stump itself because elevation can cause flexion contracture of the hip joint
12. After 24 and 48 hours postoperatively, position the client prone if prescribed to stretch the muscles and prevent flexion contractures of hip
13. In the prone position, place a pillow under the abdomen and stump and keep the legs close together to prevent abduction
14. Maintain application of an Ace wrap or elastic stump shrinker as prescribed to provide stump shrinkage
15. Remove and rewrap the Ace bandage or elastic stump shrinker three or four times daily, as prescribed
16. Wash the stump with mild soap and water and apply lanolin to the skin if prescribed
17. Massage the skin toward the suture line to increase circulation
18. Prepare for a **cast** application if prescribed to prepare the stump for prosthesis
19. Encourage the client to look at the stump
20. Encourage verbalization regarding loss of the body part, and assist the client to identify coping mechanisms to deal with the loss

C. Interventions for below-knee amputation
  1. Prevent edema
  2. Do not allow the stump to hang over the edge of the bed
  3. Do not allow the client to sit for long periods of time, to prevent contractures

D. Interventions for above-knee amputation
  1. Prevent internal or external rotation of the limb
  2. Place a sandbag or rolled towel along the outside of the thigh to prevent rotation

E. Rehabilitation
  1. Instruct the client in crutch walking
  2. Prepare the stump for prosthesis
  3. Prepare the client for the fitting of the stump for prosthesis
  4. Instruct the client in exercises to maintain range of motion
  5. Provide psychosocial support to the client

XIII. RHEUMATOID ARTHRITIS (RA)

A. Description
  1. Chronic systemic inflammatory disease (immune complex disorder); the cause may be related to a combination of environmental and genetic factors
  2. Leads to destruction of connective tissue and synovial membrane within the joints
  3. Weakens and leads to dislocation of the joint and permanent deformity
  4. Formation of pannus occurs at the junction of synovial tissue and articular cartilage, projecting into the joint cavity and causing necrosis

  5. Exacerbations are increased by physical or emotional stress
  6. Risk factors include exposure to infectious agents; fatigue and stress can exacerbate the condition
  7. Vasculitis can cause malfunction and eventual failure of an organ or system

B. Data collection
  1. Inflammation, tenderness, and stiffness of the joints
  2. Moderate to severe pain and morning stiffness lasting longer than 30 minutes
  3. Joint deformities, muscle atrophy, and decreased range of motion
  4. Spongy, soft feeling in the joints
  5. Low-grade temperature, fatigue, and weakness
  6. Anorexia, weight loss, and anemia
  7. Elevated sedimentation rate and positive rheumatoid factor
  8. X-ray shows joint deterioration
  9. Synovial tissue biopsy presents inflammation

C. Rheumatoid arthritis (RA) factor
  1. A blood test used to diagnose rheumatoid arthritis
  2. Values
    a. Nonreactive: 0 to 39 international units/mL
    b. Weakly reactive: 40 to 79 international units/mL
    c. Reactive: Higher than 80 international units/mL

D. Pain
  1. Salicylates (acetylsalicyic acid [aspirin])
    a. Monitor for side effects, including tinnitus, gastrointestinal (GI) upset, and prolonged bleeding time
    b. Administer with meals or a snack
    c. Monitor for abnormal bleeding or bruising
  2. Nonsteroidal anti-inflammatory drugs (NSAIDs)
    a. May be prescribed in combination with salicylates if pain and inflammation have not decreased within 6 to 12 weeks following salicylate therapy
    b. Monitor for side effects such as GI upset, central nervous system manifestations, skin rash, hypertension, fluid retention, and changes in renal function
  3. Corticosteroids: Administer as prescribed during exacerbations or when commonly used agents are ineffective
  4. Antineoplastic medications: Administer as prescribed in clients with life-threatening RA
  5. Gold salts: Administer as prescribed in combination with salicylates and NSAIDs to induce remission and decrease pain and inflammation

E. Physical mobility
  1. Preserve joint function
  2. Provide range-of-motion (ROM) exercises to maintain joint motion and muscle strengthening
  3. Balance rest and activity
  4. Splints during acute inflammation to prevent deformity
  5. Prevent flexion contractures

6. Apply heat or cold therapy to joints, as prescribed
7. Use paraffin baths and massage, as prescribed
8. Encourage consistency with exercise program
9. Instruct the client to stop exercise if pain increases
10. Exercise only to the point of pain
11. Avoid weight-bearing on inflamed joints

F. Self-care (Box 58-8)
1. Determine the need for assistive devices such as higher toilet seats, chairs, and wheelchairs to facilitate mobility
2. Collaborate with occupational therapy to obtain assistive or adaptive devices
3. Instruct the client in alternative strategies for providing activities of daily living

G. Fatigue
1. Identify factors that may contribute to fatigue
2. Monitor for signs of anemia
3. Administer iron, folic acid, and vitamin supplements, as prescribed
4. Monitor for drug-related blood loss by testing the stool for occult blood
5. Instruct the client in measures to conserve energy, such as pacing activities and obtaining assistance when possible

H. Body image disturbance
1. Assess the client's reaction to the body change
2. Encourage the client to verbalize feelings
3. Assist the client with self-care activities and grooming
4. Encourage the client to wear street clothes

I. Surgical interventions
1. Synovectomy: Surgical removal of the synovia to help maintain joint function
2. Arthrodesis: Bony fusion of a joint to regain some mobility

---

BOX 58-8

Client Education for Rheumatoid Arthritis (RA) and Degenerative Joint Disease (DJD)

Assist the client to identify and correct hazards in the home.
Instruct the client in the correct use of assistive or adaptive devices.
Instruct in energy conservation measures.
Review prescribed exercise program.
Instruct the client to sit in a chair with a high, straight back.
Instruct the client to use a small pillow under the head only, when lying down.
Instruct the client in measures to protect the joints.
Instruct the client regarding the prescribed medications.
Stress the importance of follow-up visits with the health care provider.

---

3. Joint replacement (arthroplasty): Surgical replacement of diseased joints with artificial joints; performed to restore motion to a joint and function to the muscles, ligaments, and other soft tissue structures that control a joint

XIV. OSTEOARTHRITIS (DEGENERATIVE JOINT DISEASE [DJD])

A. Description
1. Progressive degeneration of the joints as a result of wear and tear
2. Causes the formation of bony buildup and the loss of articular cartilage in peripheral and axial joints
3. Affects the weight-bearing joints and joints that receive the greatest stress, such as the knees, toes, and lower spine
4. The cause is unknown but may be trauma, fractures, infections, or obesity

B. Data collection
1. Dull, aching joint pain that diminishes after rest and intensifies after activity, noted early in the disease process
2. As the disease progresses, pain occurs with slight motion or even at rest
3. Symptoms are aggravated by temperature change and humidity
4. Crepitus
5. Joint enlargement
6. Presence of Heberden's nodes or Bouchard's nodes
7. Limited ROM
8. Difficulty getting up after prolonged sitting
9. Skeletal muscle atrophy
10. Inability to perform activities of daily living
11. Compression of the spine as manifested by radiating pain, stiffness, and muscle spasms in one or both extremities

C. Pain
1. Administer NSAIDs, salicylates, and muscle relaxants, as prescribed
2. Prepare the client for corticosteroid injections into joints, as prescribed
3. Place affected joint in a functional position
4. Immobilize the affected joint with a splint or brace
5. Avoid large pillows under the head or knees
6. Provide a bed or foot cradle
7. Position the client prone twice a day
8. Instruct the client in the importance of moist heat, hot packs or compresses, and paraffin dips as prescribed
9. Apply cold applications as prescribed when the joint is acutely inflamed
10. Encourage adequate rest, recommending 10 hours of sleep at night and a 1- to- 2 hour nap in the afternoon

D. Nutrition
1. Encourage a well-balanced diet
2. Encourage weight loss if necessary
E. Physical mobility
1. Reinforce the exercise program and the importance of participating in the program
2. Instruct the client that exercises should be active rather than passive and to exercise only to the point of pain
3. Instruct the client to stop exercise if pain is increased with exercising
4. Instruct the client to decrease the number of repetitions in an exercise when the inflammation is severe
F. Surgical management
1. Osteotomy: The bone is cut to correct joint deformity and promote realignment
2. Total joint replacement (TJR)
   a. Performed when all measures of pain relief have failed
   b. Hips and knees are most commonly replaced
   c. Contraindicated in the presence of infection, advanced osteoporosis, or severe inflammation

XV. OSTEOPOROSIS

A. Description
1. An age-related metabolic disease
2. Bone demineralization results in the loss of bone mass, leading to fragile and porous bones and subsequent fractures
3. Greater bone resorption than bone formation occurs
4. Occurs most commonly in the wrist, hip, and vertebral column
5. Can occur postmenopausally or as a result of a metabolic disorder or calcium deficiency
6. Client may be asymptomatic until the bones become so weak that a sudden injury causes a fracture
7. Risk factors (Box 58-9)
B. Data collection
1. May be asymptomatic
2. Back pain after lifting, bending, or stooping
3. Back pain that increases with palpation
4. Pelvic or hip pain, especially with weight-bearing
5. Problems with balance
6. Decline in height from vertebral compression
7. Kyphosis of the dorsal spine
8. Constipation, abdominal distention, and respiratory impairment as a result of movement restriction and spinal deformity
9. Pathological fractures
10. Appearance of thin porous bone on x-ray
C. Interventions
1. Assess risk for injury
2. Provide a safe and hazard-free environment; assist the client to identify hazards in the home environment
3. Use side rails to prevent falls
4. Move the client gently when turning and repositioning
5. Encourage ambulation; assist with ambulation if the client is unsteady
6. Instruct in the use of assistive devices such as a cane or walker
7. Provide ROM exercises
8. Instruct in the use of good body mechanics
9. Instruct the client in exercises to strengthen abdominal and back muscles to improve posture and provide support for the spine
10. Instruct the client to avoid activities that can cause vertebral compression
11. Apply a back brace as prescribed during an acute phase to immobilize the spine and provide spinal column support
12. Encourage the use of a firm mattress
13. Provide a diet high in protein, calcium, vitamins C and D, and iron
14. Encourage adequate fluid intake to prevent renal calculi
15. Instruct the client to avoid alcohol and coffee
16. Administer estrogen or androgens to decrease the rate of bone resorption, as prescribed
17. Administer calcium, vitamin D, and phosphorus as prescribed for bone metabolism
18. Administer calcitonin as prescribed to inhibit bone loss
19. Administer analgesics, muscle relaxants, and anti-inflammatory medications, as prescribed

XVI. GOUT

A. Description
1. A systemic disease in which urate crystals deposit in joints and other body tissues
2. Leads to abnormal amounts of uric acid in the body
3. Primary gout results from a disorder of purine metabolism
4. Secondary gout involves excessive uric acid in the blood that is caused by another disease

---

BOX 58-9

Risk Factors for Osteoporosis

Female gender
Increasing age
Family history
White (European descent) or Asian race
Thin small frame
Early menopause
Insufficient intake of calcium
Sedentary lifestyle
Excessive use of alcohol
Cigarette smoking

B. Phases
  1. Asymptomatic
    a. No symptoms
    b. Serum uric acid level is elevated
  2. Acute: Excruciating pain and inflammation of one or more small joints, especially the great toe
  3. Intermittent: Asymptomatic period between acute attacks
  4. Chronic
    a. Results from repeated episodes of acute gout
    b. Results in deposits of urate crystals under the skin and within the major organs, especially the renal system
C. Data collection
  1. Excruciating pain in the involved joints
  2. Swelling and inflammation of the joints
  3. Tophi (hard, fairly large, and irregularly shaped deposits in the skin) that may break open and discharge a yellow, gritty substance
  4. Low-grade fever
  5. Malaise and headache
  6. Pruritus
  7. Presence of renal stones
  8. Elevated uric acid levels
D. Interventions
  1. Provide a low-purine diet, as prescribed
  2. Instruct the client to avoid foods such as organ meats, wines, aged cheese
  3. Encourage a high fluid intake of 2000 mL/day to prevent stone formation
  4. Encourage weight-reduction diet if required
  5. Instruct the client to avoid alcohol and starvation diets because they may precipitate a gout attack
  6. Increase urinary pH (above 6) by eating alkaline ash foods such as citrus fruits and juices, milk, and other dairy products
  7. Provide bed rest during the acute attacks
  8. Monitor joint ROM ability and appearance of joints
  9. Position the joint in mild flexion during acute attack
  10. Elevate the affected extremity
  11. Protect the affected joint from excessive movement or direct contact with sheets or blankets
  12. Provide heat or cold for local treatments to affected joint, as prescribed
  13. Administer NSAIDs and antigout medications, as prescribed

PRACTICE QUESTIONS

1. A client is treated in the physician's office after a fall, which sprained the ankle. Radiography has ruled out fracture. Before sending the client home, the nurse would plan to teach the client about which item that is to be avoided in the next 24 hours?
   1. Application of a heating pad
   2. Application of an Ace wrap
   3. Resting the foot
   4. Elevating the ankle on a pillow while sitting or lying down

2. A nurse is collecting physical data of the musculoskeletal system on an assigned client. The nurse would document the presence of which of the following as a normal finding?
   1. Presence of fasciculations
   2. Atrophy on the client's dominant side
   3. Hypertrophy on the client's dominant side
   4. Atrophy on the client's nondominant side

3. A nurse has given dietary instructions to a client to minimize the risk of osteoporosis. The nurse determines that the client understands the recommended changes if the client verbalizes to increase intake of which of these foods?
   1. Potatoes
   2. Cheese
   3. Fish
   4. Chicken

4. A nurse is providing care of the client following a bone biopsy. Which action by the nurse is unnecessary in the care of this client?
   1. Monitoring the site for swelling, bleeding, hematoma
   2. Administering intramuscular narcotic analgesics
   3. Elevating the limb for 24 hours
   4. Monitoring vitals signs every 4 hours

5. A nurse has reinforced instructions to the client returning home after arthroscopy of the knee. The nurse determines that the client understands the instructions if the client states that he or she will:
   1. Stay off the leg entirely for the rest of the day
   2. Resume regular exercise the following day
   3. Refrain from eating food for the remainder of the day
   4. Report fever or site inflammation to the physician

6. A nurse is caring for the client who is going to have an arthrogram using a contrast medium. Which of the following data collected by the nurse would be of highest priority?
   1. Allergy to iodine or shellfish
   2. Ability of the client to remain still during the procedure
   3. Whether the client has any remaining questions about the procedure
   4. Whether the client needs to void before the procedure

7. A client with possible rib fracture has never had a chest x-ray. The nurse would plan to tell the client which of the following items about the procedure?
   1. The x-ray stimulates a small amount of pain
   2. It is necessary to remove jewelry and any other metal objects
   3. The client will be asked to breathe in and out during the x-ray
   4. The x-ray technologist will stand next to the client during the x-ray

8. A nurse is teaching the client who is to have a gallium scan about the procedure. The nurse would include which of the following items as part of the instructions?
   1. The gallium will be injected intravenously 2 to 3 hours before the procedure
   2. The procedure takes about 15 minutes to perform
   3. The client must stand erect during the filming
   4. The client should remain on bed rest for the remainder of the day after the scan

9. A client has had a bone scan procedure. The nurse determines that the client understands the elements of follow-up care if the client states that he or she will:
   1. Report any feelings of nausea or flushing
   2. Ambulate at least three times before the end of the day
   3. Eat only small meals for the remainder of the day
   4. Drink plenty of water for a day or two following the procedure

10. A client seeks treatment in the emergency room for a lower leg injury. There is visible deformity to the lower aspect of the leg, and the injured leg appears shorter than the other. The area is painful, swollen, and beginning to become ecchymotic. The nurse interprets that this client has experienced a:
    1. Contusion
    2. Fracture
    3. Sprain
    4. Strain

11. A nurse is one of several people who witness a vehicle hit a pedestrian at a fairly low speed on a small street. The individual is dazed and tries to get up, and the leg appears fractured. The nurse would plan to:
    1. Stay with the person and encourage the person to remain still
    2. Assist the person to get up and walk to the sidewalk
    3. Leave the person for a few moments to call an ambulance
    4. Try to manually reduce the fracture

12. A nurse witnesses a client sustain a fall and suspects that the client's leg may be fractured. Which action is the priority?
    1. Take a set of vital signs
    2. Call the radiology department
    3. Reassure the client that everything will be fine
    4. Immobilize the leg before moving the client

13. A nurse in the emergency room is caring for a client with a fractured arm. The nurse understands that which item is not necessary before reduction of the fracture in the casting room?
    1. Explanation of the procedure to the client
    2. Administration of an analgesic
    3. Anesthesia consent
    4. Consent for the procedure

14. A nurse provides cast application instructions to a client who is going to have a plaster cast applied. The nurse determines that the client needs further instructions if the client states that:
    1. A stockinette will be placed over the leg area to be casted
    2. The cast edges may be trimmed with a cast knife
    3. The cast will give off heat as it dries
    4. The client may bear weight on the cast in 30 minutes

15. A nurse is planning to teach the client with a left arm cast about measures to keep the left shoulder from becoming stiff. Which suggestion would the nurse include in the teaching plan?
    1. Lift the left arm up over the head
    2. Lift the right arm up over the head
    3. Make a fist with the hand of the casted arm
    4. Use a sling on the left arm

16. A client has a fiberglass (nonplaster) cast applied to the lower leg. The client asks the nurse when he will be able to walk on the cast. The nurse replies that the client will be able to bear weight on the cast:
    1. Within 20 to 30 minutes of application
    2. In approximately 8 hours
    3. In 24 hours
    4. In 48 hours

17. A nurse has reinforced instructions with the client with a nonplaster (fiberglass) leg cast about cast care at home. The nurse determines that the client needs further instructions if the client makes which statement?
    1. "I should avoid walking on wet, slippery floors."
    2. "It's all right to wipe dirt off the top of the cast with a damp cloth."
    3. "I'm not supposed to scratch the skin underneath the cast."
    4. "If the cast gets wet, I can dry it with a hair dryer turned to the warmest setting."

18. A client with a hip fracture asks the nurse why Buck's extension traction is being applied before surgery. The nurse's response is based on the understanding that Buck's extension traction primarily:
    1. Provides rigid immobilization of the fracture site
    2. Provides comfort by reducing muscle spasms and provides fracture immobilization
    3. Lengthens the fractured leg to prevent severing of blood vessels
    4. Allows bony healing to begin before surgery

19. A client in skeletal leg traction with an overbed frame is not allowed to turn from side to side. Which action by the nurse would be most useful in trying to provide good skin care to the client?
    1. Asking the client to lift up by digging into the mattress with the unaffected leg
    2. Pushing down on the mattress of the bed while administering care
    3. Having another nurse tilt the client to the side

4. Asking the client pull up on a trapeze to lift the hips off the bed

20. A nurse is evaluating the pin sites of a client in skeletal traction. The nurse would be least concerned with which finding?
    1. Purulent drainage
    2. Serous drainage
    3. Pain at a pin site
    4. Inflammation

21. A client has Buck's extension traction applied to the right leg. The nurse would plan which intervention to prevent complications of the device?
    1. Massaging the skin of the right leg with lotion every 8 hours
    2. Giving pin care once a shift
    3. Inspecting the skin on the right leg at least once every 8 hours
    4. Releasing the weights on the right leg for range-of-motion exercises daily

22. A nurse is caring for the client who has had skeletal traction applied to the left leg. The client is complaining of severe left leg pain. Which action should the nurse take first?
    1. Medicate the client with an analgesic
    2. Provide pin care
    3. Call the physician immediately
    4. Check the client's alignment in bed

23. A nurse has reinforced instructions regarding specific leg exercises for the client immobilized in right skeletal lower leg traction. The nurse determines that the client needs further instruction if the nurse observes the client:
    1. Pulling up on the trapeze
    2. Flexing and extending the feet
    3. Performing active range of motion (ROM) to the right ankle and knee
    4. Doing quadriceps-setting and gluteal-setting exercises

24. A nurse is checking the casted extremity of a client. The nurse would check for which of the following signs and symptoms indicative of infection?
    1. Coolness and pallor of the extremity
    2. Presence of a "hot spot" on the cast
    3. Diminished distal pulse
    4. Dependent edema

25. A client has sustained a closed fracture and has just had a cast applied to the affected arm. The client is complaining of intense pain. The nurse has elevated the limb, applied an ice bag, and administered an analgesic, which was ineffective in relieving the pain. The nurse interprets that this pain may be caused by:
    1. Impaired tissue perfusion
    2. The newness of the fracture
    3. The anxiety of the client
    4. Infection under the cast

26. A nurse is assigned to care for a client with multiple trauma who is admitted to the hospital. The client has a leg fracture and a plaster cast has been applied. In positioning the casted leg, the nurse should:
    1. Keep the leg in a level position
    2. Keep the leg level for 3 hours, and elevate it for 1 hour
    3. Elevate the leg on pillows continuously for 24 to 48 hours
    4. Elevate the leg for 3 hours, and put it flat for 1 hour

27. A client is complaining of skin irritation from the edges of a cast applied the previous day. The nurse should plan for which of the following actions?
    1. Massaging the skin at the rim of the cast
    2. Applying lotion to the skin at the rim of the cast
    3. Using a rough file to smooth the cast edges
    4. Petaling the cast edges with adhesive tape

28. A client is being discharged to home after application of a plaster leg cast. The nurse determines that the client understands proper care of the cast if the client states that he or she will:
    1. Avoid getting the cast wet
    2. Use the fingertips to lift and move the leg
    3. Cover the casted leg with warm blankets
    4. Use a padded coat hanger end to scratch under the cast

29. A client being measured for crutches asks the nurse why the crutches cannot rest up underneath the arm for extra support. The nurse's response is based on the understanding that this could result in:
    1. Impaired range of motion while the client ambulates
    2. Skin breakdown in the area of the axilla
    3. Injury to the brachial plexus nerves
    4. A fall and further injury

30. A nurse is planning to reinforce instructions to the client about how to stand on crutches. In the written instructions, the nurse plans to tell the client to place the crutches:
    1. 3 inches to the front and side of the client's toes
    2. 8 inches to the front and side of the client's toes
    3. 20 inches to the front and side of the client's toes
    4. 15 inches to the front and side of the client's toes

31. A nurse is giving the client with a left leg cast crutch-walking instructions using the three-point gait. The client is allowed touch-down of the affected leg. The nurse tells the client to advance the:
    1. Left leg and right crutch, then right leg and left crutch
    2. Crutches and then both legs simultaneously
    3. Crutches and the right leg, then advance the left leg
    4. Crutches and the left leg, then advance the right leg

32. A nurse has given the client instructions regarding crutch safety. The nurse determines that the client needs reinforcement of the instructions if the client states:
    1. The need to have spare crutches and tips available
    2. That crutch tips will not slip, even when wet
    3. Not to use someone else's crutches
    4. That crutch tips should be inspected periodically for wear

33. A client has slight weakness in the right leg. Based on this data, the nurse determines that the client would benefit most from the use of a:
    1. Walker
    2. Wooden crutch
    3. Lofstrand crutch
    4. Straight-leg cane

34. A client who has experienced a cerebrovascular accident (CVA) has partial hemiplegia of the left leg. The straight-leg cane formerly used by the client is not quite sufficient any longer. The nurse determines that the client could benefit from the somewhat greater support and stability provided by a:
    1. Quad cane
    2. Wooden crutch
    3. Lofstrand crutch
    4. Wheelchair

35. A client with right-sided weakness needs to learn how to use a cane. The nurse plans to teach the client to position the cane by holding it with the:
    1. Left hand, and placing the cane in front of the left foot
    2. Right hand, and placing the cane in front of the right foot
    3. Left hand, and 6 inches lateral to the left foot
    4. Right hand, and 6 inches lateral to the right foot

36. A client who is learning to use a cane is afraid it will slip with ambulation, causing a fall. The nurse provides the client with the greatest reassurance by telling the client that:
    1. Canes prevent falls, not cause them
    2. The cane has a flared tip with concentric rings to provide stability
    3. The physical therapist will determine if the cane is inadequate
    4. The cane would help to break a fall, even if the client does slip

37. A nurse is evaluating the client's use of a cane for left-sided weakness. The nurse would intervene and correct the client if the nurse observed that the client:
    1. Holds the cane on the right side
    2. Keeps the cane 6 inches out to the side of the right foot
    3. Moves the cane when the right leg is moved
    4. Leans on the cane when the right leg swings through

38. A nurse is caring for the client who has developed compartment syndrome from a severely fractured arm. The client asks the nurse how this can happen. The nurse's response is based on the understanding that:
    1. An injured artery causes impaired arterial perfusion through the compartment
    2. The fascia expands with injury, causing pressure on underlying nerves and muscles
    3. A bone fragment has injured the nerve supply in the area
    4. Bleeding and swelling cause increased pressure in an area that cannot expand

39. A nurse is caring for a client with fresh application of a plaster leg cast. The nurse plans to prevent the development of compartment syndrome by:
    1. Elevating the limb and applying ice to the affected leg
    2. Elevating the limb and covering the limb with bath blankets
    3. Placing the leg in a slightly dependent position and applying ice
    4. Keeping the leg horizontal and applying ice to the affected leg

40. A nurse is monitoring a confused older client admitted to the hospital with a hip fracture. Which of the following data obtained by the nurse would not place the client at increased risk for disturbed thought processes?
    1. Stress induced by the fracture
    2. Hearing aid available and in working order
    3. Unfamiliar hospital setting
    4. Eyeglasses left at home

41. A nurse is caring for an older client who had a hip pinned after being fractured. In planning nursing care, which of the following would the nurse avoid to minimize the chance for further injury?
    1. Side rails in the "up" position
    2. Use of night-light in hospital room and bathroom
    3. Call bell placed within reach
    4. Delays in responding to call light

42. A nurse is repositioning the client who has returned to the nursing unit following internal fixation of a fractured right hip. The nurse plans to use a:
    1. Pillow to keep the right leg abducted during turning
    2. Pillow to keep the right leg adducted during turning
    3. Trochanter roll to prevent external rotation while turning
    4. Trochanter roll to prevent abduction while turning

43. A client who has had a right total knee replacement asks the nurse how long the right leg must be kept in the continuous passive motion (CPM) machine. The nurse's response is based on the understanding that the device should be used:
    1. For 30 minutes out of every hour

2. Every other hour for 60 minutes

3. For 3 hours at a time, followed by 1 hour of rest

4. As much as the client can tolerate

44. A nurse has an order to get the client out of bed to a chair on the first postoperative day after total knee replacement. The nurse plans to do which of the following to protect the knee joint?

1. Apply a knee immobilizer before getting the client up, and elevate the client's surgical leg while sitting

2. Apply an ace wrap around the dressing, and put ice on the knee while sitting

3. Lift the client to the bedside chair, leaving the continuous passive motion (CPM) machine in place

4. Obtain a walker to minimize weight-bearing by the client on the affected leg

45. A client with diabetes mellitus has had a right below-knee amputation. The nurse would be especially vigilant in monitoring for which of the following because of the client's history of diabetes mellitus?

1. Edema of the stump

2. Hemorrhage

3. Separation of wound edges

4. Slight redness of incision

46. A client is admitted to the nursing unit after a left below-knee amputation following a crush injury to the foot and lower leg. The client tells the nurse, "I think I'm going crazy. I can feel my left foot itching." The nurse interprets the client's statement to be:

1. A normal response, and indicates the presence of phantom limb sensation

2. A normal response, and indicates the presence of phantom limb pain

3. An abnormal response, and indicates that the client needs more psychological support

4. An abnormal response, and indicates that the client is in denial about the limb loss

47. A client is complaining of low back pain, with radiation down the left posterior thigh. The nurse continues to collect data from the client to see if the pain is worsened or aggravated by:

1. Bed rest

2. Application of heat

3. Bending or lifting

4. Ibuprofen (Motrin)

48. A client has just undergone spinal fusion after suffering a herniated lumbar disk. The nurse would avoid which of the following to maintain client safety after this procedure?

1. Logrolling technique for repositioning

2. Pillows under the length of the legs

3. Head of bed flat

4. Overhead trapeze

49. A nurse has reinforced instructions with a client with a herniated lumbar disk about proper body mechanics and other items pertinent to low back care. The nurse determines that the client needs further instructions if the client verbalizes that he or she will:

1. Get out of bed by sitting straight up and swinging legs over the side of the bed

2. Increase fiber and fluids in the diet

3. Strengthen the back muscles by swimming or walking

4. Bend at the knees to pick up objects

50. A client who has had spinal fusion and insertion of hardware is extremely concerned about the perceived lengthy rehabilitation period. The client expresses concerns about finances and ability to return to prior employment. The nurse understands that the client's needs could best be addressed by referral to the:

1. Surgeon

2. Clinical nurse specialist

3. Social worker

4. Physical therapist

51. A nurse is planning to reinforce instructions to the client about proper use of a thoracolumbosacral orthosis (TLSO) after spinal fusion with instrumentation. The nurse plans to include which of the following teaching points in discussion with the client?

1. Areas of skin redness at the edges of the brace indicates a good, snug fit

2. The device is applied before getting out of bed in the morning

3. The brace should be applied directly next to the skin

4. The Velcro closures should be fairly loose to avoid constriction

52. A client is being transferred to the nursing unit from the postanesthesia care unit following spinal fusion with rod insertion. The nurse would prepare to transfer the client from the stretcher to the bed by using:

1. A bath blanket and the assistance of three people

2. A bath blanket and the assistance of four people

3. A slider board and the assistance of two people

4. A slider board and the assistance of four people

53. A client is being discharged to home following spinal fusion with insertion of rods. The nurse would suggest a consultation with the continuing care nurse regarding the need for follow-up modification of the home environment if the client states that:

1. The bedroom and bath are on the second floor of the home

2. The bathroom has hand railings in the shower

3. The family has rented a commode for use by the client

4. There are three steps to get up to the front door

54. A client with a left arm fracture exhibits loss of sensation in the left fingers, pallor, slow refill, and diminished left radial pulse. The nurse should take which of the following actions?
    1. Administer an analgesic
    2. Check the circulation again in 30 minutes
    3. Provide range-of-motion exercises to the fingers of the left hand
    4. Contact the physician

55. A client is complaining of pain underneath a cast in the area of a bony prominence. The nurse interprets that this client may need to have:
    1. The cast replaced with an air splint
    2. Extra padding put over this area of the cast
    3. The cast bivalved
    4. A window cut in the cast

56. A client is fearful about having an arm cast removed. Which of the following actions by the nurse would be the most helpful?
    1. Telling the client that the saw makes a frightening noise
    2. Reassuring the client that no one has had an arm lacerated yet
    3. Stating that the hot cutting blades cause burns only very rarely
    4. Showing the client the cast cutter and explaining how it works

57. A nursing instructor asks a nursing student about the risk factors associated with osteoporosis. The instructor tells the student that she needs to read and learn about this disorder if the student states that which of the following is an associated risk factor?
    1. High-calcium diet consumption
    2. Postmenopausal age
    3. Long-term use of corticosteroids
    4. Family history of osteoporosis

58. A nurse is providing instructions to a client with osteoporosis regarding appropriate food items to include in the diet. The nurse tells the client that which food item would provide the least amount of calcium?
    1. Plain yogurt
    2. Seafood
    3. Sardines
    4. Pork

59. A client has several fractures of the lower leg and has been placed in an external fixation device. The client is upset about the appearance of the leg, which is very edematous. The nurse suggests which of the following nursing diagnoses for the client?
    1. Disturbed Body Image
    2. Activity Intolerance
    3. Risk for Impaired Physical Mobility
    4. Social Isolation

60. A nurse is caring for a client with a diagnosis of gout. Which of the following laboratory values would the nurse expect to note in the client?
    1. Uric acid level of 8.0 mg/dL
    2. Calcium level of 9.0 mg/dL
    3. Phosphorus level of 3.0 mg/dL
    4. Potassium level of 4.0 mEq/L

61. A nurse is caring for a client with osteoarthritis. The nurse collects data, knowing that which of the following is a clinical manifestation associated with the disorder?
    1. Morning stiffness
    2. An elevated sedimentation rate
    3. Dull aching pain in the affected joints
    4. Positive rheumatoid factor

ALTERNATE FORMAT QUESTION: MULTIPLE RESPONSE

A nurse is preparing a list of cast care instructions for a client who just had a plaster cast applied to his right forearm. Select all instructions that the nurse includes on the list.

___ Keep the cast and extremity elevated
___ Allow the wet cast 24 to 48 hours to dry
___ Use a hair dryer set on a warm to hot setting to dry the cast
___ Tingling and numbness in the extremity are expected
___ Use a soft padded object that will fit under the cast to scratch the skin under the cast
___ The cast needs to be kept clean and dry

ANSWERS

1. *Answer:* **1**
Rationale: Soft tissue injuries such as sprains are treated by **RICE** (rest, ice, compression, elevation) for the first 24 hours after the injury. Ice is applied intermittently for 20 to 30 minutes at a time. Heat is not used in the first 24 hours because it could increase venous congestion, which would increase edema and pain.
Test-Taking Strategy: Note the key word, *avoided*. This word indicates a false response question and that you need to select the incorrect intervention. It is likely that sprains should be rested and elevated, so options 3 and 4 are eliminated. Use of an Ace wrap is also helpful in reducing the pain and swelling, so eliminate option 2. By the process of elimination, heat is the item to avoid in the first 24 hours. Review the measures to treat a sprain if you had difficulty with this question.
Level of Cognitive Ability: Application
Client Needs: Physiological Integrity
Integrated Process: Nursing Process/Planning
Content Area: Adult Health/Musculoskeletal

References: Christensen, B., & Kockrow, E. (2003). *Adult health nursing* (4th ed.). St. Louis: Mosby, p. 157.
Linton, A., & Maebius, N. (2003). *Introduction to medical-surgical nursing* (3rd ed.). Philadelphia: W.B. Saunders, p. 157.

2. Answer: 3
Rationale: Hypertrophy, or increased muscle size on the client's dominant side of up to 1 cm, is considered normal. Atrophy on either side is considered an abnormal finding. Fasciculations are fine muscle twitches that are not normally present.
Test-Taking Strategy: Use the process of elimination, noting the key word, *normal*. Options 2 and 4 are eliminated first because atrophy is not a normal finding. Knowing that fasciculations are not normal helps you select option 3 over option 1. Review normal musculoskeletal findings if you had difficulty with this question.
Level of Cognitive Ability: Comprehension
Client Needs: Physiological Integrity
Integrated Process: Nursing Process/Data Collection
Content Area: Adult Health/Musculoskeletal
References: Black, J., & Hawks, J. (2005). *Medical-surgical nursing: Clinical management for positive outcomes* (7th ed.). Philadelphia: W.B. Saunders, pp. 202, 569.
Jarvis, C. (2004). *Physical examination and health assessment* (4th ed.). Philadelphia: W.B. Saunders, p. 676.

3. Answer: 2
Rationale: Calcium intake is important to minimize the risk of osteoporosis. The major dietary source of calcium is from dairy foods, including milk, yogurt, and a variety of cheeses. Calcium may also be added to certain products, such as orange juice, which are then advertised as being "fortified" with calcium. Calcium supplements are also recommended to minimize the risk of osteoporosis. Options 1, 3, and 4 are foods that are not high in calcium.
Test-Taking Strategy: Use the process of elimination. Knowing that calcium is required for the client with osteoporosis and recalling the foods high in calcium will direct you to option 2. Review this content if you had difficulty with this question.
Level of Cognitive Ability: Comprehension
Client Needs: Health Promotion and Maintenance
Integrated Process: Nursing Process/Evaluation
Content Area: Adult Health/Musculoskeletal
Reference: Nix, S. (2005). *Williams basic nutrition and diet therapy* (12th ed.). St. Louis: Mosby, pp. 129-130.

4. Answer: 2
Rationale: Nursing care after bone biopsy includes monitoring the site for swelling, bleeding, and hematoma formation. The biopsy site is elevated for 24 hours to reduce edema. The vital signs are monitored every 4 hours for 24 hours. The client usually requires mild analgesics; more severe pain usually indicates that complications are arising.
Test-Taking Strategy: Note the key word, *unnecessary*. This word indicates a false response question and that you need to select the incorrect action. One way to approach this question is to look at the method of anesthesia used for this procedure. If you know that this procedure is done under

local anesthesia, it makes sense that monitoring vital signs every 4 hours is probably sufficient (option 4). The nurse would routinely monitor for complications (option 1). From the remaining options, site elevation is important to reduce edema, but narcotic administration by the intramuscular route seems excessive for a local procedure. Review care of the client following a bone biopsy if you had difficulty with this question.
Level of Cognitive Ability: Application
Client Needs: Physiological Integrity
Integrated Process: Nursing Process/Implementation
Content Area: Adult Health/Musculoskeletal
References: Black, J., & Hawks, J. (2005). *Medical-surgical nursing: Clinical management for positive outcomes* (7th ed.). Philadelphia: W.B. Saunders, pp. 2265-2267.
Chernecky, C., & Berger, B. (2004). *Laboratory tests and diagnostic procedures* (4th ed.). Philadelphia: W.B. Saunders, p. 280.

5. Answer: 4
Rationale: After arthroscopy, the client can usually walk carefully on the leg once sensation has returned. The client is instructed to avoid strenuous exercise for at least a few days. The client may resume the usual diet. Signs and symptoms of infection should be reported to the physician.
Test-Taking Strategy: Note the key words, *understands the instructions*. Remember, the client is always taught the signs and symptoms of infection to report to the physician. Review home care instructions following arthroscopy if you had difficulty with this question.
Level of Cognitive Ability: Comprehension
Client Needs: Health Promotion and Maintenance
Integrated Process: Nursing Process/Evaluation
Content Area: Adult Health/Musculoskeletal
References: Christensen, B., & Kockrow, E. (2003). *Adult health nursing* (4th ed.). St. Louis: Mosby, p. 112.
Linton, A., & Maebius, N. (2003). *Introduction to medical-surgical nursing* (3rd ed.). Philadelphia: W.B. Saunders, p. 799.

6. Answer: 1
Rationale: Because of the risk of allergy to contrast dye, the nurse places highest priority on identifying whether the client has an allergy to iodine or shellfish. The nurse also reinforces information about the test, tells the client about the need to remain still during the procedure, and encourages the client to void before the procedure for comfort.
Test-Taking Strategy: Note the key words, *highest priority*. This tells you that more than one or all of the options are correct (in fact, they all are). Although options 2, 3, and 4 all compete for priority, only option 1 (allergy to iodine or shellfish) takes first preference. The consequence of possible anaphylactic shock (physiological risk) makes this the correct option. Review care of the client scheduled for an arthrogram if you had difficulty with this question.
Level of Cognitive Ability: Application
Client Needs: Safe, Effective Care Environment
Integrated Process: Nursing Process/Data Collection
Content Area: Delegating/Prioritizing
Reference: Pagana, K., & Pagana, T. (2003). *Mosby's diagnostic and laboratory test reference* (6th ed.). St. Louis: Mosby, p. 134.

7. *Answer:* **2**

Rationale: An x-ray is a photographic image of a part of the body on a special film, which is used to diagnose a wide variety of conditions. The x-ray itself is painless; any discomfort would arise from repositioning a painful part for filming. The nurse may want to premedicate a client who is at risk for pain. Any radiopaque objects such as jewelry or other metal must be removed. The client is asked to breathe in deeply and then hold the breath while the chest x-ray is taken. To minimize risk of radiation exposure, the x-ray technologist stands in a separate area protected by a lead wall. The client also wears a lead shield over the genital area.

Test-Taking Strategy: Use the process of elimination. Visualize this procedure to eliminate options 1 and 4. From the remaining options, eliminate option 3 because the client needs to be still during the x-ray. Review this diagnostic procedure if you had difficulty with this question.

Level of Cognitive Ability: Application
Client Needs: Safe, Effective Care Environment
Integrated Process: Nursing Process/Implementation
Content Area: Adult Health/Musculoskeletal
Reference: Pagana, K., & Pagana, T. (2003). *Mosby's diagnostic and laboratory test reference* (6th ed.). St. Louis: Mosby, p. 239.

8. *Answer:* **1**

Rationale: A gallium scan is similar to a bone scan, but with an injection of gallium isotope instead of technetium Tc 99m. Gallium is injected 2 to 3 hours before the procedure. The procedure takes 30 to 60 minutes to perform. The client must lie still during the procedure. There is no special aftercare.

Test-Taking Strategy: Use the process of elimination. If you know that a gallium scan is similar to a bone scan, then you begin by eliminating options 3 and 4. The time frame in option 2 is rather short, so eliminate this option. Review this test if you had difficulty with this question.

Level of Cognitive Ability: Application
Client Needs: Physiological Integrity
Integrated Process: Nursing Process/Implementation
Content Area: Adult Health/Musculoskeletal
References: Chernecky, C., & Berger, B. (2004). *Laboratory tests and diagnostic procedures* (4th ed.). Philadelphia: W.B. Saunders, p. 572.
Pagana, K., & Pagana, T. (2003). *Mosby's diagnostic and laboratory test reference* (6th ed.). St. Louis: Mosby, p. 437.

9. *Answer:* **4**

Rationale: There are no special restrictions following a bone scan. The client is encouraged to drink large amounts of water for 24 to 48 hours to flush the radioisotope from the system. There are no hazards to the client or staff from the minimal amount of radioactivity of the isotope.

Test-Taking Strategy: Use the process of elimination. There is no purpose for options 2 or 3, which allows you to eliminate them first. Nausea and flushing could accompany dye injection during a procedure, but this procedure uses radioisotopes and the question relates to care after the procedure. Thus, option 1 is eliminated also. This leads you to option 4, which will hasten elimination of the isotope from the client's system.

Review this diagnostic procedure if you had difficulty with this question.

Level of Cognitive Ability: Comprehension
Client Needs: Physiological Integrity
Integrated Process: Nursing Process/Evaluation
Content Area: Adult Health/Musculoskeletal
Reference: Chernecky, C., & Berger, B. (2004). *Laboratory tests and diagnostic procedures* (4th ed.). Philadelphia: W.B. Saunders, p. 382.

10. *Answer:* **2**

Rationale: Typical signs and symptoms of fracture include pain, loss of function in the area, deformity, shortening of the extremity, crepitus, swelling, and ecchymosis. Not all fractures lead to the development of every sign. A contusion results from a blow to soft tissue and causes pain, swelling, and ecchymosis. A sprain is an injury to a ligament caused by a wrenching or twisting motion. Symptoms include pain, swelling, and inability to use the joint or bear weight normally. A strain results from a pulling force on the muscle. Symptoms include soreness and pain with muscle use.

Test-Taking Strategy: Use the process of elimination. Within the list of signs and symptoms in the question, note the one stating that one leg is shorter than another. Only a fractured bone (which shortens with displacement) could cause this sign. This makes it easy to eliminate each of the incorrect options. Review the signs of a fracture if you had difficulty with this question.

Level of Cognitive Ability: Comprehension
Client Needs: Physiological Integrity
Integrated Process: Nursing Process/Data Collection
Content Area: Adult Health/Musculoskeletal
Reference: Linton, A., & Maebius, N. (2003). *Introduction to medical-surgical nursing* (3rd ed.). Philadelphia: W.B. Saunders, pp. 821, 824-825.

11. *Answer:* **1**

Rationale: With a suspected fracture, the client is not moved unless it is dangerous to remain in that spot. The nurse should remain with the client, and have someone else call for emergency help. A fracture is not reduced at the scene. Before moving the client, the site of the fracture is immobilized to prevent further injury.

Test-Taking Strategy: Use the process of elimination. Eliminate options 2 and 4 first because these actions could result in further injury to the client. From the remaining options, the most prudent action would be for the nurse to remain with the client and have someone else call for emergency assistance. Review immediate care of the client with a fracture if you had difficulty with this question.

Level of Cognitive Ability: Application
Client Needs: Physiological Integrity
Integrated Process: Nursing Process/Implementation
Content Area: Adult Health/Musculoskeletal
Reference: Black, J., & Hawks, J. (2005). *Medical-surgical nursing: Clinical management for positive outcomes* (7th ed.). Philadelphia: W.B. Saunders, pp. 623, 2501.

12. *Answer:* **4**

Rationale: When a fracture is suspected, it is imperative that the area is splinted before the client is moved. Emergency help should be called for if the client is not hospitalized, and a physician is called for the hospitalized client. The nurse should remain with the client and provide realistic reassurance. The nurse does not prescribe radiology tests.

Test-Taking Strategy: Note the key word, *priority*. Eliminate option 2 because the nurse does not order x-rays. Option 3 is eliminated next, because the nurse never tells a client that "everything will be fine." From the remaining options, focus on the data in the question. Immobilizing the limb is imperative for the client's safety, which makes it a better choice than taking vital signs. Review care of the client when a fracture is suspected if you had difficulty with this question.

Level of Cognitive Ability: Application
Client Needs: Physiological Integrity
Integrated Process: Nursing Process/Implementation
Content Area: Adult Health/Musculoskeletal
Reference: Black, J., & Hawks, J. (2005). *Medical-surgical nursing: Clinical management for positive outcomes* (7th ed.). Philadelphia: W.B. Saunders, pp. 623, 2501.

13. *Answer:* **3**
Rationale: Before a fracture is reduced, the client is informed about the procedure and consent is obtained. An analgesic is given as prescribed, because the procedure is painful. Administration of anesthesia may or may not be done, depending on severity. Closed reductions may be done in the emergency room without anesthesia. If anesthesia is used, the procedure is done in the operating room.

Test-Taking Strategy: Note the key words, *not necessary* and *casting room*. Options 1 and 4 are obviously needed, so these options are eliminated first. The question specifically states that the procedure is going to be done in the casting room, which helps you select option 3 (anesthesia consent) as the unnecessary item. Review the procedure for reduction of a fracture if you had difficulty with this question.

Level of Cognitive Ability: Comprehension
Client Needs: Physiological Integrity
Integrated Process: Nursing Process/Planning
Content Area: Adult Health/Musculoskeletal
References: Black, J., & Hawks, J. (2005). *Medical-surgical nursing: Clinical management for positive outcomes* (7th ed.). Philadelphia: W.B. Saunders, pp. 623-626.
deWit, S. (2005). *Fundamental concepts and skills for nursing.* Philadelphia: W.B. Saunders, p. 33.
Linton, A., & Maebius, N. (2003). *Introduction to medical-surgical nursing* (3rd ed.). Philadelphia: W.B. Saunders, pp. 189, 825.

14. *Answer:* **4**
Rationale: The procedure for casting involves washing and drying the skin and placing a stockinette material over the area to be casted. A roll of padding is then applied smoothly and evenly. The plaster is rolled onto the padding, and the edges are trimmed or smoothed as needed. A plaster cast gives off heat as it dries. A plaster cast can tolerate weight-bearing once it is dry, which varies from 24 to 72 hours, depending on the nature and thickness of the cast.

Test-Taking Strategy: Note the key words, *needs further instructions*. These words indicate a false response question and that you need to select the incorrect client statement. Familiarity with the different types of casting materials and their differences helps you answer this question. Options 1, 2, and 3 are all true for plaster casts. Option 4 is true for nonplaster casts. Review the procedure for applying a cast if you had difficulty with this question.

Level of Cognitive Ability: Comprehension
Client Needs: Psychosocial Integrity
Integrated Process: Teaching/Learning
Content Area: Adult Health/Musculoskeletal
Reference: Christensen, B., & Kockrow, E. (2003). *Adult health nursing* (4th ed.). St. Louis: Mosby, p. 148.

15. *Answer:* **1**
Rationale: Immobility and the weight of a casted arm may cause the shoulder above an arm fracture to become stiff. The shoulder of a casted arm should be lifted over the head periodically as a preventive measure. The use of slings further immobilizes the shoulder and may be contraindicated. Making fists with the left hand provides isometric exercise to maintain muscle strength. Range of motion of the affected fingers is also a useful general measure. Lifting the right arm is of no particular value.

Test-Taking Strategy: Use the process of elimination. Visualize each of the movements and think about the muscle groups that are moved with each. Options 2 and 4 provide for no movement of the left arm and are eliminated first. Making a fist with hand on the casted arm provides good isometric exercise to the muscles surrounding the fracture but, again, does nothing for the shoulder. The only helpful suggestion is raising the arm over the head, which provides some range of motion for the shoulder joint. Review these measures if you had difficulty with this question.

Level of Cognitive Ability: Application
Client Needs: Health Promotion and Maintenance
Integrated Process: Teaching/Learning
Content Area: Adult Health/Musculoskeletal
Reference: Christensen, B., & Kockrow, E. (2003). *Adult health nursing* (4th ed.). St. Louis: Mosby, p. 150.

16. *Answer:* **1**
Rationale: A fiberglass cast is made of water-activated polyurethane materials, which are dry to the touch within minutes and reach full rigid strength in about 20 minutes. Because of this, the client can bear weight on the cast within 20 to 30 minutes.

Test-Taking Strategy: Use the process of elimination. Options 3 and 4 should be eliminated first, because these time frames are similar to the drying times for plaster casts. Knowing that the nonplaster type of cast is lighter and dries extremely quickly may help you choose the 20- to 30-minute time frame as correct. Review client teaching points related to casts if you had difficulty with this question.

Level of Cognitive Ability: Application
Client Needs: Health Promotion and Maintenance
Integrated Process: Nursing Process/Implementation
Content Area: Adult Health/Musculoskeletal

Reference: Christensen, B., & Kockrow, E. (2003). *Adult health nursing* (4th ed.). St. Louis: Mosby, p. 150.

17. *Answer:* **4**
Rationale: Client instructions should include avoidance of walking on wet, slippery floors to prevent falls. Surface soil on a cast may be removed with a damp cloth. If the cast gets wet, it can be dried with a hair dryer set to a cool setting to prevent skin breakdown. If the skin under the cast itches, cool air from a hair dryer may be used to relieve it. The client should never scratch under a cast because of risk of skin breakdown and ulcer formation.
Test-Taking Strategy: Note the key words, *needs further instructions*. These words indicate a false response question and that you need to select the incorrect client statement. Options 1 and 3 are certainly true and are therefore eliminated. Knowledge of nonplaster cast material is needed to select between the remaining options. A fiberglass cast may be wiped with a damp cloth, because it is water resistant. It may be helpful to remember never to use a hair dryer on a cast or on the skin under any cast with the dryer set at the warmest setting; only cool settings are used to prevent burns. Review client teaching points related to casts if you had difficulty with this question.
Level of Cognitive Ability: Comprehension
Client Needs: Health Promotion and Maintenance
Integrated Process: Teaching/Learning
Content Area: Adult Health/Musculoskeletal
Reference: Christensen, B., & Kockrow, E. (2003). *Adult health nursing* (4th ed.). St. Louis: Mosby, p. 150.

18. *Answer:* **2**
Rationale: Buck's extension traction is a type of skin traction often applied after hip fracture, before the fracture is reduced in surgery. It reduces muscle spasms and helps immobilize the fracture. It does not lengthen the leg for the purpose of preventing blood vessel severance. It also does not allow for bony healing to begin.
Test-Taking Strategy: Use the process of elimination. Recalling the purpose of traction will assist in eliminating options 3 and 4. From the remaining options, eliminate option 1 because of the words "rigid immobilization." Review this type of traction if you had difficulty with this question.
Level of Cognitive Ability: Application
Client Needs: Physiological Integrity
Integrated Process: Nursing Process/Implementation
Content Area: Adult Health/Musculoskeletal
Reference: Christensen, B., & Kockrow, E. (2003). *Adult health nursing* (4th ed.). St. Louis: Mosby, p. 150.

19. *Answer:* **4**
Rationale: If the client in skeletal traction may not turn from side to side, the nurse should have the client pull up on a trapeze and try to lift the hips off the bed for skin care, bed pan use, and linen changes. If the client is unable to pull up on a trapeze, the nurse can push down on the mattress with one hand while administering care with the other.
Test-Taking Strategy: Use the process of elimination. Option 3 is contraindicated because it ignores a medical order. Option 1 is not feasible as stated. The client cannot lift up from the bed using one foot only. Options 2 and 4 are both acceptable alternatives. Because the question asks which would be "most useful," the answer is option 4. Providing care for the client who can lift the hips off the bed using a trapeze is easier and more efficient than providing care to one who cannot. Review care of the client in traction if you had difficulty with this question.
Level of Cognitive Ability: Application
Client Needs: Physiological Integrity
Integrated Process: Nursing Process/Implementation
Content Area: Adult Health/Musculoskeletal
Reference: Christensen, B., & Kockrow, E. (2003). *Adult health nursing* (4th ed.). St. Louis: Mosby, p. 153.

20. *Answer:* **2**
Rationale: A small amount of serous oozing is expected at pin insertion sites. Signs of infection such as inflammation, purulent drainage, and pain at the pin site are not expected findings and should be reported.
Test-Taking Strategy: Note the key words, *least concerned with*. Options 1 and 4 seem to indicate an infectious problem, and are eliminated. To select between options 2 and 3, look at them carefully. The complaint of pain is at "a pin site" only. It gives no indication that the pain is related to the fracture or muscle spasm. Because serous drainage is an expected finding, you would select this over the complaint of pain as the answer to the question. Review care of the client in skeletal traction if you had difficulty with this question.
Level of Cognitive Ability: Analysis
Client Needs: Physiological Integrity
Integrated Process: Nursing Process/Evaluation
Content Area: Adult Health/Musculoskeletal
References: Black, J., & Hawks, J. (2005). *Medical-surgical nursing: Clinical management for positive outcomes* (7th ed.). Philadelphia: W.B. Saunders, p. 635.
Christensen, B., & Kockrow, E. (2003). *Adult health nursing* (4th ed.). St. Louis: Mosby, p. 153.

21. *Answer:* **3**
Rationale: Buck's extension traction is a type of skin traction. The nurse inspects the skin of the limb in traction at least once every 8 hours for irritation or inflammation. Massaging the skin with lotion is not indicated. The nurse never releases the weights of traction unless specifically ordered by the physician. There are no pins to care for with skin traction.
Test-Taking Strategy: Use the process of elimination. Recalling the components of Buck's extension traction allows you to eliminate options 2 and 4 easily. There are no pins, and the nurse never removes weights without a specific order to do so. Because the apparatus would have to be removed to apply lotion, which is unnecessary, then the answer is to inspect the skin. Review care of the client with Buck's extension traction if you had difficulty with this question.
Level of Cognitive Ability: Application
Client Needs: Safe, Effective Care Environment
Integrated Process: Nursing Process/Planning
Content Area: Adult Health/Musculoskeletal
Reference: Christensen, B., & Kockrow, E. (2003). *Adult health nursing* (4th ed.). St. Louis: Mosby, p. 153.

22. Answer: 4

Rationale: A client who complains of severe pain may need realignment or may have had traction weights ordered that are too heavy. The nurse realigns the client and, if ineffective, then calls the physician. Severe leg pain, once traction has been established, indicates a problem. Medicating the client should be done after trying to determine and treat the cause. Providing pin care is unrelated to the problem as described.

Test-Taking Strategy: Note the key word, *first*. Use the steps of the nursing process. Option 4 is the only option that addresses data collection. Review care of the client in skeletal traction if you had difficulty with this question.

Level of Cognitive Ability: Application
Client Needs: Physiological Integrity
Integrated Process: Nursing Process/Implementation
Content Area: Adult Health/Musculoskeletal
Reference: Christensen, B., & Kockrow, E. (2003). *Adult health nursing* (4th ed.). St. Louis: Mosby, p. 153.

23. Answer: 3

Rationale: Exercise is indicated within therapeutic limits for the client in skeletal traction to maintain muscle strength and range of motion. The client may pull up on the trapeze, perform active ROM with uninvolved joints, and do isometric muscle-setting exercises (e.g., quadriceps- and gluteal-setting exercises). The client may also flex and extend his or her feet.

Test-Taking Strategy: Note the key words, *needs further instruction*. These words indicate a false response question and that you need to select the incorrect client action. Options 1 and 4 are most easily identified as correct actions, and are therefore eliminated as possible answers to this question. To select between options 2 and 3, imagine the lines of pull on the fracture site with the movements described. Although flexing and extending the feet does not disrupt the line of pull from the traction, performing active ROM to the affected knee and ankle does. Review care of the client in traction if you had difficulty with this question.

Level of Cognitive Ability: Comprehension
Client Needs: Physiological Integrity
Integrated Process: Teaching/Learning
Content Area: Adult Health/Musculoskeletal
Reference: Black, J., & Hawks, J. (2005). *Medical-surgical nursing: Clinical management for positive outcomes* (7th ed.). Philadelphia: W.B. Saunders, p. 637.

24. Answer: 2

Rationale: Signs and symptoms of infection under a casted area include odor or purulent drainage from the cast, or the presence of "hot spots," which are areas of the cast that are warmer than others. The physician should be notified if any of these occur. Signs of impaired circulation in the distal limb include coolness and pallor of the skin, diminished arterial pulse, and edema.

Test-Taking Strategy: Begin to answer this question by thinking of what you would expect to find with infection: redness, swelling, heat, and purulent drainage. With these in mind, options 1 and 3 can be eliminated. To select between

options 2 and 4, "dependent edema" is not necessarily indicative of infection; swelling would be continuous. The "hot spot" on the cast could signify infection underneath that area. Review the complications of a cast if you had difficulty with this question.

Level of Cognitive Ability: Application
Client Needs: Physiological Integrity
Integrated Process: Nursing Process/Data Collection
Content Area: Adult Health/Musculoskeletal
References: Black, J., & Hawks, J. (2005). *Medical-surgical nursing: Clinical management for positive outcomes* (7th ed.). Philadelphia: W.B. Saunders, p. 633.
Christensen, B., & Kockrow, E. (2003). *Adult health nursing* (4th ed.). St. Louis: Mosby, p. 148.
Linton, A., & Maebius, N. (2003). *Introduction to medical-surgical nursing* (3rd ed.). Philadelphia: W.B. Saunders, p. 824.

25. Answer: 1

Rationale: Most pain associated with fractures can be minimized with rest, elevation, application of cold, and administration of analgesics. Pain that is not relieved from these measures should be reported to the physician, because it may be the result of impaired tissue perfusion, tissue breakdown, or necrosis. Because this is a new closed fracture and cast, infection would not have had time to set in.

Test-Taking Strategy: Use the process of elimination. Options 2 and 3 can be eliminated first, based on the description in the question. Because the fracture and cast are so new, it is extremely unlikely that infection could have possibly set in. The most likely option is impaired tissue perfusion, because pain from ischemia is not relieved by comfort measures and analgesics. Review the complications of a cast if you had difficulty with this question.

Level of Cognitive Ability: Analysis
Client Needs: Physiological Integrity
Integrated Process: Nursing Process/Data Collection
Content Area: Adult Health/Musculoskeletal
Reference: Black, J., & Hawks, J. (2005). *Medical-surgical nursing: Clinical management for positive outcomes* (7th ed.). Philadelphia: W.B. Saunders, pp. 633, 644.
Christensen, B., & Kockrow, E. (2003). *Adult health nursing* (4th ed.). St. Louis: Mosby, p. 151.

26. Answer: 3

Rationale: A casted extremity is elevated continuously for the first 24 to 48 hours to minimize swelling and to promote venous drainage.

Test-Taking Strategy: Use the process of elimination. Recall that edema sets in after fracture, and can be aggravated by casting. For this reason, options 1 and 2 are the least helpful, and can be eliminated first. There is no useful purpose for the timing in option 4. Review care of the client with a cast if you had difficulty with this question.

Level of Cognitive Ability: Application
Client Needs: Physiological Integrity
Integrated Process: Nursing Process/Implementation
Content Area: Adult Health/Musculoskeletal
Reference: Christensen, B., & Kockrow, E. (2003). *Adult health nursing* (4th ed). St. Louis: Mosby, p. 151.

27. Answer: 4

Rationale: The edges of the cast can be petaled with tape to minimize skin irritation. If a client has a cast applied and returns home, the client can be taught to do the same.

Test-Taking Strategy: Use the process of elimination. Options 1 and 2 are similar, and neither helps to get rid of the cause of the irritation, so they are eliminated first. Imagine the use of a "rough file"; it would create plaster chips and dust, which could go underneath the cast. Review cast petaling if you had difficulty with this question.

Level of Cognitive Ability: Application
Client Needs: Physiological Integrity
Integrated Process: Nursing Process/Planning
Content Area: Adult Health/Musculoskeletal
Reference: Linton, A., & Maebius, N. (2003). *Introduction to medical-surgical nursing* (3rd ed.). Philadelphia: W.B. Saunders, p. 827.

28. Answer: 1

Rationale: A plaster cast must remain dry to keep its strength. The cast should be handled using the palms of the hands, not the fingertips, until fully dry. Air should circulate freely around the cast to help it dry; the cast also gives off heat as it dries. The client should never scratch under the cast; a cool hair dryer may be used to eliminate itching.

Test-Taking Strategy: Knowledge of cast care is needed to answer this question. Knowing that a wet cast can be dented with the fingertips, causing pressure underneath, helps you eliminate option 2 first. Knowing that the cast needs to dry helps you eliminate option 3 next. Option 4 is dangerous to skin integrity and is also eliminated. Plaster casts, once they have dried after application, should not become wet. Review home care instructions for a client with a cast if you had difficulty with this question.

Level of Cognitive Ability: Comprehension
Client Needs: Health Promotion and Maintenance
Integrated Process: Nursing Process/Evaluation
Content Area: Adult Health/Musculoskeletal
References: Christensen, B., & Kockrow, E. (2003). *Adult health nursing* (4th ed.). St. Louis: Mosby, p. 150.
Lewis, S., Heitkemper, M., & Dirksen, S. (2004). *Medical-surgical nursing: Assessment and management of clinical problems* (6th ed.). St. Louis: Mosby, p. 1669.

29. Answer: 3

Rationale: Crutches are measured so that the tops are three or four fingerbreadths or 1 to 2 inches from the axilla. This ensures that the client's axilla are not resting on the crutch or bearing the weight of the body. This could result in injury to the nerves of the brachial plexus.

Test-Taking Strategy: Use the process of elimination, recalling the anatomy of the arm and axillary area. This will direct you to option 3. Review measures for crutch walking if you had difficulty with this question.

Level of Cognitive Ability: Comprehension
Client Needs: Physiological Integrity
Integrated Process: Nursing Process/Implementation
Content Area: Adult Health/Musculoskeletal
References: Christensen, B., & Kockrow, E. (2003). *Adult health nursing* (4th ed.). St. Louis: Mosby, p. 153.

Linton, A., & Maebius, N. (2003). *Introduction to medical-surgical nursing* (3rd ed.). Philadelphia: W.B. Saunders, p. 830.

30. Answer: 2

Rationale: The classic tripod position is taught to the client before giving instructions on gait. The crutches are placed anywhere from 6 to 10 inches in front and to the side of the client, depending on the client's body size. This provides a wide enough base of support to the client and improves balance.

Test-Taking Strategy: Use the process of elimination and visualize each position. Three inches and 20 inches seem excessively short and long, respectively. These options can be eliminated first. Of the remaining options, 8 inches seems more in keeping with the normal length of a stride than 15 inches for someone wearing a cast; this is the correct option. Review crutch walking if you had difficulty with this question.

Level of Cognitive Ability: Application
Client Needs: Health Promotion and Maintenance
Integrated Process: Nursing Process/Planning
Content Area: Adult Health/Musculoskeletal
References: Christensen, B., & Kockrow, E. (2003). *Adult health nursing* (4th ed.). St. Louis: Mosby, pp. 153-155.
Linton, A., & Maebius, N. (2003). *Introduction to medical-surgical nursing* (3rd ed.). Philadelphia: W.B. Saunders, p. 830.

31. Answer: 4

Rationale: A three-point gait requires good balance and arm strength. The crutches are advanced with the affected leg, and then the unaffected leg is moved forward. Option 1 describes a two-point gait. Option 2 describes a swing-to gait. Option 3 describes the three-point gait used for a right leg problem.

Test-Taking Strategy: Option 1 does not provide the support needed for the casted extremity described in the question and should be eliminated. Option 2 is not necessary if the client is allowed to let the extremity touch the floor. Of the remaining options, option 4 is the option that provides support to the left leg. Review crutch walking if you had difficulty with this question.

Level of Cognitive Ability: Application
Client Needs: Health Promotion and Maintenance
Integrated Process: Nursing Process/Implementation
Content Area: Adult Health/Musculoskeletal
Reference: Linton, A., & Maebius, N. (2003). *Introduction to medical-surgical nursing* (3rd ed.). Philadelphia: W.B. Saunders, p. 830.

32. Answer: 2

Rationale: Crutch tips should remain dry. Water could cause slipping by decreasing the surface friction of the rubber tip on the floor. If crutch tips get wet, the client should dry them with a cloth or paper towel. The client should use only crutches measured for the client. The tips should be inspected for wear, and spare crutches and tips should be available if needed.

Test-Taking Strategy: Note the key words, *needs reinforcement of the instructions.* These words indicate a false response

question and that you need to select the incorrect client statement. Option 3 is a correct statement, and is therefore eliminated. Options 1 and 4 are also correct. Remember, crutch tips can slip when they get wet, posing a possible threat to the unsuspecting client. Review crutch safety if you had difficulty with this question.
Level of Cognitive Ability: Comprehension
Client Needs: Health Promotion and Maintenance
Integrated Process: Teaching/Learning
Content Area: Adult Health/Musculoskeletal
Reference: Christensen, B., & Kockrow, E. (2003). *Adult health nursing* (4th ed.). St. Louis: Mosby, p. 153.

33. *Answer:* 4
Rationale: A straight-leg cane is useful for the client with slight weakness in one leg. A walker is beneficial to the client with greater or bilateral weakness or who is at risk for falls. Wooden crutches are often used by clients with a leg cast. Lofstrand crutches aid clients who need crutches, but have limited arm strength.
Test-Taking Strategy: Use the process of elimination. Giving a walker to a client with a slight leg weakness is excessive, and is eliminated first. Because there is no evidence in the situation of the question that the client has weight-bearing difficulty, crutches are not indicated either. This leaves the straight-leg cane as the correct option. Review the purpose of these various assistive devices if you had difficulty with this question.
Level of Cognitive Ability: Comprehension
Client Needs: Physiological Integrity
Integrated Process: Nursing Process/Evaluation
Content Area: Adult Health/Musculoskeletal
Reference: Linton, A., & Maebius, N. (2003). *Introduction to medical-surgical nursing* (3rd ed.). Philadelphia: W.B. Saunders, p. 831.

34. *Answer:* 1
Rationale: A quad cane may be used by the client requiring greater support and stability than is provided by a straight-leg cane. The quad cane provides a four-point base of support and is indicated for use by clients with partial or complete hemiplegia. Neither crutches nor a wheelchair are indicated for a client such as described in the question.
Test-Taking Strategy: Use the process of elimination. Giving a wheelchair to a client with partial hemiplegia is excessive, and is eliminated first. Wooden crutches are not indicated, because there is no restriction in weight-bearing. A Lofstrand crutch is useful for clients with bilateral weakness. This leaves the quad cane as the correct option. Review these various assistive devices if you had difficulty with this question.
Level of Cognitive Ability: Comprehension
Client Needs: Physiological Integrity
Integrated Process: Nursing Process/Evaluation
Content Area: Adult Health/Musculoskeletal
References: Christensen, B., & Kockrow, E. (2003). *Adult health nursing* (4th ed.). St. Louis: Mosby, pp. 154-155.
deWit, S. (2005). *Fundamental concepts and skills for nursing.* Philadelphia: W.B. Saunders, p. 807.

35. *Answer:* 3
Rationale: The client is taught to hold the cane on the opposite side of the weakness. This is done because, with normal walking, the opposite arm and leg move together (called reciprocal motion). The cane is placed 6 inches lateral to the fifth toe.
Test-Taking Strategy: Use the process of elimination. Knowing that the cane is held at the client's side, not in front, helps you eliminate options 1 and 2 first. Knowing that the preferred method is to have the cane positioned on the stronger side helps you select option 3 over option 4. Review client instructions for the use of a cane if you had difficulty with this question.
Level of Cognitive Ability: Application
Client Needs: Health Promotion and Maintenance
Integrated Process: Teaching/Learning
Content Area: Adult Health/Musculoskeletal
Reference: deWit, S. (2005). *Fundamental concepts and skills for nursing.* Philadelphia: W.B. Saunders, p. 807.

36. *Answer:* 2
Rationale: A cane should have a slightly flared tip, with flexible concentric rings. This tip acts as a shock absorber and provides optimal stability. Options 1, 3, and 4 are incorrect.
Test-Taking Strategy: Note the key words, *greatest reassurance.* Eliminate options 1 and 4 because neither of these statements provide reassurance for the client. Option 3 also provides no information to relieve the client's anxiety. Option 2 is a true statement and addresses, in a factual way, the client's concerns about safety. Review client instructions for the use of a cane if you had difficulty with this question.
Level of Cognitive Ability: Application
Client Needs: Psychosocial Integrity
Integrated Process: Nursing Process/Implementation
Content Area: Adult Health/Musculoskeletal
Reference: Christensen, B., & Kockrow, E. (2003). *Adult health nursing* (4th ed.). St. Louis: Mosby, p. 154.

37. *Answer:* 3
Rationale: The cane is held on the stronger side to minimize stress on the affected extremity and provide a wide base of support. The cane is held 6 inches lateral to the fifth great toe. The cane is moved forward with the affected leg. The client leans on the cane for added support while the stronger side swings through.
Test-Taking Strategy: Note the key word, *intervenes.* This word indicates a false response question and that you need to select the incorrect client action. Knowing that the cane is held on the stronger side helps you eliminate options 1 and 2 first. To select from the remaining options, recall that the client moves the cane with the weaker leg, and leans on it for support when the stronger leg swings through. Review client instructions for cane walking if you had difficulty with this question.
Level of Cognitive Ability: Comprehension
Client Needs: Health Promotion and Maintenance
Integrated Process: Nursing Process/Evaluation
Content Area: Adult Health/Musculoskeletal
References: deWit, S. (2005). *Fundamental concepts and skills for nursing.* Philadelphia: W.B. Saunders, p. 807.

Potter, P., & Perry, A. (2005). *Fundamentals of nursing* (6th ed.). St. Louis: Mosby, pp. 948-949.

38. *Answer: 4*
Rationale: Compartment syndrome is caused by bleeding and swelling within a compartment lined by fascia, which does not expand. The bleeding and swelling places pressure on the nerves, muscles, and blood vessels in the compartment, triggering the symptoms.
Test-Taking Strategy: A basic understanding of the concept of a compartment is needed to answer this question. Option 1 can be eliminated first because it is not the result of an arterial injury. Knowing that the fascia itself cannot expand eliminates option 2. To select from the remaining options, it is necessary to know that bleeding and swelling cause the symptoms, not a nerve injury. Review the cause of compartment syndrome if you had difficulty with this question.
Level of Cognitive Ability: Application
Client Needs: Physiological Integrity
Integrated Process: Nursing Process/Implementation
Content Area: Adult Health/Musculoskeletal
Reference: Linton, A., & Maebius, N. (2003). *Introduction to medical-surgical nursing* (3rd ed.). Philadelphia: W.B. Saunders, pp. 823-824.

39. *Answer: 1*
Rationale: Compartment syndrome is prevented by controlling edema. This is achieved most optimally with elevation and application of ice.
Test-Taking Strategy: Use the process of elimination. Recalling that edema is controlled or prevented with limb elevation helps you eliminate options 3 and 4 first. From the remaining options, think about the effects of ice versus bath blankets. Ice will further control edema, but bath blankets will produce heat and prevent air circulation needed for the cast to dry. Review measures to prevent compartment syndrome if you had difficulty with this question.
Level of Cognitive Ability: Application
Client Needs: Physiological Integrity
Integrated Process: Nursing Process/Planning
Content Area: Adult Health/Musculoskeletal
Reference: Christensen, B., & Kockrow, E. (2003). *Adult health nursing* (4th ed.). St. Louis: Mosby, pp. 143-144.

40. *Answer: 2*
Rationale: Confusion in the older client with hip fracture could result from the unfamiliar hospital setting, stress from the the fracture, concurrent systemic diseases, cerebral ischemia, or side effects of medications. Use of eyeglasses and hearing aids enhances the client's interaction with the environment, and can reduce disorientation.
Test-Taking Strategy: Note the key words, *would not place the client at increased risk.* These words indicate a false response question and that you need to select the item that would be helpful to the client. Stress from the fracture (option 1) and unfamiliar setting (option 3) are not likely to help the client's functional level, and are eliminated first. Eyeglasses and hearing aids are both useful adjuncts in communicating with a client. Because the eyeglasses were left at home, they are of no help at the current time. Review the psychosocial aspects

of care for the client with a hip fracture if you had difficulty with this question.
Level of Cognitive Ability: Comprehension
Client Needs: Psychosocial Integrity
Integrated Process: Nursing Process/Data Collection
Content Area: Adult Health/Musculoskeletal
Reference: Linton, A., & Maebius, N. (2003). *Introduction to medical-surgical nursing* (3rd ed.). Philadelphia: W.B. Saunders, p. 835.

41. *Answer: 4*
Rationale: Safe nursing actions intended to prevent injury to the client include keeping side rails up, having the bed in a low position, and providing a call bell that is within the client's reach. Responding promptly to the client's use of the call light minimizes the chance that the client will try to get up alone, which could result in a fall.
Test-Taking Strategy: Note the key word, *avoid.* Because options 1 and 3 (side rails up and call bell in reach) are standard nursing actions, they are eliminated first. Use of a night-light would help prevent falls, which is also helpful. This leaves the delay in answering the call light as the correct option. Delays will give the client reason to try to get up unattended and risk another fall and possible injury. Review safety measures for a client following hip surgery if you had difficulty with this question.
Level of Cognitive Ability: Application
Client Needs: Safe, Effective Care Environment
Integrated Process: Nursing Process/Implementation
Content Area: Adult Health/Musculoskeletal
Reference: Linton, A., & Maebius, N. (2003). *Introduction to medical-surgical nursing* (3rd ed.). Philadelphia: W.B. Saunders, p. 804.

42. *Answer: 1*
Rationale: Following internal fixation of a hip fracture, the client is turned to the affected side or the unaffected side, as prescribed by the surgeon. Before moving the client, the nurse places a pillow between the client's legs to keep the affected leg in abduction. The client is then repositioned while proper alignment and abduction are maintained. A trochanter roll is useful in preventing external rotation, but it is used once the client has been repositioned. It is not used while turning the client.
Test-Taking Strategy: Use the process of elimination. A trochanter roll is useful in preventing external rotation, but it is used once the client has been repositioned, not while turning the client. Therefore, eliminate options 3 and 4. To select between options 1 and 2, recall that use of a pillow would keep the legs abducted, not adducted. Thus, option 1 is the answer to the question. Review care of the client following hip surgery if you had difficulty with this question.
Level of Cognitive Ability: Application
Client Needs: Physiological Integrity
Integrated Process: Nursing Process/Implementation
Content Area: Adult Health/Musculoskeletal
References: Christensen, B., & Kockrow, E. (2003). *Adult health nursing* (4th ed.). St. Louis: Mosby, pp. 126-127.
Linton, A., & Maebius, N. (2003). *Introduction to medical-surgical nursing* (3rd ed.). Philadelphia: W.B. Saunders, p. 804.

43. *Answer:* 4
Rationale: The client who has received a total knee replacement often has the leg put into a CPM machine while in the postanesthesia care unit. The device increases circulation and movement of the knee joint. It should be used as much as the client can tolerate.
Test-Taking Strategy: Use the process of elimination. Recalling the purpose and effects of a CPM machine will direct you to option 4. Review the purpose and use of this machine if you had difficulty with this question.
Level of Cognitive Ability: Application
Client Needs: Physiological Integrity
Integrated Process: Nursing Process/Implementation
Content Area: Adult Health/Musculoskeletal
Reference: deWit, S. (2005). *Fundamental concepts and skills for nursing.* Philadelphia: W.B. Saunders, pp. 791-792.

44. *Answer:* 1
Rationale: The nurse assists the client to get out of bed on the first postoperative day after putting a knee immobilizer on the affected joint for stability. The surgeon orders the weight-bearing limits on the affected leg. The leg is elevated while the client is sitting in the chair to minimize edema.
Test-Taking Strategy: Use the process of elimination. A compression dressing should already be in place on the wound, so option 2 can be eliminated first. Because the CPM machine is used only while the client is in bed, option 3 is incorrect and is eliminated. From the remaining options, recalling that ambulation is not started until the second postoperative day will direct you to option 1. Also, the knee immobilizer will protect the knee joint. Review care of the client following total knee replacement if you had difficulty with this question.
Level of Cognitive Ability: Application
Client Needs: Physiological Integrity
Integrated Process: Nursing Process/Planning
Content Area: Adult Health/Musculoskeletal
Reference: Christensen, B., & Kockrow, E. (2003). *Adult health nursing* (4th ed.). St. Louis: Mosby, p. 126.

45. *Answer:* 3
Rationale: Clients with diabetes mellitus are more prone to wound infection and delayed wound healing due to the disease. Postoperative stump edema and hemorrhage are complications in the immediate postoperative period that apply to any client with an amputation. Slight redness of the incision is considered normal, as long it is dry and intact.
Test-Taking Strategy: The question guides you to look for complications that are primarily the result of the coexisting condition of diabetes mellitus. Recalling that diabetes mellitus increases the client's risk of developing infection and delayed wound healing helps eliminate options 1 and 2 first. From the remaining options, select option 3 because separation of wound edges is a more serious problem than a slight redness to the incision line, which is considered normal. Review the complications of an amputation if you had difficulty with this question.
Level of Cognitive Ability: Comprehension
Client Needs: Physiological Integrity

Integrated Process: Nursing Process/Data Collection
Content Area: Adult Health/Musculoskeletal
References: Christensen, B., & Kockrow, E. (2003). *Adult health nursing* (4th ed.). St. Louis: Mosby, p. 486.
Lewis, S., Heitkemper, M., & Dirksen, S. (2004). *Medical-surgical nursing: Assessment and management of clinical problems* (6th ed.). St. Louis: Mosby, p. 1684.

46. *Answer:* 1
Rationale: Phantom limb sensations are felt in the area of the amputated limb. These can include itching, warmth, and cold. The sensations are caused by intact peripheral nerves in the area amputated. Whenever possible, clients should be prepared for these sensations. The client may also feel painful sensations in the amputated limb, called phantom limb pain. The origin of the pain is less well understood, but the client should also be prepared for this, whenever possible.
Test-Taking Strategy: Use the process of elimination. By knowing that sensation and pain may be felt in the residual limb helps you eliminate options 3 and 4 first, because the sensations are not abnormal responses. From the remaining options, select option 1 because the client has described an itching sensation, but has not complained of pain in the residual limb. Review the expected findings following amputation if you had difficulty with this question.
Level of Cognitive Ability: Analysis
Client Needs: Psychosocial Integrity
Integrated Process: Nursing Process/Evaluation
Content Area: Adult Health/Musculoskeletal
Reference: Black, J., Hawks, J., & Keene, A. (2001). *Medical-surgical nursing: Clinical management for positive outcomes* (6th ed.). Philadelphia: W.B. Saunders, p. 1410.

47. *Answer:* 3
Rationale: Low back pain with radiation into one leg (sciatica) is consistent with herniated lumbar disk. The nurse continues to collect data from the client to see if the pain is aggravated by events that increase intraspinal pressure, such as bending, lifting, sneezing, coughing or lifting the leg straight up while supine (straight leg raising test). Options 1, 2, and 4 assist in alleviating pain.
Test-Taking Strategy: Focus on the issue, the causes of back pain and the factors that alleviate or aggravate it. Recall that bed rest, heat (or sometimes ice), and nonsteroidal anti-inflammatory agents usually relieve back pain, whereas bending, lifting and straining aggravate it. If this question was difficult, review the causes of back pain and the factors that alleviate or aggravate it.
Level of Cognitive Ability: Application
Client Needs: Physiological Integrity
Integrated Process: Nursing Process/Data Collection
Content Area: Adult Health/Musculoskeletal
Reference: Christensen, B., & Kockrow, E. (2003). *Adult health nursing* (4th ed.). St. Louis: Mosby, p. 160.

48. *Answer:* 4
Rationale: Following spinal fusion, the head of bed is generally kept in a flat position. The client is logrolled from side to side as ordered. Pillows may be placed under the entire length

of the legs by surgeon preference to relieve tension on the lower back. The use of an overhead trapeze is contraindicated because its use could promote twisting of the spine after surgery.

Test-Taking Strategy: Note the key word, *avoid*. After spinal surgery, the nurse uses positioning techniques and aids that will keep the spine in good alignment. Thus, options 1 and 3 are indicated and are therefore eliminated as items to avoid, according to the question. To select from the remaining options, recall that using pillows under the length of the legs promotes slight flexion of the spine while avoiding pressure on the popliteal space, which predisposes to thrombophlebitis. Using an overbed trapeze could allow the client to twist the spine, which is directly contraindicated. Review postoperative care following spinal fusion if you had difficulty with this question.

Level of Cognitive Ability: Application
Client Needs: Physiological Integrity
Integrated Process: Nursing Process/Implementation
Content Area: Adult Health/Musculoskeletal
Reference: Christensen, B., & Kockrow, E. (2003). *Adult health nursing* (4th ed.). St. Louis: Mosby, p. 161.

49. *Answer:* **1**
Rationale: Clients are taught to get out of bed by sliding near to the edge of the mattress. The client then rolls onto one side and pushes up from the bed using one or both arms. The back is kept straight and the legs are swung over the side. Increasing fluids and dietary fiber helps prevent straining at stool, thereby preventing increases in intraspinal pressure. Walking and swimming are excellent exercises for strengthening lower back muscles. Proper body mechanics includes bending at the knees, not the waist, to lift objects.

Test-Taking Strategy: Note the key words, *needs further instructions*. These words indicate a false response question and that you need to select the incorrect client statement. Options 3 and 4 are examples of interventions that are indicated and are eliminated first. Clients with low back pain should avoid situations that increase intraspinal pressure; option 2 prevents increases in intraspinal pressure. Option 1 causes an increase in intraspinal pressure if you think of the body mechanics involved in getting out of bed this way. Review the principles of proper body mechanics if you had difficulty with this question.

Level of Cognitive Ability: Comprehension
Client Needs: Health Promotion and Maintenance
Integrated Process: Teaching/Learning
Content Area: Adult Health/Musculoskeletal
Reference: Christensen, B., & Kockrow, E. (2003). *Adult health nursing* (4th ed.). St. Louis: Mosby, p. 161.

50. *Answer:* **3**
Rationale: Following spinal surgery, concerns about finances and employment are best handled by referral to a social worker. This individual will provide information about resources available to the client. The physical therapist has the best knowledge of techniques for increasing mobility and endurance. The clinical nurse specialist and surgeon do not have information related to financial resources.

Test-Taking Strategy: An understanding of the roles of the various members of the health care team helps you answer this question. Focusing on the data in the question and the issue, concerns about finances and ability to return to prior employment, will direct you to option 3. Review health care professional roles if you had difficulty with this question.

Level of Cognitive Ability: Comprehension
Client Needs: Safe, Effective Care Environment
Integrated Process: Nursing Process/Implementation
Content Area: Adult Health/Musculoskeletal
Reference: Linton, A., & Maebius, N. (2003). *Introduction to medical-surgical nursing* (3rd ed.). Philadelphia: W.B. Saunders, p. 449.

51. *Answer:* **2**
Rationale: A back brace or thoracolumbosacral orthosis is individually fitted to the client. The brace should not irritate the skin with proper fitting. The brace is applied in the morning before getting out of bed. The closures should be secure, but not overly loose or tight. A layer of clothing is worn between the orthosis and the skin.

Test-Taking Strategy: Use the process of elimination. Skin irritation is not likely to be a good sign, so eliminate option 1 first. Loose connections are also not likely to indicate proper fit, so option 4 should be eliminated next. From the remaining options, eliminate option 3 because the orthosis is likely to become soiled with perspiration or cause skin irritation. Review care of the client with a brace if you had difficulty with this question.

Level of Cognitive Ability: Application
Client Needs: Physiological Integrity
Integrated Process: Teaching/Learning
Content Area: Adult Health/Musculoskeletal
References: Black, J., & Hawks, J. (2005). *Medical-surgical nursing: Clinical management for positive outcomes* (7th ed.). Philadelphia: W.B. Saunders, p. 2147.
Lewis, S., Heitkemper, M., & Dirksen, S. (2004). *Medical-surgical nursing: Assessment and management of clinical problems* (6th ed.). St. Louis: Mosby, p. 1622.

52. *Answer:* **4**
Rationale: Following spinal fusion, with or without instrumentation, the client is transferred from stretcher to bed using a slider board and the assistance of four people. This permits optimal stabilization and support of the spine while allowing the client to be moved smoothly and gently.

Test-Taking Strategy: Use the process of elimination. This question can be answered by analyzing the level of comfort and stability provided to the client's spine with the amounts of assistance given in each option. Using this approach, you can eliminate each of the incorrect options. Review care of the client following rod insertion if you had difficulty with this question.

Level of Cognitive Ability: Application
Client Needs: Safe, Effective Care Environment
Integrated Process: Nursing Process/Implementation
Content Area: Adult Health/Musculoskeletal
Reference: Lewis, S., Heitkemper, M., & Dirksen, S. (2004). *Medical-surgical nursing: Assessment and management of clinical problems* (6th ed.). St. Louis: Mosby, p. 1619.

53. *Answer:* 1

Rationale: Stair climbing may be restricted or limited for several weeks following spinal fusion with instrumentation. The nurse ensures that resources are in place prior to discharge so that the client may sleep and perform all ADLs on a single living level.

Test-Taking Strategy: Use the process of elimination. Options 2 and 3 are obviously useful to the client, and can therefore be eliminated. To select between options 1 and 4 (both of which involve stairs), option 4 is the least problematic, whereas option 1 poses a significant problem to the client who is restricted from stair climbing. Review the home care needs of the client following rod insertion if you had difficulty with this question.

Level of Cognitive Ability: Comprehension
Client Needs: Safe, Effective Care Environment
Integrated Process: Nursing Process/Planning
Content Area: Adult Health/Musculoskeletal
Reference: Christensen, B., & Kockrow, E. (2003). *Adult health nursing* (4th ed.). St. Louis: Mosby, p. 161.

54. *Answer:* 4

Rationale: The client with pallor, slow capillary refill, weakened or lost pulse, and absence of sensation or motion to the distal limb may have arterial damage from a lacerated, contused, thrombosed, or severed artery. These signs can occur with constriction from a tight cast as well. Regardless of the cause, the nurse notifies the physician immediately. Emergency intervention is needed, which could include removal of the constricting bandage, fracture reduction, or surgery to repair the area.

Test-Taking Strategy: Use the process of elimination. Recall that these signs indicate insufficient arterial circulation and can lead to irreversible ischemia and damage. Because of this, eliminate options 1 and 3 first as not being helpful. Rechecking the circulation in 30 minutes loses valuable time for action to restore the impaired circulation, so eliminate option 2. The physician should be notified immediately. Review the complications of a fracture if you had difficulty with this question.

Level of Cognitive Ability: Application
Client Needs: Physiological Integrity
Integrated Process: Nursing Process/Implementation
Content Area: Adult Health/Musculoskeletal
Reference: Linton, A., & Maebius, N. (2003). *Introduction to medical-surgical nursing* (3rd ed.). Philadelphia: W.B. Saunders, pp. 832-833.

55. *Answer:* 4

Rationale: A window may be cut in a dried cast to relieve pressure, monitor pulses, relieve discomfort, or remove drains. Bivalving the cast involves splitting the cast along both sides to allow space for swelling, facilitate taking x-rays, or make a half-cast for use as an intermittent splint. Padding is not placed on top of a cast. The use of an air splint is not indicated.

Test-Taking Strategy: Note the key words, *bony prominence*. Wherever there is a bony prominence, there is a risk of pressure and skin breakdown. If the pressure area is under a cast, the cast must be removed in that area to relieve the pressure.

Therefore, options 1 and 3 can be eliminated. Because extra padding over the area of the cast does no good either, option 2 can be eliminated next. This leaves putting a window in the cast as the correct answer. This will relieve the pressure in that one area without disrupting the cast. Review the complications of a cast and the treatments for complications if you had difficulty with this question.

Level of Cognitive Ability: Analysis
Client Needs: Physiological Integrity
Integrated Process: Nursing Process/Evaluation
Content Area: Adult Health/Musculoskeletal
Reference: Christensen, B., & Kockrow, E. (2003). *Adult health nursing* (4th ed.). St. Louis: Mosby, p. 151.

56. *Answer:* 4

Rationale: Clients may be fearful of having a cast removed because of misconceptions about the cast cutting blade. The nurse should show the cast cutter to the client before it is used, and explain that the client may feel heat, vibration, and pressure. The cast cutter resembles a small electric saw with a circular blade. The nurse should reassure the client that the blade does not cut like a saw, but instead cuts the cast by vibrating side to side.

Test-Taking Strategy: Note the key words, *most helpful*. Option 2 gives no information, although it may be well-intentioned, and is eliminated first. Options 1 and 3 give accurate information, but are not reassuring. Option 4 gives the client the most reassurance because it best prepares the client for what will happen when the cast is removed. Review this procedure if you had difficulty with this question.

Level of Cognitive Ability: Application
Client Needs: Psychosocial Integrity
Integrated Process: Nursing Process/Implementation
Content Area: Adult Health/Musculoskeletal
Reference: Christensen, B., & Kockrow, E. (2003). *Adult health nursing* (4th ed.). St. Louis: Mosby, p. 149.

57. *Answer:* 1

Rationale: Risk factors associated with osteoporosis include a diet that is deficient in calcium. Options 2, 3, and 4 include risk factors associated with osteoporosis. Additional risk factors include being sedentary, cigarette smoking, excessive alcohol consumption, chronic illness, and long-term use of anticonvulsants and furosemide (Lasix).

Test-Taking Strategy: Note the key words, *needs to read and learn about this disorder*. These words indicate a false response question and that you need to select the incorrect student statement. Remember, risk factors associated with osteoporosis include a diet that is deficient in calcium. Review these risk factors if you are not familiar with them.

Level of Cognitive Ability: Comprehension
Client Needs: Health Promotion and Maintenance
Integrated Process: Teaching/Learning
Content Area: Adult Health/Musculoskeletal
References: Christensen, B., & Kockrow, E. (2003). *Adult health nursing* (4th ed.). St. Louis: Mosby, pp. 121-122.
Linton, A., & Maebius, N. (2003). *Introduction to medical-surgical nursing* (3rd ed.). Philadelphia: W.B. Saunders, pp. 812-813.

58. *Answer:* **4**
Rationale: Foods high in calcium include plain yogurt, dairy products, seafood, sardines, green vegetables, calcium-fortified orange juice, and cereal. Of the items listed in the options, option 4 would contain the least amount of calcium.
Test-Taking Strategy: Note the key words, *least amount of calcium.* Recalling the foods that are high and low in calcium will direct you to option 4. Review foods high in calcium if you had difficulty with this question.
Level of Cognitive Ability: Application
Client Needs: Health Promotion and Maintenance
Integrated Process: Teaching/Learning
Content Area: Adult Health/Musculoskeletal
Reference: Linton, A., & Maebius, N. (2003). *Introduction to medical-surgical nursing* (3rd ed.). Philadelphia: W.B. Saunders, pp. 613-614.

59. *Answer:* **1**
Rationale: In regard to nursing diagnoses, the client experiences a Disturbed Body Image related to a change in the structure and function of the affected leg. There are no data in the question to support a diagnosis of (actual) Activity Intolerance or Social Isolation. The client does have an actual Impaired Physical Mobility because of the fixation device.
Test-Taking Strategy: Note the key words, *upset about the appearance.* Next, note the relation between these words and option 1. Review the defining characteristics for Disturbed Body Image if you had difficulty with this question.
Level of Cognitive Ability: Analysis
Client Needs: Psychosocial Integrity
Integrated Process: Nursing Process/Planning
Content Area: Adult Health/Musculoskeletal
Reference: Gulanick, M., Myers, J., Klopp, A., Gradishar, D., Galanes, S., & Puzas, M. (2003). *Nursing care plans: Nursing diagnosis and intervention* (5th ed.). St. Louis: Mosby, p. 19.

60. *Answer:* **1**
Rationale: In addition to the presence of clinical manifestations, gout is diagnosed by the presence of persistent hyperuricemia, with the uric acid level higher than 7 mg/dL. Options 2, 3, and 4 all indicate normal laboratory values. Additionally, the presence of uric acid in an aspirated sample of synovial fluid confirms the diagnosis.
Test-Taking Strategy: Use the process of elimination and knowledge of normal laboratory values. Recalling that increased uric acid levels occur in gout and noting that option 1 is the only abnormal value will assist in answering the question. Review the manifestations of gout and the normal uric acid level if you had difficulty with this question.
Level of Cognitive Ability: Analysis
Client Needs: Physiological Integrity
Integrated Process: Nursing Process/Data Collection
Content Area: Adult Health/Musculoskeletal
Reference: Chernecky, C., & Berger, B. (2001). *Laboratory tests and diagnostic procedures* (3rd ed.). Philadelphia: W.B. Saunders, p. 1042.

61. *Answer:* **3**
Rationale: The stiffness and joint pain that occur in osteoarthritis diminishes after rest and intensifies after activity, and may be aggravated by cold, damp weather. No specific laboratory findings are useful in diagnosing osteoarthritis. The client may have a normal or slightly elevated sedimentation rate. Dull, aching pain occurs in the affected joints and, unlike rheumatoid arthritis, systemic manifestations are absent and joint involvement is not symmetrical. Morning stiffness, an elevated sedimentation rate, and a positive rheumatoid factor occur in rheumatoid arthritis.
Test-Taking Strategy: Use the process of elimination and knowledge about the differences between osteoarthritis and rheumatoid arthritis to answer this question. Remember, dull, aching pain occurs in the affected joints in osteoarthritis. Review the characteristics of osteoarthritis if you had difficulty with the question.
Level of Cognitive Ability: Analysis
Client Needs: Physiological Integrity
Integrated Process: Nursing Process/Data Collection
Content Area: Adult Health/Musculoskeletal
Reference: Phipps, W., Monahan, F., Sands, J., Marek, J., & Neighbors, M. (2003). *Medical-surgical nursing: Health and illness perspectives* (7th ed.). St. Louis: Mosby, p. 1523.

ALTERNATE FORMAT QUESTION: MULTIPLE RESPONSE

Answers:
Keep the cast and extremity elevated
Allow the wet cast 24 to 48 hours to dry
The cast needs to be kept clean and dry
Rationale: A plaster cast takes 24 to 48 hours to dry (synthetic casts dry in 20 minutes). The cast and extremity are elevated to prevent swelling and circulatory compromise. A wet cast is handled with the palms of the hand until it is dry and the extremity is turned (unless contraindicated) so that all sides of the wet cast will dry. A cool setting on the hair dryer can be used to dry a plaster cast (heat cannot be used on a plaster cast because the cast heats up and burns the skin). The cast needs to be kept clean and dry, and the client is instructed not to stick anything under the cast because of the risk of breaking skin integrity. The client is instructed to monitor the extremity for circulatory impairment such as pain, swelling, discoloration, tingling, numbness, coolness, or diminished pulse. The physician is notified immediately if circulatory compromise occurs.
Test-Taking Strategy: Focus on the issue, a plaster cast. Recalling that edema occurs following a fracture and recalling the complications associated with a cast will assist in answering the question. Review cast care instructions if you had difficulty with this question.
Level of Cognitive Ability: Application
Client Needs: Physiological Integrity
Integrated Process: Teaching/Learning
Content Area: Adult Health/Musculoskeletal
Reference: Black, J., & Hawks, J., (2005). *Medical-surgical nursing: Clinical management for positive outcomes* (7th ed.). Philadelphia: W.B. Saunders, pp. 631-633.

REFERENCES

Black, J., & Hawks, J. (2005). *Medical-surgical nursing: Clinical management for positive outcomes* (7th ed.). Philadelphia: W.B. Saunders.

Chernecky, C., & Berger, B. (2004). *Laboratory tests and diagnostic procedures* (4th ed.). Philadelphia: W.B. Saunders.

Christensen, B., & Kockrow, E. (2003). *Adult health nursing* (4th ed.). St. Louis: Mosby.

deWit, S. (2005). *Fundamental concepts and skills for nursing.* Philadelphia: W.B. Saunders.

Gulanick, M., Myers, J., Klopp, A., Gradishar, D., Galanes, S., & Puzas, M. (2003). *Nursing care plans: Nursing diagnosis and intervention* (5th ed.). St. Louis: Mosby.

Jarvis, C. (2004). *Physical examination and health assessment* (4th ed.). Philadelphia: W.B. Saunders.

Lewis, S., Heitkemper, M., & Dirksen, S. (2004). *Medical-surgical nursing: Assessment and management of clinical problems* (6th ed.). St. Louis: Mosby.

Linton, A., & Maebius, N. (2003). *Introduction to medical-surgical nursing* (3rd ed.). Philadelphia: W.B. Saunders.

Nix, S. (2005). *Williams basic nutrition and diet therapy* (12th ed.). St. Louis: Mosby.

Pagana, K., & Pagana, T. (2003). *Mosby's diagnostic and laboratory test reference* (6th ed.). St. Louis: Mosby.

Phipps, W., Monahan, F., Sands, J., Marek, J., & Neighbors, M. (2003). *Medical-surgical nursing: Health and illness perspectives* (7th ed.). St. Louis: Mosby.

Potter, P., & Perry, A. (2005). *Fundamentals of nursing* (6th ed.). St. Louis: Mosby.

Musculoskeletal Medications

I. SKELETAL MUSCLE RELAXANTS (Box 59-1)

A. Description
1. Act directly on the neuromuscular junction or indirectly on the central nervous system (CNS)
2. Centrally acting muscle relaxants depress neuron activity in the spinal cord or brain
3. Peripherally acting muscle relaxants act directly on the skeletal muscles
4. Used to prevent or relieve muscle spasms, to treat spasticity associated with spinal cord disease or lesions, for painful musculoskeletal conditions, and for chronic debilitating disorders, such as multiple sclerosis, cerebrovascular accident (CVA), or cerebral palsy
5. Contraindicated in severe liver, renal, or heart disease
6. Should not be taken with CNS depressants, such as barbiturates, narcotics, and alcohol, sedatives, hypnotics, or tricyclic antidepressants

---

BOX 59-1

Skeletal Muscle Relaxants

Baclofen (Lioresal)
Carisoprodol (Soma)
Cyclobenzaprine (Flexeril)
Dantrolene (Dantrium)
Diazepam (Valium)
Metaxalone (Skelaxin)
Methocarbamol (Robaxin)
Orphenadrine extended release (Norflex)
Chlorzoxazone (Paraflex, Parafon Forte)
Chlorphenesin carbamate (Maolate)
Tizanidine (Zanaflex)

B. Side effects
1. Dizziness and hypotension
2. Drowsiness
3. Dry mouth
4. Gastrointestinal (GI) upset
5. Photosensitivity
6. Liver toxicity

C. Interventions
1. Obtain a medical history
2. Monitor vital signs
3. Monitor for CNS side effects
4. Assess for risk of injury
5. Check involved joints and muscles for pain and mobility
6. Monitor liver function tests because hepatotoxicity can occur
7. Monitor renal function studies
8. Instruct the client to take the medication with food to decrease GI upset
9. Instruct the client to report side effects
10. Instruct the client to avoid alcohol and CNS depressants
11. Instruct the client to avoid activities requiring alertness

D. Nursing considerations
1. Baclofen (Lioresal)
   a. Causes CNS effects such as drowsiness, dizziness, weakness, and fatigue
   b. Frequently causes nausea, constipation, and urinary retention
   c. Can be administered by the physician through intrathecal infusion using an implantable pump
2. Dantrolene (Dantrium)
   a. Acts directly on skeletal muscles to relieve spasticity
   b. Liver damage is the most serious adverse effect

c. Liver function test results should be monitored prior to the initiation of treatment and during treatment

d. Can cause GI bleeding, urinary frequency, impotence, photosensitivity, and rash

e. Instruct the client to wear protective clothing when in the sun

f. Instruct the client to notify physician if rash, bloody or tarry stool, or yellow discoloration of the skin or eyes occurs

g. Instruct client with implantable pump to maintain medication refill appointments and to prevent pump going dry, which could to lead to sudden withdrawal symptoms (could be life-threatening)

3. Cyclobenzaprine (Flexeril)

a. Contraindicated in clients who have received monoamine oxidase inhibitors (MAOIs) within 14 days of initiation of cyclobenzaprine therapy and in clients with cardiac disorders

b. Used with caution in clients with a history of urinary retention, angle-closure glaucoma, or increased intraocular pressure

c. Should be used only short term (2 to 3 weeks of therapy)

4. Methocarbamol (Robaxin)

a. Parenteral form is contraindicated in clients with renal impairment

b. Parenteral form can cause hypotension, bradycardia, anaphylaxis, and seizures

c. May cause urine to turn brown, black, or green

d. Inform the client to notify the physician if blurred vision, nasal congestion, urticaria, or rash occurs

5. Chlorzoxazone (Paraflex, Parafon Forte)

a. Monitor for hypersensitivity reactions such as urticaria, redness or itching, and possibly angioedema

b. May cause malaise and urine discoloration

6. Carisoprodol (Soma)

a. Advise the client to take the medication with food to prevent GI upset

b. Instruct the client to report any rash or hypersensitivity to the physician

II. ANTIGOUT MEDICATIONS (Box 59-2)

A. Description

1. Decrease inflammation

2. Reduce uric acid production and increase uric acid excretion to prevent or relieve gout or to manage hyperuricemia

3. Used cautiously in clients with GI, renal, cardiac, or hepatic disease

4. Allopurinol (Zyloprim) can increase the effect of warfarin and oral hypoglycemic agents

---

BOX 59-2

Antigout Medications

Allopurinol (Zyloprim)
Colchicine
Losartan (Cozaar)
Probenecid

B. Side effects

1. Headaches

2. Nausea, vomiting, and diarrhea

3. Blood dyscrasias such as bone marrow depression

4. Flushed skin and skin rash

5. Uric acid kidney stones

6. Sore gums

7. Metallic taste

C. Interventions

1. Monitor serum uric acid levels

2. Monitor intake and output (I&O)

3. Maintain a fluid intake of at least 2000 to 3000 mL/day to avoid kidney stones

4. Monitor complete blood cell count (CBC) and renal and liver function studies

5. Instruct the client to avoid alcohol and caffeine, because these products can increase uric acid levels

6. Instruct the client not to take large doses of vitamin C while taking allopurinol (Zyloprim) because kidney stones may develop

7. Encourage the client to comply with therapy to prevent elevated uric acid levels, which can trigger a gout attack

8. Instruct the client to avoid foods high in purine, such as wine, alcohol, organ meats, sardines, salmon, and gravy

9. Instruct the client to take the medication with food

10. Instruct the client to report side effects to the physician

11. Advise the client to have a yearly eye examination, because visual changes can occur from prolonged use of allopurinol

12. Caution the client not to take aspirin with these medications, because this could trigger a gout attack

13. Concurrent use of aspirin causes elevated uric acid levels; the client should be instructed to take acetaminophen (Tylenol)

III. ANTIARTHRITIC MEDICATIONS (Box 59-3)

A. Acetylsalicylic acid (Aspirin) and nonsteroidal anti-inflammatory drugs (NSAIDs; see Chapter 57)

B. Gold therapy

1. Description

a. Referred to as chrysotherapy or gold salt therapy

b. Depresses migration of leukocytes and suppresses prostaglandin activity

BOX 59-3

Antiarthritis Medications

Auranofin (Ridaura)
Aurothioglucose (Solganal)
Azathioprine (Imuran)
Etanercept (Enbrel)
Gold sodium thiomalate (Myochrysine)
Hydroxychloroquine sulfate (Plaquenil)
Leflunomide (Avara)
Penicillamine (Cuprimine)

BOX 59-4

Contraindications to Gold Therapy

Eczema
Urticaria
Colitis
Hemorrhagic conditions
Systemic lupus erythematosus
Renal or hepatic dysfunction
Uncontrolled diabetes mellitus
Congestive heart failure
Recent radiation therapy

c. Reduces inflammation by decreasing enzyme release and altering the immune response
d. Primarily used for palliative relief of symptoms in rheumatoid arthritis
e. Contraindications: See Box 59-4
2. Side effects
   a. Dizziness
   b. Urticaria and rash
   c. Erythema and dermatitis
   d. Alopecia
   e. Stomatitis
   f. Diarrhea
   g. Hepatitis
   h. Metallic taste in the mouth
   i. Blood dyscrasias such as bone marrow suppression
   j. Photosensitivity reactions
   k. Gold toxicity
3. Interventions
   a. Obtain the client's medical history
   b. Monitor for blood dyscrasias before and during therapy
   c. Monitor for proteinuria and hematuria before and during therapy
   d. When administering the gold injection, monitor the client for 30 minutes after injection for possible allergic reaction
   e. Instruct the client to maintain good oral hygiene
   f. Instruct the client to use sunscreen and protective clothing to prevent photosensitivity reactions

BOX 59-5

Bisphosphonates Used to Treat Osteoporosis

Etidronate (Didronel)
Alendronate (Fosamax)
Pamidronate (Aredia)
Risedronate (Actonel)
Clodronate (Bonefos)
Tiludronate (Skelid)

g. Teach the client about the signs and symptoms of gold toxicity, which include pruritis, skin rash, metallic taste, stomatitis, and diarrhea
h. If toxicity occurs, dimercaprol (BAL in oil) may be prescribed to enhance gold excretion

IV. MEDICATIONS TO PREVENT AND TREAT OSTEOPOROSIS

A. Calcium and vitamin D supplementation
B. Estrogen replacement therapy after menopause may be prescribed to prevent osteoporesis
C. Calcitonin (Calcimar)
   1. Calcitonin is secreted by the thyroid gland and inhibits osteoclastic bone resorption
   2. When calcitonin is taken, calcium supplementation is necessary to prevent secondary hyperparathyroidism
D. Bisphosphonates (Box 59-5)
   1. Inhibit osteoclast-mediated bone resorption, thereby increasing total bone mass
   2. Common side effects are anorexia, weight loss, and gastritis
   3. Alendronate (Fosamax)
      a. Precautions need to be taken with administration to prevent gastrointestinal side effects (especially esophageal irritation) and increase absorption
      b. Should be taken after rising in the morning with a full glass of water
      c. Client should not eat or drink anything for 30 minutes following administration and should not lie down after taking the medication
E. Selective estrogen receptor modulators
   1. Mimic the effect of estrogen in bone by reducing bone resorption
   2. Raloxifene (Evista): Most common side effects are leg cramps and hot flashes
F. Teriparatide (Forteo)
   1. Stimulates new bone formation
   2. Is part of the human parathyroid hormone; works by increasing the action of osteoblasts
   3. Used for the treatment of osteoporosis in men and postmenopausal women who are at high risk for having a fracture

PRACTICE QUESTIONS

1. Allopurinol (Zyloprim) has been prescribed for the client and the client asks the nurse about the action of the medication. The nurse responds, knowing that it:
   1. Is used for the lysis of thrombi obstructing coronary arteries
   2. Prevents calcium ion entry across cell membranes of the cardiac smooth muscle
   3. Decreases sympathetic outflow from the central nervous system (CNS)
   4. Decreases uric acid production and reduces uric acid concentrations in both the serum and urine

2. A nurse is caring for a client who is taking allopurinol (Zyloprim). Which of the following medications, if prescribed for the client, would the nurse question?
   1. Mebendazole (Vermox)
   2. Ergonovine maleate (Ergotrate)
   3. Warfarin sodium (Coumadin)
   4. Pentazocine (Talwin)

3. A nurse prepares to reinforce instructions to a client who is taking allopurinol (Zyloprim). The nurse plans to include which of the following in the instructions?
   1. Inform the client that the effect of the medication will occur immediately
   2. Instruct the client to drink 3000 mL of fluid per day
   3. Instruct the client to take the medication on an empty stomach
   4. Instruct the client that, if swelling of the lips occur, this is a normal expected response

4. A client with rheumatoid arthritis is taking acetylsalicylic acid (aspirin) on a daily basis. Which medication dose would the nurse expect the client to be taking?
   1. 1 g daily
   2. 1000 mg daily
   3. 325 mg daily
   4. 4 g daily

5. Colchicine is prescribed for a client with a diagnosis of gout. The nurse reviews the client's medical history in the health record, knowing that the medication would be contraindicated in which disorder?
   1. Renal failure
   2. Hypothyroidism
   3. Diabetes mellitus
   4. Myxedema

6. A nurse is caring for a client with gout who is taking colchicine. The client has been instructed to restrict the diet to low-purine foods. Which of the following foods would the nurse instruct the client to avoid while taking this medication?
   1. Potatoes
   2. Ice cream
   3. Spinach
   4. Scallops

7. A physician prescribes auranofin (Ridaura) for the client with rheumatoid arthritis. Which of the following would indicate to the nurse that the client is experiencing toxicity related to the medication?
   1. Constipation
   2. Complaints of a metallic taste in the mouth
   3. Ringing in the ears
   4. Joint pain

8. A film-coated form of diflunisal (Dolobid) has been prescribed for a client for the treatment of chronic rheumatoid arthritis. The client calls the clinic nurse because of difficulty swallowing the tablets. Which initial instruction would the nurse provide to the client?
   1. Crush the tablets and mix it with food
   2. Open the tablet and mix the contents with food
   3. Swallow the tablets with large amounts of water or milk
   4. Notify the physician for a medication change

9. A physician instructs an older client with rheumatoid arthritis to take ibuprofen (Motrin). The nurse reinforces the instructions, knowing that the normal adult dose for this client is which of the following?
   1. 100 mg orally twice a day
   2. 200 mg orally twice a day
   3. 400 mg orally three times a day
   4. 1000 mg orally four times a day

10. Baclofen (Lioresal) is prescribed for the client with multiple sclerosis. The nurse assists in planning care, knowing that the primary therapeutic effect of this medication is which of the following?
    1. Increased muscle tone
    2. Decreased muscle spasms
    3. Decreased local pain and tenderness
    4. Increased range of motion

11. A nurse is monitoring a client receiving baclofen (Lioresal) for side effects related to the medication. Which of the following would indicate that the client is experiencing a side effect?
    1. Drowsiness
    2. Diarrhea
    3. Polyuria
    4. Muscular excitability

12. A nurse is reinforcing discharge instructions to a client receiving baclofen (Lioresal). Which of the following would the nurse include in the instructions?
    1. Restrict fluid intake
    2. Avoid the use of alcohol
    3. Stop the medication if diarrhea occurs
    4. Notify the physician if fatigue occurs

13. A adult client with muscle spasms is taking an oral maintenance dose of baclofen (Lioresal). The nurse reviews the medication record, expecting that which dose would be prescribed?
    1. 15 mg four times a day
    2. 25 mg four times a day

3. 30 mg four times a day
4. 40 mg four times a day

14. A client with acute muscle spasms has been taking baclofen (Lioresal). The client calls the clinic nurse because of continuous feelings of weakness and fatigue and asks the nurse about discontinuing the medication. The nurse makes which appropriate response to the client?
    1. "It is best that you taper the dose if you intend to stop the medication."
    2. "Weakness and fatigue commonly occur and will diminish with continued medication use."
    3. "It is all right to stop the medication if you think that you can tolerate the muscle spasms."
    4. "You should never stop the medication."

15. Dantrolene sodium (Dantrium) is prescribed for a client experiencing flexor spasms, and the client asks the nurse about the action of the medication. The nurse responds, knowing that the therapeutic action of this medication is which of the following?
    1. Acts within the spinal cord to suppress hyperactive reflexes
    2. Acts on the central nervous system (CNS) to suppress spasms
    3. Acts directly on the skeletal muscle to relieve spasticity
    4. Depresses spinal reflexes

16. A nurse is reviewing the laboratory studies on a client receiving dantrolene sodium (Dantrium). Which laboratory test would identify an adverse effect associated with the administration of this medication?
    1. Blood urea nitrogen (BUN)
    2. Creatinine
    3. Liver function tests
    4. Hematological function tests

17. A nurse is reviewing the record of a client who has been prescribed baclofen (Lioresal). Which of the following disorders, if noted in the client's history, would alert the nurse to contact the physician?
    1. Coronary artery disease
    2. Diabetes mellitus
    3. Seizure disorders
    4. Hyperthyroidism

18. Cyclobenzaprine hydrochloride (Flexeril) is prescribed for a client to treat muscle spasms and the nurse is reviewing the client's record. Which of the following disorders, if noted in the client's record, would indicate a need to contact the physician regarding the administration of this medication?
    1. Glaucoma
    2. Hyperthyroidism
    3. Emphysema
    4. Diabetes mellitus

19. A client receives a prescription for methocarbamol (Robaxin) and the nurse reinforces instructions to the client regarding the medication. Which client statement would indicate a need for further instructions?
    1. "My urine may turn brown or green."
    2. "If my vision becomes blurred, I don't need to be concerned about it."
    3. "I might get some nasal congestion from this medication."
    4. "This medication is prescribed to help relieve my muscle spasms."

20. The nurse is reviewing the physician's orders for an adult client who has been admitted to the hospital following a back injury. Carisoprodol (Soma) is prescribed for the client to relieve the muscle spasms; the physician has prescribed 350 mg to be administered four times a day. When preparing to give this medication, the nurse determines that this dosage is:
    1. The normal adult dosage
    2. A lower than normal dosage
    3. A higher than normal dosage
    4. A dosage requiring further clarification

ALTERNATE FORMAT QUESTION: MULTIPLE RESPONSE

Allopurinol (Zyloprim) has been prescribed for a client with a diagnosis of gout and the nurse prepares to provide instructions to the client about the medication. Select the instructions that the nurse provides to the client.

___ Limit fluid intake
___ Take the medication with food
___ Limit alcohol intake to one beer per day
___ Contact the physician if a rash develops
___ A complete blood cell count and renal and liver function studies may be prescribed

ANSWERS

1. *Answer:* 4

Rationale: Allopurinol is an antigout medication. It decreases uric acid production by inhibiting the enzyme xanthine oxidase, and reduces uric acid concentrations in both serum and urine. Options 1, 2, and 3 are not actions of this medication.

Test-Taking Strategy: Use the process of elimination. Note that options 1 and 2 are similar in that they both address a cardiac situation. This leaves option 3 and 4. Recalling that this medication is in the antigout classification will assist in directing you to the correct option from those remaining. If you had difficulty with this question, review the action of allopurinol.

Level of Cognitive Ability: Application
Client Needs: Physiological Integrity
Integrated Process: Nursing Process/Implementation
Content Area: Pharmacology
Reference: Hodgson, B., & Kizior, R. (2005). *Saunders nursing drug handbook 2005.* Philadelphia: W.B. Saunders, p. 30.

2. *Answer:* 3

Rationale: Allopurinol is an antigout medication that may increase the effect of oral anticoagulants. Warfarin sodium (Coumadin) is an anticoagulant, and if this medication was prescribed for the client, the nurse would question the order. Ergonovine maleate is an antimigraine medication. Pentazocine is an opioid analgesic. Mebendazole is an anthelmintic.

Test-Taking Strategy: Knowledge regarding the medication interactions related to allopurinol is needed to answer this question. Remember, allopurinol will increase the effect of oral anticoagulants. If you had difficulty with this question, review the interactions associated with this medication.

Level of Cognitive Ability: Analysis
Client Needs: Safe, Effective Care Environment
Integrated Process: Nursing Process/Implementation
Content Area: Pharmacology
Reference: McKenry, L., & Salerno, E. (2003). *Mosby's pharmacology in nursing* (21st ed.). St. Louis: Mosby, p. 687.

3. *Answer:* 2

Rationale: Clients taking allopurinol are encouraged to drink 3000 mL of fluid a day. A full therapeutic effect may take 1 week or longer. Allopurinol is to be given with or immediately following meals or milk to prevent gastrointestinal irritation. If the client develops a rash, irritation of the eyes, or swelling of the lips or mouth, he or she should contact the physician, because this may indicate hypersensitivity.

Test-Taking Strategy: Use the process of elimination. Option 4 can be eliminated first because it indicates a hypersensitivity, which is not a normal expected response. From the remaining options, recalling that this medication is used to treat gout will direct you to option 2. If you had difficulty with this question, review client instructions related to allopurinol.

Level of Cognitive Ability: Application
Client Needs: Health Promotion and Maintenance
Integrated Process: Nursing Process/Planning
Content Area: Pharmacology
Reference: Hodgson, B., & Kizior, R. (2005). *Saunders nursing drug handbook 2005.* Philadelphia: W.B. Saunders, p. 31.

4. *Answer:* 4

Rationale: Aspirin may be used to treat client with rheumatoid arthritis. It may also be used to reduce the risk of recurrent transient ischemic attach (TIA) or stroke or reduce the risk of myocardial infarction (MI) in clients with unstable angina or a history of a previous MI. The normal dose for clients being treated with aspirin to decrease thrombosis and MI is 300 to 325 mg/day. Clients being treated to prevent TIAs are usually prescribed 1.3 g/day in two to four divided doses. Clients with rheumatoid arthritis are treated with 3.6 to 5.4 g/day in divided doses.

Test-Taking Strategy: Use the process of elimination. Eliminate options 1 and 2 because they are similar. From the remaining options, noting the client's diagnosis will direct you to option 4. If you had difficulty with this question, review aspirin dosages.

Level of Cognitive Ability: Analysis
Client Needs: Physiological Integrity
Integrated Process: Nursing Process/Data Collection
Content Area: Pharmacology
Reference: Hodgson, B., & Kizior, R. (2005). *Saunders nursing drug handbook 2005.* Philadelphia: W.B. Saunders, p. 87.

5. *Answer:* 1

Rationale: Colchicine is contraindicated in clients with severe gastrointestinal, renal, hepatic or cardiac disorders or blood dyscrasias. Clients with impaired renal function may exhibit myopathy and neuropathy manifested as generalized weakness. This medication should be used with caution in clients with impaired hepatic function, the older client, and the debilitated.

Test-Taking Strategy: Use the process of elimination. Note that options 2, 3, and 4 are all endocrine-related disorders. Option 1, the correct option, is different from the others. Review this medication if you had difficulty with this question.

Level of Cognitive Ability: Analysis
Client Needs: Physiological Integrity
Integrated Process: Nursing Process/Data Collection
Content Area: Pharmacology
Reference: Hodgson, B., & Kizior, R. (2005). *Saunders nursing drug handbook 2005.* Philadelphia: W.B. Saunders, p. 256.

6. *Answer:* 4

Rationale: Colchicine is a medication used for clients with gout to inhibit the reabsorption of uric acid by the kidney and promote excretion of uric acid in the urine. Uric acid is produced when purine is catabolized. Clients are instructed to modify their diet and limit excessive purine intake. High-purine foods to avoid or limit include organ meats, roe, sardines, scallops, anchovies, broth, mincemeat, herring, shrimp, mackerel, gravy, and yeast.

Test-Taking Strategy: Note the key word, *avoid.* Options 1 and 3 are high-nutrient and low-purine foods, so eliminate these options first. From this point, use knowledge regarding the purpose of the medication, the treatment for gout, and food sources high in purine to select the correct option. If you had difficulty with this question, review foods that are high in purine.

Level of Cognitive Ability: Application
Client Needs: Health Promotion and Maintenance
Integrated Process: Nursing Process/Implementation

Content Area: Pharmacology
Reference: Hodgson, B., & Kizior, R. (2005). *Saunders nursing drug handbook 2005.* Philadelphia: W.B. Saunders, p. 255.

7. *Answer:* 2
Rationale: Ridaura is the one gold preparation that is given orally rather than by injection. Gastrointestinal reactions including diarrhea, abdominal pain, nausea, and loss of appetite are common early in therapy, but these usually subside in the first 3 months of therapy. Early symptoms of toxicity include a rash, purple blotches, pruritus, mouth lesions, and a metallic taste in the mouth.
Test-Taking Strategy: Use the process of elimination. Option 4, joint pain, can be eliminated because the medication is administered to reduce the joint pain. Note that the question is asking for a toxic effect; therefore, from the options remaining, you should be directed to the correct option, metallic taste. Remember, gold is a metal. If you had difficulty with this question, review toxicity related to gold compounds.
Level of Cognitive Ability: Analysis
Client Needs: Physiological Integrity
Integrated Process: Nursing Process/Data Collection
Content Area: Pharmacology
Reference: Hodgson, B., & Kizior, R. (2005). *Saunders nursing drug handbook 2005.* Philadelphia: W.B. Saunders, p. 99.

8. *Answer:* 3
Rationale: Dolobid may be given with water, milk, or meals. The tablets should not be crushed or broken open. Taking the medication with a large amount of water or milk should be tried before contacting the physician.
Test-Taking Strategy: Use the process of elimination. Eliminate option 4 first as the least likely initial instruction. Next, noting the words "film-coated" will assist in eliminating options 1 and 2. Additionally, these options are similar in that they both suggest breaking the tablets. If you had difficulty with this question, review the procedure for administration of this medication.
Level of Cognitive Ability: Application
Client Needs: Health Promotion and Maintenance
Integrated Process: Nursing Process/Implementation
Content Area: Pharmacology
Reference: Hodgson, B., & Kizior, R. (2005). *Saunders nursing drug handbook 2005.* Philadelphia: W.B. Saunders, p. 323.

9. *Answer:* 3
Rationale: For acute or chronic rheumatoid arthritis or osteoarthritis, the normal oral adult dose for an older client is 400 to 800 mg three or four times daily.
Test-Taking Strategy: Use the process of elimination. Noting the words "older client" in the question will assist in eliminating option 4. From the remaining options, it is necessary to be familiar with normal dosages. Review the normal dosage for this medication if you had difficulty with this question.
Level of Cognitive Ability: Application
Client Needs: Physiological Integrity
Integrated Process: Teaching/Learning
Content Area: Pharmacology
Reference: Hodgson, B., & Kizior, R. (2005). *Saunders nursing drug handbook 2005.* Philadelphia: W.B. Saunders, p. 549.

10. *Answer:* 2
Rationale: Baclofen is a skeletal muscle relaxant and acts at the spinal cord level to decrease the frequency and amplitude of muscle spasms in clients with spinal cord injuries or diseases and in clients with multiple sclerosis. Options 1, 3, and 4 are incorrect.
Test-Taking Strategy: Focus on the client's diagnosis. Recalling the action of this medication will direct you to option 2. Review this medication if you had difficulty with this question.
Level of Cognitive Ability: Analysis
Client Needs: Physiological Integrity
Integrated Process: Nursing Process/Planning
Content Area: Pharmacology
Reference: Hodgson, B., & Kizior, R. (2005). *Saunders nursing drug handbook 2005.* Philadelphia: W.B. Saunders, p. 107.

11. *Answer:* 1
Rationale: Baclofen is a central nervous system (CNS) depressant and frequently causes drowsiness, dizziness, weakness, and fatigue. It can also cause nausea, constipation, and urinary retention. Clients should be warned about the possible reactions. Options 2, 3, and 4 are not side effects.
Test-Taking Strategy: Use the process of elimination. Recalling that baclofen is a CNS depressant used to treat muscle spasticity will direct you to option 1. If you had difficulty with this question, review the side effects of this medication.
Level of Cognitive Ability: Analysis
Client Needs: Physiological Integrity
Integrated Process: Nursing Process/Data Collection
Content Area: Pharmacology
Reference: Hodgson, B., & Kizior, R. (2005). *Saunders nursing drug handbook 2005.* Philadelphia: W.B. Saunders, p. 108.

12. *Answer:* 2
Rationale: Baclofen is a central nervous system (CNS) depressant. The client should be cautioned against the use of alcohol and other CNS depressants, because baclofen potentiates the depressant activity of these agents. Constipation rather that diarrhea is a adverse effect of baclofen. It is not necessary to restrict fluids, but the client should be warned that urinary retention can occur. Fatigue is related to a CNS effect that is most intense during the early phase of therapy and diminishes with continued medication use. It is not necessary that the client notify the physician if fatigue occurs.
Test-Taking Strategy: Recalling that baclofen is a CNS depressant will direct you to option 2. If you were unsure of the correct option, use general principles related to medication administration. Alcohol should be avoided with the use of medications. Review this medication if you had difficulty with this question.
Level of Cognitive Ability: Application
Client Needs: Health Promotion and Maintenance
Integrated Process: Nursing Process/Implementation
Content Area: Pharmacology
Reference: Hodgson, B., & Kizior, R. (2005). *Saunders nursing drug handbook 2005.* Philadelphia: W.B. Saunders, p. 108.

13. *Answer:* 1
Rationale: Baclofen is dispensed in 10- and 20-mg tablets for oral use. Dosages are low initially and then gradually increased.

Maintenance doses range from 15 to 20 mg administered three or four times a day.

Test-Taking Strategy: Knowledge regarding the normal adult maintenance dosage is required to answer this question. Review this maintenance dosage if you had difficulty with this question.

Level of Cognitive Ability: Analysis
Client Needs: Physiological Integrity
Integrated Process: Nursing Process/Data Collection
Content Area: Pharmacology
Reference: Lehne, R. (2004). *Pharmacology for nursing care* (5th ed.). Philadelphia: W.B. Saunders, p. 209.

14. *Answer: 2*
Rationale: The client should be instructed that symptoms such as drowsiness, weakness, and fatigue are more intense in the early phase of therapy and diminish with continued medication use. The client should be instructed never to withdraw or stop the medication abruptly, because abrupt withdrawal can cause visual hallucinations, paranoid ideation, and seizures. It is best for the nurse to inform the client that these symptoms will subside and encourage the client to continue the use of the medication.

Test-Taking Strategy: Use the process of elimination. Eliminate option 4 first because it is a rather extreme nursing response. Next, eliminate options 1 and 3 because these responses do not represent the scope of nursing practice or nursing actions. Review this medication if you had difficulty with this question

Level of Cognitive Ability: Application
Client Needs: Physiological Integrity
Integrated Process: Communication and Documentation
Content Area: Pharmacology
Reference: Hodgson, B., & Kizior, R. (2005). *Saunders nursing drug handbook 2005.* Philadelphia: W.B. Saunders, p. 108.

15. *Answer: 3*
Rationale: Dantrium acts directly on skeletal muscle to relieve muscle spasticity. The primary action is the suppression of calcium release from the sarcoplasmic reticulum. This in turn decreases the ability of the skeletal muscle to contract. Options 1, 2, and 4 are not actions of the medication.

Test-Taking Strategy: Use the process of elimination. Options 1, 2, and 4 are all similar in that they address central nervous system (CNS) suppression and the depression of reflexes. Therefore, eliminate these options. Review this medication if you had difficulty with this question.

Level of Cognitive Ability: Application
Client Needs: Physiological Integrity
Integrated Process: Nursing Process/Implementation
Content Area: Pharmacology
Reference: Hodgson, B., & Kizior, R. (2005). *Saunders nursing drug handbook 2005.* Philadelphia: W.B. Saunders, p. 284.

16. *Answer: 3*
Rationale: Dose-related liver damage is the most serious adverse effect of dantrolene. To reduce the risk of liver damage, liver function tests should be performed before

treatment and periodically throughout the treatment course. It is administered in the lowest effective dosage for the shortest time necessary.

Test-Taking Strategy: Use the process of elimination. Eliminate options 1 and 2 because these tests both assess kidney function. From the remaining options, it is necessary to recall that this medication affects liver function. Review this medication if you had difficulty with this question.

Level of Cognitive Ability: Analysis
Client Needs: Physiological Integrity
Integrated Process: Nursing Process/Data Collection
Content Area: Pharmacology
Reference: Hodgson, B., & Kizior, R. (2005). *Saunders nursing drug handbook 2005.* Philadelphia: W.B. Saunders, p. 286.

17. *Answer: 3*
Rationale: Clients with seizure disorders may have a lowered seizure threshold when baclofen is administered. Concurrent therapy may require an increase in the anticonvulsive medication. The disorders in options 1, 2, and 4 are not a concern when the client is taking baclofen.

Test-Taking Strategy: Knowledge regarding the contraindications and the cautions associated with the administration of baclofen is required to answer this question. Remember, a lowered seizure threshold can occur when baclofen is administered. If you are unfamiliar with these contraindications and cautions, review this content.

Level of Cognitive Ability: Analysis
Client Needs: Safe, Effective Care Environment
Integrated Process: Nursing Process/Data Collection
Content Area: Pharmacology
Reference: Hodgson, B., & Kizior, R. (2005). *Saunders nursing drug handbook 2005.* Philadelphia: W.B. Saunders, p. 108.

18. *Answer: 1*
Rationale: Because this medication has anticholinergic effects, it should be used with caution with clients with a history of urinary retention, angle-closure glaucoma, and increased intraocular pressure. Cyclobenzaprine hydrochloride should be used only for short-term 2- to 3-week therapy.

Test-Taking Strategy: Recalling that this medication has anticholinergic effects will assist in directing you to option 1. If you are unfamiliar with this medication and the contraindications associated with its administration, review this content.

Level of Cognitive Ability: Analysis
Client Needs: Safe, Effective Care Environment
Integrated Process: Nursing Process/Data Collection
Content Area: Pharmacology
Reference: Hodgson, B., & Kizior, R. (2005). *Saunders nursing drug handbook 2005.* Philadelphia: W.B. Saunders, p. 269.

19. *Answer: 2*
Rationale: The client needs to be told that the urine may turn brown, black, or green. Other adverse effects include blurred vision, nasal congestion, urticaria, and rash. The client needs to be instructed that, if these adverse effects occur, the

physician needs to be notified. The medication is used to relieve muscle spasms.

Test-Taking Strategy: Note the key words, *need for further instructions.* These words indicate a false response question and that you need to select the incorrect client statement. Recalling the adverse effects of this medication will direct you to option 2. If you had difficulty with this question, review this medication.

Level of Cognitive Ability: Analysis
Client Needs: Health Promotion and Maintenance
Integrated Process: Teaching/Learning
Content Area: Pharmacology
Reference: Skidmore-Roth, L. (2005). *Mosby's drug guide for nurses* (6th ed.). St. Louis: Mosby, p. 542.

20. *Answer:* **1**
Rationale: The normal adult dosage for carisoprodol is 350 mg orally three or four times daily.

Test-Taking Strategy: This question may be difficult if you are not familiar with the normal medication dosage. Remember, the normal adult dosage for carisoprodol is 350 mg orally three or four times daily. Review this medication if you had difficulty with this question.

Level of Cognitive Ability: Analysis
Client Needs: Physiological Integrity
Integrated Process: Nursing Process/Evaluation
Content Area: Pharmacology
Reference: Skidmore-Roth, L. (2005). *Mosby's drug guide for nurses* (6th ed.). St. Louis: Mosby, p. 141.

ALTERNATE FORMAT QUESTION: MULTIPLE RESPONSE

Answers:
Take the medication with food
Contact the physician if a rash develops
A complete blood cell count and renal and liver function studies may be prescribed

Rationale: Allopurinol (Zyloprim) is an antigout medication. It decreases uric acid production by inhibiting xanthine oxidase, an enzyme. The medication can be taken with or immediately following food intake. The client should drink at least 2000 to 3000 mL of fluid daily to prevent the development of uric acid stones. Alcohol intake needs to be avoided (not limited), because alcohol can increase uric acid levels. The client is also instructed to report side effects such as a rash to the physician. A complete blood cell count and renal and liver function studies may be prescribed to monitor for adverse effects of the medication.

Test-Taking Strategy: Focus on the client's diagnosis and use general medication administration guidelines to answer the question. Review client teaching points related to this medication if you had difficulty with this question.

Level of Cognitive Ability: Application
Client Needs: Health Promotion and Maintenance
Integrated Process: Teaching/Learning
Content Area: Pharmacology
Reference: *Mosby's 2005 drug consult for nurses.* (2005). St. Louis: Mosby, p. 1121.

REFERENCES

Hodgson, B., & Kizior, R. (2005). *Saunders nursing drug handbook 2005.* Philadelphia: W.B. Saunders.

Lehne, R. (2004). *Pharmacology for nursing care.* (5th ed.). Philadelphia: W.B. Saunders.

McKenry, L., & Salerno, E. (2003). *Mosby's pharmacology in nursing* (21st ed.). St. Louis: Mosby.

Mosby's 2005 drug consult for nurses. (2005). St. Louis: Mosby.

Skidmore-Roth, L. (2005). *Mosby's drug guide for nurses* (6th ed.). St. Louis: Mosby.

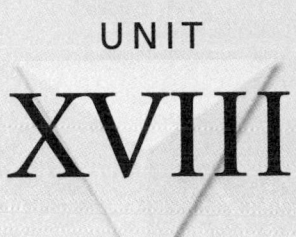
The Adult Client with an Immune Disorder

PYRAMID TERMS

acquired immunity Immunity received passively from the mother's antibodies, animal serum, or production of antibodies in response to a disease. Immunization produces active acquired immunity.

allergy An abnormal, individual response to certain substances that normally do not trigger such an exaggerated reaction.

cellular response A delayed response; also called delayed hypersensitivity. Active against slowly developing bacterial infections.

humoral response An immediate response that provides protection against acute, rapidly developing bacterial and viral infections.

immune deficiency The absence or inadequate production of immune bodies.

natural immunity Also called innate immunity; present at birth.

▲ PYRAMID TO SUCCESS

Pyramid points focus on the effects of and complications associated with an immune deficiency. Specific focus relates to the nursing care related to the disorder, the impact of the treatment or disorder, and client adaptation. Acquired immunodeficiency syndrome is a pyramid focus, along with protecting the client from infection, and preventing the transmission of infection to other individuals. Psychosocial issues relate to social isolation and the body image disturbances that can occur as a result of the immune disorder. The Integrated Processes addressed in this unit include Caring, Clinical Problem-Solving Process (Nursing Process), Communication and Documentation, and Teaching/Learning.

▲ CLIENT NEEDS
Safe, Effective Care Environment

Advance directives
Advocacy related to client's decisions
Asepsis

Client rights
Confidentiality regarding diagnosis
Consultation with members of the health care team
Establishing priorities
Handling hazardous and infectious materials
Informed consent for treatments and procedures
Standard and other precautions

Health Promotion and Maintenance

Client lifestyle choices
Data collection related to the immune system
Expected body image changes
Health promotion programs
Health screening measures
Immunizations
Prevention of disease related to infection

Psychosocial Integrity

Ability to cope, adapt, and/or problem solve during illness or stressful events
Assisting in mobilizing appropriate support and resource systems
Assisting the client and family to cope
Grief and loss related to death and the dying process
Promoting a positive environment to maintain optimal quality of life
Religious, spiritual, and cultural preferences

Physiological Integrity

Diagnostic tests and laboratory values
Managing pain
Monitoring for the expected and unexpected responses to treatments
Promoting nutrition
Protecting the client from the infection
Providing basic care and comfort

REFERENCES

Black, J., & Hawks, J. (2005). *Medical-surgical nursing: Clinical management for positive outcomes* (7th ed.). Philadelphia: W.B. Saunders.

Chernecky, C., & Berger, B. (2004). *Laboratory tests and diagnostic procedures* (4th ed.). Philadelphia: W.B. Saunders.

Christensen, B., & Kockrow, E. (2003). *Adult health nursing* (4th ed.). St. Louis: Mosby.

Christensen, B., & Kockrow, E. (2003). *Foundations of nursing* (4th ed.). St. Louis: Mosby.

Fortinash, K., & Holoday-Worret, P. (2004). *Psychiatric mental health nursing* (3rd ed.). St. Louis: Mosby.

Harkreader, H., & Hogan, M.A. (2004). *Fundamentals of nursing: Caring and clinical judgment* (2nd ed.). Philadelphia: W.B. Saunders.

Hodgson, B., & Kizior, R. (2005). *Saunders nursing drug handbook 2005.* Philadelphia: W.B. Saunders.

Lewis, S., Heitkemper, M., & Dirksen, S. (2004). *Medical-surgical nursing: Assessment and management of clinical problems* (6th ed.). St. Louis: Mosby.

Linton, A., & Maebius, N. (2003) *Introduction to medical-surgical nursing* (3rd ed.). Philadelphia: W.B. Saunders.

McKenry, L., & Salerno, E. (2003). *Mosby's pharmacology in nursing* (21st ed.). St. Louis: Mosby.

National Council of State Boards of Nursing. (2005). *Detailed test plan for the National Council licensure examination for practical/vocational nurses.* Chicago: Author.

Pagana, K., & Pagana, T. (2003). *Mosby's diagnostic and laboratory test reference* (6th ed.). St. Louis: Mosby.

Perry, A., & Potter, P. (2002). *Clinical nursing skills and techniques* (5th ed.). St. Louis: Mosby.

Phipps, W., Monahan, F., Sands, J., Marek, J., & Neighbors, M. (2003). *Medical-surgical nursing: Health and illness perspectives* (7th ed.). St. Louis: Mosby.

Potter, P., & Perry, A. (2003). *Essentials for practice* (5th ed.). St. Louis: Mosby.

Immune Disorders

I. FUNCTIONS OF THE IMMUNE SYSTEM

A. Provides protection against invasion from outside the body, such as by microorganisms
B. Protects the body from internal threats
C. Maintains the internal environment by removing dead or damaged cells

II. IMMUNE RESPONSE

A. T lymphocytes and B lymphocytes
   1. Migrate to lymphoid tissue where they remain dormant to form either sensitized lymphocytes for cellular immunity or antibodies for humoral immunity
   2. Some B lymphocytes lie dormant until a specific antigen enters the body, at which time they greatly increase in number and are available for defense
   3. T lymphocytes are responsible for rejection of transplanted tissue
   4. Both T and B lymphocytes are necessary for a normal immune response
B. **Humoral response**
   1. An immediate response
   2. Provides protection against acute, rapidly developing bacterial and viral infections
C. **Cellular response**
   1. A delayed response; also called delayed hypersensitivity
   2. Active against slowly developing bacterial infections
   3. Also involved in autoimmune response, some allergic reactions, and rejection of foreign cells

III. IMMUNITY

A. **Natural immunity**
   1. Also called innate
   2. Present at birth
B. **Acquired immunity**
   1. Received passively from the mother's antibodies, animal serum, or from the production of antibodies in response to a disease
   2. Immunization produces active **acquired immunity**

IV. IMMUNIZATIONS (See Chapter 38 regarding immunizations)

V. LABORATORY STUDIES

A. Antinuclear antibody (ANA)
   1. A blood test used in the differential diagnosis of rheumatic diseases and to detect antinucleoprotein factors and patterns associated with certain autoimmune diseases
   2. Positive at a titer of 1:20 or 1:40, depending on the laboratory
   3. A positive result does not necessarily confirm a disease
B. Anti-dsDNA (anti–double-stranded DNA) antibody test
   1. A blood test done specifically to identify or differentiate DNA antibodies found in systemic lupus erythematosus (SLE) or other rheumatic diseases
   2. Supports a diagnosis, monitors disease activity and response to therapy, and establishes a prognosis for SLE
   3. Values
      a. Negative: Lower than 70 units by enzyme-linked immunosorbent assay (ELISA)
      b. Borderline: 70 to 200 units
      c. Positive: Higher than 200 units
C. Refer to Chapter 11 for testing related to acquired immunodeficiency syndrome (AIDS)

VI. IMMUNE DEFICIENCY
A. Description
1. Absence or inadequate production of immune bodies
2. Can be congenital (primary) or acquired (secondary)
3. Treatment depends on the inadequacy of immune bodies and its primary cause
B. Data collection
1. Factors that decrease immune function
2. Frequent infections
3. Nutritional status
4. Medication history such as corticosteroids
5. History of alcohol or drug abuse
C. Interventions
1. Protect from infection
2. Promote balanced, adequate nutrition
3. Use strict aseptic technique for all procedures
4. Provide psychosocial care regarding lifestyle changes and role changes
5. Instruct the client in measures to prevent infection

VII. HYPERSENSITIVITY AND ALLERGY
A. Description
1. An **allergy** is an abnormal, individual response to certain substances that normally do not trigger such an exaggerated reaction
2. In some types of allergies, a reaction occurs on a second and subsequent contact with the allergen
3. Skin testing may be done to determine the allergen
B. Data collection
1. History of exposure to allergens
2. Itching, tearing, and burning of eyes
3. Itching and burning of the skin
4. Rashes
5. Nose twitching, nasal stuffiness
C. Interventions
1. Identification of the specific allergen
2. Managing the symptoms with the use of antihistamines, anti-inflammatory agents, or corticosteroids
3. Salves, wet compresses, and soothing baths for local reactions
4. Desensitization programs

VIII. ANAPHYLAXIS
A. Description
1. A serious and dramatic allergic reaction with the release of histamine from the damaged cells
2. Can cause shock and death if not treated immediately
B. Data collection
1. Identification of allergies
2. Difficulty breathing
3. Difficulty swallowing
4. Complaints of a swollen tongue
5. Facial edema and swelling of the lips
6. Skin redness
7. Presence of a rash
C. Interventions
1. Establish a patent airway
2. Prepare for the administration of epinephrine (Adrenalin), diphenhydramine hydrochloride (Benadryl), or corticosteroids
3. Provide measures to control shock
4. Provide emotional support
5. Instruct the client to wear a Medic-Alert bracelet
6. Instruct the client in the use of prescribed medication for immediate treatment of a reaction

IX. LATEX ALLERGY
A. Description
1. A hypersensitivity to latex
2. The source of the allergic reaction is thought to be caused by the proteins in the natural rubber latex or the various chemicals used in the manufacturing process of the latex from a liquid substance into the finished product
3. Symptoms of the **allergy** can range from mild contact dermatitis to moderately severe symptoms of rhinitis, conjunctivitis, urticaria, and bronchospasm, to severe life-threatening anaphylaxis
B. Common routes of exposure (Box 60-1)
1. Cutaneous: Wearing natural latex gloves
2. Percutaneous and parenteral: IV lines and catheters; hemodialysis equipment

---

BOX 60-1

Products that May Contain Natural Rubber Latex

Ace bandages (brown)
Adhesive bandages
Ambu bag
Balloons
Band-Aid dressings
Blood pressure cuff (tubing and bladder)
Catheters
Catheter leg bag straps
Condoms
Diaphragms
Elastic pressure stockings
Electrocardiography pads
Feminine hygiene pads
Gloves
IV catheters, tubing, and rubber injection ports
Levine tubes
Pads for crutches
Prepackaged enema kits
Rubber stoppers on medication vials
Stethoscopes
Syringes

3. Mucosal: Use of latex condoms, catheters, airways, and nipples
4. Aerosol: Aerosolization of powder from latex gloves can occur when gloves are dispensed from the box or when gloves are removed from the hands

C. At-risk individuals
1. Health care workers
2. Individuals who work with manufacturing latex products
3. Females
4. Individuals with spina bifida
5. Individuals who wear gloves frequently such as food handlers, hairdressers, and auto mechanics
6. Individuals allergic to kiwis, bananas, pineapples, tropical fruits, avocados, potatoes, and chestnuts

D. Data collection
1. Anaphylactic hypersensitivity
   a. Rapid onset
   b. Urticaria, wheezing, dyspnea, laryngeal edema, bronchospasm, tachycardia, angioedema, hypotension, and cardiac arrest
2. Delayed-type hypersensitivity: Includes symptoms of contact dermatitis, such as pruritus, edema, erythema, vesicles, papules, and crusting and thickening of the skin

E. Interventions (Box 60-2)
1. Ask the client about a known **allergy** to latex when obtaining initial data
2. Identify risk factors to a latex **allergy** in the client
3. Individuals with an **allergy**
   a. Avoid latex products
   b. Obtain an emergency medical kit that contains antihistamines and epinephrine
   c. Wear a Medic-Alert bracelet
   d. Inform health care providers and local and paramedic ambulance companies about the **allergy**
   e. Advise the individual to place a warning label in the car window to alert police and paramedics of the **allergy**, in case of a car crash
   f. Provide information about local support groups and resources of alternative products

---

BOX 60-2

Interventions for the Client with a Latex Allergy

Use nonlatex gloves and latex-safe supplies.
Keep a latex-safe supply cart near the client's room.
Apply a cloth barrier to the client's arm under a blood pressure cuff.
Use latex-free syringes, medication containers (glass ampules), and latex-safe IV equipment.

X. AUTOIMMUNE DISEASE

A. Description
1. Body is unable to recognize its own cells as part of itself
2. Can affect collagenous tissue

B. Systemic lupus erythematosus (SLE)
1. Description
   a. A chronic, progressive, systemic inflammatory disease that can cause major organs and systems to fail
   b. Connective tissue and fibrin deposits in blood vessels on collagen fibers and on organs
   c. Leads to necrosis and/or inflammation in blood vessels, lymph nodes, gastrointestinal (GI) tract, pleura
   d. There is no cure for the disease
2. Causes
   a. The cause is unknown and it is thought to be the result of a defect in the immunological mechanisms or to be of genetic origin
   b. Precipitating factors include medications, stress, genetic factors, sunlight or ultraviolet light, and pregnancy
3. Data collection
   a. Precipitating factors, such as sunlight, stress, and medications
   b. Dry scaly raised rash on the face or upper body
   c. Fever
   d. Weakness, malaise, and fatigue
   e. Anorexia
   f. Weight loss
   g. Photosensitivity
   h. Joint pain
   i. Erythema of the palms
   j. Butterfly erythema of the face
   k. Anemia
   l. Positive antinuclear antibodies (ANAs) and lupus erythematosus preparation test (LE prep)
   m. Elevated sedimentation rate
4. Interventions
   a. Monitor skin integrity and provide frequent oral care
   b. Instruct the client to clean skin with a mild soap, avoiding harsh and perfumed substances
   c. Assist with the use of ointments and creams for rash, as prescribed
   d. Identify factors contributing to fatigue
   e. Administer iron, folic acid, or vitamin supplements as prescribed if anemia occurs
   f. Provide a high-vitamin and high-iron diet
   g. Provide a high protein diet if there is no evidence of kidney disease
   h. Instruct in measures to conserve energy, such as pacing activities and balancing rest with exercise
   i. Administer topical or systemic corticosteroids, salicylates and nonsteroidal anti-inflammatory

drugs (NSAIDs) as prescribed for pain and inflammation

j. Administer hydroxychloroquine (Plaquenil) as prescribed to decrease the inflammatory response

k. Instruct the client to avoid exposure to sunlight and ultraviolet light

l. Monitor for proteinuria and red cell casts in the urine

m. Monitor for bruising, bleeding, and injury

n. Assist with plasmapheresis as prescribed to remove autoantibodies and immune complexes from the blood before organ damage occurs

o. Monitor for signs of organ involvement such as pleuritis, nephritis, pericarditis, neuritis, anemia, coronary artery disease, hypertension, and peritonitis

p. Note that lupus nephritis occurs early in the disease process

q. Provide supportive therapy as major organs become affected

r. Provide emotional support and encourage the client to verbalize feelings

s. Provide information regarding support groups and encourage utilization of community resources

C. Scleroderma (progressive systemic sclerosis)
  1. Description
    a. A chronic connective tissue disease, similar to SLE, characterized by inflammation, fibrosis, and sclerosis
    b. Affects the connective tissue throughout the body
    c. Causes fibrotic changes involving the skin, synovial membranes, esophagus, heart, lungs, kidneys, and GI tract
    d. Treatment is directed toward forcing the disease into remission and slowing its progress
  2. Data collection
    a. Pain
    b. Stiffness and muscle weakness
    c. Pitting edema of the hands and fingers, which progresses to the rest of the body
    d. Taut and shiny skin that is free from wrinkles
    e. Skin tissue is tight, hard, and thick and loses its elasticity
    f. Masklike hard skin that adheres to underlying structures
    g. Dysphagia
    h. Decreased range of motion
    i. Joint contractures
    j. Inability to perform activities of daily living
  3. Interventions
    a. Encourage activity as tolerated
    b. Maintain a constant room temperature
    c. Provide small, frequent meals, eliminating foods that stimulate gastric secretions such as spicy foods, caffeine, and alcohol

d. Advise the client to sit up for 1 to 2 hours after meals if esophageal involvement exists

e. Provide supportive therapy as the major organs become affected

f. Administer corticosteroids as prescribed for inflammation

g. Provide emotional support and encourage the use of resources as necessary

D. Polyarteritis nodosa
  1. Description
    a. A collagen disease that causes inflammation of the arteries and thickening and impairment of the circulation
    b. Treatment is similar to treatment for SLE
    c. Affects middle-aged men and involves every body system
    d. The cause is unknown and the prognosis is poor
    e. Renal disorders and cardiac involvement are the most frequent causes of death
  2. Data collection
    a. Malaise and weakness
    b. Low grade fever
    c. Severe abdominal pain
    d. Bloody diarrhea
    e. Weight loss
    f. Elevated sedimentation rate
  3. Interventions
    a. Provide supportive care as required
    b. Provide a well-balanced diet
    c. Administer corticosteroids and analgesics to control pain and inflammation
    d. Provide emotional support and encourage the client to verbalize feelings
    e. Initiate support services for the client

E. Pemphigus vulgaris
  1. Description
    a. A rare disease that occurs predominately between middle and old age
    b. The cause is unknown and the disorder is potentially fatal
    c. Initial lesions occur on the oral mucosa and then progress to a generalized distribution
    d. Treatment is aimed at suppressing the immune response that causes blister formation
  2. Data collection
    a. Lesions appear as fragile, flaccid bullae
    b. Partial-thickness wounds that bleed, weep, and form crusts when bullae are disrupted
    c. Debilitation, malaise, and pain
    d. Chewing and swallowing difficulties
    e. Nikolsky's sign: Separation of the epidermis caused by rubbing the skin
    f. Leukocytosis, eosinophilia, foul-smelling discharge from skin
  3. Interventions
    a. Provide supportive care

b. Provide oral hygiene and increase fluid intake

c. Soothe oral lesions

d. Assist with oatmeal or potassium permanganate baths as prescribed for relief of symptoms

e. Administer topical or systemic antibiotics as prescribed for secondary infections

f. Administer corticosteroids and cytotoxic agents as prescribed to bring about remission

F. Goodpasture's syndrome

1. Description

a. An autoimmune disorder; autoantibodies against the glomerular basement membrane and neutrophils are produced

b. Most common in males and young adults; exact cause is unknown

c. The lungs and the kidneys are primarily affected; disorder is usually not diagnosed until significant pulmonary or renal involvement occurs

2. Data collection

a. Clinical manifestations indicate pulmonary and renal involvement

b. Shortness of breath

c. Hemoptysis

d. Decreased urine output

e. Edema and weight gain

f. Hypertension and tachycardia

3. Interventions

a. Focus on suppressing the autoimmune response with medications such as corticosteroids and plasmapheresis (filtration of the plasma to remove some proteins) to remove the autoantibodies

b. Supportive therapy for pulmonary and renal involvement

XI. ACQUIRED IMMUNODEFICIENCY SYNDROME (AIDS)

A. Description

1. An infectious disease characterized by severe deficits in cellular function

2. Manifested clinically by opportunistic infection and/or unusual neoplasms

3. Etiology: Human immunodeficiency virus (HIV)

4. The disease has a long incubation period, sometimes up to 10 years or longer

5. Manifestations may not appear until late in the infection

B. AIDS-related complex (ARC)

1. Similar to AIDS

2. Two or more symptoms or two or more laboratory findings characteristic of immunodeficiency

3. Client is not as ill as the AIDS client

4. May lead to AIDS

C. High-risk groups

1. Male homosexuals or bisexuals

2. Intravenous drug abusers

3. Persons receiving blood transfusions (hemophiliacs, surgical clients)

4. Those individuals with frequent exposure to blood and body fluids

5. Heterosexual contact with high-risk individuals

6. Babies born to infected mothers

D. Data collection

1. Malaise, weight loss

2. Lymphadenopathy of at least 3 months

3. Leukopenia

4. Diarrhea

5. Fatigue

6. Night sweats

7. Presence of opportunistic Infections

8. *Pneumocystis jiroveci* (formerly called *Pneumocystis carinii*) pneumonia (major source of mortality)

9. Kaposi's sarcoma: Purplish-red lesions of internal organs and skin

10. Candidiasis

11. Fungal infections

12. Cytomegalovirus (CMV)

E. Interventions

1. Provide respiratory support

2. Administer respiratory treatments, as prescribed

3. Administer oxygen, as prescribed

4. Maintain fluid and electrolyte balance

5. Monitor for signs of infection

6. Prevent the spread of infection

7. Initiate standard precautions

8. Provide comfort as necessary

9. Provide meticulous skin care

10. Provide adequate nutritional support, as prescribed

11. See Chapters 22 and 38 for additional information on AIDS

PRACTICE QUESTIONS

1. A client is suspected of having systemic lupus erythematous (SLE). The nurse monitors the client, knowing that which of the following is a characteristic sign of SLE?

   1. Rash on the face across the bridge of the nose and on the cheeks

   2. Fatigue

   3. Fever

   4. Elevated red blood cell count

2. The nurse provides information to a client with systemic lupus erythematosus (SLE) about measures to manage fatigue. The nurse determines that the client needs additional information if the client states that he or she will:

   1. Avoid long periods of rest

   2. Sit whenever possible

   3. Take a hot bath in the evening

4. Engage in moderate low-impact exercise when not fatigued

3. A client has requested and undergone testing for human immunodeficiency virus (HIV). The client now asks what will be done next, because the results of two enzyme-linked immunosorbent assay (ELISA) tests have been positive. The nurse's response is based on the understanding that:
   1. The client will probably have a bone marrow biopsy done
   2. A Western blot test will be done to confirm these findings
   3. A CD4+ cell count will be obtained to measure T-helper lymphocytes
   4. The client will be definitively diagnosed as HIV-positive at this point

4. A nurse is caring for the client with acquired immunodeficiency syndrome (AIDS). The nurse detects early infection with *Pneumocystis jiroveci* (formerly called *Pneumocystis carinii*) by monitoring the client for which clinical manifestation?
   1. Dyspnea on exertion
   2. Dyspnea at rest
   3. Fever
   4. Cough

5. A client with acquired immunodeficiency syndrome (AIDS) has a concurrent diagnosis of histoplasmosis. The nurse notes during data collection that the client has enlarged lymph nodes. The nurse interprets that:
   1. The client has disseminated histoplasmosis infection
   2. This is a side effect of the medications given to treat AIDS
   3. This indicates that the histoplasmosis is resolving
   4. The client probably has yet another infection that is developing

6. A nurse is caring for the client with acquired immunodeficiency syndrome (AIDS) who is experiencing night fever and night sweats. Which nursing intervention would be least helpful in managing this symptom?
   1. Keep a change of bed linens nearby in case they are needed
   2. Administer an antipyretic after the client spikes a fever
   3. Make sure that the pillow has a plastic cover
   4. Keep liquids at the bedside

7. A client with acquired immunodeficiency syndrome (AIDS) has raised, dark purplish-colored lesions on the trunk of the body. The nurse anticipates that which procedure will be done to confirm whether these lesions are due to Kaposi's sarcoma?
   1. Enzyme-linked immunosorbent assay (ELISA)
   2. Western blot test
   3. Skin biopsy
   4. Lung biopsy

8. A nurse participating in a health fair is setting up a booth on prevention of human immunodeficiency virus (HIV) transmission. A poster is planned that will list sexual behaviors in one of two columns, rated "safe" and "not safe." Which of the following behaviors would the nurse place in the "not safe" column?
   1. Use of latex condoms
   2. Use of "natural skin" condoms
   3. Abstinence
   4. Mutual monogamy

9. A client with acquired immunodeficiency syndrome (AIDS) is experiencing nausea and vomiting. The nurse would suggest which dietary alteration for this client to enhance nutritional intake?
   1. Avoid dairy products and red meat
   2. Plan large, nutritious meals
   3. Add spices to food for added flavor
   4. Serve foods while they are very warm

10. A client with pemphigus vulgaris is being seen in the clinic on a regular basis. The nurse plans care based on which description of this condition?
   1. The presence of skin vesicles found along the nerve caused by a virus
   2. An autoimmune disorder that causes blistering in the epidermis
   3. The presence of red, raised papules and large plaques covered by silvery scales
   4. The presence of tiny red vesicles

11. A nurse is providing dietary instructions to the client with systemic lupus erythematosus (SLE). Which dietary item would the nurse instruct the client to avoid?
   1. Cantaloupe
   2. Broccoli
   3. Turkey
   4. Steak

12. A client is brought to the emergency room and is experiencing an anaphylaxis reaction from eating shellfish. The nurse prepares for which initial action?
   1. Administration of epinephrine (Adrenalin)
   2. Administration of a corticosteroid
   3. Maintaining a patent airway
   4. Instructing the client on the importance of obtaining a Medic-Alert bracelet

13. A nurse is assisting in planning care for a client with a diagnosis of immune deficiency. The nurse would incorporate which of the following as a priority in the plan of care?
   1. Emotional support to decrease fear
   2. Protecting the client from infection
   3. Encouraging discussion about lifestyle changes
   4. Identifying factors that decrease the immune function

14. A client calls the nurse in the emergency room and tells the nurse that he was just stung by a bee while gardening. The client is afraid of a severe reaction, because the client's neighbor experienced

such a reaction just 1 week ago. The appropriate nursing action is to:

1. Ask the client if he ever received a bee sting in the past
2. Tell the client to call an ambulance for transport to the emergency room
3. Advise the client to soak the site in hydrogen peroxide
4. Tell the client not to worry about the sting unless difficulty with breathing occurs

15. A nurse is assisting in administering immunizations at a health care clinic. The nurse understands that an immunization will provide:
   1. Natural immunity from disease
   2. Acquired immunity from disease
   3. Innate immunity from disease
   4. Protection from all diseases

16. A nurse is assigned to care for a client with systemic lupus erythematosus (SLE). The nurse plans care, knowing that this disorder is:
   1. A local rash that occurs as a result of allergy
   2. An inflammatory disease of collagen contained in connective tissue
   3. A disease caused by overexposure to sunlight
   4. A disease caused by the continuous release of histamine in the body

17. A nurse is providing home care instructions to a client who has been diagnosed with a latex allergy. The nurse instructs the client to avoid:
   1. Outdoor activities as much as possible
   2. Going to parties
   3. The use of condoms
   4. Sunlight

18. A nurse is collecting data on a client who has been diagnosed with an allergy to latex. In determining the client's risk factors associated with the allergy, the nurse questions the client about an allergy to which food item?
   1. Milk
   2. Bananas

3. Yogurt
4. Eggs

19. A nurse is caring for a client who has returned home from the emergency room following treatment for a sprained ankle. The nurse notes that the client was sent home with crutches and needs instructions regarding crutch walking. When collecting data from the client, the nurse discovers that the client has an allergy to latex. Before providing instructions regarding crutch walking, the nurse most appropriately:
   1. Contacts the physician
   2. Covers the crutch pads with cloth
   3. Tells the client that the crutches must be removed from the house immediately
   4. Calls the local medical supply store and asks for a cane to be delivered

20. A nurse is ordering dressing supplies for a client who has an allergy to latex. The nurse asks the medical supply personnel to deliver which of the following?
   1. Adhesive bandages
   2. Elastic bandages
   3. Cotton pads and silk tape
   4. Brown Ace bandages

ALTERNATE FORMAT QUESTION: MULTIPLE RESPONSE

Select the interventions that would apply in the care of a client at high risk for an allergic response to a latex allergy.

___ Use nonlatex gloves
___ Keep a latex-safe supply cart available in the client's area
___ Only use a blood pressure cuff from an electronic device to measure the blood pressure
___ Use medications from glass ampules
___ Do not puncture rubber stoppers with needles

ANSWERS

1. *Answer:* **1**
Rationale: Skin lesions or rash on the face across the bridge of the nose and on the cheeks is a characteristic sign of SLE. Fever and fatigue may potentially occur before and during exacerbation. Anemia is most likely to occur in SLE.
Test-Taking Strategy: Note the key words, *characteristic sign*. Remember, a characteristic sign of SLE is a butterfly rash across the face. If you are unfamiliar with this disorder, review this content.
Level of Cognitive Ability: Application
Client Needs: Physiological Integrity
Integrated Process: Nursing Process/Data Collection
Content Area: Adult Health/Immune

Reference: Linton, A., & Maebius, N. (2003). *Introduction to medical-surgical nursing* (3rd ed.). Philadelphia: W.B. Saunders, p. 548.

2. *Answer:* **3**
Rationale: To help reduce fatigue in the client with SLE, the nurse should instruct the client to sit whenever possible, to avoid hot baths, to schedule moderate low-impact exercises when not fatigued, and to maintain a balanced diet. The client is instructed not to rest for long periods because it promotes joint stiffness.
Test-Taking Strategy: Note the key words, *needs additional information*. These words indicate a false response question and that you need to select the incorrect client statement.

Focusing on the issue will direct you to option 3 as being the action that would exacerbate fatigue. If you had difficulty with this question, review measures to prevent fatigue.
Level of Cognitive Ability: Comprehension
Client Needs: Health Promotion and Maintenance
Integrated Process: Teaching/Learning
Content Area: Adult Health/Immune
References: Christensen, B., & Kockrow, E. (2003). *Adult health nursing* (4th ed.). St. Louis: Mosby, pp. 81-82.
Linton, A., & Maebius, N. (2003). *Introduction to medical-surgical nursing* (3rd ed.). Philadelphia: W.B. Saunders, pp. 341, 548.

3. *Answer: 2*
Rationale: If the results of two ELISA tests are positive, the Western blot test is done to confirm the findings. If the result of the Western blot test is positive, then the client is considered to be positive for HIV and infected with the HIV virus.
Test-Taking Strategy: Knowledge of the diagnostic tests and procedural steps in diagnosing HIV is needed to answer this question. Remember, the Western blot test is done to confirm the findings if the results of two ELISA tests are positive. Review these diagnostic tests if you had difficulty with this question.
Level of Cognitive Ability: Application
Client Needs: Physiological Integrity
Integrated Process: Nursing Process/Implementation
Content Area: Adult Health/Immune
References: Linton, A., & Maebius, N. (2003). *Introduction to medical-surgical nursing* (3rd ed.). Philadelphia: W.B. Saunders, p. 550.
Pagana, K., & Pagana, T. (2003). *Mosby's diagnostic and laboratory test reference* (6th ed.). St. Louis: Mosby, pp. 23-27.

4. *Answer: 4*
Rationale: The client with *Pneumocystis jiroveci* (formerly *P. carinii*) infection usually has a cough as the first symptom, which begins as nonproductive and then progresses to productive. Later signs include fever, dyspnea on exertion, and finally dyspnea at rest.
Test-Taking Strategy: Note the key word, *early.* Although all these symptoms may appear at some point in the client with *Pneumocystis jiroveci,* knowing that the cough appears first helps you eliminate each of the other options. Review the early signs of *Pneumocystis jiroveci* infection if you had difficulty with this question.
Level of Cognitive Ability: Application
Client Needs: Physiological Integrity
Integrated Process: Nursing Process/Data Collection
Content Area: Adult Health/Immune
Reference: Christensen, B., & Kockrow, E. (2003). *Adult health nursing* (4th ed.). St. Louis: Mosby, p. 685.

5. *Answer: 1*
Rationale: Histoplasmosis usually starts as a respiratory infection in the client with AIDS. It then becomes a disseminated infection, with enlargement of lymph nodes, spleen, and liver. Options 2, 3, and 4 are incorrect.
Test-Taking Strategy: Use the process of elimination. Knowing that lymph nodes may enlarge with generalized infection

helps you eliminate options 2 and 3. Because the question contains no information that indicates that another infection is developing (option 4), option 1 is the correct choice by elimination. Review disseminated infections in the client with AIDS if you had difficulty with this question.
Level of Cognitive Ability: Analysis
Client Needs: Physiological Integrity
Integrated Process: Nursing Process/Data Collection
Content Area: Adult Health/Immune
Reference: Christensen, B., & Kockrow, E. (2003). *Adult health nursing* (4th ed.). St. Louis: Mosby, p. 685.

6. *Answer: 2*
Rationale: For clients with AIDS who experience night fever and night sweats, it is useful to offer the client an antipyretic of choice before going to sleep. It is also helpful to keep a change of bed linens and night clothes nearby for use. The pillow should have a plastic cover, and a towel may be placed over the pillowcase if there is profuse diaphoresis. The client should have liquids at the bedside to drink.
Test-Taking Strategy: Note the key words, *least helpful.* These words indicate a false response question and that you need to select the least helpful intervention. Options 1 and 3 are helpful from an environmental viewpoint, so they are eliminated first. Knowing that liquids will help prevent dehydration assists you to eliminate option 4. This leaves option 2 as the answer. Because night fever and sweats occur serially, it is most helpful to give the antipyretic before sleep as a prophylactic measure. Review care of the client with AIDS if you had difficulty with this question.
Level of Cognitive Ability: Application
Client Needs: Physiological Integrity
Integrated Process: Nursing Process/Implementation
Content Area: Adult Health/Immune
References: Black, J., & Hawks, J. (2005). *Medical-surgical nursing: Clinical management for positive outcomes* (7th ed.). Philadelphia: W.B. Saunders, p. 2395.
Linton, A., & Maebius, N. (2003). *Introduction to medical-surgical nursing* (3rd ed.). Philadelphia: W.B. Saunders, p. 549.

7. *Answer: 3*
Rationale: The skin biopsy is the procedure of choice to diagnose Kaposi's sarcoma. Lung biopsy would confirm *Pneumocystis jiroveci* (formerly *P. carinii*) infection. The ELISA and Western blot tests are used to diagnose HIV status.
Test-Taking Strategy: Use the process of elimination. Begin to answer this question by eliminating options, 1 and 2, which are used to diagnose whether or not the client is HIV positive. Recalling the meaning of Kaposi's sarcoma, and noting the words "lesions" and "trunk" in the question, will help you choose correctly from the remaining options. Review the diagnostic testing to confirm Kaposi's sarcoma if you had difficulty with this question.
Level of Cognitive Ability: Analysis
Client Needs: Physiological Integrity
Integrated Process: Nursing Process/Data Collection
Content Area: Adult Health/Immune
Reference: Black, J., & Hawks, J. (2005). *Medical-surgical nursing: Clinical management for positive outcomes* (7th ed.). Philadelphia: W.B. Saunders, p. 2393.

8. *Answer:* 2

Rationale: Abstinence is the safest way to avoid HIV infection. The next most reliable method is participation in a mutually monogamous relationship. The use of latex condoms is considered safe, because the latex prevents the transmission of the HIV virus as long as the condom is used properly and remains in place. The use of "natural skin" condoms is not considered safe, because the pores in the condom are large enough for the virus to pass through.

Test-Taking Strategy: Note the key words, *not safe*. The wording of the question tells you that there is one option that is dissimilar from the others, which in this case is the correct answer to the question. Use knowledge of transmission of sexually transmitted diseases and standard precautions to direct you to option 2. Review these preventive measures if you had difficulty with this question.

Level of Cognitive Ability: Application
Client Needs: Health Promotion and Maintenance
Integrated Process: Teaching/Learning
Content Area: Adult Health/Immune
References: Black, J., & Hawks, J. (2005). *Medical-surgical nursing: Clinical management for positive outcomes* (7th ed.). Philadelphia: W.B. Saunders, pp. 13, 2378.
Swearingen, P. (2003). *Manual of medical-surgical nursing care* (5th ed.). St. Louis: Mosby, pp. 677-678.

9. *Answer:* 1

Rationale: The AIDS client with nausea and vomiting should avoid fatty products such as diary products and red meat. Meals should be small and frequent to lessen the chance of vomiting. Spices and odorous foods should be avoided, because they aggravate nausea. Foods are best tolerated either cold or at room temperature.

Test-Taking Strategy: Note that the client is experiencing nausea and vomiting. Use knowledge of the effects of AIDS on the gastrointestinal tract and general principles for treating nausea and vomiting to answer this question. Doing so will guide you to eliminate each of the incorrect options systematically. Review nutritional support for the client with AIDS if you had difficulty with this question.

Level of Cognitive Ability: Application
Client Needs: Physiological Integrity
Integrated Process: Nursing Process/Implementation
Content Area: Adult Health/Immune
References: Linton, A., & Maebius, N. (2003). *Introduction to medical-surgical nursing* (3rd ed.). Philadelphia: W.B. Saunders, p. 552.
Swearingen, P. (2003). *Manual of medical-surgical nursing care* (5th ed). St. Louis: Mosby, p. 687.

10. *Answer:* 2

Rationale: Pemphigus vulgaris is an autoimmune disease that causes blistering in the epidermis. The clients have large flaccid blisters (bullae). Because the blisters are in the epidermis, they have a very tiny covering of skin and break easily, leaving large denuded areas of skin. On initial examination, clients may have crusting areas instead of intact blisters. Option 1 describes herpes zoster. Option 3 describes psoriasis and option 4 describes eczema.

Test-Taking Strategy: Use the process of elimination. Recalling that pemphigus vulgaris is an autoimmune disorder will direct you to option 2. If you had difficulty with this question, review the characteristics of this disorder.

Level of Cognitive Ability: Application
Client Needs: Physiological Integrity
Integrated Process: Nursing Process/Planning
Content Area: Adult Health/Immune
References: Black, J., & Hawks, J. (2005). *Medical-surgical nursing: Clinical management for positive outcomes* (7th ed.). Philadelphia: W.B. Saunders, p. 1418.
Linton, A., & Maebius, N. (2003). *Introduction to medical-surgical nursing* (3rd ed.). Philadelphia: W.B. Saunders, p. 1029.

11. *Answer:* 4

Rationale: The client with SLE is at risk for cardiovascular disorders, such as coronary artery disease, and hypertension. The client is advised of lifestyle changes to reduce these risks, which include smoking cessation, prevention of obesity, and hyperlipidemia. The client is advised to reduce salt, fat, and cholesterol intake.

Test-Taking Strategy: Note the key word, *avoid*, in the question. Use knowledge regarding basic nutritional components of food items to help direct you to option 4. If you had difficulty with this question, review therapeutic management of SLE.

Level of Cognitive Ability: Application
Client Needs: Physiological Integrity
Integrated Process: Teaching/Learning
Content Area: Adult Health/Immune
Reference: Christensen, B., & Kockrow, E. (2003). *Adult health nursing* (4th ed.). St. Louis: Mosby, pp. 80-81.

12. *Answer:* 3

Rationale: The initial action would be to maintain a patent airway. The client would then receive epinephrine. Corticosteroids may also be prescribed. The client will need to be instructed about wearing a Medic-Alert bracelet, but this is not the initial action.

Test-Taking Strategy: Use the ABCs—airway, breathing, and circulation—to answer the question. Airway is always the priority. Review care to the client experiencing an anaphylaxis reaction if you had difficulty with this question.

Level of Cognitive Ability: Application
Client Needs: Physiological Integrity
Integrated Process: Nursing Process/Planning
Content Area: Delegating/Prioritizing
Reference: Christensen, B., & Kockrow, E. (2003). *Adult health nursing* (4th ed.). St. Louis: Mosby, p. 665.

13. *Answer:* 2

Rationale: The client with immune deficiency has inadequate or no immune bodies and is at risk for infection. The priority nursing intervention would be to protect the client from infection. Options 1, 3, and 4 may be components of care but are not the priority.

Test-Taking Strategy: Use Maslow's Hierarchy of Needs theory to answer the question. Remember that physiological needs are the priority. This will direct you to option 2. Review the care of a client with immune deficiency if you had difficulty with this question.

Level of Cognitive Ability: Application
Client Needs: Physiological Integrity
Integrated Process: Nursing Process/Implementation
Content Area: Delegating/Prioritizing
Reference: Linton, A., & Maebius, N. (2003). *Introduction to medical-surgical nursing* (3rd ed.). Philadelphia: W.B. Saunders, p. 540.

14. *Answer:* 1
Rationale: In some types of allergies, a reaction usually occurs only on second and subsequent contacts with the allergen. The appropriate action, therefore, would be to ask the client if he ever received a bee sting in the past. Option 2 is unnecessary. Option 3 is not appropriate advice. The client should not be told "not to worry."
Test-Taking Strategy: Use the steps of the nursing process to answer the question. Option 1 is the only option that addresses data collection. Review information related to allergic reactions if you had difficulty with this question.
Level of Cognitive Ability: Application
Client Needs: Physiological Integrity
Integrated Process: Nursing Process/Implementation
Content Area: Adult Health/Immune
References: Black, J., & Hawks, J. (2005). *Medical-surgical nursing: Clinical management for positive outcomes* (7th ed.). Philadelphia: W.B. Saunders, p. 2325.
Lewis, S., Heitkemper, M., & Dirksen, S. (2004). *Medical-surgical nursing: Assessment and management of clinical problems* (6th ed.). St. Louis: Mosby, p. 246.

15. *Answer:* 2
Rationale: Acquired immunity can occur by receiving an immunization that causes antibodies to a specific pathogen to form. Natural (innate) immunity is present at birth. There is no vaccine for immunization that protects the client from all diseases.
Test-Taking Strategy: Use the process of elimination and knowledge regarding immunity to disease to answer the question. Eliminate option 4 first because of the absolute word "all." Next, eliminate options 1 and 3 because they are similar. Review natural and acquired immunity if you had difficulty with this question.
Level of Cognitive Ability: Comprehension
Client Needs: Physiological Integrity
Integrated Process: Nursing Process/Implementation
Content Area: Adult Health/Immune
Reference: Linton, A., & Maebius, N. (2003). *Introduction to medical-surgical nursing* (3rd ed.). Philadelphia: W.B. Saunders, pp. 143, 533-534.

16. *Answer:* 2
Rationale: SLE is an inflammatory disease of collagen contained in connective tissue. Options 1, 3, and 4 are not associated with this disease.
Test-Taking Strategy: Knowledge regarding the characteristics of SLE is required to answer this question. Remember, SLE is an inflammatory disease of collagen contained in connective tissue. Review this disorder if you had difficulty with this question.
Level of Cognitive Ability: Comprehension

Client Needs: Physiological Integrity
Integrated Process: Nursing Process/Planning
Content Area: Adult Health/Immune
Reference: Christensen, B., & Kockrow, E. (2003). *Adult health nursing* (4th ed.). St. Louis: Mosby, p. 79.

17. *Answer:* 3
Rationale: Mucosal exposure to latex can occur on contact with latex condoms. The nurse would provide instructions to the client about the need to avoid the use of condoms, unless they are latex-free. There is no reason to avoid outdoor activities or sunlight. There is also no reason to avoid parties; however, the client should be informed that certain forms of balloons are made of latex.
Test-Taking Strategy: Note the key word, *avoid*. Eliminate options 1 and 4 first because they are similar. From the remaining options, focusing on the issue will direct you to option 3. Review instructions for the client with a latex allergy if you had difficulty with this question.
Level of Cognitive Ability: Application
Client Needs: Health Promotion and Maintenance
Integrated Process: Teaching/Learning
Content Area: Adult Health/Immune
References: Christensen, B., & Kockrow, E. (2003). *Foundations of nursing* (4th ed.). St. Louis: Mosby, pp. 242-243.
Lewis, S., Heitkemper, M., & Dirksen, S. (2004). *Medical-surgical nursing: Assessment and management of clinical problems* (6th ed.). St. Louis: Mosby, p. 253.

18. *Answer:* 2
Rationale: Individuals who are allergic to bananas, avocados, tropical fruits, kiwis, potatoes, and chestnuts are at risk for developing a latex allergy. This is thought to be caused by a possible cross-reaction between the food and the latex allergen. Options 1, 3, and 4 are unrelated to latex allergy.
Test-Taking Strategy: Use the process of elimination and knowledge regarding the food items related to a latex allergy. Eliminate options 1, 3, and 4 because they are similar and all relate to dairy products. Review the food items that are associated with a risk for latex allergy if you had difficulty with this question.
Level of Cognitive Ability: Analysis
Client Needs: Physiological Integrity
Integrated Process: Nursing Process/Data Collection
Content Area: Adult Health/Immune
Reference: Lewis, S., Heitkemper, M., & Dirksen, S. (2004). *Medical-surgical nursing: Assessment and management of clinical problems* (6th ed.). St. Louis: Mosby, p. 253.

19. *Answer:* 2
Rationale: Pads used on crutches contain latex. If the client requires the use of crutches, the nurse can cover the pads with a cloth to prevent cutaneous contact. Option 3 is inappropriate and may alarm the client. The nurse cannot order a cane for a client. Additionally, this type of assistive device may not be appropriate, considering this client's injury. There is no reason to contact the physician at this time.
Test-Taking Strategy: Use the process of elimination and knowledge regarding the alternative resources that can be used for a client with an allergy to latex. There is no information in

the question that supports the need to contact the physician. The nurse should not prescribe assistive devices for the client. Option 3 is not a therapeutic action. Review care of the client with a latex allergy if you had difficulty with this question.

Level of Cognitive Ability: Application
Client Needs: Safe, Effective Care Environment
Integrated Process: Nursing Process/Implementation
Content Area: Adult Health/Immune
References: Harkreader, H., & Hogan, M.A. (2004). *Fundamentals of nursing: Caring and clinical judgment* (2nd ed.). Philadelphia: W.B. Saunders. p. 1221.
Potter, P., & Perry, A. (2005). *Fundamentals of nursing* (6th ed.). St. Louis: Mosby, p. 1624.

20. *Answer: 3*
Rationale: Cotton pads and plastic or silk tape are latex-free products. The items identified in options 1, 2, and 4 are all products that contain latex.
Test-Taking Strategy: Use the process of elimination and knowledge regarding the products that contain latex to answer this question. Noting the words *cotton* and *silk* in option 3 may assist in answering correctly. Review the list of products that contain latex if you had difficulty with this question.
Level of Cognitive Ability: Application
Client Needs: Safe, Effective Care Environment
Integrated Process: Nursing Process/Implementation
Content Area: Adult Health/Immune
References: Phipps, W., Monahan, F., Sands, J., Marek, J., & Neighbors, M. (2003). *Medical-surgical nursing: Health and illness perspectives* (7th ed.). St. Louis: Mosby, p. 412.

Potter, P., & Perry, A. (2005). *Fundamentals of nursing* (6th ed.). St. Louis: Mosby, p. 1624.

ALTERNATE FORMAT QUESTION: MULTIPLE RESPONSE

Answers:
Use nonlatex gloves
Keep a latex-safe supply cart available in the client's area
Use medications from glass ampules
Do not puncture rubber stoppers with needles
Rationale: If a client is allergic to latex and at high risk for an allergic response, the nurse would use nonlatex gloves and latex-safe supplies and keep a latex-safe supply cart available in the client's area. Any supplies or materials that contain latex would be avoided. These include blood pressure cuffs, medications with a rubber stopper that requires puncture with a needle, latex-safe syringes, and latex-safe intravenous tubing.
Test-Taking Strategy: Focus on the issue, the client at high risk for an allergic response to a latex allergy. Recalling that items that contain rubber are likely to contain latex will direct you to the correct interventions. Review care of the client with a latex allergy if you had difficulty with this question.
Level of Cognitive Ability: Application
Client Needs: Safe, Effective Care Environment
Integrated Process: Nursing Process/Implementation
Content Area: Adult Health/Immune
Reference: Harkreader, H., & Hogan, M.A. (2004). *Fundamentals of nursing: Caring and clinical judgment* (2nd ed.). Philadelphia: W.B. Saunders, p. 1221.

REFERENCES

Black, J., & Hawks, J. (2005). *Medical-surgical nursing: Clinical management for positive outcomes* (7th ed.). Philadelphia: W.B. Saunders.

Christensen, B., & Kockrow, E. (2003). *Adult health nursing* (4th ed.). St. Louis: Mosby.

Christensen, B., & Kockrow, E. (2003). *Foundations of nursing* (4th ed.). St. Louis: Mosby.

Harkreader, H., & Hogan, M.A. (2004). *Fundamentals of nursing: Caring and clinical judgment* (2nd ed.). Philadelphia: W.B. Saunders.

Lewis, S., Heitkemper, M., & Dirksen, S. (2004). *Medical-surgical nursing: Assessment and management of clinical problems* (6th ed.). St. Louis: Mosby.

Linton, A., & Maebius, N. (2003). *Introduction to medical-surgical nursing* (3rd ed.). Philadelphia: W.B. Saunders.

Pagana, K., & Pagana, T. (2003). *Mosby's diagnostic and laboratory test reference* (6th ed.). St. Louis: Mosby.

Phipps, W., Monahan, F., Sands, J., Marek, J., & Neighbors, M. (2003). *Medical-surgical nursing: Health and illness perspectives* (7th ed.). St. Louis: Mosby.

Potter, P., & Perry, A. (2005). *Fundamentals of nursing* (6th ed.). St. Louis: Mosby.

Swearingen, P. (2003). *Manual of medical-surgical nursing care* (5th ed.). St. Louis: Mosby.

CHAPTER 61

Immunological Medications

I. HUMAN IMMUNODEFICIENCY VIRUS (HIV) AND ACQUIRED IMMUNODEFICIENCY SYNDROME (AIDS) (Box 61-1)

A. Medications include nucleoside reverse transcriptase inhibitors, non-nucleoside reverse transcriptase inhibitors, nucleotide reverse transcriptase nhibitors, protease inhibitors, and fusion inhibitors

B. Other medications include those that are used to treat complications or opportunistic infections that develop

C. Nucleoside reverse transcriptase inhibitors, non-nucleoside reverse transcriptase inhibitors, and nucleotide reverse transcriptase inhibitors work by inhibiting the activity of reverse transcriptase

D. Protease inhibitors work by interfering with the activity of the enzyme protease

E. Fusion inhibitors work by inhibiting the binding of HIV to cells

F. Nucleoside reverse transcriptase inhibitors
1. Abacavir (Ziagen): Can cause nausea; monitor for hypersensitivity reaction, including fever, nausea, vomiting, diarrhea, lethargy, malaise, sore throat, shortness of breath, cough, rash
2. Didanosine (Videx): Can cause nausea, diarrhea, peripheral neuropathy, pancreatitis
3. Lamivudine (Epivir): Causes nausea and nasal congestion
4. Stavudine (d4T, Zerit): Can cause peripheral neuropathy, pancreatitis
5. Zidovudine (Retrovir, AZT): Can cause nausea, vomiting, anemia, leukopenia, myopathy, fatigue, headache
6. Zalcitabine (ddC, Hivid): Can cause oral ulcers, peripheral neuropathy, pancreatitis

G. Non-nucleoside reverse transcriptase inhibitors
1. Nevirapine (Viramune): Can cause rash, Stevens-Johnson syndrome, hepatitis, increased transaminase levels
2. Delavirdine (Rescriptor): Can cause rash, liver function changes, pruritus
3. Efavirenz (Sustiva): Can cause rash, dizziness, confusion, difficulty concentrating, dreams, encephalopathy

H. Nucleotide reverse transcriptase inhibitors: Tenofovir disoproxil fumarate (Viread) can cause nausea and vomiting

I. Protease inhibitors
1. Amprenavir (Agenerase)
   a. Can cause nausea, vomiting, headache, altered taste sensations, perioral paresthesia, rashes, increased liver function
   b. Oral solution contains an alcohol that can interact with metronidazole (Flagyl) and can cause feelings of inebriation
2. Indinavir (Crixivan): Can cause nausea, diarrhea, hyperbilirubinemia, nephritis, kidney stones
3. Kaletra (lopinavir and ritonivir combination): Can cause nausea, diarrhea, altered taste sensations, perioral and circumoral paresthesia, hepatitis
4. Nelfinavir (Viracept): Can cause nausea, flatulence, diarrhea
5. Ritonavir (Norvir): Can cause nausea, vomiting, diarrhea, altered taste sensations, perioral and circumoral paresthesia, hepatitis, increased triglyceride levels
6. Saquinavir (Fortovase): can cause nausea, diarrhea, headache

J. Fusion inhibitor: Enfuvirtide (Fuzeon)—can cause skin irritation at injection site, fatigue, nausea, insomnia, peripheral neuropathy

K. Anti-inflammatory medication
1. Sulfasalazine (Azulfidine)
   a. Used to treat toxoplasmosis or nocardiasis
   b. Administered orally
   c. Can cause renal toxicity
   d. Suppresses bone marrow function

BOX 61-1

Medications for HIV and AIDS

NUCLEOSIDE REVERSE TRANSCRIPTASE INHIBITORS
Abacavir (Ziagen)
Didanosine (Videx)
Lamivudine (Epivir)
Lamivudine and zidovudine combination (Combivir)
Lamivudine, zidovudine, and abacavir combination
 (Trizivir)
Stavudine (d4T, Zerit)
Zidovudine (Ritrovir, AZT)
Zalcitabine (ddC, Hivid)

NON-NUCLEOSIDE REVERSE TRANSCRIPTASE INHIBITORS
Nevirapine (Viramune)
Delavirdine (Rescriptor)
Efavirenz (Sustiva)

NUCLEOTIDE REVERSE TRANSCRIPTASE INHIBITOR
Tenofovir disoproxil fumarate (Viread)

PROTEASE INHIBITORS
Amprenavir (Agenerase)
Indinavir (Crixivan)
Lopinavir and ritonivir combination (Kaletra)
Nelfinavir (Viracept)
Ritonavir (Norvir)
Saquinavir (Fortovase)

FUSION INHIBITOR
Enfuvirtide (Fuzeon)

ANTI-INFLAMMATORY MEDICATION
Sulfasalazine (Azulfidine)

ANTI-INFECTIVE MEDICATIONS
Pentamidine isethionate (Pentam 300)
Metronidazole (Flagyl)

ANTIFUNGAL MEDICATIONS
Ketonazole (Nizoral)
Fluconazole (Dilfulcan)
Amphotericin B (Fungizone)

ANTIVIRALS
Gancyclovir (Cytovene)
Acyclovir (Zovirax)
Foscarnet (Foscavir)

ANTIFUNGAL, ANTI-INFECTIVE, ANTIPROTOZOAL
Dapsone (Avlosulfon, DDS)

ANTIMALARIAL, ANTIPROTOZOAL
Pyrimethamine (Daraprim)

---

  e. Increases photosensitivity
  f. Monitor urine output and complete blood count (CBC)
  g. Monitor the client for sore throat, pallor, purpura, jaundice, and weakness
  h. Encourage fluid intake
  i. Advise the client to avoid exposure to the sun
L. Anti-infective medications
  1. Pentamidine isethionate (Pentam 300)
    a. Used to treat *Pneumocystis jiroveci* (formerly called *P. carinii*) pneumonia
    b. Administered by intramuscular (IM) or intravenous (IV) route
    c. Can cause nephrotoxicity
    d. Monitor blood pressure and heart rate (may cause hypotension)
    e. Monitor for hypoglycemia
    f. Is hepatotoxic and immunosuppressive
    g. Monitor liver function test results and CBC
  2. Metronidazole (Flagyl)
    a. Used to treat cryptosporidiosis and giardiasis
    b. Administered orally or by the IV route
    c. Administer with food or milk
    d. Monitor for dry mouth, dizziness, or fungal infection
    e. Instruct the client to avoid alcohol during treatment

M. Antifungal medications
  1. Ketonazole (Nizoral)
    a. Used in the treatment of candidiasis, coccidioidomycosis, and histoplasmosis
    b. Administered orally
    c. Administer with food or milk
    d. Instruct the client to avoid antacids for 2 hours after taking the medication because gastric acid is needed to activate the medication
    e. Is hepatotoxic
    f. Monitor hepatic function
    g. Instruct the client to avoid exposure to the sun because the medication increases photosensitivity
    h. Instruct the client to avoid alcohol during treatment
  2. Fluconazole (Dilfulcan)
    a. Used to treat candidiasis
    b. Administered orally
    c. Is hepatotoxic
    d. Monitor for abdominal pain, fever, and diarrhea
    e. Monitor hepatic function
  3. Amphotericin B (Fungizone)
    a. Used to treat candidiasis and other fungal infections
    b. Administered by the IV route
    c. Is nephrotoxic

d. Can cause thrombophlebitis
e. Suppresses bone marrow function
f. Monitor renal function
g. Monitor infusion site
h. Monitor CBC

N. Antivirals
1. Ganciclovir (Cytovene)
a. Used to treat cytomegalovirus retinitis
b. Administered orally or by the IV route
c. Suppresses bone marrow function
d. Monitor neutrophil and platelet count
e. Administer with food
2. Acyclovir (Zovirax)
a. Used to treat herpes simplex, herpes zoster, and varicella zoster
b. May be administered orally or by the IV route
c. Is nephrotoxic
d. Monitor renal function
e. Encourage fluid intake
f. Is irritating to a blood vessel when administered by the IV route
3. Foscarnet (Foscavir)
a. Used in the treatment of cytomegalovirus retinitis in human immunodeficiency virus (HIV)–infected clients
b. Administered by the IV route
c. Is nephrotoxic
d. Monitor renal function

II. SYSTEMIC LUPUS ERYTHEMATOSUS (Box 61-2)

A. Description: Used to control symptoms and to prevent or control serious complications that occur as a result of organ damage by the inflammatory process
B. Azathioprine (Imuran)
1. Glucocorticoid-sparing effect
2. Potentiates the immunosuppressive action of glucocorticoids and thereby allows a lower dose of glucocorticoid to have a greater immunosuppressive action
3. Monitor CBC and liver function test results
C. Cyclophosphamide (Cytoxan)
1. Immunosuppressive treatment of diffuse proliferative nephritis and other organ inflammation unresponsive to glucocorticoids
2. Reserved for use in severe cases because of the adverse side effects

---

BOX 61-2

Medications for Systemic Lupus Erythematosus

Azathioprine (Imuran)
Corticosteroids, such as prednisone (Deltasone)
Cyclophosphamide (Cytoxan)
Hydroxychloroquine sulfate (Plaquenil Sulfate)
Nonsteroidal anti-inflammatory drugs (NSAIDs)

D. Hydroxychloroquine sulfate (Plaquenil Sulfate)
1. An antimalarial used to prevent the recurrence of an exacerbation
2. An eye examination should be performed initially and 6 months after treatment
3. Administer with meals or a glass of milk
E. Prednisone (Deltasone)
1. Used at high doses to treat exacerbations and at low doses to control symptoms when other medications do not work
2. See Chapter 45 for information on glucocorticoids
F. Nonsteroidal anti-inflammatory drugs (NSAIDs)
1. Used to control fever and arthralgia
2. See Chapter 57 for information on NSAIDs

III. IMMUNIZATIONS (See Chapter 38)

PRACTICE QUESTIONS

1. Dapsone (DDS) is prescribed for a client with acquired immunodeficiency syndrome (AIDS) for the treatment of toxoplasmosis. The nurse reinforces medication instructions and tells the client to:
   1. Discontinue the medication if nausea and vomiting develop
   2. Plan to take the medication every 6 hours around the clock
   3. Contact the physician if fever or a sore throat occurs
   4. Report to the clinic weekly for the injections

2. Pyrimethamine (Daraprim) has been added to the medication regimen for the client with acquired immunodeficiency syndrome (AIDS). On review of the client's record, the nurse notes this new prescription and plans care, knowing that this has been prescribed for the treatment of:
   1. Toxoplasmosis
   2. Cardiac irregularities
   3. Kaposi's sarcoma
   4. Nausea and vomiting

3. Saquinavir (Fortovase) is prescribed for the client who is human immunodeficiency virus (HIV) seropositive. The nurse reinforces medication instructions and tells the client to:
   1. Take the medication on an empty stomach
   2. Eat low-calorie foods
   3. Eat foods that are low in fat
   4. Avoid sun exposure

4. A client who is seropositive for human immunodeficiency virus (HIV) has been taking Ritonavir (Norvir). The client returns to the clinic for follow-up laboratory tests. The nurse reviews the client's record and expects to note a physician's order for which of the following laboratory tests?
   1. Platelet count
   2. Triglyceride level

3. Prothrombin time (PT)

4. International normalized ratio (INR)

5. The client who is seropositive for human immunodeficiency virus (HIV) has been taking stavudine (d4T, Zerit). The nurse monitors which of the following most closely while the client is taking this medication?

1. Appetite

2. Gait

3. Gastrointestinal function

4. Level of consciousness (LOC)

6. The client who is seropositive for human immunodeficiency virus (HIV) has been taking zalcitabine (ddC, Hivid) as a component of treatment. The nurse plans to monitor which of the following most closely while the client is taking this medication?

1. Liver function studies

2. Platelet count

3. Red blood cell count

4. Glucose level

7. The nurse is assigned to care for a client with cytomegalovirus retinitis and acquired immunodeficiency syndrome (AIDS) who is receiving foscarnet (Foscavir). The nurse checks the latest results of which of the following laboratory studies while the client is taking this medication?

1. Serum albumin

2. Serum creatinine

3. CD4+ cell count

4. Lymphocyte count

8. The client with acquired immunodeficiency syndrome (AIDS) and *Pneumocystis jiroveci* (formerly called *P. carinii*) infection has been receiving pentamidine (Pentam 300). The client develops a fever of 101° F (38.3° C). The nurse does further monitoring of the client, knowing that this sign would most likely indicate that:

1. The dose of the medication is too low

2. The client is experiencing toxic effects of the medication

3. The client has developed inadequacy of thermoregulation

4. This is a result of another infection, caused by leukopenic effects of the medication

9. The client with acquired immunodeficiency syndrome (AIDS) has been started on therapy with zidovudine (Retrovir, AZT). The nurse carefully monitors which of the following laboratory results during treatment with this medication?

1. Complete blood count (CBC)

2. Blood urea nitrogen (BUN) level

3. Blood culture

4. Blood glucose level

10. The nurse is reviewing the results of serum laboratory studies drawn on a client with acquired immunodeficiency syndrome (AIDS) who is receiving didanosine (Videx). The nurse interprets that the client may have the medication discontinued by the physician if which of the following significantly elevated results is noted?

1. Serum cholesterol level

2. Serum amylase level

3. Blood glucose level

4. Serum protein level

ALTERNATE FORMAT QUESTION: MULTIPLE RESPONSE

Ketoconazole (Nizoral) is prescribed for a client with a diagnosis of candidiasis. Select the interventions that the nurse includes when administering this medication.

____ Administer the medication on an empty stomach

____ Administer the medication with an antacid

____ Monitor hepatic and liver function studies

____ Instruct the client to avoid exposure to the sun

____ Instruct the client to avoid alcohol

ANSWERS

1. *Answer: 3*

Rationale: Dapsone may be prescribed for the treatment of toxoplasmosis. The medication is taken orally on a daily basis. The medication suppresses bone marrow activity and the complete blood count (CBC) is monitored closely. If the client develops fever, sore throat, purpura, or jaundice, the physician is notified. Medications are available to treat nausea and vomiting and the client should not discontinue the medication if these symptoms occur, but should contact the physician.

Test-Taking Strategy: Use the process of elimination. Eliminate option 1 first because the nurse would not tell the client to discontinue the medication. Next, eliminate

options 2 and 4, knowing that the medication is administered orally on a daily basis. Review this medication if you had difficulty with this question.

Level of Cognitive Ability: Application

Client Needs: Physiological Integrity

Integrated Process: Teaching/Learning

Content Area: Adult Health/Immune

Reference: McKenry, L., & Salerno, E. (2003). *Mosby's pharmacology in nursing* (21st ed.). St. Louis: Mosby, p. 1070.

2. *Answer: 1*

Rationale: Daraprim is an antimalarial and an antiprotozoal medication. It is used in the treatment of toxoplasmosis or

Pneumocystis jiroveci (formerly called *P. carinii*) pneumonia. It is not used to treat nausea, vomiting, cardiac irregularities, or Kaposi's sarcoma.

Test-Taking Strategy: Use the process of elimination. If you knew that this medication was an antimalarial and an anti-protozoal medication, then you would easily be directed to option 1. Review this medication if you had difficulty with this medication.

Level of Cognitive Ability: Analysis
Client Needs: Physiological Integrity
Integrated Process: Nursing Process/Planning
Content Area: Adult Health/Immune
Reference: Skidmore-Roth, L. (2005). *Mosby's drug guide for nurses* (6th ed.). St. Louis: Mosby, p. 738.

3. *Answer:* **4**
Rationale: Saquinavir is an antiretroviral (protease inhibitor) used in combination with other antiretroviral medications in the management of HIV infection. It is administered with meals and is best absorbed if the client consumes high-calorie, high-fat meals. It can cause photosensitivity and the client is instructed to avoid sun exposure.

Test-Taking Strategy: Use the process of elimination. Options 2 and 3 can be eliminated first, knowing that these dietary measures would not likely be prescribed. From the remaining options, it is necessary to know that this medication can cause photosensitivity. Review this medication if you had difficulty with this question.

Level of Cognitive Ability: Application
Client Needs: Physiological Integrity
Integrated Process: Teaching/Learning
Content Area: Adult Health/Immune
Reference: Hodgson, B., & Kizior, R. (2005). *Saunders nursing drug handbook 2005.* Philadelphia: W.B. Saunders, p. 959.

4. *Answer:* **2**
Rationale: Ritonavir is an antiretroviral (protease inhibitor) used in combination with other antiretroviral medications in the management of HIV infection. It can increase triglyceride levels, and therefore the client's triglyceride level should be monitored. The platelet count, PT, and INR are not laboratory tests that would specifically be monitored in the client on this medication.

Test-Taking Strategy: Knowledge regarding the side effects of ritonavir is required to answer this question. Remember, this can increase triglyceride levels, and therefore the client's triglyceride level should be monitored. Review this medication if you had difficulty with this question.

Level of Cognitive Ability: Analysis
Client Needs: Physiological Integrity
Integrated Process: Nursing Process/Planning
Content Area: Adult Health/Immune
Reference: Hodgson, B., & Kizior, R. (2005). *Saunders nursing drug handbook 2005.* Philadelphia: W.B. Saunders, p. 945.

5. *Answer:* **2**
Rationale: Stavudine is an antiretroviral (protease inhibitor) used in the management of HIV infection in clients who do not respond to or who cannot tolerate conventional therapy. The medication can cause peripheral neuropathy and the

nurse should closely monitor the client's gait and ask the client about paresthesia.

Test-Taking Strategy: Use the process of elimination. Recalling that this medication causes peripheral neuropathy will direct you to the correct option. If you are not familiar with this medication, review this content.

Level of Cognitive Ability: Application
Client Needs: Physiological Integrity
Integrated Process: Nursing Process/Data Collection
Content Area: Adult Health/Immune
References: Hodgson, B., & Kizior, R. (2005). *Saunders nursing drug handbook 2005.* Philadelphia: W.B. Saunders, p. 987. Skidmore-Roth, L. (2005). *Mosby's drug guide for nurses* (6th ed.). St. Louis: Mosby, pp. 796-797.

6. *Answer:* **1**
Rationale: Zalcitabine is an antiretroviral (nucleoside reverse transcriptase inhibitor) used to manage HIV infection with other antiretrovirals. It has also been used as a single agent in clients who are intolerant of other regimens. It can cause serious liver damage, and liver function studies should be monitored closely. Options 2, 3, and 4 are not specifically associated with the use of this medication.

Test-Taking Strategy: Use the process of elimination. Recalling that this medication is hepatotoxic will direct you to option 1. If you are unfamiliar with this medication, review this content.

Level of Cognitive Ability: Application
Client Needs: Physiological Integrity
Integrated Process: Nursing Process/Data Collection
Content Area: Adult Health/Immune
Reference: Skidmore-Roth, L. (2005). *Mosby's drug guide for nurses* (6th ed.). St. Louis: Mosby, p. 908.

7. *Answer:* **2**
Rationale: Foscavir is very toxic to the kidneys. The serum creatinine level is monitored prior to therapy, two or three times per week during induction therapy, and at least weekly during maintenance therapy. It also may cause decreased levels of calcium, magnesium, phosphorus, and potassium. Thus, these levels are also measured with the same frequency.

Test Taking Strategy: Use the process of elimination. Recalling that this medication is nephrotoxic will direct you to option 2. Review this medication if you are unfamiliar with it.

Level of Cognitive Ability: Application
Client Needs: Physiological Integrity
Integrated Process: Nursing Process/Data Collection
Content Area: Adult Health/Immune
Reference: Skidmore-Roth, L. (2005). *Mosby's drug guide for nurses* (6th ed.). St. Louis: Mosby, p. 379.

8. *Answer:* **4**
Rationale: Frequent side effects of this medication include leukopenia, thrombocytopenia, and anemia. The client should be routinely monitored for signs and symptoms of infection. Options 1, 2, and 3 are inaccurate interpretations.

Test-Taking Strategy: Use the process of elimination, focusing on the key words, *develops a fever.* Note the relation between these key words and option 4. Review the side effects of this medication if you had difficulty with this question.

Level of Cognitive Ability: Analysis
Client Needs: Physiological Integrity
Integrated Process: Nursing Process/Data Collection
Content Area: Adult Health/Immune
Reference: Skidmore-Roth, L. (2005). *Mosby's drug guide for nurses* (6th ed.). St. Louis: Mosby, p. 671.

9. *Answer:* **1**
Rationale: A common side effect of this medication therapy is agranulocytopenia and anemia. The nurse monitors the CBC results for these changes. Options 2, 3, and 4 are unrelated to the use of this medication.
Test-Taking Strategy: Use the process of elimination. Recalling that AZT causes anemia will direct you to option 1. Review this medication if you had difficulty with this question.
Level of Cognitive Ability: Application
Client Needs: Physiological Integrity
Integrated Process: Nursing Process/Data Collection
Content Area: Adult Health/Immune
Reference: Skidmore-Roth, L. (2005). *Mosby's drug guide for nurses* (6th ed.). St. Louis: Mosby, p. 911.

10. *Answer:* **2**
Rationale: A serum amylase level that is increased 1.5 to 2 times normal may signify pancreatitis in the AIDS client, which is potentially fatal. The medication may have to be discontinued. The medication is also hepatotoxic and can result in liver failure.
Test-Taking Strategy: Use the process of elimination. Recalling that this medication can cause damage to the pancreas and is hepatotoxic will direct you to the correct option. Review this medication if you had difficulty with this question.

Level of Cognitive Ability: Analysis
Client Needs: Physiological Integrity
Integrated Process: Nursing Process/Data Collection
Content Area: Adult Health/Immune
Reference: Skidmore-Roth, L. (2005). *Mosby's drug guide for nurses* (6th ed.). St. Louis: Mosby, p. 264.

ALTERNATE FORMAT QUESTION: MULTIPLE RESPONSE

Answers:
Monitor hepatic and liver function studies
Instruct the client to avoid exposure to the sun
Instruct the client to avoid alcohol
Rationale: Ketoconazole (Nizoral) is an antifungal medication. It is administered with food or milk (not on an empty stomach), and antacids are avoided for 2 hours after taking the medication because gastric acid is needed to activate the medication. The medication is hepatotoxic and the nurse monitors liver function studies. The client is instructed to avoid exposure to the sun, because the medication increases photosensitivity. The client is also instructed to avoid alcohol.
Test-Taking Strategy: Use general medication guidelines to assist in selecting the correct interventions. Also, remember that this medication is administered with food or milk and that it is hepatotoxic. Review this medication if you had difficulty with this question.
Level of Cognitive Ability: Application
Client Needs: Physiological Integrity
Integrated Process: Nursing Process/Implementation
Content Area: Adult Health/Immune
Reference: *Mosby's 2005 drug consult for nurses.* (2005). St. Louis: Mosby, pp. 29-31.

REFERENCES

Hodgson, B., & Kizior, R. (2005). *Saunders nursing drug handbook 2005.* Philadelphia: W.B. Saunders.
McKenry, L., & Salerno, E. (2003). *Mosby's pharmacology in nursing* (21st ed.). St. Louis: Mosby.

Mosby's 2005 drug consult for nurses. (2005). St. Louis: Mosby.
Skidmore-Roth, L. (2005). *Mosby's drug guide for nurses* (6th ed.). St. Louis: Mosby.

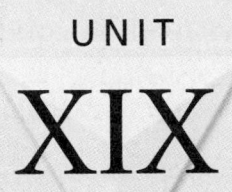

The Adult Client with a Mental Health Disorder

PYRAMID TERMS

abuse An act of misuse, deceit, or exploitation; a wrong or improper use or action toward another individual that results in injury, damage, maltreatment, or corruption.

addiction Also known as drug dependence; incorporates the concepts of loss of control with respect to the use of a drug, taking the drug despite related problems and complications, and a tendency to relapse.

coping mechanisms Methods of adjusting to environmental stress without altering one's own goals or purposes; can include both conscious and unconscious mechanisms.

crisis A temporary state of disequilibrium in which an individual's usual coping mechanisms or problem-solving methods fail. It can result in personality growth or personality disorganization.

defense mechanisms A coping mechanism (protective defense) of the ego that attempts to protect the individual from feelings of inadequacy and worthlessness and prevent awareness of anxiety. When anxiety is too painful, the individual copes by using defense mechanisms to protect the ego and decrease anxiety.

milieu The physical and social environment in which an individual lives. Milieu therapy focuses on positive physical and social environmental manipulation to produce positive change.

restraints Physical restraints include any manual method or mechanical device, material, or equipment that inhibits free movement. Chemical restraints include the administration of medications for the specific purpose of inhibiting a specific behavior or movement.

seclusion Placing a client alone in a specially designed room for protection and close supervision. It is the last measure in a process to maximize safety to the client and others.

suicide The ultimate act of self-destruction in which an individual purposefully ends his or her own life.

suicide attempt Any willful, self inflicted, or life-threatening attempt by an individual that has not led to death.

▲ PYRAMID TO SUCCESS

The Pyramid to Success focuses on the therapeutic nurse-client relationship, client rights, hospital admission procedures, the ethical and legal issues related to the care of the client with a mental health disorder, grief and loss, and end-of-life issues. Pyramid points focus on the use of restraints, seclusion, and electroconvulsive therapy (ECT). Focus on care of the client with an addiction, such as an eating disorder or drug or alcohol disorder. Additional focus areas include anxiety, depression, suicide, abuse and violence, rape crisis interventions, post-traumatic stress disorders, obsessive-compulsive disorders, schizophrenia, and bipolar disorders. Pyramid points address the use of medications prescribed for the client with a mental health disorder, particularly lithium and the benzodiazepines. The Integrated Processes addressed in this unit include Caring, the Clinical Problem-Solving Process (Nursing Process), Communication and Documentation, and Teaching/Learning.

CLIENT NEEDS
Safe, Effective Care Environment

Client advocacy
Client rights
Confidentiality
Establishing priorities
Informed consent related to treatments, such as restraints, seclusion, and electroconvulsive therapy (ECT)
Legal responsibilities related to reporting incidences of violence and abuse
Psychiatric consultations and referrals
Providing safety to client and others
Use of restraints and seclusion

Health Promotion and Maintenance

Health promotion programs related to addictions
Individual lifestyle choices
Psychosocial data collection techniques

Psychosocial Integrity

Abuse, neglect
Behavioral interventions
Chemical dependency
Coping mechanisms
Crisis intervention
Domestic violence
End-of-life issues
Grief and loss
Religious, cultural, and spiritual influences on health
Sexual abuse, rape
Stress management
Support systems
Therapeutic milieu
Therapeutic nurse-client relationship

Physiological Integrity

Abusive and self-destructive behavior
Alterations in body systems related to addictions
Elimination
Expected and untoward effects of medications
Laboratory values related to medication therapy
Medication administration
Nutrition

Personal hygiene measures
Potential complications related to medications and electroconvulsive therapy
Rest and sleep

REFERENCES

Chernecky, C., & Berger, B. (2004). *Laboratory tests and diagnostic procedures* (4th ed.). Philadelphia: W.B. Saunders.

Fortinash, K., & Holoday-Worret, P. (2004). *Psychiatric mental health nursing* (3rd ed.). St. Louis: Mosby.

Harkreader, H., & Hogan, M.A. (2004). *Fundamentals of nursing: Caring and clinical judgment* (2nd ed.). Philadelphia: W.B. Saunders.

Ignatavicius, D., & Workman, M. (2006). *Medical surgical nursing: Critical thinking for collaborative care* (5th ed.). Philadelphia: W.B. Saunders.

Keltner, N., Schwecke, L., & Bostrom, C. (2003). *Psychiatric nursing* (4th ed.). St. Louis: Mosby.

Lewis, S., Heitkemper, M., & Dirksen, S. (2004). *Medical-surgical nursing: Assessment and management of clinical problems* (6th ed.). St. Louis: Mosby.

Morrison-Valfre, M. (2005). *Foundations of mental health care* (3rd ed.). St. Louis: Mosby.

National Council of State Boards of Nursing. (2005). *Detailed test plan for the National Council licensure examination for practical/vocational nurses.* Chicago: Author.

Stuart, G., & Laraia, M. (2005). *Principles and practice of psychiatric nursing* (8th ed.). St. Louis: Mosby.

Varcarolis, E.M. (2002). *Foundations of psychiatric mental health nursing* (4th ed.). Philadelphia: W.B. Saunders.

Foundations of Psychiatric Mental Health Nursing

I. MENTAL HEALTH

A. A lifelong process of successful adaptation to a changing internal and external environment

B. The individual is in contact with reality and the environment and possesses the ability to love, work, and resolve conflicts within a framework of reasonability

C. The individual has psychobiological resilience

II. PSYCHIATRIC/MENTAL HEALTH ILLNESS

A. Description
1. Loss of the ability to respond to the environment in ways that is in accord with oneself or society's expectations
2. Characterized by thought or behavior patterns that impair functioning and cause the individual distress

B. Personality characteristics
1. Is unaccepting of self and dislikes self
2. Has an unrealistic perception of strengths and weaknesses
3. Thoughts and perceptions may not be reality-based
4. Is unable to find meaning and purpose in life
5. Lacks direction and productivity in life
6. Has difficulty in meeting own needs
7. Depends on others for thought and actions

C. Adaptations to stress
1. Feels out of control with self and with the environment
2. Has a negative perception of the environment
3. Has ineffective **coping mechanisms**

D. Interpersonal relationships
1. Is unable to love and care for others
2. Is unable to feel loved by others or accept feelings from others

III. COPING AND DEFENSE MECHANISMS

A. **Coping mechanisms**
1. Coping involves any effort to decrease the stress response
2. **Coping mechanisms** can be either constructive or destructive in nature, task-oriented and related to direct problem solving, or can be a defense-oriented regulating response to protect oneself
3. Destructive **coping mechanisms** often cause a mental health disorder because the problem that causes the disorder is avoided
4. Neurotic or psychotic behaviors can typically result when **coping mechanisms** become destructive

B. **Defense mechanisms** (Box 62-1)
1. A **coping mechanism** (protective defense) of the ego that attempts to protect the individual from feelings of inadequacy and worthlessness and prevent awareness of anxiety
2. When anxiety is too painful, the individual copes by using **defense mechanisms** to protect the ego and decrease anxiety

C. Interventions
1. Determine the client's use of the **defense mechanism**
2. Determine if the use of the **defense mechanism** characterizes unhealthy adjustment
3. Facilitate appropriate use of **defense mechanisms**
4. Avoid criticizing the behavior and the use of **defense mechanisms**
5. Assist the client to identify the source of the anxiety
6. Assist the client to explore methods to reduce the anxiety

IV. THE NURSE-CLIENT RELATIONSHIP

A. Principles
1. Maintain genuineness, respect, an empathic understanding, and concreteness with the client

BOX 62-1

Types of Defense Mechanisms

Compensation: Putting forth extra effort to achieve in areas in which one has a real or imagined deficiency

Conversion: The expression of emotional conflicts through physical symptoms

Denial: Disowning consciously intolerable thoughts and impulses

Displacement: Feelings toward one person are directed to another who is less threatening, thereby satisfying an impulse with a substitute object

Dissociation: The blocking off of an anxiety-provoking event or period of time from the conscious mind

Fantasy: Gratification by imaginary achievements and wishful thinking

Fixation: Never advancing to the next level of emotional development and organization; the persistence in later life of interests and behavior patterns appropriate to an earlier age

Identification: The unconscious attempt to change oneself to resemble an admired person

Insulation: Withdrawing into passivity and becoming inaccessible in order to avoid further threatening situations

Intellectualization: Excessive reasoning to avoid feeling; the thinking is disconnected from feelings, and situations are dealt with at a cognitive level

Introjection: A type of identification in which the individual incorporates the traits or values of another into self

Isolation: Response in which a person blocks feelings associated with an unpleasant experience

Projection: Transferring one's internal feelings, thoughts, and unacceptable ideas and traits to someone else

Rationalization: An attempt to make unacceptable feelings and behavior acceptable by justifying the behavior

Reaction formation: Developing conscious attitudes and behaviors and acting out behaviors opposite to what one really feels

Regression: Returning to an earlier developmental stage to express an impulse in order to deal with reality

Repression: An unconscious process in which the client blocks undesirable and unacceptable thoughts from conscious expression

Sublimation: Replacement of an unacceptable need, attitude, or emotion with one that is more socially acceptable

Substitution: The replacement of a valued unacceptable object with an object that is more acceptable to the ego

Suppression: The conscious, deliberate forgetting of unacceptable or painful thoughts, ideas, and feelings

Symbolization: The conscious use of an idea or object to represent another actual event or object; often, the meaning is not clear because the symbol may represent something in the unconscious

Undoing: Engaging in behavior that is considered to be opposite of a previous unacceptable behavior, thought, or feeling

2. Care for the client in a holistic manner
3. Identify religious and spiritual practices of the client because these practices may give the client hope, comfort, and support with healing
4. Identify cultural beliefs and values, including emotion-producing situations, how emotions are expressed, and what the appropriate social response to expressed emotions may be
5. Maintain appropriate limits
6. Maintain honest and open communication
7. Encourage expression of the client's feelings
8. Assist the client to develop resources

B. Phases of a therapeutic nurse-client relationship
   1. Preinteraction phase
      a. Begins before the nurse's first contact with the client
      b. The nurse's task is self-exploration about his or her values and feelings about caring for the client
   2. Orientation or introductory phase
      a. Establish boundaries, acceptance, and trust with the client
      b. Identify the expectations of the relationship (establishing a contract)
      c. Determine why the client sought help and whether it was voluntary
      d. Assess the anxiety in the client
      e. Define goals with the client
      f. Prepare the client for termination and separation of the relationship
   3. Working phase
      a. Promote an attitude of acceptance
      b. Assist the client to express feelings
      c. Identify problems (theme identification)
      d. Promote insight and the use of constructive **coping mechanisms**
      e. Increase the client's independence
   4. Termination or separation phase
      a. Prepare the client for termination and separation on initial contact
      b. Evaluate progress and achievement of goals
      c. Identify and deal with termination and separation issues
      d. Encourage the client to discuss feelings about termination
      e. Do not promise the client that the relationship will be continued
      f. Refer and transfer the client to other support systems

V. THERAPEUTIC COMMUNICATION PROCESS

A. Principles
   1. Communication includes both verbal and nonverbal expression
   2. Successful communication includes appropriateness, efficiency, flexibility, and feedback

TABLE 62-1

Therapeutic and Nontherapeutic Communication Techniques

Therapeutic Techniques	Nontherapeutic Techniques
Listening	Giving advice or approval or disapproval
Maintaining silence	Changing the subject
Maintaining neutral responses	Being defensive or challenging the client
Use of broad openings and open-ended questions	Making stereotypical comments
Focusing and refocusing	Making value judgments
Restating	Providing false reassurance
Clarifying and validating	Placing the client's feelings on hold
Sharing perceptions	Asking the client "Why?"
Reflecting	
Providing acknowledgment and feedback	
Giving information and presenting reality	
Encouraging formulation of a plan of action	
Providing nonverbal encouragement	
Summarizing	

3. Anxiety in either the nurse or client impedes communication
4. Communication needs to be goal-directed and within a professional framework
B. Therapeutic and nontherapeutic communication techniques (Table 62-1)

VI. DIAGNOSTIC AND STATISTICAL MANUAL OF MENTAL DISORDERS

A. Classifies medical diagnoses according to the American Psychiatric Association
B. A system used in clinical, research, and educational settings, in which diagnostic criteria are inclusive for each diagnosis but allow for individualized differences within a pattern of behavior
C. Includes a list of culture-bound syndromes that may or may not be associated with a particular diagnostic category
D. Knowledge of the criteria for a particular psychiatric diagnosis will assist the nurse in making a clinical decision about a nursing diagnosis

VII. TYPES OF MENTAL HEALTH ADMISSIONS AND DISCHARGES

A. Voluntary admission
   1. Any citizen of lawful age may apply in writing (usually on a standard admission form) for admission to the hospital
   2. Sought by the client, or the client's guardian if the client is too ill, and voluntarily seeks assistance
   3. Client agrees to accept treatment
   4. Civil rights are fully retained by the client (Box 62-2)
   5. Client is free to sign himself or herself out of the hospital

BOX 62-2

Client Rights

Right to accessible health care
Right to a coordination and continuity of health care
Right to courteous and individualized health care
Right to information about the qualifications, names, and titles of personnel delivering care
Right to refuse observation by those not directly involved in care
Right to privacy and confidentiality
Right to informed consent
Right to treatment
Right to refuse treatment
Right to treatment in the least restrictive setting
Right not to be subjected to unnecessary restraints
Right to habeas corpus; may request a hearing at any time to be released from the hospital
Right to information about diagnosis, prognosis, and treatment
Right to information on the charges of service
Right to communicate with people outside the hospital through written correspondence, telephone, and personal visits
Right to keep clothing and personal effects
Right to be employed
Right to religious freedom
Right to execute wills
Right to retain licenses, privileges, or permits established by the law, such as a driver's or professional license

B. Involuntary admission
   1. May be necessary when a person is mentally ill, is a danger to self or others, or is in need of psychiatric treatment or physical care
   2. An admission status in which a person who has the legal capacity to consent to mental health

treatment refuses to do so and is involuntarily detained for treatment by the state

3. The client who is involuntarily admitted does not lose his or her right of informed consent
4. The length of time for hospitalization is specified by the state; varies from state to state
5. The client is considered legally competent until he or she has been declared incompetent through a legal proceeding
6. If the nurse believes that a client lacks competency, action should be initiated to have a legal guardian appointed by the court
7. Categories
   a. Evaluation and emergency care
   b. Certification for observation and treatment
   c. Extended or indeterminate commitment

C. Release from the hospital
1. Description
   a. Depends on the client's admission status
   b. The client who sought voluntary admission has the right to demand and receive release
   c. Some states provide for conditional release of voluntary clients, which enables the treating physician or administrator to order continued treatment on an outpatient basis if the clinical needs of the client warrant further care
2. Conditional release
   a. Usually requires outpatient treatment for a specified period of time to determine the client's compliance with medication protocol, ability to meet basic needs, and ability to reintegrate into the community
   b. A voluntary client who is conditionally released cannot be reinstitutionalized without the client's consent, unless the institution complies with the procedures for involuntary admission
   c. An involuntary client who is conditionally released may be reinstitutionalized while the commitment is still in effect, without recommencement of formal admission procedures
3. Discharge
   a. Discharge (unconditional release) is the termination of the client-institution relationship
   b. This release may be ordered by the psychiatrist, court-ordered, or administratively ordered
   c. The administration officer of an institution has the discretion to discharge clients
   d. In most states, clients can institute a court proceeding to seek a judicial discharge (writ of habeas corpus)
   e. Discharge planning and follow-up care are important for the continued well-being of the client with a mental health disorder
   f. Aftercare case managers are needed to facilitate the client's adaptation back into the community and to provide early referral if the treatment plan is not followed

VIII. MILIEU THERAPY
A. Description
1. **Milieu** is the physical and social environment in which an individual lives
2. Provides a safe environment that is adapted to the individual client's needs; also provides greater comfort and freedom of expression than has been experienced in the past by the client
3. Staffed by persons trained to provide support, understanding, and individual attention
4. All members contribute to the planning and functioning of the setting
5. The power hierarchy is diminished because all members are viewed as significant and valuable members of the community

B. Focus
1. Positive environmental manipulation, both physical and social, to effect a positive change
2. Client's rights through involvement in setting goals, freedom of movement, and informal relationships with staff
3. Group and social interaction
4. Use of community meetings, activity groups, social skills groups, and physical exercise programs

IX. PSYCHOTHERAPY
A. Description
1. Use of a group of techniques to modify feelings, attitudes, and behaviors in clients
2. Therapist uses both verbal and nonverbal means of communication to build a relationship with the client

B. Focus
1. The basic concept involves understanding
2. Issues of importance to the client, purpose of the interaction, identification of the roles of the therapist and client, and the use of primarily verbal means of communication
3. Nonverbal techniques include silence, body language, facial expressions, and respect for personal space

C. Levels of psychotherapy (Box 62-3)
1. Supportive therapy: Allows the client to express feelings, explore alternatives, and make decisions in a safe, caring environment
2. Reeducative therapy: Involves learning new ways of perceiving and behaving
3. Reconstructive therapy: Involves deep psychotherapy or psychoanalysis

X. BEHAVIOR AND BEHAVIOR MODIFICATION
A. Behavior therapy
1. An approach to bring about behavioral change
2. It includes a group of diversified approaches for dealing with maladaptive behavior

---

BOX 62-3

Levels of Psychotherapy

Supportive therapy
Re-educative therapy
Reconstructive therapy

---

3. Believes that most behaviors are learned
4. Maladaptive behavior is a way of dealing with stress; the therapy is an approach for bringing about a change in the behavior

B. Self-control therapy
   1. Combination of cognitive and behavioral approaches
   2. A basic theme is that talking to oneself can direct and control actions more effectively
   3. Useful to deal with stress

C. Desensitization
   1. The reduction of intense reactions to a stimulus by repeated exposure to the stimulus in a weaker and milder form
   2. Gradually, over a period of time, exposure is increased until the fear of the object or situation has ceased

D. Aversion therapy
   1. Negative reinforcement is a technique to change behavior
   2. A stimulus attractive to the client is paired with an unpleasant event in hopes of endowing the stimulus with negative properties

E. Modeling: The therapist acts as a role model for specified identified behaviors and the client learns through imitation

F. Operant conditioning: Entails rewarding a client for desired behaviors and is the basis for behavior modification

XI. COGNITIVE THERAPY

A. An active, directed time-limited structured approach used to treat a variety of psychiatric disorders

B. Therapeutic techniques are designed to identify reality testing and correct distorted conceptualization and the dysfunctional belief underlying these cognitions

C. The client learns to master problems in situations that he or she previously considered insuperable by evaluating and correcting his or her thinking

D. The cognitive therapist helps the client think and act more realistically and adaptively about psychological problems so as to reduce symptoms

E. Various cognitive and behavioral strategies are used in cognitive therapy

XII. GROUP AND GROUP THERAPY

A. Stages of group development (Box 62-4)
   1. Initial stage

BOX 62-4

Stages of Group Development

Initial stage
Working stage
Termination stage

BOX 62-5

Self-help or Support Groups

Alcoholics Anonymous
Gamblers Anonymous
Overeaters Anonymous
Narcotics Anonymous
Co-dependents Anonymous
Adult Children of Alcoholics
Al-Alon
Bereavement
Parents without Partners
Other groups:
   Recovery groups, such as for those who have experienced trauma
   Smoking cessation
   Health conditions, such as cancer
   Unexpected body image changes, such as mastectomy or colostomy

---

   a. Involves superficial rather than open and trusting communication
   b. Members are becoming acquainted with each other and are searching for similarity between themselves and other group members
   c. Members may be unclear about the purpose or goals of the group
   d. A certain amount of structuring of group norms, roles, and responsibilities takes place

2. Working stage
   a. During this stage, the real work of the group is accomplished
   b. Members are familiar with each other, the group leader, and the group roles, and they feel free to approach their problems and to attempt to solve their problems
   c. Conflict and cooperation surface during the group's work

3. Termination stage
   a. The group evaluates the experience and explores members' feelings about it and the impending separation
   b. Provides an opportunity for members who have difficulty with termination to learn to deal more realistically and comfortably with this normal part of human experience

B. Self-help or support groups (Box 62-5)
   1. Based on the premise that people who have experienced a similar problem are able to help others who have the same problem

2. Prevent the individual member from feeling lonely and isolated
3. Help members decrease levels of stress and increase levels of self-acceptance
4. Members are better able to deal with the problems that they brought to the group and develop new or more effective patterns of behavior

C. Family therapy

1. Specific intervention mode based on the premise that the member of the family with the presenting symptoms signals the presence of pain in the entire family
2. The therapist works to assist the family to identify and express their thoughts and feelings, define family roles and rules, try new, more productive styles of relating, and restore strength to the family

PRACTICE QUESTIONS

1. A nurse assists in planning care for a client scheduled to be discharged from a mental health clinic. The nurse understands that the client's unresolved feelings related to loss may resurface during which phase of the therapeutic nurse-client relationship?
   1. Orientation phase
   2. Working phase
   3. Termination phase
   4. Trusting phase

2. A client with depression who has attempted suicide says to the nurse, "I should have died. I've always been a failure. Nothing ever goes right for me." The nurse makes which therapeutic response to the client?
   1. "I don't see you as a failure."
   2. "Feeling like this is all part of being ill."
   3. "You've been feeling like a failure for a while?"
   4. "You have everything to live for."

3. A client states to the nurse, "I haven't slept at all the last couple of nights." The nurse makes which therapeutic response to the client?
   1. "Go on ....."
   2. "Sleeping?"
   3. "The last couple of nights?"
   4. "You're having difficulty sleeping?"

4. The nurse is collecting data from a client and is attempting to obtain subjective data regarding the client's sexual-reproductive status. The client states, "I don't want to discuss this; it's private and personal." Which statement by the nurse indicates a therapeutic response?
   1. "I hate being asked these sorts of questions too."
   2. "I am a nurse and as such I'll have you know that all information is kept confidential."
   3. "I know that some of these questions are difficult for you, but as a nurse, I must legally respect your confidentiality."
   4. "This is difficult for you to speak about, but I am trying to perform a complete data collection and I need this information."

5. A nurse is caring for a client who says, "I don't want you to touch me. I'll take care of myself!" The nurse makes which therapeutic response to the client?
   1. "I will respect your feelings. I'll just leave this cup for you to collect your urine in. After breakfast, I will take more blood from you."
   2. "If you didn't want our care, why did you come here?"
   3. "Why are you being so difficult? I only want to help you."
   4. "Sounds like you're feeling pretty troubled by all of us. Let's work together so you can do everything for yourself as you request."

6. A nurse is assigned to care for a client who is experiencing disturbed thought processes. The nurse is told that the client believes that the food is being poisoned. Which communication technique does the nurse plan to use to encourage the client to eat?
   1. Open-ended questions and silence
   2. Offering opinions about the necessity of adequate nutrition
   3. Identifying the reasons that the client may not want to eat
   4. Focusing on self-disclosure regarding food preferences

7. A nurse is assigned to care for a client admitted to the hospital after sustaining an injury from a house fire. The client attempted to save a neighbor involved in the fire but, in spite of the client's efforts, the neighbor died. Which action would the nurse be engaged in with the client during the working phase of the nurse-client relationship?
   1. Identifying the client's potential for self-harm
   2. Identifying the client's ability to function
   3. Inquiring about the client's perception of the neighbor's death
   4. Inquiring about the client's feelings that may affect coping

8. A client who has just been sexually assaulted is very quiet and calm. The nurse identifies this behavior as indicative of which defense mechanism?
   1. Denial
   2. Projection
   3. Rationalization
   4. Intellectualization

9. A nurse is assisting with the data collection on a client admitted to the psychiatric unit. The nurse reviews the data obtained and identifies which of the following as a priority concern?
   1. The presence of bruises on the client's body
   2. The client's report of not eating or sleeping
   3. The client's report of suicidal thoughts
   4. The significant other disapproving of the treatment

10. Laboratory work is prescribed for a client who has been experiencing delusions. When the laboratory technician approaches the client to obtain

a specimen of the client's blood, the client begins to shout, "You're all vampires. Let me out of here!" The nurse who is present at the time would respond by stating which of the following?

1. "The technician is not going to hurt you, but is going to help you!"
2. "What makes you think that the technician is a vampire?"
3. "The technician will leave and come back later for your blood."
4. "It must be fearful to think others want to hurt you."

11. An inebriated client is brought to the emergency room by the local police. The client is told that the physician will be in to see the client in about 30 minutes. The client becomes very loud and offensive and wants to be seen by the physician immediately. The nurse assisting to care for the client would plan for which appropriate nursing intervention?
    1. Attempt to talk with the client to de-escalate the behavior
    2. Watch the behavior escalate before intervening
    3. Inform the client that he or she will be asked to leave if the behavior continues
    4. Offer to take the client to an examination room until he or she can be treated

12. A client is admitted to a psychiatric unit for treatment of psychotic behavior. The client is at the locked exit door, and is shouting, "Let me out. There's nothing wrong with me. I don't belong here." The nurse identifies this behavior as:
    1. Projection
    2. Denial
    3. Regression
    4. Rationalization

13. A client says to the nurse, "I'm going to die, and I wish my family would stop hoping for a 'cure'! I get so angry when they carry on like this! After all, I'm the one who's dying." The therapeutic response by the nurse is:
    1. "You're feeling angry that your family continues to hope for you to be 'cured'?"
    2. "I think we should talk more about your anger with your family."
    3. "Well, it sounds like you're being pretty pessimistic. After all, years ago people died of pneumonia."
    4. "Have you shared your feelings with your family?"

14. A nurse employed in a psychiatric unit is assigned to care for a client admitted to the unit 2 days ago. On review of the client's record, the nurse notes that the admission was a voluntary admission. Based on this type of admission, the nurse would expect which of the following?
    1. The client will be very resistant to treatment measures

2. The client's family will be very resistant to treatment measures
3. The client will be angry and will refuse care
4. The client will participate in the treatment plan

15. A licensed practical nurse (LPN) enters a client's room, and the client is demanding release from the hospital. The LPN reviews the client's record and notes that the client was admitted 2 days ago for treatment of an anxiety disorder, and that the admission was a voluntary admission. The LPN reports the findings to the registered nurse (RN) and expects that the RN will take which of the following actions?
    1. Tell the client that discharge is not possible at this time
    2. Call the client's family
    3. Contact the physician
    4. Persuade the client to stay a few more days

16. A client is admitted to the psychiatric nursing unit. When collecting data from the client, the nurse notes that the client was admitted by involuntary status. Based on this type of admission, the nurse most likely expects that the client:
    1. Presents a harm to self
    2. Requested the admission
    3. Consented to the admission
    4. Provided written application to the facility for admission

17. A nurse is caring for a client who is scheduled for electroconvulsive therapy (ECT). The nurse notes that an informed consent has not been obtained for the procedure. On review of the record, the nurse notes that the admission was an involuntary hospitalization. Based on this information, the nurse determines that:
    1. An informed consent does not need to be obtained
    2. An informed consent should be obtained from the family
    3. An informed consent needs to be obtained from the client
    4. The physician will obtain the informed consent

18. Following a group therapy session, a client approaches the licensed practical nurse (LPN) and verbalizes a need for seclusion because of uncontrollable feelings. The LPN reports the findings to the registered nurse (RN) and expects that the RN will take which of the following actions?
    1. Inform the client that seclusion has not been prescribed
    2. Obtain an informed consent
    3. Call the client's family
    4. Place the client in seclusion immediately

19. A nurse is providing care to a client admitted to the hospital with a diagnosis of anxiety disorder. The nurse is talking with the client and the client says,

"I have a secret that I want to tell you. You won't tell anyone about it, will you?" The appropriate nursing response is which of the following?
1. "No, I won't tell anyone."
2. "I cannot promise to keep a secret."
3. "If you tell me the secret, I will tell it to your doctor."
4. "If you tell me the secret, I will need to document it in your record."

20. A psychiatric nurse is greeted by a neighbor in a local grocery store. The neighbor says to the nurse, "How is Carol doing? She is my best friend and is seen at your clinic every week." The appropriate nursing response is which of the following?
1. "I'm not suppose to discuss this, but since you are my neighbor, I can tell you that she is doing great!"
2. "I'm not suppose to discuss this, but since you are my neighbor, I can tell you that she really has some problems!"
3. "If you want to know about Carol, you need to ask her yourself."
4. "I cannot discuss any client situation with you."

21. A client was involuntarily admitted to the psychiatric unit because of episodes of extremely violent behavior. The client is demanding to be discharged from the hospital. The licensed practical nurse (LPN) reports the information to the registered nurse (RN), and the RN does not allow the client to leave. The LPN understands that which of the following represents the legal ramifications associated with the RN's behavior?
1. The RN will be charged with imprisonment
2. The RN will be charged with assault
3. The RN will be charged with slander
4. No charge will be made against the RN because the RN's actions are reasonable

22. A nurse is preparing a client for the termination phase of the nurse-client relationship. Which nursing task would the nurse appropriately plan for this phase?
1. Identify expected outcomes
2. Plan short-term goals
3. Assist in making appropriate referrals
4. Assist in developing realistic solutions

23. During the termination phase of the nurse-client relationship, the clinic nurse observes that the client continuously demonstrates bursts of anger. The appropriate interpretation of the behavior is that the client:
1. Requires further treatment and is not ready to be discharged
2. Is displaying typical behaviors that can occur during termination

3. Needs to be admitted to the hospital
4. Needs to be referred to the psychiatrist as soon as possible

24. An 18-year-old woman is admitted to an inpatient psychiatric unit with the diagnosis of anorexia nervosa. A behavior therapy approach is used as part of her treatment plan. The nurse understands that the purpose of this approach is to:
1. Help the client identify and examine dysfunctional thoughts and beliefs
2. Emphasize social interaction with clients who withdraw
3. Provide a supportive environment
4. Examine conflicts and past issues

25. Milieu therapy is prescribed for a client. The nurse understands that this type of therapy can best be described as which of the following?
1. A form of behavior modification therapy
2. A cognitive approach to changing behavior
3. The client is involved in setting goals
4. A behavioral approach to changing behavior

26. Disulfiram (Antabuse) is prescribed for a client with a problem related to alcohol. The nurse understands that this medication works on the principle of which of the following therapies?
1. Desensitization
2. Self-control therapy
3. Milieu therapy
4. Aversion therapy

27. A nurse informs a client with an eating disorder about group meetings with Overeaters Anonymous. Which statement by the client indicates the need for additional information about this self-help group?
1. "In this self-help group, people who have a similar problem are able to help others."
2. "This self-help group is designed to serve people who have a common problem."
3. "The members of this self-help group provide support to each other."
4. "The leader of this self-help group is a nurse or psychiatrist."

28. A client is attending a Gamblers Anonymous meeting for the first time. The model used by this group is the 12-step program developed by Alcoholics Anonymous. The nurse understands that the first step in the 12-step program is which of the following?
1. Stating that the gambling will be stopped
2. Discontinuing relationships with friends who are gamblers
3. Substituting gambling for other activities
4. Admitting to having a problem

29. A nurse is assisting in conducting a group therapy session and a client with a manic disorder is

monopolizing the group. The appropriate nursing action is which of the following?
1. Suggest that the client stop talking and try listening to others
2. Ask the client to leave
3. Tell the client to stop monopolizing the group
4. Refer the client to another group

30. A nurse is assisting in monitoring a group therapy session. During this session, the members are identifying tasks and boundaries. The nurse understands that these activities are characteristic of which stage of group development?
1. Forming
2. Storming
3. Norming
4. Performing

ALTERNATE FORMAT QUESTION: MULTIPLE RESPONSE

The nurse in the mental health unit reviews the therapeutic and nontherapeutic communication techniques with a nursing student. Select all therapeutic communication techniques.
____ Making value judgments
____ Listening
____ Giving advice or approval or disapproval
____ Maintaining neutral responses
____ Providing false reassurance
____ Restating
____ Asking the client "Why?"
____ Providing acknowledgment and feedback

ANSWERS

1. *Answer:* 3
Rationale: In the termination phase, the relationship comes to a close. Ending treatment may sometimes be traumatic for clients who have come to value the relationship and the help. Because loss is an issue, any unresolved feelings related to loss may resurface during this phase. Options 1, 2, and 4 are incorrect.
Test-Taking Strategy: Note the key words *unresolved* and *loss* in the question. Consider the phases of the therapeutic nurse-client relationship to direct you to option 3. Review these phases and the nursing implications if you had difficulty with this question.
Level of Cognitive Ability: Comprehension
Client Needs: Psychosocial Integrity
Integrated Process: Caring
Content Area: Mental Health
Reference: Morrison-Valfre, M. (2005). *Foundations of mental health care* (3rd ed.). St. Louis: Mosby, pp. 105-107.

2. *Answer:* 3
Rationale: Responding to the feelings expressed by a client is an effective therapeutic communication technique. The correct option is an example of the use of restating. Options 1, 2, and 4 block communication because they minimize the client's feelings and do not facilitate exploration of the client's expressed feelings.
Test-Taking Strategy: Use therapeutic communication techniques. Select the option that directly addresses the client's feelings and concerns. Option 3 is the only option that is stated in the form of a question and is open-ended; therefore, it will encourage the verbalization of feelings. Review these techniques if you had difficulty with this question.
Level of Cognitive Ability: Application
Client Needs: Psychosocial Integrity
Integrated Process: Communication and Documentation
Content Area: Mental Health
Reference: Morrison-Valfre, M. (2005). *Foundations of mental health care* (3rd ed.). St. Louis: Mosby, p. 88.

3. *Answer:* 4
Rationale: Option 4 identifies the therapeutic communication technique of restatement. Although it is a technique that has a prompting component to it, it repeats the client's major theme and addresses the problem from the client's perspective. Option 1 allows the client to direct the discussion when it needs to be more focused at this point. Option 2 uses reflection that simply repeats the client's last words to prompt further discussion. Option 3 focuses on the number of nights rather than the specific problem of sleep.
Test-Taking Strategy: Use therapeutic communication techniques. Option 4 identifies restatement and repeats the client's major theme. Review therapeutic communication techniques if you had difficulty with this question.
Level of Cognitive Ability: Application
Client Needs: Physiological Integrity
Integrated Process: Communication and Documentation
Content Area: Mental Health
Reference: Morrison-Valfre, M. (2005). *Foundations of mental health care* (3rd ed.). St. Louis: Mosby, p. 88.

4. *Answer:* 3
Rationale: Option 3 is the only option that identifies a therapeutic response. In option 1, the nurse's feelings are the focus. This response clearly ignores the fact that the issue is about the client and the client's discomfort, not about the nurse. In option 2, the nurse becomes pompous and a little angry and supercilious, which is not therapeutic. In option 4, the nurse begins correctly with an empathic stance but then becomes demanding.
Test-Taking Strategy: Using the process of elimination and therapeutic communication techniques will easily direct you to option 3. Review therapeutic communication techniques if you had difficulty with this question.
Level of Cognitive Ability: Analysis
Client Needs: Psychosocial Integrity
Integrated Process: Communication and Documentation
Content Area: Mental Health
References: Morrison-Valfre, M. (2005). *Foundations of mental health care* (3rd ed.). St. Louis: Mosby, p. 88.

Varcarolis, E. (2002). *Foundations of psychiatric mental health nursing* (4th ed.). Philadelphia: W.B. Saunders, p. 258.

5. *Answer:* **4**
Rationale: The therapeutic response is the one that reflects the client's feelings and offers the client control of care. In option 1, the nurse uses avoidance and gives information. Option 2 is an aggressive and nontherapeutic communication technique. Option 3 is social and nontherapeutic, because it labels the client's behavior and is likely to provoke anger from the client.
Test-Taking Strategy: Focus on the client's statement and use therapeutic communication techniques. Option 4 is the only option that addresses the client's statement. Review therapeutic communication techniques if you had difficulty with this question.
Level of Cognitive Ability: Application
Client Needs: Psychosocial Integrity
Integrated Process: Communication and Documentation
Content Area: Mental Health
References: Jarvis, C. (2004). *Physical examination and health assessment* (4th ed.). Philadelphia: W.B. Saunders, pp. 40, 47-49. Morrison-Valfre, M. (2005). *Foundations of mental health care* (3rd ed.). St. Louis: Mosby, p. 88.

6. *Answer:* **1**
Rationale: Open-ended questions and silence are strategies used to encourage clients to discuss their problem. Options 2 and 3 do not encouraging the client to express feelings. The nurse should not offer opinions and should encourage the client to identify the reasons for the behavior. Option 4 is not a client-centered intervention.
Test-Taking Strategy: Use the process of elimination. Eliminate options 2 and 3 first, because they do not support client expression of feelings. Eliminate option 4 next, because it is not a client-centered intervention. Focusing on the client's feelings will direct you to option 1. Review therapeutic communication techniques if you had difficulty with this question.
Level of Cognitive Ability: Application
Client Needs: Psychosocial Integrity
Integrated Process: Caring
Content Area: Mental Health
Reference: Stuart, G., & Laraia, M. (2005). *Principles and practice of psychiatric nursing* (8th ed.). St. Louis: Mosby, pp. 30-35.

7. *Answer:* **4**
Rationale: The client must first deal with feelings and negative responses before the client is able to work through the meaning of the crisis. Option 4 pertains directly to the client's feelings. Options 1, 2, and 3 do not directly address the client's feelings.
Test-Taking Strategy: Use the process of elimination. Focusing on the feelings of the client will direct you to option 4. Review the phases of the nurse-client relationship if you had difficulty with this question.
Level of Cognitive Ability: Application
Client Needs: Psychosocial Integrity
Integrated Process: Nursing Process/Implementation
Content Area: Mental Health

Reference: Morrison-Valfre, M. (2005). *Foundations of mental health care* (3rd ed.). St. Louis: Mosby, pp. 23, 90-91.

8. *Answer:* **1**
Rationale: Denial is a common response by a victim of sexual abuse. It is described as an adaptive and protective reaction. Projection is blaming or "scapegoating." Rationalization is justifying the unacceptable attributes about him or herself. Intellectualization is the excessive use of abstract thinking or generalizations to decrease painful thinking.
Test-Taking Strategy: Use the process of elimination and knowledge regarding defense mechanisms. Note the key words, *calm* and *quiet*. These behaviors are indicative of denial in a sexually abused victim. If you had difficulty with this question, review content related to the sexually abused victim and defense mechanisms.
Level of Cognitive Ability: Comprehension
Client Needs: Psychosocial Integrity
Integrated Process: Nursing Process/Data Collection
Content Area: Mental Health
Reference: Morrison-Valfre, M. (2005). *Foundations of mental health care* (3rd ed.). St. Louis: Mosby, p. 273.

9. *Answer:* **3**
Rationale: The client's thoughts are extremely important when verbalized. Suicidal thoughts are the highest priority. Options 1, 2, and 4 will all affect the treatment of the client but are not of greatest importance at this time.
Test-Taking Strategy: The client is the focus of the question; therefore, eliminate option 4. Focus on the key words, *priority concern*, and use prioritizing skills. Remember, if the client verbalizes suicidal thoughts, it is a priority concern. Review data collection techniques related to the suicidal client if you had difficulty with this question.
Level of Cognitive Ability: Analysis
Client Needs: Psychosocial Integrity
Integrated Process: Nursing Process/Data Collection
Content Area: Mental Health
Reference: Morrison-Valfre, M. (2005). *Foundations of mental health care* (3rd ed.). St. Louis: Mosby, pp. 283, 287.

10. *Answer:* **4**
Rationale: Option 4 is the only option that recognizes the client's need. This response helps the client focus on the emotion underlying the delusion, but does not argue with it. If the nurse attempts to change the client's mind, the delusion may, in fact, be even more strongly held. Options 1, 2, and 3 do not focus on the client's feelings.
Test-Taking Strategy: Use therapeutic communication techniques and knowledge regarding the dynamics of delusions and how delusions meet the client's underlying needs. This will direct you to option 4. Additionally, option 4 focuses on the client's feelings. Review therapeutic communication techniques if you had difficulty with this question.
Level of Cognitive Ability: Application
Client Needs: Psychosocial Integrity
Integrated Process: Communication and Documentation
Content Area: Mental Health
References: Morrison-Valfre, M. (2005). *Foundations of mental health care* (3rd ed.). St. Louis: Mosby, p. 328.

Stuart, G., & Laraia, M. (2005). *Principles and practice of psychiatric nursing* (8th ed.). St. Louis: Mosby, pp. 30-35.

11. Answer: 4
Rationale: Safety of the client, other clients, and staff is of prime concern. When dealing with an impaired individual, trying to talk may be out of the question. Waiting to intervene could cause the client to become even more agitated and a threat to others. Option 3 would only further aggravate an already agitated individual. Option 4 is in effect an isolation technique that allows for separation from others and provides a less stimulating environment, where the client can maintain dignity.
Test-Taking Strategy: Focus on the issue of the question and use the process of elimination. Noting that the client is inebriated will assist in directing you to option 4. Option 4 most directly addresses the situation and the behavior and feelings of the client. Review nursing interventions for a client who is inebriated if you had difficulty with this question.
Level of Cognitive Ability: Application
Client Needs: Psychosocial Integrity
Integrated Process: Nursing Process/Planning
Content Area: Mental Health
Reference: Morrison-Valfre, M. (2005). *Foundations of mental health care* (3rd ed.). St. Louis: Mosby, pp. 71, 116.

12. Answer: 2
Rationale: Denial is refusal to admit to a painful reality and is treated as if it does not exist. In projection, a person unconsciously rejects emotionally unacceptable features and attributes them to other people, objects, or situations. In regression, the client returns to an earlier, more comforting, although less mature way of behaving. Rationalization is justifying the unacceptable attributes about oneself.
Test-Taking Strategy: Use the process of elimination. Note the key words, *"There's nothing wrong with me."* Select the option that recognizes the client's attempt to avoid looking at the reality of the situation. If you had difficulty with this question, review defense mechanisms.
Level of Cognitive Ability: Comprehension
Client Needs: Psychosocial Integrity
Integrated Process: Nursing Process/Data Collection
Content Area: Mental Health
Reference: Morrison-Valfre, M. (2005). *Foundations of mental health care* (3rd ed.). St. Louis: Mosby, p. 70.

13. Answer: 1
Rationale: Reflection is the therapeutic communication technique that redirects the client's feelings back to validate what the client is saying. In option 2, the nurse attempts to use focusing but the attempt to discuss central issues seems premature. In option 3, the nurse makes a judgment and is nontherapeutic in the one-on-one relationship. In option 4, the nurse is attempting to assess the client's ability to openly discuss feelings with family members. Although this may be appropriate, the timing is somewhat premature and closes off facilitation of the client's feelings.
Test-Taking Strategy: Use therapeutic communication techniques. Note that option 1 uses the therapeutic technique of reflection and also focuses on the client's feelings. Options 2,

3, and 4 are nontherapeutic at this time. Review therapeutic communication techniques if you had difficulty with this question.
Level of Cognitive Ability: Application
Client Needs: Psychosocial Integrity
Integrated Process: Communication and Documentation
Content Area: Mental Health
References: Morrison-Valfre, M. (2005). *Foundations of mental health care* (3rd ed.). St. Louis: Mosby, p. 88.
Stuart, G., & Laraia, M. (2005). *Principles and practice of psychiatric nursing* (8th ed.). St. Louis: Mosby, pp. 30-35.

14. Answer: 4
Rationale: Generally, voluntary admission is sought by the client or client's guardian. If the client seeks voluntary admission, the most likely expectation is that the client will participate in the treatment program.
Test-Taking Strategy: Use the process of elimination. Note the key words, *voluntary admission*. This will direct you to option 4. Additionally, note that options 1, 2, and 3 are similar. Review the various types of hospital admission processes if you had difficulty with this question.
Level of Cognitive Ability: Comprehension
Client Needs: Psychosocial Integrity
Integrated Process: Nursing Process/Planning
Content Area: Mental Health
Reference: Morrison-Valfre, M. (2005). *Foundations of mental health care* (3rd ed.). St. Louis: Mosby, p. 23.

15. Answer: 3
Rationale: Generally, voluntary admission is sought by the client or client's guardian. Voluntary clients have the right to demand and obtain release. The best nursing action is to contact the physician.
Test-Taking Strategy: Use the process of elimination. Noting the type of hospital admission will assist in eliminating option 1. It is inappropriate to "persuade" a client to stay in the hospital. Option 2 should be eliminated based simply on the issue of client rights and the issue of confidentiality. Review the various types of hospital admission and discharge processes if you had difficulty with this question.
Level of Cognitive Ability: Application
Client Needs: Safe, Effective Care Environment
Integrated Process: Nursing Process/Implementation
Content Area: Mental Health
References: Morrison-Valfre, M. (2005). *Foundations of mental health care* (3rd ed.). St. Louis: Mosby, p. 23.
Stuart, G., & Laraia, M. (2005). *Principles and practice of psychiatric nursing* (8th ed.). St. Louis: Mosby, p. 150.

16. Answer: 1
Rationale: Involuntary admission is made without the client's consent. Involuntary admission is necessary when a person is a danger to self or others or is in need of psychiatric treatment or physical care. Options 2, 3, and 4 describe the process of voluntary admission.
Test-Taking Strategy: Use the process of elimination. Note the key words, *involuntary status*. This should direct you to option 1. Also, note that options 2, 3, and 4 are similar. Review the

process of involuntary admission if you had difficulty with this question.
Level of Cognitive Ability: Comprehension
Client Needs: Psychosocial Integrity
Integrated Process: Nursing Process/Planning
Content Area: Mental Health
Reference: Stuart, G., & Laraia, M. (2005). *Principles and practice of psychiatric nursing* (8th ed.). St. Louis: Mosby, 150.

17. *Answer:* 3
Rationale: Clients who are involuntarily admitted do not lose their right to informed consent. The informed consent needs to be obtained from the client. Options 1, 2, and 4 are incorrect.
Test-Taking Strategy: Use the process of elimination and knowledge regarding the hospital admission processes and client's rights to answer this question. Focusing on the issue of client's rights will direct you to option 3. Review client's rights if you had difficulty with this question.
Level of Cognitive Ability: Comprehension
Client Needs: Safe, Effective Care Environment
Integrated Process: Nursing Process/Planning
Content Area: Mental Health
Reference: Morrison-Valfre, M. (2005). *Foundations of mental health care* (3rd ed.). St. Louis: Mosby, p. 218.

18. *Answer:* 2
Rationale: A client may request to be secluded or restrained. Federal laws require the consent of the client, unless an emergency situation exists in which an immediate risk to the client or others can be documented. The use of seclusion and restraint is permitted only on the written order of a physician, which must be reviewed and renewed every 24 hours; it also must specify the type of restraint to be used.
Test-Taking Strategy: Use the process of elimination. There is no reason to call the family at this time; therefore, eliminate option 3. Knowing that a physician's written order is necessary in this situation will assist in eliminating option 4. Option 1 is not the best choice because this information, if given to a client experiencing uncontrollable feelings, may cause escalation of the feelings. Review the procedures for seclusion if you had difficulty with this question.
Level of Cognitive Ability: Application
Client Needs: Safe, Effective Care Environment
Integrated Process: Nursing Process/Implementation
Content Area: Mental Health
Reference: Morrison-Valfre, M. (2005). *Foundations of mental health care* (3rd ed.). St. Louis: Mosby, pp. 25, 262-263.

19. *Answer:* 2
Rationale: The nurse should never promise to keep a secret. Secrets are appropriate in a social relationship, but not in a therapeutic one. The nurse needs to be honest with the client and tell the client that a promise cannot be made to keep the secret.
Test-Taking Strategy: Use the process of elimination and therapeutic communication techniques. Option 1 can be eliminated because it is inappropriate. Also, options 3 and 4 are not only inappropriate, but are to an extent threatening and may even block further communication. Review the principles

related to a therapeutic nurse-client relationship if you had difficulty with this question.
Level of Cognitive Ability: Application
Client Needs: Psychosocial Integrity
Integrated Process: Communication and Documentation
Content Area: Mental Health
References: Morrison-Valfre, M. (2005). *Foundations of mental health care* (3rd ed.). St. Louis: Mosby, p. 88.
Stuart, G., & Laraia, M. (2005). *Principles and practice of psychiatric nursing* (8th ed.). St. Louis: Mosby, pp. 30-35.

20. *Answer:* 4
Rationale: A nurse is required to maintain confidentiality regarding clients and their care. Confidentiality is basic to the therapeutic relationship and is a client's right. Option 3 is correct in a sense; however, it is a rather blunt statement. Both options 1 and 2 identify statements that do not maintain client confidentiality.
Test-Taking Strategy: Use the process of elimination. Focus on the issue of the question, maintaining confidentiality. This should assist in eliminating options 1 and 2. From the remaining options, select option 4 over option 3 because it is most direct and correct. Option 3 is a rather blunt and somewhat rude statement. Review confidentiality issues if you had difficulty with this question.
Level of Cognitive Ability: Application
Client Needs: Safe, Effective Care Environment
Integrated Process: Communication and Documentation
Content Area: Mental Health
Reference: Morrison-Valfre, M. (2005). *Foundations of mental health care* (3rd ed.). St. Louis: Mosby, p. 21.

21. *Answer:* 4
Rationale: False imprisonment is an act with the intent to confine a person to a specific area. A nurse can be charged with false imprisonment if the nurse prohibits a client from leaving the hospital if the client was voluntarily admitted and if there are no agency or legal policies for detaining the client. On the other hand, if the client has been involuntarily admitted or has agreed to an evaluation before discharge, the nurse's actions are reasonable.
Test-Taking Strategy: Use the process of elimination. Noting the key words, *involuntarily admitted*, will assist to eliminate option 1 and direct you to option 4. Options 2 and 3 are unrelated to the issue of the question and can be easily eliminated. Review the issues related to false imprisonment and hospital admissions if you had difficulty with this question.
Level of Cognitive Ability: Comprehension
Client Needs: Safe, Effective Care Environment
Integrated Process: Nursing Process/Implementation
Content Area: Mental Health
Reference: Morrison-Valfre, M. (2005). *Foundations of mental health care* (3rd ed.). St. Louis: Mosby, pp. 24-25.

22. *Answer:* 3
Rationale: Tasks of the termination phase include evaluating client performance, evaluating achievement of expected outcomes, evaluating future needs, making appropriate referrals, and dealing with the common behaviors associated

with termination. Options 1, 2, and 4 identify the tasks of the working phase of the relationship.
Test-Taking Strategy: Noting the key words, *termination phase*, should direct you to option 3. If you are unfamiliar with the appropriate tasks of the phases of the nurse-client relationship, review this content.
Level of Cognitive Ability: Application
Client Needs: Psychosocial Integrity
Integrated Process: Nursing Process/Planning
Content Area: Mental Health
Reference: Morrison-Valfre, M. (2005). *Foundations of mental health care* (3rd ed.). St. Louis: Mosby, pp. 106-107.

23. *Answer:* 2
Rationale: In the termination phase of a relationship, it is normal for a client to demonstrate a number of regressive behaviors. Typical behaviors include return of symptoms, anger, withdrawal, and minimizing the relationship. The anger that the client is experiencing is a normal behavior during the termination phase and does not necessarily indicate the need for hospitalization or treatment.
Test-Taking Strategy: Use the process of elimination. Note the key words, *termination phase*. This alone may assist in directing you to option 2. Additionally, note the similarity among options 1, 3, and 4. These options address the need for further supervised treatment. If you are unfamiliar with the client behaviors associated with the termination phase, review this content.
Level of Cognitive Ability: Analysis
Client Needs: Psychosocial Integrity
Integrated Process: Nursing Process/Evaluation
Content Area: Mental Health
Reference: Morrison-Valfre, M. (2005). *Foundations of mental health care* (3rd ed.). St. Louis: Mosby, p. 107.

24. *Answer:* 1
Rationale: Behavior therapy is used to help clients identify and examine dysfunctional thoughts as well as identify and examine values and beliefs that maintain these thoughts. Options 2, 3, and 4 are incorrect.
Test-Taking Strategy: Use the process of elimination and note the key word, *behavior*. Focusing on this key word should direct you to option 1. If you are unfamiliar with this type of therapy and its purpose, review this content.
Level of Cognitive Ability: Comprehension
Client Needs: Psychosocial Integrity
Integrated Process: Nursing Process/Implementation
Content Area: Mental Health
Reference: Morrison-Valfre, M. (2005). *Foundations of mental health care* (3rd ed.). St. Louis: Mosby, pp. 40-42.

25. *Answer:* 3
Rationale: Milieu therapy provides a safe environment that is adapted to the individual client's needs and also provides greater comfort and freedom of expression than has been experienced in the past by the client. All members contribute to the planning and functioning of the setting. Options 1, 2, and 4 are not characteristics of milieu therapy.
Test-Taking Strategy: Use the process of elimination. Note that options 1, 2, and 4 are similar and that option 3 identifies

the umbrella (global) description. Review this model of care if you had difficulty with this question.
Level of Cognitive Ability: Comprehension
Client Needs: Psychosocial Integrity
Integrated Process: Nursing Process/Implementation
Content Area: Mental Health
Reference: Stuart, G., & Laraia, M. (2005). *Principles and practice of psychiatric nursing* (8th ed.). St. Louis: Mosby, pp. 700-701.

26. *Answer:* 4
Rationale: Aversion therapy, also known as aversion conditioning or negative reinforcement, is a technique used to change behavior. In this therapy, a stimulus (alcohol) attractive to the client is paired with an unpleasant event in hopes of associating the stimulus with negative properties. Desensitization is the reduction of intense reactions to a stimulus by repeated exposure to the stimulus in a weaker and milder form. Milieu therapy provides positive environmental manipulation, both physical and social, to effect a positive change in the client. Self-control therapy combines cognitive and behavioral approaches and is useful to deal with stress.
Test-Taking Strategy: Focus on the information in the question. Recalling that aversion therapy is a form of negative reinforcement will direct you to the correct option. If you had difficulty with this question, review this form of therapy.
Level of Cognitive Ability: Comprehension
Client Needs: Psychosocial Integrity
Integrated Process: Nursing Process/Implementation
Content Area: Mental Health
Reference: Morrison-Valfre, M. (2005). *Foundations of mental health care* (3rd ed.). St. Louis: Mosby, p. 300.

27. *Answer:* 4
Rationale: The leader of a self-help group is an experienced member of the group. A nurse or psychiatrist may be asked by the group to serve as a resource but would not be the leader of the group. Options 1, 2, and 3 are characteristics of a self-help group.
Test-Taking Strategy: Use the process of elimination and note the key words, *need for additional information*, in the stem of the question. Note that options 1, 2, and 3 are similar. This should direct you to option 4. Review the characteristics of a self-help group if you had difficulty with this question.
Level of Cognitive Ability: Comprehension
Client Needs: Psychosocial Integrity
Integrated Process: Nursing Process/Evaluation
Content Area: Mental Health
Reference: Morrison-Valfre, M. (2005). *Foundations of mental health care* (3rd ed.). St. Louis: Mosby, p. 49.

28. *Answer:* 4
Rationale: The first step in the 12-step program is to admit that a problem exists. Options 1 and 2 are unrealistic as a first step in the process to recovery. Although option 3 may be a strategy, it is not the first step.
Test-Taking Strategy: Note the key words, *first step*, in the question. This will assist in directing you to option 4. If you are unfamiliar with the 12-step program, review this content.

Level of Cognitive Ability: Comprehension
Client Needs: Psychosocial Integrity
Integrated Process: Nursing Process/Implementation
Content Area: Mental Health
Reference: Stuart, G., & Laraia, M. (2005). *Principles and practice of psychiatric nursing* (8th ed.). St. Louis: Mosby, pp. 506-507.

29. Answer: 1

Rationale: If a client is monopolizing the group, it is important that the nurse be direct and decisive. The best action is to suggest that the client stop talking and try listening to others. Although option 3 may be a direct response, option 1 is the most therapeutic direct statement. Options 2 and 4 are inappropriate.

Test-Taking Strategy: Use the process of elimination. Eliminate options 2 and 4 first because they are similar. Use therapeutic communication techniques to assist in directing you to option 1. If you had difficulty with this question, review therapeutic communication techniques.

Level of Cognitive Ability: Application
Client Needs: Psychosocial Integrity
Integrated Process: Nursing Process/Implementation
Content Area: Mental Health
Reference: Morrison-Valfre, M. (2005). *Foundations of mental health care* (3rd ed.). St. Louis: Mosby, p. 88.

30. Answer: 1

Rationale: In the forming or initial stage, the members are identifying tasks and boundaries. Storming involves responding emotionally to tasks. In the norming stage, members express intimate personal opinions and feelings around personal tasks. In the performing stage, members direct group energy toward the completion of tasks.

Test-Taking Strategy: Use the process of elimination. Note the key word, *identifying*, in the question. This key word should assist in directing you to option 1. If you had difficulty with this question, review the stages of group development.

Level of Cognitive Ability: Comprehension
Client Needs: Psychosocial Integrity
Integrated Process: Nursing Process/Implementation
Content Area: Mental Health
Reference: Stuart, G., & Laraia, M. (2005). *Principles and practice of psychiatric nursing* (8th ed.). St. Louis: Mosby, p. 672.

ALTERNATE FORMAT QUESTION: MULTIPLE RESPONSE

Answers:
Listening
Maintaining neutral responses
Restating
Providing acknowledgment and feedback

Rationale: Some therapeutic communication techniques include listening, maintaining silence, maintaining neutral responses, using broad openings and open-ended questions, focusing and refocusing, restating, clarifying and validating, sharing perceptions, reflecting, providing acknowledgment and feedback, giving information and presenting reality, encouraging formulation of a plan of action, providing nonverbal encouragement, and summarizing.

Test-Taking Strategy: Focus on the issue, therapeutic communication techniques. This will assist in selecting the correct answers. Review therapeutic and nontherapeutic techniques if you had difficulty with this question.

Level of Cognitive Ability: Comprehension
Client Needs: Psychosocial Integrity
Integrated Process: Communication and Documentation
Content Area: Mental Health
Reference: Harkreader, H., & Hogan, M.A. (2004). *Fundamentals of nursing: Caring and clinical judgment* (2nd ed.). Philadelphia: W.B. Saunders, pp. 251-252.

REFERENCES

Harkreader, H., & Hogan, M.A. (2004). *Fundamentals of nursing: Caring and clinical judgment* (2nd ed.). Philadelphia: W.B. Saunders.

Jarvis, C. (2004). *Physical examination and health assessment* (4th ed.). Philadelphia: W.B. Saunders.

Morrison-Valfre, M. (2005). *Foundations of mental health care* (3rd ed.). St. Louis: Mosby.

Stuart, G., & Laraia, M. (2005). *Principles and practice of psychiatric nursing* (8th ed.). St. Louis: Mosby.

Varcarolis, E. (2002). *Foundations of psychiatric mental health nursing* (4th ed.). Philadelphia: W.B. Saunders.

Mental Health Disorders

I. ANXIETY

A. Description
1. A subjective, individual experience
2. A normal response to stress
3. A feeling of apprehension, uneasiness, uncertainty, or dread
4. Occurs as a result of threats that may be misperceived or misinterpreted
5. Occurs as a result of a threat to identity or self-esteem
6. May result when values are threatened
7. May precede new experiences

B. Types of anxiety
1. Normal: A healthy type of anxiety
2. Acute: Precipitated by imminent loss or change that threatens the sense of security
3. Chronic: Anxiety that the individual has lived with for a long time

C. Levels of anxiety
1. Mild
   a. Associated with the tension of daily life
   b. The individual is alert
   c. The perceptual field is increased
   d. Can be motivating, producing growth and creativity and increasing ability to learn
2. Moderate
   a. The focus is on immediate concerns
   b. Narrows the perceptual field
   c. Selective inattentiveness occurs
   d. Learning and problem solving still take place
3. Severe
   a. A feeling that something bad is about to happen
   b. A significant reduction in perceptual field occurs
   c. Focus is on specific details or scattered details
   d. All behavior is directed at relieving the anxiety

e. Learning and problem solving are not possible
f. The individual needs direction to focus
4. Panic
   a. Associated with dread and terror and a sense of impending doom
   b. The personality is disorganized
   c. The individual is unable to communicate or function effectively
   d. Increased motor activity occurs
   e. Loss of rational thoughts, with distorted perception
   f. Inability to concentrate
   g. If prolonged, panic can lead to exhaustion and death

D. Interventions: General nursing measures
1. Recognize the anxiety
2. Establish trust
3. Protect the client
4. Do not attack **coping mechanisms**
5. Do not force the client into situations that provoke anxiety
6. Decrease stimulation in the environment
7. Modify the environment by setting limits or limiting the interaction with others
8. Provide creative outlets
9. Provide activities that limit the amount of time for destructive behavior
10. Promote relaxation techniques
11. Administer antianxiety medications, as prescribed

E. Interventions: Mild to moderate levels
1. Help the client identify the anxiety
2. Encourage the client to talk about feelings and concerns
3. Help the client identify thoughts and feelings that occurred prior to the onset of anxiety
4. Encourage problem solving
5. Encourage gross motor exercise

F. Interventions: Severe to panic levels
  1. Reduce the anxiety quickly
  2. Use a calm manner
  3. Always remain with the client
  4. Minimize environmental stimuli
  5. Provide clear, simple statements
  6. Use a low-pitched voice
  7. Attend to the physical needs of the client
  8. Provide gross motor activity
  9. Administer antianxiety medications as prescribed

II. GENERALIZED ANXIETY DISORDER

A. Description
  1. An unrealistic anxiety in which the cause can usually be identified
  2. Physical symptoms occur
B. Data collection
  1. Restlessness and inability to relax
  2. Episodes of trembling and shakiness
  3. Chronic muscular tension
  4. Dizziness
  5. Inability to concentrate
  6. Chronic fatigue and sleep problems
  7. Inability to recognize the connection between the anxiety and physical symptoms
  8. The client is focused on the physical discomfort
C. Panic disorder
  1. Description
    a. The cause usually cannot be identified
    b. Has a sudden onset, with feelings of intense apprehension and dread
    c. Severe, recurrent, intermittent anxiety attacks, lasting 5 to 30 minutes
  2. Data collection
    a. Choking sensation
    b. Labored breathing
    c. Pounding heart
    d. Chest pain
    e. Dizziness
    f. Nausea
    g. Blurred vision
    h. Numbness or tingling of the extremities
    i. A sense of unreality and helplessness
    j. A fear of being trapped
    k. A fear of dying
  3. Interventions
    a. Attend to physical symptoms
    b. Assist the client to identify the thoughts that aroused the anxiety and identify the basis for these thoughts
    c. Assist the client to change the unrealistic thoughts to more realistic thoughts
    d. Use cognitive restructuring
    e. Administer antianxiety medications as prescribed

III. POST-TRAUMATIC STRESS DISORDER (PTSD)

A. Description: After experiencing a psychologically traumatic event, outside the range of usual experience, the individual reexperiences the event via recurrent and intrusive dreams or flashbacks
B. Stressors
  1. A natural disaster
  2. A terrorist attack
  3. Combat experiences
  4. Victim of rape
  5. Accidents
  6. Victim of crime or violence
  7. Victim of sexual, physical, and emotional **abuse**
  8. Reexperiencing the event as flashbacks
C. Data collection
  1. Emotional numbness
  2. Detachment
  3. Depression
  4. Anxiety
  5. Sleep disturbances and nightmares
  6. Flashbacks of the event
  7. Hypervigilance
  8. Guilt about surviving the event
  9. Poor concentration and avoidance of activities that trigger the memory of the event
D. Interventions
  1. Desensitization through gradual exposure to the event or situations similar to the event
  2. Instruct the client in relaxation techniques
  3. Provide individual therapy that addresses loss of control issues or anger
  4. Use of support groups
  5. Use of hypnotherapy

IV. PHOBIAS

A. Description
  1. An irrational fear of an object or situation that persists, although the person may recognize it as unreasonable
  2. Associated with panic level anxiety if the object, situation, or activity cannot be avoided
  3. **Defense mechanisms** commonly used include repression and displacement
B. Types (Box 63-1)
C. Interventions
  1. Stay with the client when the anxiety is high to promote safety and security
  2. Identify the basis of the anxiety
  3. Allow the client to verbalize feelings about the anxiety-producing object or situation; frequently talking about the feared object is the first step in the desensitization process
  4. Desensitization occurs by gradually introducing the individual to the feared object or situation in small doses

BOX 63-1

Types of Phobias

Acrophobia: Fear of heights
Agoraphobia: Fear of open spaces
Astraphobia: Fear of electrical storms
Claustrophobia: Fear of closed spaces
Hematophobia: Fear of blood
Hydrophobia: Fear of water
Monophobia: Fear of being alone
Mysophobia: Fear of dirt or germs
Nyctophobia: Fear of darkness
Pyrophobia: Fear of fires
Social phobia: Fear of situations in which one might be embarrassed or criticized and the fear of making a fool of oneself
Xenophobia: Fear of strangers
Zoophobia: Fear of animals

BOX 63-2

Types of Somatoform Disorders

Somatization disorder
Hypochondriasis
Conversion disorder

4. Provide for client safety related to the behaviors
5. Implement a schedule for the client that distracts from the behaviors
6. Set limits on the rituals that might interfere with the client's physical well-being to protect the client from physical harm
7. Encourage the client to verbalize concerns
8. Establish a written contract that will assist the client to decrease the frequency of compulsive behaviors gradually

5. Teach relaxation techniques such as breathing exercises, muscle relaxation exercises, and visualization of pleasant situations
6. Do not force contact with the phobic object or situation

V. OBSESSIVE-COMPULSIVE DISORDER (OCD)

A. Obsessions: Preoccupation with persistent intrusive thoughts and ideas
B. Compulsions
 1. Repeated performance of rituals or purposeless behaviors designed to prevent some event, divert unacceptable thoughts, and decrease anxiety
 2. Obsessions and compulsions often occur together and can disrupt normal activities
 3. Anxiety occurs if obsessions or compulsions are resisted, and from being powerless to resist the thoughts or rituals
 4. Obsessive thoughts can involve issues of violence, aggression, sexual behavior, orderliness, or religion and can uncontrollably interrupt conscious thoughts and the ability to function
C. Compulsive behavior patterns
 1. Decrease the anxiety
 2. Are associated with the obsessive thoughts
 3. Neutralize the thought
 4. During stressful times, the ritualistic behavior increases
 5. **Defense mechanisms** include repression, displacement, and undoing
D. Interventions
 1. Identify the situations that precipitate the behavior
 2. Do not interrupt the compulsive behaviors
 3. Allow time for the client to perform the compulsive rituals

VI. SOMATOFORM DISORDERS

A. Description (Box 63-2)
 1. Characterized by persistent worry or complaints regarding physical illness when there are no supporting physical findings
 2. The client focuses on the physical signs and symptoms and cannot control the signs and symptoms
 3. The physical signs and symptoms increase with psychosocial stressors
 4. The anxiety is redirected into a somatic concern
B. Somatization disorder
 1. Description
  a. The client has multiple physical complaints involving multiple body systems
  b. The emotional stress can result from anxiety, fear, depression, worry, or repressed anger
  c. The client may unconsciously use somatization for secondary gains such as increased attention and decreased responsibilities
 2. Data collection
  a. Physical complaints of abdominal pain, denial of emotional problems, signs of anxiety, fear, and low self-esteem
  b. Psychosexual symptoms
  c. Secondary gain
C. Hypochondriasis
 1. Description
  a. The preoccupation with fears of having a serious disease
  b. No evidence of physical illness exists
  c. Causes a significantly impaired social and occupational functioning
 2. Data collection
  a. Preoccupation with physical functioning
  b. Frequent somatic complaints

c. Complaints of fatigue and insomnia

d. Anxiety

e. Difficulty expressing feelings

f. Extensive use of home remedies or nonprescription medications

g. Repeatedly visiting the doctor

h. Secondary gain

D. Conversion disorder

1. Description

a. A physical symptom or a deficit suggesting loss of body function or altered body function related to psychological conflict or a neurological disorder

b. An expression of a psychological conflict or need

c. The most common conversion symptoms are blindness, deafness, paralysis, and the inability to talk

d. There is no organic cause

e. Symptoms are not intentionally produced by client

f. Symptoms are directly related to conflict and decrease anxiety

2. Data collection

a. "La belle indifference": Unconcerned with symptoms

b. Physical limitation or disability

c. Feelings of guilt, anxiety, or frustration

d. Low self-esteem and feelings of inadequacy

e. Unexpressed anger of conflict

f. Secondary gain

E. Interventions

1. Obtain a nursing history and assess for physical problems

2. Do not reinforce the sick role

3. Discourage verbalization about physical symptoms by not responding with positive reinforcement

4. Explore the needs being met by the physical symptoms with the client

5. Assist the client to identify alternative ways of meeting needs

6. Assist the client to relate feelings and conflicts to the physical symptoms

7. Allow a specific time period to discuss physical complaints, because the client will feel less threatened if this behavior is limited rather than stopped completely

8. Convey understanding that the physical symptoms are real to the client

9. Assure the client that physical illness has been ruled out

10. Explore the source of anxiety and stimulate verbalization of anxiety

11. Encourage the use of relaxation techniques as the anxiety increases

12. Implement pain reduction measures as required

13. Report and assess any new physical complaint

14. Encourage diversional activities to decrease the client's focus on himself or herself

15. Provide positive feedback for accomplishments to increase self-esteem

16. Assist the client in recognizing his or her own feelings and emotions

17. Establish a written contract with the client that will redirect the clients thoughts and feelings

18. Administer antianxiety medications, as prescribed

VII. DISSOCIATIVE DISORDER

A. Description

1. A disruption in integrative functions of memory, consciousness, or identity

2. Associated with exposure to an extremely traumatic event

B. Dissociative identity disorder (multiple personality)

1. Description

a. Two or more fully developed distinct and unique personalities within the person

b. Personalities may take full control of the client, one at a time

c. The personalities may or may not be aware of each other

2. Data collection

a. The inability to recall important information (unrelated to ordinary forgetfulness)

b. Transition from one personality to the other is related to stress and is sudden

c. Dissociation is used as a method of distancing and defending self from anxiety and traumatizing experiences

C. Dissociative amnesia

1. Description

a. Inability to recall important personal information because it provokes anxiety

b. Memory impairment may be impartial or almost complete

2. Data collection

a. Localized: The client blocks out all memories about a specified period

b. Selective: The client recalls some but not all memories about a specified period

c. Generalized: Loss of all memory about past life

D. Dissociative fugue

1. Description

a. The assumption of a new identity in a new environment

b. May occur suddenly

2. Data collection

a. May drift from place to place

b. Develops few social relationships

c. When the fugue lifts, the client returns home and is unable to recall the fugue state

E. Depersonalization disorder
1. Description: An altered self-perception in which one's own reality is temporarily lost or changed
2. Data collection
   a. Feelings of detachment
   b. Intact reality testing
F. Interventions
1. Develop a trusting relationship with the client
2. Encourage verbal expression of painful experiences, anxieties, and concerns
3. Explore methods of coping
4. Identify sources of conflict
5. Focus on the client's strengths and skills
6. Orient the client
7. Provide nondemanding simple routines
8. Allow the client to progress at his or her own pace
9. Use stress-reduction techniques
10. Plan for individual, group, and/or family psychotherapy to integrate dissociated aspects of personality or memory and to expand self-awareness

VIII. BIPOLAR DISORDER
A. Description (Box 63-3)
1. Characterized by episodes of mania and depression, with periods of normal mood and activity in between
2. The medication of choice is lithium carbonate, which can be toxic and therefore requires the regular monitoring of serum lithium levels
B. Interventions for mania (Box 63-4)
1. Remove hazardous objects from the environment
2. Monitor the client closely for fatigue
3. Use comfort measures to promote sleep
4. Provide frequent rest periods
5. Monitor the client's sleep patterns
6. Provide a private room if possible
7. Administer a hypnotic or sedative medication, as prescribed
8. Encourage the client to ventilate feelings
9. Use calm, slow interactions
10. Help the client focus on one topic during the conversation
11. Ignore or distract the client from grandiose thinking
12. Present reality to the client
13. Don't argue with the client
14. Limit group activities and assess the client's tolerance level
15. Provide high-calorie finger foods and fluids
16. Supervise the client's choice of clothing
17. Reduce environmental stimuli
18. Set limits on inappropriate behaviors
19. Provide physical activities and outlets for tension

BOX 63-3

Data Collection: Bipolar Disorder

MANIA
Inappropriate affect
Restlessness
Flight of ideas
Inability to eat or sleep because of involvement in more important things
Extroverted personality
Delusional self-confidence
Initiation of activity
High and unstable affect
Becomes angry quickly
Pressured speech
Grandiose and persecutory delusions
Inappropriate dress
Urgent motor activity
Significant decrease in appetite
Inability to sleep yet still active
Sexually promiscuous
Distracted by environmental stimuli
Unlimited energy

DEPRESSION
Decreased emotion and physical activity
Inability to make quick decisions
Introverted personality
Lack of initiative
Lack of self-confidence
Internalizing hostility
Decrease in activities of daily living (ADLs)
Lack of energy
Easily fatigued
Withdrawn from groups
Lack of sexual interest

---

20. Avoid competitive games
21. Provide gross motor activities such as walking and writing
22. Provide structured activities or one-on-one activities with the nurse
23. Provide simple and direct explanations for routine procedures
24. Supervise the administration of medication

IX. SCHIZOPHRENIA
A. Description
1. A group of mental disorders characterized by psychotic features, inability to trust others, disordered thought processes, and disrupted interpersonal relationships
2. Disturbances in affect, mood, behavior, and thought processes
B. Data collection
1. Physical characteristics
   a. Disheveled appearance
   b. Body image distortions

BOX 63-4

Dealing with Inappropriate Behaviors

AGGRESSIVE BEHAVIOR

Assist the client in identifying feelings of frustration and aggression.

Encourage the client to talk out instead of acting out feelings of frustration.

Assist the client in identifying precipitating events or situations that lead to aggressive behavior.

Describe the consequences of the behavior on self and others.

Assist in identifying previous coping mechanisms.

Assist the client in problem-solving techniques to cope with frustration or aggression.

DE-ESCALATION TECHNIQUES

Maintain safety for the client, other clients, and self.

Maintain a large personal space and use a nonaggressive posture.

Use a calm approach and communicate with a calm, clear tone of voice (be assertive, not aggressive).

Determine what the client considers to be his or her need.

Avoid verbal struggles.

Provide the client with clear options that deal with the client's behavior.

Assist the client with problem solving and decision making regarding the options.

MANIPULATIVE BEHAVIOR

Set clear, consistent, realistic, and enforceable limits and communicate expected behaviors.

Be clear about the consequences associated with exceeding set limits and follow through with the consequences in a nonpunitive manner if necessary.

Discuss the client's behavior in a nonjudgmental and nonthreatening manner.

Avoid power struggles with the client (avoid arguing with the client).

Assist the client in developing means of setting limits on his or her own behavior.

BOX 63-5

Abnormal Motor Behaviors

DESCRIPTION

Abnormal motor behavior or activity, displayed by the mentally ill client, occurring as a result of a psychiatric disorder

TYPES OF ABNORMAL MOTOR BEHAVIORS

Akathisia

Displaying motor restlessness and muscular quivering; the client is unable to sit or lie quietly

Echolalia

Repeating the speech of another person

Echopraxia

Repeating the movements of another person

Parkinson-like Symptoms

Making masklike faces, drooling, and having shuffling gait, tremors, and muscular rigidity

Waxy Flexibility

Having one's arms or legs placed in a certain position and holding that same position for hours

Dyskinesia

Impairment of the power of voluntary movements

c. Preoccupied with somatic complaints
d. Neglects eating, sleeping, and elimination
2. Motor activity (Box 63-5)
   a. Catatonic posturing: Holding bizarre postures for long periods of time
   b. Catatonic excitement: Moving excitedly with no environmental stimuli present
   c. May be totally immobilized
   d. Unable to respond to commands or, responds only to commands
   e. Waxy flexibility
   f. Movements may be repetitive or stereotyped
   g. Motor activity may be increased, as evidenced by agitation, pacing, inability to sleep, loss of appetite and weight, and impulsiveness

   h. May be unable to initiate activity, known as volition or anergia
3. Emotional characteristics
   a. Mistrust
   b. Views the world as threatening and unsafe
   c. Feelings not easily interpreted
   d. Ambivalence manifested as compulsive rituals, negativism, and overcompliance
   e. May display feelings of helplessness, anxiety, anger, guilt and depression, and decreased self-esteem
4. Compulsive rituals: Attempts to solve conflicting feelings by constant, repetitive activity, which may be stereotyped or seem meaningless
5. Overcompliance: attempts to deny responsibility for any action by doing only what another exactly instructs
6. Affective disturbances
   a. Flat affect or inappropriate affect
   b. Altered thought processes
7. Thought processes (Box 63-6)
   a. Impaired reality testing
   b. Fragmentation of thoughts
   c. Blocking
   d. Loose associations
   e. Autistic thinking
   f. Perceives environment in a totally self-centered way
   g. Neologisms
   h. Magical thinking
   i. Unable to conceptualize meaning in words or thoughts

BOX 63-6

Abnormal Thought Processes

DESCRIPTION

Abnormal thought processes, displayed by the mentally ill client, occurring as a result of a psychiatric disorder

TYPES OF ABNORMAL THOUGHT PROCESSES

Neologisms

Words that an individual makes up that only have meaning for the individual; often part of a delusional system

Looseness of Association

The individual's thinking is haphazard, illogical, and confused and connections in thought are interrupted; seen mostly in schizophrenic disorders

Flight of Ideas

A constant flow of speech in which the individual jumps from one topic to another in rapid succession; there is a connection between topics, although it is sometimes difficult to identify; seen in manic states

Blocking

A sudden cessation of a thought in the middle of a sentence; the client is unable to continue the train of thought; often, sudden, new thoughts come up that are unrelated to the topic

Circumstantiality

Before getting to the point or answering a question, the individual gets caught up in countless details and explanations

Confabulation

Filling a memory gap with detailed fantasy believed by the teller; the purpose of confabulation is to maintain self-esteem; seen in organic conditions such as Korsakoff's psychosis

Word Salad

A mixture of words and phrases that have no meaning

BOX 63-7

Delusions

DESCRIPTION

A false belief held to be true, even when there is evidence to the contrary

TYPES

Persecution

The thought that one is being singled out for harm by others

Grandeur

The false belief that one is a very powerful and important person

Jealousy

The false belief that one's partner or significant other is going out with other people

INTERVENTIONS

Ask the client to describe the delusion.

Be open and honest in interactions to reduce suspiciousness.

Focus the conversation on reality-based topics rather than on the delusion.

Encourage the client to express feelings and focus on the feelings that the delusions generate.

If the client obsesses on the delusion, set firm limits on the amount of time for talking about the delusion.

Do not dispute with the client or try to convince the client that the delusions are false.

Validate if part of the delusion is real.

---

    j. Unable to organize facts logically

    k. Delusions

  8. Types of delusions (Box 63-7)

    a. Loss of reference in which the client believes that certain events, situations, or interactions are directly related to self

    b. Delusions of persecution in which the client believes that he or she is being harassed, threatened, or persecuted by some powerful force

    c. Delusions of grandeur in which the client attaches special significance to self in relation to others or the universe and has an exaggerated sense of self that has no basis in reality

    d. Somatic delusions in which the client believes that his or her body is changing or responding in an unusual way, which has no basis in reality

  9. Perceptual distortions

    a. Illusions, which may be brief experiences that misinterpret or exaggerate reality

    b. Hallucinations—for example, perceiving objects, sensations, or images with no basis in reality (Box 63-8)

  10. Language and communication disturbances (Box 63-9)

    a. Related to disorders in thought process

    b. Unable to organize language

    c. Difficulty communicating clearly

    d. Inappropriate responses to a situation

    e. Client believes that a single word or phrase represents the whole meaning of the conversation, and may feel that he or she has communicated adequately

    f. May develop private language

C. Types of schizophrenia (Box 63-10)

  1. Paranoid schizophrenia

    a. Suspiciousness

    b. Hostility

    c. Delusions

    d. Auditory hallucinations

    e. Anxiety and anger

    f. Aloofness

    g. Persecutory themes

    h. Violence

  2. Disorganized schizophrenia

    a. Extreme social withdrawal

    b. Disorganized speech or behavior

    c. Flat or inappropriate affect

    d. Silliness unrelated to speech

    e. Stereotyped behaviors

BOX 63-8

Hallucinations

DESCRIPTION
A sense perception for which no external stimuli exist; can have an organic or functional etiology

TYPES
Visual
Seeing things that are not there
Auditory
Hearing voices when none are present
Olfactory
Smelling smells that do not exist
Tactile
Feeling touch sensations in the absence of stimuli
Gustatory
Experiencing taste in the absence of stimuli

INTERVENTIONS
Ask the client directly about the hallucination.
Avoid reacting to the hallucination as if it were real.
Decrease stimuli or move the client to another area.
Do not negate the client's experience.
Focus on reality-based topics.
Attempt to engage the client's attention through a concrete activity.
Respond verbally to anything real that the client talks about.
Avoid touching the client.
Monitor for signs of increasing anxiety or agitation, which may indicate that the hallucinations are increasing.

BOX 63-9

Language and Communication Disturbance

Neologism: A new word devised that has special meaning only to the client
Echolalia: Repetition of words or phrases heard from another person
Verbigeration: Purposeless repetition of words or phrases
Clang association: Repetition of words or phrases that are similar in sound but in no other way
Word salad: Form of speech in which words or phrases are connected meaninglessly
Pressured speech: Speaks as if the words are being forced out quickly
Mutism: Absence of verbal speech

    f. Grimacing mannerisms
    g. Inability to perform activities of daily living (ADLs)
  3. Catatonic schizophrenia
    a. Marked psychomotor disturbances
    b. Immobility
    c. Stupor
    d. Waxy flexibility
    e. Excessive purposeless motor activity

BOX 63-10

Types of Schizophrenia

Paranoid
Disorganized
Catatonic
Undifferentiated
Residual

    f. Echolalia
    g. Automatic obedience
    h. Stereotyped or repetitive behavior
  4. Undifferentiated schizophrenia
    a. Does not meet the criteria for paranoid, disorganized, or catatonic schizophrenia
    b. Delusions and hallucinations
    c. Disorganized speech
    d. Disorganized or catatonic behavior
    e. Flat affect
    f. Social withdrawal
  5. Residual schizophrenia
    a. Diagnosed as schizophrenic in the past
    b. Time limited between attacks but may last for many years
    c. The client exhibits marked social isolation and withdrawal and impaired role functioning
D. Interventions: Box 63-11
E. Interventions: active hallucinations
  1. Monitor for hallucination cues
  2. Intervene with one-on-one contact
  3. Decrease stimuli or move the client to another area
  4. Avoid conveying to the client that others are also experiencing the hallucination
  5. Respond verbally to anything real that the client talks about
  6. Avoid touching the client
  7. Encourage the client to express feelings
  8. During a hallucination, attempt to engage the client's attention through a concrete activity
  9. Accept and do not joke about or judge the client's behavior
  10. Provide easy activities and a structured environment with routine ADLs
  11. Monitor for signs of increasing fear, anxiety, or agitation
  12. Provide **seclusion** as necessary
  13. Administer medications, as prescribed
F. Interventions: Delusions
  1. Interact on the basis of reality
  2. Encourage the client to express feelings
  3. Do not dispute with the client or try to convince the client that delusions are false
  4. Initially initiate activities on a one-on-one basis
  5. Alter hospital routines as necessary, such as using canned or packaged food or food from home
  6. Recognize accomplishments and provide positive feedback for successes

BOX 63-11

Implementation for Schizophrenia

Assess the client's physical needs.

Set limits on the client's behavior when it interferes with others and becomes disruptive.

Maintain a safe environment.

Initiate one-on-one interaction and progress to small groups as tolerated.

Spend time with the client even if the client is unable to respond.

Monitor for altered thought processes.

Maintain ego boundaries and avoid touching the client.

Limit the time of interaction with the client.

Avoid an overly warm approach; a neutral approach is less threatening.

Do not make promises to the client that cannot be kept.

Establish daily routines.

Assist the client to improve grooming and accept responsibility for personal care.

Sit with the client in silence if necessary.

Provide short, brief, and frequent contact with the client.

Tell the client when you are leaving.

Tell the client when you don't understand.

Do not "go along" with the client's delusions or hallucinations.

Provide simple, concrete activities such as puzzles or word games.

Reorient the client as necessary.

Help the client establish what is real and unreal.

Stay with the client if the client is frightened.

Speak to the client in a simple direct and concise manner.

Reassure the client that the environment is safe.

Remove the client from group situations if the client's behavior is too bizarre, disturbing, or dangerous to others.

Set realistic goals.

Initially, do not offer choices to the client, but gradually assist the client in making his or her own decisions.

Use containers for food, especially with the paranoid schizophrenic client.

Provide a radio or tape or CD player at night for insomnia.

Explain to the client everything that is being done.

Set limits on the client's behavior if the client is unable to do so.

Decrease excessive stimuli in the environment.

Monitor for suicide risk.

Assist the client to use alternative means to express feelings, such as through music or art therapy or writing.

BOX 63-12

Types of Paranoid Disorders

Paranoid personality
Paranoid state
Paranoia
Paranoid schizophrenia

B. Behaviors
1. Suspicious and mistrustful
2. Emotionally distant
3. Distorts reality
4. Poor insight
5. Hypervigilance
6. Low self-esteem
7. Highly sensitive, difficulty in admitting own error, and takes pride in being correct
8. Hypercritical and intolerant of others
9. Hostile, aggressive, and quarrelsome
10. Evasive
11. Concrete thinking
C. Delusions
1. Serves a purpose in establishing identity and self-esteem
2. Grandiose and persecutory delusions
3. Process of delusion includes denial, projection, and rationalization
4. As trust in others increases, the need for delusions decreases
D. Types (Box 63-12)
1. Paranoid personality
a. Suspicious
b. Nonpsychotic
c. No hallucinations or delusions
d. No symptoms of schizophrenia
2. Paranoid state
a. Onset abrupt in response to stress and subsides when stress decreases
b. No hallucinations but experiences paranoid delusions
c. May be sensitive and suspicious before the development of delusions
d. Psychotic state
e. No symptoms of schizophrenia
3. Paranoia
a. Client appears normal except for delusional system
b. Single, highly organized delusional system
c. Not bizarre
d. No hallucinations
e. Reserved and sensitive before onset
f. Psychotic state
g. No symptoms of schizophrenia
4. Paranoid schizophrenia
a. Prior to onset, client becomes cold, withdrawn, distrustful, resentful, argumentative, sarcastic, and defiant

X. PARANOID DISORDERS

A. Description
1. The client demonstrates suspiciousness and mistrust of others
2. The client is often viewed by others as hostile, stubborn, and defensive
3. Concrete, pervasive delusional system characterized by persecutory and grandiose beliefs

BOX 63-13

Interventions for Paranoid Disorders

Assess for suicide risk.
Diminish suspicious behavior.
Avoid direct eye contact.
Establish a trusting relationship.
Promote increased self-esteem.
Remain calm, nonthreatening, and nonjudgmental.
Provide continuity of care.
Respond honestly to the client.
Follow through on commitments made to the client.
Acknowledge the client's feelings but tell the client that you do not share his or her interpretation of an event.
Provide a daily schedule of activities.
Assist the client to identify diversionary activities.
Gradually introduce the client to groups.
Refocus conversation to reality-based topics.
Use role playing to help the client identify thoughts and feelings.
Provide positive reinforcement for successes.
Do not argue with delusions.
Use concrete, specific words.
Do not be secretive with the client.
Do not whisper in the client's presence.
Assure the client he or she will be safe.
Involve the client in noncompetitive tasks.
Provide the client with the opportunity to complete small tasks.
Monitor eating, drinking, sleeping, and elimination patterns.
Limit physical contact.
Monitor for agitation and decrease stimuli as needed.

b. Bizarre, numerous, and changeable delusions
c. Delusions become less logical as the client becomes more disorganized
d. Persecutory hallucinations
e. Psychotic state
f. All symptoms of schizophrenia are present
E. Interventions (Box 63-13)

XI. PERSONALITY DISORDERS

A. Description
  1. Includes various inflexible maladaptive behavior patterns or traits that may impair functioning and relationships
  2. The individual usually remains in touch with reality and typically has a lack of insight into his or her behavior
  3. Stress exacerbates manifestations of the personality disorder
  4. In severe cases, the personality disorder may deteriorate to a psychotic state
B. Characteristics
  1. Poor impulse control
    a. Acting out to manage internal pain

b. Forms of acting out include physical and verbal attacks, manipulation, substance **abuse**, promiscuous sexual behaviors, and **suicide attempts**
  2. Mood characteristics
    a. Experiences abandonment and depression
    b. Moods include rage, guilt, fear, and emptiness
  3. Impaired judgment
    a. Has difficulty with problem solving
    b. Unable to perceive the consequences of behavior
  4. Impaired reality testing: Distorts reality and often projects own feelings onto others
  5. Impaired object relations: Rigid and inflexible and has difficulty in intimate relationships
  6. Impaired self-perception: Distorted self-perception; experiences self-hate or self-idealization
  7. Impaired thought processes
    a. Concrete or diffuse thinking
    b. Difficulty concentrating
    c. Impaired memory
  8. Impaired stimulus barrier
    a. Unable to regulate incoming sensory stimuli
    b. Increased excitability
    c. Excessive response to noise and light
    d. Poor attention span
    e. Agitated
    f. Insomnia
C. Schizoid personality disorder
  1. Description: Characterized by an inability to form warm, close social relationships
  2. Data collection
    a. Social detachment and lack of close relationships
    b. Interest in solitary activities
    c. Aloof and indifferent
    d. Restricted expression of emotions
    e. Lack of interest in others
D. Schizotypal personality disorder
  1. Description: Exhibits abnormal or highly unusual thoughts, perceptions, speech, and behavior patterns
  2. Data collection
    a. Suspicious
    b. Paranoid
    c. Magical thinking
    d. Odd thinking and speech
    e. Relationship deficits
E. Paranoid personality disorder
  1. Description: Characterized by suspiciousness and mistrust of others
  2. Data collection
    a. Suspicious and distrustful
    b. Argumentative
    c. Hostile aloofness
    d. Rigid, critical, and controlling of others
    e. Grandiosity

F. Histrionic personality disorder
1. Description
a. Characterized by overly dramatic and intensely expressive behavior
b. The client is lively and dramatic and enjoys being the center of attention
c. Interpersonal relations may be poor
2. Data collection
a. Attention seeking
b. Needs to be the center of attention
c. Sexually seductive or provocative
d. Self-dramatizing and theatrical
e. Overly concerned with appearance
f. Has romantic fantasies and controls partners
g. Bores easily
h. Displays dependency
G. Narcissistic personality disorder
1. Description
a. Characterized by an increased sense of self-importance
b. The client is preoccupied with fantasies and unlimited success and has a constant need for attention and admiration
2. Data collection
a. Grandiosity
b. Requires admiration and inflated accomplishments
c. Overestimates abilities and underestimates contributions of others
d. Lacks empathy and sensitivity to needs of others
H. Avoidant personality disorder
1. Description: Characterized by social withdrawal and extreme sensitivity to potential rejection
2. Data collection
a. Feelings of inadequacy
b. Hypersensitive to reactions of others and reacts poorly to criticism
c. Social inhibition
d. Lack of support system
I. Dependent personality disorder
1. Description
a. The individual lacks self-confidence and the ability to function independently
b. Passively allow others to make decisions and assume responsibility for major areas in his or her life
2. Data collection
a. Difficulty making decisions
b. Lacks autonomy
c. Cannot tolerate being alone and must always have a close relationship
d. Needs others to assume responsibility and make decisions
J. Obsessive-compulsive personality disorder
1. Description: The client has difficulty expressing warm and tender emotions and reflects

perfectionism, stubbornness, need to control others, and a devotion to work
2. Data collection
a. Orderliness and perfectionism
b. Overly conscientious
c. Inflexible and preoccupied with details and rules
d. Devoted to work and lacks leisure activities and friendships
e. Miserly and stubborn
f. Hoards worthless objects
K. Antisocial personality disorder
1. Description
a. A pattern of irresponsible and antisocial behavior
b. Characterized by selfishness, inability to maintain lasting relationships, poor sexual adjustment, failure to accept social norms, irritability, and aggressiveness
2. Data collection
a. Perceives the world as hostile
b. Superficial charm and hostility
c. No shame or guilt
d. Self-centered
e. Unreliable
f. Easily bored
g. Poor work history
h. Unable to tolerate frustration
i. Views others as objects to be manipulated
j. Poor judgment
k. Impulsive
L. Borderline personality disorder
1. Description
a. Characterized by instability in interpersonal relationships, mood, and self-image
b. Behavior may be impulsive and unpredictable
2. Data collection
a. Unclear identity
b. Unstable and intense
c. Extreme shifts in mood
d. Easily angered
e. Easily bored
f. Argumentative
g. Depression
h. Self-destructive behavior
i. Manipulation
j. Unable to tolerate anxiety
k. Chronic feelings of emptiness and fear of being alone
l. Splitting
M. Passive-aggressive personality disorder
1. Description
a. Characterized by passively expressing covert aggression rather than dealing with it directly
b. The behavior can interfere with both social and work activities

2. Data collection
   a. Procrastination
   b. Stubbornness
   c. Intentional inefficiency
   d. Forgetfulness
   e. Dependency

▲ N. Interventions
   1. Maintain safety against self-destructive behaviors
   2. Allow the client to make choices and be as independent as possible
   3. Encourage the client to discuss feelings rather than act them out
   4. Provide consistency in response to the client's acting-out behaviors
   5. Discuss expectations and responsibilities with the client
   6. Discuss the consequences that will follow certain behaviors
   7. Inform the client that harm to self, others, and property is unacceptable
   8. Identify splitting behavior
   9. Assist the client to deal directly with anger
   10. Develop a written contract with the client
   11. Encourage the client to keep a journal recording daily feelings
   12. Encourage the client to participate in group activities, and praise nonmanipulative behavior
   13. Set and maintain limits to decrease manipulative behavior
   14. Remove the client from group situations in which attention-seeking behaviors occur
   15. Provide realistic praise for positive behaviors in social situations

▲

XII. COGNITIVE IMPAIRMENT DISORDERS
A. Autism: See Chapter 30
B. Attention deficit hyperactivity disorder (ADHD): See Chapter 30
C. Tourette's disorder: See Chapter 30
D. Dementia and Alzheimer's disease
   1. Dementia
      a. Organic syndrome with progressive deterioration in intellectual functioning
      b. Long- and short-term memory loss occur, with impairment in judgment, abstract thinking, problem-solving ability, and behavior
      c. Results in a self-care deficit
      d. The most common type of dementia is Alzheimer's disease
   2. Alzheimer's disease (Box 63-14)
      a. An irreversible form of senile dementia resulting from nerve cell deterioration
      b. Individuals with Alzheimer's disease experience cognitive deterioration and progressive loss of ability to carry out ADLs

---

BOX 63-14

Alzheimer's Disease

Agnosia: Failure to recognize or identify objects despite intact sensory function
Amnesia: Inability to learn new information or to recall previously learned information
Aphasia: Language disturbance in understanding and expressing the spoken word
Apraxia: Inability to perform motor activities despite intact motor function

---

      c. The client experiences a steady decline in physical and mental functioning; usually requires nursing home placement in the final stages of the illness
   3. Interventions ▲
      a. Identify and reinforce retained skills
      b. Provide continuity of care
      c. Orient to the environment
      d. Furnish environment with familiar possessions
      e. Acknowledge the client's feelings
      f. Assist the client and family members to manage memory deficits and behavior changes
      g. Encourage the family members to express feelings about caregiving
      h. Provide the caregiver support and identify the resources and support groups available
      i. Monitor ADLs
      j. Remind how to perform self-care activities
      k. Maintain independence
      l. Provide consistent routines
      m. Provide exercise such as walking with an escort
      n. Avoid activities that tax the memory
      o. Allow plenty of time to complete a task
      p. Use constant encouragement in a step-by-step approach
      q. Provide activities that occupy time, such as listening to music, and watching television
      r. Provide mental stimulation with simple games or activities
   4. Wandering ▲
      a. Provide a safe environment
      b. Prevent unsafe wandering
      c. Provide close supervision
      d. Close and secure doors
      e. Use identification bracelets and electronic surveillance
   5. Communication ▲
      a. Adapt to the communication level of the client
      b. Use a firm volume and a low-pitched voice to communicate
      c. Stand directly in front of the client and maintain eye contact
      d. Call the client by name and identify yourself; wait for a response

e. Use a calm and reassuring voice

f. Use pantomime gestures if the client is unable to understand spoken words

g. Use slow, clear, verbal communication techniques

h. Use short words and simple sentences

i. Ask only one question at a time and give one direction at a time

j. Repeat questions if necessary but do not rephrase

6. Impaired judgment

   a. Remove throw rugs, toxic substances, and dangerous electrical appliances from the environment

   b. Reduce hot water heater temperature

7. Altered thought processes

   a. Call the client by name

   b. Orient the client frequently

   c. Use familiar objects in the room

   d. Place a calendar and clock in a visible place

   e. Maintain familiar routines

   f. Allow the client to reminisce

   g. Make tasks simple

   h. Allow time for the client to complete a task

   i. Provide positive reinforcement for positive behaviors

8. Altered sleep patterns

   a. Allow client to wander in a safe place until they become tired

   b. Prevent shadows in the room

   c. Avoid the use of hypnotics, because they cause confusion and aggravate the sundown effect

9. Agitation

   a. Determine the precipitant of the agitation

   b. Reassure the client

   c. Remove items that can be hazardous during the time of agitation

   d. Approach the client slowly and calmly from the front; then speak, gesture, and move slowly

   e. Remove the client to a less stressful environment

   f. Use touch gently

   g. Do not argue with the client or restrain the client

   h. Distract the client with questions about the problem and gradually turn his or her attention to something else

XIII. PSYCHOSEXUAL ALTERATIONS

A. Sexuality

1. One's sense of being a sexual individual

2. Includes how one looks, behaves, and relates to others

B. Sexual expression (Box 63-15)

C. Alterations in sexual behavior

1. Transsexualism: Feeling that one's sex is inappropriate and desiring to acquire sexual characteristics of the opposite sex

---

BOX 63-15

Sexual Expression

Bisexuality: Sexual attraction to and activity with both sexes

Heterosexuality: Male-female sexual relationships

Homosexuality: Sexual attraction to a member of the same sex

Transvestism: Obsession with wearing clothing of the opposite sex

---

2. Exhibitionism: Sexual urges and fantasies of exposing the genitals to strangers

3. Fetishism: Using nonliving objects for sexual gratification

4. Pedophilia: Desiring sexual activity with a child younger than 13 years of age

5. Sexual masochism: Sexual gratification that involves receiving pain

6. Sexual sadism: Sexual gratification that involves inflicting pain

7. Voyeurism: Sexual gratification through observing others disrobing or engaging in sexual activity

8. Zoophilia: Intense sexual arousal or desire for sexual contact with animals

9. Frotteurism: Intense sexual arousal or desire when rubbing against a nonconsenting person

D. Interventions

1. Data collection regarding sexual history and precipitating event for sexual disorder

2. Encourage the client to explore personal beliefs

3. Provide a nonjudgmental attitude

4. Provide supportive psychotherapy

PRACTICE QUESTIONS

1. A nurse collects data on a client with a diagnosis of bipolar affective disorder–mania. The finding that requires the nurse's immediate intervention is:

   1. The client's outlandish behaviors and inappropriate dress

   2. The client's grandiose delusions of being a royal descendant of King Arthur

   3. The client's nonstop physical activity and poor nutritional intake

   4. The client's constant, incessant talking that includes sexual innuendoes and teasing the staff

2. A client in a manic state emerges from her room. She is topless and is making sexual remarks and gestures toward staff and peers. The appropriate nursing action is to:

   1. Quietly approach the client, escort her to her room, and assist her in getting dressed

   2. Approach the client in the hallway and insist that she go to her room

3. Confront the client on the inappropriateness of her behaviors and offer her a time-out
4. Ask the other clients to ignore her behavior; eventually she will return to her room

3. A nurse reviews the activity schedule for the day and determines that the best activity that the manic client could participate in is:
   1. A brown bag lunch and a book review
   2. Ping-Pong
   3. A paint by number activity
   4. A deep breathing and progressive relaxation group

4. A client who is delusional says to the nurse, "The federal guards were sent to kill me." The nurse should make which appropriate response to the client?
   1. "The guards are not out to kill you."
   2. "I don't believe this is true."
   3. "I don't know anything about the guards. Do you feel afraid that people are trying to hurt you?"
   4. "What makes you think the guards were sent to hurt you?"

5. A woman comes into the emergency room in a severe state of anxiety following a car accident. The most important nursing intervention is to:
   1. Remain with the client
   2. Put the client in a quiet room
   3. Teach the client deep breathing
   4. Encourage the client to talk about her feelings and concerns

6. A male client with delirium becomes agitated and confused in his room at night. The best initial intervention by the nurse is to:
   1. Use a night-light and turn off the television
   2. Keep the television and a soft light on during the night
   3. Move the client next to the nurse's station
   4. Play soft music during the night and maintain a well-lit room

7. A nurse is collecting data on a client who is actively hallucinating. Which nursing statement would be therapeutic at this time?
   1. "I talked to the voices you're hearing and they won't hurt you now."
   2. "I can hear the voice and she wants you to come to dinner."
   3. "Sometimes people hear things or voices others can't hear."
   4. "I know you feel 'they are out to get you' but it's not true."

8. A nurse is caring for a client with a diagnosis of depression. The nurse monitors for signs of constipation and urinary retention, knowing that these problems are most likely caused by:
   1. Inadequate dietary intake and dehydration
   2. Lack of exercise and poor diet
   3. Poor dietary choices
   4. Psychomotor retardation and side effects of medication

9. A client is admitted to the inpatient unit and is being considered for electroconvulsive therapy (ECT). The client appears calm, but the family is hypervigilant and anxious. The client's mother begins to cry and states, "My son's brain will be destroyed. How can the doctor do this to him?" The nurse makes which therapeutic response?
   1. "It sounds as though you need to speak to the psychiatrist."
   2. "Your son has decided to have this treatment. You should be supportive of him."
   3. "Perhaps you'd like to see the ECT room and speak to the staff."
   4. "It sounds as though you have some concerns about the ECT procedure. Why don't we sit down together and discuss any concerns you may have."

10. A nurse is caring for a client who has been treated with long-term antipsychotic medication. As part of the nursing care plan, the nurse monitors for tardive dyskinesia. In the event that tardive dyskinesia occurs, the nurse would most likely observe:
    1. Abnormal movements and involuntary movements of the mouth, tongue, and face
    2. Abnormal breathing through the nostrils
    3. Severe headache, flushing, tremor, and ataxia
    4. Severe hypertension, migraine headache, and "marbles in the mouth" syndrome

11. A client who is diagnosed with pedophilia and has been recently paroled as a sex offender says, "I'm in treatment and I have served my time. Now this group has posters of me all over the neighborhood telling about me with my picture on it." Which of the following is an appropriate response by the nurse?
    1. "You understand that people fear for their children, but you're feeling unfairly treated?"
    2. "When children are hurt as you hurt them, people want you isolated."
    3. "You seem angry but you have committed serious crimes against several children, so your neighbors are frightened."
    4. "You're lucky it doesn't escalate into something pretty scary after your crime."

12. A nurse is preparing for the hospital discharge of a client with a history of command hallucinations to harm self or others. The nurse instructs the client about interventions for hallucinations and anxiety and determines that the client understands the interventions when the client states:
    1. "My medications won't make me anxious."
    2. "I can call my therapist when I'm hallucinating so that I can talk about my feelings and plans and not hurt anyone."
    3. "I'll go to support group and talk so that I won't hurt anyone."
    4. "I won't get anxious or hear things if I get enough sleep and eat well."

13. A nurse observes that a client is psychotic, pacing, agitated, and making aggressive gestures. The client's speech pattern is rapid and the client's affect is belligerent. Based on these observations, the nurse's immediate priority of care is to:
    1. Provide safety for the client and other clients on the unit
    2. Offer the client a less stimulated area to calm down and gain control
    3. Provide the clients on the unit with a sense of comfort and safety
    4. Assist the staff in caring for the client in a controlled environment

14. A nurse is caring for a client diagnosed with catatonic stupor. The client is lying on the bed, with the body pulled into a fetal position. The appropriate nursing intervention is which of the following?
    1. Leave the client alone and intermittently check on him
    2. Take the client into the dayroom with other clients so they can help watch him
    3. Sit beside the client in silence and verbalize occasional open-ended questions
    4. Ask direct questions to encourage talking

15. A mother of a teenage client with an anxiety disorder is concerned about her daughter's progress on discharge. She states that her daughter "stashes food, eats all the wrong things that make her hyperactive," and "hangs out with the wrong crowd." In helping the mother prepare for her daughter's discharge, the nurse advises the mother to:
    1. Restrict the daughter's socializing time with her friends
    2. Consider taking time from work to help her daughter readjust to the home environment
    3. Restrict the amount of chocolate and caffeine products in the home
    4. Keep her daughter out of school until she can adjust to the school environment

16. A client is unwilling to go out of the house for fear of "doing something crazy in public." Because of this fear, the client remains homebound except when accompanied outside by the spouse. The nurse determines that the client has:
    1. Social phobia
    2. Agoraphobia
    3. Claustrophobia
    4. Hypochondriasis

17. A client has reported that crying spells have been a major problem over the past several weeks, and that the doctor said that depression is probably the reason. The nurse observes that the client is sitting slumped in the chair and the clothes that the client is wearing don't fit well. The nurse interprets that further data collection should focus on:
    1. Sleep patterns
    2. Onset of the crying spells

3. Weight loss
4. Medication compliance

18. A client was admitted to a medical unit with acute blindness. Many tests are performed and there seems to be no organic reason why this client cannot see. The nurse later learns that the client became blind after witnessing a hit-and-run car crash, in which a family of three was killed. The nurse suspects that the client may be experiencing a:
    1. Psychosis
    2. Conversion disorder
    3. Dissociative disorder
    4. Repression

19. A manic client announces to everyone in the dayroom that a stripper is coming to perform that evening. When the psychiatric aide firmly states that this will not happen, the manic client becomes verbally abusive and threatens physical violence to the aide. Based on the analysis of this situation, the nurse determines that the most appropriate action would be to:
    1. Escort the manic client to his or her room, with assistance, and administer PRN haloperidol (Haldol)
    2. Tell the client that smoking privileges are revoked for 24 hours
    3. Orient the client to time, person, and place
    4. Tell the client that the behavior is not appropriate

20. A nurse notes documentation in a client's record that the client is experiencing delusions of persecution. The nurse understands that these types of delusions are characteristic of which of the following?
    1. The false belief that one is a very powerful person
    2. The false belief that one is a very important person
    3. The false belief that one's partner is going out with other people
    4. The false belief that one is being singled out for harm by others

ALTERNATE FORMAT QUESTION: MULTIPLE RESPONSE

Select all nursing interventions for a hospitalized client with mania who is exhibiting manipulative behavior.

___ Communicate expected behaviors to the client
___ Enforce rules and inform the client that she will not be allowed to attend therapy groups
___ Ensure that the client knows that she is not in charge of the nursing unit
___ Be clear with the client regarding the consequences of exceeding limits set regarding behavior
___ Assist client in testing out alternative behaviors for obtaining needs

ANSWERS

1. *Answer:* 3

Rationale: Mania is a mood characterized by excitement, euphoria, hyperactivity, excessive energy, decreased need for sleep, and impaired ability to concentrate or complete a single train of thought. It is a period when the mood is predominantly elevated, expansive, or irritable. Option 3 identifies a physiological need requiring immediate intervention.

Test-Taking Strategy: Use the process of elimination and note the key words, *immediate intervention.* Use Maslow's Hierarchy of Needs theory to assist in answering the question. Option 3 indicates a potential disruption in the client's physiological status. Review care of the client with mania if you had difficulty with this question.

Level of Cognitive Ability: Comprehension
Client Needs: Psychosocial Integrity
Integrated Process: Nursing Process/Data Collection
Content Area: Mental Health
Reference: Morrison-Valfre, M. (2005). *Foundations of mental health care* (3rd ed.). St. Louis: Mosby, pp. 214-215.

2. *Answer:* 1

Rationale: A person who is experiencing mania lacks insight and judgment, has poor impulse control, and is highly excitable. The nurse must take control without creating increased stress or anxiety to the client. A quiet, firm approach while distracting the client (walking her to her room and assisting her to get dressed) achieves the goal of having her being dressed appropriately and preserving her psychosocial integrity. Option 4 is inappropriate. "Insisting" that the client go to her room may meet with a great deal of resistance. Confronting the client and offering her a consequence of "time-out" may be meaningless to her.

Test-Taking Strategy: Use the process of elimination and focus on the issue of the question. Noting that the issue relates to having the client dress appropriately will direct you to option 1. Review care of the client with mania if you had difficulty with this question.

Level of Cognitive Ability: Application
Client Needs: Psychosocial Integrity
Integrated Process: Nursing Process/Implementation
Content Area: Mental Health
Reference: Morrison-Valfre, M. (2005). *Foundations of mental health care* (3rd ed.). St. Louis: Mosby, p. 221.

3. *Answer:* 2

Rationale: A person who is experiencing mania is overactive, full of energy, lacks concentration, and has poor impulse control. The client needs an activity that will allow him or her to utilize excess energy, but not endanger others during the process. Options 1, 3, and 4 are relatively sedate activities that require concentration, a quality that is lacking in the manic state. Such activities may lead to increased frustration and anxiety for the client. Ping-Pong is an activity that will help to expend the increased energy this client is experiencing.

Test-Taking Strategy: Use the process of elimination. Note the similarity in options 1, 3, and 4 in that they are relatively sedate activities that require concentration. Review the appropriate interventions for a manic client if you had difficulty with this question.

Level of Cognitive Ability: Application
Client Needs: Psychosocial Integrity
Integrated Process: Nursing Process/Implementation
Content Area: Mental Health
Reference: Stuart, G., & Laraia, M. (2005). *Principles and practice of psychiatric nursing* (8th ed.). St. Louis: Mosby, p. 355.

4. *Answer:* 3

Rationale: Disagreeing with delusions may make the client more defensive and the client may cling to the delusions even more. It is most therapeutic for the nurse to empathize with the client's experience. Options 1 and 2 are statements that disagree with the client. Option 4 encourages discussion regarding the delusion.

Test-Taking Strategy: Use therapeutic communication techniques for the client experiencing delusions. Eliminate options 1 and 2 because they are similar and are statements that disagree with the client. Option 4 encourages discussion regarding the delusion. Review communication techniques for the client experiencing delusions if you had difficulty with this question.

Level of Cognitive Ability: Application
Client Needs: Psychosocial Integrity
Integrated Process: Communication and Documentation
Content Area: Mental Health
Reference: Morrison-Valfre, M. (2005). *Foundations of mental health care* (3rd ed.). St. Louis: Mosby, pp. 88, 100.

5. *Answer:* 1

Rationale: If a client is left alone with severe anxiety, he or she may feel abandoned and become overwhelmed. Placing the client in a quiet room is also indicated, but the nurse must stay with the client. It is not possible to teach the client deep breathing until the anxiety decreases. Encouraging the client to discuss concerns and feelings would not take place until the anxiety has decreased.

Test-Taking Strategy: Use the process of elimination. Note the key words, *severe* and *most important nursing intervention.* Eliminate options 3 and 4 first, knowing that these actions are not possible when the client is in a severe state of anxiety. From the remaining options, remember the most important intervention is to remain with the client. Review care of the client with severe anxiety if you had difficulty with this question.

Level of Cognitive Ability: Application
Client Needs: Psychosocial Integrity
Integrated Process: Nursing Process/Implementation
Content Area: Mental Health
References: Morrison-Valfre, M. (2005). *Foundations of mental health care* (3rd ed.). St. Louis: Mosby, p. 189.
Stuart, G., & Laraia, M. (2005). *Principles and practice of psychiatric nursing* (8th ed.). St. Louis: Mosby, p. 278.

6. *Answer:* 1

Rationale: It is important to provide a consistent daily routine and a low-stimulation environment when the client is agitated and confused. Noise levels including a radio and television may add to the confusion and disorientation. Moving the client next to the nurses' station is not the initial intervention.

Test-Taking Strategy: Use the process of elimination and note the key word, *initial,* in the stem of the question.

Eliminate options 2 and 4 first because they are similar. From the remaining options, recalling that a low-stimulation environment is best will direct you to option 1. Review measures related to the client with agitation and confusion if you had difficulty with this question.
Level of Cognitive Ability: Application
Client Needs: Psychosocial Integrity
Integrated Process: Nursing Process/Implementation
Content Area: Mental Health
Reference: Morrison-Valfre, M. (2005). *Foundations of mental health care* (3rd ed.). St. Louis: Mosby, pp. 168-169.

7. *Answer:* **3**
Rationale: It is important for the nurse to reinforce reality with the client. Options 1, 2, and 4 do not reinforce reality but reinforce the hallucination that the voices are real.
Test-Taking Strategy: Use the process of elimination. Note that options 1, 2, and 4 all indicate reinforcement to the client that the voices are real. Option 3 is the only statement that indicates reality. Review nursing interventions related to the client who is hallucinating if you had difficulty with this question.
Level of Cognitive Ability: Application
Client Needs: Psychosocial Integrity
Integrated Process: Communication and Documentation
Content Area: Mental Health
Reference: Morrison-Valfre, M. (2005). *Foundations of mental health care* (3rd ed.). St. Louis: Mosby, pp. 88, 328.

8. *Answer:* **4**
Rationale: Constipation can be related to inadequate food intake, lack of exercise, and poor diet. In this situation, urinary retention is most likely due to medications. Option 4 is the only option that addresses both constipation and urinary retention.
Test-Taking Strategy: Use the process of elimination and focus on the data in the question. Options 1, 2, and 3 are all similar and address diet. Option 4 addresses both concerns, constipation and urinary retention. If you had difficulty with this question, review the interventions for a client with depression and the effects of medications prescribed for this disorder.
Level of Cognitive Ability: Analysis
Client Needs: Physiological Integrity
Integrated Process: Nursing Process/Data Collection
Content Area: Mental Health
Reference: Morrison-Valfre, M. (2005). *Foundations of mental health care* (3rd ed.). St. Louis: Mosby, pp. 220, 336.

9. *Answer:* **4**
Rationale: The nurse needs to encourage the family and client to verbalize their fears and concerns. Option 4 is the only option that encourages verbalization. Options 1, 2, and 3 avoid dealing with the client or family concerns.
Test-Taking Strategy: Use therapeutic communication techniques and focus on the client's feelings and concerns. This will direct you to option 4. Review these techniques if you had difficulty with this question.
Level of Cognitive Ability: Application
Client Needs: Psychosocial Integrity
Integrated Process: Nursing Process/Implementation

Content Area: Mental Health
Reference: Morrison-Valfre, M. (2005). *Foundations of mental health care* (3rd ed.). St. Louis: Mosby, pp. 88, 218.

10. *Answer:* **1**
Rationale: Tardive dyskinesia is a severe reaction associated with the long-term use of antipsychotic medication. The clinical manifestations are abnormal movements (dyskinesia) and involuntary movements of the mouth, tongue, and face. In its more severe form, tardive dyskinesia involves the fingers, arms, trunk, and respiratory muscles. When this occurs, the medication is discontinued.
Test-Taking Strategy: Knowledge regarding the clinical manifestations of tardive dyskinesia is required to answer this question. Remember, tardive dyskinesia involves abnormal and involuntary movements. If you had difficulty with this question, review the characteristics associated with this reaction.
Level of Cognitive Ability: Comprehension
Client Needs: Physiological Integrity
Integrated Process: Nursing Process/Data Collection
Content Area: Mental Health
Reference: Morrison-Valfre, M. (2005). *Foundations of mental health care* (3rd ed.). St. Louis: Mosby, pp. 334-335.

11. *Answer:* **1**
Rationale: Focusing and verbalizing the implied concern is the therapeutic response because it assists the client to clarify thinking and re-examine what the client is really saying. Option 1 is the only option that reflects the use of this therapeutic communication technique. Option 2 is insensitive and anxiety-provoking. Option 3 does not facilitate the client's expression of feelings. Option 4 gives advice and also does not facilitate the client's expression of feelings.
Test-Taking Strategy: Use therapeutic communication techniques to answer the question. Remembering to focus on the client's feelings and concerns will direct you to option 1. Review these techniques if you had difficulty with this question.
Level of Cognitive Ability: Application
Client Needs: Psychosocial Integrity
Integrated Process: Communication and Documentation
Content Area: Mental Health
Reference: Morrison-Valfre, M. (2005). *Foundations of mental health care* (3rd ed.). St. Louis: Mosby, p. 88, 310.

12. *Answer:* **2**
Rationale: There may be an increased risk for impulsive and/or aggressive behavior if a client is receiving command hallucinations to harm self or others. Talking about the auditory hallucinations can interfere with the subvocal muscular activity associated with a hallucination. Option 2 is a specific agreement to seek help and evidences self-responsible commitment and control over his or her own behavior.
Test-Taking Strategy: Use the process of elimination. Note the relation between the word "hallucinations" in the question and in the correct option. Review care of the client with command hallucinations if you had difficulty with this question.
Level of Cognitive Ability: Comprehension
Client Needs: Psychosocial Integrity
Integrated Process: Teaching/Learning

Content Area: Mental Health
Reference: Morrison-Valfre, M. (2005). *Foundations of mental health care* (3rd ed.). St. Louis: Mosby, p. 331.

13. Answer: 1
Rationale: Safety to the client and other clients is the priority. Option 1 is the only option that addresses the client and other clients' safety needs. Option 2 addresses the client's needs. Option 3 addresses other clients' needs. Option 4 is not client-centered.
Test-Taking Strategy: Use the process of elimination and focus on the issue, safety. Option 1 is the umbrella (global) option and addresses the safety of all. Review care of the psychotic client if you had difficulty with this question.
Level of Cognitive Ability: Application
Client Needs: Safe, Effective Care Environment
Integrated Process: Nursing Process/Implementation
Content Area: Mental Health
References: Morrison-Valfre, M. (2005). *Foundations of mental health care* (3rd ed.). St. Louis: Mosby, p. 116.
Stuart, G., & Laraia, M. (2005). *Principles and practice of psychiatric nursing* (8th ed.). St. Louis: Mosby, p. 721.

14. Answer: 3
Rationale: Clients with catatonic stupor may be immobile and mute and require consistent, repeated approaches. The nurse facilitates communication with the client by sitting in silence, asking open-ended questions, and pausing to provide opportunities for the client to respond. The nurse would not leave the client alone. Option 2 relies on other clients to care for this client and this is an inappropriate expectation. Asking direct questions of this client is not therapeutic. Option 3 is the best action because it provides for client supervision and communication as appropriate.
Test-Taking Strategy: Use the process of elimination. Eliminate option 1 because the nurse would not leave the client alone. Eliminate option 2 next because this action relies on other clients to care for this client. Eliminate option 4 because asking direct questions of this client is not therapeutic. Review care of the client with catatonic stupor if you had difficulty with this question.
Level of Cognitive Ability: Application
Client Needs: Psychosocial Integrity
Integrated Process: Nursing Process/Implementation
Content Area: Mental Health
References: Fortinash, K., & Holoday-Worret, P. (2004). *Psychiatric mental health nursing* (3rd ed.). St. Louis: Mosby, p. 250.
Morrison-Valfre, M. (2005). *Foundations of mental health care* (3rd ed.). St. Louis: Mosby, p. 328.

15. Answer: 3
Rationale: Clients with anxiety disorder should abstain from or limit their intake of caffeine, chocolate, and alcohol. These products have the potential of increasing anxiety. Options 1 and 4 are unreasonable and are an unhealthy approach. It may not be realistic for a family member to take time away from work.
Test-Taking Strategy: Use the process of elimination. Options 1, 2, and 4 are similar and are concerned with monitoring or curtailing the client's physical activities. Option 3 addresses preparation of the client's environment and focuses on the concern or issue expressed in the question. Review discharge planning for the client with anxiety if you had difficulty with this question.
Level of Cognitive Ability: Application
Client Needs: Health Promotion and Maintenance
Integrated Process: Teaching/Learning
Content Area: Mental Health
Reference: Stuart, G., & Laraia, M. (2005). *Principles and practice of psychiatric nursing* (8th ed.). St. Louis: Mosby, pp. 266, 487.

16. Answer: 2
Rationale: Agoraphobia is a fear of being alone in open or public places where escape might be difficult. Agoraphobia includes experiencing fear or a sense of helplessness or embarrassment if a phobic attack occurs. Avoidance of such situations usually results in the reduction of social and professional interactions. Social phobia focuses more on specific situations, such as the fear of speaking, performing, or eating in public. Claustrophobia is a fear of closed-in places. Clients with hypochondriacal symptoms focus their anxiety on physical complaints and are preoccupied with their health.
Test-Taking Strategy: Use the process of elimination and focus on the data in the question. Recalling the specific types of phobias and associated client behaviors will direct you to option 2. If you had difficulty with this question, review phobia types and associated client behaviors.
Level of Cognitive Ability: Comprehension
Client Needs: Psychosocial Integrity
Integrated Process: Nursing Process/Data Collection
Content Area: Mental Health
Reference: Morrison-Valfre, M. (2005). *Foundations of mental health care* (3rd ed.). St. Louis: Mosby, pp. 185-186.

17. Answer: 3
Rationale: All the options are possible issues to address; however, the weight loss is the first item that needs further data collection because ill-fitting clothing could indicate a problem with nutrition. The client has already told the nurse that the crying spells have been a problem. Medication or sleep patterns are not mentioned or addressed in the question.
Test-Taking Strategy: Use the process of elimination and Maslow's Hierarchy of Needs theory to answer the question. Focusing on the data in the question will assist in eliminating options 1, 2, and 4. Review the priorities of care for a client with depression if you had difficulty with this question.
Level of Cognitive Ability: Analysis
Client Needs: Physiological Integrity
Integrated Process: Nursing Process/Data Collection
Content Area: Mental Health
Reference: Morrison-Valfre, M. (2005). *Foundations of mental health care* (3rd ed.). St. Louis: Mosby, p. 215.

18. Answer: 2
Rationale: A conversion disorder is the alteration or loss of a physical function that cannot be explained by any known pathophysiological mechanism. It is thought to be an expression of a psychological need or conflict. In this situation,

the client witnessed an accident that was so psychologically painful that the client became blind. A dissociative disorder is a disturbance or alteration in the normally integrative functions of identity, memory, or consciousness. Psychosis is a state in which a person's mental capacity to recognize reality, communicate, and relate to others is impaired, thus interfering with the person's capacity to deal with life's demands. Repression is a coping mechanism in which unacceptable feelings are kept out of awareness.
Test-Taking Strategy: Use the process of elimination. Noting that the client evidences no organic reason to account for the blindness will direct you to option 2. If you had difficulty with this question, review conversion disorders and defense mechanisms.
Level of Cognitive Ability: Comprehension
Client Needs: Psychosocial Integrity
Integrated Process: Nursing Process/Data Collection
Content Area: Mental Health
Reference: Morrison-Valfre, M. (2005). *Foundations of mental health care* (3rd ed.). St. Louis: Mosby, pp. 229-230.

19. *Answer:* **1**
Rationale: The client is at risk for injury to self and others and therefore should be escorted out of the dayroom. Hyperactive and agitated behavior usually responds to haloperidol (Haldol). Option 2 may increase the agitation that already exists in this client. Orientation will not halt the behavior. Telling the client that the behavior is not appropriate has already been attempted by the psychiatric aide.
Test-Taking Strategy: Use the process of elimination and therapeutic interventions for the manic client. Options 2, 3, and 4 will not de-escalate the client's agitation. If you had difficulty with this question, review the appropriate interventions in dealing with a manic client.
Level of Cognitive Ability: Application
Client Needs: Psychosocial Integrity
Integrated Process: Nursing Process/Implementation
Content Area: Mental Health
Reference: Stuart, G., & Laraia, M. (2005). *Principles and practice of psychiatric nursing* (8th ed.). St. Louis: Mosby, p. 351.

20. *Answer:* **4**
Rationale: A delusion is a false belief held to be true even when there is evidence to the contrary. A delusion of persecution is the thought that one is being singled out for harm by others. A delusion of grandeur is the false belief that he or she is a very powerful and important person. A delusion

of jealousy is the false belief that one's partner is going out with other people.
Test-Taking Strategy: Use the process of elimination. Eliminate options 1 and 2 first, because they are similar. From the remaining options, note the relationship between the word "persecution" in the question and the description in option 4. Review the description of the types of delusions if you had difficulty with this question.
Level of Cognitive Ability: Comprehension
Client Needs: Psychosocial Integrity
Integrated Process: Nursing Process/Data Collection
Content Area: Mental Health
Reference: Mosby's medical, nursing, and allied health dictionary (6th ed.). (2005). St. Louis: Mosby, p. 490.

ALTERNATE FORMAT QUESTION: MULTIPLE RESPONSE
Answers:
Communicate expected behaviors to the client
Be clear with the client regarding the consequences of exceeding limits set regarding behavior
Assist client in testing out alternative behaviors for obtaining needs
Rationale: Interventions for dealing with the client exhibiting manipulative behavior include setting clear, consistent, and enforceable limits on manipulative behaviors; being clear with the client regarding the consequences of exceeding limits set; following through with the consequences in a nonpunitive manner; and assisting the client in identifying personal strengths and in testing out alternative behaviors for obtaining needs. Enforcing rules and informing the client that she will not be allowed to attend therapy groups is a violation of the client's rights. Ensuring that the client knows that she is not in charge of the nursing unit is inappropriate; power struggles need to be avoided.
Test-Taking Strategy: Focus on the issue, manipulative behavior. Recalling clients' rights and that power struggles need to be avoided will assist in selecting the correct interventions. Review care of the client with manipulative behavior if you had difficulty with this question.
Level of Cognitive Ability: Application
Client Needs: Psychosocial Integrity
Integrated Process: Nursing Process/Implementation
Content Area: Mental Health
Reference: Varcarolis, E. (2002). *Foundations of psychiatric mental health nursing* (4th ed.). Philadelphia: W.B. Saunders, p. 394.

REFERENCES

Fortinash, K., & Holoday-Worret, P. (2004). *Psychiatric mental health nursing* (3rd ed.). St. Louis: Mosby.
Morrison-Valfre, M. (2005). *Foundations of mental health care* (3rd ed.). St. Louis: Mosby.
Mosby's medical, nursing, and allied health dictionary (6th ed.). (2005). St. Louis: Mosby.

Potter, P., & Perry, A. (2005). *Fundamentals of nursing* (6th ed.). St. Louis: Mosby.
Stuart, G., & Laraia, M. (2005). *Principles and practice of psychiatric nursing* (8th ed.). St. Louis: Mosby.
Varcarolis, E. (2002). *Foundations of psychiatric mental health nursing* (4th ed.). Philadelphia: W.B. Saunders.

CHAPTER 64

Addictions

I. EATING DISORDERS

A. Description: Characterized by uncertain self-identification and grossly disturbed eating habits

B. Compulsive overeating
1. Bingelike overeating without purging
2. Food consumption is out of the individual's control and occurs in a stereotyped fashion
3. Client may be repulsed by eating; the eating relieves tension but does not produce pleasure
4. Is aware that eating patterns are abnormal and feels depressed after eating
5. Eats secretly during a binge and consumes high-calorie and easily digestible food
6. Repeatedly tries to diet but without success
7. Lacks interest in exercise programs and feels helpless and hopeless about weight
8. When experiencing guilt, anger, depression, boredom, loneliness, inadequacy, or ambivalence, responds by eating

C. Anorexia nervosa
1. Description
   a. The onset is often associated with a stressful life event
   b. The client intensely fears obesity
   c. Body image is distorted, and the client has a disturbed self-concept
   d. Preoccupied with foods that prevent weight gain; has a phobia against foods that produce weight gain
   e. The eating disorder can be life-threatening
   f. Death can occur from starvation, **suicide**, or electrolyte imbalance
2. Data collection
   a. Refusal to eat and appetite loss
   b. Appetite denial
   c. Feelings of lack of control
   d. Self-induced vomiting and self-administered enemas
   e. Exercises compulsively
   f. Overachiever and perfectionist
   g. Decreased temperature, pulse, and blood pressure
   h. Weight loss
   i. Gastrointestinal (GI) disturbances
   j. Constipation
   k. Electrolyte imbalances
   l. Scaly, dry skin
   m. Sleep disturbances
   n. Hormone deficiencies
   o. Amenorrhea for at least three consecutive menstrual periods
   p. Teeth and gum deterioration
   q. Cyanosis and numbness of extremities
   r. Esophageal varices from vomiting
   s. Bone degeneration

D. Bulimia nervosa
1. Description
   a. The client indulges in eating binges followed by purging behaviors
   b. Most clients remain within a normal weight range but feel that their lives are dominated by the eating-related conflict
2. Data collection
   a. Preoccupied with body shape and weight
   b. Consumes high-calorie food in secret; guilt about secretive eating
   c. Binge-purge syndrome
   d. Attempts to lose weight through diets, vomiting, enemas, cathartics, amphetamines, diuretics
   e. Need to control yet experiences feelings of powerlessness or loss of control

f. Low self-esteem

g. Poor interpersonal relationships

h. Mood swings

i. Self-mutilating behavior; suicidal thoughts, and attempts at **suicide**

j. Electrolyte imbalances

k. Loss of tooth enamel and dental decay

l. Stomach ulcers and rectal bleeding

m. Esophageal varicose from vomiting

n. Cardiac disease and hypertension

E. Interventions: Clients with an eating disorder

1. Assess the client's nutritional status

2. Establish a contract with the client concerning the diet plan for the day

3. Assist the client in identifying precipitators to the eating disorder

4. Encourage the client to state feelings about the eating behavior

5. Be accepting and nonjudgmental, expressing neither approval nor disapproval of the behavior

6. Encourage behavior modification techniques

7. Provide praise and positive reinforcement for accomplishments

8. Supervise client during mealtimes and for a specified period after meals

9. Set a time limit for each meal

10. Provide a pleasant, relaxed environment for eating

11. Monitor for signs of physical complications related to the eating disorder

12. Record intake and output (I&O)

13. Weigh the client daily at the same time, using the same scale, after the client voids

14. When weighing the client, ensure that the client is wearing the same clothing as when the previous weight was taken

15. Monitor and restore fluid and electrolyte balance

16. Monitor elimination patterns

17. Monitor and limit the client's activity level

18. Encourage the client to participate in diversional activities

19. Assess the client's **suicide** potential

20. Administer antidepressant medication, as prescribed

21. Encourage psychotherapy, as prescribed

22. Refer the client to support groups

II. SUBSTANCE ABUSE DISORDERS

A. Description: Behavioral changes associated with regular substance **abuse** that affects the central nervous system (CNS)

B. Substance dependence (Box 64-1)

1. Pattern of repeated use of a substance, which usually results in tolerance, withdrawal, and compulsive drug-taking behavior

BOX 64-1

CAGE Screening Test

C: Have you ever felt the need to cut down on your drinking or drug use?

A: Have you ever been annoyed at criticism of your drinking or drug use?

G: Have you ever felt guilty about something you have done when you have been drinking or taking drugs?

E: Have you ever had an eye opener, drinking or taking drugs first thing in the morning to get going or to avoid withdrawal symptoms?

2. Client takes substances in larger amounts and over longer periods of time than was intended

3. Client has the desire to cut down but is unsuccessful in efforts to decrease or discontinue use

4. Daily activities revolve around the use of a substance

C. Substance tolerance: The need for increased amounts of the substance to achieve the desired effect

D. Substance **abuse**

1. Client recurrently uses substances

2. Client experiences recurrent, significant harmful consequences related to the use of substances

3. Client has legal problems related to substance **abuse**

E. Substance withdrawal

1. Physiological and/or substance-specific cognitive symptoms

2. Occurs when blood levels decrease in an individual with prolonged heavy use of a substance

F. Precipitating factors of substance **abuse**

1. Rebellion and peer group pressure in adolescence

2. Pleasure-seeking experience, because the substance decreases physical and emotional pain

3. Group influence and peer pressure

4. Depression

5. Loss and grieving

G. Dysfunctional behaviors of substance **abuse**

1. Insensitive to self and others

2. Manipulative

3. Impulsiveness

4. Anger, including physical and verbal **abuse**

5. Avoidance of relationships, with physical and emotional distancing

6. Sense of self-importance and requiring special treatment

7. Denial, blaming everything but the substance

8. Uses rationalization and projection to justify unacceptable behaviors

9. Low self-esteem

10. Depression

III. ALCOHOL ABUSE

A. Description
  1. Alcohol is a central nervous system (CNS) depressant affecting all body tissues
  2. Physical dependence is a biological need for alcohol to avoid physical withdrawal symptoms
  3. Psychological dependence is a craving for the subjective effect of alcohol

B. Risk factors
  1. Biological predisposition
  2. Depressed and highly anxious characteristics
  3. Low self-esteem
  4. Poor self-control
  5. History of rebelliousness, poor school performance, delinquency
  6. Poor relationship with parent(s)

C. Data collection
  1. Slurred speech
  2. Uncoordinated movements
  3. Unsteady gait
  4. Restlessness
  5. Belligerence
  6. Confusion
  7. Sneaking drinks, drinking in the morning, and experiencing blackouts
  8. Binge drinking
  9. Arguments about drinking
  10. Missing work
  11. Increased tolerance to alcohol
  12. Intoxication, with blood alcohol levels of 0.1% (100 mg alcohol/dL blood) or higher

D. Psychological symptoms
  1. Depression
  2. Hostility
  3. Suspiciousness
  4. Rationalization
  5. Irritability
  6. Isolation
  7. Decrease in inhibitions
  8. Decrease in self-esteem
  9. Denial that a problem exists

E. Complications associated with chronic alcohol use
  1. Vitamin deficiencies
    a. Vitamin B deficiency, causing peripheral neuropathies
    b. Thiamine deficiency, causing Korsakoff's syndrome
  2. Alcoholic-induced persistent amnesiac disorder, causing severe memory problems
  3. Wernicke's encephalopathy, causing confusion, ataxia, and abnormal eye movements
  4. Hepatitis; cirrhosis of the liver
  5. Esophagitis and gastritis
  6. Pancreatitis
  7. Anemias
  8. Immune system dysfunctions
  9. Brain damage
  10. Peripheral neuropathy
  11. Cardiac disorders

IV. ALCOHOL WITHDRAWAL

A. Description
  1. Early signs develop within a few hours after cessation of alcohol intake
  2. These signs peak after 24 to 48 hours and then rapidly disappear, unless the withdrawal progresses to alcohol withdrawal delirium

B. Withdrawal (Box 64-2)

C. Withdrawal delirium (Box 64-3)
  1. A medical emergency
  2. Death can occur from myocardial infarction, fat emboli, peripheral vascular collapse, electrolyte imbalance, aspiration pneumonia, or suicide
  3. The state of delirium usually peaks 48 to 72 hours after cessation or reduction of intake (although can occur later); lasts 2 to 3 days

D. Interventions
  1. Provide care in a nonjudgmental manner
  2. Check the client frequently

BOX 64-2

Early Signs of Alcohol Withdrawal

Anxiety
Anorexia (nausea and vomiting may occur)
Insomnia
Tremors
Hyperalertness
Hypertension
Jerky movements
Irritability
Startles easily
May report a feeling of "shaking inside"
May experience hallucinations, illusions, or vivid nightmares
Tachycardia
Seizures (usually appear 7 to 48 hours after cessation of alcohol)

BOX 64-3

Manifestations of Alcohol Withdrawal Delirium

Anxiety
Insomnia
Anorexia
Agitation
Delirium
Diaphoresis
Tachycardia and hypertension
Fever (100° to 103° F [37.7° to 39.4° C])
Disorientation, with fluctuating levels of consciousness
Hallucinations and delusions

3. Monitor vital signs and neurological signs (hourly for the client with delirium)
4. Provide a quiet nonstimulating environment; encourage a family member (one at a time) to stay with the client to minimize anxiety
5. Orient the client frequently
6. Explain all treatments and procedures in a quiet and simple manner
7. Initiate seizure precautions
8. Administer sedating or anticonvulsant medication, as prescribed
9. Provide small, frequent, high-carbohydrate foods (administer antiemetic before meals as needed)
10. Monitor input and output (I&O)
11. Administer vitamins (multivitamin, vitamin B complex including thiamine, and vitamin C)
12. Assist client with activities of daily living and assist with ambulation if stable
13. Allow client to express fears

E. Disulfiram (Antabuse) therapy
1. Description
   a. An alcohol deterrent used for alcoholic dependence
   b. The medication sensitizes the client to alcohol, so a disulfiram-alcohol reaction occurs if alcohol is ingested
   c. The client must abstain from alcohol for at least 12 hours before the initial dose is administered
   d. Adverse effects usually begin within minutes to a half-hour after consuming alcohol; and may last $\frac{1}{2}$ to 2 hours
   e. The client must avoid drinking alcohol for 14 days after disulfiram therapy has been discontinued; otherwise, the client is at risk for disulfiram-alcohol reaction
2. Adverse reactions
   a. Facial flushing
   b. Sweating
   c. Throbbing headache
   d. Neck pain
   e. Nausea and vomiting
   f. Hypotension
   g. Tachycardia
   h. Respiratory distress
3. Client education
   a. Educate about the effects of the medication
   b. Ensure that the client agrees to abstain from alcohol and any alcohol-containing substances
   c. Instruct the client that the effects of the medication may occur for several days after discontinuance
   d. Instruct the client to avoid the use of substances that contain alcohol, such as cough medicine, rubbing alcohol, vinegar, mouthwash, and aftershave lotion

F. Dealing with the client who abuses alcohol (Boxes 64-4 and 64-5)

V. DRUG DEPENDENCY
A. Central nervous system (CNS) depressants
1. Can include alcohol, benzodiazepines, and barbiturates and act as a depressant, sedative, and hypnotic
2. Intoxication (Box 64-6)
3. Overdose can produce cardiovascular or respiratory depression, coma, shock, convulsions, and death

---

BOX 64-4

Dealing with the Client Who Abuses Alcohol

Direct the client's focus to the substance abuse problem.
Help the client identify those situations that precipitate angry feelings.
Set limits on manipulative behavior and verbal and physical abuse.
Hold the client firmly to reasonable limits, consistently reinforcing rules, with reasonable consequences for breaking rules.
Hold the client accountable for all behaviors.
Assist the client to explore strengths and weaknesses.
Encourage time-out if the client is losing control.
Encourage the client to participate in group therapy and support groups.

BOX 64-5

Therapies for Substance Abuse Clients and their Families

Psychotherapy (individual, group, family)
Behavior therapy, aversion conditioning with disulfiram (Antabuse)
Support groups, such as Alcoholics Anonymous, Narcotics Anonymous, Pills Anonymous, Al-Anon, Al-a-Teen, Narc-Anon (for family members and friends of alcoholics or addicts), Adult Children of Alcoholics
Transitional living programs (halfway houses)
Hospitalization

BOX 64-6

Signs of Intoxication: CNS Depressants

Slurred speech
Incoordination and unsteady gait
Drowsiness
Irritability
Hypotension
Impairment of memory, attention, judgment, and social or occupational functioning

4. Overdose: If awake, induce vomiting and administer activated charcoal; if comatose, clear airway, intubation, gastric lavage with activated charcoal, seizure precautions, possible dialysis, flumazenil (Romazicon) intravenously

5. Withdrawal: Effects include nausea, vomiting, tachycardia, diaphoresis, irritability, tremors, insomnia, seizures; treated with carefully titrated similar drug (abrupt withdrawal can lead to death)

B. Central nervous system stimulants
1. Can include amphetamines, cocaine, and crack
2. Intoxication (Box 64-7)
3. Overdose can produce respiratory distress, ataxia, hyperpyrexia, seizures, coma, cerebrovascular accident, myocardial infarction, and death
4. Overdose: Treated with antipsychotics and management of associated effects
5. Withdrawal: Effects include fatigue, depression, agitation, apathy, anxiety, insomnia, disorientation, lethargy, and craving; treated with antidepressants, dopamine agonist, or bromocriptine (Parlodel)

C. Opioids
1. Can include opium, heroin, meperidine (Demerol), morphine sulfate, codeine sulfate, methadone (Dolophine), hydromorphone (Dilaudid), or fentanyl (Sublimaze)
2. Intoxication (Box 64-8)

3. Overdose can produce respiratory depression, coma, shock, seizures, and death
4. Overdose: Treated with a narcotic antagonist such as naloxone (Narcan)
5. Withdrawal: Effects include yawning, insomnia, irritability, rhinorrhea, diaphoresis, cramps, nausea and vomiting, muscle aches, chills, fever, lacrimation, and diarrhea; treated by methadone tapering or medication detoxification

D. Hallucinogens
1. Can include lysergic acid diethylamide (LSD), mescaline (peyote), psilocybin (mushrooms), or phencyclidine (PCP)
2. Intoxication (Box 64-9)
3. Overdose: Effects of LSD, peypote, psilocybin include psychosis, brain damage, and death; effects of PCP include psychosis, hypertensive crisis, hyperthermia, seizures, respiratory arrest
4. Treatment (LSD, peypote, psilocybin): Low environmental stimuli (speak slowly, clearly, and in a low voice) and medications to treat anxiety
5. Treatment (PCP): Possible gastric lavage (if alert), acidifying urine to assist in excreting drug, and interventions to treat behavioral disturbances, hyperthermia, hypertension, respiratory distress

E. Inhalants
1. Can include gases or liquids such as butane, paint thinner, paint and wax removers, airplane glue, nail polish remover, nitrous oxide
2. Intoxication (Box 64-10)
3. Overdose: Can cause damage to the nervous system and death
4. Treatment: Interventions include treating affected body systems

---

BOX 64-7

Signs of Intoxication: CNS Stimulants

Tachycardia
Dilated pupils
Hypertension
Nausea and vomiting
Euphoria
Insomnia
Impairment of judgment and social or occupational functioning
Paranoia, delusions, hallucinations
Potential for violence

BOX 64-8

Signs of Intoxication: Opioids

Constricted pupils
Decreased respirations
Drowsiness
Hypotension
Slurred speech
Impairment of memory, attention, and judgment
Euphoria
Psychomotor retardation

BOX 64-9

Signs of Intoxication: Hallucinogens

Dilated pupils
Tachycardia
Diaphoresis
Tremors
Incoordination
Elevated vital signs, including blood pressure
Muscular rigidity and chronic jerking
Seizures
Blank stare
Impairment of judgment and social and occupational functioning
Anxiety and depression
Paranoia
Hallucinations
Agitation and belligerence
Bizarre behavior, regressive behavior, or violent behavior

F. Marijuana (*Cannabis sativa*)
   1. Generally smoked but can be ingested
   2. Causes euphoria, detachment, relaxation, talkativeness, slowed perception of time, anxiety, paranoia
   3. Long-term dependence can result in lethargy, difficulty concentrating, and memory loss
G. Other recreational drugs
   1. Can include ecstasy, GHB (gamma-hydroxybutyrate), and ketamine
   2. Effects include euphoria, increased energy, increased self-confidence, and increased sociability
   3. Adverse effects include hyperthermia, rhabdomyolysis, renal failure, hepatotoxicity, depression, panic attacks, psychosis, cardiovascular collapse, and death
II. Interventions: Withdrawal
   1. Initiate seizure precautions
   2. Hydrate the client
   3. Monitor vital signs every hour
   4. Monitor I&O
   5. Orient client frequently
   6. Maintain minimal stimuli
   7. Approach client in an accepting and nonjudgmental manner
   8. Direct client's focus to the substance **abuse** problem

---

BOX 64-10

Signs of Intoxication: Inhalants

Excitation followed by drowsiness, lightheadedness, disinhibition, agitation
Euphoria
Giggling and laughter
Enhancement of sexual pleasure

BOX 64-11

Withdrawal: Nursing Care

Obtain information regarding the drug type and amount consumed.
Monitor vital signs.
Remove unnecessary objects from the environment.
Provide one-to-one supervision if necessary.
Provide a quiet, calm environment with minimal stimuli.
Maintain client orientation.
Ensure client's safety by implementing seizure precautions.
Use restraints, if necessary and prescribed, to prevent client from harming self and others.
Provide for physical needs.
Provide food and fluids as tolerated.
Administer medications as prescribed to decrease withdrawal symptoms.
Collect blood and urine samples for drug screening.

---

9. Identify with client situations that precipitate angry feelings
10. Limit the client's placing blame or rationalizing to explain the substance **abuse** problem
11. Assist client to use assertive techniques rather than manipulation to meet needs
12. Set limits on manipulative behavior and verbal and physical **abuse**
13. Hold client firmly to reasonable limits, consistently reinforcing rules, with reasonable consequences for breaking rules
14. Hold client accountable for all behaviors
15. Assist client to explore strengths and weaknesses
16. Encourage time-out if client is losing control
17. Encourage client to participate in unit activities
18. Encourage client to participate in group therapy and support groups
19. Nursing care for clients: See Box 64-11

PRACTICE QUESTIONS

1. A nurse is caring for a female client who was recently admitted to the hospital for anorexia nervosa. The nurse enters the client's room and notes that the client is doing vigorous push-ups. Which nursing action is appropriate?
   1. Allow the client to complete her exercise program
   2. Tell the client that she is not allowed to exercise vigorously
   3. Interrupt the client and offer to take her for a walk
   4. Interrupt the client and weigh her immediately
2. A nurse is caring for a client with anorexia nervosa. The nurse is monitoring the behavior of the client and understands that the client with anorexia nervosa manages anxiety by:
   1. Always reinforcing self-approval
   2. Having the need to always make the right decision
   3. Engaging in immoral acts
   4. Observing rigid rules and regulations
3. A nursing student is developing a plan of care for the hospitalized client with bulimia nervosa. The nursing instructor intervenes if the student documents which incorrect intervention in the plan?
   1. Monitor intake and output
   2. Monitor electrolyte levels
   3. Observe for excessive exercise
   4. Check for the presence of laxatives and diuretics in the client's belongings
4. A nurse is monitoring a client who abuses alcohol for signs of alcohol withdrawal delirium. The nurse monitors for which of the following?
   1. Hypertension, disorientation, hallucinations
   2. Hypotension, ataxia, vomiting
   3. Stupor, agitation, muscular rigidity
   4. Hypotension, coarse hand tremor, agitation

5. The spouse of a client admitted to the hospital for alcohol withdrawal says to the nurse, "I should get out of this bad situation." The most helpful response by the nurse would be:

   1. "I agree with you. You should get out of this situation."
   2. "What do you find difficult about this situation?"
   3. "Why don't you tell your husband about this?"
   4. "This is not the best time to make that decision."

6. A nurse is caring for a client who is suspected of being dependent on drugs. Which question would be appropriate for the nurse to ask when collecting data from the client regarding drug abuse?

   1. "Why did you get started on these drugs?"
   2. "How long did you think you could take these drugs without someone finding out?"
   3. "How much do you use and what effect does it have on you?"
   4. The nurse does not ask any questions because of fear that the client is in denial and will throw the nurse out of the room

7. A client who has been drinking alcohol on a regular basis admits to having "a problem" and is asking for assistance with the problem. The nurse would encourage the client to attend which of the following community groups?

   1. Al-Anon
   2. Alcoholics Anonymous
   3. Families Anonymous
   4. Fresh Start

8. A client with a diagnosis of anorexia nervosa, who is in a state of starvation, is in a two-bed hospital room. A newly admitted client will be assigned to this client's room. Which client would be an appropriate choice as this client's roommate?

   1. A client with pneumonia
   2. A client receiving diagnostic tests
   3. A client who could benefit from the client's assistance at mealtime
   4. A client who thrives on managing others

9. A client has been hospitalized and has participated in substance abuse therapy group sessions. On discharge, the client has consented to participate in Alcoholics Anonymous (AA) community groups. Which statement by the client would best indicate to the nurse that the client has well assimilated therapy session topics and coping response styles, and has processed information effectively for self-use?

   1. "I know I'm ready to be discharged; I feel like I can say 'no' and leave a group of friends if they are drinking. No problem."
   2. "This group has really helped a lot. I know it will be different when I go home. But I'm sure that my family and friends will all help me like the people in this group have. They'll all help me; I know they will. They won't let me go back to my old ways."

   3. "I'm looking forward to leaving here; I know that I will miss all of you. So, I'm happy and I'm sad, I'm excited and I'm scared. I know that I have to work hard to be strong and that everyone isn't going to be as helpful as you people."
   4. "I'll keep all my appointments and go to all my AA groups. I'll do everything I'm supposed to. Nothing will go wrong that way."

10. A nurse is assigned to care for a client at risk for alcohol withdrawal. The nurse monitors the client, knowing that the early signs of withdrawal will develop within how much time after cessation or reduction of alcohol intake?

    1. Within a few hours
    2. In 7 days
    3. In 14 days
    4. In 21 days

11. A nurse determines that the wife of an alcoholic client is benefiting from attending an Al-Anon group when the nurse hears the wife say:

    1. "My attendance at the meetings has helped me to see that I provoke my husband's violence."
    2. "I no longer feel that I deserve the beatings my husband inflicts on me."
    3. "I can tolerate my husband's destructive behaviors now that I know they are common in alcoholics."
    4. "I enjoy attending the meetings because they get me out of the house and away from my husband."

12. A female client with anorexia nervosa is a member of a support group. The client has verbalized that she would like to buy some new clothes but her finances are limited. Group members have brought some used clothes for the client to replace her old clothes. The client believes that the new clothes were much too tight, so she has reduced her calorie intake to 800 calories daily. The nurse identifies this behavior as:

    1. Normal
    2. Indicative of the client's ambivalence
    3. Evidence of the client's altered and distorted body image
    4. Regression

13. A hospitalized client with a history of alcohol abuse tells the nurse, "I am leaving now. I have to go. I don't want any more treatment. I have things that I have to do right away." The client has not been discharged. In fact, the client is scheduled for an important diagnostic test to be performed in 1 hour. After the nurse discusses the client's concerns with the client, the client dresses and begins to walk out of the hospital room. The appropriate nursing action is to:

    1. Restrain the client until the physician can be reached
    2. Call security to block all exit areas

3. Tell the client that she cannot return to this hospital again if she leaves now
4. Call the nursing supervisor

14. A nursing student is asked to identify the characteristics of bulimia nervosa. The nursing instructor intervenes if the student identifies which incorrect characteristic of this disorder?
1. Enlarged parotid glands
2. Dental erosion
3. Electrolyte imbalances
4. Body weight well below ideal range

15. A nurse is caring for a client who has a history of opioid abuse and is monitoring the client for signs of withdrawal. Which clinical manifestations are associated with withdrawal from opioids?
1. Yawning, irritability, diaphoresis, cramps, and diarrhea

2. Tachycardia, hypertension, sweating, and marked tremors
3. Dilated pupils, tachycardia, and diaphoresis
4. Depressed feelings, high drug craving, fatigue, and agitation

ALTERNATE FORMAT QUESTION: MULTIPLE RESPONSE

Select the appropriate interventions for caring for the client in alcohol withdrawal.
___ Monitor vital signs
___ Provide stimulation in the environment
___ Maintain an NPO status
___ Provide reality orientation as appropriate
___ Address hallucinations therapeutically

ANSWERS

1. *Answer: 3*
Rationale: Clients with anorexia nervosa are frequently preoccupied with vigorous exercise and push themselves beyond normal limits to work off caloric intake. The nurse must provide for appropriate exercise as well as place limits on vigorous activities. Options 1, 2, and 4 are inappropriate nursing actions.
Test-Taking Strategy: Use the process of elimination. Recalling that the nurse needs to set firm limits with clients who have this disorder will direct you to option 3. If you had difficulty with this question, review interventions for the client with anorexia nervosa.
Level of Cognitive Ability: Application
Client Needs: Physiological Integrity
Integrated Process: Nursing Process/Implementation
Content Area: Mental Health
Reference: Morrison-Valfre, M. (2005). *Foundations of mental health care* (3rd ed.). St. Louis: Mosby, pp. 240-241.

2. *Answer: 4*
Rationale: Clients with anorexia nervosa have the desire to please others. Their need to be correct or perfect interferes with rational decision-making processes. These clients are moralistic. Rules and rituals help the clients manage their anxiety. Options 1, 2, and 3 are incorrect.
Test-Taking Strategy: Use the process of elimination and focus on the issue, managing anxiety. Eliminate options 1 and 2 because of the absolute word "always." Eliminate option 3 because it is not characteristic of the client with anorexia. Review the characteristics associated with this disorder if you had difficulty with this question.
Level of Cognitive Ability: Comprehension
Client Needs: Psychosocial Integrity
Integrated Process: Nursing Process/Data Collection

Content Area: Mental Health
Reference: Morrison-Valfre, M. (2005). *Foundations of mental health care* (3rd ed.). St. Louis: Mosby, p. 235.

3. *Answer: 3*
Rationale: Excessive exercise is a characteristic of anorexia nervosa, not a characteristic of clients with bulimia. Frequent vomiting, in addition to laxative and diuretic abuse may lead to dehydration and electrolyte imbalance. Monitoring for dehydration and electrolyte imbalance are important nursing actions. Option 3 is the only option that is not associated with care of the client with bulimia.
Test-Taking Strategy: Use the process of elimination. Note the key word, *incorrect*, in the stem of the question. This word indicates a false response question and that you need to select the incorrect intervention. Options 1, 2, and 4 are similar and directly or indirectly infer concern about fluid and electrolyte balance. Option 3 is different from the other options. Review the characteristics associated with bulimia nervosa if you had difficulty with this question.
Level of Cognitive Ability: Analysis
Client Needs: Physiological Integrity
Integrated Process: Nursing Process/Planning
Content Area: Mental Health
Reference: Morrison-Valfre, M. (2005). *Foundations of mental health care* (3rd ed.). St. Louis: Mosby, pp. 237-238.

4. *Answer: 1*
Rationale: The symptoms associated with alcohol withdrawal delirium typically are anxiety, insomnia, anorexia, hypertension, disorientation, visual or tactile hallucinations, changes in level of consciousness, agitation, fever, and delusions.
Test-Taking Strategy: Use the process of elimination. Review each option carefully to ensure that all the symptoms are contained in the correct option. Eliminate options 2 and 4 first,

knowing that hypertension rather than hypotension occurs. From the remaining options, recalling that the client who is stuporous is not likely to exhibit agitation will direct you to option 1. Review the symptoms associated with alcohol withdrawal if you had difficulty with this question.
Level of Cognitive Ability: Analysis
Client Needs: Physiological Integrity
Integrated Process: Nursing Process/Data Collection
Content Area: Mental Health
Reference: Stuart, G., & Laraia, M. (2005). *Principles and practice of psychiatric nursing* (8th ed.). St. Louis: Mosby, p. 491.

5. Answer: 2
Rationale: The most helpful response is the one that encourages the client to problem-solve. Giving advice implies that the nurse knows what is best and can also foster dependency. The nurse should not agree with the client nor should the nurse request that the client provide explanations.
Test-Taking Strategy: Use therapeutic communication techniques. Eliminate option 3 because of the word "Why," which should be avoided in communication. Eliminate option 1 because the nurse is agreeing with the client. Eliminate option 4 because this option places the client's feelings on hold. Option 2 is the only option that addresses the client's feelings. Review therapeutic communication techniques if you had difficulty with this question.
Level of Cognitive Ability: Application
Client Needs: Psychosocial Integrity
Integrated Process: Communication and Documentation
Content Area: Mental Health
Reference: Morrison-Valfre, M. (2005). *Foundations of mental health care* (3rd ed.). St. Louis: Mosby, p. 88.

6. Answer: 3
Rationale: Whenever the nurse collects data from a client who is dependent on drugs, it is best for the nurse to attempt to elicit information by being nonjudgmental and direct. Option 1 is incorrect because it is judgmental, off focus, and reflects the nurse's bias. Option 2 is incorrect because it is judgmental, insensitive, and aggressive, which is nontherapeutic. Option 4 is incorrect because it indicates passivity on the nurse's part and uses rationalization to avoid the therapeutic nursing intervention.
Test-Taking Strategy: Use the process of elimination and therapeutic communication techniques to answer the question. Option 3 is the statement that is nonjudgmental and direct. Review data collection of a client who is a drug abuser if you had difficulty with this question.
Level of Cognitive Ability: Application
Client Needs: Health Promotion and Maintenance
Integrated Process: Nursing Process/Data Collection
Content Area: Mental Health
Reference: Morrison-Valfre, M. (2005). *Foundations of mental health care* (3rd ed.). St. Louis: Mosby, pp. 298-299.

7. Answer: 2
Rationale: Alcoholics Anonymous is a major self-help organization for the treatment of alcoholism. Option 1 is a group for families of alcoholics. Option 3 is for parents of children who abuse substances. Option 4 is for nicotine addicts.

Test-Taking Strategy: Use the process of elimination. If you are unfamiliar with these support groups, note the relation between "drinking" in the question and "Alcoholics" in the correct option. Familiarize yourself with the purposes of specific support groups if you had difficulty with this question.
Level of Cognitive Ability: Application
Client Needs: Safe, Effective Care Environment
Integrated Process: Nursing Process/Implementation
Content Area: Mental Health
Reference: Morrison-Valfre, M. (2005). *Foundations of mental health care* (3rd ed.). St. Louis: Mosby, p. 299.

8. Answer: 2
Rationale: The client receiving diagnostic tests is an appropriate roommate. The client with anorexia is most likely experiencing hematological complications, such as leukopenia. Having a roommate with pneumonia would place the client with anorexia nervosa at risk for infection. The client with anorexia nervosa should not be put in a situation in which he or she can focus on the nutritional needs of others or be managed by others, because this may contribute to sublimation and suppression of their own hunger.
Test-Taking Strategy: Use the process of elimination and note the key words, *in a state of starvation*. Recalling the characteristics and complications associated with anorexia nervosa will direct you to option 2. Review care of the client with anorexia nervosa if you have difficulty with this question.
Level of Cognitive Ability: Analysis
Client Needs: Safe, Effective Care Environment
Integrated Process: Nursing Process/Planning
Content Area: Mental Health
Reference: Morrison-Valfre, M. (2005). *Foundations of mental health care* (3rd ed.). St. Louis: Mosby, p. 236.

9. Answer: 3
Rationale: In option 3, the client is expressing real concern and ambivalence about discharge from the hospital. The client also demonstrates reality in the statement. Option 1 indicates client denial. In option 2, the client is relying heavily on others. In option 4, the client is concrete and procedure-oriented; again, the client denies that "nothing will go wrong that way" if the client follows all the directions.
Test-Taking Strategy: Use the process of elimination and select the option that identifies the most realistic client verbalization. This will direct you to option 3. Review care of the client with a substance abuse problem if you had difficulty with this question.
Level of Cognitive Ability: Analysis
Client Needs: Psychosocial Integrity
Integrated Process: Nursing Process/Evaluation
Content Area: Mental Health
Reference: Morrison-Valfre, M. (2005). *Foundations of mental health care* (3rd ed.). St. Louis: Mosby, p. 302.

10. Answer: 1
Rationale: Early signs of alcohol withdrawal develop within a few hours after cessation or reduction of alcohol and peak after 24 to 48 hours.
Test-Taking Strategy: Use the process of elimination and note the key word, *early*. This will assist in directing you to

option 1. If you are unfamiliar with the manifestations associated with alcohol withdrawal, review this content.
Level of Cognitive Ability: Comprehension
Client Needs: Physiological Integrity
Integrated Process: Nursing Process/Data Collection
Content Area: Mental Health
Reference: Stuart, G., & Laraia, M. (2005). *Principles and practice of psychiatric nursing* (8th ed.). St. Louis: Mosby, p. 491.

11. Answer: 2
Rationale: Al-Anon support groups are a protected, supportive opportunity for spouses and significant others to learn what to expect and to obtain suggestions about successful behavioral changes. Option 2 is the healthiest response, because it exemplifies an understanding that the alcoholic partner is responsible for his behavior and cannot be allowed to blame family members for loss of control. The nonalcoholic partner should not feel responsible when the spouse loses control (option 1). Option 3 indicates that the wife remains codependent. Option 4 indicates that the group is being seen as an escape, not a place to work on issues.
Test-Taking Strategy: Use the process of elimination and focus on the issue of the question, benefiting from attending an Al-Anon group. This will direct you to option 2. Review the purpose of this type of support group if you had difficulty with this question.
Level of Cognitive Ability: Analysis
Client Needs: Psychosocial Integrity
Integrated Process: Nursing Process/Evaluation
Content Area: Mental Health
Reference: Stuart, G., & Laraia, M. (2005). *Principles and practice of psychiatric nursing* (8th ed.). St. Louis: Mosby, p. 506.

12. Answer: 3
Rationale: Altered or distorted body image is a concern with clients with anorexia nervosa. Although the client may struggle with ambivalence and present with regressed behavior, the client's coping pattern relates to the basic issue of distorted body image. The client's behavior is not normal.
Test-Taking Strategy: Use the process of elimination. Focus on the information provided in the question to determine that the issue relates to a distorted body image. This will direct you to option 3. If you had difficulty with this question, review the characteristics associated with the client with anorexia nervosa.
Level of Cognitive Ability: Comprehension
Client Needs: Psychosocial Integrity
Integrated Process: Nursing Process/Data Collection
Content Area: Mental Health
Reference: Stuart, G., & Laraia, M. (2005). *Principles and practice of psychiatric nursing* (8th ed.). St. Louis: Mosby, pp. 532-533.

13. Answer: 4
Rationale: A nurse can be charged with false imprisonment if a client is made to wrongfully believe that they cannot leave the hospital. Most health care facilities have documents that the client is asked to sign, which relate to the client's responsibilities when they leave against medical advice (AMA).

The client should be asked to sign this document before leaving. The nurse should request that the client wait to speak to the physician before leaving but, if the client refuses to do so, the nurse cannot hold the client against his or her will. Restraining the client and calling security to block exits constitutes false imprisonment. Any client has a right to health care (option 3) and cannot be told otherwise.
Test-Taking Strategy: Use the process of elimination. Keeping the concept of false imprisonment in mind, eliminate options 1 and 2 because they are similar. Eliminate option 3, knowing that any client has a right to health care. Review the points related to false imprisonment if you had difficulty with this question.
Level of Cognitive Ability: Application
Client Needs: Safe, Effective Care Environment
Integrated Process: Nursing Process/Implementation
Content Area: Mental Health
Reference: Morrison-Valfre, M. (2005). *Foundations of mental health care* (3rd ed.). St. Louis: Mosby, pp. 24-25.

14. Answer: 4
Rationale: Clients with bulimia nervosa may not initially appear to be physically or emotionally ill. They are often at or slightly below ideal body weight. On further inspection, the client demonstrates enlargement of the parotid glands with dental erosion and caries if the client has been inducing vomiting. Electrolyte imbalances are present.
Test-Taking Strategy: Use the process of elimination and note the key word, *incorrect*. Focusing on the client's diagnosis will direct you to option 4. Option 4 is a characteristic sign of anorexia nervosa, not bulimia nervosa. Review the characteristics of these disorders if you had difficulty with this question.
Level of Cognitive Ability: Comprehension
Client Needs: Physiological Integrity
Integrated Process: Nursing Process/Data Collection
Content Area: Mental Health
Reference: Morrison-Valfre, M. (2005). *Foundations of mental health care* (3rd ed.). St. Louis: Mosby, p. 237.

15. Answer: 1
Rationale: Opioids are central nervous system (CNS) depressants. Withdrawal effects include yawning, insomnia, irritability, rhinorrhea, diaphoresis, cramps, nausea and vomiting, muscle aches, chills, fever, lacrimation, and diarrhea. Withdrawal is treated by methadone tapering or medication detoxification. Option 1 identifies the clinical manifestations associated with withdrawal from opioids. Option 2 describes withdrawal from alcohol. Option 3 describes intoxication from hallucinogens. Option 4 describes withdrawal from cocaine.
Test-Taking Strategy: Focus on the issue of the question, the clinical manifestations associated with withdrawal from opioids. Recalling that opioids are central nervous system depressants will direct you to option 1. If you had difficulty with this question, review the manifestations associated with opioid withdrawal.
Level of Cognitive Ability: Analysis
Client Needs: Physiological Integrity
Integrated Process: Nursing Process/Data Collection
Content Area: Mental Health

Reference: Stuart, G., & Laraia, M. (2005). *Principles and practice of psychiatric nursing* (8th ed.). St. Louis: Mosby, p. 498.

ALTERNATE FORMAT QUESTION: MULTIPLE RESPONSE

Answers:

Monitor vital signs

Provide reality orientation as appropriate

Address hallucinations therapeutically

Rationale: When the client is experiencing withdrawal of alcohol, the priority for care is to prevent the client from harming self or others. The nurse would provide a low-stimulation environment to maintain the client in as calm a state as possible. The nurse would monitor the vital signs closely and report abnormal findings. The nurse would reorient the client to reality frequently and would address hallucinations therapeutically. Adequate nutritional and fluid intake needs to be maintained.

Test-Taking Strategy: Use therapeutic communication techniques and interventions to assist in selecting the correct interventions. Also, recalling the characteristics associated with alcohol withdrawal will assist in answering correctly. Review these interventions if you had difficulty with this question.

Level of Cognitive Ability: Application

Client Needs: Psychosocial Integrity

Integrated Process: Nursing Process/Implementation

Content Area: Mental Health

Reference: Ignatavicius, D., & Workman, M. (2006). *Medical surgical nursing: Critical thinking for collaborative care* (5th ed.). Philadelphia: W.B. Saunders, p. 101.

REFERENCES

Ignatavicius, D., & Workman, M. (2006). *Medical surgical nursing: Critical thinking for collaborative care* (5th ed.). Philadelphia: W.B. Saunders.

Morrison-Valfre, M. (2005). *Foundations of mental health care* (3rd ed.). St. Louis: Mosby.

Stuart, G., & Laraia, M. (2005). *Principles and practice of psychiatric nursing* (8th ed.). St. Louis: Mosby.

Crisis Theory and Intervention

I. CRISIS INTERVENTION

A. Description

1. Crisis is a temporary state of severe emotional disorganization resulting from failure of coping mechanisms and/or lack of support
2. Skills for decision making and problem solving are inadequate
3. Treatment is immediate, supportive, and directly responsive to the immediate **crisis** to assist the client and/or the family through the stressful situation

B. Phases of a **crisis**

1. Phase 1: External precipitating event
2. Phase 2
   a. Perception of threat
   b. Increase in anxiety
   c. Client may cope or resolve **crisis**
3. Phase 3
   a. Failure of coping
   b. Increasing disorganization
   c. Physical symptoms emerge
   d. Relationship problems
4. Phase 4
   a. Mobilization of internal and external resources
   b. Resolutions related to precrisis functioning include functioning at a higher level, at the same level, or at a lower level

C. Types of **crises** (Box 65-1)

D. **Crisis** intervention

1. Treatment is immediate, supportive, and directly responsive to the immediate **crisis**
2. Goal-directed intervention
3. Feelings of the client are acknowledged
4. Provides opportunities for expression and validation of feelings
5. Connections are made between the meaning of the event and the **crisis**

BOX 65-1

Types of Crises

Maturational: Relates to developmental stages and associated role changes

Situational: Arises from an external source; associated with a life event that upsets an individual's or group's psychological equilibrium

Adventitious: Relates to a crisis, disaster, or event that is not a part of everyday life and is unplanned and accidental

---

6. Explores alternative **coping mechanisms** and tries out new behaviors

II. GRIEF

A. The emotional responses to a loss; a process that an individual must experience to finally accept the reality of loss

B. Usually involves moving through a series of stages or tasks to help resolve the grief (Box 65-2)

C. Feelings associated with grief can include anger, frustration, loneliness, sadness, guilt, regret, or peace

D. Healing can occur when the pain of the loss has lessened and the survivor has adapted to life without the deceased; the survivor will continue to experience memories of the deceased

E. Types of grief

1. Normal grief: Physical, emotional, cognitive, or behavioral reactions can occur; the process of resolution can take months to years
2. Anticipatory grief: Occurs before the loss and is associated with an acute, chronic, or terminal illness
3. Disenfranchised grief: Occurs when a loss is experienced and cannot be openly acknowledged

BOX 65-2

The Grief Response

STAGE 1: SHOCK AND DISBELIEF

Survivor may have feelings of numbness, difficulties with decision-making, emotional outbursts, denial, and isolation.

STAGE 2: EXPERIENCING THE LOSS

Survivor may feel angry at the loved one who died or may feel guilt about the death.

Bargaining and or depression may also occur in this stage.

STAGE 3: REINTEGRATION

Survivor begins to reorganize his or her life and accepts the reality of the loss.

BOX 65-3

Children's Grief Responses to Death

BIRTH TO 1 YEAR

Has no concept of death

Reacts to the loss of mother or caregiver

ONE TO 2 YEARS

May see death as reversible

Occurs only after the death of the significant person in the child's life

May scream, withdraw, or become disinterested in environment

TWO TO 5 YEARS

May see death as reversible

Has a sense of loss and is concerned about who will care for him or her

Possible regression or aggressive behavior

FIVE TO 9 YEARS

Begins to see death as permanent

May feel responsible for the occurrence

Has difficulty concentrating

PREADOLESCENCE THROUGH ADOLESCENCE

Sees death as permanent

Experience a strong emotional reaction

May regress

(societal norms do not define the loss as a loss within its traditional definition)

4. Dysfunctional grief: Occurs when there is prolonged emotional instability and a lack of progression to successful coping with the loss
5. Children's grief: Based on their developmental level (Box 65-3)

III. LOSS

A. The absence of something desired or previously thought to be available
B. Actual loss: Can be identified by others and can arise either in response to or in anticipation of a situation
C. Perceived loss: Experienced by one person and cannot be verified by others
D. Anticipatory loss: Experienced before the loss occurs
E. Mourning
   1. The outward and social expression of loss
   2. May be dictated by cultural and religious beliefs
F. Bereavement
   1. Includes both the inner feelings and outward reactions of the survivor
   2. Includes both grief and mourning

IV. NURSE'S ROLE: GRIEF AND LOSS

A. Includes the client, family members, and significant other
B. Communicate with the client, family members, and significant other (Box 65-4)
C. Allow ongoing opportunities for fully informed choices
D. Facilitate the grief process; assess grief and assist the survivor to feel the loss and complete the tasks of the grief process
E. Consider the survivor's culture, religion, family structure, individual life experiences, coping skills, and support systems

F. Grief affects survivors physically, psychologically, socially, and spiritually; therefore, a multidisciplinary team approach, including a bereavement specialist, facilitates the grief process

V. END-OF-LIFE ISSUES

A. Description: refers to issues related to death and dying
B. Cultural and religious issues (Box 65-5; also, see Chapter 6 for additional information regarding cultural and religious issues)
   1. Hispanic and Latino groups
      a. Primary language is Spanish
      b. Predominant religion is Roman Catholic
      c. Prayer and folk remedies are common, as is the use of religious objects
      d. May avoid eye contact as a sign of respect
      e. Tend not to complain of pain
      f. The family generally makes decisions and may withhold the diagnosis or prognosis from the client
      g. Extended family members are often involved in end-of-life care (pregnant women are prohibited from caring for the dying or attending funerals)
      h. Several family members may be at the dying client's bedside

BOX 65-4

Communication Process

Determine how much the client and family want to know.

Determine if there is a spokesperson for the family.

Be aware of cultural and religious beliefs and how they may affect the communication process; consider personal space issues, eye contact, and touch.

Obtain an interpreter as necessary.

Allow opportunity for informed choices.

Assist with the decision-making process if asked; use problem solving to assist in decision making and avoid interjecting personal views or opinions.

Encourage expression of feelings, concerns, and fears.

Be honest and truthful and let the client and family know that you will not abandon them.

Ask the client and family about their expectations and needs.

Be a sensitive listener; sit in silence if necessary and appropriate.

Extend touch and hold the client's or family member's hand if appropriate.

Encourage reminiscing.

If you do not know what to do in a particular situation, seek assistance.

If you don't know what to say to a client or family who is talking about death, listen attentively and use therapeutic communication techniques such as open-ended questions or reflection.

Acknowledge your own feelings; let the client and family know that the topic of conversation is a difficult one and that you don't know what to say.

Realize that it is acceptable to cry with the client and family during the grief process.

    i. Vocal expression of grief and mourning is acceptable and expected
    j. Refuse procedures that alter the body such as organ donation or autopsy
    k. Prefer to die at home
  2. African Americans
    a. Discuss issues with the spouse or older family member (elders are held in high respect)
    b. Family is highly valued and is central to the care of the terminally ill
    c. Pain is reported openly
    d. Open displays of emotion may occur with some members of this cultural group
    e. Organ and blood donation are usually not allowed
    f. Prefer to die at home
  3. Chinese Americans
    a. Eye contact is often avoided because it represents disrespect to persons in authority
    b. Personal distance should be maintained
    c. Affection between family members is rarely exhibited in public
    d. May not report pain

BOX 65-5

Religion and End-of-Life Care

CHRISTIANITY

Catholic and Orthodox

Anointing of the sick by a priest

Other sacraments before death: Include reconciliation and holy communion

Protestant

No last rites (anointing of the sick accepted by some groups)

Prayers given to offer comfort and support

Church of Jesus Christ of Latter-Day Saints (Mormons)

May administer a sacrament if the client requests

Jehovah's Witness

Do not believe in sacraments

Will be excommunicated if they receive a blood transfusion

ISLAM

Contact person: second-degree male relative such as cousin or uncle; determines whether the client and/or family should be given information about the client

Client: May choose to face Mecca (west or southwest in the United States)

Head of deceased should be elevated above the body

Discussions about death not usually welcomed

Stopping medical treatment: Against the will of Allah (Arabic word for God)

Expressions of grief: May be through slapping or hitting the body

If possible, only a same-sex Muslim should handle the body after death; if not possible, non-Muslims should wear gloves so as not to touch the body

JUDAISM

Prolongation of life important (life support must not be discontinued until death)

Dying person should not be left alone (a rabbi's presence is desired)

Autopsy and cremation may be forbidden in some forms of Judaism

HINDUISM

Rituals: Include tying a thread around the neck or wrist of the dying person, sprinkling the person with special water, or placing a leaf of basil on their tongue

After death: Sacred threads are not removed; body is not washed

BUDDHISM

Shrine to Buddha: May be placed in the client's room

Time for meditation at the shrine is important, should be respected

Medications that could alter awareness (such as opioids) may be refused by client

Monk may recite prayers for 1 hour after death (need not be done in the presence of the body)

e. Family members may make decisions about care and often do not tell the client their diagnosis or prognosis

f. Dying at home may be considered bad luck

4. Native Americans

a. Eye contact is avoided

b. Personal distance needs to be maintained

c. Family meetings may be held to make decisions about end-of-life issues and the type of treatments that should be pursued

d. May not report pain

e. Some tribes avoid contact with the dying (may prefer to die in the hospital)

C. Legal and ethical issues

1. Outcomes related to care during illness and the dying experience should be based on the client's wishes

2. Issues for consideration may include organ and tissue donations, advance directives or other legal documents, withholding or withdrawing treatment, and cardiopulmonary resuscitation

D. Palliative care

1. Focuses on caring interventions and symptom management rather than cure for disease that no longer responds to treatment

2. A pain-controlled and symptom-controlled environment is established (the dying client should be as pain-free and as comfortable as possible)

3. Hospice care: Provides support and care for the client in the last phases of an incurable disease so that he or she might live as fully and as comfortably as possible; client and family needs are the focus of any intervention

E. Near-death physiological manifestations

1. As death approaches, metabolism is reduced and the body gradually slows down until all function ends

2. Sensory: Blurred vision, decreased sense of taste and smell, decreased pain and touch perception, loss of blink reflex; client appears to stare (hearing is believed to be the last sense lost)

3. Respirations

a. May be rapid, slow, shallow, and irregular

b. May be noisy and wet sounding (death rattle)

c. Cheyne-Stokes respiration: Alternating periods of apnea and deep, rapid breathing

4. Circulatory

a. Heart rate slows, blood pressure falls progressively

b. Skin is cool to touch and extremities become pale, mottled, and cyanotic

c. "Waxlike" skin when very near death

5. Urinary: Gradual decrease in urinary output; incontinence may occur

6. Gastrointestinal: Motility and peristalsis diminish, leading to constipation, gas accumulation, and distention; a bowel movement may occur before death or at the time of death

7. Musculoskeletal: Gradual loss of ability to move; difficulty speaking and swallowing, and loss of the gag reflex

F. Death

1. Occurs when all vital organs and body systems cease to function

2. Generally, respirations cease first; heartbeat stops a few minutes thereafter

G. Brain death: Occurs when the cerebral cortex stops functioning or is irreversibly destroyed

H. Nursing care

1. Data collection

a. Should be limited to obtaining essential data

b. Frequency depends on the client's stability (at least every 8 hours); as changes occur, assessment needs to be done more frequently

c. Avoid repeated unnecessary assessments on the dying client

2. Physical care (Box 65-6)

3. Psychosocial care

a. Monitor for anxiety and depression

b. Monitor for fear (Box 65-7)

c. Encourage the client and family to express feelings

d. Provide support and advocacy for the client and family

e. Provide privacy for the client and family

f. Provide a private room for the client

g. Maintain respect and dignity for the client

4. Postmortem care (Box 65-8)

a. Maintain respect and dignity for the client

b. Determine if the client is an organ donor; if so, follow appropriate procedures related to the donation

c. Consider cultural rituals, state laws, and agency procedures when performing postmortem care

d. Prepare the body for immediate viewing by the family

e. Provide privacy and time for the family to be with the deceased person

VI. DEPRESSION

A. Description

1. Affects feelings, thoughts, and behaviors

2. Can occur after a loss, including loss of self-esteem, the end of a significant relationship, the death of a loved one, or a traumatic event

3. The loss is followed by grief and mourning; if this process does not resolve, depression results

4. Depression may be mild, moderate, or severe

5. Treatment includes counseling, antidepressant medication, and electroconvulsive therapy (ECT) therapy

B. Mild depression

1. Triggered by an external event; follows the normal grief reaction

2. Lasts less than 2 weeks

BOX 65-6

Physical Care of the Dying Client

PAIN
Administer pain medication.
Do not delay or deny pain medication.

DYSPNEA
Elevate the head of the bed or position on the side.
Administer supplemental oxygen.
Suction as needed.

SKIN
Assess color and temperature.
Assess for breakdown.
Implement measures to prevent breakdown.

DEHYDRATION
Maintain regular oral care.
Encourage ice chips and sips of fluid.
Do not force the client to eat or drink.
Use moist cloths to provide moisture to the mouth.
Apply lubricant to the lips and oral mucous membranes.

ANOREXIA, NAUSEA, AND VOMITING
Provide antiemetics before meals.
Have family members provide the client's favorite foods.
Provide frequent small portions of favorite foods.

ELIMINATION
Monitor urinary and bowel elimination.
Place absorbent pads under the client and check frequently.

WEAKNESS AND FATIGUE
Provide rest periods.
Assess tolerance for activities.
Provide assistance and support as needed for maintaining bed or chair position.

RESTLESSNESS
Maintain a calm, soothing environment.
Do not restrain.
Limit the number of visitors at the client's bedside.
Allow a family member to stay with the client.

BOX 65-7

Fear Associated with Dying

FEAR OF PAIN
This may occur based on anxieties related to dying.
Do not delay or deny pain relief measures for a terminally ill client.

FEAR OF LONELINESS AND ABANDONMENT
Allow family members to stay with the client.
Holding hands and touching (if culturally acceptable) and listening to the client are important.

FEAR OF MEANINGLESS
Client may feel hopeless and powerless.
Encourage life reviews and focus on the client's positive aspects of their life.

Adapted from Lewis, S., Heitkemper, M., & Dirksen, S. (2004). *Medical-surgical nursing: Assessment and management of clinical problems* (6th ed.). St. Louis: Mosby, p. 168.

BOX 65-8

General Postmortem Procedures

Close the client's eyes.
Replace dentures.
Wash the body.
Place pads under the perineum.
Remove tubes and dressings.
Straighten the body and place a pillow under the head in preparation for family viewing.

6. Helplessness and powerlessness
7. May experience intense anxiety and anger
8. Diurnal variation: May feel better at a certain time of the day, such as in the morning
9. Slow thought processes and difficulty in concentrating
10. Rumination: Persistent thinking about and discussion of a particular subject
11. Negative thinking and suicidal thoughts
12. Sleep disturbances
13. Social withdrawal
14. Anorexia, weight loss, and fatigue
15. Somatic complaints
16. Menstrual changes
17. Increased use of alcohol or drugs
D. Severe depression
  1. Intense and pervasive
  2. Despair and hopelessness
  3. Feelings of guilt and worthlessness
  4. Flat affect
  5. May show agitation and pace about
  6. Poor posture and unkempt appearance
  7. Decreased speech
  8. Self-destructive thoughts; however, client may lack energy to act on thought

3. Feeling sad
4. Feeling let down or disappointed
5. Mild alterations in sleep patterns
6. Feeling less alert
7. Irritability
8. Disinterested in spending time with others
9. Increased use of alcohol or drugs
C. Moderate depression
  1. Persists over time
  2. The person experiences a sense of change and often seeks help
  3. Despondent and gloomy
  4. Feels dejected
  5. Low self-esteem

9. Social withdrawal
10. Poor concentration and overwhelmed by simple tasks
11. Severe psychomotor retardation
12. Anorexia and marked weight loss
13. Constipation and urinary retention
14. Lack of sexual interest
15. Terminal insomnia
16. Diurnal variation: The person feels worse in the morning and better as the day goes on
17. Delusions and hallucinations

E. Interventions
  1. Altered thought processes
    a. Encourage client to discuss losses or changes in life situation
    b. Encourage client to express sadness or anger; allow adequate time for verbal responses
    c. Assist in developing short-term goals
    d. Encourage the use of problem solving and positive thinking
    e. Limit decision making
    f. Spend short periods of time throughout the day with the client
    g. Be on time when a schedule is planned with the client
    h. Sit in silence with clients who are not verbalizing
    i. Use simple, concrete words when communicating
    j. Avoid a cheerful attitude
  2. Risk for self-harm
    a. Assess for **suicide** clues and intervene to provide safety precautions as necessary
    b. Ask client directly, "Have you thought of hurting yourself?"
    c. Assess lethality of plans
    d. Do not leave alone for extended periods
    e. If the client has a suicidal plan, place on one-to-one supervision
    f. Form a **suicide** contract with the client
  3. Activity intolerance
    a. Encourage daily exercise
    b. Assist with activities of daily living (ADLs) if the client is unable to perform
    c. Begin with one-to-one activities
    d. Provide activities that are easily mastered to increase self-esteem and help alleviate guilt feelings
    e. Provide activities that require little orientation (card games, drawing)
    f. Engage in gross motor activities (walking)
    g. Eventually bring the client into small group activities, then large group activities
  4. Altered nutrition
    a. Ensure adequate nutrition
    b. Offer small, high-calorie, high-protein snacks and fluids throughout the day
    c. Stay with the client during meals

d. Weigh client weekly
e. Monitor bowel patterns for constipation
  5. Sleep pattern disturbance
    a. Ensure adequate sleep
    b. Provide rest periods after activities
    c. Encourage the client to dress and stay out of bed during the day
    d. Provide relaxation measures at bedtime
    e. Decrease environmental stimuli at bedtime
    f. Spend time with the client before bedtime

VII. ELECTROCONVULSIVE THERAPY (ECT)

A. Description
  1. An effective treatment for depression that consists of inducing a grand mal (tonic-clonic) seizure by passing an electrical current through electrodes that are attached to the temples
  2. The administration of a muscle relaxant minimizes seizure activity, preventing damage to long bones and cervical vertebrae
  3. The usual course is 6 to 12 treatments given two to three times per week
  4. Maintenance ECT once a month may help decrease the relapse rate for the client with recurrent depression
  5. ECT is not a permanent cure
  6. Not necessarily effective in the client with dysrhythmic depression, depression and personality disorders, drug dependence, or depression secondary to situational or social difficulties
  7. At-risk clients include those with recent myocardial infarction, cerebrovascular accident, or cerebral vascular malformation, or clients with intracranial mass lesions

B. Uses
  1. For clients with major depressive and bipolar depressive disorders, especially when psychotic symptoms are present, such as delusions of guilt, somatic delusions, and delusions of infidelity
  2. For clients who have depression with marked psychomotor retardation and stupor
  3. For manic clients whose conditions are resistant to lithium and antipsychotic medications and clients who are rapid cyclers (a client with a bipolar disorder who has many episodes of mood swings close together)
  4. For clients with schizophrenia (especially catatonia), those with schizoaffective syndromes, and psychotic clients

C. Indications for use (Box 65-9)
D. Preprocedure
  1. Explain the procedure to the client
  2. Encourage the client to discuss feelings, including myths regarding ECT
  3. Teach the client and family what to expect

Electroconvulsive Therapy (ECT): Indications for Use

To be used when:
Antidepressant medications have no effect.
There is a need for a rapid definitive response such as when a client is suicidal or homicidal.
The client is in extreme agitation or stupor.
Risks of other treatments outweigh the risk of ECT.
The client has a history of poor medication response, a history of good ECT response, or both.
The client prefers ECT as a treatment.

4. Informed consent must be obtained when voluntary clients are being treated
5. For involuntary clients, when informed consent cannot be obtained, permission may be obtained from the next of kin, although in some states the permission for ECT must be obtained from the court
6. NPO after midnight or at least 4 hours prior to treatment
7. Baseline vital signs are taken
8. The client is requested to void
9. Hairpins, contact lenses, and dentures are removed
10. Administer preoperative medication if prescribed; glycopyrrolate (Robinul) or atropine sulfate may be prescribed to prevent the potential for aspiration and to minimize bradydysrhythmias in response to electrical stimulants

E. During the procedure
1. Place a blood pressure cuff on one of the client's arms
2. An intravenous (IV) line is inserted; electrodes are attached for electroencephalography (EEG) and electrocardiography (ECG)
3. A pulse oximeter is placed on the client's finger
4. Blood pressure is monitored throughout the treatment
5. Medications administered may include a short-acting anesthetic such as methohexital sodium (Brevital Sodium), thiopental sodium (Pentothal) and a muscle relaxant such as succinylcholine (Anectine)
6. 100% oxygen by mask via positive pressure is administered throughout the procedure
7. An airway or bite block is placed to prevent biting the tongue
8. Electrical stimulus is administered; seizure should last 30 to 60 seconds

F. Postprocedure
1. The client will be transported to a recovery room with the blood pressure cuff and oximeter in place, where oxygen, suction, and other emergency equipment are available

2. Once the client is awake, talk to the client and take vital signs
3. The client may be confused; provide frequent orientation (brief, distinct, and simple) and reassurance
4. Client returns to the nursing unit when a 90% oxygen saturation level is maintained, vital signs are stable, and mental status is satisfactory
5. Assess the gag reflex prior to giving the client fluids, food, or medication

G. Potential side effects
1. Major side effects with bilateral treatment are confusion, disorientation, and short-term memory loss
2. The client may be confused and disoriented on awakening
3. Memory deficits may occur, but memory usually recovers completely, although some clients have memory loss lasting up to 6 months

VIII. SUICIDAL BEHAVIOR
A. Description
1. Suicidal clients characteristically have feelings of worthlessness, guilt, and hopelessness that are so overwhelming that they feel unable to go on with life and unfit to live
2. The nurse caring for a depressed client always considers the possibility of **suicide**

B. High-risk groups
1. Those with a history of previous **suicide attempts**
2. Family history of **suicide attempts**
3. Adolescents
4. Older clients
5. Disabled or terminally ill adults
6. Clients with personality disorders
7. Clients with organic brain syndrome or dementia
8. Depressed or psychotic clients
9. Substance **abusers**

C. Clues (Box 65-10)
D. Data collection (Box 65-11)
E. Interventions
1. Initiate **suicide** precautions
2. Remove harmful objects
3. Do not leave the client alone
4. Provide one-to-one supervision at all times
5. Provide a nonjudgmental, caring attitude
6. Develop a contract that is written, dated, and signed and provides suggestions for alternative behavior at times of suicidal thoughts
7. Encourage the client to talk about feelings and to identify positive aspects about self
8. Encourage active participation in his or her own care
9. Keep client active by assigning simple tasks
10. Check that visitors do not leave harmful objects in the client's room

---

BOX 65-10

Suicidal Clues

Giving away personal, special, and prized possessions
Canceling social engagements
Making out or changing a will
Taking out or changing insurance policies
Positive or negative changes in behavior
Poor appetite
Sleeping difficulties
Feelings of hopelessness
Difficulty in concentrating
Loss of interest in activities
Client statements that indicate an intent to attempt suicide
Sudden calmness or improvement in a depressed client
Client asks questions about poisons, guns, other lethal objects

---

BOX 65-11

Suicidal Client: Data Collection

THE PLAN
Does the client have a plan?
What is the plan, how lethal is the plan, and how likely is death to occur?
Does the client have the means to carry out the plan?

CLIENT HISTORY OF ATTEMPTS
Were there suicide attempts in the past? If so, what were the outcomes?
Was the client accidentally rescued?
Have the past attempts and methods been the same, or have methods increased in lethality?

PSYCHOSOCIAL
Is the client alone or alienated from others?
Is hostility or depression present?
Do hallucinations exist?
Is substance abuse present?
Were there any recent losses or physical illness?
Were there any environmental or lifestyle changes?

---

11. Identify support systems
12. Do not allow the client to leave the unit unless accompanied by a staff member
13. Continue to assess the client's suicide potential

IX. ABUSIVE BEHAVIORS

A. Anger
  1. A feeling of annoyance that may be displaced onto an object or person
  2. Used to avoid anxiety; gives a feeling of power in situations in which the person feels out of control
B. Aggression: Can be harmful and destructive when not controlled

C. Violence: The physical force that is threatening to the safety of self and others
D. Data collection
  1. History of violence or self-harm
  2. Poor impulse control and low tolerance of frustration
  3. Defiant and argumentative
  4. Raises voice
  5. Makes verbal threats
  6. Paces and is agitated
  7. Muscle rigidity
  8. Flushed face
  9. Glares at others
E. Interventions
  1. Maintain safety for the client, other clients, and self
  2. Use a calm approach and communicate with a calm, clear tone of voice (be assertive, not aggressive, and avoid verbal struggles)
  3. Maintain a large personal space and use a nonaggressive posture
  4. Listen actively and acknowledge the client's anger
  5. Determine what the client considers to be his or her need
  6. Provide the client with clear options that deal with the client's behavior, set limits on behavior, and make the client aware of the consequences of anger and violence
  7. Discuss the use of restraints or seclusion if the client is unable to control angry behavior that may lead to violence
  8. Assist the client with problem-solving and decision making regarding the options
F. **Restraints** and **seclusion**
  1. Description
    a. Physical **restraints**: Any manual method or mechanical device, material, or equipment that inhibits free movement
    b. **Seclusion**: The last step in a process to maximize safety to a client and others, in which a client is placed alone in a specially designed room for protection and close supervision
    c. Chemical **restraints**: Medications given for a very specific purpose of inhibiting a specific behavior or movement; have an impact on the client's ability to relate to the environment
  2. Use of **restraints** and **seclusion**
    a. Should never be used as punishment or for the convenience of the health care staff
    b. The least restrictive means of **restraint** for the shortest duration should be used
    c. Used when behavior is physically harmful to the client or others
    d. Used when the disruptive behavior presents a danger to the facility
    e. Used when alternative or less restrictive measures are insufficient in protecting the client or others from harm

f. Used when the client anticipates that a controlled environment would be helpful and requests **seclusion**

g. Requires a written order of a physician, which must be reviewed and renewed every 24 hours and also must specify the type of **restraint** to be used

h. In an emergency, the charge nurse may place a client in **restraint** or **seclusion** and obtain a written or verbal order as soon as possible thereafter

i. Laws require the consent of the client unless an emergency situation exists and can be documented

j. The client must be removed from **restraint** or **seclusion** when safer and quieter behavior is observed

k. While in **restraint** or **seclusion**, the client must be protected from all sources of harm

l. The nurse must document the behavior leading to **restraint** or **seclusion** and the time the client is placed in and released from **restraint** or **seclusion**

m. The client in **restraint** or **seclusion** needs constant one-on-one supervision; physical, safety, and comfort needs must be assessed every 15 to 30 minutes and these observations are also documented

X. FAMILY VIOLENCE

A. Description

1. The violence begins with threats or verbal or physical minor assaults (tension building), and the victim attempts to comply with the requests of the **abuser**

2. The **abuser** loses control and becomes destructive and harmful (acute battering) while the victim attempts to protect himself or herself

3. Following the battering, the **abuser** then becomes loving and attempts to make peace (calmness and a diffusion of tension)

4. The **abuser** believes that violence is normal and that the victim is responsible for the **abuse**

5. Outsiders are usually not aware of what is happening in the family

6. Family members are socially isolated and lack autonomy and trust among each other; caring and intimacy in the family are absent

7. Family members expect other members of the family to meet their needs, but none are able to do so

8. The **abuser** threatens to abandon the family

B. Types of violence (Box 65-12)

C. The vulnerable person

1. The one in the family unit on whom violence is perpetrated

2. Those most vulnerable are children and older adults

3. Every battered person is a crime victim

BOX 65-12

Types of Violence

Physical violence: Infliction of physical pain or bodily harm

Sexual violence: Any form of sexual contact without consent

Emotional violence: Infliction of mental anguish

Physical neglect: Failure to provide health care to prevent or treat physical or emotional illnesses

Developmental neglect: Failure to provide physical and cognitive stimulation needed to prevent developmental deficits

Educational neglect: Depriving a child of education

Economic exploitation: Illegal or improper exploitation of money, funds, or other resources for one's personal gain

---

D. Characteristics of **abusers**

1. Impaired self-esteem

2. Strong dependency needs

3. Narcissistic and suspicious

4. History of **abuse** during childhood

5. Perceive victims as their property and believe that they are entitled to **abuse** them

E. Characteristics of victims

1. Feel trapped, dependent, helpless, and powerless

2. Depressed

3. Low self-esteem and blame themselves for the violence

F. Interventions

1. Report suspected or actual cases of child **abuse** or **abuse** of the older adult to appropriate authorities (follow state and agency guidelines)

2. Assess for evidence of physical injuries

3. Ensure privacy and confidentiality during data collection and provide a nonjudgmental and empathetic approach to foster trust; reassure the victim that he or she has not done anything wrong

4. Assist the victim to develop self-protective abilities and other problem-solving abilities

5. Develop a safety plan (a fast escape if the violence returns); ensure that the victim is aware of safe houses and shelters in the community

6. Assess suicidal potential of the victim

7. Assess the potential for homicide

8. Assess for the use of drugs and alcohol

9. Determine family coping patterns and support systems

10. Provide support and assistance in coping with contacting the legal system

11. Assist in resolving family dysfunction with prescribed therapies

12. Encourage individual therapy for victims that promotes coping with the trauma and prevents further psychological conflict

13. Provide individual therapy for **abusers** that focuses on preventing violent behavior and repairing relationships
14. Encourage psychotherapy, counseling, group therapy, and support groups to assist family members to develop coping strategies
15. Assist the family to identify an access to community and personal resources
16. Maintain accurate and thorough medical health records

XI. CHILD ABUSE (See Chapter 30)

A. Description: Involves physical, emotional, or sexual **abuse**; can also involve neglect
B. Data collection
   1. Physical **abuse**
      a. Unexplained bruises, burns, or fractures
      b. Bald spots on scalp
      c. Apprehensive child
      d. Extreme aggressiveness or withdrawal
      e. Fear of parents
      f. Lack of crying when approached by a stranger
   2. Physical neglect
      a. Inadequate weight gain
      b. Poor hygiene
      c. Consistent hunger (begs or steals food)
      d. Inconsistent school attendance
      e. Constant fatigue
      f. Reports of lack of child supervision
      g. Delinquency
   3. Emotional **abuse**
      a. Speech disorders
      b. Habit disorders, such as sucking, biting, rocking
      c. Learning disorders
      d. Self-harm behaviors
   4. Sexual **abuse**
      a. Difficulty walking or sitting
      b. Torn, stained, or bloody underclothing
      c. Pain, swelling, or itching of the genitals
      d. Bruises, bleeding, or lacerations in the genital or anal area
      e. Poor peer relations
      f. Delinquency
      g. Changes in sleep patterns
      h. Self-harm behaviors
   5. Shaken baby syndrome
      a. Can cause intracranial hemorrhage, leading to cerebral edema and death
      b. Baby often presents with respiratory problems
      c. Full, bulging fontanelles and a head circumference larger than expected would be noted
C. Interventions
   1. Assess injuries; support the child during a thorough physical assessment
   2. Report cases of suspected **abuse** to appropriate authorities (follow state and agency guidelines)

3. Remove the child from the abusive environment and plan to place the child in an environment that is safe (contact Child Protective Services), thereby preventing further injury
4. Move slowly and avoid any loud noises when near the child
5. Communicate with the child at the child's eye level
6. Reassure the child that he or she is not "bad" and is not responsible for the abuser's behavior
7. Document accurately and completely all information related to the suspected **abuse**
8. Assist the parents in identifying stressors and alternative ways to express feelings
9. Provide education to the parents; refer parents to **crisis** hotlines and community support systems such as Parents Anonymous (a group for parents who have abused or fear that they may abuse their child physically) or Parents United International (a group devoted to helping sexually abused families)

XII. ABUSE OF THE OLDER ADULT

A. Description
   1. Involves physical, emotional, or sexual **abuse**; can also involve neglect or economic exploitation
   2. Individuals at most risk include those who are dependent because of their immobility or altered mental status
   3. Factors that contribute to **abuse** and **neglect** include long-standing family violence, caregiver stress, and the individual's increasing dependence on others
   4. Victims may attempt to dismiss injuries as accidental; abusers may prevent victims from receiving proper medical care to avoid discovery
   5. Victims are often socially isolated by their abusers
B. Data collection
   1. Physical **abuse**
      a. Sprains, dislocations, or fractures
      b. Abrasions, bruises, or lacerations
      c. Pressure sores
      d. Puncture wounds
      e. Burns
   2. Sexual **abuse**
      a. Torn or stained underclothing
      b. Discomfort or bleeding in the genital area
      c. Difficulty in walking or sitting
      d. Unexplained genital infections or disease
   3. Emotional **abuse**
      a. Confusion
      b. Fearful and agitated
      c. Changes in appetite and weight
      d. Withdrawn and loss of interest in self and social activities

4. Neglect
   a. Disheveled appearance
   b. Dressed inadequately or inappropriately
   c. Dehydration and malnutrition
   d. Lacking in physical needs, such as glasses, hearing aids, and dentures
   e. Skin breaks
   f. Signs of medication overdose
5. Economic exploitation
   a. Inability to pay bills and fearful when discussing finances
   b. Confused, inaccurate, or no knowledge of finances

C. Interventions
   1. Assess for physical injuries and treat physical injuries
   2. Report cases of suspected **abuse** to appropriate authorities (follow state and agency guidelines)
   3. Remove the older adult from the abusive environment and contact Elderly Protective Services
   4. Explore alternative living arrangements that are least restrictive and disruptive to the victim
   5. Obtain assistance for financial matters
   6. Provide referrals to emergency community resources
   7. Assess the need for respite care; arrange counseling and treatment for the **abuser**

XIII. RAPE AND SEXUAL ASSAULT

A. Description
   1. Engaging another person in a sexual act and/or sexual intercourse through the use of force and without the consent of the sexual partner
   2. The victim is not required by law to report the rape or assault
   3. The victim is often blamed by others; often receives no support from significant others
   4. Acquaintance rape ("date rape") involves someone known to the victim
   5. Statutory rape is the act of sexual intercourse under the age of legal consent, even if there is consent from the minor
   6. Marital rape
      a. Husbands of abused women believe it is their right to have sex whenever they want
      b. Victims describe forced vaginal intercourse; anal intercourse; being physically abused during sex; having objects inserted into their vagina and anus; or being forced to have sex with animals or while their children are present

B. Data collection
   1. Female client
      a. Obtain the date of the last menstrual period
      b. Determine form of birth control used and last act of intercourse before rape
      c. Duration of intercourse, orifices violated, and penile penetration
      d. Use of condom by perpetrator

2. Shame, embarrassment, and humiliation
3. Anger and revenge
4. Fear of telling others for fear of not being believed

C. Rape trauma syndrome
   1. Sleep disturbances, nightmares
   2. Loss of appetite
   3. Fears, anxiety, phobias, suspicion
   4. Decrease in activities and motivation
   5. Disruptions in relationships with partner, family, friends
   6. Self-blame, guilt, shame
   7. Lowered self-esteem, feelings of worthlessness
   8. Somatic complaints

D. Interventions
   1. Perform data collection in a quiet, private area
   2. Stay with the victim
   3. Assess the victim's stress level before performing treatments and procedures
   4. Victim should not shower, bathe, douche (female), or change clothing until an examination is performed
   5. Obtain written consent for the examination, photographs, laboratory tests, release of information, and laboratory samples
   6. Assist with the female pelvic examination and in obtaining specimens to detect semen (the pelvic examination may trigger a flashback of the attack); a shower and fresh clothing should be made available to the client after the examination
   7. Preserve any evidence
   8. Treat physical injuries and provide client safety
   9. Document all events in the care of the victim
   10. Reinforce to the victim that surviving the assault is most important; if the victim survived the rape, then he or she did exactly what was necessary to stay alive
   11. Refer to **crisis** intervention and support groups

PRACTICE QUESTIONS

1. A nurse is reviewing the health care record of a client admitted to the psychiatric unit. The nurse notes that the admission nurse has documented that the client is experiencing anxiety as a result of a situational crisis. The nurse would determine that this type of crisis could be caused by:
   1. A fire that destroyed the client's home
   2. A recent rape episode experienced by the client
   3. The death of a loved one
   4. Witnessing a murder

2. A nurse is gathering data from a client in crisis. When determining the client's perception of the precipitating event that led to the crisis, the most appropriate question to ask is:
   1. "What leads you to seek help now?"
   2. "Who is available to help you?"
   3. "What do you usually do to feel better?"
   4. "With whom do you live?"

3. A nurse is assisting in developing a plan of care for the client in a crisis state. When developing the plan, the nurse will consider which of the following?
   1. Presenting symptoms in a crisis situation are similar for all individuals experiencing a crisis
   2. A crisis state indicates that the individual is suffering from an emotional illness
   3. A crisis state indicates that the individual is suffering from a mental illness
   4. A client's response to a crisis is individualized, and what constitutes a crisis for one person may not constitute a crisis for another person

4. A nurse observes that a client with a potential for violence is agitated, pacing up and down in the hallway, and making aggressive and belligerent gestures at other clients. Which statement would be appropriate to make to this client?
   1. "What is causing you to become agitated?"
   2. "You need to stop that behavior now!"
   3. "You will need to be restrained if you do not change your behavior."
   4. "You will need to be placed in seclusion!"

5. During a conversation with a depressed client on a psychiatric unit, the client says to the nurse, "My family would be better off without me." The nurse should make which therapeutic response to the client?
   1. "Everyone feels this way when they are depressed."
   2. "Have you talked to your family about this?"
   3. "You sound very upset. Are you thinking of hurting yourself?"
   4. "You will feel better once your medication begins to work."

6. A nurse is caring for an older adult client who has recently lost her husband. The client says, "No one cares about me anymore. All the people I loved are dead." Which response by the nurse is therapeutic?
   1. "That seems rather unlikely to me."
   2. "You must be feeling all alone at this point."
   3. "I don't believe that, and neither do you."
   4. "Right! Why not just 'pack it in'?"

7. A nurse is planning care for a client who is being hospitalized because the client has been displaying violent behavior and is at risk for potential harm to others. The nurse avoids which intervention in the plan of care?
   1. Keeping the door to the client's room open when with the client
   2. Assigning the client to a room at the end of the hall to avoid disturbing the other clients
   3. Facing the client when providing care
   4. Ensuring that a security officer is within the immediate area

8. Which behaviors observed by the nurse might lead to the suspicion that a depressed adolescent client could be suicidal?
   1. The client becomes angry while speaking on the telephone and slams the receiver down on the hook
   2. The client runs out of the therapy group swearing at the group leader, and runs to her room
   3. The client gets angry with her roommate when the roommate borrows her clothes without asking
   4. The client gives away a prized CD and a cherished autographed picture of the performer

9. A client is admitted to the psychiatric unit following a serious suicidal attempt by hanging. The nurse's most important aspect of care is to maintain client safety and plans to:
   1. Assign a staff member to the client who will remain with the client at all times
   2. Admit the client to a seclusion room where all potentially dangerous articles are removed
   3. Remove the client's clothing and place the client in a hospital gown
   4. Request that a peer remain with the client at all times

10. The police arrive at the emergency room with a client who has seriously lacerated both wrists. The initial nursing action is to:
    1. Examine and treat the wound sites
    2. Secure and record a detailed history
    3. Encourage and assist the client to ventilate feelings
    4. Administer an antianxiety agent

11. A nurse receives a telephone call from a male client who states that he wants to kill himself and has a bottle of sleeping pills in front of him. The best nursing action is to:
    1. Insist that the client give you his name and address so that you can get the police there immediately
    2. Keep the client talking and allow the client to ventilate feelings
    3. Use therapeutic communications, especially the reflection of feelings
    4. Keep the client talking and signal to another staff member to send help to the client

12. A nurse is caring for a client with severe depression. Which of the following activities would be most appropriate for this client?
    1. Paint by number
    2. A puzzle
    3. Drawing
    4. Checkers

13. A client experiencing a severe major depressive episode is unable to address activities of daily

living. The appropriate nursing intervention is to:

1. Feed, bathe, and dress the client as needed until the client can perform these activities independently
2. Structure the client's day so that adequate time can be devoted to the client's assuming responsibility for the activities of daily living
3. Offer the client choices and consequences to the failure to comply with the expectation of maintaining activities of daily living
4. Have the client's peers confront the client about how the noncompliance in addressing activities of daily living affects the milieu

14. An older male client who is a victim of elder abuse and the client's family have been attending weekly counseling sessions. Which statement by the abusive family member would indicate that he or she has learned positive coping skills?

1. "I will be more careful to make sure that my father's needs are met."
2. "I am so sorry and embarrassed that the abusive event occurred. It won't happen again."
3. "I feel better able to care for my father now that I know where to obtain assistance."
4. "Now that my father is moving into my home, I will need to change my ways."

15. A nurse is assisting in planning care for a client being admitted to the nursing unit who has attempted suicide. Which priority nursing intervention will the nurse include in the plan of care?

1. Check the whereabouts of the client every 15 minutes
2. Suicide precautions, with 30-minute checks
3. One-to-one suicide precautions
4. Ask that the client report suicidal thoughts immediately

ALTERNATE FORMAT QUESTION: MULTIPLE RESPONSE

A nurse is preparing to care for a dying client and several family members are at the client's bedside. Select the therapeutic techniques that the nurse will use when communicating with the family.

____ Be honest and truthful and let the client and family know that you will not abandon them
____ Explain everything that is happening to all family members
____ Encourage expression of feelings, concerns, and fears
____ Extend touch and hold the client's or family member's hand if appropriate
____ Make the decisions for the family
____ Discourage reminiscing

ANSWERS

1. *Answer: 3*
Rationale: A situational crisis is associated with a life event. External situations that could precipitate a situational crisis include loss or change of a job, the death of a loved one, abortion, change in financial status, divorce, addition of new family members, pregnancy, and severe illness. Options 1, 2, and 4 identify adventitious crisis. An adventitious crisis relates to a crisis, disaster, or event that is not a part of everyday life, is unplanned, and is accidental.
Test-Taking Strategy: Use the process of elimination and focus on the key words, *situational crisis*. This will assist in eliminating options 1, 2, and 4 because they are similar. If you had difficulty with this question, review the types of crisis.
Level of Cognitive Ability: Comprehension
Client Needs: Psychosocial Integrity
Integrated Process: Nursing Process/Data Collection
Content Area: Mental Health
Reference: Morrison-Valfre, M. (2005). *Foundations of mental health care* (3rd ed.). St. Louis: Mosby, p. 194.

2. *Answer: 1*
Rationale: A nurse's initial task when gathering data from a client in crisis is to assess the individual or family and the problem. The more clearly the problem can be defined, the better the chance a solution can be found. Option 1 will assist in determining data related to the precipitating event that led

to the crisis. Options 2 and 4 identify situational supports. Option 3 identifies personal coping skills.
Test-Taking Strategy: Use the process of elimination and note the key words, *precipitating event*. Focus on these key words when selecting the correct option. Eliminate options 2 and 4, because these data will determine support systems. Eliminate option 3, because this question would be asked when determining coping skills. Review data collection methods for a client in crisis if you had difficulty with this question.
Level of Cognitive Ability: Application
Client Needs: Psychosocial Integrity
Integrated Process: Nursing Process/Data Collection
Content Area: Mental Health
Reference: Morrison-Valfre, M. (2005). *Foundations of mental health care* (3rd ed.). St. Louis: Mosby, pp. 71, 197.

3. *Answer: 4*
Rationale: Although each crisis response can be described in similar terms as far as presenting symptoms are concerned, what constitutes a crisis for one person may not constitute a crisis for another person, because each is a unique individual. Being in a crisis state does not mean that the client is suffering from an emotional or mental illness
Test-Taking Strategy: Use the process of elimination. Eliminate option 1 because of the absolute word "all." Next, eliminate options 2 and 3 because a crisis does not indicate "illness." Review the characteristics of a crisis state if you had

difficulty with this question.
Level of Cognitive Ability: Comprehension
Client Needs: Psychosocial Integrity
Integrated Process: Nursing Process/Data Collection
Content Area: Mental Health
Reference: Morrison-Valfre, M. (2005). *Foundations of mental health care* (3rd ed.). St. Louis: Mosby, pp. 69-71.

4. Answer: 1
Rationale: The best statement is to ask the client what is causing the agitation. This will assist the client to become aware of the behavior and will assist the nurse in planning appropriate interventions for the client. Option 2 is demanding behavior, which could cause increased agitation in the client. Options 3 and 4 are threats to the client and are inappropriate.
Test-Taking Strategy: Use the process of elimination. Eliminate option 2 because of the demand that it places on the client. Eliminate options 3 and 4 because they indicate threats to the client. Review appropriate nursing interventions for the agitated client if you had difficulty with this question.
Level of Cognitive Ability: Application
Client Needs: Psychosocial Integrity
Integrated Process: Communication and Documentation
Content Area: Mental Health
Reference: Morrison-Valfre, M. (2005). *Foundations of mental health care* (3rd ed.). St. Louis: Mosby, pp. 88, 226.

5. Answer: 3
Rationale: Clients who are depressed may be at risk for suicide. It is critical for the nurse to assess suicidal ideation and plan. The client should be directly asked if a plan for self-harm exists. Options 1, 2, and 4 are not therapeutic responses.
Test-Taking Strategy: Use therapeutic communication techniques. Option 3 is the only option that deals directly with the client's feelings. Additionally, clients at risk for suicide need to be directly assessed regarding the potential for self-harm. Review data collection techniques for the depressed client if you had difficulty with this question.
Level of Cognitive Ability: Application
Client Needs: Psychosocial Integrity
Integrated Process: Nursing Process/Data Collection
Content Area: Mental Health
Reference: Morrison-Valfre, M. (2005). *Foundations of mental health care* (3rd ed.). St. Louis: Mosby, pp. 252-253.

6. Answer: 2
Rationale: The client is experiencing loss and is feeling hopeless. The therapeutic response by the nurse is the one that attempts to translate words into feelings. In option 1, the nurse is voicing doubt, which is often used when a client verbalizes delusional ideas. In option 3, the nurse is disagreeing with the client, which implies that the nurse has passed judgment on the client's ideas or opinions. In option 4, the nurse uses sarcasm, which gives advice and is nontherapeutic as a nursing response.
Test-Taking Strategy: Use therapeutic communication techniques. Option 2 is the only option that focuses on the client's feelings. Review therapeutic communication techniques if you had difficulty with this question.
Level of Cognitive Ability: Application

Client Needs: Psychosocial Integrity
Integrated Process: Communication and Documentation
Content Area: Mental Health
Reference: Morrison-Valfre, M. (2005). *Foundations of mental health care* (3rd ed.). St. Louis: Mosby, pp. 88, 161.

7. Answer: 2
Rationale: The client should be placed in a room near the nurses' station and not at the end of a long, relatively unprotected corridor. The nurse should not isolate himself or herself with a potentially violent client. The door to the client's room should be kept open, and the nurse should never turn away from the client. A security officer or male aide should be within immediate call in case of a suspicion of the possibility of violence.
Test-Taking Strategy: Use the process of elimination and note the key word, *avoids*. This word indicates a false response question and that you need to select the incorrect intervention. Keeping in mind that safety is the issue will direct you to option 2. If you had difficulty with this question, review guidelines for caring for the violent client.
Level of Cognitive Ability: Application
Client Needs: Safe, Effective Care Environment
Integrated Process: Nursing Process/Planning
Content Area: Mental Health
Reference: Morrison-Valfre, M. (2005). *Foundations of mental health care* (3rd ed.). St. Louis: Mosby, p. 116.

8. Answer: 4
Rationale: A depressed, suicidal client often gives away that which is of value as a way of saying "goodbye" and wanting to be remembered. Options 1, 2, and 3 identify acting-out behaviors.
Test-Taking Strategy: Use the process of elimination. Options 1, 2, and 3 are similar in that they deal with anger and "acting-out behaviors," which are often typical of some adolescents. Option 4 is different in nature and could indicate that the client may be saying good-bye. Review the clues that indicate suicide if you had difficulty with this question.
Level of Cognitive Ability: Analysis
Client Needs: Psychosocial Integrity
Integrated Process: Nursing Process/Data Collection
Content Area: Mental Health
Reference: Stuart, G., & Laraia, M. (2005). *Principles and practice of psychiatric nursing* (8th ed.). St. Louis: Mosby, p. 367.

9. Answer: 1
Rationale: Hanging is a serious suicide attempt. The plan of care must reflect action that will promote the client's safety. Constant observation status (one on one) with a staff member who is never less than an arm's length away is the safest intervention.
Test-Taking Strategy: Use the process of elimination. Eliminate option 2 because seclusion should not be the initial intervention. Eliminate option 4 next, because the responsibility to safeguard a client is not the peer's responsibility. Eliminate option 3 because removing one's clothing will not maximize all possible safety strategies. Review nursing interventions for the client at risk for suicide if you had difficulty with this question.

Level of Cognitive Ability: Application
Client Needs: Safe, Effective Care Environment
Integrated Process: Nursing Process/Implementation
Content Area: Mental Health
Reference: Morrison-Valfre, M. (2005). *Foundations of mental health care* (3rd ed.). St. Louis: Mosby, p. 288.

10. *Answer:* **1**
Rationale: The initial nursing action is to examine and treat the self-inflicted injuries. Injuries from lacerated wrists can lead to a life-threatening situation. Other interventions may follow after the client has been treated medically.
Test-Taking Strategy: Use Maslow's Hierarchy of Needs theory to prioritize. Physiological needs come first. Option 1 addresses the physiological need. Review care of the client who has attempted suicide if you had difficulty with this question.
Level of Cognitive Ability: Application
Client Needs: Physiological Integrity
Integrated Process: Nursing Process/Implementation
Content Area: Mental Health
Reference: Fortinash, K., & Holoday-Worret, P. (2004). *Psychiatric mental health nursing* (3rd ed.). St. Louis: Mosby, p. 562.

11. *Answer:* **4**
Rationale: In a crisis, the nurse must take an authoritative, active role to promote the client's safety. A bottle of sleeping pills in front of a client who verbalizes he wants to kill himself is a "crisis." The client's safety is of prime concern. Keeping the client on the phone and getting help to the client is the best intervention. The word "insist" could anger the client, and he might hang up. Option 2 lacks the authoritative action stance of securing the client's safety. Using therapeutic communication is important, but overuse of "reflection" may sound uncaring or superficial and is lacking direction and solutions to the immediate problem of the client's safety.
Test-Taking Strategy: Use the process of elimination and focus on the client's safety. Although each of the options may seem appropriate, the best option is option 4. This option encompasses every necessary action. Review interventions for the client who is suicidal if you had difficulty with this question.
Level of Cognitive Ability: Application
Client Needs: Safe, Effective Care Environment
Integrated Process: Nursing Process/Implementation
Content Area: Mental Health
References: Keltner, N., Schwecke, L., & Bostro, C. (2003). *Psychiatric nursing* (4th ed.). St. Louis: Mosby, p. 363. Stuart, G., & Laraia, M. (2005). *Principles and practice of psychiatric nursing* (8th ed.). St. Louis: Mosby, p. 233.

12. *Answer:* **3**
Rationale: Concentration and memory are poor in a client with severe depression. When a client has a diagnosis of severe depression, the nurse needs to provide activities that require little concentration. Activities that have no right or wrong choices or decisions minimize opportunities for the client to put himself or herself down.
Test-Taking Strategy: Use the process of elimination. Note the similarities in options 1, 2, and 4 in that they all require

concentration. It is important to remember that clients with depression have difficulty concentrating and need activities that require little concentration. Review care of the client with severe depression if you had difficulty with this question.
Level of Cognitive Ability: Application
Client Needs: Psychosocial Integrity
Integrated Process: Nursing Process/Implementation
Content Area: Mental Health
Reference: Stuart, G., & Laraia, M. (2005). *Principles and practice of psychiatric nursing* (8th ed.). St. Louis: Mosby, p. 353.

13. *Answer:* **1**
Rationale: The client with depression may not have the energy or interest to complete activities of daily living. Often, severely depressed clients are unable to perform even the simplest activities of daily living. The nurse assumes this role and completes these tasks with the client. Options 2 and 3 are incorrect because the client lacks the energy and motivation to perform these tasks independently. Option 4 will increase the client's feelings of poor self-esteem and unworthiness.
Test-Taking Strategy: Use the process of elimination and note the key words, *severe major depressive episode.* Eliminate options 2 and 3 because the client lacks the energy and motivation to do these independently. In addition, option 3 may lead to increased feelings of worthlessness as the client fails to meet expectations. Option 4 will increase the client's feelings of poor self-esteem and unworthiness. Review care of the client with severe depression if you had difficulty with this question.
Level of Cognitive Ability: Application
Client Needs: Physiological Integrity
Integrated Process: Nursing Process/Implementation
Content Area: Mental Health
Reference: Morrison-Valfre, M. (2005). *Foundations of mental health care* (3rd ed.). St. Louis: Mosby, p. 221.

14. *Answer:* **3**
Rationale: Elder abuse sometimes occurs with family members who are being expected to care for their aging parents. This can cause family members to become overextended, frustrated, or financially depleted. Knowing where in the community to turn for assistance in caring for aging family members can bring much needed relief. Using these alternatives is a positive alternative coping strategy, which many families use.
Test-Taking Strategy: Use the process of elimination and focus on the issue, a coping strategy. Only option 3 identifies a means of coping with the issues. The other options are statements of good faith or promises, which may or may not be kept in the future. Option 3 outlines a definitive plan for how to handle the pressure associated with the father's care. Review effective coping strategies if you had difficulty with this question.
Level of Cognitive Ability: Analysis
Client Needs: Health Promotion and Maintenance
Integrated Process: Nursing Process/Evaluation
Content Area: Mental Health
Reference: Stuart, G., & Laraia, M. (2005). *Principles and practice of psychiatric nursing* (8th ed.). St. Louis: Mosby, p. 811.

15. *Answer: 3*
Rationale: One-to-one suicide precautions are required for the client who has attempted suicide. Options 1 and 2 are not appropriate, considering the situation. Option 4 may be an appropriate nursing intervention, but the priority is stated in option 3. The best option is constant supervision so that the nurse may intervene as needed if the client attempts to cause harm to himself or herself.
Test-Taking Strategy: Use the process of elimination and note the key word, *priority*. Recalling that one-to-one suicide precautions is the priority in caring for a suicidal client will direct you to option 3. Review interventions for the suicidal client if you had difficulty with this question.
Level of Cognitive Ability: Application
Client Needs: Safe, Effective Care Environment
Integrated Process: Nursing Process/Implementation
Content Area: Mental Health
Reference: Stuart, G., & Laraia, M. (2005). *Principles and practice of psychiatric nursing* (8th ed.). St. Louis: Mosby, p. 288.

ALTERNATE FORMAT QUESTION: MULTIPLE RESPONSE

Answers:
Be honest and truthful and let the client and family know that you will not abandon them

Encourage expression of feelings, concerns, and fears
Extend touch and hold the client's or family member's hand if appropriate
Rationale: It is important for the nurse to determine if there is a spokesperson for the family and how much the client and family want to know. The nurse needs to allow the family and client the opportunity to make informed choices and assist with the decision-making process if asked. Expression of feelings, concerns, and fears should be encouraged, as should reminiscing. The nurse needs to be honest and truthful and let the client and family know that they will not be abandoned. It is appropriate to extend touch and hold the client's or family member's hand if appropriate.
Test-Taking Strategy: Recalling therapeutic communication techniques and client and family rights will assist in answering these questions. Review these techniques and care of the dying client if you had difficulty with this question.
Level of Cognitive Ability: Application
Client Needs: Psychosocial Integrity
Integrated Process: Caring
Content Area: Mental Health
Reference: Potter, P., & Perry, A. (2005). *Fundamentals of nursing* (6th ed.). St. Louis: Mosby, pp. 585, 587.

REFERENCES

Fortinash, K., & Holoday-Worret, P. (2004). *Psychiatric mental health nursing* (3rd ed.). St. Louis: Mosby.

Morrison-Valfre, M. (2005). *Foundations of mental health care* (3rd ed.). St. Louis: Mosby.

Potter, P., & Perry, A. (2005). *Fundamentals of nursing* (6th ed.). St. Louis: Mosby.

Stuart, G., & Laraia, M. (2005). *Principles and practice of psychiatric nursing* (8th ed.). St. Louis: Mosby.

Psychiatric Medications

I. SELECTIVE SEROTONIN REUPTAKE INHIBITORS (SSRIs) (Box 66-1)

A. Description
   1. Inhibit serotonin uptake
   2. Produce an antidepressant response
B. Side effects
   1. Nausea and diarrhea
   2. Dry mouth
   3. Central nervous system (CNS) stimulation
   4. Photosensitivity
   5. Insomnia, somnolence
   6. Nervousness
   7. Headache
   8. Dizziness
   9. Weight loss or gain
C. Interventions
   1. Monitor vital signs
   2. Monitor weight
   3. Initiate safety precautions, particularly if dizziness occurs
   4. Administer with a snack or with meals to reduce the risk of dizziness and lightheadedness

---

BOX 66-1

Reuptake Inhibitors

SELECTIVE SEROTONIN REUPTAKE INHIBITORS (SSRIs)
Citalopram (Celexa)
Escitalopram (Lexapro)
Fluoxetine (Prozac)
Fluvoxamine (Luvox)
Paroxetine hydrochloride (Paxil)
Sertraline hydrochloride (Zoloft)

ATYPICAL REUPTAKE INHIBITORS
Buproprion hydrochloride (Wellbutrin)
Venlafaxine hydrochloride (Effexor)

---

   5. Monitor the suicidal client, especially during improved mood and increased energy levels
   6. Instruct client on fluoxetine (Prozac) to take medication early in the day to avoid interference with sleep
   7. For the client on long-term therapy, monitor liver and renal function test results
   8. Monitor white blood cell (WBC) and neutrophil counts; discontinue the medication as prescribed if levels fall below normal
   9. If priapism (painful, prolonged penile erection) occurs, the medication is discontinued immediately and the physician is notified
   10. Inform the client about the possibility of decreased libido
   11. Instruct the client to change positions slowly to avoid hypotensive effect
   12. Instruct the client to avoid alcohol
   13. Instruct the client to report any visual changes to the physician

---

II. TRICYCLIC ANTIDEPRESSANTS (Box 66-2)

A. Description
   1. Block the reuptake of norepinephrine and serotonin at the presynaptic neuron
   2. Used to treat depression
   3. May reduce seizure threshold
   4. May reduce effectiveness of antihypertensive agents
   5. Concurrent use with alcohol or antihistamines can cause CNS depression
   6. Concurrent use with monoamine oxidase inhibitors (MAOIs) can cause hypertensive crisis
B. Side effects
   1. Anticholinergic effects
   2. Dry mouth

BOX 66-2

Tricyclic Antidepressants

Amitriptyline hydrochloride (Elavil)
Amoxapine (Asendin)
Clomipramine (Anafranil)
Desipramine hydrochloride (Norpramin)
Doxepin hydrochloride (Sinequan)
Imipramine hydrochloride (Tofranil)
Maprotiline (Ludiomil)
Mirtazapine (Remeron)
Nortriptyline hydrochloride (Aventyl)
Protriptyline hydrochloride (Vivactil)
Trazodone (Desyrel)
Trimipramine maleate (Surmontil)

3. Decreased gastrointestinal (GI) motility and constipation
4. Difficulty voiding
5. Dilated pupils and blurred vision
6. Photosensitivity
7. Cardiovascular disturbances
8. Tachycardia, dysrhythmias
9. Orthostatic hypotension
10. Sedation
11. Weight gain
12. Anxiety, restlessness, and irritability
13. Decreased or increased libido with ejaculatory and erection disturbances

C. Interventions
  1. Instruct the client that the medication may take several weeks to produce the desired effect (client response may not occur until 2 to 4 weeks after the first dose)
  2. Monitor the suicidal client, especially during improved mood and increased energy levels
  3. Instruct the client to change positions slowly to avoid hypotensive effect
  4. Monitor pattern of daily bowel activity
  5. Monitor for urinary retention
  6. For the client on long-term therapy, monitor liver and renal function tests
  7. Administer with food or milk if GI distress occurs
  8. Administer the entire daily oral dose at one time, preferably at bedtime
  9. Instruct the client to avoid alcohol and non-prescription medications to prevent adverse medication interactions
  10. Instruct the client to avoid driving and other activities requiring alertness
  11. When the medication is discontinued, it should be tapered gradually

III. MONOAMINE OXIDASE INHIBITORS
  (MAOIs) (Box 66-3)
  A. Description

BOX 66-3

Monoamine Oxidase Inhibitors (MAOIs)

Isocarboxazid (Marplan)
Phenelzine sulfate (Nardil)
Tranylcypromine sulfate (Parnate)

1. Inhibit MAO enzyme, which is present in the brain, blood platelets, liver, spleen, and kidneys
2. Inhibition of the MAO enzyme metabolizes amines, norepinephrine, and serotonin, and the concentration of these amines increases
3. Used for depression in the client who has not responded to other antidepressant therapies, including electroconvulsive therapy (ECT)
4. Concurrent use with amphetamines, antidepressants, dopamine, epinephrine, guanethidine, levodopa, methyldopa, nasal decongestants, norepinephrine, reserpine, tyramine-containing foods, or vasoconstrictors may cause hypertensive crisis
5. Concurrent use with narcotic analgesics may cause hypertension, hypotension, coma, or seizures

B. Side effects
  1. Orthostatic hypotension
  2. Restlessness
  3. Insomnia
  4. Dizziness
  5. Weakness, lethargy
  6. GI upset
  7. Dry mouth
  8. Weight gain
  9. Peripheral edema
  10. Anticholinergic effects
  11. CNS stimulation, including anxiety, agitation, and mania
  12. Delay in ejaculation

C. Hypertensive crisis
  1. Hypertension
  2. Occipital headache radiating frontally
  3. Neck stiffness and soreness
  4. Nausea and vomiting
  5. Sweating
  6. Fever and chills
  7. Clammy skin
  8. Dilated pupils
  9. Palpitations, tachycardia, or bradycardia
  10. Constricting chest pain
  11. Antidote for hypertensive crisis: 5 to 10 mg phentolamine (Regitine) by intravenous injection

D. Interventions
  1. Monitor blood pressure frequently for hypertension
  2. Monitor for signs of hypertensive crisis
  3. If palpitations or frequent headaches occur, discontinue the medication and notify the physician

4. Administer with food if GI distress occurs
5. Instruct the client that the medication effect may be noted during the first week of therapy, but maximum benefit may take up to 3 weeks
6. Instruct the client to report headache, neck stiffness, or neck soreness immediately
7. Instruct the client to change positions slowly to prevent orthostatic hypotension
8. Instruct the client to avoid caffeine or over-the-counter preparations, such as weight-reducing pills or medications for hay fever and colds
9. Monitor for client compliance with medication administration
10. Instruct the client to carry a Medic-Alert card indicating that a MAOI medication has been prescribed
11. Avoid administering the medication in the evening because insomnia may result
12. MAO inhibitors should be tapered and discontinued 7 to 14 days before surgery
13. When the medication is discontinued, it should be discontinued gradually
14. Instruct the client to avoid foods that require bacteria or molds for their preparation or preservation or those that contain tyramine (Box 66-4)

IV. MOOD STABILIZERS (Box 66-5)

A. Description
   1. Affect cellular transport mechanism by altering both the presynaptic and postsynaptic events affecting serotonin, thus enhancing serotonin function
   2. Concurrent use with diuretics, fluoxetine, methyldopa, or nonsteroidal anti-inflammatory drugs (NSAIDs) increases lithium reabsorption by the kidney or inhibits lithium excretion, either of which increases the risk of lithium toxicity
   3. Acetazolamide, aminophylline, phenothiazines, or sodium bicarbonate may increase renal excretion of lithium, reducing its effectiveness
   4. The therapeutic dose is only slightly less than the amount producing toxicity
   5. The therapeutic drug serum level of lithium is 0.6 to 1.2 mEq/L
   6. The causes of an increase in lithium level include decreased sodium intake, fluid and electrolyte loss associated with severe sweating, dehydration, diarrhea, or diuretic therapy, illness or overdose
   7. Serum lithium levels should be checked every 1 to 2 months or whenever any behavioral change suggests an altered serum level
   8. Blood samples to check serum lithium levels should be drawn in the morning, 12 hours after the last dose was taken

---

BOX 66-4

Tyramine-Containing Foods to Avoid

Cheese, especially aged cheese, except cottage cheese
Sour cream
Pickled herring
Avocados
Bananas
Papaya
Broad beans
Figs
Overripe fruit
Brewer's yeast
Meat extracts and tenderizers
Yogurt
Sausage, bologna, pepperoni, salami
Soy sauce
Raisins
Red wine, beer, sherry
Beef or chicken liver
Caffeine as coffee, tea, or chocolate

BOX 66-5

Mood Stabilizers

LITHIUM PREPARATIONS
Lithium carbonate (Eskalith, Lithane, Lithobid)
Lithium citrate (Cibalith-Si)

OTHER MOOD STABILIZERS
Carbamazepine (Tegretol)
Divalproex sodium (Depakote)
Gabapentin (Neurontin)
Lamotrigine (Lamictal)
Oxcarbazepine (Trileptal)
Topiramate (Topamax)

B. Side effects
   1. Polyuria
   2. Polydipsia
   3. Anorexia, nausea
   4. Dry mouth
   5. Mild thirst
   6. Weight gain
   7. Abdominal bloating
   8. Soft stools or diarrhea
   9. Fine hand tremors
   10. Inability to concentrate
   11. Muscle weakness
   12. Lethargy
   13. Fatigue
   14. Headache
   15. Hair loss
C. Interventions
   1. Monitor the suicidal client, especially during improved mood and increased energy levels
   2. Administer the medication with food to minimize GI irritation

3. Instruct the client to maintain a fluid intake of six to eight glasses of water a day
4. Instruct the client to avoid excessive amounts of coffee, tea, or cola, which have a diuretic effect
5. Instruct the client to maintain an adequate salt intake
6. Do not administer diuretics while the client is taking lithium
7. Instruct the client to avoid alcohol
8. Instruct the client to avoid over-the-counter medications
9. Instruct the client that they may take a missed dose within 2 hours of scheduled time; otherwise, they should skip the missed dose and take the next dose at the scheduled time
10. Instruct the client not to adjust the dosage without consulting the physician because lithium should be tapered off and not discontinued abruptly
11. Instruct the client about the signs and symptoms of lithium toxicity
12. Instruct the client to notify the physician if polyuria, prolonged vomiting, diarrhea, or fever occur
13. Instruct the client that the therapeutic response to the medication will be noted in 1 to 3 weeks
14. Monitor electrocardiography (ECG), renal function tests, and thyroid tests

D. Lithium toxicity
  1. Description
     a. Occurs when ingested lithium cannot be detoxified and excreted by the kidneys
     b. Symptoms of toxicity begin to appear when the serum lithium level is 1.5 to 2.0 mEq/L
  2. Mild toxicity
     a. Serum lithium level of 1.5 mEq/L
     b. Apathy
     c. Lethargy
     d. Diminished concentration
     e. Mild ataxia
     f. Coarse hand tremors
     g. Slight muscle weakness
  3. Moderate toxicity
     a. Serum lithium level of 1.5 to 2.5 mEq/L
     b. Nausea, vomiting
     c. Severe diarrhea
     d. Mild to moderate ataxia and incoordination
     e. Slurred speech
     f. Tinnitus
     g. Blurred vision
     h. Muscle twitching
     i. Irregular tremor
  4. Severe toxicity
     a. Serum lithium level above 2.5 mEq/L
     b. Nystagmus
     c. Muscle fasciculations
     d. Deep tendon hyperreflexia
     e. Visual or tactile hallucinations

f. Oliguria or anuria
g. Impaired level of consciousness (LOC)
h. Grand mal seizure or coma leading to death
  5. Interventions for lithium toxicity
     a. Hold lithium and notify the physician
     b. Monitor vital signs and LOC
     c. Monitor cardiac status
     d. Prepare to obtain lithium, electrolyte, blood urea nitrogen (BUN), and creatinine levels and complete blood cell (CBC) count
     e. Monitor for suicidal tendencies and institute **suicide** precautions

V. ANTIANXIETY OR ANXIOLYTIC MEDICATIONS

A. Description
  1. Depress the CNS, thereby increasing the effects of gamma-aminobutyric acid (GABA), which produces relaxation and may depress the limbic system
  2. Benzodiazepines have anxiety-reducing (anxiolytic), sedative-hypnotic, muscle-relaxing, and anticonvulsant actions (Box 66-6)
B. Side effects
  1. Daytime sedation
  2. Ataxia
  3. Dizziness
  4. Headaches
  5. Blurred or double vision
  6. Hypotension
  7. Tremor
  8. Amnesia
  9. Slurred speech
  10. Urinary incontinence
  11. Constipation
  12. Paradoxical CNS excitement
C. Acute toxicity
  1. Somnolence
  2. Confusion

BOX 66-6

Benzodiazepines

Alprazolam (Xanax)
Chlordiazepoxide (Librium)
Clonazepam (Klonopin)
Clorazepate (Tranxene)
Diazepam (Valium)
Estazolam (ProSom)
Flurazepam (Dalmane)
Halazepam (Paxipam)
Lorazepam (Ativan)
Oxazepam (Serax)
Quazepam (Doral)
Temazepam (Restoril)
Triazolam (Halcion)

3. Diminished reflexes and coma
4. Flumazenil (Romazicon), a benzodiazepine antagonist, administered IV, will reverse benzodiazepine intoxication in 5 minutes
5. The client being treated for an overdose of a benzodiazepine may experience agitation, restlessness, discomfort, and anxiety

⏏ D. Interventions
1. Monitor for motor responses such as agitation, trembling, and tension
2. Monitor for autonomic responses such as cold, clammy hands and sweating
3. Monitor for paradoxical CNS excitement during early therapy, particularly in the older client and debilitated individuals
4. Monitor for visual disturbances, because these medications can worsen glaucoma
5. Monitor liver and renal function tests and blood counts
6. Reduce the medication dose as prescribed for the older adult client and for the client with impaired liver function
7. Initiate safety precautions because the older adult client is at risk for falling when taking the medication for sleep or anxiety
8. Assist with ambulation if drowsiness or light-headedness occurs
9. Instruct the client that drowsiness usually disappears during continued therapy
10. Instruct the client to avoid tasks that require alertness until the response to the medication has been established
11. Instruct the client to avoid alcohol
12. Instruct the client not to take other medications without consulting the physician
13. Instruct the client not to withdraw the medication abruptly

⏏ E. Withdrawal
1. To lessen withdrawal symptoms, the dosage of a benzodiazepine should be tapered gradually over 2 to 6 weeks
2. Results of abrupt or too rapid withdrawal
   a. Restlessness
   b. Irritability
   c. Insomnia
   d. Hand tremors
   e. Abdominal or muscle cramps
   f. Sweating
   g. Vomiting
   h. Seizures

VI. MEDICATIONS FOR INSOMNIA AND ANXIETY (Box 66-7)

A. Description
1. Depress the reticular activating system by promoting the inhibitory synaptic action of the neurotransmitter GABA

2. Used for short-term treatment of insomnia or for sedation to relieve anxiety, tension, and apprehension

B. Side effects
1. Confusion
2. Irritability
3. Allergic reactions
4. Agranulocytosis
5. Thrombocytopenia purpura
6. Megaloblastic anemia

C. Overdose
1. Tachycardia
2. Hypotension
3. Cold and clammy skin
4. Dilated pupils
5. Weak and rapid pulse
6. Signs of shock
7. Depressed respirations
8. Absent reflexes
9. Coma and death may result from respiratory and cardiovascular collapse

D. Withdrawal
1. Severe withdrawal symptoms begin within 24 hours after the medication is discontinued in an individual with severe drug dependence
2. Gradual withdrawal is used to detoxify a dependent person
3. Anxiety
4. Insomnia
5. Nightmares
6. Daytime agitation
7. Tremors
8. Delirium
9. Seizures

E. Interventions
1. Administer lower doses as prescribed for the older client
2. Medications should be used with caution in the client who has suicidal tendencies or has a history of drug **addiction**

BOX 66-7

Barbiturates and Sedative-Hypnotic Anxiolytics

BARBITURATES
Amobarbital (Amytal)
Aprobarbital (Alurate)
Butabarbital (Butisol)
Pentobarbital (Nembutal)
Phenobarbital (Luminal)
Secobarbital (Seconal)

SEDATIVE-HYPNOTIC ANXIOLYTICS
Buspirone (BuSpar)
Chloral hydrate (Aquachloral)
Hydroxyzine hydrochloride (Atarax)
Zaleplon (Sonata)
Zolpidem tartrate (Ambien)

3. Maintain safety by supervising ambulation and using side rails at night
4. Instruct the client to take medication as directed
5. Instruct the client to avoid driving or operating hazardous equipment if drowsiness, dizziness, or unsteadiness occurs
6. Instruct the client to avoid alcohol
7. For insomnia, instruct the client to take the medication 30 minutes before bedtime
8. Instruct the client that a hangover effect may occur in the morning
9. Instruct the client not to discontinue the medication abruptly
10. Instruct the client taking chloral hydrate to take the medication with food, a full glass of water, fruit juice, or ginger ale to improve the taste and to prevent gastric irritation

VII. ANTIPSYCHOTIC MEDICATIONS (Box 66-8)

A. Description
1. Improve the thought processes and behavior of the client with psychotic symptoms, especially the client with schizophrenia
2. Block dopamine receptors in the brain, thereby reducing the psychotic symptoms
3. Block the chemoreceptor trigger zone and vomiting center in the brain, producing an antiemetic effect
4. Phenothiazines lower the seizure threshold
5. Antipsychotics should not be given with other antipsychotic or antidepressant medications

B. Side effects
1. Anticholinergic effects
2. Dry mouth

BOX 66-8

Antipsychotic Medications

TYPICAL ANTIPSYCHOTICS
Chlorpromazine hydrochloride (Thorazine)
Fluphenazine hydrochloride (Prolixin)
Perphenazine (Trilafon)
Thioridazine hydrochloride (Mellaril)
Thiothixene hydrochloride (Navane)
Trifluoperazine (Stelazine)
Triflupromazine hydrochloride (Vesprin)

ATYPICAL ANTIPSYCHOTICS
Aripiprazole (Abilify)
Clozapine (Clozaril)
Haloperidol (Haldol)
Loxapine (Loxitane)
Molindone hydrochloride (Moban)
Olanzapine (Zyprexa)
Quetiapine (Seroquel)
Risperidone (Risperdal)
Ziprasidone (Geodon)

---

3. Increased heart rate
4. Urinary retention
5. Constipation
6. Hypotension
7. Drowsiness
8. Blood dyscrasias
9. Pruritus
10. Photosensitivity

C. Extrapyramidal syndrome
1. Parkinsonism
   a. Tremors
   b. Masklike facies
   c. Rigidity
   d. Shuffling gait
2. Dystonia
   a. Facial grimacing
   b. Abnormal or involuntary eye movements
3. Akathisia
   a. Restlessness
   b. Constantly moving about
4. Tardive dyskinesia
   a. Protrusion of the tongue
   b. Chewing motion
   c. Involuntary movement of the body and extremities

D. Interventions
1. Monitor vital signs
2. Monitor for extrapyramidal syndrome
3. Monitor for symptoms of neuroleptic malignant syndrome
4. Monitor urine output
5. Monitor serum glucose level
6. Note that the client taking an antipsychotic medication may require long-term medication for parkinsonian symptoms
7. Administer the medication with food or milk to decrease gastric irritation
8. For oral use, the liquid form might be preferred, because some clients hide tablets to avoid taking them
9. Note that absorption is faster with the liquid form
10. Avoid skin contact with the liquid concentrate to prevent contact dermatitis
11. Protect the liquid concentrate from light
12. Dilute the liquid concentrate with fruit juice
13. Inform the client that a full therapeutic effect of the medication may not be evident for 3 to 6 weeks following initiation of therapy; however, an observable therapeutic response may be apparent after 7 to 10 days
14. Inform the client that phenothiazines may cause a harmless pinkish to red-brown urine color
15. Instruct the client to use sunscreen, wide-brimmed hat, and protective clothing when outdoors
16. Instruct the client to avoid alcohol or other CNS depressants

17. Instruct the client to change positions slowly to avoid orthostatic hypotension
18. Instruct the client to report signs of agranulocytosis, including sore throat, fever, and malaise
19. Instruct the client to report signs of liver dysfunction, including jaundice, malaise, fever, and right upper abdominal pain
20. When discontinuing antipsychotics, the medication dosage should be reduced gradually to avoid sudden reoccurrence of psychotic symptoms

VIII. NEUROLEPTIC MALIGNANT SYNDROME

A. Description
  1. A potentially fatal syndrome that may occur at any time during therapy with neuroleptic medications (antipsychotic or antischizophrenic medications)
  2. Although it is rare, it is more commonly seen at the initiation of therapy, after the client is changed from one medication to another, after a dosage increase, or when a combination of medications is used
B. Data collection
  1. Dyspnea or tachypnea
  2. Tachycardia or irregular pulse rate
  3. Fever
  4. High or low blood pressure
  5. Increased sweating
  6. Loss of bladder control
  7. Skeletal muscle rigidity
  8. Pale skin
  9. Excessive weakness or fatigue
  10. Altered level of consciousness
  11. Seizures
  12. Severe extrapyramidal side effects
  13. Difficulty swallowing
  14. Excessive salivation
  15. Oculogyric crisis
  16. Dyskinesia
  17. Elevated WBC count
  18. Elevated liver function test results
  19. Elevated creatinine phosphokinase (CPK) level
C. Interventions
  1. Notify the physician
  2. Monitor vital signs
  3. Initiate safety and seizure precautions
  4. Discontinue the neuroleptic medication
  5. Monitor LOC
  6. Administer antipyretics, as prescribed
  7. Use a cooling blanket to lower the body temperature
  8. Monitor electrolytes and administer IV fluids, as prescribed

IX. MEDICATIONS TO TREAT ATTENTION-DEFICIT/HYPERACTIVITY DISORDER (ADHD) (Box 66-9)

A. Children with ADHD may require medication to reduce hyperactive behavior and lengthen attention span
B. Medications that are most effective in controlling this disorder are CNS stimulants
C. CNS stimulants, which increase agitation and activity in adults, have a calming effect on children with ADHD and increase alertness and sensitivity to stimuli
D. Interventions
  1. Monitor for CNS side effects
  2. Instruct the parents that over-the-counter medications need to be avoided
  3. Instruct the parents that the last dose of the day should be taken at least 6 hours before bedtime (14 hours for extended-released forms) to prevent insomnia
  4. Monitor height and weight (particularly in children)
  5. Reinforce that several weeks of therapy may be necessary before the therapeutic effect can be evaluated
  6. Instruct the parents that a drug-free period may be prescribed to allow growth of the child if the medication has caused growth retardation

X. MEDICATIONS TO TREAT ALZHEIMER'S DISEASE

A. Acetylcholinesterase inhibitors may be used to treat Alzheimer's disease to improve cognitive functions in the early stages
B. Donepezil (Aricept)
  1. A reversible inhibitor of acetylcholinesterase
  2. Used to treat mild to moderate dementia of Alzheimer's disease
  3. Common side effects include nausea and diarrhea
  4. Can slow the heart rate through its vagotonic effect

BOX 66-9

Medications to Treat Attention-Deficit/Hyperactivity Disorder (ADHD)

Amphetamine
Atomoxetine (Strattera)
Dextroamphetamine (Dexedrine)
Dextroamphetamine and amphetamine (Adderall XR)
Methamphetamine (Desoxyn)
Methylphenidate hydrochloride (Concerta)
Methylphenidate (Ritalin)
Pemoline (Cylert)

C. Tacrine (Cognex)
   1. A centrally acting acetylcholinesterase inhibitor
   2. Used to treat mild to moderate dementia of Alzheimer's disease
   3. Side effects include ataxia, loss of appetite, nausea, vomiting, and diarrhea
   4. An adverse effect is hepatotoxicity; liver function studies need to be monitored

PRACTICE QUESTIONS

1. A nurse has administered a dose of diazepam (Valium) to the client. The nurse would take which most important action before leaving the client's room?
   1. Drawing the shades or blinds closed
   2. Putting up the side rails on the bed
   3. Giving the client a bedpan
   4. Turning down the volume on the television

2. A nurse provides medication instructions to a client who is taking lithium carbonate (Eskalith). The nurse determines that the client needs additional instructions if the client states that he or she will:
   1. Monitor lithium blood levels very closely
   2. Contact the physician if excessive diarrhea, vomiting, or diaphoresis occurs
   3. Take the lithium with meals
   4. Decrease fluid intake while taking the lithium

3. A client with a psychotic disorder is being treated with haloperidol (Haldol). Which of the following would indicate the presence of a toxic effect of this medication?
   1. Hypotension
   2. Nausea
   3. Excessive salivation
   4. Blurred vision

4. Buspirone hydrochloride (BuSpar) is prescribed for a client with an anxiety disorder. The nurse instructs the client regarding the medication and informs the client that which of the following is a characteristic of this medication?
   1. The medication can produce a sedating effect
   2. Tolerance can occur with the medication
   3. The medication is addicting
   4. Dizziness and headaches may occur

5. Neuroleptic malignant syndrome is suspected in a client who is taking chlorpromazine (Thorazine). Which medication would the nurse prepare in anticipation of being ordered to treat this adverse effect related to the use of chlorpromazine?
   1. Phytonadione (vitamin K_1)
   2. Bromocriptine (Parlodel)
   3. Enalapril maleate (Vasotec)
   4. Protamine sulfate

6. A nurse is caring for a hospitalized client who has been taking clozapine (Clozaril) for the treatment of a schizophrenic disorder. Which laboratory study prescribed for the client will the nurse specifically review to monitor for an adverse effect associated with the use of this medication?
   1. White blood cell count
   2. Platelet count
   3. Cholesterol level
   4. Blood urea nitrogen level

7. Disulfiram (Antabuse) is prescribed for a client who is seen in the psychiatric health care clinic. The nurse is collecting data on the client and is providing instructions regarding the use of this medication. Which is most important for the nurse to determine before administration of this medication?
   1. When the last alcoholic drink was consumed
   2. A history of diabetes insipidus
   3. A history of hyperthyroidism
   4. When the last full meal was consumed

8. A nurse is collecting data from a client and the client's spouse reports that the client is taking donepezil hydrochloride (Aricept). Which disorder would the nurse suspect that this client may have based on the use of this medication?
   1. Dementia
   2. Obsessive-compulsive disorder
   3. Seizure disorder
   4. Schizophrenia

9. Fluoxetine hydrochloride (Prozac) is prescribed for the client. The nurse provides instructions to the client regarding the administration of the medication. Which statement by the client indicates an understanding about administration of the medication?
   1. "I should take the medication right before bedtime with a snack."
   2. "I should take the medication with my evening meal."
   3. "I should take the medication at noon with an antacid."
   4. "I should take the medication in the morning when I first arise."

10. A nursing student is assigned to care for a client with a diagnosis of schizophrenia. Haloperidol (Haldol) is prescribed for the client. The nursing instructor asks the student to describe the action of the medication. Which statement by the nursing student indicates an understanding of the action of this medication?
   1. It blocks the uptake of norepinephrine and serotonin
   2. It blocks the binding of dopamine to the post-synaptic dopamine receptors in the brain
   3. It is a serotonin reuptake blocker
   4. It inhibits the breakdown of released acetylcholine

11. A client receiving lithium carbonate (Eskalith) complains of loose, watery stools and difficulty walking.

The nurse would expect the serum lithium level to be which of the following?

1. 0.7 mEq/L
2. 1.0 mEq/L
3. 1.2 mEq/L
4. 1.7 mEq/L

12. When teaching a client who is being started on imipramine hydrochloride (Tofranil), the nurse would inform the client that the desired effects of the medication may:
    1. Start during the first week of administration
    2. Start during the second week of administration
    3. Not occur for 2 to 3 weeks of administration
    4. Not occur until after a month of administration

13. A client receiving thioridazine (Mellaril) complains that he feels very "faint" when he tries to get out of bed in the morning, The nurse recognizes this complaint as a symptom of:
    1. Psychosomatic symptoms
    2. Cardiac dysrhythmias
    3. Respiratory insufficiency
    4. Postural hypotension

14. A client who is taking lithium carbonate (Eskalith) is scheduled for surgery. The nurse informs the client that:
    1. The medication will be discontinued several days before surgery and resumed by injection in the immediate postoperative period
    2. The medication is to be taken until the day of surgery and resumed by injection immediately postoperatively
    3. The medication will be discontinued 1 to 2 days before the surgery and resumed as soon as full oral intake is allowed
    4. The medication will be discontinued a week before the surgery and resumed 1 week post-operatively

15. A client receiving a tricyclic antidepressant arrives at the mental health clinic. Which observation indicates that the client is correctly following the medication plan?
    1. Reports sleeping 12 hours per night and 3 to 4 hours during the day
    2. Arrives at the clinic neat and appropriate in appearance
    3. Reports not going to work for this past week
    4. Complains of not being able to "do anything" anymore

16. A nurse is performing a follow-up teaching session with a client discharged 1 month ago who is taking fluoxetine (Prozac). What information would be important for the nurse to gather regarding the adverse effects related to the medication?
    1. Problems with excessive sweating
    2. Gastrointestinal dysfunctions

3. Cardiovascular symptoms
4. Problems with mouth dryness

17. A client taking buspirone hydrochloride (BuSpar) for 1 month returns to the clinic for a follow-up visit. Which of the following would indicate medication effectiveness?
    1. No reports of alcohol withdrawal symptoms
    2. No paranoid thought processes
    3. No rapid heartbeats or anxiety
    4. No thought broadcasting or delusions

18. A client taking lithium carbonate (Eskalith) reports vomiting, abdominal pain, diarrhea, blurred vision, tinnitus, and tremors. The lithium level is checked as a part of the routine follow-up and the level is 3.0 mEq/L. The nurse knows that this level is:
    1. Normal
    2. Slightly above normal
    3. Excessively below normal
    4. Toxic

19. A client is placed on chloral hydrate (Aquachloral) for short-term treatment. Which nursing action indicates an understanding of the major side effect of this medication?
    1. Monitoring neurological signs every 2 hours
    2. Monitoring the blood pressure every 4 hours
    3. Instructing the client to call for ambulation assistance
    4. Lowering the bed and clearing a path to the bathroom at bedtime

20. A client admitted to the hospital gives the nurse a bottle of clomipramine (Anafranil). The nurse notes that the medication has not been taken by the client in 2 months. What behaviors observed in the client would validate noncompliance with this medication?
    1. Frequent hand washing with hot, soapy water
    2. Complaints of hunger
    3. A pulse rate below 60 beats per minute
    4. Complaints of insomnia

21. A client in the mental health unit is administered haloperidol (Haldol) intramuscularly. The nurse would check which of the following to determine medication effectiveness?
    1. The client's vital signs
    2. The physical safety of other unit clients
    3. The client's nutritional intake
    4. The client's orientation and delusional status

22. Diphenhydramine hydrochloride (Benadryl) is used in the treatment of allergic rhinitis for a hospitalized client with a chronic psychotic disorder. The client asks the nurse why the medication is being discontinued before hospital discharge. The nurse responds, knowing that:
    1. Allergic symptoms are short term in duration
    2. Poor compliance causes this medication to fail to reach its therapeutic blood level

3. Addictive properties are enhanced in the presence of psychotropic medications
4. This medication promotes long-term extra-pyramidal symptoms

23. A client arrives at the health care clinic and tells the nurse that he has been doubling his daily dosage of bupropion (Wellbutrin) to help him get better faster. The nurse understands that the client is now at risk for which of the following?
    1. Orthostatic hypotension
    2. Seizure activity
    3. Weight gain
    4. Insomnia

24. Immediately after taking a routine evening dose of alprazolam (Xanax), a client says, "I'm not sure I should have taken that stuff." The nurse makes which appropriate statement to the client?
    1. "You are afraid of the media claims about this medication."
    2. "Your depression will fade once the medication begins to work."
    3. "Anxiety is expected with any new experience."
    4. "Let's talk about how you feel about Xanax for a while."

25. A hospitalized client is started on phenelzine sulfate (Nardil) for the treatment of depression. At lunch time, a tray is delivered to the client. Which food item, if on the client's lunch tray, will the nurse remove?
    1. Yogurt
    2. Tossed salad
    3. Crackers
    4. Oatmeal cookies

26. A client is scheduled for discharge and will be taking phenobarbital sodium (Luminal) for an extended period. The nurse would place highest priority on teaching the client which of the following points that directly relates to client safety?
    1. Avoid drinking alcohol while taking this medication
    2. Take the medication only with meals
    3. Take medication at the same time each day
    4. Always use a dose container to help prevent missed doses

27. Fluphenazine (Prolixin) is administered to a client daily. The nurse plans to monitor for the common side effects of the medication and includes which of the following in the plan of care?
    1. Monitor the blood pressure every 2 hours
    2. Review the white blood cell (WBC) count results daily

3. Offer a nutritious snack between meals
4. Offer hard candy or gum periodically

28. A depressed client who is on tranylcypromine sulfate (Parnate) has been instructed on diet. The nurse feels confident that the client understands the diet when given a choice of restaurant foods if the client selects:
    1. Pepperoni pizza, salad, and cola
    2. Roasted chicken, roasted potatoes, and beer
    3. Pickled herring, French fries, and milk
    4. Fried haddock, baked potato, and cola

29. A client is being treated for depression with amitriptyline hydrochloride (Elavil). During the initial phases of treatment, the most important nursing intervention is:
    1. Ordering the client an tyramine-free diet
    2. Monitoring blood levels frequently, because there is a narrow range between therapeutic and toxic blood levels of this medication
    3. Getting baseline postural blood pressures on the client before administering the medication and each time the medication is dispensed to the client, especially during the initial days of treatment
    4. Checking the client for anticholinergic effects

30. A client who is on lithium carbonate (Eskalith) will be discharged at the end of the week. In formulating a discharge teaching plan, the nurse will instruct the client that it is most important to:
    1. Avoid soy sauce, wine, and aged cheese
    2. Take medication only as prescribed because it can become addicting
    3. Check with the psychiatrist before using any over-the-counter medications or prescription medications
    4. Have the lithium level checked every week

ALTERNATE FORMAT QUESTION: FILL IN THE BLANK

A physician orders phenobarbital sodium (Luminal), 10 mg by mouth daily. The medication bottle is labeled 15 mg/5 mL. How many milliliters will the nurse administer? (Round the answer to the nearest tenth.)

Answer: _____

ANSWERS

1. Answer: 2

Rationale: Diazepam is a sedative-hypnotic with anticonvulsant and skeletal muscle relaxant properties. The nurse should institute safety measures before leaving the client's room to ensure that the client does not injure herself or himself. The most frequent side effects of this medication are dizziness, drowsiness, and lethargy. For this reason, the nurse puts the side rails up on the bed before leaving the room to prevent falls. Options 1, 3 and 4 may be helpful measures that provide a comfortable, restful environment. However, option 2 is the one that provides for the client's safety needs.

Test-Taking Strategy: Use the process of elimination and note the key words, *most important.* Use Maslow's Hierarchy of Needs theory to prioritize, remembering that physiological and safety needs are a priority. This will direct you to option 2. Review nursing care for a client taking diazepam if you had difficulty with this question.

Level of Cognitive Ability: Application

Client Needs: Safe, Effective Care Environment

Integrated Process: Nursing Process/Implementation

Content Area: Pharmacology

Reference: McKenry, L., & Salerno, E. (2003). *Mosby's pharmacology in nursing* (21st ed.). St. Louis: Mosby, p. 514.

2. Answer: 4

Rationale: Because therapeutic and toxic dosage ranges are so close, lithium blood levels must be monitored very closely, more frequently at first and then once every several months. The client should be instructed to contact the physician if excessive diarrhea, vomiting, or diaphoresis occurs. Lithium is irritating to the gastric mucosa; therefore, lithium should be taken with meals. A normal diet and normal salt and fluid intake (1500 to 3000 mL/day) should be maintained, because lithium decreases sodium reabsorption by the renal tubules, which could cause sodium depletion. A low sodium intake causes lithium retention and could lead to toxicity.

Test-Taking Strategy: Use the process of elimination and note the key words, *needs additional instructions.* These words indicate a false response question and that you need to select the incorrect client statement. Remember that, generally, it is important that clients be taught to maintain an adequate fluid intake. This principle will direct you to option 4. Review the client teaching points related to the administration of this medication if you had difficulty with this question.

Level of Cognitive Ability: Comprehension

Client Needs: Health Promotion and Maintenance

Integrated Process: Teaching/Learning

Content Area: Pharmacology

Reference: Hodgson, B., & Kizior, R. (2005). *Saunders nursing drug handbook 2005.* Philadelphia: W.B. Saunders, pp. 642-643.

3. Answer: 3

Rationale: Toxic effects include extrapyramidal symptoms noted as marked drowsiness and lethargy, excessive salivation, and a fixed stare. Akathisia, acute dystonias, and tardive dyskinesia are also signs of toxicity. Hypotension, nausea, and blurred vision are occasional side effects.

Test-Taking Strategy: Use the process of elimination and note the key words, *toxic effect.* Select option 3, because "excessive" salivation indicates a toxic effect. Review the toxic effects of this medication if you had difficulty with this question.

Level of Cognitive Ability: Analysis

Client Needs: Physiological Integrity

Integrated Process: Nursing Process/Data Collection

Content Area: Pharmacology

Reference: Hodgson, B., & Kizior, R. (2005). *Saunders nursing drug handbook 2005.* Philadelphia: W.B. Saunders, p. 521.

4. Answer: 4

Rationale: Buspirone hydrochloride is used in the management of anxiety disorders. The advantages of this medication are that it is not sedating, tolerance does not develop, and it is not addicting. Dizziness, nausea, headaches, nervousness, lightheadedness, and excitement, which generally are not major problems, are side effects of the medication.

Test-Taking Strategy: Knowledge regarding the side effects and the advantages of buspirone hydrochloride is needed to answer this question. Remember, this medication is not sedating or addicting, and tolerance does not develop with its use. Review this medication and its use if you had difficulty with this question.

Level of Cognitive Ability: Application

Client Needs: Physiological Integrity

Integrated Process: Nursing Process/Implementation

Content Area: Pharmacology

Reference: Hodgson, B., & Kizior, R. (2005). *Saunders nursing drug handbook 2005.* Philadelphia: W.B. Saunders, p. 146.

5. Answer: 2

Rationale: Bromocriptine is an antiparkinsonian prolactin inhibitor used in the treatment of neuroleptic malignant syndrome. Vitamin K is the antidote for warfarin (Coumadin) overdose. Protamine sulfate is the antidote for heparin overdose. Enalapril maleate is an antihypertensive used in the treatment of hypertension.

Test-Taking Strategy: Knowledge regarding the treatment for neuroleptic malignant syndrome is needed to answer this question. Remember, bromocriptine is used to treat neuroleptic malignant syndrome. If you are unfamiliar with the various medications used as antidotes or treatments for various syndromes, review this content.

Level of Cognitive Ability: Analysis

Client Needs: Physiological Integrity

Integrated Process: Nursing Process/Planning

Content Area: Pharmacology

Reference: Lehne, R. (2004). *Pharmacology for nursing care* (5th ed.). Philadelphia: W.B. Saunders, p. 180, 691.

6. Answer: 1

Rationale: Hematological reactions can occur in the client taking clozapine and include agranulocytosis and mild leukopenia. The white blood cell count should be checked before initiating treatment and should be monitored closely during the use of this medication. The client should also be monitored for signs indicating agranulocytosis, which may include sore throat, malaise, and fever. Options 2, 3, and 4 are unrelated to this medication.

Test-Taking Strategy: Knowledge regarding the adverse effects that can occur in association with the use of clozapine is required to answer this question. Remember, clozapine can cause agranulocytosis and mild leukopenia. If you are unfamiliar with these adverse effects and the laboratory studies that need to be monitored, review this content.
Level of Cognitive Ability: Analysis
Client Needs: Physiological Integrity
Integrated Process: Nursing Process/Data Collection
Content Area: Pharmacology
Reference: Hodgson, B., & Kizior, R. (2005). *Saunders nursing drug handbook 2005.* Philadelphia: W.B. Saunders, p. 252.

7. Answer: 1
Rationale: Disulfiram is used as an adjunct treatment for selective clients with chronic alcoholism who want to remain in a state of enforced sobriety. Clients must abstain from alcohol intake for at least 12 hours before the initial dose of the medication is administered. The most important data is to determine when the last alcoholic drink was consumed. The medication is used with caution in clients with diabetes mellitus, hypothyroidism, epilepsy, cerebral damage, nephritis, and hepatic disease. It is also contraindicated in severe heart disease, psychosis, or hypersensitivity related to the medication.
Test-Taking Strategy: Use the process of elimination. Recalling that the medication is used as an adjunct treatment for selective clients with chronic alcoholism will assist in directing you to option 1. Review this medication if you had difficulty with this question.
Level of Cognitive Ability: Analysis
Client Needs: Physiological Integrity
Integrated Process: Nursing Process/Data Collection
Content Area: Pharmacology
Reference: Lehne, R. (2004). *Pharmacology for nursing care* (5th ed.). Philadelphia: W.B. Saunders, p. 378.

8. Answer: 1
Rationale: Donepezil hydrochloride is a cholinergic agent used in the treatment of mild to moderate dementia of the Alzheimer type. It enhances cholinergic functions by increasing the concentration of acetylcholine. It slows the progression of Alzheimer's disease. Options 2, 3, and 4 are incorrect.
Test-Taking Strategy: Knowledge regarding the use of donepezil hydrochloride is needed to answer this question. Remember, this medication is used to treat mild to moderate dementia. Review this medication if you had difficulty with this question.
Level of Cognitive Ability: Analysis
Client Needs: Physiological Integrity
Integrated Process: Nursing Process/Data Collection
Content Area: Pharmacology
Reference: Hodgson, B., & Kizior, R. (2005). *Saunders nursing drug handbook 2005.* Philadelphia: W.B. Saunders, p. 349.

9. Answer: 4
Rationale: Fluoxetine hydrochloride is administered in the early morning without consideration to meals. Options 1, 2, and 3 are incorrect.

Test-Taking Strategy: Use the process of elimination. Eliminate options 1, 2, and 3 because they are similar and indicate taking the medication with an antacid or food. If you are unfamiliar with the use of this medication and the client teaching points, review this content.
Level of Cognitive Ability: Analysis
Client Needs: Health Promotion and Maintenance
Integrated Process: Nursing Process/Evaluation
Content Area: Pharmacology
Reference: Lehne, R. (2004). *Pharmacology for nursing care* (5th ed.). Philadelphia: W.B. Saunders, p. 319.

10. Answer: 2
Rationale: Haloperidol acts by blocking the binding of dopamine to the post synaptic dopamine receptors in the brain. Imipramine hydrochloride (Tofranil) blocks the reuptake of norepinephrine and serotonin. Donepezil hydrochloride (Aricept) inhibits the breakdown of released acetylcholine. Fluoxetine hydrochloride (Prozac) is a potent serotonin reuptake blocker.
Test-Taking Strategy: Knowledge regarding the action of haloperidol is required to answer this question. Remember, haloperidol blocks the binding of dopamine. Review this medication if you had difficulty with this question.
Level of Cognitive Ability: Comprehension
Client Needs: Physiological Integrity
Integrated Process: Teaching/Learning
Content Area: Pharmacology
Reference: Hodgson, B., & Kizior, R. (2005). *Saunders nursing drug handbook 2005.* Philadelphia: W.B. Saunders, p. 519.

11. Answer: 4
Rationale: The therapeutic serum level of lithium ranges from 0.6 to 1.2 mEq/L. Serum lithium levels above the therapeutic level will produce signs of toxicity.
Test-Taking Strategy: Focus on the data in the question, noting that the client is experiencing loose, watery stools and difficulty waking. Recalling the therapeutic serum level of lithium will direct you to option 4. Option 4 is the only serum level that is not within the therapeutic range. Review this therapeutic level and the signs of toxicity if you had difficulty with this question.
Level of Cognitive Ability: Analysis
Client Needs: Physiological Integrity
Integrated Process: Nursing Process/Data Collection
Content Area: Pharmacology
Reference: Hodgson, B., & Kizior, R. (2005). *Saunders nursing drug handbook 2005.* Philadelphia: W.B. Saunders, p. 643.

12. Answer: 3
Rationale: The therapeutic effects of administration of imipramine hydrochloride (Tofranil) may not occur for 2 to 3 weeks after the antidepressant therapy has been initiated.
Test-Taking Strategy: Knowledge regarding the therapeutic effects of imipramine hydrochloride (Tofranil) is needed to answer this question. Remember, therapeutic effects of imipramine hydrochloride (Tofranil) may not occur for 2 to 3 weeks after initiation of therapy. Review this medication if you had difficulty with this question.
Level of Cognitive Ability: Application

Client Needs: Physiological Integrity
Integrated Process: Nursing Process/Implementation
Content Area: Pharmacology
Reference: McKenry, L., & Salerno, E. (2003). *Mosby's pharmacology in nursing* (21st ed.). St. Louis: Mosby, p. 414.

13. *Answer:* 4
Rationale: Thioridazine can cause postural hypotension. The client needs to be taught to get out of bed slowly and to rise from a sitting position slowly because of this adverse effect related to the medication. Options 1, 2, and 3 are unrelated to the use of this medication.
Test-Taking Strategy: Use the process of elimination and focus on the data in the question. Noting the key word, *faint,* in the question will direct you to option 4. Review the effects of this medication if you had difficulty with this question.
Level of Cognitive Ability: Analysis
Client Needs: Psychosocial Integrity
Integrated Process: Nursing Process/Data Collection
Content Area: Pharmacology
Reference: Hodgson, B., & Kizior, R. (2005). *Saunders nursing drug handbook 2005.* Philadelphia: W.B. Saunders, p. 1030.

14. *Answer:* 3
Rationale: The client who is on lithium carbonate must be off the medication for 1 to 2 days before a scheduled surgical procedure and can resume the medication when full oral intake is ordered after the surgery. Options 1, 2, and 4 are incorrect.
Test-Taking Strategy: Use the process of elimination. Recalling that lithium carbonate is an oral medication and is not given as an injection will assist in eliminating options 1 and 2. From the remaining options, note that option 4 identifies a period of time that is unreasonable; therefore, eliminate this option. Review this medication if you had difficulty with this question.
Level of Cognitive Ability: Application
Client Needs: Physiological Integrity
Integrated Process: Nursing Process/Implementation
Content Area: Pharmacology
Reference: Morrison-Valfre, M. (2005). *Foundations of mental health care* (3rd ed.). St. Louis: Mosby, p. 58.

15. *Answer:* 2
Rationale: Depressed individuals will sleep for long periods, are not able to go to work, and feel as if they cannot "do anything." Once they have had some therapeutic effect from their medication, they will report resolution of many of these complaints as well as demonstrate an improvement in their appearance.
Test-Taking Strategy: Use the process of elimination. The observations identified in options 1, 3, and 4 are all symptoms of depression. The improvement in appearance indicates a therapeutic response to the medication, thus indicating compliance with the medication regimen. Review the expected effects of tricyclic antidepressants if you had difficulty with this question.
Level of Cognitive Ability: Analysis
Client Needs: Physiological Integrity
Integrated Process: Nursing Process/Evaluation

Content Area: Pharmacology
Reference: Morrison-Valfre, M. (2005). *Foundations of mental health care* (3rd ed.). St. Louis: Mosby, pp. 219-220.

16. *Answer:* 2
Rationale: The most common adverse effects related to fluoxetine include central nervous system (CNS) and gastrointestinal (GI) system dysfunction. This medication affects the GI system by causing nausea and vomiting, cramping, and diarrhea. Options 1, 3, and 4 are not adverse effects of this medication.
Test-Taking Strategy: Knowledge regarding the adverse effects related to fluoxetine is required to answer this question. Remember that this medication causes CNS and GI system dysfunction. Review these side effects and adverse reactions if you had difficulty with this question.
Level of Cognitive Ability: Analysis
Client Needs: Physiological Integrity
Integrated Process: Nursing Process/Data Collection
Content Area: Pharmacology
Reference: Skidmore-Roth, L. (2005). *Mosby's drug guide for nurses* (6th ed.). St. Louis: Mosby, p. 368.

17. *Answer:* 3
Rationale: Buspirone hydrochloride is not recommended for the treatment of drug or alcohol withdrawal, paranoid thought disorders, or schizophrenia (thought broadcasting or delusions). Buspirone hydrochloride is most often indicated for the treatment of anxiety and aggression.
Test-Taking Strategy: Knowledge regarding the use of buspirone hydrochloride will direct you to the correct option. Recalling that this medication is an antianxiety one will direct you to option 3. Review this medication if you had difficulty with this question.
Level of Cognitive Ability: Analysis
Client Needs: Physiological Integrity
Integrated Process: Nursing Process/Evaluation
Content Area: Pharmacology
Reference: Hodgson, B., & Kizior, R. (2005). *Saunders nursing drug handbook 2005.* Philadelphia: W.B. Saunders, p. 146.

18. *Answer:* 4
Rationale: The therapeutic serum level of lithium is 0.6 to 1.2 mEq/L. A level of 3 mEq/L indicates toxicity.
Test-Taking Strategy: Knowledge regarding the therapeutic serum level of lithium will direct you to option 4. Review this level if you had difficulty with this question.
Level of Cognitive Ability: Comprehension
Client Needs: Physiological Integrity
Integrated Process: Nursing Process/Data Collection
Content Area: Pharmacology
Reference: Skidmore-Roth, L. (2005). *Mosby's drug guide for nurses* (6th ed.). St. Louis: Mosby, p. 643.

19. *Answer:* 3
Rationale: Chloral hydrate causes sedation and impairment of motor coordination; therefore, safety measures need to be implemented. The client is instructed to call for assistance with ambulation. Options 1 and 2 are not specifically associated with the use of this medication. Although option 4

is an appropriate nursing intervention, it is most important to instruct the client to call for assistance with ambulation.

Test-Taking Strategy: Use the process of elimination and note the key words, *major side effect*. Recalling the action and effects of the medication will assist in eliminating options 1 and 2. From the remaining options, focus on the issue, client safety. Option 3 is the client-oriented action, whereas option 4 allows the client to ambulate independently, placing the client at risk for injury. Review the nursing interventions related to this medication if you had difficulty with this question.

Level of Cognitive Ability: Application
Client Needs: Safe, Effective Care Environment
Integrated Process: Nursing Process/Implementation
Content Area: Pharmacology
Reference: Skidmore-Roth, L. (2005). *Mosby's drug guide for nurses* (6th ed.). St. Louis: Mosby, p. 171.

20. *Answer:* 1
Rationale: Clomipramine is commonly used in the treatment of obsessive-compulsive disorder. Hand washing is a common obsessive-compulsive behavior. Weight gain is a common side effect of this medication. Tachycardia and sedation are side effects. Insomnia may occur as a seldom side effect.

Test-Taking Strategy: Focus on the name of the medication. Recalling that clomipramine is used to treat commonly obsessive-compulsive disorder will direct you to option 1. Review the purpose of this medication if you had difficulty with this question.

Level of Cognitive Ability: Analysis
Client Needs: Physiological Integrity
Integrated Process: Nursing Process/Evaluation
Content Area: Pharmacology
Reference: Hodgson, B., & Kizior, R. (2005). *Saunders nursing drug handbook 2005*. Philadelphia: W.B. Saunders, pp. 242-243.

21. *Answer:* 4
Rationale: Haloperidol is used to treat clients exhibiting psychotic features. Therefore, to determine medication effectiveness, the nurse would check the client's orientation and delusional status. Vital signs are routine and not specific to this situation. The physical safety of other clients is not a direct assessment of this client. Monitoring nutritional intake is not related to this situation.

Test-Taking Strategy: Use the process of elimination and eliminate option 2, because it is unrelated to the client. From the remaining options, focus on the action and use of the medication to direct you to option 4. Review the nursing interventions related to this medication if you had difficulty with this question.

Level of Cognitive Ability: Analysis
Client Needs: Physiological Integrity
Integrated Process: Nursing Process/Evaluation
Content Area: Pharmacology
Reference: Hodgson, B., & Kizior, R. (2005). *Saunders nursing drug handbook 2005*. Philadelphia: W.B. Saunders, p. 521.

22. *Answer:* 3
Rationale: The addictive properties of diphenhydramine hydrochloride are enhanced when used with psychotropic medications. Allergic symptoms may not be short term

and will occur if allergens are present in the environment. Poor compliance may be a problem with psychotic clients, but is not the issue of the question. Diphenhydramine hydrochloride may be used for extrapyramidal symptoms and mild medication-induced movement disorders.

Test-Taking Strategy: Knowledge regarding the properties of diphenhydramine hydrochloride (Benadryl) is required to answer this question. Note the relation between the words "psychotic disorder" in the question and option 3. Review this medication if you had difficulty with this question.

Level of Cognitive Ability: Analysis
Client Needs: Physiological Integrity
Integrated Process: Nursing Process/Implementation
Content Area: Pharmacology
References: Hodgson, B., & Kizior, R. (2005). *Saunders nursing drug handbook 2005*. Philadelphia: W.B. Saunders, p. 335. Skidmore-Roth, L. (2005). *Mosby's drug guide for nurses* (6th ed.). St. Louis: Mosby, p. 276.

23. *Answer:* 2
Rationale: Bupropion does not cause significant orthostatic blood pressure changes. Seizure activity is common in dosages greater than 450 mg daily. Bupropion frequently causes a drop in body weight. Insomnia is a side effect but seizure activity causes a greater client risk.

Test-Taking Strategy: Use the process of elimination. Noting that the client has been doubling the medication dose and recalling that seizure activity can occur with higher than recommended doses will direct you to option 2. Review this medication if you had difficulty with this question.

Level of Cognitive Ability: Analysis
Client Needs: Physiological Integrity
Integrated Process: Nursing Process/Data Collection
Content Area: Pharmacology
Reference: Hodgson, B., & Kizior, R. (2005). *Saunders nursing drug handbook 2005*. Philadelphia: W.B. Saunders, p. 144.

24. *Answer:* 4
Rationale: The nurse should focus on determining the reason for the client's concern. The nurse would add anxiety to the client by mentioning media concerns. Alprazolam is used to treat anxiety, not depression. Cliché responses (option 3) do not express concern.

Test-Taking Strategy: Use therapeutic communication techniques. Remembering to address the client's feelings first will direct you to option 4. Review these techniques if you had difficulty with this question.

Level of Cognitive Ability: Application
Client Needs: Psychosocial Integrity
Integrated Process: Communication and Documentation
Content Area: Pharmacology
References: Hodgson, B., & Kizior, R. (2005). *Saunders nursing drug handbook 2005*. Philadelphia: W.B. Saunders, p. 36. Morrison-Valfre, M. (2005). *Foundations of mental health care* (3rd ed.). St. Louis: Mosby, p. 88.

25. *Answer:* 1
Rationale: Phenelzine sulfate is a monoamine oxidase inhibitor (MAOI). The client should avoid taking in foods

that are high in tyramine. These foods could trigger a potentially fatal hypertensive crisis. Foods to avoid include yogurt, aged cheeses, smoked or processed meats, red wines, and fruits such as avocados, raisins, or figs.
Test-Taking Strategy: Recall that phenelzine sulfate is a MAOI and that foods high in tyramine need to be avoided. Next, from the food items listed, identify the food that contains tyramine. Review the food items to avoid with MAOIs if you had difficulty with this question.
Level of Cognitive Ability: Application
Client Needs: Physiological Integrity
Integrated Process: Nursing Process/Implementation
Content Area: Pharmacology
Reference: Hodgson, B., & Kizior, R. (2004). *Saunders nursing drug handbook 2004.* Philadelphia: W.B. Saunders, p. 799.

26. *Answer:* 1
Rationale: Phenobarbital sodium is an anticonvulsant and a hypnotic agent. The client should avoid taking any other central nervous system depressants (such as alcohol) while taking this medication. The medication may be given without regard to meals. Taking the medication at the same time each day enhances compliance and maintains more stable blood levels of the medication. Using a dose container or "pillbox" may be helpful for some clients.
Test-Taking Strategy: Use the process of elimination. Focus on the issue, client safety, and note the key words, *highest priority.* This tells you that more than one or all of the options may be partially or totally correct and that you must prioritize your answer. Eliminate options 2 and 4 because of the absolute words "only" and "always" in these options. Also, remember that alcohol should not be consumed when taking hypnotics. Review client teaching points related to this medication if you had difficulty with this question.
Level of Cognitive Ability: Application
Client Needs: Safe, Effective Care Environment
Integrated Process: Teaching/Learning
Content Area: Pharmacology
Reference: Hodgson, B., & Kizior, R. (2005). *Saunders nursing drug handbook 2005.* Philadelphia: W.B. Saunders, p. 851.

27. *Answer:* 4
Rationale: Dry mouth is a common side effect of this medication. Frequent mouth rinsing with water, sucking on hard candy, and chewing gum will alleviate this common side effect. Hypotension and hypertension are rare side effects of fluphenazine. Leukopenia is common but not viewed as a serious health threat, and the WBC count would not be obtained on a daily basis. Weight gain is a common side effect and frequent snacks will aggravate this problem.
Test-Taking Strategy: Use the process of elimination. Eliminate options 1 and 2 first. It is unlikely that the client would need blood pressure monitoring every 2 hours or that a white blood cell count will be determined daily. From the remaining options, recalling the side effects of this medication will direct you to option 4. Review the common side effects related to this medication if you had difficulty with this question.
Level of Cognitive Ability: Application
Client Needs: Physiological Integrity

Integrated Process: Nursing Process/Planning
Content Area: Pharmacology
Reference: Skidmore-Roth, L. (2005). *Mosby's drug guide for nurses* (6th ed.). St. Louis: Mosby, pp. 370-371.

28. *Answer:* 4
Rationale: Tranylcypromine sulfate is a monoamine oxidase inhibitor (MAOI) used to treat depression. A tyramine-restricted diet is required while on this medication to avoid hypertensive crisis, a life-threatening side effect of the medication. Foods to be avoided are meats prepared with tenderizer, smoked or pickled fish, beef or chicken liver, and dry sausage (salami, pepperoni, bologna). In addition, figs, bananas, aged cheese, yogurt, sour cream, beer, red wine, alcoholic beverages, soy sauce, yeast extract, chocolate, caffeine, and aged, pickled, fermented, or smoked foods need to be avoided. Many over-the-counter medications also contain tyramine and must be avoided as well.
Test-Taking Strategy: Knowledge that tranylcypromine sulfate is an MAOI medication and the foods that need to be avoided with these medications is necessary to answer this question. Review these foods if you had difficulty with this question.
Level of Cognitive Ability: Analysis
Client Needs: Health Promotion and Maintenance
Integrated Process: Nursing Process/Evaluation
Content Area: Pharmacology
Reference: Hodgson, B., & Kizior, R. (2005). *Saunders nursing drug handbook 2005.* Philadelphia: W.B. Saunders, p. 1066.

29. *Answer:* 3
Rationale: Amitriptyline hydrochloride is a tricyclic antidepressant often used to treat depression. It causes orthostatic changes and can produce hypotension and tachycardia. This can be frightening to the client and dangerous, because it could result in dizziness and client falls. The client must be instructed to move slowly from a lying to a sitting to a standing position to avoid injury if these effects are experienced. The client may also experience sedation, dry mouth, constipation, blurred vision, and other anticholinergic effects, but these are transient and will diminish with time.
Test-Taking Strategy: Use the process of elimination. Recalling the adverse effects of the tricyclic antidepressants will direct you to option 3. Review this medication if you had difficulty with this question.
Level of Cognitive Ability: Application
Client Needs: Physiological Integrity
Integrated Process: Nursing Process/Implementation
Content Area: Pharmacology
Reference: Hodgson, B., & Kizior, R. (2005). *Saunders nursing drug handbook 2005.* Philadelphia: W.B. Saunders, p. 57.

30. *Answer:* 3
Rationale: Lithium is the medication of choice to treat manic-depressive illness. Many over-the-counter (OTC) medications interact with lithium, and the client is instructed to avoid OTC medications while taking lithium. Lithium is not addicting and, although serum lithium levels need to be monitored, it is not necessary to check

these levels every week. A tyramine-free diet is associated with monoamine oxidase inhibitors.

Test-Taking Strategy: Use the process of elimination. General principles related to medication administration will direct you to option 3. Review this medication if you had difficulty with this question.

Level of Cognitive Ability: Application
Client Needs: Health Promotion and Maintenance
Integrated Process: Teaching/Learning
Content Area: Pharmacology
Reference: Skidmore-Roth, L. (2005). *Mosby's drug guide for nurses* (6th ed.). St. Louis: Mosby, p. 505.

ALTERNATE FORMAT QUESTION: FILL IN THE BLANK

Answer: 3.3 mL
Rationale: Follow the formula for the calculation of the medication dose. The physician orders 10 mg.

Formula:

$$\frac{Desired}{Available} \times volume = dose$$

$$\frac{10\ mg}{15\ mg} \times 5\ mL = 3.33\ mL$$

Test-Taking Strategy: Use the formula for medication calculations to answer the question. Note that a conversion is not necessary with this calculation problem. Use a calculator to verify the answer. Remember to round the answer to the nearest tenth. Review medication calculations if you had difficulty with this question.

Level of Cognitive Ability: Application
Client Needs: Physiological Integrity
Integrated Process: Nursing Process/Implementation
Content Area: Pharmacology
Reference: Skidmore-Roth, L. (2005). *Mosby's drug guide for nurses* (6th ed.). St. Louis: Mosby, pp. 684-685.

REFERENCES

Hodgson, B., & Kizior, R. (2004). *Saunders nursing drug handbook 2004*. Philadelphia: W.B. Saunders.

Hodgson, B., & Kizior, R. (2005). *Saunders nursing drug handbook 2005*. Philadelphia: W.B. Saunders.

Lehne, R. (2004). *Pharmacology for nursing care* (5th ed.). Philadelphia: W.B. Saunders.

McKenry, L., & Salerno, E. (2003). *Mosby's pharmacology in nursing* (21st ed.). St. Louis: Mosby.

Morrison-Valfre, M. (2005). *Foundations of mental health care* (3rd ed.). St. Louis: Mosby.

Skidmore-Roth, L. (2005). *Mosby's drug guide for nurses* (6th ed.). St. Louis: Mosby.

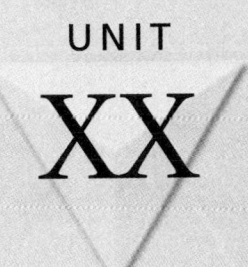
Comprehensive Test

QUESTIONS

1. Before administering an intermittent tube feeding through a nasogastric tube, the nurse checks for gastric residual. The nurse understands that the rationale for checking gastric residual before administering the tube feeding is to:
   1. Confirm proper nasogastric tube placement
   2. Observe the digestion of formula
   3. Check fluid and electrolyte status
   4. Evaluate absorption of the last feeding

2. A client is complaining of gas pains following surgery and requests medication. The nurse selects which medication from the PRN medication list to give to the client?
   1. Magnesium hydroxide (milk of magnesia, MOM)
   2. Droperidol (Inapsine)
   3. Acetaminophen (Tylenol)
   4. Simethicone (Mylicon)

3. A client is admitted to the hospital with a diagnosis of major depression. The nurse collects data on the client and determines that a major concern is the client's altered nutrition related to poor nutritional intake. The most appropriate nursing intervention related to this concern is:
   1. Explain to the client the importance of a good nutritional intake
   2. Weigh the client three times per week, before breakfast
   3. Report the nutritional concern to the psychiatrist and obtain a nutritional consult as soon as possible
   4. Consult with the nutritionist, offer the client several small, frequent meals daily, and schedule brief nursing interactions with the client during these times

4. A client received 20 units of NPH insulin subcutaneously at 8 AM. The nurse should check the client for a hypoglycemic reaction at:
   1. 10 AM
   2. 11 AM
   3. 5 PM
   4. 11 PM

5. A nurse assists in developing a plan of care for a client with hyperparathyroidism receiving calcitonin (Calcimar). Which outcome has the highest priority regarding this medication?
   1. Absence of side effects
   2. Reaching normal serum calcium levels
   3. Relief of pain
   4. Verbalization of appropriate medication knowledge

6. A nursing instructor asks a nursing student about the cause of hemophilia. The student responds by telling the instructor that:
   1. Hemophilia is a Y-linked hereditary disorder
   2. Males inherit hemophilia from their fathers
   3. Females inherit hemophilia from their mothers
   4. Hemophilia A results from deficiency of factor VIII

7. A 4-year-old child is admitted to the hospital for abdominal pain. The mother reports that the child has been pale, excessively tired, and is bruising very easily. On physical examination, lymphadenopathy and hepatosplenomegaly are noted and diagnostic studies are ordered because acute lymphocytic leukemia (ALL) is suspected. The nurse understands that which laboratory study will confirm this diagnosis?

1. White blood cell (WBC) count
2. A lumbar puncture
3. Bone marrow biopsy
4. A platelet count

8. A child with leukemia is complaining of nausea. The nurse suspects that the nausea is related to the medication therapy. The nurse, concerned about the child's nutritional status, would most appropriately offer which of the following during this episode of nausea?
    1. The child's favorite foods
    2. Cool, clear liquids
    3. Low-protein foods
    4. Low-calorie foods

9. A child with a brain tumor is admitted to the hospital for "debulking" of the tumor. To ensure a safe environment for this child, the nurse suggests to include which of the following in the plan of care?
    1. Assisting the child with ambulation at all times
    2. Avoiding contact with other children on the nursing unit
    3. Initiating seizure precautions
    4. Using a wheelchair for out-of-bed activities

10. A client is diagnosed with stage I Lyme disease. The nurse reviews the client's health record, knowing that which of the following is a characteristic of this stage?
    1. Signs of neurological disorders
    2. Enlarged and inflamed joints
    3. Arthralgias
    4. Flulike symptoms

11. A nurse is preparing to suction a client through the client's tracheostomy tube. Select all interventions that the nurse would perform for this procedure.
    _____ Set the wall suction unit pressure at 160 mm Hg
    _____ Don clean gloves before the procedure
    _____ Oxygenate the client before suctioning
    _____ Moisten the suction catheter tip in sterile saline solution before insertion
    _____ Apply suction while inserting the catheter
    _____ Advance the catheter until resistance is met and then pull the catheter back 1 cm
    _____ Apply suction while rotating and withdrawing the catheter
    _____ Allow no more than 10 seconds to suction

12. A nurse is assisting in caring for a client who has a placenta previa. The nurse understands that a cervical examination will not be performed on the client primarily because it could:
    1. Increase the chance of infection
    2. Initiate premature labor
    3. Cause profound hemorrhage
    4. Rupture the fetal membranes

13. A mother is breast-feeding her newborn infant. The mother complains to the nurse that she is experiencing nipple soreness. The nurse provides which of the following suggestions to the client?

1. Avoid rotating breast-feeding positions so that the nipple will toughen
2. Stop nursing during the period of nipple soreness to allow the nipples to heal
3. Nurse the newborn infant less frequently and substitute a bottle-feeding until the nipples become less sore
4. Position the newborn infant with the ear, shoulder, and hip in straight alignment and with the baby's stomach against the mother's

14. A nurse is caring for a client with a diagnosis of agoraphobia. Which behavior would the nurse expect the client to describe when communicating with the client about the disorder?
    1. A need to wash hands several times before eating a meal
    2. A fear of leaving the house
    3. A fear of speaking in public
    4. A fear of riding in elevators

15. A nurse is preparing to deliver a food tray to an Orthodox Jewish client. The nurse checks the food on the tray and notes that the client has received a roast beef dinner with whole milk as a beverage. Which action will the nurse take?
    1. Deliver the food tray to the client
    2. Call the dietary department and ask for a different meal
    3. Replace the whole milk with fat-free milk
    4. Ask the dietary department to replace the roast beef with pork

16. A client is brought to the emergency room by the ambulance team following collapse at home. Cardiopulmonary resuscitation is attempted but is unsuccessful. The wife of the client tells the nurse that the client is an organ donor and that his eyes are to be donated. Which of the following is the most appropriate nursing action?
    1. Place dry, sterile dressings over the eyes of the deceased
    2. Call the National Donor Association to confirm that the client is a donor
    3. Close the deceased client's eyes, elevate the head of the bed, and place wet saline gauze pads and an ice pack on the eyes
    4. Ask the wife to obtain the legal documents regarding organ donation from the lawyer

17. A nurse administers a dose of scopolamine to a preoperative client. The nurse tells the client to expect which of the following side effects of the medication?
    1. Excessive urination
    2. Diaphoresis
    3. Dry mouth
    4. Pupillary constriction

18. A nurse is reinforcing instructions to a client about methods to prevent Lyme disease. Which

statement by the client indicates the need for further instructions?

1. "I need to avoid the use of insect repellents because it will attract the ticks."
2. "I need to wear long-sleeved tops and long pants in wooded areas."
3. "I need to wear a hat in wooded areas."
4. "I need to wear closed shoes and socks that can be pulled up over my pants when walking in the woods."

19. A nurse is caring for a child diagnosed with Down syndrome. In describing the disorder to the parents, the nurse bases the explanation on the fact that Down syndrome is a:

1. Condition characterized by above-average intellectual functioning with deficits in adaptive behavior
2. Condition characterized by average intellectual functioning and the absence of deficits in adaptive behavior
3. Congenital condition that results in moderate to severe retardation and has been linked to an extra group G chromosome
4. Condition characterized by subaverage intellectual functioning with the absence of deficits in adaptive behavior

20. A client with a diagnosis of major depression becomes more anxious, reports sleeping poorly, and seems be more irritable with the nursing staff and family. The nurse interprets the client's behavior as:

1. The client is at increased risk for suicide
2. A normal response to hospitalization
3. The client is dealing with pertinent issues
4. The client may need some time off the unit

21. A client is admitted to the hospital with a venous stasis leg ulcer. The nurse inspects the ulcer, expecting to note that it:

1. Has a pale-colored base
2. Is deep, with even edges
3. Has little granulation tissue
4. Has brown pigmentation surrounding it

22. A nurse is told that a client's potassium level is 3.2 mEq/L. Which of the following would the nurse note on the cardiac monitor as a result of the laboratory value?

1. Elevated T waves
2. Absent P waves
3. Elevated ST segment
4. U waves

23. An adult client with hepatic encephalopathy has a serum ammonia level of 95 mcg/dL and receives treatment with lactulose syrup. The nurse determines that the client has the best and most optimal response if the level changes to which of the following after medication administration?

1. 80 mcg/dL
2. 40 mcg/dL

3. 10 mcg/dL
4. 5 mcg/dL

24. A nurse assists in developing a plan of care for the child with meningitis. Which of the following would be the priority problem for this child?

1. Ineffective cerebral tissue perfusion
2. Parental knowledge deficit
3. Dysfunctional family process
4. Acute pain

25. A nurse is caring for a postoperative client who has been NPO and the physician has prescribed a clear liquid diet. In planning to initiate this diet, which priority item would the nurse place at the bedside?

1. Code cart
2. A straw
3. Cardiac monitor
4. Suction equipment

26. A nurse has given the client taking ethambutol (Myambutol) information about the medication. The nurse determines that the client understands the instructions if the client states that he or she will immediately report:

1. Distressing gastrointestinal side effects
2. Impaired sense of hearing
3. Orange-red discoloration of body secretions
4. Difficulty discriminating the color red from green

27. A nurse is caring for an older client with a diagnosis of myasthenia gravis and has reinforced self-care instructions. Which statement by the client indicates that further teaching is necessary?

1. "I can change the time of my medication on the mornings that I feel strong."
2. "I rest each afternoon after my walk."
3. "If I get abdominal cramps and diarrhea, I should call my doctor."
4. "I cough and deep breathe many times during the day."

28. A nurse is preparing to take an axillary temperature using a glass thermometer. Select all interventions that apply.

_____ Shake down the mercury in the thermometer to 96° F (35.5° C) or below
_____ Ensure that the client's axilla is moist before placing the thermometer
_____ Place the thermometer in the center of the axilla
_____ Place the client's arm at his or her side after putting the thermometer in place
_____ Leave the thermometer in place for 8 to 10 minutes

29. A nurse is preparing to administer a prescribed intramuscular (IM) dose of meperidine hydrochloride (Demerol), 35 mg, to a client. The medication label reads meperidine hydrochloride, 50 mg/mL. How many milliliters will the nurse administer to the client?

Answer: _____

30. A nurse is calculating a client's 24-hour fluid intake. The client consumed coffee (8 oz), water (8 oz), and orange juice (6 oz) for breakfast; soup (4 oz) and iced tea (8 oz) for lunch; and a glass of milk (10 oz), a cup of tea (8 oz), and a glass of water (8 oz) for dinner. Additionally, the client consumed 24 oz of water during the day. How many milliliters of fluid did the client consume in the 24-hour period?

    Answer: _____

31. A nurse is preparing to provide instructions to a client with Addison's disease regarding diet therapy. The nurse understands that which of the following diets would most likely be prescribed for this client?
    1. Low-sodium diet
    2. High-sodium diet
    3. Low-protein diet
    4. Low-carbohydrate diet

32. A client with diabetes mellitus who has been controlled with daily insulin has been placed on atenolol (Tenormin) for the control of angina pectoris. Because of the effects of the medication, the nurse checks for which sign or symptom as the most reliable indicator of hypoglycemia?
    1. Tachycardia
    2. Sweating
    3. Low blood glucose level
    4. Nervousness

33. A nurse is asked to regulate the flow rate of an intravenous (IV) solution being administered to a client. The IV bag contains 50 mL of solution and the solution is to be administered over 30 minutes. The administration set has a drop factor of 10 drops (gtt)/mL. The nurse would regulate the roller clamp on the infusion set to deliver how many drops per minute? (Round to the nearest whole number.)

    Answer: _____

34. A nurse has reviewed the record of an assigned older client. Which data would indicate a potential complication associated with age-related changes in the musculoskeletal system?
    1. Decrease in height
    2. Decrease in lean body mass
    3. Overall sclerotic lesions
    4. Changes in structural bone tissue

35. A nurse reinforces home care instructions to the mother of a child with Reye's syndrome. Which statement by the mother indicates a need for further instruction?
    1. "I need to decrease the stimuli at home to prevent intracranial pressure."
    2. "I need to give frequent, small, nutritious meals if my child starts to vomit."

    3. "I need to have the child nap during the day to provide rest."
    4. "I need to check for jaundiced skin and eyes every day."

36. A physician orders potassium chloride (KCl) elixir, 20 mEq orally twice daily. The medication label states potassium chloride (KCl), 30 mEq/15 mL. The nurse prepares to administer the morning dose. How many milliliters will the nurse administer to the client?

    Answer: _____

37. A nurse is caring for a client who has bipolar disorder with aggressive social behavior. Which of the following activities would be most appropriate initially for this client?
    1. Ping-Pong
    2. Writing
    3. Chess
    4. Basketball

38. A nurse is assisting in providing surgical instructions to a preoperative client. Which instruction would be most appropriate to include in the preoperative plan of care?
    1. Wound care
    2. Activity restrictions
    3. Personal hygiene
    4. Coughing and deep breathing exercises

39. A nursing student is asked to discuss juvenile rheumatoid arthritis (JRA) at a clinical conference scheduled at the end of the clinical day. Which item indicates the need to further research this disorder?
    1. It most often occurs before the age of 16 years
    2. It is twice as likely to occur in boys rather than girls
    3. The cause is unknown
    4. Clinical manifestations include morning stiffness and painful, stiff, swollen joints

40. A nurse is caring for a child with spina bifida who has a neurogenic bladder. As part of the nursing care plan, the nurse would monitor for urinary tract infections. The nurse would anticipate that the most likely medication to be prescribed prophylactically would be:
    1. Prednisone (Deltasone)
    2. Furosemide (Lasix)
    3. Sulfisoxazole (Gantrisin)
    4. Immune globulin intravenously

41. A nurse provides medication instructions to a client with peptic ulcer disease. Which statement by the client indicates the best understanding of the medication therapy?
    1. "The cimetidine (Tagamet) will cause me to produce less stomach acid."
    2. "Sucralfate (Carafate) will change the fluid in my stomach."

3. "Antacids will coat my stomach."
4. "Omeprazole (Prilosec) will coat the ulcer and help it heal."

42. In planning activities for the depressed client, especially during the early stages of hospitalization, which of the following is best?
    1. Provide an activity that is quiet and solitary in nature to avoid increased fatigue, such as working on a puzzle or reading a book
    2. Plan nothing until the client asks to participate in the milieu
    3. Offer the client a menu of daily activities and insist that the client participate in all of them
    4. Provide a structured daily program of activities and encourage the client to participate

43. A nurse is assisting in preparing a plan of care for a 4-year-old child hospitalized with nephrotic syndrome. The nurse suggests which intervention regarding diet therapy that is most appropriate for this child?
    1. Provide a high-protein diet
    2. Discourage visitors at mealtimes
    3. Encourage the child to eat in the playroom with others
    4. Provide a high-salt diet

44. A nursing instructor asks a student to describe the pathophysiology that occurs in Cushing's disease. Which statement by the student indicates an accurate understanding of this disorder?
    1. "It is characterized by an oversecretion of glucocorticoid hormones."
    2. "It is characterized by an undersecretion of glucocorticoid hormones."
    3. "It is characterized by an oversecretion of insulin."
    4. "It is characterized by an undersecretion of corticotropic hormones."

45. The nursing instructor asks the nursing student about the physiology related to the cessation of ovulation that occurs during pregnancy. Which response by the student indicates an understanding of this physiological process?
    1. "Ovulation ceases during pregnancy because the circulating levels of estrogen and progesterone are high."
    2. "Ovulation ceases during pregnancy because the circulating levels of estrogen and progesterone are low."
    3. "The low levels of estrogen and progesterone increase the release of follicle-stimulating hormone and luteinizing hormone."
    4. "The high levels of estrogen and progesterone promote the release of follicle-stimulating hormone and luteinizing hormone."

46. A nurse is assisting in collecting data on a child with seizures. The nurse is interviewing the child's parents to establish their adjustment to caring for their child with a chronic illness. Which statement by a parent would indicate a need for further teaching?
    1. "Our child is involved in a swim program with neighbors and friends."
    2. "Our child sleeps in our bedroom at night."
    3. "Our babysitter just completed cardiopulmonary resuscitation (CPR) training."
    4. "We worry about injuries when our child has a seizure."

47. A client is taking lansoprazole (Prevacid) for the chronic management of Zollinger-Ellison syndrome. The nurse advises the client to take which of the following products if needed for a headache?
    1. Acetaminophen (Tylenol)
    2. Ibuprofen (Motrin)
    3. Naprosyn (Aleve)
    4. Acetylsalicylic acid (aspirin)

48. A depressed client verbalizes feelings of low self-esteem and self-worth typified by statements such as "I'm such a failure. I can't do anything right!" The best nursing action would be to:
    1. Tell the client that this is not true, and that we all have a purpose in life
    2. Remain with the client and sit in silence; this will encourage the client to verbalize feelings
    3. Reassure the client that you know how the client is feeling and that things will get better
    4. Identify recent behaviors or accomplishments that demonstrate skill or ability

49. A nurse is assigned to care for an infant with cryptorchidism. The nurse anticipates that the most likely diagnostic studies to be prescribed would be those that check:
    1. Kidney function
    2. Babinski reflex
    3. DNA synthesis
    4. Chromosomal analysis

50. A nurse is caring for a client with a diagnosis of pemphigus. The nurse understands that a hallmark sign characteristic of this condition is:
    1. Homans' sign
    2. Chvostek's sign
    3. Trousseau's sign
    4. Nikolsky's sign

51. A client asks the nurse about the causes of acne. The nurse most appropriately responds by telling the client:
    1. "It is caused by eating chocolate, nuts, and fatty foods."
    2. "It is caused by oily skin."
    3. "The exact cause is not known."
    4. "It is caused as a result of exposure to heat and humidity."

52. To perform cardiopulmonary resuscitation (CPR), the nurse would use the method shown in the figure below to open the airway in which of the following situations?

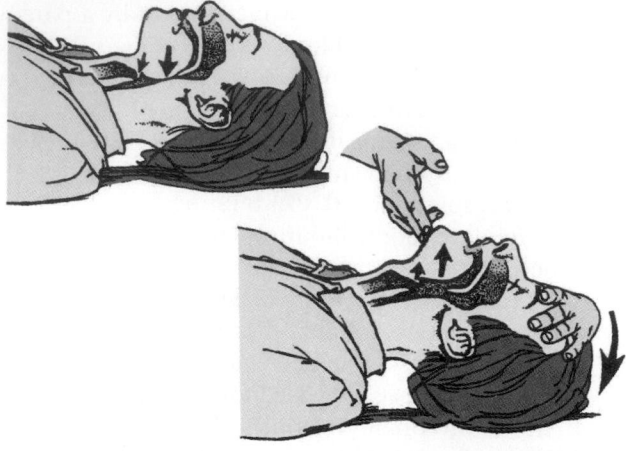

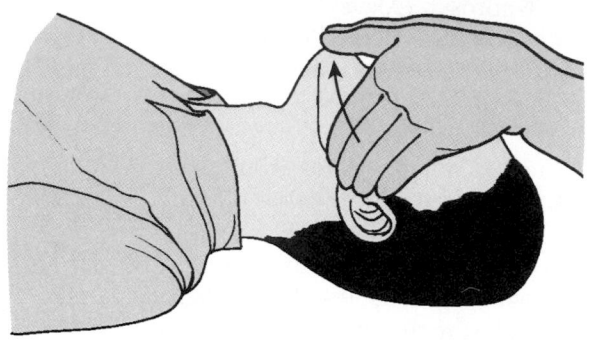

1. In all situations requiring CPR
2. If neck trauma is suspected
3. If the client is unconscious
4. If the client has a history of headaches

53. The nurse is reviewing the health record of a pregnant client at 16 weeks' gestation. The nurse would expect to note documentation that the fundus of the uterus is located at which of the following areas?
    1. Midway between the symphysis pubis and the umbilicus
    2. At the umbilicus
    3. Just above the symphysis pubis
    4. At the level of the xiphoid process

54. A nurse is assigned to care for a child with a compound (open) fracture of the arm that occurred as a result of a fall. The nurse plans care, knowing that this type of fracture involves which of the following?
    1. The bone is broken but the skin over the area of the break is not
    2. A greater risk of infection than in a simple fracture
    3. One side of the bone is broken and the other side is bent
    4. The entire bone is broken across its width

55. A nursing student is asked to discuss the topic of clubfoot at a clinical conference. The student plans to tell the group that clubfoot:
    1. Is a rare deformity of the skeletal system
    2. Always occurs bilaterally
    3. Affects girls more often than boys
    4. Is a congenital anomaly

56. A client with type 1 diabetes mellitus is to begin an exercise program and the nurse is reinforcing instructions to the client regarding the program. Which of the following should the nurse include in the teaching plan?
    1. Exercise should be performed during peak times of insulin
    2. Administer insulin after exercising
    3. Take a blood glucose test before exercising
    4. Try to exercise prior to mealtime

57. A nurse is caring for an older client who is terminally ill. Which of the following signs indicates to the nurse that death may be imminent?
    1. Cold, clammy skin and irregular, noisy breathing
    2. Eupnea and normal body temperature
    3. Presence of swallowing reflex and active bowel sounds
    4. Rubor and paresthesias

58. A nurse has given the client with tuberculosis instructions for proper handling and disposal of respiratory secretions. The nurse determines that the client understands the instructions if the client verbalizes that he or she will:
    1. Wash hands at least four times a day
    2. Turn the head to the side if coughing or sneezing
    3. Discard used tissues in a plastic bag
    4. Brush the teeth and rinse the mouth once a day

59. A client has been taking isoniazid (INH) for $1\frac{1}{2}$ months. The client complains to the nurse about numbness, paresthesias, and tingling in the extrem-ities. The nurse interprets that the client is experiencing:
    1. Small blood vessel spasm
    2. Impaired peripheral circulation
    3. Hypercalcemia
    4. Peripheral neuritis

60. A nurse is preparing a 2-year-old child with suspected nephrotic syndrome for a renal biopsy to confirm the diagnosis. The mother asks the nurse, "Will my child ever look thin again?" The nurse most appropriately responds by saying:
    1. "Wearing loose-fitting clothing should help conceal the extra weight."
    2. "In most cases, medication and diet will control fluid retention."
    3. "Do you feel guilty because you didn't notice the weight gain?"
    4. "When children are little, it's expected that they'll look a little chubby."

61. A nurse is caring for a client hospitalized with acute exacerbation of chronic obstructive pulmonary disease (COPD). Which of the following would the nurse expect to note in this client?
    1. Increased oxygen saturation with exercise
    2. A shortened expiratory phase of respiration
    3. Dyspnea on exertion
    4. Hypocapnia

62. A nurse is preparing to administer an enema to an adult client. Select all interventions that the nurse would perform for this procedure.
_____ Don gloves
_____ Place the client in the right Sims' position
_____ Ensure that the temperature of the solution is between 100° F (37.8° C) and 105° F (40.5° C)
_____ Hang the container containing the enema solution 24 inches above the client's anus
_____ Lubricate the enema tube and insert it approximately 4 inches
_____ Clamp the tubing if the client expresses discomfort during the procedure

63. A nurse is assigned to care for an adult client who had a cerebrovascular accident and is aphasic. Select all appropriate interventions for communicating with the client.
_____ Face the client when talking
_____ Give the client directions using short phrases and simple terms
_____ Avoid the use of body language when talking to the client
_____ Use pantomime when talking to enhance words
_____ Phrase what was said differently the second time, if there is a need to repeat it
_____ Speak slowly and maintain eye contact

64. A nurse is caring for a client with a nasogastric tube connected to continuous gastric suction. The nurse observes that the client is mouth breathing and has dry mucous membranes and a foul breath odor. In planning care, which nursing intervention would be appropriate to maintain the integrity of this client's oral mucosa?
    1. Offer small sips of water frequently
    2. Encourage the client to suck on sour, hard candy
    3. Brush the teeth frequently; use mouthwash and water
    4. Use lemon glycerin swabs to provide oral hygiene

65. A client is admitted to the hospital with possible rheumatic endocarditis. The nurse would check the client for signs and symptoms of concurrent:
    1. Viral infection
    2. Yeast infection
    3. Staphylococcal infection
    4. Streptococcal infection

66. A client taking hydrochlorothiazide (hydro DIURIL, HCTZ) has been started on triamterene (Dyrenium) as well. The client asks the nurse why both medications are required. The nurse formulates a response, based on the understanding that:
    1. Triamterene is a potassium-sparing diuretic, whereas hydrochlorothiazide is a potassium-losing diuretic
    2. Hydrochlorothiazide is a potassium-sparing diuretic, whereas triamterene is a potassium-losing diuretic
    3. Both are weak potassium-losing diuretics
    4. Both are weak potassium-sparing diuretics

67. A client who has begun taking fosinopril (Monopril) is very distressed, telling the nurse that he or she cannot taste food normally since beginning the medication 2 weeks ago. The nurse provides the best support to the client by:
    1. Requesting that the physician change the order to another brand of angiotensin-converting enzyme (ACE) inhibitor
    2. Reassuring the client that this is expected, and generally disappears in 2 to 3 months
    3. Telling the client not to take the medication with food
    4. Suggesting that the client taper the dose until taste returns to normal

68. A nurse is planning to administer amlodipine (Norvasc) to a client. The nurse plans to check which of the following before giving the medication?
    1. Blood pressure and heart rate
    2. Respiratory rate
    3. Heart rate and respiratory rate
    4. Level of consciousness and blood pressure

69. A client had an aortic valve replacement 2 days ago. This morning, the client says to the nurse, "I don't feel any better than I did before surgery." The appropriate response by the nurse is:
    1. "It's only the second day post-op. Cheer up."
    2. "This is a normal frustration; it'll get better."
    3. "You are concerned that you don't feel any better after surgery."
    4. "You will feel better in a week or two."

70. A nurse is assigned to care for a client admitted to the hospital with a diagnosis of systemic lupus erythematosus (SLE). The nurse reviews the physician's orders, expecting to note that which of the following medications are prescribed?
    1. Antibiotic
    2. Narcotic analgesic
    3. Antidiarrheal
    4. Corticosteroid

71. A nurse administers an injection to a client with a diagnosis of acquired immunodeficiency syndrome (AIDS). After administering the medication, the nurse disposes of the used needle by:
    1. Placing it in a puncture-resistant container
    2. Laying the needle and syringe on the bedside table and carefully recapping the needle
    3. Asking the client to recap the needle
    4. Recapping the needle before placing it in a puncture-resistant container

72. A nurse is assisting in conducting a research study and is identifying clients in the community at risk for latex allergy. Which client population is most at risk for developing this type of allergy?
    1. The homeless
    2. Individuals living in a group home
    3. Children in day care centers
    4. Hairdressers

73. A client has just had a cast removed, and the underlying skin is yellow-brown and crusted. The nurse gives the client instructions for skin care. The nurse determines that the client has misunderstood the directions if the client states that he or she will:
    1. Soak the skin and wash it gently
    2. Scrub the skin vigorously with soap and water
    3. Apply an emollient lotion to enhance softening
    4. Use a sunscreen on the skin if exposed for a period of time

74. A client has had skeletal traction applied to the right leg and has an overhead trapeze available for use. The nurse would monitor which of the following as a high-risk area for pressure and breakdown?
    1. Scapulae
    2. Back of the head
    3. Right heel
    4. Left heel

75. A client has been placed in Buck's extension traction. The nurse can provide for countertraction to reduce shear and friction by:
    1. Slightly elevating the head of the bed
    2. Slightly elevating the foot of the bed
    3. Providing an overhead trapeze
    4. Using a footboard

76. A nurse has given the client with Bell's palsy instructions on preserving muscle tone in the face and preventing denervation. The nurse determines that the client needs additional information if the client has stated that he or she will:
    1. Expose the face to cold and drafts
    2. Massage the face with a gentle upward motion
    3. Wrinkle the forehead, blow out the cheeks, and whistle
    4. Use a device for electrical stimulation of the face

77. A nurse is admitting a client with Guillain-Barré syndrome to the nursing unit. The client has an ascending paralysis to the level of the waist. Knowing the complications of the disorder, the nurse brings which of the following items into the client's room?
    1. Nebulizer and pulse oximeter
    2. Flashlight and incentive spirometer
    3. Electrocardiographic monitoring electrodes and intubation tray
    4. Blood pressure cuff and flashlight

78. A client is admitted to the hospital with an exacerbation of multiple sclerosis (MS). The nurse is assessing the client for possible precipitating risk factors. Which of the following factors, if stated by the client, would the nurse note as being unrelated to the exacerbation?
    1. A stressful week at work
    2. Ingestion of more fruits and vegetables
    3. A recent bout of the flu
    4. Inability to sleep well

79. A most common side effect associated with the administration of aluminum hydroxide (Amphojel) is:
    1. Diarrhea
    2. Constipation
    3. Muscle weakness
    4. Headache

80. A client with chronic renal failure is receiving ferrous sulfate (Feosol). Which of the following is a common side effect associated with this medication?
    1. Diarrhea
    2. Constipation
    3. Headache
    4. Weakness

81. A nurse is trying to communicate with a hearing-impaired client. Which of the following strategies by the nurse would be least helpful when talking to this client?
    1. Avoidance of showing frustration through facial expression
    2. Smiling continuously during conversation
    3. Facing the client directly while speaking
    4. Facing the client so that there is light on the nurse's face

82. A nurse is preparing to administer digoxin (Lanoxin), 0.125 mg orally, to a client with congestive heart failure. The nurse checks which most important vital sign before administering the medication?
    1. Blood pressure
    2. Heart rate
    3. Respirations
    4. Temperature

83. A postoperative client has an order to receive an intravenous (IV) infusion of 1000 mL normal saline solution over a period of 10 hours. The drop (gtt) factor for the intravenous infusion set is 15 gtt/mL. The nurse sets the flow rate at how many drops per minute?

    Answer: _____

84. A nurse is preparing to set up a sterile field using the principles of aseptic technique to perform a dressing change. Select all appropriate interventions.
    _____ Use a dry table that is below waist level
    _____ Place the sterile field 1 foot behind the working area and out of view of the client
    _____ Open the distal flap of a sterile package first
    _____ Avoid placing items within 1 inch of any area surrounding the outer edge of the sterile field
    _____ Don clean gloves before touching items on the sterile field

85. A nurse is performing nasotracheal suctioning of a client. The nurse interprets that the client is adequately tolerating the procedure if which of the following observations is made?
    1. Secretions are becoming bloody
    2. Heart rate decreases from 78 to 54 beats per minute
    3. Coughing occurs with suctioning
    4. Skin color becomes cyanotic

ANSWERS

1. Answer: 4

Rationale: All the stomach contents are aspirated and measured before administering a tube feeding. This procedure measures the gastric residual. The gastric residual is checked to confirm whether undigested formula from a previous feeding remains, and thereby evaluates the absorption of the last feeding. It is important to check the gastric residual before administration of a tube feeding. A full stomach could result in overdistention, thus predisposing the client to regurgitation and possible aspiration.

Test-Taking Strategy: Note that the issue of the question is the purpose of checking residual. Focusing on this issue should direct you to option 4. Review this procedure if you had difficulty with this question.

Level of Cognitive Ability: Comprehension
Client Needs: Physiological Integrity
Integrated Process: Nursing Process/Data Collection
Content Area: Adult Health/Gastrointestinal
Reference: deWit, S. (2005). *Fundamental concepts and skills for nursing.* Philadelphia: W.B. Saunders, p. 481.

2. Answer: 4

Rationale: Simethicone is an antiflatulent used in the relief of pain cause by excessive gas in the gastrointestinal tract. Magnesium hydroxide is an antacid and laxative. Droperidol is used to treat postoperative nausea and vomiting. Acetaminophen is a non-narcotic analgesic.

Test-Taking Strategy: Use the process of elimination and note the key words, *gas pains.* Recalling the classifications of the medications in the options will direct you to option 4. If this question was difficult, review this medication.

Level of Cognitive Ability: Application
Client Needs: Physiological Integrity
Integrated Process: Nursing Process/Implementation
Content Area: Pharmacology
Reference: Hodgson, B., & Kizior, R. (2005). *Saunders nursing drug handbook 2005.* Philadelphia: W.B. Saunders, p. 970.

3. Answer: 4

Rationale: Change in appetite is one of the major symptoms of depression. Offering the client several small, frequent meals and the nurse's presence at that time to support, encourage, or perhaps even feed the client is the most appropriate intervention. The client is experiencing poor concentration and will not understand the importance of an adequate nutritional intake. Weighing the client does not address how to increase nutritional intake. Reporting the nutritional problems to the psychiatrist is to some degree correct, but doesn't address how one might increase food intake.

Test-Taking Strategy: Use the process of elimination and focus on the issue, the poor nutritional intake. Option 4 is the only option that addresses the altered nutrition concretely and designs a method in which the client will feasibly increase the nutritional intake. Review care of the client with depression if you had difficulty with this question.

Level of Cognitive Ability: Application
Client Needs: Physiological Integrity
Integrated Process: Nursing Process/Implementation
Content Area: Mental Health

Reference: Morrison-Valfre, M. (2005). *Foundations of mental health care* (3rd ed.). St. Louis: Mosby, p. 215.

4. Answer: 3

Rationale: NPH is an intermediate-acting insulin. Its onset of action is 1 to 2 hours, it peaks in 6 to 14 hours, and its duration of action is 24 hours. Hypoglycemic reactions most likely occur during peak time.

Test-Taking Strategy: Knowledge regarding the onset, peak, and duration of action for NPH insulin is required to answer this question. Recalling that peak action is between 6 and 14 hours will direct you to option 3. Review the characteristics of NPH insulin if you had difficulty with this question.

Level of Cognitive Ability: Application
Client Needs: Physiological Integrity
Integrated Process: Nursing Process/Implementation
Content Area: Pharmacology
Reference: Linton, A., & Maebius, N. (2003). *Introduction to medical-surgical nursing* (3rd ed.). Philadelphia: W.B. Saunders, p. 908.

5. Answer: 2

Rationale: Hypercalcemia can occur in clients with hyperparathyroidism and calcitonin is used to lower plasma calcium level. The highest priority outcome in this client situation would be a reduction in serum calcium level. Option 3 is unrelated to this medication. Although options 1 and 4 are expected outcomes, they are not the priority.

Test-Taking Strategy: Use the process of elimination. Noting the client diagnosis will assist in directing you to option 2. Additionally, note the relation between the name of the medication and the word "calcium" in option 2. Review this medication if you had difficulty with this question.

Level of Cognitive Ability: Analysis
Client Needs: Physiological Integrity
Integrated Process: Nursing Process/Evaluation
Content Area: Adult Health/Endocrine
Reference: Skidmore-Roth, L. (2005). *Mosby's drug guide for nurses* (6th ed.). St. Louis: Mosby, p. 125.

6. Answer: 4

Rationale: Males inherit hemophilia from their mothers and females inherit the carrier status from their fathers. Some females who are carriers have an increased tendency to bleed and, although it is rare, females can have hemophilia if their fathers have the disorder and their mothers are carriers of the genetic disorder. Hemophilia is inherited in a recessive manner via a genetic defect on the X chromosome. Hemophilia A results from a deficiency of factor VIII. Hemophilia B (Christmas disease) is a deficiency of factor IX.

Test-Taking Strategy: Knowledge regarding hemophilia and related causes is needed to answer the question. Remember, hemophilia A results from a deficiency of factor VIII. Review this disorder if you had difficulty with this question.

Level of Cognitive Ability: Comprehension
Client Needs: Physiological Integrity
Integrated Process: Teaching/Learning
Content Area: Child Health
Reference: Price, D., & Gwin, J. (2005). *Thompson's pediatric nursing* (9th ed.). Philadelphia: W.B. Saunders, p. 234.

7. Answer: 3
Rationale: The confirmatory test for leukemia is microscopic examination of bone marrow obtained by bone marrow aspirate and biopsy. A lumbar puncture may be done to look for blast cells in the spinal fluid that are indicative of central nervous system disease. The WBC count may be high or low in leukemia. An altered platelet count occurs as a result of chemotherapy.
Test-Taking Strategy: Use the process of elimination and note the key word, *confirm*. This key word and recalling that the bone marrow is affected in leukemia will direct you to option 3. Review diagnostic studies related to leukemia if you had difficulty with this question.
Level of Cognitive Ability: Comprehension
Client Needs: Physiological Integrity
Integrated Process: Nursing Process/Planning
Content Area: Child Health
Reference: Price, D., & Gwin, J. (2005). *Thompson's pediatric nursing* (9th ed.). Philadelphia: W.B. Saunders, p. 231.

8. Answer: 2
Rationale: When the child is nauseated, it is best to offer cool, clear liquids because they are soothing and better tolerated. It is best not to offer favorite foods when the child is nauseated because foods eaten during times of nausea will be associated with being sick. It is best to offer small, frequent meals of high-protein and high-calorie content.
Test-Taking Strategy: The issue of the question relates to nutritional status in a child with nausea. You should easily be able to eliminate options 3 and 4 because of the word "low" in these options. From the remaining options, recalling that the issue is related to nausea will assist in directing you to option 2. Review interventions related to these issues if you had difficulty with this question.
Level of Cognitive Ability: Application
Client Needs: Physiological Integrity
Integrated Process: Nursing Process/Implementation
Content Area: Child Health
Reference: Price, D., & Gwin, J. (2005). *Thompson's pediatric nursing* (9th ed.). Philadelphia: W.B. Saunders, pp. 157, 233.

9. Answer: 3
Rationale: Seizure precautions should be considered for any child with a brain tumor, both preoperatively and postoperatively. A thorough neurological assessment should be performed on the child and the child's safety should be assessed before allowing the child to get out of bed without help. Options 1 and 4 are not required unless functional deficits exist. Option 2 is not necessary.
Test-Taking Strategy: Use the process of elimination and note the key words, *safe environment*. Eliminate options 1 and 4 first because they are similar. Additionally, note the absolute word "all" in option 1. Eliminate option 2 because it is unnecessary. Review care of the child with a brain tumor if you had difficulty with this question.
Level of Cognitive Ability: Application
Client Needs: Safe, Effective Care Environment
Integrated Process: Nursing Process/Planning
Content Area: Child Health

Reference: Leifer, G. (2003). *Introduction to maternity and pediatric nandrsing* (4th ed.). Philadelphia: W.B. Saunders, p. 553.

10. Answer: 4
Rationale: The hallmark of stage I is the development of a skin rash at the site of the tick bite. The rash develops into a concentric ring, giving it a bull's eye appearance. The lesion enlarges up to 50 to 60 cm, and smaller lesions develop farther away from the original tick bite. In stage I, most infected persons develop flulike symptoms that last 7 to 10 days, and these symptoms may recur later.
Test-Taking Strategy: Use the process of elimination and eliminate options 2 and 3 first because they are similar. Next, note that the question asks for the characteristic of stage I. From the remaining options, select the least serious characteristic, because the issue of the question relates to stage I. If you had difficulty with this question, review the stages of Lyme disease.
Level of Cognitive Ability: Comprehension
Client Needs: Physiological Integrity
Integrated Process: Nursing Process/Data Collection
Content Area: Adult Health/Integumentary
Reference: Linton, A., & Maebius, N. (2003). *Introduction to medical-surgical nursing* (3rd ed.). Philadelphia: W.B. Saunders, p. 202.

11. Answer:
Oxygenate the client before suctioning
Moisten the suction catheter tip in sterile saline solution before insertion
Advance the catheter until resistance is met and then pull the catheter back 1 cm
Apply suction while rotating and withdrawing the catheter
Allow no more than 10 seconds to suction
Rationale: Wall suction unit pressure is set between 80 and 120 mm Hg maximum. Pressure set at a higher level can cause trauma to respiratory tract tissues. Strict asepsis needs to be maintained, and the nurse would wear sterile gloves to perform this procedure. The client should be preoxygenated using a resuscitator bag to prevent hypoxia during suctioning. Moistening the suction catheter tip in sterile saline solution before insertion lubricates the catheter and makes it easier to introduce. Suction is not applied on insertion of the catheter because it will deplete oxygen and can traumatize tissues. When inserting the catheter, resistance will occur when the catheter reaches the carina (junction of the main bronchi). At this point, the nurse pulls the catheter back 1 cm. The nurse applies suction while rotating and withdrawing the catheter to remove secretions around the circumference of the trachea. Suctioning for more than 10 seconds depletes the client's oxygen.
Test-Taking Strategy: Focus on the issue, suctioning procedure through a tracheostomy. The priority issues to think about when answering this question include maintaining oxygenation, maintaining asepsis, and preventing tissue trauma. This will assist in selecting the correct interventions. Review suctioning procedure if you had difficulty with this question.
Level of Cognitive Ability: Application
Client Needs: Physiological Integrity
Integrated Process: Nursing Process/Implementation

Content Area: Adult Health/Respiratory
Reference: deWit, S. (2005). *Fundamental concepts and skills for nursing.* Philadelphia: W.B. Saunders, pp. 517-520.

12. *Answer:* 3
Rationale: Because the placenta is implanted low in the uterus, cervical examination could cause the disruption of the placenta and initiate profound hemorrhage. The other options are also correct, but the profound hemorrhage is of the greatest concern in this case.
Test-Taking Strategy: Use the process of elimination and note the key word, *primarily.* Recalling that bleeding is a primary concern will direct you to option 3. Review care of the client with placenta previa if you had difficulty with this question.
Level of Cognitive Ability: Comprehension
Client Needs: Physiological Integrity
Integrated Process: Nursing Process/Implementation
Content Area: Maternity/Antepartum
Reference: Leifer, G. (2003). *Introduction to maternity and pediatric nursing* (4th ed.). Philadelphia: W.B. Saunders, pp. 91-92.

13. *Answer:* 4
Rationale: Comfort measures for nipple soreness include positioning the newborn with the ear, shoulder, and hip in straight alignment and with the baby's stomach against the mother's. Options 1, 2, and 3 do not identify measures that will alleviate the nipple soreness.
Test-Taking Strategy: Use the process of elimination to answer the question. Eliminate options 2 and 3 because they are similar. From the remaining options, careful reading of option 1 will assist in eliminating this option. Review these measures if you had difficulty with this question.
Level of Cognitive Ability: Application
Client Needs: Health Promotion and Maintenance
Integrated Process: Teaching/Learning
Content Area: Maternity/Postpartum
Reference: Leifer, G. (2005). *Maternity nursing* (9th ed.). Philadelphia: W.B. Saunders, pp. 178, 186.

14. *Answer:* 2
Rationale: Agoraphobia is a fear of leaving the house; panic attacks occur when doing so. Option 1 describes an obsessive-compulsive behavior. Option 3 describes a social phobia. Option 4 describes claustrophobia.
Test-Taking Strategy: Use the process of elimination and focus on the key word, *agoraphobia.* Recalling the definition of agoraphobia will assist in directing you to option 2. If you had difficulty with this question, review the various types of phobias.
Level of Cognitive Ability: Comprehension
Client Needs: Psychosocial Integrity
Integrated Process: Nursing Process/Data Collection
Content Area: Mental Health
Reference: Morrison-Valfre, M. (2005). *Foundations of mental health care* (3rd ed.). St. Louis: Mosby, pp. 185-186.

15. *Answer:* 2
Rationale: In the Orthodox Jewish tradition, the dairy-meat combination is not acceptable. Pork and pork products are also not allowed in the diet. The nurse would not deliver the food tray to the client and would ask the dietary department to deliver a different meal.
Test-Taking Strategy: Use the process of elimination. Recalling that the dairy-meat combination is not acceptable in the Orthodox Jewish tradition will direct you to option 2. Review the dietary rules of this religious group if you had difficulty with this question.
Level of Cognitive Ability: Application
Client Needs: Psychosocial Integrity
Integrated Process: Nursing Process/Implementation
Content Area: Fundamental Skills
Reference: Nix, S. (2005). *Williams basic nutrition and diet therapy* (12th ed.). St. Louis: Mosby, p. 249.

16. *Answer:* 3
Rationale: When a corneal donor dies, the eyes are closed and gauze pads wet with saline are placed over them, along with a small ice pack. Within 2 to 4 hours, the eyes are enucleated. The cornea is usually transplanted within 24 to 48 hours. The head of the bed should also be elevated.
Test-Taking Strategy: Use the process of elimination. Note that the issue relates to donation of the eyes. This should assist in eliminating options 2 and 4. From the remaining options, recalling that the head of the bed should be elevated will direct you to option 3. Review this procedure if you had difficulty with the question.
Level of Cognitive Ability: Application
Client Needs: Safe, Effective Care Environment
Integrated Process: Nursing Process/Implementation
Content Area: Fundamental Skills
Reference: Black, J., & Hawks, J. (2005). *Medical-surgical nursing: Clinical management for positive outcomes* (7th ed.). Philadelphia: W.B. Saunders, p. 1958.

17. *Answer:* 3
Rationale: Scopolamine is an anticholinergic medication that causes the frequent side effects of dry mouth, urinary retention, decreased sweating, and dilation of the pupils. The other options are incorrect.
Test-Taking Strategy: Use the process of elimination. Recalling that this medication is an anticholinergic will direct you to option 3. If this medication is unfamiliar to you, review the side effects associated with anticholinergics.
Level of Cognitive Ability: Application
Client Needs: Physiological Integrity
Integrated Process: Nursing Process/Implementation
Content Area: Pharmacology
Reference: Hodgson, B., & Kizior, R. (2005). *Saunders nursing drug handbook 2005.* Philadelphia: W.B. Saunders, p. 962.

18. *Answer:* 1
Rationale: In the prevention of Lyme disease, individuals need to be instructed to use an insect repellent on the skin and clothes when in an area where ticks are likely to be found. Long-sleeved tops, long pants, closed shoes, and a hat or cap should be worn. If possible, heavily wooded areas or areas with thick underbrush should be avoided. Socks can be pulled up and over the pant legs to the prevent ticks from entering under clothing.

Test-Taking Strategy: Note the key words, *need for further instructions.* These words indicate a false response question and that you need to select the incorrect client statement. Noting the word "avoid" in option 1 will direct you to this option. If you had difficulty with this question, review measures to prevent contact with ticks.
Level of Cognitive Ability: Comprehension
Client Needs: Safe, Effective Care Environment
Integrated Process: Teaching/Learning
Content Area: Adult Health/Integumentary
References: Linton, A., & Maebius, N. (2003). *Introduction to medical-surgical nursing* (3rd ed.). Philadelphia: W.B. Saunders, p. 202.
Phipps, W., Monahan, F., Sands, J., Marek, J., & Neighbors, M. (2003). *Medical-surgical nursing: Health and illness perspectives* (7th ed.). St. Louis: Mosby, p. 1544.

19. *Answer:* 3
Rationale: Down syndrome is a form of mental retardation. It is a congenital condition that results in moderate to severe mental retardation. The syndrome has been linked to an extra group G chromosome, chromosome 21 (trisomy 21). Options 1, 2, and 4 are incorrect descriptions.
Test-Taking Strategy: Use the process of elimination. Eliminate options 1 and 2 first because average and above-average intelligence are not associated with this disorder. Eliminate option 4 because deficits in adaptive behavior do occur with Down syndrome. Recalling that Down syndrome is associated with an extra chromosome will help direct you to the correct option. Review the characteristics of this syndrome if you had difficulty with this question.
Level of Cognitive Ability: Comprehension
Client Needs: Physiological Integrity
Integrated Process: Nursing Process/Implementation
Content Area: Child Health
Reference: Price, D., & Gwin, J. (2005). *Thompson's pediatric nursing* (9th ed.). Philadelphia: W.B. Saunders, p. 104.

20. *Answer:* 1
Rationale: The behaviors identified in the question may be manifested by the client who is contemplating suicide. Many of these symptoms are symptoms of the depressed client; however, with this client, these behaviors have increased. Hospitalization may actually lessen these symptoms in the depressed client, because a feeling of hope or relief may occur once treatment begins. Dealing with pertinent issues may be traumatic, but this is not the best interpretation of the behavior. Time off the unit for this client could put the client at risk for injury.
Test-Taking Strategy: Use the process of elimination and focus on the client behaviors addressed in the question. Noting the client's diagnosis and the words "becomes more anxious" will direct you to option 1. If you had difficulty with this question, review the characteristics and client behaviors related to suicide.
Level of Cognitive Ability: Analysis
Client Needs: Psychosocial Integrity
Integrated Process: Nursing Process/Data Collection
Content Area: Mental Health

Reference: Morrison-Valfre, M. (2005). *Foundations of mental health care* (3rd ed.). St. Louis: Mosby, p. 287.

21. *Answer:* 4
Rationale: Venous leg ulcers, also called stasis ulcers, tend to be more superficial than arterial ulcers, and the ulcer bed is pink. The edges of the ulcer are uneven, and there is evidence of granulation tissue. There is a brown pigmentation to the skin, from the accumulation of metabolic waste products due to venous stasis. The client also exhibits peripheral edema.
Test-Taking Strategy: Use the process of elimination and knowledge of the differences between signs and symptoms of arterial and venous leg ulcers. Knowing that the information in options 1, 2, and 3 are caused by tissue malnutrition (and thus represents an arterial problem), will assist in answering the question. Review the characteristics of a venous stasis ulcer if you had difficulty with this question.
Level of Cognitive Ability: Comprehension
Client Needs: Physiological Integrity
Integrated Process: Nursing Process/Data Collection
Content Area: Adult Health/Cardiovascular
Reference: Christensen, B., & Kockrow, E. (2003). *Adult health nursing* (4th ed.). St. Louis: Mosby, p. 345.

22. *Answer:* 4
Rationale: A serum potassium level below 3.5 mEq/L is indicative of hypokalemia. Potassium deficit is the most common electrolyte imbalance and is potentially life-threatening. Cardiac changes include peaked P waves, flat T waves, depressed ST segment, and prominent U waves.
Test-Taking Strategy: Use the process of elimination. From the information in the question, you need to determine that this condition is a hypokalemic one. From this point, it is necessary to know the cardiac changes that are expected when hypokalemia exists. Review these cardiac effects if you had difficulty with this question.
Level of Cognitive Ability: Analysis
Client Needs: Physiological Integrity
Integrated Process: Nursing Process/Data Collection
Content Area: Fundamental Skills
Reference: deWit, S. (2005). *Fundamental concepts and skills for nursing.* Philadelphia: W.B. Saunders, p. 426.

23. *Answer:* 2
Rationale: The normal serum ammonia level is 35 to 65 mcg/dL. In the client with hepatic encephalopathy, the serum level is not likely to drop below normal. The most optimal yet realistic change from the options provided would be to 40 mcg/dL, which falls in the normal range. A level of 80 mcg/dL represents an insufficient effect of the medication.
Test-Taking Strategy: Familiarity with the normal serum ammonia level is needed to answer this question. It is also necessary to understand the association between hepatic encephalopathy and this laboratory value. Recalling that the normal level is 35 to 65 mcg/dL will direct you to option 2. Review this test and the desirable effects of this medication if you had difficulty with this question.
Level of Cognitive Ability: Analysis
Client Needs: Physiological Integrity
Integrated Process: Nursing Process/Data Collection

Content Area: Adult Health/Gastrointestinal
References: Chernecky, C., & Berger, B. (2004). *Laboratory tests and diagnostic procedures* (4th ed.). Philadelphia: W.B. Saunders, p. 163.
Pagana, K., & Pagana, T. (2003). *Mosby's diagnostic and laboratory test reference* (6th ed.). St. Louis: Mosby, p. 49.
Skidmore-Roth, L. (2005). *Mosby's drug guide for nurses* (6th ed.). St. Louis: Mosby, p. 478.

24. **Answer: 1**
Rationale: Ineffective cerebral tissue perfusion is the priority problem for the child with meningitis. Pain related to meningeal irritation may also be an appropriate problem, but is not the priority. There is no data in the question to indicate that options 2 and 3 are a problem.
Test-Taking Strategy: Use Maslow's Hierarchy of Needs theory to assist in eliminating options 2 and 3 because they are psychosocial problems. Next, use the ABCs—airway, breathing and circulation—to direct you to option 1. Tissue perfusion relates to circulation. Review care of the child with meningitis if you had difficulty with this question.
Level of Cognitive Ability: Analysis
Client Needs: Physiological Integrity
Integrated Process: Nursing Process/Planning
Content Area: Child Health
Reference: Leifer, G. (2003). *Introduction to maternity and pediatric nursing* (4th ed.). Philadelphia: W.B. Saunders, p. 547.

25. **Answer: 4**
Rationale: In a postoperative client, a concern related to initiating a diet is aspiration. Suction equipment must be available. A cardiac monitor and a code cart are unnecessary. A straw may help the client sip fluids, but is not necessary.
Test-Taking Strategy: Note the key words, *postoperative* and *priority*. Use the ABCs—airway, breathing, and circulation—to answer this question. Option 4 will maintain airway clearance. If you had difficulty with this question, review care to the postoperative client.
Level of Cognitive Ability: Application
Client Needs: Physiological Integrity
Integrated Process: Nursing Process/Planning
Content Area: Fundamental Skills
Reference: deWit, S. (2005). *Fundamental concepts and skills for nursing.* Philadelphia: W.B. Saunders, pp. 469, 745.

26. **Answer: 4**
Rationale: Ethambutol causes optic neuritis, which decreases visual acuity and the ability to discriminate between the colors red and green. This poses a potential safety hazard when driving a motor vehicle. The client is taught to report this symptom immediately. The client is also taught to take the medication with food if gastrointestinal upset occurs. Impaired hearing results from antitubercular therapy with streptomycin. Orange-red discoloration of secretions occurs with rifampin (Rifadin).
Test-Taking Strategy: Use the process of elimination. Option 1 is the least likely symptom to report; rather, it should be managed by taking the medication with food. Thus, this option can be eliminated first. From the remaining options,

it is necessary to know that this medication causes optic neuritis and difficulty with red-green discrimination. If this question was difficult, review the side effects of this medication.
Level of Cognitive Ability: Analysis
Client Needs: Health Promotion and Maintenance
Integrated Process: Nursing Process/Evaluation
Content Area: Adult Health/Respiratory
Reference: Hodgson, B., & Kizior, R. (2005). *Saunders nursing drug handbook 2005.* Philadelphia: W.B. Saunders, p. 412.

27. **Answer: 1**
Rationale: The client with myasthenia gravis should be taught that timing of anticholinesterase medication is critical. It is important to instruct the client to administer the medication on time to maintain a chemical balance at the neuromuscular junction. If not given on time, the client may become too weak to swallow. Options 2, 3, and 4 include the necessary information that the client needs to understand to maintain health with this neurological degenerative disease.
Test-Taking Strategy: Use the process of elimination and note the key words, *further teaching is necessary*. These words indicate a false response question and that you need to select the incorrect client statement. Basic principles related to medication administration will direct you to option 1. Remember, clients should not adjust dosage and medication times. If you had difficulty with this question, review the guidelines related to medication administration.
Level of Cognitive Ability: Analysis
Client Needs: Physiological Integrity
Integrated Concept/Process: Teaching/Learning
Content Area: Adult Health/Neurological
References: deWit, S. (2005). *Fundamental concepts and skills for nursing* Philadelphia: W.B. Saunders, pp. 643, 645.
Linton, A., & Maebius, N. (2003). *Introduction to medical-surgical nursing* (3rd ed.). Philadelphia: W.B. Saunders, p. 404.

28. **Answer:**
Shake down the mercury in the thermometer to 96° F (35.5° C) or below
Place the thermometer in the center of the axilla
Leave the thermometer in place for 8 to 10 minutes
Rationale: If the mercury in the thermometer is above 96° F (35.5° C), the nurse would shake down the mercury with a flick action of the wrist. The nurse places the thermometer in the client's dry axilla because a wet axilla will give a false reading of body temperature. The nurse asks the client to hold the arm tightly against the chest (not at his or her side), resting the arm on the chest. When taking an axillary temperature, longer contact is needed than with an oral temperature to obtain an accurate reading, and the thermometer is left in place for 8 to 10 minutes.
Test-Taking Strategy: Focus on the issue, taking an axillary temperature using a glass thermometer. Visualize each of the interventions to assist in identifying the correct actions. Review the procedure for taking an axillary temperature if you had difficulty with this question.
Level of Cognitive Ability: Application
Client Needs: Physiological Integrity
Integrated Process: Nursing Process/Implementation

Content Area: Fundamental Skills
Reference: deWit, S. (2005). *Fundamental concepts and skills for nursing.* Philadelphia: W.B. Saunders, pp. 330-331.

29. *Answer:* **0.7 mL**
Rationale: Use the medication calculation formula and note the prescribed dose (35 mg) and the available dose (50 mg/mL).
Formula:

$$\frac{\text{Desired}}{\text{Available}} \times 1\ \text{mL} = \text{mL per dose}$$

$$\frac{35\ \text{mg}}{50\ \text{mg}} \times 1\ \text{mL} = 0.7\ \text{mL}$$

Test-Taking Strategy: Follow the formula for the calculation of the correct dose, noting the prescribed dose and the available dose. Note that the prescribed dose is a smaller amount than the dose available. This indicates that the amount to be given will be less than 1 mL. Once you have done the calculation, use a calculator to verify the answer. If you had difficulty with this question, review medication calculation problems.
Level of Cognitive Ability: Application
Client Needs: Physiological Integrity
Integrated Process: Nursing Process/Implementation
Content Area: Fundamental Skills
Reference: Kee, J., & Marshall, S. (2004). *Clinical calculations: With applications to general and specialty areas* (5th ed.). Philadelphia: W.B. Saunders, p. 80.

30. *Answer:* **2520 mL**
Rationale: The client consumed a total of 84 oz of fluid. Because 1 oz is equal to 30 mL, multiply 84 oz by 30 mL/oz. This yields 2520 mL.
Test-Taking Strategy: Focus on the issue, the total milliliters that the client consumed in a 24-hour period. Recalling that 1 oz equals 30 mL will assist in answering the question. Use a calculator to verify the amount. Review the procedure for changing ounces to milliliters if you had difficulty with this question.
Level of Cognitive Ability: Comprehension
Client Needs: Physiological Integrity
Integrated Process: Nursing Process/Data Collection
Content Area: Fundamental Skills
Reference: Potter, P., & Perry, A. (2005). *Fundamentals of nursing* (6th ed.). St. Louis: Mosby, pp. 1149-1152.

31. *Answer:* **2**
Rationale: A high-sodium, high–complex carbohydrate, and high-protein diet will be prescribed for the client with Addison's disease. To prevent excess fluid and sodium loss, the client is instructed to maintain an adequate salt intake of up to 8 g of sodium daily and to increase salt intake during hot weather, before strenuous exercise, and in response to fever, vomiting, or diarrhea.
Test-Taking Strategy: Knowledge regarding the pathophysiology associated with Addison's disease will assist in answering this question. Noting that options 1 and 2 are opposite will assist in determining that one of these options is correct. Remember, a high-sodium, high–complex carbohydrate, and high-protein diet will be prescribed for the client with

Addison's disease. If you were unfamiliar with this disorder, review this content.
Level of Cognitive Ability: Comprehension
Client Needs: Physiological Integrity
Integrated Process: Nursing Process/Planning
Content Area: Adult Health/Endocrine
Reference: Christensen, B., & Kockrow, E. (2003). *Adult health nursing* (4th ed.). St. Louis: Mosby, p. 472.

32. *Answer:* **3**
Rationale: Beta-adrenergic blocking agents, such as atenolol, inhibit the appearance of signs and symptoms of acute hypoglycemia, which would include nervousness, increased heart rate, and sweating. Therefore, the client receiving this medication should adhere to the therapeutic regimen and monitor blood glucose levels carefully. Option 3 is the most reliable indicator of hypoglycemia.
Test-Taking Strategy: Note the key words, *most reliable*, in the stem of the question. This indicates that more than one option could be partially or completely correct. Each option is, in fact, a sign or symptom of hypoglycemia. Recalling the masking effects of beta-adrenergic blocking agents helps you to choose the blood glucose level as the most reliable indicator. Review this medication if you had difficulty with this question.
Level of Cognitive Ability: Application
Client Needs: Physiological Integrity
Integrated Process: Nursing Process/Data Collection
Content Area: Pharmacology
Reference: Skidmore-Roth, L. (2005). *Mosby's drug guide for nurses* (6th ed.). St. Louis: Mosby, p. 78.

33. *Answer:* **17 gtt/minute**
Rationale: The formula and calculation for this IV flow rate is:

$$\text{gtt/minute} = \frac{\text{Volume (mL)} \times \text{drop factor (gtt/mL)}}{\text{time (in minutes)}}$$

$$= \frac{50\ \text{mL} \times 10\ \text{gtt/mL}}{30\ \text{minutes}} = \frac{500}{30} = 16.66, \text{ or } 17\ \text{gtt/minute}$$

Test-Taking Strategy: To calculate the answer to this question correctly, you must be familiar with the standard formula for calculating IV flow rates. Use the formula and check your answer with a calculator. Remember to round to the nearest whole number. Review this formula if you had difficulty with this question.
Level of Cognitive Ability: Application
Client Needs: Physiological Integrity
Integrated Process: Nursing Process/Implementation
Content Area: Fundamental Skills
Reference: Kee, J., & Marshall, S. (2004). *Clinical calculations: With applications to general and specialty areas* (5th ed.). Philadelphia: W.B. Saunders, p. 80.

34. *Answer:* **3**
Rationale: Sclerotic lesions occur as bone resorption increases and results in replacement of original bone with fibrous material. This condition occurs in Paget's disease, an age-related disorder. Options 1, 2, and 4 identify normal age-related changes in the musculoskeletal system.
Test-Taking Strategy: Use the process of elimination. Note the key words, *potential complication*. Recalling the normal age-related musculoskeletal findings will assist in directing

you to the correct option. Review these normal findings and those that indicate a complication if you had difficulty with this question.
Level of Cognitive Ability: Comprehension
Client Needs: Physiological Integrity
Integrated Process: Nursing Process/Data Collection
Content Area: Adult Health/Musculoskeletal
Reference: Black, J., & Hawks, J. (2005). *Medical-surgical nursing: Clinical management for positive outcomes* (7th ed.). Philadelphia: W.B. Saunders, pp. 605-606.

35. *Answer:* **2**
Rationale: The vomiting that occurs in Reye's syndrome is caused by cerebral edema and is a symptom of intracranial pressure. Small, frequent meals will not affect the amount of vomiting and if vomiting occurs the physician is notified. Options 1, 3, and 4 are all correct statements. Decreasing stimuli and providing rest decrease stress on the brain tissue. Checking for jaundice will assist in identifying the presence of liver complications, which are characteristic of Reye's syndrome.
Test-Taking Strategy: Note the key words, *need for further instruction.* These words indicate a false response question and that you need to select the incorrect client statement. Recalling the causes of vomiting with Reye's syndrome will direct you to option 2. Review the pathophysiology associated with Reye's syndrome if you had difficulty with this question.
Level of Cognitive Ability: Comprehension
Client Needs: Health Promotion and Maintenance
Integrated Process: Teaching/Learning
Content Area: Child Health
Reference: Price, D., & Gwin, J. (2005). *Thompson's pediatric nursing* (9th ed.). Philadelphia: W.B. Saunders, p. 304.

36. *Answer:* **10**
Rationale: Follow the formula for dosage calculation.
Formula:

$$\frac{\text{Desired}}{\text{Available}} \times \text{mL} = \text{mL per dose}$$

$$\frac{20 \text{ mEq}}{30 \text{ mEq}} \times 15 \text{ mL} = 10 \text{ mL}$$

Test-Taking Strategy: Follow the formula for the calculation of the correct dose and focus on the key information, 30 mEq/15 mL. Verify the answer with a calculator. Review medication calculations if you had difficulty with this question.
Level of Cognitive Ability: Application
Client Needs: Physiological Integrity
Integrated Process: Nursing Process/Planning
Content Area: Fundamental Skills
Reference: Kee, J., & Marshall, S. (2004). *Clinical calculations: With applications to general and specialty areas* (5th ed.). Philadelphia: W.B. Saunders, p. 80.

37. *Answer:* **2**
Rationale: Solitary activities that require a short attention span with mild physical exertion are the most appropriate activities initially for a client who is aggressive. Writing (journaling), walks with staff, and finger painting are activities that minimize stimuli and provide a constructive release for tension.

Competitive games (options 1, 3, and 4) should be avoided because they can stimulate aggression and increase psychomotor activity.
Test-Taking Strategy: Use the process of elimination. Options 1, 3, and 4 are similar in that they are activities that the client cannot do alone and that are competitive. Review care of the client with aggressive behavior if you had difficulty with this question.
Level of Cognitive Ability: Application
Client Needs: Psychosocial Integrity
Integrated Process: Nursing Process/Implementation
Content Area: Mental Health
References: Keltner, N., Schwecke, L., & Bostro, C. (2003). *Psychiatric nursing* (4th ed.). St. Louis: Mosby, p. 378. Stuart, G., & Laraia, M. (2005). *Principles and practice of psychiatric nursing* (8th ed.). St. Louis: Mosby, p. 355.

38. *Answer:* **4**
Rationale: The type of planning and instruction required vary with each individual and type of surgery. Coughing and deep breathing are taught in the preoperative period. Specific instructions that the client needs to receive prior to discharge should include wound care, activity restrictions, dietary instructions, postoperative medication instructions, personal hygiene, and follow-up appointments.
Test-Taking Strategy: Use the process of elimination and note the key words, *preoperative client.* Options 1, 2, and 3 refer to information that needs to be taught postoperatively. Option 4 refers to information that should be taught preoperatively. Review instructions related to the preoperative and postoperative period if you had difficulty with this question.
Level of Cognitive Ability: Application
Client Needs: Health Promotion and Maintenance
Integrated Process: Nursing Process/Planning
Content Area: Fundamental Skills
Reference: Christensen, B., & Kockrow, E. (2003). *Adult health nursing* (4th ed.). St. Louis: Mosby, pp. 50-52.

39. *Answer:* **2**
Rationale: JRA is twice as likely to occur in girls than boys. Options 1, 3, and 4 are accurate regarding this disorder.
Test-Taking Strategy: Note the key words, *the need to further research.* These words indicate a false response question and that you need to select the incorrect statement. Knowledge regarding the cause and clinical manifestations associated with JRA will direct you to option 2. Remember, JRA is twice as likely to occur in girls. Review this disorder if you are unfamiliar with JRA.
Level of Cognitive Ability: Comprehension
Client Needs: Physiological Integrity
Integrated Process: Teaching/Learning
Content Area: Child Health
Reference: Leifer, G. (2003). *Introduction to maternity and pediatric nursing* (4th ed.). Philadelphia: W.B. Saunders, p. 580.

40. *Answer:* **3**
Rationale: A neurogenic bladder prevents the bladder from completely emptying because of the decrease in muscle tone. The most likely medication to be prescribed to prevent urinary tract infection would be an antibiotic. A common

prescribed medication is sulfisoxazole (Gantrisin). Prednisone relieves allergic reactions and inflammation rather than preventing infection. Furosemide promotes diuresis and decreases edema caused by congestive heart failure. Intravenous immune globulin assists with antibody production with immunocompromised clients.

Test-Taking Strategy: Knowledge of the actions and uses of these medications is required to answer this question. Focusing on the data in the question and the medications in the options will assist in directing you to option 3. Review these medications if you had difficulty with this question.

Level of Cognitive Ability: Analysis
Client Needs: Physiological Integrity
Integrated Process: Nursing Process/Planning
Content Area: Pharmacology
References: Lilley, L., Harrington, S., & Snyder, J. (2005). *Pharmacology and the nursing process* (4th ed.). St. Louis: Mosby, pp. 626-627.
Skidmore-Roth, L. (2005). *Mosby's drug guide for nurses* (6th ed.). St. Louis: Mosby, p. 807.

41. Answer: 1
Rationale: Cimetidine, a histamine H₂-receptor antagonist, will decrease the secretion of gastric acid. Sucralfate promotes healing by coating the ulcer. Antacids neutralize acid in the stomach. Omeprazole inhibits gastric acid secretion.

Test-Taking Strategy: Knowledge regarding the actions of the medications used to treat peptic ulcers is required to answer this question. If you are unfamiliar with these medications or their actions, review this content.

Level of Cognitive Ability: Analysis
Client Needs: Physiological Integrity
Integrated Process: Nursing Process/Evaluation
Content Area: Adult Health/Gastrointestinal
Reference: Skidmore-Roth, L. (2005). *Mosby's drug guide for nurses* (6th ed.). St. Louis: Mosby, pp. 192-193.

42. Answer: 4
Rationale: A depressed person suffers with depressed mood and is often withdrawn. Also, the person experiences difficulty concentrating, loss of interest or pleasure, low energy, fatigue, and feelings of worthlessness and poor self-esteem. The plan of care needs to provide successful experiences in a stimulating yet structured environment.

Test-Taking Strategy: Use the process of elimination. Options 1 and 2 are eliminated first because they are too restrictive and offer little or no structure and stimulation. Option 3 is eliminated next because of the word "insist" and the absolute word "all" in this option. Review care of the client with depression if you had difficulty with this question.

Level of Cognitive Ability: Application
Client Needs: Psychosocial Integrity
Integrated Process: Nursing Process/Planning
Content Area: Mental Health
Reference: Stuart, G., & Laraia, M. (2005). *Principles and practice of psychiatric nursing* (8th ed.). St. Louis: Mosby, p. 351.

43. Answer: 3
Rationale: Mealtimes should center on pleasurable socialization. The child is encouraged to eat meals with other children

on the unit. A diet that is normal in protein with a sodium restriction is normally prescribed.

Test-Taking Strategy: Use the process of elimination. Eliminate options 1 and 4 first. A diet that is normal in protein with a sodium restriction is normally prescribed. Option 2 diminishes the importance of socialization at mealtime. This leaves option 3 as the correct option. Review dietary recommendations for the child with nephrotic syndrome if you had difficulty with this question.

Level of Cognitive Ability: Application
Client Needs: Physiological Integrity
Integrated Process: Nursing Process/Planning
Content Area: Child Health
References: Leifer, G. (2003). *Introduction to maternity and pediatric nursing* (4th ed.). Philadelphia: W.B. Saunders, p. 690.
Price, D., & Gwin, J. (2005). *Thompson's pediatric nursing* (9th ed.). Philadelphia: W.B. Saunders, p. 247.

44. Answer: 1
Rationale: Cushing's syndrome is characterized by an over-secretion of glucocorticoid hormones. Addison's disease is characterized by the failure of the adrenal cortex to produce and secrete adrenalcorticol hormones. Options 3 and 4 are inaccurate regarding Cushing's syndrome.

Test-Taking Strategy: Use the process of elimination. Option 3 can be eliminated first because it is not associated with Cushing's syndrome. Remembering that in Cushing's ("u" as in "up") syndrome, there is an oversecretion and in Addison's ("d" as in "down"), there is an undersecretion will direct you to option 1. Review this disorder if you had difficulty with this question.

Level of Cognitive Ability: Comprehension
Client Needs: Physiological Integrity
Integrated Process: Teaching/Learning
Content Area: Adult Health/Endocrine
Reference: Linton, A., & Maebius, N. (2003). *Introduction to medical-surgical nursing* (3rd ed.). Philadelphia: W.B. Saunders, p. 874.

45. Answer: 1
Rationale: Ovulation ceases during pregnancy because the circulating levels of estrogen and progesterone are high, thus inhibiting the release of follicle-stimulating hormone and luteinizing hormone, which are necessary for ovulation. Options 2, 3, and 4 are incorrect.

Test-Taking Strategy: Knowledge regarding the hormonal changes that occur during the menstrual cycle and during pregnancy is required to answer this question. Remember, ovulation ceases during pregnancy because the circulating levels of estrogen and progesterone are high. Review these hormonal changes if you had difficulty with this question.

Level of Cognitive Ability: Comprehension
Client Needs: Physiological Integrity
Integrated Process: Teaching/Learning
Content Area: Maternity/Antepartum
Reference: Leifer, G. (2003). *Introduction to maternity and pediatric nursing* (4th ed.). Philadelphia: W.B. Saunders, pp. 29, 313.

46. *Answer:* 2

Rationale: Parents are especially concerned about seizures that might go undetected at night time. The nurse should suggest a baby monitor. Reassurance by the nurse should ensure parental confidence and decrease parental overprotection. Options 1 and 3 demonstrate the parents' ability to choose respite care and activities appropriately. Option 4 is a common concern. The parents need to be reminded that, as the child grows, they cannot always observe their child, but that their knowledge of seizure activity and care are appropriate to minimize complications.

Test-Taking Strategy: Use the process of elimination and note the key words, *need for further teaching.* These words indicate a false response question and that you need to select the incorrect client statement. Option 2 identifies a need to provide the parents with an alternate method to monitor for night seizures. Review parent teaching regarding seizures if you had difficulty with this question.

Level of Cognitive Ability: Comprehension
Client Needs: Psychosocial Integrity
Integrated Process: Teaching/Learning
Content Area: Child Health
Reference: Price, D., & Gwin, J. (2005). *Thompson's pediatric nursing* (9th ed.). Philadelphia: W.B. Saunders, p. 244.

47. *Answer:* 1

Rationale: Zollinger-Ellison syndrome is a hypersecretory condition of the stomach. The client should avoid taking medications that are irritating to the stomach lining. Irritants would include aspirin and nonsteroidal anti-inflammatory drugs (naprosyn, ibuprofen). The client should be advised to take acetaminophen for headache.

Test-Taking Strategy: Use the process of elimination. Remember that options that are similar are not likely to be correct. With this in mind, eliminate options 2 and 3 first. Choose acetaminophen over aspirin because is least irritating to the stomach. Review this medication and this disorder if you had difficulty with this question.

Level of Cognitive Ability: Application
Client Needs: Physiological Integrity
Integrated Process: Nursing Process/Implementation
Content Area: Pharmacology
Reference: Skidmore-Roth, L. (2005). *Mosby's drug guide for nurses* (6th ed.). St. Louis: Mosby, p. 482.

48. *Answer:* 4

Rationale: Feelings of low self-esteem and worthlessness are common symptoms of the depressed client. An effective plan of care is to provide successful experiences for the client that are challenging but will not be met with failure to enhance the client's personal self-esteem. Reminders of the client's past accomplishments or personal successes are ways to interrupt the client's negative self-talk and distorted cognitive view of themselves.

Test-Taking Strategy: Use the process of elimination and therapeutic communication techniques. Eliminate options 1 and 3 because the nurse is offering an opinion and devaluing the client's feelings. Eliminate option 2 because, in this situation, silence can be interpreted as agreeing with the client's feelings. Review care of the client with depression if you had difficulty with this question.

Level of Cognitive Ability: Application
Client Needs: Psychosocial Integrity
Integrated Process: Nursing Process/Implementation
Content Area: Mental Health
Reference: Morrison-Valfre, M. (2005). *Foundations of mental health care* (3rd ed.). St. Louis: Mosby, pp. 220-223.

49. *Answer:* 1

Rationale: Cryptorchidism may be the result of hormone deficiency, intrinsic abnormality of a testis, or a structural problem. Diagnostic tests would assess kidney function, because the kidneys and testes arise from the same germ tissue. Babinski's reflex tests neurological function. DNA synthesis and a chromosomal analysis are unrelated to this diagnosis.

Test-Taking Strategy: Use the process of elimination and knowledge regarding the anatomical occurrence of cryptorchidism. Cryptorchidism, undescended or hidden testicles, relates to the genitourinary system. Option 2 relates to neurological function. Options 3 and 4 relate to the structure of cells. Option 1 is the only option that relates to the genitourinary system. Review this disorder if you had difficulty with this question.

Level of Cognitive Ability: Comprehension
Client Needs: Physiological Integrity
Integrated Process: Nursing Process/Planning
Content Area: Child Health
Reference: Leifer, G. (2003). *Introduction to maternity and pediatric nursing* (4th ed.). Philadelphia: W.B. Saunders, p. 697.

50. *Answer:* 4

Rationale: A hallmark sign of pemphigus is Nikolsky's sign. Nikolsky's sign is when the epidermis can be rubbed off by slight friction or injury. Trousseau's sign is a sign for tetany, in which carpal spasm can be elicited by compressing the upper arm and causing ischemia to the nerves distally. Chvostek's sign, seen in tetany, is a spasm of the facial muscles elicited by tapping the facial nerve in the region of the parotid gland. Homans' sign, a sign of thrombosis in the leg, is discomfort behind the knee on forced dorsiflexion of the foot.

Test-Taking Strategy: Use the process of elimination. If you knew that Homans' sign was related to thrombophlebitis and that Chvostek's sign and Trousseau's sign are related to tetany, then, by the process of elimination, you would select option 4. If you had difficulty with this question, review these various signs.

Level of Cognitive Ability: Comprehension
Client Needs: Physiological Integrity
Integrated Process: Nursing Process/Data Collection
Content Area: Adult Health/Integumentary
Reference: Black, J., & Hawks, J. (2005). *Medical-surgical nursing: Clinical management for positive outcomes* (7th ed.). Philadelphia: W.B. Saunders, p. 1418.

51. *Answer:* 3

Rationale: The exact cause of acne is unknown. There is no evidence that consumption of foods such as chocolate, nuts, or fatty foods affects acne. Exacerbations that coincide with the menstrual cycle results from hormonal activity.

Heat, humidity, and excessive perspiration also play a role in exacerbation of acne.

Test-Taking Strategy: Use the process of elimination. Note the key words, *most appropriate*, and focus on the issue, the causes of acne. Options 1, 2, and 4 relate specifically to factors that exacerbate acne. Review this disorder and its causes if you had difficulty with this question.

Level of Cognitive Ability: Application
Client Needs: Physiological Integrity
Integrated Process: Nursing Process/Implementation
Content Area: Adult Health/Integumentary
Reference: Leifer, G. (2003). *Introduction to maternity and pediatric nursing* (4th ed.). Philadelphia: W.B. Saunders, p. 705.

52. *Answer: 2*

Rationale: The jaw thrust without the head tilt maneuver is used when head and/or neck trauma is suspected. This maneuver opens the airway while maintaining proper head and neck alignment, thus reducing the risk of further damage to the neck. Option 1 is incorrect. In situations requiring CPR, the client will be unconscious. Option 4 is also incorrect. Additionally, it is unlikely that the nurse will be able to obtain this data.

Test-Taking Strategy: Focus on the data in the question. Eliminate option 1 because of the absolute word "all." Noting that the client requires CPR will assist in eliminating options 3 and 4. Review CPR guidelines and the various test-taking strategies if you had difficulty with this question.

Level of Cognitive Ability: Application
Client Needs: Physiological Integrity
Integrated Process: Nursing Process/Implementation
Content Area: Adult Health/Cardiovascular
Reference: Harkreader, H. & Hogan, M.A. (2004) *Fundamentals of nursing: Caring and clinical judgment* (2nd ed.). Philadelphia: W.B. Saunders, p. 909.

53. *Answer: 1*

Rationale: At 12 weeks' gestation, the uterus extends out of the maternal pelvis and can be palpated above the symphysis pubis. At 16 weeks, the fundus reaches midway between the symphysis pubis and the umbilicus. At 20 weeks, the fundus is located at the umbilicus. By 36 weeks, the fundus reaches its highest level at the xiphoid process.

Test-Taking Strategy: Knowledge regarding the patterns of uterine growth is required to answer this question. Focus on the weeks of gestation identified in the question to assist in directing you to the correct option. Review this uterine growth pattern if you had difficulty with this question.

Level of Cognitive Ability: Comprehension
Client Needs: Physiological Integrity
Integrated Process: Nursing Process/Data Collection
Content Area: Maternity/Antepartum
Reference: Leifer, G. (2003). *Introduction to maternity and pediatric nursing* (4th ed.). Philadelphia: W.B. Saunders, p. 192.

54. *Answer: 2*

Rationale: In a compound (open) fracture, a wound in the skin leads to the broken bone, and there is an added danger of infection. Option 1 describes a simple fracture. Option 3

describes a greenstick fracture. Option 4 describes a complete fracture.

Test-Taking Strategy: Use the process of elimination. Noting the key word, *open*, will assist in directing you to option 2. Review the various types of fractures if you had difficulty with this question.

Level of Cognitive Ability: Comprehension
Client Needs: Physiological Integrity
Integrated Process: Nursing Process/Planning
Content Area: Child Health
Reference: Price, D., & Gwin, J. (2005). *Thompson's pediatric nursing* (9th ed.). Philadelphia: W.B. Saunders, pp. 192-193.

55. *Answer: 4*

Rationale: Clubfoot, one of the most common deformities of the skeletal system, is a congenital anomaly characterized by a foot that has been twisted inward or outward. The condition generally affects both feet, and boys are affected twice as often as girls.

Test-Taking Strategy: Use the process of elimination. Eliminate option 1 because of the word "rare" and option 2 because of the word "always." From the remaining options, it is necessary to know that this disorder is a congenital anomaly. Review this disorder if you had difficulty with this question.

Level of Cognitive Ability: Comprehension
Client Needs: Physiological Integrity
Integrated Process: Nursing Process/Planning
Content Area: Child Health
Reference: Price, D., & Gwin, J. (2005). *Thompson's pediatric nursing* (9th ed.). Philadelphia: W.B. Saunders, p. 100.

56. *Answer: 3*

Rationale: A blood glucose test performed before exercising provides information to the client regarding the need to eat a snack first. Exercising during the peak times of insulin effect or prior to mealtime places the client at risk for hypoglycemia. Insulin should be administered as prescribed.

Test-Taking Strategy: The issue of the question relates to the occurrence of a hypoglycemic reaction. Use the process of elimination, keeping in mind this issue and the effects of insulin and exercise on the blood glucose level. You should easily be able to eliminate options 1, 2, and 4. Review the effects of exercise if you had difficulty with this question.

Level of Cognitive Ability: Application
Client Needs: Health Promotion and Maintenance
Integrated Process: Nursing Process/Data Collection
Content Area: Adult Health/Endocrine
Reference: Linton, A., & Maebius, N. (2003). *Introduction to medical-surgical nursing* (3rd ed.). Philadelphia: W.B. Saunders, p. 908.

57. *Answer: 1*

Rationale: The clinical signs of impending or approaching death include inability to swallow, pitting edema, decreased gastrointestinal and urinary tract activity, bowel and bladder incontinence, loss of motion, sensation, and reflexes, cold or clammy skin, cyanosis, lowered blood pressure, noisy or irregular respiration, and Cheyne-Stokes respirations.

Test-Taking Strategy: Use the process of elimination and eliminate options 2 and 3 because these identify normal findings.

Option 4 does not identify signs of approaching death. If you had difficulty with this question, review the signs associated with impending or approaching death.
Level of Cognitive Ability: Comprehension
Client Needs: Physiological Integrity
Integrated Process: Nursing Process/Data Collection
Content Area: Fundamental Skills
References: Lewis, S., Heitkemper, M., & Dirksen, S. (2004). *Medical-surgical nursing: Assessment and management of clinical problems* (6th ed.). St. Louis: Mosby, p. 161.
Wold, G. (2004). *Basic geriatric nursing* (3rd ed.). St. Louis: Mosby, p. 198.

58. *Answer: 3*
Rationale: The client with tuberculosis should wash the hands carefully after each contact with respiratory secretions. The client should cover the mouth and nose when laughing, sneezing, or coughing. Used tissues are discarded in a plastic bag. Oral care should be performed more than once a day.
Test-Taking Strategy: Use the process of elimination. Note that the question specifically relates to information about handling and disposal of secretions. The only options that address this topic directly are options 2 and 3. Because turning the head to the side for coughing and sneezing does not specifically address the handling of secretions, eliminate option 2. Disposal of tissues in a plastic bag is correct. Review home care instructions related to TB if you had difficulty with this question.
Level of Cognitive Ability: Comprehension
Client Needs: Safe, Effective Care Environment
Integrated Process: Nursing Process/Evaluation
Content Area: Adult Health/Respiratory
References: Linton, A., & Maebius, N. (2003). *Introduction to medical-surgical nursing* (3rd ed.). Philadelphia: W.B. Saunders, p. 506.
Swearingen, P. (2003). *Manual of medical-surgical nursing care* (5th ed.). St. Louis: Mosby, p. 124.

59. *Answer: 4*
Rationale: A common side effect of isoniazid (INH) is peripheral neuritis. This is manifested by numbness, tingling, and paresthesias in the extremities. This side effect can be minimized with pyridoxine (vitamin B₆) intake.
Test-Taking Strategy: Use the process of elimination. Options 1 and 2 would not cause the signs and symptoms presented in the question, but instead would be manifested by pallor and coolness. Thus, options 1 and 2 can be eliminated first. From the remaining options, it is necessary to know either that peripheral neuritis is a side effect of the medication or that these signs and symptoms do not correlate with hypercalcemia. Review the side effects associated with isoniazid if you had difficulty with this question.
Level of Cognitive Ability: Analysis
Client Needs: Physiological Integrity
Integrated Process: Nursing Process/Data Collection
Content Area: Adult Health/Respiratory
References: Hodgson, B., & Kizior, R. (2005). *Saunders nursing drug handbook 2005*. Philadelphia: W.B. Saunders, p. 593.
Skidmore-Roth, L. (2005). *Mosby's drug guide for nurses* (6th ed.). St. Louis: Mosby, p. 465.

60. *Answer: 2*
Rationale: It is important to give the mother information that addresses the issue that is the parent's concern. Most children experience remission with treatment. Options 1 and 3 are nontherapeutic and may add to the mother's guilt. Option 4 does not acknowledge the concern and is a stereotypical response.
Test-Taking Strategy: Use therapeutic communication techniques and focus on the mother's concern. Options 1, 3, and 4 do not address the mother's concern and are inappropriate and nontherapeutic responses. Remember, always address the mother's feelings and concerns. Review this disorder and therapeutic communication techniques if you had difficulty with this question.
Level of Cognitive Ability: Application
Client Needs: Physiological Integrity
Integrated Process: Communication and Documentation
Content Area: Child Health
References: Leifer, G. (2005). *Maternity nursing* (9th ed.). Philadelphia: W.B. Saunders, p. 690.
Price, D., & Gwin, J. (2005). *Thompson's pediatric nursing* (9th ed.). Philadelphia: W.B. Saunders, p. 250.

61. *Answer: 3*
Rationale: Clinical manifestations of COPD include hypoxemia, hypercapnia, dyspnea on exertion and at rest, oxygen desaturation with exercise, use of accessory muscles of respiration, and a prolonged expiratory phase of respiration. The chest x-ray will reveal a hyperinflated chest and a flattened diaphragm if the disease is advanced.
Test-Taking Strategy: Use the process of elimination. Eliminate option 1 because oxygen desaturation rather than saturation would occur. Next, eliminate option 2 because, in the client with COPD, a prolonged expiratory phase of respiration would be noted. From the remaining options, reading carefully will assist in directing you to option 3 as the correct option. If you are unfamiliar with the manifestations associated with COPD, review this content.
Level of Cognitive Ability: Comprehension
Client Needs: Physiological Integrity
Integrated Process: Nursing Process/Data Collection
Content Area: Adult Health/Respiratory
Reference: Linton, A., & Maebius, N. (2003). *Introduction to medical-surgical nursing* (3rd ed.). Philadelphia: W.B. Saunders, p. 497.

62. *Answer:*
Don gloves
Ensure that the temperature of the solution is between 100° F (37.8° C) and 105° F (40.5° C)
Lubricate the enema tube and insert it approximately 4 inches
Clamp the tubing if the client expresses discomfort during the procedure
Rationale: The nurse wears gloves when administering an enema to prevent the transfer of microorganisms. To administer an enema, the nurse places the client in the left Sims' position because the enema solution will travel up the colon more easily in this position. The temperature of the solution should be between 100° F (37.8° C) and 105° F (40.5° C). Solution that is too hot will burn the client and solution that is too cool

will cause cramping. The container containing the enema solution is hung about 12 to 18 inches above the client's anus. A flow of solution that is too forceful can damage the bowel. The tube is lubricated for easy insertion and is inserted approximately 4 inches in an adult. If the client complains of cramping or discomfort during the procedure, the nurse clamps the tubing until the discomfort subsides.

Test-Taking Strategy: Visualize the procedure for administering an enema. Thinking about the anatomy of the bowel and the precautions that need to be taken to prevent trauma to rectal tissue will assist in identifying the correct interventions. Review the procedure for administering an enema if you had difficulty with this question.

Level of Cognitive Ability: Application
Client Needs: Physiological Integrity
Integrated Process: Nursing Process/Implementation
Content Area: Fundamental Skills
Reference: deWit, S. (2005). *Fundamental concepts and skills for nursing.* Philadelphia: W.B. Saunders, pp. 568-572.

63. *Answer:*
Face the client when talking
Give the client directions using short phrases and simple terms
Use pantomime when talking to enhance words
Speak slowly and maintain eye contact

Rationale: A client who is aphasic has difficulty expressing or understanding language. The nurse would face the client when talking, establish and maintain eye contact, and speak slowly and distinctly. The nurse should use pantomime when talking to enhance words and body language to enhance the message. The nurse would give the client directions using short phrases and simple terms, and phrase questions so that they can be answered with a yes or no. If there is a need to repeat something, the nurse should use the same words a second time.

Test-Taking Strategy: Recall that a client who is aphasic has difficulty expressing or understanding language. Using the principles related to communicating to a client who is hearing-impaired will assist in identifying the correct interventions. Review the guidelines for communicating with an aphasic client if you had difficulty with this question.

Level of Cognitive Ability: Application
Client Needs: Physiological Integrity
Integrated Process: Communication and Documentation
Content Area: Fundamental Skills
Reference: deWit, S. (2005). *Fundamental concepts and skills for nursing.* Philadelphia: W.B. Saunders, pp. 107-108.

64. *Answer:* 3
Rationale: After the nasogastric tube is in place, mouth care is extremely important. With one naris occluded, the client tends to mouth breathe, drying the mucous membranes. Frequent small sips of water would be contraindicated when the client is on gastric suction. The hard candy would increase the salivation, but would not be useful in cleaning the oral cavity. Lemon glycerin swabs have a drying or irritating effect on the mucous membranes.

Test-Taking Strategy: Use the process of elimination and focus on the issue, maintain the integrity of the oral mucosa.

Recalling that a client on gastric suction will be NPO and swallowing water or other liquids would be prohibited will assist in eliminating options 1 and 2. From the remaining options, eliminate option 4 because lemon glycerin swabs are drying to the mucosa. Review care of the client with a nasogastric tube if you had difficulty with this question.

Level of Cognitive Ability: Application
Client Needs: Physiological Integrity
Integrated Process: Nursing Process/Implementation
Content Area: Adult Health/Gastrointestinal
Reference: Christensen, B., & Kockrow, E. (2003). *Foundations of nursing* (4th ed). St. Louis: Mosby, pp. 477, 480.

65. *Answer:* 4
Rationale: Rheumatic endocarditis is a major indicator of rheumatic fever, which is a complication of infection with group A beta-hemolytic streptococcal infections. It is frequently triggered by streptococcal pharyngitis. Options 1, 2, and 3 are incorrect.

Test-Taking Strategy: Use the process of elimination. Recalling that streptococcal infections are largely responsible for rheumatic heart disease will direct you to option 4. Review the causes of endocarditis if you had difficulty with this question.

Level of Cognitive Ability: Application
Client Needs: Physiological Integrity
Integrated Process: Nursing Process/Data Collection
Content Area: Adult Health/Cardiovascular
Reference: Christensen, B., & Kockrow, E. (2003). *Adult health nursing* (4th ed). St. Louis: Mosby, pp. 326-327.

66. *Answer:* 1
Rationale: Potassium-sparing diuretics include amiloride (Midamor), spironolactone (Aldactone) and triamterene (Dyrenium). They are weak diuretics that are of particular use when combined with potassium-losing diuretics. This is especially useful when medication and dietary supplement of potassium is not appropriate.

Test-Taking Strategy: From the construct of this question, the options are visually divided into two sets: options 1 and 2, and options 3 and 4. Neither 3 nor 4 makes sense, so eliminate these first. From the remaining options, it is especially helpful to remember that hydrochlorothiazide is potassium-losing. This will help you answer correctly using the process of elimination. Review this medication if you had difficulty with this question.

Level of Cognitive Ability: Application
Client Needs: Physiological Integrity
Integrated Process: Nursing Process/Implementation
Content Area: Pharmacology
Reference: Hodgson, B., & Kizior, R. (2005). *Saunders nursing drug handbook 2005.* Philadelphia: W.B. Saunders, p. 1075.

67. *Answer:* 2
Rationale: ACE inhibitors, such as fosinopril, cause temporary impairment of taste (dysgeusia). The nurse can tell the client that this effect usually disappears in 2 to 3 months, even with continued therapy, and provide nutritional counseling if appropriate to avoid weight loss. Options 1, 3, and 4 are inappropriate actions.

Test-Taking Strategy: Use the process of elimination. Eliminate option 4 first because it is an inappropriate nursing action. The nurse does not encourage dosage changes for any prescribed medication. Taking the medication with food is not going to change the taste of the food, so option 3 can be eliminated next. From the remaining options, you need to know that this effect occurs with medications in the ACE inhibitor group. Thus, you are left with the correct option, which is supporting the client through teaching. Review the effects of ACE inhibitors if you had difficulty with this question.
Level of Cognitive Ability: Application
Client Needs: Psychosocial Integrity
Integrated Process: Nursing Process/Implementation
Content Area: Pharmacology
Reference: Skidmore-Roth, L. (2005). *Mosby's drug guide for nurses* (6th ed.). St. Louis: Mosby, p. 381.

68. *Answer:* **1**
Rationale: Prior to administering a calcium channel blocking agent, the nurse should check the blood pressure and heart rate, which could both decrease in response to the action of this medication.
Test-Taking Strategy: To answer this question, you must know that amlodipine is a calcium channel blocker, and that this group of medications decreases the rate and force of cardiac contraction. This in turn lowers the pulse rate and blood pressure. Option 2 can be eliminated first because it is unrelated to the medication. With options 3 and 4, note that only half of the option is correct. When answering questions such as these, with two items per option, both of the items must be correct for that option to be correct. Review this medication if you had difficulty with this question.
Level of Cognitive Ability: Application
Client Needs: Physiological Integrity
Integrated Process: Nursing Process/Data Collection
Content Area: Pharmacology
Reference: Hodgson, B., & Kizior, R. (2005). *Saunders nursing drug handbook 2005.* Philadelphia: W.B. Saunders, p. 57.

69. *Answer:* **3**
Rationale: Paraphrasing is restating the client's message in the nurse's own words. Option 3 uses the therapeutic communication technique of paraphrasing. The client is frustrated and is searching for understanding. Options 1, 2, and 4 are inappropriate communication techniques. Option 1 belittles the client's concerns. Option 2 and 4 offer false reassurance by the nurse.
Test-Taking Strategy: Use therapeutic communication techniques to answer the question. Option 3 focuses on the client's feelings. Review therapeutic communication techniques if you had difficulty with this question.
Level of Cognitive Ability: Application
Client Needs: Psychosocial Integrity
Integrated Process: Communication and Documentation
Content Area: Adult Health/Cardiovascular
Reference: Potter, P., & Perry, A. (2005). *Fundamentals of nursing* (6th ed.). St. Louis: Mosby, pp. 437-440.

70. *Answer:* **4**
Rationale: Treatment of SLE is based on the systems involved and symptoms. Treatment normally consists of anti-inflammatories, corticosteroids, and immunosuppressants. Options 1, 2, and 3 are not a standard component of medication therapy.
Test-Taking Strategy: Knowledge regarding the treatment for SLE is required to answer the question. If you are unfamiliar with the treatments normally prescribed in this disease, review this content.
Level of Cognitive Ability: Analysis
Client Needs: Physiological Integrity
Integrated Process: Nursing Process/Planning
Content Area: Adult Health/Immune
Reference: Christensen, B., & Kockrow, E. (2003). *Adult health nursing* (4th ed). St. Louis: Mosby, p. 80.

71. *Answer:* **1**
Rationale: The correct procedure for needle disposal is to dispose of uncapped needles and sharps in a hard-walled, puncture-resistant container immediately after use. Needles are not recapped.
Test-Taking Strategy: Use the process of elimination and principles related to the safe disposal of needles and syringes to answer the question. Note that options 2, 3, and 4 are similar in that they all address recapping the needle. Review these principles if you had difficulty with this question.
Level of Cognitive Ability: Application
Client Needs: Safe, Effective Care Environment
Integrated Process: Nursing Process/Implementation
Content Area: Adult Health/Immune
Reference: deWit, S. (2005). *Fundamental concepts and skills for nursing.* Philadelphia: W.B. Saunders, p. 217.

72. *Answer:* **4**
Rationale: Individuals at risk for developing a latex allergy include health care workers; individuals who work with manufacturing latex products; females; individuals with spina bifida; individuals who wear gloves frequently such as food handlers, hairdressers, and auto mechanics; and individuals allergic to kiwis, bananas, pineapples, passion fruits, avocados, and chestnuts.
Test-Taking Strategy: Focus on the issue, a latex allergy. Recalling the cause and the source of the allergic reaction will easily direct you to option 4. Review the cause of this type of allergy and the individuals at risk if you had difficulty with this question.
Level of Cognitive Ability: Analysis
Client Needs: Health Promotion and Maintenance
Integrated Process: Nursing Process/Data Collection
Content Area: Adult Health/Immune
References: Christensen, B., & Kockrow, E. (2003). *Foundations of nursing* (4th ed.). St. Louis: Mosby, pp. 242-243.
Phipps, W., Monahan, F., Sands, J., Marek, J., & Neighbors, M. (2003). *Medical-surgical nursing: Health and illness perspectives* (7th ed.). St. Louis: Mosby, p. 412.

73. *Answer:* **2**
Rationale: The skin under a casted area may be discolored and crusted with dead skin layers. The client should gently soak

and wash the skin for the first few days. The skin should be patted dry, and a lubricating lotion should be applied. Clients often want to scrub the dead skin away, which irritates the skin. The client should avoid overexposing the skin to the sunlight.

Test-Taking Strategy: Note the key word, *misunderstood.* Option 3 is obviously helpful, and therefore cannot be the answer to the question as stated. Option 4 is good advice if the skin has been covered, and is eliminated next. Options 1 and 2 seem to oppose each other, making it likely that one of them is correct. Because vigorous scrubbing is more likely to be irritating than providing gentle soaking, it is the most likely choice as the answer to the question. Review skin care measures following cast removal if you had difficulty with this question.

Level of Cognitive Ability: Comprehension
Client Needs: Health Promotion and Maintenance
Integrated Process: Teaching/Learning
Content Area: Adult Health/Musculoskeletal
Reference: Christensen, B., & Kockrow, E. (2003). *Adult health nursing* (4th ed). St. Louis: Mosby, p. 149.

74. Answer: 4

Rationale: Common areas that are under pressure and are at risk for breakdown include the elbows (if they are used for repositioning instead of a trapeze) and the heel of the good leg (which is used as a brace when pushing up in bed). Other pressure points caused by the traction include the ischial tuberosity, popliteal space and Achilles tendon.

Test-Taking Strategy: Note the key words, *high-risk area.* Thus, you would compare each of the options in terms of their relative risk, and choose the one that is highest. The right heel is eliminated first because it is off the bed in the traction setup. The overhead trapeze would diminish the likelihood that the scapulae and back of the head would be immobile. This leaves the left heel as the answer to the question. This makes sense, given that the client would use the unaffected heel to push into the mattress during repositioning. With repeated use, this could cause the left heel to become reddened and break down. Review the complications of skeletal traction if you had difficulty with this question.

Level of Cognitive Ability: Application
Client Needs: Physiological Integrity
Integrated Process: Nursing Process/Data Collection
Content Area: Adult Health/Musculoskeletal
References: Christensen, B., & Kockrow, E. (2003). *Adult health nursing* (4th ed). St. Louis: Mosby, p. 153.
Linton, A., & Maebius, N. (2003). *Introduction to medical-surgical nursing* (3rd ed.). Philadelphia: W.B. Saunders, p. 830.

75. Answer: 2

Rationale: The part of the bed under an area in traction is usually elevated to aid in countertraction. For the client in Buck's extension traction (which is applied to a leg), the foot of the bed is elevated.

Test-Taking Strategy: To answer this question accurately, you need to understand the principles of traction and countertraction, and be familiar with Buck's extension traction. Option 3 is not used for the purpose of countertraction and is

eliminated first. Knowing that Buck's extension traction is applied to the leg helps you eliminate option 1. Of the two remaining choices, option 4 places undue pressure on the client's unaffected foot. Furthermore, a footboard is not used for the purpose of providing countertraction. Option 2 provides a force that opposes the traction force effectively without harming the client. Review care of the client in Buck's extension traction if you had difficulty with this question.

Level of Cognitive Ability: Application
Client Needs: Physiological Integrity
Integrated Process: Nursing Process/Implementation
Content Area: Adult Health/Musculoskeletal
Reference: Christensen, B., & Kockrow, E. (2003). *Adult health nursing* (4th ed.). St. Louis: Mosby, p. 153.

76. Answer: 1

Rationale: Prevention of muscle atrophy with Bell's palsy is accomplished with the use of facial massage, facial exercises, and electrical stimulation of the nerves if prescribed. Exposure to cold or drafts is avoided. Local application of heat to the face may improve blood flow and provide comfort.

Test-Taking Strategy: Use the process of elimination. Evaluate each of the options with regard to their effect on preserving muscle tone in the face. Options 2, 3, and 4 affect muscle tone. Option 1 is unrelated to muscle tone and is also contraindicated in clients with this condition. Because of this, option 1 is the answer to this question as stated. Review this disorder if you had difficulty with this question.

Level of Cognitive Ability: Comprehension
Client Needs: Health Promotion and Maintenance
Integrated Process: Teaching/Learning
Content Area: Adult Health/Neurological
Reference: Christensen, B., & Kockrow, E. (2003). *Adult health nursing* (4th ed.). St. Louis: Mosby, p. 643.

77. Answer: 3

Rationale: The client with Guillain-Barré syndrome is at risk for respiratory failure because of ascending paralysis. An intubation tray should be available for use. Another complication of this syndrome is cardiac dysrhythmia, which necessitates the use of ECG monitoring. Because the client is immobilized, the nurse should routinely assess for deep vein thrombosis and pulmonary embolism.

Test-Taking Strategy: Use the process of elimination. With an ascending paralysis, the client is at risk for involvement of respiratory muscles and subsequent respiratory failure. This knowledge makes you look for an option that coincides with this line of thought. Option 3 is the only option that includes an intubation tray, which would be needed if the client's status deteriorated to needing intubation and mechanical ventilation. This option most directly addresses airway. Review care of the client with Guillain-Barré syndrome if you had difficulty with this question.

Level of Cognitive Ability: Application
Client Needs: Physiological Integrity
Integrated Process: Nursing Process/Implementation
Content Area: Adult Health/Neurological
Reference: Linton, A., & Maebius, N. (2003). *Introduction to medical-surgical nursing* (3rd ed.). Philadelphia: W.B. Saunders, p. 394.

78. *Answer:* **2**
Rationale: The onset or exacerbation of MS is preceded by a number of different factors. These include emotional stress, fatigue, infection, physical injury and pregnancy. There are no known methods of primary prevention. Intake of fruit and vegetables is an unrelated item.
Test-Taking Strategy: Use the process of elimination. If you examine each of the options, all but the fruit and vegetables option involve physiological or psychological stress. Because this is the option that is different than the others, it is a likely choice for being the correct answer. Review the precipitating risk factors associated with MS if you had difficulty with this question.
Level of Cognitive Ability: Comprehension
Client Needs: Physiological Integrity
Integrated Process: Nursing Process/Data Collection
Content Area: Adult Health/Neurological
Reference: Christensen, B., & Kockrow, E. (2003). *Adult health nursing* (4th ed.). St. Louis: Mosby, p. 626.

79. *Answer:* **2**
Rationale: Aluminum-containing antacids are constipating and the client should be instructed to take a stool softener or additional bulk-type laxative to relieve this uncomfortable side effect. Options 1, 3, and 4 are not side effects of this medication.
Test-Taking Strategy: Use the process of elimination, and remember that aluminum-containing antacids are constipating. If you are unfamiliar with this medication, review this medication.
Level of Cognitive Ability: Comprehension
Client Needs: Physiological Integrity
Integrated Process: Nursing Process/Data Collection
Content Area: Pharmacology
Reference: Hodgson, B., & Kizior, R. (2005). *Saunders nursing drug handbook 2005*. Philadelphia: W.B. Saunders, p. 42.

80. *Answer:* **2**
Rationale: Feosol is an iron supplement used to treat anemia. Constipation is a frequent and uncomfortable side effect associated with the administration of oral iron supplements. Stool softeners are often prescribed to prevent constipation.
Test-Taking Strategy: Recalling that oral iron can cause constipation will easily direct you to option 2. If you had difficulty with this question, review the side effects of Feosol.
Level of Cognitive Ability: Comprehension
Client Needs: Physiological Integrity
Integrated Process: Nursing Process/Data Collection
Content Area: Pharmacology
Reference: Skidmore-Roth, L. (2005). *Mosby's drug guide for nurses* (6th ed.). St. Louis: Mosby, p. 356.

81. *Answer:* **2**
Rationale: Clients who are hearing-impaired rely on visual cues to help them comprehend the conversation of others. Smiling continuously is the least helpful strategy, because the smile distorts the appearance of the mouth if the client is trying to read lips. Facing the client and standing so that there is light on the nurse's face are helpful, because it assists the client to lip read. Taking care not to show frustration or annoyance with the client's impairment is also helpful to preserve the client's self-esteem.
Test-Taking Strategy: Note the key words, *least helpful*. Noting the words "smiling continuously" in option 2 will direct you to this option. If this question was difficult, review these communication strategies.
Level of Cognitive Ability: Application
Client Needs: Psychosocial Integrity
Integrated Process: Nursing Process/Implementation
Content Area: Adult Health/Ear
Reference: deWit, S. (2005). *Fundamental concepts and skills for nursing*. Philadelphia: W.B. Saunders, p. 108.

82. *Answer:* **2**
Rationale: Digoxin is a cardiac glycoside that is used to treat congestive heart failure and acts by increasing the force of myocardial contraction. Because bradycardia may be a clinical sign of toxicity, the nurse counts the apical heart rate for 1 full minute before administering the medication. If the pulse rate is below 60 beats per minute in an adult client, the nurse would withhold the medication and report the pulse rate to the registered nurse, who would then contact the physician.
Test-Taking Strategy: Noting that the client has congestive heart failure and recalling the action and nursing interventions related to administering this medication will assist in answering this question. Review nursing interventions related to the administration of digoxin if you had difficulty with this question.
Level of Cognitive Ability: Application
Client Needs: Physiological Integrity
Integrated Process: Nursing Process/Implementation
Content Area: Pharmacology
Reference: Skidmore-Roth, L. (2005). *Mosby's drug guide for nurses* (6th ed.). St. Louis: Mosby, p. 266.

83. *Answer:* **25 gtt/minute**
Rationale: Use the formula for calculating IV flow rates.
Formula:

$$\frac{\text{Total volume to infuse} \times \text{gtt factor}}{\text{Time in minutes}} = \text{gtt/minute}$$

$$\frac{1000 \text{ mL} \times 15 \text{ gtt/mL}}{10 \text{ hours} \times 60 \text{ minutes}} = \frac{15,000}{600} = 25 \text{ gtt/min}$$

Test-Taking Strategy: Follow the formula for calculating an IV flow rate and remember to change hours to minutes. Once you have done the calculation, recheck your work and make sure that the answer makes sense. If you had difficulty with this question, review IV flow rates.
Level of Cognitive Ability: Application
Client Needs: Physiological Integrity
Integrated Process: Nursing Process/Implementation
Content Area: Fundamental Skills
Reference: Kee, J., & Marshall, S. (2004). *Clinical calculations: With applications to general and specialty areas* (5th ed.). Philadelphia: W.B. Saunders, p. 202.

84. *Answers:*
Open the distal flap of a sterile package first
Avoid placing items within 1 inch of any area surrounding the outer edge of the sterile field

Rationale: A dry table that is above waist level is used to set up a sterile field. Moisture will contaminate the sterile field and anything below waist level is considered contaminated, according to the principles of surgical asepsis. The sterile field must be kept in sight at all times and the nurse should not turn away from it. If this happens, the nurse cannot be sure that it is still sterile. Sterile packages are opened away from the nurse's body, and the distal flap of a sterile package is opened first. This prevents contaminating the pack by reaching over the exposed sterile contents after the other flaps are opened. The outer 1-inch border of the sterile field must be considered unsterile, and sterile items are not placed within this 1-inch area. Sterile gloves, not clean gloves, are used. An unsterile item touching a sterile item contaminates the sterile item.

Test-Taking Strategy: Focus on the issue, the principles of aseptic technique. Thinking about these principles and visualizing each intervention will assist in identifying those that are appropriate. Review the principles of aseptic technique if you had difficulty with this question.

Level of Cognitive Ability: Application
Client Needs: Safe, Effective Care Environment
Integrated Process: Nursing Process/Implementation
Content Area: Fundamental Skills
Reference: deWit, S. (2005). *Fundamental concepts and skills for nursing.* Philadelphia: W.B. Saunders, pp. 768-770.

85. *Answer:* **3**
Rationale: The nurse monitors for the adverse effects of suctioning, which include cyanosis, excessively rapid or slow heart rate, or the sudden development of bloody secretions. If they occur, the nurse stops suctioning and reports these signs to the physician immediately. Coughing is a normal response to suctioning for the client with an intact cough reflex, and does not indicate that the client is not tolerating the procedure.

Test Taking Strategy: Use the process of elimination and note the key words, *adequately tolerating.* Cyanosis (option 4) and bradycardia (option 2) are abnormal findings and are eliminated first. From the remaining options, the use of the word "becoming" in association with bloody secretions tells you that this has not been an ongoing problem, making this an incorrect option also. Because the cough reflex is normally present, and suction triggers coughing, this is the preferable option. Review this procedure if you had difficulty with this question.

Level of Cognitive Ability: Analysis
Client Needs: Physiological Integrity
Integrated Process: Nursing Process/Evaluation
Content Area: Adult Health/Respiratory
Reference: Potter, P., & Perry, A. (2003) *Essentials for practice* (5th ed.). St. Louis: Mosby, p. 665.

REFERENCES

Black, J., & Hawks, J. (2005). *Medical-surgical nursing: Clinical management for positive outcomes* (7th ed.). Philadelphia: W.B. Saunders.

Chernecky, C., & Berger, B. (2004). *Laboratory tests and diagnostic procedures* (4th ed.). Philadelphia: W.B. Saunders.

Christensen, B., & Kockrow, E. (2003). *Adult health nursing* (4th ed.). St. Louis: Mosby.

Christensen, B., & Kockrow, E. (2003). *Foundations of nursing* (4th ed.). St. Louis: Mosby.

deWit, S. (2005). *Fundamental concepts and skills for nursing.* Philadelphia: W.B. Saunders.

Harkreader, H., & Hogan, M.A. (2004). *Fundamentals of nursing: Caring and clinical judgment.* (2nd ed.). Philadelphia: W.B. Saunders.

Hodgson, B., & Kizior, R. (2005). *Saunders nursing drug handbook 2005.* Philadelphia: W.B. Saunders.

Kee, J., & Marshall, S. (2004). *Clinical calculations: With applications to general and specialty areas* (5th ed.). Philadelphia: W.B. Saunders.

Keltner, N., Schwecke, L., & Bostro, C. (2003). *Psychiatric nursing* (4th ed.). St. Louis: Mosby.

Leifer, G. (2003). *Introduction to maternity and pediatric nursing* (4th ed.). Philadelphia: W.B. Saunders.

Leifer, G. (2005). *Maternity nursing* (9th ed.). Philadelphia: W.B. Saunders.

Lewis, S., Heitkemper, M., & Dirksen, S. (2004). *Medical-surgical nursing: Assessment and management of clinical problems* (6th ed.). St. Louis: Mosby.

Lilley, L., Harrington, S., & Snyder, J. (2005). *Pharmacology and the nursing process* (4th ed.). St. Louis: Mosby.

Linton, A., & Maebius, N. (2003). *Introduction to medical-surgical nursing* (3rd ed.). Philadelphia: W.B. Saunders.

Nix, S. (2005). *Williams basic nutrition and diet therapy* (12th ed.). St. Louis: Mosby.

Morrison-Valfre, M. (2005). *Foundations of mental health care* (3rd ed.). St. Louis: Mosby.

Pagana, K., & Pagana, T. (2003). *Mosby's diagnostic and laboratory test reference* (6th ed.). St. Louis: Mosby.

Phipps, W., Monahan, F., Sands, J., Marek, J., & Neighbors, M. (2003). *Medical-surgical nursing: Health and illness perspectives* (7th ed.). St. Louis: Mosby.

Potter, P., & Perry, A. (2003). *Essentials for practice* (5th ed.). St. Louis: Mosby.

Potter, P., & Perry, A. (2005). *Fundamentals of nursing* (6th ed.). St. Louis: Mosby.

Price, D., & Gwin, J. (2005). *Thompson's pediatric nursing* (9th ed.). Philadelphia: W.B. Saunders.

Skidmore-Roth, L. (2005). *Mosby's drug guide for nurses* (6th ed.). St. Louis: Mosby.

Stuart, G., & Laraia, M. (2005). *Principles and practice of psychiatric nursing* (8th ed.). St. Louis: Mosby.

Swearingen, P. (2003). *Manual of medical-surgical nursing care* (5th ed.). St. Louis: Mosby.

Wold, G. (2004). *Basic geriatric nursing* (3rd ed.). St. Louis: Mosby.

Index

Note: Page numbers followed by f indicate figures;
those followed by t indicate tables; those followed
by b indicate boxed material.